Immunology IV

Clinical Applications in Health and Disease

The illustration on the cover is an adaptation of a figure, "***The total immune capability of the host based upon efficiency of elimination of foreign matter***" that initially appears in ***Chapter 1*** and is used continuously throughout the book as a central unifying mantra to denote the capacity of the immune system to maintain a balance between the internal and external environments. It symbolizes both the beneficial outcomes of the immune encounter seen in health with successful elimination of foreignness by the innate and adaptive immune systems as well as those where failure of elimination and persistence of foreignness seen in chronic infection, allergic diseases, the autoimmune disorders and malignancy result in the most deleterious outcomes of the immune encounter. The image of *The Creation of Adam*, by Michelangelo, as it appears in the Sistine Chapel is superimposed on the cover figure and is reproduced with the permission from the Director of the Vatican Museums, "in light of the special nature of the book and of the spiritual relevance of the topic."

Immunology IV

Clinical Applications in Health and Disease

Editor

Joseph A. Bellanti, MD
Professor of Pediatrics and Microbiology-Immunology
Director, International Center for Interdisciplinary
Studies of immunology
Georgetown University School of Medicine
Washington, DC

Associate Editors

Alejandro Escobar-Gutiérrez, PhD
Professor of Immunology
Escuela Nacional de Ciencias Biológicas, IPN
Jefe del Departamento de Investigaciones Inmunológicas,
Instituto de Diagnóstico y Referencia Epidemiológicos,
Secretaría de Salud,
México, DF, México

George C. Tsokos, MD
Professor of Medicine
Harvard Medical School
Chief, Rheumatology Division
Department of Medicine
Beth Israel Deaconess Medical Center
Boston, Massachusetts

I Care Press
Bethesda, Maryland

Published by I Care Press
Bethesda, Maryland 20816
P.O. Box 40902
Washington, DC 20016

Library of Congress Cataloging-in-Publication Data has been applied for.

ISBN: 978-0-692-01160-7

With the purchase of this book, you are granted access to the Immunology IV website which contains the entire text, illustrations and 7 animations. The removable label containing the access code found on the inside of the cover is your password to the online version.

The previous three editions of *Immunology* (1971), *Immunology II* (1978) and *Immunology III* (1985) were published by W.B. Saunders.

Printed in the United States
1 2 3 4 14 13 12 11

Contents

Preface

Immunology as both a science and a field of medicine has undergone extraordinary changes over the last 40 years since the publication of the first edition of *Immunology* in 1971. What was once a discipline defined in descriptive terms is now becoming better understood at the genomic and molecular levels. This has made the writing of the fourth edition, *Immunology IV: Clinical Applications in Health and Disease,* a formidable task and a colossal undertaking.

This fourth edition has been completely rewritten to reflect the latest research findings and clinical applications of immunology. The work retains the same general three-section format of the previous three editions—*principles, mechanisms of response,* and *clinical applications*—but is enhanced both by the expansion of topic content as well as the sequential order of information presented. A deliberate strategy in the preparation of this book has been to take a departure from the more traditional approaches of textbook writing that would provide a more structured and pedagogically unified presentation of this complex and rapidly changing field of science using concepts and technologies that have only recently been developed to achieve maximal translation of basic immunology to clinical application. Accordingly, the following features are presented:

- A visual glossary appearing at the beginning of the book containing newly created images of classic structures and products of the immune system is used continually throughout each chapter to maintain consistency of style.
- Each chapter opens with a case study selected on the basis of its relevance to the chapter content.
- A list of concise learning objectives follows that provides the reader with a framework of key information to be acquired.
- Boxes appear throughout all chapters that enrich, engage, and deepen the discussion of subject material to assist those readers interested in further in-depth learning.
- Each time an acronym is initially used within a chapter, it is defined and revisited in Appendix 1.
- At the conclusion of each chapter, the case study is revisited for a summation of information presented earlier with a more robust discussion of diagnostic, therapeutic, and preventative procedures thus enabling the reader to directly relate the increased body of scientific knowledge to clinical relevance.
- Key points at the end of each chapter are reprised in a bulleted list of concepts and take home ideas that could help readers assimilate the basic science material in a clinical context.
- Study questions/critical thinking (five to 10 per chapter) are provided that query the reader on some key areas of content reinforced with critical thinking opportunities.
- A list of Suggested Readings then closes out each chapter, providing the key references along with bibliographic information that are compatible with National Library of Medicine search functions.

In addition to the printed version of *Immunology IV*, an interactive online version accompanies the edition to keep the book at the cutting edge of developments in immunology that offers the following features:

- A Web site is provided that will be continually updated that contains an online interactive multi-level teaching format with complete XML text, embedded with over 800 colorful illustrations to help readers visualize complex physiologic and pathophysiologic processes associated with basic and clinical aspects of immunology in health and disease.
- To help readers master key concepts of immunology, we offer a series of high-end state-of-the-art computer-generated animations that vividly portray the movement of cells and their interactions with key extracellular products; readers will find these animations designated in the margins of the text via the icon where they will help contribute to a deeper understanding of the content.

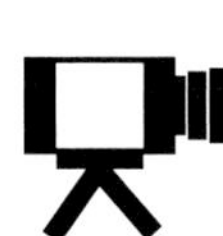

- In addition to the Questions/Critical Thinking section in the printed version, the online version expands this learning tool with a unique interactive Q & A assessment section at the end of each chapter that queries and leads the reader to the correct responses through the use of descriptive material and illustrations that enhance the learning process.
- The online version also contains hyperlinks with other learning sources and opportunities for direct queries in an "Ask the Professor" format.

The following is a brief description of the content of the three sections of the book.

Section 1 (Chapters 1–10) sets the stage for an understanding of the major principles of immunology in health and disease. Chapter 1 begins with an overview of the immune system that utilizes a unique building-block format in which individual components of the innate and adaptive immune systems are introduced individually and in a sequential fashion. In this chapter, a central unifying theme of immune responsiveness is presented as an expression of the effectiveness of elimination of foreignness and reappears throughout the book. The efficient removal of these foreign substances by the innate and adaptive immune responses are defined as expressions of the immune system in health, and those with failure of elimination or persistence of foreignness, representing the most serious sequela of immune-mediated disorders, are seen as expressions of the immune system in disease that take the form of chronic infectious diseases, allergic diseases, autoimmune disorders, or malignancy. Chapter 1 is intended as an overture or synthesizing introduction comparable to an overture in music that contains several expressive melodies or themes. Each of these themes is then expanded in greater detail in subsequent chapters. The first group of chapters in Section 1 focuses on developmental immunology and various components of the innate immune system, i.e., innate immunity, complement, and inflammation. The remaining chapters in this section center on the major constituents of the adaptive immune system and include B cell lymphocytes and immunoglobulin structure and function, T lymphocytes and cell-mediated immunity, and the mucosal immune system in health and disease. The section continues with a comprehensive chapter on cytokines and chemokines that focuses on structure/function relationships of these molecules with those of the receptors to which they bind. The use of innovative illustrations that depict the complex and redundant properties of these components will help the reader better understand how these important communication molecules function in health and in immune-mediated diseases. Section 1 ends with a chapter that describes the principles and important role of immunogenetics in regulation of the immune response in health and disease.

Section 2 (Chapters 11–15) presets the mechanisms of immune modulation, which include descriptions of current molecular, cellular, and genomic concepts involved in normal immune physiology as well as those implicated in the pathogenesis of immune-mediated disorders. The section begins with a chapter defining the mechanisms of immunodulation and the role they play in the three commonly expressed clinical forms of immunodulation, i.e., immunopotentiation, immunosuppression, and immune tolerance. Also found within this chapter are defining features of monoclonal antibody products and therapeutic fusion products together with current lists of FDA-approved immunologically relevant biologic response modifiers. The section continues with chapters describing immune mechanisms involved in bacterial, viral, fungal, and parasitic infections. The pervasive theme in each of these chapters is a return to the central unifying theme of immune responsiveness as an expression of the effectiveness of elimination of foreignness presented in Chapter 1. The consequence of the struggle between the evasion mechanisms displayed by these invading microbial agents and efficiency with which the innate and adaptive immune responses can overcome these is the single most important factor determining the outcome of the interaction either as an expression of protective immunity in health or a manifestation of disease as seen in chronic infectious diseases, autoimmune disorders, or malignancy.

Section 3 (Chapters 16–25) contains a group of chapters that describe pathophysiologic, diagnostic, and therapeutic aspects of the major clinical applications of the immune system (Chapters 16–25). The section begins with a comprehensive presentation of the greater than 150 immune deficiency disorders focusing on the vast array of causal molecular deficiencies of cytokines, receptors, and signaling pathways that are responsible for the clinical manifestations of susceptibility to infection, autoimmune disease, or malignancy that characterize these disorders. The section continues with a chapter presenting a restructured Gell and Coombs classification of adaptive immune system-related mechanisms of immunologic injury together with a proposed new classification system for disorders of innate immune function. Next presented is a chapter describing current concepts and etiologic factors underlying the allergic diseases and asthma together with a presentation of diagnostic and therapeutic procedures used in the management of these disorders. The section continues with a chapter describing current concepts of disordered adaptive immunity and immunologic tolerance as a basis for the autoimmune disorders with an annex that introduces the newly recognized monogenic and polygenic autoinflammatory diseases as expressions of disordered innate immunity. Next described are the immune responses to solid tumor malignancies with a focus on the critical interplay between immune system evasion mechanisms of the tumor that are countered by immune response strategies offered by the host. The presentation of antitumor mechanisms is next extended in a chapter describing pathogenesis and management of the lymphoproliferative disorders, including both T and B cell malignancies exemplified by the monoclonal gammopathies and the lymphomas and leukemias. The practical aspects of solid organ and stem cell transplantation are next described together with current diagnostic testing procedures and contemporary immunosuppressive treatment modalities. The clinical applications of the immunology section continues with a description of the current status and use of vaccines including their beneficial protective aspects as well as some of the real and perceived adverse untoward reactions that accompany their usage. The section ends with two chapters focusing on the use of immunologic procedures used in diagnostic testing; the first presents a practical description of laboratory procedures used in the diagnosis of the immune deficiency diseases, the allergic diseases, and the autoimmune disorders, and the second describes current and emerging basic molecular biologic methodologies and their current and potential future clinical applications. At the end of these sections are three practical appendices to assist the reader as quick reference material for the unending list of memory hooks and acronyms (Appendix 1), cytokines and chemokines (Appendix 2), and CD molecules (Appendix 3).

The major challenge in the writing of any textbook, particularly one in immunology whose title broadly purports "clinical applications in health and disease," is to define the audience for whom the book is written. This burdensome task then becomes the challenge of deciding on material to be *included* in the text—and perhaps, more importantly, the material to be *excluded.* Although we do not claim to have the only one correct approach to the teaching of immunology (there is truly no one perfect approach to teaching), but rather, we have based the writing of *Immunology IV* on our experience gained through years of teaching medical and graduate students, residents, fellows-in-training, colleagues in the medical specialties, and the practicing physicians and those preparing for certifying, recertifying, and maintenance of certification (MOC) examinations. Why did we choose to write this book with its online interactive version using the format described above? It was our intent to write a book presenting basic and clinical aspects of immunology clearly and succinctly in a manner that not only addresses different levels of learning, but also maintains a fidelity to a clinical theme without complex explanations of difficult concepts. A concerted effort was made to not overburden the writing with complicated facts but to summarize details in tabular form rather than in lengthy text. Accompanying the text is the addition of over 800 colorful illustrations in the hard copy and seven illustrative animations in the online version, all of which have been painstakingly created for the visual learner.

A two-year subscription of the online version of *Immunology IV* comes with every new copy of the book, which contains a variety of useful tools for additional study, review, and exploration. These include the online interactive multi-level teaching and clinical case study and interactive Q & A formats together with other ancillary teaching tools and related hyperlinks to help readers visualize physiologic and pathophysiologic processes associated with basic and clinical aspects of immunology in health and disease. One of the major challenges of immunology textbooks is the struggle to remain current in a field in which the accretion of new knowledge is occurring continuously and rapidly. To counterbalance this problem, the online version will be continuously updated and will be available by subscription.

Acknowledgments

No project of this magnitude would be possible without the contributions of numerous individuals to whom I wish to express my sincere gratitude. Although it is exceedingly difficult to know how to adequately acknowledge the creative and helpful efforts that each has made, I would like to recognize the tremendous dedication of the contributing authors, reviewers, associate editors, project managers, and artists who gave generously of their time to write the text, create the illustrations, and generate the animations. I am particularly indebted to the many thoughtful experts who gave of their time to read and critique manuscripts to help ensure excellence in chapter content and accuracy.

I would like to specifically recognize those who provided these many contributions not only in guidance and initial creation and review of content, but also in direction and maintenance of the project: Dr. Alejandro Escobar, Dr. George Tsokos, the late Father Joseph V. Kadlec, SJ, Dr. Noel R. Rose, Dr. Yehuda Shoenfeld, Dr. Laritta Paolini, Dr. Giorgio Trinchieri, Alison Harrison, Walter Peter, Dr. Nafees Ahmad, Dr. Rajeev Aurora, Dr. Sameh Basta, Dr. Nancy Jane Bigley, Dr. Rebecca Blackstoc, Dr. Molly Hill, Dr. Benjamin Bonavida, Dr. Jerome Zack, Dr. Carie Micelli, Dr. Sheire Morrison, Dr. Lee Goodglick, Dr. John Braun, Dr. David S. Bradley, Dr. Robert K. Bright, Dr. Peter Burrows, Dr. Sandra P. Chang, Dr. Edmund Choi, Dr. Richard A. Calderone, Dr. Richard P. Ciavarra, Dr. Michael Cole, Dr. Carolyn Hurley, Dr. Janet Decker, Dr. Peter B. Dent, Dr. James R. Drake, Dr. Kristen Drescher, Dr. Patrick Swanson, Dr. Wesley Dunnick, Dr. Thomas A. Fleisher, Dr. Linda M. Forsyth, Dr. Lawrence D. Frenkel, Dr. Rachel Gerstein, Dr. Steven Greenberg, Dr. Stephen Canfield, Dr. Daila S. Dr. Penelope Duerksen-Hughes, Dr. Susan Richards, Dr. Kevin V. Hackshaw, Dr Bruce Hofkin, Dr. Dorothy Hudig, Dr. Mark A. James, Dr. Lucy Freytag, Dr. James McLachlan, Dr. Lucia Freytag, Dr. Patric Lundberg, Dr. Neil Krishner, Dr. Lena Galkina, Dr. Peter Hotez, Dr. Julio A. Lavergne, Dr. Deborah A. Lebman, Dr. Maria F. Lima, Dr. Joaquin Madrenas, Dr. Christine Milcarek, Dr. Frederick Miller, Dr. Robert D. Miller, Dr. Bruce Hofkin, Dr. Michael L. Misfeldt, Dr. Federico Montealegre, Dr. Vanessa Rivera Amill, Dr. Lee Schein, Dr. Michael C. Newlon, Dr. Michael J. Parmely, Dr. Janet F. Piskurich, Dr. Rob McKallip, Dr. Ron Garner, Dr. Michael Radcliffe, Dr. Eddy Rios-Olivares, Dr. José Rodriguez, Dr. James W. Rohrer, Dr. Joseph Brewer, Dr. Robert Barrington, Dr. Robert Lausch, Dr. Edmund Choi, Dr. Catharine B. Saelinger, Dr. Patrick M. Schlievert, Dr. William T. Shearer, Dr. Yufang Shi, Dr. Lee S.F. Soderberg, Dr. Judy Van de Water, Dr. Luc Van Kaer, Dr. Jerrold Weiss, Dr. John Colgan, Dr. Stephen Wikel, Dr. William E. Winter, Dr. Henry Wortis, Dr. Karen Yamaga, Dr. Sandra Chang, Dr. German Benavides, Dr. Stephen M. Peters, Dr. Thomas R. Cupps and Dr. Sean Whelton.

My appreciation is also extended to other colleagues at Georgetown and to my students, clinical and research fellows, and house staff who have contributed to my intellectual life and to the life of the Immunology Center. I owe a special debt of gratitude to all students I have taught and from whom I have learned. Learning represents a great joy of discovery shared between the student and the teacher, and it is in this spirit that *Immunology IV* was written. The book is a product of conversations that I have had with every student I have met. It is the questions that they ask in the lecture hall, the laboratory, in the clinic, and at the bedside that have provided the incentive to write. Although many individuals have contributed to this textbook, I alone assume responsibility for any errors or omissions found within these pages.

I wish to particularly express my sincere gratitude to Susan Graham, who as project manager was a vital component of innumerable aspects of the project since its inception. Her extraordinary publishing and organizational talents have not only assisted in the creation of the text, illustrations, and animations, but also in bringing the mission to a successful conclusion. A special debt of gratitude is owed to Fiona Montgomery of Manchester, England, whose extraordinary artistic skills have contributed to the creation of the beautiful and colorful figures found within the pages of *Immunology IV* and whose contributions were particularly significant since they were accomplished entirely by transoceanic cybernetic communication. We wish to thank Graceway Pharmaceuticals for the educational grant that partially contributed to these figures. Particular appreciation is owed to Jane Hurd, who not only contributed to the development of the illustrative figures of the first three editions of *Immunology,* but who, together with her associates at the world-premier Hurd Studios in New York, created the exceptional state-of-the art 3-D animations that appear in the online version. A special appreciation is owing to Genentech for their generous grant in support of the animations and illustrations.

I wish to especially express my thanks to Imran Aftab and his associates at TenPearls, LLC, for their exquisite development of the online version of the book together with the mobile-enabled Web site, to John Shoemaker for his inventive development of our immunologycenter.org Web site and e-commerce capability, and to Dennis Carson, president of DC Carson, LLC, for his creative assistance in the development of marketing strategies.

Finally, I wish to express my thanks and appreciation to Laura Smith, Manager, Books Publishing, and her colleagues at Cenveo Publisher Services for their dedicated support of the project and for many helpful suggestions, services, and assistance they provided in the editing, composition, and printing of *Immunology IV.*

Joseph A. Bellanti, MD
Georgetown University Medical Center
Washington, DC

Contributors

Doru T. Alexandrescu, MD
Hematologist-Oncologist
University of California at San Diego
San Diego, CA

Mark Ballow, MD
Chief, Division of Allergy, Clinical Immunology, and Pediatric Rheumatology
Women & Children's Hospital of Buffalo
SUNY Buffalo School of Medicine and Biomedical Sciences
Buffalo, NY

José Roberto Bastarrachea-Rivera, MD
Intensive Care Unit, Hospital de la Mujer de Aguascalientes
Aguascalientes, Ags, Mexico

Joseph A. Bellanti, MD
Professor of Pediatrics and Microbiology-Immunology
Director, International Center for Interdisciplinary Studies of Immunology
Georgetown University Medical Center
Washington, DC

German A. Benavides, MD
Research Associate
International Center for Interdisciplinary Studies of Immunology
Georgetown University Medical Center
Washington, DC

Melvin Berger, MD, PhD
Adjunct Professor of Pediatrics and Pathology
Case Western Reserve University
Cleveland, OH

Rita Carsetti, PhD
Head Immunology Research Area
B Cell Laboratory
Diagnostic Immunology Unit
Research Center Bambino Gesù Children Hospital
Rome, Italy

Michael F. Cole, BDS, MSc, PhD
Professor of Microbiology and Immunology
Department of Microbiology and Immunology
Georgetown University School of Medicine
Washington, DC

Stephen J. Di Martino, MD, PhD
Assistant Attending Physician
Hospital for Special Surgery
New York, NY

Khaled el-Shami, MD, PhD
Assistant Professor of Medicine
Division of Hematology and Oncology
George Washington University Medical Center
Washington, DC

Alejandro Escobar-Gutiérrez, PhD
Head and Investigator
Department of Immunological Research
Instituto de Diagnóstico y Referencia Epidemiológicos
Secretaría de Salud
Mexico City, Mexico
Professor of Immunology, National School of Biological Sciences
Instituto Politécnico Nacional
Mexico City, Mexico

Donna L. Farber, PhD
Professor of Surgical Sciences
Columbia University
New York, NY

Dr. James D. Folds, PhD
Professor Emeritus
The University of North Carolina School of Medicine
Department of Pathology and Laboratory Medicine
Chapel Hill, NC

Alexandra F. Freeman, MD
Staff Clinician
Laboratory of Clinical Infectious Diseases
National Institute of Allergy and Infectious Diseases, NIH
Bethesda, MD

Ricardo T. Fujiwara, PhD
Departamento de Parasitologia
Instituto de Ciências Biológicas
Belo Horizonte, MG, Brasil

Steven M. Holland, MD
Chief, Laboratory of Clinical Infectious Diseases
National Institute of Allergy and Infectious Diseases, NIH
Bethesda, MD

Jimmy Hwang, MD
Associate Professor of Medicine
Lombardi Cancer Center
Georgetown University Medical Center
Washington, DC

Lionel B. Ivashkiv, MD
David H. Koch Chair in Arthritis Research
Hospital for Special Surgery
New York, NY

Vasileios C. Kyttaris, MD
Assistant Professor of Medicine
Harvard Medical School
Division of Rheumatology
Boston, MA

Maria Lattanzi, MD
Cluster Physician
Novartis Vaccines and Diagnostics
Siena, Italy

Stefano Luccioli, MD
Senior Medical Advisor, Office of Food Additive Safety
Center for Food Safety and Applied Nutrition
Food and Drug Administration
College Park, MD
Senior Associate, International Center for Interdisciplinary Studies of Immunology
Georgetown University Medical Center
Washington, DC

Eleni E. Magira, MD, PhD
Lecturer at the University of Athens Medical School
Critical Care Medicine Department
Evangelismos General Hospital
Athens, Greece

Catalin Marian, MD, PhD
Assistant Professor of Oncology
Director, Genomics and Epigenomics Shared Resource
Lombardi Comprehensive Cancer Center
Georgetown University Medical Center
Washington, DC

John L Marshall, MD
Professor of Medicine and Oncology
Georgetown University
Washington DC

Blanche Mavromatis, MD
Braddock Oncology Associates
Cumberland, MD

Susana Mendez, DVM, PhD
Assistant Professor
Baker Institute for Animal Health
Cornell University
Ithaca, NY

Robert P. Nelson Jr., MD
Professor of Medicine and Pediatrics
Divisions of Hematology/Oncology
Indianapolis, IN

Joost J. Oppenheim, MD
Chief, Laboratory of Molecular Immunoregulation
National Cancer Institute, NIH
Frederick, MD

Susan M. Orton, PhD
Associate Professor
The University of North Carolina School of Medicine
Department of Allied Health Sciences
Chapel Hill, NC

Sigifredo Pedraza-Sánchez, PhD
Medical Sciences Investigator
Unit of Biochemistry
Instituto Nacional de Ciencias Médica y Nutrición "Salvador Zubirán"
Secretaría de Salud
Mexico City, Mexico

Alessandro Plebani, MD, PhD
Professor of Pediatrics
University of Brescia School of Medicine
Chief of Pediatrics
Children's Hospital, Spedali Civili
Brescia, Italy

Rino Rappuoli, PhD
Global Head, Vaccines Research
Novartis Vaccines and Diagnostics
Siena, Italy

Luigina Romani, MD, PhD
Professor of Microbiology
University of Perugia
School of Medicine
Perugia, Italy

Sandra Rosen-Bronson, PhD
Director, Histocompatibility Laboratory
Georgetown University Hospital
Washington, DC

Barry T. Rouse, DVM, PhD, DSc
Distinguished Professor
College of Veterinary Medicine
University of Tennessee
Knoxville, TN

Kondrad Stadler, PhD
Senior Scientist
Novartis Vaccines and Diagnostics
Siena, Italy

Kathleen E. Sullivan, MD, PhD
Professor of Pediatrics
University of Pennsylvania School of Medicine
Philadelphia, PA

George C. Tsokos, MD
Professor of Medicine
Harvard Medical School
Chief, Division of Rheumatology
Beth Israel Deaconess Medical Center
Boston, MA

Alberto G. Ugazio, MD
Chairman, Department of Medical Pediatrics
Professor of Pediatrics
Ospedale Pediatrico Bambino Gesù
Rome, Italy

Marco A. Vega-López, BSc, PhD
Research Scientist
Center for Research and Advanced Studies
National Polytechnic Institute
Infectomics and Molecular Pathogenesis Department
Mucosal Immunobiology Laboratory
México City, México

Louis M. Weiner, MD
Director, Georgetown Lombardi Cancer Center
Chair, Department of Oncology
Georgetown University School of Medicine
Washington, DC

Visual Glossary

Environment

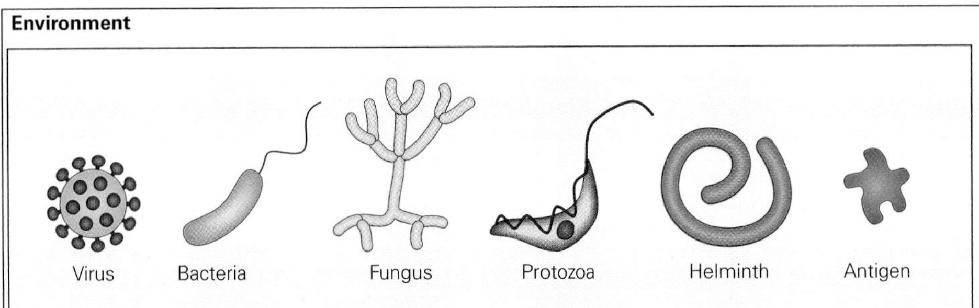

Virus
Bacteria
Fungus
Protozoa
Helminth
Antigen

Target cells

Target cell
Apoptotic cell
Virus infected cell
Cancer cell

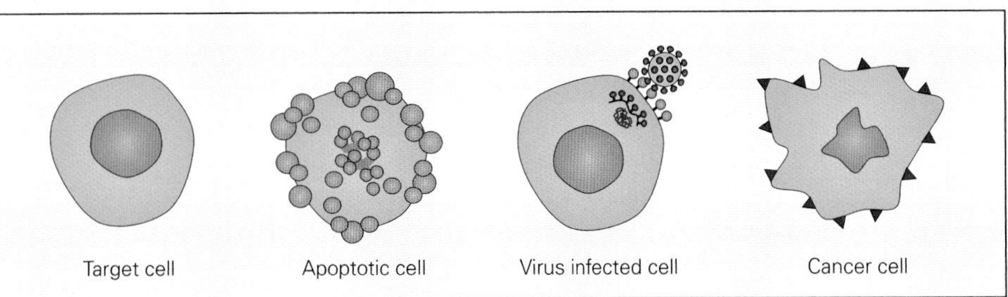

Cells of the innate immune system and complement

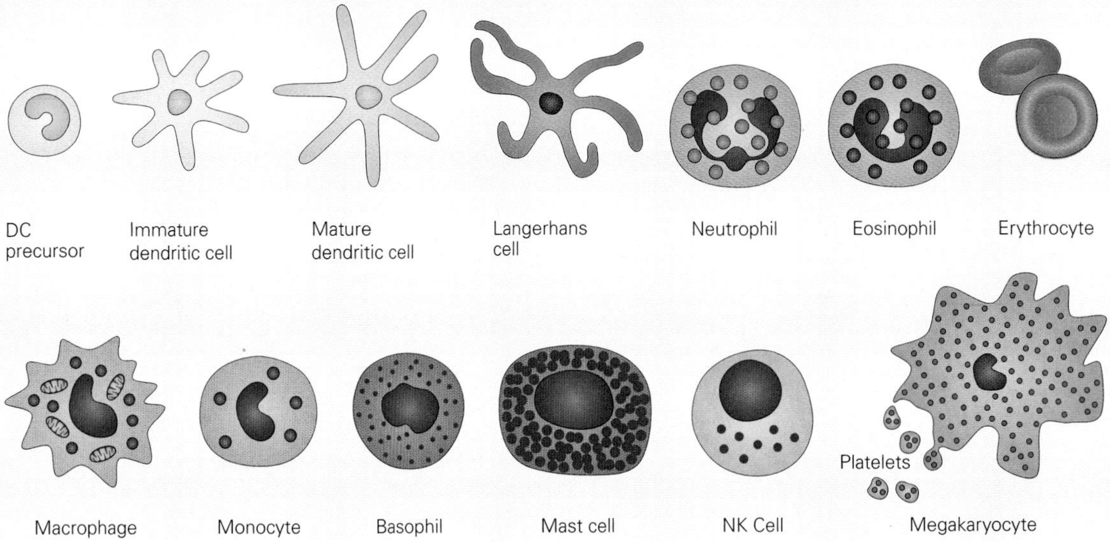

DC precursor
Immature dendritic cell
Mature dendritic cell
Langerhans cell
Neutrophil
Eosinophil
Erythrocyte
Macrophage
Monocyte
Basophil
Mast cell
NK Cell
Platelets
Megakaryocyte

Complement: Classic pathway

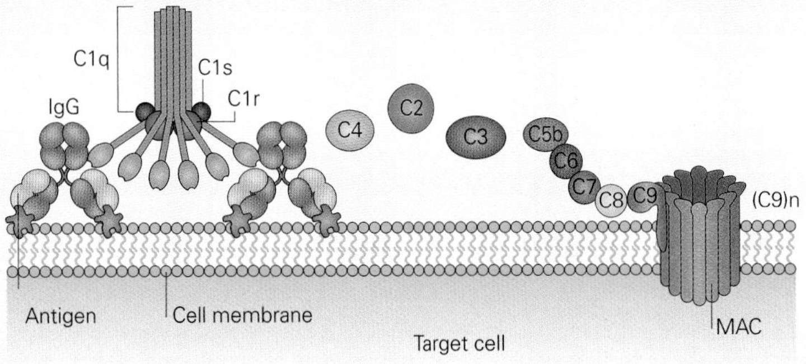

C1q
C1s
C1r
IgG
C4
C2
C3
C5b
C6
C7
C8
C9
(C9)n
Antigen
Cell membrane
Target cell
MAC

Cells and cell products of the adaptive immune system

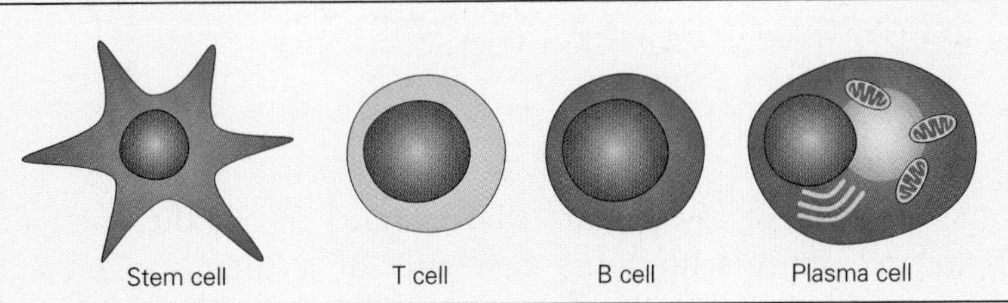

Immunoglobulins

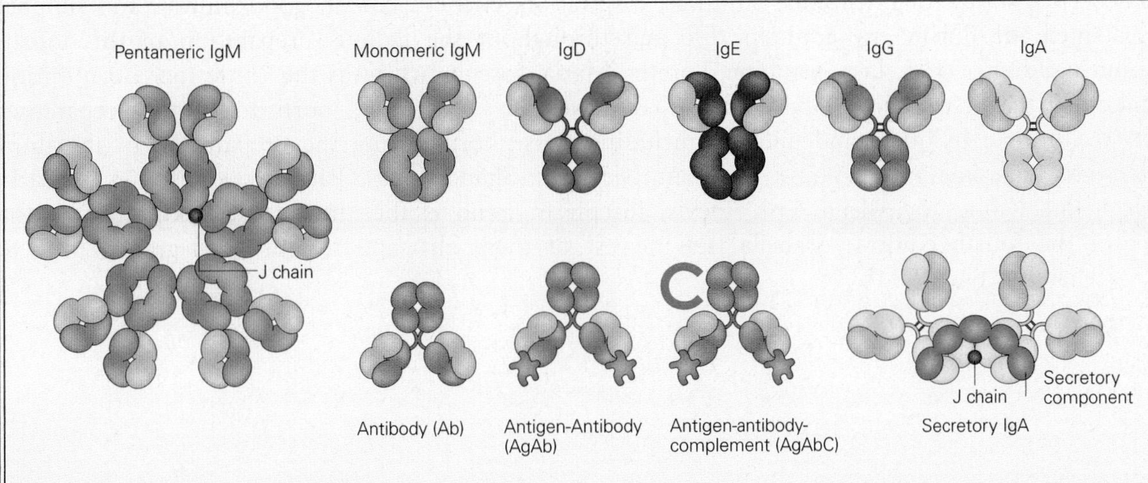

Cell receptors

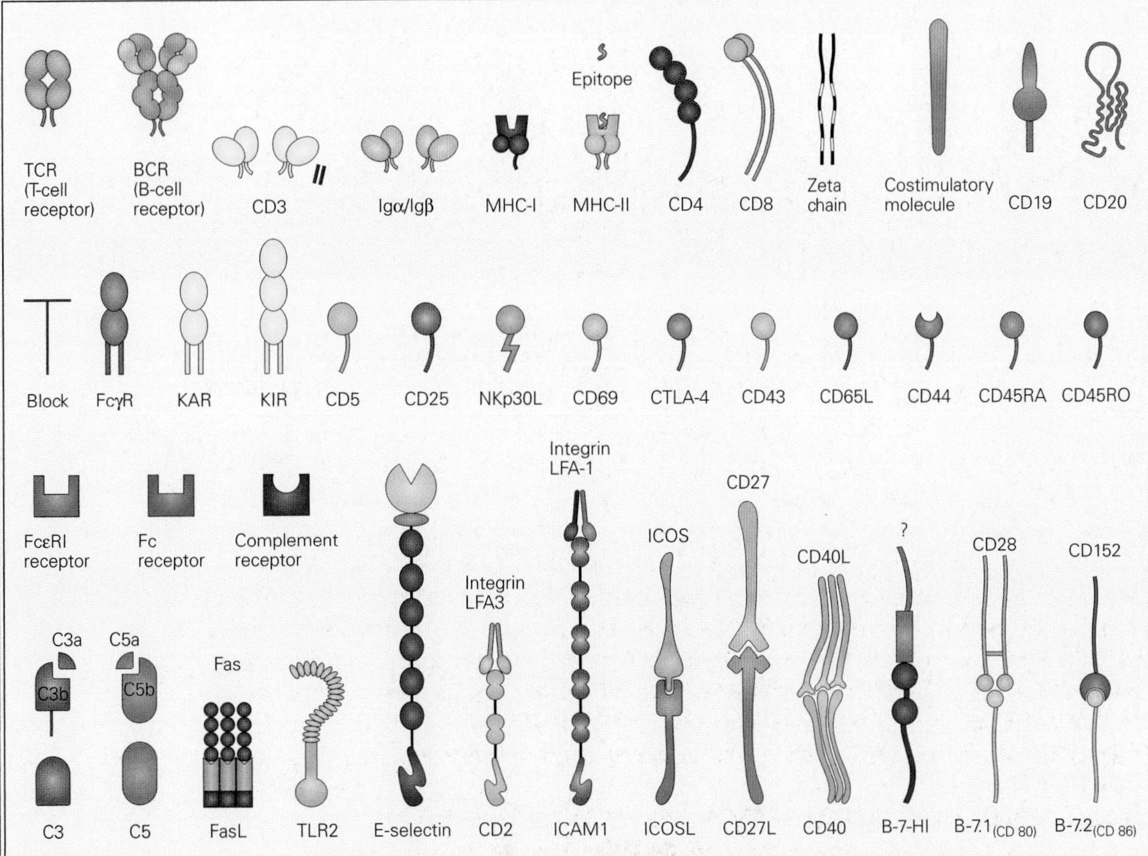

This edition is dedicated with affection to the memory of my parents who instilled in me the quest for excellence; to my brother who introduced me to science with those first gifts of a chemistry set and microscope; to my teachers who inspired in me what joy the discovery of learning could bring; and to those members of my family closest to me—to my wife Jacqueline, who during all our happy 53 years together has been a source of intellectual stimulus, inspiration, encouragement, good humor, and support that has sustained me during my academic life and throughout the tedious preparation of this fourth edition; to our children, Dawn, Lisa, Jeannine, Loretta, Maria, Joseph (who was the "little Joe" born during the preparation of the first edition), and Anthony (who was the "little Tony," born during the preparation of the second edition); to our grandchildren (including those born during the preparation of the third edition), Kristen, Julia, Johnny, Jeannine, Shannan, Mark Jr., Shane, Leesa, Patrick, Donovan, Chadwick, Gabriel, Jacqueline, Gina, Nic, Siena, Erik, Elexis, Joseph Jr. (who is the "littlest Joe," born during the preparation of the fourth edition), Isabella (the newest of them all); and to our great-grand children, Catherine, Aleena, and Elley.

Section One

THE PRINCIPLES OF IMMUMOLOGY

Chapter 1

Overview of Immunology

Joseph A. Bellanti, MD

Case Study

An eleven-year-old boy presents to his pediatrician with a circular erythematous (red) rash on the skin of his posterior right shoulder. The rash was first observed by his parents three days after returning from a four-day summer camp in Maryland and has now progressed to 10 cm in diameter with central clearing and a bull's-eye appearance. The patient has not experienced pain, tenderness, or pruritis at the site and has not noted any associated symptoms such as fever, headache, fatigue, joint pain, abdominal pain, nausea, vomiting, or diarrhea. He does not recall being bitten by any insects or ticks in the last few weeks, and his parents report that their son has been eating well and has displayed his normal activity level since returning from summer camp.

The clinician should consider Lyme disease (Box 1-1) as a possible cause of this boy's rash, as the disease is more common in the summer months, more prevalent in the northeastern United States, and often presents with a classic rash called erythema migrans (Figure 1-1). In this case, the diagnosis of early localized Lyme disease was established by the detection of serum IgM Lyme antibody reported in a serum specimen obtained one week following his return from summer camp. A subsequent blood specimen obtained four weeks later revealed significant elevation of IgG Lyme antibody. He was treated with antibiotics and did not experience further sequelae. This case is an excellent example of how our immune defenses provide barriers to foreign invaders in the environment, how these barriers may be breached by pathogens, and how the immune system reacts to such breaches. The goal of this case study is to illustrate the complex interplay between the innate and adaptive elements of the immune system in both health and disease. An understanding of the body's response to pathogens such as *B. burgdorferi* is essential to the diagnosis and management of many other diseases. The discussion of Lyme disease in Box 1-1 provides an overview of this complex process.

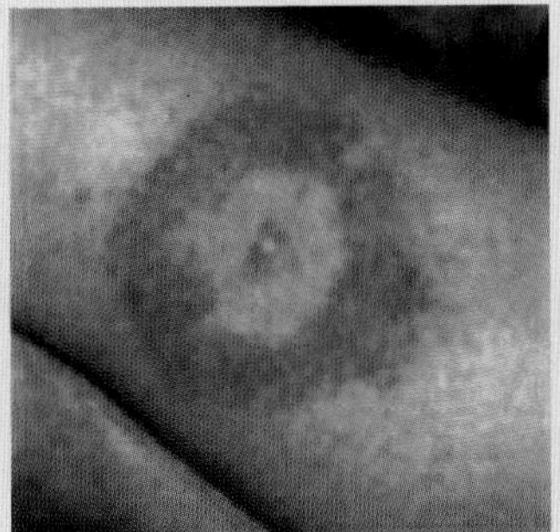

Figure 1-1. Typical bull's-eye appearance of the rash of erythema migrans seen in Lyme disease. (As seen on Wikipedia.)

LEARNING OBJECTIVES

When you have completed this chapter, you should be able to:

- Recognize the importance of the immune system in health and disease
- Identify the role of the immune system in maintaining a balance between the internal environment of the host and the external environment in which we live
- Distinguish between nonspecific (innate) and specific (adaptive) immune systems
- Identify the key cellular and molecular components of innate immunity
- Identify the key cellular and molecular components of adaptive immunity
- Explain how the mechanisms combating infection/disease (killing pathogens) can also result in tissue damage, allergic disease, graft rejection, and antitumor responses
- Summarize the concept of immune balance in health and disease

Box 1-1

Lyme disease (borreliosis) is a bacterial infection caused by the spirochete *Borrelia burgdorferi*, which is most often acquired from the bite of an infected *Ixodes*, a black-legged tick also known as a deer tick. The disease varies widely in its presentation, which may include a rash and flu-like symptoms in its initial stage, followed by the possibility of musculoskeletal, arthritic, neurologic, psychiatric, and cardiac manifestations in later stages. In most cases of Lyme disease, symptoms can be eliminated with antibiotics, especially if treatment is begun early in the course of illness. In most cases, the immune system eliminates the infection without harmful sequelae. If the infection is not treated promptly and the organism is not eliminated, the more deleterious immunopathologic effects of the immune response are seen that are expressed as the late manifestations of the disease, e.g., arthritis.

Overview of the Immune System

The Immune System Recognizes and Eliminates Pathogens

In today's usage, immunology may be described as the summation of all those physiologic processes that endow the host with the capacity to recognize materials as foreign to itself and to neutralize, eliminate, or metabolize them with or without injury to its own tissue(s). This ability to differentiate "self" from "nonself" constitutes the basic hallmark of the immune response and the basis for an understanding of clinical immunology in health and disease.

For ease of discussion, the possible outcome of an encounter of the host's immune response with a foreign substance is shown schematically in Figure 1-2.

If the foreign substance cannot be blocked by natural barriers such as skin and mucous secretions, the substance comes into contact with the immune system (Figure 1-2). This encounter with a foreign substance can either lead to an immune response or to no response, a condition referred to as **immune tolerance**. The mechanisms permitting recognition of foreign structures leading to an immune response can be broken down into two general categories: innate immunity and adaptive immunity. **Innate immunity**, previously referred to as nonspecific immunity, is a set of fixed responses activated by receptors that are encoded by genes in the host's germ line. These receptors recognize molecular patterns shared by many foreign substances that are not present in the mammalian host (*Chapter 3*). **Adaptive immunity**, formerly called specific immunity, is a set of responses to unique foreign structures (**antigens** or **immunogens**). Antigen receptors are encoded by relatively few gene elements that are somatically rearranged to result in the assembly of antigen-binding molecules with exquisite specificity for individual immunogens. These antigen-binding structures consist of both cell receptors located on specialized immune lymphoid cells (B and T lymphocytes) as well as extracellular secreted products known as antibodies (*Chapters 6 and 7*). The general characteristics of innate and adaptive immune responses are shown in Box 1-2 and Figure 1-3.

Anatomic Organization of the Immune System

In order to carry out the functions of immunity, an ubiquitous system of cells and cell products has appeared within the vertebrates containing elements of both the innate and adaptive immune systems. For ease of discussion, this system can be divided into **external** and **internal immune systems** (Figure 1-4). Foreign substances that enter the body through the natural portals of entry, i.e., skin, respiratory, gastrointestinal, or genitourinary tracts, encounter components of the external immune system found in collections of lymphoid elements found at these sites. Since most of these organ systems are lined by mucosa, this system is referred to as the mucosa-associated lymphoid tissues (**MALT**) (*Chapter 8*). An important part of this system that occurred during phylogeny is the addition of the mammary glands, which provide protective immunity at mucosal surfaces of the neonate during breast-feeding (*Chapter 2*). Foreign substances that penetrate these mucosal and skin-site barriers enter the body through the blood or lymphatics and encounter components of the internal immune system found in the lymph nodes, thymus, and spleen.

Mechanical Barriers and External Secretions

Before the activation of the innate and adaptive immune systems takes place, there are a number of natural barriers consisting of anatomic structures and physiologic mechanisms that limit the access and progression of a foreign invader (Figure 1-5). The initial entry of an infectious agent or its secreted products first encounters the mechanical

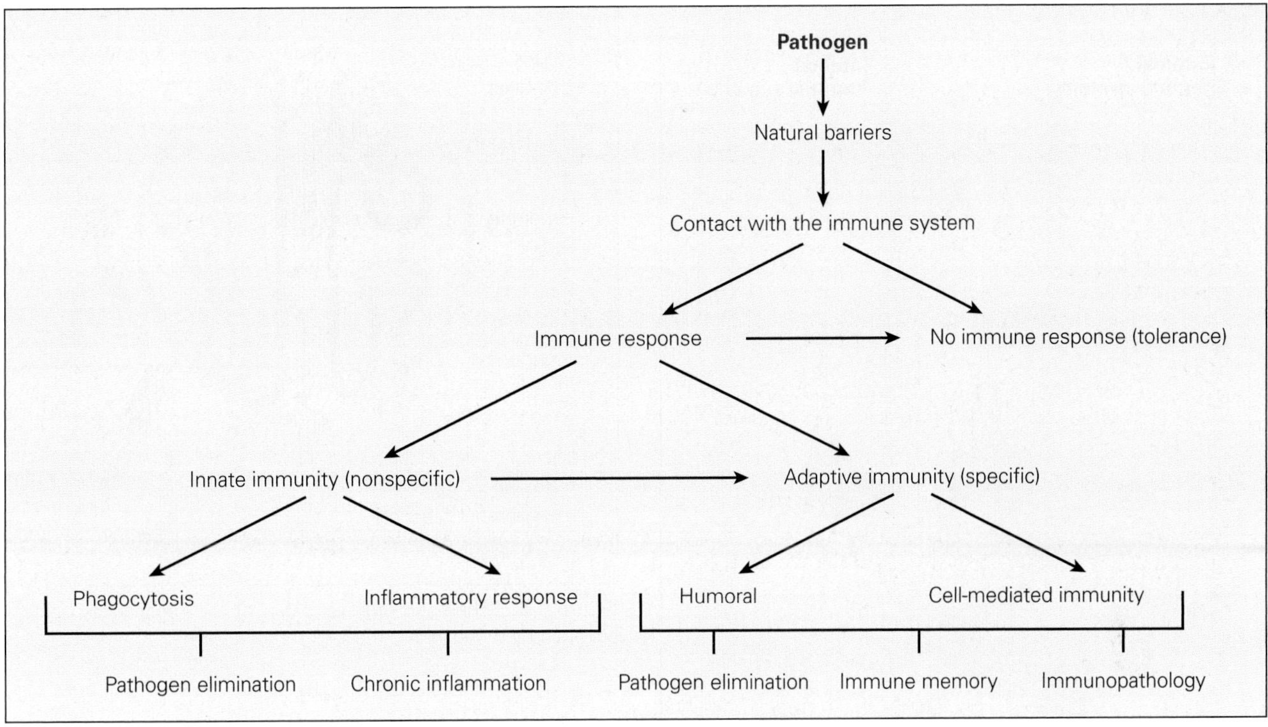

Figure 1-2. Possible outcomes of an encounter of the host with a foreign configuration.

barriers provided by the skin, the largest external protective outer covering of the body, and the mucous membranes, which line all body passages that communicate with the external environment (Figures 1-5 and 1-6).

The external secretions of the skin and mucous membranes contain a large number of substances that are detrimental to the growth of microorganisms (Table 1-1). These include a wide variety of metabolites, such as acids, peptides, and proteins.

Innate Immunity Responds Quickly to Conserved Pathogen Structures

The first set of responses to foreign substances are called innate (*innatus*, from Latin, meaning present at birth) immune responses because they are present

Box 1-2

General Characteristics of the Immune Response

The innate and adaptive immune systems both recognize foreign substances by surface receptors on cells of each system. They differ, however, in the genetic control of the synthesis of these receptors. The innate immune system uses a relatively large number of germ line genes (10^{2-3}) that are already programmed in the genome. In contrast, although the adaptive immune system utilizes fewer initial inherited preprogrammed genes, they result in an intense expansion (10^{13-24}) through a variety of complex processes involving somatic recombination and mutation, e.g., VDJ recombination, class switch recombinatorial, and somatic hypermutational events (*Chapters 6 and 7*).

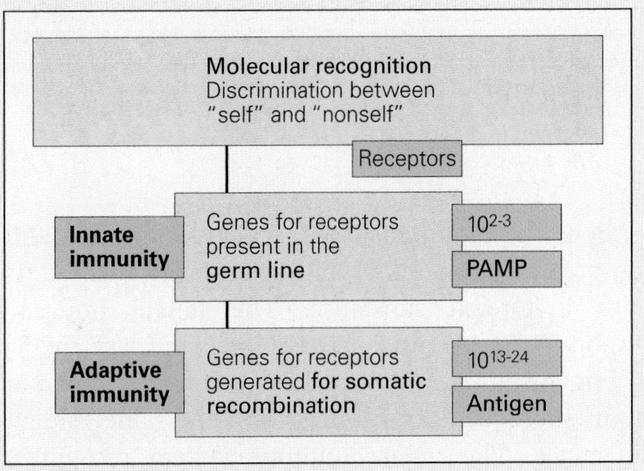

Figure 1-3. Characteristics of the immune response.

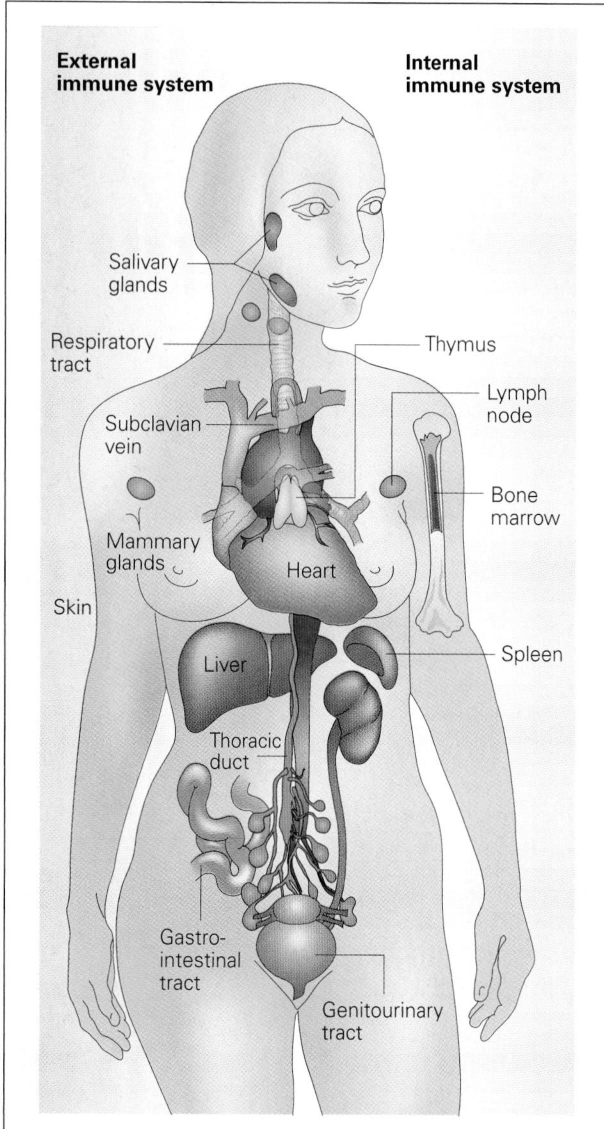

Figure 1-4. Schematic representation of the organization of the immune system into an external system consisting of the mucosal associated lymphoid tissues that encounter foreign substances at body surfaces, and an internal immune system responding to foreign substances that enter the body by breaching the skin, and mucosal barriers consisting of lymphoid tissues, lymph nodes, and spleen.

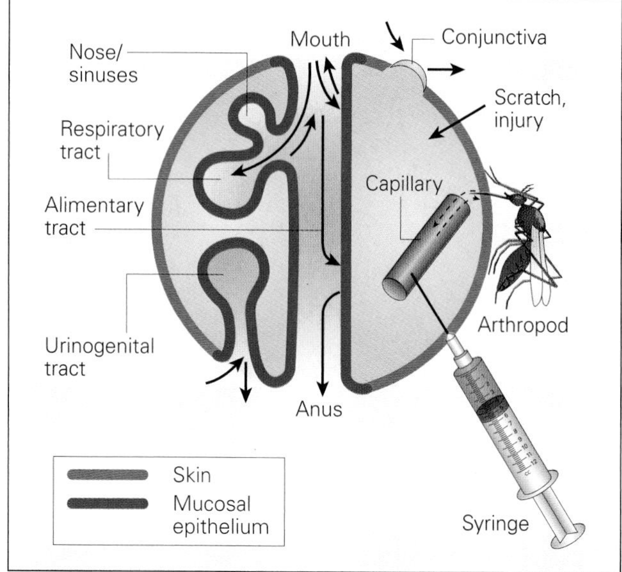

Figure 1-5. Schematic representation of the mechanical barriers provided by the skin and mucous membranes.

without the requirement for specific induction and are present upon initial and subsequent encounters with a foreign substance. The innate immune responses are primitive, stereotyped, and lack memory or the ability to respond in an enhanced manner upon subsequent encounters with the same foreign substance. The innate immune system recognizes certain structures on a foreign substance—referred to as pathogen-associated molecular patterns (**PAMPs**) that are mediated utilizing receptors called pattern-recognition receptors (**PRRs**) located on the surfaces of a variety of cells of the innate immune system, e.g., macrophages and other cells (*Chapter 3*). Because these recognition molecules used by the innate system are expressed broadly on a large number of cells and remain ready to be set off, this system is poised to act rapidly after an encounter with a foreign substance and thus constitutes the initial host immune response. The innate immune responses consist of three major mechanisms: (1) **phagocytosis** (*Chapter 5*), the ability of certain cells to ingest foreign substances; (2) **inflammation** (*Chapter 5*), the body's response to injury; and (3) **cytotoxicity**, the elimination of infected or transformed cells via apoptosis, a cellular process involving a genetically controlled series of events leading to noninflammatory programmed cell death (*Chapter 9*).

Adaptive Immunity Is More Specific and Generates Immune Memory

The second major branch of the immune system includes a complex set of genetically controlled, interdependent, and interactive responses referred to as **adaptive** or acquired (specific) immune responses. In contrast to the innate immune system, the adaptive immune system is more expansive and diverse and is characterized by:

1. **Specificity:** The recognition of the foreign substance (i.e., antigen or immunogen) by antigen-recognition molecules on the surfaces of lymphocytes in a highly precise and selective manner;

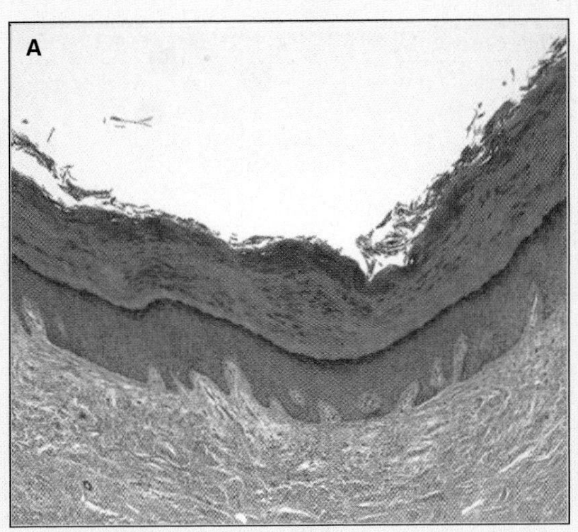

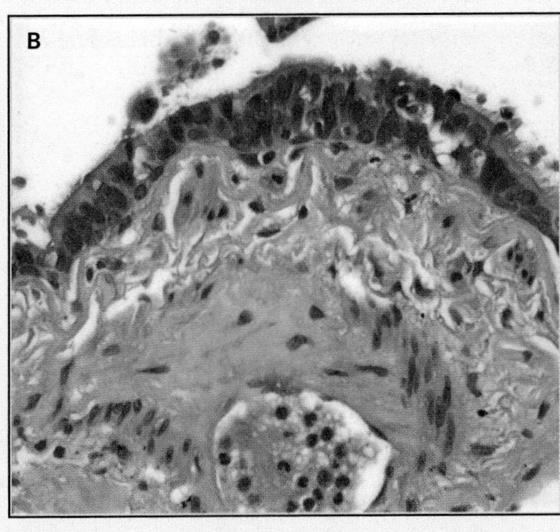

Figure 1-6. Panel A: Histopathologic sections of skin showing the keratinized squamous epithelium. Panel B: Bronchial mucous membrane with its ciliated epithelium and mucus layer. Both provide the body's first protective barrier to invasion by a foreign invader. *(Courtesy of Dr. Norio Azumi.)*

2. **Heterogeneity:** The cells and cell products that comprise the adaptive immune system consist of a variety of different types; and
3. **Memory:** The ability to recognize an antigen upon subsequent encounters with the foreign substance in a more rapid and highly augmented fashion.

Because the adaptive immune system is composed of relatively small numbers of cells with specificity to recognize an individual immunogen, the responding cells must proliferate, forming a cell clone, and differentiate into effector cells after encountering a foreign substance to attain sufficient numbers to mount an effective response commensurate with the quantity of the foreign agent being presented. Thus, the adaptive immune response generally expresses itself temporally, usually several days after the innate response, in the encounter with foreignness. A key feature of the adaptive immune response is that it produces large quantities of long-lived cells (i.e., memory cells, as described below) that persist in an apparently dormant state, but that can re-express effector functions rapidly after subsequent encounters with the same antigen. This provides the adaptive immune response with the ability to manifest immune memory, permitting it to contribute to a more effective host response against specific pathogens when they are encountered a second time, even decades after the initial sensitizing encounter.

Table 1-1. Soluble factors in secretions and sweat

Factors	Locations	Functions
Acidic pH	Skin, stomach, vagina	Inhibit bacterial growth
Fatty acids	Sweat	Inhibit bacterial growth
Mucins and agglutinins	Secretions	Aggregate bacteria
Peroxidases	Secretions	Catalyze oxidation of lipid membranes of bacteria
Protease inhibitors	Secretions	Inhibit bacterial function by inhibiting protease activity
Lysozymes	Sweat and secretions	Destroy bacteria by hydrolyzing the polysaccharide component of the cell wall.
Lactoferrin	Secretions	Inhibit bacterial growth by binding iron
Histidine-rich proteins (histatins)	Saliva	Exert antifungal properties by disrupting mitochondrial function
Cationic proteins	Sweat and secretions	Exert antibacterial activity by binding to lipid cellular membranes
Defensins and other antibacterial peptides	Secretions	Secreted by leukocytes and active against bacteria, fungi, and enveloped viruses

Table 1-2. The two major components of the adaptive immune system

Type	Effector cells	Effector mechanism(s)	Outcome
Humoral	B cells	Antibody	Neutralization of foreign antigen and coating substances for opsonization
Cell-mediated	T cells	Cytokines, cell-cell interaction Cytotoxic activity	Promotion or inhibition of inflammation, and/or humoral function Lysis of infected cells

The two major components of the adaptive immune response are (1) **humoral immunity** and (2) cell-mediated immunity (**CMI**). Humoral immunity is a process carried out by proteins called **antibodies** that belong to the family of immunoglobulins, produced by a subset of lymphocytes (B cells) in response to and capable of reacting with antigen (*Chapter 6*). Cell-mediated immunity is the other arm of the adaptive immune response carried out by another subset of lymphocytes referred to as T lymphocytes (*Chapter 7*).

Antibodies are proteins produced by and secreted from B cells and specifically bind extracellular antigen. In humans, there are five major classes (i.e., isotypes) of immunoglobulins: IgM, IgG, IgA, IgD, and IgE, each differing in physical, chemical, and biologic properties (*Chapter 6*). The primary function of antibody is to directly bind with the foreign substance/pathogen. As will be described subsequently, there are a number of other interactions of antibody with other cells and components of the innate immune system.

T cells are capable of recognizing intracellular infections (viruses and bacteria that can survive inside the cells that have ingested them). Cell-mediated immunity is a process carried out by T cells through the production of cell-regulating molecules (cytokines) or through inducing cell death (cytotoxicity) without the participation of antibody (*Chapters 7* and *9*).

Innate and Adaptive Immune Responses Act Together to Eliminate Pathogens

Traditionally, the innate and adaptive immune responses were thought to act independently. It is now clear, however, that the two arms of the immune system work together and should be viewed as interactive and interdependent rather than isolated systems. As will be described throughout this book, the innate immune system is operative on initial and subsequent encounters with foreignness and instructs the type of adaptive immune response that follows. The adaptive immune response, in turn, works intimately with components of the innate immune system. The innate immune system in essence "tells" the cells of the adaptive immune system what sort of reaction is needed and therefore is central to both the generation of an effective and appropriate immune response and the regulation of the entire immune system (Figure 1-7).

The Immune System Can Also Cause Disease (Immunopathology)

In classical usage, the term immunity referred to the beneficial relative resistance of the host to reinfection by a given microbe. The immune system is equipped, however, not only to perform a **defense function** against infectious agents, but also to concern itself with more diverse biologic functions of homeostasis and surveillance (Table 1-3). It is now evident, however, that immune responses are not always beneficial and associated with resistance to infection; they sometimes are detrimental and can confer unpleasant and harmful effects on the host in the form of immune-mediated disorders. These noxious effects are seen in such clinical entities as allergy, autoimmune disorders, and malignancy (*Chapters 18, 19,* and *20*).

As shown in Table 1-3, although the removal of exogenous microbes provides the normal primordial function of defense, this role may be exaggerated as in the case of patients with allergic disease who manifest with severe asthma (*Chapter 18*). Alternatively, this defense function may be diminished, e.g., in patients with immune deficiencies who suffer

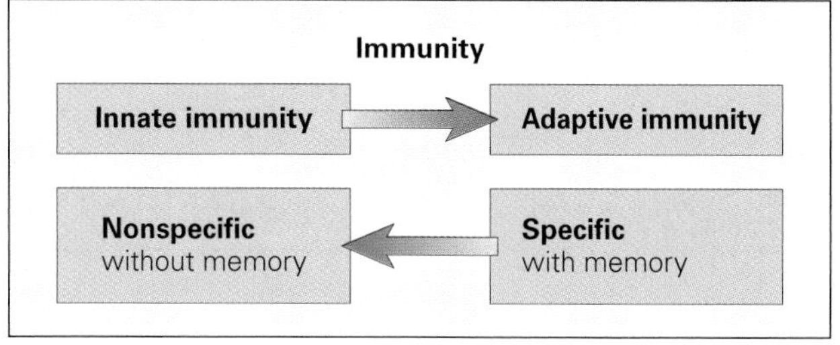

Figure 1-7. Schematic representation of the interactive nature of the innate and adaptive immune systems.

Table 1-3. Functions of the immune system in health and disease

Function	Nature of immune stimulus	Example	Aberrations	
			Hyper-	Hypo-
Defense	Exogenous	Infectious agents	Allergy	Immune deficiency
Homeostasis	Endogenous or exogenous	Removal of effete or damaged cells	Autoimmune diseases	—
Surveillance	Endogenous or exogenous	Removal of cell mutants	—	Malignant disease

Note: — = not applicable.

from undue susceptibility to recurrent infections (*Chapter 16*). A second function is **homeostasis**, i.e., the function of maintaining a balance between the internal and external environments. This is exemplified normally by removal of worn-out cells, e.g., senescent erythrocytes. This normal function may be exaggerated in autoimmune disorders (*Chapter 19*) as in the case of autoimmune hemolytic anemia, where the destruction of erythrocytes is excessive and may lead to severe anemia. A third recognized function of the immune system is **surveillance**, which normally provides the host with the ability to recognize and destroy altered self-components, e.g., cell mutants. Reduced capacity of this function has been associated with a propensity for development of malignant diseases (*Chapters 20* and *21*).

A Unifying Model of Immunology

In order to better understand the expressions of the immune system in health and disease, the immune system may be viewed as a dynamic multi-compartmental network of cellular and humoral elements with ever-changing morphologic components and functions. As with all physiologic mechanisms, immune response(s) may be viewed as an adaptive system in which the body attempts to maintain homeostasis between its internal environment and the external environment.

For ease of presentation of the complex processes that characterize the totality of the immune response, a unifying model of immune processes has been developed and found to be useful. This will serve as a framework for further descriptions of the clinical applications of immunology that will be presented in greater detail in subsequent chapters of this text. The model has been adapted from one originally suggested by Talmage, which we have used in the previous editions of *Immunology*. Various sections of this overview model will be expanded in greater detail in subsequent chapters, as well as in the online version, and its broad presentation in this chapter is intended to frame a general portrait of "the forest" before a detailed description of "the individual trees." In general, it is possible to identify five major components of the host's encounter with foreignness: (1) the environment; (2) the target cells; (3) the physiologic and anatomic barriers; (4) cells and cell products of the innate immune system; and (5) cells and cell products of the adaptive immune system (Box 1-3).

The External Environment Is the Source of Most Pathogens and Other Foreign Substances

Most substances that confront, and ultimately activate, the host's immune system arise from the exterior world. Therefore, the place to begin any discussion of the immune system is with the myriad foreign substances that comprise the external environment (Figure 1-8).

Box 1-3

Elements of the Host's Encounter with Foreignness

Environment
Target Cells
The Physiologic and Anatomic Barriers
The Innate Immune System

- Phagocytic cells
- Mediator cells and mediator products
- Soluble plasma/tissue fluid components
- Natural killer cells

The Adaptive Immune System

- Antigen-presenting cells
- T-lymphocytes
- B-lymphocytes
- Antibodies

The Cytokines

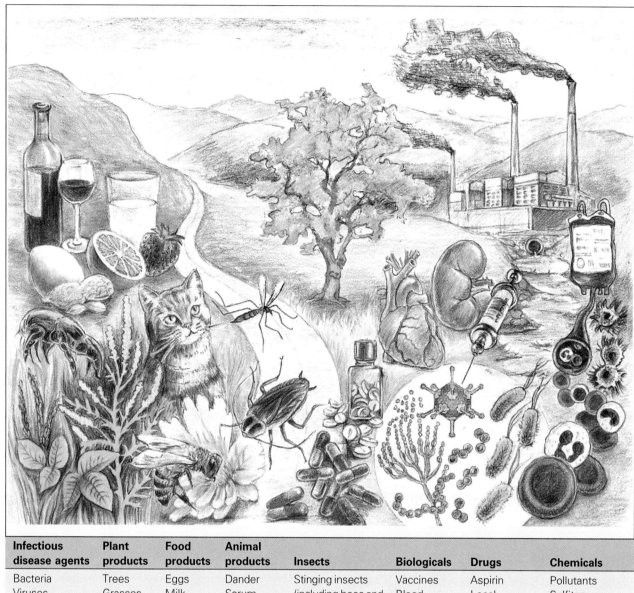

Infectious disease agents	Plant products	Food products	Animal products	Insects	Biologicals	Drugs	Chemicals
Bacteria Viruses Fungi Protozoan and helminthic parasites	Trees Grasses Pollens Poison ivy Molds and spores	Eggs Milk Nuts Peanuts Fruit	Dander Serum Dust mites Pet epithelial cells	Stinging insects (including bees and mosquitoes) Cockroaches	Vaccines Blood products Transplanted organs Malignant cells	Aspirin Local anesthetics Penicillin	Pollutants Sulfites Radiocontrast media Dioxins Dyes Food additives and preservatives Metals

Figure 1-8. Examples of infectious and noninfectious environmental agents that activate the immunologic system.

Most prominent among these environmental substances are the microbial agents, e.g., bacteria, viruses, fungi, and protozoan parasites, as well as the macroscopic helminth (worm) parasites. Infectious organisms pose the most serious threats to the individual and to society. The emergence of new infectious diseases—e.g., acquired immune deficiency syndrome (**AIDS**) caused by the human immunodeficiency virus (**HIV**); severe acute respiratory syndrome (**SARS**) caused by the SARS coronavirus (**SARS-CoV**); and avian epidemic influenza infections caused by periodic antigenic shifts of influenza viruses—exemplify this continuing and ever-present threat to individual and global health. Other foreign environmental components range from the simplest, low molecular chemicals to the most complex, naturally occurring, and human-produced biological agents (Figure 1-8). In addition to the traditional list of plant, food, animal, and man-made products that trigger allergic diseases, the catalog of environmental agents that activate the immune response has been greatly expanded in recent years by the ever-increasing number of drugs and biologicals that have become available for clinical use as a result of modern molecular and cellular biology. Continuing evidence suggests that a number of diseases may result from the direct toxic effects of the introduction of inorganic and complex organic compounds into our external environment. Collectively, the adverse effects of these toxic substances on the immune system fall under the heading of immunotoxicology and are becoming increasingly important as our environment becomes more polluted and complex. It should also be emphasized that the immune system may be activated not only by foreign substances that arise from the external environment, but also by those present in the internal environment, e.g., foreign cells arising from a transplanted organ, or virally or chemically induced or spontaneously arising malignant cells.

Shown in Table 1-4 are common terms used to define various noninfectious foreign substances found in the external environment that may be recognized as "nonself" and initiate responses can give rise to immune-mediated diseases, or may be tolerated as "self" and elicit no immune response. Those substances that share the characteristic of being recognized as foreign and have the capacity to evoke the immune responses of adaptive immunity are referred to as **immunogens** or **antigens**. Although these terms are commonly used interchangeably, some immunologists restrict the use of the word "immunogen" to those substances that have the capacity to induce the immune response; the term "antigen" to those substances that react with the specific products of B cells (i.e., antibodies) or receptors on the surface of T cells and B cells (i.e., T cell receptor [**TCR**] and B cell receptor [**BCR**]). 6
Antigens are composed of **epitopes** (i.e., antigenic determinants), which are the small regions of the immunogen that are the sites recognized by antibodies or by TCR and BCR. In specific circumstances (e.g., antigen interaction with immature B or T cells), the encounter with a foreign substance may lead to an inability of the immune system to respond to that specific substance, a state that is called **immune tolerance**; such configurations are referred to as **tolerogens** and have the capacity to "silence" the critical cells involved in the induction of the immune response (*Chapter 19*). **Allergens** are a specialized class of immunogens that take part in the pathogenesis of allergic (i.e., immediate hypersensitivity) reactions in certain genetically predisposed (**atopic**) individuals (*Chapter 18*). Therefore, all allergens are immunogens, but not all immunogens are allergens. Immunogens may be complete and may lead to an immune response *per se*, or they may be low molecular weight, incomplete immunogens (usually chemical substances) called **haptens** and require prior attachment to a carrier molecule to become fully immunogenic (e.g., penicillin). As described below, this process involves the critical collaboration of antigen-presenting cells (**APCs**), T cells, and B cells.

Table 1-4. Types of foreign substances that may initiate immune responses in the normal host or produce immune-mediated diseases or no response

Classification	Definition	Mechanism of action	Examples
Immunogen, antigen	Substance capable of evoking an adaptive immune response	Recognition as foreign; processing by antigen-presenting cells, (APCs), activation of T and B cells	Diphtheria vaccine in a healthy subject
Tolerogen	Substance capable of evoking no immune response	Silencing of antigen-presenting cells, inactivation of T and B cells	Food protein in a normal host
Allergen	A specialized class of immunogen capable of eliciting an allergic response	Immune imbalance of T cell subpopulations with excessive IgE production in a susceptible (atopic) host	Ragweed allergen that causes allergic rhinitis (hay fever) in an atopic individual
Hapten	Low molecular weight chemical substances that function as "incomplete" immunogens	Requires attachment to a carrier molecule to become fully immunogenic	Penicillin causing urticaria (hives) in a patient being treated for an infection

Host Cells Are the Targets of Environmental Agents

The introduction of an environmental agent into a host may have an adverse effect on any of a wide variety of **target cells** (Figure 1-9, Table 1-5). These target cells vary according to their type and location as well as the portal of entry of the foreign substance. It is important to emphasize that the target cell may be a normal host cell that can be modified through its interaction with an environmental agent (e.g., chemical), or by an infectious agent (such as a virus), or by malignant transformation of the target cell itself (e.g., a tumor cell). Alternatively, the target cell may be a foreign cell introduced by the transplantation of tissue from another member of the same species (e.g., a kidney transplant [**allogeneic**]) or from another species (e.g., a heart transplant from a baboon [**xenogeneic**]) (*Chapter 22*). In any of these scenarios, the target cell may sustain direct injury by the environmental agent or when recognized as foreign, may be destroyed by an adaptive immune response. In either case, the injury may be mild and reversible, with minimal signs and symptoms of disease, or may be more severe, with cell death and more serious consequences. Some examples of the more common target cells that may sustain injury are shown in Table 1-5 together with mechanisms of injury and clinical sequelae. Included are cells of the skin, gastrointestinal, genitourinary, respiratory, circulatory, and central nervous systems.

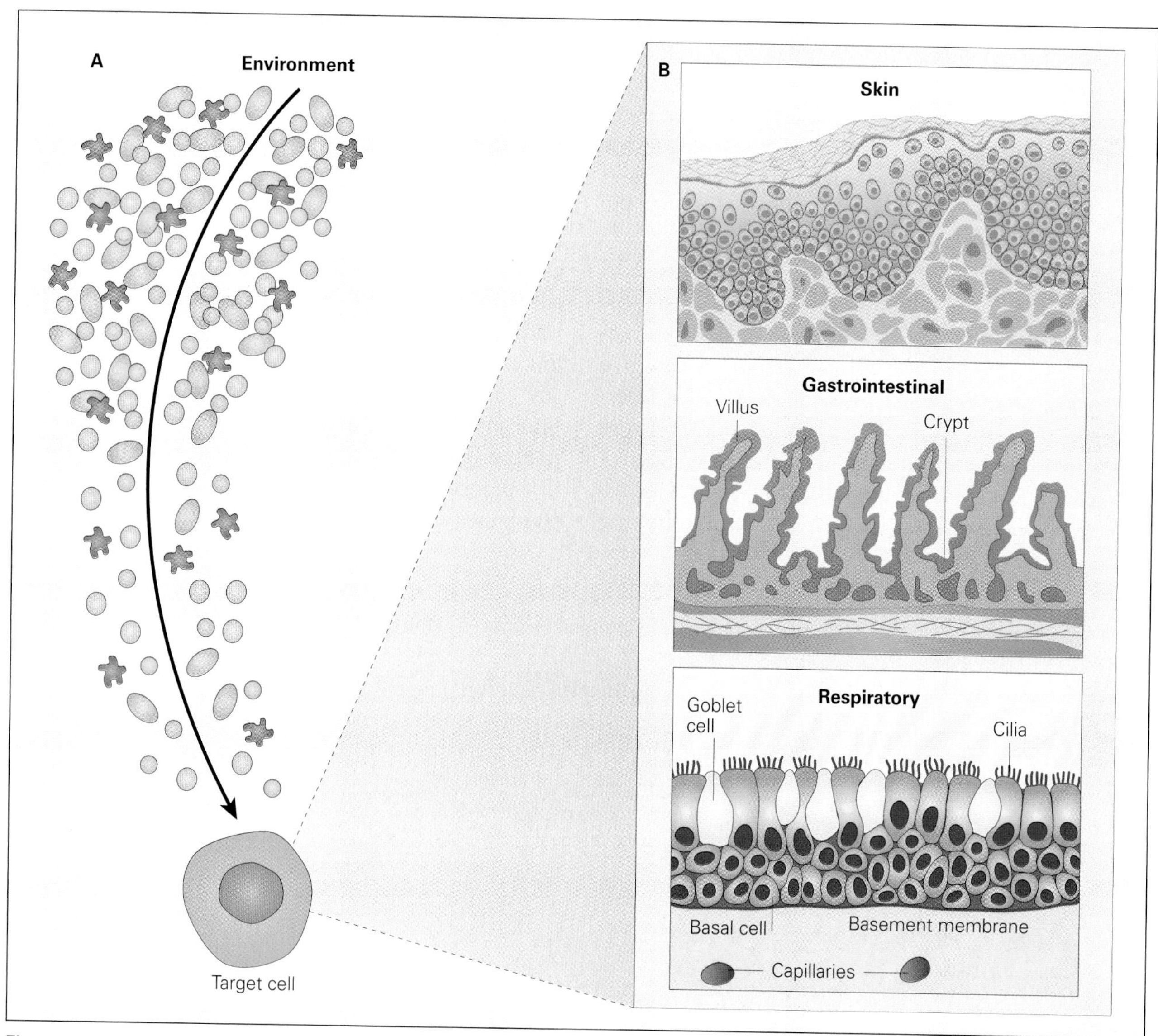

Figure 1-9. Panel A: Target cells are host cells affected by environmental agents. Panel B: Examples of target cells are presented.

Table 1-5. Examples of effects of environmental agents on target cells and their clinical sequelae

Location of target cell	Mechanism of injury	Example of environmental agent	Clinical sequelae
Skin	Disruption of epidermal cells	Oil of poison ivy	Dermatitis
Gastrointestinal tract			
Mucosal cell	Destruction	Cow's milk	Gastrointestinal bleeding
Smooth muscle	Increased contractility		Diarrhea, vomiting
Glandular cell	Increased secretion		Increased mucus production in asthma
Liver parenchymal cell	Destruction	Liver transplant	Hypoproteinemia
Genitourinary tract			
Renal glomerulus	Disruption	β-hemolytic *Streptococcus pyogenes* group A	Acute glomerulonephritis; hematuria, proteinuria
Respiratory tract			
Smooth muscle	Increased contraction	Grass pollen	Asthma; bronchospasm
Glandular cell	Increased secretion; allergic inflammation		Increased mucus production and inflammation
Circulatory system			
Endothelial cell	Increased intercellular pore size	Shellfish	Edema
Formed elements	Destruction of erythrocytes	α-methyldopa	Anemia
Nervous system			
Central	Destruction of myelin and neurons	Measles virus	Encephalomyelitis
Peripheral	Destruction of myelin and neural axons	Influenza virus	Peripheral neuritis

Contact of the skin with the haptenic structures in the oil of poison ivy may trigger an immune attack, with disruption of epidermal cells and severe dermatitis. Ingestion of an offending food substance, e.g., cow's milk in a cow milk–allergic infant, may lead to an immune attack on the mucosal cells, smooth muscle cells, and mucous glandular cells of the gastrointestinal tract, with accompanying gastrointestinal bleeding, diarrhea, vomiting, and mucus production characteristic of the severely milk-allergic infant. An immune attack on liver parenchymal cells in a patient receiving a liver transplant may lead to destruction of hepatic parenchymal cells, with severe hypoproteinemia due to impaired protein synthesis characteristic of liver failure. Infection with β-hemolytic *Streptococcus pyogenes* group A may lead to immune injury of the glomerulus, with resultant hematuria and proteinuria. The impact of the inhalation of grass pollen on the smooth muscle and mucous glands of the respiratory tract in a highly allergic patient may lead to increased contractility, with bronchospasm and increased secretion of mucus and allergic inflammation characteristic of bronchial asthma. Alternatively, a patient highly allergic to shellfish may sustain immune injury to endothelial target cells of blood vessels and may manifest clinical urticaria (hives) resulting from the leakage of edema fluid into tissues from blood vessels as a consequence of increased interendothelial pore size. A patient receiving a drug for control of hypertension, e.g., α-methyldopa, may evidence immune injury of the formed elements of the blood, such as erythrocytes, which is manifest clinically with anemia. The impact of viruses, e.g., measles, or protozoans like falciparum malaria, on cells and lining tissues (i.e., myelin sheaths of the neurologic system) may lead to tissue destruction, with resultant neurologic dysfunction characteristic of the demyelinating diseases of the neurologic system, e.g., multiple sclerosis, encephalomyelitis, peripheral neuritis, or the symptoms of cerebral malaria.

Physiologic and Anatomic Barriers Block the Entry of Most Environmental Agents

As described previously, most foreign substances, including microbial pathogens, enter the body through the natural portals of entry, e.g., the respiratory (nose and mouth), gastrointestinal (mouth), and genitourinary (urethra, vagina) tracts, where

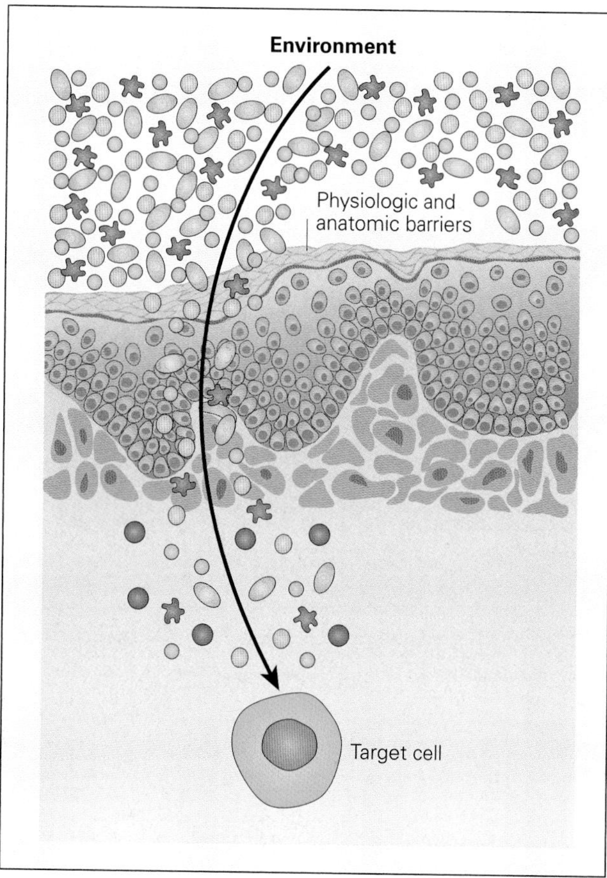

Figure 1-10. The physiologic and anatomic barriers provide initial protection between the environment and the target cell.

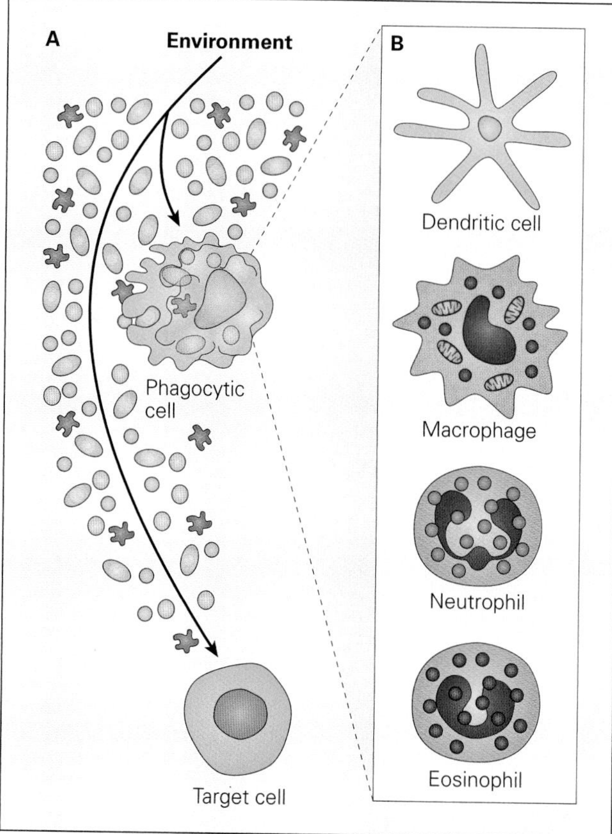

Figure 1-11. Panel A: The phagocytic cell is the first element of the innate immune system and forms a barrier between the external environment and target cells. Panel B: Examples of phagocytic cells.

initial barriers like the skin and mucous membranes or acid pH of the stomach provide blockage to entry of the foreign substance into the body (Figure 1-10).

Elements of Innate Immunity

Phagocytes Engulf and Destroy Pathogens

During the course of evolution, a number of elements of the innate immune system developed within vertebrates and are referred to as **phagocytic cells** (*Chapter 2*). They are involved in the process of uptake and engulfment of particles from the external environment, i.e., **phagocytosis**; complete digestion of these ingested particles may lead to their elimination. These cells participate both in phagocytosis and inflammation, which constitute the body's first line of inducible defense and represent the most primitive of the responses of the innate immune system (*Chapter 5*). The phagocytic cell may be considered, then, as another barrier between the external environment and the target cell, protecting the target cell from subsequent injury (Figure 1-11). Phagocytosis is carried out primarily by mononuclear phagocytes (monocytes in the blood and macrophages in tissues), dendritic cells, neutrophils (polymorphonuclear leukocytes), and, to a lesser degree, eosinophils.

How Phagocytes Recognize Pathogens

The innate immune response is triggered by common structural components found on or within a wide variety of microorganisms and other foreign substances and function as signaling molecules by which phagocytes recognize pathogens. These signaling molecules on pathogens are generically called PAMPs (*Chapter 3*). Other molecules on cells of the innate immune system function to recognize PAMPs and are referred to as PRRs. They are found either as soluble molecules in diverse body fluids, or as membrane-associated sensors expressed on cell surfaces, which are exemplified by a group of molecules referred to as the toll-like receptors (**TLRs**). An example of one of the important PAMPs is the lipopolysaccharide (**LPS**) of gram-negative bacteria that is recognized by the TLR4 member of the toll-like receptor family. These signaling molecules will be described in greater detail in Chapter 3.

Phagocytes Are Attracted to Sites of Tissue Injury as Part of Inflammation: The Body's Reaction to Injury

Following any of several causes of tissue injury, e.g., trauma, burns, or infection, there occurs a variety of tissue responses referred to as inflammation, i.e., the body's response to injury, in which the migration of phagocytic cells from the blood to the tissues is critical (*Chapter 5*). The phagocytic cells can be mobilized to sites of inflammation by damaged tissue, products of bacteria, or soluble plasma protein components called *complement* by the process of directed cell migration called **chemotaxis** (*Chapter 4*). The neutrophils comprise the major component of acute inflammation, whereas macrophages and other cells, e.g., lymphocytes, are found accumulated at tissue sites undergoing chronic inflammation (Figure 1-11).

The process of phagocytosis itself can contribute to tissue injury-mediated inflammation by the release of intracellular products, e.g., lysosomal enzymes and cytokines, as seen in certain autoimmune diseases (*Chapter 19*). Phagocytic cells use several mechanisms to enhance the uptake of particles from the external environment; such mechanisms include a variety of membrane-associated receptors on the surface of phagocytes that can bind specific components of immunoglobulins (Fc receptors) and of complement (complement receptor) as described below. Shown in Box 1-4 are some examples of cases that illustrate the clinical relevance of inflammation.

Mediators Produced by a Variety of Cells Promote Inflammation

The term *mediators* encompasses a group of pharmacologically active macromolecular and low molecular weight substances produced by specialized cells referred to as **mediator cells** (Table 1-6) 7 following their interaction with environmental agents (Figure 1-14A). These mediator substances are produced by several types of mediator cells but primarily by circulating basophils and tissue mast cells (Figure 1-14B) and promote inflammation as part of the healing processes in the normal host (Figure 1-15A) but can also contribute to the deleterious effects of the inflammatory process on target cells, as seen in the patient with allergic disease(s) (Figure 1-15B). Mediators are either preformed or newly synthesized in mediator cells in response to an

Box 1-4

A Case Study Illustrating Acute Inflammation

A ten-month-old female presented with a one-day history of fever and red, tender lesions on the right side of the face. Seven days prior, while playing near a coffee table, she sustained injury to the head and presented one week later with irritability, fever, redness, swelling, and tenderness over the right side of the face and two localized 2 × 2 and 4 × 4 cm fluctuant masses with overlying redness of the skin over the right side of the face (Figure 1-12). A CBC revealed a WBC of 29,800/mm^3 with 77 percent PMNs and 2 percent bands. A soft tissue CT scan showed swelling but no fractures were evident. A nasal pharyngeal culture was obtained and revealed a heavy growth of *Staphylococcus aureus*, coagulase+. Drainage of the two masses revealed purulent material containing a predominance of neutrophils and a heavy growth of *Staphylococcus aureus*, coagulase+. The child was treated with clindamycin and ceftriaxone and recovered without subsequent events. This case illustrates how the innate immune system responds to an acute bacterial infection with acute localized inflammatory subcutaneous abscesses with hematologic responses of elevated numbers of mature and immature myeloid cells consisting of PMNs and band forms, important cellular components of the host response to bacterial infections in acute inflammation and a valuable diagnostic test (*Chapter 12*).

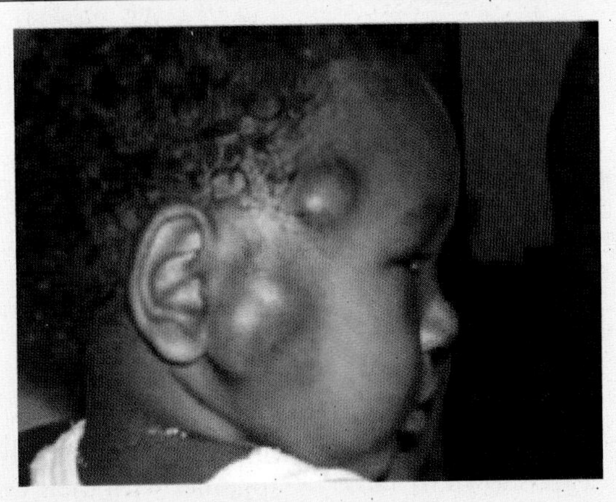

Figure 1-12. Photograph of a ten-month-old child with tender, localized soft tissue abscesses on the right side of the face. (As seen on Wikipedia.)

(continued)

Box 1-4 (continued)

A Case Study Illustrating Chronic Inflammation

During the course of routine pediatric care, a pediatrician administered a tuberculin skin test to a twelve-month-old male infant. The infant was found to manifest a 20 × 20 mm positive TST at forty-eight to seventy-two hours, and a positive right lobe pulmonary infiltrate with mediastinal lymphadenopathy was revealed by chest X-ray and computerized tomography (**CT**) scan (Figure 1-13). Gastric lavage and bronchial alveolar lavage specimens were obtained for culture, and the child was started on isoniazid, rifampin, ethambutol, pyrazinamide, and prednisolone. The bronchial lavage cells consisted primarily of alveolar macrophages and lymphocytes. At twenty-nine days, the hospital laboratory reported that a mycobacterial agent was growing in culture and the isolate was subjected to further identification. At fifty days, the organism was identified as *M. avium*, an organism found in birds closely related to the *M. tuberculosis* agent causing tuberculosis in humans. The prednisolone was discontinued, and the antibiotic regimen was changed to rifampin, ethambutol, and clarithromycin. This case illustrates how the innate immune system responds to a chronic bacterial infection with pulmonary lesions consisting primarily of macrophages and lymphocytes, i.e., granuloma (*Chapter 12*).

This case study also illustrates the host immune response to a mycobacterial organism which evokes a chronic inflammatory response consisting of macrophages and lymphocytes, important cellular components of the host response to bacterial infections which establish chronic infections (*Chapter 12*). The chest X-ray findings and observation of macrophages and lymphocytes in the BAL specimen is consistent with a chronic inflammatory response to a bacterial agent known to cause chronic infection and because of the seriousness of the infection the anti-inflammatory corticosteroids were added to the therapeutic regimen.

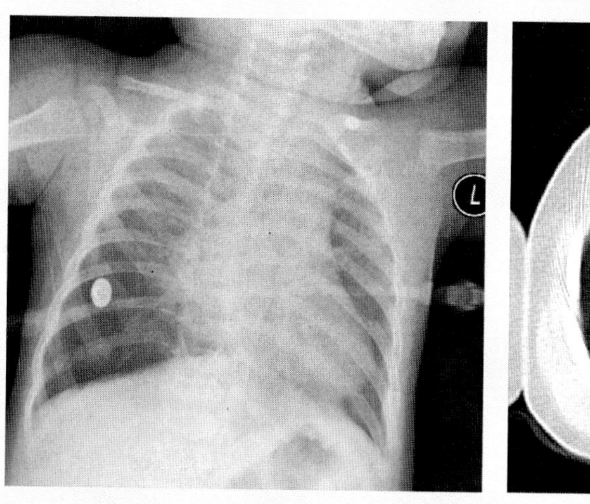

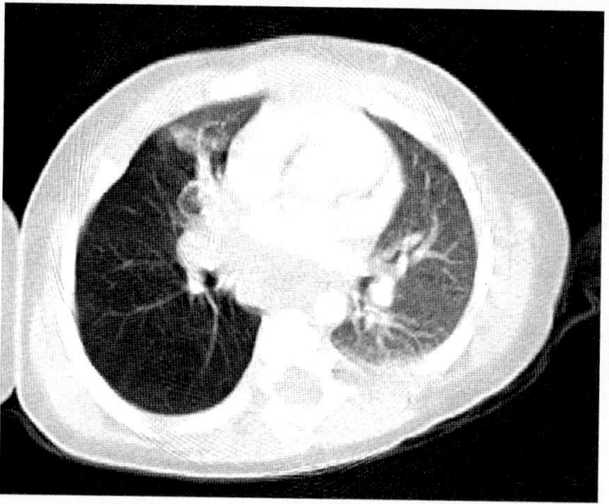

Figure 1-13. Panel A: X-ray of the chest and CT chest scan showing right upper lobe infiltrate. Panel B: Shows enlarged mediastinal lymph nodes in a twelve-month-old infant with pneumonia caused by *M. avium*. This illustrates a chronic inflammatory response to this intracellular bacterial infection. *(Courtesy of Dr. Thomas Rubio.)*

environmental agent. The best studied of these substances are shown in Table 1-6 together with their cellular sources and biologic functions and include histamine, serotonin, kinins, and products of the arachidonic acid (eicosanoid) system, including leukotrienes C_4, D_4, E_4, platelet-activating factor (**PAF**), cytokines, and chemokines.

Mediator cells consist of a heterogeneous collection of morphologic types that include primarily tissue mast cells, circulating basophils, and eosinophils, but also platelets, enterochromaffin cells, monocytes/macrophages, and neutrophils. The best studied of these are the basophils, mast cells, and eosinophils, which are important sources of mediator substances that perform a normal function of promoting inflammation in the healthy host (Figure 1-15A) as well as contributing to allergic inflammation when produced in large quantities in the allergic patient (Figure 1-15B)

Table 1-6. Mediator cells and mediators: types, products, and functions

Mediator cell	Types	Products	Action
Mast cells	Preformed	Histamine, serine proteases (chymase, tryptase), carboxypeptidase A, and proteoglycans (heparin and chondroitin sulfate E).	Smooth muscle contraction, enhanced vascular permeability, neural stimulation, mucus secretion storage, anticoagulation
	Newly synthesized (lipid)	Prostaglandin (PG) D_2 and leukotrienes (LT), C_4, D_4, E_4	Bronchoconstrictors enhance vascular permeability
	Cytokines	IL-4	Th2 cell differentiation and IgE synthesis
		IL-3, GM-CSF, IL-5, IL-6, and IL-16	Eosinophil and basophil development, activation, and survival
		TNF-α	Up-regulates endothelial and epithelial adhesion molecules, increases bronchial responsiveness, and has anti-tumor effects
	Chemokines	IL-8 (CXCL-8), MIP-1a (CCL-3)	Leukocyte chemotaxis
Basophils	Similar to those produced by mast cells	Histamine, leukotrienes, and cytokines, e.g., IL-4 and IL-13 (PGD_2 and IL-5 not produced by basophils)	Immediate hypersensitivity and allergic inflammation; basophil expression of IL-4 and CD40L induces B-cell IgE switching; IL-4 could further drive Th2 cell differentiation
		Chondroitin sulfate, major basic protein, and Charcot-Leyden crystal protein, small amounts of tryptase	
Eosinophils	Granule stored	Cationic proteins, major basic protein (MBP), eosinophil-derived neurotoxin (EDN), and eosinophil peroxidase (EPO)	Host defense and pathogenesis of eosinophil-mediated diseases; neurologic manifestations
	Eiconasoids	LTC_4, LTD_4, and LTE_4	
	Cytokines	IL-1, transforming growth factor , IL-3, IL-4, IL-5, IL-8	
	Chemokines	TNF-α	Leukocyte chemotaxis

Source: Adapted from Prussin, C., and Metcalfe, D. *Journal of Allergy and Clinical Immunology* 11 (2003): S486.

(*Chapter 17*). Principal among the cells drawn to sites of allergic inflammation is the eosinophil, which exerts its cardinal effects through mediator release in certain of the immediate hypersensitivity diseases associated with allergy in the human (*Chapter 18*). The presence of elevated quantities of eosinophils in the nasal secretions of a patient with allergic rhinitis or in the sputum of a patient with allergic asthma provides the clinician with useful information for the diagnosis of these conditions.

Soluble Plasma Tissue Fluid Components: Complement and Acute Phase Proteins Promote Inflammation and Phagocytosis

In addition to mediators generated or released from mediator cells, a wide variety of other soluble plasma protein components function as biologic amplification systems augmenting the functions of both the innate and adaptive immune systems (*Chapter 2*). These include the complement (*Chapter 4*) and coagulation systems that are commonly activated during inflammation (*Chapter 5*) and the acute phase proteins, mannose-binding lectin, and C-reactive protein (Table 1-7). The components of these systems are synthesized in other tissues, e.g., the liver, and are found predominantly as plasma components.

Complement consists of a collection of cascading plasma proteins that may be activated by three pathways: (1) the **lectin**, (2) **alternative**, and (3) **classical** pathways (*Chapter 4*) (Figure 1-16). The lectin and alternative pathways are initiated by PAMPs located on the surface of infectious agents as part of the innate immune response. The classical pathway is activated by the specific interaction of a specific component of complement with antibody fixed to antigen as part of the adaptive immune response. The products of the complement cascade may facilitate certain immune functions in the defense of the host as the lysis of certain viruses, bacteria, or foreign cells, chemotaxis of phagocytic cells, promotion of phagocytosis (opsonization), and mediation of the inflammatory process (*Chapter 4*).

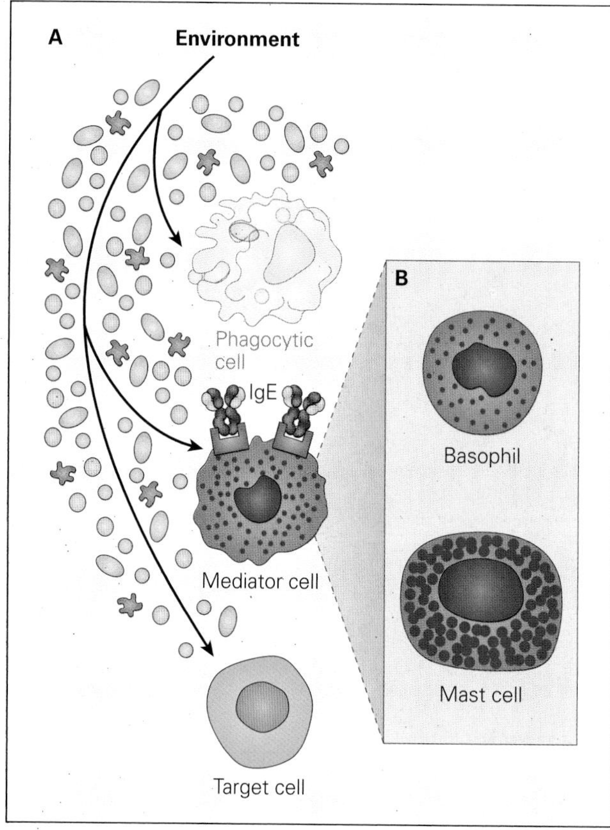

Figure 1-14. Panel A: Mediator cells responding to an environmental agent. Panel B: Basophils and mast cells are the two most important examples of mediator cells.

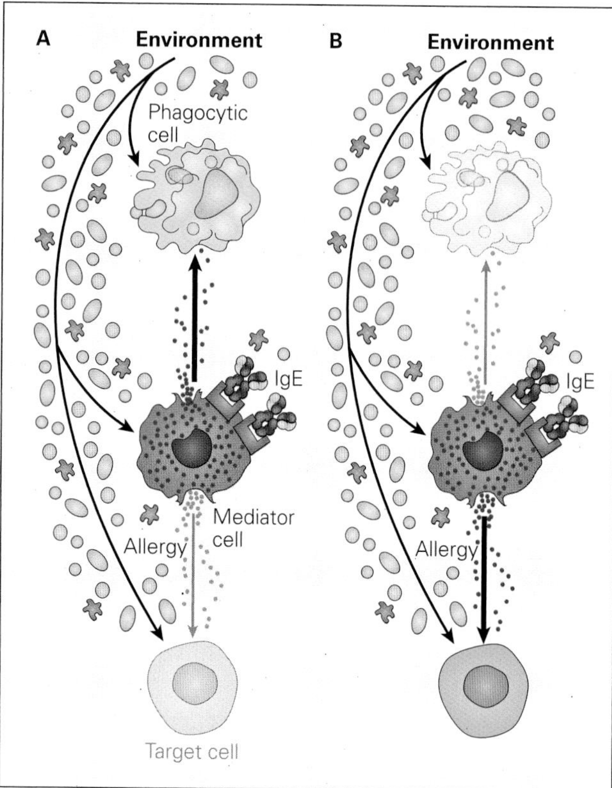

Figure 1-15. Panel A: Mediator cells responding to an environmental agent with mediator products being released from mediator cells showing their beneficial effects on phagocytic cells in the promotion of inflammation in the normal host. Panel B: Mediator cells' deleterious effects on target cells of the allergic patient (e.g., allergy).

Natural Killer Cells Recognize and Eliminate Infected and Cancerous Host Cells

The natural killer (**NK**) cells (Figure 1-17A) belong to the innate immune system and are specialized to kill target cells that are infected with viruses (*Chapter 13*) or host cells that have become cancerous (*Chapter 20*). These cells are called "natural" killers because they are normally found in great numbers at birth in the cord blood of neonatal infants and do not need additional stimulation to recognize a specific antigen in order to attack and kill target cells. The NK cell is a type of large granular lymphocyte arising from a lymphoid precursor (*Chapter 2*) that does not express markers of either the T or B cell lineage but which possesses Fc receptors for IgG and complement. The interaction of an NK cell with a target cell can occur in two ways: (1) by a direct cell-to-cell interaction through the ligation of a variety of NK receptors (Figure 1-17B); or (2) by the bridging of both cells through an immunoglobulin

Table 1-7. Soluble plasma/tissue fluid components and their immune functions

Acute phase proteins	
Mannose-binding lectin	Activates complement
C-reactive protein	Promotes phagocytosis
Complement proteins	
C3b (opsonin)	Promotes phagocytosis
C3a, C4a, C5a (anaphylatoxins)	Stimulates inflammation
C5a (chemotactic factor)	Attracts neutrophils
Coagulation/Kinin proteins	
Plasmin	Degrades blood clots
Thrombin	Part of clotting cascade
Kinins	Cause vasodilation and smooth muscle contraction

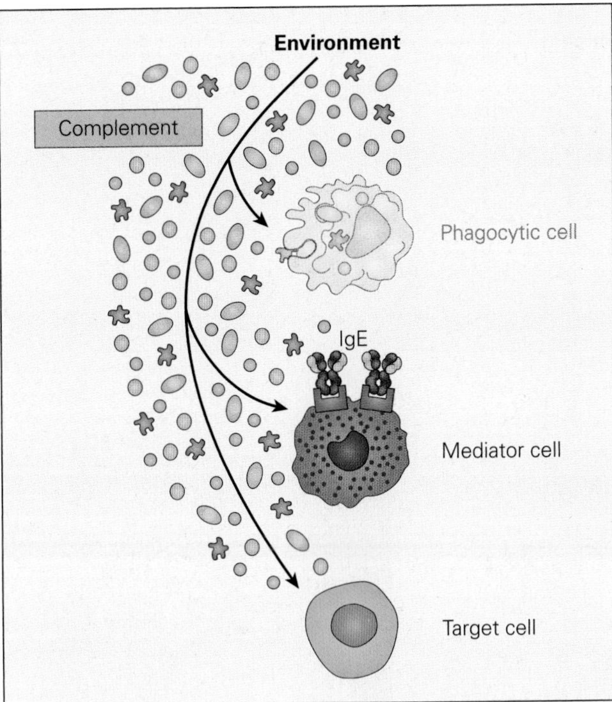

Figure 1-16. Complement is one of several soluble plasma/tissue fluid components, e.g., acute phase reactants, complement, and coagulation components, which also participate in innate immunity.

molecule by a process referred to as antibody-dependent cell-mediated cytotoxicity (**ADCC**) (Figure 1-17C). When the NK cell kills a target cell by direct contact, it does so as part of the innate immune response by releasing cytotoxic granules containing perforin and granzymes (Figure 1-17B). Upon degranulation, perforin first inserts itself into the target cell's plasma membrane, forming a pore through which granzymes next enter with subsequent release of intracellular contents. This direct method of target cell killing utilizes a complex balance of signalling through killer inhibitory receptors (**KIRs**) and killer activating receptors (**KARs**) that are described in Chapter 3. Alternatively, when the NK cell kills a target cell with the facilitation of immunoglobulin (i.e., ADCC), it therefore is seen as part of the adaptive immune response (Figure 1-17C). The end result of killing by NK cells by either pathway is programmed death of the cell by apoptosis (*Chapter 9*). There is a subset of invariant NK T cells that contain a T cell receptor that may provide a mechanism for specific recognition of antigen (*Chapter 3*) that will be described below under the T cell section. Patients with some immunodeficiencies, such as those caused by HIV infection, have a decrease in NK cell activity.

Elements of Adaptive Immunity

Lymphocytes Perform Adaptive Immune Functions

As described previously, the cells of the adaptive immune system, in contrast to those of the innate immune system, interact with the environmental agent in a highly discriminative way, i.e., they display **specificity, heterogeneity**, and **memory**. These functions are primarily carried out by two types of cells that are involved in the recognition of antigen: (1) the thymus-dependent or T lymphocytes, which participate in CMI against intracellular pathogens, organ transplants, and malignant cells; and (2) the bone marrow or bursal-dependent B lymphocytes, which provide humoral immunity, i.e., antibody-mediated immunity against extracellular pathogens, their toxins, and other environmental substances. A third group of cells involved in the presentation of antigen to T cells, i.e., APCs, include dendritic cells, macrophages, and B cells (Table 1-8). APCs take up predominantly protein antigens, cut them into peptides, bind the peptides to major histocompatibility complex (**MHC**) molecules, and display these presented antigens on their cell surface, where they can be recognized and bound by antigen receptors on T lymphocytes.

As will be described in greater detail below, the T lymphocytes are identified by a surface cluster of differentiation (**CD**) molecule named CD3 and are comprised of two major groups: the CD4 and CD8 populations (Table 1-8). The CD4 cells display helper activities on other populations of cells, and in turn are subdivided into Th1, Th2, a T regulatory (**Treg**) group, and, in addition, a recently described T cell subset called Th17, each with a characteristic profile of production of proinflammatory cytokines (*Chapter 9*). The CD8 T cytotoxic population is the second major group of T lymphocytes that function in killing target cells; they are comprised of Tc1 and Tc2 subpopulations with similar cytokine profiles as Th1 and Th2 cells. Collectively, the T lymphocytes play or facilitate a central role in the orchestration of all functions of the adaptive immune system and perform four important tasks: (1) promotion of inflammation by cytokine production (Th1 and Th17 cells), (2) helping B lymphocytes (Th2 cells), (3) regulating immunosuppressive responses (T regulatory cells), and (4) killing of unwanted target cells (Tc1 and Tc2 cells) (Table 1-8).

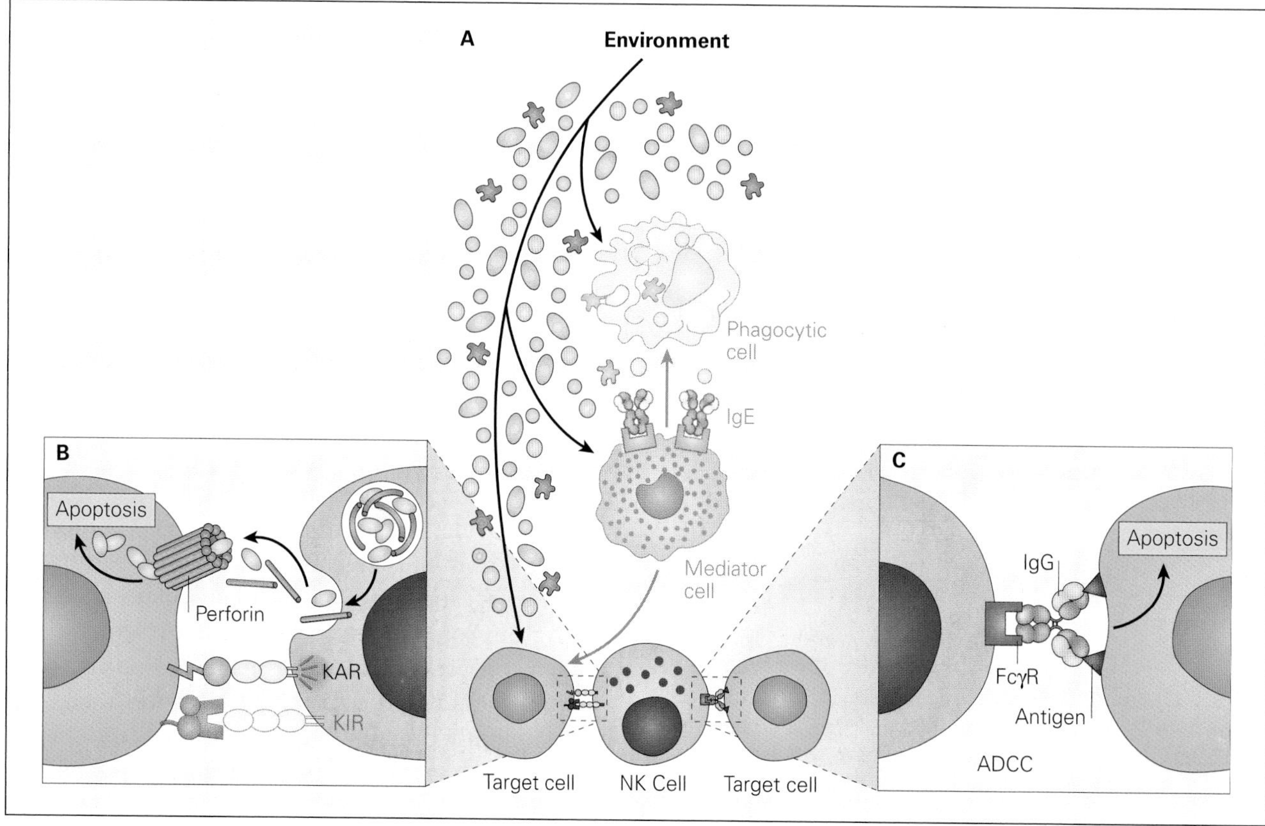

Figure 1-17. Panel A: Schematic representation of the NK cell and its role in innate and adaptive immunity showing the two ways it can kill target cells. Panel B: Shows direct killing when KAR > KIR, during which release of perforins and granzymes lead to cell death by apoptosis (innate immunity). Panel C: Shows killing by ADCC by utilizing an immunoglobulin molecule to bridge the NK cell with a target cell (adaptive immunity). KAR = killer activating receptor; KIR = killer inhibitory receptor.

The adaptive immune system, unlike the innate immune system, which displays a relatively stereotyped and limited response to foreignness, has developed an extensive inventory of unique genetic recombination mechanisms that produce a virtually unlimited repertoire of cells and cell products, each interacting with one another to accomplish the task of recognizing "self" from "nonself" that comprise the antigen recognition system. For versatility, adaptivity, and sophistication, this system remains unparalleled to all other biological systems.

Table 1-8. Cellular components, functions, and mechanisms of the antigen recognition system

Cellular component	Functions	Examples of effector cell types	Mechanisms
Antigen-presenting cells	Antigen presentation	Macrophages, dendritic cells, B lymphocytes	Uptake, digestion, and antigen display on cell surface MHC
T lymphocytes	Cell-mediated immunity	CD4 helper lymphocytes	
		• Th1 cells	Promotion of inflammation by cytokine production
		• Th2 cells	Helping B lymphocytes proliferate, produce antibody, and become memory B cells
		• T regulatory cells	Regulating immunosuppressive responses
		• Th17 cells	Promotion of inflammation by cytokine production
		CD8 cytotoxic lymphocytes • Tc1 cells • Tc2 cells	Killing of unwanted target cells
B lymphocytes	Humoral immunity	Plasma cells	Antibody synthesis

Table 1-9. Various types of antigen-presenting cells

Type	Location
Macrophages	Widely dispersed in tissues
Alveolar macrophages	Lung
Langerhans	Skin
Kuppfer cells	Liver
Microglial	Central nervous system
Dendritic cells	Widely dispersed in tissues
B lymphocytes	Lymph nodes and other lymphoid tissues

Because the role of T lymphocytes is to deal with intracellular infections and "altered self" cells (tumor cells), they must have a way to recognize intracellular antigen. In addition to their role in innate immunity, dendritic cells and macrophages also play a major collaborative role in the presentation of antigen to T lymphocytes of the adaptive immune system and are therefore referred to as APCs (Table 1-9). Following the uptake and digestion by APCs, foreign substances, usually proteins, are processed by proteolysis into peptide fragments that are later presented to T cells in a highly discriminative manner. This process employs cell receptors consisting of molecules on both the surface of the APC membrane (i.e., MHC proteins) (*Chapter 10*) (Table 1-10) as well as a specific antigen-binding receptor on the T cell membrane, the TCR (*Chapter 7*). Of these, the dendritic cells are the most potent APCs, and are particularly important in initiation and promotion of subsequent adaptive immune responses. In addition to these cells of the innate immune system, B cells of the adaptive immune system, as described below, can also serve as APCs (Table 1-10).

Antigen Processing and Presentation Follows Different Pathways for Cytosolic (Endogenous) and Vesicular (Exogenous) Antigen

T lymphocytes play a pivotal role in both cell-mediated and humoral immune responses of the adaptive immune system. These functions are carried out by T lymphocytes that interact with antigen through the TCR. The processing of antigen can occur at two sites: (1) at the level of APCs or (2) at the target cell site. As described above, the phagocytes and other APCs play major roles in internalizing, processing, and presentation of "processed antigen" to T lymphocytes for induction of immune responses carried out by both CD4 and CD8 lymphocyte populations. Antigen can also be processed and presented to T lymphocytes at the target cell site in a cell that has been infected with a virus, for example, or modified by a chemical or by malignant transformation. Shown in Figure 1-18 is a schematic representation of the two modes of antigen processing at these two sites that determines which MHC the processed antigen will react with. These events are described in greater detail in Chapter 10.

In the case of antigens processed by APCs by the exogenous pathway, CD4 T cells recognize antigen that has been processed into peptide fragments (epitopes) that are then placed in a groove of the MHC-II molecule, and presented to the TCR on subsets of helper T cells (called CD4+ cells). Other antigens found within cells, e.g., target cells, are processed through an endogenous pathway and are delivered by MHC-I to TCR of "cytotoxic" T cells (called CD8+ cells). Shown in Table 1-11 and Box 1-5 is a comparison of the MHC-I and MHC-II molecules and their roles in the endogenous and exogenous pathways.

A useful mnemonic in remembering which MHC molecules associate with their corresponding T cells is the "rule of eights" (Box 1-6).

The Interaction Between APC and T Cells Influences Which T Cells Are Activated

The interaction between the T cell and the APC is very complex, since naive antigen-specific lymphocytes are difficult to activate by antigen alone. Thus, several other receptor/ligand interactions called co-stimulatory molecules, e.g., CD28 and CD80, must occur in a regulated order before the T cell is activated and starts to proliferate into armed effector T cells (*Chapter 7*).

Table 1-10. Antigen-presenting molecules

Molecule	Cell location	Function
MHC-I	All nucleated cells	Presents peptides synthesized within virus-infected and tumor cells to cytotoxic (CD8) T lymphocytes
MHC-II	Professional antigen-presenting cells: dendritic cells, macrophages, B cells	Presents peptides from engulfed pathogens and antigens to helper (CD4) T lymphocytes

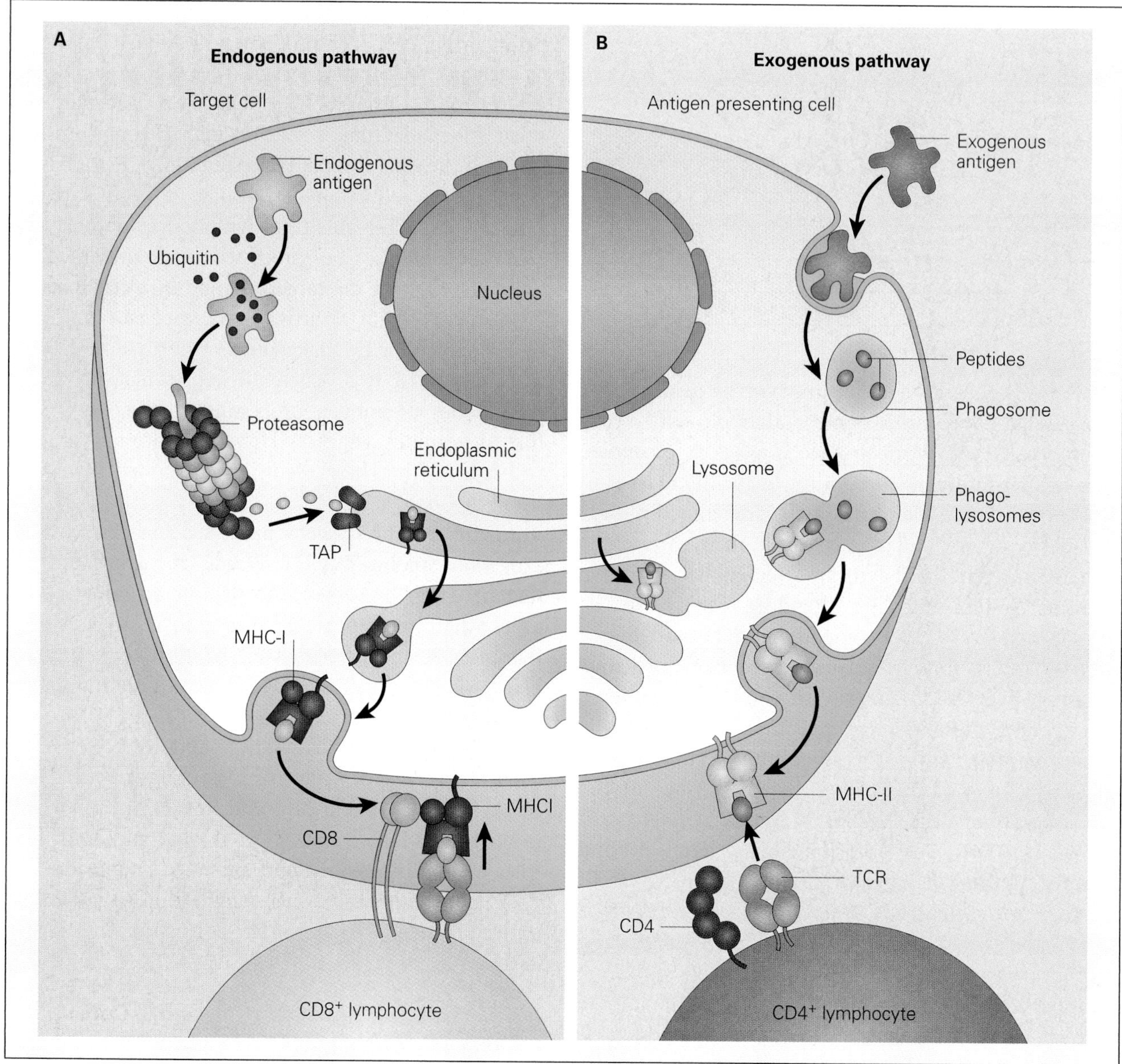

Figure 1-18. Schematic representation of the two modes of antigen processing. Panel A: Shows the endogenous pathway, which presents processed antigen (i.e., peptides) from a target cell to a CD8+ lymphocyte in the context of MHC-I. Panel B: Shows the exogenous pathway, which presents the peptide products from an APC to a CD4+ lymphocyte in the context of MHC-II.

CD4+ T cell activation results in the secretion of cytokines that help and regulate other cells (*Chapter 9*). The pattern of cytokine expression defines the subsets of CD4+ T cells: Th1, Th2, Treg1, Th3, and Th17 cells.

- Th1 cells secrete interferon gamma (**IFN-γ**) and create a milieu in which key cytotoxic effectors—macrophages, natural killer cells, and cytotoxic CD8+ T lymphocytes—are activated, generating cell-mediated immunity.
- Th2 cells secrete IL-4 and IL-10 (and other cytokines) and help antigen-primed B lymphocytes differentiate into plasma cells and secrete antibodies, the effector molecules of humoral responses.
- A third category of T cells, Treg cells, with the phenotype CD4+CD25+, express the signature transcription factor FOXP3 and usually secrete IL-10 and transforming growth factor beta (**TGF-β**). Cells with this phenotype are thought to recognize self-antigens and function to prevent autoimmunity and are also involved in chronic viral infections, allergy, transplantation, and malignancy.
- Th17 cells represent a wide variety of recently described cells involved in inflammation through the elaboration of pro-inflammatory cytokines and interact with IL-23 (*Chapter 9*).

Following the interaction of an environmental agent with the T cell, a series of morphologic, biologic, and

Table 1-11. Comparison of MHC molecules and their roles in the endogenous and exogenous pathways

	MHC-I	MHC-II
Genes	**HLA-A, B, C**	**HLA-DP, DQ, DR**
Structure	Transmembrane α chain bound to β 2-microglobulin	Transmembrane α and β chains
Presented peptide	Peptides derived from self/nonself intracellular proteins, e.g., viral peptides	Peptides derived from extracellular proteins, e.g., bacterial peptides
Mechanism of presentation	Endogenous Pathway Intracellular proteins are degraded by the ubiquitin/proteasome pathway in the cytosol; transported by TAP[a] to endoplasmic reticulum and loaded onto MHC-I; the MHC-I/peptide complex translocates to the cell membrane	Exogenous Pathway Extracellular proteins are endocytosed and degraded by lysosomal proteases; subsequently peptide-containing endosomes are fused to MHC-II-containing vesicles; peptides are loaded onto MHC-II and the MHC-II/peptide complex translocates to the cell membrane
Presenting cells	All nucleated cells, including APC; modified "target cell"	APC: DC, B cells, macrophages
Interacting T cell	CD8 T cell	CD4 T cell

a.TAP: Transporter-associated antigen processing.

biochemical events occur in which the cell may display a wide set of functions either directly or indirectly through the elaboration of a potent group of protein molecules with diverse immunoregulatory activities, i.e., the cytokines (*Chapter 9*). The T cell may interact with three components of the immune network: (1) APC, in a T cell/APC interaction; (2) B cells, in a T cell/B cell interaction; and (3) target cells, in a T cell/target cell interaction.

As described above, T cells can recognize only peptide fragments that have been processed and presented by APC, i.e., dendritic cells (**DC**), macrophages, and B cells. Shown in Figure 1-19 is a schematic representation of the processing of antigen by a dendritic cell and presentation of the processed peptides to a CD4+ T cell through its TCR.

T and B Lymphocytes Have Uniquely Generated Cell Surface Receptors for Recognition of a Specific Antigen

Antigen recognition by cells of the adaptive immune system is due to specific membrane-associated receptors (Table 1-12). These receptors are generated by a unique process of gene segment recombination

Box 1-5

Antigen Processing and MHC-I and MHC-II Molecules and Their Roles in Endogenous and Exogenous Pathways

Antigen processing prepares peptides for presentation to specialized cells of the immune system called T lymphocytes. This process involves two distinct pathways: (1) the endogenous pathway, for processing of antigens from an organism's own (self) proteins or intracellular pathogens (e.g., viruses), or (2) the exogenous pathway, for processing phagocytosed pathogens (e.g., bacteria). Subsequent presentation of peptides on class I or class II MHC molecules is dependent on which pathway is used. The endogenous pathway is used to present cellular peptide fragments on the cell surface on MHC-I molecules. The exogenous pathway is utilized by professional antigen-presenting cells to present peptides on MHC-II molecules. Both MHC-I and II molecules are required to bind peptides before they are stably expressed on a cell surface.

In the **endogenous pathway**, viral proteins or worn-out proteins within the cell are first ubiquitinated (i.e., a post-translational modification of a protein preparing them for degradation by proteasomes). The peptides are transported into the rough endoplasmic reticulum by a transporter protein called TAP (transporter associated with antigen processing) that transports the peptides into the lumen of the endoplasmic reticulum and then are presented on the surface of the cell with MHC-I (Figure 1-18) (*Chapter 10*).

In the **exogenous pathway**, Endocytosed proteins are digested by acid-dependent proteases in endosomes, and the resultant peptides are presented on the surface of the cell together with MHC-II molecules (Figure 1-18).

Box 1-6

The "Rule of Eights"

A useful mnemonic in remembering which MHC molecules associate with which T cells is the "rule of eights." Molecules processed by APCs through the exogenous pathway present peptides in association with MHC-II and CD4 lymphocytes ($2 \times 4 = 8$). Peptide fragments of proteins that have been produced within the cell through the endogenous pathway are presented in association with MHC-I and CD8 lymphocytes ($1 \times 8 = 8$).

within each developing B and T lymphocyte. BCR are membrane-bound antibody molecules, while TCR are related but smaller molecules are not secreted. The structural similarities of the antigen-binding molecules (BCR, TCR, MHC-I, and MHC-II) suggest a common ancestral origin and have led to their grouping as part of the immunoglobulin supergene family (*Chapter 6*).

Leukocytes Are Characterized by Distinct Cell Surface Proteins

In addition to antigen receptors, white blood cells possess a variety of cell surface molecules referred to as the CD molecules (*Appendix 4*). The knowledge gained from the composition of these molecular structures made possible by the availability of specific monoclonal antibodies to the CD markers has allowed the identification of the lineages of many other cells of the immune system. Shown in Table 1-13 are some clinically relevant CD markers on immune cells. Shown in Box 1-7 and Figure 1-20 are some of the major distinguishing features of B and T lymphocytes, including the specific BCR and TCR molecules, respectively, together with the MHC and CD molecules.

Cell-Mediated Immunity

In contrast to B lymphocytes, which through the production of antibody (i.e., humoral immunity) are well-suited to identify and react with extracellular antigens, the T lymphocytes are those cells of the adaptive immune system that have emerged during the course of evolution to handle intracellular

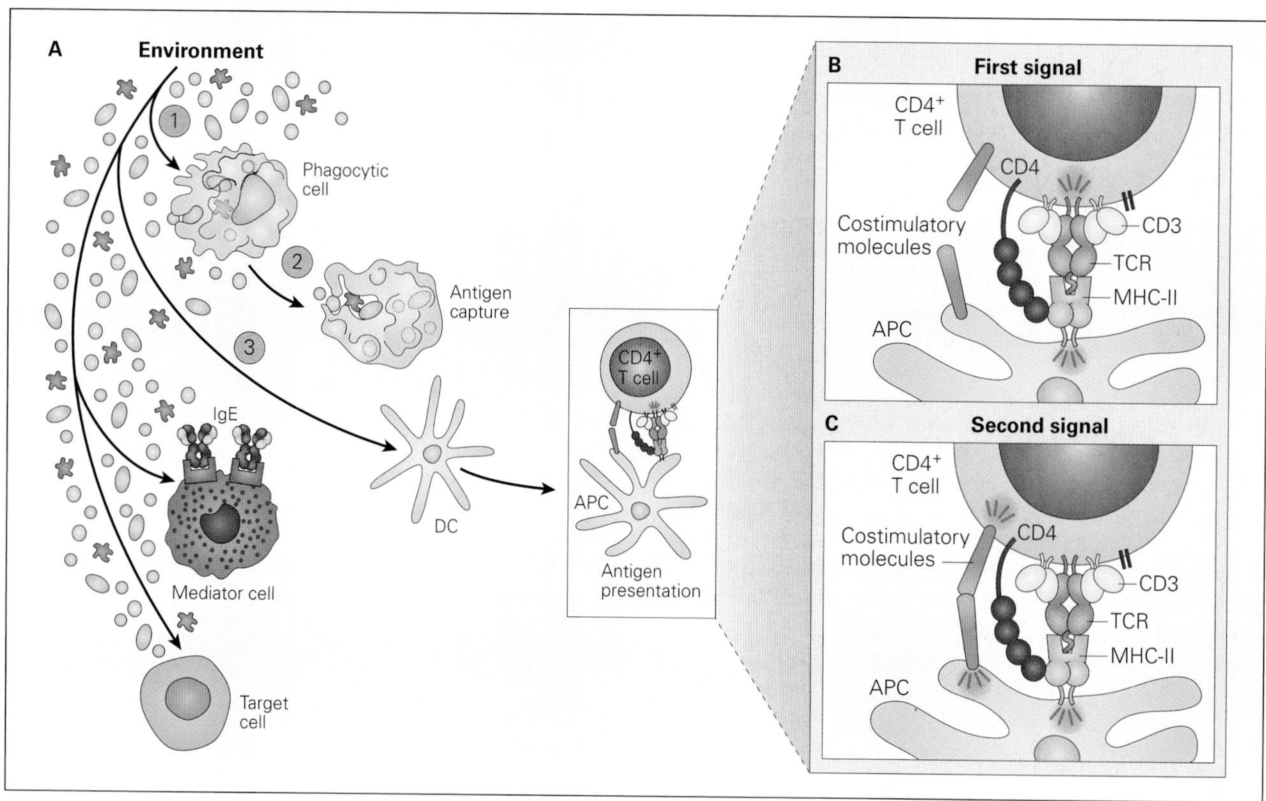

Figure 1-19. Panel A: Schematic representation of the processing of antigen by a macrophage (steps 1 and 2) or by a dendritic cell (as in 3). Panel B: Presents peptides to a T cell through its TCR, showing generation of signal 1. Panel C: Shows signal 2.

Table 1-12. Antigen receptors of T and B cells

Component	Receptor	Site	Action
T lymphocytes	TCR	Cell membranes of all T lymphocytes	Binding of processed antigen on MHC-I or MHC-II
B lymphocytes	BCR	Cell membranes of all B lymphocytes	Binding of whole unprocessed antigen

antigens and to dispose of them by cell-mediated immunity (*Chapter 7*). A major role of the T cell arm is to identify and destroy infected cells or foreign cells which have appeared as a result of modification of normal host cells into foreign target cells, e.g., viral and other intracellular microbial infections or chemical transformation, transplantation, or malignant transformation, and to do so without injury to one's own tissues. The T cell accomplishes this task through a set of cellular responses that are collectively referred to as CMI.

As described above, T cells through their TCR not only can recognize peptide fragments that have been processed and presented by APCs, i.e., DCs, macrophages, and B cells, but also have developed an extraordinary method of identifying and disposing of unwanted or potentially inimical cell-associated antigens that have an intracellular domicile. This is accomplished through the second arm of adaptive immunity, CMI. As in the case of humoral immunity, which will be described below, the outcome of CMI can either be beneficial or detrimental. Shown in Table 1-14 are some examples of beneficial and injurious outcomes of CMI.

The way that the T cell system has evolved to perform the tasks of CMI involves two pathways mediated by T lymphocytes. T cells, as described previously, consist of two types, CD4 and CD8 populations. Further differentiation of the CD4 T helper population occurs with the production of Th1, Th2, Th17, and two populations of Treg cells Th3 and TR1 (Figure 1-21), which have a variety of interactions with other cells in performing the following functions: (1) promotion of inflammation by cytokine production (Th1 lymphocytes); (2) helping B lymphocytes (Th2 lymphocytes); and (3) regulating immunosuppressive responses (Treg lymphocytes). Similarly, the CD8 cells differentiate into T cytotoxic cells capable of reaction with target cells and performing the fourth function of killing unwanted target cells.

Cell-mediated immune responses can be separated into two major types: (1) delayed hypersensitivity inflammatory reaction (Figure 1-22) (mediated by the release of inflammatory cytokines from the Th1 and Th17 pathways (Box 1-8, Figure 1-21); and (2) CMI that involves direct cytotoxicity mediated by CD8 Tc cells (Figure 1-23).

Th1 Cells Signal Macrophages to Kill Engulfed Intracellular Bacterial Pathogens

Mycobacterium tuberculosis is an example of a bacterium that can be phagocytosed by macrophages and is able to protect itself from being killed by virtue of its intracellular location within the phagolysosome (Figure 1-24). The organism can now replicate in the phagosome, protected from the harmful effects of the

Table 1-13. Some clinically relevant cluster of differentiation (CD) markers for immune system cells

Antigen	Distribution	Function
CD3	T cells	Part of CD3/TCR complex; specific marker for T cells
CD4	Helper T cells (Th), some monocytes	MHC-II interaction (co-receptor for TCR); HIV receptor
CD8	Cytotoxic T cells (Tc)	MHC-I interaction (co-receptor for TCR)
CD19/20	B cells	Specific marker for B cells
CD56/161	NK cells	Specific markers for NK cells
CD14	Monocytes, macrophages	Receptor for gram-negative LPS; specific marker for monocytes
CD40L	T cells	Binds to the CD40 on B cells for IgM to IgG switching
CD64	Phagocytes	FcγRI (high-affinity receptor for the IgG Fc)
CD32	Phagocytes, eosinophils	FcγRII (low-affinity receptor for the IgG Fc)
CD16	Neutrophils, macrophages, NK cells	FcγRIII (lower-affinity receptor for the IgG Fc)

Box 1-7

Distinguishing Features Between B and T Lymphocytes: The CD System

Immune cells cannot be identified by their appearance under a microscope, but can be distinguished from one another by cell surface proteins that are detected in the laboratory by antibodies. The naming system used to standardize these cell surface markers is referred to as the CD system. About 250 cell surface molecules have been assigned different CD numbers, and each of these molecules has a function (i.e., signaling, antigen binding, or adhesion) (*Appendix 4*). For example, CD3 is part of the antigen-binding receptor on T cells (i.e., the TCR) and is involved in signaling. T lymphocytes also carry CD4 or CD8, which functions as adhesion molecules as well as many other cell surface molecules, such as CD40 ligand (CD40L or CD154) found on activated CD4 positive T lymphocytes. In contrast, B lymphocytes carry CD19, CD20 molecules, and a CD40-signaling molecule that helps with B cell activation as well as cell surface immunoglobulin (Ig or antibody Ab), which binds antigen. MHC molecules also bind antigen and interact with the TCR and CD4 or CD8.

Shown in Figure 1-20 is a schematic representation of the key distinguishing features of B and T lymphocytes.

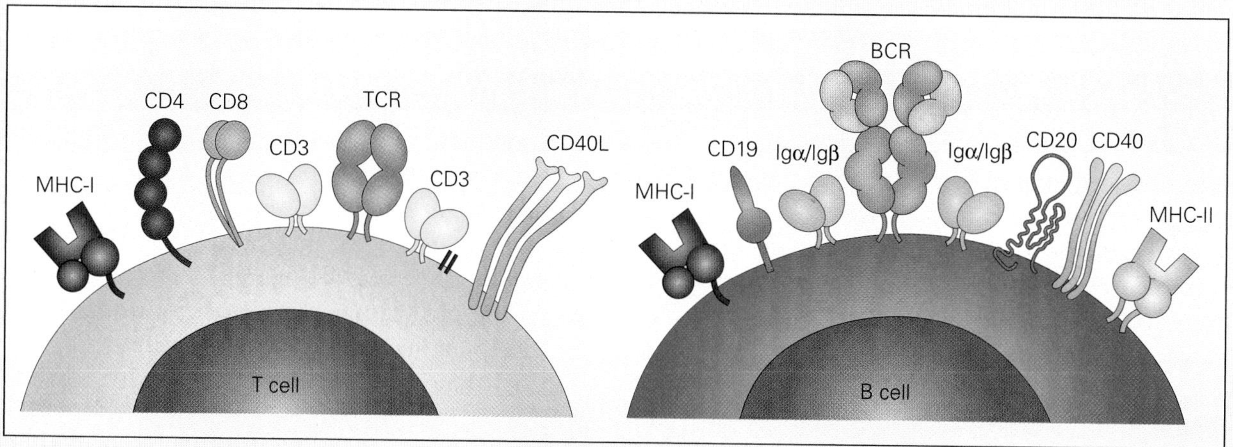

Figure 1-20. A schematic representation of the key distinguishing features of B and T lymphocytes. The receptors on T and B cells, i.e., the TCR and BCR, respectively, require different forms of the antigen for the binding reaction to occur. B cells primarily recognize native unaltered antigen; in contrast, the T cell only recognizes antigen determinants that have been processed by APCs and that are presented to the T cell in the context of either MHC-I or MHC-II molecules. As will be described below, the B lymphocytes are the cells that ultimately produce antibody. Note that although T cells bind peptide antigen on either MHC-I (cytotoxic T cells) or MHC-II (helper T cells), as nucleated cells, all T cells have MHC-I and can present virus peptide to cytotoxic T cells should they become infected.

humoral antibody immune response. Th1 cells recognize peptides on the macrophage membrane in association with MHC-II, produce cytokines, and signal the macrophage with IFN-γ together with other cytokines to kill the bacteria (Figure 1-24, step 1). Other Th1 cytokines also attract more macrophages to the infection site and activate them to produce inflammatory cytokines that result in delayed-type hypersensitivity, e.g., the TST. Figure 1-24 shows various outcomes of the host-microbial interaction between the macrophage and the intracellular location of the tubercle bacillus (steps 1–2). One outcome shows the killing of the tubercle bacillus resulting from enhanced macrophage killing of the bacillus by activation by IL-12 and later Th1 production of IFN-γ (steps 3–5) or failure of killing when the replication of the tubercle bacillus overwhelms the macrophage capacity (steps 6–7).

Table 1-14. Examples of beneficial and detrimental outcomes of cell-mediated immunity

Outcome	Example
Beneficial	Elimination of intracellular pathogens (e.g., tuberculosis) Resistance against tumors
Detrimental	Graft rejection Autoimmune tissue injury

Another type of cell-mediated immune response that involves direct cytotoxicity mediated by CD8 Tc cells can be found with viruses, especially the nonenveloped (nonlipid containing) type which again, because of their intracellular location, are

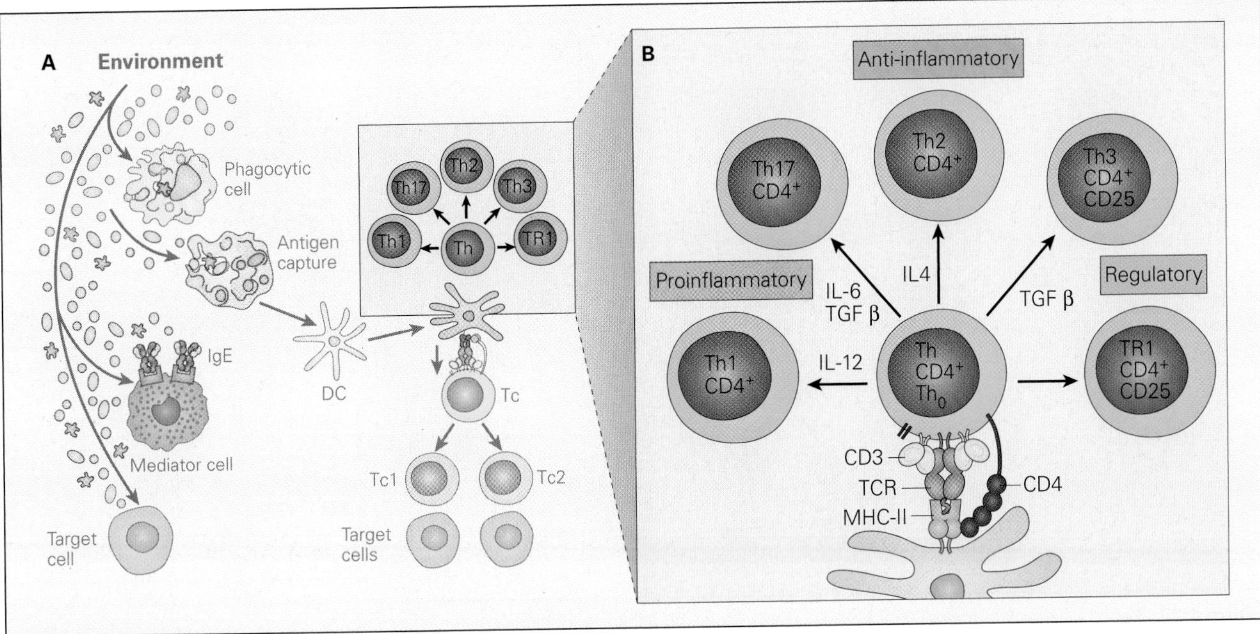

Figure 1-21. Panel A: The two main T cell populations are named CD4+ and CD8+ cells. The CD4 are helper T cells and are shown highlighted with the CD4+ subsets Th1, Th17, Th2, Th3, and Tr1 and shown below are the CD8 cytotoxic T cells (faded). Panel B: Shows the molecular events in the immunologic synapse at the CD4+/dendritic cell interface together with the cytokines that induce the Th0 differentiation into each of the subsets.

Box 1-8

The Delayed Hypersensitivity Skin Reaction: Historical and Clinical Considerations

The prototype of the delayed hypersensitivity reaction is the tuberculin skin test (TST), a localized inflammatory skin reaction originally described by the brilliant German microbiologist Robert Koch in the 1890s. Following the intradermal injection of a small quantity of a component of the tubercle bacillus called tuberculin into a subject who has been previously sensitized to the tubercle bacillus, a positive skin reaction is seen within forty-eight to seventy-two hours. It consists of redness (erythema) and induration (hardness) at the site of the injection (Figure 1-22).

Because of the delayed evolution and appearance of the reaction, it was designated *delayed hypersensitivity* to distinguish it from another form of dermal reactivity seen in allergic individuals mediated by one of the serum immunoglobulin IgE and that occurs within minutes following the introduction of antigen into the skin; thus it is referred to as *immediate hypersensitivity* (*Chapter 17*). Microscopically, there is an influx of macrophages and lymphocytes brought into the area where the tuberculin was injected. It is now recognized that the reaction is produced primarily by sensitized Th1 and Th17 lymphocytes (although CD8 and NK cells may also participate) through the release of pro-inflammatory cytokines that bring in lymphocytes and macrophages and are responsible for the erythema and induration characteristic of the delayed hypersensitivity reaction.

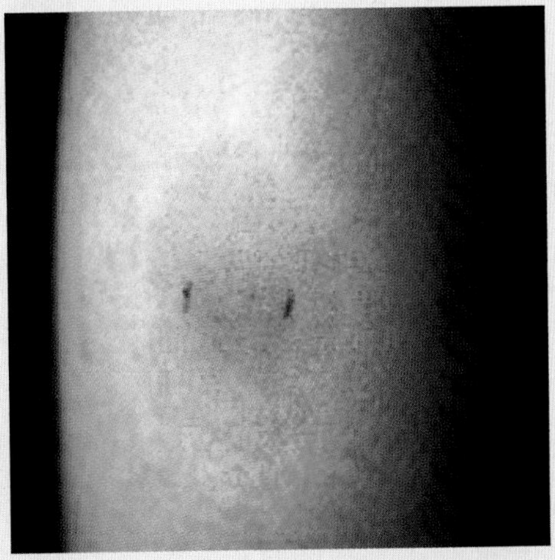

Figure 1-22. A photograph of a positive intradermal TST showing erythema and induration (indicated by the two vertical lines). (As seen on Wikipedia.)

hidden from the deleterious effects of antibody (*Chapter 13*). They can, however, be detected by their peptides, which are expressed in association with the MHC-I on the cell membrane of the infected cell. Shown in Figure 1-25 is a schematic representation of the interaction of a CD8+ cytotoxic cell with a virus-infected target cell, which is subsequently killed by apoptosis using perforin and granzyme or

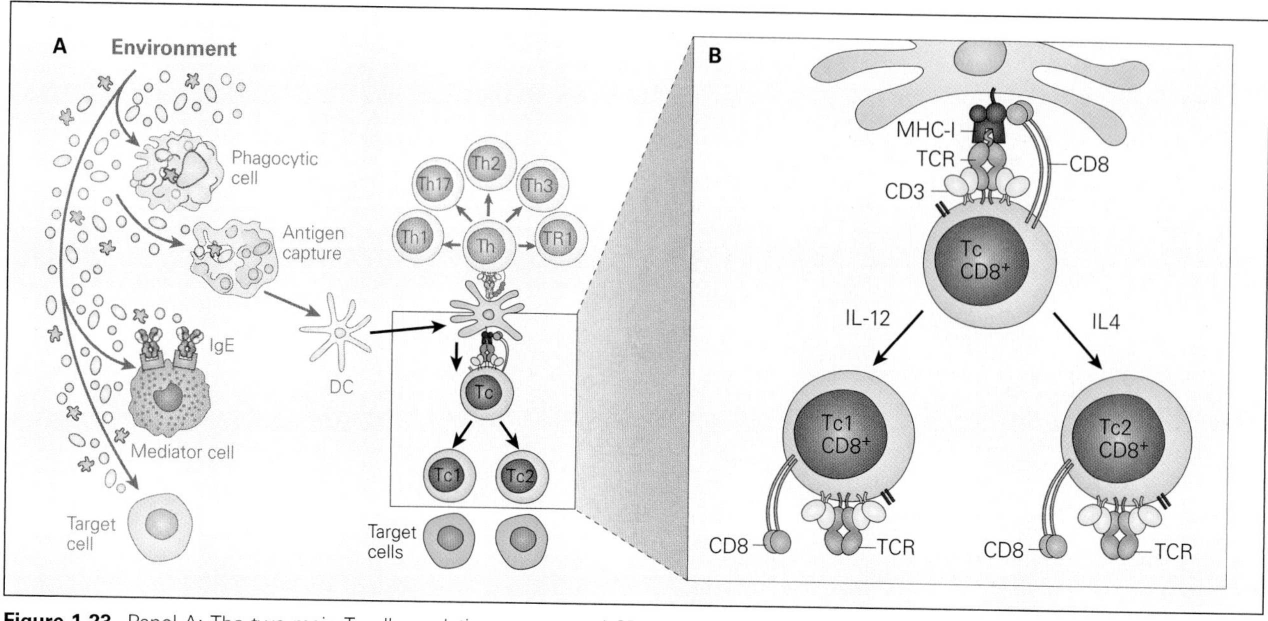

Figure 1-23. Panel A: The two main T cell populations are named CD4+ and CD8+ cells. The CD8+ are cytotoxic T cells and are shown highlighted with the CD4+ cells shown faded (above). Panel B: Shows the molecular events in the immunologic synapse at the CD8+/target cell interface, including the cytokines, which lead to differentiation into CD8+ Tc1 and Tc2 cytotoxic cells.

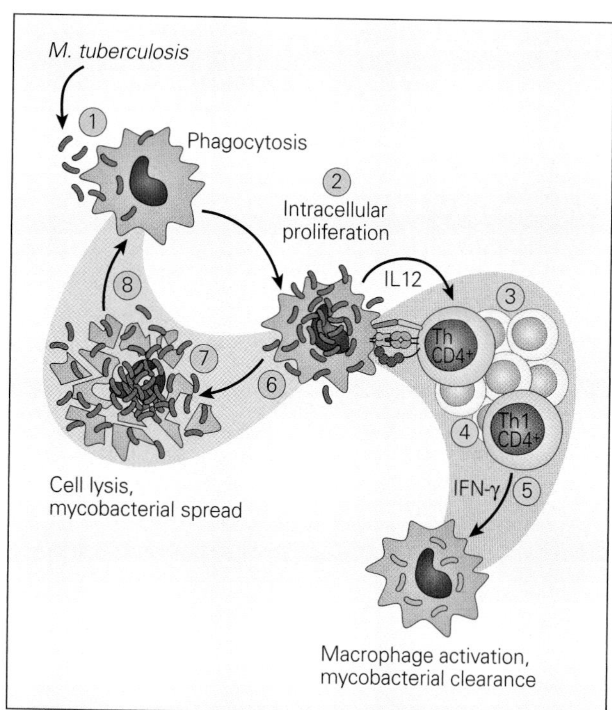

Figure 1-24. Schematic representation of the host-microbial interaction between the macrophage and the intracellular location of the tubercle bacillus (steps 1–2) showing the various outcomes of either killing the tubercle bacillus resulting from enhanced macrophage killing of the bacillus by activation by IL-12 and later Th1 production of IFN-γ (steps 3–5), or failure of killing when the replication of the tubercle bacillus overwhelms the macrophage capacity (steps 6–7).

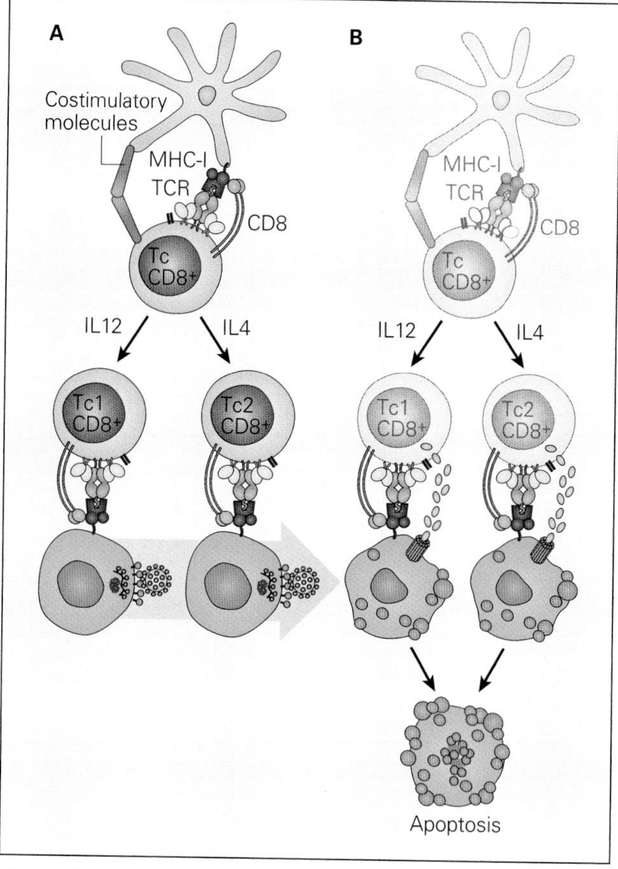

Figure 1-25. Panel A: Schematic representation of the interaction of a CD8$^+$ Tc cytotoxic cell with a virus-infected target cell. Panel B: Shows subsequent killing of the cell by apoptosis using perforin and granzyme or other signals.

other signals. Cytotoxic cells can also recognize and kill tumor cells and transplanted allogeneic cells in the same way.

Humoral Immunity

B lymphocytes are those cells that ultimately respond to environmental immunogens (or antigens) with the production of protein molecules identified as immunoglobulins, which function as antibody and which can react specifically with antigen (*Chapter 6*). Because these effector molecules circulate in the blood and tissues, they were designated by the ancient term "humors" and were assigned a role in humoral immunity, in contrast to those carried by cells, i.e., cell-mediated immunity. The synthesis of these molecules occurs in the terminally differentiated form of the B cell, the plasma cell, with the collaboration of the Th2 helper lymphocyte (Figure 1-26).

Th2 Cells Activate B Cells to Secrete Antibody and Become Memory B Cells

Following antigen processing by antigen-presenting cells, the processed antigenic peptide MHC-II complex is transported to the cell membrane, where it is recognized by the $CD4^+$ Th2 cells. The Th2 cells can now signal the production of IgM by B cells, which then switch to secrete IgG, IgA, or IgE, depending on the type and location of the antigen (Figure 1-26). The primary effect of these antibodies is to directly interact with antigen in various sites: IgG in blood and tissues; IgA and IgE at mucosal surfaces; and IgM in blood and lymph. Following clearance of the antigen, a bank of resting B cells remains referred to as *memory cells* that can survive for years, or even a lifetime, and which can undergo proliferation and differentiation with augmented antibody production when antigen is re-encountered (Figure 1-26). These memory cells are responsible for the so-called secondary or anamnestic immune response that forms the basis for the booster effect of repeated doses of vaccine used in routine immunization programs (*Chapter 23*).

B Lymphocytes Act as Both Antigen-Presenting Cells and the Producers of Immunoglobulins

Paradoxically, the B lymphocyte can function as an APC and as the cell that ultimately synthesizes immunoglobulin (Figure 1-26). The exquisite specificity of recognition of antigen by the B cell is a function of the immunoglobulins that are found both on the surface of these cells as well as a secreted product. The cell surface immunoglobulins of the B cell that recognize antigen consist of monomeric IgM and IgD. As a consequence of the binding of antigen with the BCR (Figure 1-27), four processes are triggered: (1) antigen processing and presentation to CD4+ cells, which in turn enhance the activation of B cells; (2) B cell proliferation and differentiation, primarily in germinal centers of the spleen or lymph node (*Chapter 2*) into clones of antibody-secreting plasma cells; (3) each of which secretes immunoglobulins that are specific for the antigen; and (4) memory formation, with the creation and retention of a bank of recall lymphocytes capable of expansion when antigen is re-encountered (Figures 1-26 and 1-27). The molecular bases of these cellular interactions are

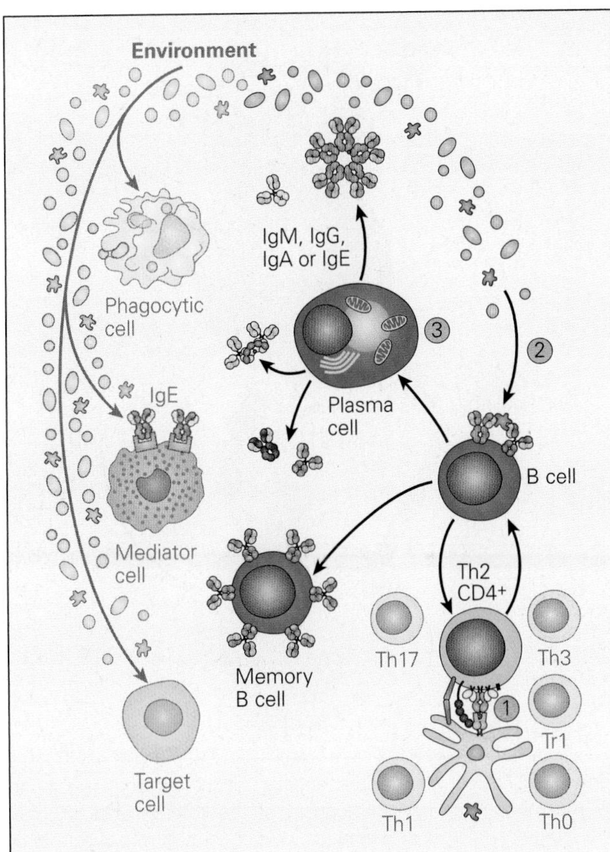

Figure 1-26. A schematic representation of Th2 cell/B cell interaction showing the processing and presentation of antigen from a dendritic cell to a Th2 cell (1) or processing of antigen by a B cell (2) followed by cooperation of the Th2 cell with the B cell which differentiates into a plasma cell with resultant production of antibody (3) (IgG, IgM, IgA, or IgE). The B cell functions not only as an antigen-presenting cell but as an antibody-forming plasma cell and a long-lived memory B cell.

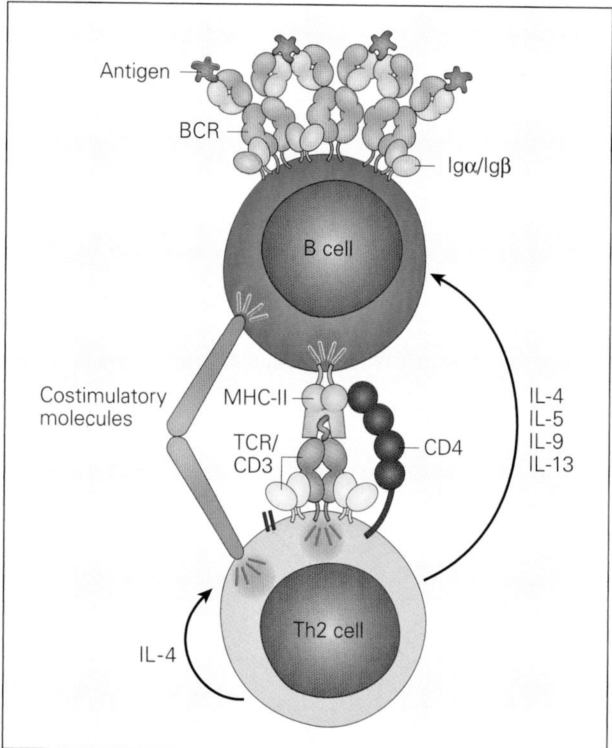

Figure 1-27. Schematic representation of the binding of antigen by the monomeric IgM component of the BCR on a B lymphocyte, digestion, and presentation of peptides in the context of MHC-II to the TCR of a Th2 cell followed by the release of cytokines responsible for T cell and B cell activation and division and ultimately by the production of immunoglobulins by the B cell.

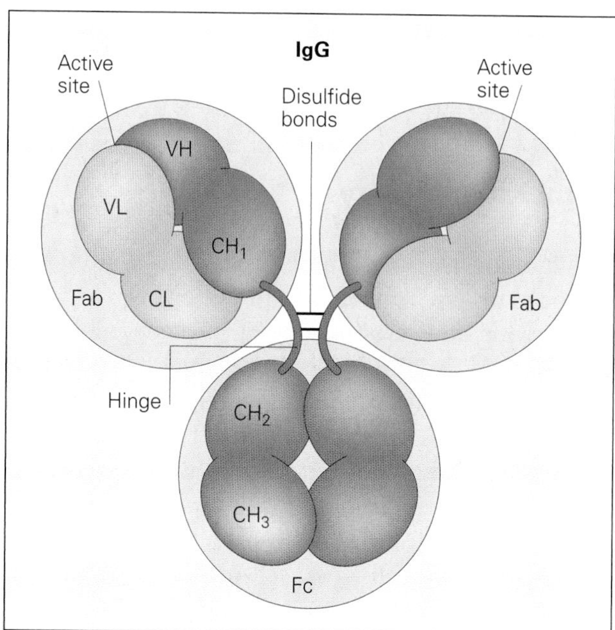

Figure 1-28. A schematic representation of an IgG molecule showing a four-chain structure with the antigen-binding Fab regions and the Fc constant region. Each of the chains are arranged in bulk-like regions called domains.

described more fully in Chapters 6 and 7 and involve signal transduction; the process is enhanced by the action of co-stimulatory molecules on the surface of the B cell (*Chapter 6*). Following binding of antigens to surface BCR, B cells internalize, process, and express the epitopes of the processed antigen in a groove of the MHC-II molecule, and present them to the TCR on CD4+ cells. This T-B cell interaction is modulated in a number of ways that include T cell-derived cytokines and IFN-γ, which enhance B cell proliferation and differentiation into antibody-secreting plasma cells. The physical interaction of T cells with B cells also plays an essential role in the sequential switch in production of immunoglobulins from more primitive IgM molecules to IgG, IgA, and IgE, a process referred to as **immunoglobulin class switching** (*Chapter 6*).

Antibodies Are Specific Antigen-Binding Immunoglobulin Molecules

Antibodies are Y-shaped proteins that are found in the blood or other bodily fluids of vertebrates that are used by the immune system to identify and neutralize foreign objects, such as bacteria and viruses. (The structure and functions of the immunoglobulin molecules are described in greater detail in Chapter 6.) Shown in Figure 1-28 is a schematic representation of an IgG molecule to illustrate the basic general structure of all immunoglobulin isotypes, i.e., classes. The basic molecule consists of four polypeptide chains: two identical heavy chains and two identical light chains connected by disulfide bonds and arranged in regions called domains (Figure 1-28). Each heavy and light chain has two regions, the constant (**C**) region and the variable (**V**) region. Some parts of an antibody have unique functions. The tip of the Y contains the site that recognizes and binds antigen and is called the fragment, antigen-binding (**Fab**) region. It is composed of one constant and one variable domain from each heavy and light chain of the antibody. The base of the Y plays a role in modulating immune cell activity. This region is called the fragment, crystallizable (**Fc**) region and is composed of two heavy chains. The Fc region determines the IgG isotype and the effector biological functions (as described below).

The primary function of antibody is to bind directly with antigen and to neutralize its effects. In addition to its primary effect of direct binding with antigen, antibody has a number of secondary effects and may interact with any or all of the three following cells: the phagocytic cells, the mediator cells, and the NK cells (Figure 1-29).

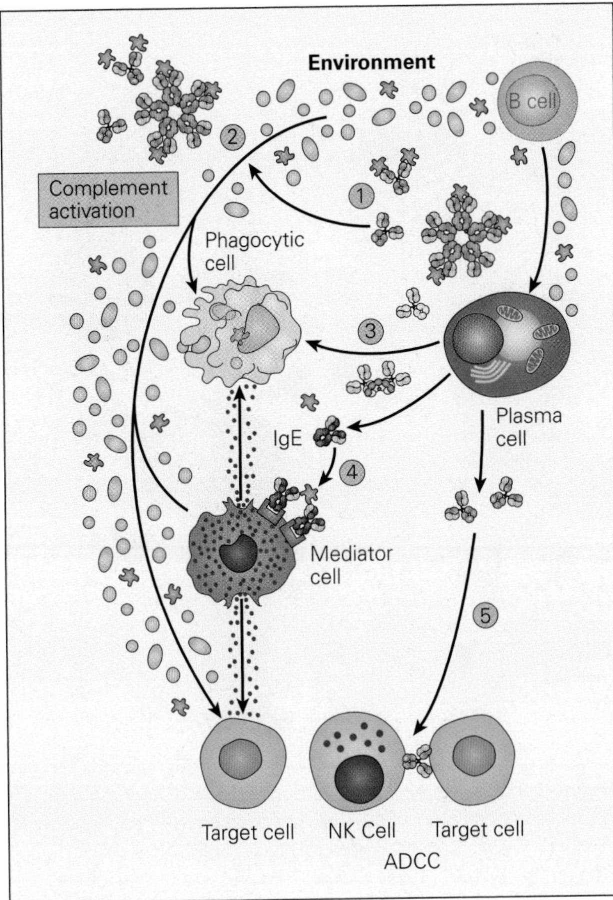

Figure 1-29. The primary functions of antibody include (1) neutralization of antigen in extracellular fluids; (2) activation of complement by either IgG or IgM; (3) facilitating uptake of antigen (osonization) by phagocytic cells; (4) binding of IgE with mediator cells; and (5) the targeting of antibody-dependent cellular cytotoxicity with ADCC interaction.

Physiologic Antibody Production Is Polyclonal

There are two categories of antibody responses elicited in this process: (1) polyclonal antibody formation, which represents the production of several families of antibodies directed at different parts of an immunogen (i.e., epitopes) produced by many different B cell clones; and (2) monoclonal antibody formation, representing a singular population of antibody directed at a distinct epitope produced by the progeny of a single B cell clone (Table 1-15, Box 1-9). The concept of monoclonal antibody has found clinical application in certain diseases, including multiple myeloma (*Chapter 21*, Box 1-9) and in the development of monoclonal antibodies useful in treatment and diagnosis of several allergic, autoimmune, and malignant diseases (*Chapter 11*).

Antibodies Promote Phagocytosis

The effects of antibody on phagocytic cells are shown in Figure 1-31. Three types of interactions are seen: (1) the direct binding of antibody to the surface of the phagocytic cells (cytophilic antibody); (2) the uptake of antigen-antibody (**Ag-Ab**) complexes through the Fc receptor of the immunoglobulin molecule; and (3) the uptake of antigen-antibody-complement (**Ag-Ab-C**) complexes through a complement receptor on the cell membrane of the phagocyte called the C3b receptor (*Chapter 4*). The coating of certain encapsulated bacterial organisms, e.g., *Streptococcus pneumoniae*, by antibody associated with certain classes of immunoglobulin (IgG or IgM), or by certain complement components, such as C3b, facilitates their uptake by phagocytic cells through the Fc or the C3b receptors, respectively; collectively, these antibody or complement components are referred to as **opsonins** for antibodies that promote phagocytosis.

Antibodies Signal Mediator Cells to Release Immune Mediators

The effects of antibody on mediator cells are shown schematically in Figure 1-32. Certain classes of immunoglobulin, e.g., IgE, can attach to mediator cells by virtue of their Fc fragments. This occurs by binding to a specific high-affinity IgE Fc receptor (**FcεRI**) on the cell membrane of a mast cell or basophil (*Chapter 17*). Following the interaction of at least two of these membrane-bound IgE molecules with antigen, a biochemical cascade of events occurs, with decreased cyclic adenosine monophospate (**cAMP**) resulting in the release of a wide variety of mediators that can have a direct effect on a target cell, e.g., bronchoconstriction, or that can initiate an inflammatory response. This response is most accentuated in patients with allergic disease and accounts for the symptomatology seen in these disorders (*Chapter 18*).

Table 1-15. Differences between polyclonal and monoclonal antibody formation

Type of antibody response	Number of antibody families of antibody produced	Number of epitopes to which antibody is directed	Number of B cell clones involved in antibody production
Polyclonal	Several	Several epitopes	Many
Monoclonal	Single	A single epitope	A single clone

Box 1-9

Types of Antibody Responses

The differences between the concept of polyclonal and monoclonal production of antibody is best illustrated by differences in the electrophoretic properties of serum gamma globulins from a normal individual and from a patient with multiple myeloma (Figure 1-30).

This differentiation between polyclonal and monoclonal production of antibody has great clinical significance and is seen in two clinical applications. The first is in a group of malignant lymphoproliferative disorders of B cells in which an abnormal proliferation of a single B cell clone leads to the production of monoclonal immunoglobulins in the condition referred to as multiple myeloma (*Chapter 21*). The second application is seen in the development of technology that derives from this clinical disorder in which specific monoclonal antibody reagents have been developed both for diagnostic and therapeutic purposes (*Chapters 6, 11,* and *24*) by hybridoma technology.

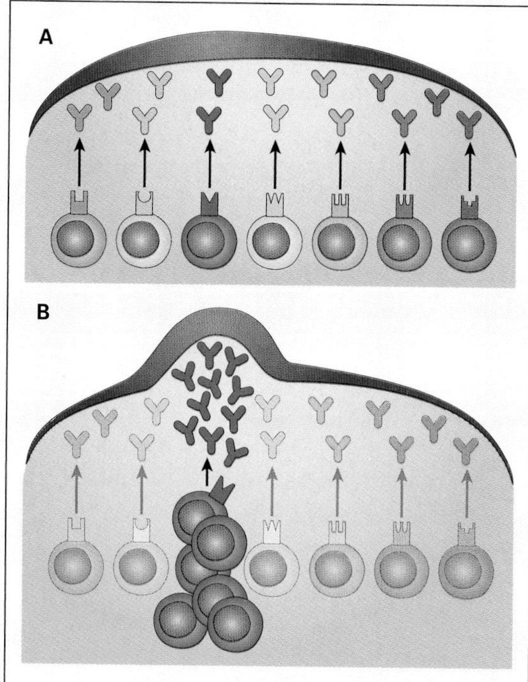

Figure 1-30. Panel A: Immunoelectrophoretic patterns of serum from a normal individual. Panel B: A patient with multiple myeloma. It can be seen that the gamma globulin from a normal individual is composed of several populations of gamma globulins produced by many B cell clones giving a homogeneous, smooth linear pattern to the arc (polyclonal), in contrast to the highly restrictive population of gamma globulin produced by a single B cell clone (monoclonal), which appears as a dense blob.

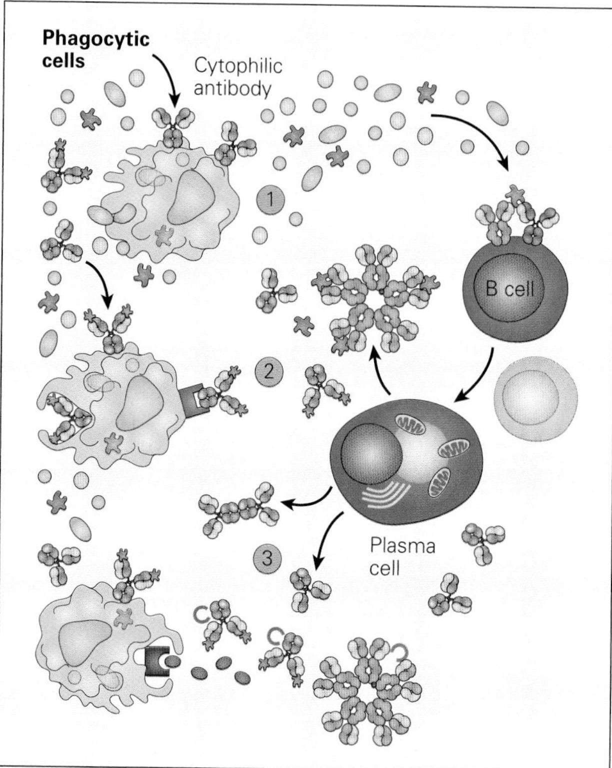

Figure 1-31. The three effects of antibody on phagocytic cells: (1) cytophilic antibody; (2) uptake of Ag-Ab complexes through the Fc receptor; and (3) uptake of Ag-Ab-C IgG and IgM complexes through the C3b receptor.

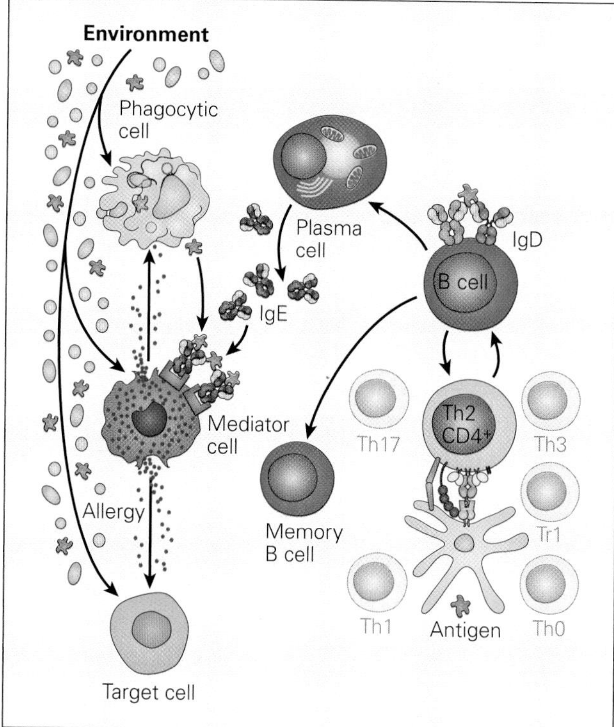

Figure 1-32. Reaction of binding of two molecules of IgE to cell membrane of mast cells or basophils with resultant release of mediators following the interaction of membrane-bound IgE with antigen.

Killing of Target Cells by NK Cells or Cytotoxic T Cells

Antibodies can also participate in NK activity. Two of the major cellular-killing mechanisms of target cells are by NK cells or by cytotoxic T cells. As described previously, there are two ways in which NK cells can kill target cells: (1) directly through the innate immune system, and (2) indirectly, where antibody can participate in ADCC as part of the adaptive immune response. Therefore the ADCC mechanism represents a response that bridges both the innate and adaptive immune systems. Shown in Figure 1-33 is a comparison of the two methods by which these two populations of cells kill target cells.

Antibodies Signal Phagocytes and NK Cells to Kill Target Cells

Occasionally, antibody may be directed against one's own target cells (Figure 1-34). This can represent a breakdown of immune tolerance with an inability of the host to differentiate "self" from "nonself." Both antibody and CD8 T cytotoxic cells may destroy target cells (Figure 1-34A). This occurs as a deleterious event in the rejection of transplanted organs and in some immune-mediated diseases, referred to as autoimmune diseases (Figure 1-34A) (*Chapter 19*), or as a beneficial event in which a malignant tumor or a chronic viral infected cell is destroyed (Figure 1-34B) (*Chapter 20*). A more deleterious outcome is seen when a chronic viral-infected cell or a malignant cell evades the immune system (Figure 1-34C).

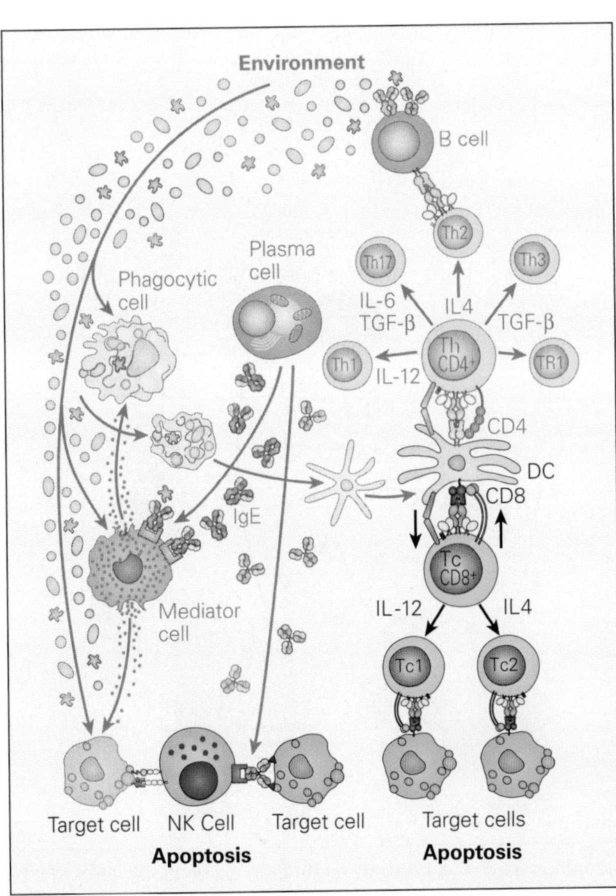

Figure 1-33. Schematic representation of the killing of target cells by either NK cells or cytotoxic T cells.

As we will see in subsequent chapters, occasionally a viral infection or a tumor may evade the deleterious effects of CD8 killing by deleting the MHC-I antigen (*Chapters 13* and *20*). In this case, the immune system may compensate by use of killing of the target cells by NK killing.

The Cytokines

Another group of important key protein and peptide molecules that orchestrate the entire functions of both the innate and the adaptive immune systems are the cytokines (*Chapter 9*). These molecules comprise the vital intercellular communication network of every cell system in the body and function as signaling molecules to regulate the growth, differentiation, activation and inhibition of all cellular aspects of the immune system.

T Cells Orchestrate and Regulate the Immune Response

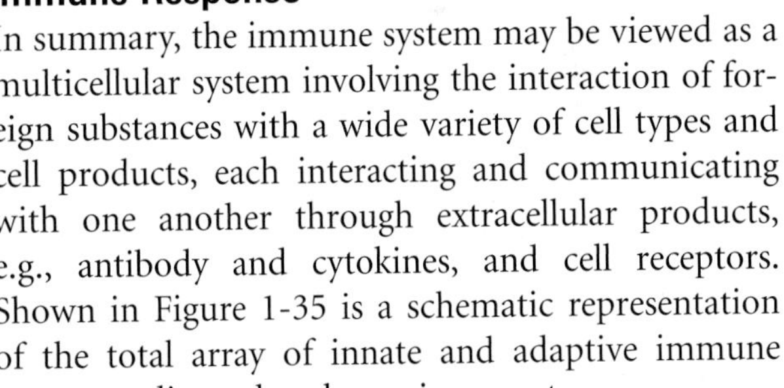

In summary, the immune system may be viewed as a multicellular system involving the interaction of foreign substances with a wide variety of cell types and cell products, each interacting and communicating with one another through extracellular products, e.g., antibody and cytokines, and cell receptors. Shown in Figure 1-35 is a schematic representation of the total array of innate and adaptive immune responses directed at the environment.

Shown in Table 1-16 are the range of interactions a T cell can have with various elements of the immune response. For ease of discussion, these are grouped according to three basic T cell directed functions: (1) immunoregulation, (2) immunocytotoxicity, and (3) immunosuppression.

The Neuroendocrine-Immune Network

It is now generally accepted that the immune system is part of a broader tripartite system referred to as the neuroendocrine-immune (**NEI**) network (Figure 1-36), which represents a system of interdependent and interrelated responses of the neurological, endocrine, and immunologic systems in response to external and internal stimuli. An understanding of

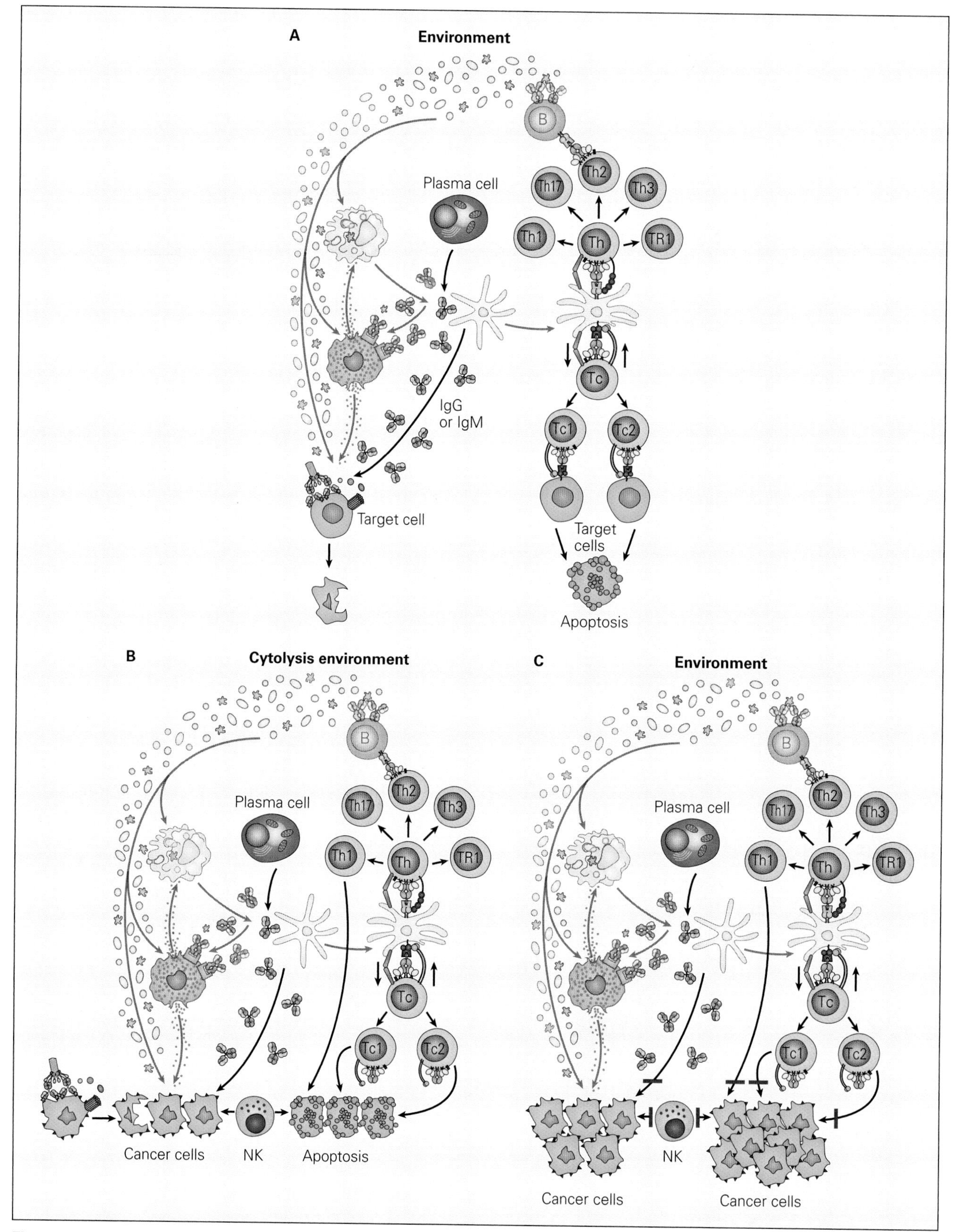

Figure 1-34. Schematic representation of the beneficial and detrimental outcomes of the killing of target cells by antibody, NK cells, or cytotoxic T cells. Panel A: This occurs as a deleterious event in graft rejection and the autoimmune diseases with destructive effects of antibody and CD8+ cell reaction directed to target cells. Panel B: A beneficial killing of a cancer cell or a chronic virally infected cell by antibody, NK cell, or cytotoxic T cells. Panel C: The detrimental outcome when the immune system is evaded by a cancer cell and the antitumor mechanisms are blocked or suppressed showing growth of the tumor.

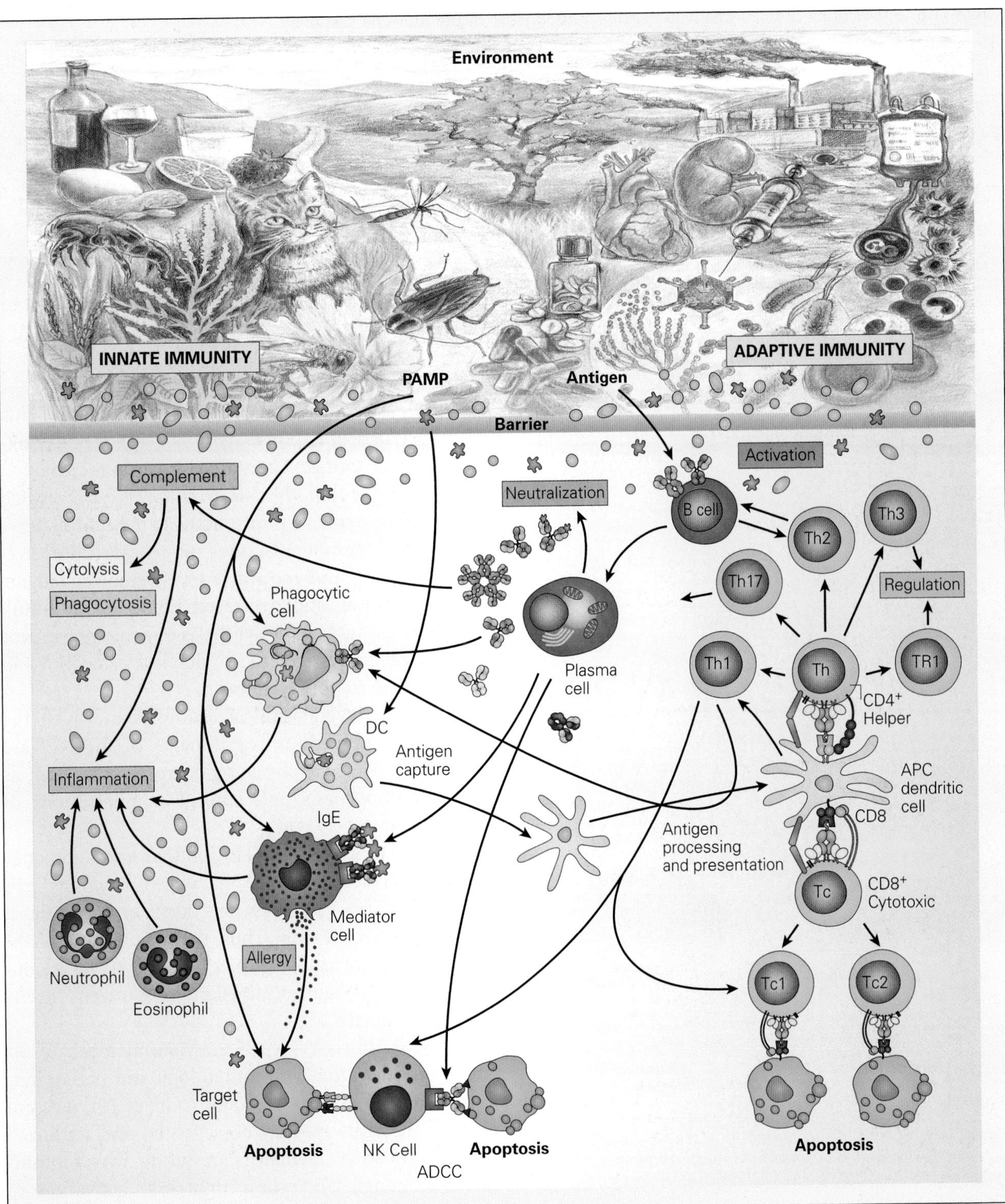

Figure 1-35. Summation of the total array of innate and adaptive immune responses to the environment.

these interactive responses is essential for comprehension of the total functioning of the immune system in health and disease.

The immunologic, endocrine, and neurologic systems work in tandem and influence one another's functions in the NEI interaction.

The central nervous system affects the immune system through the neuroendocrine humoral outflow via the pituitary, and through direct neuronal influences via the sympathetic, parasympathetic (cholinergic), and peptidergic/sensory innervation of peripheral tissues (Figure 1-35).

Table 1-16. Interactions of the T cell with various components of the immune response

Function	Effector cells	Involved cells	Effector molecules/cells	Immune principle(s)	Clinical significance	
					Health	Disease
Immunoregulation	Th_0 (CD4$^+$) Th1 Th2	Th_0-APC Th1-T Th2-B	MIF, TNF-β, IFN-γ, IL-2 IL-4, IL-13	Activation CMI Humoral	Antimicrobial immunity	Immune deficiency, autoimmune disease, cancer, allergy
Immunocytotoxicity	T_c (CD8$^+$)	T_c (CD8)/ target cell	K, NK, ADCC	Target cell destruction	Antiviral immunity	Autoimmune disease
Immunosuppression	Th3 lymphocytes	Th3-T(CD4)	IL-10, TGF-β	Immune tolerance	Maintenance of homeostasis (tolerance of foods, allergens)	Autoimmune disease

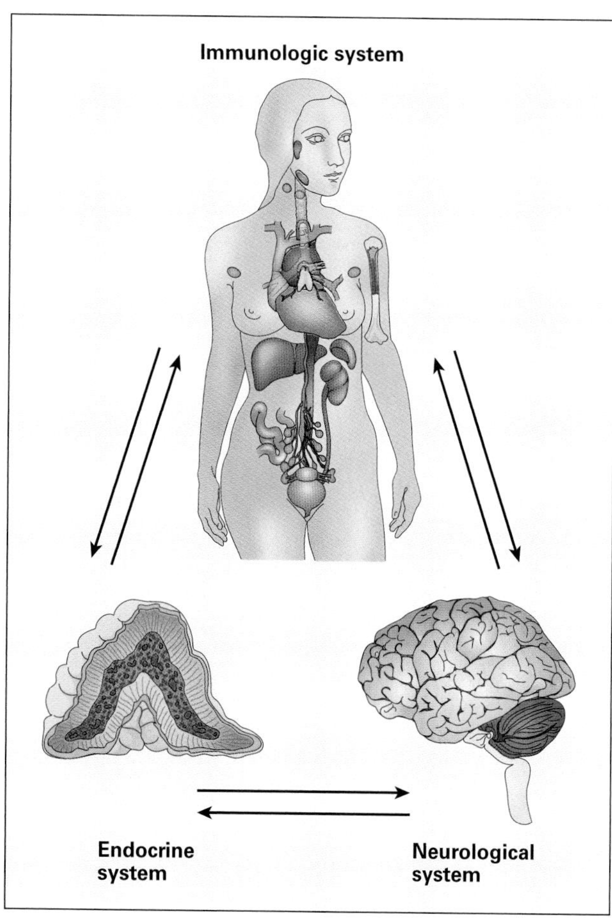

Figure 1-36. Schematic representation of the NEI network showing the bidirectional and interactive responses of the three components of the network: the neurologic, the endocrine, and the immunologic systems.

Thus, circulating hormones, e.g., corticosteroids, thyroid hormone, and sex hormones, or locally released neurotransmitters, such as norepinephrine, dopamine, and serotonin, and neuropeptides (e.g., substance P) regulate major immune functions, such as antigen presentation, secretion of cytokines, chemokines, and antibodies, selection of Th1, Th2, Th17, Tr1, or Th3 responses, lymphocyte activity, proliferation, and traffic. Alternatively, certain cytokines, such as interleukin IL-1, IL-6, and TNF-α, released during an immune response, activate the central nervous system components, alter neurotransmitter networks activity, and induce fever, sleepiness, fatigue, loss of appetite, and decreased libido. In addition, they activate the hepatic synthesis of acute phase proteins—changes referred to as "sickness behavior" and "acute-phase response," respectively.

There are several clinical examples in which the interactions of various components of the NEI are involved in normal physiologic processes as well as in the pathogenesis and clinical manifestations of disease (Table 1-17).

In pregnancy, estrogen (E2)-induced immunomodulation involves dual effects on antigen-presenting cells and CD4$^+$CD25$^+$ Treg cells, but does not have a direct effect on effector T cells. Thus, the maintenance of the fetus during normal pregnancy appears to be modulated by the Treg-enhancing effects of estrogens on the immune response.

There is much evidence that neural mechanisms are involved in the symptomatology and pathophysiology of asthma (Box 1-10 and *Chapter 18*). Afferent neurologic pathways may be activated and sensitized by inflammatory mediators, resulting in symptoms such as cough and chest tightness, activation of cholinergic reflexes, and the release of inflammatory neuropeptides. Cholinergic mechanisms are the predominant bronchoconstrictor neural pathway and may be enhanced in asthma, particularly during exacerbations, through several mechanisms, including impaired function of muscarinic autoreceptors on cholinergic nerve terminals. There may also be abnormalities in adrenergic control and in the function of

Table 1-17. Examples of clinical conditions or diseases involving the neuroendocrine-immune network

Condition or disease	Proposed pathogenic mechanism	Outcome
Pregnancy	Increased estrogen and progesterone-induced Th2 skewing and increased Th3	Retention of the fetus during pregnancy
Asthma	Activation of cholinergic reflexes by inflammatory mediators	Refractory asthma
Autoimmune disease, e.g., systemic lupus erythematosus	Estrogen-induced Th2 activity	Increased female predominance
Osteoporosis	Estrogen deficiency increases TNF-α production and osteoclastogenesis	Increased frequency of postmenopausal loss of bone matrix
Increased susceptibility to chronic infections	Chronic stress-induced Th2 shift	Increase in intracellular bacterial and viral diseases

Box 1-10

Asthma is a syndrome characterized by reversible episodes of wheezing, cough, and sensations of chest tightness and breathlessness. These symptoms are secondary to changes in the activity of the nervous system. The mechanisms by which the nervous system is altered to promote the symptoms of asthma have not yet been elucidated. Airway inflammation associated with asthma may affect neuronal activity at several points along the neural reflex pathway, including the function of the primary afferent (sensory) nerves, integration within the central nervous system, synaptic transmission within autonomic ganglia, and transmission at the level of the postganglionic neuroeffector junction. A brief overview of these interactions and the relevance they may have to asthma are provided in Chapter 18.

beta-adrenoceptors, particularly in severe asthma. The neurotransmitter of bronchodilator nerves is now identified as nitric oxide, and this mechanism may be impaired during asthma exacerbations. Finally, neurogenic inflammation may contribute to and amplify allergic inflammation in asthmatic airways by the release of neuropeptides from sensory nerves (*Chapter 18*).

Immune Balance: The Immune System in Health and Disease

From what has been described in this chapter, the immune system is clearly a physiologic system of lymphoid organs, cells and cell products designed to recognize and remove foreignness; as with all physiologic systems, it may be viewed as an adaptive system in which the body attempts to maintain homeostasis between the internal and external environments. The summation of the total immune capability of the host to all foreign matter is shown schematically in Figure 1-37. This model is based upon the following assumptions concerning the immune response: (1) the foreign substance, e.g., immunogen (antigen), drives the system, i.e., active immune responses occur only as long as the foreign substance is present and will cease after it is removed; (2) there are three responses through which all foreign substances are removed; and (3) the extent of the progression through these three phases will be determined by the efficiency of elimination of the foreign substance.

The first phase involves the innate (primary) immune response and consists of those ancient responses to first encounters with a foreign configuration—phagocytosis and the inflammatory response. If the substance (e.g., carbon particles) is completely eliminated at this stage, the host's immune response terminates and there is no further progression. Because of its primitive structure, carbon particles taken up by phagocytic cells will not require processing and delivery to the T-Ball network and the adaptive immune response will not be initiated.

If this primary encounter occurs with a more complex foreign substance, e.g., a bacterium, and leads to a processed product, e.g., "processed antigen," the more sophisticated immune adaptive responses are stimulated (Figure 1-37). These consist of two basic effector systems: (1) B lymphocyte–mediated humoral immunity with the elaboration

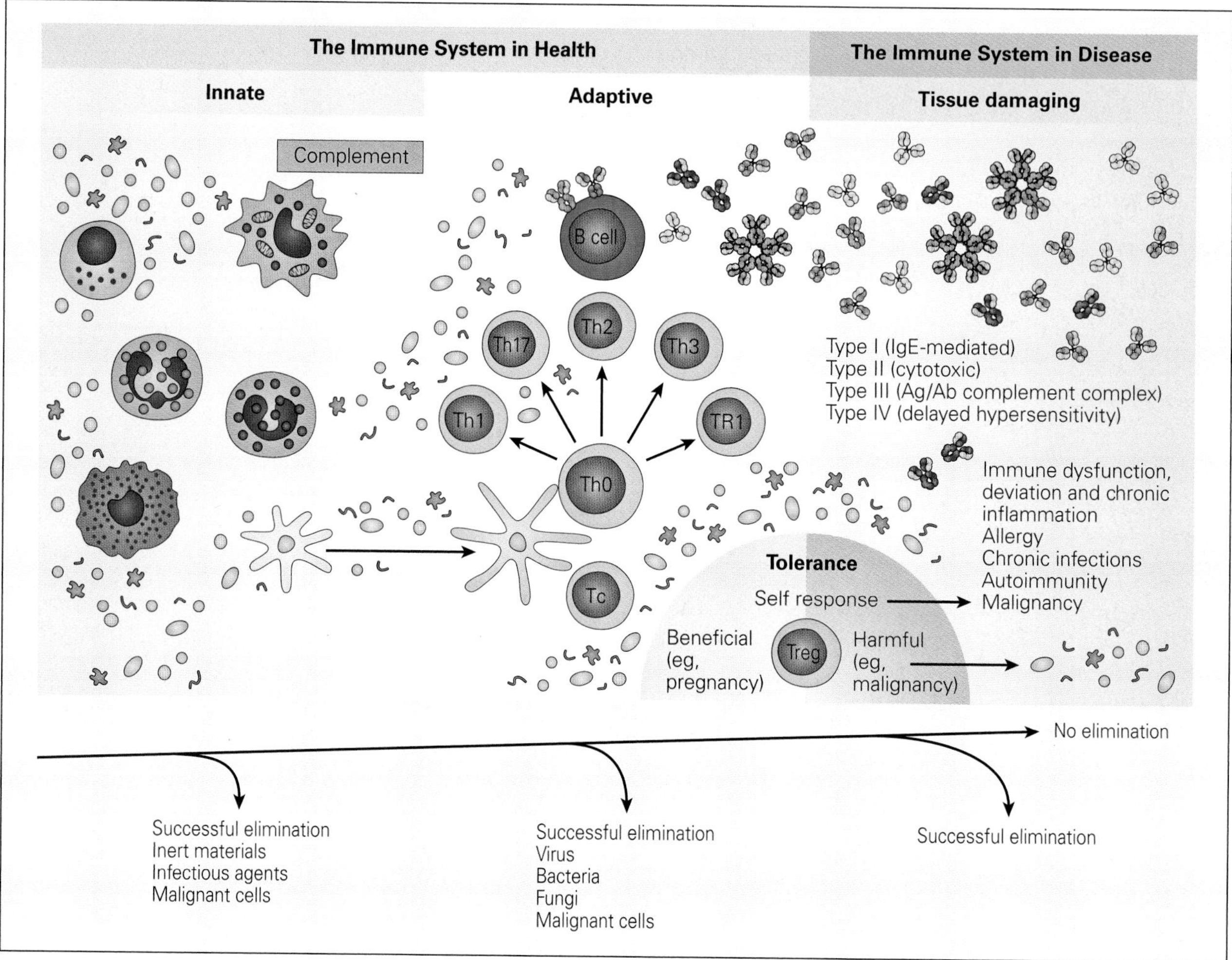

Figure 1-37. Schematic representation of the total immune capability of the host based upon efficiency of elimination of foreign matter.

of antibody associated with five major classes of immunoglobulin (IgE, IgM, IgG, IgA, and IgD) and (2) T lymphocyte-mediated antigen elimination. A sophisticated addition to these systems is the capacity to enhance these immune responses through the action of the biologic amplification system(s) of cytokines, chemokines, complement, and the coagulation cascade (*Chapter 4*) and a bank of "memory cells" that can expand rapidly when antigen is re-encountered. If antigen is successfully eliminated at this phase, the immune response terminates. Normally, most foreign substances are successfully eliminated in these first two stages, and this beneficial outcome characterizes the immune system in health.

If antigen cannot be eliminated at these first two stages and continues to persist, two outcomes may occur: suppression or the development of tissue-damaging responses. In some situations, the persistence of an antigen can lead to the silencing of an immune response, i.e., immune suppression, where the immunosuppressive role of Treg cells appears to be prominent. These responses can either be beneficial, as in the case of the retention of the fetus during pregnancy, allowing for a successful birth, or deleterious, as in the case of suppression of immunity to a malignant tumor that has successfully evaded immune surveillance and where the active mechanisms of tumor rejection are no longer operative (*Chapter 20*).

Alternatively, the persistence of antigen can lead to the development of the tissue-damaging responses (*Chapter 17*). The induction of antigen persistence in this tertiary stage may result either from the nature of the antigen itself, which, because of its adapted state, may resist degradation, e.g., the tubercle bacillus or from some genetic defect in antigen processing, such as the immune-deficiency diseases. As a result of either of these possibilities, if antigen persists, four types of immunopathologic interactions of the Gell and Coombs classification

Case Study: Clinical Relevance

Let us return to the case study of Lyme disease presented earlier and review some of the major points of the clinical presentation and how they relate to the immune system:

- Although there was no definite history of a tick bite, the diagnosis of Lyme disease was established by the presence of the bull's-eye rash and the positive, confirmatory antibody test; the exposure of the child in summer months in a Lyme disease–prevalent area further supports the diagnosis. Unfortunately, nearly 80 percent of patients with Lyme disease have no recollection of a tick bite, presumably because of the small size of the tick.
- The skin and mucous membranes normally provide the first natural barriers limiting entry of pathogens; once the skin is breached, in this case by the bite of an infected Ixodes deer tick, *B. burgdorferi* is introduced into local subcutaneous tissues. Subsequent activation of the innate immune system produces a localized inflammatory response consisting of the redness (erythema), swelling (edema), and increased warmth (calor) of the typical hallmark bull's eye lesion of erythema migrans. A second aspect of the innate immune response involves phagocytosis of the organism by localized macrophages and dendritic cells, which also function as APCs. Thus, the adaptive immune system is initiated.
- Within the APCs in local lymphoid tissues and draining lymph nodes, the organism is digested into fragments that are next presented to T cells. Subsequent interaction between T and B cells during the adaptive immune response leads to the production of antibody.
- The detection of an IgM antibody response to *B. burgdorferi* confirmed the diagnosis of recent infection. This IgM response seen in a serum specimen obtained within two weeks of infection in this particular child is consistent with the early phase of infection with Lyme disease. A specimen taken four weeks later revealed antibody of the IgG class. This observation of IgM followed by IgG antibody illustrates the isotypic switch mechanism of the immune system and is important diagnostically by allowing the differentiation of an early infection from a late infection.
- The early diagnosis and prompt treatment of Lyme disease in children most often leads to resolution without late sequelae, in contrast to adults wherein the persistence of antigen can lead to immunopathology with chronic forms of disease,

can be elicited: Types I, II, III, and IV (*Chapter 17*). These responses are no longer beneficial to the host and are manifested as the immune-mediated disorders (*Chapter 18*) that represent the immune system in disease. The duration of this tissue-damaging phase will vary according to the efficiency of antigen elimination (Figure 1-37) and may be temporary (if the antigen can be removed) or more protracted (if the antigen persists). If antigen can be removed or eliminated, the tertiary response will be terminated with minimal discomfort to the patient (e.g., discontinuation of penicillin therapy in a penicillin-allergic patient). However, if the tertiary response is ineffective and antigen continues to persist, more harmful expressions of the immune response emerge and can manifest clinically as allergic disease, autoimmune disorders, or malignancy (Figure 1-37). This represents the most harmful expression of immune imbalance and symbolizes a maximal, deleterious, self-perpetuating attack of an aberrant immune response on a host who sustains injury.

Key Points

- The immune system provides the body's primary defense against infectious organisms and other environmental substances. It also has homeostatic and tumor-surveillance functions.
- The innate immune response recognizes conserved pathogen molecules and responds rapidly to contain pathogens at their entry site.
- The adaptive immune response recognizes very specific and varying pathogen antigens and responds more slowly but with the generation of immunologic memory.
- Humoral immune responses eliminate extracellular pathogens and toxins, while cellular immune responses eliminate intracellular pathogens and tumor cells.
- The innate immune response is necessary to initiate the adaptive response, and both function together to eliminate pathogen.

- T cells orchestrate and regulate the immune response. The immune system is also regulated by (and influences) the neuroendocrine system.
- The immune mechanisms that can successfully eliminate pathogen can also cause immunopathology.

Study Questions/Critical Thinking

1. Identify each of these immune mechanisms as part of the innate immune response (I), adaptive immune response (A), or a combination of both (C).

   a. A macrophage uses its TLR to bind *E. coli* LPS and engulf the bacterium.
   b. A neutrophil uses its Fc receptors to bind IgG-coated *Staphylococcus aureus* and engulf the bacterium.
   c. An NK cell binds a virus-infected cell and induces apoptosis.
   d. A cytotoxic T cell binds a virus-infected cell and induces apoptosis.
   e. An NK cell uses its Fc receptors to bind an IgG-coated virus-infected cell and induces apoptosis.
   f. A mast cell is stimulated by the presence of tissue damage to release histamine.
   g. A mast cell is stimulated by pollen binding to IgE on its Fc receptors to release histamine.

2. Identify each of these immune responses as humoral (H) or cellular (C) immunity.

   a. Antibody to diphtheria toxin binds the toxin and blocks toxin bindng to target cells (neutralization).
   b. Cytotoxic T cells recognize and kill virus-infected cells.
   c. Helper T cells (Th2) signal B cells to secrete IgA.
   d. Helper T cells (Th1) signal macrophages to kill phagocytosed pathogen.
   e. An NK cell uses its Fc receptors to bind antibody bound to HIV gp120 on the membrane of an infected CD4 T cell; the NK cell induces apoptosis in the CD4 T cell.

3. Compare the antigen-recognition systems of the innate and adaptive immune responses. What are the advantages and disadvantages of each?
4. Discuss the multiple roles of T cells in the immune system.
5. Explain why the finding of a monoclonal antibody in patient serum could not be due to a normal immune response.
6. Explain how the immune system can cause tissue damage during the course of an immune response. Is tissue damage from the immune response inevitable for any pathogen?

Suggested Reading

Bellanti J. Immunology II. Philadelphia: W. B. Saunders; 1978.

Bellanti J. Immunology III. Philadelphia: W. B. Saunders; 1985.

Cools N, Ponsaerts P, Van Tendeloo VF, et al. Regulatory T cells and human disease. Clin Dev Immunol. ePub Jan 1, 2008: 89195.

Dinarello CA. Historical insights into cytokines. Eur J Immunol. 2007; 37 Suppl 1: S34–45.

Feig C, Peter ME. How apoptosis got the immune system in shape. Eur J Immunol. 2007; 37 Suppl 1: S61–70.

Goodarzi H, Trowbridge J, Gallo RL. Innate immunology: a cutaneous perspective. Clin Rev Allerg Immu. 2007; 33: 15–26.

Gordon S. The macrophage: past, present and future. Eur J Immunol. 2007; 37 Suppl 1: S9–17.

Lauzon NM, Mian F, Ashkar AA. Toll-like receptors, natural killer cells and innate immunity. Adv Exp Med Biol. 2007: 598: 1–11.

Lehner T. Special regulatory T cell review: the resurgence of the concept of contrasuppression in the immunoregulation. Immunology. 2008; 123: 40–4.

Mak TW. The T cell antigen receptor: 'the hunting of the snark.' Eur J Immunol. 2007; 37 Suppl 1: S83–93.

Masopust D, Vezys V, Wherry EJ, et al. A brief history of CD8 T cells. Eur J Immunol. 2007; 37 Suppl 1: S103–110.

Journal of Allergy and Clinical Immunology. Primer on allergy and immunology. 2003: 11: S486.

Sojka DK, Huang YH, Fowell DJ. Mechanisms of regulatory T-cell suppression—a diverse arsenal for a moving target. Immunology. 2008; 14; 13–22.

Steinman RM. Dendritic cells: understanding immunogenicity. Eur J Immunol. 2007; 37 Suppl 1: S53–60.

Vondenhoff MF, Kraal G, Mebius RE. Lymphoid organogensis in brief. Eur J Immunol. 2007; 37 Suppl 1: S46–52.

Zola H, Swart B, Nicholson I, et al. CD molecules 2005: human cell differentiation molecules. Blood. 2005; Nov: 106: 3,123–6.

Chapter 2

Developmental Immunology: The Changing Immune System and Its Clinical Applications

Joseph A. Bellanti, MD

Case Study

An eleven-year-old female presents to her pediatrician with fatigue and lethargy of two weeks duration. Past history revealed that she was the product of a full-term uncomplicated pregnancy and at birth weighed 3.3 kg. The initial physical examination and her three-day nursery stay were described as unremarkable. At five to six days of age, after returning home, the infant was observed by the mother to have "twisting and jerking motions" of the extremities, and at twelve days developed two generalized seizures and was subsequently hospitalized. Physical examination disclosed a lethargic infant with hypertelorism (excessive width between the eyes), low-set ears and a grade three pansystolic murmur. Laboratory evaluation revealed hypocalcemia with a serum calcium value of 6.2 mg/dL and a mild decrease in the mean number of CD3+ T cells and CD4+ T helper cells. The infant was diagnosed with hypoparathyroidism and a ventriculoseptal defect and was treated initially with intramuscular parathyroid hormone and subsequently with oral vitamin D.

The infant showed slow growth with developmental delay during the first two years, and at three years of age she began to have a history of recurrent upper respiratory infections consisting of repeated bouts of otitis media and sinusitis that continued over the next several years, requiring almost continuous antibiotic therapy. Because of her developmental delay and learning difficulties, special educational programs were required when the child entered school.

The child was brought to her pediatrician for further evaluation of the recent onset of fatigue and lethargy, which began two weeks prior to the present visit. In addition to the facial appearance and cardiac murmur found earlier, she was found to have a symmetrical, nontender enlargement of both lobes of the thyroid gland. Laboratory examination revealed a serum T4 thyroid hormone concentration of 0.4 ng/dL (normal values range from 0.8 to 2.0 ng/dL) and a thyroid-stimulating hormone (TSH) value of 6.5 μU/mL (normal values range from 0.5 to 5.0 ng/dL). Elevated serum levels of autoantibodies to thyroid were also detected, i.e., anti-thyroglobulin 5.1 U/ml (normal < 0.3 U/ml), anti-microsomal > 30.0 U/ml (normal < 0.3 U/ml).

LEARNING OBJECTIVES

When you have completed this chapter, you should be able to:

- Contrast the evolution of the innate and adaptive immune systems
- Summarize the antigen-independent and antigen-dependent development of T and B cells
- Identify the role of the thymus and the bone marrow as important central organs of development of the immune system
- Describe the organization and function of the immune organs
- Explain the significance and mechanism of lymphocyte recirculation
- Summarize the ontogeny of the adaptive immune system and its clinical applications

Case Study (continued)

The clinician should consider the deletion syndrome now referred to as the chromosome **22q11.2 deletion (CH22qD) syndrome** in any child who manifests the facial, cardiac, and hypocalcemic endocrine abnormalities as presented in this case study. The chromosome CH22qD syndrome consists of a chromosomal alteration resulting in the loss of the proximal long arm of chromosome 22 and includes several overlapping syndromes, primarily the **DiGeorge syndrome**, the **velocardiofacial** (or Shprintzen's syndrome), and the **conotruncal anomaly face (CTAF)** syndrome (Box 2-1).

In this case, the diagnosis of DiGeorge syndrome was initially made based upon the classic findings in the newborn period. Subsequently, the onset of recurrent upper respiratory infections and the recent development of autoimmune thyroiditis (Hashimoto's thyroiditis) led to the diagnosis of the CH22qD syndrome on the basis of a positive fluorescence in situ hybridization (FISH) assay (Figure 2-1). The goal of this case study is to illustrate the critical role of the thymus in the development of the immune system and how its defective development can lead to both the manifestations of recurrent infection as well as autoimmune disease.

Box 2-1

The Chromosome 22q11.2 Deletion (CH22qD) Syndrome: Historical Aspects

The DiGeorge syndrome was first described in 1968 in young infants as a rare developmental defect affecting structures derived from the third and fourth embryonic pharyngeal arches. The three principal organs derived from these embryonic structures that were affected included the thymus, the parathyroid glands, and the heart, and gave rise to the characteristic clinical findings of the disorder, which included distinct facial features of hypertelorism, low-set ears and mouth deformities, hypoplasia or aplasia of the thymus, hypoplasia or aplasia of the parathyroid glands, and conotruncal cardiac defects. Infants presented with hypocalcemia, recurrent respiratory infections resulting from immunodeficiency, and cardiac failure, which, at the time, were often incompatible with life. Subsequent to the description of the DiGeorge syndrome, two other entities were identified that shared common features with it and included the velocardiofacial (or Shprintzen's) syndrome and the conotruncal anomaly face (CTAF) syndrome. Because these three clinical syndromes were later found to share a common genetic cause in most cases, i.e., a chromosome 22q11 deletion, they were subsequently reclassified together as the chromosome 22q11.2 deletion (CH22qD) syndrome, which represents the most common deletion syndrome currently known—estimated to occur in approximately one in 4,000 to 6,000 live births. In addition to the classic findings of the DiGeorge syndrome, several additional features of the CH22qD syndrome have been identified, which collectively include:

- Congenital heart disease
- Immunodeficiency
- Hypocalcemia
- Autoimmune disorders
- Palatal anomalies
- Velopharyngeal dysfunction and other speech disorders
- Feeding disorders and growth retardation
- Otorhinolaryngologic issues
- Dysmorphic facies
- Renal anomalies
- Skeletal anomalies
- Cognitive or learning disabilities
- Behavioral or psychiatric disorders

The CH22qD syndrome is now diagnosed by fluorescence in situ hybridization (FISH) using DNA probes from the DiGeorge chromosomal region (DGCR) (Figure 2-1). Such genetic testing is widely available for the clinical and prenatal testing of the CH22qD syndrome.

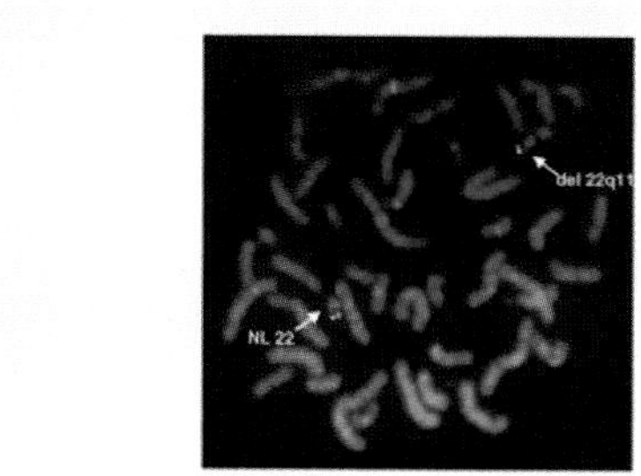

Figure 2-1. FISH of metaphase chromosomes with fluorescently labeled probes to detect a deletion of chromosome 22q11. The green signal control is seen at the distal end of both homologues of chromosome 22; note the presence of the red signal for the test probe on one homologue of chromosome 22 (NL 22) and the absence of the test probe on the other homologue (del 22q11), implying a deletion of that locus on one chromosome. Goldmuntz E. DiGeorge syndrome: new insights. Clin Perinatol. 2005;32:963–78.

The Developing Immune System

The development of the immune system into the highly complex and intricate structure we know today occurred over a span of 400 million years of evolution in response to an ever-changing and potentially hostile environment to which antecedent life forms were exposed. With the continuous introduction of new foreign agents into today's environment, brought about by modern biotechnology and industrial expansion, there is every reason to predict that the immune system of future generations of mankind will continue to change and adapt to these new environments (Figure 2-2).

As described in Chapter 1, the distinguishing hallmark of the immune system is its ability to maintain a homeostatic balance between the external and internal environments; to identify, neutralize, and eliminate foreignness; and to discriminate self from nonself. The cells and cell products of the immune system at differing stages of life manifest a striking variability in their capacity to respond to the environment and show an ever-changing capability of responsiveness from fetal life to the senescent periods. Not only is this illustrated by the striking susceptibility to infectious agents seen in the fetal and neonatal periods and in the elderly, which are related to maturational decreases of immune function, but also by the increased frequency of autoimmune disease and malignancy seen in the older adult that appear to be related to a waning immunity during this period of life. Moreover, in recent years, increasingly larger segments of the population are developing weakened immune systems not only as a result of new medical advances (e.g., transplantation, infection, such as HIV infection or malignancy), but also as a result of the accompanying drug-related immunosuppressive properties of pharmacotherapeutic agents required for the treatment or management of these conditions. All of these are expressions of the changing immune system during development or treatment on disease expression. It is therefore incumbent on those entrusted with the care of patients of all ages to have a clear understanding of the development and expressions of the immune system at different stages of life, ranging from fetal life to senescence, for improved diagnosis and therapy.

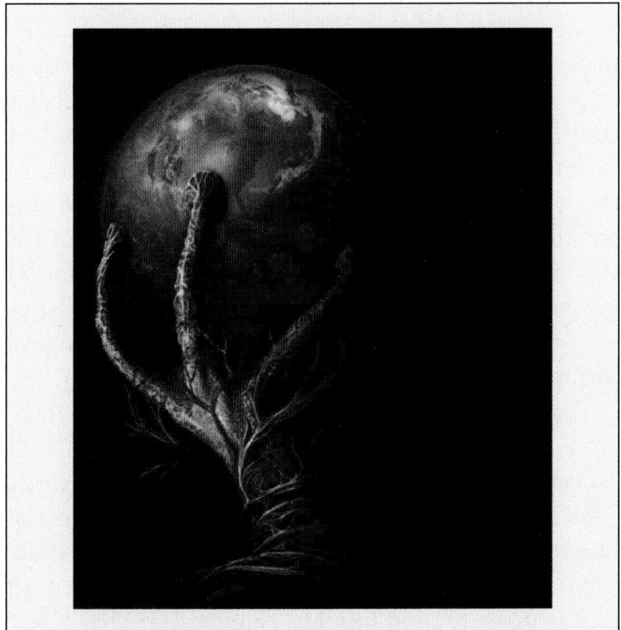

Figure 2-2. A foreign alien invading the Earth from Steven Spielberg's *War of the Worlds*, starring Tom Cruise, the film based on the classic H. G. Wells novel of the same name. Spielberg may have been drawn to the idea of an alien menace lurking just out of view on our Earth these many millennia, biding its time, awaiting the right trigger. (Courtesy of Paramount Pictures.)

The Immune System Has Evolved and Continues to Differentiate in Response to Environmental Signals

The development of the immune system at all levels may be considered as a series of genetically determined adaptive cellular transformations that occur in the species (**phylogeny**), the individual (**ontogeny**), or at the cellular level (**differentiation**) in response to an ever-changing and potentially hostile environment. In each of these situations, the best adapted form that can survive in its environment is the one selected for its survival. Thus the development of all *innate* and *adaptive* immune responses can be best considered as a continuing set of adaptive responses to the extant environment.

Shown in Table 2-1 are the evolutionary pressures exerted by the environment on the development of the immune response in the species, the individual, or at the cellular level. From an evolutionary standpoint, the effect of a hostile macroenvironment provided the selective pressures leading to the survival of those life forms within the developing species that were best adapted to that environment (i.e., phylogeny). Within the developing fetus, the microenvironment of cytokines and growth-enhancing factors in which undifferentiated progenitor cells exist (e.g., thymus or bone marrow) provides yet another type of inductive environment leading to the full expression

Table 2-1. Effect of environment on the development of the immune response

Target	Inductive environment	Process	Selected form
Species	Macroenvironment	Phylogeny	Existing life forms
Individual	Microenvironment (thymus, bone marrow)	Ontogeny	Immunologically mature individual
Cell	Molecular (immunogen)	Postnatal cellular expression of the immune response	"Memory" cells

of immunity within the developing host (i.e., ontogeny). The immunologically mature individual may be considered as the best selected form resulting from this type of ontogenetic development. The molecular environment at the cellular level, i.e., immunogen, in which immunologically reactive cells exist, provides the inductive stimulus leading to the proliferative and growth-differentiating events that are characteristic of the adaptive (specific) immune response. This leads to the synthesis of cell products such as antibody (*Chapter 6*) or mediators of cell-mediated immunity, i.e., the cytokines (*Chapter 9*). The "memory" cells that result from this process may be considered as those cellular forms that are best adapted to an environment characterized by diminishing quantities of immunogen. The interaction of the antigen-presenting cells (APCs), T cells, B cells, and natural killer (NK) cells involved in immune processes is under strict genetic control (*Chapter 10*).

Development of the Immune System at the Cellular Level

Antigen itself may be considered a part of the environment that induces the development of an immune responsiveness at the cellular level (Table 2-1). During the induction of an immune response, immunogen comes in contact with an appropriate collection of antigen-presenting cells and lymphoid cells (B and T cells), after which a series of proliferative and differentiative steps are initiated. As described in Chapter 1, there are at least three cells involved: (1) the APCs, i.e., macrophages, B lymphocytes, and dendritic cells; (2) the thymus-dependent or T lymphocytes, which participate in cell-mediated immunity (**CMI**); and (3) the bone marrow or bursal-dependent B lymphocytes, which provide humoral immunity, i.e., antibody-mediated immunity. Thus the inductive stimulus for the development of the immune response at the cellular level is immunogen; i.e., "immunogen drives the system." Once the immunogen is removed, there is an involution of this population of immunocompetent cells. However, some cells that have been selectively adapted to this changing environment remain as "memory cells" capable of carrying out specific immune events of acquired immunity during any future encounter with the same or a related antigen. These consist of either B or T lymphocytes. The whole cellular burst of activity seen in the induction of an immune response may be analogous to genetically controlled differentiation seen in the development of the species or during ontogeny of the individual. The "memory cells" may be considered the best adapted cells for this type of environment (Table 2-1). Antigen-dependent development of B and T cells is discussed in *Chapters 6* and *7*.

Phylogeny: The Development of the Immune System in Evolving Species

Innate Immunity Is an Evolutionarily Ancient Defense System

The evolution of the immune system is best studied by observing elements of immune defenses in animals and plants living today. Antimicrobial peptides, cell-surface microbial recognition molecules (toll-like receptors), and phagocytosis are found in invertebrates. The most primitive manifestation of 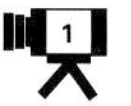 the resistance mechanism of the innate immune system is phagocytosis, recorded by Mechnikov in his writings (*Chapter 1*). **Phagocytosis**, which is found in the most ancient of the unicellular organisms, originally served a *nutritive* function. In higher forms, the process evolved to a *defense* function.

From the currently identifiable life forms, there arose an increasingly complex immune system that ranged from the primitive defense of phagocytosis seen in unicellular eukaryotes (e.g., amebae) to the humoral and cell-mediated immune responses characteristic of the adaptive immune system seen in higher primates and humans (Figure 2-3).

As cellular life differentiated into more complex forms, there developed an increasing specialization and sophistication of the systems concerned with recognition of foreignness so that the immune

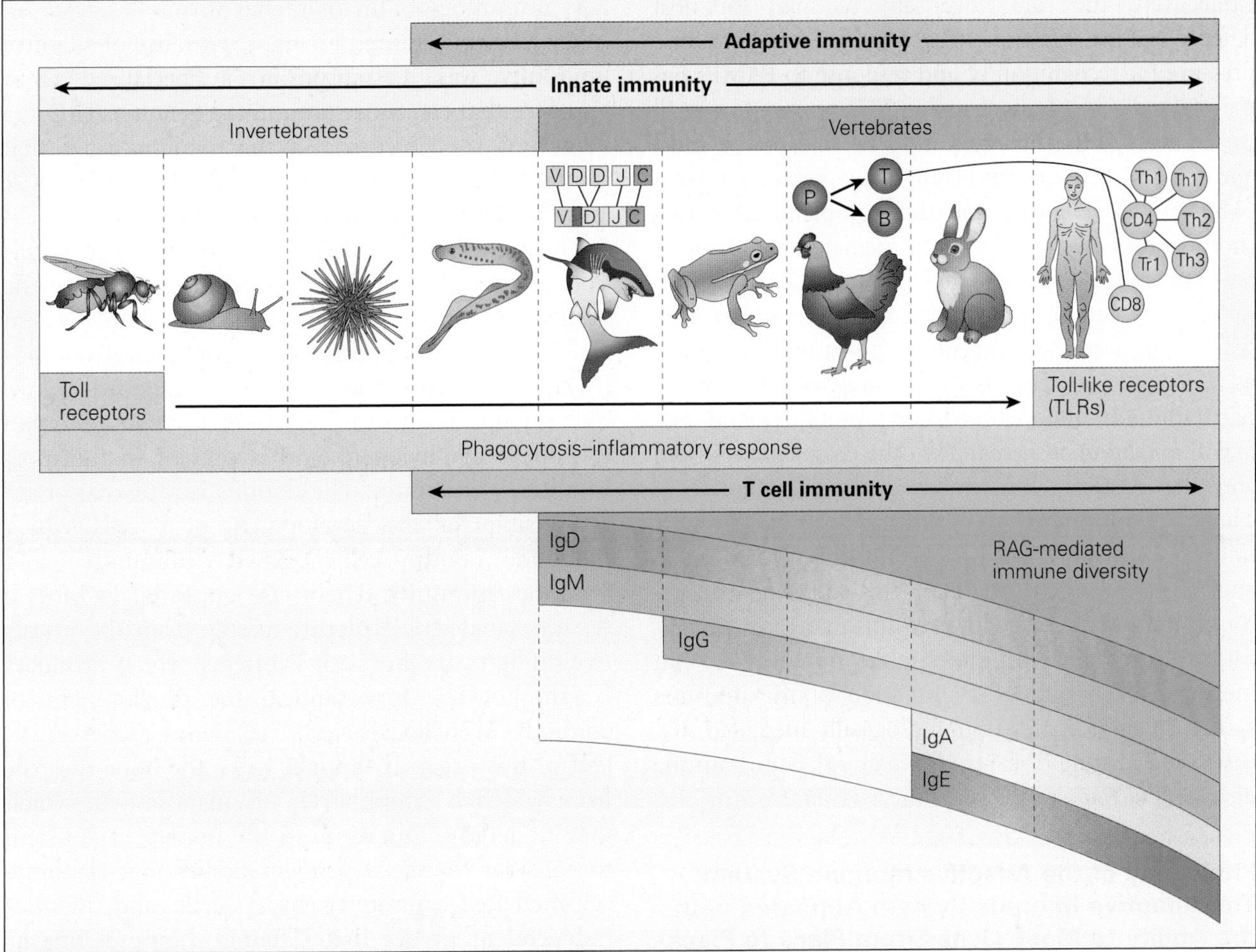

Figure 2-3. Schematic representation of the phylogeny of the immune system.

responses could be performed with increasing efficiency and with ever-increasing complexity. Although phagocytosis was continued as a nutritive function by endodermal cells (i.e., sponges) the addition of a newly acquired mesodermal layer added a defense function. It is the development and specialization of this mesodermal layer in higher life forms, beginning with vertebrates, in which specialization of cells destined for immune function, is seen.

In higher invertebrates, a vascular system developed that allowed phagocytosis to proceed by both *fixed* and *circulating cells* (Figure 2-3). In horseshoe crabs, e.g., one of the major defense systems is carried out by the hemolymph, which contains at least two types of hemocytes, granular and non-granular cells, based on cell morphology. In humans, on the other hand, there are five circulating white blood cells, three of which are phagocytic (monocytes, polymorphonuclear cells, and eosinophils) (*Chapter 1*). Thus in phylogeny, the two most important elements of the innate immune system are *phagocytosis* and *the inflammatory response*, which were found in primitive life forms.

The evolution and phylogeny of the innate immune system is now better understood in molecular terms beginning in the lowest invertebrates and continuing into higher forms. The toll-like receptors (**TLRs**) (*Chapter 3*), i.e., the type I transmembrane proteins that recognize microbes once they have breached physical barriers such as the skin or intestinal tract mucosa and activate immune cell responses, are believed to play a key role in the innate immune system. TLRs are a type of pattern-recognition receptors (**PRRs**) that recognize molecules that are broadly shared by pathogens, but distinguishable from host molecules, and are collectively referred to as pathogen-associated molecular patterns (**PAMPs**). TLRs are present in vertebrates (including fish, amphibians, reptiles, birds, and mammals) as well as in invertebrates (such as the insect drosophila), in which they were first identified and extensively studied. TLRs are also widely represented in bacteria and plants.

Collectively, they are universally required for host defense against infection (*Chapter 12*). Strong selective pressure for recognition of and response to PAMPs has maintained a largely unchanging TLR recognition in all vertebrates. TLRs thus appear to be one of the most ancient, conserved components of the immune system (*Chapter 3*). Elements of the complement system (homologues of C3 and a lectin-mediated complement pathway) are also found in invertebrates (*Chapter 4*).

With evolution, innate defense mechanisms persisted, and were supplemented and amplified by the addition of new elements of the *adaptive immune system* (antibody and cell-mediated immunity) and *biological amplification systems* (i.e., the coagulation system and the classical complement system) (Figure 2-3). Thus these older mechanisms of innate immunity were not replaced with evolution, but rather were continued and reinforced as evolving life forms added new adaptive immune responses. However, this increased specialization also has the undesirable outcome of an increased likelihood of malfunction of the immune system in the form of immunologically mediated diseases, i.e., allergic diseases (*Chapter 18*), autoimmune disorders (*Chapter 19*), and cancer (*Chapter 20*).

Phylogeny of the Adaptive Immune System: The Adaptive Immune System Appeared with the Ability to Move Genes from Place to Place in the Genome

The first evidence of the adaptive immune system appeared in primitive chordates, such as the jawed fishes. Shown in Figure 2-3 and Table 2-2 are the phylogenetic relationships among the chordates and the first appearance of the adaptive immune system in the jawed vertebrates (gnathostomes) as indicated by the expression of rearranged antigen receptor genes in the immunoglobulin superfamily and by the major histocompatibility complex. In these forms, it consists of a disseminated lymphoid system, rather than the specialized lymphoid structures that are seen in higher forms; however, both humoral and cellular immune elements are present. In these early species there existed a primitive high-molecular-weight antibody analogous to IgM and cells comparable to T cells in higher forms that could manifest some primitive expressions of cell-mediated immunity. In elasmobranches, e.g., in sharks, a tissue transplant consisting of skins or scales would be promptly rejected. Similarly, the introduction of immunogens into these species will elicit a high-molecular-weight antibody response analogous to IgM immunoglobulin of higher forms (*Chapter 6*). A key element required for the appearance of adaptive immunity was a transposon, a specialized DNA sequence that can move around the genome. This element was the precursor of the modern genes that recombine gene segments to encode the diverse BCR and TCR antigen receptors (*Chapters 6* and *7*).

During evolution, there also occurred specialization of cells and supporting structures to house the tissues and organs of the adaptive immune system which include both central and peripheral components of the immune system as described below. The thymus is the earliest central lymphoid organ to appear in phylogeny and is present in the most primitive vertebrates. The thymus is a pivotal organ responsible for the development of T cells, which modulate both cell-mediated immunity and humoral immunity. There also appeared in birds a separate anatomic structure arising from the primitive hindgut, the bursa of Fabricius, which produces B lymphocytes important in the development of antibody in avian species. The mammalian equivalent of this organ is thought to be the bone marrow from which B lymphocytes originate and in which they undergo maturation. In the human, it is useful to consider thymic-dependent tissues that elaborate cell-mediated immunity by T cells and thymic-independent tissues that elaborate humoral immunity by B cells alone. This division of the immune system into T cells and B cells has formed the seminal infrastructure of our knowledge of the immunopathogenesis of many diseases in the human.

The evolutionary order of appearance of immunoglobulin classes in many respects parallels that seen during ontogeny in the maturing individual ("ontogeny recapitulates phylogeny"). Shown in Figure 2-3, the predominant antibody in most primitive vertebrates is a high-molecular-weight molecule, analogous to the IgM immunoglobulins of the human. In higher life forms during phylogeny, a second class of antibody is elaborated with properties similar to the IgG immunoglobulins. In still higher life forms, the IgA immunoglobulins appear as rather late evolutionary events and, in mammals, the development of a novel form of a dimeric molecular form of IgA appears at mucosal surfaces, i.e., the secretory IgA immunoglobulins (*Chapter 8*). These molecules, which are produced in the mucosa-associated lymphoid tissues (**MALT**), have proven to be of immense importance in bodily defense at mucosal surfaces and appear to be a mechanism by which lower forms, such as the ungulates, receive passive antibody via colostrum. The major antibody transferred from mother to infant in the human is IgG and occurs primarily via placental transfer; however, breast milk continues to be an important source of secretory IgA antibody for the breast-fed infant and, although not absorbed by the infant's gastrointestinal tract, appears to be active locally at mucosal surfaces of the gastrointestinal tract and to be important for the infant in antimicrobial defense and in the prevention of allergic disease (*Chapters 8* and *18*). The IgE antibodies represent still later additions. The IgE immunoglobulins, seen in mammals, are a unique class of antibody involved in immediate-type hypersensitivity diseases (*Chapter 17*). It has been suggested that the IgE immunoglobulins first made their appearance in response to the defense against parasitic infection as a mechanism to expel the parasite from the body in addition to their pathogenic role in immediate hypersensitivity to these organisms (*Chapter 15*). The sequential appearance of immunoglobulin molecular forms that appear during the development of the immune response in the maturing individual (ontogeny) also repeats, to a large extent, the order seen in phylogeny, i.e., IgM→IgG→IgA→IgE (*Chapter 6*). While this is a generally true statement, more recent data suggest that, in lower forms, this proposed evolutionary progression may not be strictly the case. Sharks, e.g., have multiple isotypes including IgM, and IgD is now being recognized as a primordially ancient isotype.

Some Elements of Innate and Adaptive Immunity Appear throughout Phylogeny

Shown in Figure 2-4 and Table 2-2 are schematic representations of the appearance of immune

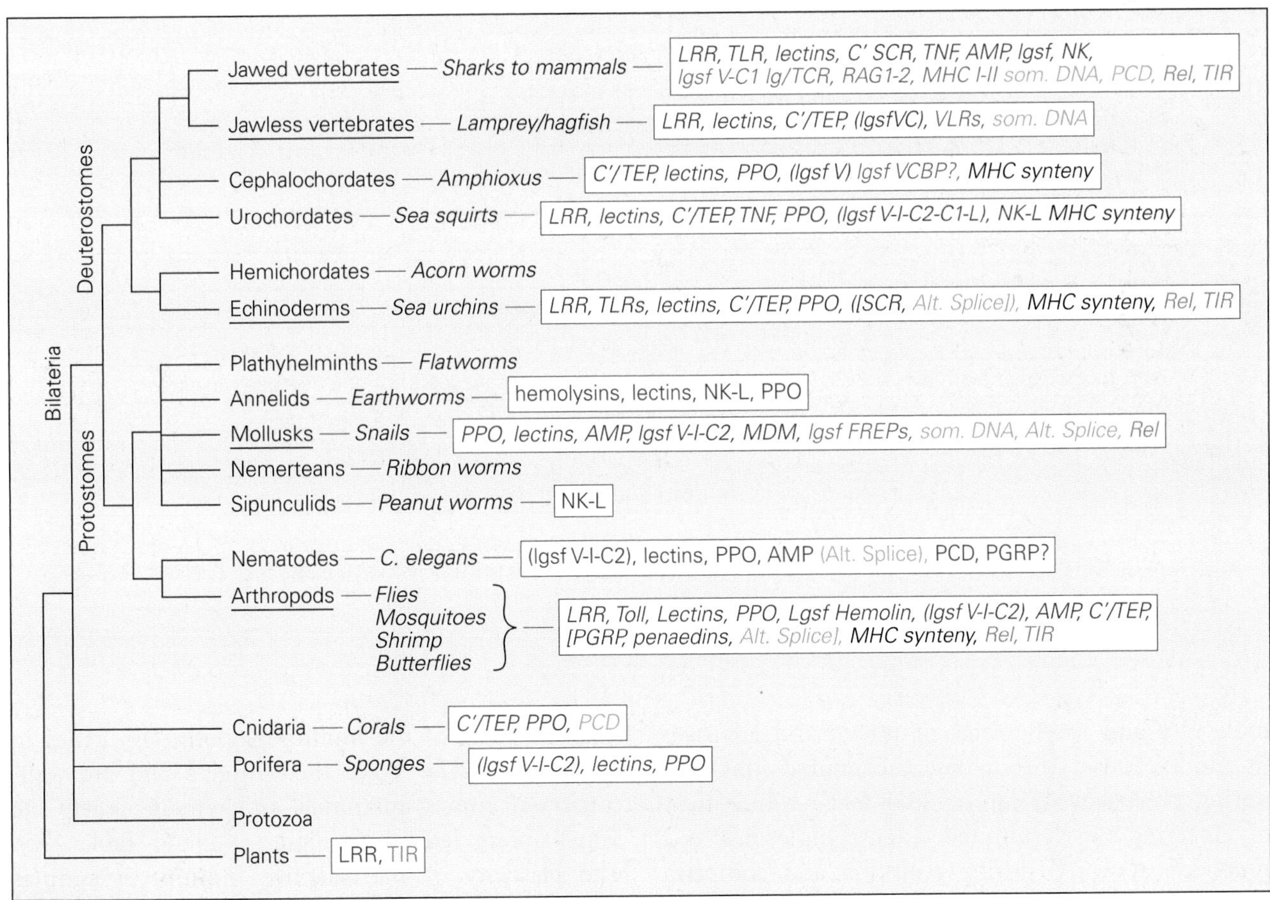

Figure 2-4. Immune molecules and mechanisms found throughout (primarily) the animal kingdom. Red indicates molecules or mechanisms involved in innate immunity. Blue indicates molecules whose genes diversify somatically and are involved (or believed to be involved) in adaptive immunity. Orange indicates somatic mechanisms at the DNA or RNA level to generate or maximize immune diversity (underlined taxa indicate that representatives in these groups have diversification mechanisms of immune genes). Green indicates conserved signaling pathways. Black indicates that genes have been found in linkage groups similar to those in the jawed vertebrate MHC. Abbreviations and short descriptions of each category are found in Table 2-2. (Adapted from Flajnik MF, Du Pasquier L. Evolution of innate and adaptive immunity: can we draw a line? Trends Immunol. 2004;25:640–4.)

Table 2-2. Immune defense molecules and functions found throughout the animal kingdom

Molecule/mechanism	Function (or example)
Leucine-rich repeat (LRR)	Various (e.g., TLR, VLR)
Toll-like receptor (TLR)	Signal innate and alert adaptive immunity
Variable lymphocyte receptor (VLR)	Lamprey (potential adaptive) defense molecules
Pattern recognition receptor (PRR)	Defense molecule recognizing conserved molecules on pathogens or PAMPs Various (e.g., NK receptors, selectins)
Lectins (galectin, C-type, or S-type lectin)	Opsonization, lysis, inflammation
Complement (C′)	Opsonization
C3-factor B/thioester-containing protein (C′/TEP)	Various (e.g., PRR)
Scavenger receptor (SCR)	Proinflammatory cytokine
Tumor necrosis factor (TNF)	Various (e.g., defensins)
Antimicrobial peptides (AMP)	Various (e.g., Ig, fibrinogen-related protein [FREP]—see below)
Immunoglobulin superfamily (Igsf)	Amphioxus Igsf member related to Ig/TCR
V region chitin-binding protein (VCBP)	Kill virally infected cells (Igsf and lectin)
Natural killer (NK) cell; NK-L (NK-like)	Invertebrate defense molecules
Prophenoloxidase (PPO)	Mollusk (potential adaptive) defense molecules
Fibrinogen-related proteins (FREPs)	Cell lysis
Hemolysin	Defense molecules
Penaedin	Igsf defense molecules
Mollusk defense molecule (MDM); Hemolin	Igsf domain types
Variable (V); Constant-1 (C-1); Constant-2 (C2); Intermediate (I)	Humoral adaptive defense
Immunoglobulin (Ig)	Adaptive defense
T cell receptor (TCR)	Enzyme required for VDJ rearrangement
Recombination-activating gene (RAG 1-2)	Antigen (peptide) presentation
MHC- I or -I/II	VDJ gene rearrangement, hypermutation, or conversion
Somatic DNA modification (Som. DNA)	Generation of multiple transcripts for one defense molecule
Alternative splicing (Alt. splice)	Induction of suicide or apoptosis in a target cell
Programmed cell death (PCD)	Conserved signaling pathway (e.g., NF-kB)
Rel	Conserved signaling pathway
Toll-interleukin 1 receptor domain (TIR)	

(Adapted from Flajnik MF, Du Pasquier L. Evolution of innate and adaptive immunity: can we draw a line? Trends Immunol. 2004;25:640–4.)

molecules and mechanisms of innate and adaptive immunity found throughout the animal kingdom during phylogeny. It can be seen that a whole host of emerging novel immune defense molecules and functions appeared during evolution and comprise both the innate and adaptive immune systems throughout the animal kingdom to counter those foreign and potentially inimical configurations found in the ever-changing external environment. Similarly, the structure, organization, and expression patterns of molecular configurations which comprise our understanding of the immunoglobulin (Ig) genes in the human today trace their origins and are well-conserved among mammals and remain largely the same among tetrapods (Figure 2-4 and Table 2-2). The plasticity of the adaptive immune system, as defined by rearranging antigen receptor genes in the immunoglobulin superfamily (*Chapter 6*), begins with the jawed vertebrates (gnathostomes) (Figure 2-4).

With evolution of the immune system during phylogeny, there also occurred the development of an elaborate system of substances that could augment

Box 2-2

Evolution of the Complement System

The evolution of the complement system in the developing species has been studied by genomic analysis in lower animals, where it has been possible to trace the presence or absence of each complement gene in the analyzed genomes. The data show that bony fish and higher vertebrates share practically the same set of complement genes with the chicken, clawed frog, a few bony fish, sea squirt, fruit fly, nematoda, and sea anemone, suggesting that most of the gene duplications that played an essential role in establishing the mammalian complement system had occurred by the time the teleost/mammalian divergence appeared around 500 million years ago. The C3 and factor B genes, but probably not the other complement genes, are present in the genome of the cnidaria, i.e., sea nettles and some protostomes, indicating that the origin of the central part of the complement system was established more than a billion years ago. In the human, the fetal liver has been shown to be capable of synthesizing the biologically active form of the second (C2) and fourth (C4) components of complement as early as eight weeks after conception, and the inhibitor of C1 (C1 INH) as early as eleven weeks after conception. Biologically active C3 is produced in vitro by fetal liver, presumably in macrophages obtained at fourteen weeks gestation.

and enhance the efficiency of the immune responses. These are referred to as biologic amplification systems and consist primarily of the coagulation and complement systems (Box 2-2 and *Chapters 4* and *5*). Although these substances are commonly assigned to the innate immune system, they function to augment and enhance the efficiency of both the innate and the adaptive immune responses.

Lymphocyte Development: Ontogeny of the Immune System

Available evidence suggests that the lymphoid system consists of two compartments: (1) a *central* compartment in which stem cells originating in the bone marrow proliferate and differentiate in the bone marrow and thymus independent of antigen contact (i.e., antigen-independent differentiation); and (2) a *peripheral* compartment consisting of lymph nodes, spleen, and MALT (*Chapter 8*), sites in which these cells can react with antigen (i.e., antigen-dependent differentiation) (Figure 2-5).

Hematopoiesis Occurs in Human Bone Marrow

The differentiation of cells destined to perform innate and acquired immune functions in the developing human have a common ancestral origin with cells of the hematopoietic system (Figure 2-6). Both cell types destined for hematopoiesis or lymphopoiesis appear to arise from a common population of pluripotent CD34+ hematopoietic stem cells (**HSCs**) of the bone marrow. Depending upon the type of microchemical environment surrounding the cells, development will occur along two avenues: the *myelocytic* and the *lymphocytic* (Figure 2-6).

All hematopoietic cells differentiate into mature cells with the aid of soluble mediators (i.e., cytokines) and contact signals from stromal cells, through various intermediate cell types that are defined by expression of cell surface antigens (*Chapter 9*). The first step in hematopoietic development is differentiation of HSCs into myeloid and lymphocyte precursors. Myeloid precursors differentiate into erythroid, megakaryocytic, and granulocytic/monocytic (**GM**) lineages, whereas lymphoid precursors develop into NK, T, and B cells (Figure 2-6). The lymphoid precursors can differentiate along two additional pathways. T cell development requires the influence of the thymus, while B cells develop in the microenvironment of the bursal-equivalent, the bone marrow in the human from the common lymphoid progenitor (**CLP**) (Figure 2-6).

In response to danger signals produced when the host encounters a foreign invader, e.g., microbes, allergens, transplants, or tumor cells, soluble mediators called cytokines and chemokines are released which cause many of the circulating leukocytes to migrate from the bone marrow into the blood and from the blood into the tissues, where they can remove these foreign agents that induce inflammation and can begin to repair the damaged tissues (*Chapter 5*). Most of the blood leukocytes that emigrate into tissues are end-stage cells of development and do not replicate, e.g., neutrophils and eosinophils, with the notable exception of monocytes, which, after migration, differentiate into tissue macrophages.

The plasticity of stem cells in ontogeny reflects that seen during phylogeny as described previously. When present in specialized microenvironments in tissues, the pluripotent CD34+ hematopoietic stem cells can differentiate into various other tissue-specific cells such as hepatocytes, neurons, muscle cells, or endothelial cells. However, the signals that

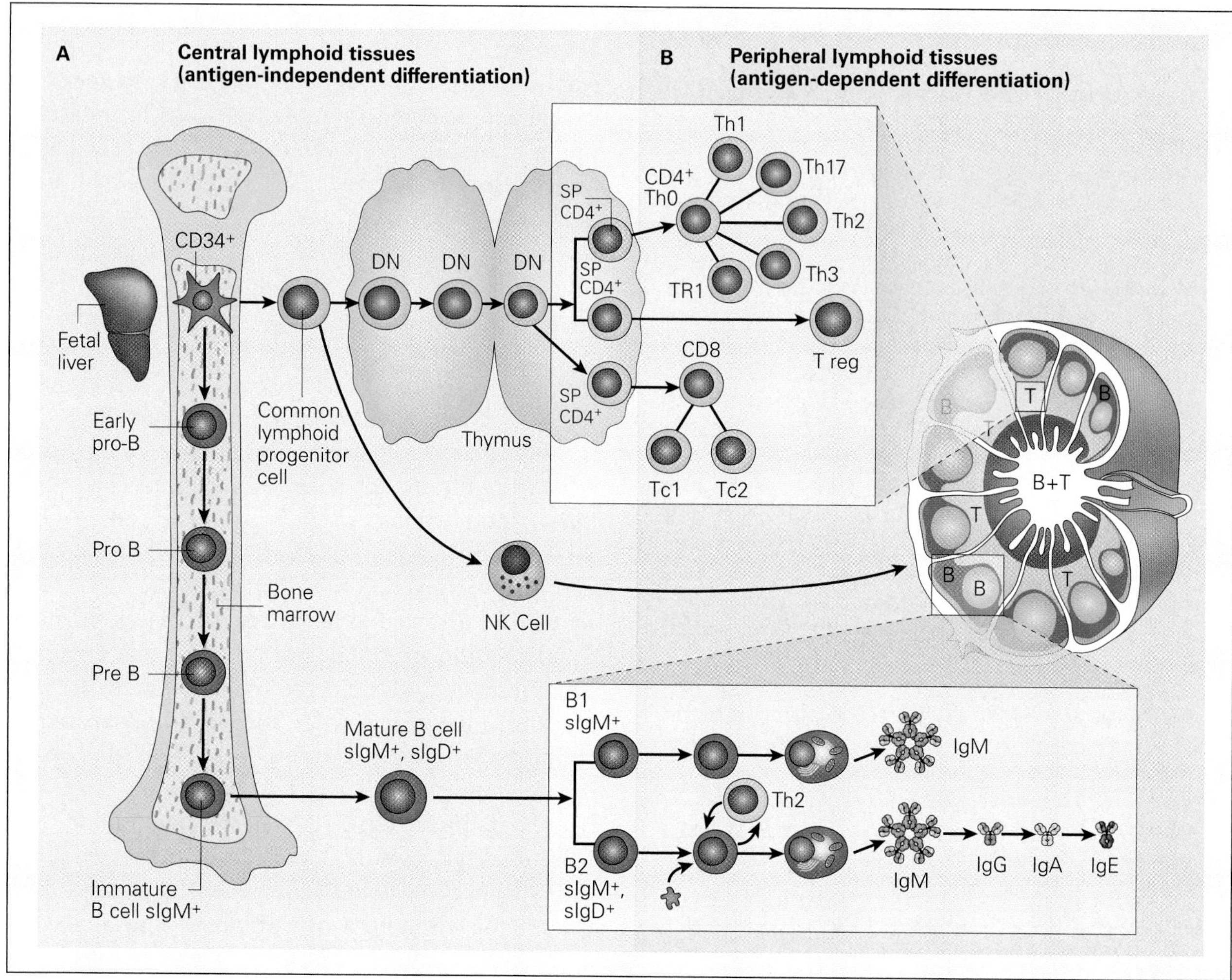

Figure 2-5. Schematic representation of the two compartments of lymphoid differentiation: central and peripheral compartments. Panel A: Development of the immune system from stem cells originating in bone marrow, fetal yolk sac or liver, and differentiating in central lymphoid tissues, i.e., bone marrow and thymus independent of antigen contact. Panel B: Migration of cells into peripheral lymphoid tissues in lymph nodes, spleen, and mucosa-associated lymphoid tissues at sites where these cells can react with antigen (i.e., antigen-dependent differentiation). B cells migrate to outer regions of lymph nodes in germinal centers; T cells migrate in inner paracortical areas; B and T cells are found in medullary cords. The insets show the location of the various subsets of T cells in the paracortical areas (upper inset) and B cells in the germinal centers of a lymph node. B cells respond to polysaccharides with the production of IgM antibodies, and B2 lymphocytes respond to protein antigens and with the help of Th2 lymphocytes lead to the sequential production of IgM, IgG, IgA, and IgE antibody.

regulate this differentiation are unknown. The HSCs also circulate in small numbers in the peripheral blood and can be harvested as a source of progenitor cells for use in the reconstitution of patients receiving bone marrow transplantation (*Chapter 20*).

While it is generally agreed that T and B lymphocytes and NK cells originate from a common lymphoid progenitor, referred to as a CLP, some researchers maintain that T and B cells are derived from separate T/macrophage and B/macrophage precursors (Figure 2-7). The developmental status of dendritic cells (**DCs**) is more complicated. The DC lineages consist of several often not clearly defined populations that seem to have either a single HSC origin or a myeloid, lymphoid, or mixed lymphoid/myeloid origin (Figure 2-7) DCs are commonly divided into "myeloid" and "plasmacytoid" types, i.e., MDCs and pDCs (*Chapter 5*).

Production of Specific T and B Lymphocytes Occurs in Antigen-Independent and Antigen-Dependent Phases

Because of the complexity of the various developmental steps involved in the ontogeny of the adaptive immune system in the human, it may be useful to begin with a summary narrative of these events followed by a more detailed description of specific events in subsequent sections of this chapter (Figure 2-8). T and B lymphocytes are characterized and defined

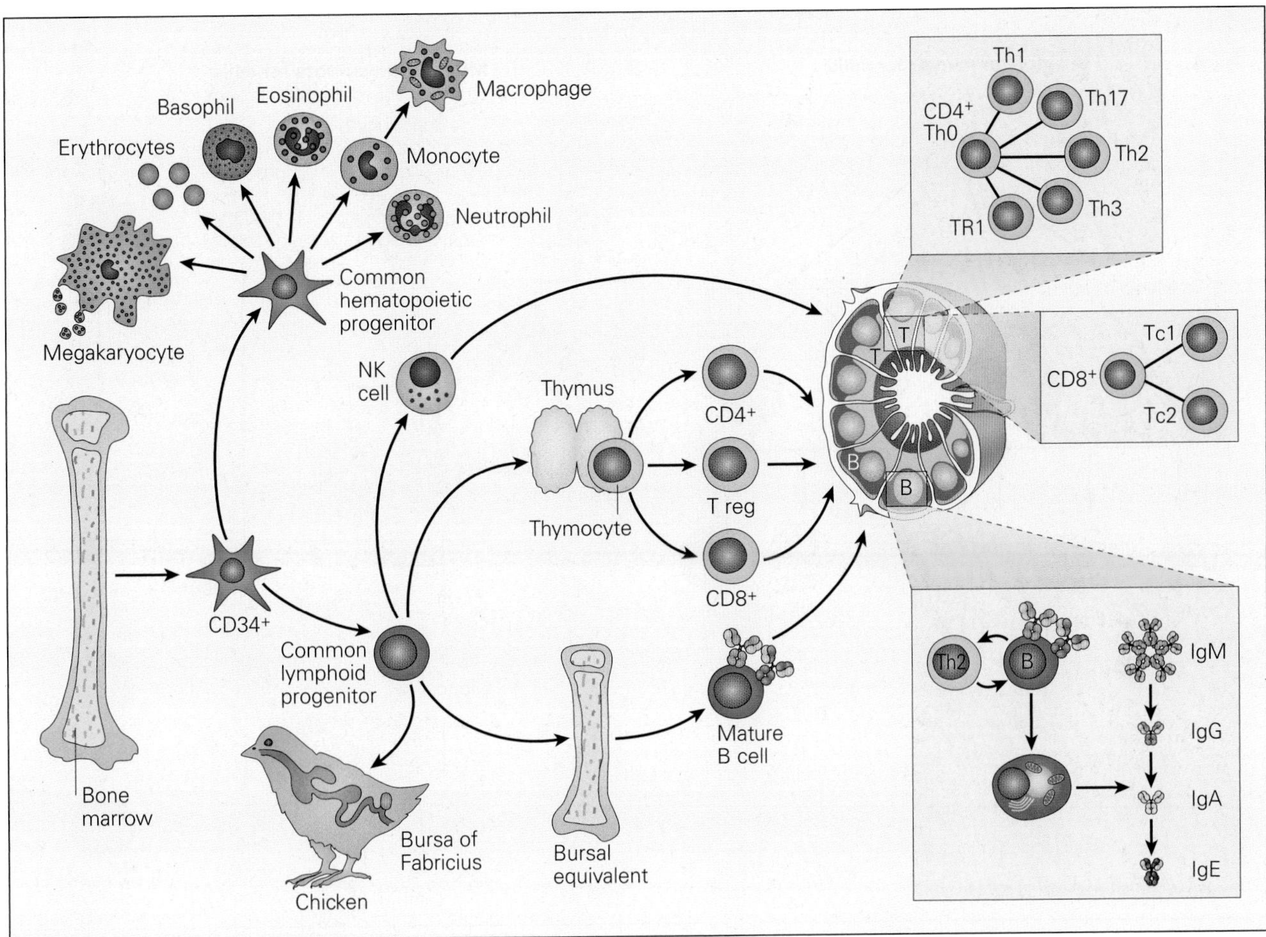

Figure 2-6. Schematic representation of the ontogeny of the immune system showing differentiation of progenitor cells into hematopoietic and immunocompetent lymphopoietic cells from a common population of pluripotent CD34+ hematopoietic stem cells of the bone marrow. Myeloid precursors differentiate into erythroid, megakaryocytic, and granulocytic/monocytic lineages, whereas lymphoid precursors develop into NK, T, and B cells. The common lymphoid progenitor cells can differentiate along two additional pathways. T cell development requires the influence of the thymus, while B cells develop in the microenvironment of the bursal-equivalent, the bone marrow in the human. Following differentiation, T and B cells populate distinct T and B cell regions in lymph nodes, respectively.

by their randomly generated and vastly diverse antigen receptors, i.e., the T cell receptor (**TCR**) and the B cell receptor (**BCR**) (*Chapters 6* and *7*). These receptors are generated in each developing lymphocyte through a process called somatic recombination, in which enzymes encoded by recombination-activating genes (**RAGs**) splice gene segments to generate unique variable (antigen-binding) regions of the BCR (immunoglobulin) and TCR molecules (*Chapters 6* and *7*). This process is unique to lymphocyte development, and from a few hundred available gene segments can generate large numbers (potentially 10^{15} to 10^{18}) of different antigen specificities. Somatic recombination occurs in the bone marrow (B cells) and thymus (T cells) in the absence of antigen, i.e., the antigen-independent phase. If a B cell or T cell then encounters its specific antigen in the peripheral lymphoid tissue (along with other appropriate stimuli), the cell proliferates and differentiates into a clone of specific effector cells (antibody-secreting plasma cells, cytotoxic T cells, or helper T cells); memory cells specific for the same antigen are also produced, i.e., the antigen-dependent phase. Although the ancestral home of the lymphocyte precursor cell for both T and B cells is the bone marrow, T cells carry out their maturation in the thymus, in contrast to B cells, which continue their development in the bone marrow.

Shown in Figure 2-8 is a schematic summary representation of both the antigen-independent central sites of differentiation for T, B, and NK lymphocytes and their subsequent antigen-dependent sites of differentiation in peripheral tissues showing the various stages of maturation that these cellular lineages undergo. In this scheme, the state of maturation of the cells undergoing progressive development is

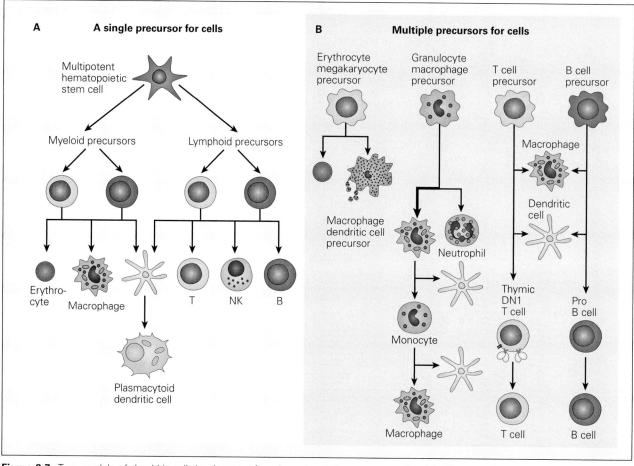

Figure 2-7. Two models of dendritic-cell development from hematopoietic precursors. Panel A: Shows a single hematopoietic stem cell. Panel B: Shows the multiple myeloid, lymphoid, or mixed lymphoid/myeloid origin. (Adapted from Shortman, K., and Naik, S. H. "Steady-state and inflammatory dendritic-cell development." *Nat Rev Immunol.* 2007;7:19–30.)

characterized by the acquisition of cell surface antigen receptors and molecules referred to as the cluster of differentiation (**CD**) molecules (Box 2-3).

T Cell Development Originates in Thymus; Functional Effector Cells and Memory Cells Are Produced in Peripheral Lymphoid Tissues

T cells are identified by the presence of CD3, a signal transduction molecule that is expressed with TCR, and the lineage specific CD4 (T helper) or CD8 (T cytotoxic) markers (*Chapter 7*). Most T cells express a TCR composed of one alpha and one beta chain (αβ TCR), each of which has a V and a C region, and which together resemble one "arm" of the immunoglobulin Y-shaped molecule. A small minority of T cells have a TCR composed of one gamma and one delta chain (γδ TCR) (Figure 2-8).

Following migration of CD34+ stem cells from the bone marrow to the thymus, a series of intrathymic maturational steps occurs, including somatic recombination of the TCR genes, that result in the transformation of a CD3+, CD4− CD8− double negative (**DN**) cell into a major population of CD3+ CD4+, CD8+ double positive (**DP**) αβ TCR-expressing T cells and a minor population of CD3+ CD4−, CD8− DN γδ T cells. The γδ T cells ultimately function as intraepithelial lymphocytes (**IEL**) at mucosal sites (Figure 2-8 and *Chapter 8*). The CD3+ CD4+, CD8+ DP population further differentiates into three (1) a CD3+, CD4−, CD8+ single positive (**SP**) T cell that migrates to the peripheral tissues as a CD8+ T cytotoxic (**Tc**) population; (2) a CD3+, CD4+, CD25+ SP T cell that migrates to the peripheral tissues as a T regulatory (**Treg**) population; and (3) a CD3+, CD4+, CD8− SP T cell that migrates to the peripheral tissues as a CD4+ T helper (**Th**) population. The transformation of these precursor cells into Tc, Treg, and Th subpopulations each involve signals provided by cytokines (*Chapter 9*) and by binding to either MHC-I or MHC-II on thymus epithelial cells. T cells that have generated self-specific TCR undergo apoptosis in the thymus (*Chapters 6* and *7*).

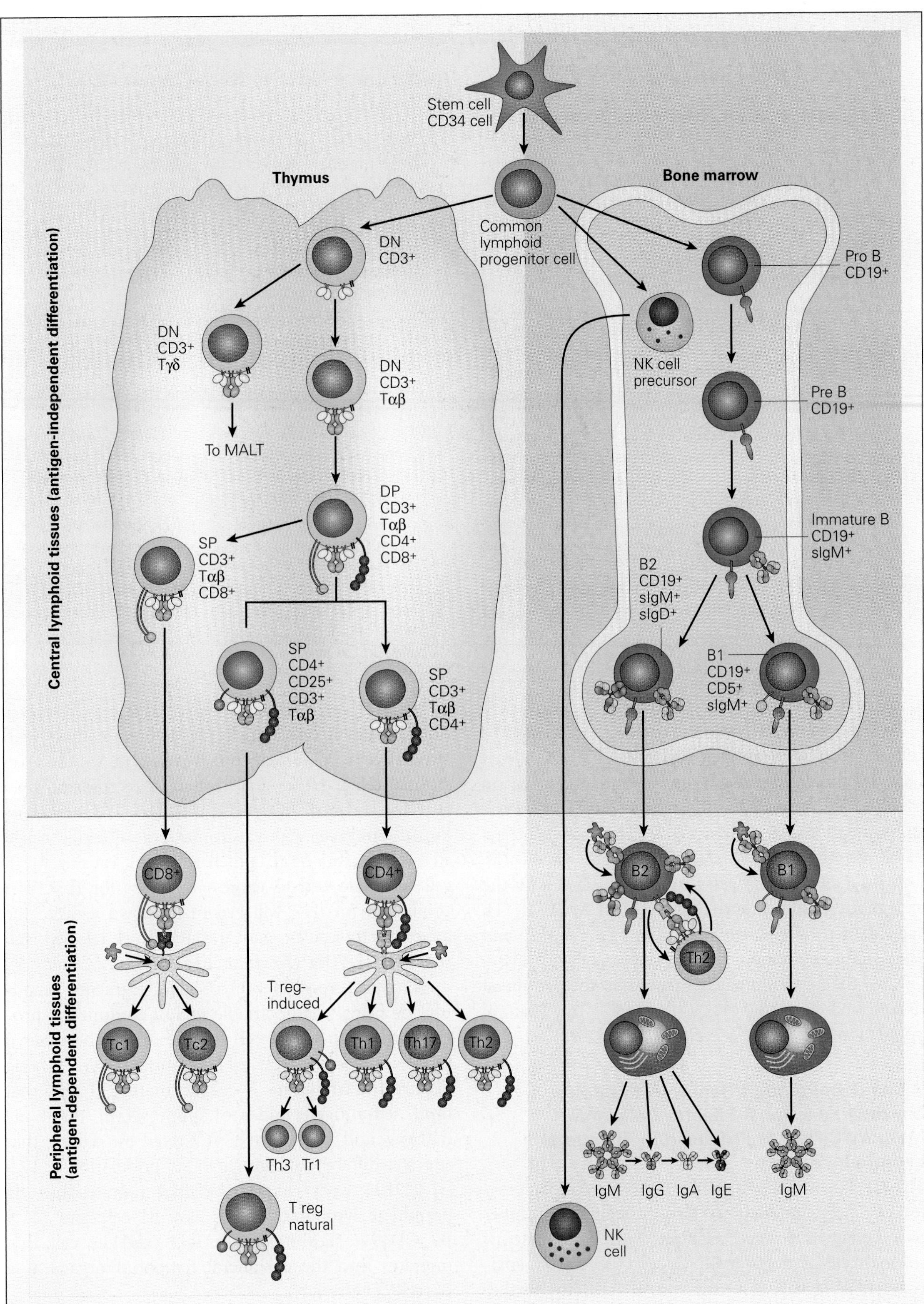

Figure 2-8. Schematic representation of the antigen-independent central sites of differentiation for T, B, and NK lymphocytes in the thymus and bone marrow and their subsequent antigen-dependent sites of differentiation in peripheral lymphoid tissues.

Box 2-3

Cluster of Differentiation (CD) Molecules

CD molecules are a set of immunologically significant cell surface molecules. They are found on the surfaces of many cells, most primarily on leukocytes. CD molecules can either function as ligands or receptors. A ligand binds to a receptor, following which there occurs a conformational change, or change in shape, in the receptor molecule leading to the initiation of a signal cascade ultimately altering the behavior of the receptor cell. Examples of CD molecules are CD4 and CD8, which define the functions of Th cells and Tc cells, respectively.

The CD nomenclature was proposed and established in the First International Workshop and Conference on Human Leukocyte Differentiation Antigens (HLDA), which was held in Paris in 1982. This system was intended for the classification of the many monoclonal antibodies, generated by different laboratories around the world, against various cell surface molecules on leukocytes. Since then, the use has expanded to the classification of many other cell types, and more than 250 CD clusters and subclusters have been identified (*Appendix 3*). The HLDA workshops assign each CD based on the same reactivity to one human antigen by at least two mAbs; the provisional indicator "w" (as in "CDw186") is sometimes given to a cluster not well characterized or represented by only one mAb.

Important Points to Know about CD Molecules

- CD molecules, as used in this chapter and elsewhere, are commonly identified by sorting cells by flow cytometry. A "+" or a "–" symbol is used to indicate if a certain fraction of cells possesses or lacks a CD molecule; e.g., a "CD34+, CD31–" cell is one that expresses CD34 but not CD31. This would typically correspond to a stem cell rather than a fully differentiated endothelial cell.
- The most commonly referred to CD molecules are CD4 and CD8, which are markers for the two major subtypes of T lymphocytes (dendritic cells also express CD8).
- CD4 is specifically recognized and bound by the human immunodeficiency virus (HIV), following which the CD4+ T cell is infected and subsequently destroyed (*Chapter 13*). The relative abundance of CD4+ and CD8+ T cells (expressed as the CD4/CD8 ratio) is often used to monitor the progression of an HIV infection.
- CD molecules are not merely markers on the cell surface but also function as cell receptors to which specific ligands bind. Not every CD molecule has been thoroughly characterized, but most of them provide important features to the cells that carry them. In the case of the pivotal CD4 and CD8, these molecules are critical in the antigen-recognition pathway.

In the peripheral lymphoid tissues, the CD8+ Tc cells interact with antigen processed by APCs, e.g., DCs, by the endogenous pathway and presented on MHC-I. Tc can further differentiate into T cytotoxic subpopulations, e.g., Tc1, Tc2, Th17, and others based on their cytokine secretion. The CD4+ Th cells interact with antigen processed by APCs by the exogenous pathway and presented on MHC-II. Th can further differentiate into Th1, Th2, Th17, and Treg (induced) subpopulations. The CD3+, CD4+, CD25+ SP T cell ultimately migrates to the peripheral tissues and functions as a "natural" Treg natural population.

B Cell Development Begins in the Bone Marrow; Functional Effector Cells and Memory Cells Are Produced in Peripheral Lymphoid Tissues

The CD34+ stem cells in the bone marrow destined for B cell production go through a number of differentiative steps. Contact with bone marrow stromal cells is necessary to supply the correct environmental signals for the pro-B cell to further differentiate. B cells initially need direct contact with stromal cells (VLA-4 on pro-B cells and VCAM-1 on stromal cells). After initial contact, a receptor on pro-B cells encoded by c-Kit, called KIT (a tyrosine kinase) interacts with a stromal cell molecule called stem-cell factor; c-Kit is then activated, causing the B cell to divide and to express receptors for IL-7. The production of IL-7 will eventually down-regulate the adhesion molecules, and the B cell is released still requiring IL-7 for growth and maturation (*Chapter 9*).

Somatic recombination of gene segments encoding the heavy chain variable region commit the progenitor cell to the B cell lineage and it becomes a pre-B cell; expression of membrane IgM (sIgM) defines the immature B cell. Immature B cells that bind self-antigen undergo apoptosis in the bone marrow and are deleted (*Chapter 6*). Those that survive, differentiate into two subpopulations: (1) a B1 CD19+ CD5+ sIgM+ cell that migrates into the peripheral lymphoid organs as a B1 cell; and (2) a B2 CD19+ sIgM+ surface IgD (sIgD+) cell that migrates into the peripheral lymphoid organs as a B2 cell (Figure 2-5).

The functional significance of B and T lymphocyte development is important to clinical medicine. It provides a useful basis upon which our understanding of immune deficiency disorders rests (*Chapter 16*). Thus, individuals displaying selective disorders of B lymphocytes, the so-called agammaglobulinemias or dysgammaglobulinemias, present with recurrent bacterial infections. Selective deficiencies of the thymic-dependent tissues, on the other hand, are also seen and manifest with other types of infections, such as fungal and viral diseases. Still a third type of patient presents with combined deficiency of both thymic-dependent and thymic-independent tissues. These individuals, suffering from the so-called severe combined immune deficiency (**SCID**) syndrome, have profound deficiencies in both cell-mediated and antibody-mediated immune functions, have the most serious sequelae of all immune deficiency syndromes, and present with a diversity of viral, bacterial, fungal, and parasitic infections. This

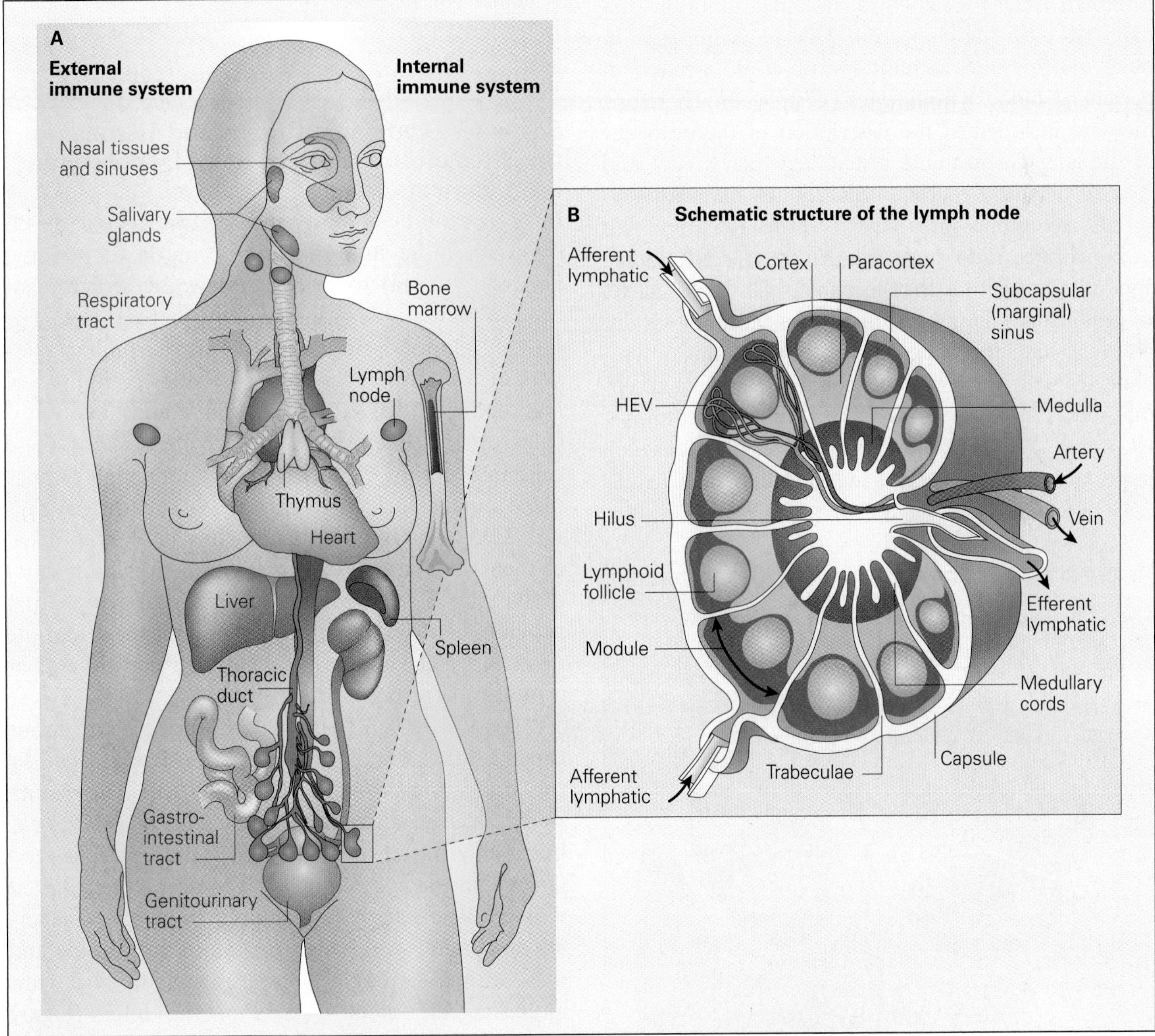

Figure 2-9. Panel A: Schematic representation of the fully developed immune system in the human in the external immune, or MALT, or the internal immune system; both consist of a network of lymphoid tissues composed of macrophages, dendritic cells, and T and B lymphocytes organized either as loose collections of these cells in lymphoid follicles or as more highly organized organs such as lymph nodes and spleen. Panel B: Schematic structure of a lymph node showing its organization into a cortex, paracortex, and medulla with primary and secondary follicles in the cortex and medullary cords in the medulla and a lymphatic supply (entering through afferent vessels in the cortex and exiting through a single efferent lymphatic vessel in the hilus) and an afferent and efferent blood supply entering and leaving through the hilus.

has also provided a basis for the new discipline of molecular profiling of disease processes, such as the autoimmune diseases (*Chapter 19*) and the lymphoproliferative diseases (*Chapter 21*). This has not only allowed a clearer understanding of the molecular origins and fundamental relationships of these disorders for more precise diagnosis but also has opened new therapeutic approaches tailored to the treatment of these diseases.

Natural Killer Cells Also Develop in the Bone Marrow

Although usually assigned to the innate immune system, NK cells develop from CD34+ stem cells in bone marrow and account for up to 15 percent of peripheral blood lymphocytes (*Chapter 3*). Therefore, they are included in the description of the ontogeny of the adaptive immune system together with T and B cells (Figure 2-6). NK cells do not have antigen-specific receptors; they have receptors that bind self carbohydrates onto host cells to activate NK killing and other receptors that recognize self MHC alleles to inhibit the killing of normal cells. Morphologically, NK cells have the appearance of large granular lymphocytes with neither T cell nor B cell antigen receptors. NK cells do express CD16 (an Fc receptor for IgG) and CD56 (an NK-specific adhesion molecule), important markers for the identification of NK cells in the peripheral circulation. NK cells are involved in a variety of immune reactions in the recognition and killing of target cells utilizing direct and antibody-dependent cellular cytotoxicity (**ADCC**) mechanisms (*Chapter 1*). They are believed to be particularly important in the destruction of virus-infected cells (*Chapter 13*) and certain tumor cells (*Chapter 20*) via apoptosis. A recently recognized induced NK cell has been identified which bears an invariant T cell receptor (NK-T cell), responds to carbohydrate antigens, and appears to play an important role in the pathogenesis of chronic forms of asthma in the human (*Chapter 18*).

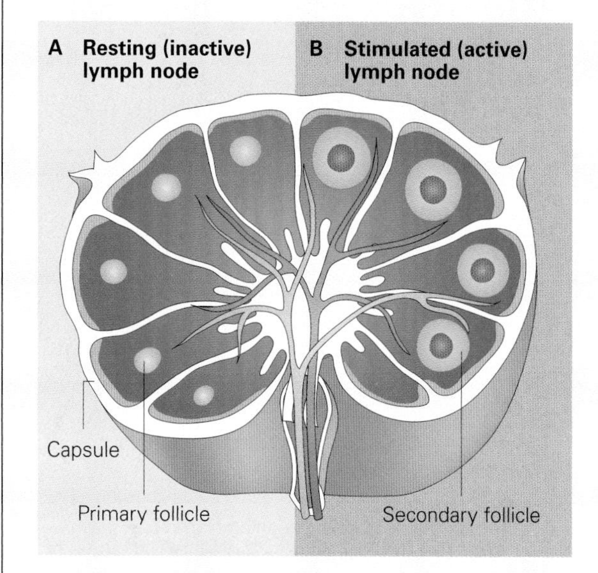

Figure 2-10. Schematic structure of a lymph node. Panel A: Shows the appearance of primary follicles in a resting (inactive) lymph node. Panel B: Shows the appearance of prominent secondary follicles in a stimulated (active) lymph node.

Organization of the Immune System

Secondary Lymphoid Organs and Tissues Are the Sites of Antigen-Dependent Lymphocyte Development

In order to fully comprehend the ontogenetic development of the immune system in the developing host, it is useful to briefly review the structure of the lymphoid system in the fully mature host. The fully developed immune system in the human consists of a network of lymphoid tissues composed of macrophages, dendritic cells, and T and B lymphocytes organized either as loose collections of these cells in lymphoid follicles or as more highly organized organs such as lymph nodes and spleen (Figure 2-9A). Lymphoid tissues consist of both fixed elements but also a continuously recirculating pool of lymphoid cells from the blood and lymph that provide continuous immune surveillance for the detection and elimination of foreign constituents at a multitude of body sites.

A typical lymph node is surrounded by a fibrous capsule that extends into the parenchyma, dividing the node into nodules (Figure 2-9B). The lymph node receives afferent and efferent blood vessels, both entering through a lymphatic arteriole and leaving through a lymphatic venule in the hilus; it also receives a lymphatic supply from several afferent lymphatic vessels that penetrate the capsule and exit through a single efferent lymphatic that runs alongside the blood vessels in the hilus (Figure 2-9B). After entering the lymph node, the lymphatics form the *marginal sinuses* in the subcapsular region and the *interfollicular sinuses* in the deeper zones and then merge to form the central *medullary sinuses* which drain the lymph via the single efferent lymphatic vessel.

Table 2-3. Structural and functional properties of cortex and medulla of a lymph node

Location	Region	Predominant lymphocyte type	Nodular structure
Cortex			
Outer cortex	Nodular cortex	B cells	Present
Inner cortex	Juxtamedullary cortex or paracortex	T cells	Not present
Medulla			
Medullary cords	Plasma cells and T cells	B and T cells	Not present

The parenchyma of a lymph node consists of a cortex and a medulla (Table 2-3). The cortex is divided into an outer cortex containing B cells and an inner cortex (paracortex) containing T cells. In the medulla are found medullary *cords*, rope-like structures of lymphatic tissue, which contain both B and T cells in addition to most of the lymph node plasma cells (Table 2-3). The subcapsular sinus, which is lined by endothelial and phagocytic cells, receives lymphocytes and antigens in lymph from surrounding tissue spaces or adjacent nodes via the afferent lymphatics. The B cells in the cortex are organized into loose collections of cells referred to as *primary follicles* (when the lymph node is inactive) (Figure 2-10A). Following antigen stimulation, these give rise to *secondary follicles*, which consist of a germinal center composed of dividing cells (centrocytes and centroblasts) and a mantle zone comprised of small lymphocytes (Figure 2-10B).

Shown in Figure 2-10 is a comparison of the structure of a typical lymph node in both the resting (inactive) state and stimulated (active) state. The resting lymph node consists of smaller primary lymphoid follicles; following stimulation, there appear prominent secondary follicles.

T and B Lymphocytes Recirculate Between Blood, Lymph, and Lymphoid Tissues

One of the distinguishing features of the lymphoid system is its unique ability to recirculate T and B lymphocytes from the blood to the lymph as well as from the lymph to the blood in what is referred to as the recirculating pool of lymphocytes (Figure 2-11).

As previously described, the lymph circulates through the lymph nodes via the *afferent lymphatic vessels* and drains through the *subcapsular sinuses*, trabecular sinuses, and medullary sinuses and leaves the node through a lymphocyte-enriched efferent lymphatic vessel. The sinus spaces are crisscrossed by pseudopods of macrophages and dendritic cells that act not only to trap foreign particles and filter the lymph into the medullary sinuses but also function as potent APCs that process and present antigen to T lymphocytes for full expression of the immune response. Lymphocytes, both B cells and T

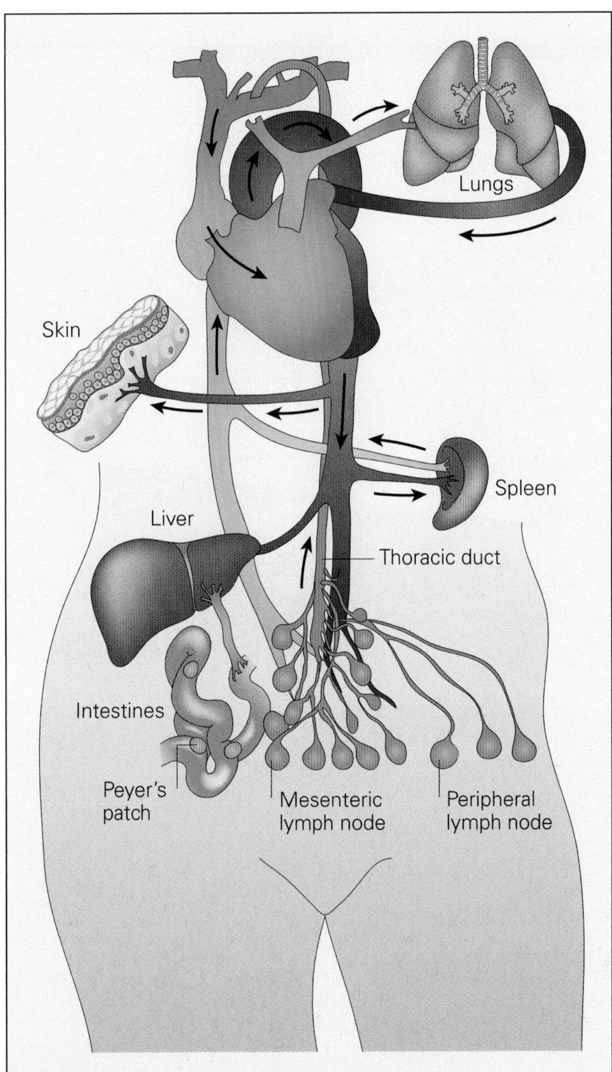

Figure 2-11. Schematic representation of the recirculating pool of the lymphoid system showing the recirculation of blood to the lymph as well as from the lymph to the blood. Blood containing elements of the innate and adaptive immune systems is brought to various organs via the arterial system and returns through the venous system; lymphoid elements that arise in the mesenteric and peripheral lymphoid tissues reenter the blood through the thoracic duct.

cells, not only enter and constantly circulate through the lymph nodes via the lymphatics but they can also enter the lymph node via the bloodstream. Lymphocytes that enter the node from the circulation pass through a set of unique and highly specialized structures referred to as the high endothelial venules (**HEVs**) found in the paracortex (Figure 2-12).

Adhesion molecules on the lymphocytes (homing receptors) and their corresponding ligands (addressins) on HEVs signal the lymphocytes to enter the lymphoid tissue (*Chapter 5*). The close proximity of T and B lymphocytes, antigen, and antigen-presenting cells in the lymphoid tissue increases the chances of contact between T and B cells specific for the same antigen and lymphocyte activation (Figure 2-13).

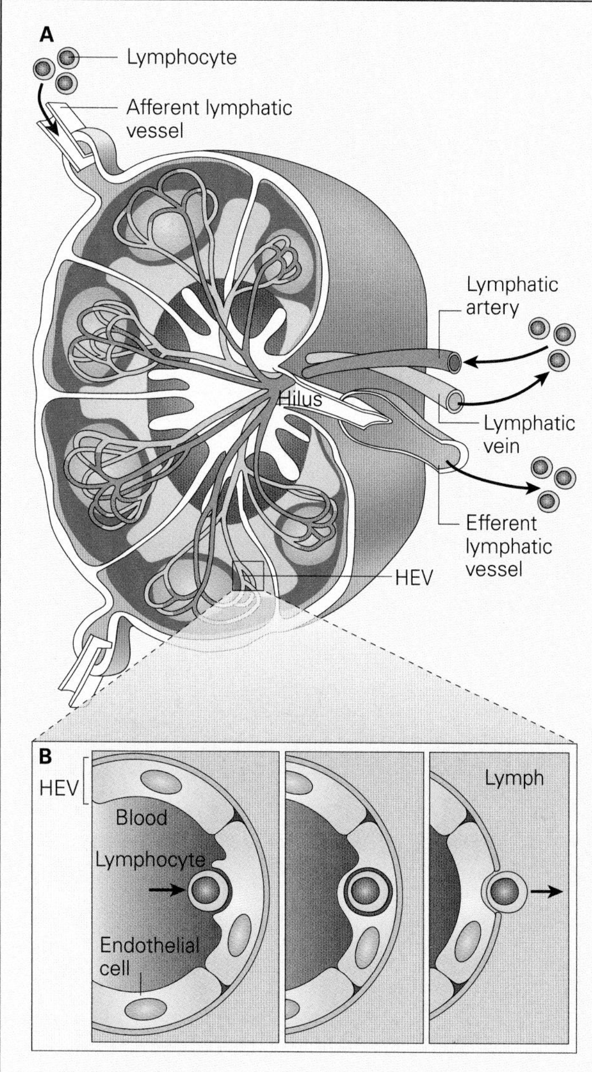

Figure 2-12. Panel A: Schematic representation of the recirculating pool showing the dual lymphatic and blood supply of a lymph node. Panel B: Lymphocytes that enter the node from the circulation pass through a set of unique and highly specialized structures referred to as the HEVs found in the paracortex.

The HEVs allow blood lymphocytes to migrate by direct intraepithelial passage from the blood into the lymphatic parenchyma and then leave the lymph node in a similar manner through the efferent lymphatic vessel and can reenter the blood through the thoracic duct (Figure 2-11). This is in contrast to the interepithelial passage of neutrophils from blood to tissues (Figure 2-14).

The Spleen Filters Blood Rather Than Lymph

The spleen is the other major lymphoid organ that serves similar functions as lymph nodes, although the spleen is the only lymphoid organ that selectively filters blood rather than lymph. The spleen has a number of *immune* and *nonimmune* functions. It removes effete or worn-out cells from the circulatory system (i.e., its homeostatic function), converts hemoglobin to bilirubin, and releases iron into the circulation and body stores for reutilization. Like the lymph nodes, the spleen is a component of the peripheral lymphoid system and is important in the mediation of immune events of adaptive immunity. This organ is particularly important in early life when other elements of the immune system are incompletely developed and are undergoing further maturation. Physical removal of the spleen following surgery or trauma as well as its functional incapacitation, as in the case of the thrombotic sequelae of hemolytic anemias, e.g., sickle-cell disease, has been shown to be associated with overwhelming bacterial infection not only in infants and children but also in young adults. People without a spleen must take prophylactic antibiotics before dental work to prevent infections.

Similar to the structure of a lymph node, the spleen is surrounded by a capsule from which trabeculae extend into its interior (Figure 2-15). The interior of the spleen consists of: (1) the white pulp, containing lymphoid nodules and is the chief site of lymphocyte production in the spleen; (2) the red pulp, which surrounds the white pulp and contains large numbers of erythrocytes consonant with its filtration function; and (3) a marginal zone, surrounding the white pulp and containing unique subsets of resident cells (B cells, macrophages, and dendritic cells). Shown in Figure 2-16 is a photomicrograph illustrating these three areas.

Lymphocytes surrounding the follicles and periarteriolar sheaths of the white pulp are referred to as the periarteriolar lymphoid sheaths (**PALS**) and

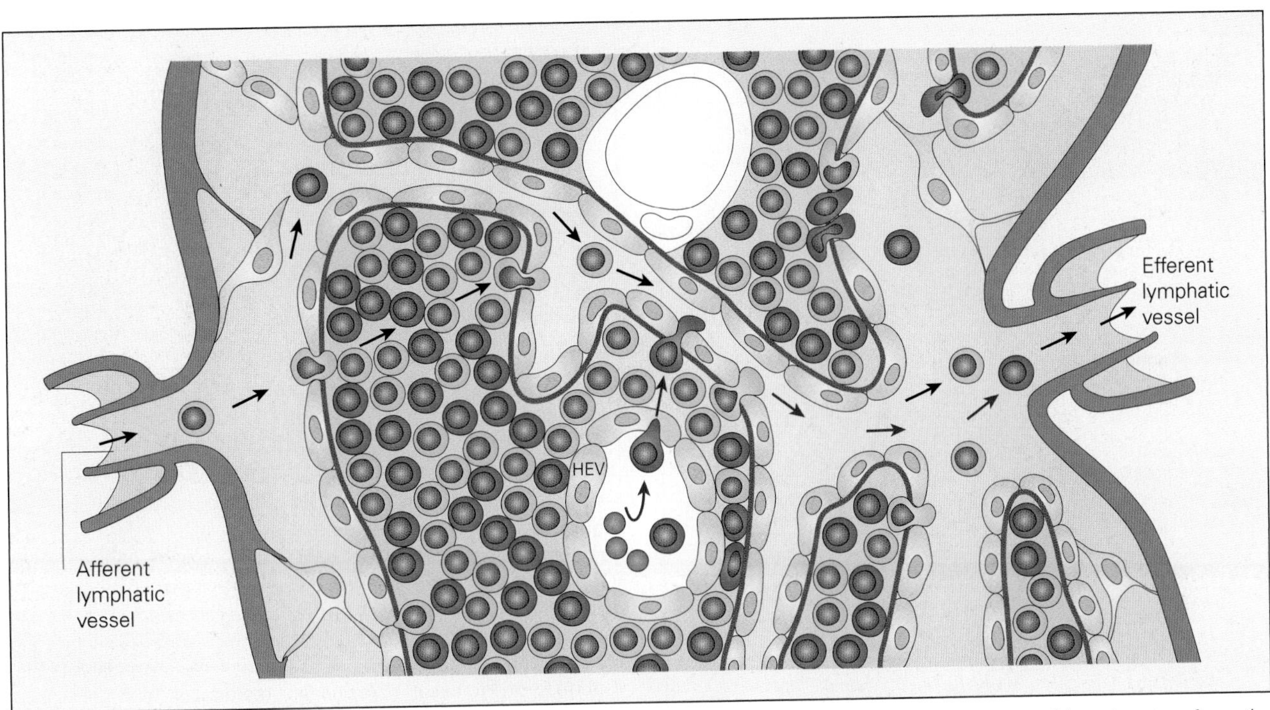

Figure 2-13. Schematic representation of circulation of lymphocytes within a lymph node. Note the dual entry of lymphocytes: from the afferent lymphatic vessel (on the left) through the lymphoid parenchyma, leaving the lymph node from the efferent lymphatic vessel (on the right); and from a post-capillary HEV found in the paracortex (in the center), migrating through the HEV into the lymphatic parenchyma and then leaving the lymph node in a similar manner through the efferent lymphatic vessel and reentering the blood through the thoracic duct as shown in Figure 2-11. Note the close proximity of T and B lymphocytes, antigen, and antigen-presenting cells in the lymphoid tissue.

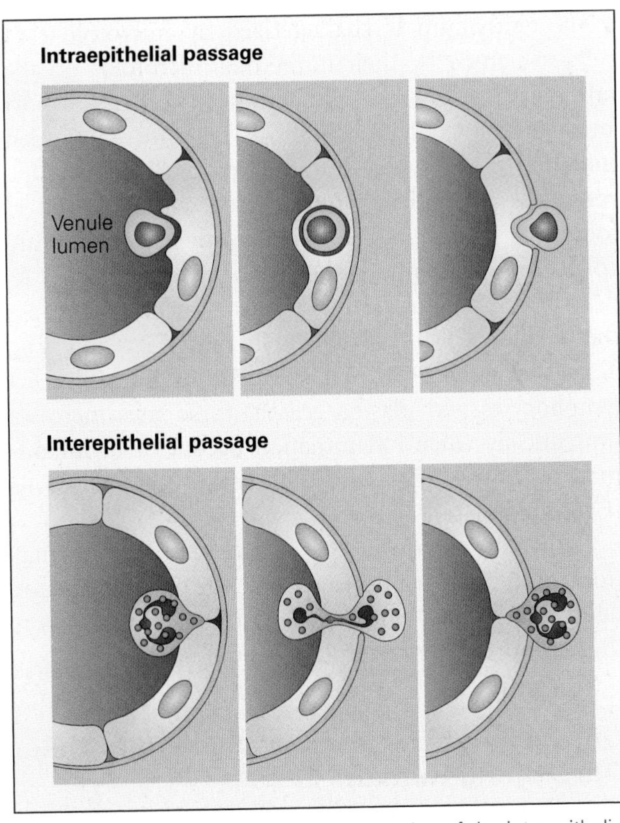

Figure 2-14. Panel A: Schematic presentation of the intraepithelial passage of a lymphocyte through the HEV into the lymph node parenchyma. Panel B: Schematic presentation of the interepithelial passage of a polymorphonuclear leukocyte from a small blood vessel into the tissues.

consist of both T and B lymphocytes. These consist of T cells that are found around the central arteriole and B cells that may be organized (as in the case of lymph nodes) into either "unstimulated" primary follicles (aggregates of "virgin" B cells) or "stimulated" secondary follicles (which possess a germinal center with memory cells).

The arterial blood supply enters through the hilus of the spleen and follows along trabeculae until the small arterioles become surrounded by collars of lymphocytes (white pulp) which constitute the PALS (Figures 2-15 and 2-16). The artery then bifurcates into smaller "arterial" capillaries and eventually into venous sinuses and exits through the trabecular veins. In the past, there were two theories (Figure 2-15) to explain how blood progresses from the arterial capillaries into the venous blood, i.e., the "closed theory" in which the capillary and sinus endothelia are contiguous and blood is emptied directly into the sinuses and then into the trabecular veins versus the "open theory" in which the arterial capillaries do not terminate directly into the sinuses but rather empty blood into the red pulp and then into the venous sinuses after percolating through the red pulp. Studies have now shown that blood flows from "arterial" capillaries lined with

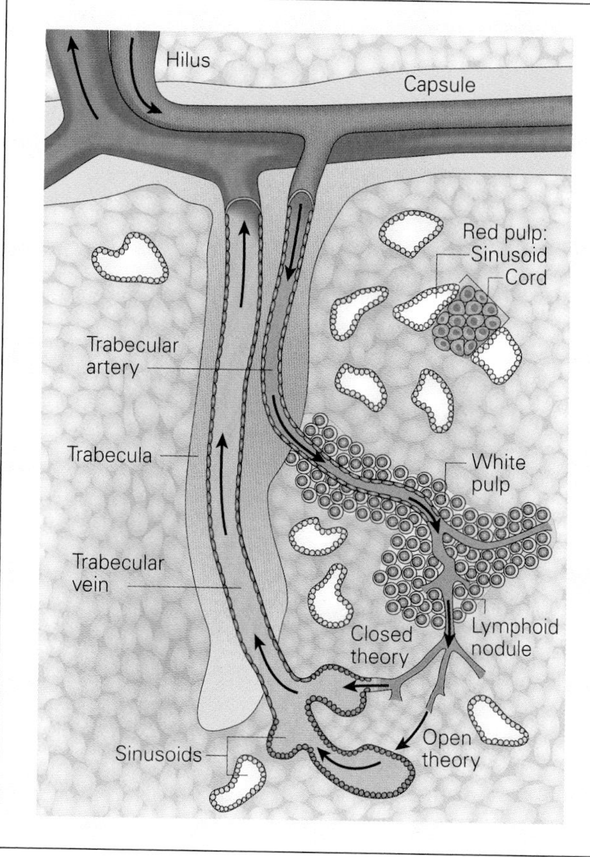

Figure 2-15. Schematic representation of the structure of the spleen. Note the two theories of the splenic blood circulation, i.e., the "closed" and the "open" theories.

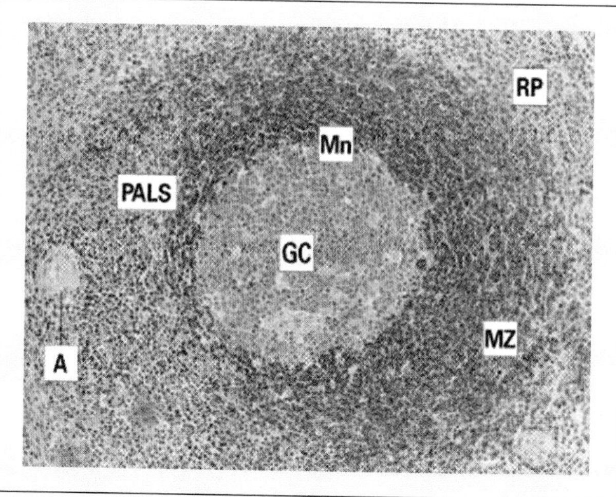

Figure 2-16. Spleen section showing a white pulp lymphoid aggregate. A secondary lymphoid follicle, with germinal center (GC) and mantle (Mn), is surrounded by the marginal zone (MZ) and red pulp (RP). Adjacent to the follicle, an arteriole (A) is surrounded by the PALS consisting mainly of T cells. Note that the marginal zone is present only at one side of the secondary follicle. (Courtesy of Professor I Maclennan; reproduced with permission from Male, D., Brostoff, J., Roth, D. B., and Roitt, I., *Immunology*, 7th ed. Mosby-Elsevier, 2006.)

endothelium into channels within the red pulp formed by the cytoplasmic processes of reticular cells, findings that favor the "open theory."

Mucosa-associated Lymphoid Tissues Promote Immune Responses to Pathogens That Enter the Body at Mucosal Sites

In contrast to the structure of lymph nodes and spleen, the mucosa-associated lymphoid tissues located in the submucosa of tissues lining the mucosal surfaces, which include the gastrointestinal tract, respiratory tract, lacrimal glands, and genitourinary system, consist of small aggregates of T cells, B cells, and plasma cells (mainly of the IgA type) (*Chapter 8*). The gastrointestinal tract also contains additional complex structures including the tonsils, which are similar to lymph nodes, and Peyer's patches, which consist of follicles with germinal centers and mantle zones and are found in the ileum.

Shown in Figure 2-17 is a schematic representation of the structure of the lymphoid tissues in the small intestine. A large number of antigen-presenting cells are found in the region between the follicle and the follicle-associated intestinal epithelium in an area referred to as the dome area (Figure 2-17B). The dome epithelium is characterized by microfold (M) cells so-named by their numerous microfolds on the luminal side of the epithelium. M cells transport small amounts of antigen from the mucosal lumen into the MALT, where humoral and cellular immune responses are initiated. Interspersed within the interfollicular tissues and the intraepithelial region are collections of intraepithelial T lymphocytes. As described previously, the IEL at mucosal sites are the CD3+ CD4−, CD8− DN $\gamma\delta$ TCR-expressing T cells (Figure 2-10). The number of intraepithelial lymphocytes and plasma cells at these sites increases dramatically when inflammation occurs, as in inflammatory bowel disease (IBD), e.g., regional ileitis (Crohn's disease).

Shown in Figure 2-18 is a schematic representation of global relationships of the MALT in the ileum with the blood and lymph compartments that comprise the recirculating pool.

Ontogeny of the Immune System in the Developing Human

Having summarized the general aspects of the overall development of the cellular components of the

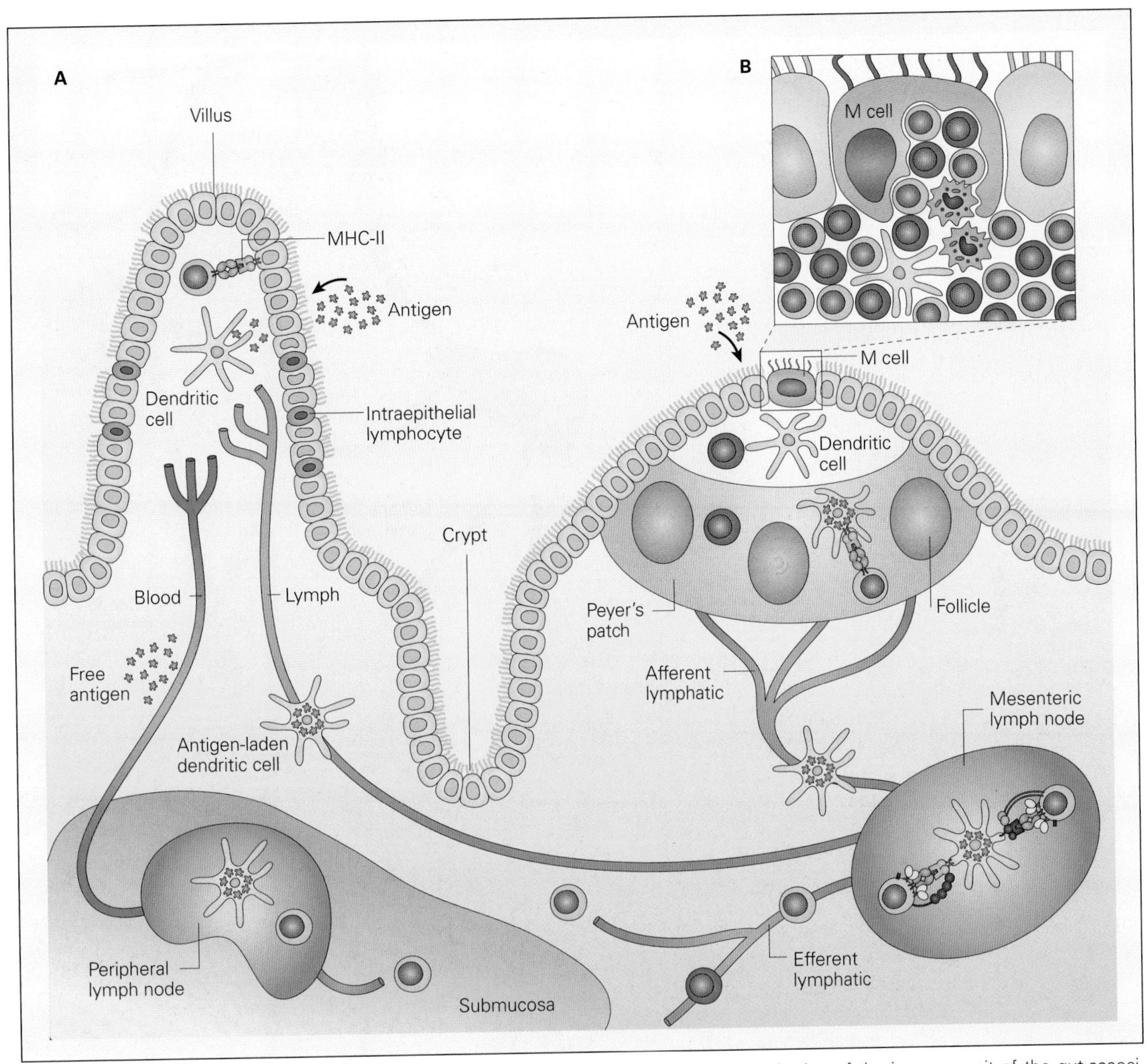

Figure 2-17. Panel A: The structure of the MALT in the small intestine showing the organization of the immune unit of the gut-associated lymphoid tissues (GALT) in the Peyer's patch. Antigen-presenting M cells take up antigen from the luminal side and present processed antigen to the dendritic cells, T cells, and B cells in the follicle which then enter the lymphatic drainage to mesenteric lymph nodes, referred to as the done area. Panel B: Note the lymphocytes and occasional macrophages in the pocket formed by the invagination of the basolateral membrane of the M cell. Antigens endocytosed by the M cell are passed via this pocket into subepithelial tissues.

immune system, it is now possible to describe in greater detail the ontogeny of the immune system in the developing human. The maturation of the immune response in the human begins in utero during the early weeks of gestation. As in all mammals, the beginnings of the innate (nonspecific) and adaptive (specific) immune systems start simultaneously with those of the hematopoietic system in the mesoderm of the primitive yolk sac as early as three to four weeks of gestation. A movement of progenitor cells to the liver occurs at five to six weeks of gestation, following which further development leads to seeding of the thymus and bone marrow at eleven to twelve weeks of gestation. The thymus and the bone marrow, thus, establish their primacy as the principal organs of immune function in utero, the thymus giving rise to thymic-dependent T lymphocytes important in CMI and the bone marrow giving rise to the bone marrow-dependent (or bursal equivalent in birds) B lymphocytes responsible for humoral immunity. Concomitant with these maturational events is the simultaneous development of antigen-presenting

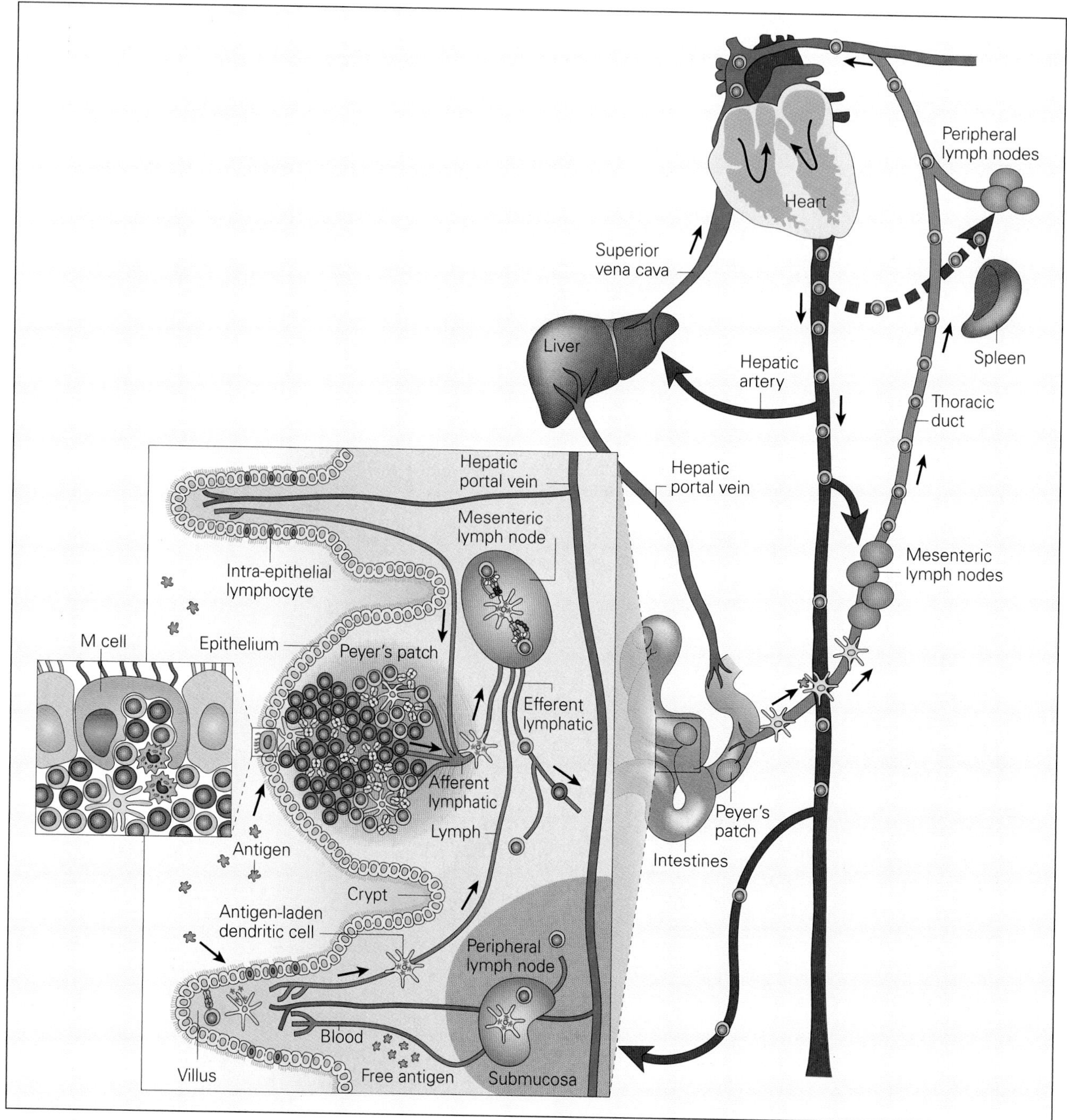

Figure 2-18. Schematic representation of the structure of the MALT in the ileum showing the relationship of localized immunologic events taking place in the GALT with the recirculating pool of lymphoid elements in the blood and lymph.

cells, which include macrophages and dendritic cells which, together with B lymphocytes, play a critical role in antigen presentation to the T lymphocytes (*Chapter 1*).

Maximal Thymus Function Occurs from Fourteen Weeks Gestation through Puberty

The thymus develops as an outgrowth of the third and fourth pharyngeal pouches and later migrates through the anterior mediastinum to its final location between the sternum and the great vessels (Figure 2-19A). The thymus acquires its functioning ability only when the cortex and medulla have differentiated. The first indications of this differentiation in a fetus occur after twelve weeks; it is completed at approximately four months of gestational age. With this differentiation the young thymocytes settle into the cortex region.

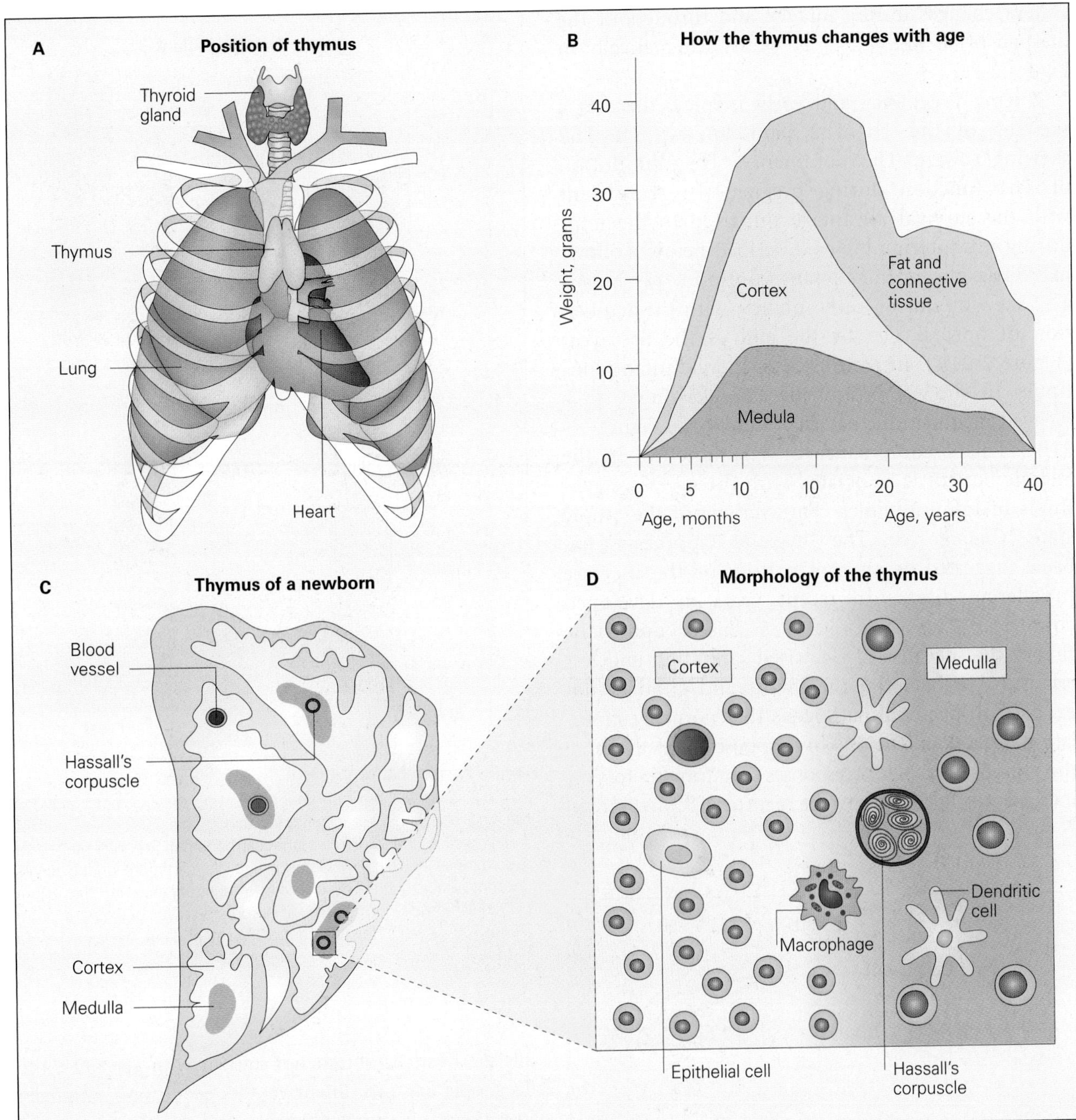

Figure 2-19. Schematic representation of the structural and functional aspects of the thymus during development. Panel A: Anatomy and development of the thymus. Panel B: Maturational changes of the thymus with age. Panel C: Total anatomy of the thymus. Panel D: Cellular morphology of a newborn's thymus. (Adapted from Burmester, G., Pezzutto, A., Wandrey, S., and Ulrichs, T., *Color Atlas of Immunology*. Stuttgart and New York: Thieme, 2003.)

The size of the thymus is age-dependent and reaches a maximum weight of approximately 40 grams at ten years of age and then undergoes a continuous process of involution (Figure 2-19A). As a result, the parenchyma of the thymus consists almost entirely of fat and fibrous issue in the elderly, when only a few clusters of parenchyma and lymphocytes remain intact. It is often not possible to differentiate between the involuted organ and the surrounding mediastinal fat by macroscopic means.

The Th1/Th2 Ratio Changes during the Lifespan of an Individual

Following birth, continued maturation of the immune system occurs. The balance of the parts of the T cell components of the adaptive immune system changes during infancy and throughout the lifespan of an individual, as shown schematically in Figure 2-20.

During pregnancy and early infancy, there is a skewing of the Th1/Th2 paradigm with a Th2 skewing toward Th2 dominance. The diminution of Th1 function during pregnancy is consistent with the survival advantage imparted to the fetus during intrauterine life as described below. Following birth, the normal infant continues to show a Th2 skewing during early infancy, with the acquisition of normal Th1 by the end of the first year (Figure 2-21A). In contrast, the allergic infant continues to show a prominent Th2 skewing with a delayed acquisition of Th1 function (Figure 2-21B). This predominance of Th2 function in the allergic patient is associated with the excessive synthesis of IgE antibodies characteristic of the atopic state (*Chapter 18*). The "hygiene hypothesis" has been suggested as an explanation for the increase in allergic disease in recent years in developed countries. This hypothesis is based upon the theory that because of increased sanitation and less exposure to bacteria, the infant and child is not exposed to bacterial pathogens that normally stimulate the development of Th1 responses, and therefore the unopposed Th2 responses contribute to the increase in IgE seen in the genetically predisposed allergic host. Although not known with certainty, the Treg cells are prominent in the young and gradually lose their function with aging and are thought to be associated with the development of autoimmune diseases and cancer in this age group.

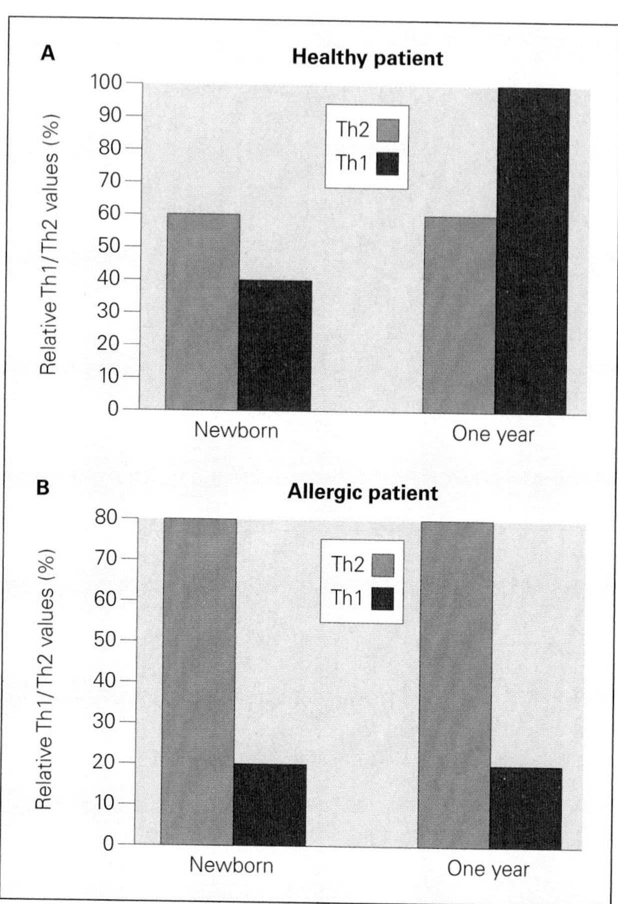

Figure 2-21. Panel A: Schematic representation of the changes in Th1/Th2 values in the normal infant during development showing the Th2 skewing of early infancy and the acquisition of normal Th1 with age. Panel B: Hypothetical schematic representation of the changes in Th1/Th2 values in the allergic infant during development showing the Th2 skewing of early infancy and the failure of acquisition of normal Th1. (Reproduced with permission from Bellanti JA, Malka-Rais J, Castro HJ, et al. Ann Allergy Asthma Immunol. 2003;90:2–6.)

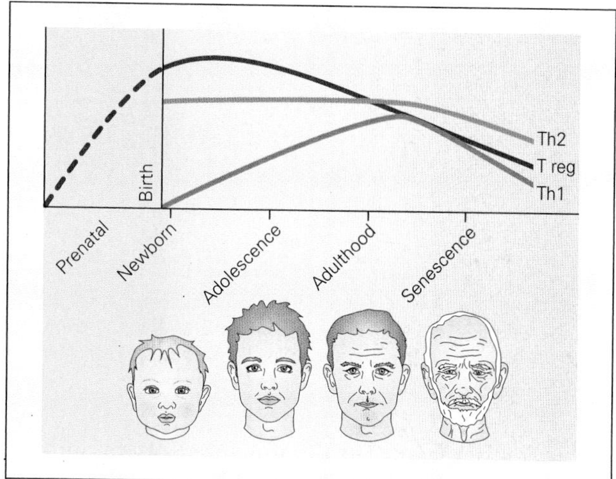

Figure 2-20. Schematic representation of the developmental changes in T cell function showing the paucity of Th1 cells in early infancy with a Th2 skewing. With increasing age, there is a maturation of the Th1 system until midlife, followed by a variable decrease with old age. Although not known with certainty, the Treg cells are prominent in the young and gradually lose their function with aging and are thought to be associated with the development of autoimmune diseases and cancer in this age group.

B Cell Development and Differentiation Differ in the Fetus and the Adult

There are significant differences in B cell development in the neonatal and the adult hosts. In adult mice and humans, B cells are generated in the bone marrow and exit from it as immature (IgM+IgD−) B cells. In the neonatal mouse, adult-type progenitors appear in the bone marrow in the first week of life; prior to this, B cells are generated in the fetal liver and spleen from fetal-type precursors. These remain active in the developing spleen until at least four weeks after birth, generating fetal-wave B cells.

Events in the spleen further differentiate adult and neonatal responses. In the adult spleen, immature B cells undergo maturation to become mature IgM−IgD+ B cells. Some cells are driven (possibly by antigen) to become marginal-zone B cells that reside in the marginal zone. In contrast, in neonatal mice, mature B cells are essentially absent until after the first week of life, when they can be found in discrete clusters close to the central arteriole. The marginal zone and its populating B cells in the neonate are not found until one to two weeks after birth.

In the adult and neonate, mature B cells can home in to other lymphoid structures, e.g., lymph nodes, where entry is controlled by expression of homing molecules such as L-selectin. In the neonatal period of both humans and mice, at least a portion of neonatal B cells either lack L-selectin or express it at low levels. B cells do gain entry to lymph nodes, however, possibly by the use of other molecular signals. In the adult, however, mature B cells can enter B cell follicles, which are crucial structures for T cell–B cell interactions. In the follicles, activation by antigen drives B cells to differentiate with the formation of germinal centers, which provide the microenvironment to support isotype class switching and further differentiation into long-lived plasma cells or memory B cells. In contrast, in the neonatal mouse, organized B cell follicles are first found seven to ten days after birth and germinal centers are absent until week three. Both plasma cells and memory B cells can home back to the bone marrow, where they are responsible for long-term antibody production. This homing process is less efficient in neonates.

The Transplacental Transfer of Antibody from the Maternal Circulation to the Fetus Has Both Beneficial and Harmful Outcomes

One of the most significant developments in phylogeny is the appearance of placentation in species with the ability to bear live young (viviparity). This occurred in higher forms with the development of the multilayered placenta. One of the challenging problems in biology is the question of how a fetus, who inherits one-half of its histocompatibility antigens from paternally controlled genes foreign to the mother, can be tolerated successfully during pregnancy. This has been classically attributed largely to a barrier function of the placenta (Box 2-4).

Although the placenta usually effectively separates the formed elements of the blood of the mother from that of the fetus, some elements, however, do gain access to the fetus and provide protection—i.e., antibodies. Conversely, some fetal cells gain access to the maternal immune system and can lead to the production of maternal antibodies against paternally derived foreign elements of fetal cells, as described below, which after their passage to the fetus can have a deleterious effect.

In the human, the predominant transfer of antibody occurs by passage of the IgG immunoglobulins from the maternal circulation to that of the fetus. This is accomplished by active transport of this immunoglobulin by a receptor located on one portion of the molecule, i.e., the Fc fragment (*Chapter 6*). In this manner, the fetus receives a library of preformed antibody from its mother, reflecting most of her experiences with infectious agents. These antibodies protect the fetus and young infant from infectious disease while its own immune system is still immature.

The development of serum immunoglobulins during intrauterine and postnatal life is shown schematically in Figure 2-22. The amount and type of antibody in the blood of the newborn infant at birth are equivalent to those of the mother and are made up almost exclusively of the IgG immunoglobulins. There are virtually no IgA, IgM, or IgE immunoglobulins present in the cord sera of healthy newborn infants. This is related to the fact that the Fc transport molecule is found only on IgG. In addition, because the fetus is usually protected in utero from antigenic stimuli, there is no active stimulation of the B cell system responsible for the production of other immunoglobulin-associated antibody. If the fetus is challenged in utero as a consequence of immunization or infection, e.g., infection with agents of the **TORCHS** syndrome (toxoplasmosis, rubella, cytomegalovirus, herpes simplex, and syphilis) or HIV, it will respond with antibody production largely of the IgM variety.

The exclusion of other classes of antibody is beneficial to the fetus in many cases. For example, the exclusion of the IgM isohemagglutinins, leukoagglutinins, or the IgE antibodies of allergy prevents disease that may be produced by the passive transfer of these antibodies. However, it also prevents the passage of other maternal antibodies that would be

Box 2-4

Why Is the Fetal Allograft Not Rejected?

In all viviparous species, the conceptus must be protected from a potentially hostile maternal immune system. As described in *Chapter 10*, the major histocompatibility complex (MHC) is comprised of a genetic region that encodes for both MHC-I and MHC-II proteins, which present peptide antigens to T lymphocytes and induce graft rejection (*Chapter 20*). In contrast to the MHC-II proteins, which are expressed only on professional antigen-presenting cells, the classical MHC-I proteins are expressed on all nucleated somatic cells. It has recently been shown that protection of the fetus from immune-mediated rejection involves down-regulation of classical MHC-I antigen expression on trophoblast cells, which form the external epithelial layer of the placenta, and therefore the maintenance of an immunologically favorable immunosuppressive environment in the uterus, a form of immune tolerance is necessary to allow the pregnancy to continue through its forty weeks of gestation with a favorable outcome. In the human, a nonclassical MHC-I antigen, human leukocyte antigen G (HLA-G), has been shown to be an important immunoregulatory factor required for maintenance of pregnancy. The reappearance of the MHC-I during later aspects of pregnancy in the last weeks of gestation contributes to placental separation and may be the basis for the onset of labor during normal parturition. The appearance of MHC-I expression earlier in gestation, on the other hand, may contribute to earlier-onset immune-mediated placental rejection and premature labor with miscarriage and fetal loss. Thus, appropriate regulation of MHC-I gene expression is critical for immunological acceptance of an allogeneic conceptus. During pregnancy, a balance of the Th1/Th2/Th3/Tr1 and CD4+CD25+. Treg paradigm is adapted to maintain a normal pregnancy, and Treg cells have been suggested as playing a major role.

Another cell type that has been the focus of intense current research in reproductive failure is the NK cell. In addition to Treg cells, NK regulatory cells have been shown to also play an important role in the maintenance of a normal pregnancy. Maternal uterine natural killer (uNK) cells are the most abundant leukocytes in preimplantation endometrium and early pregnancy deciduas and are adjacent to, and have the ability to interact directly with, fetal trophoblasts. Moreover, these cells have been shown to secrete a large assortment of cytokines that are important in angiogenesis and normal placental development and the establishment of pregnancy. When increased in number, uNK cells have been associated with reproductive failure. However, despite these exciting advances in understanding Treg and uNK cells, considerably more work needs to be done to establish a specific role of these cells and their use in the diagnosis and future treatment of reproductive failure with cytokine modification or the use of intravenous immunoglobulin, which is currently being evaluated in several clinical trials.

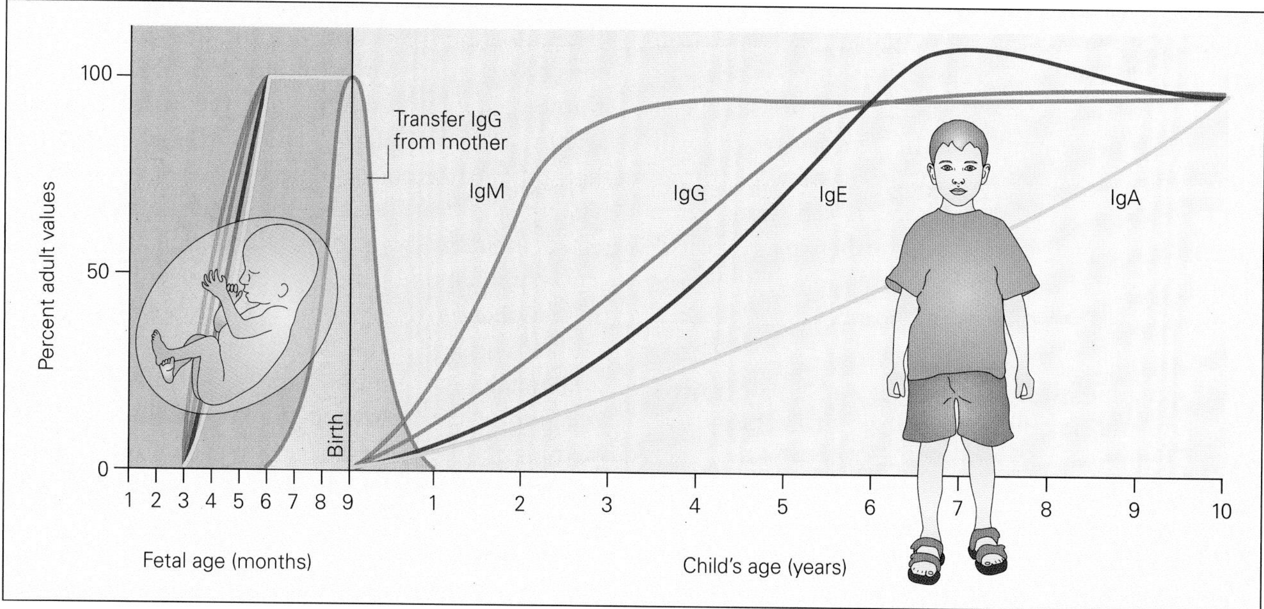

Figure 2-22. Schematic representation of the development of serum immunoglobulins in the human during infancy and childhood. Serum IgG, IgA, IgM, and IgE are presented as percentages of the normal adult values in the fetus, child, adolescent, and adult. Most of the transplacental transfer of maternal IgG to the fetus occurs during the last trimester of pregnancy. At birth, the newborn infant receives only IgG, and in full-term infants, the IgG levels are equivalent to those of the mother. After birth, the appearance of the various immunoglobulin isotypes follows the order that occurred during phylogeny. The IgM attains adult levels at one year, the IgG at five to six years, and the IgA by ten years. (Adapted from Fireman, P., ed. "*Chapter 21*: Primary immunodeficiency disease," *Atlas of Allergies and Clinical Immunology*. Philadelphia, PA: Mosby, Inc., 2006, 332.)

beneficial to the newborn, such as the IgM antibodies important in bacterial defense against gram-negative bacteria (opsonins, agglutinins, and other bacterial antibodies). This may explain, in part, the increased susceptibility of the newborn to infection with gram-negative organisms like *Escherichia coli.*

There is great variability in the types of antibodies that are obtained transplacentally by the fetus. This reflects the quantity of antibodies in the maternal circulation and of their molecular sizes. For example, low-molecular-weight IgG antibodies (e.g., rubeola antibody), present in high concentrations in maternal serum, are readily transferred. IgG antibodies in lower concentrations (such as *Bordetella pertussis*) are poorly transferred, and macroglobulin antibodies (e.g., Wassermann antibody) are completely excluded.

Since the IgG immunoglobulins are passively transferred, they have a finite half-life of between twenty to thirty days, and therefore their concentration in serum falls rapidly within the first few months of life, reaching the lowest levels between the second and fourth months. This period is referred to as *physiologic hypogammaglobulinemia* (*Chapter 16*). During the course of the first few years of life, the levels of gamma globulin increase because of exposure of the maturing infant to

Table 2-4. Examples of clinical applications of the changing immune system during the lifespan of the individual

Example	Pathogenetic mechanism	Resolution
INNATE IMMUNITY		
Inflammation/phagocytosis		
Increased susceptibility of newborn to bacterial infection	Decreased inflammatory response of the newborn; decreased microbicidal activity of phagocytic cells; decreased complement activity C3	Encourage breast-feeding; white blood cell transfusions; plasma infusions; use of recombinant GCSF or GMSF
Increased susceptibility of newborn to viral infection	Decreased inflammatory response of the newborn; decreased T cell activity (cytokines IFN-γ)	Encourage breast-feeding; investigational use of cytokine therapy, e.g., IFN-γ
Increased susceptibility of newborn to fungal infection	Decreased inflammatory response of the newborn; decreased T cell activity (cytokines IFN-γ)	Encourage breast-feeding; investigational use of cytokine therapy, e.g., IFN-γ
Increased susceptibility of newborn to parasitic infection	Decreased inflammatory response of the newborn; decreased T cell activity (cytokines IFN-γ)	Encourage breast-feeding; investigational use of cytokine therapy, e.g., IFN-γ
Increased susceptibility of elderly to infection	Decreased inflammatory response; decreased T cell activity (↓ IFN-γ)	Prophylactic immunization (influenza and pneumococcal vaccines)
ADAPTIVE IMMUNITY		
B cell		
Predominant IgM response of the newborn	Immaturity of B cell system (e.g., CD40L)	Self-resolving
Transient (two to four months) hypogammaglobulinemia of the newborn	Decreasing maternal transplacental gift of IgG	Self-resolving except more prolonged in transient hypogammaglobulinemia of infancy
Lack of response to polysaccharide antigens	Immature B cell system and T helper function	Use of protein-polysaccharide conjugate vaccines
T cell		
Lack of response to viral infection in newborns, e.g., *H simplex*; seen again in senescent adults	Deficient Th1 cytotoxic responses, e.g., diminished cytokine production, e.g., IFN-γ and IL-2	Use of immunomodulatory and antiviral drugs
Atopic disease	Imbalance of Th1 < Th2 characteristic of atopy	Immunotherapy or immunomodulatory agents
Propensity to autoimmune disease or cancer in adults	Senescence of T cell system with aging	Possible use of immunomodulatory agents

Case Study: Clinical Relevance

Let us now return to the case study of the 22q11.2 deletion syndrome presented earlier and review some of the major points of the clinical presentation and how they relate to the immune system:

- The clinical features and presentation of signs and symptoms by the infant in the newborn period—i.e., dysmorphic facies, cardiac defect, and hypoparathyroidism with hypocalcemic seizures—together with deficiencies of CD3+ and CD4+ T cell populations illustrate how the genetic 22q11.2 deletion and defective embryonic pharyngeal pouch development affected led to faulty development of the thymus, parathyroid glands, and heart and gave rise to the characteristic clinical findings of the disorder.
- The subsequent increased susceptibility to infections of the respiratory tract characterized by recurrent otitis media and sinusitis presumably by viral infection and later with bacterial infection illustrate the important role of T cell-mediated immunity in antiviral protection.
- The recent development of autoimmune thyroiditis illustrates how faulty T cell development and particularly defective Treg development in the syndrome can lead to immune dysregulation with abnormal, uncontrolled, and unleashed T cell cytotoxic destruction of the thyroid and can occur with subsequent hypofunctioning of the gland as illustrated by its physical enlargement and deficient T4 production and reciprocal hyperproduction of TSH (*Chapter 19*).

antigens in the environment. There appears to be a sequential development in gamma globulin at differing rates. The IgM immunoglobulins attain adult levels by one year of age, the IgG immunoglobulins by five or six years of age, and the IgA globulins by ten years of age. In the normal nonallergic infant, IgE immunoglobulins develop slowly over the first ten years of age. This pattern of appearance of immunoglobulin recapitulates that seen in phylogeny and also appears to parallel that seen following an antigenic exposure during the "primary" immune response (*Chapter 1*).

At times, maternal antibodies can have harmful effects, as seen in Rh isoimmunization (*Chapter 22*). Occasionally, fetal cells or other proteins may gain access to the maternal circulation and actively immunize the mother to the paternal allotypes found on these substances. This process, referred to as *isoimmunization*, may lead to serious disease in the infant, such as hemolytic disease of the newborn, thrombocytopenia, and leukopenia.

Summary of the Changing Immune System

From what has been described in this chapter, the changing immune system affects the expressions of health and disease throughout the life span of the individual. Shown in Table 2-4 are some examples of the clinical applications of the changing immune system throughout life.

Key Points

- The environment has shaped the evolving immune system at the level of the species (phylogeny), the developing individual (ontogeny), and the cell (the postnatal cellular expression of the immune response).
- Elements of innate immunity are present in plants and invertebrate animals.
- Elements of adaptive immunity are found only in vertebrates and depend on the ability to undergo somatic recombination.
- Hematopoiesis occurs in the bone marrow and is antigen independent.
- T cells must finish their development in the thymus microenvironment.
- Antigen signals naive B and T cells to become mature effector cells.
- The architecture of the secondary lymphoid organs and lymphocyte recirculation facilitate activation of the adaptive immune response.
- Hematopoietic precursors originate in the yolk sac and the fetal liver early in ontogeny.
- Thymus function peaks at puberty and declines thereafter. Th1 and Th2 ratios change over time.
- Passive immunity transfer from mother to infant offers protection from infectious disease but

can interfere with immunization and result in hypersensitivity.

Study Questions/Critical Thinking

1. Why is the adaptive immune system phylogenetically younger than the innate immune system?
2. How does the structure of the immune system contribute to its function?
3. Would it be advantageous to have lymphocytes exposed to mucosal pathogens recirculate among all lymphoid organs or to remain within the mucosal system? Explain your answer.

Suggested Reading

Adinolfi M. Ontogeny of human natural and acquired immunity. Curr Top Microbiol Immunol. 1997; 222: 67–102.

Adkins B, Leclerc C, Marshall-Clarke S. Neonatal adaptive immunity comes of age. Nat Rev Immunol. 2004; 4: 553–64.

Blackburn CC, Manley NR. Developing a new paradigm for thymus organogenesis. Nat Rev Immunol. 2004; 4: 278–89.

Blom B, Spits H. Development of human lymphoid cells. Annu Rev Immunol. 2006: 24; 287–320.

Burmester G, Pezzutto A, Wandrey S, et al. Color atlas of immunology. Stuttgart and New York: Thieme; 2003.

Colten HR. Navigating the maze of complement genetics: a guide for clinicians. Curr Allergy Asthma Rev. 2002; 2: 379–84.

Colten HR. Ontogeny of the human complement system: in vitro biosynthesis of individual complement components by fetal tissues. J Clin Invest. 1972; 51: 725–30.

Cooper MD, Alder MN. The evolution of adaptive immune systems. Cell. 2006; 124: 815–22.

Davies CJ. Why is the fetal allograft not rejected? J Anim Sci. 2007; 85(13 Suppl): E32–5.

De Paula PF, Barbosa JE, Junior PR, et al. Ontogeny of complement regulatory proteins—concentrations of factor h, factor I, c4b-binding proteins, properdin and vitronectin in healthy children of different ages and in adults. Scand J Immunol. 2003; 53: 572–7.

Fireman P, (Ed). In: Atlas of allergies and clinical immunology. Philadelphia: Mosby, Inc; 2006.

Flajnik MF, Du Pasquier L. Evolution of innate and adaptive immunity: can we draw a line? Trends Immunol. 2004; 25: 640–4.

Hsu E, Pulham N, Rumfelt LL, et al. The plasticity of immunoglobulin gene systems in evolution. Immunol Rev. 2006; 210: 8–26.

Litman GW, Cooper MD. Why study the evolution of immunity? Nat Immunol. 2007; 8: 547–8.

Moffett A, Loke C. Implantation, embryo-maternal interactions, immunology and modulation of the uterine environment—a workshop report. Placenta. 2006; 27 Suppl A: S54–5.

Moretta A, Bottino C, Mingari MC, et al. What is a natural killer cell. Nat Immunol. 2002; 3: 6–8.

Nonaka M, Kimura A. Genomic view of the evolution of the complement system. Immunogenetics. 2006; 58: 701–13.

Ohta T, Flajnik M. IgD, like IgM is a primordial immunoglobulin class perpetuated in most jawed vertebrates. Proc Natl Acad Sci. 2006; 103: 10723–8.

Pancer Z, Cooper MD. The evolution of adaptive immunity. Annu Rev Immunol. 2006; 24: 497–518.

Quenby S, Farquharson R. Uterine natural killer cells, implantation failure, and recurrent miscarriage. Reprod Biomed Online. 2006; 13: 24–8.

Shortman K, Naik SH. Steady-state and inflammatory dendritic-cell development. Nat Rev Immunol. 2007; 7: 19–30.

Chapter 3

Innate Immunity

Alejandro Escobar-Gutiérrez, PhD
Sigifredo Pedraza-Sánchez, PhD
José Roberto Bastarrachea-Rivera, MD

Case Study

A fifty-seven-year-old man was hospitalized because of dyspnea, dry cough, and fever of eight days duration. Prior to admission, he developed general symptoms of malaise, anorexia, weakness, difficulty breathing, chills, mild headache, low-grade fever, tachycardia, and tachypnea. There was also a several day history of mild night sweats, diminished urine output described by the patient as yellowish and concentrated, as well as a productive cough and hemoptysis. A history of progressive respiratory failure and hypertension for ten years was elicited; however, he denied a history of diabetes, allergies, or prior surgeries. At the time of admission, the patient appeared apprehensive and disoriented with a low-grade fever (37.8°C), cyanosis, and audible rales over the left lower lung. The blood pressure was 70/50 mm. The chest X-ray showed bilateral diffuse alveolar-interstitial infiltrates. At the time of admission, arterial blood gas analysis showed a moderate hypoxemia with non-compensated respiratory acidosis compatible with acute respiratory insufficiency. Routine laboratory analysis showed anemia with a hemoglobin concentration of 10 g/dL and a leukocytosis of 17,500/mm^3 with 95 percent neutrophils. Additional laboratory results showed intravascular coagulation, acute kidney insufficiency with elevated serum creatinine of 3.4 mg/dL, and elevated direct bilirubin of 3.4 mg/dL. Other indirect data showed evidence of a systemic inflammatory response consistent with sepsis. Since the patient's oxygenation progressively deteriorated with increasing confusion, intubation and mechanical ventilator support were required.

Blood cultures obtained on admission showed growth of *Pseudomonas aeruginosa* and intravenous imipenem and ceftazidime were initiated. Bronchoalveolar lavage fluid (BALF) was negative for *Pneumocystis jiroveci, Mycobacterium tuberculosis*, or pyogenic bacteria. No malignant cells were found. There were 2,000 cells/mm^3 in the BALF mostly consisting of alveolar macrophages (78 percent) compatible with an infectious process. Based on these findings, a diagnosis of septic shock with multiple organ failure was made. The patient was treated with intravenous fluids, whole blood transfusions, and vasopressor medications. Although he was persistently febrile for several days, his hemodynamics, gas exchange, lung function, and renal function gradually improved and, after fifteen days, he was weaned from mechanical ventilation. Cognitive

LEARNING OBJECTIVES

When you have completed this chapter, you should be able to:

- Describe the constitutive and induced elements of the innate immune system
- Identify the cellular and molecular components of the innate immune response
- Distinguish between pathogen-associated molecular patterns (PAMPs) on pathogens and pattern-recognition receptors (PRRs) on cells and products of the innate immune system
- Recognize the role of soluble mediators such as cytokines and chemokines and complement components that control the innate immune response
- Explain how these various cellular and soluble factors of the innate immune response contribute to inflammation that could have either a beneficial effect in host protection against invading pathogens or a detrimental effect in tissue injury and disease
- Summarize the clinical relevance of the innate immune response in health and disease

Case Study (continued)

function returned to normal and renal function eventually recovered after twenty days of dialysis support. Manifestations of sepsis subsided gradually with progressive decrease in white cell count, increase in platelet count, and negative blood cultures. Antibiotics were continued for fourteen days. Following rehabilitation for severe muscle wasting, the patient recuperated rapidly and was discharged from the hospital thirty days later in excellent condition.

The Role of Innate Immunity in the Immune System

Immunity Is Due to Both Constitutive and Induced Elements

Throughout their lives, humans are immersed in a sea of microorganisms consisting of viruses, bacteria, fungi, and parasites. In addition, they are exposed to transformed cells and a myriad of other foreign biological and inert components in the environment that are potentially harmful and can cause disease. The maintenance of health in such situations is provided mainly by the presence of appropriate physiological host mechanisms that limit the access or spreading of the foreign material or infectious agent by neutralizing or eliminating it. Such states of freedom from symptoms or disease are the consequence of a complex series of processes collectively known as immunity, which constitute one of the cornerstones of the homeostatic mechanisms that the host employs in maintaining a balance between the external and internal environments (*Chapter 1*). Immunity can be *constitutive* (natural immunity) or *inducible* (the innate and adaptive immune responses). Working together, these responses are capable of keeping individuals free of disease when confronting microorganisms or malignant transformed cells (Figure 3-1 and Box 3-1).

The induced immune response is comprised of two arms: (1) the innate immune response, which is characterized by a rapid and effective stereotyped activation of cellular and inflammatory products directed to a wide variety of microorganisms, and (2) the adaptive immune response, a set of highly specific lymphocytic defense mechanisms directed against particular molecular components called antigens but which require a relatively longer period of time for their activation and amplification. In any host-parasite relationship, the success of the infectious agent as invader depends on its ability to evade both arms of the immune response; full evasion is expressed as the establishment of a chronic infection. Figure 3-2 and Table 3-1 summarize the interactions

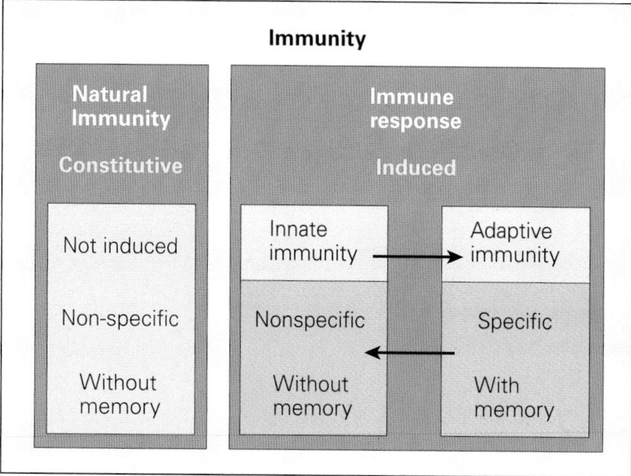

Figure 3-1. Schematic representation of natural (constitutive) and induced (innate and adaptive) immune responses. The arrows indicate the interrelationships between innate and adaptive immunity.

Box 3-1

Defense mechanisms can be divided into two groups according to the manner in which they are stimulated by foreign substances:

1. **Constitutive defenses**: These are present in all animals and provide nonspecific, generalized, and permanent protection against invasion by normal flora, or colonization, infection, and infectious disease caused by pathogens. The constitutive defenses have also been referred to as "natural" immunity, since they are inborn in a specific host and consist largely of anatomic and physiologic barriers, e.g., skin and mucous membranes (*Chapter 1*).
2. **Inducible defenses**: These are triggered by the host following exposure to a pathogen (as during an infection), malignant cells, or after allogeneic transplantation and consist of the many interactive components of innate and adaptive immunity. Unlike the constitutive defenses, the inducible are not immediately prepared to come into play until after the host has been appropriately exposed to and activated by a foreign intruder, e.g., a pathogen, or an internal component, e.g., a cancer cell.

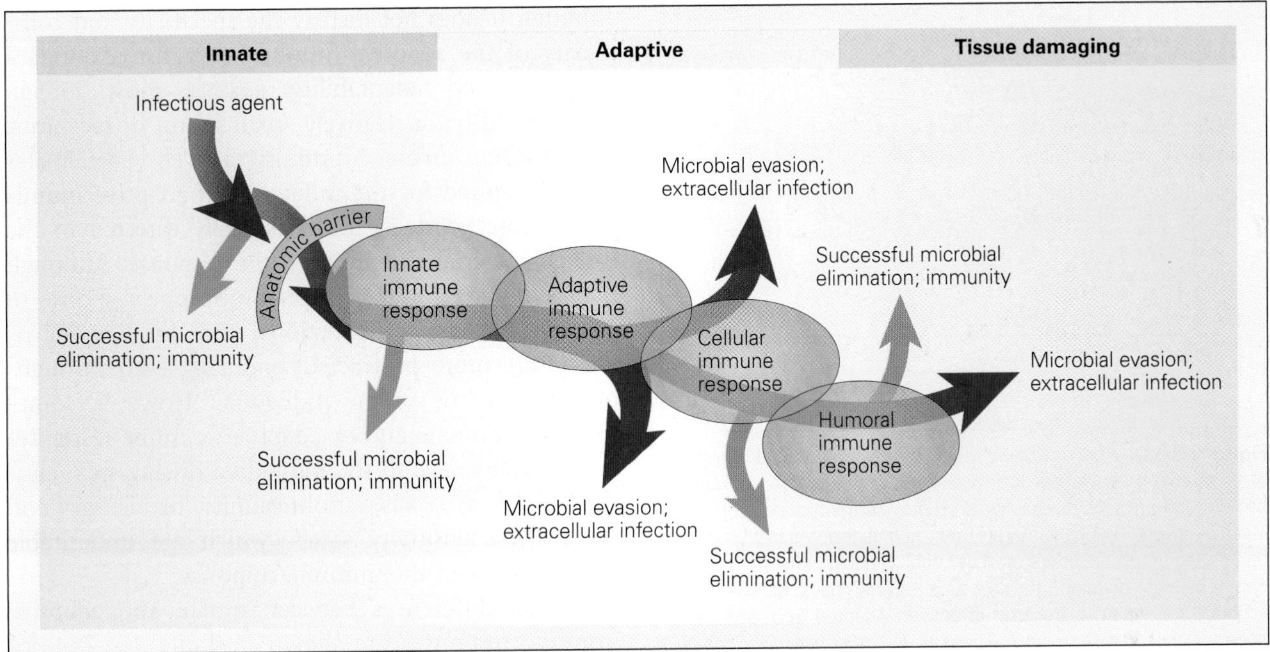

Figure 3-2. Schematic representation of the progressive steps in the immune response to microbial pathogens by cellular and humoral components of both the innate and adaptive immune systems. Immunity occurs as a coordinated set of sequential overlapping steps, each triggered by the interaction of these components in response to all foreign substances such as infectious agents. Each step of the immune process interacts with the next one (overlapping circles), and depending on the virulence of the agent and its ability to evade the effectiveness of the immune response, the agent can be either eliminated (green arrows) with a successful outcome or persist (red arrows) with microbial evasion.

of various components of constitutive and induced (adaptive) immune responses to an infectious agent and give examples of clinical outcomes depending upon the successful elimination or evasion of the agent with failure of elimination.

Anatomical barriers and physiologic mechanisms of natural immunity, provide immediate protection against penetration of many exogenous agents and consist of intact skin and mucous membranes, antimicrobial substances, stomach acidity, and physiological reflexes, e.g., coughing, sneezing, vomiting, or diarrhea (Table 3-1 and *Chapter 1*). These static and constant barriers are then followed by the inducible elements of both innate and adaptive (acquired) immune reactions in response to distinct exogenous and endogenous insults to the host. The time course sequence of events of these protective mechanisms is shown schematically in Figure 3-3.

This chapter will explore the elements and mechanisms of innate immunity in humans and will describe how these contribute to both the beneficial aspects of antimicrobial host protection as well as the deleterious features of disease-related events occurring during bacterial infection. It will be seen that a major part of the pathology of certain diseases, such as sepsis and septic shock, are triggered by exaggerated innate immune responses. The chapter will describe the general characteristics of innate immunity including the families of receptors involved in recognition of microorganisms, comparisons of this

Table 3-1. Examples of interactions of various components of constitutive and induced immune responses to an infectious agent with successful or detrimental outcomes depending upon elimination or evasion of the agent with failure of elimination.

Immune response	Successful outcome	Microbial evasion
Constitutive immunity: Anatomic barriers, physiologic reflexes (e.g., coughing, vomiting)	Microbial elimination	Infection
Induced immunity: Innate response	Microbial elimination	Colonization
Adaptive response: Humoral (antibodies)	Microbial elimination; immunity	Chronic infection (extracellular)
Adaptive response: Cellular (Tc, Th1)	Microbial elimination; immunity	Chronic infection (intracellular)

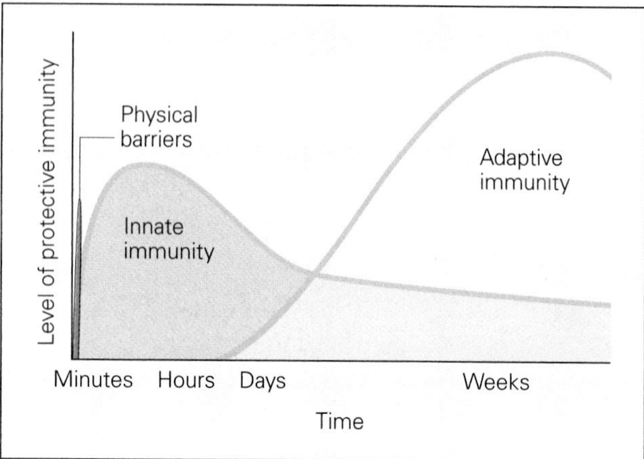

Figure 3-3. Schematic representation of the time course sequence of protective mechanisms to invasion by a foreign invader. Surface barriers and physiologic mechanisms provide immediate protection. Innate immune mechanisms are next stimulated within minutes to hours and keep invaders at bay until mechanisms of adaptive immunity can develop. It may take several days or weeks for acquired immunity to become effective. (Adapted from and reproduced with permission from Tizard, I. R. *Veterinary Immunology: An Introduction*, 8th Ed. Philadelphia: Elsevier, 2008.)

system with adaptive immunity, and the involvement of the innate immune response during bacterial sepsis and its complications.

Innate and Adaptive Immune Responses Have Distinct Recognition Molecules and Mechanisms for Pathogen Elimination

As described in Chapter 1, the immune response basically consists of a set of highly integrated reaction(s) involved in the twofold function of: (1) *recognition* and (2) *elimination* of a foreign substance. The innate immune response (from Latin, *innatus*, possessed at birth; inborn) constitutes the first line of the inducible defenses by which many of the potentially harmful exogenous invaders are rapidly controlled or eliminated by this phylogenetically ancient reaction (*Chapter 2*). Unlike the adaptive immune response, however, which represents a recognition system of antigen-specific receptors found exclusively on lymphocytes in higher life forms, the innate immune response has evolved as an alternate set of pathogen-detecting molecules found on a wider variety of cells which first appeared in lower life forms, even in plants, and which have been retained in all animal kingdoms, including higher vertebrates. The hallmark of innate immunity lies in its immediacy and swiftness of response which allow the system to react quickly during infections, and although it does not display the specificity and complexity of the adaptive immune response, exhibits a flexibility and adaptability against most foreign intruders, using a relatively small group of receptors. In addition, innate immunity actively participates and is required for the induction of adaptive immunity, whose products are specifically directed to the foreign material that induced the response. Although it takes longer for the adaptive immune response to perform its effector functions, the duration of its effects are more protracted, enduring even throughout the lifetime of the individual. However, sometimes both innate and/or adaptive immune responses can cause damage to the individual during such clinical entities as sepsis, autoimmunity, or allergies and other hypersensitivity states, which are undesirable consequences of the immune response.

Several differences between innate and adaptive immune responses are shown in Table 3-2. One of the most fundamental differences is the more limited specificity of the innate immune response to recognize individual components of particular infectious agents in contrast to that seen with adaptive immunity. The targets of adaptive immune responses are the antigens, very specific structures that induce cell-mediated immunity or antibody synthesis upon interaction with and activation of specific T or B cells, respectively. In contrast, the innate immune response is triggered by common structural components found on or within a wide variety of microorganisms, which are generically called pathogen-associated molecular patterns (**PAMPs**) (*Chapter 12*). The second difference is related to the diversity of the receptors involved in the recognition of PAMPs and antigens; the receptors for innate responses display a relatively low diversity and are generically called pattern-recognition receptors (**PRRs**), consisting of germ-line encoded molecules that are inherited and do not change during any developmental stage of the individual (*Chapter 9*). In contrast, the receptors for the adaptive immune responses are the T cell receptor (**TCR**) and the B cell receptor (**BCR**) (*Chapters 6 and 7*), which are genetically encoded proteins somatically diversified through genetic recombination and mutation, thus providing a vastly changing and extensive repertoire of antigen-detecting molecules selectively found on lymphocytes during the lifespan of the individual. The third difference is the timing and strength of both responses (Figure 3-3). Innate immune responses occur rapidly in terms of

Table 3-2. Major differences between innate and adaptive immune responses

Characteristic	Innate immune response	Adaptive immune response
Timing	Rapid response usually between minutes to hours	Primary response seen in three to ten days; memory response in one to two days
Molecular inductors	PAMPs: common structures found on many infectious agents, mostly absent in host	Antigens: macromolecules (mainly proteins and polysaccharides), formed by epitopes, present in foreign molecules but sometimes shared by hosts
Receptors	PRRs encoded in germ-line genes	Specific receptors (T cell receptor and B cell receptor) genes in low number that somatically rearrange
Phylogenetic distribution	In some plants, invertebrates, and vertebrates	Mainly in vertebrates
Number of receptors	Between 10^2 and 10^3	Between 10^{14} and 10^{18}
Affinity of receptors	Low affinity $Ka = 10^5$	High affinity $Ka = 10^8$
Cells	Neutrophils, monocytes/macrophages, eosinophils, basophils, epithelial, endothelial, dendritic, NK, and mast cells	T and B lymphocytes
Effector mechanisms	Cytokine and chemokine production, phagocytic killing, inflammation, cell-mediated apoptosis	Cytokine production, cell cytotoxicity, neutralizing, opsonizing, and complement activating antibodies

minutes to hours and consistently display the same strength, regardless whether in response to a first stimulation or after a subsequent encounter with the foreign configuration, whereas adaptive immune responses take longer to be mounted (three to ten days) after the first contact with the antigen. The response, however, is more rapid and stronger after a second or third stimulus (one to two days), a phenomenon associated with immunological memory and which characterizes the secondary immune response (*Chapters 1* and *6*). Finally, the phylogenetic distribution of these two kinds of immune responses is distinct: innate immunity consists of a collection of very primitive defense systems, present in some plants, invertebrates, and vertebrates, whereas adaptive immunity is apparently restricted mainly to vertebrates (Table 3-2).

The power of the adaptive immune response is related to its exquisite antigenic specificity, as will be described in *Chapters 6* and *7*. However, the induction of this response is made possible only by its dependence on the innate response through a series of sequential steps including antigen presentation with involvement of co-stimulatory molecules. Antigen uptake, processing, and presentation follow as a consequence of stimulation of dendritic cells and macrophages with PAMPs. These cells express on their membrane more antigen-presenting molecules as well as co-stimulatory molecules (CD40, CD80/CD86) required for the stimulation of T lymphocytes through their binding with CD40L and CD28, respectively, thus complementing T cell activation. In addition, activation of the complement system provides C3d, a fragment of the C3 molecule (*Chapter 4*), which plays a key role in B cell activation (*Chapter 6*). Another important consideration in the relationship between innate and adaptive immunity is the preferential induction of Th1 responsible for cell-mediated immunity (**CMI**) that are described in greater detail in Chapter 7. Th1 responses are induced by dendritic cells or macrophages when they are stimulated by microbial products and produce IL-12. This observation has served to support the possible use of microbial products as adjuvants to reduce the detrimental Th2 responses that predominate in diseases as, e.g., allergies (*Chapter 18*).

As will be described below, the receptors, cells, molecules, and mechanisms participating in the two branches of the immune response converge and interact with each other at critical points providing a unique and highly discriminative capacity of the whole immune response to eliminate potentially harmful foreign substances including microorganisms, allergens, eukaryotic parasites, or their products, and even some altered self-components, e.g., transformed or malignant cells.

The Role of Inflammation in Innate Immunity

The innate immune response constitutes the first response to a foreign molecule or an infectious agent. When constitutive anatomical and physiological barriers are overcome, the invader next encounters in plasma and tissue fluids a variety of soluble molecules whose immediate activation generates new antimicrobial components that can provide a protective defense bulwark. These include molecules from the coagulation (thrombin), fibrinolytic (plasmin), and kinin (bradkinin) cascades, as well as from complement activation (anaphylatoxins C3a, C4a, and C5a, the chemotactic factor C5a, and the opsonizing C3b fragment), which in turn is initiated by the mannose-binding lectin (lectin pathway) (*Chapter 4*).

Activation of the Innate Immune Response Results in Inflammation

The next defensive component of innate immunity occurs within a period of one to four hours and is provided by the production of a family of signaling molecules that initiates the inflammatory influx and activation of the inflammatory response with major involvement of epithelial cells, endothelial cells, dendritic cells, and mast cells. This includes the up-regulation of adhesion molecules on endothelial cells of blood vessels and on various phagocytic cells (neutrophils, monocytes, and eosinophils) which not only leads to the activation of these and other inflammatory cells (mast cells and basophils) and recruitment of cytotoxic cells (NK cells) but also facilitates the migration of some of these cells from the blood into the tissues (*Chapter 5*). Activation of these cells by phagocytosis, for example, leads to the rapid secretion of soluble mediators, mainly cytokines, chemokines, oxygen and nitrogen cytotoxic metabolites, and antimicrobial peptides (*Chapter 5*). Usually, the innate immune response is adequate to eliminate the foreign invader, leaving only those agents whose intrinsic pathogenic properties evade the immune response allowing them to further progress in the infectious process. Within a relatively brief time (~96 hours), the adaptive immune response will ensue, with the activation of antigen-specific effector cells and memory cells that can respond faster upon subsequent encounters with the same or a closely related foreign substance.

The interactive relationships between innate and adaptive immune responses are shown schematically in Figure 3-4. Although the reaction to a foreign agent by the innate immune response usually progresses to an adaptive immune response, innate immunity can and often does result in pathogen elimination at this stage without activation of adaptive immunity.

Complement Activation Enhances Inflammation and Pathogen Destruction

Complement is a complex molecular system consisting of approximately forty factors and components (glycoproteins and proteins) present in plasma or as receptors on the surface of many cells of the innate and adaptive immune systems (*Chapter 4*). It functions as a biologic amplification system to enhance many of the functions of the

immune system involved in the control of inflammation, activation of phagocytes, and lytic attack of target cells. The soluble components are present in an inactive state in the blood and interstitial fluids and their activation occurs as a successive set of sequential reactions referred to as the *complement cascade.* There are three distinct pathways of complement cascade activation that converge in a final common pathway: (1) the alternative pathway induced by molecular components present in bacteria and fungi; (2) the lectin pathway, which is triggered by certain carbohydrates, e.g., mannose, on microorganism surfaces; and (3) the classical pathway, which is initiated by soluble or pathogen-bound antigen-antibody complexes (Table 3-3). The final common pathway of the activated complement system is the formation of a cytolytic structure—a membrane attack complex (**MAC**), which leads to perforation of cell membranes and osmotic disruption of cells. In addition and no less important, are the enzymatically cleaved components (i.e., sub-products of the complement cascade) released throughout the process. These, then, become biologically active following their interaction with cells and tissues through specific cell-associated receptors.

Complement promotes the inflammatory response (*Chapter 5*), eliminates pathogens through opsonization and lysis (*Chapter 12*), and enhances the adaptive immune response. Consequently, deficiencies in complement elements are known to both predispose patients to infection (*Chapter 16*) but also can contribute to the pathogenesis of sepsis and immune complex mediated diseases, such as systemic lupus erythematosus (**SLE**). These concepts are described in greater detail in Chapters 4 and 19.

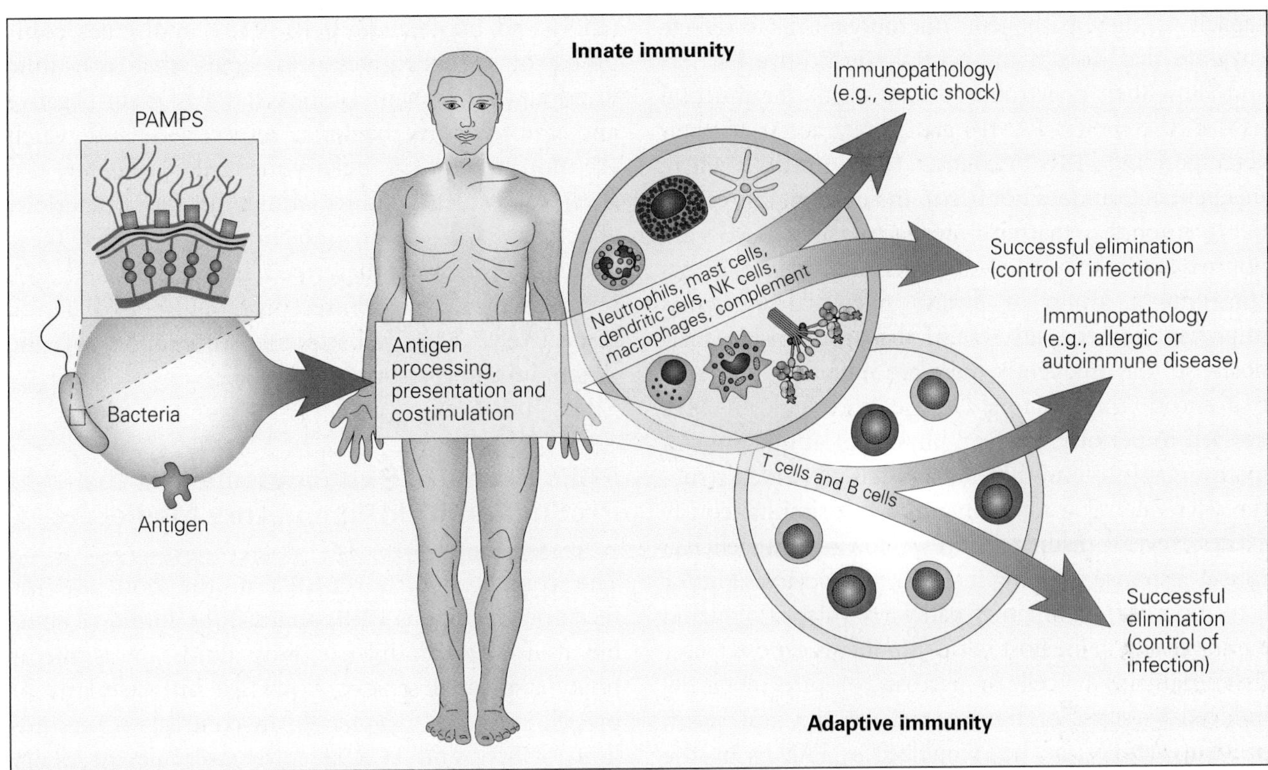

Figure 3-4. Schematic representation of the interactive relationships between the innate and adaptive immune responses to microbial infection. Infectious agents can be considered as mosaics of PAMPs and antigens. The innate immune response is induced early by PAMPs and assists the antigen-driven adaptive immune responses through antigen processing, presentation, and co-stimulation. Although both immune responses are usually effective in controlling infections, at times an uncontrolled or exaggerated response can result in self-damage from an uninhibited innate immune response (e.g., the systemic inflammatory response syndrome [SIRS]) or can lead to immunopathology from an unrestrained adaptive immune response (e.g., autoimmune disease).

The Innate Immune System Recognizes PAMPs

Chief among the identity molecules on microorganisms are the PAMPs, which are recognized by the PRRs on cells of the innate and adaptive immune systems. This section will give a more detailed description of the properties and functions of these important foreignness-sensing molecules and their role in innate immunity.

Table 3-3. Summary of the three major pathways of complement activation together with their effector functions and outcomes of each

Pathway	Alternative	Lectin	Classical
Effector functions	Binding to pathogen surface	Binding to Mannose-Binding Lectin	Binding to Pathogen-bound antibody
	Complement activation		
Outcomes	Pathogen opsonization	Inflammation	Effector functions

PAMPs are very conserved molecular structures located on microbes without major variations in their composition. Usually these structures are essential for the survival of the microorganism and they must remain constant or the microbe will die. PAMPs represent molecular motifs shared by large groups of microorganisms but absent in the host. When a potential infectious agent confronts the host, these components are responsible for triggering the innate immune response. The term PAMP was coined by Dr. Charles A. Janeway, Jr.; however, these structures are not exclusive of pathogenic microorganisms but are also shared by commensal microorganisms; in this case, the term microbe-associated molecular pattern (**MAMP**) has been suggested (*Chapter 12*). It is unclear why PAMPs found in commensal microorganisms usually fail to elicit an immune response, while the same motifs contained within more invasive microbes do not. One possible explanation may be related to the capacity of these pathogenic microorganisms to secrete enzymes that disrupt the natural constitutive barriers and allow their penetration deeper inside the mucosal tissues where their PAMPs gain direct access to their corresponding PRRs in contrast to commensals where this penetration does not occur. In addition, it is essential to emphasize that virulence factors and PAMPs are not necessarily the same (*Chapter 12*). Virulence factors constitute a group of diverse microbial molecules important for the survival of the agent inside their hosts, so that frequently there are mutations in genes that encode these factors. On the other hand, PAMPs evolved to perform essential physiological functions in microorganisms and therefore exist as conserved structures. Frequently a microorganism can simultaneously express several distinct PAMPs, allowing it to elicit a robust response resulting in either phagocytosis and/or activation of inflammatory pathways. Interestingly and paradoxically, some host self-components exposed after tissue damage, or cellular necrosis, or physiologically induced by stress or trauma, such as the heat shock proteins (**HSP**), can be recognized as PAMPs by the receptors of the innate immune system. These are sometimes referred to as danger-associated molecular patterns (**DAMPs**).

The molecular structure of PAMPs is quite variable and includes proteins, polysaccharides, and glycolipids expressed on the surface of viruses and microorganisms (*Chapter 12*). They can also be released and recognized in soluble form or exist as intracellular moieties as in the case of nucleic acids. For example, viral single- or double-stranded RNA, bacterial unmethylated DNA sequences rich in CpG, and even some synthetic compounds have been identified as PAMPs.

A partial list of the best-known PAMPs is shown in Table 3-4. These include lipopolysaccharides (**LPS**) and lipoteichoic acid (**LTA**), molecules composed of carbohydrates and lipids that constitute important components of the cell wall of gram-negative and gram-positive bacteria, respectively, and which are not present in eukaryotic cells (*Chapter 12*). Both molecules produce much of the deleterious effects attributable to infections caused by these bacteria. As will be described below, LPS and LTA are recognized by cell receptors TLR4 and TLR2, respectively, with subsequent stimulation of the innate immune response.

PRRs Promote Phagocytosis and the Production of Inflammatory Mediators

The counterparts of PAMPs in the host are the receptors known as PRRs that can be found as soluble molecules in diverse body fluids or as membrane-associated sensors expressed intracellularly or on cell surfaces (*Chapter 9*). In contrast to the millions of BCR and TCR receptor molecules necessary for clearance of the great diversity of infecting agents by the adaptive immune system, only a few hundred PRRs are required to achieve the same goal by the innate immune system. Soluble PRRs—e.g., C-reactive protein (**CRP**) or mannose-binding protein (**MBP**)—participate mainly as opsonins (facilitating phagocytosis) and as activators of a variety of enzymes found in plasma. The interaction of PRRs with their PAMPs initiates a cascading set of intracellular events resulting in cell activation through the production of a variety of molecules, e.g., cytokines, which directly or indirectly participate in the elimination of the invading agent. Some specific membrane receptors of the innate immune system

Table 3-4. Examples of some major PAMPs/DAMPs

Exogenous (PAMPs)
Viruses: single stranded RNA, double stranded RNA, unmethylated DNA
All bacteria: cell wall peptidoglycan, glycolipids, lipoproteins, lipopeptides, diacyl and triacyl lipopeptides (DLP, TLP), formulated proteins, flagellin, unmethylated CpG nucleotides
Gram-positive bacteria: lipoteichoic acid (LTA)
Gram-nagative bacteria: lipopoplysaccharides (LPS), porins
Mycobacteria: lipoarabinomannan (LAM), mycolic acids
Fungi: zymosan
Protozoa: glycophosphatidylinositol (GPI), lipophosphoglycan (LPG), profilin
Endogenous (DAMPs)
Necrosis and tissue damage products: High-mobility group protein B1 (HGM-1), S100 family members, amyloid-beta, 60 and 70 kDa heat-shock proteins (hsp60, hsp70), hyaluronic acid, heparan sulphate, fibronectin, fibrinogen

participate in phagocytosis, e.g., members of the scavenger receptor (**SR**) family. These also participate in the elimination of "self cells" that already have been killed by apoptosis and are called apoptotic bodies (*Chapter 9*). A list of the major PRRs is shown in Table 3-5.

The interest in innate immunity started just after the discovery of Toll-like receptors (**TLRs**), an important family of cell-surface molecules able to recognize many different PAMPs and therefore involved in immunity as well as in distinct diseases. Toll was initially discovered in *Drosophila melanogaster* as an important molecule for the embryonic development of their larvae. Later, it became evident that Toll molecules were also important for antifungal defenses in these insects. Bioinformatic analyses identified equivalent receptors to Toll, i.e., Toll-like receptors, as conserved molecules involved in antimicrobial responses present in many other biological species, including mammals.

In the human, there are ten known TLRs (Table 3-6), all of which are membrane-associated proteins with a characteristic structure formed by extracellular leucine-rich repeats (**LRRs**) with intracytoplasmic tails or domains involved in signaling, similar to the intracellular domain of the interleukin-1 (**IL-1**) receptor, therefore named Toll-IL-1-related (**TIR**) domain (*Chapter 9*). Shown in Figure 3-5 is a schematic representation of cellular locations of TLRs, some of which are located on the cell surface while others have an intracellular location. Most TLRs form heterodimers. The engagement of a TLR by its ligand activates intracellular signaling pathways using the adaptor molecule MyD88 and downstream, distinct kinases; these pathways end with the activation of stress-activated protein kinases, the nuclear factor κB (**NF-κB**), and transcription of distinct genes of inflammation (TNF-α, IL-1, IL-6, IL-8, etc.) (*Chapter 9*). Major participation of TLRs occurs by triggering innate response and enhancing adaptive immunity; however, they are also involved in the pathogenesis of autoimmune, chronic inflammatory, and infectious diseases (*Chapter 12*). It seems possible that most inflammatory and immune-mediated diseases will have a TLR component identified at some level in the future.

TLR4 is expressed predominantly on myeloid cells, i.e., monocytes/macrophages, neutrophils, and dendritic cells, and recognizes LPS from gram-negative bacteria in association with at least other two molecules, CD14 and MD-2, that participate in the complex of recognition-signaling induced by LPS. In addition to LPS recognition, TLR4 can also recognize

Table 3-5. Some examples of major PRRs

Soluble
Pentraxins: C-reactive protein (CRP), serum amyloid P (SAP), pentraxin-related protein (PTX3)
Collectins: surfactant proteins A and D (SP-A, SP-D), mannose-binding lectin (MBL), MBL-associated proteins (MASP)
Complement: C3b
LPS-recognition proteins: soluble CD14, LPS-binding protein (LBP)
Cell-bound
Toll-like receptors (TLR): seven molecules TLR1, TLR2, TLR4, TLR5, TLR6, TLR10, TLR11
Scavenger receptors: macrophage scavenger receptor (MSR), scavenger receptors AI, AII (SR-AI, -AII), macrophage receptor with collagenous structure (MARCO)
Complement receptors (CR): four recognized molecules (CR1-CR4)
C-type lectin receptors: macrophage mannose receptor (MMR), dendritic-cell specific ICAM-3 binding non-integrin (DC-SIGN), Dectin-1
Others: CD14, N-formylmethionyl-leucyl-phenylalanine residues receptor (fMLF)
Intracellular
Toll-like receptors (TLR): four molecules TLR3, TLR7, TLR8, TLR9
CARD (Caspase-recruited domain) helicases: Retinoic acid-inducible gene I (RIG-I), melanoma differentiation-associated gene 5 (MDA5)
Interferon (IFN)-inducible proteins: dsRNA-dependent protein kinase (PKR), 2′,5-oligoadenylate synthetase (OAS)
NOD (Nucleotide-binding oligomerization domains)-like receptors (NLR): NOD1, NOD2, NOD3
PYD (Pyrin domain)-containing receptors: Pyrin and NACHT domain-containing proteins (PAN), NACHT-LRR and Pyrin domain-containing proteins (NALP), Pyrin domain-containing Apaf1-like proteins (PYPAF)

Table 3-6. Summary of human TLRs

Receptor	Ligand(s)	Pathogen
TLR 1	Triacyl lipoproteins	Gram-negative bacteria, mycobacteria
	Lipoproteins	All bacteria
	Lipoteichoic acids	Gram-positive bacteria
TLR 2	Lipoarabinomannan	Mycobacteria
	Zymosan	Fungi
	Glycosylphosphatidylinositol	Protozoans
TLR 3	Double-stranded RNA	Viruses
	Lipopolysaccharides	Gram-negative bacteria
TLR 4	Lipopeptides	Gram-negative bacteria
	Viral glycoproteins	Viruses
TLR 5	Flagellin	Bacteria
	Diacyl lipoproteins	Mycobacteria
TLR 6	Zymosan	Fungi
TLR 7	Single-stranded RNA	Viruses
TLR 8	Single-stranded RNA	Viruses
TLR 9	Unmethylated CpG DNA	Bacteria
TLR 10	Unknown	Unknown
TLR 11	Profilin	Protozoans

some host stress proteins such as heat shock proteins (e.g., hsp60 and hsp70 in the human). In some cases, association of two different TLRs constitutes the active recognition complex; e.g., bacterial triacylated lipopeptides are recognized by TLR1-TLR2 complexes and diacylated lipopeptides by TLR2-TLR6 dimers. TLR2 is also able to recognize gram-positive cell-wall peptidoglycan, mycobacterial lipoarabinomannan (**LAM**), and other products such as "atypical" LPS from *Porphyromonas gingivalis*, which causes periodontal disease. Mutations on TLR2 have also been correlated with susceptibility to lepromatous leprosy and staphylococcal septicemia. TLR5 recognizes flagellin, the principal component of bacterial flagella in bacteria such as *Salmonella*. Although the ligand for TLR10, present mainly on B cells, has not yet been identified, the ligand for TLR11 was found to be profilin, an actin-binding protein associated with cellular cytoskeleton.

In contrast, other TLRs are known to be localized within intracellular endosomes and are able to recognize viral nucleic acids (double-stranded RNA by TLR3, single-stranded RNA by TLR7 and TLR8) or bacterial unmethylated CpG, i.e., by TLR9 (Box 3-2). In every case, type I interferons (**IFN-α, -β**, and **-λ**), as well as pro-inflammatory cytokines or defensins, are induced upon their engagement with their specific receptors (*Chapter 13*).

TLRs recognize exogenous and endogenous PAMPs (indicated in the light yellow boxes) and trigger innate immune responses. TLRs are transmembrane proteins with an extracellular domain formed by leucine-rich repeats, and an intracellular domain with a structure very similar to IL-1 receptor. After ligand stimulation, TLRs are dimerized, and intracellular TIR domain joins to myeloid differentiation primary-response protein 88 (**MyD88**), a cytoplasmic adapter protein with two recognition sites, one for TIR and the other for the cytoplasmic enzyme IL-1R-associated kinase (**IRAK**). Kinases activate other proteins by binding a phosphate group to them. Once recruited, IRAK suffers a further activation by autophosphorylation, and binds to the TNF-receptor-associated factor 6 (**TRAF-6**). The IRAK-1/TRAF-6 complex dissociates from the membrane and associates with another complex formed by TGF-β-activated kinase-1 (**TAK-1**) and TAK-1-binding proteins (**TABs**). After activation, TAK-1 phosphorylates both the inhibitor of the NF-κB (**IκB**) kinase (**IKK**) and the mitogen-activated protein kinase (**MAPK**), leading to reaction cascades that culminate with the activation of the transcription factors NF-κB and c-Jun N-terminal kinase (**JNK**), respectively. In cytoplasm, NF-κB is sequestered by its specific inhibitory protein (**IκB**). IKK phosphorylates IκB and it is released from NF-κB. Then, free NF-κB is finally translocated to the nucleus of the cell, allowing its binding to the promoter regions of genes for cytokines, inducible nitric

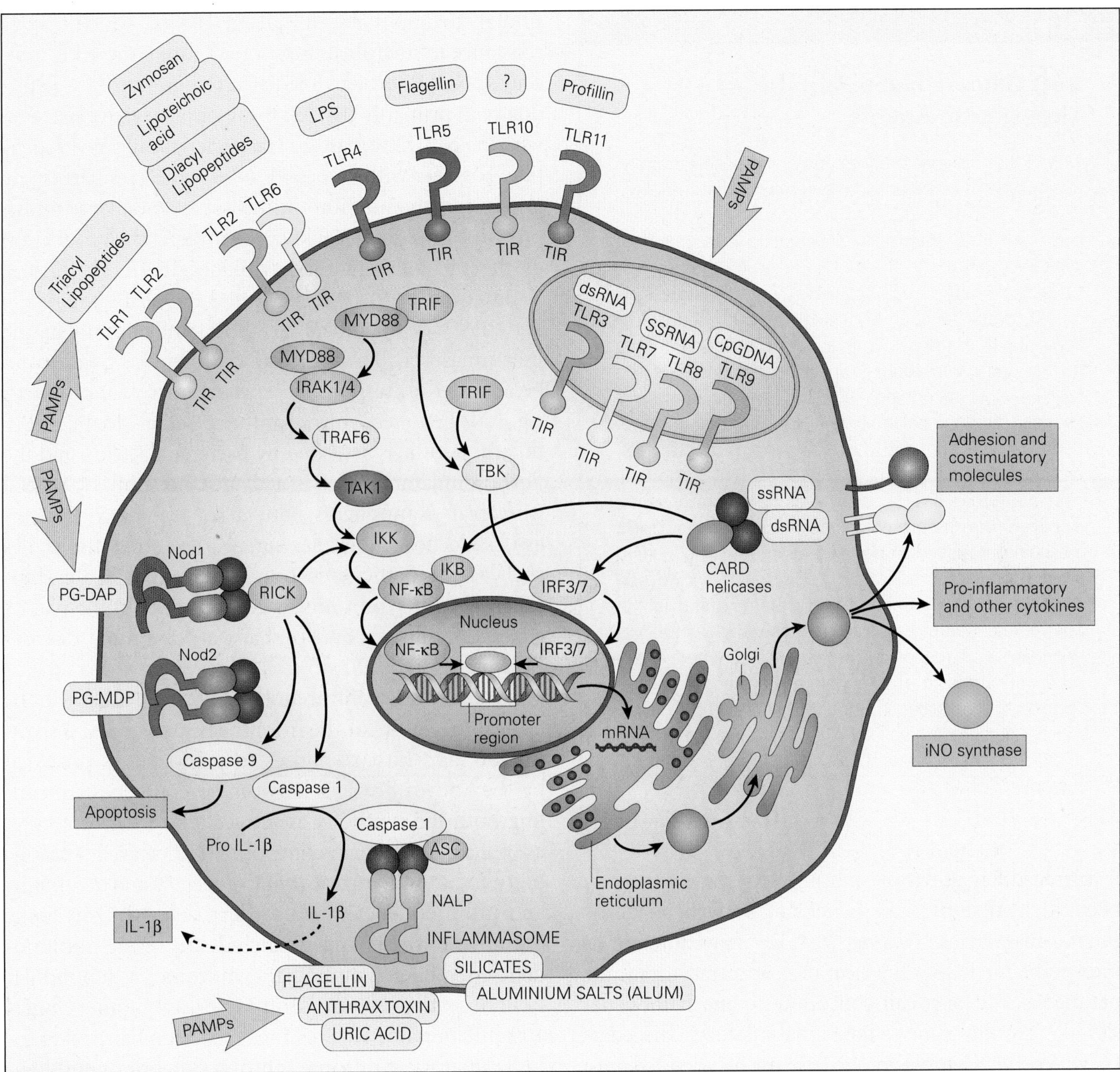

Figure 3-5. Schematic representation of the membrane-associated and intracytoplasmic location of the toll-like receptors (TLRs) and the critical role of the recognition and signaling pathways of the TLRs and the inflammasome.

oxide synthase, and co-stimulatory molecules of the adaptive response (Figure 3-5).

Although it is not the purpose of this chapter to give an exhaustive review of the different families of PRRs that participate in innate immunity, some important receptors are briefly described below.

Dendritic cell–specific, intercellular adhesion molecule-3 (ICAM-3) grabbing non-integrin (**DC-SIGN**) CD209 is another cell-surface PRR that belongs to the C-lectin family of receptors and is expressed on dendritic cells (**DCs**). This molecule participates in the interaction between DCs and T cells, as well as in DC migration, but more importantly is its capacity to recognize PAMPs of different viruses and microorganisms, as HIV, dengue virus, mycobacteria, or yeast. DC-SIGN engagement can, in fact, either promote phagocytosis of microorganisms or paradoxically facilitate the entry of HIV to T cells; however, it also mediates the phagosome maturation as well as the production of nitric oxide and oxygen metabolites. However, the role of DC-SIGN and other molecules of the C-lectin family (e.g., dectin-1) is not well understood in innate immunity, but it is thought that these could play a role in the interaction between innate and adaptive immunity because of their participation in the relationships among DC and T cells.

Box 3-2

CpG Oligodeoxynucleotides as Therapeutic Agents

One of the major differences between CpG oligodeoxynucleotides in bacteria and the human is that the oligodeoxynucleotides in bacteria contain unmethylated cytosine and guanosine dinucleotide (CpG) repeat motifs in contrast to the human in which these structures are methylated. Only the unmethylated CpG repeat motifs function as PAMPs and are capable of activating both the systemic and mucosal components of the innate and acquired immune responses of the human. CpG recognition by TLR9 mainly in macrophages, dendritic cells, and NK cells induces the production of IL-12 and IL-18 (which promote IFN-production), the inflammatory cytokine TNF-α, the antiviral interferons IFN-α/β, as well as defensins (*Chapter 9*). Therefore, as promoters of Th1 responses, CpGs are being proposed to be used as immunomodulating agents for use as adjuvants, to improve vaccine efficacy, to enhance cancer immunotherapy, and in the control and treatment of allergic diseases where predominant Th2 responses are seen and where CpG-mediated shifts to Th1 responses can lead to better control of the disease. Recent studies using CpG motifs conjugated to specific allergens has been shown to offer a new approach to allergen immunotherapy (*Chapter 18*).

Intracellular (cytoplasmic) PRRs have recently been identified to have beneficial as well as detrimental properties (*Chapter 9*). They may function as important mediators for clearance of intracytoplasmic pathogens, but also can contribute to the pathogenesis of autoimmune and inflammatory disorders (*Chapter 19*). Cytoplasmic PRRs can be grouped into three families: IFN-inducible proteins, caspase-recruiting domain (**CARD**) helicases, and nucleotide-binding oligomerization domain (**NOD**)-like receptors (**NLRs**) (Figure 3-5).

The best known of these molecules belonging to the IFN-inducible family of proteins is the interferon-inducible double-stranded-RNA-dependent protein kinase (**PKR**), whereas retinoic-acid-inducible gene I (**RIG-I**) is the typical example of a CARD helicase. Both types of molecules recognize viral nucleic acids, and there is evidence suggesting their participation in the homeostatic controls of inflammatory reactions in diseases such as asthma or inflammatory bowel disease.

The NLR- and the PYD- (Pyrin domain) containing receptor families of intracellular PRRs in vertebrates are similar to molecules found in plants, which confer resistance to microbial infections. Among the NLR molecules, NOD1 protein mediates recognition of a peptidoglycan primarily derived from gram-negative bacteria, whereas NOD2 recognizes the bacterial muramyl dipeptide. Together with caspase-1, NLR molecules participate also in the organization of inflammasomes, large multiprotein complexes (700 kDa) controlling the production of the pro-inflammatory cytokines IL-1β, IL-18, and IL-33 (*Chapter 9*) (Box 3-3). NALP1, NALP2, NALP3, and IPAF are members of NLR family found in the inflammasome. These cytosolic protein complexes can be activated in response to specific microbial products; e.g., NALP1 recognizes anthrax lethal toxin, IPAF inflammasome is activated by bacterial flagellin, and the NALP3 inflammasome is activated not only by several microbial components, but also by many danger-associated host molecular signals, i.e., stress molecules such as the pathogenic role of uric acid in development of joint symptoms in gout or silica in the pathogenesis of silicosis and perhaps autoimmune diseases (*Chapters 5* and *19*).

Evidence that intracellular PRRs are likely to be critical regulators of the immune response, i.e., inflammation, and host responses to pathogens is provided by the known linkages between several genes controlling both the synthesis of intracellular PRR molecules as well as those which contribute to increased susceptibility to autoinflammatory (*Chapter 19* and *19 Annex*) and immunodeficiency disorders (*Chapter 16*). Some examples of these linkages include the severe immunodeficiency bare lymphocyte syndrome, a subpopulation of patients with Crohn's disease, some clinical autoinflammatory syndromes (e.g., familial cold autoinflammatory syndrome, chronic infantile neurological cutaneous and articular syndrome), neonatal-onset multisystem inflammatory disease, and Muckle-Wells syndrome. These findings support the concept that cytoplasmic PRRs constitute intracellular sensors of autologous and bacterial products and that mutational alterations of their genes can lead to ineffective receptors and, consequently, a dysregulated inflammatory response (*Chapter 5*).

In summary, distinct families of receptors of innate immunity serve to identify different microorganisms through their PAMPs, in soluble form, on membranes or even intracellular, starting immediate effector responses as well as cooperation in the induction of adaptive response; this in turn guarantees an efficient primary response able to cope with the driving microorganisms, limiting its load, invasiveness, or eliminating them.

Box 3-3

The Inflammasome

The Inflammasome is a large multiprotein (700 kDa), cytosolic complex capable of activating the protease caspase-1 responsible for secretion of the proinflammatory cytokines interleukin-1beta (IL-1β) and IL-18, as well as the induction of pyroptosis, an inflammatory form of cell death induced by a variety of ***external*** or ***internal stimuli*** (*Chapters 5* and *9*). Inflammasomes act as sensors formed in response to a wide range of stimuli including microbial (i.e., pattern-associated molecular patterns or PAMPs), foreign and self-molecules, (i.e., danger- or damage-associated molecular patterns or DAMPs) that not only mediate protective innate immune responses towards invading pathogens and deleterious cellular damage, but also regulate adaptive immune response. Inflammasomes are comprised of cytosolic pattern-recognition receptors of the nucleotide-binding oligomerization domain (Nod)-like receptor (NLR) family and the oligomerization of several NLR proteins with other adapter molecules results in the generation of the active inflammasome (*Chapter 9*). Although inflammasomes are comprised of a variety of diverse constitutive monomeric parts, their basic structure consists of a central nucleotide-binding domain (NBD). Formed by self-oligomerization, these pivotal structured sensors are located between an aminoterminal protein-protein interaction domain (caspase recruitment domain [CARD], pyrin [PYD] or baculovirus inhibitor of apoptosis repeat [BIR]), and a carboxy-terminal leucine-rich repeat (LRR) domain responsible for the recognition of particular ligands. The most important inflammasomes identified, thus far in humans, are IPAF (ICE protease-activating factor), typically activated by ***external microbial PAMP stimuli*** including bacterial flagellins; NLRP1 (NLR related protein 1), activated by the *Bacillus anthracis* lethal toxin; and the NLRP3/cryopyrin, activated by bacterial peptidoglycans and lipopolysaccharides, viral and bacterial RNA and DNA as well as by ***other DAMP stimuli***, e.g., serum amyloid A (SAA) or cholesterol crystals, and inorganic materials as urate (gout), calcium pyrophosphate (pseudogout) crystals asbestos (asbestosis), silica (silicosis) and aluminum adjuvant (vaccines). Mutations and polymorphisms in inflammasome-related proteins have been recently identified in a variety of autoinflammatory diseases which are assuming great clinical importance (*Chapter 19 Annex*). The effector molecule of the inflammasome is the active caspase-1, a cysteine protease dimetric complex that is formed after the combination of two CARD domain-containing precursor procaspase molecules. The final functional consequence of inflammasome activation is a form of programmed cell death called *pyroptosis* resulting in cell death, necrosis and inflammation, in contrast to *apoptosis* that represents a normal homeostatic mechanism of programmed cell death without necrosis and inflammation (*Chapters 5* and *9*). Pyroptotic cell death can be considered a generalized protective host response mechanism triggered by microbial infectious agents e.g., *Salmonella* and *Shigella* species, as well as a deleterious response leading to pathologic inflammatory conditions, e.g., gout, stroke, heart attack or cancer.

Elements of Innate Immunity

A Variety of Leukocytes Participate in Innate Immunity by Producing Inflammatory Mediators

When the innate immune response is triggered, a wide variety of cells from both the immune system and other tissues participate in the body's response to injury, which is referred to as the inflammatory response (*Chapter 5*). These include epithelial and endothelial cells, neutrophils, mononuclear phagocytes, dendritic cells, mast cells, NK cells, and other cells (Table 3-7) which bring about their inflammatory effects through the production of substances referred to as mediators (*Chapter 1*) and are therefore referred to as pro-inflammatory cells. Inflammation is the collective term for the tissue, cellular, and molecular consequences of such responses.

Soluble Mediators Control the Innate Immune Response

As described previously, cells produce various soluble molecules, collectively known as mediators, which control the activation, direction, magnitude, and duration of the innate and inflammatory responses. Mediators can be preformed and accumulated within storage granules in the cells, whereas others, as required, are synthesized *de novo* or derived from inactive soluble precursors normally found in plasma. When neutralization or elimination of the inductive stimuli occurs, resolution of the response is the healing process. Chronic inflammation results from failure in controlling mediator production by cells of the innate immune system, so the uncontrolled production of pro-inflammatory molecules is responsible for tissue damage in the host (*Chapter 5*).

The development of inflammatory reactions is mediated by protein products of the plasma enzyme systems (complement, coagulation, fibrinolytic, and kinin pathways), by vasoactive mediators released from mast cells, basophils, and platelets (histamine) by lipid mediators (prostaglandins [**PG**], leukotrienes [**LTs**], and platelet-activating factor [**PAF**]) as well as by peptides (cytokines and chemokines) released from different cells. At the beginning of the

Table 3-7. Principal cells involved in the innate immune response

Cell	Examples/location	Products/mechanisms	Function
Epithelial	Skin, mucous membranes	Chemokines, cytokines, defensins, and cathelicidins	Mechanical barrier and active producer of protective mediators
Endothelial	Blood vessels	Up-regulate adhesion molecules and produce nitric oxide, cytokines, chemokines, and other inflammatory mediators	Clearance of foreign substances
Neutrophils	Blood	Microbicidal activity using oxidative and nonoxidative processes Neutrophil extracellular traps (NETs)	Phagocytosis/intracellular digestion Antimicrobial defense
Mononuclear phagocytes	Blood, tissues	Secretion of cytokines and chemokines, e.g., TNF-α, IL-1β, IL-6, IL-8, type I interferons (IFN-α, β, γ),	Phagocytosis and intracellular digestion Production of cytokines Antigen processing and presentation
Dendritic cells	Plasmacytoid (pDCs) Myeloid (mDCs) Tissues	Type I interferons (IFN-α, β, γ), Th1 polarizing cytokines (IL-12 family [IL-12, IL-23, and IL-27]). Treg-polarizing cytokines (IL-10 and TGF-β)	Antigen-presenting cells, co-stimulation for T cells, Th1, and Treg polarization
Mast cells	TC type in skin and intestinal submucosa, T type in intestinal mucosa and lung alveolar walls	Tryptase, chymase, cathepsin G-like protease, carboxypeptidase, histamine, leukotrienes, platelet-activating factor, TNF-α, IL-4	Promote inflammation important in allergic and parasitic diseases
Natural killer (NK)	Blood, liver, spleen, bone marrow	IFN-γ	Elimination of virally infected cells or malignant cells
Basophils	Blood	Similar to mast cells	Similar to mast cells
Eosinophils	Blood	Major basic protein, eosinophil cationic protein, eosinophil peroxidase, eosinophil neurotoxin, prostaglandin E2, leukotrienes, PAF, metalloproteinases, cytokines, chemokines	Important in allergic and parasitic diseases

inflammatory reaction triggered by a microbe, bradkinin in plasma, and histamine and proteases released by mast cells in the tissues are the main mediators produced. Later, complement-system-derived anaphylatoxins and cell products such as chemokines, cytokines, PGs, LTs, and PAF, are responsible for the accumulation and/or activation of epithelial and endothelial cells and neutrophils, macrophages, and other leukocytes. Once leukocytes have arrived at a site of injury, they release other mediators such as reactive oxygen intermediates (**ROIs**) and nitric oxide (**NO**) as well as proteolytic enzymes, which participate in the inactivation and removal of invading infectious agents, whereas cytokines and chemokines are active in controlling the recruitment and activation of cells and in the reconstruction of the damaged tissue. Other participating cells, such as lymphocytes, dendritic cells, and NK cells, mainly release cytokines and chemokines.

Because most of the mediators of inflammation will be described in Chapter 5, only a brief summary of the participation of cytokines and chemokines is included here (*Chapters* 5 and *9*).

Cytokines and Chemokines Are Soluble Cell-Cell Communication Molecules

As described in Chapter 9, cytokines are a heterogeneous group of cell-derived peptides with low

molecular weight (8–45 kDa) that function as the cell-cell messengers that exert their effects by binding to specific high-affinity receptors on cell surfaces. Cytokines comprise the interleukins (**ILs**), interferons (**IFNs**), growth factors (**GFs**), colony-stimulating factors (**CSFs**), and chemokines, a particular family of small polypeptide cytokines that function as chemoattractants for migrating cells. Virtually all cells of the body produce and respond to a wide variety of cytokines due to the highly complex nature of the cytokine network which not only influences their own expression (self-regulation) but also their production and activity on other regulatory cytokines. These responses are evident at different levels of organization, ranging from individual cells to the level of the complete organism and depend upon timing, concentration of cytokines, and distribution of their receptors. Individual cytokines are **pleiotropic** in their functions, i.e., acting on multiple target cells, and **redundant**, meaning that there are different molecules producing similar effects. This pleiotropism and redundancy in the network of cytokines guarantees its complete and efficient performance, since even under pathological conditions, if there is a missing or deficient cytokine, others can substitute or compensate for its deficient function. Another noteworthy characteristic of cytokines is their **synergy**, so that the effects observed with a single cytokine are markedly enhanced when two or more are simultaneously produced. The response to cytokines can be **autocrine** when its effect occurs on the same cell producing the cytokine, **paracrine** if it influences another cell at a short distance, and **endocrine** when its actions are systemic at distal sites to their production. Functionally, cytokines are not only mediators of both innate and adaptive immune responses but also participate in the regulation of other body functions, such as temperature, appetite, and sleep patterns.

There are two main groups of cytokines with respect to their role in inflammation: (1) **pro-inflammatory cytokines** and (2) **anti-inflammatory cytokines**. The pro-inflammatory cytokines carry out diverse activities such as cell activation, up-regulation of the synthesis of other cytokines, enhancement of chemotaxis of inflammatory cells, stimulation of leukopoiesis, synthesis of acute phase proteins, and the induction of fever and other systemic manifestations. Major participating pro-inflammatory cytokines in innate immunity include tumor necrosis factor-alpha (**TNF-α**), several interleukins (IL-1β, IL-6, IL-8, and IL-33), and type I (IFN-α and IFN-β) and type III (IFN-λ) interferons. TNF-α constitutes the most important cytokine in inflammation, and IL-6 to a lesser extent, since several of the main physiological changes observed in experimental models of sepsis (e.g., fever and wasting) have been shown to be associated with these cytokines. As an example, the most important biological characteristics of TNF-α are summarized in Box 3-4. Conversely, anti-inflammatory cytokines control the magnitude of the inflammatory process by counteracting

Box 3-4

Tumor Necrosis Factor Alpha (TNF-α)

Origin. Activated mononuclear phagocytes, neutrophils, mast cells, NK cells, activated T cells, B cells, vascular endothelial cells, smooth muscle cells, keratinocytes. Most of the TNF-α remains expressed on the cell membrane where extracellular proteases cleave the molecule into the free form.

Receptors. Two cellular TNF receptors (TNF-R1 and TNF-R2) in all cell types except for the red blood cells. Soluble TNF receptors (sTNFRs) are also found in plasma and may function to block the effectiveness of TNF-α in cancer (Chapter 20).

Autocrine activities. *On macrophages*: enhancement of phagocytosis and other inflammatory mediators, up-regulation of MHC-II molecules, TNF-α production. *On neutrophils*: up-regulation of adhesion molecules.

Paracrine activities. Apoptotic cell death, cellular proliferation, differentiation, inhibition of viral replication.

Endocrine activities. *On hypothalamus:* fever, appetite suppression, release of corticotropin-releasing hormone (CRH), release of hypothalamic monoamines and peptides. *On liver*: stimulating production of acute phase proteins. *On endothelial cells*: up-regulation of adhesion molecules expression, prostaglandin PGI, and coagulation factors synthesis. *On bone marrow*: hematopoiesis. *On muscle cells*: protein breakdown. *On endothelial cells*: up-regulation of adhesion molecules expression, prostaglandin PGI, and coagulation factors synthesis. *On fibroblasts*: cell proliferation, collagen synthesis.

Synergism. With IL-1β, IL-6, type I IFNs (IFN-α and INF-β).

Other activities. At high concentrations induce endotoxic shock-like symptoms; stimulation of endothelial cells for the production of tissue factor that may trigger the extrinsic pathway of the coagulation; hypotension resulting from the inhibition of myocardial contractility and vascular smooth muscle tone. Prolonged low concentrations result in cachexia, a wasting syndrome, and suppression of T cell functions.

Pharmacological control. Monoclonal antibodies: infliximab, adalimumab. Soluble TNF-α receptor fusion protein (etanercept).

various aspects of this process. This category includes IL-10, transforming growth factor-beta (**TGF-β**), and the IL-1 receptor antagonist (**IL-1ra**). In addition to their classification as pro- and anti-inflammatory activities, some cytokines can play different roles depending on the environment, e.g., IL-6, IL-10, and IFN-γ, displaying one or another property depending upon the sites of their synthesis or the magnitude of their response.

Inflammatory Mediators Attract Leukocytes into the Infection Site

Some pro-inflammatory cells, i.e., the epithelial and endothelial cells, are fixed in organ structures and remain *in situ* after activation, while others, such as the circulating leukocytes, migrate from the blood into tissues in response to activating stimuli provoked by the mediator substances (Figure 3-6). The directed movement and cellular influx into tissues of leukocytes, referred to as chemotaxis, is mediated by a group of proteins and peptides that are used by the host as signaling compounds. These include the participation of chemokines (*Chapter 9*) and C5a (a component of complement, *Chapter 4*) and occurs through interactions between cell-surface adhesion molecules on leukocytes and endothelial cells (Table 3-8).

The Cellular and Molecular Events Associated with the Inflammatory Response

The cellular and molecular events associated with the inflammatory response comprise a set of highly

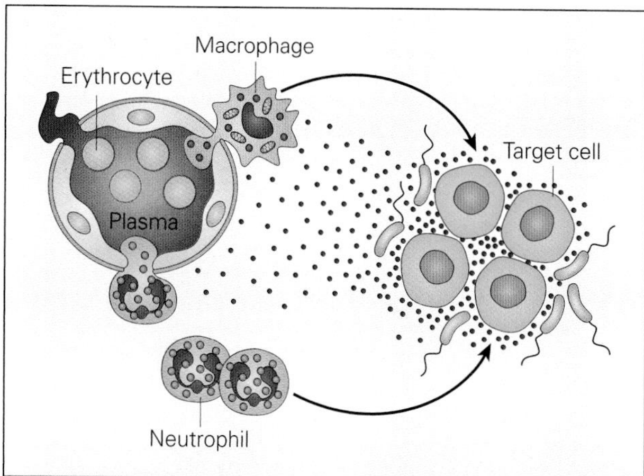

Figure 3-6. Schematic representation of the chemotaxis of phagocytic cells. After bacterial infection or injury of target cells, chemokines (as depicted as a gradient of red dots) are produced that recruit the egress of circulating monocytes that differentiate into tissue macrophages as well as neutrophils from the vascular compartment to the affected tissue site. The complement-derived fragment C5a (not shown) also displays chemotactic capacity.

integrated events between inflammatory cells and vascular endothelium mediated by a set of highly specialized adhesion molecules that include selectins, Ig superfamily molecules, and integrins that are described in greater detail in Chapter 5 and are summarized in Table 3-8.

Initial contact is performed by molecules from the selectin family (L-, E-, and P-selectins) and their glycoprotein ligands; these molecules lead to the initial loose and transient adherence of inflammatory cells to vascular endothelium. In later phases, the Ig superfamily molecules and integrins play major roles and are associated with firmer adhesion, locomotion, and transendothelial migration of inflammatory cells. These events are mediated by integrins (leukocyte function-associate antigens [**LFA-1** and **-3**]; very late antigens [**VLA-1** to **-6**]) and their ligands from the immunoglobulin superfamily molecules (intercellular adhesion molecules [**ICAM-1**, **-2**, **-3**], vascular cell adhesion molecules [**VCAM-1 to -4**], and others [Table 3-8]). Several other mediators, mainly cytokines, mediate local cell activation, and other molecules can participate significantly in the amplification and permanence of the cell response. Among these mediators, the most important are proteolytic enzymes, active peptides (the anaphylatoxins C3a, C4a, and C5a, and kinins), histamine, biolipids (prostaglandins, leukotrienes, and platelet activation factor), ROIs, and NO. They are released by activation of the complement cascade found in plasma, degranulation of mast cells, secretion by other inflammatory cells upon stimulation, or derived from damaged endothelial cells in blood vessels at the site of inflammation (*Chapter 4*). All participating cells have PRRs and receptors for Fc fragments of immunoglobulins and for complement components.

Epithelial Cells Provide the First Line of Defense Against Pathogens

Epithelial cells are found on the external surfaces of the body, primarily on the skin, the conjunctival surfaces of the eyes, the internal surfaces of the digestive, respiratory, reproductive, and urinary tracts, and the ducts of various glands and provide the first anatomic barriers to penetration of inimical substances into the host (*Chapter 1*). Epithelial surfaces not only constitute the first anatomical barrier to infectious agents but also actively participate in innate immune responses through the generation of products that initiate inflammation. These cells are joined and maintained together by tight junctional attachments

Table 3-8. Adhesion molecules involved in leukocyte traffic

Family/molecules	Distribution	Cell ligand
Selectins (transient interaction)		
Selectin L (CD62L)	Leukocytes	Glycoproteins
Selectin E (CD62E)	Endothelium	Glycoproteins
Selectin P (CD62P)	Endothelium, platelets	Glycoproteins
Ig superfamily (strong interaction)		
CD2	T cells	LFA-3
ICAM-1(CD54)	Endothelium (activated), dendritic cells, lymphocytes	LFA-1, CR3
ICAM-2(CD102)	Endothelium (non-activated), dendritic cells	LFA-1, CR3
ICAM-3(CD50)	Lymphocytes	LFA-1
ICAM-4(CD242)	Erythrocytes	LFA-1, CR3
VCAM-1(CD106)	Endothelium (activated)	VLA-4
LFA-3	Dendritic cells, lymphocytes	CD2
Integrins (strong interaction)		
LFA-1	Monocytes/macrophages neutrophils, T cells, dendritic cells	ICAM-1, ICAM-2, ICAM-3, ICAM-4
CR3 (Mac-1)	Monocytes/macrophages, neutrophils	ICAM-1, ICAM-2
VLA-4	Monocytes/macrophages, eosinophils, lymphocytes	VCAM-1

on the basolateral membranes that provide a protective barrier to the passage of substances from the external environment to the interior milieu of the cell. In the skin, the epithelium is composed by several layers of cells with dead cells in the outermost layer (Figure 3-7). In mucous membranes, some of the epithelial cells have cilia, which through their undulating action facilitate the removal of foreign particles, including infectious agents. Epithelial cells are not simply physical barriers, however, but play a very active role in local host defense by synthesizing a wide variety of antimicrobial molecules. These include antimicrobial peptides, i.e., defensins and cathelicidins (Box 3-5) with additional chemotactic activity for phagocytes, mucus, and enzymes that kill or limit the spread of most invaders as well as chemokines and cytokines that recruit and activate phagocytic cells (*Chapter 12*). The antimicrobial peptides act by disrupting the integrity of the microbial membranes through their net-positive charge and their ability to fold into amphipathic structures (i.e., relating to molecules which are hydrophobic at one end and hydrophilic at the other). The recognition of the important role of inflammatory substances produced by epithelial and endothelial cells is becoming increasingly apparent in the pathogenesis of asthma (*Chapter 18*).

The mucus layer over mucosal epithelia is composed of mucins associated with other proteins and lipids and forms a continuous gel into which a bicarbonate-rich fluid is secreted, maintaining a neutral pH at the epithelial surface. Mucins are synthesized and secreted by local goblet cells and are composed of protein backbone subunits to which a large number of carbohydrate side chains are attached. They represent active

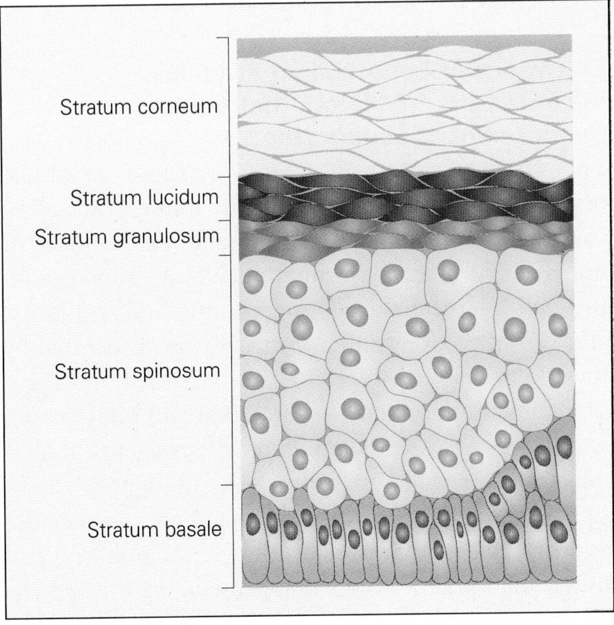

Figure 3-7. Schematic representation of the various layers of skin showing the metabolically more active cells in the stratum basale and dead cells in the stratum corneum.

Box 3-5

Antimicrobial Peptides

Defensins are a family of small (fifteen to thirty amino acids) cysteine-rich cationic amphipathic peptides. Defensins are essentially conserved natural antibiotics with antimicrobial activity against a range of microorganisms: gram-positive and gram-negative bacteria (*Chapter 12*), fungi (*Chapter 14*), and some viruses. Almost all the known defensins are multiple-disulfide bonded peptides with a cationic charge and are amphipathic. Human defensins comprise two subfamilies: α- and β-defensins, produced by different cell types including epithelial cells, macrophages, and neutrophils. The main antimicrobial mechanism of defensins is mediated through their ability to perforate viral and microbial membranes; once defensins are embedded at these sites, they form a pore in the membrane, allowing efflux of substances and the death of invaders. Defensins also serve as signals that initiate and amplify adaptive immune host defenses and may participate in tissue inflammation and endocrine regulation during infection.

The **cathelicidin** family of antimicrobial peptides includes a group of cationic and usually amphipathic peptides that display a variety of activities related to host defense functions, among which the most well known is a direct, broad-spectrum antimicrobial activity. Although the cytoplasmic granules of circulating neutrophils are the main source of cathelicidins, they also are produced by non-myeloid cells, particularly at sites such as skin and mucosal surfaces that are exposed to the external environment. In humans, only one cathelicidin, designated hCAP18/LL-37, has been identified. Cathelicidins rapidly kill a broad range of microorganisms using a mechanism that appears to be mediated by recognition of molecular patterns on the microbial surface with subsequent insertion into the lipid moiety thereby adversely affecting the integrity of microbial membranes. Cathelicidins may also provide protection against the detrimental effects of microbial invasion by binding and neutralizing potentially harmful microbial components such as endotoxin, lipoteichoic acid, and lipoarabinomannan. Another antimicrobial mechanism of cathelicidins is mediated indirectly through their ability to recruit inflammatory and immune cells by up-regulating the expression of chemokines and receptors in macrophages, neutrophils, and CD4+ T cells. Cathelicidins also display chemotactic effects inducing selective migration of human peripheral blood monocytes and may play a role in the repair of damaged tissue and wound closure by promoting wound neovascularization and re-epithelialization of healing skin.

components of the local immune response at mucosal surfaces because of their ability to fix commensal bacteria and interact with other components of the mucosal immune system, e.g., IgA (*Chapter 8*).

The Vascular Endothelium Produces Inflammatory Mediators that Enhance Recruitment of Leukocytes

The vascular endothelium is a dynamic metabolic organ that plays a major role in homeostasis. The endothelium regulates the flow and distribution of nutrient substances from the blood into tissues through the production of hemostatic, inflammatory, and vasoactive molecules, which are also generated by the blood cells themselves. The endothelium represents the interface between the blood and body tissues and is exposed to circulating infectious agents, malignant cells, or inflammatory mediators. Upon activation, endothelial cells up-regulate adhesion molecules and produce nitric oxide, cytokines, chemokines, and other inflammatory mediators, enhancing the recruitment and activation of circulating leukocytes to sites of intravascular infection. Leukocyte migration is controlled by these adhesion molecules that are expressed primarily on the endothelial surface of venules (Table 3-8). As described in Chapter 2, the high endothelial venules (**HEVs**) found in the paracortex of lymph nodes are key structures responsible for the recirculation of lymphocytes from the blood to the lymph. Lymphocytes that enter the lymph node from the circulation pass through these unique and highly specialized structures.

Phagocytosis Is the Major Cellular Mechanism for Pathogen Elimination

As described in Chapters 1 and 5, the term phagocytosis refers to the endocytosis of large particles, including infectious agents, mainly bacteria, fungi, and protozoans, performed by phagocytic cells which represent a distinctive group of specialized migratory cells derived from precursor CD34+ stem cells (*Chapter 2*). Phagocytic cells are comprised of two major groups: the neutrophils and the macrophages. Both are attracted to sites of injured or infected tissues by (1) chemokines secreted by these affected cells or (2) chemoattractants generated from soluble plasma-derived precursors, e.g., C5a complement.

Neutrophils Are the Predominant Pathogen-Killing Leukocytes

Neutrophils, also known as polymorphonuclear leukocytes (**PMNs**), are the most abundant white cells in the blood. Following an acute inflammatory stimulus, these cells are the first to migrate from the blood to peripheral tissues toward the site of inflammation, where they are sequestered, accumulated, and activated into the microvasculature. Activated neutrophils can eliminate foreign materials and invading microorganisms by several mechanisms. The first is through phagocytosis, engulfing and destructing inert particles and microorganisms using a combination of oxidative and nonoxidative processes (*Chapter 5*). A second mechanism is carried out by antimicrobial peptides (defensins and cathelicidins, Box 3-5), as described previously. A third defense mechanism utilizes neutrophil extracellular traps (**NETs**, Box 3-6), a web of secreted fibers composed of DNA, histones, and granule products produced by inflammatory stimuli or phagocytosis of infectious agents. These NETs have the potential risk of triggering local damage when they are released in an uncontrolled manner, leading to tissue or organ injury and dysfunction. Many microbial pathogens evolved to circumvent the attack of neutrophils through several protective mechanisms such as: (1) depressing the innate response, (2) interfering with their recognition, (3) inhibiting phagocytosis, (4) surviving intracellularly, (5) inducing the death of the neutrophil, and (6) evading killing by NETs.

Mononuclear Phagocytes Produce Key Inflammatory Cytokines and Chemokines

Mononuclear phagocytes (monocytes and macrophages) are essential for the development of inflammation and together with neutrophils are the phagocytic cells involved in the clearance of inert particles and microbial agents. Monocytes are bone marrow-derived cells and are continuously released into the blood. When these cells are recruited by chemotactic molecules and leave the circulation, they become activated and differentiate into macrophages. Other names have been applied to tissue macrophages such as Kupffer cells in the liver, histiocytes in connective tissues, mesangial cells in the kidneys, osteoclasts and condroclasts in bones and cartilage, alveolar macrophages in the lungs, and microglial cells in the brain. In contrast to neutrophils, which are end-stage nonreplicating cells continually replaced from the bone marrow, mononuclear phagocytes can proliferate *in situ* and are long-lived (i.e., months to years). Macrophages actually have a number of important functions in body defense such as (1) capture by phagocytosis and intracellular killing of microorganisms, infected cells, and tumor cells through PAMP recognition; (2) scavenging of worn-out cells, apoptotic bodies, and other debris potentially harmful to tissues; (3) processing and presentation of antigens for recognition by T cells, expressing co-stimulatory molecules, mainly during secondary adaptive immune responses (*Chapter 7*); and (4) releasing cytokines and chemokines that play

Box 3-6

Neutrophil Extracellular Traps

Neutrophil extracellular traps (NETs) are considered to be part of innate immunity because they ensnare and kill pathogens. Upon in-vitro activation with the pharmacological agent phorbol myristate acetate (PMA), IL-8, or LPS, neutrophils release granule proteins and chromatin to form an extracellular fibril matrix through an active process. Bacteria and some pathogenic fungi such as *Candida albicans* induce neutrophils to form NETs. Thus, NETs disarm pathogens with antimicrobial proteins such as neutrophil elastase and histones that are bound to the DNA, providing for a high local concentration of antimicrobial components and can bind, inactivate, and even kill microbes extracellularly independent of phagocytic uptake. NETs are known to be involved in host defense during pneumococcal pneumonia, streptococcal necrotizing fasciitis, and appendicitis. In addition to their antimicrobial properties, NETs may serve as a physical barrier that prevents further spread of pathogens. Furthermore, delivering the granule proteins of neutrophils into NETs may keep potentially injurious proteins like proteases from diffusing away and inducing damage in tissue adjacent to the site of inflammation. Paradoxically, NETs may also have a deleterious effect on the host because the exposure of extracellular histone complexes could potentially induce the development of autoimmune diseases like systemic lupus erythematosus (SLE) (*Chapter 19*). NETs have also been identified in preeclampsia, a pregnancy-related inflammatory disorder in which neutrophils are known to be activated. These observations suggest that NETs play an important role in the pathogenesis of infectious and inflammatory disorders.

a major role in innate immune responses. The major cytokines produced by macrophages are TNF-α, IL-1β, IL-6, and IL-8 (a CXCL chemokine) and IL-33 (*Chapter 9*), all of which are involved in local and systemic responses depending on the magnitude of the stimulus for their production, while interferons type I (IFN-α and β) and type III (IFN-λ) induce other viral-infected cells to arrest viral proliferation, activate NK cells, or increase the expression of MHC-I molecules on cell surfaces (*Chapter 9*). Some important systemic effects of cytokines produced by macrophages are fever induced by IL-1, wasting (i.e., cachexia) caused by TNF-α, production of acute phase proteins by liver induced by IL-6, and an increase in the maturation and release of neutrophils from bone marrow by IL-3. Although phagocytosis and cytokine/chemokine production are the two key effector functions of macrophages in the innate immune response, these cells also have a role in adaptive responses as antigen-presenting cells and as targets of the effector components of the cellular and humoral adaptive responses, being activated by T cell-derived cytokines and antibodies. Macrophage capacity to kill pathogenic microorganisms also can be overcome by microbes that are able to survive inside cells, establishing an intracellular infection, such as *Salmonella* spp, *Mycobacterium tuberculosis, Cryptococcus neoformans*, or *Toxoplasma gondii.* Macrophage activation by soluble products, e.g., IFN-γ, of the T cell arm of adaptive immunity, is the ultimate defense mechanism capable of terminating intracellular infection.

Dendritic Cells Produce Inflammatory Cytokines and Initiate Adaptive Immunity by Presenting Antigens to T Cells

Dendritic cells (DCs) are a sparsely distributed, migratory group of cells that are specialized to sample the sites of entry of infectious agents. Dendritic cells are not only important elements of the innate immune system but also constitute the most efficient antigen-presenting cells for T cell activation, thus linking innate and adaptive immune responses. There are two subsets of DCs: (1) plasmacytoid (pDCs) and (2) myeloid (mDCs), derived from lymphoid or myeloid precursors, respectively (*Chapter 2*). A distinguishing feature of pDCs is their capacity to produce large amounts of type I interferons, i.e., IFN-α and IFN-β, during the course of viral infection driven by activation via the endosomal TLR7 and TLR9 pathways, while mDCs respond best to bacterial infection, recognizing LPS via the cell-surface TLR4 together with the production of IL-12 and TNF-α. Both types of DCs circulate in the blood prior to migration into epithelial sites of skin and mucosal tissues, where they remain as immature DCs. These cells utilize the mechanisms of pinocytosis (i.e., "cell-drinking," a form of endocytosis in which small droplets of liquids are brought into the cell suspended within small vesicles) and phagocytosis for the uptake of a wide variety of foreign proteins and infectious agents. This results in the activation of DCs during which the maturation of the cells is promoted with the expression of the chemokine receptor CCR7 allowing the cells to migrate from the periphery to secondary lymphoid organs. During emigration, the captured molecules are processed into small peptides, linked to the grooves of MHC-II molecules, and expressed on the cell surface of DCs (*Chapter 7*). By the time DCs reach secondary lymphoid organs, they are able to present antigens to populations of naïve and memory T cells. Activated DCs also produce cytokines of the IL-12 family (IL-12, IL-23, and IL-27) with Th1-cell polarizing capacity and IL-6, IL-10, and TGF-β with regulatory T cell polarizing effects (*Chapter 9*). Therefore, DCs play a dual role in immune responses, first as an important component of the innate immune response activated by a variety of foreign agents and secondarily as the major bridge between innate and adaptive immune responses. This twofold function of DCs is accomplished not only through their role as the most efficient antigen-presenting cells of the innate immune system but also through their obligatory association with Th-cell subsets of the adaptive immune system.

Mast Cell Mediators Regulate a Variety of Physiological Systems

Mast cells (**MCs**) originate in bone marrow and circulate as CD34+ progenitor cells, differentiating into mature mast cells under the influence of cytokines only after entry into tissues. They are distributed throughout the body as resident cells, particularly in association with blood vessels and nerves, and in close proximity to mucosal surfaces that interface with the external environment (such as those found within the respiratory and gastrointestinal systems) and function in a variety of ways in the healthy individual.

After their development from bone marrow-derived progenitor cells that are primed with stem cell factor (**SCF**) (*Chapter 9*), mast cells continue their maturation and differentiation in peripheral tissue, developing into two well-described subsets of mast cells, MC(T) and MC(TC) on the basis on their enzyme content. The first subset consists of MCs containing tryptase (T), i.e., MC(T); the second are mast cells containing both trypsin (T) and chymotrypsin (C), i.e., MC(TC). The TC type predominates in normal skin and intestinal submucosa, and contains tryptase, chymotryptase, a cathepsin G-like protease, and a carboxypeptidase, whereas the trypsin-containing T type MC(T) is found in intestinal mucosa and lung alveolar wall. Mast cells are particularly important in innate immune responses because they are capable of detecting infectious agents and initiating an acute inflammatory response through the secretion of mediators. These cells recognize microbial PAMPs through TLR1, -2, -4, and -6 and the complement-derived molecules iC3b, and anaphylatoxins (C4a, C3a, and C5a) through their respective receptors. After activation, mast cells immediately extrude granule-stored preformed mediators (histamine, tryptase, chymase, and carboxypeptidase) and, in minutes, generate lipid-derived substances PG D_2 and the LTC_4, LTD_4, and LTE_4); and later, within hours, synthesize chemokines (CCL3, CCL4, and CCL5) and cytokines (TNF-α, IL-4, IL-5, and IL-6) (*Chapter 9*). The rapid release of these mediators promotes vascular permeability, induces vasoconstriction, and recruits eosinophils, neutrophils, and other cells within a very short time. Therefore, mediators released from MCs are among the main participants in the innate immune response, while chemokines and cytokines derived from them are also active in the adaptive immune response. However, mast cell activity does not end with this initial response; they continue to elaborate cytokines for hours after a single stimulus, expanding their participation in chronic inflammation. Other MC functions, such as their involvement in allergy or host defense mechanisms against parasitic infections, immunomodulation, and tissue repair and angiogenesis, will be described in Chapter 17.

Basophils and Eosinophils Also Participate in Innate Immunity

Basophils are granulocytes derived from bone marrow precursor cells and released into the blood circulation. Their characteristics and functions are similar to those described for mast cells. Eosinophils are another kind of blood granulocyte that can be recruited to sites of innate immune reactions, where their number can be 100 times higher than in the blood. Eosinophil cytoplasmic granules contain a variety of cationic proteins that exert several biological effects on normal cells and infectious agents, and these include: major basic protein (**MBP**), eosinophil cationic protein (**ECP**), eosinophil-derived neurotoxin (**EDN**), and eosinophil peroxidase (**EPO**). During the innate immune responses, and induced by phagocytosis of opsonized particles, the eosinophil granule content is released, acting mainly on extracellular helminthic parasites and contributing to tissue damage in inflammatory diseases. Other eosinophil products also participate in acute and chronic inflammatory reactions, particularly in allergic diseases (*Chapter 18*). These include LT, PAF, and cytokines such as granulocyte-macrophage colony-stimulating factor (**GM-CSF**), IL-3, IL-5, IL-6, IL-8, TNF-α, and TGF-β.

Natural Killer Cells Recognize and Kill Virus-Infected and Tumor Cells

Natural killer (NK) cells are large granular lymphocytes derived from bone marrow precursors and are found mainly in peripheral circulation (5 to 20 percent of total lymphocytes), spleen, liver, and bone marrow. The term "natural killer" was coined in the mid-1970s to indicate their natural occurrence and their capacity to kill tumor cells without prior sensitization. Although NK cells belong to the lymphoid lineage, they express neither T (TCR/CD3 complex) nor B (CD19) cell surface markers and are considered the third most important lymphocyte subset (*Chapter 2*). NK cells have a morphology similar to that of activated cytotoxic lymphocytes, i.e., a large size, an abundant endoplasmic reticulum (**ER**), and the presence of preformed granules containing perforins and granzymes.

Because they express CD16 (Fc-γRIII) and CD56, NK cells are usually identified as CD3−/CD56+/CD16+ cells. The role of NK cells in the innate immune response is remarkable because of their nonspecific capacity to eliminate target cells, e.g., virus-infected or malignant cells, through apoptosis independently of T or B cells. NK cells also stimulate inflammatory responses through secretion of IFN-γ, TNF-α, GM-CSF, and chemokines (CCL4, CCL5, CCL22) (*Chapter 9*).

NK cells recognize and kill target cells by apoptosis basically in two ways using an array of different cell surface receptors. The first method is part of the innate immune response and utilizes the complex balance between activating and inhibitory signals that the NK cell generates to either activate or inhibit their killing activity, respectively (Figure 3-8). Some NK cells have receptors generically called killer inhibitory receptors (**KIRs**) that belong to at least two groups of unrelated molecule structures (C-type lectin and immunoglobulin superfamily), which recognize MHC-I molecules on normal self cells and which, in the normal state, inhibit activation and killing due to the presence in their intracytoplasmatic tail of immunoreceptor tyrosine-based inhibitory motifs (**ITIMs**) (Figure 3-9 and *Chapter 5*). Another diverse set of lectin-type receptors, generically referred to as killer activating receptors (**KARs**), detect other molecules on altered target cells, e.g., malignant or virus-infected cells, which can provide an activation signal for the NK cell via immunoreceptor tyrosine-based activation motifs (**ITAMs**) (Figure 3-9). If a target cell has decreased expression of MHC-I (*Chapter 20*), the inhibitory signal from KIR will be decreased, shifting the signal balance towards activation of the NK cell and initiating the process of target cell death by apoptosis. Once the signal balance is tipped toward activation rather than inhibition, the killing mechanism is initiated, and the NK cells utilize their intracellular granules perforin and granzymes to kill the target cells by inducing apoptosis (Figure 3-8B). Upon release, perforin in close proximity to a cell slated for killing, first forms pores in the cell membrane of the target cell through which the granzymes and associated molecules then enter, inducing apoptosis (Figure 3-8B and *Chapter 9*). The NK cell may also utilize another innate immune response pathway leading to target cell death by apoptosis through the engagement of a surface molecule called Fas ligand (FasL, CD178) found on the NK cell with a Fas (CD 95) receptor on a target cell. Upon being activated, NK cells proliferate and produce IFN-γ, TNF-α, and several chemokines, which not only have important effects on other immune cells such as macrophages and T cells but which, in the case of TNF-α, can induce apoptotic cell death.

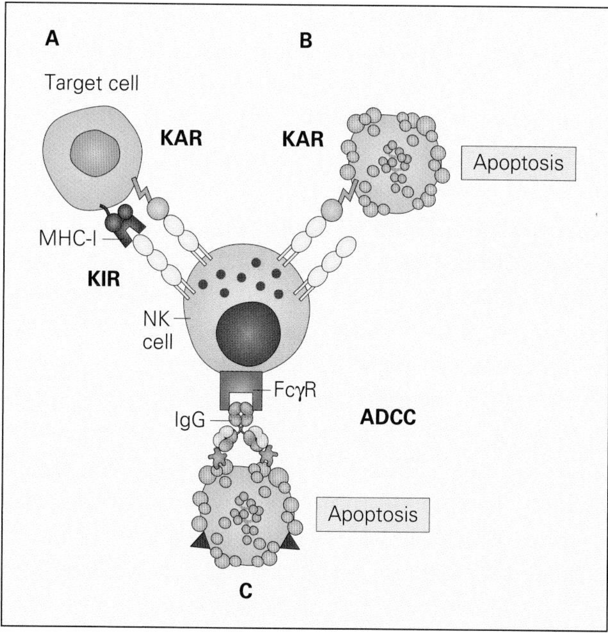

Figure 3-8. Natural killer cell activation. NK cells recognize and kill target cells by innate and adaptive immune mechanisms. In the innate response, without the participation of adaptive elements, activation or inhibition of NK cells is the result of a balance between positive and negative signals: Panel A: The activation signal is provided by activation of the killer activating receptor (KAR) and restrained by a negative signal provided by engagement of the killer inhibitory receptor (KIR) which normally overrides KAR and prevents NK cell-mediated apoptosis. This negative signal is provided by the recognition of self-MHC class I molecules Panel B: When target cells down-regulate or lack MHC class I molecules (mediated by viral infection or malignant transformation), the target cell becomes susceptible to NK cell-mediated killing by apoptosis. Panel C: In the adaptive response, NK cells kill target cells through the antibody-dependent cellular cytotoxicity (ADCC) mechanism: the FcγR on the NK cell engages the IgG molecule through its Fc fragment and the target cell is recognized by the Fab'2 portion of the molecule initiating the cascade of intracellular events which culminate with the apoptosis of the target cell.

The second method whereby NK cells kill target cells is through a hybrid mechanism in which the IgG molecule links the innate and adaptive immune systems and is referred to as antibody-dependent cellular cytotoxicity (**ADCC**) (Figure 3-8). In this scenario, the NK cell recognizes target cells to which IgG antibody has been attached through its Fab regions. At the same time, the Fc portion of the IgG antibody engages the NK cell through its Fc receptor referred to as CD16 (Fc-γRIII), thus linking the NK cell with the target cell (Figure 3-9). Following this linkage, the NK cell can destroy the target cell through induction of the apoptotic pathway as described above. The ability to utilize a variety of cytotoxic mechanisms makes the NK cell an essential combatant of the immune response in the struggle against malignant and virus-infected cells.

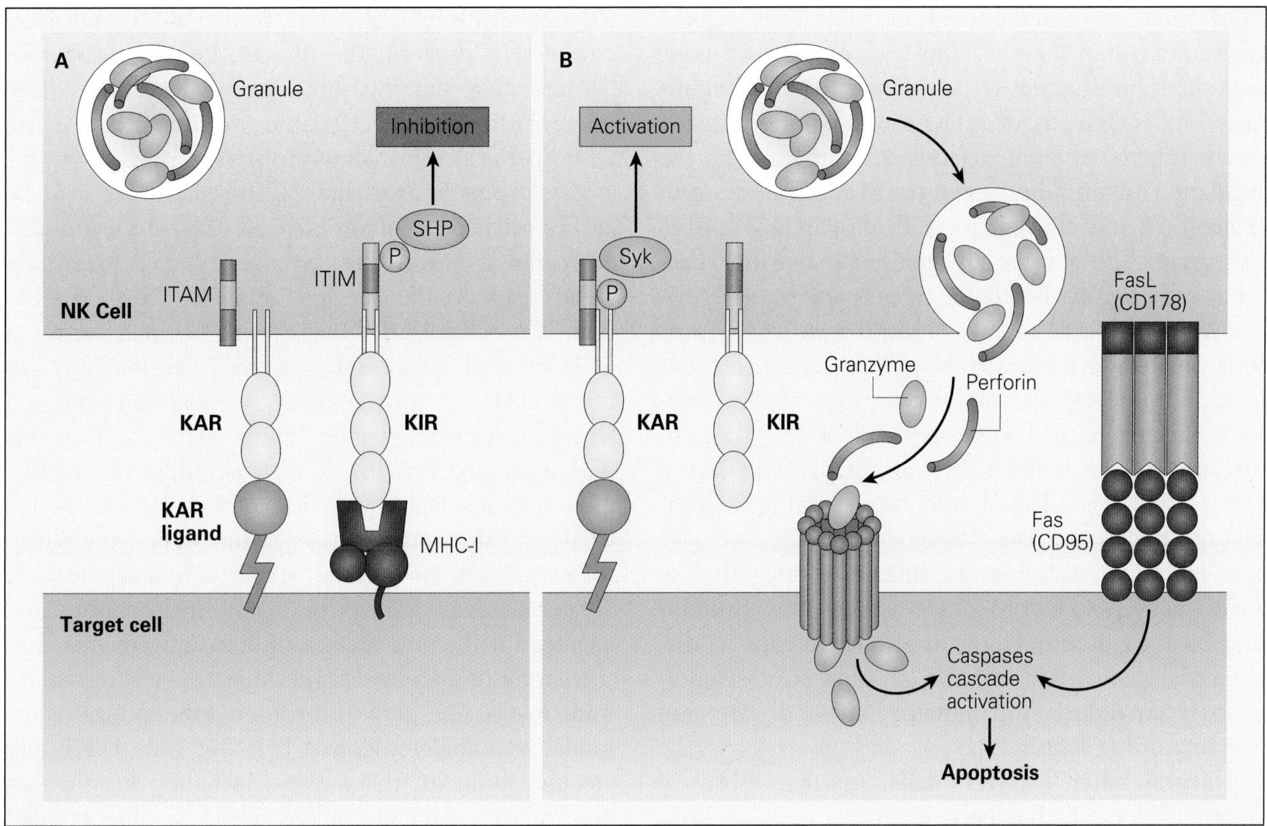

Figure 3-9. Schematic representation of the mechanism of cytotoxic action of NK cells. The NK cell displays 2 types of cell receptors, KAR which is stimulatory and KIR which is inhibitory. Panel A: Under normal conditions, the KIR molecules interact with MHC-I normally expressed on the target cell providing an inhibitory signal mediated by ITIM, overriding the stimulatory signal for NK cell activation by KAR; Panel B: NK cell activation is elicited by activation of the KAR mediated by ITAM when the target cell is not engaging KIR due to the failure of expression of MHC-I on the target cell. NK cell-mediated cytotoxicity is elicited by the release of granules containing perforin and granzymes that result in target cell apoptosis and release of cytokines and chemokines. The apoptotic cascade can also be triggered by the interaction of FasL (CD178) and Fas (CD95) molecules expressed on NK cells and target cells, respectively.

Some Lymphocytes Behave Like Innate Immune Cells

There are several subsets of thymus and bone marrow-derived cells that display characteristics of innate immunity, and therefore are referred to as *innate lymphocytes* or *innate-like lymphocytes*. These cell subsets express TCRs and BCRs with limited diversity, usually directed to the recognition of conserved antigenic structures up-regulated in stressed, infected, or transformed cells, and are protective against infection and cancer. The immediate mode of action of innate lymphocytes is a consequence of effector functions acquired during their maturation, rather than as a result of their activation after an encounter with their cognate antigen. Innate-like lymphocytes can therefore be considered bridges between the innate and the adaptive immune systems.

Gamma-delta T (γδT) cells. As described in *Chapters 2* and *7*, during thymopoiesis, two major types of mature T cells are generated from a common CD4– CD8– double-negative (**DN**) precursor: αβT cells and γδT cells, distinguished by the protein chains contained within their TCR complexes. Interestingly, γδT cells are the only cells that use somatic rearrangement to generate their antigen receptor repertoire. As mature cells, they are a minor population in the peripheral blood (1 percent to 15 percent of total lymphocytes); however, they are notably increased in the blood of patients during viral and bacterial infections and among the cells that infiltrate autoimmune target tissues. They also play an important role in mucosal immunity (*Chapter 8*). In the intestine, γδT cells are the major population of intraepithelial lymphocytes and they also constitute an important subset—although to a lesser extent—in the lungs.

The majority of γδT cells express neither CD4 nor CD8 markers, i.e., DN cells, and their TCRs have restricted recognition capacities for (1) some native

MHC molecules and the stress-inducible MHC-related molecules MICA/B and (2) host self or bacterial non-peptidic phosphorylated compounds (phosphoantigens), independently of MHC molecule presentation. At the functional level, γδT cells are implicated in the regulation of immune responses at mucosal surfaces (*Chapter 8*) and as a first line of defense in host epithelial surfaces in the response against some viruses, bacteria, and parasites before the recruitment of αβT cells. Activated γδT cells rapidly produce a variety of pro-inflammatory cytokines (IFN-γ, TNF-α) and chemokines, kill infected and tumor cells using similar cytotoxic effector mechanisms as NK and CD8+ αβT cells, and also behave as APCs through the participation of MHC-I and MHC-II molecules, as well as the co-stimulatory molecules. The pathologic relevance of γδT cells in human autoimmune diseases is suggested by their reactivity to highly conserved host stress proteins and by their accumulation in affected organs in diseases like rheumatoid arthritis, multiple sclerosis, pulmonary sarcoidosis, inflammatory bowel disease, and polymyositis (*Chapter 19*).

Natural killer T (NKT) cells. Another subset of natural killer cells has been identified as NKT cells, which were originally defined by the co-expression of T cell markers (CD3/TCR complex) along with characteristic surface receptors for NK cells (CD56, CD58, and CD161), indicating a dual nature of this subset. NKT cells can either express or not express CD4 or CD8 molecules and, similar to NK cells, are considered part of the innate immune response because they act swiftly during infections, killing microorganisms or cells and producing cytokines without the need of slower differentiation or proliferative processes as with T and B cells.

The original definition of NKT cells, which included a broader group of cells, is now restricted to a more specific subset, the so-called invariant NKT (**iNKT**) cells. They characteristically express on their surface a TCR invariant or constant region (Vα24/J18/Vβ11 in the human) able to recognize glycolipids presented on CD1d molecules (Figure 3-10). The CD1 family (CD1a through CD1d) consists of antigen-presenting molecules encoded by genes located outside of the MHC and structurally similar to the MHC-I molecules. In comparison to classical MHC molecules, the CD1 antigen-binding groove is highly hydrophobic and adapted for the presentation of lipid antigens that consist largely of glycolipids. The cognate α-galactosylceramide (α-Gal Cer, derived from a marine sponge) is the model glycolipid recognized by iNKT cells. iNKT cells are present in internal organs, including the thymus, bone marrow, liver, and spleen. There are other populations of cells expressing T and NK membrane markers differing from the iTCR cells, but showing variable TCRs, which are able to recognize a broader set of structures in microorganisms, and these are generically called NKT-like cells.

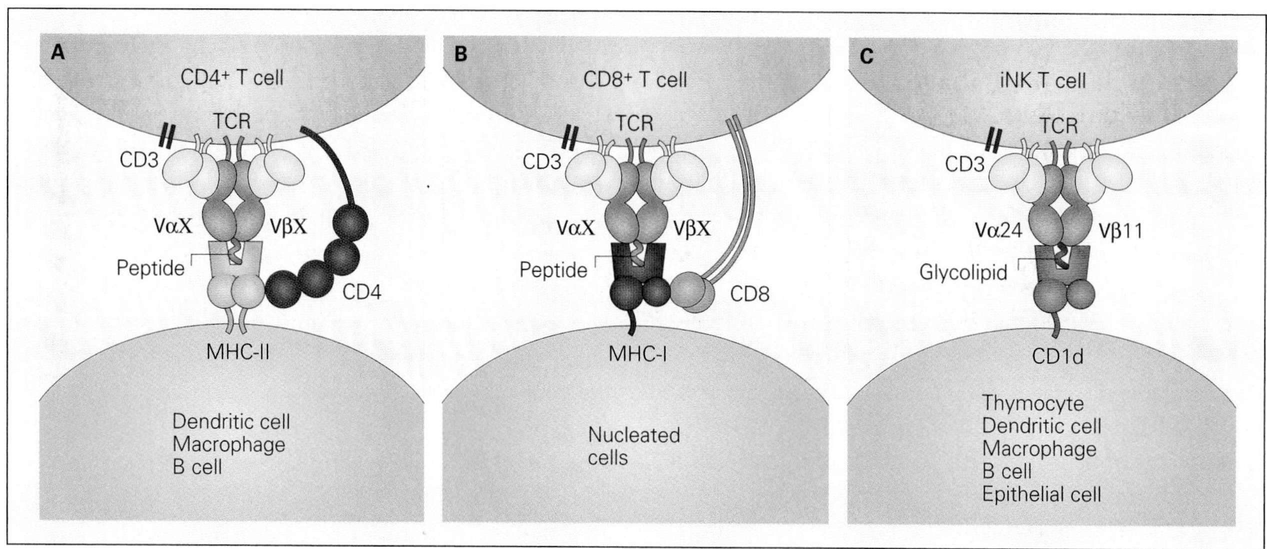

Figure 3-10. iNKT cells recognize antigen differently than T cells. Panel A: Peptides resulting from the antigen processing by "professional" antigen-presenting cells (mainly dendritic cells or macrophages) are presented on MHC-II molecules to highly variable specific TCRs expressed on helper CD4+ T cells. Panel B: In a similar fashion to A, nucleated cells are able to process proteins, and their peptides are presented on MHC-I molecules to CD8+ T cells, also expressing variable TCRs. Panel C: In contrast, iNKT cells express only a constant or invariant TCR (Vα24, Vβ11), which recognizes glycolipid molecules presented on MHC-I–like CD1d molecules on thymocytes, dendritic cells, macrophages, epithelial, and B cells.

After activation, iNKT cells quickly produce polarizing Th1- and Th2-type cytokines, such as IFN-γ and IL-4, respectively, suggesting an early role in immunoregulation of adaptive immune responses. There are data supporting the involvement of iNKT cells in autoimmune diseases, infectious diseases (viral, bacterial, fungal, protozoan, and helminthic), and asthma, both for improving the outcome as well as for impairing the course of the diseases, and also in the antitumor immune responses in experimental models and in humans.

In summary, NKT cells constitute a heterogeneous group of cells which form part of the innate immunity, involved in the early response to distinct insults. Their role in the entire immune response, particularly their functions in homeostasis is currently under intense study.

Mucosa-associated invariant T (MAIT) cells. These cells are found in low numbers in the intestinal lamina propria of humans and require commensal flora to expand and/or persist. They express a semi-invariant TCR (Vα7.2-Jβ33 chain), are double negative CD4– and CD8–, recognize hydrophilic antigens presented in MR1 (MHC-I–related (1) molecules present in B cells, and upon antigen activation, produce IFN-γ, IL-4, IL-5, and IL-10. Probably MAIT cells are the gut equivalent to internal NKT cells and may participate in protection of the gut and in the regulation of local immune responses.

B-1 cells. The B-1 cells are a phenotypically and functionally distinct subset of B cells, which spontaneously secrete "natural" IgM antibodies in the absence of any apparent stimulation by specific antigens (*Chapter 2*). Accordingly with the expression of CD5 molecules, B-1 cells are subdivided into B-1a that carry the CD5 molecule and B-1b that do not; B-1a cells represent the majority of B-lineage cells during neonatal life but decline thereafter. The repertoire of natural antibodies is much more restricted than those produced by conventional B cells and a large proportion are polyreactive to phylogenetically conserved structures such as nucleic acids, heat shock proteins, carbohydrates, and phospholipids. The antibodies produced by B-1 cells may participate as a bridge between innate and adaptive immunity and make an optimal transition between the two immune responses by producing the first wave of antibodies required for antigenic clearance of viruses, bacteria, and certain parasites. Other functions performed by these cells are in the immune regulation through the synthesis of IL-10 and in the clearance of senescent and apoptotic cells. It has been suggested that they are also involved in autoimmunity as increases in CD5+ B cell frequency have been reported in patients suffering from rheumatoid arthritis, Sjögren's syndrome, myasthenia gravis, insulin-dependent diabetes mellitus, and Hashimoto's thyroiditis (*Chapter 19*).

Marginal zone B (MZ B) cells. MZ B cells are a rare nonrecirculating subset of mature peripheral B cells exclusively located in the spleen, different from the more abundant recirculating follicular B cell subset. MZ B cell population is separated from the B cell follicle by the marginal sinus. MZ B cells express high levels of CD1d and CD21 molecules. They are quick and easily activated by low levels of antigen, are potent antigen-presenting cells for naive T cells, and produce short-lived IgM antibody-forming cells involved in the early defense against blood-borne pathogens, as well as in autoreactive B cell responses.

Immunological Principles Suggest New Treatments for Sepsis

Although it is beyond the scope of this textbook to present detailed descriptions of the treatment of sepsis and septic shock, it may be possible to construct a central unifying paradigm based upon immunologic principles outlined in this chapter. The overall strategy in dealing with sepsis is based primarily on counterattacking the deleterious effects caused by the strong innate immune responses unleashed against the invading microorganism as previously described in this chapter.

Antibiotics cannot completely reverse the sequelae of sepsis because the immunopathology of the syndrome is not simply caused by the infecting microorganism itself but primarily by the overwhelming uncontrolled inflammatory response initiated by the host against the microorganism. The ultimate rationale of treatment should therefore be directed to lessen as much as possible the detrimental effects of the inflammatory response and to attempt to reestablish the internal physiological equilibrium that existed in the host prior to infection. As described previously, during sepsis, vascular and hemodynamic equilibrium is lost owing to vascular clogging and leakage of blood vessels with resultant hypovolemia and hypotension. The basic strategy of treatment of the patient with severe sepsis, therefore, is directed to preventing the damage to vital organs and supporting vital signs using specific strategies including intravenous fluid replacement and trying to reverse the effects of hypotension with mechanical ventilation and cardiovascular support with vasopressors.

Several experimental models have been developed for the study of innate immune responses to bacterial infection and sepsis, particularly those caused by LPS released from gram-negative bacteria. An important contribution of this research was the observation that the TNF-α produced as a consequence of LPS injection was an important mediator causing much of the effects and symptoms present in sepsis. Based upon these observations, a novel approach for the treatment of sepsis in the human has been the use of neutralizing antibodies against TNF-α. In mice, the use of anti-TNF-α monoclonal antibodies (prior to LPS challenge) protected animals and abrogated the harmful or fatal effects of LPS with increased survival. The use of anti-TNF-α monoclonal antibodies in human clinical trials, however, has failed to ameliorate sepsis symptoms and in some cases actually worsened symptoms, with an increase in frequency of septicemia as a result of neutralizing TNF-α. There are several reasons for this failure, including the fact that the mice were pretreated with antibodies prior to LPS challenge, in contrast to humans, wherein the anti-TNF-α preparations were administered once the sepsis had begun. Another possibility is that the antibodies used in the human studies were incapable of completely neutralizing TNF-α. It is evident that the syndrome is so complex that many factors influence the symptoms, and trying to eliminate just one of these factors is not enough to reverse it. Moreover, patients chosen for the trials were clinically very heterogeneous; therefore, results obtained from several centers could not be compared. These findings suggest that: (1) animal models cannot always predict results in human trials, and (2) there is a need for more precise clinical criteria, definitions, and classification of sepsis, severe sepsis, or septic shock.

A second therapeutic approach for sepsis has been the possible therapeutic benefits offered by the anti-inflammatory effects of corticosteroids since many of the manifestations of sepsis result from the overwhelming inflammatory response of the host to microbial invasion. However, in several clinical studies, the only therapeutic benefit of corticosteroids in sepsis was seen in patients with secondary adrenal insufficiency using low doses of these agents.

Other approaches for treatment of sepsis with anti-inflammatory strategies have been suggested and include neutralizing IL-1 (with the IL-1 receptor antagonist anakinra (*Chapter 9*)), use of bradykinin antagonists, reducing PAF (e.g., the use of a phospholipase A2 antagonist), inhibiting arachidonic acid metabolites (use of prostaglandin E1 and thromboxane inhibitors), restoring the antioxidant potential of cells with N-acetylcysteine (for reactive oxygen species), inhibiting the enzymes for the nitric oxide synthesis, and neutralizing complement and coagulation factors. These treatment strategies have seen only varying degrees of success, possibly again due to the heterogeneity of clinical subjects included in these studies.

The best therapeutic results for the treatment of sepsis have been achieved through the use of activated protein C (**aPC**), a major physiological anticoagulant recently approved by the Food and Drug Administration. The mechanism of action of aPC is achieved by its ability to degrade factor Va and factor VIIIa, which not only provides physiologic antithrombotic activity but also anti-inflammatory and anti-apoptotic effects. Since plasma concentrations of aPC and protein S are reduced in severe sepsis, the rationale for aPC replacement therapy is to address the deficiency, believed to be the major cause of the hypercoagulability and resultant mortality seen in patients. Its use in severe sepsis has been shown to reduce mortality by 13 percent in patients with the highest risk of death.

Other possible therapeutic approaches to inhibit or control the harmful effects of the inflammatory response include: (1) control of apoptosis; (2) inhibition or control of the macrophage migration inhibition factor (**MIF**), which induces production of inflammatory cytokines and is increased in septic patients; (3) blockage of the complement factors C5a/C5aR; and (4) since severe inflammation occurs as result of an exaggerated response induced by PAMPs—involving different TLRs and/or NDLs—inhibiting or controlling this interaction would be desirable. It is obvious that owing to our incomplete understanding of the biology of the complex processes involved in such physiologic responses, we are far from being able to successfully treat, cure, or at least reduce significantly the death rate in patients with severe sepsis. More research will be required to fully understand the pathogenetic intervention points that can be used clinically to control the innate immune response when it is uncontrolled and life-threatening.

Conclusions

Evolution has provided vertebrates with a very complex set of biologic systems, among them the immune system, an intricate structure of interactive and interdependent cells and cellular products whose primary function is the recognition and disposal of foreign configurations which enter into or arise within the internal milieu. Innate immunity is the most primitive branch of this defensive protective network, formed by a cluster of soluble and membrane-associated receptors able to recognize a great diversity of infectious agents sharing common molecular structures called PAMPs. In addition, the efficiency with which the mechanisms of innate immunity are initiated allow them to rapidly proceed before an infecting microorganism reaches a critical infection-producing threshold (in minutes to hours) and does not need the "learning" experience required by the adaptive immune response (which requires days to mount an effective response and is dependent on prior experience with the microorganism). Thus, microbicidal mechanisms triggered by innate immunity can control most infections or at least reduce microorganism loads before adaptive responses start. However, innate immunity can sometimes result in harmful sequelae because of the resultant overwhelming and uncontrolled inflammatory response, which is initiated against the infection and can sometimes be the ultimate cause of death, as seen in severe sepsis and its complications.

Modern molecular biology together with many other scientific disciplines have revealed important elements of innate immunity such as TLRs and NLRs but more research will be required to fully understand and apply them to the management of human diseases. Further research will undoubtedly divulge possible new strategic intervention points that can be used clinically to control the innate immune response when it is unfavorably unleashed and becomes a life threat. Therefore, the efforts to deal with severe sepsis and related syndromes must be viewed from both the clinical and basic aspects of research and recognition that their interaction should increase the likelihood of success in tilting the host-parasite balance in favor of the host rather than the pathogen.

Case Study: Clinical Relevance

Let us now return to the case study of sepsis presented earlier and review some of the major points of the clinical presentation and how they relate to the immune system:

- The clinical case illustrates the pathophysiology of inflammation in a patient who presented with septic shock with multiple organ failure.
- The major clinical manifestations seen in the patient were initiated by the responses of the innate immune system to a gram-negative bacterial infection by Pseudomonas aeruginosa and the associated release of endotoxin and other PAMPs.
- These PAMPs then lead to stimulation of a specific set pattern-recognition receptors (PRRs) of the innate immune system referred to as TLRs found on the surface of many inflammatory cells, e.g., macrophages, and then endotoxin specifically leads to the stimulation of TLR-4.
- Other frequent microbial-related causes of sepsis are the lipoteichoic acids from gram-positive bacteria. In most situations, infections are usually controlled or completely cleared efficiently by the innate and adaptive responses without detriment.
- Sometimes, as demonstrated in this case, systemic disturbances are the culmination of a strong innate immune response together with inflammatory and coagulation responses.
- LPS-induced inflammation is often protective but also could be the cause of disease manifestations ranging from fever to shock and rapid death. The primary pathogenic effects in sepsis include production of fever (caused by fever-producing effects on the hypothalamus by the release of IL-1), an elevation of the number of circulating neutrophils, complement activation, activation of macrophages, aggregation of platelets, endothelium injury with increase of capillary permeability, and the release of nitric oxide.
- The presence of bacteria in blood is called bacteremia, and when clinical evidence of infection and signs of systemic response (fever, tachycardia, tachypnea, leukocytosis) are present, the term sepsis is applied. Moreover, sepsis syndrome is sepsis plus the evidence of altered organ perfusion together with at least one of the following findings: hypoxemia, oliguria, lactic acidosis, or alteration in mental status. All of these symptoms were present in the patient at the time of hospital admission.
- Since the terminology used to define the systemic response to infection has varied widely, a consensus conference committee met in 1992 to standardize the nomenclature used to define the following commonly used terms: systemic inflammatory response syndrome (SIRS), sepsis, severe sepsis, and septic shock. The committee defined sepsis as a systemic inflammatory response syndrome due to presumed

Case Study: Clinical Relevance (continued)

or confirmed infection and as shown in Table 3-9 produced specific definitions for each of the common and sometimes confusing terms used to describe these conditions.

- The generic term used to describe the constellation of clinical manifestations associated with systemic infection is the systemic inflammatory response syndrome (SIRS), which is defined as a generalized complex response that results from the activity of cells of the immune system (largely from the innate immune response) and their pro-inflammatory products; this response is usually triggered by an exacerbated host response to an infection, but it also can be initiated by a variety of other severe insults, including trauma, burns, and acute pancreatitis. Clinically, SIRS is characterized by the clinical findings shown in Table 3-9.
- The term sepsis should be applied only when infection is the suspected or proven cause of SIRS (up to 95 percent of cases).
- Severe sepsis is the term used when sepsis is associated with multiple organ dysfunction resulting from disordered organ perfusion and oxygenation.
- Septic shock occurs when the sepsis syndrome is associated with hypotension, defined as arterial blood pressure < 50 mm Hg, despite adequate fluid restoration. Other manifestations of sepsis include edema or positive fluid balance, hyperglycemia, elevated levels of plasma C-reactive protein (CRP) and procalcitonin, acute oliguria, thrombocytopenia (< 100,000 platelets/mL), coagulation abnormalities (present in the case study), microvascular abnormalities, and hyperbilirubinemia. Despite therapeutic interventions, the mortality rate in septic shock can be as high as 46 percent.
- The burden of sepsis and septic shock is highlighted by the 750,000 cases of sepsis that occur in the United States annually. Sepsis is involved in approximately 2 percent of all hospitalizations. It is estimated that there will be more than 1 million cases per year in the United States by 2020 as the population ages.
- The case illustrated here showed many of the characteristics of severe sepsis, septic shock, and SIRS: bacteremia was confirmed, the patient had fever, vascular (hypotension) and coagulation abnormalities, thrombocytopenia, multiple organ damage with dysfunction, or failure of several organs including kidney and lung (which are the two most commonly affected organs), and at the end, against all odds, the patient survived with the help of antibiotics, fluid resuscitation, mechanical respiratory ventilation, and immunosuppressive agents.

Table 3-9. Consensus conference definitions of systemic inflammatory response syndrome (SIRS), sepsis, severe sepsis, and septic shock

Syndrome	Definition
Systemic inflammatory response syndrome (SIRS)	Two or more of the following: Temperature > 38°C (100.4°F) or < 36°C (96.8°F) Pulse > 90 beats per minute Respiratory rate > 20 breaths per minute or $PaCO_2$ < 32 mm Hg White blood cells > 12,000/mm^3 or < 4,000/mm^3 or > 10 percent immature ("band") forms
Sepsis	SIRS due to suspected or confirmed infection
Severe sepsis	Sepsis associated with organ dysfunction, hypoperfusion, or hypotension
Septic shock	Sepsis-induced hypotension despite adequate fluid resuscitation along with the presence of perfusion abnormalities

Key Points

- Constitutive physical and chemical barriers block most pathogen entry.
- Innate responses occur within a few hours of pathogen contact and are no faster on repeat contact. Adaptive responses occur within a few days and generate immune memory (immunity).
- Inflammation is defined as the movement of cells and mediators from the circulation (chemotaxis) into an infection site. This can be brought about by microbial products, chemokines, and complement activation. Inflammation can be both protective and destructive.
- The innate immune response is initiated by contact with conserved pathogen structures the PAMPs.

- Following PAMP binding to membrane or intracellular PRRs, phagocytes are signaled to engulf pathogens, and APCs (macrophages and dendritic cells) are activated to stimulate adaptive immunity.
- Epithelial cells provide both a physical barrier and source of chemical protection against pathogens.
- Neutrophils are the predominant phagocytic and pathogen-killing cells. Macrophages secrete inflammatory cytokines in addition to engulfing and destroying pathogens. Dendritic cells are the principal APCs. Mast cells produce a variety of inflammatory mediators. Natural killer cells recognize and kill virus-infected and malignant target cells.

Study Questions/Critical Thinking

1. Does an infection where the pathogen crosses the skin or mucous membranes always result in adaptive immunity and immune memory? Explain your answer.
2. How are PAMPs recognized by innate immune cells related to antigens recognized by B and T lymphocytes? List some examples of PAMPs and explain why they are good targets for innate immunity.
3. How do leukocytes find and enter the site of infection? Why is it advantageous to keep leukocytes out of healthy tissue?
4. Anti-inflammatory medications are available in pharmacies. What are the reasons for and against using these medications?
5. In what ways can a pathogen avoid elimination by the innate immune system?

Suggested Reading

Akira S, Takeda K. Toll-like receptor signaling. Nar Rev Immunol. 2004; 4: 499–511.

Akira S, Uematsu S, Takeuchi O. Pathogen recognition and innate immunity. Cell. 2006; 124: 783–801.

American College of Chest Physicians; (1992;). Society of Critical Care Medicine Consensus Conference. Definitions for sepsis and organ failure and guidelines for the use of innovative therapies in sepsis. 1992; 20: 864–74.

Athman R, Philpott D. Innate immunity via Toll-like receptors and Nod proteins. Curr Opin Microbiol. 2004; 7: 25–32.

Bendelac A, Bonneville M, Kearney JE. Autoreactivity by design: innate B and T lymphocytes. Nature Rev Immunol. 2001; 1: 177–92.

Bergman IM. Toll-like receptors (TLR) and mannan-binding lectin (MBL): on constant alert in a hostile environment. Ups J Med Sci. 2011; 116: 90–9.

Bianchi ME. DAMPs, PAMPs and alarmins: all we need to know about danger. J Leukoc Biol. 2007; 81: 1–5.

Bone RC, Balk RA, Cerra FB,, et al. ACCP/SCCM Consensus Conference Committee. Definitions for sepsis and organ failure and guidelines for the use of innovative therapies in sepsis. The ACCP/SCCM Consensus Conference Committee. American College of Chest Physicians/Society of Critical Care Medicine. Chest. 2009; 136 Suppl 5:e28.

Born WK, Reardon CL, O'Brien RL. The function of $\gamma\delta$ T cells in innate immunity. Curr Op Immunol. 2006; 18: 31–38.

Creticos PS, Schroeder JT, Hamilton RG,, et al. Immune tolerance network group: immunotherapy with ragweed-toll-like receptors against vaccine for allergic rhinitis. N Engl J Med. 2006; 355: 1445–55.

Cristofaro P, Opal SM. Roll of Toll-like receptors in infection and immunity. Clinical implications. Drugs. 2006; 66: 15–29.

Janeway CA Jr, Medzhitov R. Innate immune recognition. Annu Rev Immunol. 2002; 20: 197–216.

Khare S, Luc N, Dorfleutner A, Stehlik C. Inflammasomes and their activation. Crit Rev Immunol. 2010; 30: 463–87.

Kumar H, Kawai T, Akira S. Pathogen recognition in the innate immune response. Biochem J. 2009; 420: 1–16.

Lee MS, Kim YJ. Pattern-recognition receptor signaling initiated from extracellular, membrane, and cytoplasmic space. Mol Cells. 2007: 23: 1–10.

McGuinness DH, Dehal PK, Pleass RJ. Pattern recognition molecules and innate immunity to parasites. Trends Parasitol. 2003; 19: 312–9.

Medzhitov R. Toll-like receptors and innate immunity. Nature Rev Immunol. 2001; 1: 135–45.

Muller WA. Sorting the signals from the signals in the noisy environment of inflammation. Sci Signal. 2011; 4: 1–3.

O'Brien JM Jr, Ali NA, Aberegg SK,, et al. Sepsis. Am J Med. 2007; 120; 1012–22.

Russell JA. Management of sepsis. N Engl J Med. 2006; 355: 1699–713.

Sansonetti PJ. The innate signaling of dangers and the dangers of innate signaling. Nat Immunol. 2006; 7: 1237–42.

Schnare M, Rollinghoff M, Qureshi S. Toll-like receptors: sentinels of host defence against bacterial infection. Int Arch Allergy Immunol. 2006; 139: 75–85.

Stearns-Kurosawa DJ, Osuchowski MF, Valentine C,, et al. The pathogenesis of sepsis. Annu Rev Pathol. 2011; 6: 19–48.

Tosi MF. Innate Immunity response to infection. J Allergy Clin Immunol. 2005; 116: 241–49.

Wiesner J, Vilcinskas A. Antimicrobial peptides: the ancient arm of the human immune system. Virulence. 2010; 1: 440–64.

Zhu J, Mohan C. Toll-like receptor signaling pathways—therapeutic opportunities. Mediators Inflamm. 2010; 2010: 781235.

Chapter 4

Complement

Melvin Berger, MD

Case Study

An eleven-year-old white girl presented with a one-month history of progressive fatigue, decreased appetite, and general malaise. She had intermittent low-grade fevers and nasal congestion, with coughing that was often worse in the morning. She complained of headache and pain around the eyes, which varied with changing positions, especially during gymnastics. The past history was remarkable for repeated episodes of otitis media and respiratory infections in early childhood, but she had been given chronic antibiotic prophylaxis, and these infections had become less problematic in recent years. She was an adopted child and the biologic family history was unknown. Her growth and development were normal and she was regarded as a good student and was active in extracurricular activities.

On physical examination, she appeared tired but not uncomfortable. The vital signs were normal. The height and weight were in the twenty-fifth to thirtieth percentiles. The eyes, ears, nose, and throat were normal except for erythema of the nasal mucosa with mucoid secretions and the presence of similar secretions in the posterior pharynx. The neck, thyroid, and cervical lymph nodes were normal, the chest was clear, and the cardiac exam was normal. The abdomen was non-tender and no hepatosplenomegaly or abnormal masses were palpable. The extremities were normal with no arthritis. There was no rash.

Screening laboratory studies revealed a hematocrit of 30 percent (normal range 40 to 51 percent) with indices consistent with mild iron deficiency, a white cell count of 8000/mm^3 (nl 4.4–10.8), a normal platelet count, and an erythrocyte sedimentation rate of 80 mm/hr (nl <20). Blood chemistries were normal except that the serum albumin was 3.3 grams/dL (nl 3.5–5.0). Multiple cultures were negative, but the urine showed 4+ protein and red blood cells and the sediment contained coarse granular and red blood cell casts. A twenty-four-hour urine collection contained 2 grams of protein. The creatinine clearance was normal. Cultures of blood, urine, and a swab of the pharynx were negative. X-rays of the chest were normal but sinus radiographs showed opacification of all of the sinuses. Treatment with decongestants and oral antibiotics led to symptomatic improvement and normalization of the sedimentation rate, but the proteinuria and hematuria persisted.

LEARNING OBJECTIVES

When you have completed this chapter, you should be able to:

- Describe the complement system
- Explain the three complement-activation pathways
- Compare and contrast the three C3 convertases and describe the shared activities of the three pathways
- Discuss the importance and mechanisms of complement regulation
- Describe the biological functions of activated complement
- Discuss the importance of complement in the defense against infectious diseases
- Explain the role of complement and complement deficiency in immunopathology
- Describe how complement activity is measured
- Summarize the clinical significance of the complement system in health and disease

Case Study (continued)

Additional laboratory studies showed normal serum immunoglobulins and a negative antinuclear antibody test. Tests for circulating immune complexes by the C1q binding assay showed markedly elevated results, but the Raji cell-binding assay was negative. Results of tests for total hemolytic complement showed undetectable activity. The serum concentrations of the C1, C4, and C2 were markedly reduced, and C3 was undetectable, but the concentration of C5 was normal. A renal biopsy was performed, and the results showed type I membranoproliferative glomerulonephritis with irregular granular deposits, which had positive immunofluorescence for IgG, IgM, and C1q, but which were negative for C3b.

The Complement System

As described in Chapter 1, the innate and adaptive immune systems are no longer considered as distinct separate entities but are now recognized to be closely linked and interrelated. Nowhere is this interrelationship between the innate and adaptive immune systems better illustrated than with the **complement system**; a bioamplification system of more than thirty distinct proteins, including soluble enzymatic components and regulatory factors in serum as well as cell receptors of both the innate and adaptive immune systems. Although the major function of the complement system is antimicrobial defense, it is also involved in homeostasis and surveillance. Failure of these functions is expressed clinically as susceptibility to infection, hypersensitivity, or autoimmunity. Because the complement system is so potentially destructive, however, it must be carefully regulated. This, in turn, adds to the great complexity of the system. The vast array of components of the complement system is commensurate with its many physiologic and pathologic functions in health and disease.

Table 4-1. Complement components

Component	Molecular weight	Serum concentration (ug/ml)
Classical pathway		
C1	570,000	370
C4	209,000	430
C2	117,000	30
C3	190,000	1,400
C5	206,000	75
C6	95,000	60
C7	120,000	55
C8	163,000	80
C9	79,000	160
Lectin pathway		
Mannose-binding lectin	32,000	0.5 to 5.0
MASP 1	90,000	1.6–7.5
MASP 2	74,000	NC*
Alternative pathway		
B	100,000	200
D	25,000	1–5
P (properdin)	223,000	25

Note: NC* = not known with certainty.

The Complement Components

Shown in Table 4-1 are the major components of the complement system together with their molecular weights and serum concentrations. The proteins that comprise the complement system are either labeled 1 through 9 numerically with the prefix "C" or designated by letters of the alphabet (e.g., B, D, or P). Although the components generally are activated in a sequential order from 1 through 9, the notable exception is with C4, which comes before C2. The reason for this inconsistency is related to the fact that the components were numbered in the order in which they were discovered rather than the order in which they act, hence C4 comes before C2. Several complement components are cleaved during activation of the system, and the resultant fragments are designated with lowercase suffixes, e.g., C3a and C3b. Normally, the larger fragment is designated "b" and the smaller "a," with the notable sole exception of the cleavage products of C2, wherein the larger fragment is designated C2a and the smaller C2b. Many of the steps of the complement system function as enzymatic molecules and act in a cascading fashion, with each product activating the next component. Once a given set of components is activated, it is designated as a **complex** with a bar over the composite, e.g., $\overline{\text{C3bC2a}}$.

Complement Is Activated by One of Three Pathways

Normally, the complement components exist in an inactive form and must be first activated in order to function. There are three major pathways by which the complement system may be activated: (1) the classical pathway, (2) the mannose-binding or lectin pathway, and (3) the alternative pathway (Figure 4-1). The **classical pathway**, so-named because it was the first described, is dependent upon antibody to be functional; in contrast, the lectin and alternative pathways are antibody independent. All three of these pathways ultimately result in the activation of C3 and the formation of a C5 convertase, which leads to the activation of C5 and the lytic pathway. C5 activation is a common step at which the activation pathways converge. Each of these pathways proceeds as a series of sequential steps that progress in a cascading fashion. Since some of the steps are enzymatic in nature, there is amplification as the pathways proceed.

The subsequent steps of each pathway move ultimately toward assembly of a membrane attack complex (**MAC**) that can perforate holes in cell membranes and serves as a common final cytolytic pathway regardless of which activation pathway initiated the process (Figure 4-1). Although the early activation stages of each pathway are initiated in different ways, each involves similar sequential steps of proteolytic cleavage, followed by conformational changes in the larger fragment of the cleaved protein, which acquires the ability to combine with the components that cleaved it. This leads to a progressive set of changes in which each emerging cleavage product then acquires enzymatic activity allowing it to act upon the next protein in the sequence. Since each step involves formation of an enzyme that can cleave many molecules of the next component, the system serves as a forward amplifying cascade.

The Classical Pathway Is Activated When Complement C1 Binds IgM or IgG Bound to Antigen

2 The classical pathway was the first to be discovered and was identified initially as a heat-labile component in serum that "complemented" the function of antibodies in killing bacteria (*Chapter 12*). This pathway is activated when one part of the C1 component of complement, called C1q, binds to the Fc region of an IgM or IgG antibody bound to an antigen on the surface of a target cell and ends with the lysis of the cell (Figure 4-2). Since this pathway is linked to antibody, unlike the other two, it is considered part of the adaptive immune system.

The C1 component exists as a C1 complex consisting of C1q, two molecules of C1r, and two molecules of C1s (Figure 4-2). The C1q component circulates in the blood as an inactive macromolecular complex consisting of six subunit structures (protomers), each of which is made up of a collagen-like stalk at the end of which is a globular immunoglobulin-binding domain. Two each of both the C1r and C1s molecules are intertwined around the stalks (Figure 4-3). Each C1q subunit protomer consists of three protein chains called alpha (α), beta (β), and gamma (γ) (Figure 4-3A and Figure 4-3B).

The C1r/C1s subunits of the C1 complex are held together within the C1q hexamer in an inactive form with a circular inactive head-to-tail configuration (Figure 4-4A). When two or more of the globular heads of C1q attach to antigen-bound IgG or IgM molecules, internal rearrangements in the C1r/C1s complex occur and the molecule assumes a linear C1s-C1r-C1r-C1s tetrameric configuration (Figure 4-4B). Associated with this molecular change, C1r develops proteolytic activity and cleaves and activates the C1s molecules, resulting in exposed activated C1s components at each end capable of interacting with the next two components of the classical pathway, i.e., C4 and C2.

Electron micrographs of the C1 complex show the six trimers arranged with their stalks together and the globular heads all at the same end, giving the appearance of a bouquet of tulips. Around each stalk are wrapped the two molecules each of C1r and C1s, so that all together the macromolecular C1 complex is comprised of twenty-two protein chains (Figure 4-4). Because of the requirement for two of the heads of C1q to be engaged with the Fc region of either an IgM or IgG antibody for activation to begin, IgM, which has five Fc regions attached together, is a very efficient activator of the classical pathway. In contrast, many molecules of IgG must be bound to the surface of a target cell or bacterium in order for two of the IgG molecules to find themselves in close enough proximity to bridge a single C1q. The other classes of immunoglobulins, IgD, IgA, and IgE, do not bind to C1q and hence do not activate the classical pathway. C1s, when activated, i.e., $\overline{\text{C1s}}$, not only exhibits proteolytic activity, but it can cleave synthetic esters in vitro as well, and is hence often referred to as "C1 esterase."

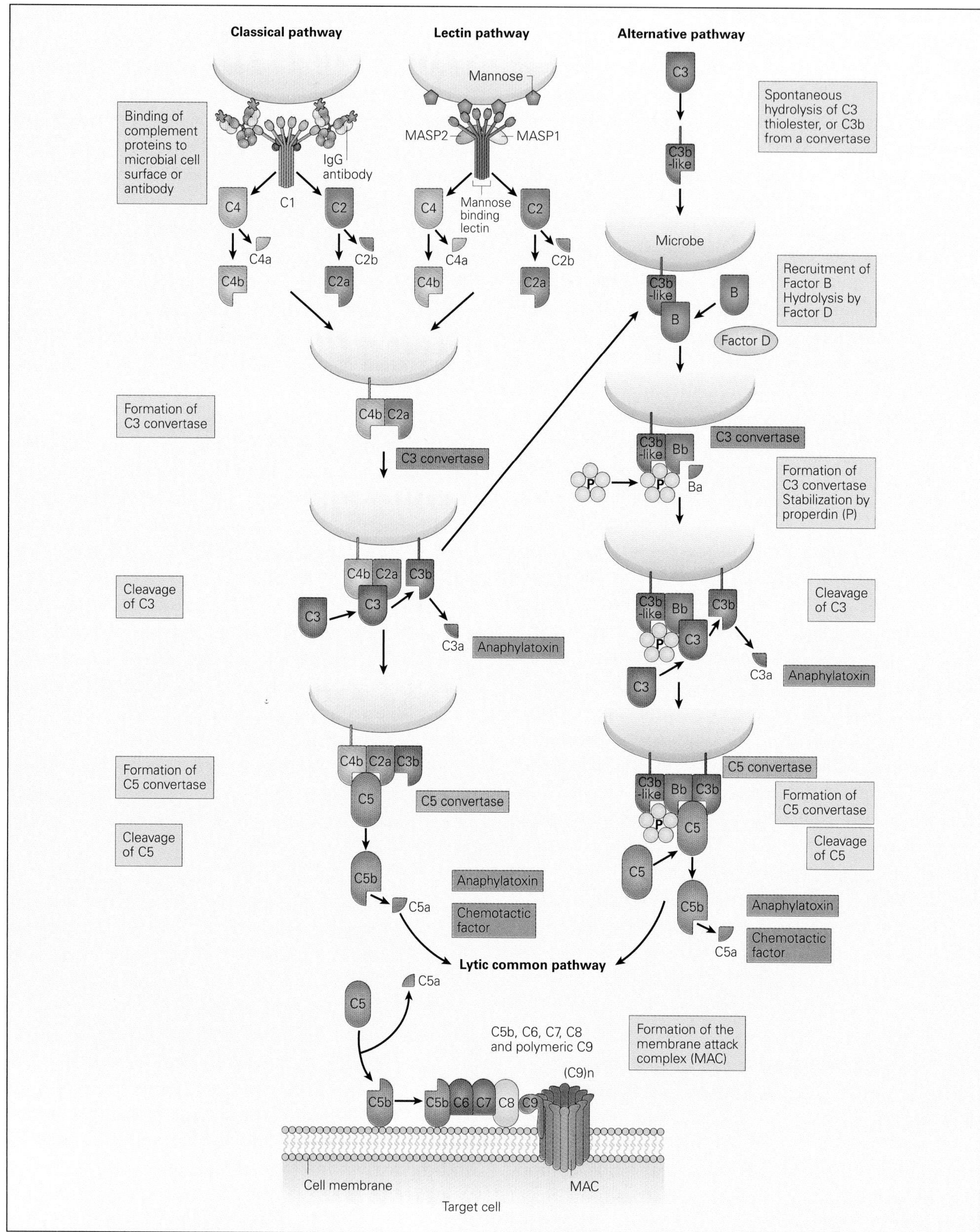

Figure 4-1. Three pathways of complement activation. Panel A: Classical pathway activation is initiated by engagement of globular domains of C1 with two or more Fc domains of IgG or IgM. Panel B: Lectin pathway is activated by binding of ligands to mannose-binding lectin (MBL). Note analogous function of MBL-associated serine proteases (MASPs) and C1r and C1s. Active convertases are denoted by bars over their components. Classical and lectin pathways both employ $\overline{\text{C4b2a}}$ as their C3 convertase. Panel C: Alternative pathway is activated when Factor B binds to C3b-like C3 or to C3b formed by one of the other pathways. Factor D, which circulates in its active form, carries out the cleavage of B, which is analogous to the cleavage of C2 by C1s or MASP. The alternative pathway C3 convertase is $\overline{\text{C3bBb}}$. Addition of a molecule of C3b to the C3 convertases forms the C5 convertases. Note that after C5 is cleaved, there are no further proteolytic steps. Multiple molecules of C9 may join the full membrane attack complex.

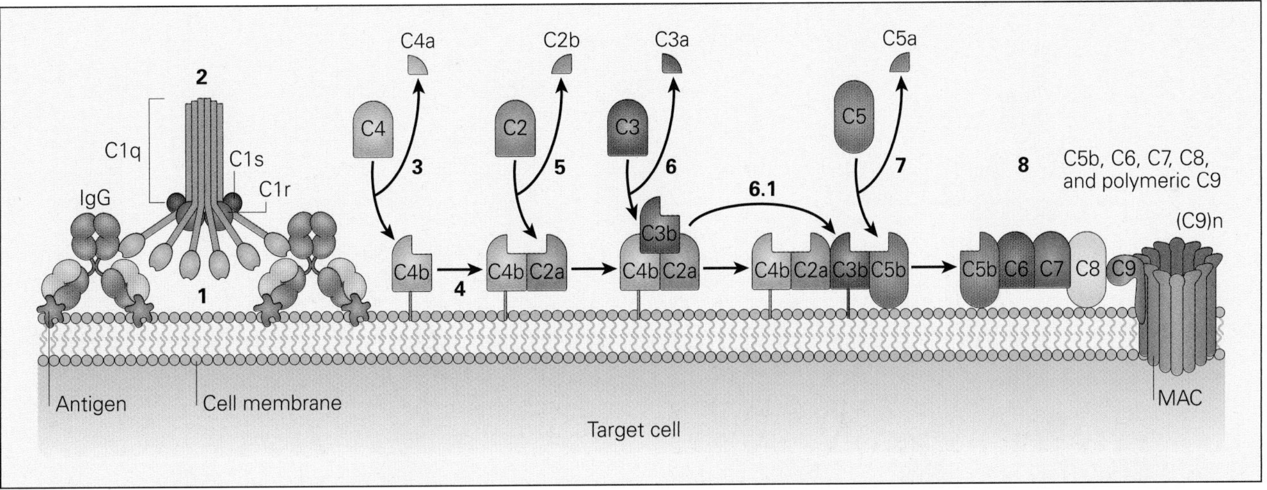

Figure 4-2. Schematic representation of the classical complement cascade showing the initiation of the pathway by binding of the C1q component of C1 binding to the Fc region of an IgG antibody molecule bound to an antigen on the surface of a target cell. The numbers in bold indicate the sequential steps which are involved in the activation of each of the components leading to the final lytic event carried out by the MAC. Some sources now use a revised nomenclature for the fragment of C2, in which C2a is the small fragment which diffuse away and C2b is the larger fragment that binds with C4b and acts in the convertase, $\overline{\text{C4b2b}}$.

Activated $\overline{\text{C1s}}$ Cleaves C4 and C2

The physiologic role of activated $\overline{\text{C1s}}$ is to carry out limited proteolytic cleavage of C4 and C2, the next two components in the reaction sequence (Figure 4-5A). $\overline{\text{C1s}}$ first cleaves the largest of the three chains of C4 at a single site, liberating a small peptide (C4a) and leaving the larger fragment (C4b) with a transient ability to form covalent bonds to the target cell. The resulting C4b fragment also takes on a new conformation allowing it to bind a molecule of C2, so that it can be cleaved by $\overline{\text{C1s}}$ as well, resulting in a smaller fragment (C2b), which is released and diffuses away and a larger fragment (C2a) whose conformation and activity are changed to acquire a proteolytic active site. These changes allow C2a to adhere to C4b, forming a $\overline{\text{C4bC2a}}$ complex capable of cleaving and activating C3. This $\overline{\text{C4bC2a}}$ complex is therefore called "C3 convertase."

The Binding of C4b with C2a Forms $\overline{\text{C4b2a}}$, the C3 Convertase

The binding of one molecule of C4b covalently attached to the target cell surface with one molecule of C2a loosely bound to it results in the formation

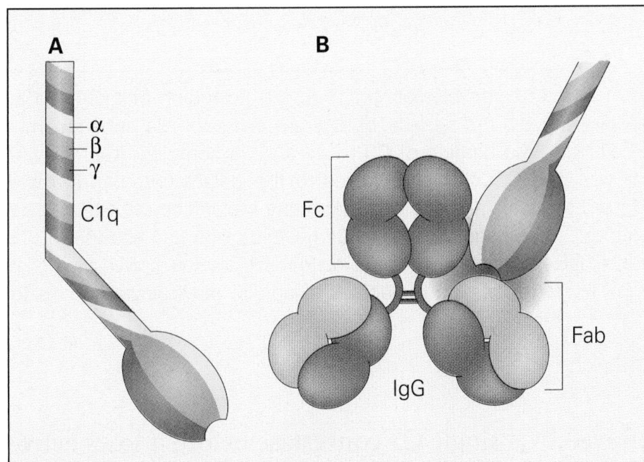

Figure 4-3. Schematic representation of the structure of the C1q component. Panel A: Each individual unit (protomer) of C1q is composed of three similar, but not identical alpha (α), beta (β), and gamma (γ) protein chains (shown colored yellow, beige, and orange, respectively) that are twisted into a collagen-like stalk and a globular domain that forms the binding site for the Fc of IgG or IgM. Panel B: Schematic representation of the interaction of the globular end of one C1q protomer binding to an immunoglobulin in a groove between the Fc and Fab regions.

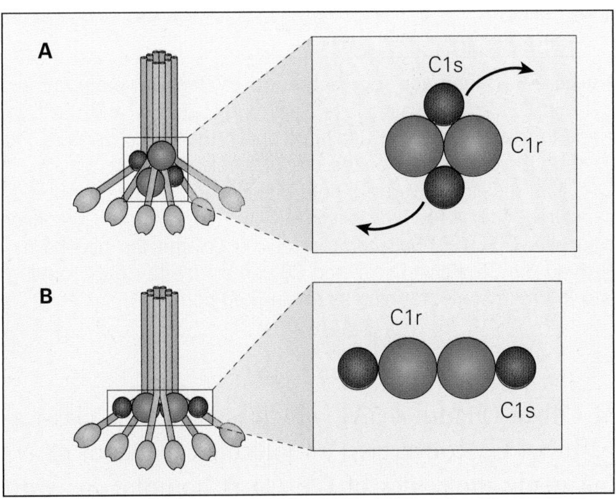

Figure 4-4. Schematic representation of the composition of the C1 component made up of a C1q subunit composed of a 6-membered hexameric structure together with a C1r/C1s complex. Panel A: shows the head-to-tail configuration in the inactive state. Panel B: shows the linear tetrameric C1s-C1r-C1r-C1s structure when activated. Since each stalk consists of 3 protein chains (α, β, γ) the entire C1 complex consists of 22 proteins.

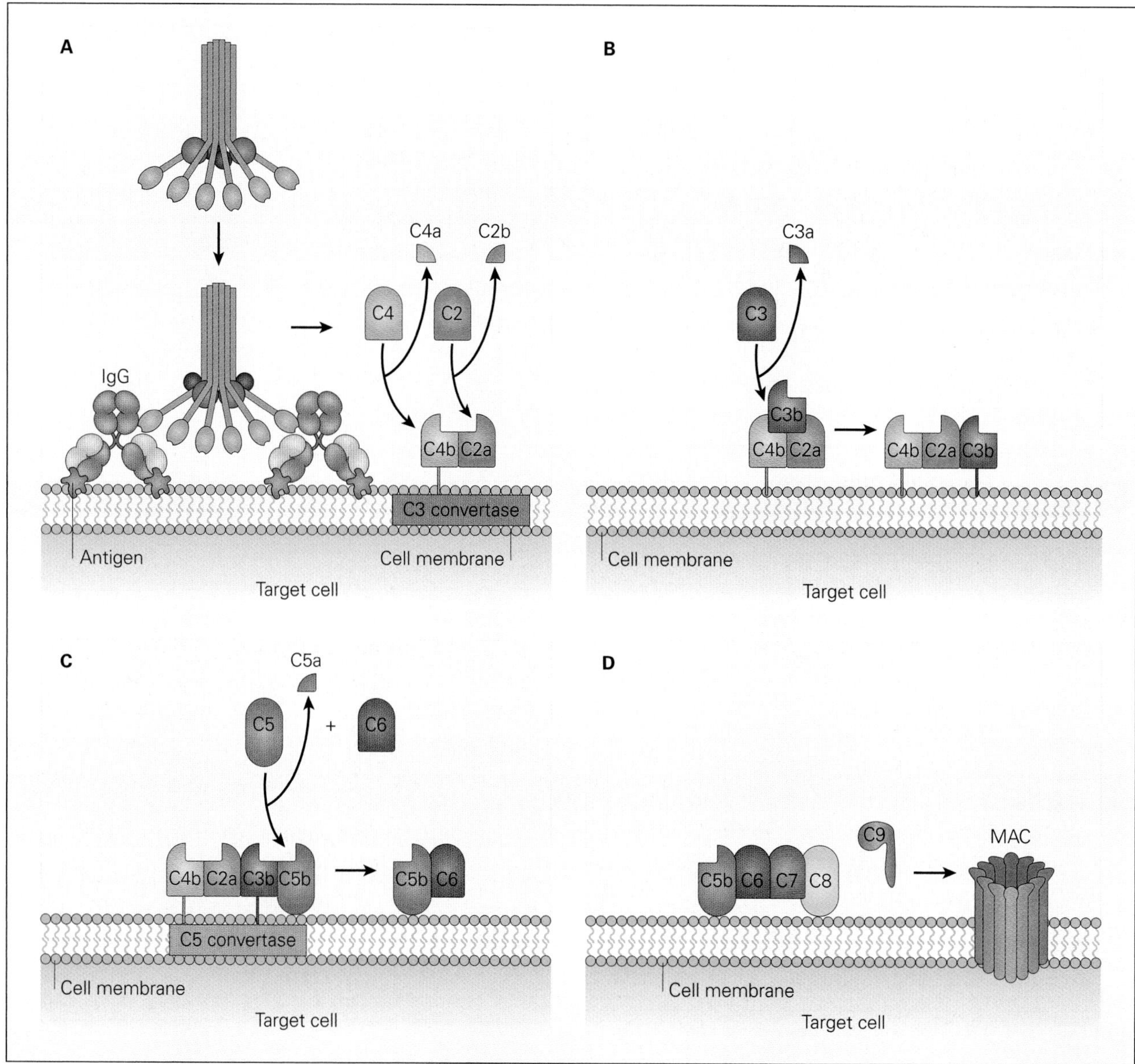

Figure 4-5. **Schematic representation of classical pathway activation.** Panel A: Upon binding of C1 to the Fc region of IgG or IgM, C1r and C1s are activated. $\overline{\text{C1s}}$ cleaves C4 and C2, and the C4b binds covalently to the surface of a target cell and C2a subsequently binds to the C4b forming $\overline{\text{C4b2a}}$ complex, the C3 convertase. Panel B: Following the binding of C3 to the $\overline{\text{C4b2a}}$ complex, it is cleaved by the C2a component of the complex releasing C3a, which diffuses away, and C3b, which adheres to the $\overline{\text{C4b2a}}$ complex forming $\overline{\text{C4b2a3b}}$, the C5 convertase; note that $\overline{\text{C4b2a}}$ may deposit at a distance from the initial C1 site and that many molecules of C3b may be deposited. Only a few will join with $\overline{\text{C4b2a}}$ to form the C5 convertase. Panel C: Cleavage of C5 by C2a releases C5a and allows C5b to bind with C6. The C5b6 complex can insert into the plasma membrane; C5b6 can also insert at a distance from the convertase that cleaved the C5. Panel D: C7 and C8 can bind with C5b6, forming a complex that causes C9 molecules to unfold, polymerize, and insert into the membrane, forming a protein-lined pore.

of $\overline{\text{C4b2a}}$ (Figure 4-5A), which is called the classical pathway C3 convertase, a molecule capable of cleaving many molecules of C3. C3 is homologous with C4, and upon cleavage, the larger fragment (C3b) also transiently has the ability to bind covalently to the surface of the target on which activation is occurring (Figure 4-5B). Many molecules of C3 can be cleaved by a single C3 convertase before it loses activity when the C2a subunit diffuses or is pushed away. Some of the newly formed C3b molecules will diffuse away before they can bind to the surface. Many others will bind to the surface at short distances around the convertase—these may serve to opsonize (i.e., facilitate phagocytosis) the target.

The Binding of $\overline{\text{C4b2a}}$ with C3b Forms $\overline{\text{C4b2a3b}}$, the C5 Convertase

Some of the C3b molecules may deposit in very close proximity to the C4b2a complex and actually join with it (Figure 4-5B). These C3b molecules can provide binding sites for C5 molecules, which will be cleaved by the C2a (Figure 4-5C). Thus, the complex C4b2a3b serves as the classical pathway C5 convertase.

The Binding of C5b with C6 Initiates the Terminal Addition of C7, C8, and C9 to Form the Membrane Attack Complex C5b6789

Like C4 and C3, the cleavage of C5 liberates a small fragment (C5a), but unlike C4 and C3, C5 cannot form a covalent bond with the surface. The larger fragment, C5b, however, undergoes a conformational change that allows it to bind C6 (Figure 4-5C). This leads toward formation of the lipid soluble C5b6789 membrane attack complex (Figure 4-5D), in which C7 and C8 can bind with C5b6, forming a complex that causes C9 molecules to unfold, polymerize, and insert into the cell membrane of a target cell, forming a protein-lined pore leading to cytolysis of the target cell. These events will be described in greater detail below.

The Mannose-Binding Lectin Pathway Is Activated When Complement Binds the Acute Phase Protein to Cell Surface Mannose Molecules

The mannose-binding lectin (**MBL**) pathway is the most recent pathway to be elucidated at a molecular level. Activation by this route begins with the MBL, which has a structure similar to C1, binding to mannose residues on the surface of a target cell (Figure 4-6).

Like C1, this multichain molecule is made up of several subunits, including MBL, a hexameric structure analogous to the C1q molecule with six collagen-like stalks, each of which ends with a globular domain that contains its binding sites. However, in the case of MBL, the binding sites recognize polysaccharides containing mannose, in contrast to the C1q, which recognizes the Fc domain of an IgM or IgG antibody. Hence, this component is referred to as the MBL. Because MBL, C1q, and other similar molecules have collagen-like regions and binding sites that often have lectin-like activity in recognizing polysaccharides, they are often considered to be members of the same family of collagen-like lectins, or "collectins." The lung-surfactant proteins A and D are also members of this collectin family. Different isoforms of MBL may contain between two and eight of the basic protomer subunits, each of which itself is a trimer.

Since many bacteria and fungi are coated with mannose-containing polysaccharides, and antibody is not required for MBL to bind to these moieties, the MBL pathway of complement activation is considered part of the innate immune system, as is the alternative pathway, which will be described below. Evolutionarily speaking, the alternative and lectin pathways are likely older than the classical pathway, and C1 may be considered as an adaptor molecule which appeared later in phylogeny (*Chapter 2*), allowing this important part of the innate immune system to be used to enhance the activity of antibody produced by the adaptive immune system. The ability of the lectin and alternative pathways to activate complement in the absence of antibody may be important early in life, i.e., during the

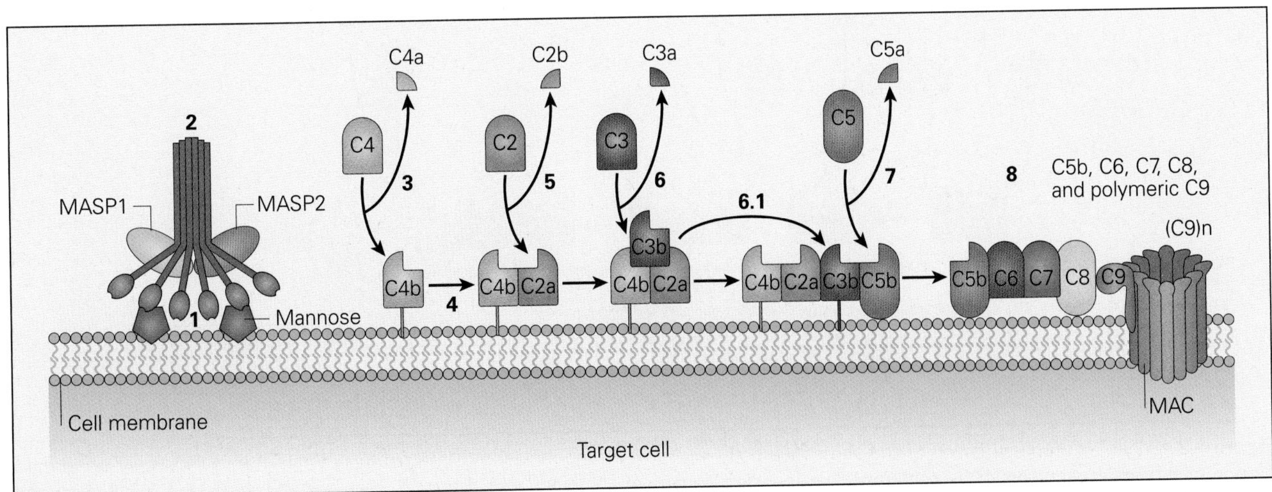

Figure 4-6. Schematic representation of the mannose-binding lectin pathway showing the initiation of the pathway by binding of the mannose-binding lectin (a structure similar to the C1q component of the classical pathway) to mannose molecules on the surface of a target cell.

newborn period, at a time when the adaptive immune system is immature, as well as early in the course of infections, before antibody production and other effector mechanisms of the specific immune system are able to participate.

Like the binding of C1, through C1q, to the Fc regions of IgG or IgM, the binding of MBL to mannose containing polysaccharides leads to activation of nascent proteases. In this pathway, the proteases that are analogous to C1r and C1s are termed MBL-associated serine proteases (**MASPs**). Three different MASPs have been identified and may circulate in the plasma as a large complex together with MBL and another protein component whose function has yet to be determined. When MBL is engaged with polysaccharides, MASP 1 becomes activated and cleaves MASP 2. This activation sequence of MASP 1 → MASP 2 is analogous to the structural/functional changes associated with activation of the C1r/C1s complex described previously in the classical pathway and are shown schematically in Figure 4-7.

Both MASP 1 and MASP 2 have been shown to be capable of cleaving C3, but some studies suggest that they actually act more like C1r and C1s in cleaving C4 and C2 and that the larger fragments of those components actually form the C3 convertase, just as in classical pathway activation. The physiologic importance of the lectin pathway is illustrated by the occurrence of an increased susceptibility to infections and also to autoimmune diseases like lupus in patients with MBL deficiency.

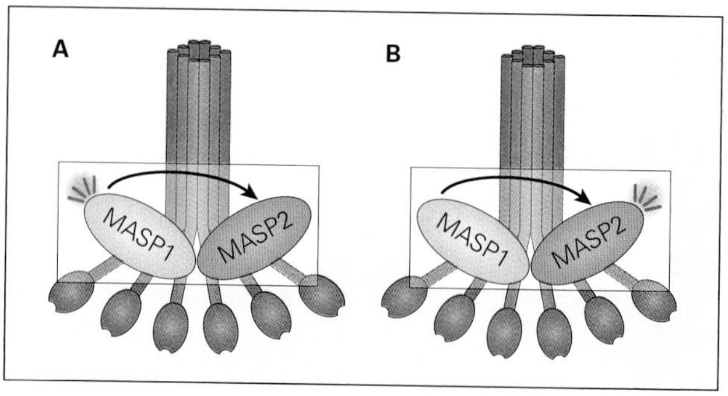

Figure 4-7. Schematic representation of the activation of MASP 2 by MASP 1. Panel A: When MBL is engaged with polysaccharides, MASP 1 becomes activated and cleaves MASP 2. Panel B: This activation sequence of MASP 1 → MASP 2 is analogous to the structural/functional changes associated with activation of the C1r/C1s complex in the classical pathway. The glow on MASP1 in A and on MASP2 in B indicate the state of activation of these molecules during the lectin pathway cascade.

The Alternative Pathway Is Activated When C3b Binds to the Pathogen Surface

The **alternative pathway**, also known as the properdin pathway, shares with the lectin pathway the ability to activate complement without antibody (Figure 4-8). Alternative pathway activation is initiated when C3b, which may be formed by one of the other pathways or by nonspecific proteolytic cleavage of C3, binds with Factor B, which is analogous to C2. When bound to C3b, B acquires a conformation that allows it to be cleaved by the protease D, as will be described below. B also acquires this conformation when it binds with a molecule of uncleaved C3 that has undergone a conformational change to resemble C3b. This is referred to as "C3b-like C3."

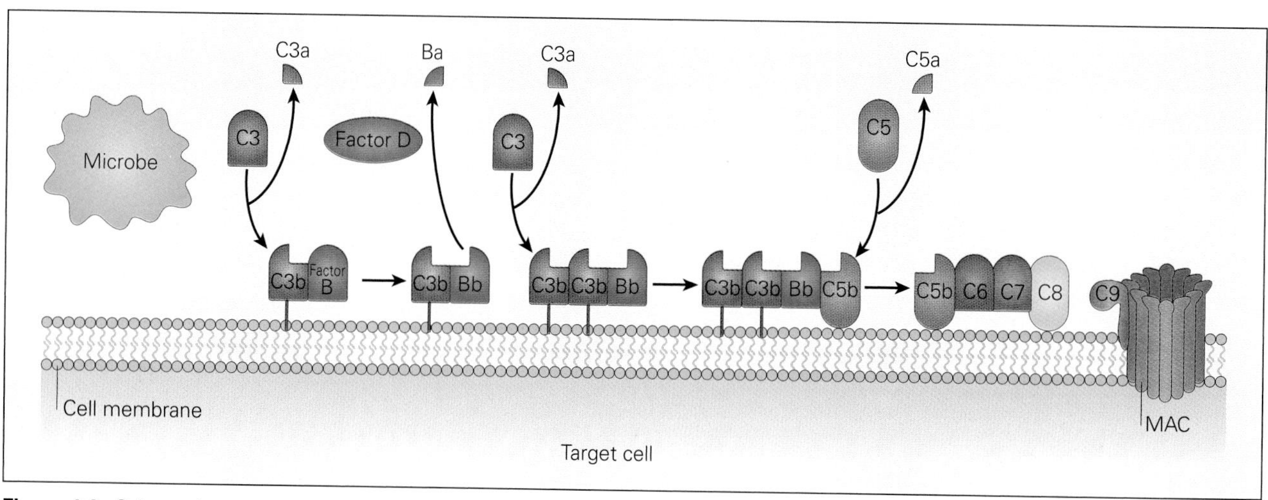

Figure 4-8. Schematic representation of the alternative pathway showing the initiation of the pathway when C3b, which may be formed by one of the other pathways or by nonspecific proteolytic cleavage of C3, binds with Factor B, which is analogous to C2. When bound to C3b, B acquires a conformation that allows it to be cleaved by the protease D following which the subsequent steps of the pathway are similar to those of the other two pathways.

Most investigators visualize native C3 in the circulation as a kind of coiled spring that holds a unique structure called a thioester in an internal hydrophobic pocket (Figure 4-9).

This highly unusual chemical structure is formed by the binding of a thiol on the side chain of one of the protein's cysteine residues with the carboxyl on the side chain of a glutamate three residues away in the polypeptide. C4 also contains this internal thioester. Upon cleavage of the protein chain containing the thioester by a convertase or a nonspecific protease, the coiled spring is released, the thioester is transiently

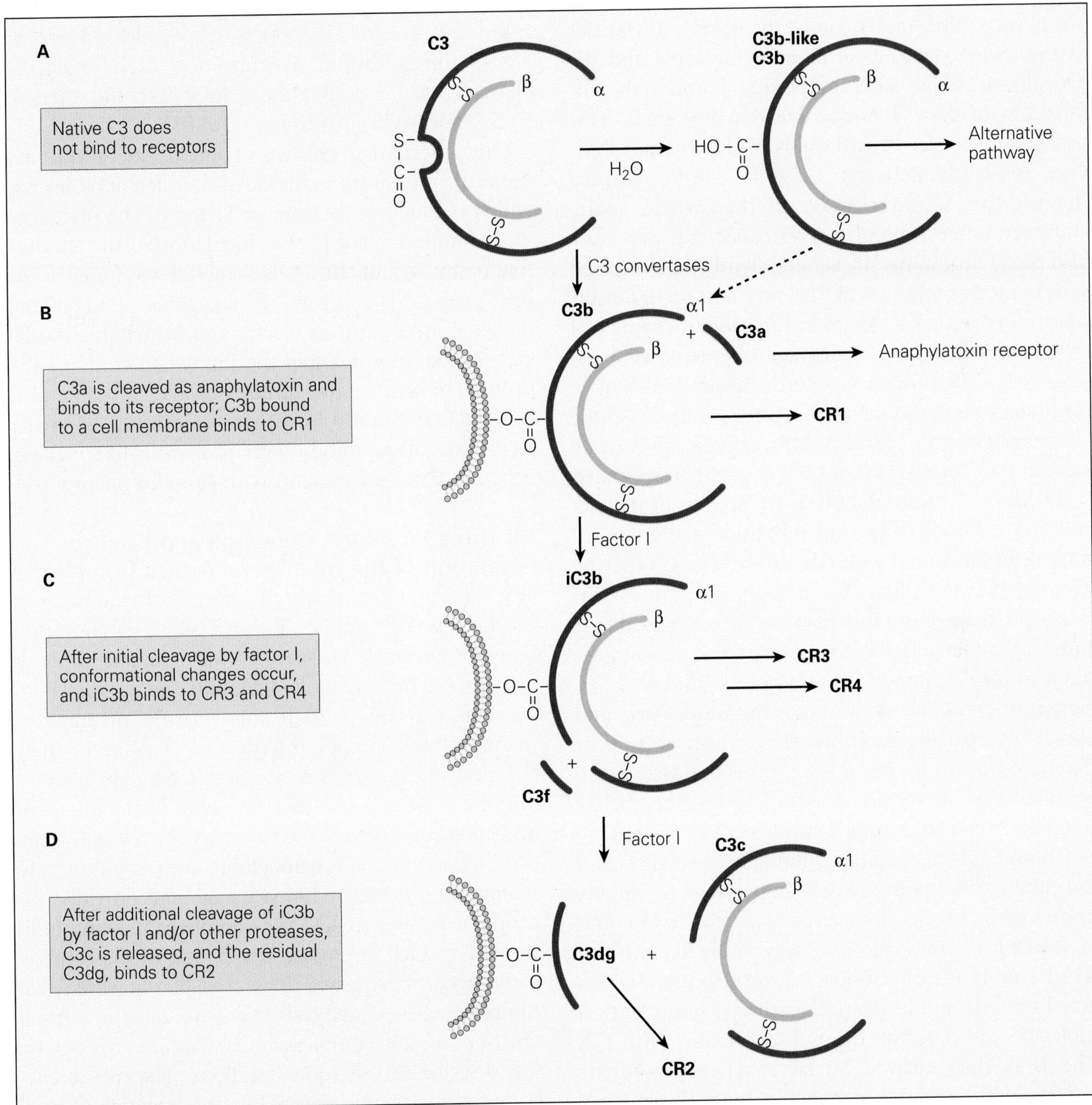

Figure 4-9. Conformations of C3 at different states of cleavage. Panel A, left: Intact native C3 in the circulation is shown tightly wound with an internal thioester. Panel A, right: Infiltration of a water molecule into this structure can hydrolyze that bond which allows the "spring to uncoil," and the molecule assumes a conformation like that of C3b, which can activate the alternative pathway. Panel B: Cleavage near the N-terminal of the α (largest) chain releases C3a and leads to the same conformational change. Panel B, middle: The thioester may transfer to another acceptor at this time, giving surface-bound C3b that may participate in convertases and/or serve as an opsonin since it can be recognized by CR1. Panel B: Initial cleavage by I in the presence of a cofactor gives iC3b, which is inactive in convertases. Panel C: This also changes the conformation, reducing the affinity for CR1 but increasing the affinity for CR3. However, no part of the C3b molecule has been removed from the cell. Panel D: Additional cleavages by I in the presence of cofactors lead to release of C3c, with C3dg bound to the surface; C3dg can be cleaved further to C3d. Both C3dg and C3d bind to CR2.

exposed, and the carbon on the glutamate can transfer one of its bonds from the sulfur of the cysteine to another acceptor. It is the ability of these molecules to transfer a carbon bond to hydroxyl or amino groups on other proteins or to sugar molecules that allows C3 and C4 to bind covalently during complement activation. If the transfer to another protein or sugar does not occur within milliseconds, the bond will transfer to the hydroxyl group of a water molecule and the hydrogen from the water molecule will bind to the sulfur atom of the cysteine to create a free thiol. This process of transfer or hydrolysis of the internal thioester is greatly accelerated by the conformational changes that follow cleavage of the protein chain. However, water molecules may occasionally penetrate into the hydrophobic pocket and hydrolyze this bond even in intact molecules of C3. Once that occurs, similar conformational changes in the protein chains will follow, even though no cleavage fragment has been removed. That process goes on constantly at a slow rate, hence there is always some turnover of C3. These C3 molecules with hydrolyzed thioester bonds assume a conformation like that of C3b, hence they are called "C3b-like C3" molecules. About 1 percent of the circulating C3 molecules undergo this reaction every hour. This constant low-grade turnover of C3 may be thought of as the idling of a car engine, i.e., the system is always turned on and ready to accelerate at any time. This allows the alternative pathway of complement to play an important role in recognition of foreign invaders as part of the innate immune system and allows it to participate in the elimination of dead or damaged body cells. But it also means that the system must be carefully regulated, as will be described below in the section on control of complement activation.

C3 and C4 are highly homologous proteins, and the alternative pathway C3 convertase is highly homologous to the classical pathway convertase and is formed in an analogous way. This is initiated when a molecule of C3b-like C3, or C3b itself, which acts like C4b in the classical pathway, binds with a molecule called factor B i.e., homologous with C2. The B is then cleaved by factor D, a proteolytic enzyme that circulates in its active form all the time, but can act on factor B only when it is held in the proper configuration by C3b. Cleavage of factor B is analogous to cleavage of C2, but the large fragment is named Bb. Like C2, factor B is a nascent protease, and the Bb fragment that results from cleavage by factor D is an active enzyme that can cleave C3 and C5. The C3b or C3b-like C3 molecule that initiated the pathway also serves the same role as the C4b in the classical pathway C3 convertase in holding additional molecules of C3 substrate in place, which are then cleaved by Bb. Just as in the classical pathway, some of the newly cleaved C3b molecules will deposit sufficiently close to the $\overline{\text{C3bBb}}$ enzyme to join with it. This new molecule of C3b can provide a binding site for C5, which will be cleaved by Bb. Thus, the addition of this new C3b molecule changes the C3 convertase $\overline{\text{C3bBb}}$ into the alternative pathway C5 convertase, $\overline{\text{C3bBb3b}}$.

The alternative pathway contains an additional molecule not found in the classical or lectin pathways, which is called properdin, or factor P. The discovery of this molecule led to the elucidation of the alternative pathway and thus it is sometimes referred to as the "properdin pathway." P is capable of stabilizing the alternative pathway convertases, which might otherwise lose activity when the Bb, which contains the proteolytic active site, diffuses away. This may also occur pathologically in the presence of C3 nephritic factor, an autoantibody with properdin-like properties found in some patients with glomerulonepritis.

All Three Pathways Converge and Lead to Formation of the Membrane Attack Complex

One of the most dramatic aspects of complement function is the ability of this system to convert a series of separate, circulating, water-soluble proteins into a large multisubunit, lipophilic membrane channel that can insert itself into plasma membranes, spanning both leaflets. Insertion of just one of these channels into an erythrocyte allows enough water to rush into the cell to cause explosive lysis. This phenomenon of lysis of erythrocytes by complement, with release of their hemoglobin into solution, was recognized more than 100 years ago and provided the endpoint for assays, i.e., the complement fixing (**CF**) antibody, which led to the elucidation of the complement reaction sequence. It is arguable, however, that complement-mediated lysis is not the most important function of the complement system in vivo, as we will describe in subsequent sections. The membrane-bound water channel formed by the assembly of C5-9 is called the membrane attack complex, and its formation is described in the next paragraph.

Once C5 has been activated, regardless of which pathway was responsible, the remaining steps of activation of C6 through C9 follow the same sequence. Unlike the early activation pathways, however, activation beyond C5 and formation of the membrane attack complex does not involve proteolytic cleavages or other enzymatic activity. C5 does not contain the same internal thioester as its homologs C3 and C4, and C5b cannot form covalent bonds with the target. However, just after cleavage, C5b gains the ability to interact with C6. Interaction with C6 increases the lipophilicity of C5b, and the C5b6 complex can insert into lipid membranes at some distance from the C5 convertase, even on adjacent cells. The C5b6 complex can then attract and bind a molecule of C7. The complex of C5b67 is highly lipophilic and, if formed in the fluid phase, will rapidly insert into plasma membranes, where it will serve as a binding site for C8. Binding of C8 to C5b67 creates an active complex, which can disrupt the phospholipids of a target cell membrane and can cause lysis of erythrocytes, even without the addition of C9. The C5b-8 complex can induce conformational changes in soluble C9 molecules. These conformational changes include elongation and unfolding of the C9 molecules, exposing previously protected hydrophobic regions as well as potential sites for disulfide bonding between chains. These changes, in turn, give the C9 molecules the ability to polymerize and cause their addition to the complex. Isolated C9 can also be induced to undergo these conformational changes and polymerize under laboratory conditions. These polymers may contain up to twelve molecules of C9 linked in dimers by disulfide bonds. Electron micrographs of these C9 polymers appear like grommets or donuts that resemble membrane attack complexes isolated from cells or artificial membranes that have been attacked by complement (Figure 4-10). The top ring of these structures has been estimated to be 15–20 nm in diameter, and it sits above a cylindrical stalk, 15–16 nm in length, which spans the plasma membrane. The conformational changes that accompany C9 activation and polymerization may be recognized by monoclonal antibodies that do not recognize the native C9 molecule in the circulation. These antibodies to the C9 "neoantigen" i.e., formed upon activation, may be used to identify sites of MAC deposition in pathology specimens and can be used for in vitro assays of complement activation.

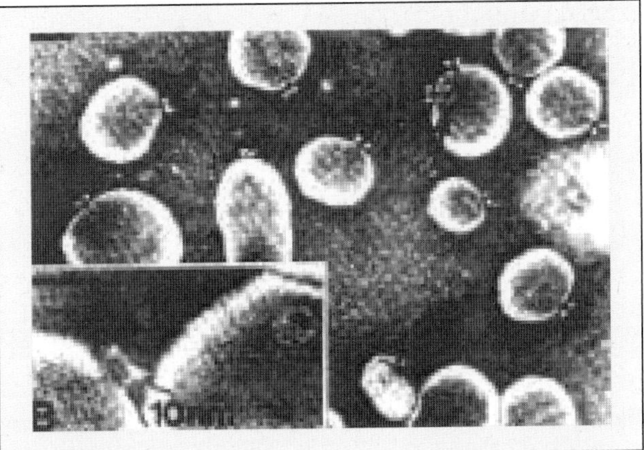

Figure 4-10. Electron micrographs of complement membrane attack complexes in membranes of liposomes. Note that polymerized C9 appears to form a protein-lined grommet, channel, or pore in the membrane. (Reproduced with permission from Bhakdi S, Tranum-Jensen J. Mechanism of complement cytolysis and the concept of channel-forming proteins. Philos Trans R Soc Lond B Biol Sci. 1984;306:311–24.)

Regulation of Complement Activation

In addition to its ability to cause cell lysis, complement activation gives rise to the fragments C3a and C5a, which are potent mediators of inflammation. The deposition of large amounts of C3b and other fragments is important for opsonization of invading microorganisms as well as proper clearance and disposal of antigen-antibody complexes. The apparent dichotomy between complement's role as a part of the innate immune system, which is always turned on to detect foreign invaders, and its potential for tissue damage and destruction, if inappropriately unleashed, suggests that a delicate balance must be maintained at all times. This balance depends on a set of control mechanisms no less intricate and complicated than the activation pathways described above.

Another way of understanding the need to control complement activation becomes readily apparent when one considers the possibility that the alternative pathway can be initiated wherever C3b has been deposited spontaneously or by another pathway, and visualizes the alternative pathway as an amplification loop (Figure 4-11). Why then, isn't all of the C3 in the body activated and deposited every time a complex gets started? The answer to this dilemma depends on knowledge of the specific proteins that control complement activation, which are discussed below. However, an illustration of the importance of these proteins is provided by the case of a patient with congenital deficiency of the complement regulatory protein, C3 inactivator (Factor I presented earlier). This patient lacked detectable C3 activity in his serum, giving him an increased

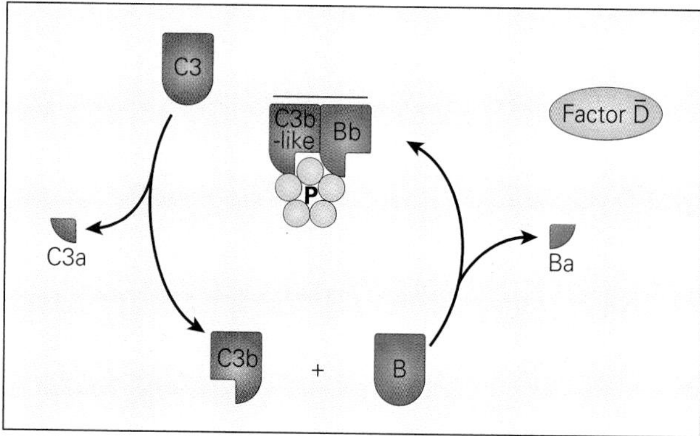

Figure 4-11. Schematic representation of the alternative pathway as an "amplification loop." C3, in its "C3b-like" conformation after hydrolysis of the internal thioester by water or C3b formed by cleavage of the α chain, can bind with B, promoting its cleavage by D. Addition of Bb to the C3b forms the alternative pathway convertase C3bBb, which cleaves more C3 to C3b, feeding the cycle. Stabilization of the convertase by properdin (P) increases activation by this loop.

susceptibility to infection; but he did have C3b deposited on his red blood cells, causing mild but chronic hemolytic anemia due to complement-mediated destruction of his red blood cells. Thus, the illustration shown in Figure 4-11 most likely depicts the ongoing pathophysiology in this patient in whom in fact most of the C3 was continuously consumed by nonspecific activation as quickly as it was synthesized. How do the rest of us maintain a system that is able to quickly recognize and destroy invaders but leave our own cells unaffected? Common themes in regulation of activation and function of the components are summarized in Table 4-2.

Complement Activity Is Controlled by Rates of Synthesis and Decay of Activated Proteins

The circulating concentrations of the complement proteins themselves may be regulated systemically, since many are acute phase reactants whose synthesis by the liver can be increased rapidly in response to cytokines, hormones, and other signals. Local synthesis as well as changes in vascular permeability can also contribute to regulation of the amounts of the components available at any site or time.

Activation of the cascades of the early activation pathways described above is also inherently regulated by the limited stability of the multisubunit convertase enzymes. The proteolytic active sites of these complexes are on the C2a and Bb subunits, which are neither covalently bound to the subunit that provides the binding site for the next component, which is the substrate, nor to the target. Dissociation of the active subunit causes loss, or decay, of the convertase activity. This happens spontaneously by diffusion, or may be accelerated by proteins that bind to the covalently attached member of the convertase and push away the proteolytically active subunit. Several proteins have this function; some are soluble and some are membrane-bound. They are listed in Table 4-3.

Many of these proteins share homology with each other. This is not unexpected since they bind to C3 and/or C4, which are themselves homologous. These proteins are part of a family called regulators of complement activation (**RCA**) and are encoded by the RCA family of genes on

Table 4-2. Complement regulatory proteins

Name(s)	Abbreviation or symbol	Family	Function
C1 inhibitor (C1 esterase inhibitor)	C1 INH	Serpin	Inhibits C1r, C1s, MASPs, noncomplement proteases
C4 binding protein	C4bp	RCA[a]	Binds to C4, inhibits classical pathway
Factor H (b-1-H)	H	RCA	Binds to C3b, inhibits alternative pathway
Properdin	P		Stabilizes alternative pathway convertases
C3b/C4b inactivator (Factor I)	I		Cleaves C4b and C3b
Decay accelerating factor	DAF, CD55	RCA	Destabilizes all convertases
Complement receptor Type I	CR1, CD35	RCA	Binds to C3b, destabilizes covertases and acts as cofactor for cleavage by I
Membrane cofactor protein	MCP, CD46	RCA	Cofactor for cleavage of C4b and C3b by I
S protein (Vitronectin)			Inhibits insertion of C5b67
C8 binding protein (homologous restriction factor)			Inhibits addition and action of C8
Protectin (membrane inhibitor of reactive lysis)	CD59		Inhibits binding and polymerization of C9

a. RCA = Regulators of complement activation.

Table 4-3. Major mechanisms of regulation of complement activation and function

Mechanism	Examples
Inhibition of active proteases	C1 inhibitor (C1 INH)
Dissociation of convertases	DAF, CR1
Stabilization of convertases	Properdin (P)
Cleavage of active convertase subunits	Factor I
Promoters of cleavage by factor I	Factor H, C4 binding protein, CR1, membrane cofactor protein
Binding of lipophilic intermediates	S-protein (vitronectin), C8 binding protein (aka: homologous restriction factor, HRF), protectin (CD59)

chromosome 1. A prototypic member of this family is called decay accelerating factor (**DAF**). This is a protein bound to the plasma membrane by a glycolipid anchor, which is believed to give it increased mobility to move laterally across the membrane to prevent attack of complement on our own cells. The major function of DAF is to bind to C3b and C4b molecules and push off Bb or C2a. DAF is present on most cells in the body and, as a membrane protein, it is also designated as CD55.

In addition to their ability to bind to and push off (or block binding of) associated subunits of convertases, some of the regulatory proteins also facilitate degradation of the C4b or C3b to which they bind. There is a circulating protease, called Factor I or C3b/C4b inactivator, which can cleave C3b and C4b into forms that will no longer bind other components of the convertases, even though they can still serve as opsonins. This cleavage can only occur, however, when an additional cofactor is present. Such cofactors include the soluble proteins C4 binding protein (**C4bp**) and Factor H (formerly termed β-1-H globulin). Several integral membrane proteins also have this kind of "cofactor" activity, including complement receptor type 1 (CR1, CD35), commonly considered the C3b receptor, and a separate membrane cofactor protein or MCP (CD 46). DAF and MCP can bind to C3b and C4b only on the same cell on which they are found, which is why they are not considered receptors, but CR1 can also bind C3b on other cells or circulating complexes.

Competition for Binding to C3b Regulates Activation of the Alternative Pathway

From the viewpoint of a C3b molecule, regulation of alternative pathway activation might be seen as competition between binding of Factor B, which would lead to additional activation, versus Factor H, which would lead to inactivation. The enzymes that execute those actions, Factor D and Factor I, respectively, are both present in their active forms in the circulation at all times (Figure 4-12). What then determines the fate of that C3b molecule? The chemical nature of the surface on which the C3b is bound has an important role in influencing the binding of B versus H. Surfaces that are rich in sialic acid, like our own normal cells, favor the binding of H and thus promote the action of I. These surfaces are thus poor activators of the alternative pathway. In contrast, many bacteria and cells from some other species of mammals lack sialic acid. On these surfaces, binding of B is favored. Those cells are good activators of the alternative pathway. This provides another illustration of how complement functions as part of the innate immune system, providing a way to distinguish self from not-self even in the absence of antibody or a rearranged T-cell receptor. It is interesting in this context that bacteria such as K1 *E. coli* and type III group B streptococcus, which have adapted by adding sialic acid to their surface carbohydrates or capsules, become dangerous pathogens, especially for newborns who lack specific antibody. Related bacteria without the sialic acid pose little threat. Antibody molecules provide good acceptor sites for C3b deposition, on which B is favored over H and the C3b is protected against inactivation. This allows the alternative pathway to amplify initial signals generated by antibody and the classical pathway. Besides their coating with sialic acid, our own cells are protected from amplification of the alternative pathway by the presence of DAF and MCP, as well as by CR1, on cells that carry this receptor.

C1 Inhibitor Blocks Enzyme Activity of C1r, C1s, and MASPs; a Deficiency of C1 INH Is Responsible for Hereditary Angioedema

In addition to these critical mechanisms of regulation of the activation of the alternative pathway, there is a specific plasma protein, called C1 inhibitor

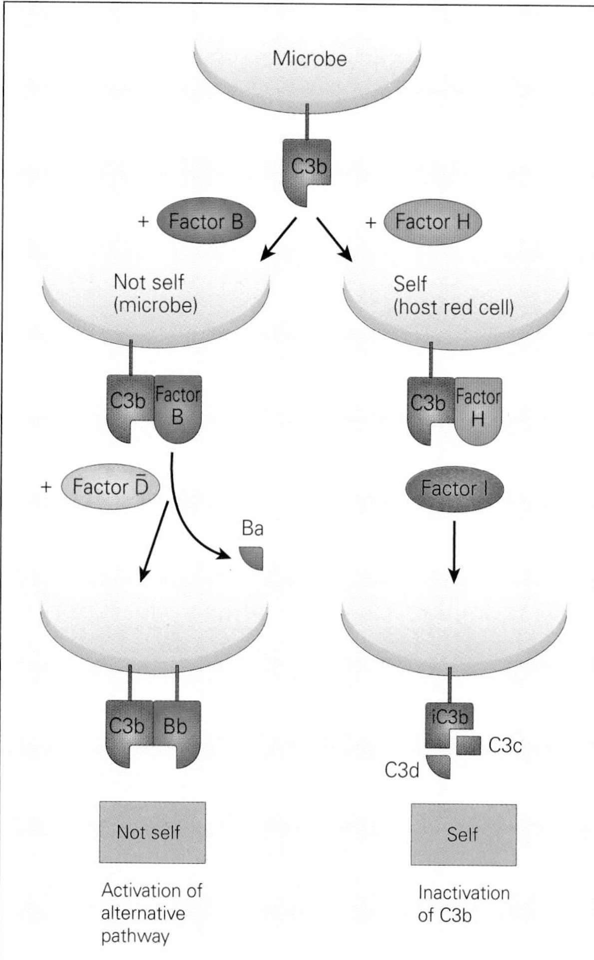

Figure 4-12. Competition between B and H for bound C3b is a major determinant of activation versus inactivation of the alternative pathway. Binding of B is favored in the absence of sialic acid, and will lead to cleavage of B by D and cycling of the alternative pathway as shown in Figure 4-8. The absence of sialic acid is characteristic of bacteria that are weak pathogens and serves as an important way the innate immune system distinguishes not-self from self. The presence of sialic acid is characteristic of human cell surfaces. This promotes binding of H, which can serve as a cofactor for I. Like D, I always circulates in its active form. Cleavage of C3b by I results in formation of iC3b, which can no longer act in convertases. Further cleavages by I may result in removal of C3c, with the small fragment C3d remaining on the cell surface (Figure 4-9).

(**C1 INH**) or C1 esterase inhibitor, which can complex with C1r and C1s and terminate their activity. This protein has also been shown to inhibit MASPs. The proteolytic activity of all of these enzymes depends on a serine in their active site, and C1 INH is a member of the serine protease inhibitor or the serpin family of proteins. C1 INH can also inhibit serine proteases in the clotting and kallikrein-kinin systems. Congenital deficiency of this protein results in the condition hereditary angioedema (**HAE**), which is manifest clinically in repeated attacks of swelling (Figure 4-13 and *Chapter 16*). Acquired forms of C1 esterase inhibitor deficiency may also occur, particularly in association with chronic lymphocytic leukemia. Laryngeal edema due to C1 esterase inhibitor deficiency can be fatal.

Specialized Inhibitors Block Membrane Attack Complex Formation

As described above, activation of the complement system beyond C5 involves conversion of individual soluble protein molecules into a large, multimeric transmembrane complex. There are several circulating molecules that are capable of interacting with the newly developing lipophilic sites on C5b-6 and C5-7, which prevent attachment of these intermediate complexes to plasma membranes. These include some of the lipoproteins; a specialized protein called S-protein or vitronectin, which also inhibits the blood-clotting system; and others. Besides these plasma proteins, which inhibit the formation of membrane attack complexes before they insert, there are membrane proteins that protect the cells on which they reside. These include homologous restriction factor (**HRF**), also known as C8-binding protein, which is believed to inhibit further actions of C8 once it has become complexed with C5-7 in the membrane, and an additional protein called "protectin" or CD59. CD59 inhibits polymerization of C9 and its incorporation into complexes containing C8. This

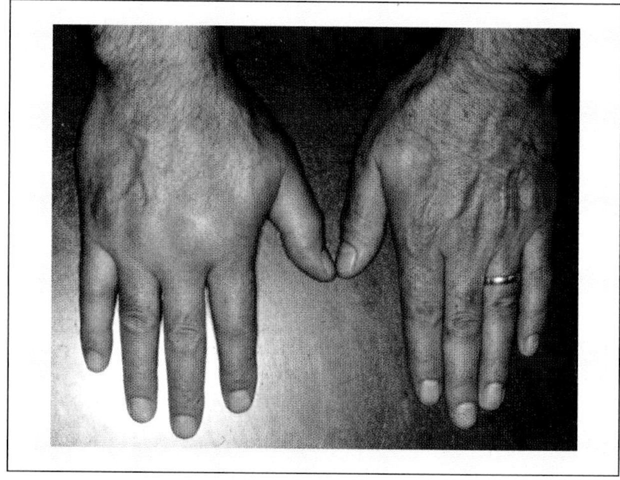

Figure 4-13. Photograph of the hands of a patient with hereditary angioedema showing swelling of the dorsum of the right hand during an attack. (*Courtesy of Dr. Fred S. Rosen.*)

inhibits development of the full lytic activity of the membrane attack complex. Like DAF (CD55), HRF and CD59 are not true transmembrane proteins, but are linked to the cell membrane by phosphatidyl inositol glycolipid anchors. An inability to form this linkage in clonal descendants of affected hematopoietic stem cells results in populations of erythrocytes with increased susceptibility to lysis by complement. At night, when the respiratory rate decreases and the plasma becomes slightly acidified, spontaneous activation of the alternative pathway may increase and result in the lysis of erythrocytes that lack these complement control proteins. This condition is known as paroxysmal nocturnal hemoglobinuria (**PNH**), which is notable for the dark color of the urine (due to its content of free hemoglobin) in the late night or upon arising, which clears as the day goes on.

Therapeutic Complement Regulators Are Being Developed as Inhibitors of Complement Activity in Disease

Besides those rare disorders in which disease results from pathologic complement activation due to congenital or acquired deficiency of complement control proteins, like C1 esterase inhibitor deficiency or PNH, complement activation may contribute to other diseases as well. Complement activation may increase tissue damage after burns and ischemia (see below). In addition, in many diseases that involve autoantibodies, complement activation may physiologically follow antibody binding, but because the antigen is a normal body constituent, complement activation contributes to the pathology. In all of those situations, it may be desirable to inhibit complement activation as part of the therapy. Several approaches to treatment of hereditary angioedema are currently in clinical trials, and it is possible that augmentation of normal C1 esterase inhibitor activity may be beneficial in other conditions and disease states because of the broad range of activity of this inhibitor. Small molecule inhibitors of the complement convertases are under development, but they have not yet come into use clinically.

As described above, by binding to C3b, CR1 can inhibit both the classical and alternative pathways. A recombinant form of soluble CR1 has been prepared and has shown promising activity in animal models and in preliminary clinical trials (see Complement in Ischemia/Reperfusion Injury, below). A monoclonal antibody against C5 has been developed which has shown very promising results in treatment of PNH and may prove useful in other disorders in which membrane attack complex formation participates.

Therapeutic Effects of IGIV as an Inhibitor of C3 Deposition

IgG antibody molecules provide very good acceptors for the nascent covalent binding site i.e., exposed during C3 activation. Activating complement in the presence of increased concentrations of IgG results in distraction of some of the C3b molecules from the target on which the C1 is being activated to some of the extra IgG molecules in solution. In this way, excess IgG can decrease C3b deposition and can prevent hemolysis of sensitized erythrocytes and other forms of tissue damage. Therapeutically, administration of high doses of IGIV (one to two grams per kilogram) has this effect in vivo, and inhibition of complement deposition is one of the major mechanisms by which this treatment decreases tissue damage in autoantibody-mediated diseases (*Chapter 11*). Data showing decreased deposition of membrane attack complexes in the muscle capillaries of dermatomyositis patients treated with IGIV provides an example of this mechanism of action of IGIV in vivo.

Complement Receptors

In addition to the complement components themselves, and the control proteins, there are at least seven distinct proteins that serve as cell membrane receptors for different fragments of the complement system. These important proteins mediate many of the physiologic effects of complement.

Complement Binding to C1q Receptors on Phagocytes Enhances Phagocytosis

Following activation of C1, the active C1r and C1s are pulled off and inactivated by binding to C1 INH. This leaves the stalks of C1q sticking up from the IgG and IgM molecules bound to their antigen. Incubation of monocytes and macrophages with antigen-antibody complexes bearing C1q enhances the phagocytosis of other particles by these cells. The receptor which mediates this effect on the cells is believed to be a heavily glycosylated protein with 631 amino acids that can also bind to other members of the collectin family, such as MBL and pulmonary surfactant proteins A and D.

Anaphylotoxins C3a and C5a, When Bound to Receptors on Mast Cells and Basophils, Stimulate Mediator Release

In describing the complement activation pathways above, reference was made to the liberation of small fragments from C4, C3, and C5 upon their cleavage by the respective convertases. However, most of the attention was given to the larger fragments, which continue the activation cascades. These three components all share considerable homology and they are all activated by cleavage just after an arginine 74-77 residues from the N-terminal of the α chain of the respective molecules. C4a has little biologic activity and will not be described further. However, C3a and C5a have distinct receptors on mast cells, which are members of the family of seven-membrane spanners or "g-protein coupled receptors" because they have seven transmembrane domains and send intracellular signals by associating with intracellular transducers called g-proteins. Binding of C3a and also of C5a to their receptors on mast cells and basophils activates the cells and causes the release of their intracellular storage granules, which are rich in histamine. The effects of this mast cell degranulation and histamine release resemble those of the IgE-mediated histamine release that occurs during anaphylaxis. The anaphylotoxins can also cause smooth muscle contraction and mucous secretion, independently from their actions on mast cells. Thus, the ability of these complement fragments to mimic allergen-induced anaphylaxis gave them their designation as anaphylotoxins. It is important to recognize that release of these anaphylotoxins after reaction of IgG or IgM with the classical pathway may result in increased vascular permeability and other pro-inflammatory effects at sites of antigen-antibody complex formation or deposition, including the binding of autoantibodies to vascular endothelial cells or of antigen-antibody complexes to basement membranes. In this way, the complement anaphylotoxins are probably responsible for the itching and hives seen in the condition hypocomplementemic (urticarial) vasculitis.

Plasma Protein Carboxypeptidase B Inactivates Anaphylotoxins

As noted above, the anaphylotoxins are cleavage fragments that include the N-terminal of the respective protein chains. The cleavage occurs just past an arginine residue, so the C-terminal amino acid of the anaphylotoxins is arginine. This residue may be removed by the plasma protein carboxypeptidase-B, now also known as anaphylotoxin inactivator. As its name implies, removal of the arginine residue greatly reduces the ability of C3a and C5a to activate mast cells and basophils. The fragments remaining after the arginine has been removed are called C3a-desArg and C5a-desArg, respectively.

C5a and C5a-desArg Are Potent Chemoattractants

C5a differs from C4a and C3a in that it has a considerably higher molecular weight, approximately 11,000 daltons, compared to 8,650 and 9,000 for C4a and C3a, respectively. This difference in molecular weight is due to the presence of a sugar side chain on C5a. This side chain gives C5a the unique ability to interact with a distinct receptor (CD 88), which is found on phagocytes: including polymorphonuclear leukocytes, monocytes, and macrophages. C5a as well as C5a-desArg are potent chemoattractants and activators of these phagocytes, and also prime them for increased bactericidal activity and secretion. Attraction and activation of phagocytes by C5a and C5a-desArg are among the most important contributions of the complement system to host defense against bacterial infection. Some research suggests that C5a receptors are present on non-myeloid parenchymal cells in different tissues and that binding of C5a to these cells may induce secretion of IL-6 and other cytokines. Since IL-6 itself is a potent inducer of acute phase reactant proteins, this may provide a pathway for systemic amplification of local inflammatory responses.

Binding of Activated C3 to Its Receptors Stimulates Phagocytosis, Immune Complex Clearance, and B Cell Activation

C3 is present in the circulation at the highest concentration of any of the complement components, approximately 1 mg/ml. As noted above, there are three different pathways by which C3 can be activated and deposited on a surface or target of complement activation, and there is a whole family of proteins that function to regulate the deposition of C3 and the form and fate of the bound fragments. Many of the biologic functions of C3 are subserved by the interaction of bound C3 fragments with different receptors on different cell types. The properties of these are summarized in Table 4-4. It can be argued that the most important roles of the complement system really involve these interactions of C3 with its receptors, which are involved in opsonization of bacteria, clearance of immune complexes, and regulation of the adaptive immune response to antigens. The importance of these interactions is emphasized by the presence of three distinct major receptors for different fragments of bound C3. In the complement nomenclature, these are termed CR1, CR2, CR3, and CR4; referring to CD35, CD21, and CD11b/CD18, respectively. The presence of these different receptors for varying fragments of C3 on different types of cells means that controlling the form of C3 on any given target of complement activation will play an important role in determining the destination and effects of that target in the host.

Native C3 in the circulation does not bind to receptors, but the conformational changes that occur after cleavage markedly increase the affinity with which the large fragment, C3b, binds to the type 1 complement receptor, or CR1 (CD 35). CR1 can also bind C4b. CR1 is a member of the RCA family of proteins and is comprised of twenty-eight or more short consensus repeats of about sixty-eight amino acids each, which are organized into four long, homologus repeats that actually form the binding sites characteristic of this family.

CR1 is present on neutrophils, other granulocytes, and monocytes and plays an important role in promoting phagocytosis. The increase in binding of a target particle, such as a bacterium, to a phagocyte that may be mediated by the deposition of C3b, is termed **opsonization** and may be considered roughly analogous to putting ketchup on French fries. Molecularly, the interaction of multiple C3b molecules on the target with multiple CR1 receptors on the phagocyte is important in increasing the adherence of the particle to the phagocyte. In most situations, the actual signal to begin the ingestion of the particle—phagocytosis, per se—is provided by the interaction of the Fc domain of IgG with a receptor for that antibody. Those types of receptors do not exist for IgM. Thus, particles opsonized with IgM and C3b may be bound to but not ingested by phagocytes, unless they receive some additional activating signal. As noted above, CR1 can also act as a regulator of complement activation, which has both decay-accelerating and cofactor activity. Erythrocytes also carry CR1, which plays an important role in the transport and clearance of C3b-coated antigen-antibody complexes (see "Role of Complement in Trafficking and Disposal of Antigen-Antibody Complexes" on the next page). In addition, CR1 is also expressed on glomerular podocytes, where it plays a role in directing the deposition of immune complexes. CR1 is also expressed on antigen-presenting dendritic cells, B lymphocytes, and some subpopulations of T lymphocytes.

Factor I initially carries out a single cleavage on C3b, but because there are disulfide bonds between the two chains of C3b that sit on both sides of this cleavage, the protein remains bound to the target, although its conformation changes. This new form of C3b is inactive in convertases; hence, it is called iC3b. This no longer binds to CR1 but can still serve as an opsonin by binding to a different receptor called complement receptor type 3 (CD11b/CD18). This molecule is a member of the family of leukocyte β-integrins and has multiple additional functions besides binding iC3b (*Chapter 5*). It is one of the leukocytes' most important adherence molecules: its ability to bind to intracellular adhesion molecule type 1 (**ICAM-1**) on endothelial cells is critically important in allowing neutrophils to exit from the circulation and crawl into the tissues at sites of infection. Mutations in CD18 may prevent the neutrophils from reaching sites of infection, leaving the host extremely susceptible to pneumonia and other bacterial infections which

Table 4-4. Major membrane receptors for C3 fragments bound to targets

Complement designation	CD designation	Protein family	Ligand-binding specificity	Cellular expression
CR1	CD35	RCA	C4b, C3b	RBCs, PMNs, monocytes, some macrophages, lymphocytes, glomerular podocytes
CR2	CD21	RCA	C3d	B-lymphocytes, dendritic cells
CR3	CD11b/CD18	β2 Integrins	iC3b, β-glucans, ICAM-1	PNMs, monocytes
CR4	CD11c/CD18	β2 Integrins	iC3b	Macrophages, PMNs, dendritic cells

occur paradoxically in the face of extremely high white blood cell counts (since the marrow is signaled to release additional cells but they cannot get out of the circulation). This situation is recognized as leukocyte adherence deficiency (**LAD**) type 1 (*Chapter 16*). CR3 also has lectin-like activity and can bind bacterial polysaccharides even in the absence of complement. Like CR1, this important adherence molecule and receptor is stored inside circulating cells and is rapidly brought to the surface when the cells are activated, e.g., by chemoattractants such as C5a and C5a-desArg. Its binding activity is also increased when the cells are activated, and expression of the activated adherence molecule on the surface of neutrophils by intravascular C5a can lead to neutrophil aggregation. Plugging of pulmonary capillaries by neutrophil aggregates is believed to be the cause of the tachypnea and/or hypoxia which often accompanies large scale complement activation induced when blood comes into contact with artificial materials such as the membranes in oxygenators used for cardiopulmonary bypasses and in dialysis machines. CR4 (CD11c/CD18), a related member of the same family i.e., found on tissue macrophages, may bind iC3b and/or C3d.

After Factor I cleaves iC3b at an additional site, the bulk of the molecule separates from a small fragment that remains covalently bound to the target (Figure 4-9). The large fragment, C3c, diffuses away, and the small fragment that remains bound is termed C3dg. This is often cleaved even further to give C3d. Both C3d and C3dg can bind to complement receptor type 2 (CR2, CD 21). This distinct receptor is also a member of the RCA family, and serves its most important functions on B lymphocytes, where it is generally found in close association with CD19. The presence of C3d on an antigen allows co-engagement of the CD19-CD21 complex and the antigen receptor (surface immunoglobulin) at the same time. This co-engagement enhances and prolongs antigen signaling, providing one way in which complement acts in the afferent as well as the effector arms of the immune response.

Role of Complement in Defense against Infection and Immunopathology

Complement Enhances Phagocytosis of Bacteria and Can Lyse Some Bacterial Cells

The pyogenic infections suffered by the child described in the case study at the beginning of this chapter illustrates one of the most important physiologic functions of the complement system: enhancing defenses against bacterial infection. In the case of Gram-positive bacteria, whose thick cell walls protect them from lysis by the membrane attack complex, the deposition of large amounts of C3b and iC3b play a critical role in opsonization, ingestion, and intracellular killing of the organisms by phagocytes (*Chapter 12*). Any or all of the activation pathways may be involved in this. If the bacteria do not inhibit alternative pathway activation, the feedback loop of that pathway will result in deposition of so much C3 that the strain of bacteria will often be considered a not very virulent pathogen. In contrast, bacteria that have adapted to human host defenses by putting sialic acid in their capsules and/or by developing membrane proteins which help them evade C3 deposition will generally be more virulent. Streptococcal M-proteins are good examples of this type of evasion of host defenses by virulent bacteria. Electron microscopic localization studies have shown that anti-capsular antibodies lead to the deposition of complement on the capsule if there is one, while C3b deposited below the capsule, on the cell wall, by alternative pathway activation, may not be accessible to receptors on the surface of phagocytes. In general, antibodies, particularly of the IgG class, work synergistically with complement in promoting phagocytosis. The presence of antibody that can activate complement by the classical pathway will accelerate initial deposition of C3b. C3b molecules bound to IgG and IgM molecules will be protected from H and I and will thus accelerate amplification by the alternative pathway. The simultaneous interaction of IgG with Fc receptors and C3b and iC3b with their receptors will greatly enhance clearance of opsonized bacteria from the bloodstream by macrophages of the reticuloendothelial system, as well as phagocytosis of bacteria at peripheral sites of infection by neutrophils. The ability of C5a and C5a-desArg to attract and activate the neutrophils also plays an important role in the latter process. MBL and the lectin pathway of complement activation are important in host defenses against infection with pyogenic bacteria as well as yeasts and other types of organisms, and deficiency of MBL also results in an increased incidence of infection (*Chapter 16*).

In general, Gram-negative bacteria are susceptible to lysis by the membrane attack complex of complement, since they lack the protection conferred on

Gram-positives by the thick cell wall. However, some virulent strains of Gram-negative bacteria have developed mechanisms to evade complement attack that may include the presence of sialic acid in their capsules and/or long polysaccharide side chains on their LPS. In some cases, there are also specific outer membrane proteins that inhibit complement activation or cause deposition at sites that do not damage the bacterial membrane itself. Neisseria, in particular, may be resistant to intracellular killing following opsonization and phagocytosis, and assembly of the membrane attack complex is necessary for adequate defense against these types of organisms. Meningococcal meningitis and disseminated gonococcal infection are particularly problematic in patients with deficiencies of components C5 through C8.

Complement Can Neutralize Viruses and Lyse Viral Envelopes

In addition to its protective role against bacteria, complement also plays a role in antiviral defense (*Chapter 13*). Viruses are intracellular pathogens and must interact with specific sites on host cells in order to gain entry into the cells and subvert their mechanisms for viral replication (*Chapter 13*). Deposition of early components of the classical pathway and/or C3b molecules on the surface of the virus may block the proteins on the virus that are necessary for entry into host cells and thus neutralize the virus. It is also possible for antibodies to viral antigens on the surface of enveloped viruses to activate the classical pathway and lead to membrane attack complex-mediated lysis of the envelopes. On the other hand, the envelopes, which are formed from the plasma membranes of the infected cells, may continue to bear complement control proteins from those cells, which then inhibit complement attack on the viruses. Several viruses have incorporated portions of the host genome into their own, and may have proteins or protein domains that protect them for complement attack. Furthermore, some viruses, most notably the Epstein-Barr virus (**EBV**), have subverted complement receptors for entry into the host cells. A large surface molecule on EBV contains a stretch of nine amino acids that also is found in C3d and enables to virus to enter and infect B cells by binding to CR2.

Complement in Ischemia/Reperfusion Injury and Cell Necrosis

In addition to its multiple roles in recognizing a wide variety of foreign invaders, the innate immune system helps prevent autoimmunity by recognizing and removing injured cells that might otherwise be seen as antigens by the adaptive immune system. Following any of a number of injuries, there may be deprivation of blood supply to the affected tissues, i.e., ischemia, followed by an attempt to reestablish a blood supply, i.e., reperfusion. Complement plays a role in each of these processes. Ischemia and cell death lead to exposure of basement membranes and other extra- and intracellular structures that would not normally be accessible to plasma proteins or lymphocytes. Burns and infection may also alter the structures of normal cellular proteins. These exposed surfaces and/or altered proteins may lead to activation of the alternative pathway, and the other pathways as well, by binding of MBL and/or weakly reactive natural antibodies of the IgM class, which can then activate C1. Complement activation at sites of ischemia and tissue injury, including after thermal burns, can lead to local deposition of C3 fragments and membrane attack complexes (detectable by binding of antibodies to neoantigens on C9), as well as generation of C5a and C5a-desArg. Upon reperfusion, the locally produced C5a and C5a-desArg can cause neutrophil aggregation with plugging of capillaries and aggravation of the local tissue damage. A particularly illustrative example of this is provided by studies of the induction of ischemia/reperfusion injury by experimental temporary ligation of the coronary arteries in animals. In that type of model, treatment of the animals with a recombinant, soluble form of CR1, which can inhibit both the classical and alternative pathways of complement activation, resulted in decreased deposition of membrane attack complexes, decreased capillary plugging by neutrophil aggregates, and a markedly decreased area of infarction. Unfortunately, the form of CR1 used in those studies has not yet proved applicable for human treatment, but is in clinical trials. However, those studies do illustrate the role of complement in ischemia/reperfusion injury and the potential for complement inhibition as a therapeutic modality in a wide variety of diseases.

Complement Is Important for Removal of Dead Host Cells

On a cellular level, upon apoptosis, complement control proteins are likely internalized or lost as cell membrane lipids invert, promoting activation of the alternative pathway. Opsonization of apoptotic cells by deposition of C3b and other fragments may facilitate the removal of dead cells by macrophages. Nonimmunologic activation of the classical pathway may follow the binding of C1q to mitochondrial proteins and other, normally intracellular, structures that become exposed during apoptosis and/or necrosis of cells. The deposition of complement-derived opsonins likely contributes to the safe disposal of these damaged cells and constituents. The absence of these mechanisms in patients with deficiencies of MBL or the subcomponents of C1 is believed to be important in the formation of autoantibodies, particularly to nuclear antigens, and to the development of systemic lupus erythematosus (*Chapter 19*), which occurs with a very high incidence in patients with deficiency of MBL or C1q, as well in patients who are deficient in other early acting components of the classical pathway. Thus, one of the normal functions of complement is to promote the disposal of dead cells and their contents. A failure or incapacity of this function has generated a theory for the development of autoimmune disease, i.e., the **waste disposal hypothesis** (described below Box 4-1 and Figure 4-14), which is based upon the accumulation of ineffectively removed celluar debris resulting from this failed complement function.

Complement Is Responsible for Solubilization, Trafficking, and Disposal of Antigen-Antibody Complexes

Our case study may be considered one of those experiments of nature that illustrates by its absence an important normal function of the complement system in the proper disposal of antigen-antibody complexes formed as a result of a common infection. The occurrence of pathologic immune complexes in chronic infections, such as chronic active hepatitis or subacute bacterial endocarditis, as well as in autoimmune diseases, had long been recognized as a consequence of prolonged antigen production. It had also been recognized that this might lead to nephritis or other secondary complications, but recognition of the role of

Box 4-1

The Waste-Disposal Hypothesis and Systemic Lupus Erythematosus

It is now clearly established that complement can have both pro- and anti-inflammatory activities. Normal functioning of the complement system may actually reduce inflammation by promoting prompt killing and removal of infecting organisms, solubilizing antigen-antibody precipitates, clearing immune complexes from the circulation, and promoting disposal of apoptotic cells and debris. Normal cells constantly undergo apoptosis and must be removed and digested without being presented as antigens and evoking harmful immunologic responses (*Chapter 19*). If this normal clearing mechanism does not occur efficiently, intracellular components can accumulate and initiate autoimmune responses. This may explain the very high frequency of systemic lupus erythematosus (SLE) in patients with early complement component deficiencies. Shown in Figure 4-14 are three variations of the waste-disposal hypothesis together with consequences of its failure. Panel A shows the normal functioning of complement in facilitating the removal of an apoptotic cell without antigen presentation and inflammation. This is the major step which would fail to occur with an early complement component defect and/or if the system were overwhelmed. In panel B, as a result of complement deficiency, the apoptotic cell is not ingested normally by macrophages and instead results in maturation of a dendritic cell that then, together with the stimulatory cytokines IL-4 and IL-12, can present antigen to T cells with resultant enhanced autoreactivity. Other receptor-ligand systems, particularly those involving phosphoserine, may also contribute to suppression of the inflammatory/immunostimulatory consequences of phagocytosis of apoptotic cells. In panel C, a self-reactive B cell that has bound intracellular antigens is stimulated to differentiate into an autoantibody-secreting plasma cell. Since most patients with SLE do not have a complete deficiency of any individual complement component, it is presumed that partial abnormalities in regulatory mechanisms may contribute to the expression of the final disease phenotype. However, the occurrence of SLE in more than 90 percent of patients with C1q deficiency strongly suggests that this defect alone is sufficient to cause this multisystem autoimmune disease. It is remarkable that the spectrum of autoantibodies in patients with SLE is typically directed to proteins and nucleic acid antigens present in virtually every cell in the body. Experiments in mice suggest that in addition to complement deficiency, deficiencies in proteins that complex with or degrade chromatin are also associated with SLE-like syndromes.

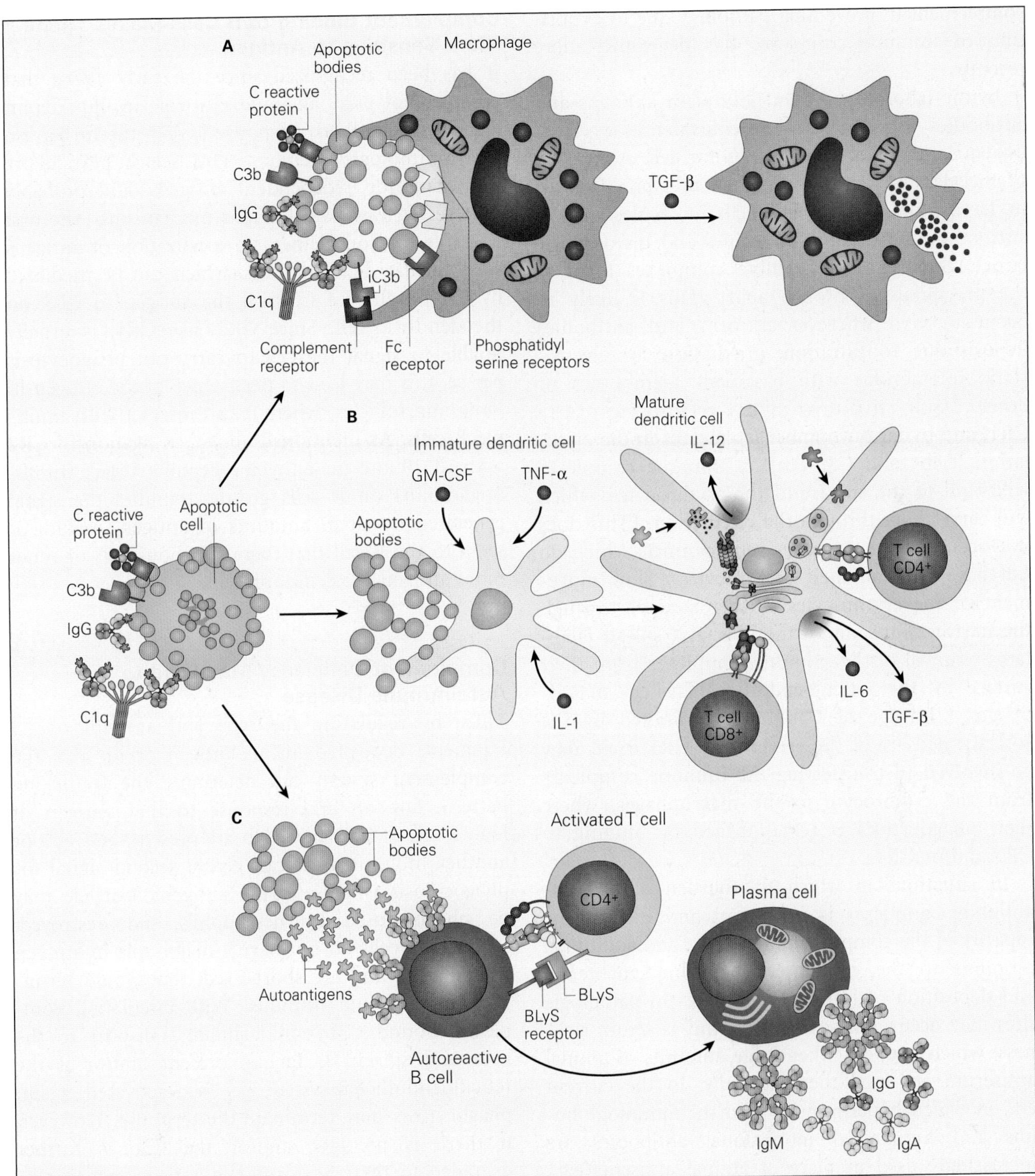

Figure 4-14. The waste-disposal hypothesis for systemic lupus erythematosus. Panel A: A macrophage is shown engulfing apoptotic bodies released from an apoptotic cell. There are a variety of ligands on apoptotic cells and receptors on macrophages that make this process extremely efficient. The binding of C1q, C-reactive protein, and IgG to apoptotic cells may promote the activation of complement, leading to the clearance of apoptotic cells by ligation of complement receptors. Once the macrophage has engulfed the apoptotic cell, it secretes the anti-inflammatory cytokine transforming growth factor *b* (TGF-β). Panel B: When there is an excess of apoptotic cells and the failure of one or more of the normal systems of receptor-ligand recognition for the uptake of apoptotic cells, immature dendritic cells may take up apoptotic bodies. If this occurs in the presence of inflammatory cytokines such as granulocyte-macrophage colony-stimulating factor (GM-CSF), tumor necrosis factor *a* (TNF-α), and interleukin-1, the dendritic cell may mature into an autoantigen-presenting cell. The dendritic cell is shown presenting autoantigens to a T cell in the presence of costimulatory molecules and cytokines. Panel C: Shows an autoreactive B cell that has taken up autoantigens from an apoptotic cell through its antibody receptors. The B cell is receiving help from an activated T cell, which is expressing co-stimulatory molecules and cytokines involved in the maturation of B cells, including an important member of the tumor necrosis family, B lymphocyte stimulator (BLyS), also referred to as zTNF-4. The autoreactive B cell divides and matures into a plasma cell that secretes autoantibodies. It is likely that in the majority of patients, systemic lupus erythematosus develops only in the presence of abnormalities in more than one of these steps. (Adapted from Walport MJ. Complement. Second of two parts. N Engl J Med. 2001;344:1140–4.)

complement in preventing pathology due to deposition of immune complexes has developed more recently.

In the laboratory, when polyvalent antigens and antibodies are combined at equivalence, a cross-linked, lattice-like precipitate is formed. Activation of the classical pathway by such precipitates leads to deposition of C4b and C3b molecules on the antibodies and antigen molecules and disrupts the lattice. Smaller, more soluble complexes form as the precipitate is broken apart. This is likely to occur in vivo wherever antigens and antibodies deposit due to filtration, gravitation, or electrostatic interactions with basement membranes or other tissue structures. Since erythrocytes carry CR1, and by far outnumber leukocytes in the circulation, C4b- and C3b-bearing immune complexes will bind to the surface of the erythrocytes, which will carry them through the circulation. (This does not occur in non-primates such as mice, which do not have CR1 on their erythrocytes.) Slow movement of the erythrocytes as they squeeze through the narrow sinusoids of the liver and spleen facilitates removal of the immune complexes from their surface by the reticuloendothelial system macrophages. Cleavage of C3b by I, promoted by the cofactor activity of the erythrocyte CR1 itself, may be involved in transferring the immune complexes from the erythrocyte to the macrophages, where their phagocytosis is accomplished by binding to CR3 and/or CR4.

In situations in which the burden of antigen-antibody complexes is very great and exceeds the capacity of the complement system to add additional opsonins to the complexes, hypocomplementemia and deposition of immune complexes in pathologic sites may occur. One example of this is serum sickness, which happens when large amounts of animal antiserum are used therapeutically. In the current era, in which hyperimmune human immunoglobulins and humanized monoclonal antibodies are increasingly used in place of animal antisera (e.g., using monoclonal anti-T cell antibodies in place of horse antithymocyte globulin to prevent transplant rejection), this condition is being seen with decreasing frequency. However, serum-sickness-like reactions still occur in some viral diseases and in drug reactions in which a small molecule given therapeutically can bind to circulating proteins and be recognized by the immune system as a hapten (*Chapter 18*).

Complement Binding to B Cells Makes Them More Sensitive to Antigen

It has been recognized since the early 1970s that complement plays an important role in the afferent arm of the antibody response and in the formation of immunologic memory. This seems particularly important for T-dependent antigens, and probably involves at least two different mechanisms. The first is a role for complement in localization of antigens on follicular dendritic cells, which can be mediated by the binding of C3d on the antigen to CR2 on the dendritic cell. Since CR2, like CR1, is usually unable to signal the cell to carry out phagocytosis per se, this may lead to persistence of the antigen in lymphoid follicles, where it can interact with multiple B cells. As mentioned above, co-ligation of CR2 with CD19 and the antigen receptor (surface immunoglobulin) on B cells greatly amplifies the signal generated by small amounts of antigen, making it seem to the B cell that there are thousands of times more antigen molecules present.

Complement Deficiency May Lead to Autoimmune Disease

Thus, by regulating the type and amount of C3 fragments deposited on an antigen or invader, the complement system can determine the trafficking pattern, fate of, and response to that antigen. If high levels of C3b and iC3b are present, and IgG or another molecule that can give a second signal for phagocytosis is present, the antigenic particle may be phagocytosed by neutrophils and destroyed. Since these cells do not have a major role in antigen presentation and are short-lived, that would terminate an antigenic stimulus. With circulating complexes, bound C3b will facilitate transport to the liver and spleen. If IgG is present and/or if the reticuloendothelial system has been activated, again, phagocytosis may terminate the response. However, if there is no IgG, and/or the C3b is further degraded to the C3d form, the antigen may persist on dendritic cells and stimulate further antibody responses. Obviously, if there is a congenital complement deficiency, if there has been excessive consumption of C3, or if the capacity of the complement or reticuloendothelial systems has been exceeded, then the immune complexes may deposit in tissues where secondary pathology may result. The role of complement in modulation of antibody synthesis and immunologic homeostasis and its implications in autoimmune disease has given rise to the concept of the waste-disposal hypothesis (Box 4-1).

Clinical Significance of Complement Functions

From what has been described in this chapter, it may be possible now to summarize the basic four biologic properties of complement that have the greatest clinical relevance for an understanding of the role of complement in the immune response in health and disease. These four key biologic properties are shown in Table 4-5 and Figures 4-15 to 4-18, together with examples of their clinical significance, and include: (1) opsonization, (2) anaphylatoxin activity, (3) chemotactic activity, and (4) cytotoxic activity.

Assays of Complement Function

The release of hemoglobin from antibody-sensitized animal erythrocytes upon complement lysis formed the basis of most early complement assays and led to the concept of measurement of the hemolytic activity of the intact classical complement pathway. The dilution of serum that resulted in lysis of 50 percent of a standardized suspension of erythrocytes was usually taken as the endpoint, and hence the assay was termed CH50, for complement hemolysis, 50 percent. This term is still used for assays of the total activity of the classical pathway, but the animal cells have been replaced by liposomes containing enzymes that can easily be quantitated by automated instruments used for other enzyme-linked immunoassays. Other commercial assay systems use antigen- and antibody-coated plates, which measure the binding of monoclonal antibodies to the C9 neoantigen. An assay for the intact function of the alternative pathway, called the AH50, is frequently performed using lysis of rabbit erythrocytes, which lack sialic acid and are thus good activators of the alternative pathway. Assays of the CH50 and AH50 are useful as screening tests for complete deficiency of any given component of the respective pathway, but may not be sufficiently sensitive for detecting partial consumption of a given component. For example, since C3 is present in much higher concentrations than any other component in normal serum, it would not be the rate-limiting step in an assay of either whole pathway unless it was seriously depleted. Assays of the individual components may be performed by direct quantitation of the amount of that protein present, which is usually done using monoclonal antibodies in enzyme-linked immunosorbent assays (**ELISA**) or

Table 4-5. Biologic activities and clinical significance of the major complement system

Biologic activity	Complement component	Mechanism of action
Host defense against infection		
Opsonization	C3b	C3b binds to the surface of pathogens, leading to greater internalization by phagocytic cells by opsonization.
Anaphylatoxin activity	C3a, C4a, C5a	Mast cell degranulation, increased vascular permeability, smooth muscle contraction.
Chemotactic activity	C5a	Helps recruit inflammatory cells from vascular sites into tissues.
Cytotoxicity	C5b, C6, C7, C8, and polymeric C9	The membrane attack complex (MAC) is the cytolytic end product of the complement cascade; it forms a transmembrane channel, which causes osmotic lysis of the target cell.
Interface between innate and adaptive immunity		
Augmentation of B cell responses	C3b and C4b bound to immune complexes and antigen; C3 receptors on B cells and APCs	These complexes and receptors can augment antibody responses by enhancing uptake of antigen or antigen-antibody complexes.
Enhancement of immunogenicity	C3b and C4b bound to immune complexes and antigen; C3 receptors on follicular DCs	These complexes and receptors can enhance immunologic memory.
Disposal of waste		
Removal of immune complexes	C1q; covalently bound fragments of C3 and C4	Clearance of immune complexes from tissues.
Removal of apoptotic cells	C1q; covalently bound fragments of C3 and C4	Clearance of apoptotic cells.

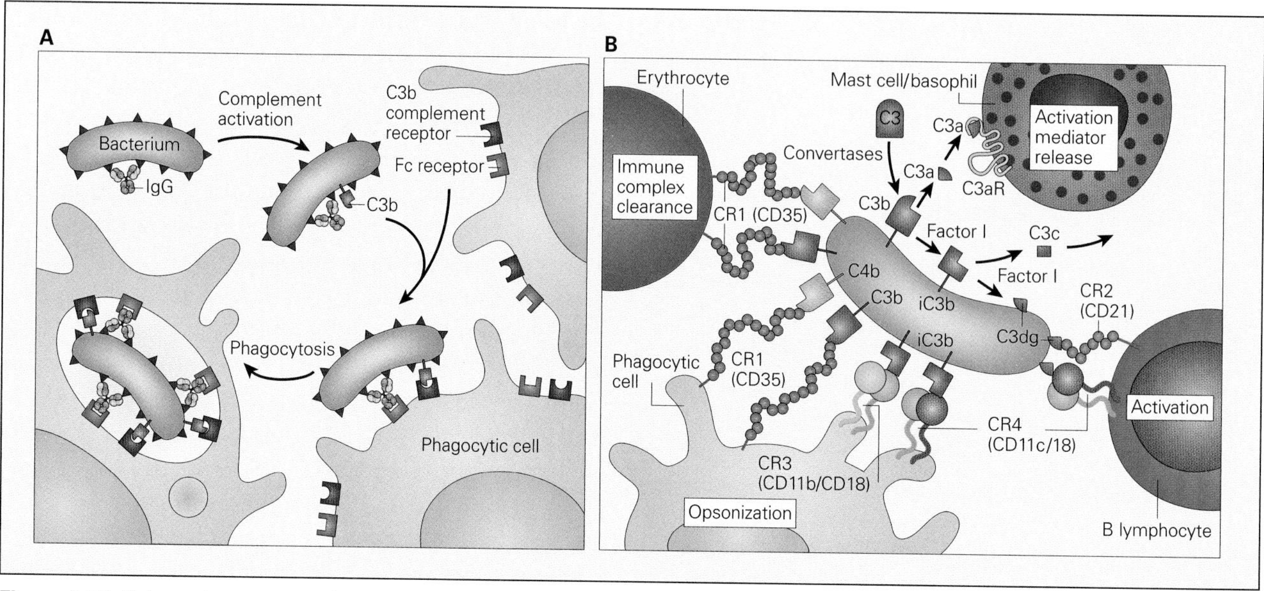

Figure 4-15. Schematic representation of the phagocytic-promoting activity (opsonic function) of complement, associated with the binding of C3b to its cell surface receptor. Panel A: Illustrates the opsonic activity of C3b; Panel B: Represents a more contemporary view of the multiple complement components involved in the opsonization of a bacterial cell.

automated nephelometry systems. Despite the above caveats, involvement of complement in a disease process such as SLE is frequently detected by measuring the serum C4 and C3 concentrations, and serial determinations of C4 and C3 over time are often used to monitor disease activity.

Often, immunohistochemical or immunofluorescent staining of a tissue section will be used to determine whether complement is involved in pathophysiology of a disease process. This is particularly applicable in skin biopsies used to diagnose SLE, and for understanding the pathogenesis and prognosis of different forms of glomerulonephritis. If C3 fragments are detected, staining for factor B and/or P, versus for C4b, may reveal whether local complement activation involves the alternative versus the classical pathway. Similarly, determination of whether decreased serum concentrations

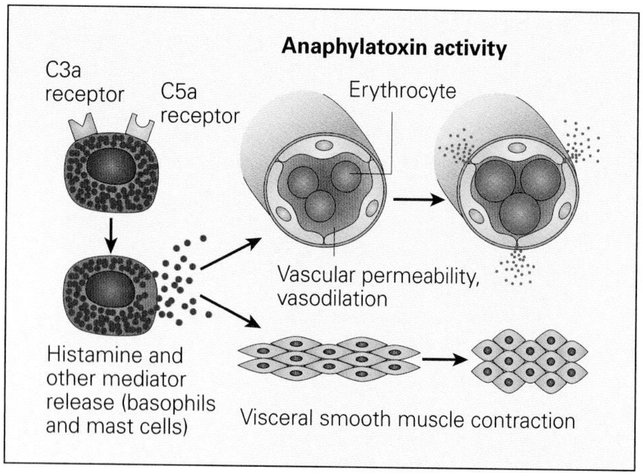

Figure 4-16. Schematic representation of the anaphylatoxin activity associated with C3a, C4a, and C5a, causing mediator release from mediator cells (primarily basophils and mast cells) with subsequent smooth muscle contraction and alterations in vascular permeability. Anaphylatoxins can also directly stimulate smooth muscle contraction and mucus secretion.

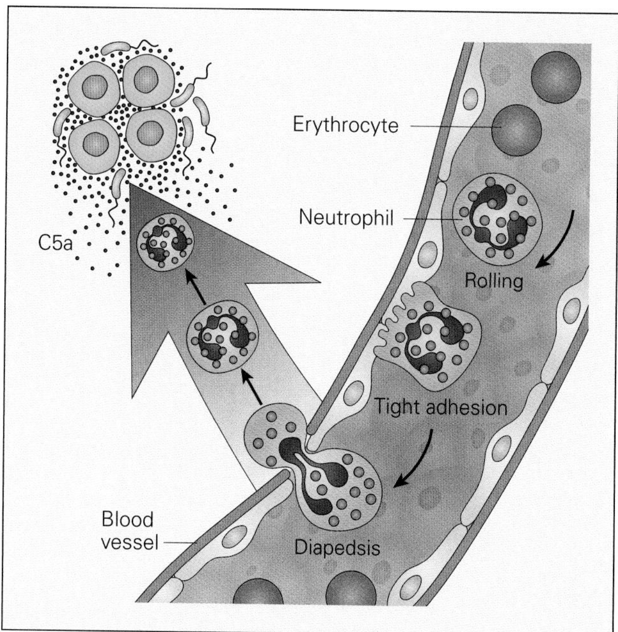

Figure 4-17. Schematic representation of unidirectional movement of neutrophils from the vascular compartment (chemotactic response) to chemoattractant stimuli in tissue C5a generated by complement activation.

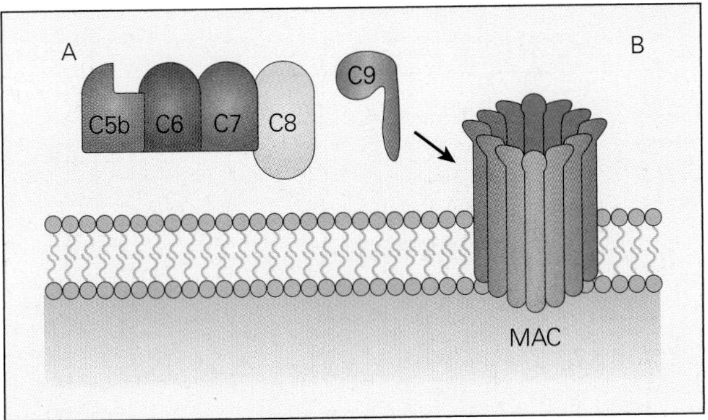

Figure 4-18. Panel A: Schematic representation of the sequential binding of the terminal complement components (C5b, C6, C7, C8, and C9). Panel B: The insertion of the assembled MAC into a cell membrane.

of Factor B versus C4 accompany decreased concentrations of C3 in serum may help determine which pathway of complement activation is involved. Frequently, however, both Factor B and C4 may be depleted from serum and/or deposited together in tissues, since the alternative pathway may be recruited by initial activation of the classical pathway. Drawing conclusions about the involvement of complement in any given pathologic process and/or determining which pathway might be involved can be further complicated by the fact that many of the components are acute phase reactants whose synthesis and serum concentrations increase dramatically when there is infection with fever or significant inflammation. In these situations, increased synthesis may result in serum values that are within the normal range, even though marked consumption is occurring. This dilemma can be solved by the use of assays for fragments that are released during complement activation, such as C3c or C3a-desArg, whose concentrations will reflect their production independently of the serum concentration of the intact component from which they were derived. The affinities with which C5a and C5a-desArg are bound by their receptor are so high that measurement of serum levels of this fragment are not useful. Besides the use of antibodies for immunolocalization of complement fragments or neoantigens in tissue, another method for detecting the involvement of complement in one set of autoimmune diseases is the Coombs' test in autoimmune hemolytic anemia. Agglutination of a patient's red blood cells by a so-called non-gamma Coombs' reagent indicates the presence of C3b and/or C3d fragments on the erythrocytes. Often, specific sera are available that can identify exactly which fragment of C3 is present.

Circulating antigen-antibody complexes may be assayed by their ability to bind to radioactively labeled, purified C1q. This C1q binding assay will detect only complexes that contain IgG and/or IgM. The Raji cell assay employs an immortalized lymphoblastoid cell line that bears CR2. The absence of C3 fragments on the circulating immune complexes in our case study patient explains why she had positive results in the C1q binding assay but negative results in the Raji cell assay.

In the current era, a wide variety of monoclonal antibody-based assays are available to directly detect an array of infectious pathogens and/or their antigens or antibodies to these antigens. In the past, however, ELISAs and similar systems that allow direct readouts of antibody concentrations were not available. If an antigen preparation was available, however, it could be incubated with serum that was to be tested for the presence of antibody. A standard serum with known hemolytic complement activity could then be added and allowed to react with the antibodies bound to the antigen. This process would activate some of the complement, which would then become bound or fixed to the antigen, and therefore unavailable to cause lysis of subsequently added sensitized animal erythrocytes. These complement fixation assays for antibody are not as widely employed in current practice as they were in the past, but infectious disease literature often still refers to "complement fixation titers" of antibodies against specific pathogens.

Case Study: Clinical Relevance

Let us now return to the case study of congenital C3 deficiency presented earlier and review some of the major points of the clinical presentation and how they relate to the immune system:

C3 Deficiency Impairs Disposal of Antigen-Antibody Complexes

- This well-studied and previously reported case illustrates two of the most important sets of functions of the complement system in vivo: its roles in host defense against infection, and in solubilization,

Case Study: Clinical Relevance (continued)

trafficking, and disposal of antigen-antibody complexes.

- The patient had originally presented in infancy with pyogenic bacterial infections, particularly involving the ears and sinopulmonary tract. In fact, these infections prompted an immunologic evaluation at the age of four years, which had shown the complete absence of serum C3 and of hemolytic complement activity.
- Another clinical manifestation of patients with C3 deficiency is the occurrence of rashes that occur intermittently, often with a relationship to the infections (Figure 4-19).
- The detailed laboratory data (for actual numerical values, see reference 2) illustrates how the C3 deficiency impairs the proper disposal of the antigen-antibody complexes that are presumably formed as a result of the sinusitis. The presence of circulating antigen-antibody complexes that can activate the early components of complement is revealed by the positive results on the C1q binding assay and the decreased serum concentrations of C1, C4, and C2.
- However, since there is no C3 available to promote clearance of the circulating antigen-antibody complexes by receptors in the reticuloendothelial system, the complexes are not detected by the Raji cell assay, which depends on binding of C3 fragments on the complexes to specific receptors on this cultured cell line from a lymphoma patient.
- As a result of the lack of C3 fragments, the complexes deposit in an abnormal site, the glomerulus, where they cause inflammation and destruction of the normal architecture of the tissues. Eventually, this patient required renal transplantation.
- Understanding the pathophysiology of this patient's tendency to develop infections, especially with bacteria, which seems to have been worse when she was an infant and became less problematic as her adaptive immune system matured, only to then develop glomerulonephritis associated with immune complex deposition, requires knowledge of the complex system we know as complement.

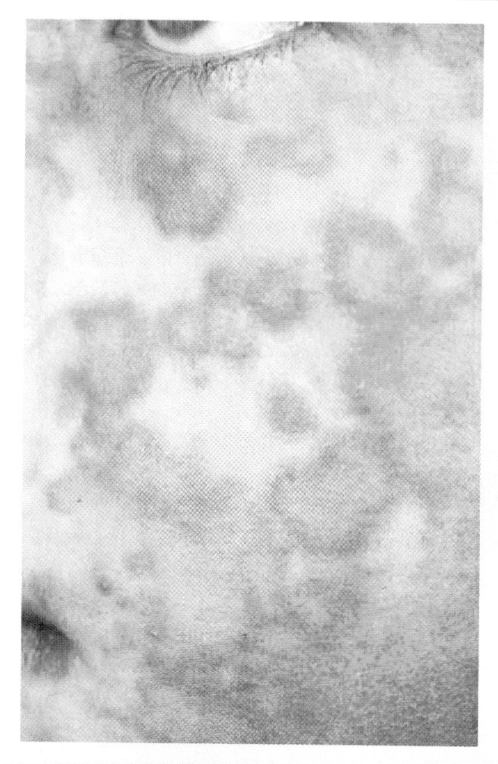

Figure 4-19. Facial rash in a patient with a hereditary C3 deficiency. This rash occurred each time the patient had a pyogenic infection of the respiratory tract, and in each instance, the rash lasted a few days. (Reproduced with permission from Walport MJ. Complement. Second of two parts. N Engl J Med. 2001;344:1140–4.)

Conclusions

There are more than thirty distinct proteins in the complement system. Understanding the activation, control, and cellular interactions of these proteins provides a basis for realizing their importance in maintaining normal physiologic homeostasis and their contributions to normal host defenses as well as prevention of immune complex and autoimmune disease. Participation of complement in inflammation and disease often represents a breakdown or an overwhelming of these normal activities. We continue to learn more about the roles played by complement in tying together the innate and adaptive immune systems and in normal physiology, and we are at the dawn of therapeutic manipulation of this important system.

Key Points

- Complement proteins are present in the circulation and can be activated rapidly upon infection. Since some active complement proteins are enzymes, each molecule can produce many activated products.
- Complement can be activated by contact with pathogen surface (alternative pathway), binding to

the acute phase protein MBP on the pathogen surface (lectin pathway), or binding to antigen-bound IgM or IgG on the pathogen surface (classical pathway).

- Complement activated by all three pathways promotes phagocytosis, attracts leukocytes to the infection site, increases inflammation, and can cause pathogen lysis.
- Complement activity is regulated by soluble and cell-surface molecules that inactivate many of the activated complement proteins or block their binding to host cell membranes.
- Receptors for active complement proteins signal leukocytes to engulf pathogens, remove immune complexes, enter infection sites, and make B cells more sensitive to antigen stimulation.
- Complement activation plays a role in the immune defense to bacteria and viruses. It is also important for removal of dead cells and immune complexes.
- Complement deficiencies are usually associated with increased bacterial infections and may result in kidney disease or autoimmunity.

Study Questions/Critical Thinking

1. The complement system includes more than thirty proteins. Why is it so complex?
2. Can the inactivation or removal of any one complement protein block all biological functions of complement?
3. Describe the morphological features that influence bacterial sensitivity to complement opsonization and lysis.
4. How does the presence of antibody improve the function of complement?
5. What protects our cells from complement damage? How can this protection be overcome?
6. Explain how a deficiency in C1 inhibitor can lead to some of the same symptoms as a deficiency in C1.
7. What cells have complement receptors, and what biological functions are stimulated by binding? Are these cells part of the innate or adaptive immune response?

Suggested Reading

Alper CA, Abramson N, Johnson RB Jr, et al. Increased susceptibility to infection associated with abnormalities of complement-mediated functions and of the third component of complement. N Engl J Med. 1970; 282: 349–54.

Anderson DC, Springer TA. The leukocyte adhesion deficiency: an inherited defect in the Mac-1, LFA1, and P150,95 glycoproteins. Ann Rev Med. 1987; 38: 175–94.

Arumugam TV, Shiels IA, Woodruff TM, et al. The role of the complement system in ischemia-reperfusion injury. Shock. 2004; 21: 401–9.

Ballow M, Shira JE, Harden L, et al. Complete absence of the third component of complement in man. J Clin Invest. 1975; 56: 703–10.

Basta M, Dalakas MC. High-dose intravenous immunoglobulin exerts its beneficial effect in patients with dermatomyositis by blocking endomysial deposition of activated complement fragments. J Clin Invest. 1994; 94: 1729–35.

Basta M, Kirshbom P, Frank MM, et al. Mechanism of therapeutic effect of high-dose intravenous immunoglobulin: attenuation of acute, complement-dependent immune damage in a guinea pig model. J Clin Invest. 1989; 84: 1974–81.

Berger M, Balow JE, Wilson CB, et al. Circulating immune complexes and glomerulonephritis in a patient with congenital absence of the third component of complement. N Engl J Med. 1983; 308: 1009–12.

Bhakdi S, Käflein R, Halsensen TS, et al. Complement S-protein (vitronectin) is associated with cytolytic membrane-bound C5b-9 complexes. Clin Exp Immunol. 1998; 74: 459–64.

Bhakdi S, Tranum-Jensen J. Membrane damage by channel-forming proteins. Trends in Biochem Sci. 1983; 8: 134–46.

Bhakdi S, Tranum-Jensen J. Molecular nature of the complement lesion. Proc Natl Acad Sci (USA). 1979; 74: 5655–9.

Bora NS, Lublin DM, Kumar VB, et al. Structural gene for human membrane cofactor protein (MCP) of complement maps to within 100 kb of the 3' end of the C3b/C4b receptor gene. J Exp Med. 1989; 169: 597–602.

Caliezi C, Wuillemin WA, Zeerleder S, et al. C1-esterase inhibitor: an anti-inflammatory agent and its potential use in the treatment of diseases other than hereditary angioedema. Pharmacol Rev. 2000; 52: 91–112.

Carroll MC, Alicot EM, Katzman PJ, et al. Organization of the genes encoding complement receptors type 1 and 2, decay-accelerating factor, and the C4-binding protein in the RCA locus on human chromosome 1. J Exp Med. 1988; 167: 1271–80.

Cherukuri A, Cheng PC, Pierce SK. The role of the CD19/CD21 complex in B cell processing and presentation of complement-tagged antigens. J Immunol. 2001; 167: 163–72.

Cooper NR. Complement evasion strategies of microorganisms. Immunol Today. 1991; 12: 327–31.

Cornacoff JB, Hebert LA, Smead WL, et al. Primate erythrocyte-immune complex clearing mechanism. J Clin Invest. 1983; 71: 236–47.

Davies A, Lachmann PJ. Membrane defence against complement lysis: the structure and biological properties of CD59. Immunol Res. 1993; 12: 258–75.

Davis AE , III. The pathophysiology of hereditary angioedema. Clin Immunol. 2005; 114: 3–9.

Edwards MS, Kasper DL, Jennings HJ, et al. Capsular sialic acid prevents activation of the alternative complement pathway by type III, group B streptococci. J Immunol. 1982; 128: 1278–83.

Endo L, Corman LC, Panush RS. Clinical utility of assays for circulating immune complexes. Med Clin N Amer. 1985; 69: 623–36.

Falk RJ, Dalmass AP, Kim Y, et al. Neoantigen of the polymerized ninth component of complement: characterization of a monoclonal antibody and histochemical localization in renal disease. J Clin Invest. 1983; 72: 560–73.

Fearon DT, Austen KF. The alternative pathway of complement: a system for host resistance to microbial infection. N Engl J Med. 1980; 303: 259–263.

Fearon DT, Carroll MC. Regulation of B lymphocyte responses to foreign and self-antigens by the CD19/CD21 complex. Annu Rev Immunol. 2000; 18: 393–422.

Fries LF, Gaither TA, Hammer CH, et al. C3b covalently bound to IgG demonstrates a reduced rate of inactivavtion by factors H and I. J Exp Med. 1984; 160: 1640–55.

Goldstein IM, Perez HD. Biologically active peptides derived from the fifth component of complement. Prog Hemost Thromb. 1980; 5: 41–79.

Harrison RA, Lachmann PJ. The physiological breakdown of the third component of complement. Mol Immunol. 1980; 17: 9–20.

Hillmen P, Hall C, Marsh JC, et al. Effect of eculizumab on hemolysis and transfusion requirements in patients with paroxysmal nocturnal hemoglobinuria. N Engl J Med. 2004; 350: 552–9.

Holers VM. Complement deficiency states, disease susceptibility, and infection risk in system lupus erythematosus. Arthritis Rheum. 1999; 42: 2023–5.

Hostetter MK, Thomas ML, Rosen FS, et al. Binding of C3b proceeds by a transesterification reaction at the thiolester site. Nature. 1982; 298: 72–5.

Hugli TE. Structure and function of the anaphylatoxins. Springer Semin Immunopathol. 1984; 7: 193–220.

Jacob HS, Craddock PR, Hammerschmidt DE, et al. Complement-induced granulocyte aggregation. N Engl J Med. 1980; 302: 789–94.

Jarva H, Jokiranta TS, Wurzner R, et al. Complement resistance mechanisms of streptococci. Mol Immunol. 2003; 40: 95–107.

Jenne D, Stanley KK. Molecular cloning of S-protein, a link between complement, coagulation, and cell-substrate adhesion. EMBO J. 1985; 412: 3151–7.

Joiner KA, Brown EJ, Frank MM. Complement and bacteria: chemistry and biology in host defense. Annu Rev Immunol. 1984; 2: 461–91.

Lachmann PJ. The control of homologous lysis. Immunol Today. 1991; 12: 312–5.

Lawley TJ, Bielory L, Gascon P, et al. A prospective clinical and immunologic analysis of patients with serum sickness. N Engl J Med. 1984; 311: 1407–13.

Matsushita M, Theil S, Jensenius JC, et al. Proteolytic activities of two types of mannose-binding lectin-associated serine protease. J Immunol. 2000; 165: 2637–42.

Mayer MM, Michaels DW, Ramm LE, et al. Membrane damage by complement. CRC Crit Rev Immunol. 1981; 2: 133–66.

Miller GW, Nussenzweig V. A new complement function: solubilization of antigen-antibody aggregates. Proc Natl Acad Sci USA. 1975; 72: 418–22.

Morgan BP, Meri S. Membrane proteins that protect against complement lysis. Springer Semin Immunopathol. 1994; 15: 369–96.

Müller-Eberhard HJ, Schreiber RD. Molecular biology and chemistry of the alternative pathway of complement. Adv Immunol. 1980; 29: 1–53.

Müller-Eberhard HJ. Complement. Springer Semin Immunopathol. 1983; 6: 117–258, 1983; 7: 259–390, and 1984; 7: 93–270.

Nicholson-Weller A. Decay-accelerating factor (CD55). Curr Top Microbiol Immunol. 1992; 178: 7–30.

Parker CJ. Paroxysmal nocturnal hemoglobinuria and glycosyl phosphatidylinositol anchored proteins that regulate complement. Clin Exp Immunol. 1991; 86 Suppl 1: 36–42.

Pepys MB. Role of complement in the induction of immunological responses. Transplant Rev. 1976; 32: 93–120.

Petersen SV, Thiel S, Jensen L, et al. Contron of the classical and the MBL pathway of complement activation. Mol Immunol. 2000; 37: 803–11.

Pillemer L, Blum L, Lepow IH, et al. The properdin system and the immunity I. Demonstration and Isolation of a new serum properdin, and its role in immune phenomena. Science. 1954; 120: 279–85.

Podack ER, Tschopp J. Membrane attack by complement. Molec Immunol. 1984; 21: 589–603.

Podack ER, Tschopp J, Muller-Eberhard HJ. Molecular Organization of C9 within the membrane attack complex of complement: induction of circular C9 polymerization by the C5b-8 assembly. J Exp Med. 1982; 156: 268–82.

Ross GD, Newman SL, Lambris JD, et al. Generation of three different fragments of bound C3 with purified Factor I or serum; II. Location of binding sites in C3 fragments for factors B and H, complement receptors, and bovine conglutinin. J Exp Med. 1983; 158: 334–52.

Ross SC, Densen P. Complement deficiency states and infection: epidemiology, pathogenesis, and consequences of neisserial and other infections in an immune deficiency. Medicine. 1984; 63: 243–73.

Rosse WF. Paroxysmal nocturnal hemoglobinuria as a molecular disease. Medicine. 1997; 76: 63–93.

Schifferli JA, Ng YC, Peters DK. The role of complement and its receptor in the elimination of immune complexes. N Engl J Med. 1986; 315: 488–95.

Stevens P, Huang SNY, Welch WD, et al. Restricted complement activation by e. coli with the K-1 capsular serotype: possible role in pathogenicity. J Immunol. 1978; 121: 2174–80.

Tanner J, Weiss J, Fearon D, et al. Epstein-Barr virus Gp350/220 binding to the B Lymphocyte C3d receptor mediates adsorption, capping and endocytosis. Cell. 1987; 50: 203–13.

Tenner AJ. Membrane receptors for soluble defense collagens. Curr Opin Immunol. 1999; 11: 34–41.

Theil S, Reid KBM. Structures and functions associated with the group of mammalian lectins containing collage-like sequences. FEBS Lett. 1989; 250: 78.

Turner MW, Hamvas RM. Mannose-binding lectin: structure, function, genetics, and disease associations. Rev Immunogenet. 2000; 2: 305–22.

Volanakis JE, Frank MM. The human complement system in health and disease. New York: Marcel Dekker; 1998.

Wagner E, Jang H, Frank MM. Complement and kinins: mediators of inflammation. In JB, Henry's Clinical Diagnosis and Management by Laboratory Methods, 20th ed. (pp 892–913). Philadelphia: WB Saunders; 2001.

Walport MJ. Complement. New Engl J Med. 2001; 344: 1058–66, 1140–4.

Ware CF, Kolb WP. Assembly of the functional membrane attack complex of human complement: formation of disulfide-linked C9 dimers. Proc Natl Acad (USA). 1981; 78: 6426–30.

Weisman HF, Bartow T, Leppo MK, et al. Soluble human complement receptor type 1: in vivo inhibitor of complement suppressing post-ischemic myocardial inflammation and necrosis. Science. 1990; 249: 146–51.

Wen L, Atkinson JP, Giclas PC. Clinical and laboratory evaluation of complement deficiency. J Allergy Clin Immunol. 2004; 113: 585–93.

Wetsel RA. Structure, function and cellular expression of complement anaphylatoxin receptors. Curr Opin Immunol. 1995; 7: 48–53.

Zuraw BL. Current and future therapy for hereditary angioedema. Clin Immunol. 2005; 114: 10–6.

Chapter 5

Inflammation

Lionel B. Ivashkiv, MD, PhD
Stephen J. Di Martino, MD, PhD

Case Studies

Case Study 1

A forty-five-year-old man with a history of hypertension presents to the emergency room at 3 AM with a history of acute onset of severe pain in the right great toe. The pain began the previous afternoon, mild at first, but then rapidly increased in severity. The pain is constant and throbbing, as if "some big-toothed rat was gnawing" on his toe. He cannot bear weight on the right foot, nor could he bear the weight of the sheet against his toe when he went to bed that night. The patient does not recall trauma, but two days prior, he played in a two-hand-touch football game with his nephews at a family barbeque, where he consumed three or four beers, several burgers, and grilled swordfish. The next morning, the patient took his thiazide diuretic, as prescribed, and two aspirins for a headache. On physical examination, the patient has redness and swelling of his right first metatarsophalangeal (MTP) joint, which is very warm to light touch. When the first MTP joint is palpated to assess for an effusion, the patient screams and says, "If you know what's good for you, you won't do that again."

Case Study 2

A fifty-four-year-old woman presents with several months of pain and swelling in both hands and feet. At first, she noted pain located under the plantar aspect of both feet for which she took over-the-counter non-steroidal anti-inflammatory drugs (NSAIDs). During the next several weeks, she developed worsening pain, swelling, and stiffness in her wrists and in the small joints of her hands. Recently, the NSAIDs have not been relieving her symptoms. She has been unable to get out of bed in the morning for two hours because of severe pain and stiffness as well as debilitating fatigue. On physical examination, she has warmth, swelling, tenderness, and decreased range of motion in both wrists. Several metacarpophalangeal (MCP) and proximal interphalangeal (PIP) joints of both hands are swollen and tender; the patient has a weak grasp secondary to pain. Laboratory findings include the following: erythrocyte sedimentation rate (ESR) 80 mm/hr (normal = 1 – 25 mm/hr), hemoglobin 10.1 g/dl (normal = 13 – 18 g/dl), and rheumatoid factor 120 IU/ml (normal $<$30 IU/ml).

LEARNING OBJECTIVES

When you have completed this chapter, you should be able to:

- List the causes of inflammation
- Describe the process of inflammation
- Explain the role of inflammation in the normal defense against infectious pathogens
- Explain the mechanisms by which inflammation causes disease
- Summarize the role of inflammation in health and disease

Case Studies (continued)

Case Study 3

A sixty-five-year-old man is sent to the emergency room from his dialysis facility with a fever of 39.0°C and a swollen left knee. The patient looks ill and states that his knee has been hurting for the past few days. At first, he used a topical ointment and wrapped the knee in a compressive bandage, but the pain worsened, and it no longer can bear weight. On examination, his left knee is warm, has a large effusion, and is tender to palpation; there is extreme pain with even minimal knee flexion or extension. The knee is aspirated, yielding 60 ml of purulent fluid. The synovial fluid has a white blood cell (WBC) count of 95,000/mm^3 and no crystals are observed on microscopic examination.

The Physiology of Inflammation

The Clinical Signs of Inflammation Are *Tumor, Rubor, Calor, Dolor,* and *Functio Laesa*

Although the etiology of inflammation differs in the cases described above, each patient displays many, if not all, of the classic clinical hallmarks of inflammation first described almost 2,000 years ago: the first four are attributed to Celsus: **heat** (*calor*), **pain** (*dolor*), **redness** (*rubor*), and **swelling** (*tumor*). Galen later added **loss of function** (*functio laesa*) (Figure 5-1).

Any vascularized tissue has the potential to become inflamed, and the clinical signs will vary among organ systems. The suffix "itis" denotes inflammation of a particular structure (e.g., arthritis: inflammation of a joint; pericarditis: inflammation of the pericardium). Inflammation is a normal physiological response—not a disease—that eliminates or contains an injurious agent (e.g., bacterial, chemical, foreign body), clears cellular debris, and prepares the injured tissue for healing. Unfortunately, the same cells and mediators that participate in the beneficial aspects of the inflammatory response also have the potential to damage or even destroy normal tissue. For this reason, inflammation is controlled by tightly regulated mechanisms; however, in disease states such as gout, rheumatoid arthritis (**RA**), and septic arthritis, the inflammatory process becomes poorly controlled and may lead to the destruction of host tissue with resultant clinical symptomatology.

What Is Inflammation?

Inflammation (Latin, *inflammatio*, to set on fire) is the complex biological response of vascular tissues to injury or harmful stimuli, such as those caused by pathogens, damaged cells, or irritants. In general, whatever the cause, the following events occur during an inflammatory response: (1) vascular changes: blood flow increases and fluid and plasma proteins leak into the inflamed tissue; (2) cellular infiltration: leukocytes adhere to vascular endothelium and migrate through the endothelial layer to gain access to surrounding tissue; and (3) chemotaxis: leukocytes follow a chemical gradient to the site of insult and unleash potent killing mechanisms.

Inflammation can be classified as either **acute** or **chronic**. Both are characterized by the classic events described above, but acute inflammation takes place

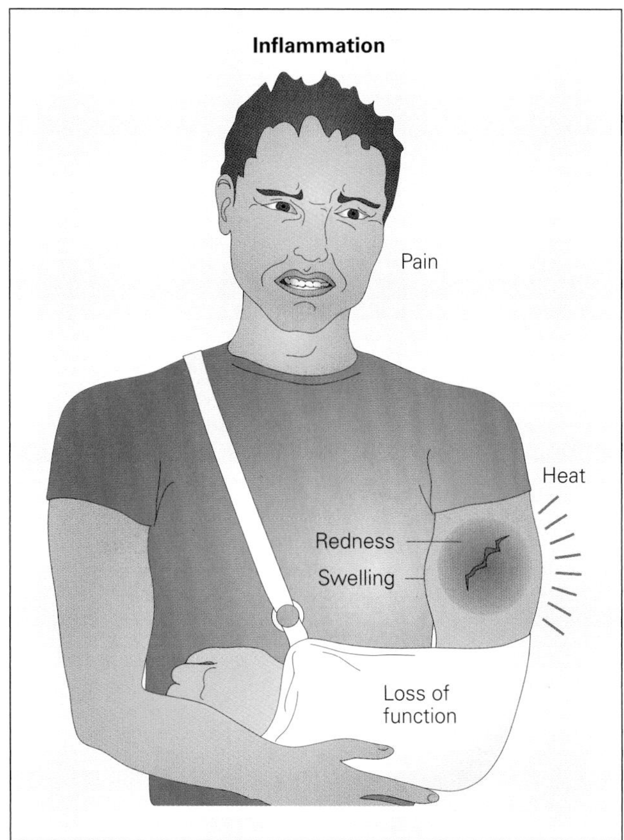

Figure 5-1. Cartoon illustrating the cardinal signs of inflammation—heat, redness, swelling, pain, and loss of function—first described by Celsus and Galen more than 2,000 years ago. These symptoms are largely caused by a combination of vasodilation, vascular leakage, and tissue damage.

over minutes to days and histologically is characterized by accumulation of neutrophils. Acute inflammation may either lead to healing by a process referred to as resolution or, if the insult cannot be eliminated, progress to chronic inflammation. In contrast, chronic inflammation continues for more than a few days and usually is associated with an influx of monocytes, lymphocytes, and other immune cells. Chronic inflammation can represent either a progression from acute inflammation, with no resolution phase, or may also arise from a mild acute response or as a repeated low-level inflammation where no resolution phase is initiated. In either case, it is the persistence and failure of elimination of the foreign invader that drives the immune response to chronic inflammation as described in Chapter 1, i.e., the concept of "immunologic balance."

Where Does Inflammation Fit into the Spectrum of Innate and Acquired Immune Responses?

Inflammation is widely regarded as the fundamental mechanism by which multicellular organisms deal with injury caused either by infection-related or non-infection-related insults.

Since the primary force shaping the evolution of the immune system is defense against microorganisms, it is not surprising that the mechanisms of inflammation were initially discovered and promulgated in the context of the study of infectious diseases. However, it is now recognized that inflammation plays a central role not only in infectious diseases but also in noninfectious disease insults. As described in Chapter 1, the principal function of the immune response is the recognition of foreign substances with or without injury to its own tissue(s) and is carried out by both innate and adaptive immune responses. Inflammation plays a central role in initiating the innate immune response. One cardinal aspect of innate immunity is that it is intrinsic to a given species and displays neither specificity nor memory; in humans, this includes constitutive physical barriers such as skin and mucosa, physiologic barriers such as temperature (i.e., development of fever) and pH (i.e., many organisms are killed by the low pH of the stomach), and soluble antimicrobial factors such as complement and lysozyme (*Chapters 1* and *4*). In addition, cells of the innate immune system (i.e., phagocytic cells such as macrophages and neutrophils, dendritic cells, and NK cells) recognize conserved molecular patterns expressed by microbes and react rapidly, usually within minutes (*Chapter 3*).

Adaptive or acquired immunity, on the other hand, refers to that part of the immune response that can more specifically recognize, neutralize, and eradicate foreign invaders, e.g., viruses, bacteria, fungi, protozoans, and even helminths (*Chapter 1*) using a massive array of recombinatorial and mutational events carried out by antigen-presenting cells, T cells and B cells (*Chapters 6* and *7*). Lymphocytes and antibodies are key products of the adaptive immune response and not only endow this system with specificity to a particular pathogen but also provide long-lived memory for that organism so that upon subsequent encounter it can be readily recognized and eliminated more rapidly.

The inflammatory process is, therefore, an important part of both arms of the immune system. Acute inflammation, characterized by influx of neutrophils into injured tissue, is one of the earliest events in an innate immune response.  It is important to stress, however, that this process may be enhanced by components of the adaptive immune response, such as antibodies and cytokines. Inflammation can be thought as central to maintaining tissue homeostasis. While some degree of inflammatory responses limiting the progression of an insult is beneficial, exaggerated or prolonged inflammation or the lack of an adequate inflammatory response can lead to disease.

Inflammation as a Response to "Danger Signals" (Microbial versus Nonmicrobial)

When an inciting agent causes inflammation, the inflammatory response can generate danger signals that are critical for progressive immune reactivity against that particular inciting agent. In recent years, there has been a major paradigm shift away from the classic dogma of inflammation as a response to nonself to one which defines inflammation more broadly as a response to "danger signals" triggered by tissue injury resulting from exposure to microorganisms or nonmicrobial-related insults. Although the roles of inflammatory responses to microbial invasion are well recognized, the means by which nonmicrobial insults can injure and be recognized by the host's inflammatory response are less well understood. For example, exposure to an allergen can cause allergic disease because the immune system recognizes the allergen as nonself. But how is this accomplished? The immune system has evolved to identify the nonself using pattern-recognition receptors (**PRRs**), which are receptors on host immune cells that can identify repeating patterns of molecular structures, common to most microorganisms referred to as pathogen-associated molecular patterns (**PAMPs**) (*Chapter 3*). Although the first PRRs identified were Toll-like receptors (**TLRs**) and the ligands for these receptors were originally thought to be exclusively of microbial origin (e.g., endotoxin, peptidoglycans, viral RNA, etc.), it is now known that TLRs can also recognize "danger signals" arising from a wide variety of nonmicrobial agents, which has given rise to a much broader model of inflammation as a response to these warning sentinels. Recent studies have shown that uric acid crystals, for example, can act as a danger signal to promote inflammation seen in the acute manifestations of gout through a NALP3 inflammasome, whose subsequent activation leads to interleukin-1 beta secretion (*Chapter 3*). Similarly, the inhalation of airborne pollutants, such as asbestos or silica, well recognized to be linked to inflammation of the lung, fibrosis, and lung cancer, appear to be mediated by similar IL-1β mechanisms triggered by the activated NALP3 inflammasome. The basic premise of the "danger signal model" is that the immune system is more concerned with damage than with foreignness ("nonself"), set into action because of "alarm signals" called danger-associated molecular patterns (**DAMPs**) from injured tissues rather than by the recognition of nonself. Thus, the danger model of immunity provides a framework to better understand the nature of the immune response and releases it from the previously held paradigm, which was dependent solely on the self versus nonself concept.

Inflammation Can Result from Many Diverse Causes

Diverse agents, both foreign or derived from self, can cause inflammation, most of which induce cellular injury or death (Table 5-1). Each may act through a different mechanism. For example, in adaptive immunity, immune complexes can activate leukocytes either directly through Fc receptors or indirectly by activating the complement cascade (*Chapter 4*), which then stimulates both endothelial cells and leukocytes (*Chapter 3*). In another example of innate immunity, bacterial products, such as endotoxin, can bind to Toll-like receptors on leukocytes and endothelial cells, triggering activation as well as synthesis of proinflammatory cytokines and chemokines (*Chapter 9*).

Table 5-1. Causes of inflammation

Category	Examples
Infections	Bacteria Viruses Fungi Parasites
Immune-mediated factors	Immune complexes Cytokines
Hypoxia	Loss of blood supply (ischemia) Oxygen deprivation
Physical events	Trauma (wound) Temperature extremes Pressure Radiation Electric shock
Chemical agents	Drugs Environmental toxins Endogenous toxins

Cellular and Molecular Elements of Inflammation

Inflammation generally proceeds through the following stages: change in vascular flow, increased vascular permeability, leukocyte adhesion to the endothelium, transendothelial migration (extravasation) of leukocytes, chemotaxis, and, in the case of microorganisms, killing (phagocytosis and production of toxic metabolites). These steps require a variety of soluble inflammatory mediators that can activate cells, upregulate adhesion molecules on both endothelium and leukocytes, and stimulate cellular migration (i.e., chemoattractants). The specifics of this paradigm that determine which particular adhesion molecules, chemoattractants, or cytokines that predominate will vary according to the tissue or organ in question, the subset of leukocyte, and the underlying inflammatory etiology. Before addressing the stages of inflammation, the cellular and molecular participants in the inflammatory response will be briefly reviewed.

Cells of the Inflammatory Response: Inflammation Results in the Importation and Activation of Effector Cells at the Infection Site

Shown in Figure 5-2 is a schematic representation of the components and sequential involvement of cells that participate in the inflammatory response together with their known functions.

Endothelial cells regulate leukocyte access to the tissues (Figure 5-2A). During an acute or chronic inflammatory response, leukocytes usually exit the circulation and enter surrounding tissue via postcapillary venules (this may vary from tissue to tissue). The endothelial cells that line the lumen of these vessels are active participants in this process. The endothelial cell layer is one cell thick, and tight junctions exist along the borders of each cell which, under normal circumstances in the healthy state, prevent the leakage of fluid into surrounding tissues. Following activation, endothelial cells undergo structural and functional changes that allow leakage of fluid and plasma proteins into the surrounding tissue (Figure 5-2). In addition, they upregulate cytokines and adhesion molecules that are important for the tethering and tight adhesion of leukocytes.

Neutrophils are the most abundant leukocytes and are the first to arrive during an acute inflammatory response (Figure 5-2B). These cells are potent killers. Microscopically, they are easy to identify because of their multi-lobed nuclei, few organelles, and abundant granules. On activation, the various granule populations found within the cytoplasm can be rapidly mobilized to the cell surface, simultaneously releasing their contents into the microenvironment and dramatically changing the array of receptors on the cell surface (Figure 5-2B). The granules contain large quantities of degradative enzymes such as elastase, cathepsin, and proteinase 3, as well as other antimicrobial products. In addition, separate granule populations contain different components of the molecular machinery used to generate toxic oxygen radicals commonly referred to as reactive oxygen species (**ROS**). The machinery functions only after the separate components of the NADPH oxidase system, described below, are brought together on the cell surface following degranulation. The ROS cited above not only destroy foreign invaders, but also may damage host tissue. Neutrophils also can engulf foreign microbes and cellular debris, i.e., phagocytosis, and this function can be enhanced by opsonins, i.e., C3b and antibody. Neutrophils are activated by cytokines and by immune complexes, which have the ability to enhance their killing mechanisms.

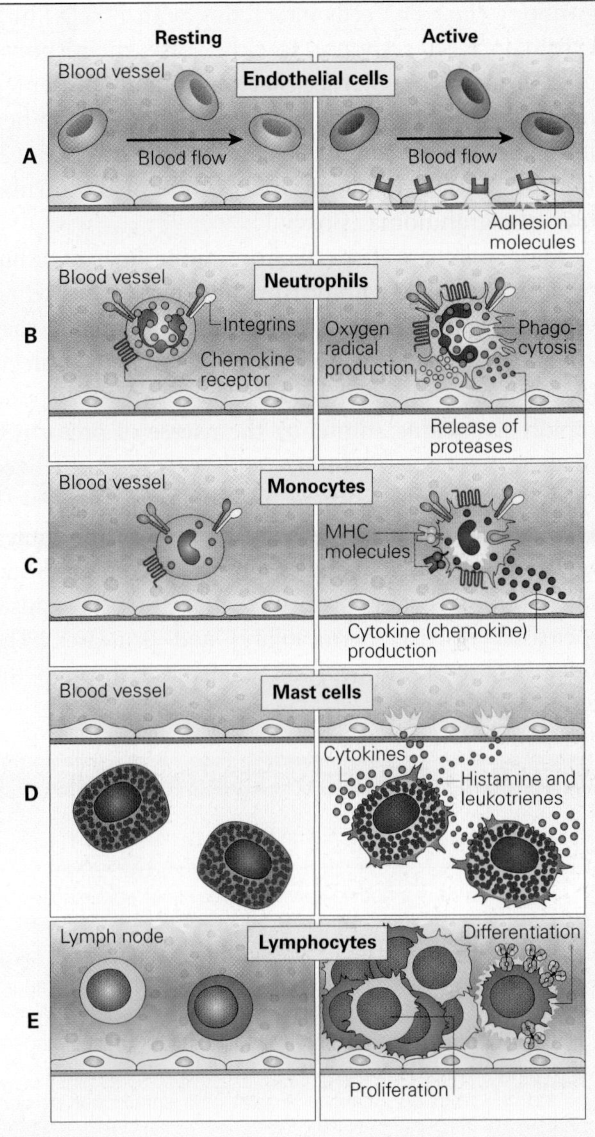

Figure 5-2. Schematic representation of cells involved in the inflammatory response and their functions. Panel A: Endothelial cells; Panel B: Neutrophils; Panel C: Monocytes; Panel D: Mast cells; and Panel E: Lymphocytes. (Adapted from a figure kindly provided by Peter Gentile).

Monocyte/macrophages play a key role in chronic inflammatory responses (Figure 5-2C). Once a monocyte leaves the circulation and becomes activated, it differentiates into a highly phagocytic cell called a **macrophage**. Some examples of specialized macrophages include Kupffer's cells in the liver, microglia in the CNS, and alveolar macrophages in the lungs. Like neutrophils, monocytes can phagocytose microbes and cellular debris, release degradative enzymes (they possess some granules that are similar to neutrophil's, albeit fewer in number), and produce toxic oxygen radicals, i.e., the ROS. However, macrophages are also highly anabolic cells that synthesize large quantities of many products such as cytokines and growth factors (Figure 5-2C). Furthermore, macrophages play an important role in the development of specific immunity during an adaptive immune response. Following the phagocytosis and breakdown of microbes, macrophages can function as antigen-presenting cells (**APCs**) and present the microbial fragments (in the context of MHC molecules) to T lymphocytes. Activated T lymphocytes can then help generate an

antibody (i.e., Th2 cells interacting with B cells) or a 6 cytotoxic T cell response. In either case, the response is specific for the microbe that was initially presented in the MHC of the macrophage (*Chapter 1*). When foreign materials cannot be eliminated, macrophages together with lymphocytes participate in the formation of a granuloma (Box 5-1).

Mast cells are derived from bone marrow, but when mature, live within tissue near nerves and blood vessels (Figure 5-2D). Together with basophils, they are referred to as mediator cells, and their strategic 7 locations in tissue and blood allow them to respond rapidly to inciting stimuli by the release of preformed mediators, e.g., histamine and newly synthesized mediators, e.g., leukotriene metabolites (*Chapter 1*). Like neutrophils, these cells are packed with granules; however, mast cell granules primarily contain histamine (an important preformed mediator that causes increased vascular permeability) and proteases. The inflammatory response is also enhanced through the activity of leukotrienes and cytokines such as TNF-α (Figure 5-4). Mast cells and basophils express the high affinity IgE receptor—Fc epsilon receptor I (FcεRI)—on their surface, and have been most extensively studied regarding their role in allergy; the binding of an allergen complexed with IgE to the cell-surface IgE receptor will cause the mast cell to degranulate (*Chapter 18*). However, mast cells also actively produce mediators that participate in the inflammatory response. Many inflammatory stimuli such as complement activation products, bacterial surfaces, and chemokines stimulate mast cell degranulation.

Lymphocytes also participate in chronic inflammation (Figure 5-2E). Although the proliferation and differentiation of lymphocytes, especially B cells, occurs primarily in lymphoid tissues rather than the infection site, lymphocytes play important roles in inflammation, particularly in chronic inflammation. Some subsets of lymphocytes carry out cytotoxicty (CD8+T cells and natural killer

Box 5-1

Granuloma

A granuloma is a nodule consisting mainly of epithelioid macrophages and other inflammatory and immune cells as well as an extracellular matrix and is often surrounded by a lymphocyte cuff or fibrosis (Figure 5-3). Often found in granulomas are Langhans giant cells which represent multinucleated cells formed by the fusion of epithelioid cells (macrophages), that contain nuclei arranged in a horseshoe-shaped pattern in the cell periphery. (Langhans giant cells should not be confused with Langerhans cells, which are mononuclear dendritic cells derived from monocytes or the insulin-producing Islets of Langerhans found in the pancreas.)

Granulomas form when the immune system attempts to fend off and isolate a foreign substance but is unable to or has limited capacity to do so. The substance can be an infectious disease pathogen, e.g., the tubercle bacillus, or a foreign body or splinter but in many cases granulomas form without apparent cause, as in autoimmune disorders. Granulomas are seen in a variety of diseases such as Crohn's disease, tuberculosis, leprosy, sarcoidosis, berylliosis, and syphilis. They are also the hallmark lesion of Wegener's granulomatosis and Churg-Strauss syndrome, two related autoimmune disorders (*Chapter 19*).

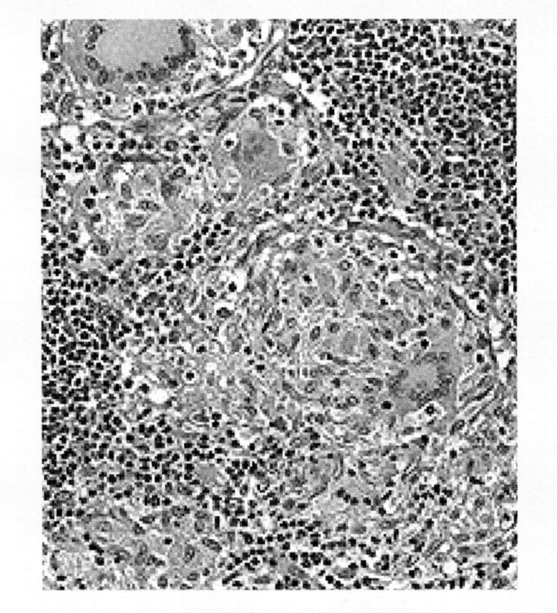

Figure 5-3. H&E (hematoxylin and eosin) section of a non-caseating granuloma seen in the colon of a patient with Crohn's disease showing a Langhans giant cell in the upper left. (As seen on Wikipedia.)

An important distinction of granulomas is whether they are caseating or non-caseating. Caseation (literally, turning to cheese) is a form of necrosis at the center of a granuloma and is a feature of the granulomas of tuberculosis and is related to the destructive action of pro-inflammatory cytokines, e.g., TNF-α. Granulomas can be also classified as infectious or noninfectious. Granulomas caused in reaction to infectious pathogens tend to be caseating, while granulomas in autoimmune and auto-inflammatory conditions, e.g., sarcoidosis, are mostly non-caseating.

[**NK**] cells) while others are important for cytokine production, e.g., Th1 cells (interleukin-2 [**IL-2**], Interferon-gamma [**IFN-γ**], and tumor necrosis factor beta [**TNF-β**]) or Th17 cells (interleukin-17, -21, and -22 [**IL-17, IL-21**, and **IL-22**]). The primary function of cytotoxic cells is to seek out and destroy virus-infected cells and cancerous cells at the infection or tumor site. The production of pro-inflammatory cytokines by the Th1 and Th17 subpopulations results in the up-regulation of a variety of cellular events (e.g., chemotaxis and activation of macrophages), allowing them to kill phagocytosed pathogens more effectively. The production of IL-4, IL-5, IL-6, IL-9, and IL-13 by CD4+ Th2 cells leads to activation of B cells with subsequent antibody production or can result in recruitment of eosinophils (i.e., IL-5) (*Chapter 9*).

Soluble Mediators Regulate the Inflammatory Response

In addition to cell-associated mediators, there are several substances that circulate in the blood as soluble mediators of inflammation. Shown in Table 5-2 is a list of soluble mediators that regulate the inflammatory response together with their specific functions. Cytokines are a large group of proteins that regulate the activation, proliferation, and differentiation of immune cells (*Chapter 9*). Although leukocytes are the major sources of cytokines, many other cell types can also synthesize cytokines as well. Figure 5-4 illustrates some of the leukocyte-derived cytokines involved in inflammatory arthritis.

Some cytokines, such as tumor necrosis factor alpha (**TNF-α**), IFN-γ, interleukin-6 (**IL-6**), and interleukin-1 (**IL-1**), are thought to have predominantly pro-inflammatory effects, while other cytokines, such as interleukin-4 (**IL-4**), interleukin-10 (**IL-10**), and transforming growth factor-beta (**TGF–β**), are thought to have predominantly anti-inflammatory effects (Table 5-2 and *Chapter 9*). Currently, a paradigm exists in rheumatology stating that an imbalance between the relative amounts of "pro-inflammatory" and "anti-inflammatory" cytokines can trigger the development of inflammatory/autoimmune diseases (*Chapter 19*). This paradigm, however, may be oversimplified as it has become clear that whether or not any particular cytokine exhibits pro- or anti-inflammatory properties depends largely upon the timing and context of its appearance during the immune response.

Immune complexes are heterogeneous structures comprised of antibodies either bound to their specific antigen alone as antigen-antibody (**Ag-Ab**) complexes or together with complement, as antigen-antibody-complement (**AgAbC**) complexes (Figure 5-5).

Table 5-2. Soluble mediators of inflammation

Mediator	Examples	Functions
Cytokines	IL-1, IL-6, TNF-α	Vasodilatation, increased endothelial cell adhesion molecule expression Fever, acute phase protein release from liver, neutrophil release from bone marrow
	IFN-γ	More efficient macrophage killing of phagocytosed pathogens Increased MHC expression
	IL-10, TGF-β	Anti-inflammatory effects
Immune complexes	Antigen bound to IgM or IgG	Complement activation Macrophage and neutrophil production and release of toxic metabolites Increased phagocytosis
Complement anaphylatoxins	C5a	Mast cell degranulation, chemotaxis, and activation of leukocytes
Proteases	Serine proteases Metalloproteases Thiolproteases Acid proteases	Catabolize microbial proteins Digest host proteins
Chemokines	IL-8, macrophage chemotactic protein (MCP)	Leukocyte chemotaxis
Arachadonic acid metabolites	Thromboxane Prostaglandins Leukotrienes	Platelet aggregation Vasodilation Pain stimulation Leukocyte chemotaxis

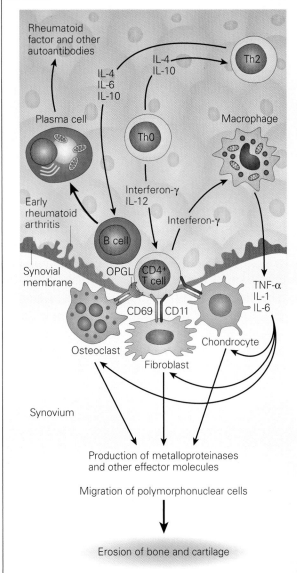

Figure 5-4. Schematic representation of cytokine signaling pathways involved in inflammatory arthritis. Antigen-activated CD4+ T cells stimulate macrophages to produce interleukin-1 (IL-1), interleukin-6 (IL-6), and TNF-α and synovial fibroblasts to secrete matrix metalloproteinases and other effector molecules. This occurs through signaling pathways mediated by the cell-surface receptors CD69 and CD11 as well as through the release of soluble mediators such as interferon-γ. IL-1, IL-6, and TNF-α are the principal cytokines that drive inflammation in rheumatoid arthritis. Activated CD4+ T cells also stimulate B cells through cell-surface contact with the cytokines IL-4, IL-6, and IL-10 released from Th2 helper lymphocytes. Although rheumatoid factor and other autoantibodies are known to be produced by plasma cells, their precise pathogenic role in RA is unknown but may participate in inflammation through the activation of complement and formation of immune complexes. Activated CD4+ T cells also express osteoprotegerin ligands (OPGL) that stimulate osteoclastogenesis that may participate in the joint damage of rheumatoid arthritis. (Adapted from Choy EH, Panayi GS. Cytokine pathways and joint inflammation in rheumatoid arthritis. N Engl J Med. 200;344: 907–16.)

Immune complexes may be small or large, soluble or insoluble; they may form within the circulation and then deposit in tissue or they may form within the tissue itself (Table 5-2). Once an antibody forms an immune complex, it can participate in destructive processes, such as activating the complement cascade, assisting with phagocytosis, as well as stimulating degranulation and production of toxic oxygen metabolites by macrophages and neutrophils. Many inflammatory/autoimmune diseases are characterized by the deposition of immune complexes within various organs (*Chapter 17*).

Complement is a group of plasma proteins that can be activated by several stimuli: immune complexes, microbial surfaces, and bacterial sugars (Table 5-2 and *Chapter 4*). Once activated, the complement cascade culminates in the formation of both the membrane attack complex as well as several potent pro-inflammatory products, e.g., anaphylatoxins, chemoattractants C3a, and C5a. The membrane attack complex is a group of proteins that forms a channel that inserts itself into the wall of invading microorganisms, causing the organism's intracellular contents to leak out. C5a is the most potent pro-inflammatory product formed during complement activation. Its activities include triggering mast cell degranulation, upregulation of adhesion molecules on endothelium and leukocytes, stimulation of chemotaxis in all leukocytes, and induction of oxygen radical production and degranulation in neutrophils and monocytes. Complement activation products have been found in the synovial fluid of RA patients, the blood of lupus patients, and in the skin lesions of patients with psoriasis.

Proteases are enzymes that break down other proteins (Table 5-2). There are four types: serine, metallo-, thiol, and acid proteases, each named for the active

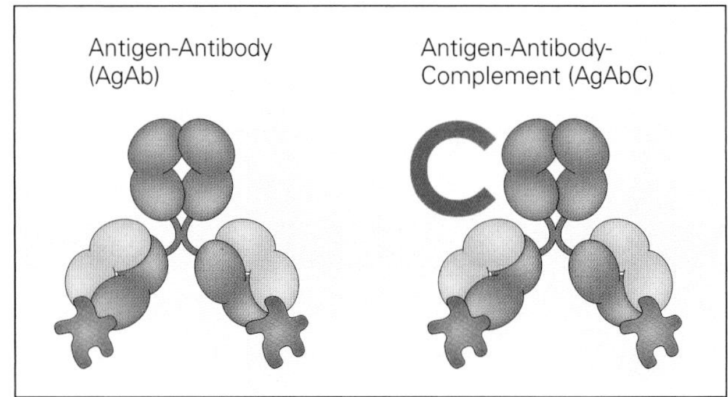

Figure 5-5. Schematic representation of the structure of antigen-antibody (Ag-Ab) complexes and antigen-antibody-complement (AgAbC) complexes.

moiety in their catalytic site. Many proteases are presynthesized and packaged within granules ready for quick release from leukocytes (e.g., elastase, cathepsin, proteinase 3, and type IV gelatinase), while others are synthesized at the site of inflammation (e.g., some matrix metalloproteases). During an inflammatory response, proteases catabolize microbial proteins and damaged host tissue proteins, including collagen, elastin, and proteoglycans. Because proteases have no way of distinguishing foreign from host proteins, they have the potential to damage normal tissue when inflammatory responses are poorly controlled. Because proteases are so destructive, many have naturally occurring inhibitors such as alpha-1-antiproteinase, which inhibits human leukocytes elastase, and the tissue inhibitors of metalloproteinase (**TIMPs**), which inhibit some collagenases and gelatinases.

Chemokines are a specialized group of cytokines consisting of more than forty small, related proteins, each of which can form a chemical gradient that can be sensed and tracked by leukocytes and which result in directed cell movement, i.e., chemotaxis, as described below (Table 5-2 and *Chapter 9*). Each chemokine triggers cell migration by binding to a specific cell surface receptor. Because each leukocyte population has a different panel of chemokine receptors on their surface, the pattern of chemokine production during an inflammatory response can help dictate the composition of the cellular infiltrate. For example, interleukin-8 (**IL-8**) will attract neutrophils but not monocytes; in contrast, IP-10 will attract activated T cells but not neutrophils.

Arachidonic acid metabolites are another group of mediators that regulate the inflammatory response (Table 5-2 and *Chapters 1* and *18*). Many cells, utilizing the enzyme phospholipase A, can convert membrane phospholipids to arachidonic acid. Cyclooxygenase (**COX**), an enzyme targeted by nonsteroidal anti-inflammatory drugs (**NSAIDs**), converts arachidonic acid to thromboxane and several types of prostaglandins. These mediators are important for platelet aggregation, vasodilation, and stimulation of pain. Another enzyme, lipooxygenase (**LOX**), converts arachidonic acid to the leukotrienes. LTB4 is a potent chemoattractant for all leukocytes.

The Inflammatory Process

It may now be possible to summarize the cellular and molecular events associated with the inflammatory response to tissue damage or injury. Although these events have been best studied following infection, similar reactions occur in response to the myriad of agents that trigger inflammation.

The following is a description of a generic inflammatory response of which variations may occur depending upon the inciting agent and the organ involved. The inflammatory response involves three major stages: first, dilation of capillaries to increase blood flow; second, microvascular structural changes and escape of plasma proteins from the bloodstream; and third, leukocyte transmigration through the endothelium and accumulation at the site of injury.

Vascular Changes Increase Blood Flow at the Infection Site

Within minutes of exposure to an inflammatory agent, local arterioles and capillaries dilate in response to the cellular and soluble mediator substances described previously. This increases blood flow and is responsible for the warmth and redness of inflammation evidenced by calor. Some triggers of this event include histamine released from mast cells, serotonin released from platelets, and prostaglandins, which can be synthesized by many cell types. Next, protein-rich fluid begins to leak into surrounding tissue at the level of the post-capillary venules. Collectively, these changes produce a slowing of blood flow in the microvasculature and a local increase in osmotic pressure. As normal laminar flow of blood slows, leukocytes, which travel in the central portion of the bloodstream, are able to tether or marginate to the blood vessel's wall.

Vascular Permeability Increases in Response to Inflammatory Mediators

Inflammatory mediators increase vascular permeability by causing cytoskeletal rearrangements within endothelial cells that result in the opening of tight junctions between cells and retraction of the cells themselves. This process can be stimulated by histamine, bradykinin, and ligands for Toll-like receptors, as well as cytokines such as TNF-α and IL-1. The openings between endothelial cells combined with the increased osmotic pressure cause fluid to leak into surrounding tissues. This protein-rich fluid is called an exudate and is responsible for some of the swelling observed in inflammation. The exudate also serves to dilute the inciting inflammatory agent and provides key immunologic proteins such as antibodies and complement to the site of tissue injury.

Leukocytes Adhere to Endothelial Cells and Migrate into the Infection Site

This stage of inflammation is itself divided into several steps: endothelial cell activation, rolling, capture, tight adhesion, and diapedesis (Figure 5-6). In the absence of inflammation, resting endothelial cells and leukocytes do not adhere strongly to each other. However, when various pro-inflammatory stimuli (e.g., histamine, C5a, ligands for TLRs, and cytokines such as TNF-α and IL-1) activate either or both of these cell types, intracellular vesicles that contain adhesion molecules (as described below) are released onto the cell surface.

Adhesion Molecules

There are three major families of adhesive molecules responsible for the bulk of leukocyte-endothelial interactions. These include: (1) selectins—located on leukocytes and endothelial cells; (2) members of the immunoglobulin superfamily of proteins—largely expressed on endothelial cells; and (3) integrins—located on leukocytes (Table 5-3). All three of these families of adhesive molecules interact with each other and are responsible for the various phases of the endothelial-leukocyte interaction of inflammation described previously. Endothelial selectins interact with glycoproteins located on leukocyte surfaces and, conversely, leukocyte selectins interact with glycoproteins located on endothelial cell surfaces. Members of the immunoglobulin superfamily expressed primarily on endothelial cells, in turn, interact with integrins located on the surface of leukocytes (Figure 5-6).

Initial Phase of Loose Adhesion of Leukocytes to Endothelial Cells by Selectins: Capture and Rolling

Following the deceleration of blood flow, leukocytes come into contact with the vascular luminal wall and initially adhere loosely. Specific members of the selectin family expressed either on endothelial cells or leukocytes are critical to the rolling and capture of leukocytes along the blood vessel wall (Table 5-3, Box 5-2, and Figures 5-7 and 5-8). All selectins bind to the sialyated carbohydrates of glycoproteins found on the opposing surface of a cell in close proximity. Because the bond between selectins and their carbohydrate ligands is transient and of low affinity, the leukocytes are actually rolled over the vessel wall by the force of blood flow passing over (Figure 5-6). The next phase of inflammation is characterized by the capture of leukocytes by loose bonding of the leukocyte to the

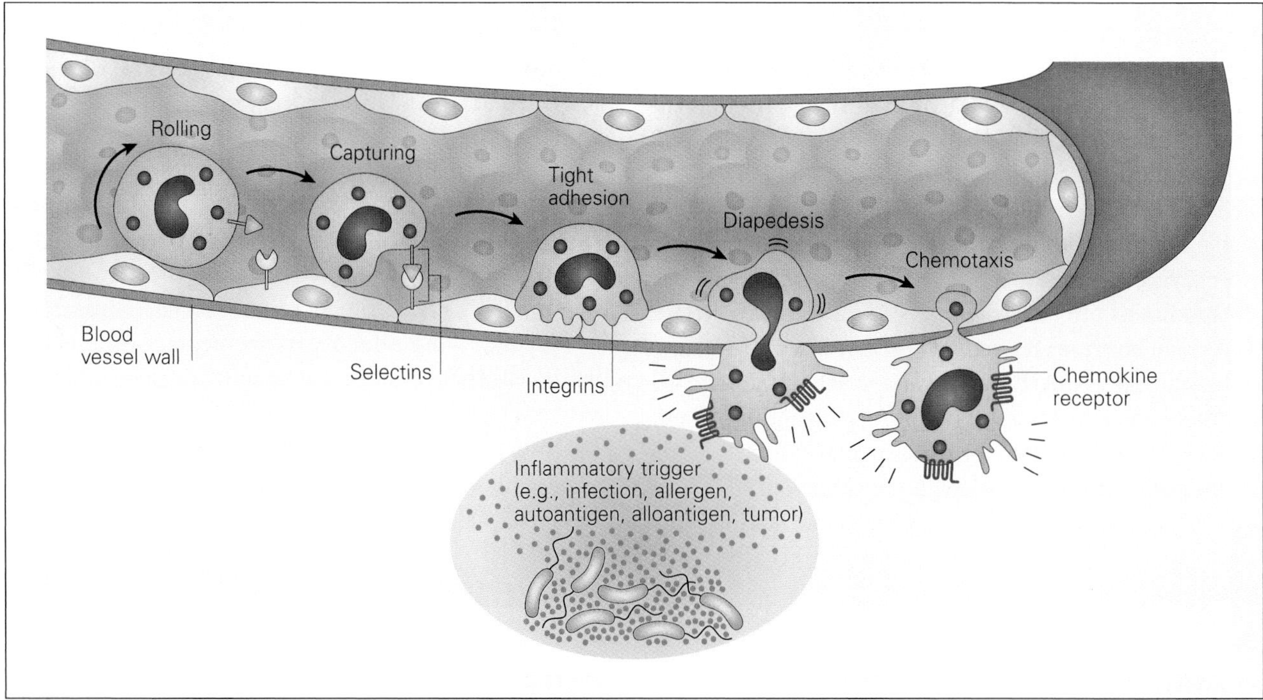

Figure 5-6. Schematic representation of the various stages of leukocyte adhesion and transendothelial migration. Slowing blood flow due to capillary dilation allows transient attachment between leukocyte selectins and endothelial cell glycoproteins and vice versa. Tighter adhesion between leukocyte integrins and endothelial cell ICAMs and VCAM (see Figure 5-10), supported by chemokine stimulation, allows the leukocyte to leave the capillary by squeezing between endothelial cells and enter the infection site (extravasation).

Table 5-3. Various integrins, selectins, and members of the immunoglobulin superfamily of proteins are involved in the leukocyte endothelial interactions of inflammation

Adhesion molecule	Specific cellular location	Ligand(s)	Primary function
Selectins (transient interaction)			
P-selectin	Platelet and endothelial cell surface expression after stimulation	Glycoproteins	Mediate cellular margination and rolling
E-selectin	Exclusively expressed on stimulated endothelial cells	Glycoproteins	
L-selectin	Constitutively expressed on neutrophils, monocytes, and a T cell subset Shed from neutrophils after stimulation with chemoattractants	Glycoproteins	
Immunoglobulin superfamily (strong interaction)			
ICAM-1 (CD54)	Low-level constitutive endothelial cell expression Increased endothelial cell expression with stimulation	LFA-1, Mac-1	Play a major role in leukocyte-endothelial adhesion
ICAM-2 (CD102)	High-level constitutive endothelial cell expression No increase with stimulation	LFA-1, Mac-1	
ICAM-3 (CD50)	Lymphocytes	LFA-1	
ICAM-4 (CD242)	Erythrocytes	LFA-1, Mac-1	
VCAM-1 (CD106)	No constitutive endothelial cell expression Increased endothelial cell expression with stimulation	VLA-4	
Integrins (strong interaction)			
LFA-1 (CD11a/CD18b)	Lymphocytes	ICAM-1, ICAM-2, ICAM-3, ICAM-4	Leukocyte migration, phagocytosis, and growth and development
Mac-1 (CR3, CD11b/CD18b)	Neutrophils and monocytes	ICAM-1, ICAM-2	
gp 150/95 (CD11c/CD18b)	Neutrophils and monocytes	ICAM-1, ICAM-2	
VLA-4 (very late antigen-4)	Lymphocytes, monocytes, and eosinophils	VCAM-1	

endothelial cell (Figure 5-8). This is brought about by the binding of L-selectins on the leukocyte to glycoproteins on the endothelial cell and, conversely, by the binding of E and P selectins on the endothelial surface with glycoproteins of the leukocyte membrane.

Immunoglobulin Superfamily of Adhesion Molecules: Tight Adhesion

Another set of adhesion molecules that participate in the leukocyte-endothelial interaction involved in inflammation is the immunoglobulin superfamily of molecules (Table 5-3, Box 5-3, Table 5-4, and Figure 5-9). The defining structural characteristic in this family of molecules is characterized by the presence of a variable number of intramolecular loop-like structures linked by disulfide bonds that are homologous to those present in immunoglobulins (**Igs**) (*Chapter 6*) and are referred to as Ig loops (Figure 5-9). While many members of the immunoglobulin superfamily of adhesion molecules bind to extracellular matrix proteins, the predominant molecules of this family that play a role in leukocyte endothelial adhesion are intercellular adhesion molecules 1 and 2 (**ICAM-1**, and **ICAM-2**), and vascular cell adhesion molecule 1 (**VCAM-1**) (Table 5-3 and Figure 5-10). Variable numbers of these molecules are expressed on the surface both constituitively and after cellular stimulation. For these molecules to function properly and bind to integrin ligands, integrins first need to become activated; this occurs when the cell that bears the integrin is stimulated sufficiently by one of the proinflammatory mediators or chemoattractants described previously (Box 5-4). When activated, the integrins can form a high affinity bond with its counterligand, the strength of which causes the leukocyte to stop rolling and adhere tightly.

- Low levels of ICAM-1 are constitutively expressed on endothelial cells. Increased surface expression of ICAM-1 can result from cellular stimulation due to

Box 5-2

Selectins

Selectins represent a group of cell adhesion molecules that participate in the inflammatory response and comprise a family of single chain transmembrane glycoproteins that function as lectins with properties that allow them to bind sugar polymers. Their protein structure is characterized by variable numbers of short, cysteine-rich repeats (related to complement regulatory proteins), an epithelial growth factor-like domain, and a C-type (calcium-dependent) lectin domain (Figure 5-7). The lectin domain of the selectins mediates their adhesive properties by binding to sialylated Lewis X (a complex sugar moiety), which is covalently linked to a variety of mucin-like proteins on the surface of other cells. Selectins primarily mediate cellular margination and rolling. Three selectins are known to exist: P-selectin, E-selectin, and L-selectin.

The selectins are expressed on the surface of some cells and have a carbohydrate-recognition-domain (CRD) or lectin at (N-terminal) end of a flexible "stalk" connected by an epidermal growth factor-like (EGF)-domain, retained by a single transmembrane helix, and a small C-terminal cytosolic domain. These proteins are thought to be involved in the "homing" of leukocytes to the lymphatic glands.

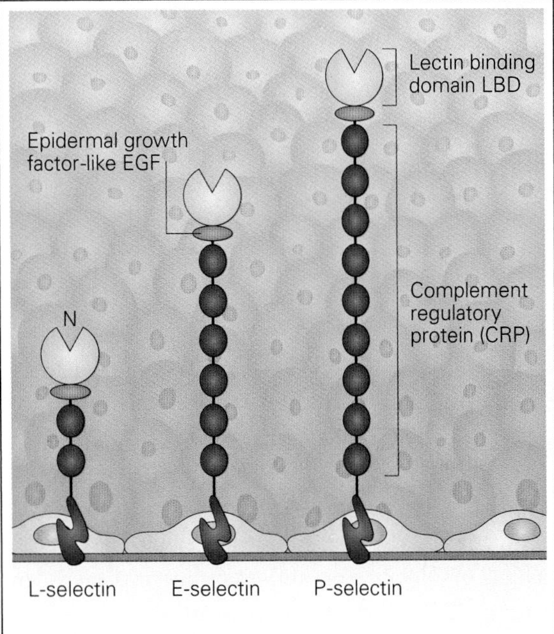

Figure 5-7. Schematic representation of the structure of selectins. The protein structure of selectins is characterized by variable numbers of short consensus repeats (related to complement regulatory proteins), an epithelial growth factor-like domain, and a C-type (calcium-dependent) lectin domain. Through their lectin domain, selectins interact with sugar residues present on cell surface glycoproteins and glycol lipids. Three selectins are known to exist: P-selectin, E-selectin, and L-selectin.

E-selectin, or ELAM-1 as it used to be called, is of considerable pharmaceutical interest as it is involved, along with ICAM-1, in recruiting leukocytes and macrophages into sites of inflammation. E-selectin and ICAM-1 are transiently expressed on endothelial cells lining the microvasculature when they are exposed to certain cytokines.

The counter-ligand to E-selectin is a complex oligosaccharide, known as sialyl Lewis X, which is found on the surfaces of leukocytes (especially neutrophils), and it is the "stickiness" of endothelial cells that are expressing E-selectin that induces a temporary slowing down, or rolling action, as these cells of the lymphatic fluid float past.

P-selectin: P-selectin (previously known as PADGEM, GMP140) is present in the dense granules of platelets and in the Weibel-Palade bodies (granules) of endothelial cells. Upon aggregation of platelets or stimulation of the endothelial cell by thrombin, histamine, or C5a, the granule-associated P-selectin is translocated to the surface. In vitro, this process is very rapid (minutes) and expression is short-lived (< thirty minutes). P-selectin expression persists longer when examined in vivo. Its ligands are glycoproteins expressed on the surface of neutrophils.

E-selectin: E-selectin, also known as CD62E, is a cell adhesion molecule expressed only on endothelial cells activated by cytokines. Like other selectins, it plays an important part in inflammation. E-selectin is expressed exclusively on endothelial cells that have been stimulated by IL-1, TNF-α, endotoxin, or C1q-immune complex aggregates. Expression of E-selectin requires de novo protein synthesis and takes several hours for maximal expression. Expression is transient (< twenty-four hours) both in vitro and in vivo. E-selectin binds to glycoproteins expressed on the surface of neutrophils. In addition to its role in promoting neutrophil attachment to the endothelial surface, binding of E-selectin to its glycoprotein ligand stimulates transcription by endothelial cells of c-fos, an immediate early response gene.

E-selectin recognizes and binds to sialylated carbohydrates present on the surface proteins of certain leukocytes. These carbohydrates include members of the Lewis X and Lewis A families found on monocytes, granulocytes, and T-lymphocytes.

Role of Selectins in Inflammation

During inflammation, E-selectin plays an important part in recruiting leukocytes to the site of injury. The local release of cytokines IL-1 and TNF by damaged cells induces the overexpression of E-selectin on endothelial cells of nearby blood vessels. Leukocytes in the blood expressing the correct ligand will bind with low affinity to E-selectin, causing the leukocytes to "roll" along the

(continued)

Box 5-2 (continued)

internal surface of the blood vessel as temporary interactions are made and broken.

As the inflammatory response progresses, chemokines released by injured tissue enter the blood vessels and activate the rolling leukocytes, which are now able to tightly bind to the endothelial surface and begin making their way into the tissue.

P-selectin has a similar function, but is expressed on the endothelial cell surface within minutes as it is stored within the cell rather than produced on demand.

L-selectin: L-selectin is expressed on neutrophils, a subset of T cells, and monocytes. Unlike either P-selectin and E-selectin, L-selectin is constitutively expressed. In addition, neutrophils shed L-selectin in response to chemotactic stimuli (including IL-8, C5a, and the surrogate bacterial chemoattractant N-formyl-methionyl-leucyl-phenylalanine), but not in response to immune complexes. L-selectin binds to CD34 and other glycosylated proteins on the surface of vascular endothelial cells.

multiple agents, including IL-1, TNF-α, endotoxin, or C1q-immune complex aggregates.

- ICAM-2 is constitutively expressed at high levels on endothelial cells. Unlike ICAM-1, the expression of this receptor does not increase on the surface of stimulated endothelial cells.
- VCAM-1 is not expressed on resting endothelial cells. However, after stimulation with IL-1, TNF-α, endotoxin, or C1q-immune complex aggregates, endothelial cells synthesize and express VCAM-1 on their surface; the ligand for VCAM-1 is very late antigen four (**VLA-4**).

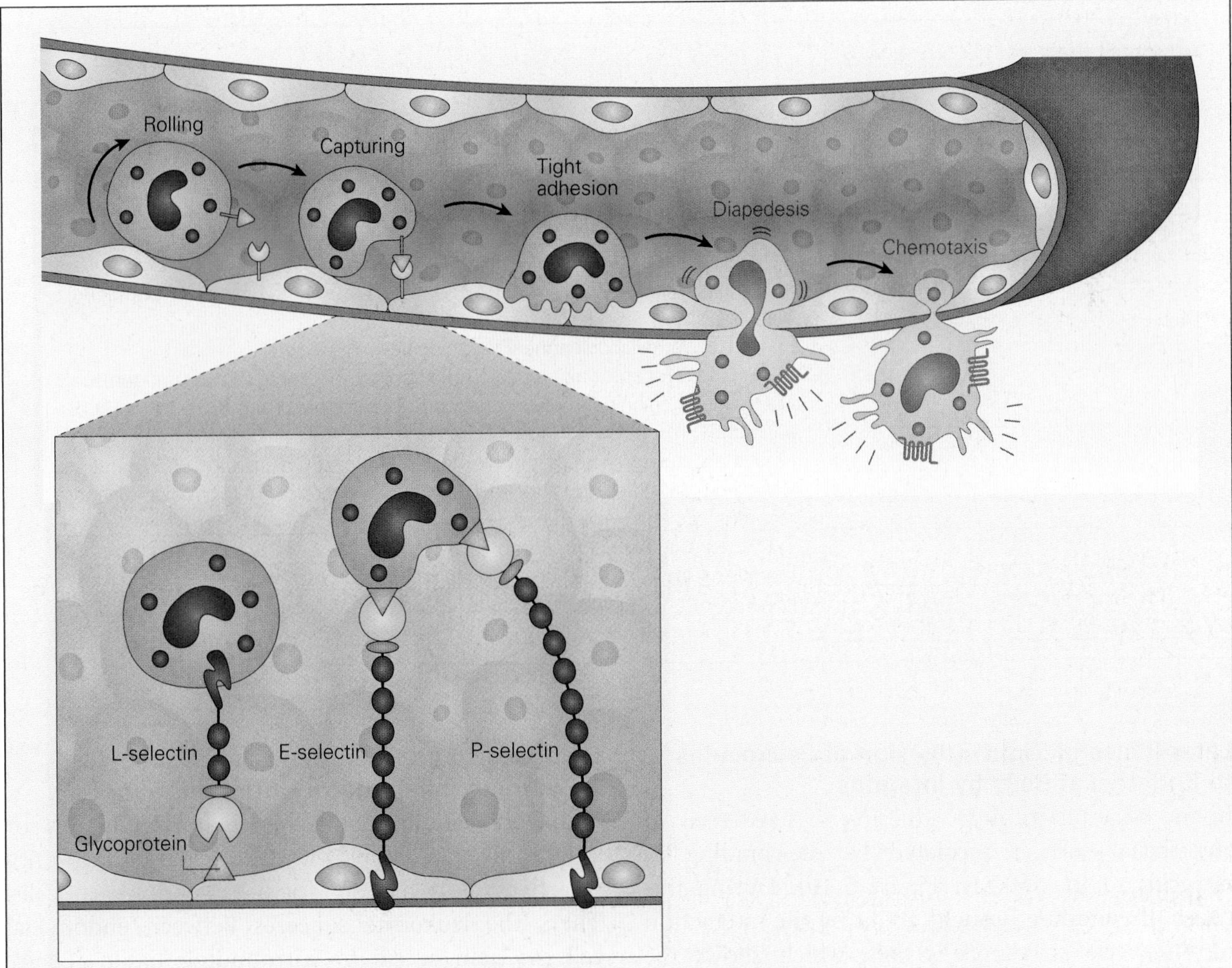

Figure 5-8. Schematic representation of the capture phase of the leukocyte-endothelial interaction showing the loose binding of selectins to glycoproteins.

Box 5-3

The Immunoglobulin Superfamily

The immunoglobulin superfamily (IgSF) is a large group of cell surface and soluble proteins that are involved in the recognition, binding, or adhesion processes of cells. Molecules are categorized as members of this superfamily based on shared structural features with immunoglobulins (*Chapter 6*). The defining structural characteristic of this family of molecules is the presence of an immunoglobulin domain or fold. In addition to the cell adhesion molecules, members of the IgSF also include other cell surface antigen receptors, co-receptors, co-stimulatory molecules, and certain cytokine receptors involved in antigen presentation to lymphocytes (Table 5-4).

Table 5-4. Members of the immunoglobulin superfamily

Molecule function/category	Examples
Adhesion molecules	CD2 CD48 CD22, CD83 Intercellular adhesion molecules (ICAMs) Vascular cell adhesion molecules (e.g., VCAM-1)
Antigen receptors	B cell receptor (BCR) and antibodies or immunoglobulins T cell receptor (TCR) chains
Antigen-presenting molecules	MHC-I MHC-II Beta-2 microglobulin
Co-receptors	CD4 CD8 CD19
Antigen receptor accessory molecules	CD3-γ, -δ and -ε chains CD79a and CD79b
Co-stimulatory or inhibitory molecules	CD28 CD80 and CD86 (also known as B7.1 and B7.2 molecules)
Receptors on natural killer (NK) cells	Killer-cell immunoglobulin-like receptors (KIR)
Cytokine and growth factor receptors	Interleukin-1 receptor type I Interleukin-1 receptor type II precursor (IL-1R-2, IL-1R-beta, CD121b antigen) Platelet-derived growth factor receptor (PDGFR) Platelet endothelial cell adhesion molecule-1 (PECAM-1) Interleukin-6 receptor alpha chain precursor (IL-6R-alpha, CD126 antigen) Macrophage colony-stimulating factor 1 receptor precursor (CSF-1-R, CD115 antigen) Mast/stem cell growth factor receptor precursor (SCFR, c-kit, CD117 antigen) Basic fibroblast growth factor receptor 1 precursor (FGFR-1, tyrosine kinase receptor CEK1)
Receptor tyrosine kinases/ phosphatases	Tyrosine-protein kinase receptor Tie-1 precursor Receptor-type tyrosine-protein phosphatase mu precursor
Ig binding receptors	Polymeric immunoglobulin receptor (PIGR) Some Fc receptors

Later Phase of Tight Adhesion of Leukocytes to Endothelial Cells by Integrins

In the next phase, tight adhesion of leukocytes to endothelial cells is mediated by the binding of integrins to the ICAMs (Figure 5-10). During this phase, the binding brought about by the interaction of these two structures is taut, which allows the subsequent phases of egress of the leukocytes from the vascular compartment into tissues to occur.

Diapedesis and Chemotaxis of Leukocytes Toward an Inflammatory Stimulus

Following tight adhesion, the leukocyte migrates for a short distance along the endothelial surface until it arrives at a junction between endothelial cells. Then, the leukocyte squeezes between endothelial cells to gain access to surrounding tissue (Figure 5-12). This process, called diapedesis, is thought to be mediated by adhesion molecules named platelet/

endothelial cell adhesion molecule-1 (**PECAM-1**) and CD99. This movement of cells is part of the overall process of chemotaxis in which the movement of cells is directed by chemoattractants such as products of bacterial invasion or the complement components C3a and C5a (*Chapter 4*).

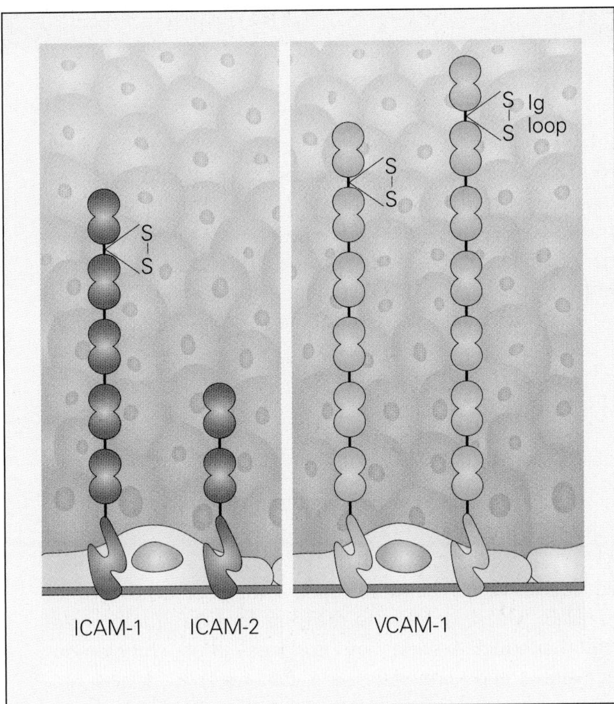

Figure 5-9. Schematic representation of the immunoglobulin family of adhesion proteins that play a role in leukocyte-endothelial adhesion: ICAM-1, ICAM-2, and VCAM-1. ICAM-1 has five extracellular domains, ICAM-2 has two domains, and VCAM-1 can have either six or seven domains.

Leukocytes Migrate Toward the Infection Site by Following a Chemoattractant Gradient

Chemotaxis is the directed movement of a cell as it follows a chemical gradient from a lower to a higher concentration of chemoattractant (Figure 5-12). It depends upon a cell's ability to sense the difference in the fraction of chemoattractant receptors occupied at the leading edge of the cell compared to the trailing end. In an inflammatory response, the highest concentration of chemoattractant is usually found immediately surrounding the inciting agent itself or is synthesized by cells within the immediate vicinity of the inciting agent. At extremely high concentrations of chemoattractant, cells stop migrating; this allows leukocytes to unleash their killing mechanisms in the proper place, as will be described in the next section under phagocytosis. Classic chemoattractants

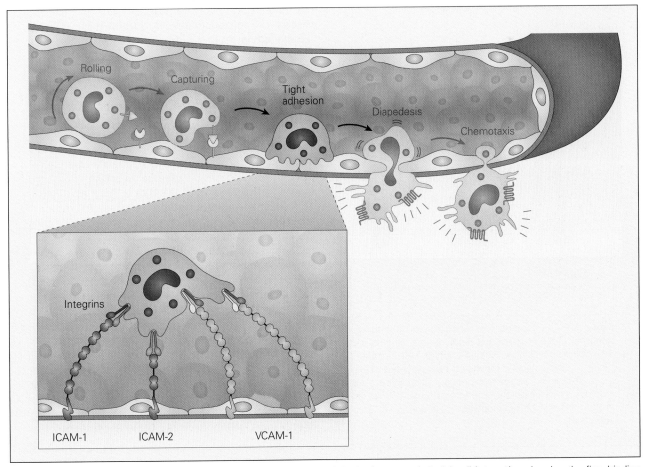

Figure 5-10. Schematic representation of the tight adhesion phase of the leukocyte-endothelial cell interaction showing the firm binding brought about by the interaction of integrins on the leukocyte membrane with ICAMs on the endothelium.

Box 5-4

Integrins

The integrins are a family of heterodimeric adhesive molecules found on all cell types and which regulate a wide variety of cellular processes such as cell migration, phagocytosis, and growth and development. They represent the most dynamic and versatile of all the adhesion molecules. Integrins are composed of a transmembrane alpha and a beta protein chain structure (Figure 5-11). Among the integrins, members differing by either a beta 1 or beta 2 chain comprise subclasses and are primarily responsible for the migration of hematopoietic cells into areas of inflammation. These integrins include lymphocyte function-associated antigen-1 (LFA-1), a beta 2, alpha L heterodimer; macrophage-1 antigen (Mac-1), a beta 2, alpha M heterodimer and a complement receptor 3 (CR3); and very late antigen-4 (VLA-4), a beta 1, alpha 4 heterodimer (Table 5-1 and Figure 5-11).

The Two Types of Integrins: Beta 1 and Beta 2

Beta 2 integrins: The leukocyte integrins are the only integrins that share the beta 2 subunit i.e., also designated by the cluster of differentiation antigen CD18. There are three beta 2 integrins that are known as LFA-1 (CD11a/CD18), Mac-1 (CD11b/CD18), and gp150/95 (CD11c/CD18). All three of the integrins are expressed constitutively and must be activated in order to become adhesive for their ligands.

LFA-1 is constitutively expressed on lymphocytes and is critical for the interaction of lymphocytes with the endothelium and, more importantly, for adhesion of lymphocytes to antigen-presenting cells. LFA-1 binds to intercellular adhesion molecule-1 (ICAM-1), ICAM-2, and ICAM-3 on endothelial and other cells.

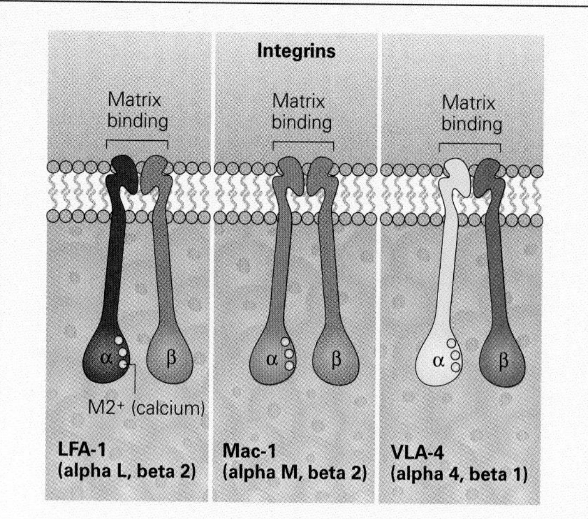

Figure 5-11. Schematic representation of structures of integrins. The integrins are heterodimers of two transmembrane subunits, designated α and β, held together by metal binding. Integrins regulate a wide variety of cellular processes such as cell migration, phagocytosis, and growth and development. The integrins primarily involved in the migration of hematopoietic cells are LFA-1, Mac-1, and VLA-4.

Mac-1 is expressed on neutrophils and monocytes. Specific granules in the neutrophil contain stores of Mac-1 and are mobilized to the surface after neutrophil activation. Mac-1 binds to ICAM-1, but not to ICAM-2 or ICAM-3. Mac-1 is also the receptor for C3bi (the complement product present on surfaces after complement activation) and fibrinogen. As a C3bi receptor, Mac-1 promotes phagocytosis of microorganisms and other particulates (*Chapter 4*). The precise role of gp150/95 (which is found on neutrophils and monocytes) has not been precisely defined.

Beta 1 integrins: VLA-4 is a beta 1 integrin whose expression is confined to eosinophils, lymphocytes, and monocytes (Table 5-3). This molecule binds to endothelial vascular cell adhesion molecule-1 (VCAM-1) and is critical for the accumulation of mononuclear cells at sites of chronic infection.

Clinical Significance of Beta 2 Integrins: Leukocyte Adhesion Deficiency Type I

The importance of the beta integrins is seen by the manifestations of leukocyte adhesion deficiency type I, a primary immunodeficiency disease resulting from the absence of expression of the beta 2 integrins (*Chapter 16*). Patients with this disorder have severe, recurrent infections and die in childhood due to overwhelming infections because of the defective beta 2 subunit, and thus almost no CD18 will be expressed on the leukocyte surface membrane. This will eventually lead to severe defects in the firm adhesion of leukocytes on endothelial cells and thus to the defective inflammatory response leading to infections. Although affected individuals have very high peripheral white cell counts, white blood cells are unable to migrate into infected sites owing to the beta 2 integrin deficiency. Leukocytes are also less capable of phagocytosing C3bi-opsonized particles than leukocytes from unaffected individuals. Thus, this molecular lesion is responsible for the inability of leukocytes to adhere tightly to the endothelium or particulates resulting directly to an inability to contain bacterial infections.

(continued)

Box 5-4 (continued)

Other Clinical Applications of Integrins

In addition to the clinical relevance of integrins in the leukocyte adhesion deficiency type I syndrome, there are several other rapidly occurring clinical applications of integrin antagonists that are being tested in clinical studies (*Chapter 11*). These include three groups of products: (1) humanized antibodies, (2) synthetic peptides, and (3) nonpeptide small molecules. All target the extracellular region of integrins and interfere with binding of the ligand to its substrate. Antibodies have been developed that target several different integrins, including Efalizumab (Raptiva®), which antagonizes αLβ2 and is used in the treatment of psoriasis, and Natalizumab (Tysabri or Antegren®), which binds to the α4 chain and antagonizes α4β1 and α4β7 integrins and is used to treat multiple sclerosis and Crohn's disease. The antibodies MEDI-522 (Vitaxin or Abegrin) and CNTO95 target integrin αV and are currently being tested as inhibitors of angiogenesis in several cancer clinical trials (*Chapter 20*). Abciximab (ReoPro®) is a Fab fragment that binds αIIbβ3 and is used to inhibit platelet aggregation. Examples of synthetic peptides that mimic their natural peptide counterparts include Cilengitide that inhibits αVβ3 and αVβ5 and Eptifibatide (Integrilin®) that inhibits αIIbβ3. Examples of nonpeptide inhibitors include Tirofiban (Aggrostat®), which targets αIIbβ3 and is also used to inhibit platelet aggregation, and Valategrast, a small molecule inhibitor of α4β1 for treatment of asthma. With the increased knowledge of integrin structure and function, other biologic response modifiers of the integrin families are being generated and tested in preclinical models and clinical studies.

include C5a, formylated peptides (bacterial in origin), leukotriene B4, and platelet-activating factor. In addition, chemokines, a specialized class of cytokines (*Chapter 9*), which tend to be more selective in the type of leukocyte they attract, may be synthesized at the focus of an inflammatory response. As leukocytes migrate from the vasculature to the focus of an inflammatory response, they must break down components of the extracellular matrix that block their path. Leukocytes achieve this by a gradual, focused release of granule contents, which contain proteases, at their leading front as they migrate.

Phagocytosis and Killing Eliminate the Infectious Agent

Phagocytosis is the process by which neutrophils and macrophages engulf microbes or cellular debris (*Chapter 1*). Before a phagocyte can engulf a target, it must first recognize and attach to a target. Recognition molecules include TLRs, scavenger receptors, and lipopolysaccharide (**LPS**) receptors (*Chapter 3*). Opsonins are soluble factors that coat the surface of a potential target, allowing a phagocyte to recognize it. Opsonization usually occurs by one or both of the following mechanisms: (1) antibodies that are specific to a particular target bind to and coat its surface; the Fc portions of the antibodies then can bind to and activate Fc receptors on the phagocyte; (2) microbial surfaces can activate the complement cascade, even in the absence of antibodies. During complement activation, a product called C3b is generated that can then bind to bacterial surfaces (*Chapter 4*). Phagocytes express several receptors for C3b called complement receptors 1 through 4 (CR1, CR2, etc.).

Following recognition of a pathogen, the phagocyte engulfs it by extending protrusions of its cytoplasm and cell membrane that envelop and incorporate the pathogen within an intracellular membrane-bound structure called the phagosome or phagocytic vacuole (Figure 5-13). Degradation of the target takes place within this structure as the phagocyte's granules (i.e., lysosomes) fuse with the phagocytic vacuole to form a phagolysosome, a process called degranulation.

During degranulation, the granules of a phagocyte fuse with either the phagocytic vacuole or the plasma membrane. (In the latter case, the granule's contents are released into the extracellular space.) The granules contain many factors that can damage or kill microorganisms; these factors include proteases, antimicrobial proteins such as bactericidal/permeability increasing protein (**BPI**) and the defensins (these factors insert into microbial membranes and cause their intracellular contents to leak out), and the components of the nicotinamide adenine dinucleotide phosphate (**NADPH**) oxidase system.

Metabolic Pathways Employed by the Phagocytic Cell in Microbicidal Activity

Following uptake of a foreign substance and the formation of the phagocytic vacuole, a series of biochemical reactions is initiated in phagocytic cells.

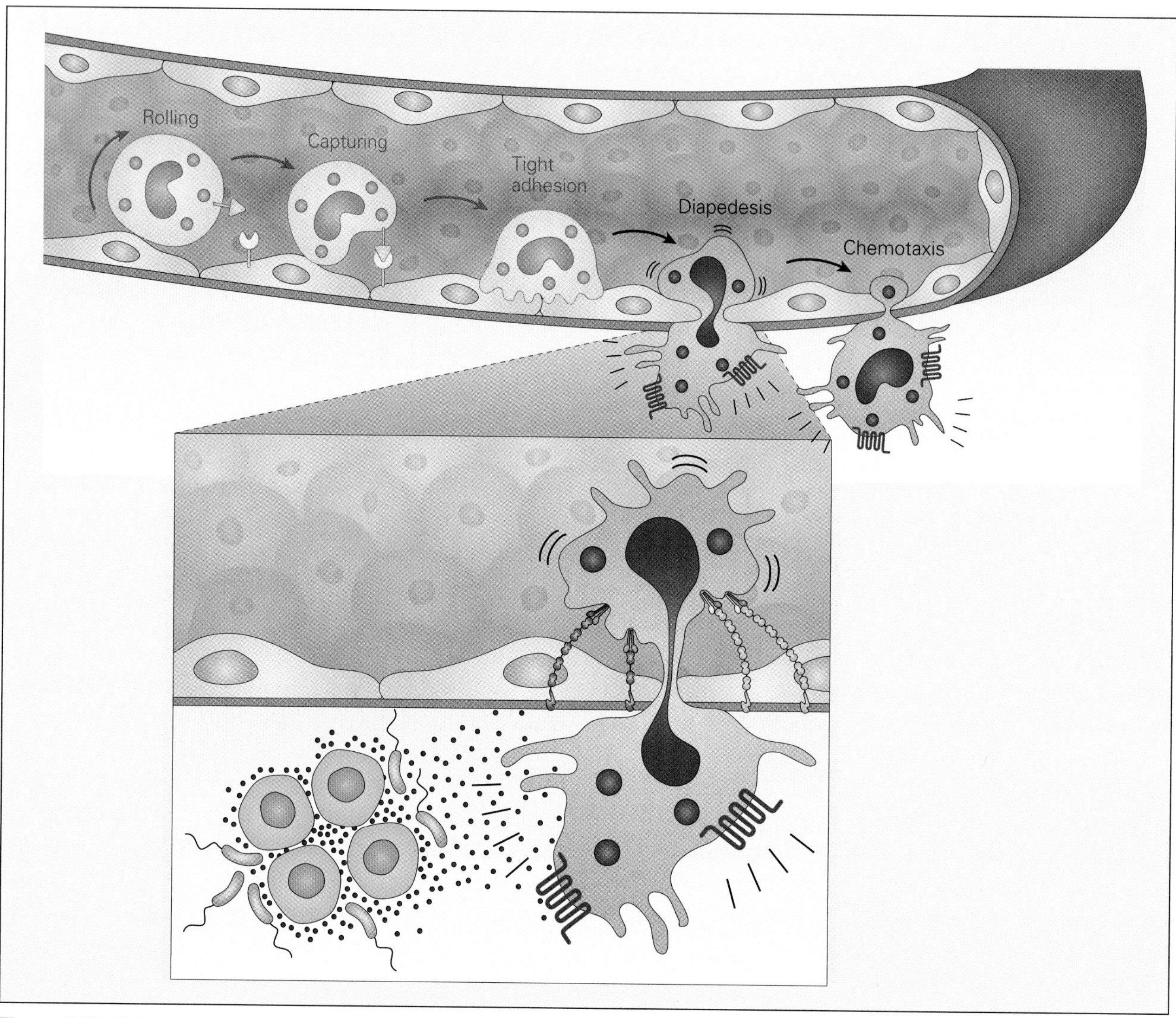

Figure 5-12. Schematic representation of subsequent phases of the leukocyte-endothelial cell interaction in which leukocytes squeeze through in between endothelial cells (diapedesis) into tissues and subsequently display directed cell movement to inflammatory stimuli (chemotaxis).

This is referred to as the "respiratory burst," during which an increase in glucose and oxygen consumption occurs. The end result of the respiratory burst is that several activated forms of oxygen are produced that participate in the bacterial killing by three major pathways: (1) the oxygen-dependent pathway, (2) the oxygen-independent pathway, and (3) the nitric oxide (**NO**) pathway (Box 5-5). The metabolic pathways that are primarily involved include the glycolytic pathway and the hexose monophosphate (**HMP**) shunt. The NADPH oxidase system, together with the enzymes superoxide dismutase (SOD) and myeloperoxidase (**MPO**), allows phagocytes to produce toxic oxygen metabolites, i.e., O_2^-, hydroxyl (OH^-) anion, and hydrogen peroxide (H_2O_2), which are the critically important microbicidal products employed by the phagocytic cell during phagocytosis and intracellular killing of bacteria. A genetic deficiency of the NADPH oxidase system is seen in the primary immunodeficiency disorder, chronic granulomatous disease (**CGD**) (*Chapter 16*). The NADPH oxidase system is a group of coenzymes that are kept physically separated from one another while a phagocyte is at rest. Because different granule populations contain different components of the NADPH oxidase system, degranulation into the same compartment allows the separated components to come together and become a functional unit (either on the cell membrane or within a phagocytic vacuole).

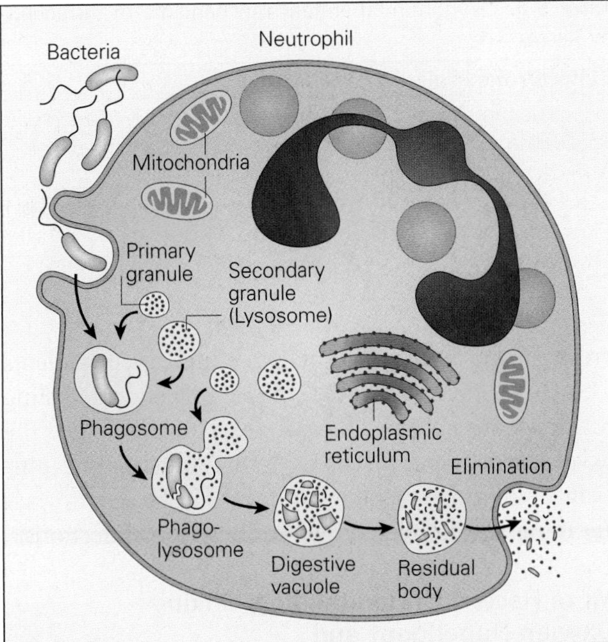

Figure 5-13. Schematic representation of phagocytosis. Pathogen binding to phagocyte membrane receptors signals the phagocyte to form a phagocytic vacuole (phagosome) and fuse the phagosome with a lysosome to form a phagolysosome. Degradation of the organism takes place within the phagolysosome. Under some conditions, the phagocyte releases its lysosomal enzymes and toxic oxygen products into the surrounding fluid.

Box 5-5

Microbicidal Metabolic Pathways of the Phagocytic Cell

Bacterial killing by three major pathways:

1. **Oxygen-dependent intracellular killing** results from the increase in glucose and oxygen consumption during phagocytosis referred to as the respiratory burst. The consequence of the respiratory burst is that a number of oxygen-containing compounds are produced, which contribute to killing of the microbe being phagocytosed. The oxygen-dependent pathway has been further subdivided into:
   - those that have been thought to kill bacteria directly (oxygen-dependent myeloperoxidase-independent intracellular killing) (Figure 5-14); and
   - those that utilize myeloperoxidase (MPO) (the oxygen-dependent myeloperoxidase-dependent intracellular killing) (Figure 5-15).
2. In addition, bacteria can be killed by **oxygen-independent intracellular killing** using preformed substances released from granules or lysosomes when they fuse with the phagosome.
3. A third mechanism of bacterial killing by phagocytic cells involves the production of nitric oxide (**nitric oxide-dependent killing**).

Oxygen-Dependent Intracellular Killing

Oxygen-Dependent Myeloperoxidase-Independent Intracellular Killing

During oxygen-dependent myeloperoxidase-independent intracellular killing of bacteria by phagocytes, glucose is metabolized via the hexose monophosphate shunt and NADPH is formed (Figure 5-14). Cytochrome B, which is part of the specific granule, combines with the plasma membrane NADPH oxidase and activates it. The activated NADPH oxidase uses oxygen to oxidize the NADPH. The result is the production of superoxide anion (O_2^-) and NAPD. Some of the superoxide anion is converted to H_2O_2 and singlet oxygen ($^1O_2$) by superoxide dismutase. In addition, superoxide anion can react with H_2O_2, resulting in the formation of hydroxyl radical (OH^-) and more singlet oxygen. The result of all of these reactions is the production of the toxic oxygen compounds O_2^-, H_2O_2, $^1O_2$, and OH^-.

Oxygen-Dependent Myeloperoxidase-Dependent Intracellular Killing

A second form of oxygen-dependent bactericidal mechanisms of phagocytic cells relies on the enzyme myeloperoxidase (**MPO**). As the azurophilic granules fuse with the phagosome, myeloperoxidase is released into the phagolysosome. Myeloperoxidase utilizes H_2O_2 and halide ions (usually Cl^-) to produce hypochlorite, a highly toxic substance (Figure 5-15). Some of the hypochlorite can spontaneously break down

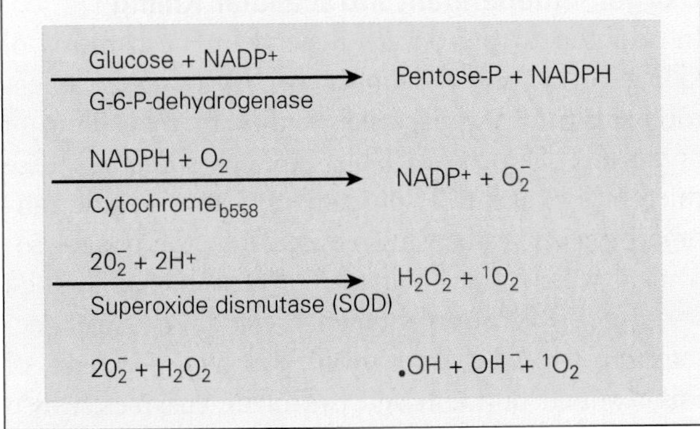

Figure 5-14. Production of activated forms of oxygen via the oxygen-dependent myeloperoxidase-independent pathway. The G-6-PD is required for the production of NADPH, an essential component of the NADPH oxidase system that generates O_2^- by transferring 2 electrons from NADPH to molecular oxygen (O_2). O_2^- is metabolized to H_2O_2 and singlet oxygen ($^1O_2$) by SOD. The O_2^- can react with H_2O_2 forming hydroxyl radicals (OH^-) and more $^1O_2$.

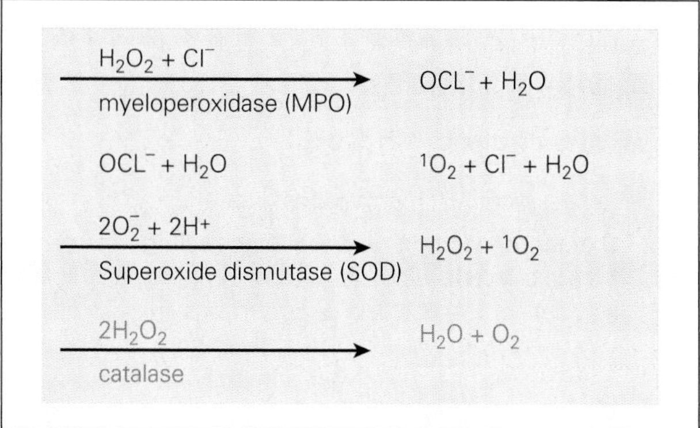

Figure 5-15. Production of activated forms of oxygen via the oxygen-dependent myeloperoxidase-dependent pathway. MPO utilizes H_2O_2 and halide ions (usually Cl^-) to produce hypochlorite (OCl^-) that can break down to form $^1O_2$. The H_2O_2 formed from O_2^- by SOD is then broken down by catalase.

to yield singlet oxygen. The result of these reactions is the production of toxic hypochlorite (OCl^-) and $^1O_2$.

Detoxification Mechanisms Used by Phagocytic Cells

Polymorphonuclear leukocytes (**PMNs**) and macrophages have means to protect themselves from the toxic oxygen intermediates that are being generated in these oxygen-dependent pathways (Table 5-5). These reactions involve two enzymes: (1) superoxide dismutase (**SOD**) and (2) catalase. SOD catalyzes the dismutation of O_2^- into O_2 and H_2O_2. As such, it is an important antioxidant defense in nearly all cells exposed to oxygen. Catalase converts hydrogen peroxide to water and oxygen thereby avoiding its deleterious effects on the cell (Table 5-5).

Oxygen-Independent Intracellular Killing

In addition to the oxygen-dependent mechanisms of killing, there are a number of oxygen-independent mechanisms that phagocytes utilize in the killing of organisms. Shown in Table 5-6 are some of these microbicidal agents of phagocytes. These include cationic proteins (cathepsin) released into the phagolysosome, which can damage bacterial membranes; lysozyme, which breaks down bacterial cell walls; lactoferrin, which chelates iron, depriving bacteria of this required nutrient; and hydrolytic enzymes, which

Table 5-5. Detoxification mechanisms used by phagocytic cells

Reaction	Detoxifying enzyme
$2O_2^- + 2H^+ \rightarrow O_2 + H_2O_2$	Superoxide dismutase
$2H_2O_2 \rightarrow 2H_2O + O_2$	Catalase

Table 5-6. Oxygen-independent mechanisms of intracellular killing

Effector molecule	Function
Cationic proteins (including cathepsin)	Damage to microbial membranes
Lysozyme	Splits mucopeptide in bacterial cell wall
Lactoferrin	Deprives proliferating bacteria of iron
Proteolytic and hydrolytic enzymes	Digestion of killed organisms

break down bacterial proteins. Thus, even patients who have defects in the oxygen-dependent killing pathways are able to kill bacteria. However, since the oxygen-dependent mechanisms are much more efficient in killing, patients with defects in these pathways are more susceptible and get more serious infections.

More Recent Understanding Linking Oxygen-Dependent and Oxygen-Independent Pathways

The various stages involved in the uptake of organisms by phagocytic cells and their subsequent killing by intracellular mechanisms are shown in Figures 5-16, 5-17, and 5-18. The initial steps involve the formation of a phagosome, which later fuses with the primary and secondary granule of the lysosome (Figure 5-16). Following generation of the NADPH oxidase complex and stimulation of the oxidative pathways involving the generation of oxygen radicals, the organism is killed (Figure 5-17). The results of recent studies have bridged the apparent gap between oxygen-dependent and oxygen-independent killing by showing that the generation of superoxide leads to a high level potassium influx into the phagolysosome, which in turn leads to activation of intraphagolysosomal enzymes like elastase and cathepsin G (Figure 5-18). Therefore, the pathways present in phagocytes are actually synergistic, with the oxygen-consuming NADPH oxidase further activating the granule proteins to kill pathogens. Although killing was previously believed to be accomplished by reactive oxygen radicals generated by the NADPH oxidase, and by the hypohalous acid produced by MPO, more recent findings focus on the oxidase activity delivering electrons into the phagocytic vacuole, thereby inducing a charge across the membrane that must be compensated. The need for compensating ions then opens up potassium channels that then liberate the granulocyte elastase (**GE**) and cathepsin G (**CG**) from a glycocalyx, allowing them to ultimately kill the ingested bacteria or fungi (Figure 5-18).

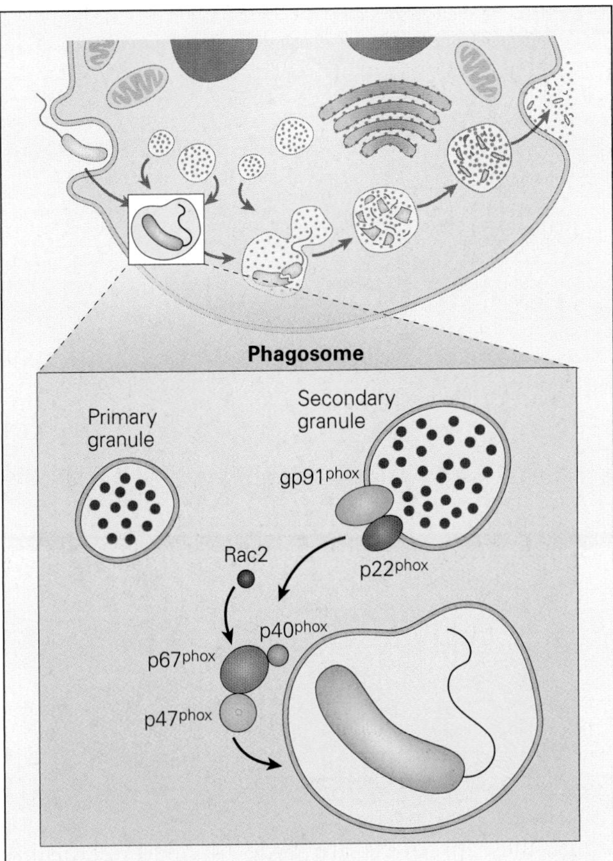

Figure 5-16. Schematic representation of uptake of a bacterium to form a phagocytic vacuole (phagosome). The primary granules are the first to be produced in the bone marrow and contain myeloperoxidase (MPO), granulocyte elastase (GE), cathepsin G (CG), and proteinase 3 (PR3). The secondary granules arise later in bone marrow development and contain lactoferrin and the cytochrome b complex (gp91phox and p22phox). p47phox and p67phox are found as isolated components in the cytosol. The NADPH oxidase is assembled on either the wall of the phagolysosome or the plasma membrane. Initially, cytochrome b is composed of the dimer gp91phox and p22phox and later by the addition of p47phox and p67phox. When p40phox and rac join the complex, the mature NADPH oxidase is formed.

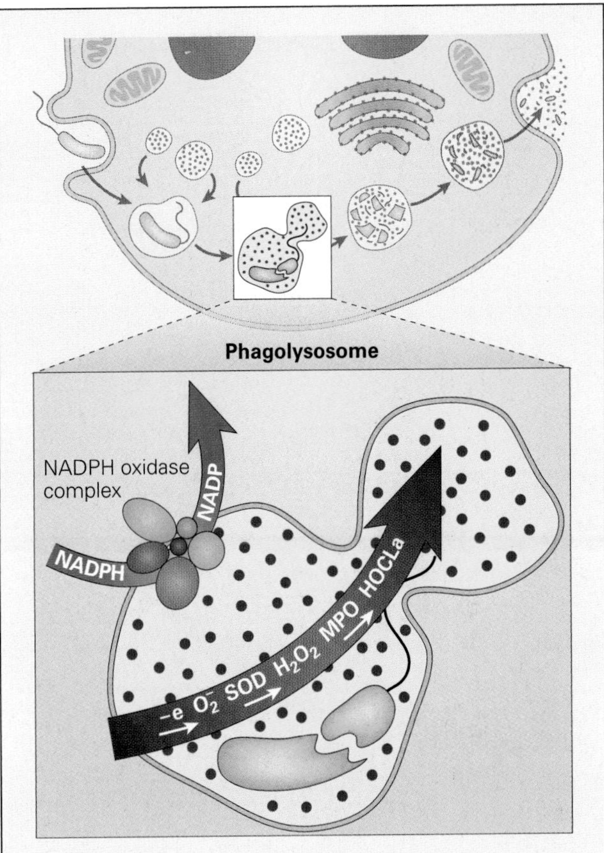

Figure 5-17. Schematic representation of fusion of the phagosome with a lysosome to form a phagolysosome. The NADPH oxidase complex harvests an electron from NADPH, oxidizing it to NADP+, and delivers that electron to molecular oxygen in the phagosome, generating superoxide (O_2^-). Superoxide is converted to hydrogen peroxide (H_2O_2) by superoxide dismutase (SOD); this in turn is converted to hypohalous acid (HOCl or bleach) by myeloperoxidase (MPO). Degradation of the organism begins to take place within the phagolysosome. Under some conditions, the phagocyte releases its lysosomal enzymes and toxic oxygen products into the surrounding fluid with resultant inflammation and tissue injury.

Nitric Oxide–Dependent Killing

Another mechanism by which phagocytic cells kill microorganisms is by the production of NO. This has been demonstrated primarily by macrophages. Binding of bacteria to macrophages, particularly binding via Toll-like receptors, results in the production of TNF-α, which acts in an autocrine manner to induce the expression of the inducible nitric oxide synthetase gene (**i-nos**) resulting in the production of NO (*Chapter 11*). If the cell is also exposed to interferon gamma (IFN-γ), additional NO will be produced (Figure 5-19). NO released by the cell is toxic and can kill microorganisms in the vicinity of the macrophage.

Clinical Significance of Understanding the Metabolic Pathways Employed by the Phagocytic Cell in Microbicidal Activity

The NADPH oxidase system, together with the enzymes superoxide dismutase and myeloperoxidase, allows phagocytes to produce toxic oxygen metabolites, i.e., O_2^-, OH^- anion, and H_2O_2, which are the critically important microbicidal products employed by the phagocytic cell during phagocytosis and intracellular killing of bacteria (Table 5-7). A genetic deficiency of the NADPH oxidase system is seen in the primary immunodeficiency disorder, chronic granulomatous disease (**CGD**) (*Chapter 16*). The NADPH oxidase system is a unique group of coenzymes that are kept physically separated from one another while a phagocyte is at rest. Because

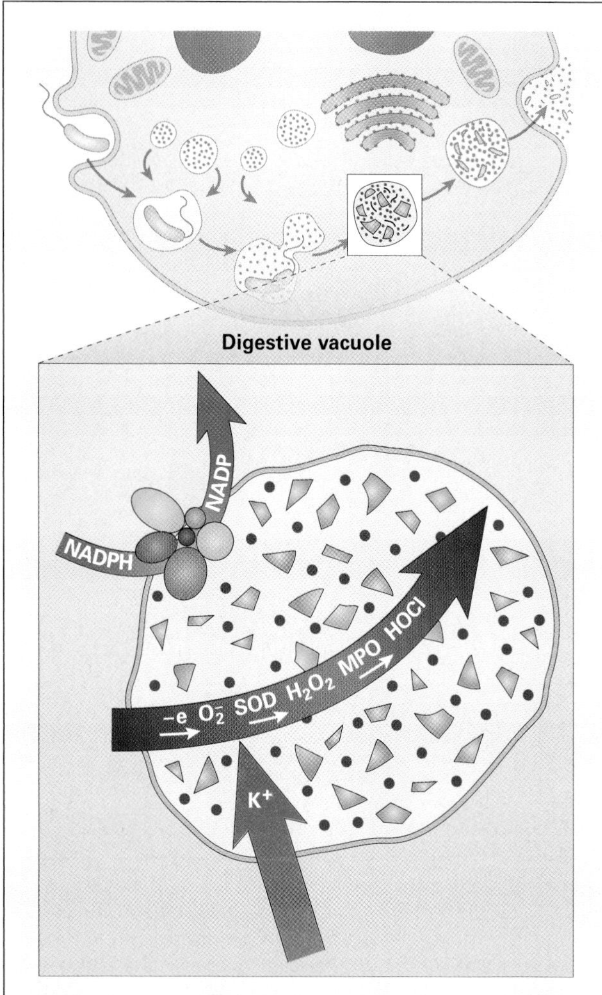

Figure 5-18. Schematic representation of the final degradation of the organism within the phagolysosome. Killing was previously believed to be accomplished by reactive oxygen radicals generated by the NADPH oxidase, and by the hypohalous acid produced by MPO. More recent findings focus on the oxidase activity delivering electrons into the phagocytic vacuole, thereby inducing a charge across the membrane that must be compensated. The need for compensating ions opens up potassium channels that then liberate the granulocyte elastase and cathepsin G from a glycocalyx, allowing them to ultimately kill the ingested organism.

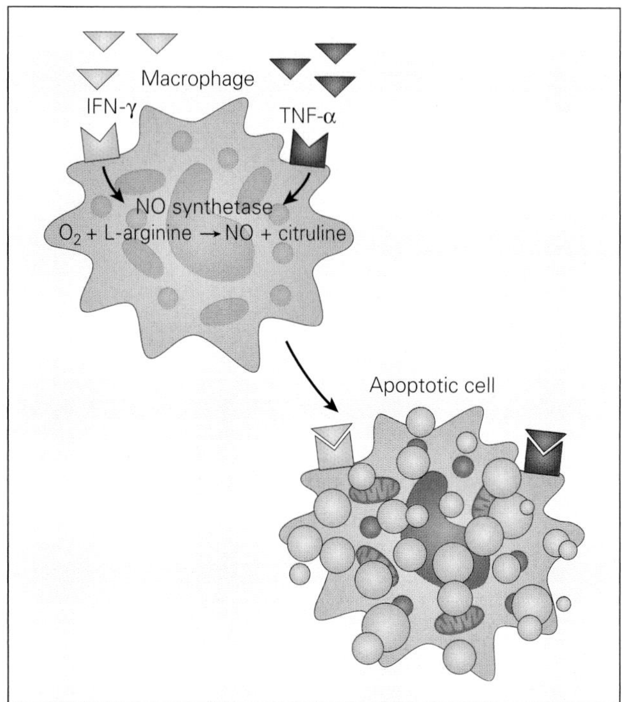

Figure 5-19. Schematic representation of the nitric oxide-dependent killing mechanism showing the bridging of the innate and adaptive immune systems by tumor necrosis factor and IFN-γ.

different granule populations contain different components of the NADPH oxidase system, degranulation into the same compartment allows the separated components to come together and become a functional unit (either on the cell membrane or within a phagocytic vacuole). Once assembled, the complex transfers electrons from NADPH to oxygen, forming O_2^-. Rapidly, O_2^- is converted to H_2O_2 by superoxide dismutase and to hypochlorous acid (HOCl) by myeloperoxidase. These toxic oxygen metabolites indiscriminately oxidize proteins and cause them to lose their function. While these products are toxic to microorganisms, they are also toxic to host tissue.

Immune Evasion by Bacteria: How Do Bacteria Circumvent the Immune System?

If the immune system is successful in recognizing, taking up, and destroying an invading bacterial invader, the organism will not be able to establish itself in the body and thus cannot cause disease. However, the immune system does not always succeed in its task, and often the reason for this failure is that the invading organism has evolved a strategy for evading or suppressing the host's immune response to it (*Chapter 12*). There are many different strategies that have evolved in different organisms to evade antimicrobial mechanisms. Shown in Table 5-8 are some of these strategies with examples of each.

Avoiding Contact with Phagocytes

Bacteria can avoid the attention of phagocytes in a number of ways. Some bacteria or their products inhibit phagocyte chemotaxis. For example, Streptococcal streptolysin (which also kills phagocytes) suppresses neutrophil chemotaxis, even in very low concentrations. Fractions of *Mycobacterium tuberculosis* are known to inhibit leukocyte migration, and *Clostridium* ø toxin also inhibits neutrophil chemotaxis.

Table 5-7. Microbicidal agents of phagocytes

Mechanism	Examples
Acidification	pH 3.5-4 kills microbes, activates digestive enzymes
Toxic oxygen products	O_2^-, H_2O_2, $^1O_2^{\cdot}$, OH^-, HOCl
Toxic nitrogen oxides	NO
Antimicrobial peptides (see also *Box 3-3*)	Bactericidal permeability increasing protein (BPI), defensins, cationic proteins
Enzymes	Lysozyme, acid hydrolases
Competitors	Lactoferrin (binds iron) Vitamin B_{12}-binding protein

Inhibition of Phagocytic Engulfment

Some bacteria employ strategies to avoid engulfment (ingestion) if phagocytes do make contact with them. Many important pathogenic bacteria bear on their surfaces, substances that inhibit phagocytic adsorption or engulfment such as capsules, e.g., *Streptococcus pneumoniae,* which prevents phagocytosis.

Survival Inside of Phagocytes

Some bacteria that can resist killing inside of phagocytes are considered intracellular parasites and can survive inside of phagocytic cells, in either neutrophils or macrophages. Intracellular parasites survive inside of phagocytes by virtue of mechanisms that interfere with the bactericidal activities of the host cell. Some of these bacterial mechanisms include:

Inhibition of Fusion of the Phagocytic Lysosomes (Granules) with the Phagosome

The bacteria survive inside of phagosomes because they prevent the discharge of lysosomal contents into the phagosome environment. Specifically, phagolysosome formation is inhibited in the phagocyte. This is the strategy employed by *Salmonella, M. tuberculosis, Legionella,* and the chlamydiae.

Survival Inside the Phagolysosome

With some intracellular parasites, phagosome-lysosome fusion occurs, but the bacteria are resistant to inhibition and killing by the lysosomal constituents. *Mycobacterium leprae* grows inside phagocytic vacuoles even after extensive fusion with lysosomes. Other mycobacteria (including *M. tuberculosis*) have waxy, hydrophobic cell walls and capsule components (mycolic acids) that are not easily attacked by lysosomal enzymes.

Products of Bacteria That Kill or Damage Phagocytes

Many Gram-positive pathogens, particularly the pyogenic cocci, secrete extracellular enzymes that kill phagocytes. Many of these enzymes are called hemolysins because their activity in the presence of red blood cells results in their lysis. Pathogenic streptococci produce streptolysin. Streptolysin O binds to cholesterol in membranes. The effect on neutrophils is to cause lysosomal granules to explode, releasing their contents into the cell cytoplasm. Pathogenic staphylococci produce leukocidin, which also acts on the neutrophil membrane and causes discharge of lysosomal granules. Extracellular proteins that inhibit phagocytosis include the Exotoxin A of *Pseudomonas aeruginosa,* which kills macrophages, and the bacterial exotoxins that are adenylate cyclases (e.g., anthrax toxin edema factor (**EF**) and pertussis toxin AC) that decrease phagocytic activity.

Production of Products That Interfere with or Destroy Activated Oxygen Molecules

Some bacteria avoid being killed by phagocytes by the production of enzymes that can destroy some

Table 5-8. Some of the evasion strategies, mechanisms, and examples used by bacteria

Evasion strategy	Mechanism	Examples
Avoiding contact with phagocytes	Inhibition of chemotaxis	Streptococcal streptolysin, *Mycobacterium tuberculosis, Clostridium* ø toxin
Inhibition of phagocytic engulfment	Production of capsules	*S. pneumoniae*
Survival inside of phagocytes	Blocking phagosome-lysosome fusion	*Salmonella, M. tuberculosis, Legionella,* and the chlamydiae
	Survival inside the phagolysosome	*Mycobacterium leprae, M. tuberculosis, Bacillus anthracis*
Products of bacteria that kill or damage phagocytes	Production of enzyme	Hemolysins, streptolysins
Production of products that interfere or destroy activated oxygen molecules	Production of bacterial enzymes	Peroxidases, catalases, superoxide dismutase

of the activated forms of oxygen important in microbicidal activity, e.g., peroxidase, catalase, and SOD.

Inflammation Has Systemic as well as Local Effects

Inflammation not only consists of a local, protective response to microbial invasion or injury, but is also encompassed of a broader set interrelated and interdependent responses that comprise the neurologic endocrine immunologic (**NEI**) network (*Chapter 1*). For example, cytokines produced in macrophages, i.e., IL-1, can exert an effect on hypothalamus with fever, acute phase protein release from the liver produced during inflammation that can lead to release/production of more phagocytes from the bone marrow, and the production of adrenocortico tropic hormone (**ACTH**) from hypothalamic stimulation, which can lead to the immunosuppressive effects of corticosteroids released from the adrenal gland. Moreover, the discovery that cholinergic neurons inhibit acute inflammation has qualitatively expanded understanding of how the nervous system modulates immune responses. Stimulation of the nervous system reflexively regulates the inflammatory response in real time, just as it controls the heart rate and other vital functions. The opportunity now exists to apply these observations to the treatment of inflammation by modifying selective and reversible hardwired neural systems, e.g., biofeedback systems and acupuncture.

Inflammation Is Normally Controlled by Negative Feedback Mechanisms

From what has been described thus far, inflammation clearly represents a complex set of interactions among soluble factors and cells that can arise in any tissue in response to tissue damage resulting from trauma, infection, ischemia, toxins, or autoimmune injury. The process normally leads to recovery and healing. However, if targeted destruction and assisted repair are not properly phased, acute inflammation can lead to persistent chronic tissue damage mediated by leukocytes, lymphocytes, or collagen. Inflammation may be considered in terms of its checkpoints, where a cascading set of signals drives each to escalate. However, these "go" signals trigger "stop" signals, and, paradoxically, molecules responsible for mediating the inflammatory response can also suppress it, depending on timing and context. Some examples of these inhibitory mechanisms include delayed macrophage production of an IL-1 receptor antagonist (**IL-1ra**), TNF induction of TNF receptor (**TNFR**), shedding and competition of the released receptors with cell surface receptors for TNF, production of anti-inflammatory cytokines IL-10 and TGF-β, and CNS suppression of inflammation (*Chapter 9*). The non-inflammatory state does not arise passively from an absence of inflammatory stimuli; rather, maintenance of homeostatic balance in health requires the positive actions of specific gene products to suppress reactions to potentially inflammatory stimuli that do not warrant a full response.

Cell Death and Inflammation: Apoptosis, Autophagy, Oncosis and Pyroptosis

One of the outcomes of inflammation is cell death. Cells can die through distinct biochemical pathways that produce different morphological and physiological outcomes. There are four basic terms that have been used to describe these various outcomes: **apoptosis, autophagy, oncosis** and **pyroptosis** (Figure 5-20). Apoptosis and autophagy are mechanisms that maintain normal intracellular homeostasis and do not lead to inflammation in contrast to oncosis and pyroptosis, which are associated with release of intracellular contents, necrosis and inflammation. The stimulation of inflammation by pyroptosis is mediated by activation of the inflammasome (*Chapter 9* and *Chapter 19 Annex).*

Apoptosis

Apoptosis (from the Greek, denotes a "falling off," as leaves from a tree) is perhaps the most widely recognized term to describe programmed cell death without inflammation. In this scenario, cells die as a result of the requirement for particular cysteine dependent aspartate-specific proteases (**caspases**) which produce an orchestrated disassembly of the cell (Figure 5-20). In standard cell conditions, caspases are present in the cytoplasm in an inactive form. Several external stimuli are able to activate these enzymes that now cleave cellular substrates, resulting in the characteristic features of apoptosis, which include cytoplasmic and nuclear condensation and fragmentation, DNA cleavage and maintenance of an intact plasma membrane. The contents of apoptotic cells are packaged into membrane-enclosed structures called **apoptotic bodies**, which are recognized and taken up by macrophages, i.e., phagocytosis, and removed in vivo, resulting in an absence of inflammation (Figure 5-20). Apoptosis is the physiological mechanism by which most normal cells are regularly removed and eliminated, including those processes during which unwanted or autoreactive cells are removed

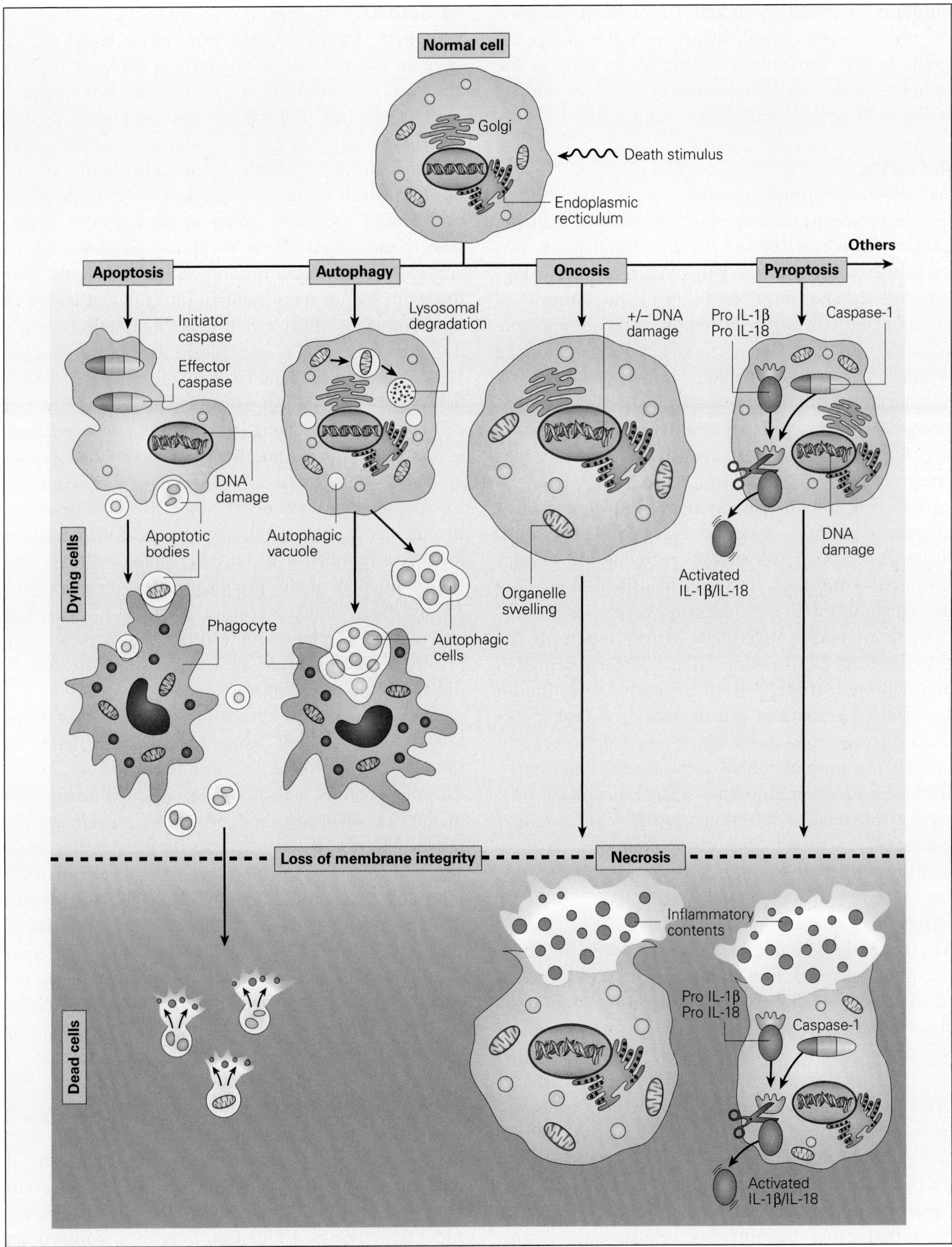

Figure 5-20. Schematic representation of the four pathways leading to cell death: apoptosis, autophagy, oncosis and pyroptosis, apoptosis, autophagy represent normal homeostatic mechanism of cell death without necrosis and inflammation in contrast to oncosis and pyroptosis which lead to cell death necrosis and inflammation (Adapted with permission from Fink SL, Cookson BT. Apoptosis, pyroptosis, and necrosis: mechanistic description of dead and dying eukaryotic cells. Infect Immun. 2005;73:1907-16.)

during ontogeny of the B and T systems in the bone marrow (*Chapter 6*) and thymus (*Chapter 7*), respectively, as well as the death-dealing system used by the immune system in the destruction of virally-infected (*Chapter 13*) or malignant cells (*Chapter 20*).

Autophagy

Autophagy, or autophagocytosis (from the Greek, to denote self-eating) is a second non-necrosis inducing pathway in which the cell literally degrades its own components through the lysosomal machinery (Figure 5-20). The most well-known mechanism of autophagy involves the formation of membrane-surrounded structures enclosing targeted regions of the cell called autophagic vacuoles, which separate their contents from the rest of the cytoplasm. The resultant vesicle then fuses with a lysosome and subsequently degrades its contents. Like apoptosis, autophagy represents a tightly-regulated process that plays a normal part in cell growth, development, and homeostasis, helping to maintain a balance between the synthesis, degradation, and subsequent recycling of cellular products. Autophagy has been identified as a route by which intracellular infectious agents or tumor-derived and self antigens are transferred from the cytoplasm to the lysosome where they are degraded and delivered to MHC-II molecules for presentation to CD4+ T cells. The precise role of autophagy in disease is not well known but it may help to prevent or halt the progression of some diseases associated with neurodegeneration and cancer, and play a protective role against infection caused by intracellular pathogens; however, in other situations, it may actually contribute to disease development.

Oncosis

The term oncosis is a type of cell death in which the cell undergoes swelling (from the Greek, *onkos*, which means swelling) as a counterpoint to apoptosis. Oncosis is defined as a prelethal pathway leading to cell death accompanied by cellular swelling, organelle swelling, blebbing, and increased membrane permeability (Figure 5-20). The process of oncosis ultimately leads to depletion of cellular energy stores and failure of the ionic pumps in the plasma membrane. Oncosis may result from toxic agents that interfere with ATP generation or processes that cause uncontrolled cellular energy consumption. It is now being recognized that the changes accompanying oncosis may result from active enzyme-catalyzed biochemical processes.

Pyroptosis

Pyroptosis (from the Greek *pyro*, which relates to fire or fever, and *ptosis*, a "falling off") is the most recently described mechanism of cell death associated with features of cell lysis and release of inflammatory cellular contents (Figure 5-20). It is a pathway morphologically and mechanistically distinct from other forms of cell death in which caspase 1 dependence is a defining feature. Unlike apoptosis, which involves caspase 3, caspase 6 and caspase 8, in pyroptosis caspase 1 is the enzyme that mediates this process of cell death. Furthermore, loss of mitochondrial integrity and release of cytochrome *c*, which can activate apoptotic caspases, do not occur during pyroptosis. Pyroptosis features rapid plasma-membrane rupture and release of proinflammatory intracellular contents. This is in marked contrast to the packaging of cellular contents and non-inflammatory phagocytic uptake of membrane-bound apoptotic bodies or autophagic vacuoles that characterize apoptosis and autophagy, respectively. As described in Chapter 3, the activation of the inflammasome involves a number of key caspase linked pathways and the production of the proinflammatory cytokines IL-1β and IL-18 undergo caspase 1-dependent activation and secretion during pyroptosis. Pyroptosis is not only involved in host protects against infection but can also induces pathological inflammation.

In summary, eukaryotic cells can initiate several distinct pathways of self-destruction, and the nature of the cell death process i.e., non-inflammatory in the case of apoptosis and autophagy or proinflammatory in the case of oncosis and pyroptosis provide specific instructions for tissue responses of neighboring cells, which in turn dictates important systemic physiological outcomes. Apoptosis and autophagy are the noninflammatory physiologic mechanisms of homeostasis employed by the immune system for cellular education and deletion of autoreactive unwanted cells during the developing immune system but also in destruction of infected or malignant cells in disease processes. Oncosis (a prelethal phase) and later pyroptosis (caspase 1-dependent cell death), are inherently inflammatory and are triggered by various pathological stimuli, such as stroke, heart attack, or cancer, and are crucial for controlling microbial infections. Pathogens have evolved mechanisms to inhibit the proinflammatory mechanisms, i.e., pyroptosis, enhancing their ability to persist and cause disease. Ultimately, there is a competition between host and pathogen to regulate anti-inflammatory and proinflammatory mechanisms and the outcome dictates life or death of the host.

Case Studies: Clinical Relevance

Let us now return to the case studies of gout, rheumatoid arthritis, and septic arthritis that we presented earlier and review some of the major points of the clinical presentation and how they relate to the immune system:

Case Study 1: Acute Gout

- Gout is an inflammatory response to monosodium urate crystals. Either overproduction or underexcretion will elevate the plasma levels of uric acid and may lead to formation of urate crystals. These crystals have a predilection for depositing within joints and periarticular structures such as tendons. (Figure 5-21).
- Acute attacks usually come about quickly in one or a few joints, and exhibit redness, warmth, and swelling, as well as severe pain and tenderness. Monosodium urate crystals trigger an inflammatory response by more than one mechanism. They can either activate the complement cascade, or form intracellular crystals that interact with inflammasomes (cytoplasmic molecular associations formed by innate receptors [NALP] and the enzyme caspase-1), which facilitates overproduction and secretion of IL-1 (*Chapter 3*), or they may directly stimulate synovial lining cells as well as other local cell populations to produce cytokines, chemokines, and arachidonic acid metabolites. Both mechanisms culminate in the activation of mast cells and endothelial cells followed by increased vascular permeability and leukocyte emigration. This process quickly produces a neutrophilic infiltrate. During an acute gout attack, when aspirated synovial fluid is examined by microscopy, neutrophils that are engulfing urate crystals can be observed.
- While the inflammatory response triggered by uric acid crystals may be severe, the course is usually short. Therefore, medical therapy of an acute attack is aimed at limiting the inflammatory response; rheumatologists usually employ NSAIDS, corticosteroids, or colchicine.
- Colchicine is a very old drug that binds to the microtubules of neutrophils and prevents their migration

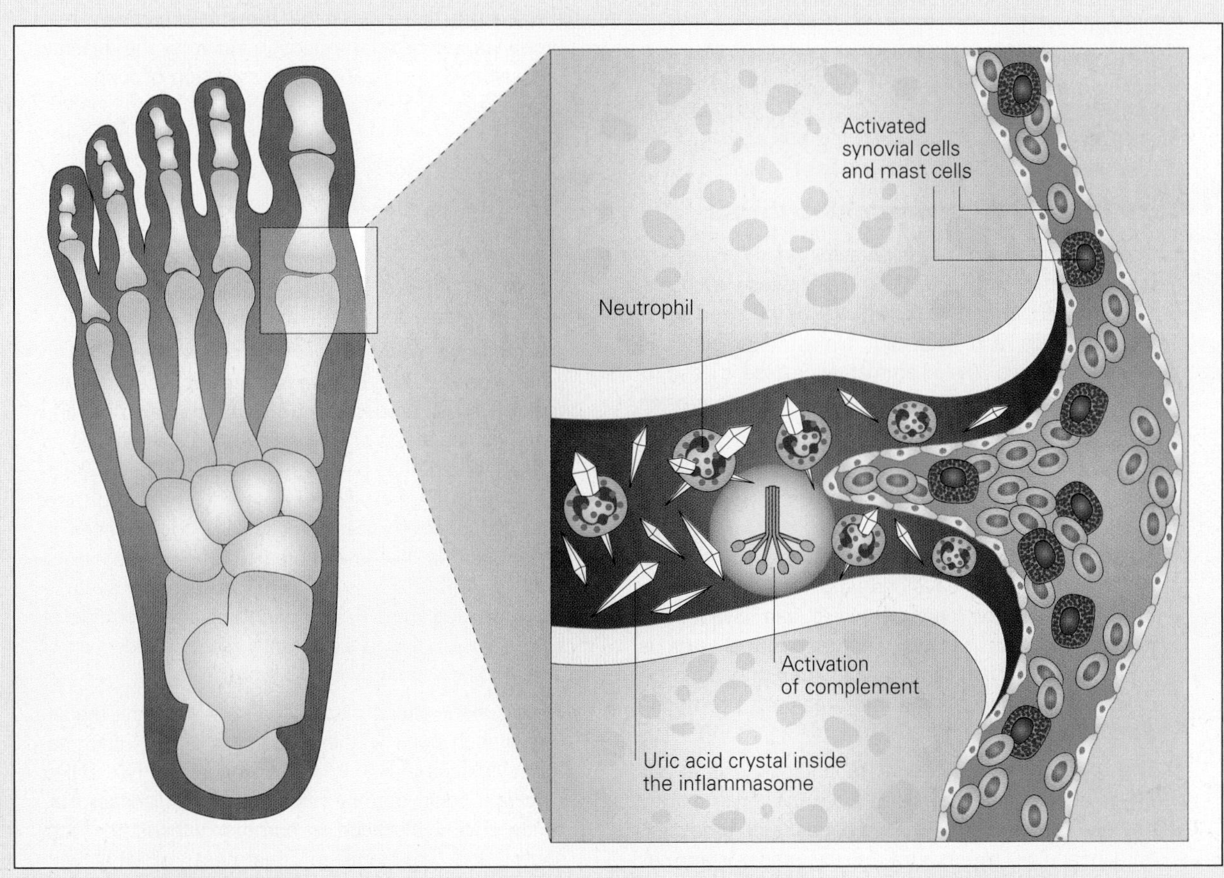

Case Studies: Clinical Relevance (continued)

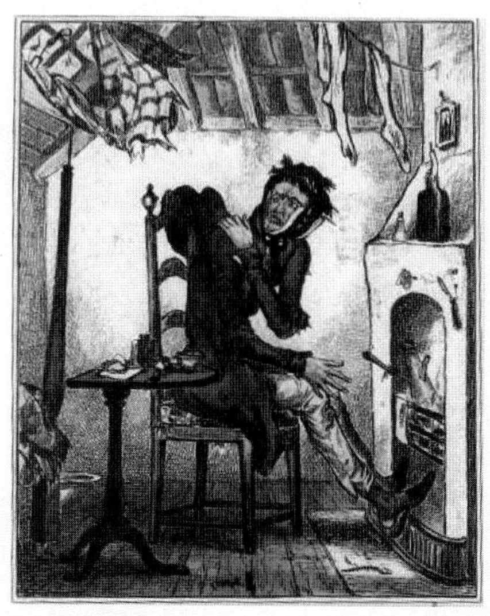

Figure 5-22. Caricature of a patient with "rheum-atick," "that mortal man should ever be obliged to exist under such panes." (Courtesy of the National Library of Medicine.)

into tissues, in part by interfering with the necessary cytoskeletal rearrangements that take place as the cell squeezes through the endothelium and crawls through surrounding tissue. Colchicine is used predominantly for the treatment of gout and pseudogout, but also has been used for other inflammatory conditions such as SLE pericarditis, amyloidosis, familial Mediterranean fever, and Behcet's disease.

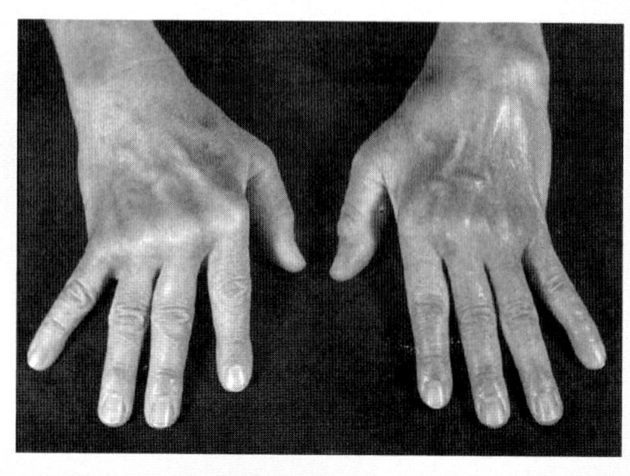

Figure 5-23. Photograph of the hands of a patient with moderately advanced rheumatoid arthritis. Note the deformities of the metacarpophalangeal joints, with atrophy of the hypothenar muscles and ulnar deviation. (Courtesy of F. Paul Alepa.)

- Gout can evolve into a more chronic form. Patients may develop numerous attacks timed closely together, prolonged attacks, the deposition of uric acid crystals in the kidneys, or the formation of large urate crystal deposits called tophi. In these circumstances, it may be necessary to treat with allopurinol, a drug that blocks the metabolic pathway that produces uric acid production, lowers the plasma uric acid level, and can cause resorption of tophi.

Case Study 2: Rheumatoid Arthritis

- Rheumatoid arthritis (RA) is an autoimmune disease of unknown etiology (Figure 5-22). The disease is characterized by a symmetric, polyarthritis of the small joints of the hands and feet, but almost any joint can become involved. The inflammatory process is destructive, and if the patient is not treated, leads to erosion and eventual deformity of the joints (Figure 5-23).
- Pathologically, the synovial tissue becomes hypertrophied, highly vascularized, and infiltrated with leukocytes (Figure 5-24). The synovial lining, comprised predominantly of proliferating fibroblasts and infiltrating macrophages, develops into an inflammatory mass, termed the pannus, which can invade and destroy adjacent tissues. The subsynovial area is comprised of infiltrating macrophages and dendritic cells and lymphocytes that are organized into aggregates in a subset of patients.
- The role of lymphocytes in RA pathogenesis is still under debate, but they likely drive the inflammatory process by activating macrophages and producing autoantibodies. Neutrophils are the predominant cell type in the synovial fluid, where they can incite damage to the superficial areas of articular cartilage.
- Of the various inflammatory cells in RA synovium, macrophages have been most clearly implicated in pathogenesis. This is because macrophages are the major synovial producers of TNF-α. The role of TNF-α in the pathogenesis of RA deserves special mention as TNF-α blockade has been a major advance in the treatment of RA (Figure 5-4). An excellent example of how scientific discovery can directly lead to advances in patient care is the development of TNF-α antagonists. Not only was TNF-α found to be produced by synoviocytes isolated from RA patients, but also blockade of TNF-α was shown to significantly reduce production of other pro-inflammatory cytokines (*Chapter 11*).
- These observations placed TNF-α at a critical regulatory branch point in the production of pro-inflammatory cytokines in RA. In animal models of RA, TNF-α blockade could dramatically ameliorate disease. Currently, TNF-α blockade is commonly used for both acute and maintenance treatment of RA with

Case Studies: Clinical Relevance (continued)

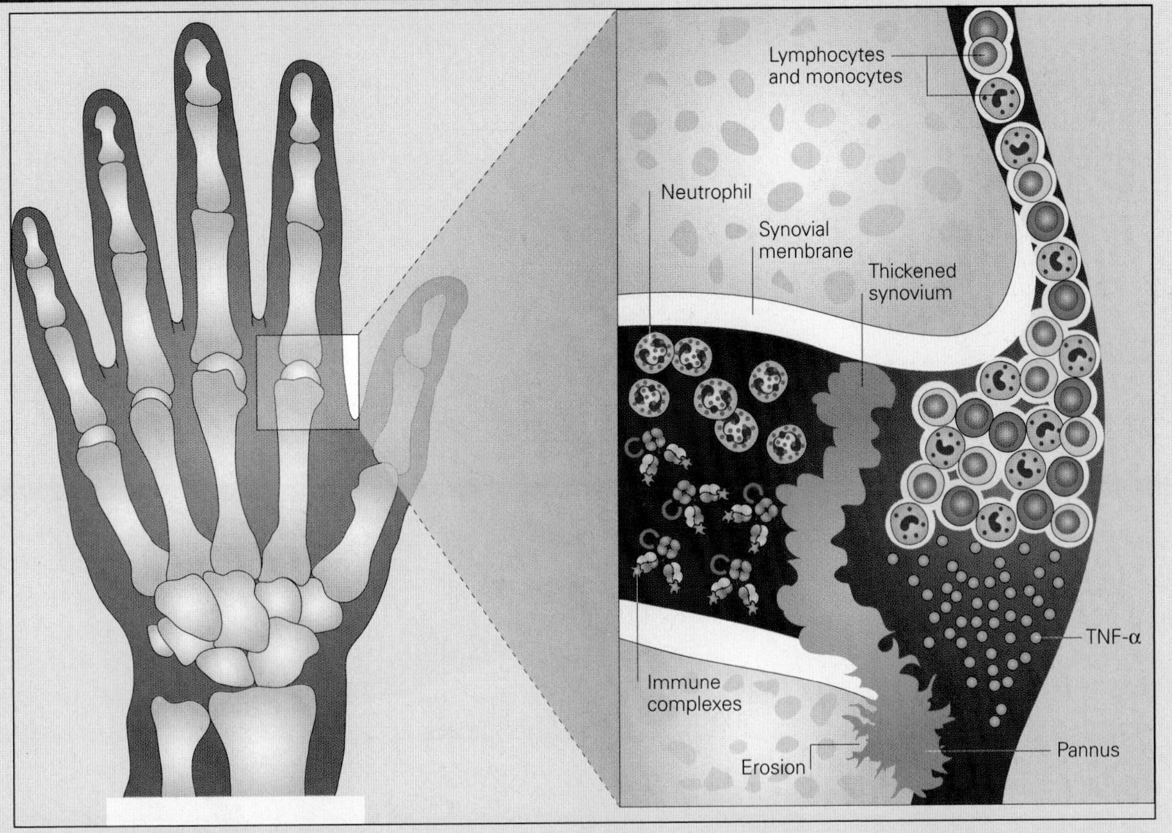

Figure 5-24. Schematic representation of the role of inflammation in the pathogenesis of rheumatoid arthritis seen in the metacarpophalangeal (MCP) joint of the hand of the patient in Case 2. Shown in the inset, the synovium consists of a synovial membrane and underlying loose connective tissue. In early rheumatoid arthritis, the synovial membrane becomes thickened because of hyperplasia and hypertrophy of the synovial lining cells and begins to invade the cartilage. An extensive network of new blood vessels is formed in the synovium bringing in monocytes and lymphocytes comprised predominantly of Cd4+ T cells and B cells (plasma cells) which infiltrate the synovial membrane and synovial fluid. The production of antibody by plasma cells and subsequent formation of antigen-antibody-complement, i.e., immune complexes leads to the chemotactic influx of neutrophils. In established rheumatoid arthritis, the synovial membrane becomes transformed into inflammatory tissue, the pannus, and the production of TNF-α by macrophages and lymphocytes by this invading tissue destroys adjacent cartilage and bone.

excellent clinical efficacy. It has also shown benefit for the treatment of seronegative spondyloarthropaties as well as Crohn's disease.

- In addition, autoantibodies, which include rheumatoid factor and anti-cyclic citrullinated protein, can be found in the blood of most patients. Although the reason for formation of autoantibodies is unknown, it is thought that they may form immune complexes within joints or within other tissues (RA is a systemic disease, not only affecting joints). These complexes may activate of the complement system or inflammatory cells directly, causing a burst of cytokine production. Indeed, both complement split products and many pro-inflammatory cytokines have been found in either the blood or synovial fluid of active RA patients.

Case Study 3: Septic Arthritis

- Risk factors for developing a bacterial infection within a joint include advanced age, multiple comorbidities, rheumatoid arthritis, the presence of a prosthetic joint, and immunosuppression. The source of the infection is usually seeding from the blood in a previously damaged joint, but infections may also follow puncture wounds or surgical procedures. Staphylococcus aureus is the most common nongonococcal organism found in septic joints. However, Gram-negative organisms, anaerobes, and fungi

Case Studies: Clinical Relevance (continued)

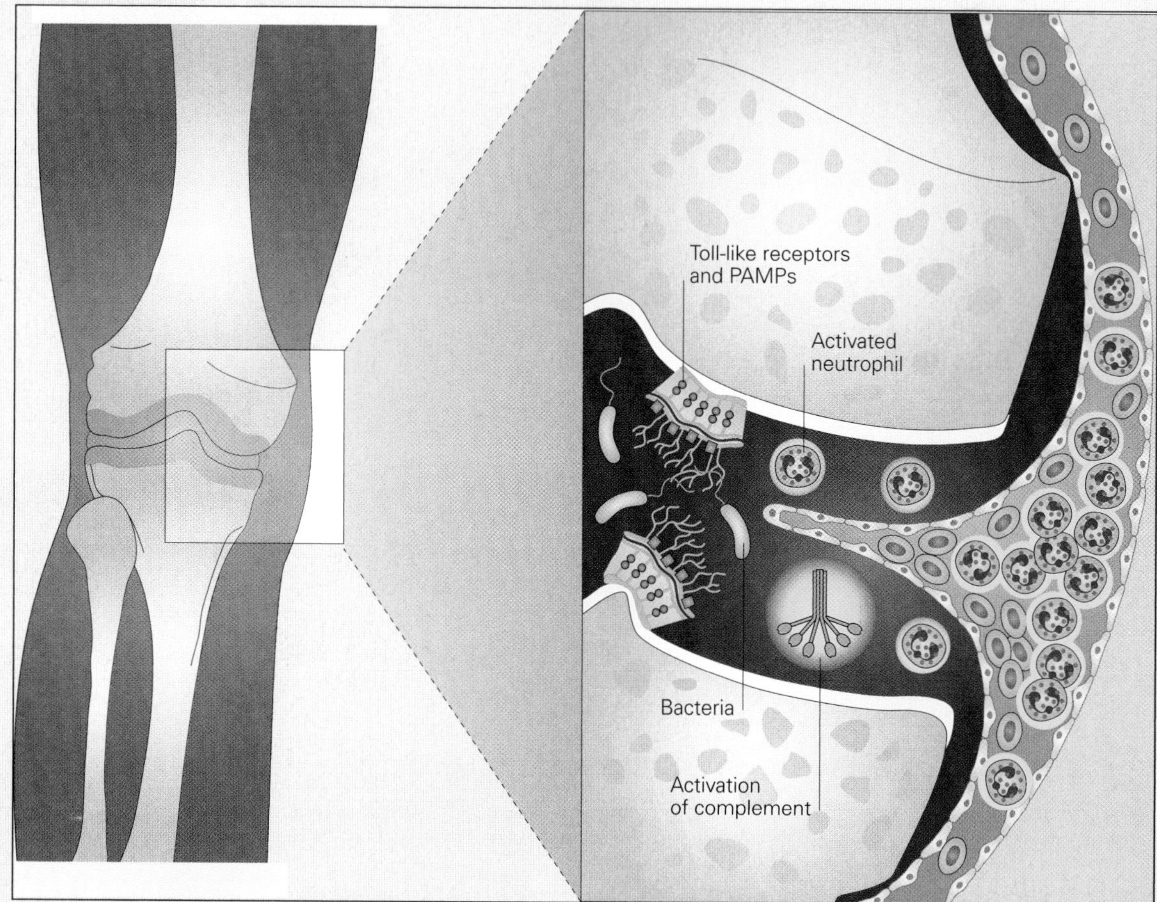

Figure 5-25. Schematic representation of the inflammatory responses in the joint of a patient with septic arthritis (Case 3).

may also cause infection, especially in immunocompromised patients. Clinical presentation is usually that of a monoarticular joint swelling associated with warmth, redness, tenderness, and pain with even minimal movement of the joint through its normal arc of motion. Fever and malaise are often present, and arthrocentesis usually yields a high white blood cell count (> 100,000 cells/microliter).

- Microorganisms can activate the inflammatory response through any of the following mechanisms: previously formed antibodies may cause immune complex formation; the complement cascade may be directly activated by a bacterial or fungal surface; bacterial products called formylated peptides are potent chemoattractants and may cause leukocyte accumulation; and finally, many cells of the immune system possess an array of evolutionarily determined cell surface receptors called TLRs that recognize highly conserved components of microbial origin (Figure 5-25).
- At least ten TLRs have been identified in mammals and each recognizes a unique set of ligands (*Chapters 3* and *12*). For example, TLR4 is activated by LPS from Gram-negative organisms, while TLR2 recognizes cell wall components from Gram-positive organisms. Once ligated, TLRs cause cellular activation, upregulation of adhesion molecules, and robust production of cytokines.
- Treatment of septic arthritis is aimed at identification and elimination of the organism. Rapid therapy is necessary as the arthritis is quite destructive. In addition to proper antibiotic coverage, the joint space must be drained. This can be accomplished by either repeated needle aspirations or surgical debridement.

Key Points

- The key signs of inflammation are swelling, redness, heat, pain, and loss of function.
- Inflammation can be triggered by infection, immune complexes, cytokines, trauma, loss of oxygen, and toxins.
- Vascular changes at the infection or trauma site result in fluid and cells leaving the circulation and entering the tissues.
- Adhesion molecule expression and chemokine secretion in response to inflammatory mediators signal leukocytes where to leave the circulation.
- Pathogen binding to phagocytes signals the phagocytes to engulf and kill the pathogens.
- Fever, increased leukocyte counts, and acute phase protein synthesis also occur in response to inflammatory mediators.
- Inflammation damages host tissues.

Study Questions/Critical Thinking

1. Explain the causes of each of the five key signs of inflammation.
2. Macrophages and neutrophils are both phagocytic cells. Compare and contrast their roles in inflammation.
3. How is inflammation normally confined to the infection site?
4. Inflammation is a potentially very damaging process; how is it controlled?

Suggested Reading

Abram CL, Lowell CA. The ins and outs of leukocyte integrin signaling. Annu Rev Immunol. 2009; 27: 339–362.

Bergman IM. Toll-like receptors (TLR) and mannan-binding lectin (MBL): on constant alert in a hostile environment. Ups J Med Sci. 2011; 116: 90–9.

Bieber JD, Terkeltaub RA. Gout: on the brink of novel therapeutic options for an ancient disease. Arthritis Rheum. 2004: 50: 2400–14.

Borregaard N, et al. Human neutrophil granules and secretory vesicles. Eur J Haematol. 1993; 51: 187–98.

Choy EH, Panayi GS. Cytokine pathways and joint inflammation in rheumatoid arthritis. New Engl J Med. 2001; 344: 907–16.

Cotran RS, Kumar V, Robbins SL. In FJ Schoen, Cellular Injury and Cellular Death 5th ed. Philadelphia: W.B. Saunders.

Cotran RS, Kumar V, Robbins SL. In FJ Schoen, Inflammation and repair, in pathologic basis of disease. Philadelphia: W.B. Saunders, 1994.

Kuby, J. Cytokines. In J Kuby, Immunology (pp. 297-322). New York: W.H. Freeman and Company; 1996.

Liu L, Kubes P. Molecular mechanisms of leukocyte recruitment: organ-specific mechanisms of action. Thromb Haemostasis. 2003; 89: 213–220.

Luster AD. Chemokines—chemotactic cytokines that mediate inflammation. New Eng J Med. 1998; 338: 436–45.

McIntyre TM, et al. Cell-cell interactions: leukocyte-endothelial interactions. Curr Opin Hematol. 2003; 10: 150–8.

Medzhitov R, Janeway C , Jr. Innate immunity. New Engl J Med. 2000; 343: 338–44.

Muller WA. Leukocyte-endothelial cell interactions in the inflammatory response. Lab Invest. 2002; 82: 521–33.

Nathan C. Points of control in inflammation. Nature. 2002; 420: 846–52.

Puxeddu I, et al. Mast cells in allergy and beyond. Int J Biochem Cell B. 2003; 35: 1601–7.

Segal AW. How superoxide production by neutrophil leukocytes kills microbes. Novart Fdn Sym. 2006; 279: 92–8.

Takeda K, Kaisho T, Akira S. Toll-like receptors. Ann Rev Immunol. 2003; 21: 335–76.

Tracey KJ. The inflammatory reflex. Nature. 2002; 420: 853–9.

Chapter 6

B Lymphocytes and Immunoglobulins

Rita Carsetti, PhD
Alessandro Plebani, MD
Alberto G. Ugazio, MD
Joseph A. Bellanti, MD

Case Study

A twenty-three-year-old white male presented with symptoms of a sore throat, high fever, and fatigue, which began three weeks previously and has become progressively more severe. Physical examination revealed enlarged, inflamed tonsils with exudates (Figure 6-1) and large anterior cervical lymph nodes. Penicillin was administered with little clinical improvement, and the patient was seen again a few days later because of the persistence of fever and continuing fatigue.

A mono spot test was positive (Box 6-1), the hemoglobin was 15 g/dl, and the leukocyte count was 23,000/mm^3 (normal = 4,500 – 11,000/mm^3) with 23 percent neutrophils (normal 45 – 75 percent), 57 percent lymphocytes (normal 16 – 46 percent), and > 20 percent atypical lymphocytes (Figure 6-2).

The patient was treated conservatively with bed rest and supportive therapy and gradually recovered over a six-week period.

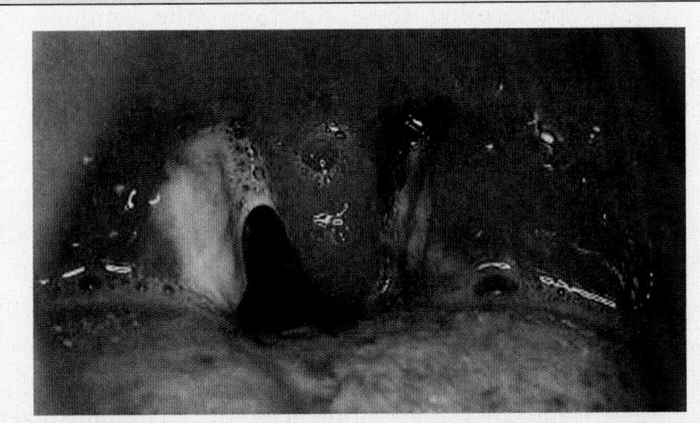

Figure 6-1. Pharyngotonsillitis and enlarged inflamed tonsils with exudates on right tonsil. (As seen on Wikipedia.)

LEARNING OBJECTIVES

When you have completed this chapter, you should be able to:

- Describe the basic structure of the immunoglobulin molecule
- Explain the functions of antibodies and the role of humoral immunity in preventing and eliminating infectious disease
- List the immunoglobulin isotypes and describe the relationship between their structure, body locations, and functions
- Discuss how somatic recombination of immunoglobulin genes results in the generation of diversity in antigen recognition
- Describe antigen-independent development of B cells and explain the steps that result in allotype restriction, expression of IgM and IgD membrane receptors with identical antigen-combining regions, and removal of self-specific B cells
- Describe antigen-dependent development of B cells and explain the steps that result in selection and proliferation of antigen-specific B cells, isotype switching, affinity maturation, and B cell memory
- Utilize this information to recognize the importance of the role of immunoglobulins in health and disease

Box 6-1

A mono spot test, also known as the mononucleosis spot test, mononuclear heterophile test, heterophile antibody test, is a laboratory assay which measures a heterophile antibody (i.e., a human antibody that reacts with proteins from another species) performed in patients with symptoms such as exudative pharyngotonsillitis, fever, headache, enlarged lymph nodes, and fatigue that are suspected to be due to infectious mononucleosis. The test is nonspecific and may also be positive in patients with other infections; false-negative results may be observed in 10 percent to 15 percent of patients, primarily in children younger than ten years of age.

Introduction

As described in Chapter 1, B lymphocytes, together with T lymphocytes, comprise the two arms of the adaptive immune system involved in the specific recognition of antigen. The B lymphocytes perform this function by producing a wide array of protein molecules referred to as immunoglobulins that function as antigen recognition units called antibodies, which are found both as membrane-bound molecules on the surface of the B cell referred to as the B cell receptor (**BCR**) or as secreted extracellular antigen-binding products in the serum and body fluids. The recognition of antigen by T cells is also carried out in a highly specific manner by an antigen-recognition molecule on the T cell surface structurally similar to immunoglobulin referred to as the T cell receptor (**TCR**) (*Chapter 7*). Prior to their identification as immunoglobulins, these products were referred to as "humors," a term derived from the humoral medicine of the ancient Greeks, which stated that a mixture of fluids known as humors (Greek: *chymos*, i.e., juice or sap) controlled human health and emotion. For this reason, the B cell system and its secreted products are sometimes referred to as the humoral immune limb of the adaptive immune system, in contrast to the T cell system and its products, which carry out a cell-mediated immunity (**CMI**) function (*Chapter 7*). The B designation term derives from the origin of these cells in the bone marrow of higher vertebrates and in the bursa of Fabricius in birds (*Chapter 2*). Shown in Figure 6-3 is a separation of the serum proteins by electrophoresis, illustrating the location of the slowest migrating serum proteins, the gamma globulins, that contain most of the immunoglobulins.

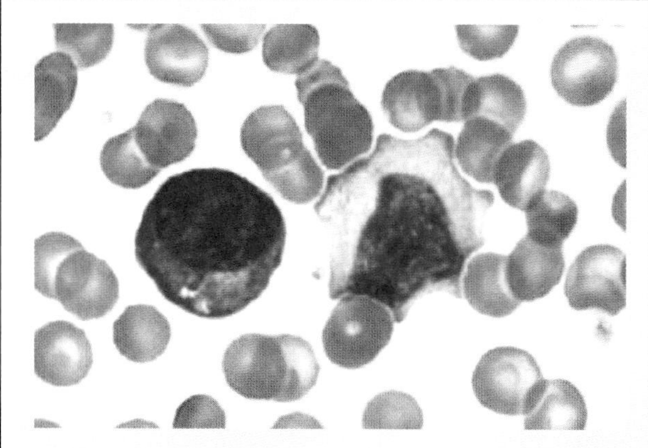

Figure 6-2. Peripheral blood smear of a patient with infectious mononucleosis showing atypical lymphocytes characterized by cytoplasmic vacuoles and cell membrane indentations. (Reproduced with permission by the Clinical Chemistry and Hematology Laboratory, Wadsworth Center, New York State Department of Health, http://www.wadsworth.org.)

Immunoglobulins evolved for the purpose of specific recognition and neutralization of pathogens, resulting in the limitation, clearance, and prevention of infection as well as the elimination of other potentially noxious material. In addition to this direct function of immunoglobulin binding to extracellular antigens, the molecule is also involved in several indirect interactions with other cells of the immune system through binding with receptors on phagocytes, mediator cells, natural killer (**NK**) cells, and the complement system (*Chapter 1*). In performing these functions, the immunoglobulins are found in blood and interstitial tissues as part of the **internal immune system** as well as in external secretions of the respiratory, gastrointestinal, genitourinary systems, and breast milk as part of the **external immune system**, i.e., the mucosa-associated lymphoid tissues (**MALT**) (*Chapter 1* and *Chapter 8*). As described in Chapter 2, the development of the immune system in the species (i.e., **phylogeny**), the individual (i.e., **ontogeny**), or the cell (i.e., **cellular expression of the immune response**) occurs under the inductive influences of changing macro- or microenvironments and results in the selection of the best adapted form which could survive in these new

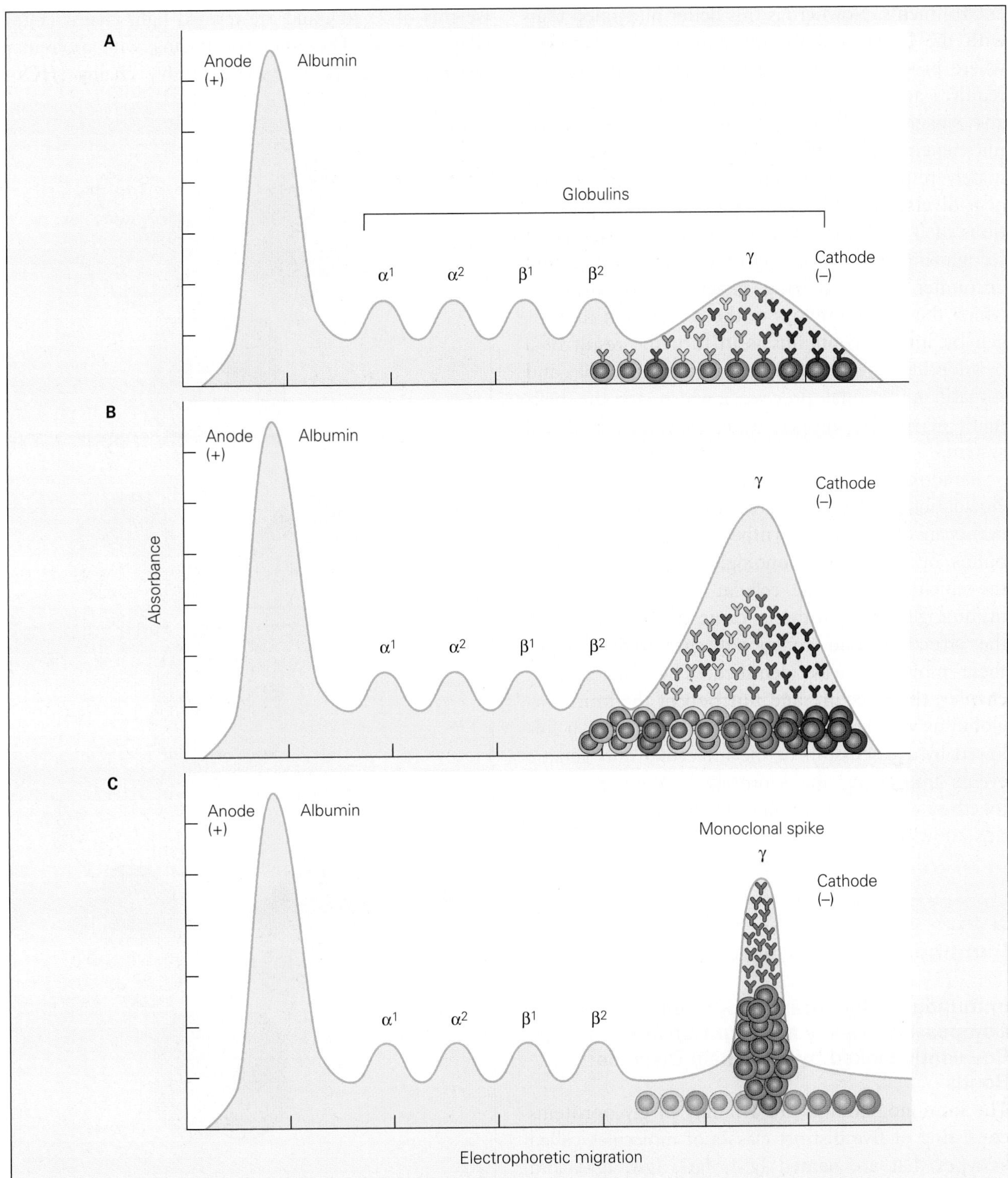

Figure 6-3. Various patterns of distribution of serum proteins as determined by protein electrophoresis. Albumin, the largest peak, lies closest to the positive electrode (anode). The next components (globulins) are labeled alpha-1 (α1), alpha-2 (α2), beta-1 (β1), beta-2 (β2), and gamma (γ) and lie toward the negative electrode (cathode), with the gamma peak being the slowest migrating globulin closest to the cathode. Panel A: The gamma globulin content of serum from a healthy adult showing a normal symmetrical polyclonal distribution resulting from production of gamma globulin by various clones of unstimulated B cells. Panel B: A polyclonal increase in gamma globulin from a patient undergoing infection showing the stimulation of a wide variety of B cells producing several families of gamma globulin resulting in a broad gamma peak. Panel C: A monoclonal M spike of gamma globulins from a patient with multiple myeloma showing a highly limited increase in gamma globulin from a single clone of B cells resulting in a highly restricted monoclonal peak.

environments. Nowhere is this better illustrated than with the B cell and its immunoglobulin products, where progression along its differentiation pathway requires adaptation of the B cell lineage to factors and signals of increasing complexity found in the microenvironment of the cell. These processes ultimately result in and assure the remarkable survival of a diverse repertoire of antigen-detecting populations of B cells, each with a unique BCR capable of recognizing and responding to any antigen it should encounter. This amazing generation of diversity which the B cell employs in the recognition of antigen by immunoglobulins is in turn the result of a bewildering array of gene recombinatorial and somatic mutational processes, which are the hallmark of specific antigen recognition by the B cell system.

Paradoxically, the discovery of the B cell and the elucidation of the intricate intracellular molecular events involved in the synthesis of its immunoglobulins occurred in chronologic reverse order, and the elucidation of the cellular events involved in immunoglobulin synthesis came about only after the structural and functional characterization of these molecules was identified. Therefore in this chapter, the structure and function of the immunoglobulins will be described first and will be then followed by a discussion of the molecular and genetic events underlying the synthesis of these proteins, together with some of the clinical applications of this knowledge.

Immunoglobulin Structure

Immunoglobulins Are Glycoproteins Composed of Heavy and Light Chains Covalently Linked by Interchain Disulfide Bonds

The immunoglobulins are a family of glycoproteins consisting of five distinct classes of molecules called isotypes that are named IgM, IgG, IgA, IgD, and IgE. The classification of immunoglobulins into these various groups is based on chemical and structural differences among the various isotypes. The IgG molecule, for example, is made up of four polypeptide chains held together by disulfide bonds (Figure 6-4).

Two of the chains in each of the five immunoglobulin isotypes are relatively small, with molecular weights of 22 kD, and are termed light chains (**LCs**) (Figure 6-4A). The other two chains, with molecular weights of 55 kD, are called heavy chains (**HCs**).

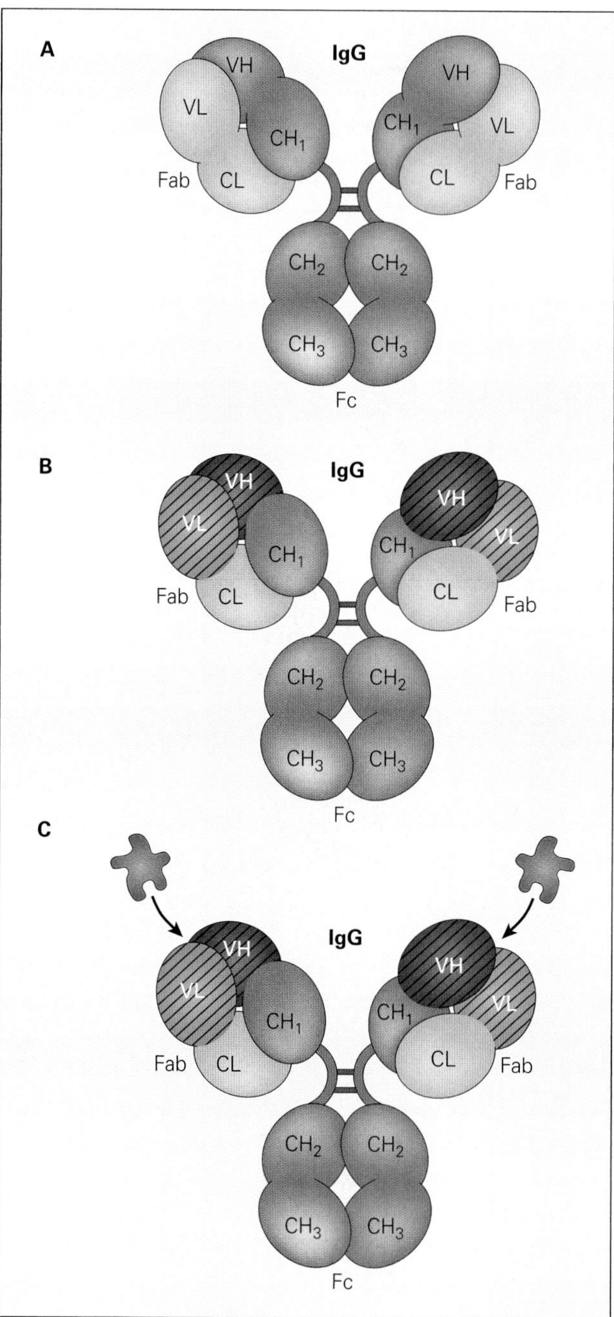

Figure 6-4. Panel A: A schematic representation of the IgG molecule showing the two light chains and the two heavy chains and the location of interchain disulfide bonds in the hinge region. The amino terminal end is at the top and the carboxyl terminal end is on the bottom. Panel B: The variable regions of the light and heavy chains (i.e., VL and VH, respectively, crosshatched) that, together with the constant regions of the light (CL) and the heavy (CH_1), make up the antigen-binding region (Fab) of the molecule. Panel C: The binding of antigen with the antigen-binding region (Fab).

Each immunoglobulin G molecule is composed of two identical light chains and two identical heavy chains which form a Y-shaped structure, with two of the upper arms each made up of light and heavy chains containing the amino terminal end and the lower stem composed only of the heavy chains containing the carboxyl end of the molecule (Figure 6-4). As will be described in greater detail, there are two major functions that an antibody molecule performs, each of which is related to this immunoglobulin structure; the upper two arms perform an **antigen-recognition function**, which endows the molecule with the capacity to bind uniquely with an individual antigen through this end of the molecule, which is referred to as the antigen-binding fragment (**Fab**), while the lower stem of the molecule displays an **effector function** that relates to how this region of the molecule interacts with other components of the immune system such as complement (*Chapter 4*) and cell receptors specific for this part of the molecule, which is referred to as the crystallizable fragment (**Fc**) (Figure 6-4).

Variable and Constant Regions

Both light and heavy chains of the immunoglobulin molecule are further divided into regions referred to as variable (**V**) and constant (**C**) regions (Figure 6-4B). The variable region (shown crosshatched) consists of the first 110 amino acids of the light and heavy chains at the amino terminal end of the immunoglobulin molecule, which vary extensively in amino acid composition (Figure 6-4B). This variation is responsible for the highly specific antigen-recognition function of an individual antibody molecule for its antigen (Figure 6-4C). Within the variable regions of both light and heavy chains, some polypeptide segments show exceptional variability in their amino acid composition and are called hypervariable regions (**HVR**) or complementarity determining regions (**CDRs**). The amino acid sequence of the remaining portions of the LC and HC do not differ within a given isotype class and are therefore called the constant heavy (**CH**) or **Fc regions** of the molecule (Figure 6-4).

Both light and heavy chains are further divided into segments of approximately 110 amino acids called **domains**. The light chains contain two domains, i.e., the variable light (**VL**) and the constant light (**CL**); the heavy chains contain one variable heavy (**VH**) domain and either three or four constant CH domains depending on the immunoglobulin isotype (Figure 6-4). The constant region of the IgG, IgA, and IgD HCs contain three domains called CH1, CH2, and CH3; the constant regions of IgM and IgE have an extra domain resulting in four domains named CH1, CH2, CH3, and CH4. Figure 6-5 shows the light and heavy chain composition of each of the five immunoglobulin isotypes showing the differences in the number of domains in each of the molecules. The IgM exists in both a monomeric form found on the surface of B cells and a pentameric form found in serum made up of five of the individual monomers. Similarly, IgA exists as a monomeric form in serum and as a dimeric form in external secretions made up of two of the monomers.

The Hinge Region Gives Flexibility to the Immunoglobulin Molecule

Another important structural feature of the Y-shaped immunoglobulin molecule is a proline-rich region between the CH1 and CH2 domains of the heavy chain called the **hinge region**. This region contains cysteine residues that allow linkage of the HC polypeptides to each other by S-S bonds. As its name implies, this region of the immunoglobulin confers flexibility to the molecule by providing mobility of the two upper arms of the molecule, thus enhancing their antigen-binding potential. As will be described in greater detail, the disulfide bonds that characterize this region allow interchain linkages of the HCs with one another and differ in number among the various immunoglobulin isotypes, resulting in hinge regions of varying lengths. Two immunoglobulin isotypes, IgM and IgE, do not have hinge regions and lack interchain disulfide bonds in this region; however, their CH2 regions perform a hinge-like function (Figure 6-5).

Immunoglobulin Isotypes Are Named by Their Heavy Chains and Contain Two Types of Light Chains

The various light and heavy chains of the five isotypes which comprise their immunoglobulin structure are different from one another. A chemically different kind of heavy chain exists for each of the five classes of immunoglobulins and is responsible for the antigenic differences that have been observed among classes. More importantly, it is the heavy chain that is responsible for the observed biologic differences, i.e., the **effector function**, among the

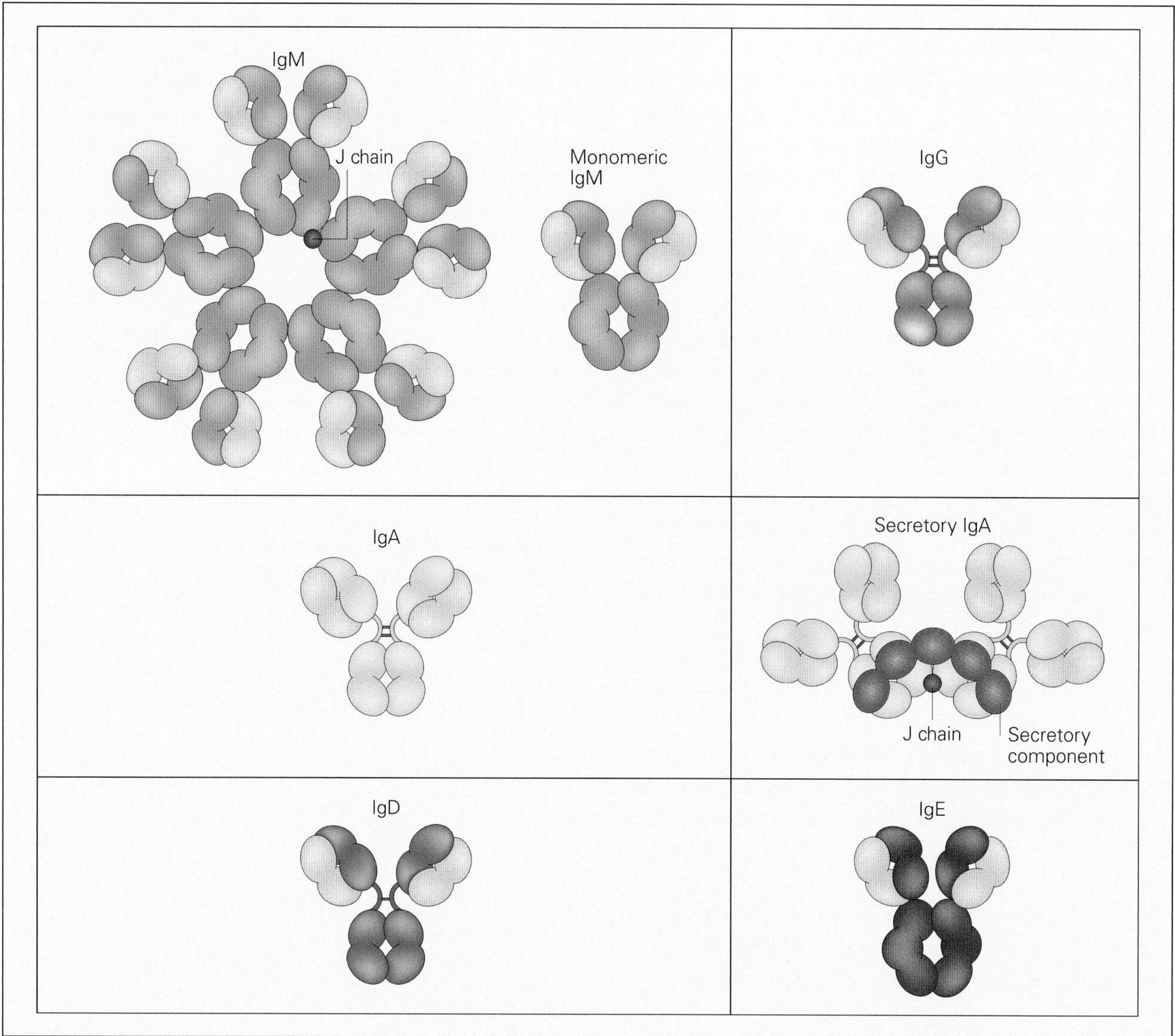

Figure 6-5. Schematic representation of the chain structure of each of the five immunoglobulin isotypes arranged into domains. The IgM and IgA exist in a monomeric form and a pentameric and dimeric form, respectively. Each immunoglobulin light chain contains two domains; in each heavy chain of IgG, IgA, and IgD, there are four domains, and in IgM and IgE there are five domains.

various classes or isotypes of immunoglobulin. As shown in Table 6-1, there are five kinds of heavy chains identified by the Greek equivalent of their class name—**γ**, **α**, **μ**, **δ**, and **ε**, each specific for IgG, IgA, IgM, IgD, and IgE, respectively.

Just as there are five heavy chains that are each specific for a specific isotype, there are also two different types of light chains in each of the isotypes, kappa (κ) and lambda (λ) (named for the pair of investigators who first identified the two types—Korngold and Lipari) (Figure 6-6). Each immunoglobulin has either two identical κ or two identical λ light chains; no immunoglobulin consists of a mixed molecule containing both chains. In humans, approximately 60 percent of the serum immunoglobulins are of the kappa variety and 40 percent of the lambda isotype. The identity of the light chain as either kappa or lambda is determined by the amino acid sequence of the constant region. In contrast to the kappa isotype, which is of only one type, there are four slightly different constant region sequences of the lambda LC, forming four subclasses (subtypes). Each type of light chain can be found in association with each kind of heavy chain, i.e., in each of the five classes of immunoglobulin, but a given immunoglobulin will be exclusively of the κ or λ type; there are no mixed molecules. There are ten possible combinations of heavy and light chains, and all ten are normally found

Table 6-1. Some physical and biologic properties of human immunoglobulin classes and subclasses

Class	Mean serum concentration (mg/dL)	Molecular weight (kDa)	Mean survival $t^{1/2}$ (days)	Biologic function	Fc receptors found on	No. of subclasses/ designation	Molecular designation
IgG	1,240	150,000	23	Major component of the secondary immune response; complement activation (classical pathway); function in neutralization and opsonization; placental transfer	PMNs lymphocytes macrophages, monocytes, dendritic cells, NK cells, mast cells, and trophoblast	(4) IgG1 IgG2 IgG3 IgG4	$\gamma2\kappa2$, $\gamma2\lambda2$
IgA	280	170,000	6	Present in serum and external secretions as secretory IgA, function in neutralization	PMNs, monocytes	(2) IgA1 IgA2	$\alpha2\kappa2$, $\alpha2\lambda2$
IgM	120	890,000	5	Principal molecule in primary immune response; lymphocyte surface receptor; complement fixation (classical pathway)	Not described	(1) IgM	$\mu2\kappa2$, $\mu2\lambda2$
IgD	3	150,000	2.8	Lymphocyte surface receptor	Not described	(1) IgD	$\delta2\kappa2$, $\delta2\lambda2$
IgE	0.03	196,000	1.5	Reaginic[a] (allergic) antibody	Mast cells, basophils, B cells, platelets, DCs, and eosinophils	(1) IgE	$\varepsilon2\kappa2$, $\varepsilon2\lambda2$

a. Reagin was the earlier descriptive term used for the skin-sensitizing antibody found in allergic (atopic) patients prior to its identification with IgE antibody (*Chapter 18*).

in any individual (Table 6-1). Any immunoglobulin may therefore be designated by its heavy- and light-chain composition, in a manner analogous to the hemoglobin nomenclature. An IgG molecule, for example, would have a formula of $\gamma_2\kappa_2$ or $\gamma_2\lambda_2$.

This information is clinically relevant for the diagnosis of one of the lymphoproliferative diseases in the human, multiple myeloma (*Chapter 21*). This disorder is characterized by a malignant proliferation of a single clone of B cells (i.e., a monoclonal proliferation), which in turn produces a single clone of immunoglobulin molecule (i.e., a monoclonal gammopathy of either a kappa or lambda light-chain type). The identification of an exclusive kappa or lambda light chain either on the intact immunoglobulin or as isolated polypeptide chains in the urine (i.e., Bence Jones protein) provides the basis for diagnostic confirmation of the disease.

Some Immunoglobulins Are Polymerized into Larger Molecules by the J Chain

Serum IgG, IgA, IgD, and IgE exist in this basic four-chain structural unit as monomers, and the same unit is repeated in the higher molecular weight immunoglobulins in two of the isotypes, i.e., IgM and IgA. In the case of IgM, the basic unit structure of the molecule is a monomeric subunit made up two heavy chains and two light chains and is the form of the molecule found on the surface of the B cell as the BCR (Figure 6-5). In the serum, however, IgM generally exists as a pentamer of five of these basic four-chain monomeric subunits, each held together by disulfide bonds (Figure 6-5). A relatively small molecule with high sulfydryl content, the joining (J) **chain**, participates in the polymerization of IgM into its pentameric form.

Similar to IgM, IgA also exists in a monomeric form in serum and a polymeric form in external

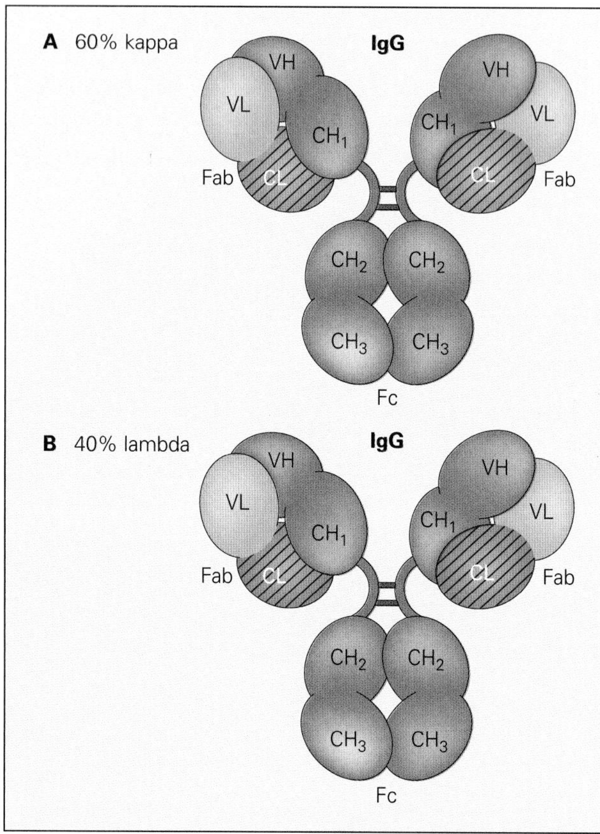

Figure 6-6. Schematic representation of the two light-chain isotypes kappa (κ) and lambda (λ) based on different light-chain constant region (CL) sequences (crosshatched). In humans, approximately 60 percent of the serum immunoglobulins are of the kappa and 40 percent of the lambda isotype.

secretions. IgA, like IgM, can be polymerized through a sulfhydryl residue near the carboxyl terminus of the molecule, with the participation of the J chain. As will be described in greater detail, in secretions, two IgA monomers are linked by the J chain and the secretory component (**SC**), another nonimmunoglobulin protein, to produce a bimolecular complex of high molecular weight found in external secretions called secretory IgA (sIgA) (Figure 6-5). At these sites, the IgA is synthesized as a dimer together with a J chain within B lymphocytes (i.e., plasma cells) contiguous with epithelial cells, and after transepithelial passage, the secretory component is added to form the complete secretory IgA molecule.

Immunoglobulin G and Immunoglobulin A Have Subclasses

There are four subclasses of IgG called IgG1, IgG2, IgG3, and IgG4, and two subclasses of IgA named IgA1 and IgA2 (Table 6-1). As will be described in greater detail, the relative concentrations of these immunoglobulin and subclasses found in serum and external secretions vary. For example, the serum concentrations of individual IgG subclasses are mercifully directly proportional to their numerical nomenclature, i.e., IgG1 > IgG2 > IgG3 > IgG4. Additionally, differences exist between the ratio of the two IgA subclass concentrations in serum and in external secretions. Approximately 95% of the IgA found in serum is of the IgA1 subclass variety and 5 percent of the IgA2; in contrast, there is a relative enrichment of the IgA2 subclass in external secretions, where almost equal proportions of IgA1 and IgA2 are found (*Chapter 8*).

In addition to differences in their heavy chains, the other major distinguishing features among the various classes and subclasses of the immunoglobulins are found in the hinge regions, where differences in the number and arrangement of interchain disulfide bonds exist (Figure 6-7). As previously noted, there are no hinge regions in the IgM and IgE and the number of interheavy chain disulfide bonds is different in the other immunoglobulin isotypes and subclasses. For example, the largest number of disulfide bonds in the various IgG subclasses is found in IgG3, and the IgA2 subclass in external secretions has a shorter hinge region than the IgA1, and it has fewer disulfide bonds between the H and L chains than in the IgA1 (Figure 6-7). The biologic significance of these differences is not readily apparent, but may account for known differences in diverse biologic functions of these molecules, such as life span or susceptibility to proteolytic degradation. For example, the IgG2 subclass has four heavy-heavy interchain bonds and is quite resistant to papain hydrolysis, as will be described later; the unusually long hinge region of the IgG3 molecule is responsible for the relatively shorter half-life of this IgG subclass compared to the other three (Table 6-5). The properties of abnormal IgG subclasses seen in pathologic conditions may also have clinical relevance. Myeloma globulins of the IgG3 subclass, for example, have an asymmetric structure because of the unusually long hinge region that contributes to the abnormal viscosity in the blood of individuals with myeloma involving this immunoglobulin subclass, which may create serious vaso-occlusive problems (Figure 6-7) (*Chapter 21*).

Antigen-Binding Specificity Resides in the Amino Terminal Variable Region of the Immunoglobulin

An antibody produced in response to one antigen obviously must have structural features that are different from an antibody produced in response to any

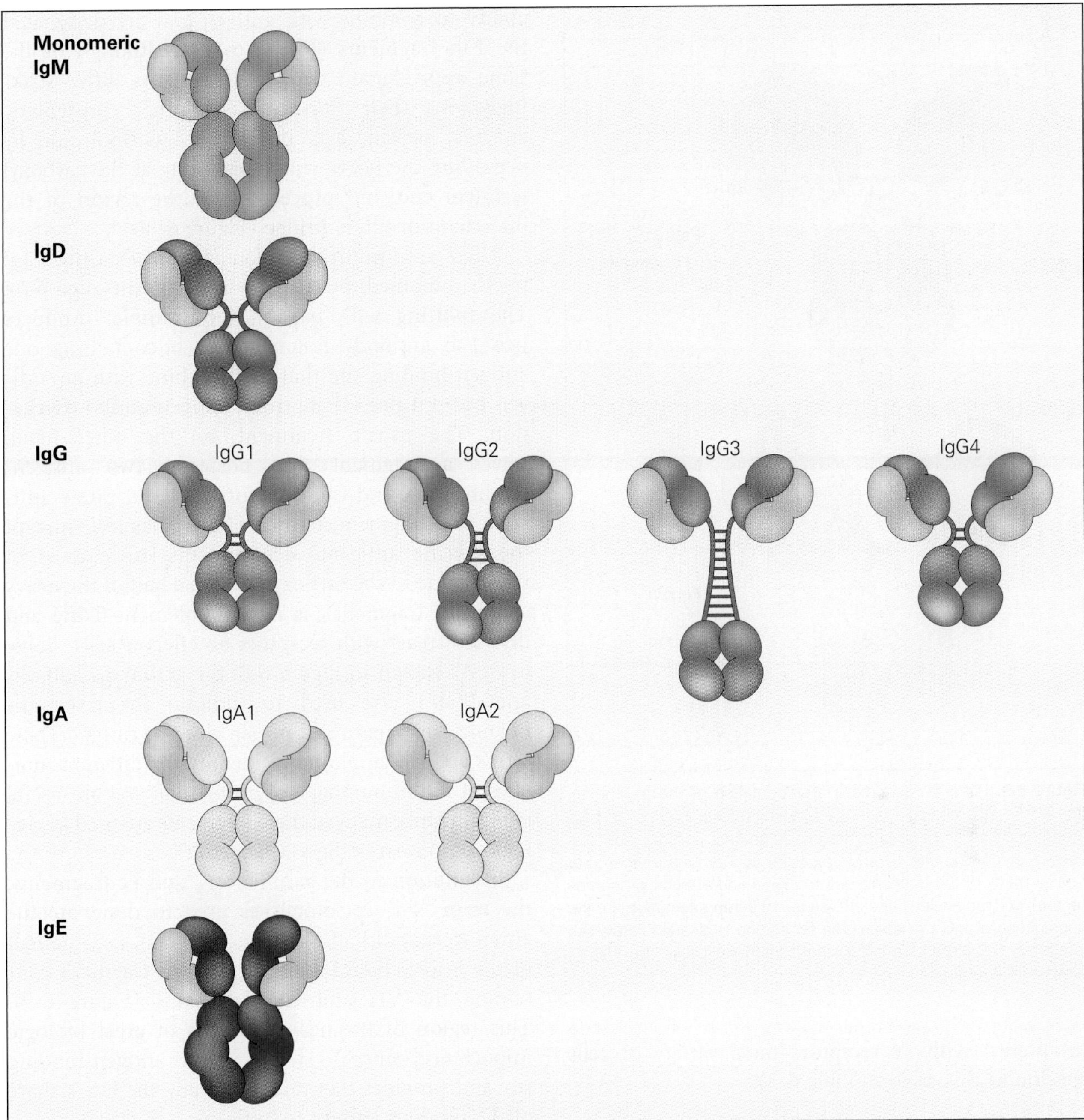

Figure 6-7. Schematic representation of the arrangement of peptide chains and disulfide bonds in various classes and subclasses of immunoglobulins. Disulfide bonds are represented by red bars. Note the large numbers of disulfide bonds in IgG3, the IgG subclass with the shortest half-life. Although IgA1 and IgA2 are shown here with two inter-heavy chain disulfide bonds and appear identical, in one of the allotypes of IgA2 (A2m(1)), the disulfide bonds between the H and the L chains are missing (not shown in this figure).

other antigen. Antibody to tetanus toxoid, for example, must differ in some chemically defined way from antibody to diphtheria toxoid since both antibodies can be shown to combine only with their homologous antigens. This property, known as specificity, resides in the primary amino acid structure of the antibody molecule in the region referred to as the antigen-binding site located in the Fab region.

Effector Functions of Antibodies Are Determined by Their Constant Region Domains

As will be described in greater detail, the constant regions of the heavy chain of the molecule, i.e., the Fc segment, carry out several effector functions. These include its ability to interact with complement, to cross the placenta in the case of IgG, and

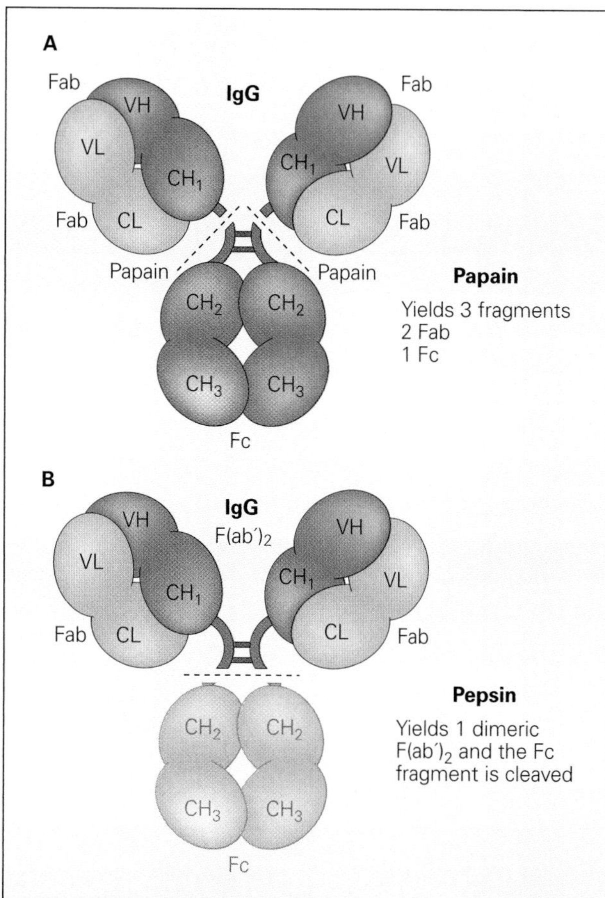

Figure 6-8. Panel A: Schematic representation of the fragmentation of the IgG molecule by papain, which results in two Fab fragments and one Fc fragment. The Fab fragments possess only one antigen-combining site. The Fc fragment cannot bind antigen, but retains many of the antigenic determinants and effector properties of the IgG molecule. Panel B: Schematic representation of the degradation of IgG by pepsin. The Fc portion is cleaved below the interchain S-S bonds leaving a single fragment called the F(ab′)$_2$, which has two antigen-binding sites.

to interact with Fc receptors on a variety of cells specific to this region (Table 6-3).

Immunoglobulins Can Be Cleaved by Proteolytic Enzymes into Antigen-Binding (Fab) and Constant (Fc) Fragments

Knowledge of the structure of the immunoglobulins has been greatly enhanced by the use of proteolytic enzymes, which degrade the molecule into definable fragments (Figure 6-8). Papain splits the heavy chains of IgG in the hinge region, the area of the interchain disulfide bonds, yielding three fragments (Figure 6-8A). One fragment, which can be crystallized, contains most of the IgG-specific antigenic determinants of the molecule and is designated the Fc fragment; the other two fragments retain the ability to combine with antigen and are designated the Fab fragments (Figure 6-8A). Although of the same approximate size, the fragments differ strikingly in their functions. Another proteolytic enzyme, pepsin, acts upon the IgG molecule by degrading the heavy chain beginning at the carboxyl terminal end and proceeding to the region of the interchain disulfide bridge (Figure 6-8B).

There are important differences between the fragments obtained by papain and pepsin digestion. The splitting with papain, for example, produces two Fab antibody fragments, each containing one antigen-binding site that can combine with an antigen but not precipitate in an antigen-antibody reaction. The pepsin treatment, on the other hand, leaves a fragment that possesses two antigen-binding sites and can therefore still precipitate antigen. This fragment, termed F(ab′)$_2$, has lost most of the specific antigenic determinants, since most of these reside in the carboxyl-terminal half of the heavy chain (Fc fragment), is not complement-fixing and does not react with receptors on effector cells (Table 6-3). As shown in Figure 6-8, the acronyms Fab, Fc, and F(ab′)$_2$ are used to indicate the fragments obtained by papain and pepsin cleavage of IgG. These terms are still employed to identify the different moieties of the immunoglobulin molecule and are useful clinically since many of these fragments are used as biologic response modifiers (*Chapter 11*).

In addition to the Fab, F(ab′)$_2$, and Fc fragments, the term "Fd" is sometimes used to designate the amino-terminal half of the heavy chain, i.e., the half of the heavy chain located in the Fab fragment containing the VH and CH1 domains (Figure 6-9). This region of the heavy chain is of great biologic importance, since it shares in the antigen-binding site and provides thermodynamically the lion's share of the binding affinity to antigen.

Enzymes Affect Immunoglobulins *In Vivo* as well as *In Vitro*

Knowledge of how enzymes modify immunoglobulins *in vitro* is not only important in determining immunoglobulin structure but also has clinical relevance *in vivo* (*Chapters 8* and *12*). Enzymes produced by some bacteria living on mucous epithelia, including the gonococcus, meningococcus, and some alpha-hemolytic streptococci, have been found to produce enzymes that have proteolytic activity capable of degrading the IgA1 subclass. These enzymes cleave IgA1 molecules in the hinge region and produce fragments quite similar in

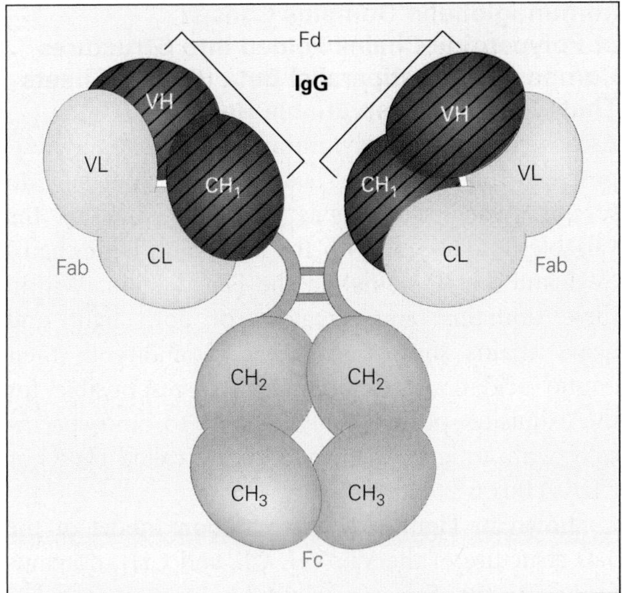

Figure 6-9. The Fd fragments (hatch-marked) of the heavy chain of an immunoglobulin represent the variable domain (VH) and first constant domain (CH1) of a heavy chain located in the Fab fragment.

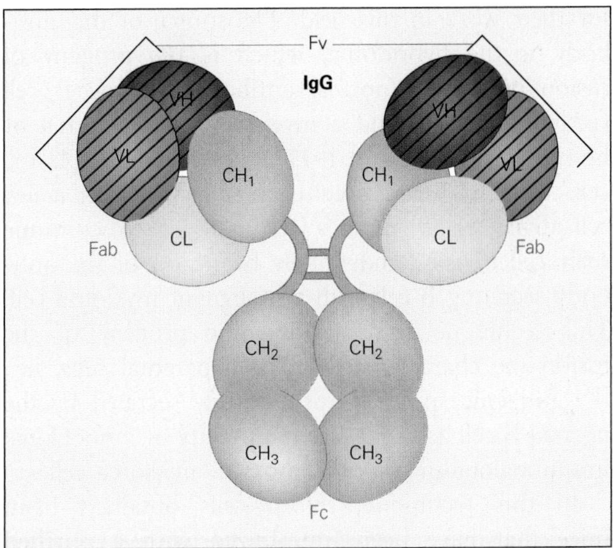

Figure 6-10. The Fv fragments (crosshatched) are made up of a dimer composed of the variable regions of both H and L chains, i.e., the VL and VH domains.

size to the Fab and Fc fragments of IgG. In contrast, the IgA2 that predominates in external secretions, and which is deficient in disulfide bonds between the H and L chains, is somewhat impervious to the proteolytic effects of these proteases. The relative enrichment of IgA2 in external secretions may therefore represent a mechanism of evolutionary adaptation of the host immune response to counter this enzymatic defense mechanism of the bacteria (*Chapter 12*). Table 6-2 lists the composition and biologic activities associated with each fragment in a format that might lend a memory assist for the reader through the use of the mnemonic **A's** and **C's** (A's for the Fab and C's for the Fc fragments, respectively).

Modified Immunoglobulins Have Been Created in the Laboratory for Clinical Use

Another fragment of immunoglobulin, referred to as the Fv fragment, has been generated either from more extensive pepsin degradation or from the use of a DNA recombinant expression system (Figure 6-10 and *Chapter 25*). The Fv fragment retains the complete antibody-binding sites and consists of the variable regions of both heavy and light chains containing the N-terminal half of the Fab, i.e., the VH and VL domains (Figure 6-10). These fragments are used clinically, for example, when treating cancer patients with mouse monoclonal antibodies specific for tumor antigens (*Chapter 11*). The efficacy of these monoclonal fragments, however, is diminished from whole immunoglobulin preparations since they lack the constant regions essential for many of the effector functions.

Hybridoma Technology as a Source of Monoclonal Antibody

One of the most important advances in immunology that has had great clinical significance has been the development of a method for the *in vitro* production of large quantities of homogenous antibody to a single antigenic specificity, i.e., monoclonal antibody. In 1984, Kohler and Milstein received the Nobel Prize

Table 6-2. Fragments of IgG produced by papain cleavage; the A's and C's acronym

	Fab (A's)	Fc (C's)
Composition:	Amino-terminal half of heavy chain and one light chain Aberrated amino acid sequence	Carboxyl-terminal half of heavy chain dimer Carbohydrate Crystallizable Constant amino acid sequence
Function:	Antigen-binding or antibody active fragment	Complement fixation Cross placenta Cellular attachment through Fc receptors

for their work in this field. The source of this antibody is the hybridoma, which is the progeny of fusion between a normal antibody-secreting B cell (i.e., plasma cell) and a myeloma cell of animal or human origin (Figure 6-11). Since normal plasma cells usually die when cultivated in vitro after a few cell divisions, there is a requirement to continue their cell division indefinitely by fusion of the antibody-secreting B cell with a malignant myeloma cell. This technique confers upon the progeny of the fusion the characteristics of both parental cells, i.e., the antigenic specificity of antibody secreted by the normal B cell as well as the perpetuity of monoclonal immunoglobulin production by the myeloma cell.

In this technique, spleen cells obtained from mice that have been immunized with a purified protein or a suspension of cells are the most commonly used sources of antibody-secreting B cells (Figure 6-11). To extend the biologic life of the normal B cells indefinitely, they are exposed to an agent that promotes cell fusion, such as polyethylene glycol, when mixed with a suspension of myeloma cells in tissue culture. Following fusion, a number of clones of hybrids appear, which are capable of producing various monoclonal antibodies to any of the antigenic specificities found on the immunogen. Clones of hybridomas of the desired antibody specificity are then selected from the pool to remove unfused or unwanted hybrids. The preferred antibody-producing hybridoma cell line can be injected back into ascitic-producing mice or expanded by tissue culture techniques to provide an unlimited source of monoclonal antibody for use in the diagnosis and treatment of a wide variety of allergic and infectious diseases, autoimmune disorders, and cancer (*Chapter 11*).

With the advent of recombinant DNA technology (*Chapter 25*), more modern methods to generate or alter monoclonal antibodies have been developed. These methods are targeted at making the monoclonal antibodies from a mouse more human-like in order to lessen any adverse immune responses to therapy with these preparations in the human. The rapidly emerging availability of monoclonal antibody represents a major advance in the diagnosis and therapy of a wide variety of immunologically mediated diseases, such as allergic diseases, autoimmune disorders, and malignancy. The classification and use of these monoclonal antibody preparations in these disorders are described more extensively in Chapter 11.

Immunoglobulin Domains Consist of Polypeptide Chains Folded into Structures Composed of Antiparallel Beta Pleated Sheets That Contain Hypervariable Regions

As described previously, immunoglobulins are composed of both light and heavy chains arranged into several domains. Antigens are recognized by the variable domains of both the heavy and light chains (VH and VL domains) in the Fab portion. Within these domains, some regions of both light and heavy chains show exceptional variability in their amino acid composition, which is responsible for the exquisite specificity of antibody to bind specifically with antigen; these regions are called HVRs or CDRs (Box 6-2, Figure 6-12).

Shown in Figure 6-13 is a ribbon model of the 3-D structure of the VL, VH, CL, and CH_1, domains found in the Fab region of an immunoglobulin. Each domain in an antibody molecule has a similar structure of two beta sheets packed tightly against each other and folded in a compressed antiparallel beta structure called an immunoglobulin fold (Figure 6-13A). This fold consists of two antiparallel beta pleated sheets held together by the intrachain S-S. It is analogous to a sandwich held together with a toothpick. The heavy and light chains associate through interactions between the Ig domains. The framework regions form the beta-pleated sheets, and the HVRs in the VH and VL regions form some of the loops that link the beta strands and are clustered at one end of the Fab region (Figure 6-13B). Domains with a very similar structure are present in many other proteins of the body and together constitute the **immunoglobulin superfamily of molecules** (*Chapter 5*).

Biological Functions of Immunoglobulins

Antibodies Have Both Antigen-Recognition and Effector Functions

Immunoglobulins can either be found as transmembrane proteins on the surface of the B cell or they can be secreted by the terminal cell of B cell differentiation, i.e., the plasma cell (Figure 6-14).

Immunoglobulins function as antibodies and have the property to combine with the antigen (i.e., immunogen) that triggered their production. This unique property of recognition, referred to as specificity (*Chapter 1*), is controlled by an amazing assortment of genes that regulate the production of

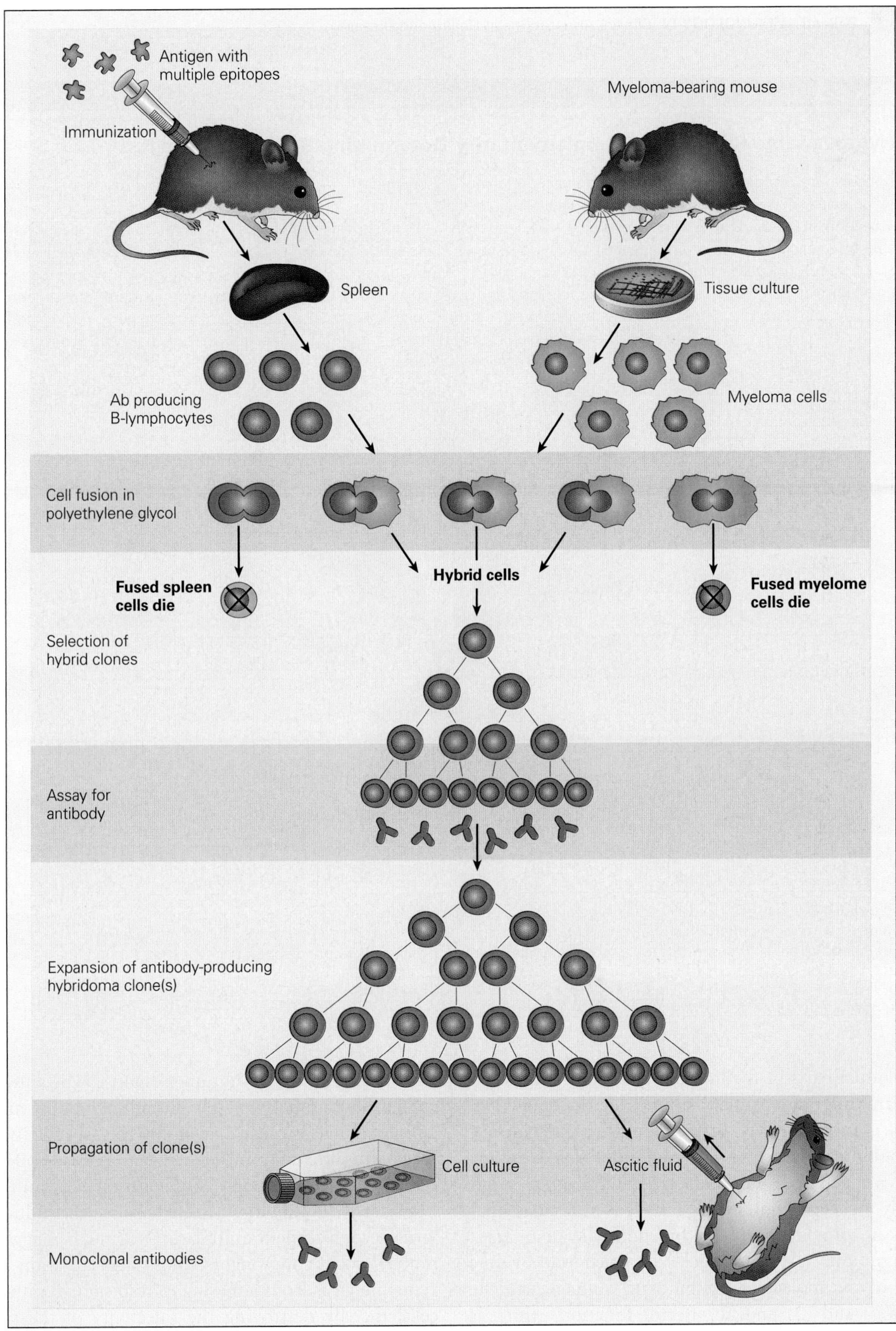

Figure 6-11. Schematic representation of the hybridoma technique for the production of monoclonal antibody. Spleen cells from mice that have been immunized with a desired antigen serve as a source of the antibody-secreting B cells and are fused to myeloma cells from a myeloma-bearing mouse. Following fusion, a number of hybrid clones appear, and the desired antibody-producing clones of interest are selected and expanded in cell culture to produce large quantities of monoclonal antibody. The older method of obtaining monoclonal antibody from ascitic fluid of animals injected with the antibody-producing hybrid clones is only of historic interest and is no longer commercially used.

Box 6-2

Hypervariable Regions or Complementarity Determining Regions of the Fab

Antigens are recognized by the variable domains (VH and VL domains) in the Fab portion of an immunoglobulin or the T cell receptor (*Chapter 7*). When the amino acid sequences of variable regions from antibodies with different antigen-binding specificities are compared, variability is unevenly distributed throughout the variable regions (Figure 6-12). At some positions, the same amino acids are found in most variable regions. These conserved regions are termed "framework regions," which are shown in yellow and light blue. At other positions, many possible amino acids might be found when different variable region sequences are compared. This sequence variation is concentrated in three regions in the LC and three regions in the HC shown as red loops. These regions are called hypervariable regions (HVRs) because of their great variability in amino acid composition or complementarity determining regions (CDRs) because they "complement" an antigen. Since an immunoglobulin has two antigen-binding sites, there are six CDRs for each Fab (each heavy and light chain contains three CDRs), twelve CDRs on a single antibody molecule, and sixty CDRs on a pentameric IgM molecule. Among the CDRs, CDR3 shows the greatest variability.

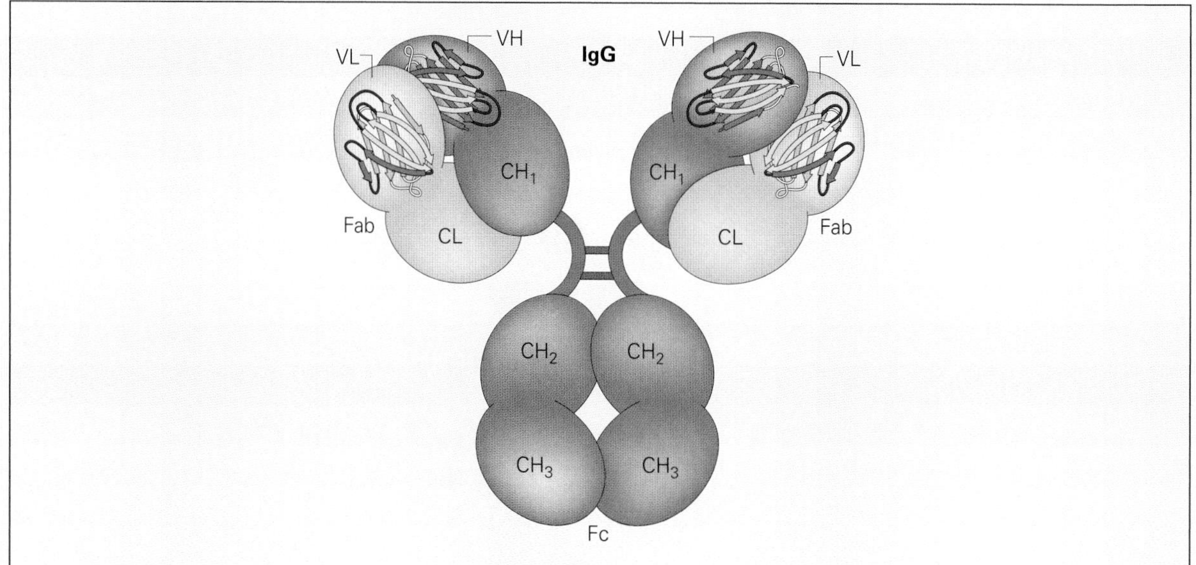

Figure 6-12. Schematic representation of the hypervariable regions (HVRs) or complementarity determining regions (CDRs) and framework regions in the VH and VL domains. Some positions with a high degree of variability of the amino acid sequence are referred to as the HVRs or CDRs (shown as red loops). In other positions where the same amino acids are found, these conserved regions are termed "framework regions," shown in yellow.

individual parts of the immunoglobulin molecule by determining the primary amino acid sequence of these components. As described in Chapter 1, immunoglobulins are not simply molecules that combine with antigen in a "lock and key" fashion, as was originally believed, but are specialized molecules that basically provide two sets of functions: (1) an antigen-recognition function, which is carried out by one end of the molecule that binds to antigen, i.e., the $F(ab')_2$; and (2) and an effector function, which is performed by the other end of the molecule by interaction with phagocytic cells, other effector cells, and mediator molecules, e.g., complement, i.e., the Fc (*Chapter 4*). Both these functions are extremely important during the immune response. The antigen-recognition property of the immunoglobulin molecule confers its exquisite capability (i.e., specificity) to react with different molecular structures, i.e., epitopes (*Chapter 1*) of a foreign configuration, i.e., antigen. For example, antibodies directed against the influenza virus recognize neuraminidase (**N**) and hemagglutinin (**H**), viral components whose neutralization prevents the virus from adhering to respiratory epithelial cells, thereby destroying the infectivity of the virus (*Chapter 13*). This is achieved by producing two separate sets of antibodies, one directed at the N and the other at the H, with different amino acid sequences, each recognizing one of the two unrelated target

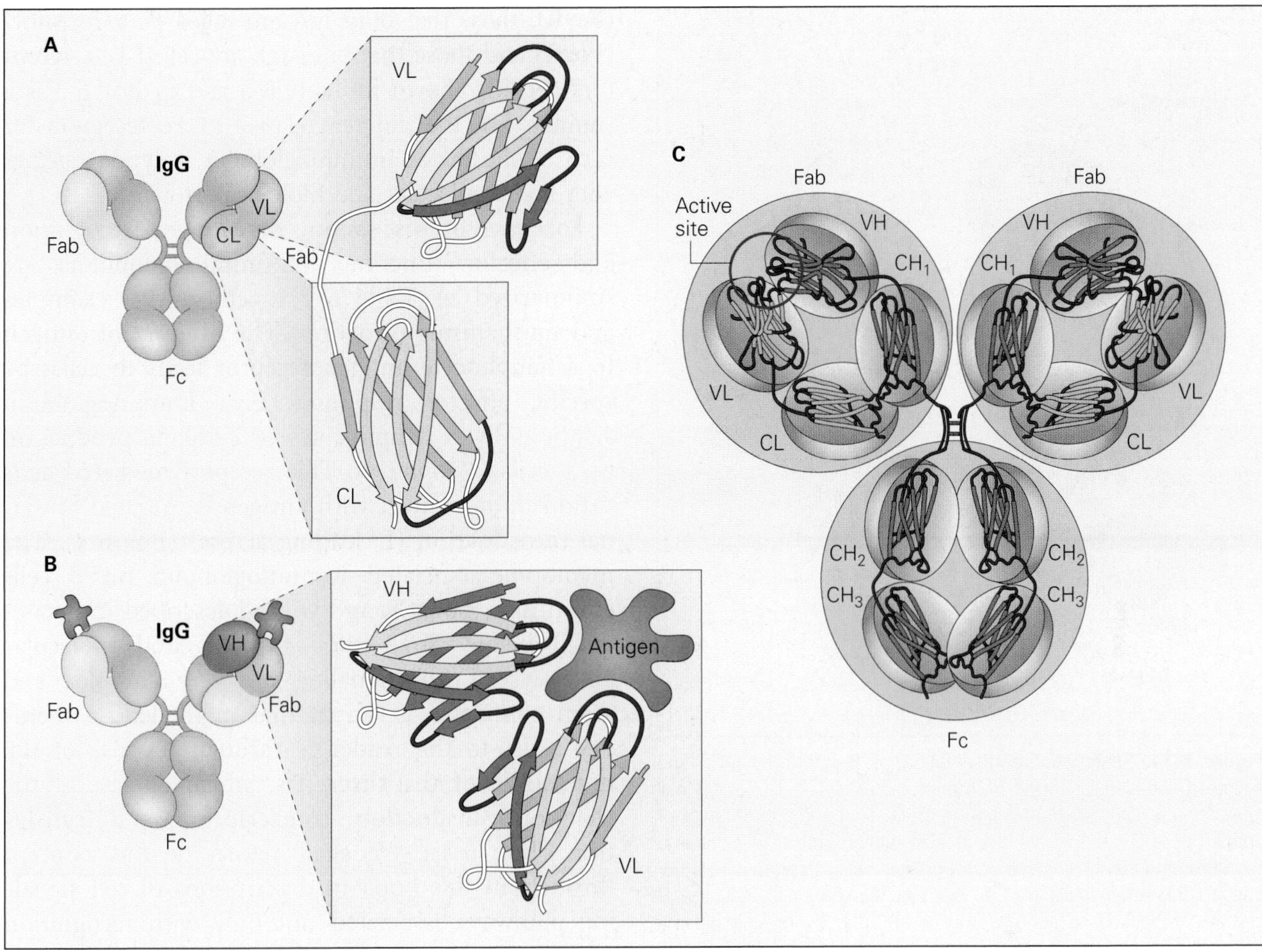

Figure 6-13. Schematic representation of the beta-pleated sheet structures of various domains in the IgG molecule. Panel A: The structure of the VL and CL domains in the Fab region showing the hypervariable portions in the loops (shown in red). Panel B: The structure of the VH and VL domains from a top view showing the insertion of an antigen in the cleft between the two domains. Panel C: The beta-pleated structures of all the domains in the IgG.

antigens. As will be described in greater detail below and in Chapter 7, antigen recognition by the B cell occurs both at its cell surface through the BCR and by its secreted immunoglobulin product; in contrast, antigen recognition by the T cell occurs only through its surface receptor, i.e., the TCR (*Chapter 7*).

During the course of an immune response to an immunogen specific classes of antibodies are generated at temporally different time periods, e.g., IgM antibody is synthesized early and IgG later by a process referred to as **immunoglobulin class switching** or **isotype switching**. The genetic mechanism by which this class switching occurs is referred to as **somatic recombination** or **V(D)J recombination** that will be described in greater detail below. The effector function of an immunoglobulin is related to the specific isotype produced. For example, IgM antibodies synthesized early in the immune response because of their large molecular size are found and function best within the vascular system. Other immunoglobulins of lower molecular weight, e.g., the IgG antibodies, produced later in the immune response can readily diffuse between the intravascular and interstitial tissues where they function most effectively. Still other antibody molecules, i.e., the secretory IgA, are found at mucosal surfaces where they are produced and function as first lines of defense against pathogens that enter through the mucosal route, as exemplified by influenza, rhinoviruses, and HIV (*Chapter 8*).

The family of Fc receptors

Fc receptors are molecules found on the surface of many cells, including NK cells, macrophages, neutrophils, mast cells, smooth muscle cells, epithelial cells and B cells, which contribute to both the protective and deleterious functions of the immune system by engaging the Fc region of antibody (Table 6-3). The binding of the unattached $F(ab')_2$ portions of various isotype molecules with

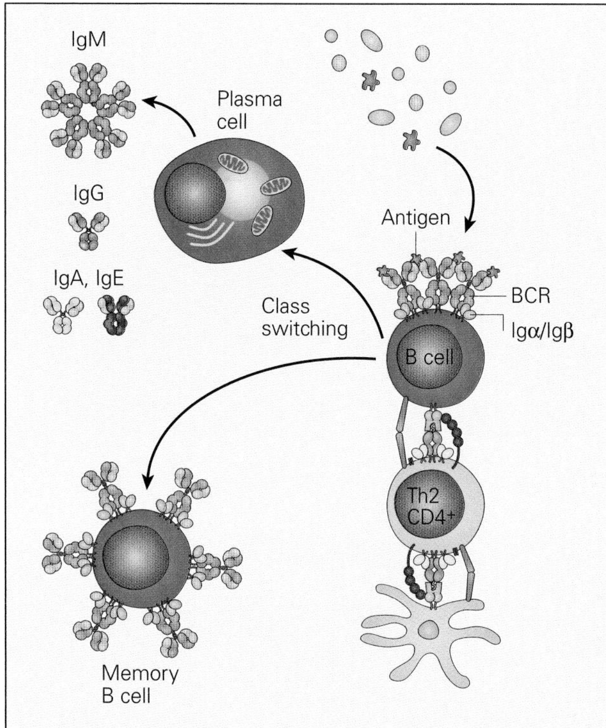

Figure 6-14. Schematic representation of membrane-bound and secreted extracellular forms of immunoglobulin. The Th2 cell/B cell interaction is illustrated showing the processing and presentation of antigen by a B cell followed by its cooperation with a Th2 cell and the differentiation of a B cell into a plasma cell. In contrast to other antigen-presenting cells (APCs), such as the dendritic cell, the B cell also functions as an APC and as an antibody-forming plasma cell with resultant production of antibody (IgG, IgM, IgA, or IgE) and differentiation into a long-lived memory B cell.

epitopes of an invading microbe or foreign substance leads to stimulation of phagocytic or cytotoxic activity of the cell to destroy microbes, or infected cells by antibody-mediated phagocytosis or antibody-dependent cell-mediated cytotoxicity (**ADCC**), respectively. The cross-linking of allergens to IgE antibody attached to specific FceR1 receptors on mast cells or basophils leads to the release of potent vasoactive and proinflammatory mediators important in augmenting both beneficial inflammatory responses as well as promoting allergic inflammation in the allergy-prone (atopic) individual (*Chapter 18*).

Classes of Fc receptors

There are several different classes of Fc receptors, which are classified based on the type of antibody that they recognize. The Latin letter used to identify a type of antibody is converted into the corresponding Greek letter, which is placed after the 'Fc' part of the name. For example, those that bind the most common class of antibody, IgG, are called Fc-γ receptors (**FcγR**), those that bind IgA are called Fc-α receptors (**FcαR**) and those that bind IgE are called Fc-ε receptors (**FcεR**). Shown in Table 6-3 and in Box 6-3 is a summary of the different classes of Fc receptors for each of the major immunoglobulin isotypes together with their molecular and biological properties.

For ease of discussion, the antigen recognition and effector functions of immunoglobulins are summarized in Table 6-4 together with examples and mechanisms of action. The binding of antigen to a lymphocyte antigen receptor leads to cell-type specific effector responses, e.g., immunoglobulin synthesis by B lymphocytes or cytokine production by T cells (*Chapter 9*). This receptor-mediated activation upon contact with antigen is initiated by signal **transduction** (L, leading across) (Box 6-4). The membrane-associated immunoglobulin on B cells constitutes the BCR and will be described in greater detail below. Since the acronyms and molecular pathways of cell signaling are very complex and often confusing, a format that might lend a memory assist to the reader is through the use of the mnemonic of the **three T's**, which consist of the triad of **transduction, transcription**, and **translation** (Box 6-4). We shall return to this concept throughout this book in descriptions of cell signaling pathways associated not only with recognition of antigen by B and T cells but also recognition of all ligands responsible for cellular activation and function, i.e, cytokines and hormones (*Chapter 9*).

The Family of Immunoglobulins Includes Five Functional Classes of Antibodies

As described previously, the five different isotypes constitute a family of immunoglobulins, each with a different structure and a different function (Table 6-1). The individual classes also referred to as isotypes are designated IgG, IgA, IgM, IgD, and IgE.

IgM Is Produced Rapidly Early in the Humoral Response

IgM is the largest of the immunoglobulin molecules, present in the serum as a pentamer with ten antigen-binding sites and, because of its large size, is restricted almost entirely to the intravascular space. These macromolecules are highly efficient agglutinators of particulate antigens, e.g., bacteria and red blood cells, and they activate complement through the classical pathway with a high degree of efficiency (*Chapter 4*). This class of immunoglobulin appears to be of greatest importance early in the

Table 6-3. Summary of the different classes of Fc receptors for each of the major immunoglobulin isotypes together with their molecular and biological properties.

Receptor name	Principal antibody ligand	Affinity for ligand	Cell distribution	Effect(s) following binding to antibody
FcγRI (CD64)	IgG1 and IgG3	High (Kd ~ 10^{-9} M)	Macrophages Neutrophils Eosinophils Dendritic cells	Phagocytosis Cell activation Activation of respiratory burst Induction of microbe killing
FcγRIIA (CD32)	IgG	Low (Kd > 10^{-7} M)	Macrophages Neutrophils Eosinophils Platelets Langerhans cells	Phagocytosis Degranulation (eosinophils)
FcγRIIB1 (CD32)	IgG	Low (Kd > 10^{-7} M)	B Cells Mast cells	No phagocytosis Inhibition of cell activity
FcγRIIB2 (CD32)	IgG	Low (Kd > 10^{-7} M)	Macrophages Neutrophils Eosinophils	Phagocytosis Inhibition of cell activity
FcγRIIIA (CD16a)	IgG	Low (Kd > 10^{-6} M)	NK cells Macrophages (certain tissues)	Induction of antibody-dependent cell-mediated cytotoxicity (ADCC) Induction of cytokine release by macrophages
FcγRIIIB (CD16b)	IgG	Low (Kd > 10^{-6} M)	Eosinophils Macrophages Neutrophils Mast cells Follicular dendritic cells	Induction of microbe killing
FcεRI (high affinity)	IgE	High (Kd ~ 10^{-10} M)	Mast cells Eosinophils Basophils Langerhans cells Smooth muscle	Degranulation
FcεRII (CD23) (low affinity)	IgE	Low (Kd > 10^{-7} M)	B cells T cells (on activated cells) Eosinophils Langerhans cells Epithelial cells	Functions as a possible adhesion molecule
FcαRI (CD89)	IgA	Low (Kd > 10^{-6} M)	Monocytes Macrophages Neutrophils Eosinophils	Phagocytosis Induction of microbe killing
Fcα/μR	IgA and IgM	High for IgM, Mid for IgA	B cells Mesangial cells Macrophages	Endocytosis Induction of microbe killing
FcRn	IgG		Monocytes Macrophages Dendritic cells Epithelial cells Endothelial cells Hepatocytes	Transfers IgG from a mother to fetus through the placenta Transfers IgG from a mother to infant in milk Protects IgG from degradation

Box 6-3

The Family of Fc Receptors

Fc-gamma receptors (FcγR)

All Fcγ receptors (FcγR) belong to the immunoglobulin superfamily (*Chapter 5*) and are the most important Fc receptors for inducing phagocytosis of opsonized (coated) microbes. This family includes several members, FcγRI (CD64), FcγRIIA (CD32), FcγRIIB (CD32), FcγRIIIA (CD16a), FcγRIIIB (CD16b), which differ in their antibody affinities due to their different molecular structure (Table 6-3). For example, FcγRI binds to IgG more strongly than FcγRII or FcγRIII. FcγRI also has an extracellular portion composed of three immunoglobulin (Ig)-like domains, one more domain than FcγRII or FcγRIII. This property allows activation of FcγRI by a sole IgG molecule (or monomer), while the latter two Fcγ receptors must bind multiple IgG molecules within an immune complex to be activated.

Fc-alpha receptors (FcαR)

Only one Fc receptor belongs to the FcαR subgroup, which is called FcαRI (or CD89). FcαRI is found on the surface of neutrophils, eosinophils, monocytes, some macrophages (including Kupffer cells), and some dendritic cells. It is composed of two extracellular Ig-like domains, and is a member of both the immunoglobulin superfamily and the multi-chain immune recognition receptor (MIRR) family. It signals by associating with two FcRγ signaling chains. Another receptor can also bind IgA, although it has higher affinity for another antibody called IgM. This receptor is called the Fc-α/μ receptor (Fcα/μR) and is a type I transmembrane protein. With one Ig-like domain in its extracellular portion, this Fc receptor is also a member of the immunoglobulin superfamily.

Fc-epsilon receptors (FcεR)

Two types of FcεR are known: (*Chapter 18*)

- the high-affinity receptor FcεRI is a member of the immunoglobulin superfamily (it has two Ig-like domains). FcεRI is found on epidermal Langerhans cells, eosinophils, smooth muscle cells, mast cells, and basophils. As a result of its cellular distribution, this receptor plays a major role in controlling allergic responses. FcεRI is also expressed on antigen-presenting cells, and controls the production of important immune mediators called cytokines, which promote inflammation (*Chapter 9*).
- the low-affinity receptor FcεRII (CD23) is a C-type lectin found on B cells, activated T cells, eosinophils, Langerhans cells, and epithelial cells. FcεRII has multiple functions as a membrane-bound or soluble receptor adhesion molecule; it controls B cell growth and differentiation and blocks IgE-binding of eosinophils, monocytes, and basophils (*Chapter 18*).

Neonatal Fc receptor (FcRn)

Another FcR is expressed on multiple cell types and is similar in structure to MHC-I. This receptor also binds IgG and is involved in preservation of this antibody. However, since this Fc receptor is also involved in transferring IgG from a mother either via the placenta to her fetus or in milk to her suckling infant, it is called the *neonatal Fc receptor* (FcRn). Recent research suggests that this receptor plays a role in the homeostasis of IgG serum levels.

---

primary immune response. When a foreign antigen is introduced into a host for the first time, the rapid synthesis of IgM antibodies ensures protection before IgG are produced. The transition from the production of IgM to IgG and the other isotypes occurs through a "class switch mechanism" involving the interaction of a cascading set of hypermutational events that will be described below. The duration of IgM synthesis peaks within a few days and the level of specific serum IgM declines more rapidly than the level of IgG antibodies. In one of the primary immune deficiencies, hyperimmunoglobulinemia M syndrome (**HIGM**), described in Chapter 16, the congenital absence of the CD40 ligand on T cells or of the CD40 molecule on B cells results in the failure of the switch from IgM to IgG, causing the hyperproduction of IgM antibody with diminished production of IgG and the other isotypes, resulting in susceptibility to recurrent bacterial infection. A maturational delay in the development of the CD40 receptor in the immature fetus and infant is thought to account for the prominent IgM production characteristic of the fetal and newborn immune responses (*Chapter 2*).

IgG Is the Predominant Serum Antibody

The IgG are the most abundant of the immunoglobulins and achieve significant concentrations in both the vascular and extravascular spaces. They have a relatively long half-life ($t^1/_2$) of ~23 days, cross the placenta, and are able to activate complement through the classical pathway (*Chapter 4*). This class

Table 6-4. Antigen recognition and effector functions of immunoglobulin

Function	Portion of immunoglobulin which carries out function	Target of function or cellular site of action	Example	Mechanism of action
Antigen recognition	$F(ab')_2$	Toxins, bacteria, viruses, parasites, fungi, and all extracellular foreign configurations	Protective immunity	Direct binding
Effector function	Fc region of IgG (FcγRI, FcγRII, and FcγRIII)	Phagocytes (PMNs, macrophages, NK cells, eosinophils, and DCs)	Opsonization Enhanced intracellular microbicidal activity	Binding of Fc to surface of target cell
	Fc region of IgE (FcεRI) FcεRII	Mast cells and basophils (FcεRI) B cells	Allergic inflammation	Release of mediators
	Fc region of IgG and IgM	Complement	Opsonization Lysis of cells	Binding of C3b to complement receptor Membrane attack complex
Other roles	Fc region of IgG	Placenta	Maternal-fetal transfer of IgG	Specific placental IgG Fc receptor (FcRn)
	Fc region of IgA	Poly IgG receptor on epithelial cells at body surface (MALT)	Transport of sIgA into external secretions, e.g., breast milk	Binding of Fc of IgA to secretory component (SC)

of immunoglobulin, through its antigen-recognition function, is thought to contribute to protective immunity against many infectious agents, including bacteria, viruses, parasites, and some fungi. In addition to its role in the blood, IgG also provides antibody activity in tissues by exerting its effector

Box 6-4

The Concept of the Three T's: Transduction, Transcription, and Translation

The "3T's" is a useful mnemonic to provide a framework to assist the reader in understanding the cascading set of molecular reactions involved in the signaling pathways used by cells to sense a wide variety of stimuli triggered by ligands in the external environment, e.g., hormones, antigens, cytokines, etc. Ligands first bind to cells through surface membrane receptors, then generate and transmit signals through the cytosol into the nuclear DNA and then transcribe them into messenger molecules (mRNA) that ultimately produce proteins and export them from the cell (*Chapter 9*). The 3T's consist of the following:

- Transduction begins the signaling pathway by the binding of a ligand to a cell receptor following which a sequential set of activating factors are generated through a cascading series of enzymatic reactions involving primarily the addition of phosphate groups through phosphorylation (kinase) reactions, leading to a penultimate activating product that initiates the next step;
- Transcription is initiated when one or more of the penultimate activating factors binds to a promoter region of the DNA within the nucleus following which a messenger RNA (mRNA) is generated that provides the "blueprint" for the construction of the protein in the next step;
- Translation is next set in motion when the mRNA aligns itself atop of the ribosome in the endoplasmic reticulum and then engages the assembly of amino acids attached to and brought in by transfer RNAs (tRNAs), which are specified by the codons of the mRNA leading to the synthesis of intact protein which after passage and glycosylation through the Golgi apparatus is released from the cell into the extracellular environment.

Table 6-5. Properties of human IgG subclasses

Property	IgG1	IgG2	IgG3	IgG4
Normal serum concentration (mg/dL)	540	210	58	60
Serum half-life ($t^1/_2$) days	21	20	7	21
Fc binding capacity on phagocytes	+	–	+	+/–
Activation of classical complement pathway	++	+	+++	–
Capacity to cross placenta	+++	+	++	+/–
Antibody activity	Protein antigens (e.g., diphtheria and tetanus)	Polysaccharide antigens (e.g., pneumococcal and *H. influenzae*)	Protein antigens (e.g., diphtheria and tetanus)	Polysaccharide antigens (e.g., pneumococcal and *H. influenzae*)

Note: + and – represent the degree of indicated function

function. In the human, receptors for the Fc region exist on several types of phagocytic cells, including monocytes, macrophages, dendritic cells, neutrophils, and some lymphocyte subsets, such as NK cells (i.e., lymphocytes that carry out ADCC) (*Chapter 1* and Table 6-3). Target cells coated with IgG antibodies directed against cell surface antigens may be eliminated through this ADCC mechanism. This occurs through the action of cytotoxic NK cells, which bind to the surface-coated IgG antibodies through their Fc receptor, thus allowing these cells to come into close contact with and kill the target cells by apoptosis (*Chapter 3*).

Subclasses of IgG Differ Somewhat in Their Biological Properties

By antigenic analysis, it has been possible to detect relatively minor differences between molecules within a given class of immunoglobulin (Table 6-1 and Table 6-5). In this way, four different subclasses of IgG have been identified and designated IgG1, IgG2, IgG3, and IgG4, and two subclasses for IgA, named IgA1 and IgA2.

Subsequent chemical analysis has shown that subclass antigenic differences reflect substantial differences in amino acid sequence. As indicated in Table 6-5, important biologic distinctions have been correlated with the various subclasses of IgG. For example, IgG4 does not activate complement whereas the other three IgG subclasses do, and IgG3 has a significantly shorter half-life compared with the other three subclasses, which appears to be related to its longer hinge region. A major biochemical difference between subclasses is the location and number of interchain disulfide bridges. Of clinical significance is the recognition that certain IgG subclasses (i.e., IgG1 and IgG3) are associated with antibody activity directed at protein antigens, e.g., diphtheria and tetanus toxoids, while other subclasses (i.e., IgG2 and IgG4) contain antibody directed at polysaccharide antigens, e.g., pneumococcal and *H. influenzae* antigens. Measurement of pre-immunization antibody levels and responses to immunization with these vaccines provide the most valuable diagnostic tool in the workup of the patient with an undue susceptibility to recurrent infection suspected of having an immune deficiency (*Chapter 16* and *Chapter 24*). Since IgG subclass deficiencies are being identified with increasing frequency as a cause of recurrent infections, knowledge of the properties and functions of the IgG subclasses has assumed increasing importance. Although measurements of serum of IgG subclass levels could be included in the evaluation of patients with recurrent infections suspected to have humoral immune deficiencies, they should not be used alone and should always include demonstration of inadequate specific antibody resources (*Chapter 16*).

IgA Is the Predominant Antibody at Mucosal Tissue Sites

IgA is the second most abundant serum immunoglobulin and although functional in the serum, its most important contribution to protective immunity is located on mucosal surfaces (*Chapter 8*). IgA forms an important component of the MALT, where it is produced in high concentrations by lymphoid tissues found at these sites (Table 6-6 and *Chapter 8*).

In the secretions found at these sites, IgA is combined with a protein termed SC that facilitates the

Table 6-6. Components of MALT, major inductive tissues, and examples of clinical involvement

Anatomic site	Major inductive tissues	Example of clinical involvement
Gut-associated lymphoid tissues (GALT)	Jejunum (Peyer's patches) Ileum (M cells[a])	Celiac disease Food allergy Mucosal infections
Skin-associated lymphoid tissues (SALT)	Dermal lymphoid tissue	Atopic eczema
Mammary-associated lymphoid tissues	Mammary lymphoid tissues	Protective immunity for newborn
Mucous gland tissues	Lachrymal lymphoid tissues Genitourinary tissues	Allergic conjunctivitis Protective immunity (?)
Bronchus-associated lymphoid tissues (BALT) Nasopharyngeal-associated lymphoid tissues (NALT)	Peribronchial lymphoid tissue Palatine tonsils and adenoids	Asthma Allergic rhinitis

a. M cells = Microvillus cells, which overlay Peyer's patches in the ileum.

transport of the molecule into secretions and protects it against the effects of proteolytic enzymes (Figure 6-15). IgA does not activate complement by the classical pathway but may do so by the alternative pathway (i.e., the properdin system) (*Chapter 4*). IgA does not cross the placenta but it contributes to the protective immunity of the breast-fed newborn by virtue of its high concentration in the colostrum. Receptors for IgA are found on lymphocytes, polymorphonuclear cells, and monocytes (Table 6-3).

It has been possible to classify IgA into two subclasses, IgA1 and IgA2, based upon differences in antigenic structure and variation in the arrangement of interchain disulfide bridges. Although IgA2 is a minor component of serum IgA, this subclass is the dominant form in secretions. No covalent bonding exists between light and heavy chains in a common genetic variant of this IgA2 subclass i.e., the $A_2m(1)$ allotype.

IgD Is a B Cell Membrane Receptor Whose Humoral Function Is Unclear

The IgD was discovered by Rowe and Fahey in 1960; they encountered a myeloma protein antigenically and chemically different from the then-known immunoglobulins. Immunoglobulin D (**IgD**) is an antibody isotype that makes up about 1 percent of proteins in the plasma membranes of immature B lymphocytes, where it is usually coexpressed with monomeric IgM and the two function as B cell receptors as described below. IgD is also produced in a secreted form that is found in very small amounts in the blood. Secreted IgD is produced as a monomeric antibody with two heavy chains of the delta (δ) class and two Ig light chains. IgD is found on the surface of lymphocytes and is thought to represent a transitional immunoglobulin receptor, which participates as a specific surface receptor in the initiation of the adaptive immune response (*Chapter 2*).

Although IgD has not been assigned a specific antibody role as a humoral antibody, some cases of penicillin hypersensitivity have been associated with this immunoglobulin class. Hyperimmunoglobulinemia D syndrome (**HIDS**) is a newly recognized autoinflammatory disease resembling familial Mediterranean fever (**FMF**) (*Chapter 19 Annex*). Both entities are characterized by recurrent febrile attacks with abdominal distress, joint involvement (arthralgias/arthritis), headache, skin lesions, and an elevated serum IgD level (>100 U/ml). HIDS is inherited as an autosomal recessive trait and mutations of the gene coding for mevalonate kinase are responsible for the disease. The gene is located at chromosome 12q24 in contrast to the gene causing FMF that has been located on chromosome 16p.

IgE Protects Against Helminth Infections and Mediates Allergic Responses

In 1968, the description of a fifth class of immunoglobulin, IgE, was reported by two groups of investigators, Johansson and his colleagues and the Ishizakas (*Chapter 18*). Similar to the IgD, the identification of IgE was facilitated by the discovery by Johansson of a myeloma protein dissimilar to any of the known immunoglobulin classes. Formerly referred to as a reaginic antibody with skin-sensitizing properties, IgE is produced at least in part in the linings of the respiratory and gastrointestinal tracts within the MALT (*Chapter 8*). IgE is secreted in response to helminth (worm) infections. It coats the surface of the parasites, which are too large to be phagocytosed, and stimulates eosinophils to release mediators that kill the parasites (*Chapter 15*).

Although present only in trace amounts in the normal human, IgE is produced in excessive quantities in the allergic patient who demonstrates a genetic susceptibility for the development of allergy,

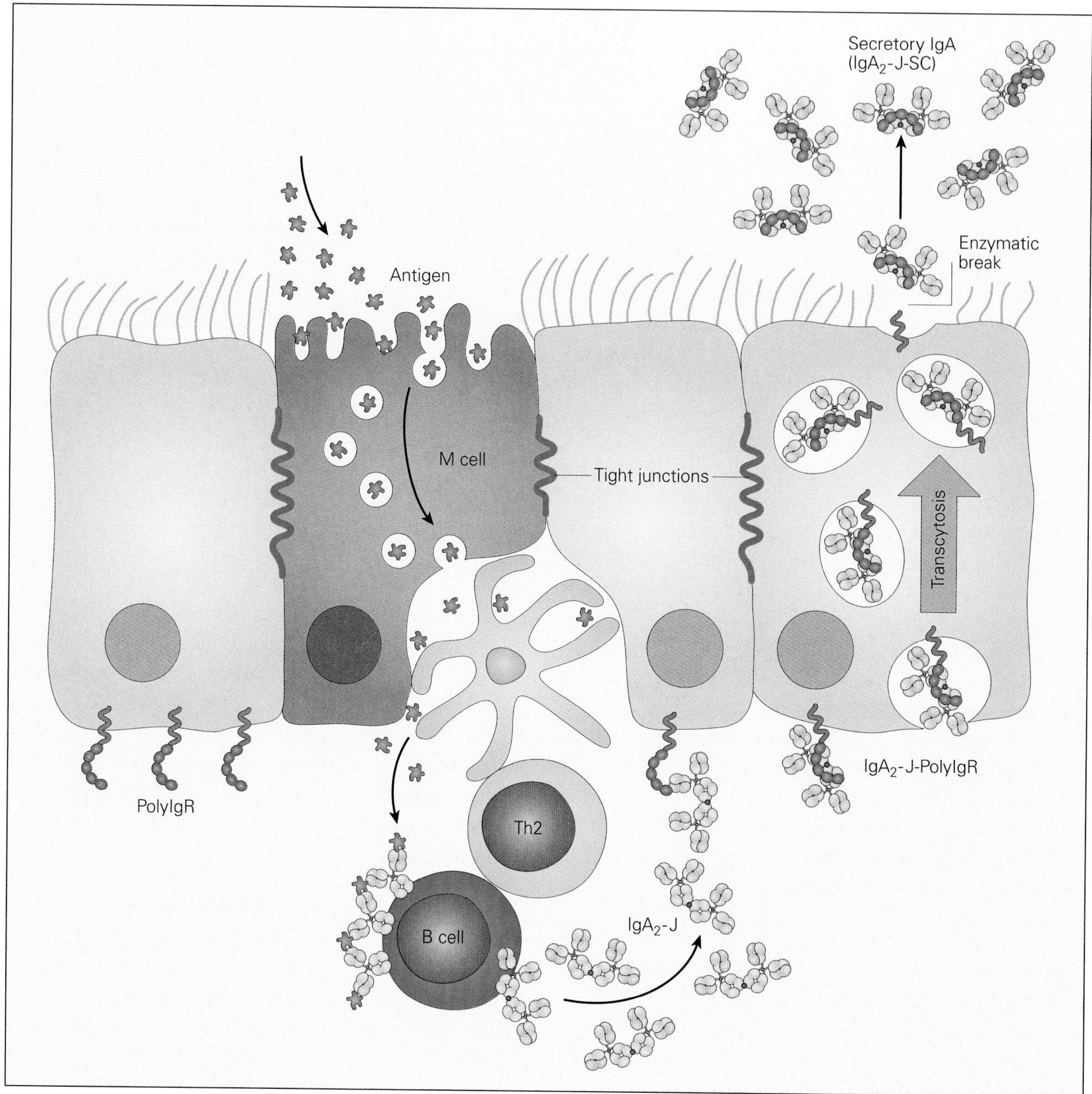

Figure 6-15. Schematic representation of the generation of secretory IgA. Plasma cells together with the influence of antigen-presenting cells and Th2 helper cells in the submucosa secrete the J chain-containing dimeric IgA, which then binds to the polymeric Ig receptor (polyIgR) on the basolateral surface of epithelial cells. The complex is then transported through the epithelial cell and at the apical surface partial enzymatic digestion of the IgA_2-J polyIgR complex occurs and the cleaved product forms a product with the secretory component (SC) attached to the dimeric IgA which is then released into the mucosal secretions as the secretory form of IgA (sIgA). The residual part of the polyIgR remains attached to the epithelial surface after the sIgA is released.

i.e., atopy (*Chapter 18*). However, it is not the amount of IgE present in the system that determines whether a patient will be allergic, but rather it is the specificity (i.e., antibody content) of the IgE that is important (i.e., excessive amounts of nonallergen-specific IgE, as in the case of an IgE myeloma patient, can actually relieve an allergic response by displacing the allergen-specific IgE loaded onto IgE FcRs).

At Times, Immunoglobulins Can Be Recognized as Foreign and Elicit Anti-Immunoglobulin Antibody Responses

Since immunoglobulin molecules are structurally glycoproteins, they can at times be immunogenic and, paradoxically, stimulate the production of antibodies directed at various components of their molecular structure. There are three types of

Table 6-7. Classification of anti-immunoglobulin responses and their clinical significance

		Molecular targets: Differences in			
		Variable		Constant	
Type	Host involvement	L	H	L	H
Isotypic	Different species	−	−	+	+
Allotypic	Same species	+	+	+	+
Idiotypic	Same individual	+	+	−	−

Note: + = difference; − = no different.

antibody responses to immunoglobulins that have been classified according to the antigenic determinants to which the antibody is directed: (1) isotypic responses; (2) allotypic responses; and (3) idiotypic responses (Table 6-7).

Isotypic Responses

Isotypic (Greek, from *iso*, equal, and *typos*, model, type) responses represent a reaction to species-specific determinants on the constant regions of the heavy and light chains of an immunoglobulin that are recognized as foreign when immunoglobulin from one species is injected into a different species. A good example of this was seen in the past when serum from horses who had been hyperimmunized with tetanus or diphtheria toxin was injected into humans as a form of treatment referred to as passive immunity (*Chapter 23*). Since the horse serum that was injected into the human was recognized as foreign, the recipient often produced antibody to many components of the serum, some of which were directed at antigen determinants localized to the constant regions of the light and heavy chains of the horse immunoglobulin molecule (Table 6-7). Although horse serum is no longer used in passive immunity, there are other diagnostic and therapeutic applications of isotypic antibody. The generation of large quantities of monoclonal antibody produced by injecting a mouse with a human IgE immunoglobulin for the continuous production of anti-IgE by the hybridoma technique, as described previously, represents an example of a diagnostic and therapeutic use of isotypic responses in the human (*Chapter 11*).

Allotypic Responses

A second type of serologic response to immunoglobulin is seen when immunoglobulin from one member of the species is introduced into another member of the same species (Table 6-7). Although humans share similar genes that specify light and heavy chains of the various immunoglobulin classes and subclasses, the genes of one individual vary in sequence from the same genes of another person. These are termed alleles and represent actual differences in the genes carried by individuals. When an individual carrying one allele is immunized with immunoglobulins synthesized in another person with a different allele, these subtle amino acid differences can be recognized as foreign, stimulating an immune response. The region of the antibody recognized in this immune response is termed an allotypic (from the Greek word *allos*, which means another, and *typos*, or model type) determinant and represents an immune response of one member of a species directed at another member. These differences can reside on both the heavy and light chains and can be found in both the variable and constant regions (Table 6-7). The most important types are Gm found on the heavy chain and Km found on the light chain. In humans, this type of immune response can occur following exposure to different allelic products in blood after transfusion or to exposure of the mother to fetal immunoglobulins during pregnancy or exposure to a therapeutic antibody. Antibodies that detect allotypes could theoretically identify donor B cells in a bone marrow graft recipient or determine identity in forensic or paternity testing. These applications, however, are not commonly used today since genetic identity testing now employs other strategies such as detection of variation in short nucleotide repeats in the DNA (*Chapter 25*).

Idiotypic Responses

An **idiotype** is defined as a serologic determinant located in the antigen-combining site of an antibody that is unique to each individual antibody within a person (Table 6-7). The unique determinant of an individual antibody molecule is called an idiotope, and all antibody molecules that share an idiotope are said to belong to the same idiotype.

The word idiotype (from the Greek prefix *idio-*, *idi-*, which means one's own or pertaining to one's self, and *typos*, which means model, type) and is an abbreviation of "individual type." As described previously, the variable region of an immunoglobulin molecule contains a unique amino acid structure that differentiates one immunoglobulin molecule from all other molecules within the same individual. An antibody recognizing the binding site is termed an anti-idiotypic antibody response. For example, anti-idiotypic antibodies can be made by a person if the individual is exposed to a monoclonal antibody (**moab**) in sufficient concentration following which the immune system recognizes the antigen-combining site as foreign. This might happen in two ways: a person is given a monoclonal antibody as a therapeutic treatment or an individual might respond to an increased concentration of a particular antibody following an immune response in an idiotypic response. Following the administration of a humanized monoclonal preparation, for example (*Chapter 11*), antibodies can be produced in the immunized host that react with the unique hypervariable loops of that antibody. The region of the moab recognized is termed an idiotypic determinant. There are several theoretical and clinical applications of the use of idiotypic antibody. First, it has been hypothesized that this type of recognition may play a negative feedback role in controlling the immune response by removing antibodies once they are no longer required. This theory of lymphocyte regulation occurs through idiotopes of antigen receptors and is called the network hypothesis. Although an anti-idiotypic response can theoretically occur when an idiotypic antibody is introduced into an individual, thereby reducing its effectiveness, human monoclonal antibodies are preferable for clinical use in passive immunization (*Chapter 23*) over preparations made from other (i.e., isotypic) or the same (i.e., allotypic) species because the chances of an anti-idiotypic response occurring is much less than an anti-isotypic or anti-allotypic response. Patients treated with mouse monoclonal antibody preparations may make antibodies against the residual amounts of mouse Ig in these products a phenomenon sometimes referred to as a human anti-mouse antibody (**HAMA**) response, which reduces their clinical effectiveness (*Chapter 11*). Humanized antibodies have been developed to circumvent this problem, but even humanized antibodies derived from the original monoclonal antibody contain hypervariable regions that can be immunogenic and elicit an immune response in treated patients. In addition to experimentally induced anti-idiotypic antibodies, these also can be seen as part of autoimmune disease processes in the human (*Chapter 19*). An IgM antibody that reacts with the constant regions of one's own IgG, called rheumatoid factor (**RF**), occurs in rheumatoid arthritis. Although the basis for its production is not known, the measurement of RF in this disorder is clinically useful (*Chapter 24*). Finally, one of the major current uses of anti-idiotypic reagents is being utilized as a treatment for B cell malignancies targeting the antibody found on the malignant B cell clone (*Chapter 21*).

Monomeric IgM and IgD Serve as BCRs

Lymphocyte antigen receptors take the form of intact immunoglobulins on B cells and are the means by which B lymphocytes sense the presence of antigen in their environments. Each lymphocyte expresses multiple copies of a unique antigen receptor with the ability to bind to a single antigen. The capacity to respond to a variety of antigens depends on the antibody repertoire of the billions of lymphocytes in our body fluids and tissues. As described previously, the wide range of antigen specificities is due to the variation in the amino-acid sequence at the antigen-binding site in the VL and VH regions of the receptor.

Shown in Figure 6-16 is a schematic representation of the BCR. The receptor consists of a monomeric IgM molecule and two additional polypeptide chains referred to as Igα and Igβ, which are now identified by their cluster of differentiation (**CD**) nomenclature, CD79a and CD79b, respectively (*Appendix 3*). The carboxyl-terminal tails of HCs of the IgM vary depending on whether they are inserted into the B cell membrane or secreted. If the antibody is expressed at the cell surface, the molecule contains a tail that has both a transmembrane region and a portion that extends into the cytoplasm, in contrast to the secreted form of IgM, which has no tail. Since the intracytoplasmic tail of the IgM is too short to transmit signals, immunoglobulin-mediated signals are transduced by the Igα and Igβ that are disulfide linked to one another and noncovalently expressed on the B cell surface associated with the membrane IgM. Within the intracytoplasmic tail region of the Igα and Igβ there is a small conserved segment rich in tyrosine called the immunoreceptor tyrosine-based activation motif

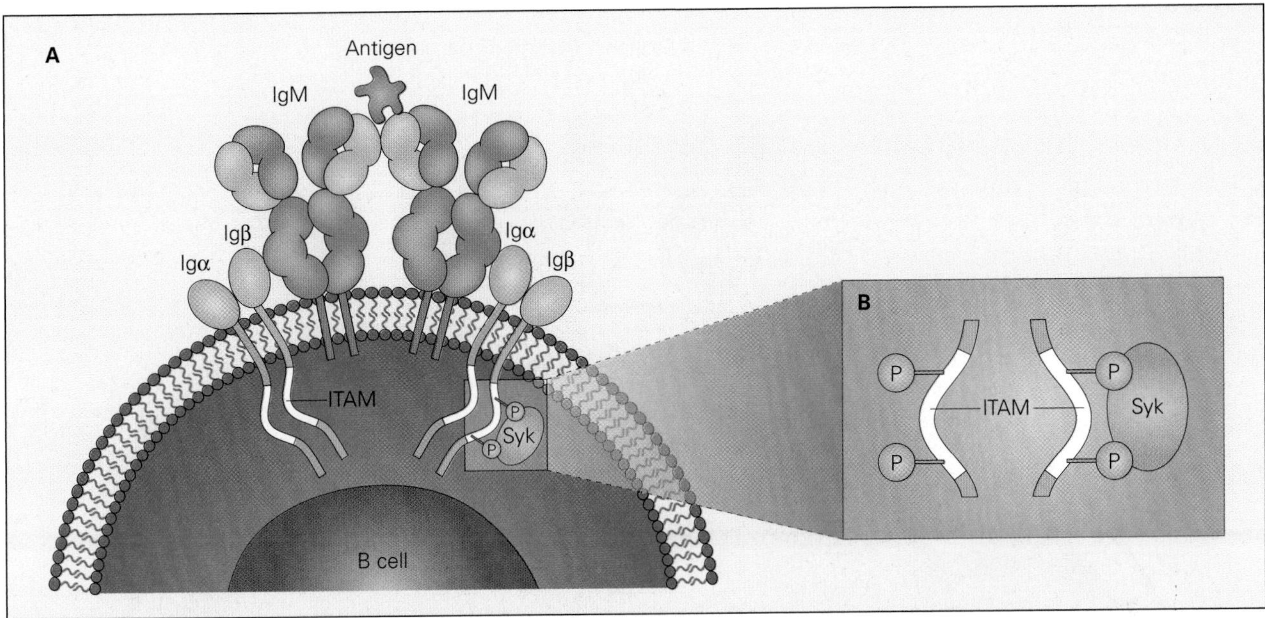

Figure 6-16. Panel A: The BCR is composed of the IgM monomer associated with the Ig-α/Ig-β heterodimer. The Ig-α/Ig-β is also referred to as the CD79a/CD79b, respectively. The tyrosine kinase Syk, docking to the BCR through the immunoreceptor tyrosine-based activation motif (ITAM) in the cytoplasmic tail of the Ig-α/Ig-β initiates the signaling cascade. Panel B: The inset, shows the addition of phosphate groups to the ITAM by the Syk tyrosine kinase and the docking of the Syk to the phosphorylated ITAM.

(**ITAM**), which after phosphorylation by a tyrosine kinase is importantly involved in the signalling pathway of the B cell. It also plays an important signalling role with T cells (*Chapter 7*). Igα and Igβ serve the same function in the BCR as CD3 and ζ-chains of the T cell receptor complex (*Chapter 7*) and certain Fc receptors. The tyrosine residues within these motifs become phosphorylated following interaction of the receptor molecules with their ligands and form docking sites for other proteins involved in the signaling pathways of the cell.

Antigen Binding to BCR Regulates B Cell Function: Transduction, Transcription, and Translation

As described previously, the signaling pathways underlying B cell function follow the triad of the 3Ts, i.e., transduction, transcription, and translation (Box 6-4). Transduction is initiated when two or more IgM molecules of the B cell receptor are brought together or cross-linked by multivalent antigen. Following the binding of antigen with the BCR, a number of important signalling pathways are stimulated by a multitude of substrates that have been phosphorylated by a cascading set of kinases (Figure 6-17). Signalling is initiated as described above when specific amino acid regions of the Igα and Igβ molecules rich in tyrosine residues, i.e., ITAMs are phosphorylated. A pivotal family of tyrosine kinase enzymes next activates their substrates by phosphorylation. These have a variety of names and sequential functions (Box 6-5). After initial binding of antigen with the BCR, a first set of enzymes (blk, fyn, or lyn) act to phosphorylate the tyrosine residues in the ITAMs. These phosphorylated residues are then able to bind to a second set of protein tyrosine kinases, Syk in B cells and ZAP-70 in T cells, which then transduce the signal onward. The end result of BCR transduction is that transcription factors are generated which then interact with the B cell DNA in the promotor region(s) and genes are expressed that result in functional changes in the B cell, which leads to the synthesis of a protein by translation (i.e., immunoglobulin in the case of the B cell) and release from the cell.

Genesis of Antibody Variability

The Two Phases of Immunoglobulin Generation in B Cells: The Antigen-Independent Phase and the Antigen-Dependent Phase

As described in Chapter 2, the development of B cells in ontogeny occurs as a series of genetically determined adaptive cellular transformations in response to an ever-changing environment. B cell development occurs in two phases: (1) in uterine development prior to exposure to foreign antigens and, subsequently, (2) after birth following exposure

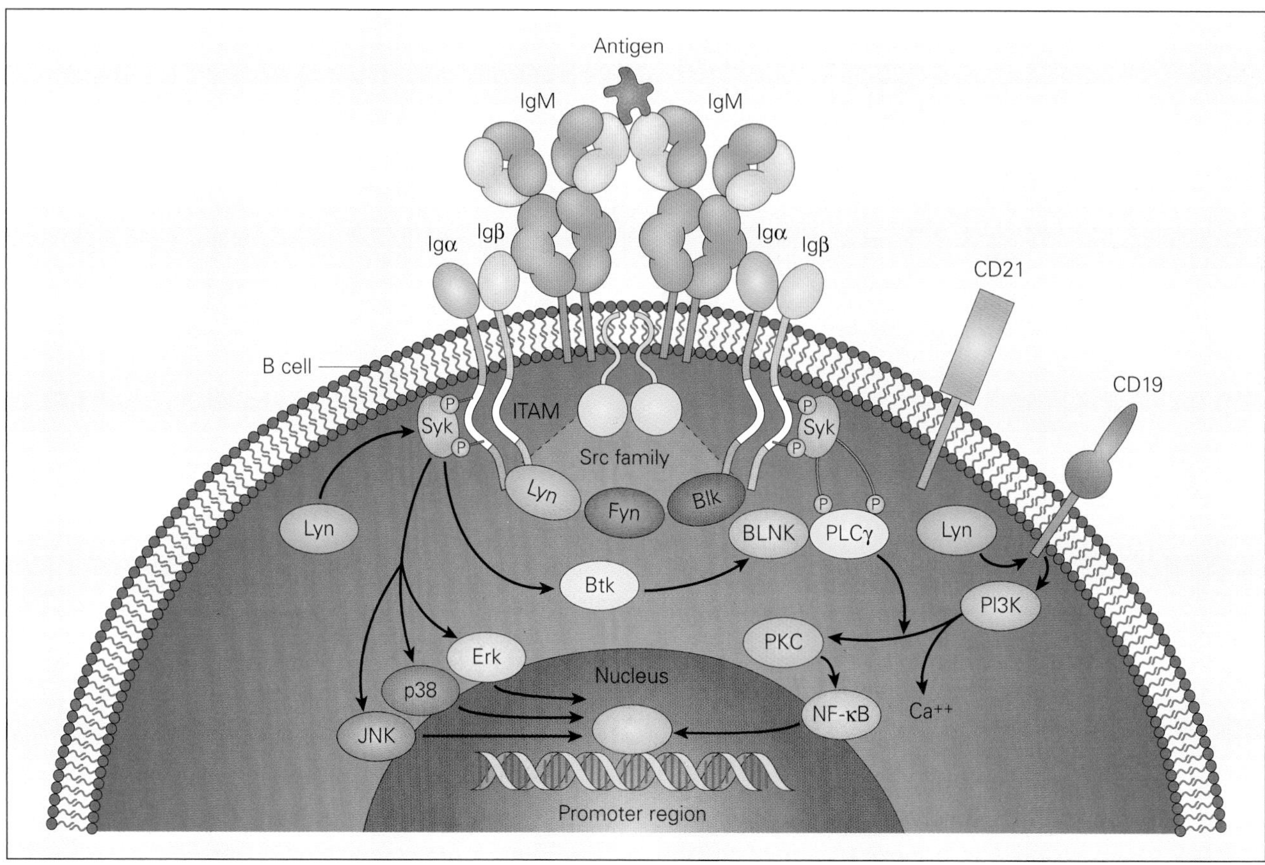

Figure 6-17. Schematic representation of the initial signaling pathways involved in B cell activation by binding of multivalent antigen with the BCR. These signalling pathways involve the phosphorylation of key substrates by a cascading set of kinases.

to the myriad of foreign substances that comprise the external environment. Figure 6-18 portrays a schematic representation of the total cellular events occurring during B cell development prior to and after birth showing the division of the lifespan of a B cell into these two phases, which are called (1) the antigen-independent phase and (2) the antigen-dependent phase.

In the human, B lymphocytes are generated from hematopoietic stem cells (**HSC**) in the bone marrow (*Chapter 2*). Here, B cells in different stages of development can be identified based upon their phenotype and function. The progression from one stage of B cell differentiation to the next is tightly regulated and, as will be described below, early B cell development is dependent on the orchestrated control of sequential immunoglobulin gene rearrangements and the expression of receptors, cell surface markers, and other gene products leading to survival, proliferation, and further differentiation. As knowledge of the structure of the immunoglobulins rapidly developed over the past several decades, an equally impressive body of information on the genetic basis of antibody production has been gained in more recent years.

Antigen-Independent B Cell Development

B Cells Are Generated in the Bone Marrow in the Absence of Specific Antigen

In the **antigen-independent phase**, a hematopoietic stem cell undergoes a series of divisions, giving rise to the generation of a large and diverse repertoire of daughter clones of B cells of increasing maturity, i.e., pro-B cell, pre-B cell, and immature B cell, characterized by the acquisition of certain surface markers, e.g., CD19 (*Appendix 3*) and ultimately with the expression of a cell surface IgM receptor (Figure 6-18). This sets the stage for the **antigen-dependent phase**, during which the binding of antigen to the surface immunoglobulin in peripheral lymphoid tissues leads to a series of proliferative and differentiative

Box 6-5

Various Types of Tyrosine Kinase Molecules Found in B Cells and T Cells

Kinases are enzymes that are phosphorylases that catalyze phosphorylation reactions (of amino acids) and fall into several groups and families, e.g., those that phosphorylate the amino acids serine and threonine, those that phosphorylate tyrosine, and some that can phosphorylate both. A tyrosine kinase is an enzyme that functions as a phosphorylase that can transfer a phosphate group from ATP to a tyrosine residue in a protein. By regulating critical enzyme activities, phosphorylation of proteins by kinases is an important mechanism in signal transduction for critical cellular processes. Tyrosine kinases are a subgroup of more than 1,000 protein kinases encoded within seven major groups recently mapped within the the "human kinome" (i.e., the set of protein kinases contained within the genome of an organism). Prominent among these are the Src family kinases (SFKs), a group of signaling enzymes originally described as a viral oncogene harbored within the Rous sarcoma virus that are now recognized to regulate critical cellular processes such as proliferation, survival, migration, and metastasis. SFKs are comprised of nine structurally related molecules, viz., Src, Blk, Fyn, Yes, Lyn, Lck, Hck, Fgr, and Yrk, with conserved peptide domains, termed Src homology (SH) domains. These kinases are not only important in the signaling pathways of B cells (Figure 6-17) but also for T cells (*Chapter 7*). The clinical relevance of these molecules has become particularly apparent in the last decade, as numerous examples of the aberrant activation of "normal" Src proteins have been associated with pathologic processes seen originally in malignancy but also in allergic diseases and autoimmune disorders and immune deficiencies. Since the kinases are a major control point in cell behavior, they have become a major target for new drug development not only in cancer therapeutics but also in these other immunologically mediated diseases. A number of specific tyrosine kinase inhibitors have been identified with the potential to interrupt signaling pathways and thus limit the proliferation of aberrant or dysfunctional cells as well as their activation through specific receptors (*Chapter 11*). A deficiency of a Bruton tyrosine kinase was identified as the cause of x-linked agammaglobulinemia (*Chapter 16*).

steps leading ultimately to the terminal differentiation of the B cell into plasma cell, the source of secreted immunoglobulin (Figure 6-18). Deletion of autoreactive B lymphocytes and tolerance induction occurs during B cell development during the antigen-independent phase (*Chapter 19*).

The B Cell is Both an Antigen Presenting Cell (APC) and an Immunoglobulin-Secreting Effector Cell

In the antigen-dependent phases of the immunoglobulin production, the B cell displays an extraordinarily unique two-fold function: 1) as an antigen presenting cell (APC) that can process antigen without T cell help (e.g., polysaccharide antigens) or with T cell help (e.g., protein antigens); and 2) in its terminally-differentiated plasma cell form, it functions as an immunoglobulin secreting cell (Figure 6-14).

The Genes Responsible for Immunoglobulin Synthesis Must Be First Assembled in the Developing B Cell

The genes responsible for immunoglobulin synthesis are found in all cells of the body arranged in **gene segments**, sequentially situated along the chromosome, each of which is responsible for the synthesis of a specific piece of the immunoglobulin molecule, i.e., the V and C portions of both the light and heavy chains. These segments occur at considerable distance from one another and therefore cannot be readily joined and be functionally expressed. The immunoglobulin genes found in these segments are inherited through a germ line configuration. It is during the **antigen-independent phase** seen in the B cell that the process of gene rearrangement of the scattered gene segments into a functional gene (i.e., **gene rearrangement, somatic recombination**) occurs which is required for expression of the gene product, i.e., surface IgM and IgD. This process of gene rearrangement continues into the antigen-dependent phase, when antigen is encountered during which immunoglobulin genes undergo additional genetic modifications (**somatic mutation and isotype switching**) (Figure 6-18).

During the antigen-independent phase, a library of antigen-binding sites on B cells is actually generated by the process of immunoglobulin gene rearrangement prior to any antigen encounter (Figure 6-18). Each B lymphocyte produces antibodies of single epitope specificity dictated by the sequence of rearranged genes. The size of the library of antigen-binding sites is limited both by the number of B cells as well as by the variety of rearranged immunoglobulin genes found in the body at any one time. As new B cells replace old B cells, the antigen-binding sites found in the library change. Clones of B cells bearing BCRs specific for a particular antigen are then stimulated to proliferate upon exposure to that antigen during the **antigen-specific phase**, which ultimately culminates in the sequential

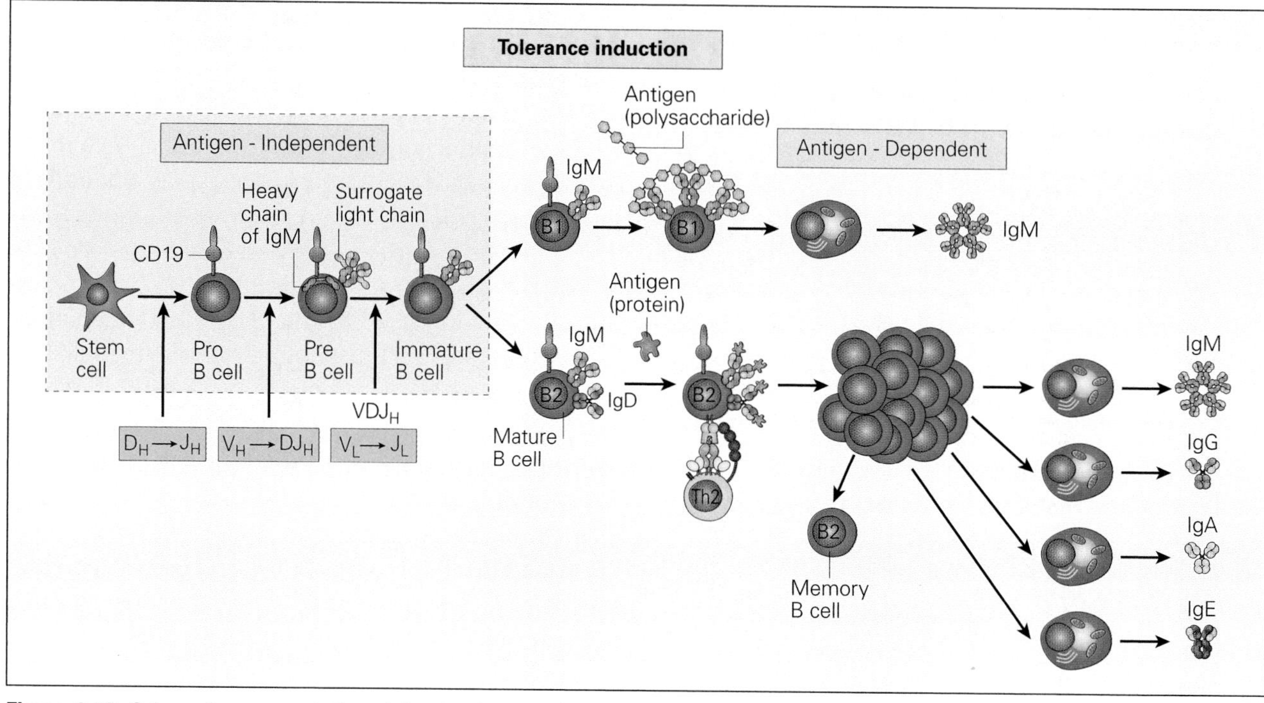

Figure 6-18. Schematic representation of the developmental stages of B cells showing the antigen-independent and antigen-dependent phases. Deletion of autoreactive B lymphocytes and tolerance induction occurs during B cell development. During the antigen-independent phase, gene rearrangement ($D_H \rightarrow J_H$; $V_H \rightarrow DJ_H$; and $V_L \rightarrow J_L$) occurs prior to any antigen encounter. During the antigen-dependent phase, thymic-independent antigens (i.e., polysaccharides) react with B1 lymphocytes without Th2 help to form predominantly IgM antibody; the B2 lymphocytes that react with thymic-dependent antigens (i.e., proteins) require Th2 help for isotype switching and somatic mutation of V_H/V_L genes to produce switching from IgM→IgG→IgA→IgE antibody.

production of IgM, IgG, IgA, and IgE during isotype switching, as will be described below. How is the immune system able to generate literally millions of different antigen-binding sites during the antigen-independent phase? The answer lies in the genes that specify the light and the heavy chain genes.

Genes for Heavy, Kappa, and Lambda Chains Are Located on Three Separate Human Chromosomes

In humans, the immunoglobulin genes are found at three chromosomal locations: (1) the κ LC locus on chromosome 2; (2) the λ LC on chromosome 22; and (3) the HC locus found on chromosome 14. Shown in Figure 6-19 is a schematic representation of chromosomal locations of these various gene loci together with the chromosomal arrangement of gene loci in the germ line, followed by gene rearrangement and protein synthesis of the immunoglobulin molecule in the subsequent antigen-dependent phase.

Shown in Table 6-8 are the major genetic loci that control the synthesis of various segments of the immunoglobulin globulin. These include heavy chain, light chain kappa, and lambda chain loci. Also shown in this table is the paired box5 (**PAX5**) gene, which is a member of the paired box (**PAX**) family of transcription factors, a set of a novel, highly conserved DNA-binding motifs that encode proteins that are important regulators in early development, and which when altered are thought to contribute to neoplastic transformation, e.g., lymphomas. The PAX5 gene encodes the B cell lineage specific activator protein (**BSAP**) that is expressed at early, but not at late stages of B cell differentiation. Its expression not only is important in B cell differentiation, but also in neural development and spermatogenesis.

The Genes That Encode the Light Chains

The genes that encode the antibody LC are located on chromosomes 2 and 22 within the immunoglobulin kappa locus (**IGK@**) and immunoglobulin lambda locus (**IGL@**), respectively, and are shown in Table 6-8 and Figure 6-19. Within the gene encoding a light chain, the genetic information is divided into segments called exons. One exon contains the genetic information that specifies the leader [L] (or signal) peptide. The two types of gene segments that encode the light-chain V region are called V_L and J gene segments. The V exon or

Table 6-8. Major gene loci, chromosomal locations, and functions of gene products involved in immunoglobulin synthesis

Locus	Name	Chromosomal location	Gene product/function
IGH@	Immunoglobulin heavy locus	14	Encodes heavy chains of human Ig
IGK@	Immunoglobulin kappa locus	2	Encodes kappa (κ) light chains of Ig
IGKC	Immunoglobulin kappa constant group		Encodes kappa (C) constant chains of Ig
IGKJ@	Immunoglobulin kappa joining group		Encodes kappa (J) joining chains of Ig
IGKV@	Immunoglobulin kappa variable group		Encodes kappa (V) variable chains of Ig
IGL@	Immunoglobulin lambda locus	22	Encodes lambda (λ) light chains of Ig
IGLC@	Immunoglobulin lambda constant group		Encodes lambda (C) constant chains of Ig
IGLJ@	Immunoglobulin lambda joining group		Encodes lambda (J) joining chains of Ig
IGLV@	Immunoglobulin lambda variable group		Encodes lambda (V) variable chains of Ig

segment specifies most of the V region of the LC, a small exon called the J exon specifies the last approximately ten amino acids of the V region, and a C exon specifies the constant region of the LC. The exons are separated by introns.

The Genes That Encode the Heavy Chains

The gene segments encoding the HC are found on chromosome 14 within the immunoglobulin heavy chain locus (**IGH@**) (shown in Table 6-8 and Figure 6-19) and are similar to those encoding the light chain. As with the light chain gene loci, there are multiple gene segments that encode the variable region of heavy chains (V_H). The heavy chain locus, however, includes an additional set of diversity (**D**) gene segments that are found between the V and J gene segments. The HC locus contains approximately fifty-one V gene segments each also preceded by a leader exon. There are about twenty-seven D segments, and six J segments that are followed by the constant region exons of each of the classes and subclasses of heavy chain beginning with mu (μ), then delta (δ), and then followed by the others. This is the germ line gene organization (Figure 6-19).

The Diversity of Antibody Variable Regions Is Generated by Somatic Recombination

During the development of B cells in the antigen-independent phase, the arrays of V, D, and J segments are cut and joined by DNA recombination (Figure 6-19). This process is called somatic recombination because it occurs in cells of the soma (from the Greek word *soma*, which means body) a term that encompasses all of the body cells except the germ cells. Outlined in Figure 6-19 are the events occurring during the synthesis of an immunoglobulin molecule showing both the germ line genes and the phases of rearrangement at both the LC and HC loci.

Temporal Order of Gene Rearrangement for Light and Heavy Chains

The rearrangement of gene segments required for the synthesis of light and heavy chains of an immunoglobulin follows an ordered process and occurs in a sequential fashion (Figure 6-19). Rearrangement at the HC locus (chromosome 14) takes place first prior to rearrangement of the LC locus. Rearrangement starts at the LC only after a complete HC is produced. The process begins at the pro-B cell stage with the joining of one D and one J_H gene segment at the heavy-chain locus on chromosome 14 to form a DJ_H gene. Any residual DNA between these two genes is deleted. Rearrangement occurs randomly and can engage any of several combinatorial possibilities involving the joining of any of the twenty-seven D segments with one of the six J joining segments. This is next followed by the joining of one of the fifty-one upstream V_H segments with the DJ_H complex, forming a rearranged VDJ_H gene. All other genes between the V and D segments of the newly formed VDJ_H gene are removed. A primary transcript is next generated containing the VDJ region of the heavy chain and both the constant mu (μ) and delta (δ) chains (C_μ and C_δ) (i.e., the primary transcript contains the segments V-D-J-C_μ-C_δ). The primary RNA is processed to not only add a polyadenylation (**poly-A**) tail at the end of the C_μ chain but also to remove sequence between the VDJ segment and this constant gene segment. Translation of this mRNA leads to the production of the Ig μ heavy chain protein.

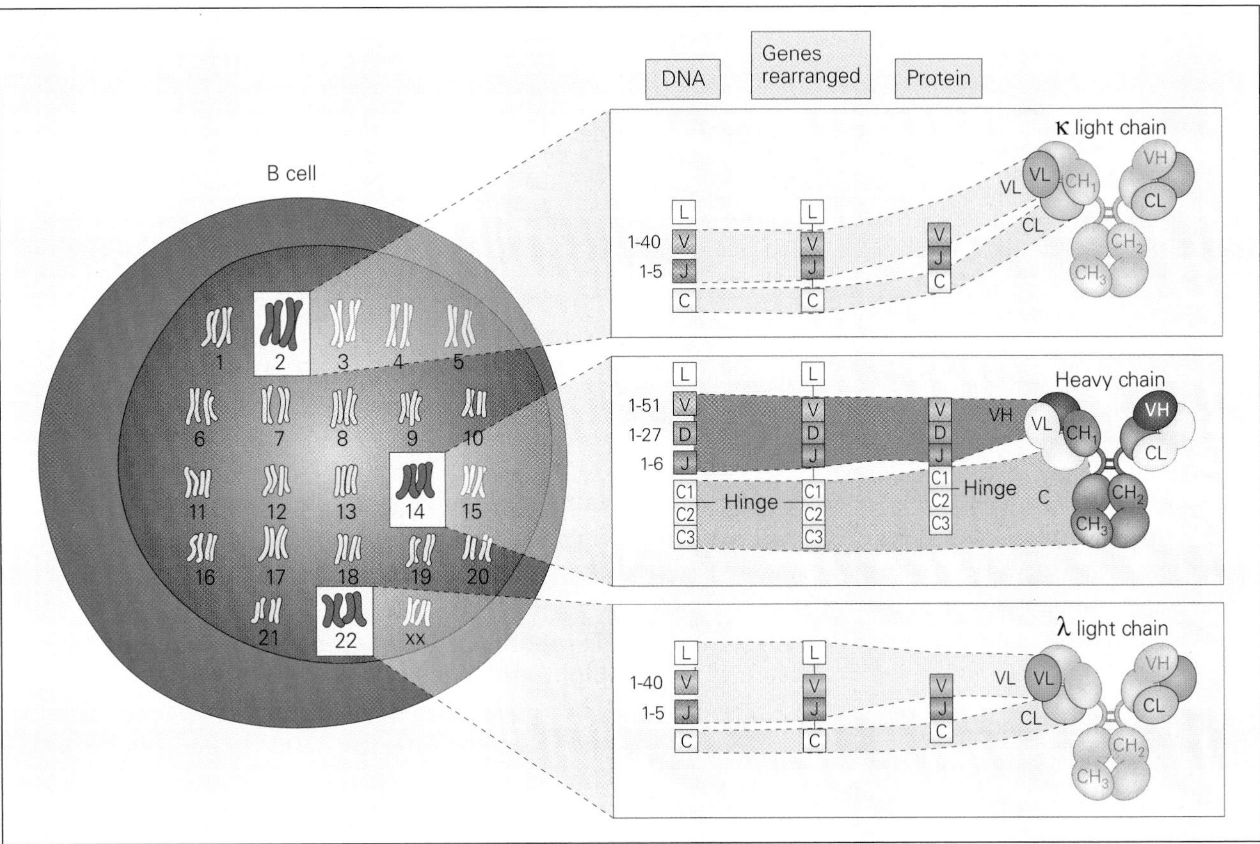

Figure 6-19. Schematic representation of the chromosomal locations of genetic loci, which control immunoglobulin synthesis together with the progressive steps of gene rearrangement, transcription, and translation involved in the synthesis and assembly of the various parts of an immunoglobulin molecule. The loci for light chains are found on chromosome 2 (kappa) and chromosome 22 (lambda) and for the heavy chain on chromosome 14.

The rearrangement at the LC loci takes place next, first at the kappa (chromosome 2) and later at the lambda locus (chromosome 22). The kappa (κ) and lambda (λ) chains of the immunoglobulin light chain loci rearrange in a very similar way, except the light chains lack a D segment. The first step of recombination for the light chains involves the joining of the V and J_L chains to give a VJ_L complex before the addition of the constant chain gene during primary transcription. Translation of the spliced mRNA for either the kappa or lambda chains results in the formation of the Igκ or Igλ light chain protein, respectively. Assembly of the Ig μ heavy chain and one of the light chains results in the formation of the fully assembled membrane bound form of the immunoglobulin IgM that is expressed on the surface of the immature B cell (Figure 6-18). A schematic representation of the temporal order by which these events occur in the synthesis of immunoglobulins and class switching is summarized in Figure 6-27.

Mechanisms of Recombination

Somatic recombination of specific DNA sequences that encode the synthesis of the various components of the light and heavy chains is carried out by an amazing sequence of enzymatic events that cuts and joins the DNA employing many of the mechanisms more ubiquitously utilized by cells in general for DNA recombination and repair.

Recombination Enzymes Recognize Specific DNA Sequences Adjoining the V, D, and J Segments

The recombination of V, D, and J gene segments is carried out by a process called variable (diversity) joining [**V(D)J**] recombination and is directed by sequences called recombination signal sequences (**RSSs**) that flank the 3′ side of V segment, both sides of the D segment, and the 5′ side of the J segment (Figure 6-20).

The RSSs that flank these segments are of two types: (1) a heptamer of seven conserved nucleotides that are found directly next to each of the V, D, and

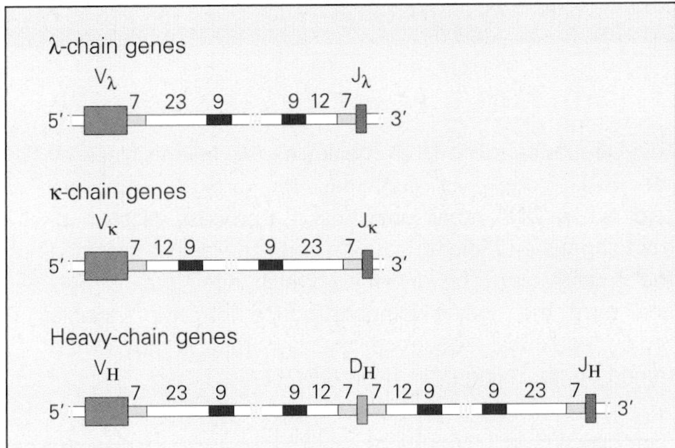

Figure 6-20. Each V, D, or J gene segment is flanked by recombination signal sequences (RSSs). Two types of RSS exist. One RSS consists of a nonamer (9 bp, shown in red) and a heptamer (7 bp, shown in yellow) separated by a spacer of 12 bp (white). The other RSS consists of the same 9- and 7- nucleotide sequences separated by a 23 bp spacer (white).

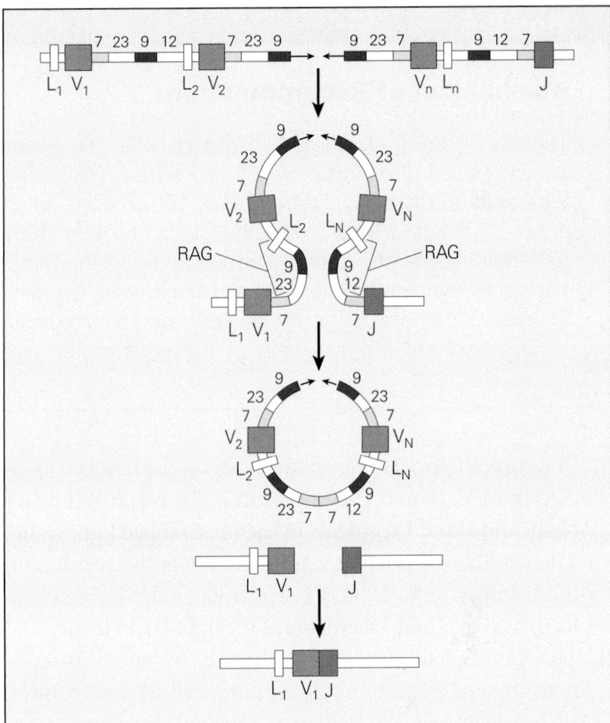

Figure 6-21. Gene segments encoding the variable region are joined to a segment containing a joining (J) region by recombination at RSSs following the formation of a hairpin loop and subsequent excision of a circular segment.

J genes encoding both light chains and heavy chains; followed by (2) a nonamer composed of nine conserved nucleotides separated by a spacer region containing either twelve or twenty-three unconserved nucleotides (Figure 6-21). The spacers are found regularly alternating and in between the heptamers and nonamers of the V, D, and J, and this molecular configuration directs and assures that the recombination of gene segments will occur efficiently and without error. Thus, only a pair of RSSs with a dissimilar spacer can be recombined, i.e., an RSS with a spacer of twelve nucleotides can only be recombined with an RSS containing twenty-three nucleotides. This is known as the **12/23 rule of recombination.**

V(D)J Recombinase

The set of enzymes needed to recombine V, D, and J segments is generically called V(D)J recombinase. Some of these enzymes are lymphocyte-specific, and others are expressed in many cell types. Two of the key enzymes made only in lymphocytes and which are critical for V(D)J recombination are recombination activating gene-1 and recombination activating gene-2 (**RAG-1** and **RAG-2**). These enzymes associate with each other to recognize the RSS sequences and induce DNA cleavage at the RSS sequences. This cleavage takes place on only one strand of DNA, which leads to a nucleotide attack and creation of a hairpin loop (Figure 6-21). The mechanism of recombination is shown in Box 6-6. The other component enzymes are present in all nucleated cells and include enzymatic activities to repair double-stranded DNA, bend DNA, or modify the ends of broken DNA strands. They include the enzymes DNA ligase IV, DNA-dependent protein kinase (**DNA-PK**), and the Ku protein associated with DNA-PK. Both in the human and mice, deficiency of RAG-1 or RAG-2 results in the inability to rearrange Ig and TCR genes, causing a severe combined immunodeficiency characterized by absence of B and T cells called the Omenn syndrome (*Chapter 16*).

Generation of the Antibody Repertoire Is Accomplished by Combinatorial and Junctional Diversity Produced During Gene Rearrangement

The diversity of the antibody repertoire is an indispensable requirement for B cells, which have the function to recognize all the possible antigens that they may encounter in the periphery. This variability in immunoglobulin generation is caused by differences occurring during V–J, V–D, and J–J joining and is referred to as junctional diversity (Figure 6-22). Several mechanisms contribute to the diversity of the antibody repertoire generated in the bone marrow, including:

Box 6-6

Mechanism of Recombination

The first step of recombination occurs when one RAG complex binds to one type of RSS and another RAG complex binds to the second type of RSS (Figure 6-21). Interaction of the two RAG complexes aligns the two RSSs and then cleaves the DNA within the ends of the immunoglobulin gene segments. This process creates a single-stranded DNA "hairpin" at the end of each immunoglobulin segment and a clean break at the ends of the two RSS sequences. The DNA molecules are held in place by the RAG complexes, whereas the broken ends are rejoined by DNA repair enzymes in a process called non-homologous-end joining to form both the signal joint and the coding joint. The enzymes, which open the hairpins and form the coding joint, introduce into the variable region additional sequence diversity that is not determined by germ line DNA (Figure 6-21).

1. The combinatorial diversity depends on the random association of V, D, and J segments in each rearranged heavy chain and V and J segments in each rearranged light chain. The number of possible combinations is the product of the number of V, D, and J segments at the heavy chain locus and of V and J segments at the light chain locus.
2. The junctional diversity, generated by the imprecise rearrangement and to the addition of N nucleotides, adds a factor of 3×10^7 to the overall diversity.
3. In addition to the mechanisms described above, which act at the genetic level, the combination of the recombined heavy and light chains into an antigen-bindng site contributes to the generation of antibody diversity. This is an important source of immunoglobulin variability, adding a factor of 3×10^7 to the overall diversity. It can, however, result in frame-shift mutations that introduce stop codons and no synthesis of functional Ig chains, called nonproductive

A Lymphoid Progenitor Cell Becomes Committed to the B Cell Lineage When It Recombines Immunoglobulin Genes

The generation of cells of the B lineage from HSC is controlled by the combined action of transcription factors, which act in a precise temporal order, regulating distinct developmental aspects. Several transcription factors cooperate to activate the B cell gene expression program and HC locus rearrangement and, at the same time, inhibit the expression of non-B cell molecules (Figure 6-23).

The PAX5 gene is a member of the PAX family of transcription factors. PAX5 is expressed at early stages of B cell differentiation. Its expression is also detected in developing CNS and testis. PAX5 may not only play an important role in B cell differentiation, but also in neural development and spermatogenesis. This gene is located in chromosome 9p13 region, which is involved in t(9;14)(p13;q32) translocations recurring in small lymphocytic lymphomas of the plasmacytoid subtype, and in derived large-cell lymphomas. This translocation brings the potent E-mu enhancer of the IgH gene into close proximity of the PAX5 promoters. Deregulation of PAX5 gene transcription may contribute to the pathogenesis of these lymphomas.

The binding of the available transcription factors to their target DNA sequences is also regulated and dependent upon the structure of the local chromatin, which controls the accessibility of the transcription factor's binding sites.

The Developing B Cell Must Express a Pre-B Cell Receptor to Continue B Cell Development

B cell development is a process tightly regulated by the orchestrated signalling of cytokine receptors, the pre-B cell receptor, and the BCR. It commences with common lymphoid progenitors (**CLP**) up-regulating the expression of B cell-related genes and committing to the B cell lineage. Cytokine signalling (IL-7, stem cell factor, and FLT3-L) is essential at this stage of development, as it suppresses cell death, sustains proliferation, and facilitates heavy-chain rearrangements. As a result of heavy-chain recombination, the pre-BCR is expressed (Figure 6-24). Since the light-chain genes have not yet been recombined, the heavy chain is expressed on the B cell surface with **surrogate light chain**, a non-disulfide linked molecule of VpreB and λ5, as well as the signal transduction molecules Igα and Igβ.

Expression of a pre-BCR determines whether somatic recombination will stop or proceed. A successful (productive) heavy-chain gene rearrangement resulting in the synthesis of a functional pre-BCR stops VH to DJH rearrangement, and the pre-B cell begins to divide into a clone of cells, all expressing the same H chain. Pro-B cells, in which

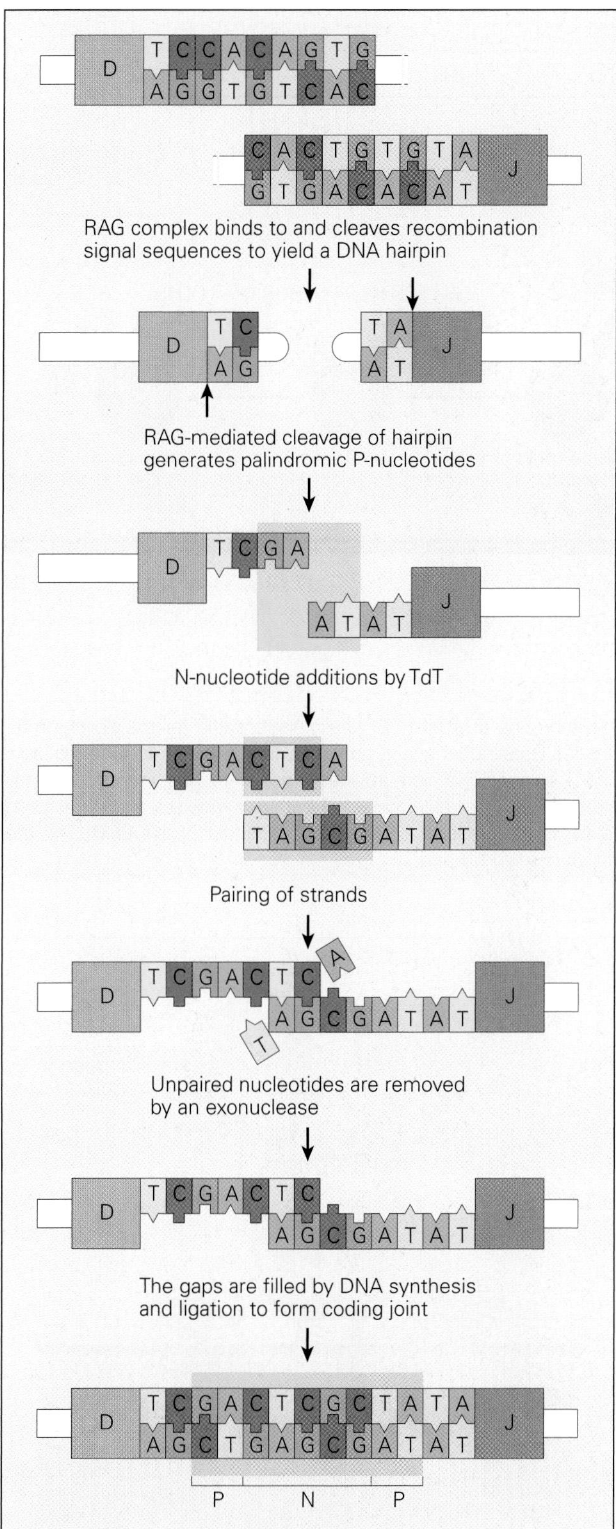
D
J
RAG complex binds to and cleaves recombination signal sequences to yield a DNA hairpin
RAG-mediated cleavage of hairpin generates palindromic P-nucleotides
N-nucleotide additions by TdT
Pairing of strands
Unpaired nucleotides are removed by an exonuclease
The gaps are filled by DNA synthesis and ligation to form coding joint
P
N
P

Figure 6-22. Schematc representation of the generation of junctional diversity during gene rearrangement.

Box 6-7

Lineage Specificity

The generation of cells of the B lineage from HSC is controlled by the combined action of several transcription factors, which act in a precise temporal order, regulating distinct developmental aspects. The generation of the earliest B cell progenitor, the pro-B cell, depends on the cooperation of the transcription factors E2A and EBF, which activate the B cell gene expression program and HC locus rearrangement (Figure 6-23). Therefore, effective rearrangement of Ig genes only occurs in cells of the B lineage. Strong molecular and genetic evidence indicates that E2A and EBF cooperatively regulate the expression of molecules indispensable for rearrangement, assembling, and signaling function of the BCR. These molecules include the RAG-1 and RAG-2 enzymes, the surrogate light chains (λ5 and VpreB), which substitute the LC in the pre-BCR, and the BCR signaling components Igα and Igβ (Figure 6-24). In addition, E2A and EBF function in concert with RAG-1 and RAG-2 to activate DH to JH rearrangement. The events induced by E2A and EBF are not sufficient to determine the commitment of progenitors to the B lineage. The critical commitment factor is another transcription factor, PAX5, also known as B cell specific activator protein (BSAP). PAX5 restricts the developmental options of early progenitors to the B cell pathway. Pro-B cells deficient for PAX5 express B cell-specific protein and initiate D_H-J_H recombination, but retain the potential to differentiate into NK cells, macrophages, dendritic cells, osteoclasts, and granulocytes *in vitro* and even T cells *in vivo*. PAX5 maintains B cell identity from the pro-B to the mature B cell stage by two mechanisms. On one side, it represses the expression of lineage-inappropriate genes, and on the other, activates genes encoding signaling molecules indispensable for B cells, such as the BCR signaling component Igα, the adaptor molecule BLNK, and the co-stimulatory receptor CD19. In addition, PAX5 plays a role in the V_H-to-DJ_H recombination process by promoting the contraction of chromatin, which results in the juxtaposition of distal V_H genes to proximal D_HJ_H rearranged gene segments. PAX5 expression terminates at the plasma cell stage, when the BCR and its signal transduction machinery are not necessary anymore and the function of B cells is restricted to antibody secretion (Figure 6-23).

the rearrangements at the heavy region locus are nonproductive (no heavy chain is synthesized, perhaps because of an introduced stop codon), can undergo somatic recombination at the H chain locus of the other chromosome. Cells with non-productive rearrangements at both H chain loci cannot produce H chain and pre-BCR, are unable to receive this signal, and are eliminated by apoptosis.

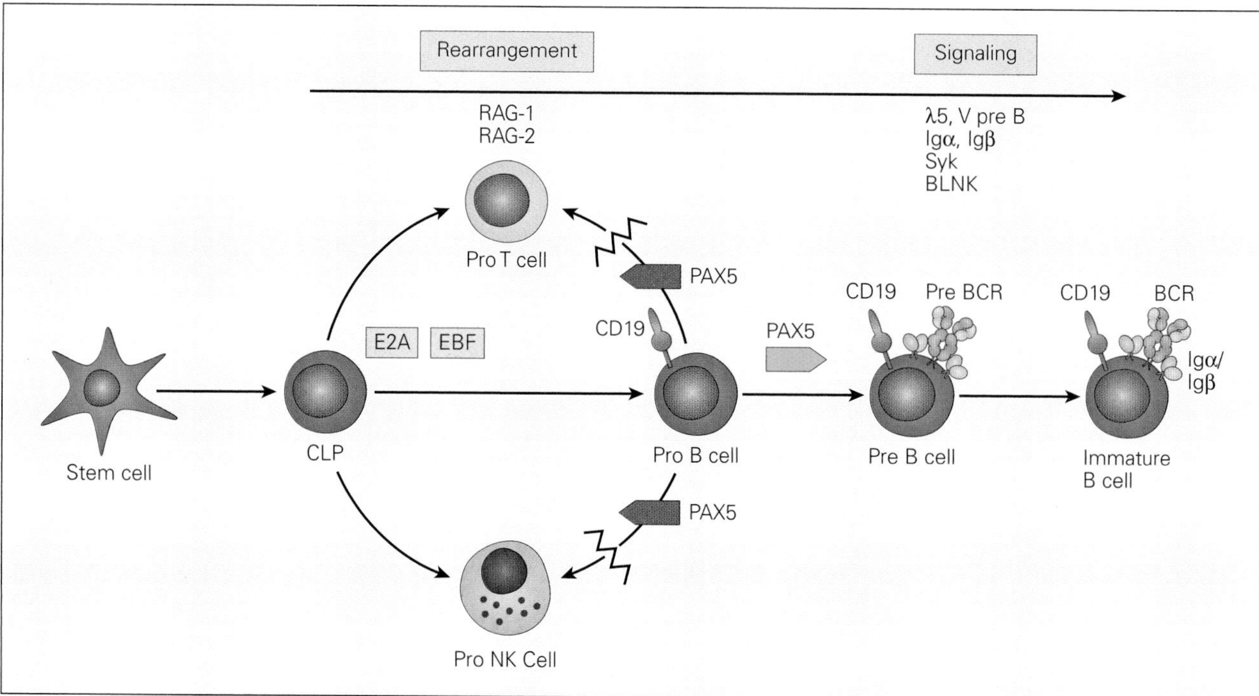

Figure 6-23. Transcription factors regulate the early stages of B cell development. E2A and EBF are indispensable for the development of pro-B cells from the common lymphocyte precursor (CLP). PAX5 maintains B cell identity and prevents differentiation to other lineages by inhibiting (red arrow) the expression of non-B cell molecules at the pro-B stage. PAX5 also provides a positive signal in the differentiation of the pro-B cell to the mature B cell stage (green arrow). Progression along the developmental pathway requires the induction of factors necessary for the rearrangement of immunoglobulin genes and for the expression and signaling function of the BCR. The pre-BCR is composed of a rearranged HC associated with the surrogate light chains, VpreB and λ5.

Allelic Exclusion Results from the Expression of Only One Parental H Chain Locus and One Parental Light-Chain Locus in Each B Cell

One of the most interesting features of immunoglobulin synthesis is that only one immunoglobulin heavy-chain gene (located on chromosome 14) or light-chain gene (located on chromosome 2 or 22) from one of the two homologous parental chromosomes in a B lymphocyte is functional at any given time, a phenomenon referred to as allelic exclusion (Figure 6-25). Recombination of V(D)J gene segments, described previously, takes place initially on only one of the two homologous alleles on chromosome 14 and is followed by the rearrangement of a functional light-chain gene from either chromosome 2 or 22. When rearrangement of one heavy gene occurs productively, the other allele on the second chromosome is silenced. If no successful rearrangement occurs, rearrangement takes place on the second chromosome. If no successful rearrangement occurs on either chromosome, the cell dies by apoptosis. Involvement of the chromosomes is random; in one cell, the paternal allele may be active, and in another, it may be the maternal allele. The

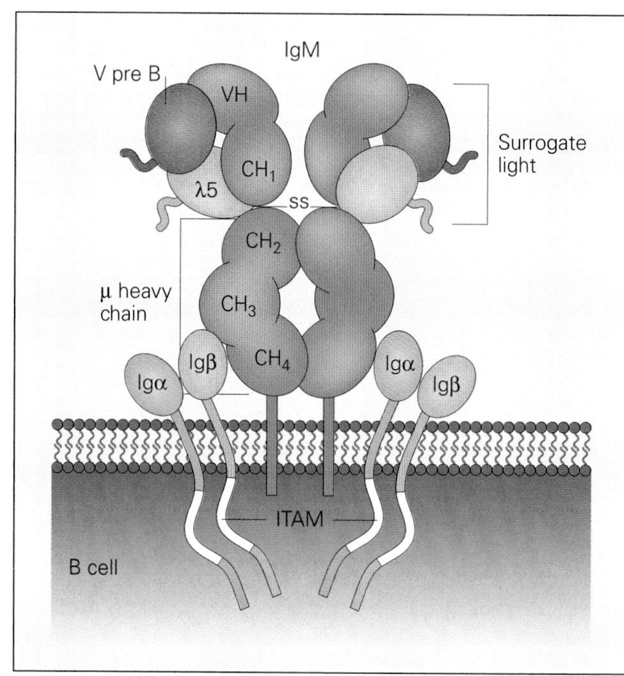

Figure 6-24. Schematic representation of the pre-B receptor structure. Since the light chain genes have not yet been recombined, the heavy chain is expressed on the B cell surface with the surrogate light chain (shown in red), a non-disulfide-linked molecule of VpreB, and λ5, as well as with the signal transduction molecules Igα and Igβ.

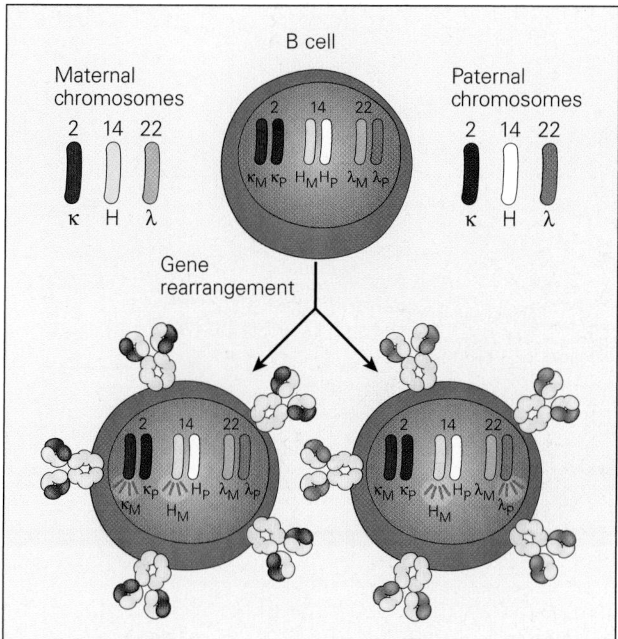

Figure 6-25. Schematic representation of allelic exclusion showing the restriction of membrane-associated immunoglobulin produced by a single B cell derived from maternal and paternal gene segments encoding κ, λ, and heavy-chain segments. The restriction is illustrated by the requirement of the association of the product of only one functionally rearranged LC locus with the product of one functionally rearranged HC locus (represented by glowing of the activated alleles on chromosomes 2, 22, and 14, respectively). If more than one locus would be rearranged functionally, then each B cell would express a mixture of antibodies. This is prevented by allelic exclusion.

process of allelic exclusion results in the synthesis of immunoglobulin molecules with identical V regions in each single plasma cell because all of the expressed mRNA will have been derived from a single rearranged chromosome 14 and from a single rearranged chromosome 2 or 22. Therefore, the antibodies produced by each lymphocyte will be of a single specificity.

Light Chain VJ Recombination Follows Successful H Chain Recombination

Once a cell has successfully expressed pre-BCR and proliferated into clone of pre-B cells with productively recombined H chain genes, recombinases are again re-expressed and the cells randomly join V and J gene segments on the kappa chain locus. Expression of a light chain with the H chain signals the B cell to stop expressing recombinase; at this stage it is called an **immature B cell** and has expressed IgM on its membrane. If the VJ joining is nonproductive at the first kappa locus, the kappa locus on the other chromosome is recombined. If that too is nonproductive (no kappa chain is synthesized), recombination occurs on one (and if necessary, the second) lambda chain locus. The cell may either express μ2κ2 IgM or μ2λ2 IgM. In humans, roughly half of antibodies have kappa chains and half have lambda light chains. The expression of the same μ chain variable region with different κ or λ chain variable regions results in many different antigen-combining regions resulting from the original successful H chain recombination.

Tolerance Induction Results from Self-Antigen Binding to the Immature B Cell IgM

Although there are beneficial effects of somatic recombination at several stages of B cell development from a wide range of possibilities leading to the large diversity of the antibody repertoire which determines the specificity of the BCR, the random events occurring during rearrangement and assembling of the BCR are not always useful and, at times, are dangerous, and may lead to the production of autoreactive B cells responsible for autoimmune disease (*Chapter 19*). Elimination of these potentially damaging specificities (negative selection) is ensured by two mechanisms: (1) clonal deletion and (2) receptor editing (Figure 6-26). The first consists of apoptosis, the mechanism by which clonal deletion of unwanted autoreactive B cells occurs and which is the main mechanism regulating tolerance to membrane-bound antigens. Ligation of the BCR on an immature B cell associated with a strong BCR-mediated signal at the immature B cell stage causes apoptosis and eliminates dangerous clonal autoreactive B cells, resulting in the prevention of autoimmunity.

Receptor editing is the second mechanism that eliminates auto-reactivity without cell loss. It has been demonstrated that secondary rearrangements occurring at the kappa locus can produce a new LC, able to replace an autoreactive one. If the rearrangement is still not productive or again generates autoreactivity, the kappa locus is inactivated and recombination starts on the lambda locus. The relative contribution of clonal deletion and editing to the establishment of tolerance is still a matter of debate.

As shown in Figure 6-26, the development of B cells proceeds by a series of defined steps, from progenitor to pro-B cell to pre-B cell to immature B cells. The parenchyma of the bone marrow consists of a dense stromal cell network extending from the endosteum to the endothelial cell basement membrane of the sinusoids, in which developing

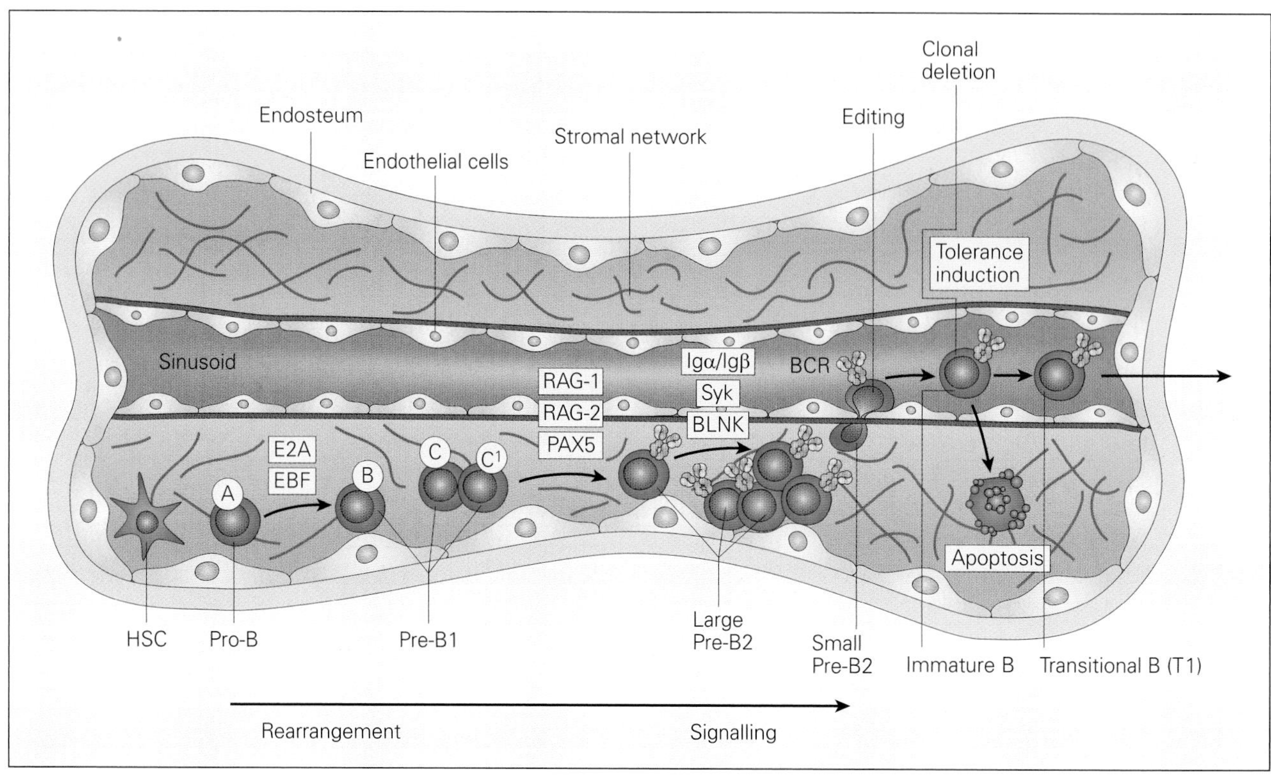

Stage of development	Pro-B cell Part A	Pre-B1 cell Part B	Pre-B1 cell Part C-C′	Large Pre-B2	Small Pre-B2	Immature B	Transitional B (T1)
HC locus	GL	DJ	VDJ	VDJ	VDJ	VDJ	VDJ
LC locus	GL	GL	GL	GL	J	VJ	VJ
BCR expression	None	None	None	Pre-BCR	Pre-BCR	BCR low	BCR high

Figure 6-26. The progression of B cells during their developmental pathway, from HSC to transitional 1 (T1) B cells, is shown. Cells of the B lineage in different stages of development are depicted on the stromal cell network. The vertical lines indicate selection checkpoints identified by the use of mice that are genetically deficient for the indicated molecules. The initiation and success of rearrangement are indispensable requirements at the pro- and pre-B1 stage; the expression and signaling functions of the BCR become the most important criteria of selection at the pre-B2 stage and thereafter. After editing, clonal deletion with elimination of autoreactive B cells by apoptosis takes place, resulting in tolerance induction. The rearrangement status at the heavy (HC) and light-chain (LC) loci are indicated. The pre-BCR is composed of the μHC associated to the surrogate LCs Vpre-B and λ5. Interleukin 7 is the most important cytokine in the bone marrow, regulating survival at the pro-B stage, and survival and proliferation of large pre-B2 cells.

cells of all hematopoietic lineages find their niches for differentiation and expansion. At their earliest stages of development, cells of the B lineage are located close to the endosteum, near the HSC from which they derive. Progenitor B cells developing toward the immature B cell stages progressively move in the direction of the central sinus, which represents the highway to the periphery. Immature B cells, which have survived negative selection, upregulate surface IgM, move inside the central sinus, and are transported with the blood to the periphery. At this stage of development, they are called transitional B cells. It has been suggested that negative selection by clonal deletion occurs only at this stage, whereas receptor editing is the mechanism of choice for the removal of autoreactive receptors in the parenchyma of the bone marrow (Figure 6-26).

B Cell Development Continues in the Periphery

It has been demonstrated that in the mouse, the late phases of B cell differentiation, from transitional to mature-naive B cells, take place in the spleen. This organ consists of two tissues, the red and the white pulp (*Chapter 2*). The red pulp is a reservoir of blood cells and the site where aged, damaged, or abnormal cells are removed. The white pulp consists of lymphoid tissue. Here, T cells are arranged in the T cell area around a central arteriole and make up the periarterial lymphatic sheath (**PALS**). B cells collect in the primary follicles surrounding the PALS and, externally to the follicles, in the marginal zone (**MZ**). Transitional B cells are found in the outer PALS, and mature B cells are located in the primary follicles. Differentiation, therefore, is associated with the acquisition of the ability to migrate to specialized lymphoid areas and is directed by different chemokines produced by the splenic microenvironment.

Transitional B cells are passively transported to the spleen and enter the red pulp via the terminal branches of the central arterioles. They rapidly move to the outer PALS, but are unable to enter the lymphoid follicle. B cells can enter the follicle at the next stage of maturation, the mature naive B cell stage. Mature B cells express a second membrane-bound immunoglobulin, IgD, in addition to IgM. Transitional B cells, as all their precursors in the bone marrow, are short-lived and functionally immature. Both longevity and functional competence are progressively acquired during the development of the transitional to the mature-naive stage.

As in the bone marrow, the signaling function of the BCR remains one of the most important criteria of selection also in the periphery. Analysis of mice with genetic mutations of various components of the BCR-signaling complex has demonstrated that an adequate BcR signal is indispensable for the development of transitional B cells and their further progression to the mature B cell stage. In general, mutation of the BCR proximal signal transduction **components** (**Igα, syk**) severely impairs signaling and causes a block of development in the bone marrow, with a severe reduction in the number of transitional B cells. In the human, this results in a severe form of agammaglobulinemia closely resembling X-linked agammaglobulinemia but inherited as an autosomal recessive disease (*Chapter 16*).

Antigen-Dependent B Cell Development

The second phase of B cell development is dependent on the interaction of B cells that emerge from the bone marrow with antigen in peripheral lymphoid tissues and is therefore referred to as the antigen-dependent phase (Figure 6-18). The introduction of an antigen (immunogen) into a host leads to the synthesis of antibody associated with various classes of immunoglobulin that make their appearance in a sequential, time-dependent manner. The antibodies formed early in the immune response are of IgM isotype, followed by IgG, IgA, or IgE antibody. Which isotype is produced depends on the nature of the antigen involved as well as the site of the antigen-lymphoid interaction in peripheral lymphoid tissues and the T cell signals received by the B cell.

The innate immune response (*Chapter 3*) and the process of inflammation (*Chapter 5*) result in antigen movement from the infection site to the draining lymph nodes as soluble antigen and also on the surface of dendritic cells. As the B cells enter the lymph nodes via the T cell areas, they encounter antigen, which binds to their BCR. BCR cross-linking by multiple repeating epitopes on the pathogen stimulates the B cell to begin proliferating. Some B cells at this stage become short-lived IgM secreting plasma cells. Most B cells endocytose their antigen-BCR complexes, process the antigen, and present it on their membranes in combination with MHC-II. In the same area of the lymph node, B cells encounter activated Th2 cells (*Chapter 7*). Antigen-stimulated B cells express membrane CD40; Th2 effector cells express membrane CD40L (ligand). The interaction of B cells and Th2 cells via the MHC-II/peptide complex of the APC with TCR/CD4 complexes on the Th2 cell (Figure 6-18) and the CD40/CD40 ligand costimulatory signal cause the Th2 cells to secrete cytokines that stimulate the B cell to proliferate and move to the B cell areas of the lymph nodes. There they form **germinal centers** of rapidly dividing B cells and, in response to cytokine signals from Th2 cells, undergo somatic hypermutation and isotype class switching (Box 6-8).

B Cell Activation May Occur in a T Cell–Dependent or T Cell–Independent Manner

In humoral immune responses, the activation of B lymphocytes can occur with or without the contribution of $CD4^+$ Th2 helper T cells (Figure 6-18). These responses are influenced by the nature of the antigens involved. Although both protein and nonprotein antigens can stimulate antibody responses, protein antigens require the participation of Th2 cells, whereas nonprotein antigens do not. Protein antigens are therefore referred to as T-dependent (**TD**)

Box 6-8

The Mechanism of Somatic Hypermutation and Class-Switch Recombination

The mechanism of SHM has remained elusive for many years. The long search for the "mutator" has lead to the discovery of activation-induced cytidine deaminase (AID). AID is specifically induced in activated B lymphocytes in the germinal centers and, surprisingly, carries out two entirely different reactions: somatic hypermutation (SHM) and class-switch recombination (CSR). AID acts on DNA of Ig variable regions and deaminates cytosine residues to uracil. As uracils are not normal constituents of DNA, during replication they are read as mistakes that have to be repaired. The result of the repair mechanism is a mutation. If the DNA-polymerase simply reads uracil as a thymine, there will be a C-to-T transition. The uracil can also be removed by the uracil DNA glycosylase (UNG), creating an abasic site that will be repaired creating transversions and transitions. If the mismatch repair is carried out by an error-prone patch-repair process, additional mutations are targeted to nearby sequences. During CSR, DNA lesions induced by AID are processed to induce double-strand breaks that are recognized by the cellular DNA damage-signaling pathway, including ATM, H2AX, and 53BP1. Blunt double-strand breaks can be ligated to similarly created breaks on downstream S-region DNA to complete class-switch recombination.

antigens, in contrast to nonprotein antigens, which are referred to as T-independent (**TI**) antigens. The most important TI antigens are polysaccharides, membrane glycolipids, and nucleic acids, all of which cannot be processed and presented by APCs in association with MHC molecules (*Chapter 10*); therefore, they cannot be recognized by helper T cells.

The clinical significance of these differences between TI and TD antibody responses is seen in several clinical applications. Since TI antigens comprise many bacterial cell-wall polysaccharides, humoral immunity to these antigens forms the major mechanism of protective immunity against infections caused by encapsulated bacteria such as the pneumococci, meningococci, and *Haemophilus influenzae* (*Chapter 12*). For this reason, individuals with congenital or acquired deficiencies of humoral immunity are especially susceptible to life-threatening infections caused by these encapsulated bacteria (*Chapter 16*). In addition, TI antigens contribute to the generation of **natural antibodies,** which are present in the circulation of normal individuals and are apparently produced without overt exposure to pathogens without the participation of Th2 cells. Antibodies to the A and B glycolipid blood group antigens are examples of these natural antibodies. Another clinical application of this knowledge is seen in the development and use of vaccines for the prevention of infections caused by bacterial pathogens (*Chapter 23*). Purified pneumococcal vaccines in clincal use are recommended for routine immunization of certain populations of children and adults. Although vaccines containing these purified TI polysaccharide antigens are capable of inducing protective antibody in older children and adults, they are not as effective in infants less than two years of age. In order to address this problem, the polysaccharides have been conjugated to protein antigens, thereby converting the TI polysaccharide-containing vaccine to a TD-conjugated vaccine. The use of these polysaccharide/proteins vaccines has shown great effectiveness in these younger, previously nonresponsive infants, and has represented a major technologic advance in the prevention of serious and often fatal infectons caused by these pathogenic bacteria.

Somatic Hypermutation Results in B Cells with Higher Affinity Antibodies for Antigen, Resulting in Affinity Maturation

The process of Ig gene rearrangement in the bone marrow generates approximately 10^{12} different specificities, which constitute the germ line repertoire. Several elements contribute to the variability of this repertoire, including the large number of V, D, and J genes, their random rearrangement, the additional sequences created by the DNA repair mechanisms, and finally the combination of HC and LC. The germ line repertoire is not selected and, therefore, is assumed to have a low affinity for antigen. During the immune response, few B cells, reacting to the antigen, will start to proliferate in the germinal centers. At this time, the introduction of random mutations into the variable region of Ig genes (somatic hypermutation, **SHM**) results in the generation of B cells carrying a new BCR, which may have a lower or higher affinity for the stimulating antigen or have acquired self-reactivity. The interaction with the antigen, trapped in immune complexes on the surface of follicular dendritic cells, selects the cells with the highest affinity, useful to the ongoing immune reaction. Only B cells able to bind the antigen will survive. All the other B cells, which are either useless because they are unable to bind antigen or are dangerous because they are autoreactive, will die in the germinal center. The germinal center reaction will generate plasma cells producing high affinity antibodies first of IgM and later of switched isotypes. Memory B cells carrying mutated and selected Ig genes will remain in the organism for a long time to prevent reinfection with the same pathogen.

This phenomenon of production of antibody of increased capacity for antigen binding is referred to as affinity maturation. The process of affinity maturation generates antibodies with increasing capacity to bind antigens and thus to more efficiently bind to, neutralize, and eliminate microbes. CD40:CD40L and helper Th2 cell interactions and cytokine production are required for affinity maturation to proceed, and therefore affinity maturation occurs only in antibody responses to helper T cell-dependent protein antigens. The contribution of CD40:CD40L interactions is described more fully in *Chapter 7*.

Isotype Class Switch Recombination Is Driven by T Cell Cytokines and Antigen

As described previously, the V_H-region exons expressed by a B cell are determined during early differentiation in the bone marrow in the antigen-independent phase, and no further V(D)J recombination occurs except for that which may happen by somatic hypermutation. In contrast, when B cell progeny mature and proliferate in lymphoid tissues during the antigen-dependent phase, different C-region genes can be expressed allowing for the synthesis of various immunoglobulin isotypes. This latter process occurs in a sequentially ordered fashion ultimately resulting in immunoglobulin production by plasma cells beginning with IgM synthesis followed by IgG, IgA, and IgE, a progression referred to as **isotype class switching**, which is dependent on the interaction with antigen and signals received through cytokines (*Chapter 9*). Shown in Figure 6-27 is a schematic representation of the mechanism of isotypic class switching, beginning with the binding of antigen to the surface IgM receptor, followed by signaling through a cascading set of transcription factors which then activate the expression of gene transcripts through DNA interactions to begin the synthesis of H chains on chromosome 14 and L chains on chromosomes 2 and 22 and final assembly and release of the component parts of the molecule into a complete immunoglobulin. The B cell begins this progression by expressing IgM as its B cell receptor together with IgD, which is expressed simultaneously in naive B cells but later deleted. IgM is the first antibody produced in an immune response that can occur with or without the help of Th2 cells. When antigen interacts with a B1 cell without Th2 cell help, a continued synthesis of IgM alone occurs with no isotype switching, in contrast to that which occurs when B2 cells receive signals through Th2 help, where the subsequent IgG, IgA IgE progression is seen (Figure 6-27).

Switching to other isotypes occurs through a specialized DNA recombination mechanism guided by stretches of repetitive DNA segments known as switch (S) regions which are found between the J_H and C_μ gene segments and at equivalent upstream sites for each of the other heavy-chain sites, with the exception of the δ gene (Figure 6-28). The absence of a switch region in the δ gene region site provides an explanation of why IgD switching does not occur during isotype switching. When a B cell switches from coexpression of IgM and IgD to the subsequent expression of an IgG subtype, DNA recombination occurs between the S_μ and S_γ and the C_μ and C_δ coding regions are deleted.

B Cell Activation and Antibody Production and the Antigen Antibody Reaction

Having described the structural features of immunoglobulins and the molecular events involved in their production in B cells at a cellular level, it may now be possible to briefly describe how these events relate to the production of antibody in the whole individual, together with the consequences of the antigen-antibody reaction.

General Features of Antibody Production in the Whole Individual

The Primary Immune Response

The introduction of an immunogen into a host may be the result of exposure to and subsequent infection by a microbe, a response to a vaccine, an encounter with an allergen responsible for allergic disease, a reaction to a self-antigen resulting in autoimmune disease, or to a cancer cell, all of which may lead to the production of antibody in the responding host

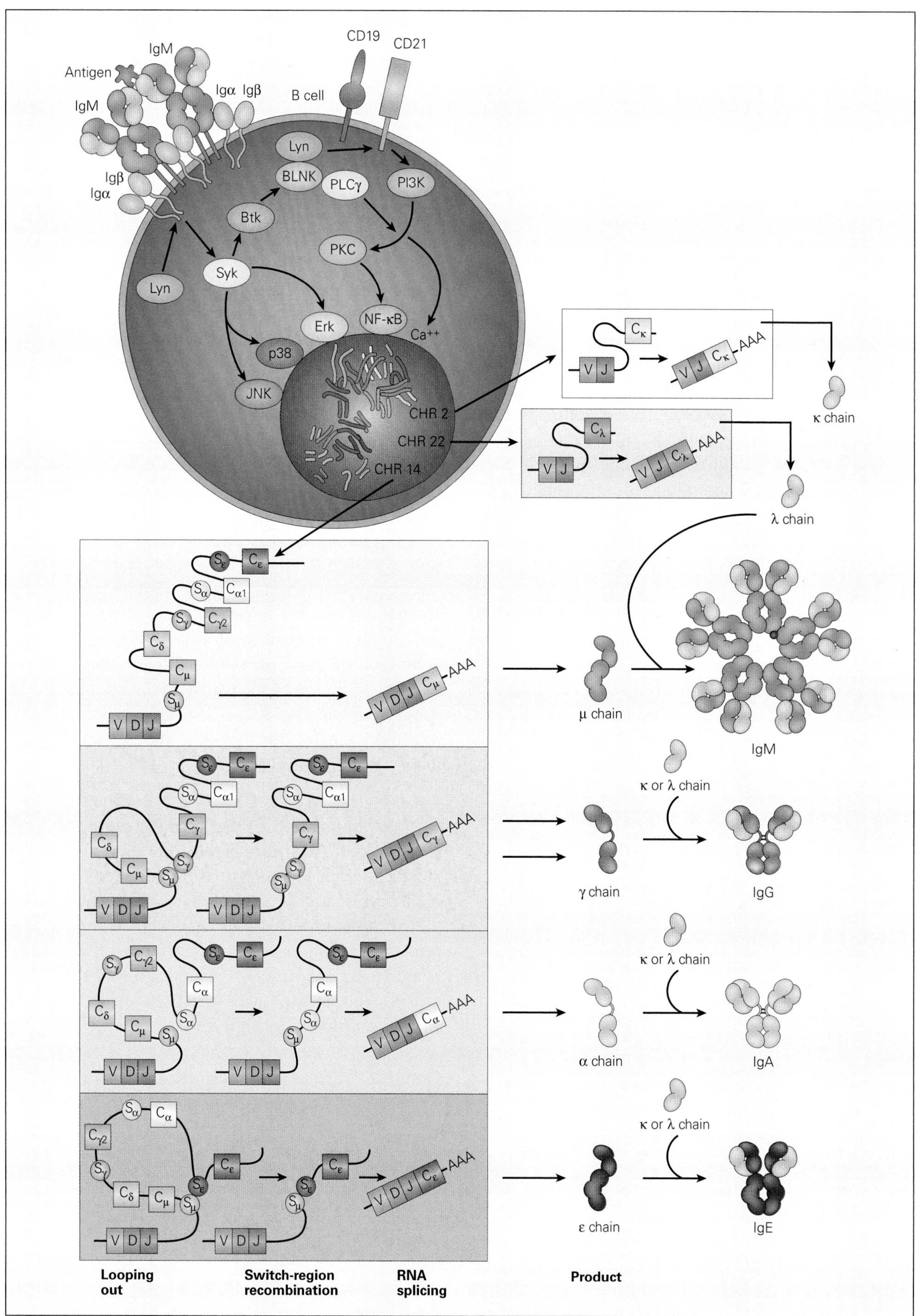

Figure 6-27. Schematic representation of the mechanism of isotype class-switching in B cells, resulting in the sequentially ordered production of immunoglobulins by plasma cells, beginning with IgM synthesis, followed by IgG, IgA, and IgE. All immunoglobulins are not produced by a single plasma cell; rather, each switched immunoglobulin is produced by an individual cell.

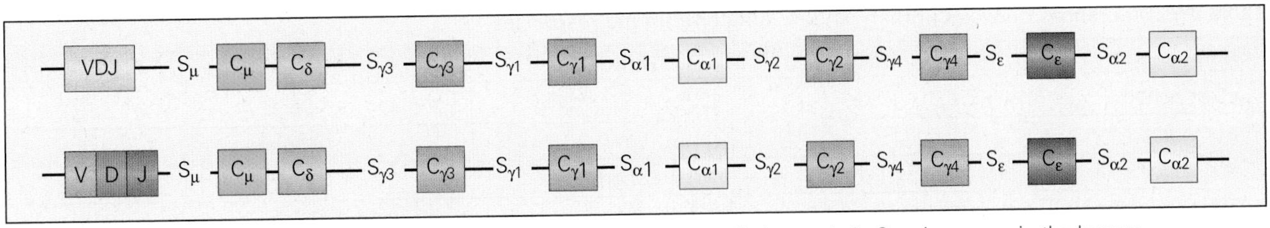

Figure 6-28. Schematic representation of the organization of the immunoglobulin heavy-chain C-region genes in the human.

after a definite time lapse. The first encounter with the immunogen in each of these cases evokes the *primary* immune response (Figure 6-29).

Immediately after the initial introduction of the immunogen, little or no antibody is detected in the serum. This period is referred to as the *inductive* or *latent period* (Table 6-9). It is during this time that the antigen is recognized as foreign and is processed by APCs, e.g., dendritic cells, macrophages, or B cells. Then the processed antigen is presented to appropriate T cells for interaction with T or B cells for subsequent cell-mediated or humoral antibody production (*Chapter 1*). This period is characterized by cellular proliferation and differentiation of responding T and B lymphocyte populations that ultimately give rise to antibody production by B cells. The duration of this period is variable and is dependent upon the following factors:

- The immunogenicity, quantity, form, and solubility of the inducing immunogen;
- The genetic variability of the host into which the immunogen is introduced;
- The route of immunization, i.e., via injection or through the oral or respiratory mucosal route;

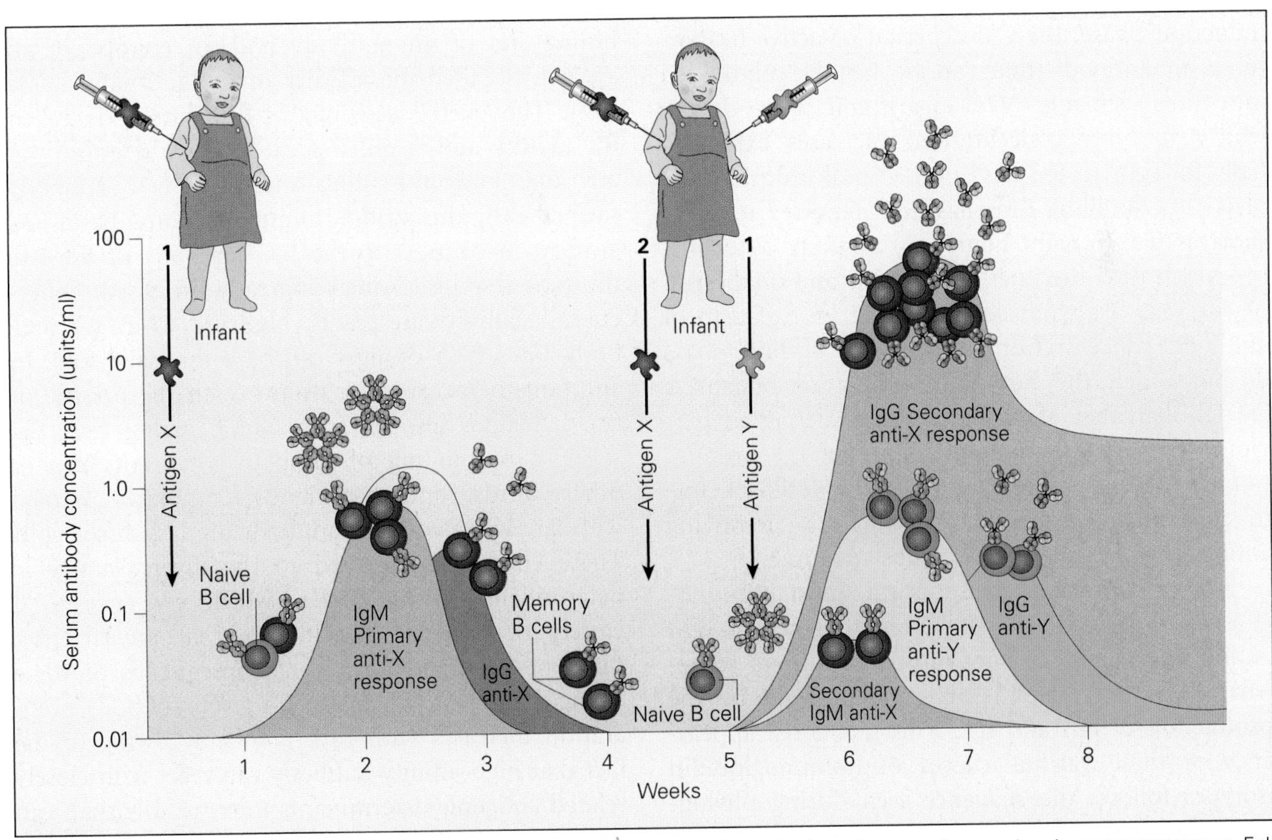

Figure 6-29. Schematic representation of humoral and B cell maturational events in the primary and secondary immune responses. Following initial immunization with antigen X (shown in red), there is initial production of IgM antibody production (light red) within the weeks one to three, followed by IgG production (dark red) within two to four weeks in a primary immune response. Following a second encounter with antigen X, there is a brief production of IgM within weeks five to seven, followed by a heightened production of IgG from five to eight weeks and clonal expansion of the x-sensitized memory B cells, characteristic of the secondary or anamnestic response. If a second antigen Y is co-administered at this time (green), a prmary immune response is seen with the same sequential steps of IgM (light green) and IgG (dark green) production as with antigen X during its previous primary immune response encounter.

Table 6-9. Differences between primary and secondary immune responses

Characteristic	Primary	Secondary
Latent period	Long	Short
Peak antibody titer	Low	High
Persistence of antibody titer	Short	Long
Affinity of antibody	Low	High
Cross reactivity of antibody	Low	High
Presence of memory cells	Few (?)	Many
Predominating Ig class	IgM	IgG
Dose of immunogen required to elicit antibody	High	Low

- The sensitivity of the immunologic assay used to detect the newly formed antibody.

For example, antibody can be detected three to four days after immunization with foreign erythrocytes introduced via transfusion, five to seven days after administration of a soluble protein, and ten to fourteen days after bacterial infection. Following the initial appearance of antibody at the end of the induction phase, there is a period of active biosynthesis of antibody that can be further subdivided into three segments: (1) a logarithmic phase during which antibody concentration increases exponentially for four to ten days until it peaks; during this phase the doubling time has been reported to be as short as five to eight hours; (2) a steady state during which time the rates of synthesis and catabolism of antibody are equivalent resulting in a plateau of antibody concentrations; and (3) a decline phase during which the rate of antibody catabolism is greater than that of its synthesis. As described previously, it has been hypothesized that the production of idiotypes may play a negative feedback role in controlling the immune response by removing antibodies once they are no longer required.

The earliest primary response to most immunogens is characterized by the predominance of IgM antibody; the IgG class of antibody appears somewhat later and is followed even later still by the production of IgA and IgE. This sequential appearance of these various classes of immunoglobulin isotypes follows the sequence seen during phylogeny, ontogeny, and at the cellular level (*Chapter 2*). IgM antibody production is usually transient, and within two weeks after the initiation of the immune response, IgG antibody predominates. The administration of the immunogen in combination with an adjuvant usually results in the continued synthesis of both IgM and IgG antibody for more extended periods of time (*Chapter 23*).

Antibody Affinity, the Binding of Antigen with a Single Antibody Combining Site Versus Antibody Avidity, and the Overall Strength of Binding of Antigen with Several Antibody-Combining Sites

The strength of the binding between a single combining site of an antibody and an epitope of an antigen is called the **affinity** of the antibody (Table 6-9). The overall strength of attachment is called the **avidity** and is much greater than the affinity of any one antigen-binding site. The IgM antibody formed early during the immune response has a low affinity, in contrast to the IgG antibody of the late immune response, which is greatly increased. Differences in affinity are readily observed with IgG antibody since such changes can be a thousand-fold. In addition to increases in affinity with the passage of time, there is also an increase of avidity (i.e., the strength of binding of antibody with antigen); in other words, antigen-antibody complexes formed with late IgG-associated antibody are less dissociable. These changes are related to the diverse antigenic determinants, i.e., epitopes, which give rise to a variety of antibody specificities that appear after different latent periods. As a consequence of these changes, the *cross reactivity* of a given antibody preparation increases with time, probably owing to the fact that high-affinity antibody can react with closely related antigenic determinants more readily than can their low-affinity counterparts. Collectively, all of these factors influencing the binding of antigen with antibody reflect the heterogeneity of the humoral immune response that is brought about by diverse populations of antibody molecules which differ in isotypic class, affinity, avidity, and specificity.

The Secondary Immune Response

Upon a subsequent exposure of a previously immunized host to the same immunogen, weeks, months, or even years later, there is a markedly enhanced response that is characterized by the accelerated appearance of immunocompetent T and B cells referred to as "memory" cells that collaborate to generate an enhanced production of antibody. The latent period is much shorter during the secondary immune response since memory cells are present at a higher frequency and are available to be stimulated quickly, in contrast to the primary immune response, where a longer period of time is required for the critical cellular steps involved in antibody production or induction of a T cell response within the germinal centers of peripheral lymphoid tissues. Although IgM is produced initially in both the primary and secondary immune responses, the duration and magnitude of IgM production in the secondary immune response is transient and is associated with a greatly enhanced production of antibody that is primarily of the IgG isotype. Subsequent antibody production is then converted from IgG to other immunoglobulin isotypes by the previously described mechanism of the immunoglobulin isotype switch. In the secondary immune response, the memory B cells that have already switched their Ig isotype immediately begin to secrete that isotype. This enhanced production of antibody during the secondary immune response is sometimes referred to as the anamnestic or recall phenomenon and forms the basis for giving booster doses of vaccines. Since IgM antibody appears in the course of infection near the beginning, its measurement can provide a predictive marker of early infection, which is useful in distinguishing whether the presence of antibody represesents intercurrent infection or is the result of prior infection. The production of the IgM antibody is also more prolonged in the fetus and the newborn infant and is thought to be related, in part, to an immaturity of immunologic mechanisms important for the switch, e.g., an immature CD40L on T cells (*Chapter 2*). Since the IgM antibody is not transferred across the placenta, this predominance of IgM antibody in early life provides an important diagnostic marker to distinguish if the presence of antibody represents active infection from other confounding possibilities during this period, i.e., passively transferred maternal IgG antibody (*Chapter 19*). A comparison of the responses seen in the primary and secondary immune responses is shown in Table 6-9.

Case Study: Clinical Relevance

Let us now return to the case study of infectious mononucleosis presented earlier and review some of the major points of the clinical presentation and how they relate to the immune system:

- Infectious mononucleosis (also called "the kissing disease" or Pfeiffer's disease, known in North America as mono and more commonly as glandular fever in other English-speaking countries) is an infectious disease caused by the Epstein-Barr virus (EBV), a member of the herpes family. Mononucleosis is seen most commonly in adolescents and young adults and is characterized by fever, sore throat, muscle soreness, fatigue, and sometimes an enlarged spleen (splenomegaly) that is susceptible to rupture.
- Infectious mononucleosis is a relatively noncommunicable infectious disease and requires intimate contact and transmission of the virus in saliva from either a symptomatic or asymptomatic individual (hence, "the kissing disease"). It may also be transmitted through blood.
- Complications include hemolytic anemia, thrombocytopenia, aplastic anemia, myocarditis, hepatitis, genital ulcers, splenic rupture, rash, and neurologic complications such as Guillain–Barre syndrome, encephalitis, and meningitis.
- Mononucleosis usually produces a very mild illness in young children. White patches on the tonsils or in the back of the throat may also be seen (resembling a streptococcal infection).
- Mononucleosis is usually caused by the Epstein-Barr virus, which infects B cells (B lymphocytes), causing them to proliferate. The disease is so-named because the count of mononuclear leukocytes in the blood, i.e., monocytes and lymphocytes, rises significantly. The reaction of T cells (especially the CD8+ lymphocytes) to the EBV-infected B cells gives rise to atypical forms of T cells known as Downey bodies.
- Most of the symptoms of infectious mononucleosis are attributed to the proliferation and activation of T cells in response to infection. Up to a few percent of the peripheral B cells may be infected with EBV in infectious mononucleosis. Activation of B cells by EBV, with resultant production of polyclonal antibodies, causes elevated titers of heterophile antibodies and occasionally causes increases in cold agglutinins,

Case Study: Clinical Relevance (continued)

cryoglobulins, antinuclear antibodies, or rheumatoid factor.

- In most cases of infectious mononucleosis, the clinical diagnosis can be made from the characteristic triad of fever, pharyngitis, and lymphadenopathy lasting from one to four weeks. Serologic test results include a normal to moderately elevated white blood cell count, an increased total number of lymphocytes, greater than 10 percent atypical lymphocytes, and a positive reaction to a mono spot test in patients with symptoms compatible with infectious mononucleosis (this is diagnostic, and no further testing is necessary).
- Because of the nonspecificity of the mono spot test, more effective laboratory diagnosis can be performed by the use of more specific tests for the measurement of EBV. EBV-specific laboratory tests include the measurement of antibodies directed to the following EBV viral antigens: the viral capsid antigen (VCA), the early antigen (EA), and the EBV nuclear antigen (EBNA). In addition, differentiation of immunoglobulin G and M antibody classes to the VCA can often be helpful for confirmation. When the mono spot test is negative, the presence of IgM antibody indicates recent infection and IgG past infection; the optimal combination of EBV serologic testing consists of the measurement of these markers: IgM and IgG to the VCA, IgM to the EA, and antibody to the EBNA.
- In addition to its ability to produce acute and chronic viral infection, EBV has been implicated in the pathogenesis of autoimmune diseases, e.g., systemic lupus erythematosus (*Chapter 19*), and has been linked to many human neoplasms, including hematopoietic, epithelial, and mesenchymal tumors (*Chapters 20* and *21*). These include nasopharyngeal carcinoma, a variety of B cell lymphomas, including Burkitt's lymphoma and Hodgkin's disease, as well as lymphoproliferative disease seen in patients with congenital or acquired immunodeficiencies.

Key Points

- The variable regions at the amino termini of immunoglobulin heavy and light chains bind specific antigen, while the constant regions of the heavy chains determine antibody biological functions. Each antibody isotype (IgM, IgD, IgG, IgA, and IgE) is found in particular body locations and has distinct biological functions.
- Monomeric IgM and IgD serve as BCR on the B cell membrane. Pentameric IgM is the first antibody secreted in response to antigen and functions primarily in the circulation to agglutinate antigen and activate complement.
- IgG is the most prevalent serum antibody with the longest half-life. It enters the tissues to neutralize and opsonize antigen and activate complement and crosses the placenta to protect the fetus and newborn.
- IgA functions at mucous membranes to neutralize antigen and block infection; secretory component protects it from mucosal proteases.
- IgE binds helminthic parasites and promotes eosinophil ADCC. It is also the antibody that mediates allergies.
- Immunoglobulins serve as B cell receptors to respond to specific antigen binding by stimulating the B cell to proliferate and differentiate into antibody-secreting plasma cells and long-lived memory B cells.
- Secreted antibody binds antigen to agglutinate and opsonizes it to promote phagocytosis, to neutralize toxins and viruses by blocking their entry into host cells, activating complement and signaling killer cells to bind and kill antibody-coated cells (e.g., ADCC).
- Immunoglobulin antigen-binding diversity is achieved by the random somatic recombination of gene segments into unique VH and VL sequences during B cell development in the bone marrow.
- B cell development is controlled by signals transmitted through the pre-BCR and BCR that result in apoptosis of cells with nonproductive somatic recombination or self-specific B cells, while allowing the survival of non-self-specific B cells that produce functional BCR.
- Antigen selects the B cells binding it and, with helper T cell cytokines, results in B cell proliferation, somatic hypermutation and affinity maturation, isotype switching, and differentiation of plasma cells and memory B cells.

Study Questions/Critical Thinking

1. Identify each of these immune mechanisms as part of the innate immune response (I), adaptive immune response (A), or a combination of both (C).
   a. A macrophage uses its TLR to bind *E. coli* LPS and engulf the bacterium.

b. A neutrophil uses its Fc receptors to bind IgG-coated *Staphylococcus aureus* and engulf the bacterium.
c. An NK cell binds a virus-infected cell and induces apoptosis.
d. A cytotoxic T cell binds a virus-infected cell and induces apoptosis.
e. An NK cell uses its Fc receptors to bind IgG-coated a virus-infected cell and induces apoptosis.
f. A mast cell is stimulated by the presence of tissue damage to release histamine.
g. A mast cell is stimulated by pollen binding to IgE on its Fc receptors to release histamine.

2. Identify each of these immune responses as humoral (H) or cellular (C) immunity.
   a. Antibody to diphtheria toxin binds the toxin and blocks toxin bindng to target cells (neutralization).
   b. Cytotoxic T cells recognize and kill virus-infected cells.
   c. Helper T cells (Th2) signal B cells to secrete IgA.
   d. Helper T cells (Th1) signal macrophages to kill phagocytosed pathogen.
   e. An NK cell uses its Fc receptors to bind antibody that is bound to HIV gp120 on the membrane of an infected CD4 T cell; the NK cell induces apoptosis in the CD4 T cell.
3. Compare the antigen-recognition systems of the innate and adaptive immune responses. What are the advantages and disadvantages of each?
4. Discuss the multiple roles of T cells in the immune system.
5. Explain why the finding of a monoclonal antibody in patient serum could not be due to a normal immune response.
6. Explain how the immune system can cause tissue damage during the course of an immune response. Is tissue damage from the immune response inevitable for any pathogen?
7. If antibody diversity is so great that we can respond to epitopes on any antigen, why is it that we still get infectious diseases?
8. Make sure you are capable of completing the following tasks.

- Draw a picture of an immunoglobulin monomer and add labels to all of the structural features.
- Describe the light chain locus organization in a hematopoietic stem cell.
- Describe the kappa light chain locus organization in a hematopoietic stem cell.
- Describe how the locus changes as the stem cell matures to a B cell. (Include the following terms: somatic recombination, germ line configuration, and V and J segments.)
- Name three ways in which the heavy chain locus differs from the light chain locus.
- Explain how somatic mutation might increase the affinity of an antibody. (Include the following terms in your answer: framework, hypervariable region).
- What is the most common Ig in serum?
- What is the Ig transferred to a baby by breast milk?
- What is the first Ig made by a B lymphocyte?
- Which Ig(s) activate classical complement cascade?
- Which Ig is involved in allergic responses?
- Which Ig determinants are detected by immunizing a patient with murine monoclonal antibody?
- Which Ig determinants are detected by immunizing a patient with a humanized monoclonal antibody?

Suggested Reading

Alam R, Gorska M. Lymphocytes. J Allergy Clin Immun. 2003; 111 Suppl 2; S476–85.

Brugnoni D, Airo P, Graf D, et al. Ontogeny of CD40L expression by activated peripheral blood lymphocytes in humans. Immunol Lett. 1996; 49: 27–30.

Brugnoni D, Airo P, Graf D, et al. Ineffective expression of CD40 ligand on cord blood T cells may contribute to poor immunoglobulin production in the newborn. Eur J Immunol. 1994; 24: 1919-24.

Conley ME, Dobbs AK, Farmer KM, et al. Primary B cell immunodeficiencies: comparisons and contrasts. Annu Rev Immunol. 2009; 27: 199–227.

Flajnik MF. Comparative analyses of immunoglobulin genes: surprises and portents. Nat Rev Immunol. 2002; 2: 688–98.

Harris LJ, Larsen SB, McPherson A. Comparison of intact antibody structures and the implications for effector functions. Adv Immunol. 1999; 72: 191–208.

Huston JS, George AJ. Engineered antibodies take center stage. Hum Antibodies. 2001; 10: 127–42.

Köhler G, Milstein C. Continuous cultures of fused cells secreting antibody of predefined specificity. Nature. 1975; 256: 495–7.

Küppers R. B cells under influence: transformation of B cells by Epstein-Barr virus. Nat Rev Immunol. 2003; 3: 801–12.

Kurosaki T. Regulation of B cell signal transduction by adaptor proteins. Nat Rev Immunol. 2002; 2: 354–63.

Kutok JL, Wang F. Spectrum of Epstein-Barr virus-associated diseases. Annu Rev Pathol. 2006; 1: 375–404.

LeBien TW, Tedder TF. B lymphocytes: how they develop and function. Blood. 2008; 112: 1570–80.

Mårtensson IL, Keenan RA, Licence S. The pre-B cell receptor. Curr Opin Immunol. 2007; 19: 137–42.

Matthias P, Rolink AG. Transcriptional networks in developing and mature B cells. Nat Rev Immunol. 2005; 5: 497–508.

Melchers F. The pre-B cell receptor: selector of fitting immunoglobulin heavy chains for the B cell receptor. Nat Rev Immunol. 2005; 5: 578–84.

Niiro H, Clark EA. Regulations of B cell fate by antigen-receptor signals. Nat Rev Immunol. 2002; 2: 945–56.

Preud'homme JL, Petit I, Barra A, et al. Structural and functional properties of membrane and secreted IgD. Mol Immunol. 2000; 37: 871–87.

Sleckman BP. Lymphocyte antigen receptor gene assembly: multiple layers of regulation. Immunol Res. 2005; 32: 253–8.

Sorensen V, Rasmussen EB, Sundvoid V, et al. Structural requirements for incorporation of J chain into human IgM and IgA. Int Immunol. 2000; 12: 19–27.

Stavnezer J, Guikema JE, Schrader CE. Mechanism and regulation of class switch recombination. Annu Rev Immunol. 2008; 26: 261–92.

Thorley-Lawson DA, Allday MJ. The curious case of the tumour virus: 50 years of Burkitt's lymphoma. Nat Rev Microbiol. 2008; 6: 913–24.

Thorley-Lawson DA, Duca KA, Shapiro M. Epstein-Barr virus; a paradigm for persistent infection—for real and in virtual reality. Trends Immunol. 2008; 29: 195–201.

Thorley-Lawson DA. Epstein-Barr virus: exploiting the immune system. Nat Rev Immunol. 2001; 1: 75–82.

von Mehren M, Adams GP, Weiner LM. Monoclonal antibody therapy for cancer. Annu Rev Med. 2003; 54: 343–369.

Welner RS, Pelayo R, Kincade PW. Evolving views on the genealogy of B cells. Nat Rev Immunol. 2008: 8; 95–106.

Yoo EM, Morrison SL. IgA: an immune glycoprotein. Clin Immunol. 2005; 116: 3–10.

Zola H, Swart B, Nicholson T, et al. CD molecules 2005: human cell differentiation molecules. Blood Journal. 2005; 106: 3123–6.

Chapter 7

T Lymphocytes and Cell-Mediated Immunity

Donna L. Farber, PhD

Case Study

On October 21, 1983, a twelve-year-old male with a rare immunodeficiency disease received a bone marrow transplant from his older sister, a treatment that seemed like the best hope for his survival. Because his older brother had died from complications of the same disease, his parents arranged for a germ-free delivery on September 21, 1971, at Texas Children's Hospital in Houston. Once it was determined that the newborn's disease was the same as that which afflicted his brother, he was placed in a plastic isolation system (a "bubble") to protect him from microbes that his body could not fend off while waiting for a matching bone marrow donor or a cure for his ailment. Because of an inability to find a suitable donor, the wait in the bubble lasted almost the entire twelve years of his life. It was finally decided to take the patient out of the bubble and to transplant bone marrow from a histoincompatible sister using recently developed techniques to deplete the bone marrow transplant of T cells that would otherwise have caused a life-threatening complication in the patient after transplantation, referred to as graft-versus-host disease (GVHD). GVHD is a common complication of allogeneic bone marrow transplantation, i.e., a transplant from a genetically non-identical member of the same species, in which functional immune T cells in the transplanted marrow recognize the recipient as "foreign" and mount an immunologic attack against the recipient host (*Chapters 10* and *22*).

On the day of the bone marrow transplant, the patient showed the following immunologic findings: WBC = 5,100/mm^3, lymphocytes 4% (n = 28 – 48%), CD3 = 11% (n = 38 – 86%), CD4 = 13% (n = 23 – 58%), CD8 = 4% (n = 13 – 33%), IgM < 60 mg/dL, IgA < 154 mg/dL, and IgG > 7 mg/dL. Sixty days after transplantation, the patient continued his isolation in a relatively sterile environment and spent Christmas 1983 at home. After his return to the hospital two weeks later, he became sick for the first time in his life on the eightieth post-transplantation day, with temperatures spiking to 105°F, vomiting, and bloody diarrhea. Although the doctors' initial fear was that GVHD had begun and was responsible for his symptoms, the condition never developed. However, unbeknownst to the doctors, the Epstein-Barr virus (EBV), which had not been screened from his sister's marrow, was inducing

LEARNING OBJECTIVES

When you have completed this chapter, you should be able to:

- Explain the functions of T cells and the role of cell-mediated immunity in eliminating infectious disease caused by intracellular pathogens
- Describe the basic structure of the T cell receptor complex
- Discuss how somatic recombination of TCR genes results in the generation of diversity in antigen recognition and discuss the functions of gamma delta T cells
- Describe antigen-independent development of alpha/beta T cells and explain the steps that result in commitment to the CD4 or CD8 T cell lineage (positive selection) and removal of self-specific T cells (negative selection)
- Describe antigen-dependent activation of T cells by APC and the functions of Th1, Th2, Th17, Th3, Tr1, and Tc cells
- Summarize the clinical relevance of T cells and cell-mediated immunity in health and disease

Case Study: (continued)

a lymphoma in her brother. Repeat immunologic testing after transplantation revealed no evidence of immunologic reconstitution by donor marrow. Over the next month, his clinical course deteriorated, with increased gastrointestinal bleeding and dehydration. Despite aggressive treatments, "David the Bubble Boy," who was born with severe combined immunodeficiency (SCID), died on February 22, 1984, on the 124th posttransplantation day. Yet his legacy would live on for many years in numerous ways.

Autopsy Findings

Postmortem examination revealed multiple tumor-like B cell proliferations in several organs that originated from David's cells and not from those of his sister. Fully infectious EBV was isolated from pharyngeal secretions and EBV nuclear antigen (EBNA) was found in transformed peripheral lymphocytes, peritoneal inflammatory cells, and bone marrow cells and EBV genomes were found in all tumor tissues. Analysis of cellular immunoglobulin and immunoglobulin gene DNA from the tumors indicated both monoclonal and oligoclonal B cell proliferations. Collectively, these findings provided evidence for a progressive evolution of EBV-induced changes of B cells from polyclonal activation to oligoclonal B cell proliferation and finally to a monoclonal B cell lymphoma, which ultimately caused his death (*Chapter 21*).

Severe Combined Immunodeficiency: A Model for Understanding T Cell Development

Babies with SCID are healthy at birth but die of recurrent, severe infections in infancy unless they are provided with a functional immune system (*Chapter 16*). Most affected infants are not brought to medical attention until they develop serious infectious complications, and the condition is fatal if untreated. The diagnosis of SCID in David was made appropriately early and an attempt at allogeneic bone marrow stem cell transplantation was made. Tragically, his death occurred from complications of a bone marrow transplant from his sister at a time when neither the currently utilized and improved technologies for tissue typing and donor-recipient matching nor appropriate screening of donor cell preparations for oncogenic potential were available (*Chapter 22*). Effective treatment with allogeneic hematopoietic stem cell transplantation is now widely established. Because of the severity of the condition and the availability of a curative therapy, it has been suggested recently that screening for SCID be included in the panel of diseases now being performed on the newborn. The best outcome for SCID, as with many other conditions for which newborn screening is now done, is achieved if hematopoietic stem cell transplantation is performed in the first months of life, ideally before the clinical presentation of infections or the failure to thrive.

In this classic case of "David the Bubble Boy," the diagnosis of SCID was initially made based on a family history in a deceased male sibling together with immunologic findings of decreased T cell and B cell function in the patient. Because David's environment was so controlled, he was protected from infection in his microbe-free bubble. The goal of this case study is to illustrate the clinical importance of an understanding of the molecular events underlying T cell development in the normal host. The knowledge gained from this tragic case of "David the Bubble Boy" has had great application to other children with immune deficiency as well as to a wide variety of patients who suffer from acquired defects of immune function and hematologic malignancies. David's life and death have led to two major scientific advances in understanding the molecular basis of T cell signalling, the use of gene therapy, and the nature of cancer immunity.

Molecular Basis of T Cell Signaling and the Use of Gene Therapy

In 1993, analysis of blood samples taken from David identified the precise genetic site where his congenital disease was located. As we shall learn from this chapter, one of the molecules that make up the IL-2 cytokine receptor, called the γc chain, was found to be deficient in the T lymphocytes of David's immune system (*Chapter 9*). The discovery was a breakthrough and has led to a better understanding of how different parts of the immune system communicate with one another; it has not only led to the identification of the molecular bases for other immune deficiencies but also new strategies for gene therapy for children afflicted with inherited immune deficiencies as well as for a whole host of other acquired immunologic disorders, including cancer in both children and adults (*Chapters 20* and *21*).

The most common treatment for SCID continues to be bone marrow transplantation, which requires matching donors (a sibling is generally best). Since David's death, at least two new therapies have been developed for children born with SCID. In one procedure, their blood is drawn, the white blood cells are altered with repaired genes, and then the cells are reinjected into the patient. The second procedure involves the use of stem cells in gene therapy whereby the missing gene is transduced into hematopoietic stem cells using viral vectors. Stem cells from the umbilical cords of infants born with SCID are altered by inserting a retrovirus carrying the deficicent gene to repair the gene that carries the disease. The altered cells are then reintroduced into the patient. The first gene therapy trials were performed in 1990, with modified peripheral T cells in ten patients with SCID. This process was historic as the first attempt to cure a disease through gene therapy. Although every patient who received this therapy was initially cured of SCID, these trials were stopped when it was discovered

Case Study: (continued)

that two of ten patients in one trial had developed leukemia resulting from the insertion of the gene-carrying retrovirus near an oncogene. In 2007, four of the ten patients were reported to have developed leukemias.

Nature of Cancer and Cancer Immunity: The Cancer Link

Because David's environment was so controlled, it was possible to link the origin of the cancerous lymphoma that killed him to the Epstein-Barr virus (EBV) present in a latent form in his sister's donated bone marrow but which underwent malignant transformation to a B cell lymphoma in the patient, since he was never exposed to the virus in his contained environment (*Chapter 13*). Epstein-Barr virus has now been identified in a variety of other EBV-associated malignant lymphoproliferative diseases seen in AIDS-associated B cell lymphomas, the post-transplantation lymphoproliferative disorder (PTLD), and a variety of B and T cell lymphomas (*Chapter 21*). The study of David and other infants with SCID has thus provided cancer links with the development of lymphomas/leukemias related not only to the EBV, as in the case of David, but also to retroviral insertional mutagenesis, as seen in other studies.

Introduction

As described in Chapters 1 and 2, the two major lymphocyte populations of the adaptive immune system include the T lymphocytes (named "T" after their maturation in the thymus) and the B lymphocytes (named "B" after their maturation in the bone marrow), the former concerned with cell-mediated immunity and the latter with antibody production. Of the two arms, the T lymphocytes are the primary initiators, coordinators, and regulators of the adaptive immune response. Both humoral and cellular aspects of the adaptive immune response depend on the coordinated activation of T cells. T lymphocytes help B cells make most antibodies, mediate direct apoptosis of virally infected cells and tumor cells, and secrete a myriad of soluble factors called cytokines that mediate the recruitment and activation of many immune and nonimmune cell types to clear the body of unwanted antigens (*Chapter 9*). T lymphocytes also enhance the innate immune response by promoting antigen clearance via phagocytes and antigen presentation by many cell types. In addition to their multiple roles in promoting immune responses, T cells are also the master regulators that prevent immunopathology and act to dampen immune responses via direct cell-cell interaction and through the secretion of regulatory cytokines. In this chapter, we will introduce developmental, cellular, molecular, and biochemical aspects of T lymphocytes, and the clinical features of conditions in which these aspects are deficient, dysregulated, or dysfunctional. We will also discuss how targeting of T lymphocytes has great therapeutic potential for augmenting antipathogen and antitumor immunity, and abrogating autoimmunity (*Chapter 19*).

T Lymphocytes: Basic Properties and Antigen Recognition

T Cells Are Key Mediators of Adaptive Immunity

T lymphocytes are small (<10 nm), resting cells that primarily reside in peripheral blood and secondary lymphoid tissue, but are also found in bone marrow and a host of peripheral organs (Figure 7-1).

For many years, there was no function ascribed to this cell that appeared unremarkable in morphology

A. Hematologic picture of small, medium and large lymphocytes

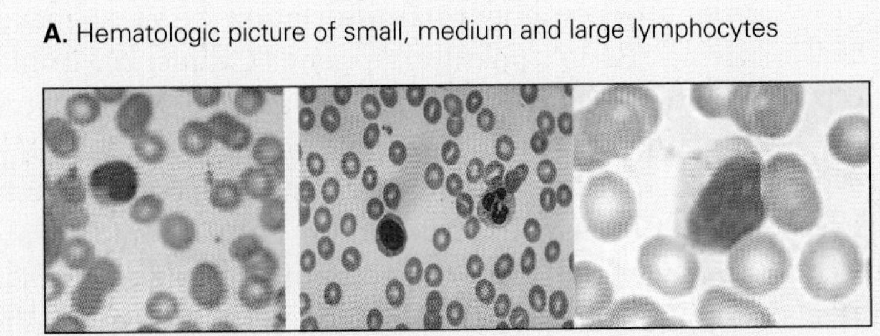

B. Electron micrograph of a lymphocyte

Scanning micrograph of a lymphocyte

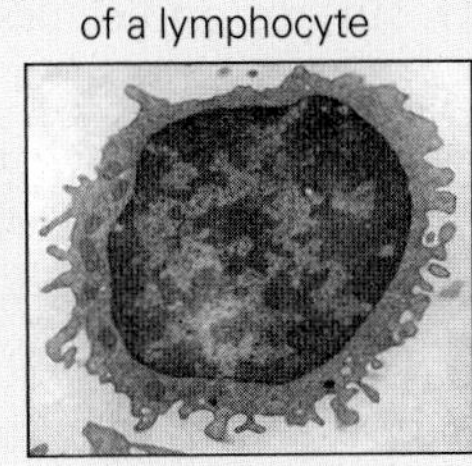

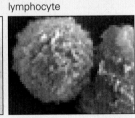

Figure 7-1. Panel A: Photomicrograph of small, medium, and large lymphocytes from a peripheral blood smear. Panel B: Electron and scanning electron micrographs of a lymphocyte. (As seen on Wikipedia.)

with a high nuclear to cytoplasmic ratio and small size, and the major players of the immune response were thought to be the more interesting polymorphonuclear leukocytes (**PMNs**) and antibodies. However, after their discovery in the late 1960s, it gradually became apparent that T lymphocytes are the key mediators of adaptive immunity. T cells comprise approximately 30 percent of white blood cells in human peripheral blood, with normal T lymphocyte counts in the range of 3–5 billion cells/L. Peripheral blood T cells account for only 2 percent of the total T cell complement of 380 billion cells, with 98 percent of T cells residing in lymphoid tissue, including peripheral lymph nodes, mucosa-associated lymphoid tissue (**MALT**), and spleen.

There are two major types of T lymphocytes, classified according to the expression of the cell surface co-receptors, CD4 and CD8 that are non-covalently associated with the TCR (*Chapter 1*). CD4+ T cells are generally referred to as "helper T cells" or Th cells, because they secrete a multitude of cytokines that help or coordinate cellular and humoral immunity. CD8+ T cells are generally referred to as cytotoxic T lymphocytes (**CTL**) or Tc cells, because when activated by antigen, they can mediate direct destruction of cellular targets by the process of apoptosis (*Chapter 9*). In humans, circulating CD4+ T cells outnumber CD8+ T cells by approximately 2:1. One of the most clinically significant aberrations of this cellular distribution was observed with the emergence of HIV/AIDS in 1981 as a reversal of the CD4/CD8 ratio owing to the selective destruction of the CD4 cells by HIV. While CD4+ and CD8+ T cells can act independently of each other, the activation and function of CD8 responses against many different antigens and pathogens requires the coordinated involvement of CD4+ T cells. There are a variety of T cells, mainly in the mucosa, which lack both CD4 and CD8 co-receptor molecules and, as will be described in greater detail below, are referred to as double negative (**DN**) T cells.

All T cells express CD3 surface molecules that define the T cell repertoire. In addition, T cells express surface antigen receptors, called T cell receptors (**TCRs**), which are exclusively found inserted in the T cell surface and are never secreted. As will be described below, the receptor has two forms based on different polypeptide chains. The most common form is made up of alpha (α) and beta (β) chains and is found on about 95 percent of circulating T cells. A second type of TCR has gamma (γ) and delta (δ) chains and is found on about 5 percent of circulating T cells, but is the predominate cell type in the MALT (*Chapter 8*). The TCR is a multimeric cell-surfacecomplex comprised of the antigen-binding heterodimer αβ or γδ and the CD3 conserved signal transducing molecules: two heterodimers (CD3-εγ and CD3-εδ and one homodimer (CD3-ζ), all of which are required for the TCR structural and functional integrity. Collectively, the CD3- and ζ-chains, together with the TCR, form what is known as the T cell receptor complex (Box 7-1, Figure 7-2).

TCR Resembles the Antibody Fab Regions and Binds MHC as well as Antigen Peptides

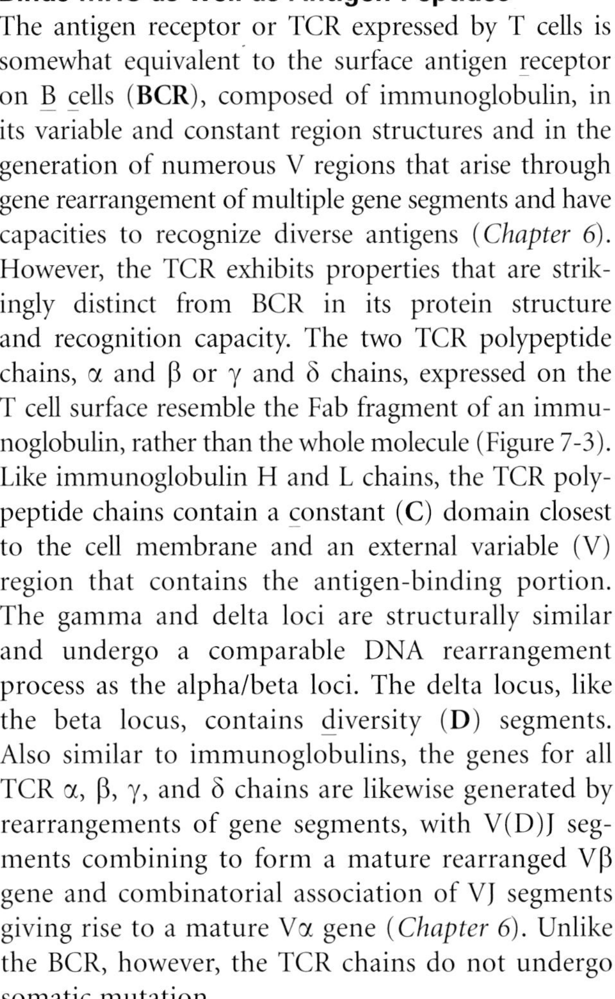

The antigen receptor or TCR expressed by T cells is somewhat equivalent to the surface antigen receptor on B cells (**BCR**), composed of immunoglobulin, in its variable and constant region structures and in the generation of numerous V regions that arise through gene rearrangement of multiple gene segments and have capacities to recognize diverse antigens (*Chapter 6*). However, the TCR exhibits properties that are strikingly distinct from BCR in its protein structure and recognition capacity. The two TCR polypeptide chains, α and β or γ and δ chains, expressed on the T cell surface resemble the Fab fragment of an immunoglobulin, rather than the whole molecule (Figure 7-3). Like immunoglobulin H and L chains, the TCR polypeptide chains contain a constant (**C**) domain closest to the cell membrane and an external variable (V) region that contains the antigen-binding portion. The gamma and delta loci are structurally similar and undergo a comparable DNA rearrangement process as the alpha/beta loci. The delta locus, like the beta locus, contains diversity (**D**) segments. Also similar to immunoglobulins, the genes for all TCR α, β, γ, and δ chains are likewise generated by rearrangements of gene segments, with V(D)J segments combining to form a mature rearranged Vβ gene and combinatorial association of VJ segments giving rise to a mature Vα gene (*Chapter 6*). Unlike the BCR, however, the TCR chains do not undergo somatic mutation.

Despite these similarities in domain structure, the TCR exhibits recognition properties that are strikingly distinct from immunoglobulin. Unlike immunoglobulin, the TCR does not recognize the whole intact antigen, but rather a portion of an

Box 7-1

The TCR Complex

The TCR Complex consists of the CD3- and ζ-chains, together with the TCR. The signal from the T cell complex is enhanced by simultaneous binding of the MHC molecules by specific co-receptors CD4 or CD8 (Figure 7-2).

The T cell receptor or TCR is a molecule found on the surface of T lymphocytes (or T cells) that is generally responsible for recognizing antigens bound to major histocompatibility complex (MHC) molecules (*Chapter 10*). It is a heterodimer consisting of an alpha and beta chain in 95 percent of T cells, while 5 percent of T cells have TCRs consisting of gamma and delta chains. Engagement of the TCR with antigen and MHC results in activation of its T lymphocyte, ie., transduction, through a series of biochemical events mediated by associated enzymes, co-receptors, and specialized accessory molecules.

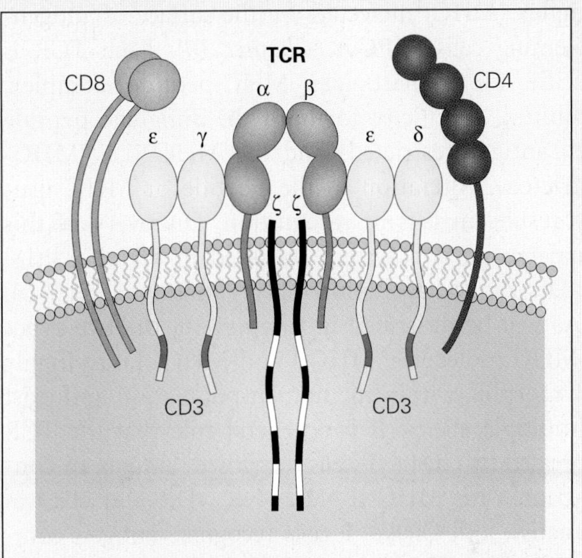

Figure 7-2. The T cell receptor complex with TCR-α and TCR-β chains, CD3 and ζ-chain accessory molecules, and the co-receptors CD4 and CD8.

TCR Co-Receptors

The signal from the T cell complex is enhanced by simultaneous binding of the MHC molecules by a specific co-receptor. On helper T cells, this coreceptor is CD4, which exclusively binds to MHC-II. On cytotoxic T cells, this co-receptor is CD8 that is specific for MHC-I. The co-receptor not only ensures the specificity of the TCR for the correctly presented antigen, it also allows prolonged engagement between the antigen-presenting cell and the T cell and recruits essential molecules (e.g., the leukocyte-specific protein tyrosine kinase [LCK]) inside the cell that are involved in the signaling of that activated T lymphocyte.

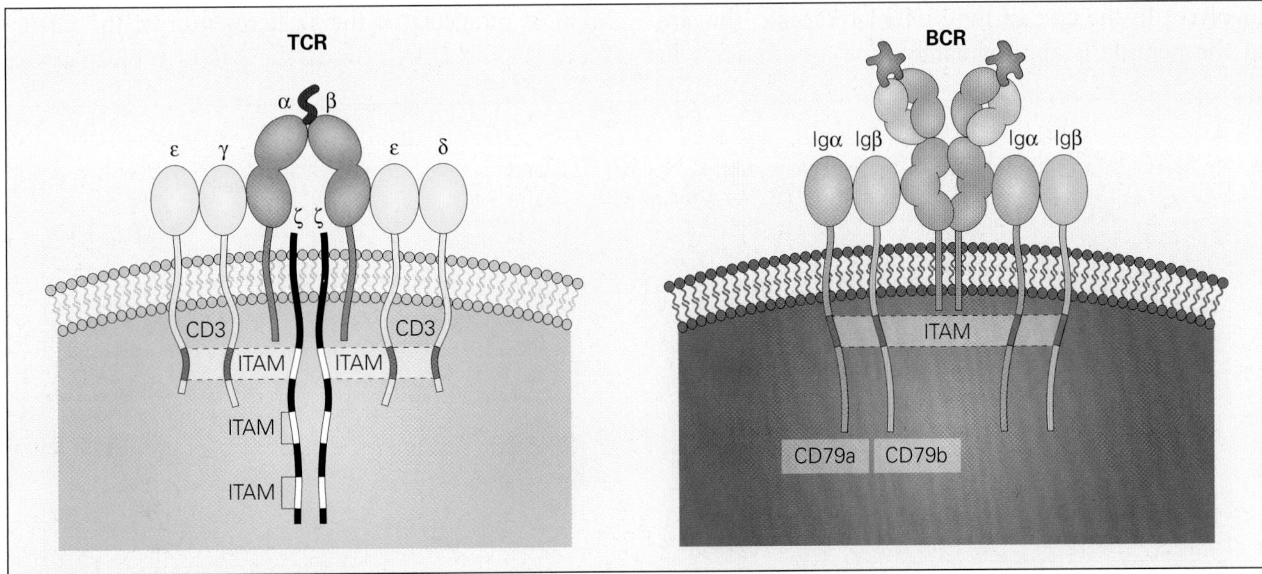

Figure 7-3. Schematic representation of the T cell receptor (TCR) and the B cell receptor (BCR). CD3 is the signal transduction molecule for TCR and is composed of six polypeptide chains. Shaded areas in both the TCR and BCR intracytoplasmic domains indicate the immunoreceptor tyrosine activation motifs (ITAMs). Each T cell has approximately 10^5 identical TCR molecules. Note that the TCR recognizes peptide processed by APCs while the BCR can recognize unprocessed protein.

antigen or an antigenic peptide (epitope) that is presented in a complex with major histocompatibility complex (**MHC**) molecules on the surface of antigen-presenting cells (**APCs**) (*Chapter 10*). Each TCR is specific for a particular MHC-peptide complex, exhibiting specificity for both the antigenic peptide (i.e., antigen-restricted) and the MHC (i.e., MHC-restricted). Alteration of the peptide or MHC usually results in loss of recognition. Discovery of this "dual recognition system" resulted in a Nobel Prize for Drs Zinkernagel and Doherty in 1996 (Box 7-2).

As will be described in Chapter 10, the two types of MHC molecules, MHC-I and MHC-II, are highly polymorphic within the human population and exist in multiple alleles. It is a general rule that the TCR expressed by CD4+ T cells recognizes antigen in conjunction with MHC-II (HLA-DR, -DP, and -DQ in humans), and CD8+ T cells recognize antigen complexed with MHC-I (HLA-A, -B, and -C in humans), "the rules of eight" (*Chapter 1*). MHC-I is found on all nucleated cells of the body. In contrast, MHC-II is expressed by a limited set of immune cell types that process antigen and present peptides to T lymphocytes and are therefore referred to as APCs. These include dendritic cells, macrophages, and B cells, and are referred to as professional APCs. Since MHC-I is expressed by all nucleated cells, many more cell types can potentially be recognized by CD8 T cells. There is also a difference in the size of the peptide presented to the TCR depending on the MHC molecule involved. In the case of the MHC-I molecule, the size of the peptide is approximately nine amino acids in length (Figure 7-4B); in contrast, a larger peptide of approximately fifteen amino acids is presented by the MHC-II molecule to the TCR receptor of the CD4+ T cell (Figure 7-4A). Since the MHC molecules are

Box 7-2

The Dual Recognition System

Drs Peter Doherty and Rolf Zinkernagel were awarded the 1996 Nobel Prize in Physiology or Medicine for their discovery of how the immune system recognizes virus-infected cells (*Chapter 13*). Their work laid a foundation for an understanding of general mechanisms used by the cellular immune system to recognize both foreign microorganisms and self molecules. This discovery has had great relevance to clinical medicine since it relates both to efforts to strengthen the immune response against invading microorganisms and certain forms of cancer, as well as efforts to diminish the effects of autoimmune reactions in inflammatory diseases, such as rheumatoid arthritis, multiple sclerosis, and diabetes.

The two Nobel laureates carried out their research at the John Curtin School of Medical Research in Canberra, Australia. During their studies of the response of mice to viruses, they found that white blood cells (lymphocytes) must recognize both the virus and certain self molecules—the so-called major histocompatibility antigens (*Chapter 10*)—in order to kill the virus-infected cells. This principle of simultaneous recognition of both self and foreign molecules or the "dual recognition system" has since then constituted a foundation for the further understanding of the specificity of the cellular immune system.

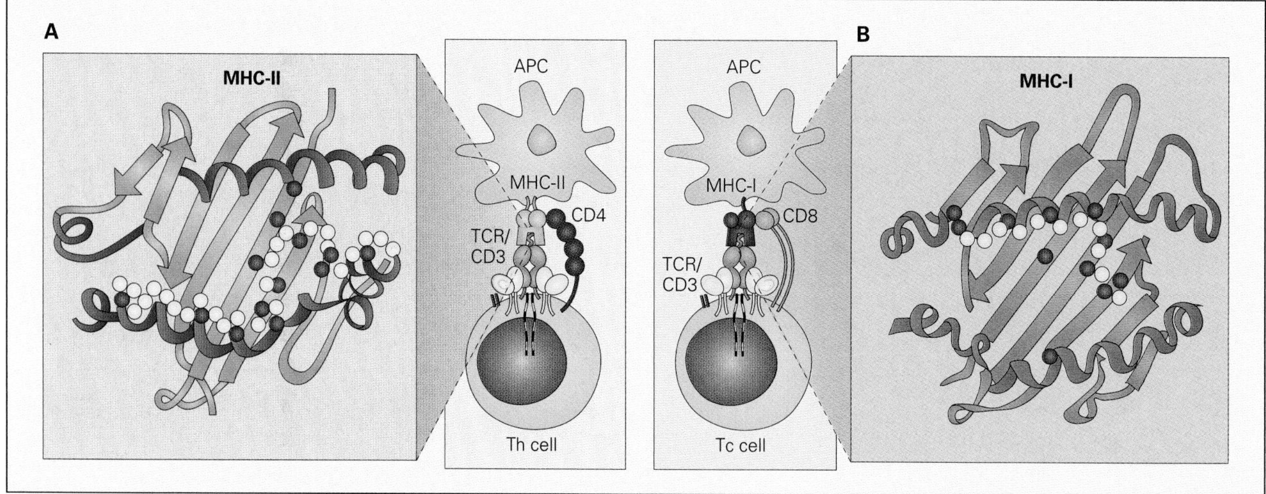

Figure 7-4. Schematic representation of the interaction between the TCR of Th (CD4+) and Tc (CD8+) cells with the two types of MHC molecules. Differences in the size of the peptide presented to the TcR depend on the MHC molecule involved. Panel B: MHC-I molecules present peptides of approximately nine amino acids (right panel), in contrast to MHC-II molecules shown in Panel A, which present peptides on the order of fifteen amino acids in length (left panel). Yellow areas represent the hypervariable regions of the MHC molecules to which the peptides (shown in red) preferentially attach.

part of the superfamily of immunoglobulin molecules (*Chapter 5*), they have a beta-pleated structure similar to that described for the variable regions of the immunoglobulin molecule and have sections of greater amino acid variability called hypervariable regions, where the MHC-peptide interaction occurs (Figure 7-4). In addition to the primary binding of the peptide through the interaction of the TCR with its respective MHC molecule, there is also the participation of co-receptor molecules, e.g., CD4 with MHC-II and CD8 with MHC-I, as will be described in greater detail below.

T Cell Receptor Gene Expression and Gene Rearrangement

The processes involved in gene expression, gene rearrangement, and protein synthesis leading to the formation of the TCR are similar to those described for the BCR and immunoglobulin synthesis (*Chapter 6*). In humans, the genes for the TCR are found on chromosome 7 and chromosome 14 (Figure 7-5)

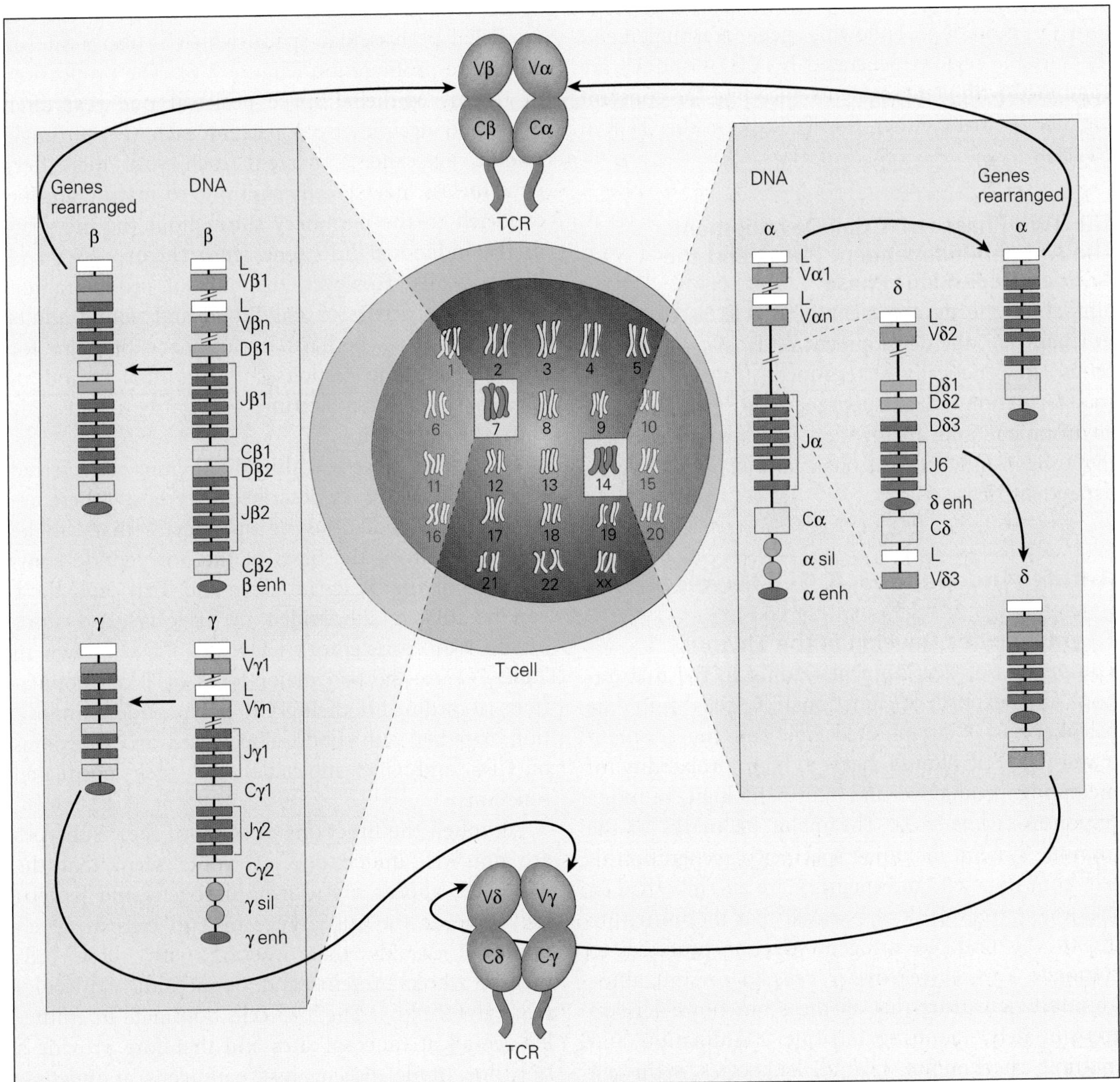

Figure 7-5. A schematic representation of the chromosomal locations of genetic loci that control the synthesis of the TCRαβ and the TCRγδ. The genes encoding the TCR α chain map to a single locus on chromosome 14 within which is embedded the locus for the TCR δ chain; the genes encoding the TCR β chain and the TCR γ chain map to two separate loci on chromosome 7. Following gene rearrangement of the variable and constant regions of the α, β, γ, and δ chains, they are joined to form the TCRαβ and the TCRγδ.

and are located on three loci. The genes encoding the TCR α chain map to a single locus on chromosome 14 within which is embedded the locus for the TCR δ chain; the genes encoding the TCR β chain and the TCR γ chain map to two separate loci on chromosome 7. Unlike the alpha and gamma loci, the delta and the beta loci contain diversity (**D**) segments. The genes for all TCR α, β, γ, and δ chains are all generated by rearrangements of gene segments, with V(D)J segments combining to form a mature rearranged Vβ gene and combinatorial association of VJ segments giving rise to a mature Vα gene (*Chapter 6*). Unlike the BCR, however, the TCR chains do not undergo somatic mutation. Following gene rearrangement, the variable regions generated by V(D)J and VJ are combined with gene segments encoding the constant regions to form either the TCRαβ or the TCRγδ receptor.

The Two Phases of T Cell Development: The Antigen-Independent Phase and the Antigen-Dependent Phase

Similar to the development of B cells as described in Chapter 6, the development of T cells occurs as a series of genetically determined adaptive cellular transformations in response to an ever-changing environment and are divided into two phases: (1) the antigen-independent phase and (2) the antigen-dependent phase.

Antigen-Independent T Cell Development

T Lymphocytes Develop in the Thymus

The process of development leading to the maturation and export of functional T cells into the periphery is a complicated one and the resultant mature T cell should have a high probability of mediating productive and non-pathologic immune responses (*Chapter 2*). The major hallmarks of the immune system, including specificity, recognition of self from non-self, and memory are all embodied in the T lymphocytes. It is essential that the immature thymocytes undergo stringent selection processes to eliminate any self-reactive T cells to prevent autoimmunity, ensuring that all these functions develop appropriately, requiring intricate coordination and multiple checkpoints. Like all leukocytes, stem cell progenitor T lymphocytes derive from the bone marrow, yet all T cell maturation and production occurs in the thymus, an organ located in the anterior mediastinum (*Chapter 2*). The human thymus consists of two main parts. The thymic epithelial space in the cortex is where the development of mature T cells from immature lymphocytes occurs under the influence of several lymphocyte growth and differentiative factors, e.g., thymic hormones and IL-7 (a process called thymopoiesis). The non-epithelial perivascular space in the medulla of the thymus is not a site of T lymphocyte maturation. The morphology and size of the thymus changes dynamically as the individual matures, with a progressive loss and involution of the thymic epithelial space and a compensatory increase in the non-epithelial perivascular space, which is also a site of adipocyte proliferation (Figure 7-6). The proportion of thymic epithelial space peaks at one year after birth and declines by 3 percent each year through middle age and 1 percent each year thereafter; nevertheless, new T cells continue to mature and be exported to the periphery throughout the life span of the individual into senescence (Figure 7-6A and Figure 7-6B). However, the bulk of production of new T cells occurs in childhood and young adulthood, reflecting perhaps evolutionary pressure for optimal immune responses during this period of life, as the human lifetime previously lasted only thirty to forty years.

Developing T cells within the thymus are referred to as thymocytes. As described previously, there are two major populations of thymocytes that can be distinguished on the basis of the polypeptide composition of the TCR (i.e., Tγδ and Tαβ) and these can be further subdivided by various expressions of the two co-receptors CD4 and CD8. Shown in Table 7-1 are the two major types of T cell populations according to their TCR polypeptide composition, together with subdivisions based on expressions of CD4 and CD8 molecules and their postulated functions.

Although the functions of some of these subtypes are not well understood, it would seem that the T γδ cells appear first during ontogeny and temporally precede the appearance of Tαβ cells in development. Ligands that interact with these cells include whole proteins and nonpeptidic molecules (e.g., glycolipids). The Tγδ cells dominate in epithelial tissues at mucosal sites and therefore provide a first line of defense against pathogens at mucosa-associated lymphoid tissues, e.g., MALT (*Chapter 8*). Moreover, since Tγδ cells are non-HLA-restricted, they are ready to function at the initial stages of

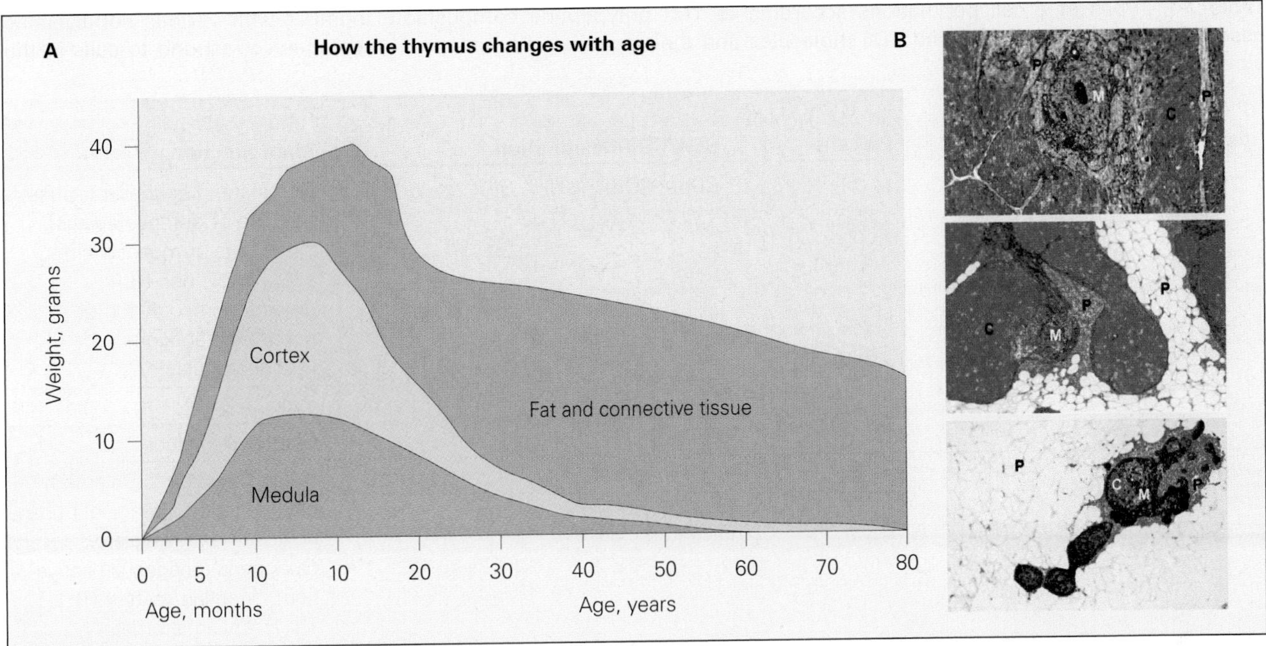

Figure 7-6. Panel A: Schematic representation of changes in weight and composition of thymus gland with maturation showing involution of the gland with age. (Hammar, J. A. "Die normal morphologische Thymusforschung im letzten," *Vierteljahrhundert*. Leipzig: Barth, 1936). Panel B: Thymus histology at different ages. A = two months of age; B = thirty-six years of age; C = sixty years of age. (P = perivascular spaces; C = cortex; M = medulla; white areas = adipocytes. (Reproduced with permission from Haynes BF, Markert ML, Sempowski GD, et al. The role of the thymus in immune reconstitution in aging, bone marrow transplantation, and HIV-1 infection. Annu Rev Immunol. 2000;18:529-60.)

infection without the need for prior antigen processing and presentation of peptides by APCs. Moreover, a number of additional immunoregulatory activities have been attributed to this class of cells. On the other hand, the majority of T cells in the systemic compartment of the body are comprised of the better-studied Tαβ population. These cells perform a wide variety of the helper, cytotoxic, and regulatory functions described below.

T Lymphocyte Development in the Thymus

The process of T lymphocyte development within the thymus leading to maturation and export of functionally mature T cells into the peripheral lymphoid tissues was described in general terms in *Chapter 2*. After migrating from the bone marrow to the thymus via a common lymphocyte precursor (**CLP**) cell, a primitive thymocyte with no CD3, CD4, or CD8 markers changes to an initial set of cells expressing only the CD3 molecule, which represents the distinguishing marker of the T cell population and which remains expressed throughout the various subsequent stages of the life span of the T cell (Figure 7-7). The next stage of development, where the TCR first appears, is characterized by cells with no CD4 or CD8 markers, referred to as double negative (**DN**) TCR+ cells, which then transition to cells with both CD4 and CD8 co-receptors, referred to as double positive (**DP**) thymocytes. The final stage of development is characterized by cells single positive (**SP**) for either CD4 or CD8 molecules that are expressed as CD4+, CD8− ("helper") and CD4−, and CD8+ ("cytotoxic") cells that leave the thymus, circulate in the recirculating lymphocyte pool, and populate peripheral lymphoid tissues (*Chapter 2*).

Shown in Figure 7-7B and 7-7C is a schematic representation of a flow cytometric analysis (*Chapter 24*) of CD4 and CD8 expression on total thymocytes obtained from thymus tissue at varying stages of development. The flow cytometric pattern resembles a swallow in flight (Figure 7-7B). The tail of the swallow, in the lower left quadrant, represents the DN T cells. The DN cells do not express a fully rearranged TCR. Following DN production, thymocytes mature to the next stage, which is represented by cells that appear at the head of the swallow or upper-right quadrant (Figure 7-7B, arrow #1), where DP T cells are found. These DP cells express a fully rearranged TCR and at this stage undergo rigorous selection to ensure that the TCR expressed exhibits appropriate modes of recognition and does not react to self proteins. If the DP cell survives, in a process referred to as "positive selection" (as described below), it will mature either into a

Table 7-1. Types of T cell populations according to TCR polypeptide composition, together with various subdivisions based on expressions of CD4 and CD8 molecules and their postulated functions. Percentages correspond to cells in the bloodstream.

T cell populations defined by the TCR	Percent	CD4/CD8 designation	Main function
Tγδ cells	5	CD4−/CD8− (DN)	Dominate in epithelial tissues; first line of defense against pathogens at mucosal sites, e.g., MALT; non-HLA-restricted; recognition of nonprotein antigens. Immunoregulatory?
		CD4+/CD8− (SN)	Function?
		CD4−/CD8+ (SN)	Cytotoxic function.
Tαβ cells	95	CD4+/CD8− (SN)	Helper function: cellular immunity, antimicrobial against phagocytosed extracellular pathogens (phagocytic activation), proinflammatory (Th1, Th17), anti-inflammatory, antibody production (Th2), immunoregulatory (Th3, Tr1).
		CD4−/CD8+ (SN)	Cytotoxic function: cellular immunity, antimicrobial against intracellular pathogens by the destruction of target cells (infected cell), tumor immunity, transplantation, autoimmunity.
		CD4−/CD8− (DN) CD4+/CD8+ (DP)	Only present in the thymus. Earliest thymocytes in development.

CD4+ (Figure 7-7B, arrow #2) or a CD8+ T cell (Figure 7-7B, arrow #3), represented by the wings of the swallow, and also referred to as SP T cells. These SP T cells are then exported and "fly out" of the thymus to the periphery, where they can circulate as mature, naïve T cells until they encounter their specific antigen in lymphoid tissues. In the peripheral lymphoid organs and blood, there are mainly SP T lymphocytes and very few DN or DP progenitors.

Thymocyte Selection Depends on TCR Binding to Self Peptide on MHC

The critical steps in T cell maturation that occur in the thymus involve T cell "education," in which T cells learn to distinguish self from nonself, deleting self-reactive T cells and expressing the appropriate CD4 or CD8 co-receptor. The learning process is also referred to as T cell selection, and depends on the characteristics of the TCR expressed by the developing T cell. In order for T cells to function properly in an immune response, the TCR must recognize antigen + self [MHC] and must not bind self peptide too tightly during T cell development. The processes that are involved in T cell selection in the thymus form the basis of central tolerance; another form of tolerance also takes place in the peripheral lymphoid tissues, referred to as peripheral tolerance; the failure of either forms of tolerance is importantly involved in the pathogenesis of autoimmune diseases. The mechanisms of both central and peripheral tolerance together with the clinical expressions of the autoimmune disorders are described in greater detail in Chapter 19.

Since the variable regions of the TCR have been generated by V(D)J and VJ joining of gene segments, many of the resulting variable regions will not be able to bind peptide on self MHC. Each developing T cell is subjected to vigorous examination for which more than 95 percent will fail and as a consequence will die by apoptosis. Those T cells

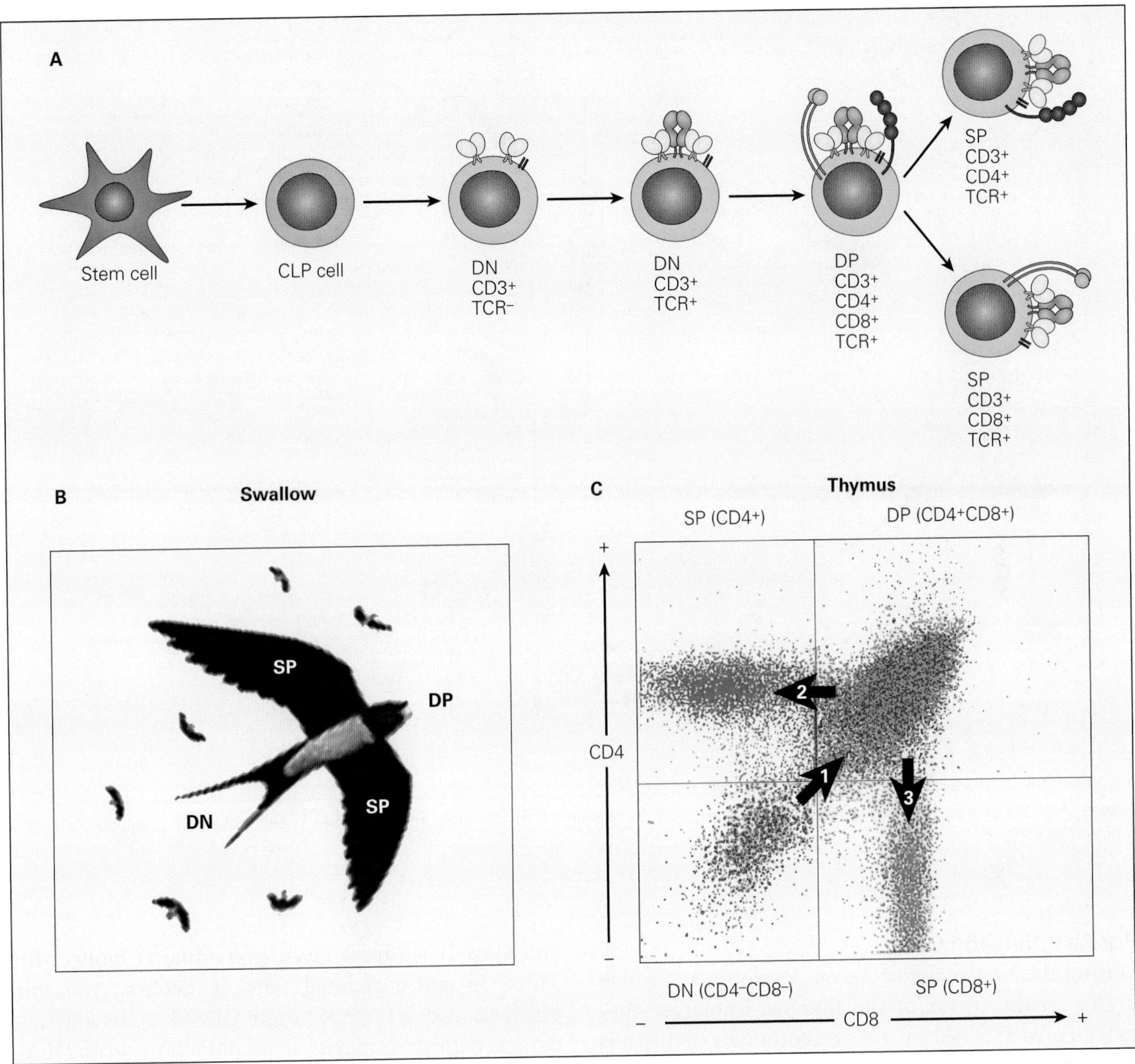

Figure 7-7. Panel A: Schematic representation of various stages of T cell maturation showing transition from a stem cell through a common lymphocyte precursor (CLP) to a mature SP CD4+ or CD8+ T cell. Panels B and C: Flow cytometric analysis of CD4 and CD8 expression on total thymocytes obtained from thymus tissue at varying stages of development, resembling a swallow in flight.

that "pass the exams" and can demonstrate self-knowledge, but not self-reactivity, will express an appropriate CD4 or CD8 co-receptor and emerge into the periphery. Thus, of the total lymphocyte repertoire of T cells in the thymus, most die by apoptosis and fewer than 5 percent emerge into the periphery. How is self-reactivity and knowledge tested?

Positive and Negative Selection

T cell selection in the thymus occurs in two phases during which a developing thymocyte undergoes positive selection and negative selection (Figure 7-8). During these phases, the outcome of whether a developing thymocyte will survive (positive selection) or die by apoptosis (negative selection) is determined not only by whether the TCR recognizes antigen + self [MHC] but also by the quantitative degree of binding or avidity of interaction of the TCR with the self-peptide MHC complex. As will be described below, the degree of binding avidity that results in the selected form of T cell resulting from the TCR/self-peptide/MHC complex interaction is determined by a type of "Goldilocks" analogy, in which binding may be too strong, too weak, or just right during T cell development.

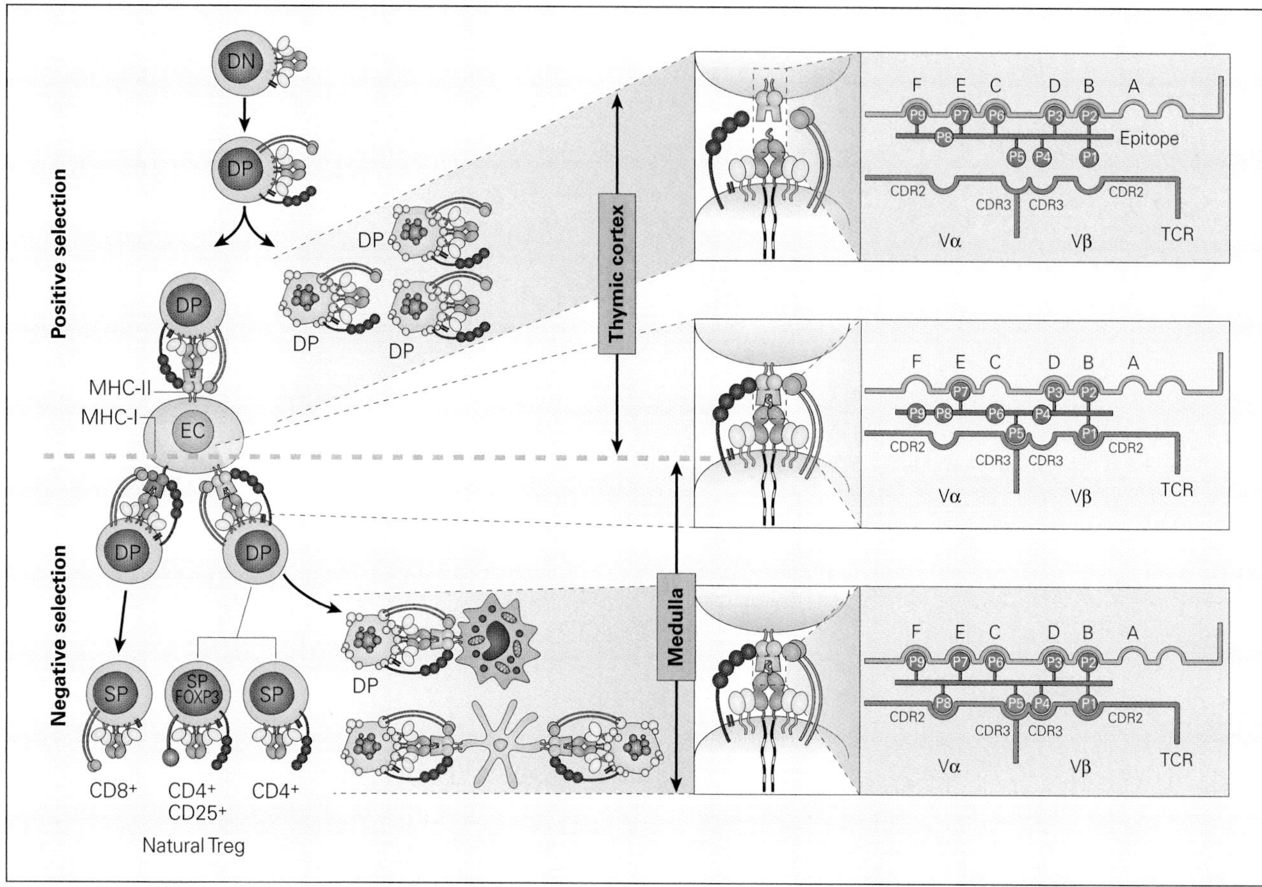

Figure 7-8. Schematic representation of the intrathymic mechanisms of positive and negative T cell selection involved in T cell maturation.

Positive Selection

During the first phase of T cell development, which occurs in the cortex of the thymus, immature thymocytes each make T cell receptors by a process of gene rearrangement similar to that of B cells described above (Figure 7-8). This process is error-prone, however, and some thymocytes fail to make functional T cell receptors, whereas other thymocytes make T cell receptors that are dysfunctional and cannot interact with one's own MHC molecules. Since the recognition of a foreign peptide must take place in the context of self MHC (this is referred to as MHC restriction), those thymocytes that express MHC-recognizable TCRs must be retained and those that are dysfunctional removed. The process by which MHC-functional thymocytes are selectively retained is called positive selection, during which developing T cells are tested for their potential ability to recognize a foreign peptide in the context of self MHC (Figure 7-8). "Self MHC" refers to all allelic forms or allotypes of HLA class I and class II within a given individual (*Chapter 10*). Thus, in an individual who is heterozygous for HLA-A2 and HLA-A37, their CD8 T cells will recognize peptide antigens in conjunction with HLA-A2 or with HLA-A37, but not with a nonself MHC molecule, such as HLA-A4 or HLA-A12, from another individual. In the thymus, this recognition process is accomplished via interaction of DP thymocytes with MHC-I or MHC-II on thymic epithelial cells within the cortex of the thymus, with two possible outcomes. If no interaction occurs, because the TCR cannot recognize self MHC, then the thymocyte will die from neglect (Figure 7-8). If the TCR and the MHC establish an effective interaction, the thymocyte survives by positive selection; conversely, if an interaction between the thymocyte TCR and MHC cannot be established, the thymocytes die by apoptosis. This first phase of T cell selection is followed by a second phase of the selection process that occurs in the medulla of the thymus, determined by the degree of interaction between TCRs and epitopes presented by MHC molecules on the surface of dendritic cells (**DCs**) or macrophages (Figure 7-8).

Negative Selection

This second stage of the selective process occurs through interactions of developing thymocytes (already previously selected to interact with self MHC molecules by positive selection) with epitopes presented by MHC molecules expressed by thymic dendritic cells or macrophages, and occurs at the DP stage at the corticomedullary junction of the thymus. In contrast to the earlier thymocyte-epithelial phase, at this stage of development not only do dendritic cells and macrophages express higher levels of MHC molecules, but also there is greater degree of TCR expression on the developing thymocytes. If the TCR expressed by a DP cell fully interacts with the epitope presented by the MHC molecule with high avidity, it will die by apoptosis or by programmed cell death by a process called negative selection (Figure 7-8). Because in the thymus no foreign antigens are present and only self antigens can be expressed, every T cell with a TCR able to recognize a self antigen is eliminated. A small minority of the surviving cells is selected to become natural regulatory T cells that acquire the CD25 (the alpha chain of the IL-2 receptor) and the FOXP3 transcription factor. The surviving selected T cells will then exit the thymus as mature, naïve T regulatory cells.

Although the mechanisms underlying positive and negative selection are not well defined, they appear to be governed by the affinity of interaction with the self-peptide MHC complex. The prevailing theory is that three outcomes may be seen that are dependent on the degree of binding or avidity of epitopes presented by MHC molecules to the TCRs: (1) T cells with strong or high avidity interaction of the TCR with MHC lead to negative selection and will undergo apoptotic death and deletion; (2) an absolute failure of interaction between the components also leads to death by neglect; and (3) an interaction that is somewhere in between and has the appropriate avidity—not too weak or too strong—promotes thymocyte survival and maturation to SP T effector (**Teff**) cells and T regulatory (**Treg**) cells (Figure 7-8). Due to the random nature of the process of T cell activation, all T cell populations with a given TCR will end up with a mixture of Teff and Treg cells—the relative proportions of which appear to be determined by the avidities of the T cell for the self peptide MHC. Negative selection, however, is not 100 percent complete, and some autoreactive T cells escape thymic censorship and are released into the circulation. Additional mechanisms of tolerance, active in the periphery, exist to silence these cells, such as anergy, deletion, and regulatory T cells. If these peripheral tolerance mechanisms also fail, autoimmunity may arise (*Chapter 19*).

The T cells that survive positive and negative selection subsequently downregulate expression of one of their two expressed co-receptors and become SP thymocytes (CD4+ or CD8+ cells), poised for export into the peripheral lymphoid system. Whether a DP thymocyte will differentiate into a CD4+ SP or a CD8+ SP depends on the MHC bound by the DP thymocyte; if the MHC is class II, then the cells will differentiate into CD4+ T cells, but if the MHC is class I, then differentiation to CD8+ T cells will occur. These new thymic emigrants take up residence in local lymph tissues, MALT, and lymphoid organs, and circulate through the blood and lymph. In the periphery, new thymic emigrants are referred to as naïve T cells because they have not yet seen the antigen for which their TCR is specific. The rate of thymic export in a young, healthy adult is approximately 600 million new T cells each day. One very innovative way that has been recently used to monitor thymic output into the periphery is by measuring the presence of T cell receptor-excision circles, or TRECs, in peripheral T cells (Box 7-3, Figure 7-9). The measurement of these TREC molecules has been found to be clinically useful in the management of patients undergoing transplantation or with infection, immunodeficiency, and malignancy (Box 7-3).

Alloreactivity Is a Consequence of Positive T Cell Selection

The T lymphocytes that have undergone positive T cell selection in the thymus emerge with no self-reactivity, yet retain a potential for recognizing antigen plus self MHC. In addition, a high proportion of peripheral T cells (>10 percent) has the capacity to bind to and react with foreign MHC or MHC of a different allotype than an individual—a phenomenon referred to as alloreactivity (*Chapter 22*). Alloreactivity is a particular problem for recipients of transplanted organs or bone marrow grafts from unrelated individuals, as in the case of "David the Bubble Boy." Unless one has a twin—or perhaps in

Box 7-3

T Cell Receptor-Excision Circles in Peripheral T Cells and their Clinical Significance

T cell receptor–excision circles (TRECs) are the leftover products of TCR rearrangement during the DP stage that consist of circular DNA containing spliced-out intervening D, J, and C segments. Thymic output can be monitored by a PCR-based assay that is sensitive enough to detect TRECs from low numbers of cells. TRECs can also be used diagnostically to monitor T cell maturation after bone marrow transplantation/reconstitution in treatments for immunodeficiencies and malignancies, to measure replenishment in infectious diseases such as in HIV infection, and in understanding the dynamics of lymphocyte homeostasis in aging. Measurement of TRECs has also been recommended as one of the predictive markers for identification of affected infants in the proposed newborn screening program for SCID.

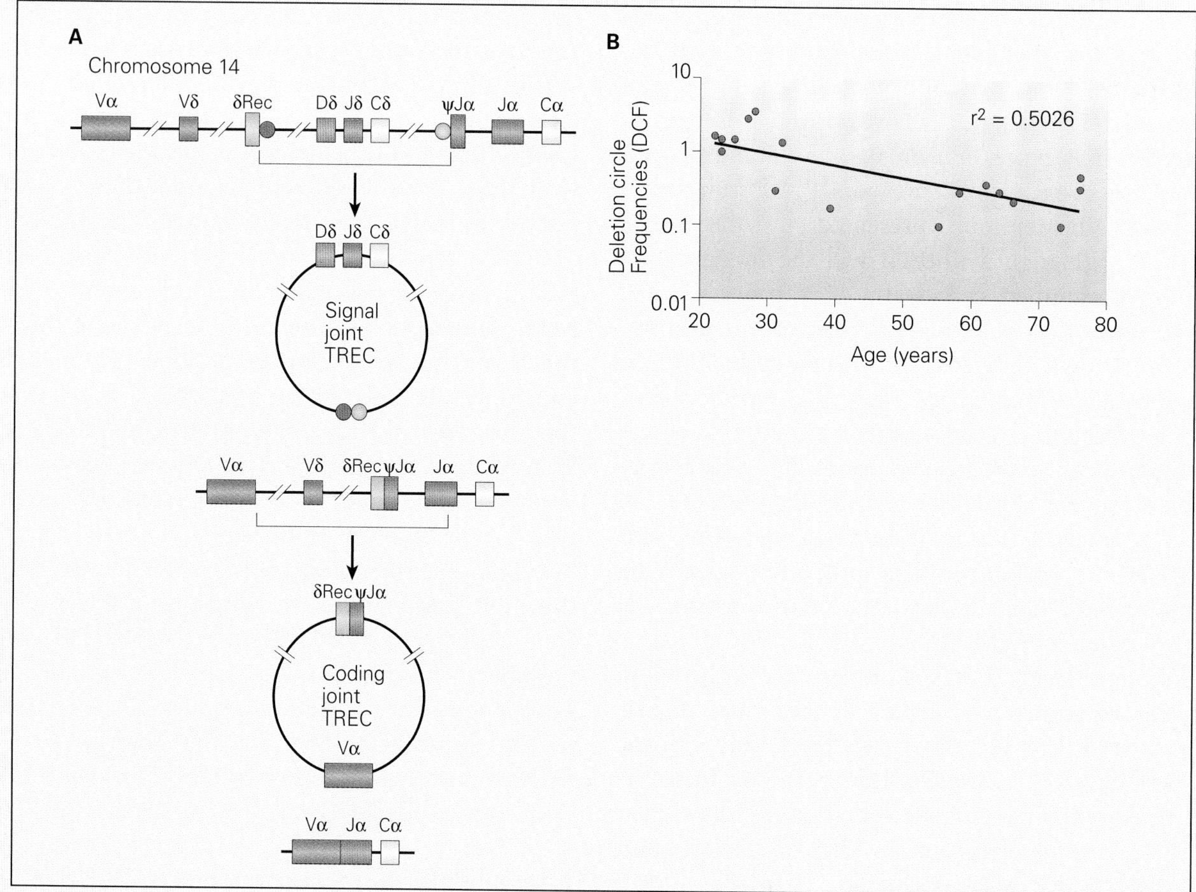

Figure 7-9. Panel A: T cell receptor-excision circles, or TRECs. Panel B: TREC content in peripheral blood at various ages. (Reproduced with permission from Poulin JF, Viswanathan MN, Harris JM, et al. Direct evidence for thymic function in adult humans. J. Exp. Med. 1999;190:479-86.)

the future, a clone—and one needs a bone marrow or an organ transplant such as a kidney, liver, heart, or lung, the only other option is to receive a cadaver organ from an unrelated individual (and for kidneys and livers, another option is to receive organs from a living relative). Unfortunately, the immune response is quite robust against alloantigens that pervade an organ, and will rapidly destroy the allograft unless potent immunosuppression is given that prevents T cell activation (*Chapter 11*). In the case of bone marrow transplantation, a unique problem is graft-versus-host disease (**GVHD**), which will be described below. Transplantation and alloreactivity will be described in greater detail in Chapter 22.

Clinical Pathologies That Result from Defects in T Cell Development

As described previously, severe combined immunodeficiency (**SCID**), or "David the Bubble Boy syndrome," is a genetic disorder in which both "arms" (B cells and T cells) of the adaptive immune system are crippled due to a defect in one of several possible genes that govern T cell development (*Chapter 16*). SCID is a severe form of heritable immunodeficiency. It is also known as the "bubble boy" disease because its victims are extremely vulnerable to infectious diseases; the most famous case is David Vetter, who is the patient presented in the case study in this chapter.

DiGeorge Syndrome

An equally devastating immune deficiency is the rare congenital condition called DiGeorge syndrome, a developmental lack of the third and fourth pharyngeal pouches that results in absence of thymus and parathyroid glands (*Chapter 2* and *Chapter 16*). These infants present with profound T cell deficiency, and most DiGeorge infants die at several months of age. In these cases, bone marrow transplantation will not reconstitute T cell numbers because no thymus is present and the patient's bone marrow lymphoid progenitors have nowhere to go to be selected and mature. The only known treatment is to perform a thymus transplant, and this approach has been used successfully in several cases. Donor thymuses are obtained from fetuses or from infants who undergo heart transplants (the thymus is removed in these cases to make room for the heart surgery, with no known deleterious consequences). Interestingly, although no histocompatibility pretesting of thymus tissue administered to patients with DiGeorge syndrome has been performed, reconstitution and restoration of immune responses has been observed, presumably due not only to the presence of T cell precursors but also to the lack of mature T lymphocytes in the transplanted thymus, which would have otherwise caused a GVHD.

Bare Lymphocyte Syndrome

Infants with bare lymphocyte syndrome (**BLS**), a rare syndrome, display an absence of MHC-II expression (*Chapter 16*). This loss of MHC-II impairs the normal positive selection of CD4+ T cells in the thymus, and these patients have dramatically reduced numbers of peripheral CD4 T cells with normal numbers of CD8 T cells and B cells. Therefore, total lymphocyte numbers do not differ significantly from those of healthy infants. Infants with BLS generally present with persistent diarrhea and chronic bacterial and viral infections, frequently with severe pneumonia. The condition is known to arise not from the direct mutation of MHC-II genes (since there are three MHC-II genes in humans, it would be a rare event for three to be mutated), but rather from mutations in genes that regulate the coordinate transcription of all MHC-II genes (*Chapter 10*). An analogous defect in MHC-I expression has also been observed in individuals who lack expression of genes involved in the MHC-I processing pathway, specifically the TAP molecules (*Chapter 10*). As expected from what we know about positive selection, MHC-I deficiency results in the absence of CD8 T cells. This immunodeficiency is less severe than MHC-II deficiency, mostly because CD4 T cells are more pivotal coordinators of both humoral and cellular immune responses, whereas CD8 T cells primarily serve as effectors for antigen clearance, as described below.

Antigen-Dependent T Cell Activation, Differentiation, and Effector Functions

T Cells Are Activated by Specialized Cells in Lymphoid Tissues

The newly exported CD4+ and CD8+ T cells from the thymus migrate to lymphoid organs and recirculate through peripheral blood and lymph, as described previously in Chapter 2. In the periphery, a naïve T cell will meet its cognate (i.e., TCR-specific) antigen in a lymph node, spleen, or the MALT and will become activated. In response to newly encountered antigens, components of the innate immune system constitute the first line of defense against pathogens at their portal of entry, as described in Chapter 3. APCs bind antigen and migrate to local lymphoid tissues, draining the site of antigen encounter. Naïve T lymphocytes become activated by contact of their TCRs with APCs bearing the cognate antigen in conjunction with MHC-I or MHC-II, and at least two types of signals are generated: (1) the first signal is generated following the interaction of the TCR with MHC/peptide, and (2) signal 2 is generated following the interaction of co-stimulatory molecules between the T cell and the APC. APCs that can activate naïve T cells, specifically naïve CD4 and CD8 T cells, have been referred to as "professional" APCs. Dendritic cells are in fact the most effective activators that can potentially stimulate

naïve T cells. Other professional APCs include macrophages, involved mostly in secondary responses, and activated B cells. Once a naïve T cell binds antigen presented by a professional APC together with the participation of costimulatory molecules and the CD4 or CD8 coreceptors, the T cell becomes activated to proliferate and differentiate into subsets of CD4+ helper or CD8+ cytotoxic effector T cells, respectively.

The primary role of effector cells is to clear the antigen or pathogen, and different types of effector T cells use various and directed means to accomplish this goal, such as the secretion of effector chemokines and cytokines (*Chapter 9*) for the recruitment and activation of additional immune and/or nonimmune cells for antigen clearance, e.g., macrophages, natural killer (**NK**) cells, neutrophils, or via direct cytotoxic effects on infected cells or directly on pathogens. After several days to weeks, most of the expanded population of effector T cells dies, leading to a contraction of the immune response. However, antigen activation also results in the production of a population of long-lived memory T cells that can be activated more quickly and efficiently on repeat contact with the same antigen (Figure 7-10). When reactivated by a new wave of the specific (cognate) antigen, memory T cells mediate the enhanced recall response that can mount immediate effector responses and mediate protective immunity. In the following sections, how each stage of this activation/differentiation process occurs, where it goes wrong in pathological manifestations, and how it can be manipulated in immunotherapy will be described below.

T Cell Activation Requires Adhesion to APC

The interaction of the T cell with an APC resulting in T cell activation and differentiation involves multiple molecular contacts. As described previously, in order for a naïve T cell to become activated, it requires interaction of the antigen-specific TCR with cognate peptide complexed with self MHC-I or MHC-II expressed on the surface of a professional APC. In addition to TCR contacting antigen/MHC, there are two other critical interactions between a T cell and APC that are required for naïve T cell activation. The first type of interaction occurs even before the TCR/MHC contact each other and represents a cell adhesive interaction. The second type of interaction is via contact of co-stimulatory receptors of T cells with their co-stimulatory ligands on APCs. The first accessory interaction via cell adhesion molecules is necessary because cells carry electrostatic charges on their membranes that will naturally repel cells as they approach in close proximity (Figure 7-11). In order for two cells to come together in a specific fashion, there needs to be molecular points of contact of sufficient affinity to overcome these natural electrostatic repulsive forces. One class of adhesion molecules is the leukocyte integrins, e.g., LFA-1 (*Chapter 5*). Integrins are a family of molecules with common structural features that consist of two polypeptide chains, α and β, and a cysteine-rich region that mediate cell-cell contact (Figure 7-11A). Different immune cell types express distinct combinations of α and β chain types. On T lymphocytes, the integrin LFA-1 is particularly important in initial interactions between a naïve T cell and APC. It is the interaction of LFA-1 on T cells with its ligand ICAM-1 expressed by APC that enables the T cell and APC to maintain sufficient proximity to test whether the TCR can bind to the antigen/MHC complex on the surface (Figure 7-11B).

The Immunological Synapse Is the Sum of Contacts Between APCs and T Cells

In recent years, there has been intense study of the macromolecular changes in the T cell that occur during the course of T cell activation, which has led to a better understanding of how T cell activation is regulated. The region of contact between a T cell and an APC is referred to as the immunological synapse (**IS**), by analogy to the neuronal synapse, the region of contact between neuronal cells (Figure 7-12).

The IS is formed early in T cell activation, but only after TCR-signaling events have occurred. After an immunologic synapse forms, many identical TCRs on the T cell surface recognize multiple MHC-peptide targets, with the participation of the co-receptors CD4 or CD8, which cluster on the cell surface (shown as a red bull's-eye in the bottom box of Figure 7-13); other cell surface molecules involved in signaling and adhesion (the yellow outer ring at the bottom of Figure 7-13) coalesce to form the outer ring.

As shown in Figure 7-13A, formation of the IS involves a reorganization of the membrane distribution of TCR and LFA-1, along with a number of accessory molecules, to form the mature IS as schematically depicted in Figure 7-13B. When the T cell initially approaches an APC through the LFA-1-ICAM adhesive interaction, the contact zone between the T cell and APC consists of LFA-1 molecules at the center and the TCR around the periphery.

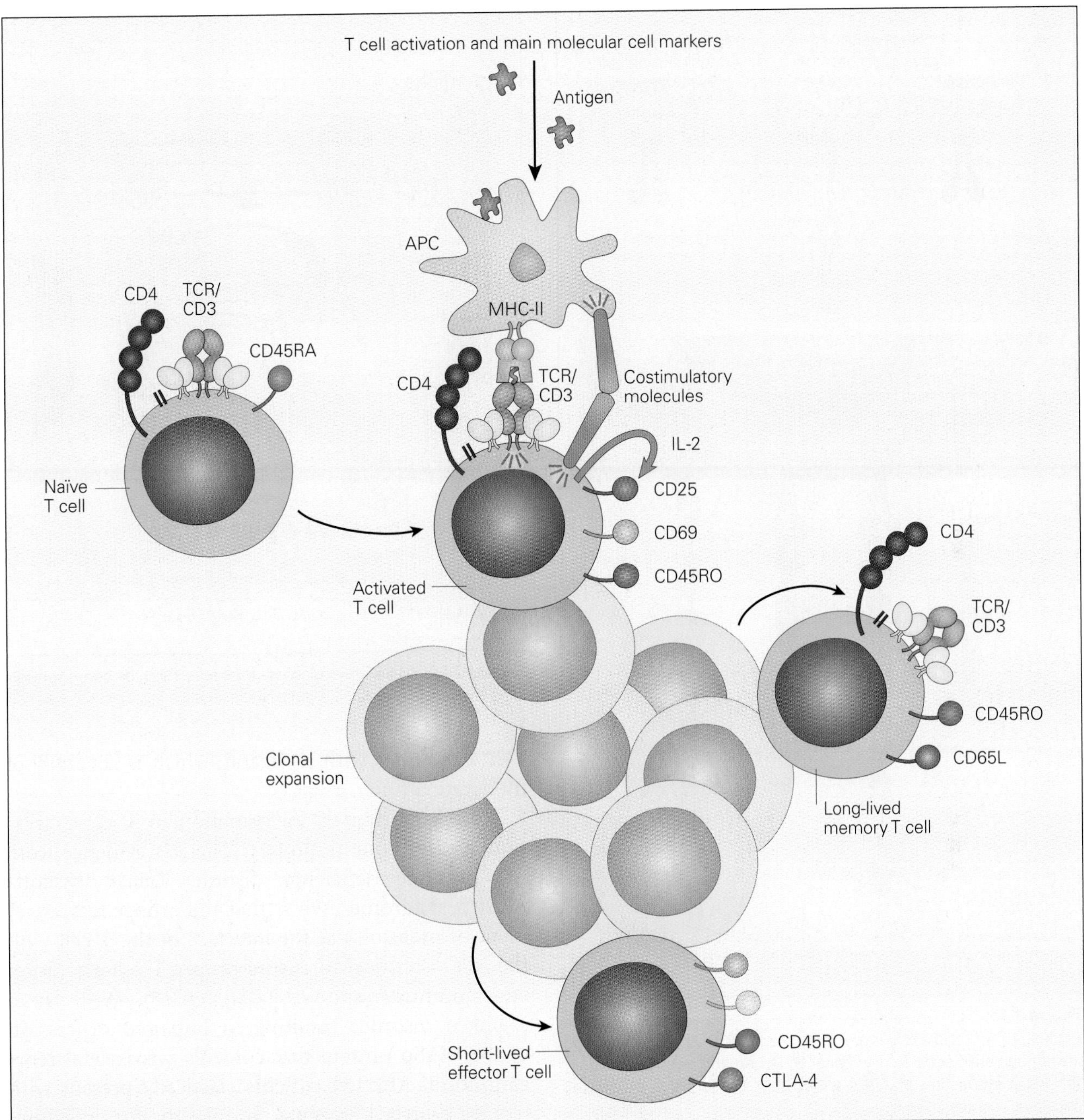

Figure 7-10. Antigen-driven clonal expansion of T cells into long-lived memory cells and short-lived effector cells.

However, as the TCR becomes activated and signaling occurs, there is a redistribution of the TCR and LFA-1, with the TCR-antigen/MHC contacts in the center and LFA-1/ICAM interactions organized around this central cluster of TCR molecules. It takes between thirty and sixty minutes for a mature synapse to form, whereas early proximal signaling occurs seconds to minutes following T cell contact with its ligand. Coincident with the formation of the synapse is a reorganization of cytoskeletal components. Prolonged cell-cell contact that is mediated by multiple molecular interactions results in profound alterations in the cellular structure that is mediated by cytoskeletal proteins, including constituents of microfilaments such as actin, talin, ezrin, Wiskott-Aldrich syndrome protein (**WASp**), microtubules (**MT**), and MT-associated proteins. These cytoskeletal rearrangements form the scaffold upon which signaling molecules can likewise assemble, promoting delivery of signals via cell surface molecules.

The mature IS is comprised of three regions, each with a characteristic arrangement of molecules

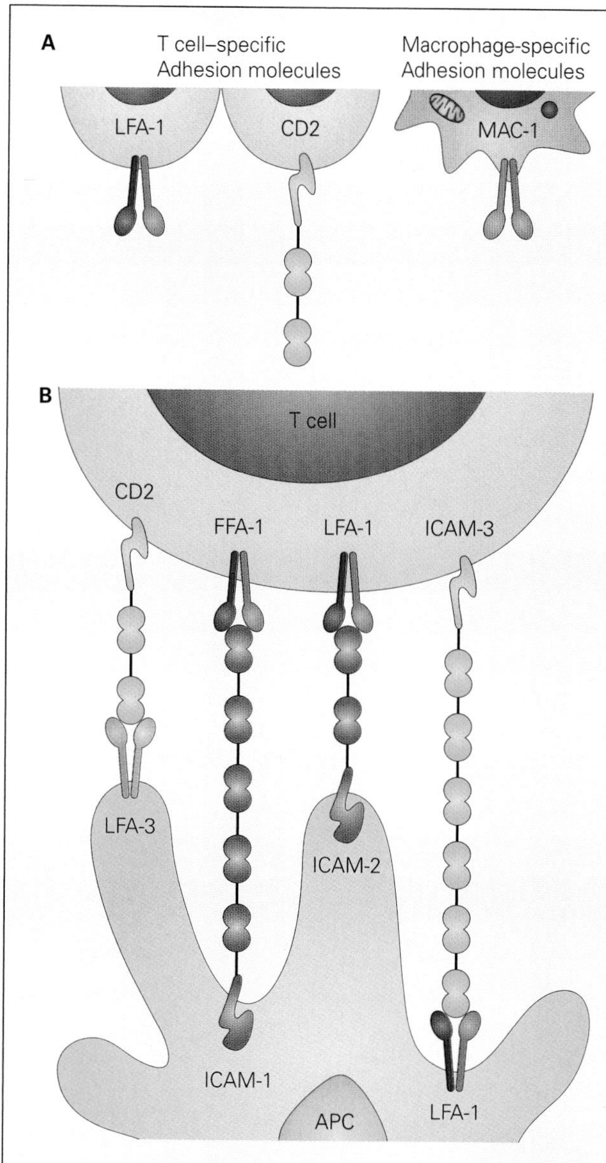

Figure 7-11. Panel A: General structure of the main adhesion molecules. LFA-1 and Mac-1 are integrins, and CD2 is part of the immunoglobulin superfamily. Panel B: Schematic representation of the initial interaction of APCs and T cells by adhesion molecules and their ligands.

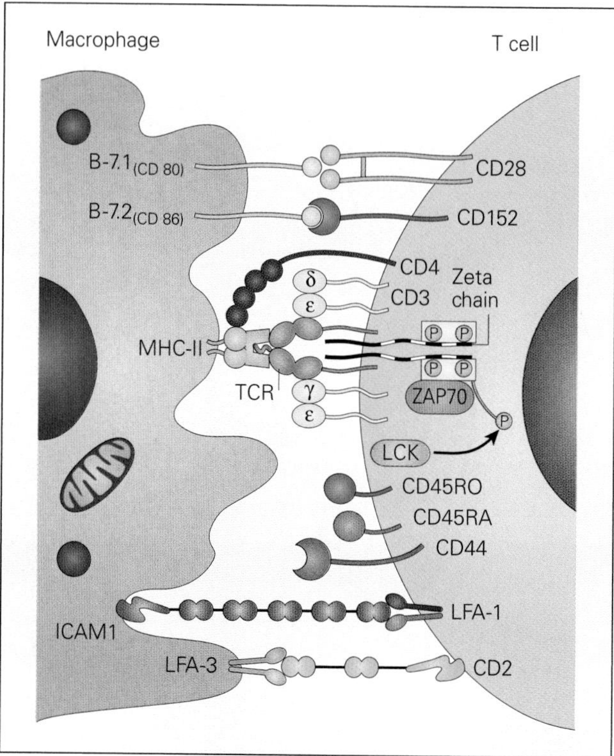

Figure 7-12. Main physiological characteristics of the immunologic synapse.

in supramolecular activation complexes (**SMACs**) (Figure 7-13B). The central core of the IS, designated the cSMAC, contains the TCR, CD28, and certain signaling molecules, such as PKC̃θ; Surrounding the cSMAC is the peripheral SMAC, or pSMAC, that contains CD4, LFA-1, and talin, a cytoskeletal component. On the outer rim of the cSMAC and the pSMAC is the distal SMAC (**dsSMAC**) that contains the larger, more highly charged molecules CD45 and CD43 that participate in T cell activation but are excluded from the inner SMAC, which may be necessary to optimize the TCR encounter with its ligand, which is generally of moderate affinity.

How important is IS formation in T cell activation and immune responses? There is evidence from the immune deficiency disorder called Wiskott-Aldrich syndrome (**WAS**) that the proper rearrangement of molecules at the interface of the T cell with the APC is critical to ensure proper T cell activation and immune responses (*Chapter 16*). WAS is an X-linked disorder resulting in impaired expression of the WASp protein that controls cytoskeletal reorganization. Affected patients classically present with bloody diarrhea, eczema, propensity for infection, and thrombocytopenia. A hallmark of WAS, in addition to the immune-mediated dysfunctions, is small platelets and a defect in platelet production and destruction. WAS sufferers have normal circulating numbers of T and B lymphocytes, yet the T lymphocytes exhibit profound defects in activation. If untreated, most individuals with WAS die before age ten. Bone marrow transplantation has proved an effective treatment for severe WAS, and splenectomy has proven effective in managing the platelet abnormalities. This syndrome highlights the importance of molecular reorganization in T cell activation (*Chapter 16*).

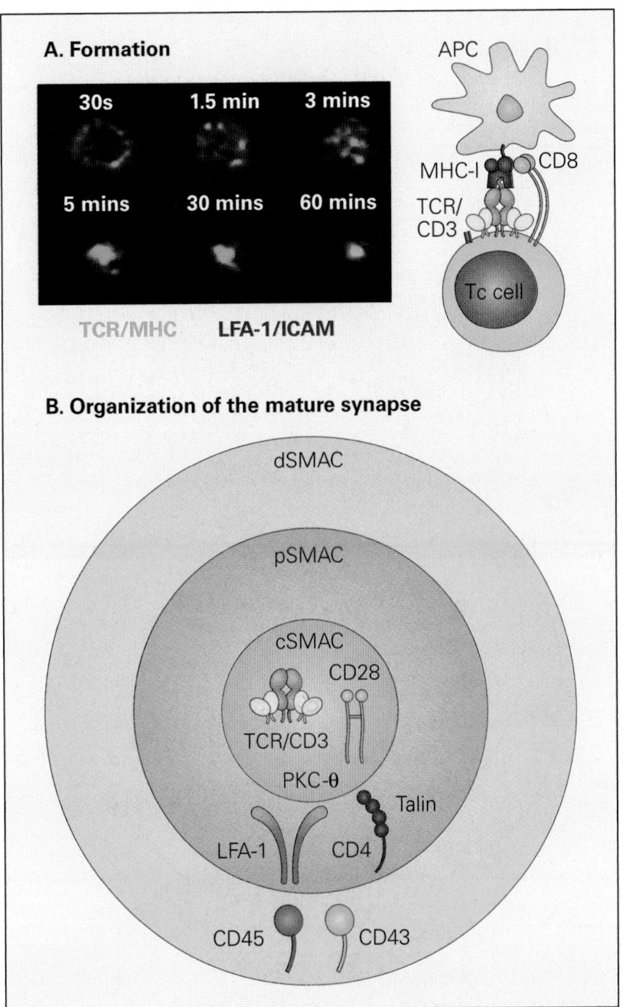

Figure 7-13. Panel A: Schematic representation of the formation of the immunologic synapse. Panel B: The organization of the mature synapse. SMAC is the supramolecular activation complex, c is central, p is peripheral, and ds is distal.

T Cell Receptor-Mediated Signaling Initiates T Cell Activation: The TCR Receptor Complex

When the TCR meets its cognate antigen/MHC (Figure 7-14), a number of early activation and signaling events are triggered through the TCR.

The cell surface TCR serves to bind antigen/MHC and CD4 co-receptor but does not directly transmit activation signals through the cytoplasm into the nucleus due to its short cytoplasmic portion. For transmission of activation signals, the TCR relies on the set of cell surface protein subunits referred to as the CD3 complex and are non-covalently associated with the TCR. The CD3 subunits, known as CD3 ε,δ,γ and CD3ζ, have extended cytoplasmic domains that enable efficient coupling of extracellular TCR-delivered signals through the cytoplasm to the nucleus (Figure 7-14A). The CD3 chains thus initiate the cascade of molecular signaling driven by sequential coupling of different kinases, adaptor molecules, and G proteins to mobilize transcription factor activation in the nucleus. The leukocyte-specific protein tyrosine kinase (**LCK**) p56 associates with the cytoplasmic portion of CD4 or CD8 molecules and helps to initiate signals through the TCR as described below.

The sequence of TCR-coupled signaling events leading to transcription of the gene encoding interleukin-2 (**IL-2**) has been identified. IL-2 is a T cell growth factor that is the first type of cytokine produced after T cell activation and promotes proliferative expansion of T cells (*Chapter 9*). The signals that are delivered following TCR ligation by antigen to IL-2 gene transcription can be grouped into three sequential classes: (1) proximal events, (2) linker/adaptor coupling, and (3) distal events. A detailed depiction of these events is shown in Figure 7-14. The proximal events comprise the earliest biochemical triggers that are activated within seconds following interaction of TCR/CD3 complex with antigen/MHC ligands (Figure 7-14A, step 1). This earliest event involves the phosphorylation of the CD3 signaling chains themselves by co-receptor-associated p56lck tyrosine kinase on specific tyrosines located in specific protein sequence motifs called immunoreceptor tyrosine-based activation motifs (**ITAMS**) in the cytoplasmic domain of each CD3 chain (Figure 7-14A, step 2). Phosphorylation of CD3 chains, and specifically the CD3ζ chain, then triggers the recruitment and activation of the tyrosine kinase zeta-associated protein of 70 kDa (**ZAP70**) (Figure 7-14B, step 3). The ZAP70 kinase, once recruited to the TCR/CD3 complex, will then phosphorylate a number of substrates, importantly the linker/adaptor molecules, linker for activated T cells (**LAT**) and SH2-containing linking protein of 76 kDa (**SLP-76**) (Figure 7-14B, step 4). Phosphorylated LAT and SLP-76 participate in the linker/adaptor phase of the signaling cascade. These molecules serve as molecular scaffolds upon which additional signaling intermediates are recruited and act to couple proximal to distal signaling events (Figure 7-14C, step 5). The complexes formed by LAT and SLP-76 include other components associated with G-protein activation such as grb2 and SOS, and the guanine nucleotide exchange factor, vav, and also additional linker molecules (GADS, SLAP), and phospholipase C (**PLC-γ**). Different components of these linker complexes serve to turn on distal signaling events. These distal

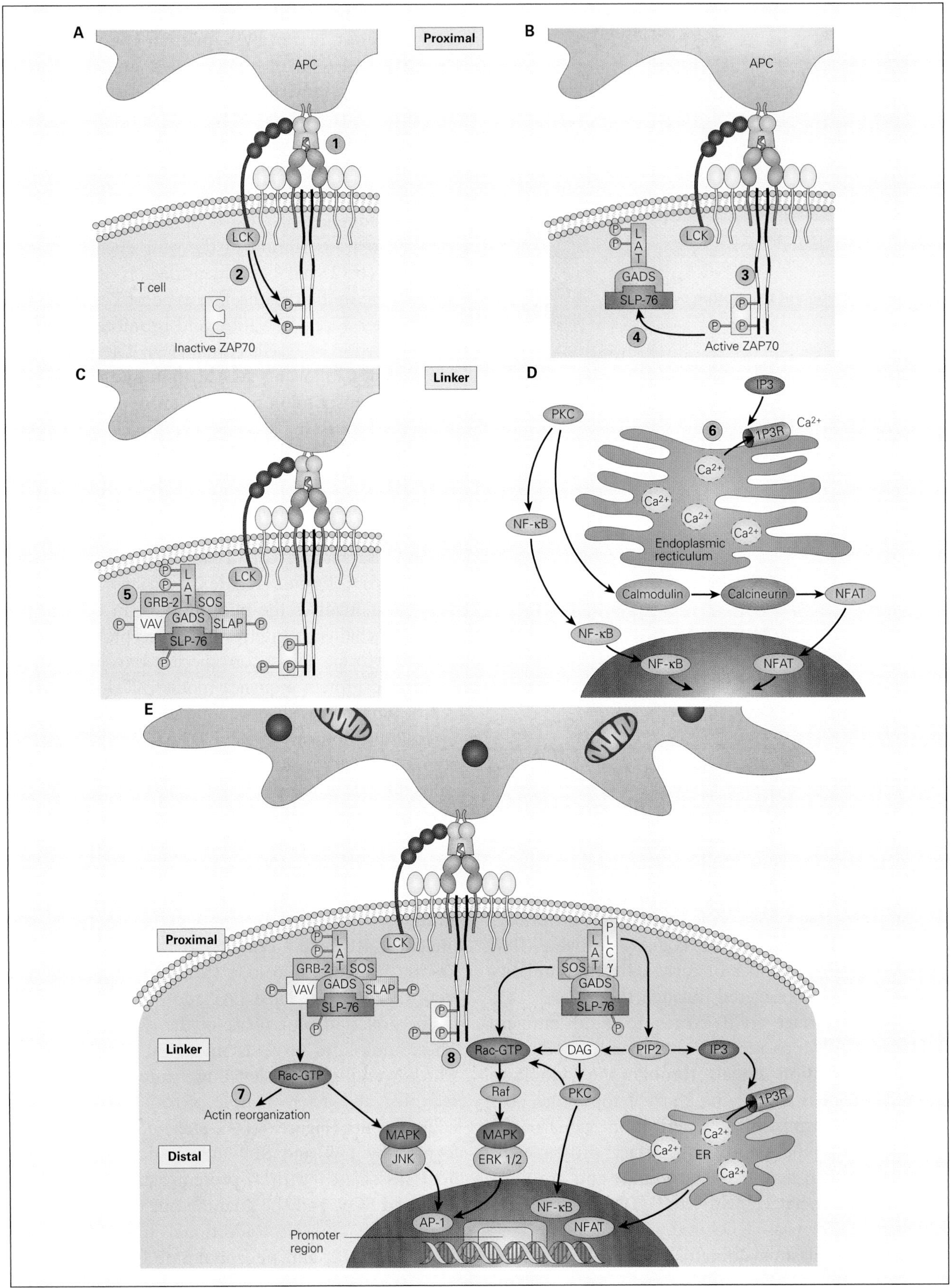
A
Proximal
B
APC
APC
1
LCK
2
T cell
Inactive ZAP70
LAT
LCK
GADS
SLP-76
3
4
Active ZAP70
C
Linker
D
IP3
PKC
6
1P3R
Ca2+
Endoplasmic
recticulum
NF-κB
LCK
5
GRB-2
SOS
VAV
GADS
SLAP
SLP-76
Calmodulin
Calcineurin
NFAT
NF-κB
NF-κB
NFAT
E
Proximal
LCK
PLCγ
SOS
Linker
Rac-GTP
DAG
PIP2
IP3
8
Raf
PKC
1P3R
7
Actin reorganization
Distal
MAPK
JNK
MAPK
ERK 1/2
ER
AP-1
NF-κB
NFAT
Promoter
region

events include the mobilization of calcium by promoting calcium release from intracellular stores, the activation of small GTP-binding proteins such as ras and rac, and the activation of a class of serine/threonine kinases known as mitogen-activated protein (**MAP**) kinases (Figure 7-14D). These distal events coordinate to activate transcription factors such as the nuclear factor of activated T cells (**NFAT**), nuclear factor κ B (**NF-κB**), and AP-1 that all control transcription of the IL-2 gene (Figure 7-14E).

Costimulation Is Required for T Cell Activation

In the previous sections, we have learned that T cells need to encounter antigen presented by an antigen-presenting cell, or APC. This binding of TCR with its ligand on APC is referred to as signal 1 (Figure 7-15). Additional adhesive contacts achieved by adhesion molecules are necessary to stabilize the interaction of the TCR with its ligand. Shown in Box 7-4 are some clinical applications resulting from defects in T cell adhesion and signaling. There is also a critical accessory interaction, called costimulation, that is absolutely essential for the activation of naïve T cells. Several decades ago, Bretscher and Cohn proposed a "two signal hypothesis," which stated that T lymphocytes could not be fully activated by TCR ligation (signal 1) alone, and that there must be a second signal (signal 2) required for T cell activation that would alert the body to the presence of a foreign invader and prevent self-reactivity in the periphery. The identity of this second signal was discovered in the early 1990s in the guise of a T cell-specific cell surface molecule called CD28 (Figure 7-15).

CD28 binds to two different molecules on the surface of APC, designated B7-1 or CD80, and B7-2 or CD86, and together represent costimulatory ligands, whereas CD28 in T cells is a costimulatory receptor. The interaction of CD28 with CD80/CD86 and other molecular costimulatory pairs, e.g., ICOS and ICOS ligand, are referred to as signal 2.

As shown in Figure 7-15, T cell activation is now known to require both interaction of the TCR with antigen/MHC (signal 1) and interaction of CD28 with CD80/86 (signal 2). This two-signal recognition leads directly to IL-2 production and initiates the T cell activation process characterized by proliferation and differentiation to effector cells (Figure 7-16).

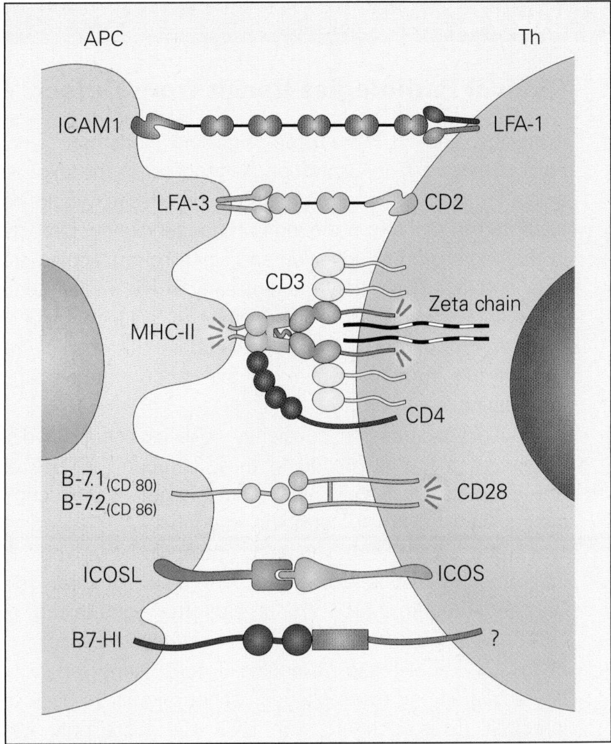

Figure 7-15. Schematic representation of signal I resulting from the binding of the TCR with its ligand on an APC. The second signal is carried out by the interaction of the costimulatory molecules B-7.1 and B-7.2 on the APC and the costimulatory receptor CD28 on the T cell.

Figure 7-14. Schematic representation of the overall steps involved in TCR-coupled signaling pathways associated with IL-2 transcription. Panel A: The proximal events are initiated by the interaction of the TCR/CD3 complex with antigen/MHC ligands that subsequently activate the LCK enzyme (step 1). The activated LCK then phosphorylates tyrosine residues located on the immunoreceptor tyrosine-based activation motifs (ITAMs) of the CD3 ζ chain (step 2). Panel B: The phosphorylated tyrosine motifs on the ITAMs then act as docking sites for the recruitment and activation of the tyrosine kinase zeta-associated protein of 70 kDa (ZAP70) (step 3). The phosphorylated ZAP70 induces the phosphorylation of the signal transducing adaptor (LAT/GADS/SLP-76) complex (step 4) that then serves as a molecular scaffold. Panel C: Additional signaling intermediates are then recruited and phosphorylated, linking proximal with distal signaling events (step 5). Panel D: These linker events include the activation of IP3 that leads to the mobilization of calcium (step 6) by promoting calcium release from intracellular stores and the sequential stimulation of calmodulin, calcineurin, and NFAT, as well as the activation of PKC that activates NF-κB; the activated NF-κB and NFAT then translocate to the nucleus. Panel E: The sequential activation of the 2 signal transducing adaptor complexes (LAT/GADS/SLP76) and (PLCγ/LAT/SOS/GADS/SLP76) and the generation of the small GTP-binding proteins Rac-GTP (step 7) and Ras-GTP (step 8) coupled with the activation of serine/threonine kinases known as MAP (mitogen-activated protein) kinases, induces the translocation of AP-1, which together with NF-κB and NFAT control the transcription of the IL-2 gene.

Box 7-4

Clinical Pathologies Result from Defects in T Cell Adhesion and Signaling

Adhesion and TCR-mediated signaling constitute very early events in T cell activation. Any defect in the expression of molecules controlling these processes would be expected to result in profound immunodeficiency. Defects in the expression of adhesion and signaling molecules are rare, and like SCID, they present early in life, usually during infancy (*Chapter 16*). Also, similar to SCID conditions, bone marrow transplantation to reconstitute the T cell arm of the immune system is the most effective and long-lasting treatment.

Leukocyte adhesion deficiency (LAD) arises from disruption of the gene encoding the β2 subunit (CD18) of the integrins of T cells and macrophages. CD18 complexes with CD11a to form the integrin LFA-1, an adhesion and signal transduction molecule involved in inflammation that is expressed by T cells (*Chapter 16*). Another integrin, Mac-1, represents the complexing of CD18 with CD11b (CD11b/CD18) expressed by macrophages. Without these molecules, T cells cannot be properly activated and macrophages cannot migrate to sites of infection. Thus, patients with LAD (there are only 200 reported patients worldwide) present with recurrent infections and persistent diarrhea, both of which can have fatal sequelae if untreated. Another interesting clinical clue for the diagnosis of the condition in the newborn is that many patients with LAD present with the finding of delayed rejection of the umbilical cord beyond the normal time of seven to ten days, presumably due to the defective inflammatory response. There are different gradations of LAD, from moderate, with some expression of CD18, to severe, connoting a total lack of CD18. As with SCID, bone marrow transplantation is the best therapy, whereas prophylactic use of antibiotics can be effective for more moderate cases. Gene therapy to replenish CD18 in bone marrow leukocyte progenitors theoretically constitutes the best cure, although it has not been attempted with these patients.

Defects in signaling molecules result in primary immunodeficiencies that also affect the development of T cells due to the requirement for TCR-mediated signaling during positive selection. Deficiencies in the ZAP-70 kinase, an early event in T cell signaling, results in a complete lack of CD8 T cells, yet CD4 T cells are present in normal numbers in the periphery (*Chapter 16*). However, the CD4 T cells that do develop exhibit defects in activation, as one would expect, given the early role of ZAP70 in TCR-mediated signaling. Patients with this CD8-lymphopenia and CD4 dysfunction also present with recurrent infections. These clinical results suggest that signaling through the TCR via ZAP70 is not as critical for the positive selection of CD4 T cells as it is for CD8 T cells. There is one additional case of a primary immunodeficiency caused by a signaling molecule defect—a SCID-like syndrome caused by a disruption in the gene encoding p56lck. Without the lck kinase, no signals can be triggered through the TCR, and T cell positive selection cannot occur, resulting in a lack of peripheral T cells. Defects in signaling molecules are fortunately rare, most likely because components of the TCR signaling pathway such as the ras pathway, PKC, calcium flux, and certain linker/adaptor molecules are also important in biochemical signaling in other cell types; therefore, mutations in these critical molecules would have potential pleiotropic effects that would have been selected against.

Although the conventional concept of cell signaling considers only two signals, IL-2 release with subsequent cytokine-mediated cell activation may be considered as a third signal. Shown in Figure 7-16 is a schematic representation of the T cell activation by antigen with the classic two signals with the participation of the cytokine-mediated third signal. As will be described below, the subsequent differentiation of the CD4 T helper population into its Th1, Th2, Th17, and inducible Treg subsets requires the participation of other cytokines, e.g., IL-12, IL-4, TGF-ß/IL-6, and TGF-ß, respectively.

If a T cell receives the two signals, the cell will be activated (Figure 7-16A). In contrast, if a T cell sees only signal 1 and not signal 2 (Figure 7-16B), then it is not activated and acquires a state of anergy (*Chapter 19*). Anergy (from the Greek prefix *an*, which means without, and *ergos*, which means force) is the opposite of energy, and refers to a state in which the T cell is recalcitrant to further stimulation. It is seen in many advanced chronic infectious or hypersensitivity diseases, e.g., tuberculosis, AIDS, and sarcoidosis.

How is this second signal generated? Because CD28 is expressed constitutively by T cells, the second signal for T cell activation is controlled at the APC level. CD80/CD86 is not present on immature DCs, resting B cells, or macrophages, and is upregulated only in mature or activated cells. Several years ago, Janeway and Medzidhov at Yale University discovered that the signal for upregulation of B7 molecules is delivered through Toll-like receptors (**TLRs**) expressed by APC. TLRs (described in detail in *Chapter 3*) recognize invariant constituents of pathogens called pathogen-associated molecular patterns

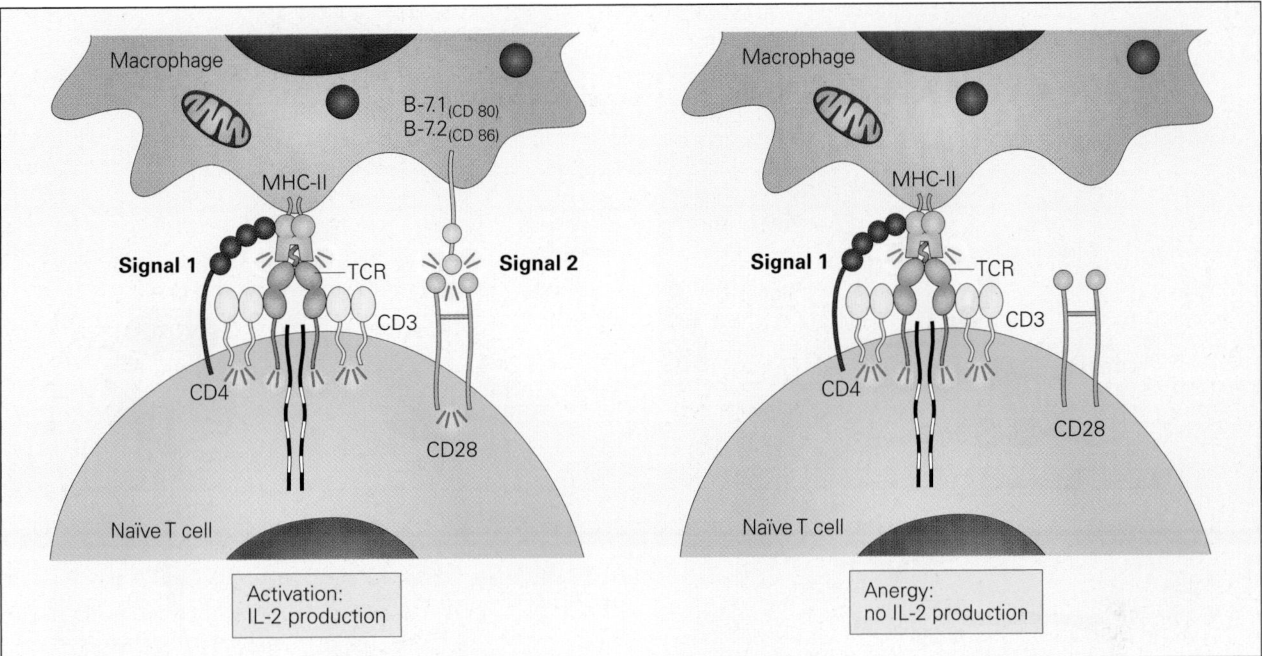

Figure 7-16. Panel A: Schematic representation of activation of a T cell producing IL-2 when it receives two signals. Panel B: In contrast, a T cell receiving only signal 1 and not signal 2 acquires a state of anergy with no production of IL-2.

(**PAMPs**) and constitute the link between innate and adaptive immunity. When a pathogen component such as LPS or teichoic acid (components of cell walls from Gram-negative and Gram-positive bacteria, respectively, that are not found on eukaryotic cells) contacts a specific TLR on the surface of the APC, this triggers a cascade of TLR-coupled signaling leading to the activation of the transcription factor NF-κB and the upregulation of CD80 and CD86 expression. TLR signaling also triggers DC maturation. These mature DCs and activated APCs can now present antigens to activate naïve T cells. The link of CD80/86 upregulation to the recognition of a pathogen is the key control point that prevents potential activation of self-reactive T cells. If T cells only required antigen-MHC, then a self-reactive T cell that may have accidentally emerged into the periphery despite T cell selection could become activated in situations where no pathogen is present. However, the requirement for two signals not only prevents the activation of T cells in the absence of antigenic trespass but also actively turns off those T cells that recognize signal 1 in the absence of signal 2. Therefore, the combination of rigorous selection during T cell development and peripheral control of T cell activation via signal 2 act together to enable appropriate immune responses and prevent immunopathology.

Additional Membrane Molecules Regulate T Cell Function

While the CD28:CD80/86 pathway is required to activate naïve T cells, there is a growing family of additional signaling molecules that serve to both negatively and positively regulate T cell activation at different stages. Once a T cell is activated by signal 1 and signal 2, fundamental changes occur to amplify the responses (Figure 7-17). In the inactive state, the IL-2 receptor only expresses the IL-2Rβ and γc components of the receptor. Following production of IL-2, there is upregulation of the third component of the IL-2 receptor, the high affinity IL-2 receptor alpha chain (**IL-2Rα**), also known as CD25, and additional regulatory molecules are expressed (*Chapter 9*). Figure 7-17 shows the different regulatory molecules that are expressed on T cells following activation with the corresponding receptor/ligand pairs on APC.

Although the list continues to grow, the major regulatory molecules that are induced by activation are ICOS, PD-1, CD40 ligand (CD40L, also known as CD154), and CTLA4 (CD152). An immune deficiency disorder has been identified and referred to as X-linked hyper IgM syndrome, in which a deficiency of the CD40L leads to a failure of the IgM/IgG switch to occur (*Chapter 16*), resulting in the excessive production of IgM but no IgG (Box 7-5 and

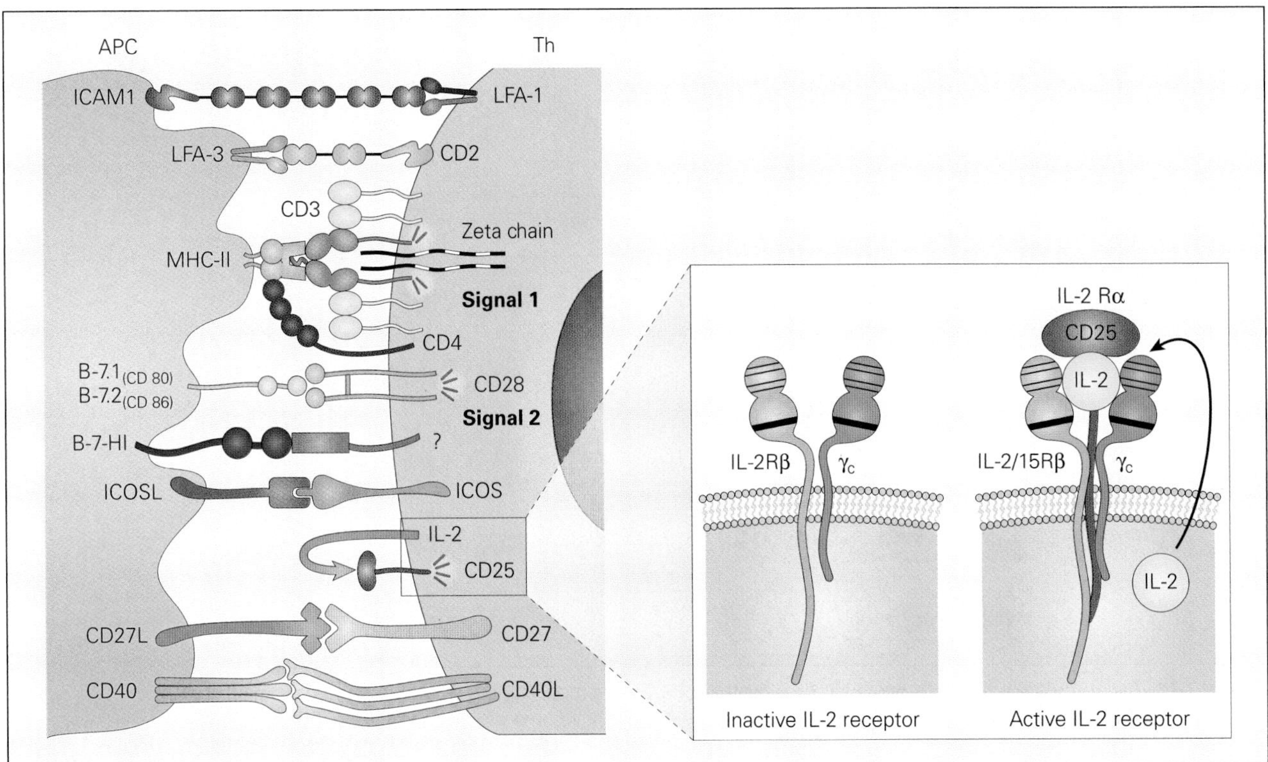

Figure 7-17. Schematic representation of the amplification of T cell responses showing the "third signal" provided by the production of IL-2 and the upregulation of the high affinity IL-2 receptor alpha chain (CD25) and additional regulatory molecules.

Figure 7-18). Interestingly, these inducible regulatory molecules can have either positive or negative effects on activation and differentiation to T cell effector functions. Two regulatory molecules expressed on activated T cells, ICOS and CD154 (CD40L), promote T cell effector functions. CD154 is expressed fairly rapidly (within twelve to twenty-four hours) following initial T cell activation and mediates interactions with APC, such as B cells and macrophages. CD154 is expressed constitutively by B cells and triggers immunoglobulin class switching (*Chapter 6*). In addition, interaction of CD154 with CD40 on DC can stimulate DCs to upregulate expression of CD80/86, a phenomenon known as "DC licensing." Finally, T cells can also activate macrophages via the CD154/CD40 interaction. ICOS has been more recently identified and appears to promote T cell effector function, particularly IL-4 production. ICOS binds to its ligand ICOS-L (B7-H) expressed by activated APCs.

Negative Regulators Prevent T Cell Overreactivity

The negative regulators of the costimulatory molecule family act to prevent unchecked activation (Figure 7-19). The most important negative regulator for global T cell activation is the CTLA4 (CD152) molecule, the high avidity receptor for CD80/86 (also referred to as B-7.1/B-7.2). CTLA4 is upregulated soon after activation (around eight hours) and binds to CD80 and CD86—the same molecules that serve as co-stimulatory ligands for CD28. However, binding of CTLA4 to CD80/86 differs from CD28 binding to these ligands in two important ways. First, CTLA4 binds with much greater avidity (i.e., more tightly) to CD80/86 compared to CD28. Second, binding of CTLA4 to its ligands shuts down T cell activation, whereas binding of CD80/86 to CD28 promotes activation. The most striking evidence that CTLA4 acts as a negative regulator of T cell activation and proliferation is derived from mice genetically manipulated to lack CTLA4 expression. These mice developed massive lymphoproliferation and lymphocytic infiltration into all major organs as a manifestation of autoimmunity, resulting in death at four weeks of age. These results established that lack of CTLA4 removes a key negative regulator of unchecked T cell activation and proliferation. Without proper regulation, T cell activation is unchecked, and this can lead to

Box 7-5

CD40L Deficiency (X-Linked Hyper IgM Syndrome)

An example of the clinical importance of the costimulatory interactions is seen in an X-linked immunodeficiency referred to as hyper-IgM syndrome, in which patients present with elevated IgM, absent IgG and other immunoglobulins, and recurrent bacterial pyogenic infections. This disorder traces its origins to the lack of CD154 (CD40L) expression on the T cell and its subsequent interaction with the CD40 on the B cell, which is required for IgM/IgG class switching (Figure 7-18). Hyper-IgM syndrome (*Chapter 16*) occurs due to a genetic mutation in the gene for CD154, located on the X chromosome, thus disrupting CD154 (CD40L) expression. This clinical profile is due to the fact that in the absence of T cell help via CD154/CD40, B cells can produce IgM only upon activation and cannot class switch immunoglobulins. Individuals with hyper-IgM syndrome also exhibit defects in cellular immunity, including defects in macrophage activation; however, treatment with intravenous immunoglobulin usually resolves most cases.

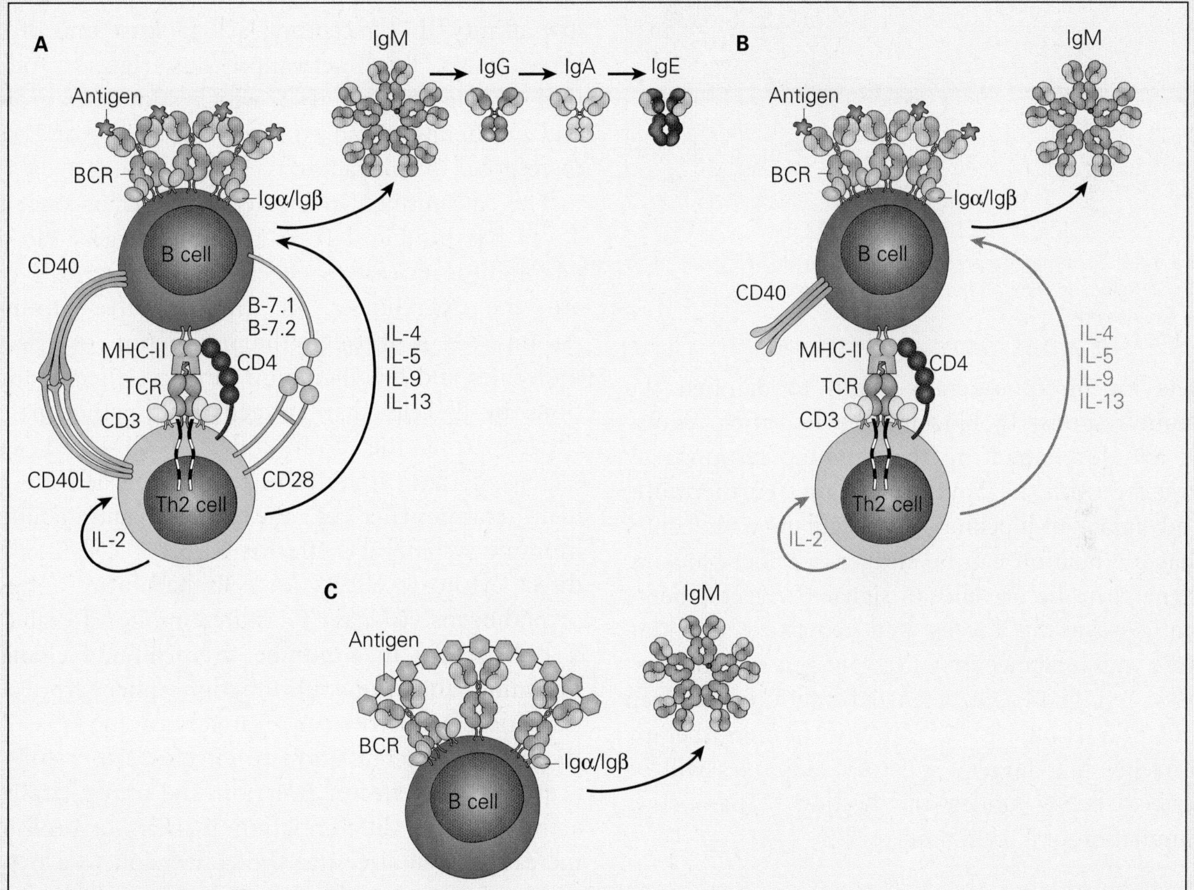

Figure 7-18. Schematic representation of the critical interaction of CD154 (CD40L) expression on the T cell, with the CD40 on the B cell that is required for IgM/IgG class switching. Panel A: Shows the full expression of the interaction of the Th2 and B lymphocyte, with CD40L-CD40 binding leading to class switching from IgM→IgG→IgA→IgE production by the B cell. Panel B: Shows that with the absence of CD40L, there is no interaction with the CD40, precluding the class switch and synthesis only of IgM. Panel C: Shows that the interaction of a B cell with a thymic-independent antigen (i.e., polysaccharide) leads only to the synthesis of IgM.

autoimmunity and pathological lymphoproliferation. Some newer regulatory molecules that also have negative effects on activation have been identified and include the molecules PD-1 and PD-2 with corresponding ligands PD-L1 and PD-L2. The precise roles of these molecules in mediating negative regulation are not yet known, but it is clear that multiple negative regulatory pathways exist to control T cell activation.

Due to their critical roles in controlling T cell activation, regulatory molecules are important

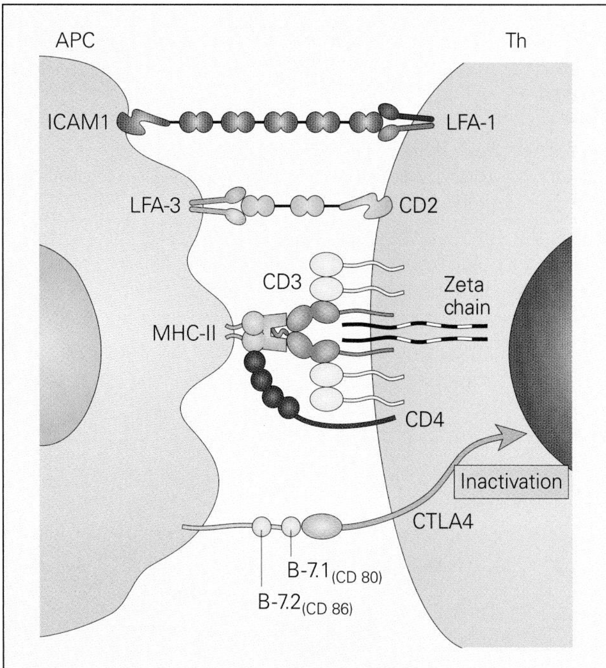

Figure 7-19. Schematic representation of the downregulation of the T cell response through the negative regulation of CTLA4 molecule expression.

targets for immunotherapy—both to dampen the immune response by blocking the activating regulators, and for enhancing the immune response by interfering with negative regulation. Furthermore, the advantage of blocking these regulatory molecules is that modulation can be antigen-specific; blocking of signal 2 in the presence of signal 1 triggers anergy of antigen-specific T cells, and conversely, blocking CTLA4 can enhance ongoing antigen-specific responses, as CTLA4 is upregulated only upon antigen stimulation (*Chapter 19*). Specific immunotherapy approaches that target regulatory molecules will be described below under the section "Therapeutic Manipulation of T Lymphocytes."

T Cell Effector Functions

Effector T Cells Are Phenotypically and Functionally Distinct from Naïve Resting T Cells

As described previously, a number of events must occur in the initial stages of T cell activation, including establishing T cell-APC contact via adhesion molecules, the engagement of signal 1 and signal 2 between the T cell and APC, the formation of the immunological synapse, and the transduction of intracellular signals for T cell activation. All of these events participate in the first stage of the activation process, which results in IL-2 production by the activated T cells, providing signal 3. IL-2 was discovered in the 1970s and was initially named T cell growth factor due to its proliferative effects on T cells (*Chapter 9*). There are three chains that assemble in various combinations to produce three functional forms of the IL-2 receptors, which differ in their affinity to bind IL-2. They are (1) the beta chain (IL-2Rβ); (2) the gamma chain (IL2-Rγ or γc); and (3) the alpha chain (IL2-Rα), also referred to as CD25. While the high affinity IL-2-R is composed of all three peptides, the intermediate and low-affinity IL-2 receptors lack at least one of the three chains. T cell activation thus triggers production of a factor, i.e., IL-2, which stimulates growth and proliferation and enhances the ability of T cells to respond to this factor.

The commitment to be activated occurs once the T cell has produced IL-2, and this triggers the differentiation process to effector cells. Effector T cells are the workhorses of the adaptive immune response. It is through the production of effector molecules and the elicitation of direct effector functions by T cells that antigens and pathogens are cleared from the body. Effector CD4+ T cells secrete myriad cytokines to recruit and activate cellular components of the innate and adaptive immune system, and effector CD8+ T cells mediate direct cytotoxic effects on cells harboring antigens or pathogens (*Chapter 9*). Differentiation to effector T cells results in a number of profound changes, including alterations in function, phenotype, and migration properties, as summarized in Table 7-2. In general, differentiation to effector cells results in acquisition of effector function, the upregulation of activation and differentiation markers, a profound increase in cell size, and the conversion to a hyperactivated state in which the resultant effector cells are more responsive to low doses of antigen and no longer require CD28/B7-derived costimulation to mediate their effector function (Table 7-2).

Effector cells are also relatively short-lived, lasting from days to weeks *in vivo*. This is why detection of effector cells in the blood of a healthy individual is difficult. However, if that same person is experiencing an infection or is suffering from an acute or chronic disease, effector T cells can be detected based on a characteristic phenotypic profile, including expression of the differentiation marker CD45RO, upregulation of the CD25 IL-2R, the

Table 7-2. Distinguishing features of naïve and effector T cells

Property	Naïve T cells	Effector T cells
Size	Small	Large
Life span	Long	Short
Phenotype	CD45RBhi	CD45RBlo/hi
	CD44lo	CD44hi
	CD62Lhi	CD62Llo
	LFA-1lo	LFA-1hi
	CD25−	CD25+
	CD69−	CD69+
Function (CD4 T cells)	Primarily IL-2	Effector cytokines
Function (CD8 T cells)	Primarily IL-2; no cytolysis	IFN-γ; cytolytic function
Costimulation requirements	High	Low–none
Location	Lymphoid tissue, blood	Lymphoid and other body tissues
Activation kinetics	Slow	Fast

Note: "hi" and "lo" refer to high and low intensity, respectively.

activation marker CD69, and/or HLA-DR (as MHC-II molecules are known to be upregulated on human effector T cells), and downregulation of the lymph node homing receptor CD62L. This effector-specific phenotype contrasts the phenotype of naïve and resting T cells that lack expression of activation markers CD25, CD69, and HLA-DR, express CD45RA, and also uniformly express CD62L, which confines their migration and distribution to lymphoid tissue and blood. The downregulation of CD62L expression by effector T cells enables their migration to peripheral tissue sites, so that the presence of antigen in any tissue or site, be it lung, liver, kidney, skin, or gut, is receptive to the influx of effector T cells. Described below is the nature of the effector-specific functions in immune responses and how certain diseases and immunopathology are specifically mediated by effector T cells.

CD4 T Cells Secrete Cytokines That Stimulate or Inhibit Immune Responses

CD4 T lymphocytes differentiate into cytokine-producing effector cells following activation. It is through the production of effector cytokines that effector CD4 T cells mediate antigen clearance via the recruitment and activation of additional immune cells (*Chapter 9*). Originally, two main types of effector CD4+ T cells, called T-helper 1 (**Th1**) and T-helper 2 (**Th2**) cells that mediate effector functions to promote an immune response, were differentiated by the pattern of their cytokine secretion. Th1 cells secrete IL-2, IFN-γ, and TNF-β (also called lymphotoxin or LT), and Th2 cells secrete IL-4, IL-5, IL-6, IL-10, and IL-13 (*Chapter 9*). This simplistic, dichotomous view of T cell differentiation has recently been challenged by the discovery of a new lineage of T cells characterized by their ability to preferentially secrete a proinflammatory cytokine, IL-17, and thus designated Th17 cells. Another type of antigen-differentiated CD4+ T cells, named "induced" regulatory T cells, acts to dampen or regulate immune responses. To date, at least two induced regulatory cells have been described: Th3 cells that secrete TGF-β and Treg1 (**TR1**) cells that produce IL-10. The properties that distinguish Th cell subsets and their cellular targets are summarized in Table 7-3.

Th1 Cells Help Macrophages Kill Pathogens That Resist Destruction in the Phagolysosome

Th1 cells act to coordinate constituents of cellular immunity and inflammation and are referred to as inflammatory T cells because they promote macrophage functions and the inflammatory response. The production of IFN-γ and TNF-ß by Th1 cells stimulates macrophages to more efficiently engulf pathogens and antigens via phagocytosis and also activates the release of reactive oxygen intermediates and other bactericidal compounds that hasten pathogen destruction (*Chapter 1* and *Chapter 5*). They stimulate the macrophages and other APCs to express more MHC, increasing antigen presentation. Th1 cells also help CD8 T cells and mediate

Table 7-3. Types of antigen-differentiated CD4 T cells and their properties

Effector cell type	Cytokines produced	Transcription factors	Cellular targets
T-helper 1 (Th1)	IL-2, IFN-γ, TNF-β	T-bet, STAT4	Macrophages, CD8 T cells
T-helper 2 (Th2)	IL-4, IL-5, IL-6, IL-10, IL-13	GATA-3, c-Maf, STAT6	B cells, mast cells, eosinophils
T-helper 17 (Th17)	IL-17, IL-21, IL-22	RORγt, STAT3	Fibroblast, endothelia, epithelium
T-helper 3 (Th3)	TGF-β	FOXP3	Th1, Th17, Th2
T-regulatory 1 (TR1, TRI)	IL-10		Th1, Th17, Th2

delayed-type hypersensitivity (**DTH**) reactions, such as those seen with the skin test for tuberculosis also referred to as the tuberculin skin test (**TST**) (Figure 7-20) and the response of many individuals to poison oak or poison ivy (*Chapter 18*). This skin reaction is characterized by local inflammation at the site of antigen entry, and a raised, red, and inflamed lesion. Th1 cells also produce IL-3 and GM-CSF that promote hematopoeisis to replenish the immune system with an influx of new T cells.

Th17 Cells Are also Proinflammatory and Are Involved in Autoimmune Diseases

Th17 effector cells are characterized by the production of the proinflammatory cytokines IL-17, IL-21, and IL-22 (*Chapter 9*). Differentiation of IL-17-producing T cells from naïve T cells is the result of the combined activity of IL-6 and TGF-ß, while IL-23, a dendritic cell-derived cytokine, may expand or stabilize previously differentiated Th17 cells. IL-17 enhances T cell priming and stimulates fibroblasts, endothelial cells, macrophages, and epithelial cells to produce multiple mediators involved in inflammatory cell infiltration and tissue destruction, including IL-1, IL-6, TNF-α, NOS-2, metalloproteases, and chemokines like KC, MCP-1, and MIP-2. IL-17 expression is increased in patients with a variety of autoimmune and allergic diseases, such as rheumatoid arthritis, multiple sclerosis, inflammatory bowel disease, and asthma, suggesting the contribution of IL-17 to the induction and/or development of these diseases. The involvement of this cytokine in such responses has also been demonstrated in animal models of autoimmune disorders. It has been shown that IL-22, an IL-10 family member also produced by NK cells, promotes antimicrobial defenses as well as inflammation. Since cell-surface receptors for IL-17 and IL-22 are expressed in tissue-resident cells, including fibroblasts, epithelial cells, and astrocytes, these two cytokines together may coordinately promote tissue inflammation and tissue destruction. IL-21 is a member of the common gamma chain family of cytokines with effects on the growth of CD8+ cells and in the transition of B cells to plasma cells. Remarkably, IL-21 acts on Th17 cells in an autocrine manner, sustaining their differentiation.

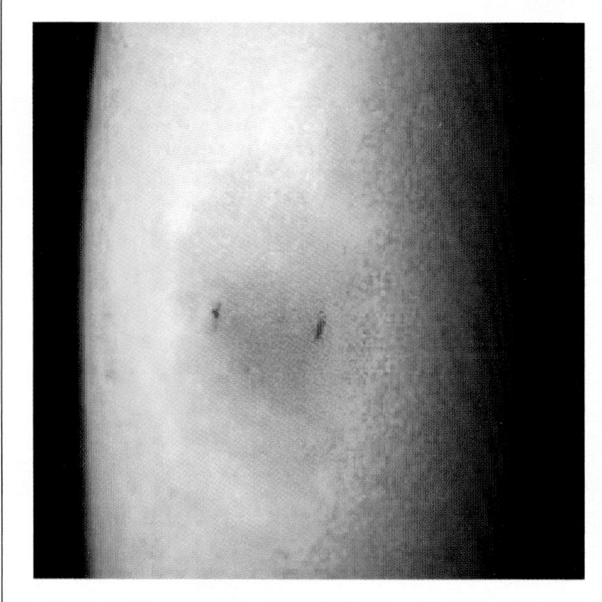

Figure 7-20. Photograph of a positive PPD skin test, i.e., a positive tuberculin skin test (TST). (As seen on Wikipedia.)

Th2 Cells Help B Cells Switch Ig Isotypes, Undergo Affinity Maturation, and Differentiate into Memory B Cells

Th2 effector cells primarily activate cells involved in humoral immunity and allergic-type inflammation with the production of IgE (*Chapter 18*). Th2 cells are particularly important in promoting B cell activation and differentiation (*Chapter 6*) in the presence of many protein antigens, the so-called "T-dependent antigens" (*Chapter 2*). IL-4 produced by Th2 cells binds to the IL-4R on B cells and acts as a B cell growth factor to stimulate their proliferation and differentiation to antibody-secreting plasma cells or to memory B cells. *In vitro*, B cells require both ligation of the surface antigen receptor and IL-4 to proliferate, which is why IL-4 (and other T cell-derived factors) can be thought of as the second signal for B cell activation. The combination of IL-4 and IL-5 produced by Th2 cells also promotes inflammation, particularly that mediated by mast cells (via IL-4) and eosinophils (via IL-5) (*Chapter 9*). Th2 effector cells are associated with allergy, not only due to their direct effects on mast cells, but also because Th2-derived cytokines tend to promote immunoglobulin class switching to IgE, which also binds to and triggers degranulation of mast cells, resulting in allergic-type hypersensitivity (*Chapter 18*). Certain cytokines produced by Th2 cells are also produced by either Th1 cells (e.g., IL-3 and GM-CSF) or Treg cells (e.g., IL-10 and TGF-β), suggesting that Th2 can have both promoting and regulatory roles in immune responses.

The Cytokine Environment Influences T Cell Differentiation into Th1, Th17, Th2, and Induced Treg Cells

What governs the generation of Th subset cells? This question is an important one that has been actively investigated to define specific roles of the different populations of effector T cells in diseases as described below. It has been difficult to isolate Th1 and Th2 effector cells from human peripheral T cells *in vitro*, since neither subset appears to express distinct cell surface markers, although mouse Th1 effector cells have been found to express the receptor for IL-12. Indeed, the widely cited and
5 currently accepted Th1/Th2 paradigm is now being disputed particularly in light of the discovery of newer subsets of the CD4 population, e.g., Th17 and Treg cells. What is now being generally agreed upon for both human and mouse T cells is that the inductive stimulus for generation of Th1, Th17, or Th2 effector cells, as well as the induced Treg phenotypes, is provided by the local cytokine milieu. The presence of IL-12 induces the differentiation of naïve CD4+ T cells into IFN-γ-producing Th1 cells through activation of signal transduction and activator of transcription-4 (**STAT4**). IFN-γ signals are transduced by STAT1, which in turn activates the transcription factor T-bet that enhances the expression of Th1 genes. IL-4 signaling through STAT-6 promotes the expression of the transcriptional factor GATA3, which skews the differentiation toward Th2 cells. The presence of TGF-β and IL-6 activates the transcription factor RAR-related orphan receptor gamma transcription factor (**RORγt**), and the retinoic acid-binding receptor (**RAR**), which leads to Th17 differentiation. Antigen-induced regulatory T cell production depends on the presence of TGF-β and the activation of the transcription factor FOXP3. It is now clear that the transcription factors T-bet in Th1 cells, RORγt in Th17 cells, GATA-3 in Th2 cells, and FOXP3 in Treg cells are potential targets for modulating production of specific effector cytokines in immunotherapy. Other factors, such as antigen dose, the type of antigen-presenting cells used to initiate T cell activation, and the type of antigen, protein or peptide, or pathogen have also been shown to affect Th1, Th17, and Th2 generation; however, varying results have been obtained in different experimental systems. While the cytokine environment and the expression of specific transcription factors affect the differentiation of T naïve cells into Th1, Th17, or Th2 effector cells, other multiple factors also influence their capacity for differentiation.

The Balance between Th1 and Th2 Responses Can Affect the Clinical Outcome of an Immune Response

A given immune response to a complex pathogen or antigen generally involves the participation of Th1, Th17, and Th2 effector cells, initiating cellular, humoral, and inflammatory cascades to efficaciously rid the body of unwanted foreign invaders. However, a biased Th1 or Th2 effector response has been found in reactions to certain types of pathogens, in various autoimmune disease conditions, and in individuals with allergic and asthmatic conditions. Although both Th1 and Th2 responses will act together in immune responses to pathogens, Th1 responses are generally more effective against viral, bacterial, and protozoan intracellular pathogens, and Th2 responses are more efficient in mediating clearance of extracellular pathogens such as bacteria, fungi, some protozoans or parasitic helminths, or removing extracellular toxins. Intracellular pathogens promote the production of IL-12 by dendritic cells. In concert with antigen stimulation, IL-12 acting via the transcription factor STAT-4 induces the development of a Th1 cell that produces the signature cytokine IFN-γ. Furthermore,

IFN-γ acting via STAT-1 also promotes the expression of the transcription factor T-bet, which is important for Th1 differentiation. In contrast, helminthic pathogens promote the generation of Th2 cells that produce the key cytokine IL-4, which activates STAT-6. IL-4 has pleiotropic effects, but a key effect is the promotion of Th2 differentiation and antagonism of IFN-γ production. Thus, a classic feature of Th cells is their production of cytokines that promote their own differentiation and antagonize the differentiation to the other lineage. Therefore, in any immune response, the balance between a productive immune response that efficaciously clears a pathogen from one that results in immune pathology such as tissue destruction is a fine one. This balance between immunity and pathology often involves the appropriate combination of Th1, Th17, and Th2 responses; any disruption of this balance can result in deleterious immune responses.

One particularly striking example of T cell-mediated pathology caused by biased T-helper immune responses occurs in individuals infected with *Mycobacterium leprae*, the etiologic agent of leprosy. Leprosy is a chronic and debilitating disease characterized by massive tissue destruction and peripheral nerve damage leading to loss of limbs and facial disfigurement. This severe form of leprosy is referred to as lepromatous leprosy (**LL**). Not all individuals infected with *M. leprae* present with these devastating symptoms, and some develop a less severe illness called tuberculoid leprosy (**TL**) that is effectively cleared by the immune system. In 1991, Barry Bloom and colleagues found that individuals with the less severe tuberculoid leprosy had a Th1-biased response predominated by IFN-γ, IL-2, and TNF-β production, whereas those with chronic lepromatous leprosy had a Th2-biased response characterized by IL-4 and IL-10 production.

These results indicate that generation of a Th1 immune response that stimulated mechanisms for clearance of intracellular pathogens resulted in less severe disease, whereas generation of a Th2-based humoral response was ineffective at clearing an intracellular pathogen, resulting in persistence of the organism, disease chronicity, and devastating pathology. More recent studies have shown that a transition from the tuberculoid to the lepromatous form of the disease occurs in various stages and a five subgroup classification for this transition has been developed (Box 7-6 and Figure 7-21). This correlation of disease severity, immunopathology, and outcome with Th1 versus Th2 responses underscores the importance of T cell differentiation in directing an overall immune response.

Other clinical manifestations of biased Th1/Th2 generation occur in autoimmune diseases. For example, Type I diabetes mellitus (**T1DM**) and multiple sclerosis (**MS**) were associated with Th1 responses since their disease pathology results from T cell-mediated destruction of islet cells in T1DM, and cells that make up the myelin sheath in MS. Studies using *in vivo* animal models of these diseases demonstrated that the autoantigen-specific T cells predominantly produce IFN-γ. Moreover, *in vivo* manipulations that result in a switch in cytokine profile of the autoreactive T cells from Th1 to Th2 are associated with protection from disease in these animal models. Similar strategies to promote switches in effector T cell responses in humans with T1DM and MS have not proved effective in controlling disease severity. However, unexpectedly, loss of IFN-γ signaling in mice deficient in IFN-γ or the IFN-γ receptor does not confer resistance to autoimmunity; in contrast, such mice are even more susceptible to autoimmunity. Those observations suggested that there may be an additional T cell subset, distinct from IFN-γ-producing Th1 cells, that is capable of inducing tissue inflammation and autoimmunity. This led to the identification of IL-17-producing cells or Th17 cells that produce IL-17, a cytokine recruiting other immune cells to peripheral tissues, leading to the enhancement of inflammation. Evidence suggesting rheumatoid arthritis and MS as primarily IL-17 autoimmune inflammatory-mediated diseases is rapidly accumulating. Moreover, inhibition or deletion of these cells in the corresponding animal models has provided a varying degree of protection. Other autoimmune diseases are mediated by pathogenic Th2 responses in which autoantibody production is a prominent feature, such as in myasthenia gravis. In this disorder, the characteristic muscular weakness seen is caused by the inhibitory effects of neuromuscular transmission produced by anti-acetylcholine receptor autoantibodies. Thus, the distinct roles of Th1, Th17, and Th2 cells in immune responses designed to rid pathogens may likewise govern a biased immune pathology when directed against self-antigens.

Box 7-6

Clinical Immunopathological Range of Leprosy

Leprosy is a chronic granulomatous disease caused by *Mycobacterium leprae* that was once widely found in Europe and Asia but now occurs primarily in developing countries in tropical and warm temperate regions. Since patients may present with manifestations of leprosy long after leaving an endemic region, clinicians must be aware of the possibility of the Leprosy displays an immunological spectrum ranging from tuberculoid (TT) leprosy, with strong cell-mediated immunity (CMI) against *Mycobacterium leprae*, to lepromatous (LL) leprosy, showing a complete absence of *M. leprae*-specific CMI. This spectral clinical-immunopathological range of leprosy is associated with differential activation of immune cells in parallel with the production of the wide variety of proinflammatory and immunoregulatory cytokines, which are the key signaling molecules between the immune and the resident cells responsible for disease expression. These findings suggest that identifying cytokine profiles associated with the various forms of leprosy may help in the early diagnosis of the disease and eventual monitoring of treatment efficacy.

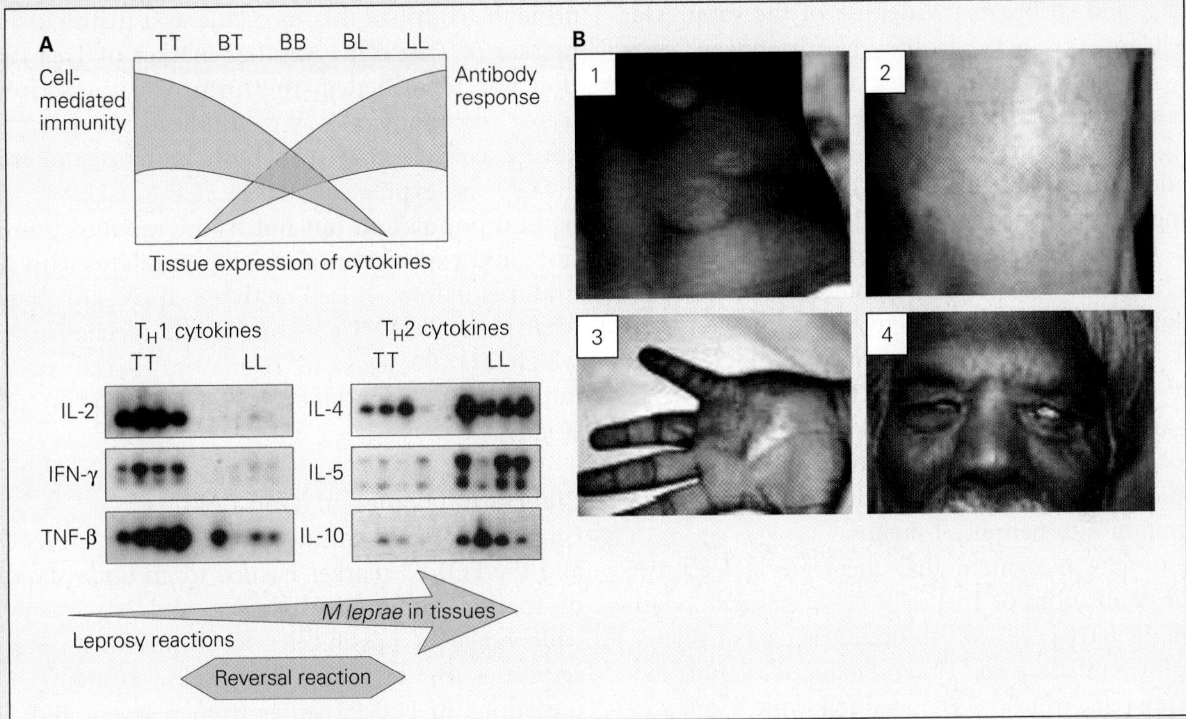

Figure 7-21. Clinical-immunopathological range of leprosy. Panel A: Schematic representation of the transition of tuberculoid leprosy to lepromatous leprosy progressing through borderline tuberculoid (BT), mid-borderline (BB), borderline lepromatous (BL), and fully lepromatous leprosy (LL) phases. Panel B: Photographs of patients with various forms of leprosy. (1) BT leprosy, showing many clear-edged, anesthetic lesions on the trunk and buttocks. (2) LL leprosy, showing widespread, non-anesthetic plaques and early nodules. (3) BT leprosy in a reversal reaction (RR), showing the patient with two lesions on his hand and a tender painful ulnar nerve; the skin lesions had been anesthetic and had recently become erythematous. (4) A patient with bilateral lagophthalmos (an inability to close the eyelids completely) secondary to the involvement of the VIIth nerve with leprosy. (Reproduced with permission from Britton WJ, Lockwood DN. Leprosy. Lancet. 2004;363:1209–19.)

Regulatory T Cells (Treg) Suppress T Cell Responses

Th1, Th17, and Th2 effector cells promote immune reactions. The cytokines produced by these effector CD4 T cell types act as growth, activation, and recruitment factors for other immune cell types that drive the immune response to clear and destroy pathogens wherever they reside. However, if unchecked, an immune response can lead to immunopathology, as the cytokines produced by effector

T cells are beneficial when produced locally in discrete quantities. Moreover, the presence of effector T cells in peripheral organs with enhanced activation properties has the potential to lead to autoimmunity. Thus, immunity without regulation cannot be tolerated. More than two decades ago, Richard Gershon identified a specific subset of CD8+ T cells with the ability to suppress an ongoing T cell response and called these T cell "suppressor cells," or Ts cells. These Ts cells were able to suppress immune responses in an antigen-nonspecific manner, and their TCR were thought to recognize a unique class of MHC molecules. However, this MHC molecule ended up being an artifact, and so began the demise of the suppressor T cell for the next decade. Nearly fifteen years later, however, another T cell that could suppress immune responses was identified by Shimon Sakaguchi, this time in the guise of a CD4+ T cell, and was designated a regulatory T cell, or Treg cell, to distinguish it from the blighted Ts cell. These Treg CD4 T cells bear the CD25 surface marker and do not have the capacity to proliferate or produce cytokines in response to activation, but can suppress T cell activation *in vitro* and *in vivo*. The most striking evidence that CD25+ CD4 T cells play an integral role in suppressing unwanted T cell responses is that *in vivo* depletion of CD25+ cells in mice results in autoimmunity and lymphocytic infiltration into peripheral organs.

It is now recognized that there are at least two major populations of Treg cells: (1) a "natural" population, or **nTreg** cells, which occurs as part of thymocyte differentiation; and (2) an "induced" population, or **iTreg** cells, which is generated following T cell activation in peripheral lymphoid tissues during the course of an antigen-driven adaptive immune response (*Chapters 2* and *19*, and Figure 7-22).

How do natural Treg cells arise? As described previously, there is evidence that nTreg cells are selected for in the thymus, based on the interaction of high affinity self antigens presented by MHC molecules expressed on epithelial cells to immature thymocytes. Instead of the normal deletion of T cells exposed to self antigens, there is an unusual survival of these cells, which constitute the natural population of Treg cells. Why this particular subset is not deleted is not well understood. Induction of iTreg cells is driven by TGF-β, in the absence of IL-6, suggesting a new dichotomy in helper T cell differentiation, and IL-6 might be a crucial polarizing factor to increase Th17 cells and to inhibit regulatory T cells, leading to autoimmunity. As previously mentioned, IL-6, together with TGF-β, is involved in the differentiation of Th17 cells, and blockade of IL-6 signaling results in suppression of the development of Th17 cells in mice.

Treg Cells Are CD4+CD25+ Cells

Treg cells have been found to express a CD4+CD25+ phenotypic profile. Due to the fact that CD25 (IL-2Rα) molecules are upregulated on all activated effector cells, however, it has been difficult to utilize this molecule as a distinguishing marker of Treg cells. Another marker of Treg function was identified in the form of a transcription factor belonging to the forkhead transcription family, called FOXP3. In both humans and mice, FOXP3 is expressed in the CD4+CD25+ Treg natural population but not in the induced population, and expression of FOXP3 correlates with natural regulatory T cell activity. It is not known what genes FOXP3 acts on, or the mechanisms by which FOXP3 leads to regulatory T cell activity, but these are important areas of research for future studies.

Clinical Relevance of Treg Cells

Clinically, the identification of natural Treg cells and the FOXP3 marker has led to an understanding of specific immunopathologies, and has opened a wide range of possibilities for controlling immune responses by targeting Treg cells. Humans with mutations in FOXP3 suffer from a severe and rapidly fatal autoimmune disorder called IPEX, for immunodysregulation, polyendocrinopathy, enteropathy, X-linked syndrome (*Chapter 16*). Similar to immunodeficiency disorders described previously, IPEX is seen during infancy; however, in stark contrast to immunodeficiencies, IPEX results in profound lymphocyte proliferation and lymphocytic infiltration into peripheral organs, leading to death after several months. The only viable treatment for IPEX is bone marrow transplantation, although this fails to be effective long-term, and the malignant type of lymphoproliferation eventually prevails. Fortunately, IPEX is an extremely rare disorder, as it has proved fatal is all but two known cases. This clinical syndrome underscores the importance of

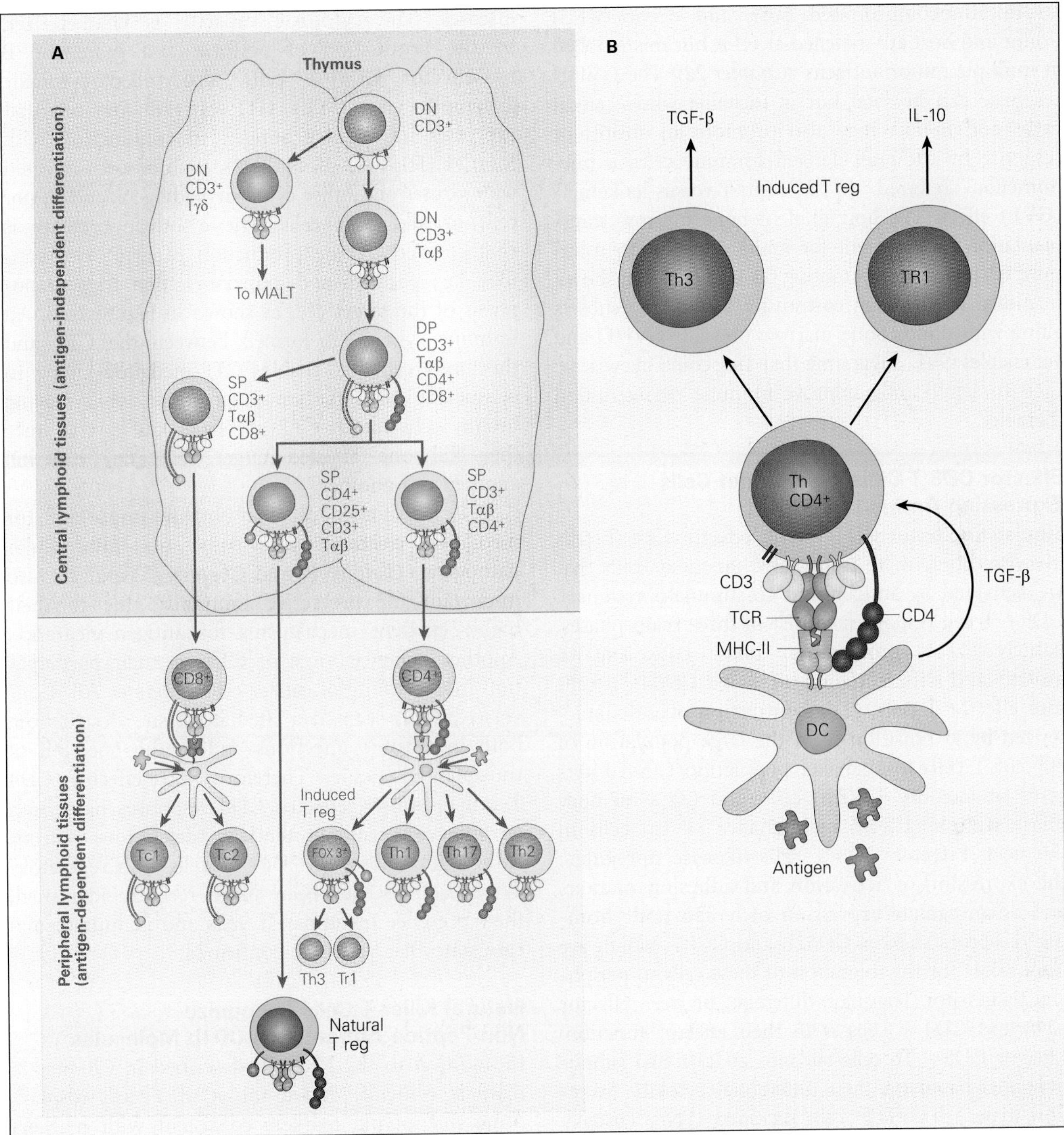

Figure 7-22. Schematic representation of the generation of Panel A: Natural Treg cell. Panel B: Induced Treg cells.

ongoing regulation in keeping immune responses healthy and preventing immunopathology.

The presence of Treg cells opens a vast array of possibilities for targeting their generation or promoting their reduction in diseases ranging from viral infection, allergy, autoimmunity, and cancer. Harnessing Treg cells can be potentially beneficial in autoimmunity, and removing the possible involvement/generation of Tregs in an antitumor response may be useful to promote antitumor immunity. Another important clinical application for Tregs is in bone marrow transplantation. One complication of bone marrow transplantation, particularly when used as therapy for cancer in otherwise immunocompetent individuals, is GVHD. GVHD occurs when immunocompetent T cells are transferred into an immunocompromised host, and occurs when donor and host are matched at HLA but mismatched at multiple minor antigens (*Chapter 22*). The GVHD response can be fatal but is treatable when caught early, and in fact may also promote an antitumor response by the graft-derived immune cells, a phenomenon referred to as "graft-versus-leukemia" (**GVL**) effect. The holy grail of bone marrow transplantation as treatment for malignancies is to minimize GVHD while promoting GVL. It has been shown in mouse models that co-transfer of the Treg subsets along with donor bone marrow prevents GVHD and yet enables GVL, suggesting that Treg could likewise be used to significantly improve immune reconstitution therapies.

Effector CD8 T Cells Lyse Target Cells Expressing Antigen on MHC-I

Similar to effector CD4 T cells, effector CD8 T cells likewise differentiate from naïve precursor cells that are activated by antigen and co-stimulatory signals. CD8+ T cell responses consist of three main phases, namely (1) a proliferation phase consisting of growth and differentiation of naïve CD8+ T cells into effector T cells; (2) a contraction phase characterized by a transition from the large population of effector T cells to a smaller population (~5–10 percent) of memory T (**Tm**) cells; and (3) a memory phase with long-term maintenance of Tm cells in the host. Effector CD8 T cells likewise upregulate the expression of activation and adhesion markers and downregulate expression of lymph node homing receptors such as CD62L and CCR7, which are responsible for the migration of these cells to peripheral tissue sites. The main difference between effector CD8 and CD4 T cells is in their effector function. Effector CD8+ Tc cells fall into at least two subpopulations based on their differential cytokine secretion, type 1 Tc (Tc1) cells secreting IFN-γ (usually in significantly greater amounts compared to CD4 T cells) and type 2 Tc (Tc2) cells secreting IL-4, IL-5, and IL-10. However, unlike CD4 T cell counterparts, both effector CD8 T cells are able to perform direct cytototoxic capability through the induction of apoptosis (*Chapter 9*). Tc1 cells, because of their capacity of efficiently migrating to inflamed tissues where they secrete IFN-γ and kill their targets, are a major defense against virus-infected cells. Tc2 cells were found in chronic human pathologies such as viral infections, malignancies, and neurologic and autoimmune diseases. The cytotoxic capacity is characterized by the production of perforin and granzyme B by effector CD8 T cells, also called cytotoxic T lymphocytes (**CTL**). CTL can kill any cell that expresses its cognate antigen in conjunction with MHC-I (HLA-A, -B, and -C), such as cells infected with viruses and other cytosolic pathogens and tumor cells or allogeneic cells. The cytotoxic capacity is characterized by the production of cytotoxic granules, i.e., perform and granzymes, that trigger apoptosis of the target cell, as shown in Figure 7-23. An immune synapse is formed between the CTL and the target cell that enables CTL-mediated killing to be specific for a particular target cell while leaving healthy cells intact. CTL are serial killers, and once they kill one affected target cell, they can kill another and another.

CD8 effector T cells are highly important for mediating clearance of viruses and intracellular pathogens (*Chapter 12* and *Chapter 13*) and are also important for protective immunity due to their highly efficient mechanisms for antigen clearance. Another beneficial role of CTLs is their participation in the killing of cancer cells (*Chapter 20*). Conversely, CTLs can also mediate tissue destruction, both in chronic infections and in the rejection of transplanted tissue. Therefore, like effector CD4 T cell responses, effector CD8 responses have both advantageous and potentially deleterious effects. Although a subset of CD8+ T cells with regulatory T cell activity has been more recently identified, their presence in human T cells and in human disease states has yet to be confirmed.

Natural Killer T Cells Recognize Non-Peptide Antigens on CD1b Molecules

In addition to the NK cells described in Chapter 3, there is evidence that a subset of T cells displays some phenotypic markers consistent with markers found on NK cells (CD161, CD56). However, the most characteristic feature of the **NKT** cell in the human is the presence of an invariant TCR consisting of Vα24-Jα18:Vβ11, in contrast to the wide diversity of the TCR in all other populations of T cells. In humans, NKT cells express CD4, CD8 (a small subgroup), or neither (DN), and on activation produce large quantities of both Th1 (IFN-γ) and Th2 (IL-4) cytokines, which enhance the function of dendritic cells, NK cells, and B cells, as well as conventional CD4+ and CD8+ cells. This rapid

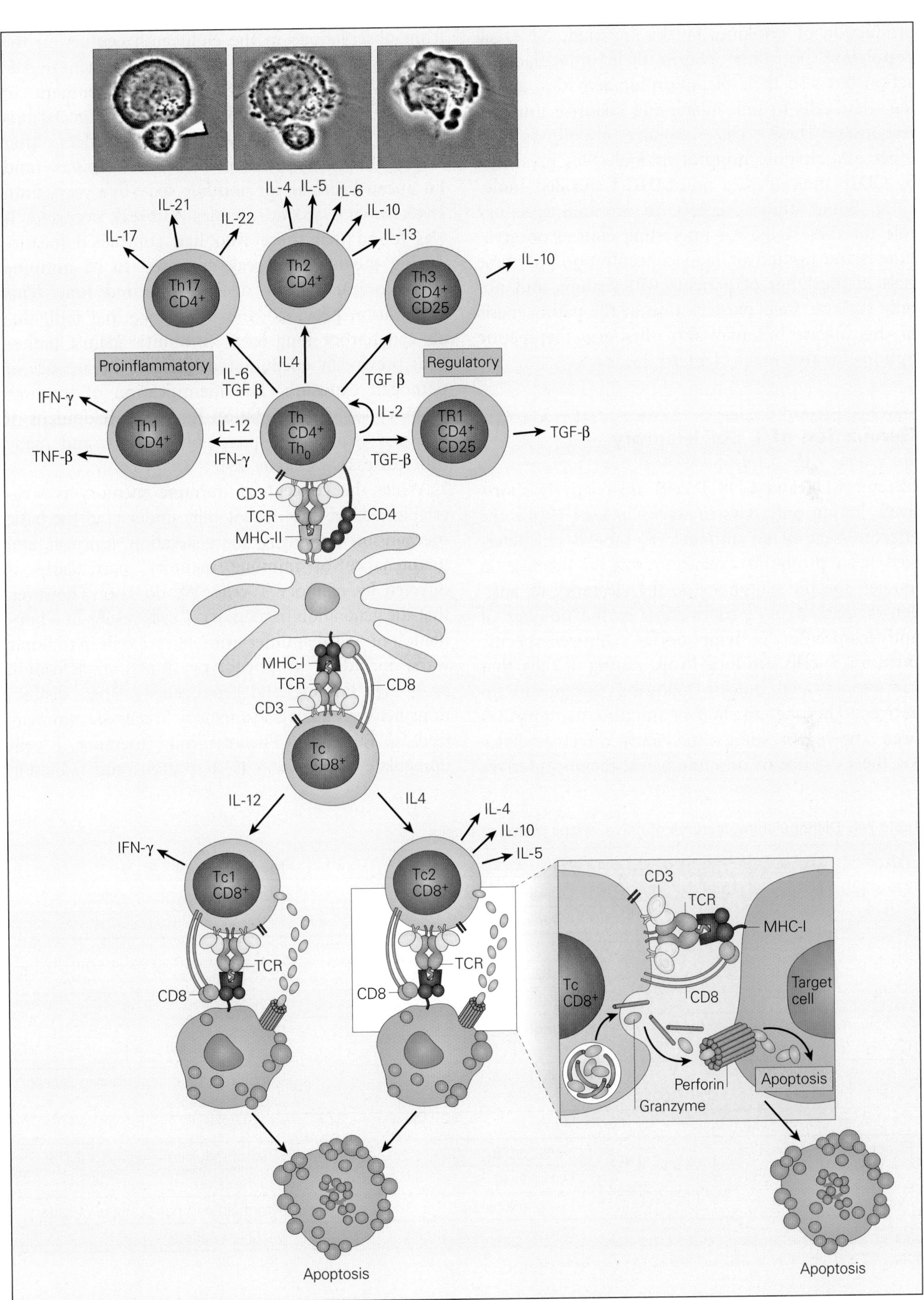

Figure 7-23. Panel A: Phase microscopy of killing of a target cell by a cytotoxic lymphocyte. Panel B: CD8 cytotoxic T cells involved in cell killing of target cells through apoptosis similar to that seen with natural killer (NK) cytotoxic activity showing the formation of a perforin-containing cylindrical structure through which granzymes enter, triggering apoptotic cell death.

production of cytokines by this invariant NKT cell population not only assures their immediacy of action but also their pleiomorphic activities, allowing these cells to link innate and adaptive immune responses. These cells recognize glycolipids and other amphipathic nonprotein molecules presented by CD1b molecules (a non-MHC-I encoded molecule). Some studies suggest an immunoregulatory role for these cells. An interesting clinical observation is the finding of high concentrations of these cells in the lungs of patients with asthma and not only suggests their participation in the pathogenesis of this disease but may also offer new therapeutic options for treatment (*Chapter 18*).

Generation of T Cell Memory

Effector CD4 and CD8 T cells are relatively short-lived, lasting only days to weeks *in vivo*. While the effector stage of an immune response is characterized by a profound expansion and an increase in antigen-specific lymphocytes, the clearance of antigen is marked by a contraction in the number of antigen-specific T lymphocytes. Antigen-specific memory T cells are long-lived, resting T cells that can be activated quickly following re-exposure to antigen. The phenomenon of immune memory has been known for some time. Early direct evidence for the existence of immunological memory derives from observations in the eighteenth century in the Faroe Islands, a remote group of islands in the North Atlantic between Scotland and Denmark. In 1781, a measles outbreak occurred on the islands due to encounter with European settlers, after which the island remained free of measles (and European visitors) for another sixty-five years until 1846, when a second measles outbreak occurred. It was found that those who had contracted measles during the first outbreak appeared to be immune from contracting the disease a second time. This observation provided direct evidence that individuals can harbor long-term immunity against pathogens previously encountered, even in the absence of pathogen exposure. The identification of immune memory set the foundation for the development of vaccines against smallpox, poliomyelitis, and many other diseases (*Chapter 23*).

While the concept of immune memory is well-established, we still do not fully understand the basic mechanisms underlying the generation, function, and maintenance of immune memory, particularly as directed by memory T cells. We do know, however, that the generation of memory T cells results in a population of cells that differ from naïve T cells in multiple ways, including in phenotype, function, activation properties, homing, and heterogeneity. These distinctions between naïve and memory T cells are summarized in Table 7-4. Phenotypically, memory T cells upregulate expression of activation and adhesion

Table 7-4. Distinguishing features of naïve versus memory T cells

Property	Naïve T cell	Memory T cell
Phenotype	CD45RBhi (mo)/CD45RA(hu)	CD45RBlo(mo)/CD45RO(hu)
	CD44lo	CD44hi
	CD11alo	CD11ahi
	CD62Lhi	CD62Llo/hi
	CCR7hi(hu)	CCR7lo/hi
Activation requirements: Co-stimulation (CD28/B7)	Mandatory	Dispensable
Antigen-presenting cells	Professional (dendritic cells)	Nonprofessional: e.g., resting B cells, endothelial cells
Responses to low antigen dose	Weak	Strong
Effector function kinetics	None (produce IL-2)	Effector cytokines, cytolysis (CD8)
	Slow (days)	Rapid (hours)
Homing	Lymphoid tissue	Lymphoid and non-lymphoid tissue
Heterogeneity	Unknown, homogenous	Multiple subsets

Note: "hi" and "lo" refer to high and low intensity, respectively.

markers such as CD44, LFA-1, and CD45RO, similar to effector cells. Functionally, memory T cells are characterized by an ability to produce effector cytokines with rapid kinetics. Memory T cells are also easier to activate compared to naïve T cells. They respond to lower disease of antigen, can be activated by a broader range of APC types (such as resting B cells and endothelial cells that fail to stimulate naïve T cells), and do not require CD28/B7-derived co-stimulation for activation. All of these factors, such as enhanced functional responses, rapid activation kinetics, and increased expression of adhesion markers, contribute to the ability of memory T cells to mediate protective immunity.

Another main distinction between naïve and memory T cells is in their homing capacity and tissue distribution. Naïve T cells primarily reside in lymphoid tissue such as lymph nodes and spleen and traffic between blood and lymph. They are drawn to lymph nodes via their expression of the lymph node homing receptor L-selectin, also known as CD62L, which permits their binding to mucin-like addressins on the surface of high endothelial venules (**HEVs**) found on postcapillary venules in the lymph node (*Chapter 2*). Another receptor that acts to drive T cells into lymph nodes is the chemokine receptor CCR7 (*Chapter 9*). Upon activation, CD62L and CCR7 expression is downregulated, enabling lymphocyte egress into peripheral non-lymphoid organs. Interestingly, memory T cells are heterogeneous for expression of lymph node homing receptors CD62L and CCR7, reflecting their distribution in both lymphoid and non-lymphoid tissue (Figure 7-24). Two subsets of memory T cells have been defined in humans and mice, based on homing receptor expression with the CD62L+/CCR7+ memory subset designated as "central memory," or lymphoid memory, and the CD62L−/CCR7− subset designated as "effector-memory," or non-lymphoid memory. In human blood, CD4 T cells can be subdivided into naïve (CD45RA/CCR7+), central memory (CD45RO/CCR7+), and effector memory (CD45RO/CCR7−). Functionally, central and effector memory subsets exhibit distinct capacities, with the CCR7− effector-memory subset primarily producing effector cytokines, and the CCR7+ central memory subset producing predominantly IL-2, and not effector cytokines. This functional dichotomy observed in polyclonal T cells is not necessarily found in antigen-specific central and effector memory T cells. For example, human HIV-

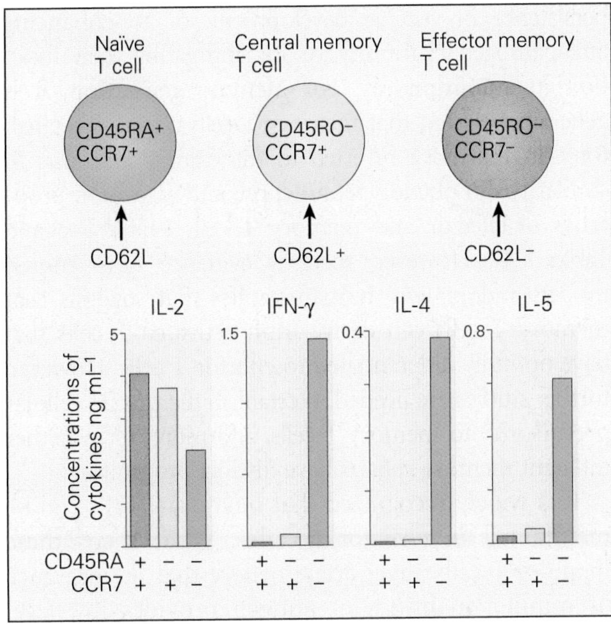

Figure 7-24. Differential functions of human central and effector memory CD4 T cells. In human blood, CD4 T cells can be subdivided into naïve (CD45RA/CCR7+), central memory (CD45RO/CCR7+), and effector memory (CD45RO/CCR7−) The most important marker of memory is L-selectin. Naïve cells are drawn to lymph nodes via their expression of the lymph node homing receptor L-selectin, also known as CD62L, that permits their binding to mucin-like addressins on the surface of high endothelial venules (HEV) found on postcapillary venules in the lymph node. Another receptor that acts to drive naïve T cells into lymph nodes is the chemokine receptor CCR7. Upon activation, CD62L and CCR7 expression is downregulated, enabling the activated lymphocyte egress into peripheral non-lymphoid organs.

specific central and effector memory subsets from peripheral blood both produce effector cytokines, suggesting that the functional capacity of memory subsets may differ for diverse antigens. Memory T cell heterogeneity in tissue distribution may also contribute to enhanced recall responses, as memory T cells can be activated directly at the site of antigen or pathogen entry. Naïve T cells, by contrast, must wait for the antigen to be transported to local lymphoid tissue via dendritic cells or other antigen-presenting cells.

Memory T cells are important for mediating long-term protective immunity, yet can also be generated in autoimmune diseases, where their presence can be deleterious. Critical questions in the study of T cell memory are how memory T cells are generated and how they are maintained over the long term. Understanding these basic properties of memory T cells is critical to designing strategies to either promote their generation and persistence in vaccine development, or to enhancing anti-pathogen immunity, or for abrogating their function in autoimmunity. For memory generation, it is generally believed that memory T cells arise from effector cells that have reverted to the resting state due to similarities in phenotype, function, and activation properties of effector and memory T cells (Table 7-2 and Table 7-4). However, there is evidence from mouse models and *in vitro* human studies that suggests that memory T cells can derive from activated T cells that have not fully differentiated to effector T cells. However, further studies are needed to establish the precise cellular precursor(s) to memory T cells, and moreover, whether different memory subsets have distinct progenitors.

It is widely recognized that memory T cells can be maintained *in vivo* for decades. What keeps these memory T cells alive? Some believe that the presence of minute quantities of antigen provides low-level stimulation of memory T cells over time. However, in animal models, antigen-specific memory T cells have been shown to persist when transferred into antigen-free hosts. Memory T cells could similarly be maintained based on cross-reactions to peptide/MHC complexes. While memory CD8 T cells appear to functionally persist in the absence of MHC-I, memory CD4 T cells lose functionality in hosts devoid of MHC-I. Another survival factor for memory T cells is cytokines. For memory CD8 T cells, the cytokines IL-7 and IL-15 have been shown to promote survival and turnover, respectively. Similarly, memory CD4 T cells require IL-7 for survival. IL-7 is a cytokine produced by most cells and is required for naïve T cell survival as well, and recall that a lack of IL-7R and IL-7 responses in human T cells leads to a lack of peripheral lymphocytes and a SCID phenotype. It is likely that a combination of antigen persistence, interactions with MHC on accessory cells, and cytokines all contribute to memory T cell survival.

Homeostasis and Aging

During the lifetime of an individual, many antigens are encountered from multiple sources and via multiple routes of entry. The immune system responds to these antigens by generating expanded populations of effector T cells that may give rise to memory T cells. At the same time, new T cells are being manufactured and matured through the thymus (*Chapter 2*). Despite these dynamic and sometimes dramatic changes in T cell composition, the absolute number of peripheral T cells within an individual remains constant over time via a phenomenon termed homeostasis. Homeostasis is maintained in the presence of new T cell production and antigen-driven T cell expansion by the continual turnover and death of peripheral T cells. Through unknown mechanisms, T cells have the ability to sense when they are low or overabundant. In situations of low T cell numbers, or lymphopenia, T cells undergo rapid proliferative expansion in an attempt to fill up the empty lymphocyte space. This has been observed in patients who are treated with cytotoxic conditioning therapy prior to bone marrow transplantation and in those with SCID prior to treatment by bone marrow transplantation. In situations of elevated T cell numbers, such as that observed in conditions of bacterial or viral infections, there is contraction of T cells mediated by apoptotic death to maintain constant numbers of T cells in the body. Disruption of immune cell homeostasis may be a central mechanism by which the balance is tipped between a healthy immune system and one characterized by immunopathology, such as autoimmunity. As a person ages, there are both dynamic and gradual changes in T cell composition and homeostasis. As described earlier, decreased thymopoiesis results in proportionally diminished thymic output with age, so by an advanced age, production of new T cells is quite low. Aging also results in the accumulation of antigenic experiences, reflected by an increase in memory T cells. Interestingly, the proportion of memory T cells changes linearly in the first decade of life, but after age 20, the ratio of naïve to memory T cells remains constant, until at advanced age (ages 70–100), when memory T cells predominate. This changing ratio of naïve memory T cells with age is assessed by measuring the proportion of naïve (CD45RA) phenotype and memory (CD45RO) phenotype cells in newborns to centenarians (Figure 7-25). The stable proportion of naïve and memory subsets through most of adult life reflects homeostatic maintenance, balancing both thymic output and antigenic-driven expansion *in vivo*. Homeostatic maintenance does break down in advanced age, as revealed by multiple immune dysfunctions seen in the elderly. Aged individuals can also lose their immune memory to previously encountered pathogens and also respond less well

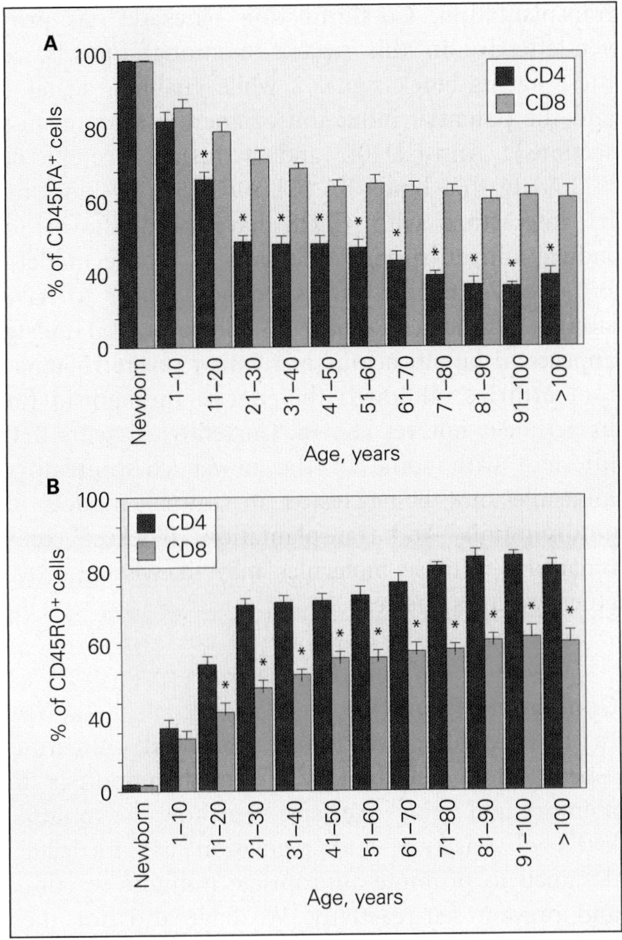

Figure 7-25. Changes in the proportion of naïve and memory T cells in aging. Panel A: Naïve cells demonstrated by the expression of the CD45RA cell marker. Panel B: Memory cells demonstrated by the CD45RO cell marker.

to vaccines. In addition, T cells from aged (> seventy years) individuals tend to produce less IL-2 and proliferate less well. Whether these defects are due to T cell-mediated senescent changes, or global disruptions in homeostasis due to lagging thymic output, and increases in the memory: naïve subset ratio has not been elucidated. As our population ages, understanding age-related immune dysfunctions takes on broader importance.

Therapeutic Manipulation of T Lymphocytes

The central role of T cells in immune responses and the multiple levels of control, from development to activation to differentiation, have great potential for targeted therapies for enhancing immunity in anti-pathogen and antitumor responses, for ablating immunity in autoimmune diseases in and in transplantation (*Chapter 11*). Over the past fifteen years, the identification of molecules involved in T cell activation, including molecules involved in signaling, co-stimulation, and cytokine regulation, has revealed new targets for the manipulation of T cell responses. Nevertheless, T cell-targeted immunotherapies remain largely experimental and are still not accepted treatments for diseases such as cancer or autoimmunity. In this last section, we will briefly describe some current and emerging T cell-targeted therapies for enhancing and abrogating immune responses.

Strategies for enhancing T cell responses have used cytokines and manipulation of co-stimulatory molecules. In the late 1970s, Stephen Rosenberg used IL-2 infusion to enhance tumor immunity by promoting the activation of tumor-specific T lymphocytes (*Chapter 20*). Many early recipients of IL-2 experienced serious complications of systemic cytokine administration, such as edema and shock, although some also experienced remission of specific tumors. IL-2 treatment was not found to be effective for most cancers and is used today primarily for treatment of renal cell carcinoma. This use of IL-2 treatment to boost existing T cell responses did not prove as efficacious as originally hoped. More recent strategies for boosting T cell immunity have focused on blocking negative regulators of T cell activation, such as the negative co-stimulator CTLA4. Treatment of melanoma patients with anti-CTLA4 antibody to block negative regulation of T cell activation was found to cause remission in some individuals. This treatment is currently in expanded clinical trials to assess its overall efficacy. Other approaches to boosting T cell responses are mostly antigen-based and relate more to vaccine design. Different strategies for priming and boosting the immune system to pathogen-related antigens using viral vectors, plasmid DNA, and protein subunits are currently being tried in vaccines against malaria, tuberculosis, and HIV infection. However, there is still no known vaccine that generates protective immunity by promoting T cell responses. The enhancement of T cell responses via immunological approaches remains a formidable challenge to medicine in the twenty-first century, with high-impact potential.

Immunotherapies designed to suppress T cell-mediated immune responses, at least globally, have proven more successful, although definitive dampening of antigen-specific T cell responses has been more elusive. Pharmacological agents of T cell-specific immunosuppression that target signaling intermediates are widely used for recipients of transplanted organs. The agents cyclosporine and FK506, or tacrolimus, are known as calcineurin-based immunosuppressives since they both target the signaling pathway coupling calcium flux to induction of the transcription factor NFAT, which is critical for IL-2 production in activated T cells (*Chapter 11*). These drugs are administered systemically and act to globally block T cell activation and must be taken for the duration of a transplant recipient's life. Due to their nonspecific effects, complications such as recurrent infections are often presented. T cell depletion therapies using anti-lymphocyte antibodies such as thymoglobulin, or using depleting anti-CD3 antibodies, are also administered prior to transplantation to clear out T cells that could potentially attack an allogeneic organ graft. Like the pharmacologic agents, these antibodies deplete all T cells and are not specific for antigen-specific T cells.

The deletion or inactivation of antigen-specific T lymphocytes remains the holy grail for targeted immunosuppression in autoimmunity and transplantation. Co-stimulation blockade has proven effective in this regard in animal models, as these agents block signal 2 while enabling signal 1 and the potential induction of anergy (see previous sections). Anti-CD40L and a fusion protein of CTLA4-Ig that binds B7 (CD80/CD86) by blocking its interaction with CD28 have been shown to induce antigen-specific tolerance in mouse models. But these same treatments do not appear to have similar efficacy in humans. However, CTLA4-Ig appears to be efficacious in treating severe rheumatoid arthritis, although the precise mechanism for its action is not yet known. Currently, reagents that interfere with some of the newer co-stimulatory molecules are being tested in animal models of autoimmunity and transplantation. Blocking combinations of these molecules may likewise improve efficacy across species.

Concluding Remarks

In this chapter, we have introduced numerous aspects of T cell biology, from thymopoiesis to memory and aging. We have seen how the multiple levels of selection and regulation are intricately designed to promote appropriate immune reactions and prevent self-reactivity. We have also described the clinical conditions that result from disruptions in these processes. Finally, we have introduced how the molecular regulators of T cell activation can be exploited in therapies to manipulate T cell-mediated immunity.

Case Study: Clinical Relevance

Let us now return to the case study of severe combined immunodeficiency (SCID) presented earlier and review some of the major points of the clinical presentation and how they relate to the immune system:

- As described in Chapter 2, the encounter of the newborn with the myriad of antigens in the external environment shortly after birth provides the inductive stimulus for development of a normal immune system. Because of his underlying immune deficiency, David was placed in a sterile environment that protected him from microbes that would have caused fatal infection.
- There are more than 150 different genetically transmitted immunodeficiency disorders (*Chapter 16*) that generally present in childhood or shortly after birth that become manifest upon contact with the microbial world. One of the most serious immunodeficiencies is SCID, thus designated due to profound deficiencies in both T and B lymphocyte maturation.
- There are several types of SCID that arise from different genetic mutations, which are shown in Table 7-5 and described in greater detail in Chapter 16. Many of the SCID types involve a specific lack of T cells, while B lymphocytes can be present in normal

Case Study: Clinical Relevance (continued)

Table 7-5. Different genetic forms of severe combined immunodeficiency

Genetic lesion	Deficient protein product	Phenotype	Frequency of SCID patients
X-linked	γc chain of the IL-2 receptor	Lacks T cells, NK cells Has B cells	45 percent
Autosomal recessive	IL-7R	Lacks T cells, NK cells Has B cells	1.4 percent
Autosomal recessive	JAK3 kinase	Lacks T cells, NK cells Has B cells	6.4 percent
Autosomal recessive	Recombinase activating protein (RAG)	Lacks T, B cells Has NK cells	rare
Autosomal recessive	Adenosine deaminase (ADA)	No T, B, or NK cells	16 percent

(Data from Buckley, RH. N Engl J Med. 2000;1,313–24.)

or elevated numbers. The most common form of SCID, accounting for 45 percent of reported cases, is the X-linked form of SCID. It connotes a deficiency in a protein known as the common gamma chain or γc of the receptor for the IL-2 family of cytokines that is critically important for the development of the immune system (Box 7-7).

- The γc protein is a signaling molecule that controls responses to many cytokines, including factors that mediate the survival of lymphocytes. Since the common gamma chain (γc) of the receptor for IL-2 is shared by the receptors for interleukins IL-2, important for T cell expansion as well as other cytokines involved in B cell differentiation, e.g., IL-4 (Figure 7-28A), the deficiency of this molecular moiety explains why both T and B cell activities are affected in the X-linked form of SCID (Figure 7-26). Patients with X-linked SCID have a complete absence of T cells and NK cells, while B lymphocytes are present but may be functionally deficient, as in the case of David (Table 7-5).
- The next most common forms of SCID are autosomal recessive variants (Table 7-5). These include defects in the gene encoding the interleukin-7 receptor that is expressed by T cells (*Chapter 9*) and is essential for their survival *in vivo*, defects in the JAK3 kinase (which is also involved in IL-7-mediated responses and signaling), and defects in the recombinase-activating gene (RAG) that mediates gene rearrangements of the TCR and the BCR (*Chapter 7*). Both JAK3- and IL-7R-deficient individuals exhibit a profound lack of T cells, while B cells are present, whereas RAG-deficiency leads to losses of both T and B cells. Finally, another genetic lesion that leads to SCID results from the absence of a metabolic enzyme involved in the purine salvage pathway, called adenosine deaminase (ADA). ADA-deficiency results in a complete lack of T cells, B cells, and NK cells due to the accumulation of deoxyadenine nucleotides that are particularly toxic to lymphocytes. Absolute lymphocyte counts of ADA children are typically less than 500/mm^3. This immune deficiency disorder has been successfully treated by genetic reconstitution of the defective ADA (*Chapter 16*).
- Infants with SCID generally present with multiple infections, including recurrent bacterial and viral infections, pneumonia, persistent diarrhea, and fungal

Box 7-7

Common Gamma Chain (X-linked Severe Combined Immunodeficiency)

Most cases of SCID are due to mutations in the gene encoding the common gamma chain (γc) of the receptor for the IL-2 family of cytokines (also known as CD132), a protein that is shared by the receptors for interleukins IL-2, IL-4, IL-7, IL-9, IL-15, and IL-21 (*Chapter 9*). These interleukins and their receptors are involved in the development and differentiation of T and B cells. Because the common gamma chain is shared by many interleukin receptors, mutations that result in a nonfunctional common gamma chain cause widespread defects in interleukin signalling. The result is a near-complete failure of the immune system to develop and function, with low or absent T cells and NK cells and nonfunctional B cells.

Case Study: Clinical Relevance (continued)

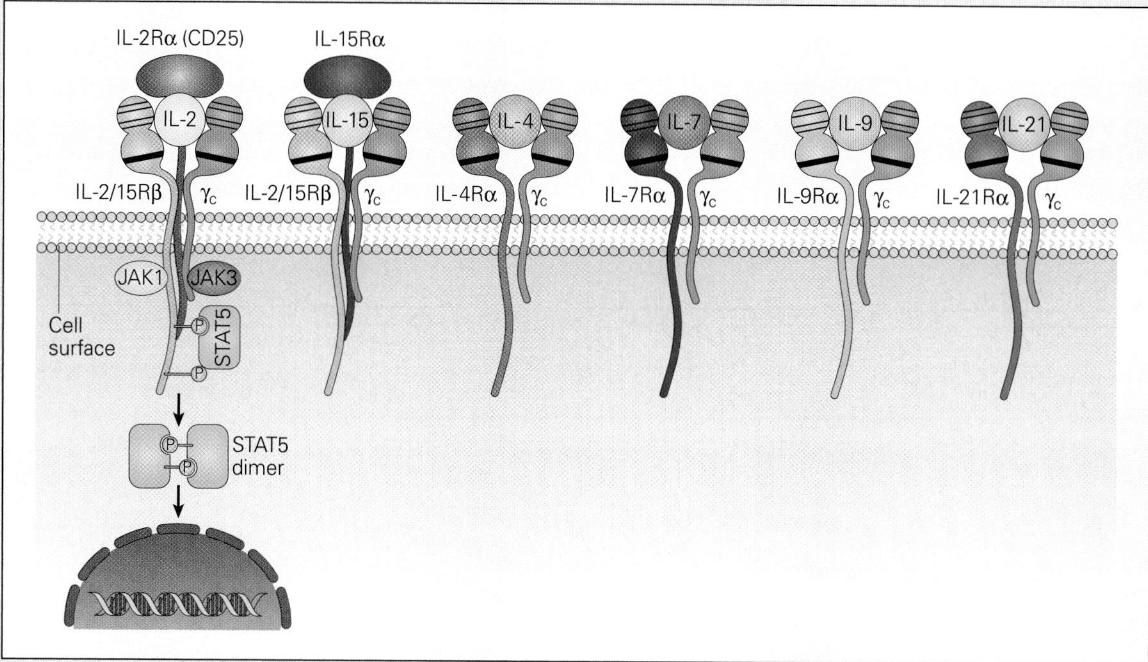

Figure 7-26. Schematic representation of the sharing of the IL-2 γc protein with several members of the IL-2 family of cytokines, including IL-2, IL-4, IL-7, IL-9, IL-15, and IL-21. This figure shows how deficiency of the IL-2 γc protein affects the critical activities of all members of the IL-2 family of cytokines on T and B cell development.

infections such as thrush, a white, purulent infection that occurs in the mouth of affected babies. The total lymphocyte counts in SCID are far below the normal range for infants (SCID patients = < 1,000/mm^3; normal is 2,000 to 11,000/mm^3). If untreated, SCID-afflicted infants will die within several months. The most famous case of SCID was "David the Bubble Boy," so named because his survival required that he live in a sterile enclosed environment with no direct contact with people—even his parents. Remarkably, he lived until age twelve in a four-room isolation unit equipped with sterile toys, books, and food that was connected through an airlock, and he was able to venture out in later years in a spacesuit provided by NASA. Tragically, his death occurred from complications of a bone marrow transplant from a sister at a time when new and improved technologies for tissue typing, donor-recipient matching, and donor-cell preparations were being developed and the oncogenic effects of the Epstein-Barr virus were only beginning to be understood.

- Currently, the best treatment and cure for SCID is bone marrow transplantation to reconstitute the defective immune system with genetically healthy lymphoid progenitors. For successful reconstitution of T cell immunity in SCID patients, it is essential that the bone marrow donor match with the SCID recipient at least one HLA allele for MHC-I and one allele for MHC-II (*Chapters 10, 16,* and *22*). The reasons for this are twofold: firstly, we know that T cells are positively selected on thymic epithelial cells that are not derived from bone marrow and are present in SCID patients (the thymus is intact in SCID individuals), and, therefore, proper positive selection must occur on the host MHC allotypes. Secondly, the antigen-presenting cells necessary for T cell activation in the periphery and B lymphocytes also derive from donor bone marrow, so in order for a donor-derived APC to activate a donor-derived T cell that has been positively selected on host MHC, both donor and host HLA allotypes must match. SCID patients do not have their own functioning immune system, so they will not reject unrelated donor bone marrow cells. Thus far, several hundred infants with SCID have been treated by bone marrow transplantation, and more recently, this procedure has even been performed in the first few weeks of life. These patients have been treated at several centers throughout the world and continue to survive into their teen years. Figure 7-27 shows the total T, B,

Case Study: Clinical Relevance (continued)

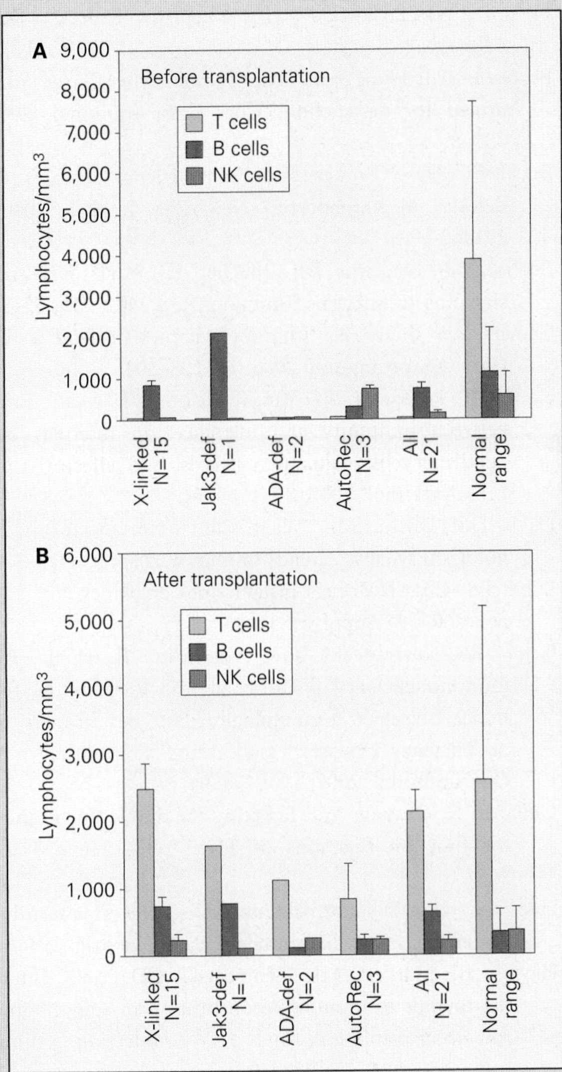

Figure 7-27. The total T, B, and NK cell counts of different SCID patients before and after bone marrow transplantation.

While T cell numbers are reconstituted, B cells are not effectively replenished by this treatment; however, a lack of B cells is easily remedied by regular administration of intravenous immunoglobulin (*Chapter 11*). The immune reconstitution of these patients inspired the conduct of valuable studies of the human immune system, particularly in the area of T cell maturation and homeostasis. While bone marrow transplantation has proved an effective treatment for SCID, there may not always be a suitable bone marrow donor available, as in the case of David. Moreover, the T cell numbers in treated SCID patients tend to decrease over many years, and B cell numbers are not always effectively reconstituted. Thus, bone marrow transplantation is not a perfect solution. Because the genetic lesions for many forms of SCID have been identified, gene therapy would provide the optimal and ultimate cure. Indeed, the first and only successful gene therapy trials were conducted in France in infants with X-linked SCID and who lack the γc chain. In these studies, the bone marrow progenitor cells were harvested from an infant with SCID, cultured with stromal factors *in vitro* to allow proliferative expansion, and then infected with retroviral vectors encoding a fully functional gene for the γc protein. These gene-transfected stem cells were then reinfused into the SCID infants. The initial results from this trial were extremely encouraging—twelve infants exhibited reconstitution of a functioning immune system and grew up in normal family environments, having normal childhoods. However, after several years, two of the treated patients developed T cell malignancies due to proliferative expansion of a clone of transfected cells (*Chapter 21*). Although these individuals were treated for the malignancy, this complication precludes vast application of gene therapy for treatment of SCID at this particular time.

Key Points

- T cells are key mediators of adaptive immunity.
- T cells exert their effects by surface receptors referred to as the TCR complex, a combination of molecules found on the surface of T lymphocytes (or T cells) generally responsible for recognizing antigens bound to MHC molecules.
- The TCR complex consists of a combination of the TCR and other accessory molecules called CD3- and ζ-chains.
- Somatic recombination of TCR genes results in the generation of diversity in antigen recognition and result in two TCRs referred to as Tαβ and Tγδ receptors.
- The Tαβ receptor consists of an alpha and beta chain in 95 percent of T cells, while 5 percent of T cells have TCRs consisting of gamma and delta chains. The TCR associates with other accessory molecules like CD3 that possess three distinct chains (γ, δ, and ε) in mammals and the ζ-chain.
- Tαβ cells comprise 95 percent of T cells and function as either helper CD4+ cells or cytotoxic CD8+ effector cells.

- CD4+ cells participate in cellular immunity, with antimicrobial activity against phagocytized extracellular pathogens (phagocytic activation), proinflammatory activity (Th1, Th17), anti-inflammatory antibody production (Th2), and immunoregulatory activity (Th3, Tr1).
- CD8+ cells participate in cytotoxic function, cellular immunity, antimicrobial against intracellular pathogens by the destruction of target cells (infected cells), tumor immunity, transplantation, and autoimmunity.
- Tγδ cells comprise 5 percent of T cells and predominate in epithelial tissues; first line of defense against pathogens at mucosal sites, e.g., MALT; non-HLA-restricted; and the recognition of nonprotein antigens. May have immunoregulatory function?
- In the thymus, antigen-independent development of alpha/beta T cells occurs and involves a number of steps that result in a commitment to the CD4 or CD8 T cell lineage (positive selection) and the removal of self-specific T cells (negative selection).
- Aberrations of T cell immunity are seen in both congenital and acquired forms of immune deficiency.

Study Questions/Critical Thinking

1. Why did the T cell system evolve to include a complex repertoire of molecules that function in T cell recognition?
2. How does the structure of the TCR complex differ from the B cell receptor recognition system?
3. Would it be advantageous to have Tγδ cell lymphocytes at mucosal sites exposed to mucosal pathogens coordinate with Tαβ cells at peripheral sites? Explain your answer.

Suggested Reading

Bacchetta R, Gambineri E, Roncarolo MG. Role of regulatory T cells and FOXP3 in human diseases. J Allergy Clin Immunol. 2007; 120: 227–35.

Beetz S, Marischen L, Kabelitz D, et al. Human gamma delta T cells: candidates for the development of immunolo-therapeutic strategies. Immunol Res. 2007; 37: 97–111.

Bendelac A, Savage PH, Teyton L. The biology of NKT cells. Annu Rev Immunol. 2007; 25: 297–336.

Blümer N, Pfefferle PI, Renz H. Development of mucosal immune function in the intrauterine and early postnatal environment. Curr Opin Gastroen. 2007; 23: 655–60.

Britton WJ, Lockwood HG. Leprosy. Lancet. 2004; 363: 1209–19.

Bryceson YT, Ljunggren HG. Lymphocyte effector functions: armed for destruction? Curr Opin Immunol. 2007; 19: 337–8.

Buckley RH. Primary immunodeficiency diseases due to defects in lymphocytes. New Eng J Med. 2000; 343: 1313–24.

Burbach BJ, Medeiros RB, Mueller KL, et al. T-cell receptor signaling to integrins. Immunol Rev. 2007; 218: 65–81.

Cemerski S, Shaw A. Immune synapses in T-cell activation. Curr Opin Immunol. 2006; 18: 298–304.

Cools N, Ponsaerts P, Van Tendeloo VF, et al. Balancing between immunity and tolerance: an interplay between dendritic cells, regulatory T cells, and effector T cells. J Leukocyte Biol. 2007; 82: 1365–74.

Davis DM, Dustin ML. What is the importance of the immunological synapse? Trends Immunol. 2004; 25: 323–7.

Dinarello CA. Historical insights into cytokines. Eur J Immunol. 2007; 37 Suppl 1: S34–45.

Geha RS, Notarangelo LD, Casanova JL, et al. Primary immunodeficiency diseases: an update from the International Union of Immunological Societies Primary Immunodeficiency Diseases Classification Committee. J Allergy Clin Immunol. 2007; 120: 776–94.

Ghilardi N, Ouyang W. Targeting the development and effector function functions of TH17 cells. Semin Immunol. 2007.

Hammar JA. Die normal morphologische Thymusforschung im letzten. Vierteljahrhundert. Barth: Leipzig: 1936.

Haynes BF, Markert ML, Sempowski GD, et al. The role of the thymus in immune reconstitution in aging, bone marrow transplantation, and HIV-1 infection. Annu Rev Immunol. 2000; 18: 529–60.

Haynes BF, Sempowski GD, Wells AF, et al. The human thymus during aging. Immunol Res. 2000; 22: 253–61.

Ivanov II, Zhou L, Littman DR. Transcriptional regulation of TH17 cell differentiation. Semin Immunol. 2007.

Iyer A, Hatta M, Usman R, et al. Serum levels of interferon-gamma, tumor necrosis factor-alpha, soluble interleukin-6R and soluble cell activation markers for monitoring response to treatment of leprosy reactions. Clin Exp Immunol. 2007; 150: 210–6.

Kunisawa J, Takahashi I, Kiyono H, Intraepithelial lymphocytes: their shared and divergent immunological behaviors in the small and large intestine. Immunol Rev. 2007; 217: 136–53.

Lehner T. Special regulatory T cell review: the resurgence of the concept of contrasuppression in immunoregulation. Immunology. 2008; 123: 40–4.

Lu B. The molecular mechanisms that control function and death of effector CD4+ T cells. Immunol Res. 2006; 36: 275–82.

Macdonald HR. NKT cells: in the beginning.... Eur J Immunol. 2007; 37 Suppl 1: S111–5.

Mak TW. The T cell antigen receptor: 'the hunting of the snark.' Eur J Immunol. 2007; 37 Suppl 1: S83–93.

Masopust D, Vezys V, Wherry EJ, et al. A brief history of CD8 T cells. Eur J Immunol. 2007; Nov; 37 Suppl 1: S103–10.

Mohty M, Gaugler B. Inflammatory cytokines and dendritic cells in acute graft-versus-host disease after allogeneic stem cell transplantation. Cytokine Growth F R. 2007.

Myers LA, Patel DD, Puck JM, et al. Hematopoietic stem cell transplantation for severe combined immunodeficiency in the neonatal period leads to superior thymic output and improved survival. Blood. 2002; 99: 872–8.

Natkunam Y. The biology of the germinal center. Hematology Am Soc Hematol Educ Program. 2007; 210–5.

Posadas SJ, Pichler WH. Delayed drug hypersensitivity reactions—new concepts. Clin Exp Allergy. 2007; 37: 989–99.

Poulin JF, Viswanathan MN, Harris JM, et al. Direct evidence for thymic function in adult humans. J Exp Med. 1999; 190: 479–86.

Sakaguchi S, Wing K, Miyara M. Regulatory T cells—a brief history and perspective. Eur J Immunol. 2007; 37 Suppl 1: 116–23.

Schoenborn JR, Wilson CB. Regulation of interferom-gamma during innate and adaptive immune responses. Advanced Immunol. 2007; 96: 41–101.

Shearer WT, Ritz J, Finegold MJ, et al. Epstein-Barr virus-associated B-cell proliferations of diverse clonal origins after bone marrow transplantation in 12-year-old patient with severe combined immunodeficiency. New Eng J Med. 1985; 312: 1151–9.

Sigal LH. Basic science for the clinician 45: CD4+ T-cell subsets of probably clinical consequence. J Clin Rheumatol. 2007; 13: 229–33.

Steele RW, Limas C, Thurman GB, et al. Familial thymic aplasia: attempted reconstiution with fetal thymus in a Millipore diffusion chamber. New Eng J Med. 1972; 287: 787–91.

Sundrud MS, Rao A. New twists of T cell fate: control of T cell activation and tolerance by TGF-beta and NFAT. Curr Opin Immunol. 2007; 19: 287–93.

Chapter 8

The Mucosal Immune System in Health and Disease

Marco A. Vega-López, BSc, PhD
Michael F. Cole, BDS, MSc, PhD
Joseph A. Bellanti, MD

Case Study

A sixty-nine-year-old male who had recently completed a course of chemotherapy for prostate cancer was recommended to receive a unit of whole blood for treatment of a related anemia. Within minutes of the start of the transfusion, the patient developed acute dyspnea, hypotension, sweating, and a feeling of impending doom. The transfusion was terminated and the patient was treated with epinephrine, intravenous fluids, and corticosteroids and recovered after several hours.

His past medical history was unremarkable except for multiple episodes of bronchitis and otitis media in childhood. There was no family history of frequent or unusual infections, allergic disease, rheumatoid or autoimmune disorders. The patient's blood type was A positive, and further communication with the laboratory confirmed that the transfused blood was also A positive and compatible with the patient's blood by cross-matching assays.

Because of the patient's recent history, an immunologic evaluation was performed that revealed a serum IgG of 960 mg/dl (normal values are 614–1,295 mg/dl), undetectable IgA (normal values are 60–309 mg/dl), and IgM of 670 mg/dl (normal values are 53–334 mg/dl). The diagnosis of selective IgA deficiency was made and the patient was counseled against receiving whole blood transfusions, intravenous gamma globulin, or other blood protein products in the future.

IgA deficiency is the most common primary immune deficiency disorder, occurring at a frequency of 1:300 to 1:500 in the population (*Chapter 16*). Although most individuals with this disorder are clinically asymptomatic, some present with symptoms of sinopulmonary or gastrointestinal infections and others with a propensity to develop autoimmune disorders. This is presumably due to the fact that IgA is produced predominantly in the mucosal immune system at body surfaces, where it conveys local protection. A deficiency of IgA therefore may have been responsible for the patient's prior history of bronchitis and otitis media in childhood.

The patient's reaction during the transfusion is considered a nonhemolytic, anaphylactoid hypersensitivity reaction (*Chapter 18*) related to the combination of IgA in the transfused blood with the patient's anti-IgA antibodies present in his serum. This pathogenetic mechanism was confirmed by the finding of an IgG anti-IgA titer of 1:400 in the patient's blood.

LEARNING OBJECTIVES

When you have completed this chapter, you should be able to:

- Compare and contrast the structures and functions of the mucosal immune system with the peripheral immune system
- Explain the importance of lymphocyte recirculation in mucosal immunity
- Describe the inductive and effector sites of the mucosa-associated lymphoid tissues
- Describe the roles of intraepithelial lymphocytes, gamma-delta T cells, and B1 B cells in the mucosal immune system
- Explain the roles of IgA in mucosal immunity
- Explain the importance of T regulatory T lymphocytes and limiting inflammation in mucosal immunity
- Discuss mucosal immunization routes and their current level of effectiveness
- Describe mucosal immunopathologies and their possible causes
- Summarize the clinical relevance of the mucosal immune system in health and disease

Introduction: Systemic Versus Mucosal Immune Responses

It has become increasingly apparent that from a structural and functional standpoint, the immunologic system consists of two major divisions: (1) an *internal system* that deals with foreign substances that have breached the anatomic barriers of skin and mucous membranes and that consist of lymphoid organs found within the interior and that are accountable for systemic immune responses, and (2) an *external system* consisting of lymphoid elements found at body surfaces that come into contact with and respond to foreign substances in the external environment and that are responsible for mucosal immune responses (inducing immune exclusion) (Figure 8-1).

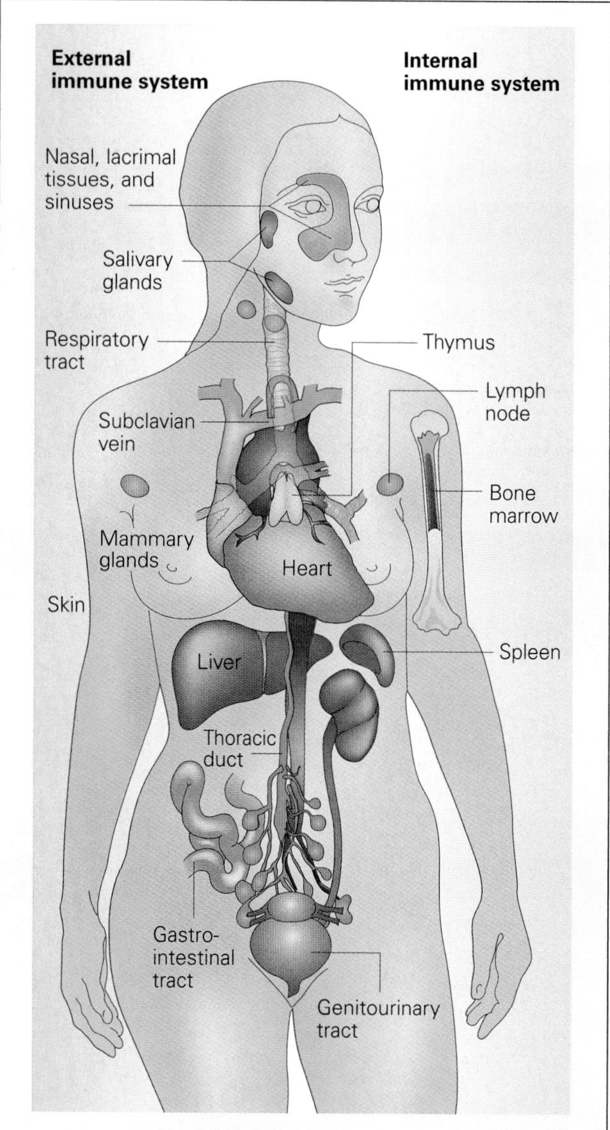

Figure 8-1. Schematic representation of the functional division of the immune system into internal and external systems.

The external immunologic system is commonly referred to as the mucosa-associated lymphoid tissues (**MALT**) and consists of an extensive network of cells and cell products of both the innate and the adaptive immune systems found within the vast domain of mucosal surfaces that interface with the external environment and that function to exclude the penetration of foreign and potentially inimical substances from entry into the internal milieu. These mucosal surfaces of the human body comprise the gastrointestinal (**GI**), respiratory, and genitourinary (**GU**) tracts, the eyes, and the mammary glands. They encompass a surface area of more than 400 m^2 and contain the portals of entry through which the vast majority of pathogens enter the body. The mucosae are thin, flexible, and permeable epithelial surfaces, unlike the skin, because they are required to uptake nutrients, excrete wastes, and exchange gases. In consequence, almost two-thirds of microbial agents that infect humans enter the body via the respiratory tract alone, and a variety of bacteria, viruses, and other parasites infect via the mucosal surfaces, accounting for a significant number of deaths in the world each year (Figure 8-2). It is not then surprising that mammals and birds have evolved an immune system dedicated to the protection of these susceptible surfaces (*Chapter 2*).

The mucosal and skin surfaces are colonized by complex commensal microbiota that, for the most part, exist in a state of homeostasis with the host and serve to protect these surfaces from colonization by pathogenic microorganisms (*Chapter 12*). Indeed, it is the colonization of the mucosal surfaces by indigenous microorganisms immediately postpartum that drives the development of the mucosal immune system in early life (*Chapter 2*). The dilemma for the mucosal immune system is how to discriminate between commensal microorganisms that protect host body surfaces and must be controlled, but not displaced, while at the same time eliminating pathogens, and to accomplish this without engendering an inflammatory response that may disrupt the barrier epithelia. An example of this dilemma is demonstrated by viridans streptococci, *S. pneumoniae*, a respiratory pathogen, and *S. mitis*, a commensal of the oropharynx. Genetic analyses indicate that these bacteria are 99 percent similar. Both share the same group antigen, both have phosphocholine

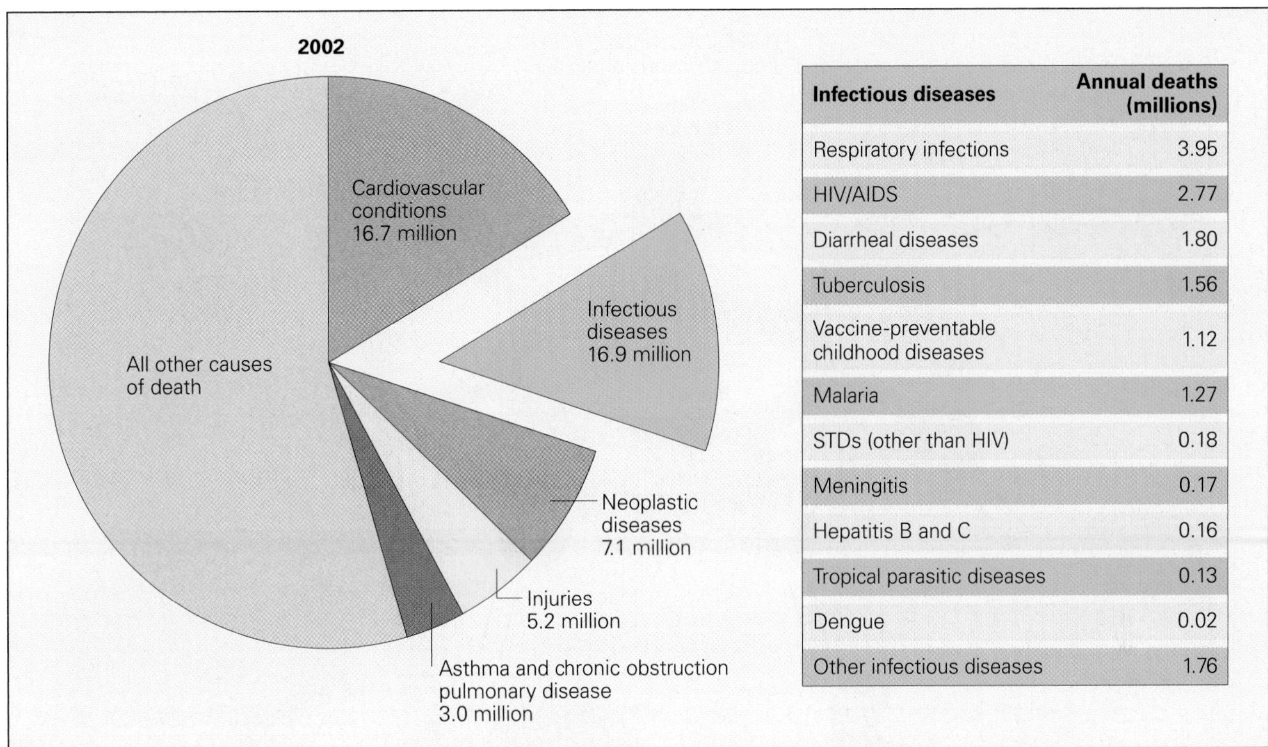

Infectious diseases	Annual deaths (millions)
Respiratory infections	3.95
HIV/AIDS	2.77
Diarrheal diseases	1.80
Tuberculosis	1.56
Vaccine-preventable childhood diseases	1.12
Malaria	1.27
STDs (other than HIV)	0.18
Meningitis	0.17
Hepatitis B and C	0.16
Tropical parasitic diseases	0.13
Dengue	0.02
Other infectious diseases	1.76

Figure 8-2. Total annual deaths in the world. Every segment of the pie shows the proportion of mortality due to a particular cause. Diseases involving mucosae account for up to 25 percent of the total death toll.

Source: http://www.who.int/whr/en.

in the cell wall, and both produce IgA1 protease and neuraminidase, yet the mucosal immune system must eliminate the former and preserve the latter. A similar situation pertains for soluble antigens; the mucosal immune system, for example, must ignore harmless food antigens but eliminate toxins and other noxious products produced by pathogenic microorganisms. Hence, tolerance, i.e., immunological unresponsiveness, and a specialized "limited" noninflammatory immune response, termed "immune exclusion" and mediated by secretory immunoglobulin A (**sIgA**) antibodies, operate at mucosal surfaces (*Chapters 6* and *19*). Although our knowledge of the mucosal immune system has increased markedly in recent years, relatively less is currently known about the mechanisms involved in immune regulation at mucosal surfaces.

Structure and Development of the Mucosal Immune System: The Mucosa-Associated Lymphoid Tissues

As described in Chapter 1, the immune system consists of the two interactive arms responsible for *innate immunity* and *adaptive immunity* concerned with the recognition and disposal of foreign substances that impinge upon it. The mucosal immune system, in contrast to the internal immune system, however, is unique in that it is the only part of the immune system that directly interfaces with the external environment as it employs components of both the innate and adaptive immune systems in performing its function of recognition and elimination of foreignness. Moreover, as stated previously, it must distinguish those foreign agents that are detrimental and that require a robust immune response, e.g., pathogenic bacteria, from those that are less harmful and even beneficial, e.g., commensal bacteria, which require a silencing of the immune response. As will be described in greater detail below, this dichotomy of immune requirements is carried out by the diversity of regulatory and stimulatory immune cells that comprise the innate and adaptive immune components of the mucosa-associated lymphoid tissues.

Mucosa-Associated Lymphoid Tissues

Included within the MALT are the mucosal surfaces of the gastrointestinal, respiratory, and genitourinary systems, as well as all tissues that interface with the external environment (Figure 8-3). In the

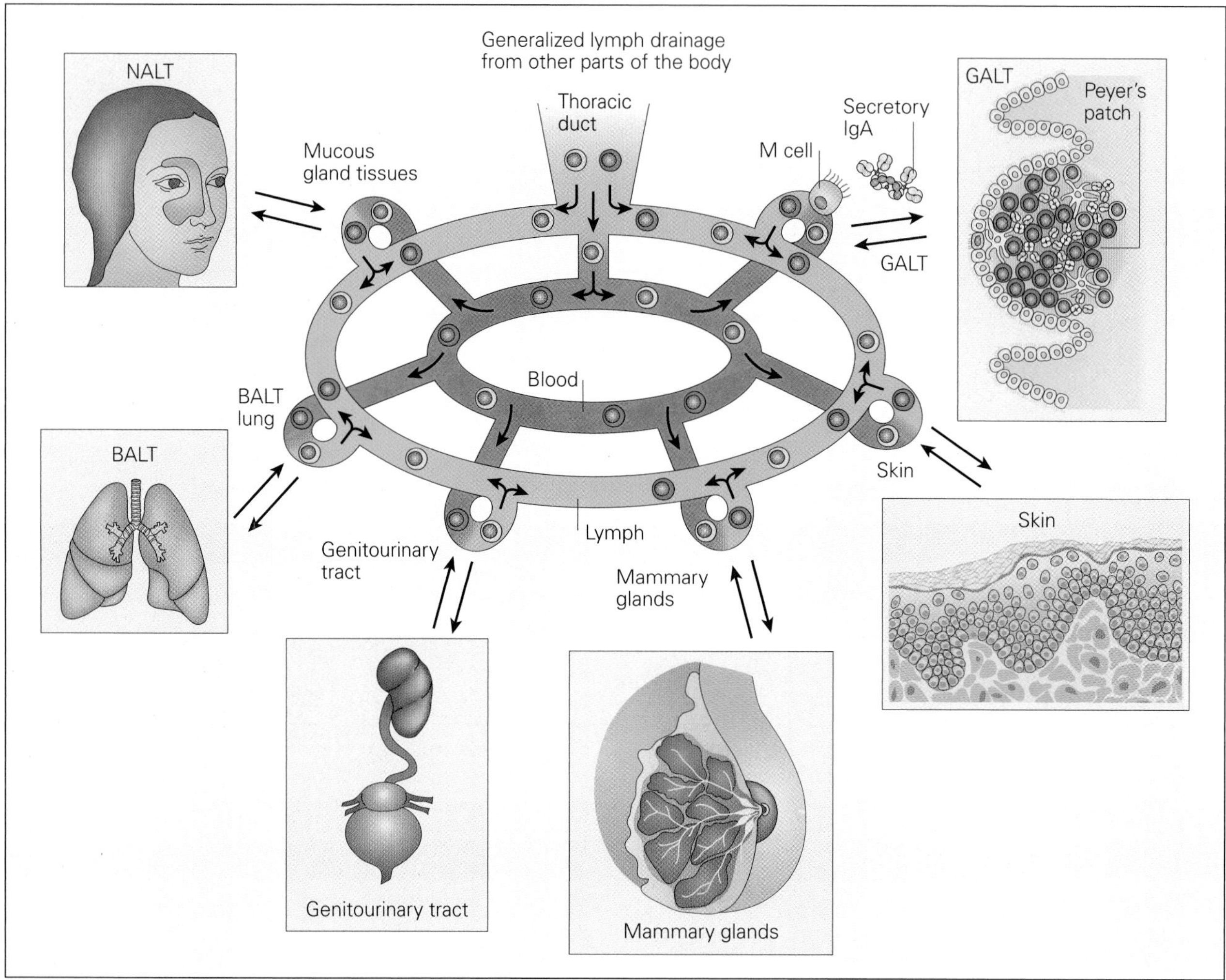

Figure 8-3. Schematic representation of the features of the MALT and its relationship to the total immunologic system. Immunologically activated T and B lymphocytes derived from the generalized lymphatic drainage comingled in the lymph with counterpart T and B lymphocytes derived from stimulation at mucosal and skin sites together with macrophages and dendritic cells (DCs) enter the blood through the thoracic duct. From there, this collection of lymphocytes forms a recirculating pool that can "home" back to their original mucosal sites of sensitization or to other mucosal sites. This recirculating pool of sensitized T and B lymphocytes in the blood can also percolate back into the lymph in primary lymphoid tissues in lymph nodes and other secondary lymphoid tissues at mucosal sites through postcapillary venules. Thus, lymphocytes enter the lymph through both the vascular as well as the lymphatic channels and form a continuously recirculating pool of lymphocytes prepared to function at internal sites as well as at mucosal surfaces.

gastrointestinal tract, these mucosal sites contain lymphoid tissues that are distributed throughout the lamina propria of the mucosal surfaces, either as discrete lymphoid tissues similar to lymph nodes such as the Peyer's patches (**PP**) in the ileum, or as more diffuse lymphoid aggregates. For ease of discussion, the various components of the MALT have been classified into clusters of anatomically organized sites shown in Table 8-1 and which include: (1) the nasopharyngeal-associated lymphoid tissues (**NALT**); (2) the bronchus-associated lymphoid tissues (**BALT**); (3) the genitourinary systems and other mucous gland-secreting tissues, e.g., lacrimal; (4) the mammary-associated lymphoid tissues; (5) the skin-associated lymphoid tissues (**SALT**); and (6) the gut-associated lymphoid tissues (**GALT**). Shown in Table 8-1 are the major components of the MALT together with tissue localizations and examples of clinical involvement in various diseases affecting each component.

The MALT is further organized into discrete lymphoid organs found at the various portals of entry to the body. Thus, at the entry to the aerodigestive tract is found a ring of lymphoid organs,

Table 8-1. Components of the MALT, major tissues, and examples of clinical involvement

Component	Major tissues	Example of clinical involvement
Nasopharyngeal-associated lymphoid tissues (NALT)	Palatine tonsils and adenoids	Allergic rhinitis
Bronchus-associated lymphoid tissues (BALT)	Peribronchial lymphoid tissues	Asthma
Mucous gland tissues	Genitourinary tissues	Protective immunity (?)
	Lacrimal lymphoid tissues	Allergic conjunctivitis
Mammary-associated lymphoid tissues	Mammary lymphoid tissues	Protective immunity for newborns
Skin-associated lymphoid tissues (SALT)	Dermal lymphoid tissues	Atopic eczema
Gut-associated lymphoid tissues (GALT)	Jejunum (PP)	Celiac disease
	Ileum (M cells)	Food allergy

termed Waldeyer's ring, comprising the lingual tonsil, the palatine tonsils, the nasopharyngeal tonsils, and the tubal tonsils at the opening of the auditory tubes. This is termed the NALT. Similar discrete and diffuse lymphoid tissues are found in the bronchi in the form of the BALT and the GALT. Of these, the GALT comprising the PP in the ileum, the appendix, and lymphoid aggregates in the large intestine and rectum are the best studied. The concept of a unified MALT, referred to as the *common mucosal immune system*, has been proposed that includes the NALT, BALT, GALT, etc. This concept is derived from findings that immune cells, activated at one particular mucosal site, i.e., the *inductive site*, home to the same or other mucosal sites via the lymphatics and bloodstream, i.e., the *effector site*, resulting in general protection of the mucosal surfaces (Figure 8-3 and *Chapter 2*).

The mucosal immune system is, therefore, responsible both for mediating the symbiotic relationship between the host and endogenous microorganisms, i.e., commensal bacteria, as well as for functioning as a first line of physical and immunological defense against invading pathogens. Through innate and acquired immunity, the mucosal immune system maintains immunological homeostasis along the vast expanse of the epithelial surface area, ranging from the oral and nasal cavities to the respiratory, intestinal, and genitourinary tracts.

The Organizational Structure of the Mucosal Immune System

Of all the components of the mucosa-associated lymphoid tissues, the gut-associated lymphoid tissues have been the most extensively studied. Shown in Figure 8-4 is a schematic representation of the most important structures of the GALT. Its features include a characteristic architecture of the epithelium, the presence of antigen-presenting cells (**APCs**) consisting of dendritic cells (**DCs**) and macrophages, T-cell areas, and B-cell areas with germinal centers in the lamina propria, where switches of IgM- to IgA-bearing B cells predominate. The columnar epithelium that covers the lymphoid follicles is infiltrated with lymphocytes and DCs, giving rise to the term follicle-associated epithelium (**FAE**). The FAE lacks goblet cells and is therefore covered with far less mucus than normal enterocytes. Of particular importance within the mucosal surface are specialized epithelial cells, called microfold (**M**) cells, located in the epithelium overlying follicles of the Peyer's patches. The M cells are characterized by an invagination at the basolateral membrane, which forms a "pocket" normally occupied by lymphocytes and APCs referred to as the subepithelial dome (**SED**) (Figure 8-4). These contain all of the immunocompetent cells that are required for the initial generation of an immune response, i.e., T cells, B cells, and APCs. Soluble and particulate luminal antigens are taken up by M cells and are delivered to adjacent APCs. M cells have been described in Peyer's patches, the appendix, and the tonsils, and represent 10 to 15 percent of the cells within the FAE. M cells are also found in isolated lymphoid follicles (**ILFs**) and at the tips of the villus, where they are termed villous M cells. The microvilli of these cells, which are less dense than those of adjacent enterocytes (Figure 8-4), provide a portal of entry into the MALT.

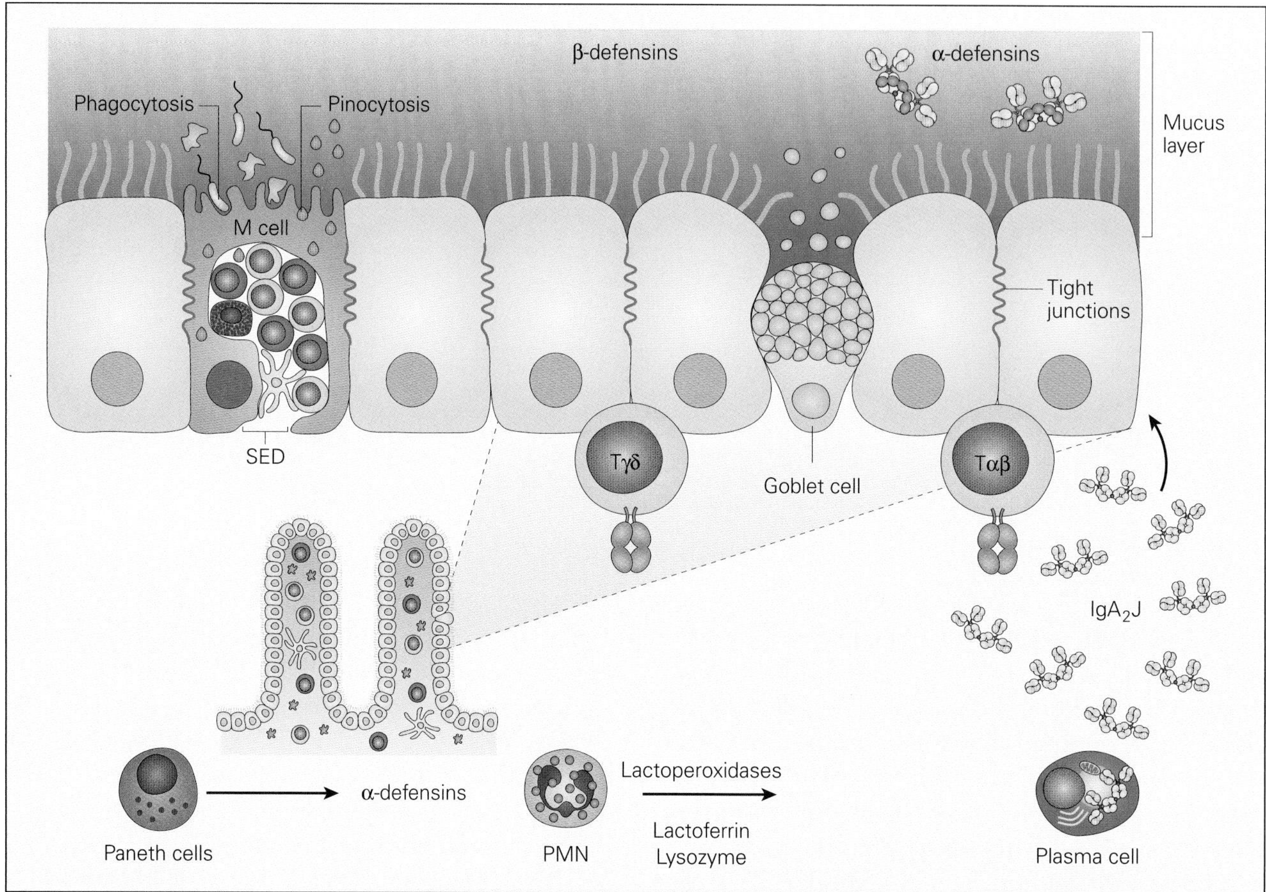

Figure 8-4. Schematic representation of the most important structures of the GALT. The GALT contain components of the innate immune system, including a thick coat of mucus on the surface of epithelial cells that prevents the penetration of deleterious macromolecules and potential pathogens. The mucus layer also contains α-defensins produced by Paneth cells, β-defensins produced by epithelial cells, as well as other innate factors, such as lysozyme, lactoperoxidase, lactoferrin phospholipases, and mucin produced by goblet cells, all serve in antimicrobial defense. The epithelial cells are connected via tight junctions and also contain components of the adaptive immune system, including both αβ and γδ intraepithelial T lymphocytes (IELs). Of particular importance within the mucosal surface are specialized epithelial cells, M cells, located in the epithelium overlying follicles of the Peyer's patches. The M cell actively pinocytoses soluble antigens and phagocytoses particulates such as viruses, bacteria, and microspheres. The M cells are characterized by an invagination at the basolateral membrane, which forms a "pocket" normally occupied by lymphocytes and APCs, referred to as the subepithelial dome (SED). The production of secretory IgA by plasma cells represents one of the major hallmarks of the MALT. Polymorphonuclear neutrophils are normally not found in healthy mucosal tissues but under inflammatory conditions may be recruited from the blood at these sites.

The Innate Immune Mucosal Defense System

The innate immune component of the mucosal immune system has features in common with those of the systemic innate immune system described in Chapter 1. Shown in Figure 8-4 are the major components together with some of the interacting components of the adaptive immune system. These include the physical barrier provided by the epithelial cells lining the mucosal surfaces together with the rhythmic wavelike activity of the ciliated epithelial cells, the production of mucus by goblet cells, the secretion of antimicrobial molecules from epithelial cells, the participation of mediator cells, i.e., mast cells, and the cytolytic activity of natural killer (**NK**) cells in the submucosa. Complement also plays a limited role in the innate immune mucosal immune responses, but since many of the cleavage products of complement promote inflammation (*Chapter 4*), they must be carefully regulated to prevent tissue damage while they promote antimicrobial defense. Collectively, these innate immune mechanisms of the mucosal immune system are operative on mucosal surfaces of the body and provide the first line of defense against exogenous substances and invading pathogens.

The Physical Barrier Provided by Epithelial Cells of the Mucosal Immune System

Similar to the skin, the mucosal surfaces are covered by a layer of epithelial cells that provide a physical barrier to the entry of exogenous substances into the host and at the same time permit their normal functioning, e.g., gas exchange in the lungs and absorption of nutrients from the gastrointestinal tract. The thickness of the epithelial mucosal cells varies in different locations. For example, in some locations, e.g., the respiratory tract, the surface lining consists of a single layer of respiratory epithelium, which facilitates gas exchange, while in other sites, the lining may be multilayered and differentiated into squamous epithelial cells, as in the oral cavity, the pharynx, the tonsils, the urethra, and the vagina, permitting greater protection at these sites. In the small intestine, the barrier function is accomplished by epithelial cells, termed enterocytes, tightly joined by interepithelial junctions and facilitated by a blanket of mucus that covers these cells (Figure 8-4). The mucus is secreted by goblet cells located beneath the epithelium and consists of glycoconjugates of various molecular sizes that function to interfere with the attachment of microorganisms to epithelial surfaces.

As described previously, located within the epithelium of several regions of the GALT are the specialized microfold M cells that function to facilitate the uptake of soluble and particulate antigens from the lumen of the intestine to APCs and T and B lymphocytes in regions below the surface of the epithelial layer. Also interspersed within the epithelial layer (Figure 8-4) are intraepithelial mast cells and intraepithelial NK cells as well as T lymphocytes expressing both types of T cell receptors, i.e., Tαβ and Tγδ lymphocytes of the adaptive immune system (*Chapter 7*).

Although formerly considered to play a passive role, recent studies suggest that intestinal epithelial cells are actively involved in host defense. As will be described in greater detail below, intestinal epithelial cells play a central role in sampling the intestinal microenvironment, discriminating pathogenic from commensal microorganisms, and influencing the function of APCs and lymphocytes.

Defensins and Other Extracellular Antimicrobial Mucosal Peptides Found in Secretions Bathing Mucosal Surfaces of the Mucosal Immune System

As described in Chapter 1, there are a number of extracellular peptides found in external secretions of the mucosal immune system that provide antimicrobial defense (Figure 8-4). These include alpha and beta defensins, which are produced by Paneth cells and epithelial cells, respectively, and which together provide a protective defensin network against most bacteria and many viruses. Although the precise mechanisms that control the production of defensins are poorly understood, proinflammatory cytokines such as interleukin-1 (**IL-1**), tumor necrosis factor-α (**TNF-α**), and bacterial lipopolysaccharide (**LPS**) play a role in their activation. Other innate immune factors such as lysozyme, lactoperoxidase, lactoferrin, and phospholipases are also found in external secretions and serve in antimicrobial defense. Although some are secreted by intestinal Paneth cells, e.g., alpha-defensins, all are produced by polymorphonuclear leukocytes (**PMNs**), e.g., lysozyme, lactoperoxidase, lactoferrin, and phospholipases. Lactoferrin, a member of the transferrin family, and lysozyme are found in high concentrations in breast milk; they exert their antimicrobial effects by binding iron or by hydrolyzing β1-4 linkages between the component sugars of peptidoglycans of the bacterial cell wall, respectively. Lactoferrin has also been shown to have antiviral activity to many viruses, including HIV, and may play a role in decreasing maternal-infant viral transmission from HIV-positive mothers to infants who are breast-fed.

Dendritic Cells and Other Antigen-Presenting Cells Within the MALT

Of particular importance in mucosal immunity are the DCs, which are found as a pleomorphic set of several populations of APCs in several sites of the intestine and associated lymphoid tissues. In the GALT, DCs are found in at least three separate locations: (1) in a region of the Peyer's patch immediately below the M cells, referred to as the SED (Figures 8-4 and 8-5); (2) in an intraepithelial location as a set of specialized DC subsets that extend

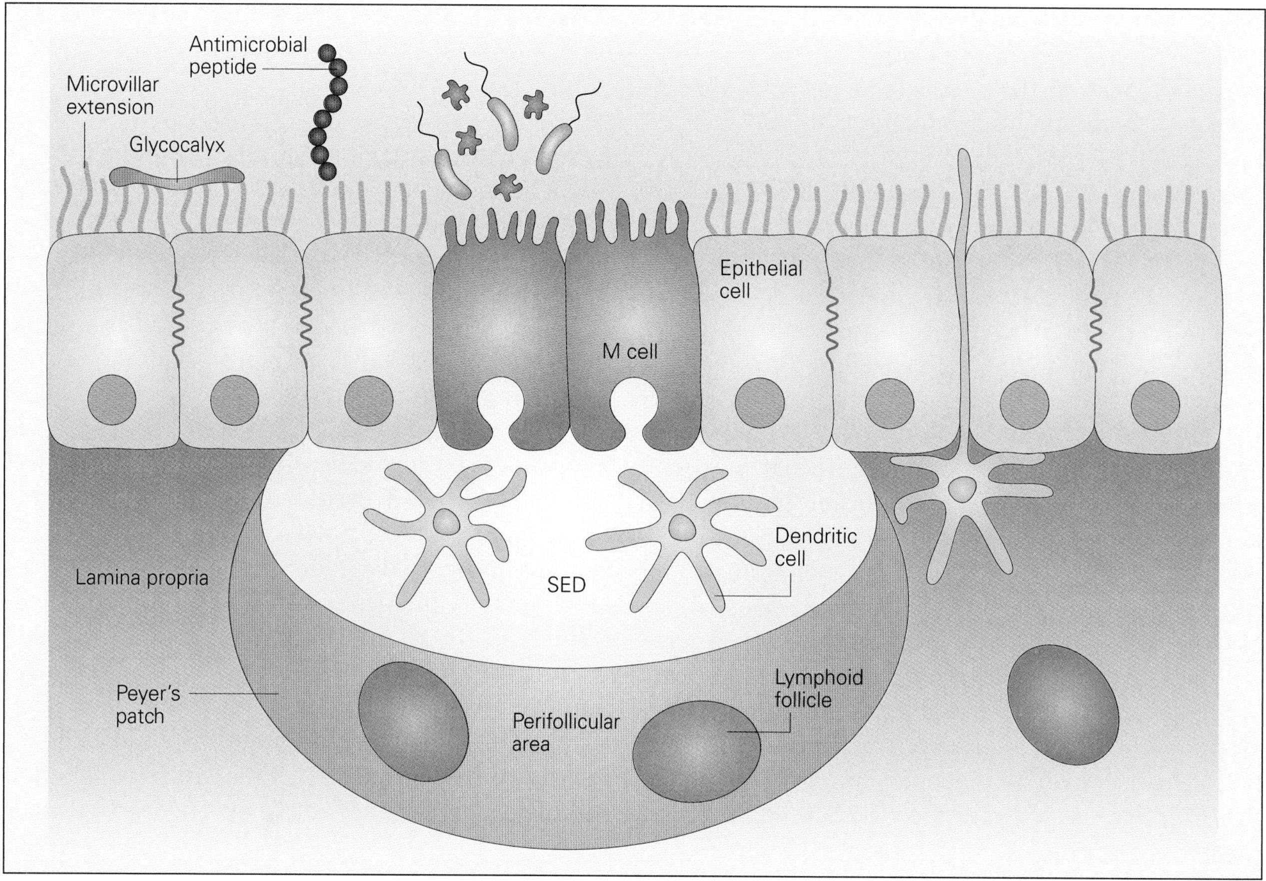

Figure 8-5. Microanatomical features of dendritic cells showing their location in the SED and in an intraepithelial location as a set of specialized DC subsets that extend dendrites between the tight junctions of enterocytes that can sample luminal contents.

dendrites between the tight junctions of enterocytes that can sample luminal contents (Figure 8-5); and (3) in lymphoid follicles scattered throughout the lamina propria. The functional properties of intestinal DCs have been found to be altered by factors present in the local environment. Many of these factors include bacteria and other microbes that contain pathogen-associated molecular patterns (**PAMPs**) that are sensed by pattern-recognition receptors (**PRRs**), i.e., Toll-like receptors (**TLRs**) on the DCs (*Chapter 3*). This alteration of DCs is sometimes referred to as "conditioning of DCs." These cells have been implicated both in the maintenance of tolerance toward the commensal microflora as well as in the generation of protective immune responses against pathogens through signalling pathways, which will be described in greater detail below. The impressive flexibility in the function of these intestinal DCs is commensurate with their unique capacity to accurately sense their local environment and to use generated signals to shape the nature of the ensuing immune response. The unique functional properties of populations of intestinal DCs and the type of signals that are required for them to mediate these functions represent an area of current intensive research and have clinical applicability to an understanding of the pathogenesis of many of the immunologically mediated diseases affecting the gastrointestinal tract, e.g., regional ileitis (Crohn's disease) and ulcerative colitis.

The Influence of the Environment on Intestinal DC Function

In light of the unique multifunctional properties described for intestinal DCs, an important question is whether this is related to adaptation of DCs to the effects of the local environment or to a pleomorphic array of DC subsets. Recent evidence demonstrating that DCs undergo conditioning in their local tissue environment suggests that the milieu may play a greater role rather than the existence of functionally distinct DC subsets. Communication between the intestinal epithelium and DCs is likely to be essential for this type of conditioning. As will be described in greater detail below, intestinal epithelial cells (**IECs**) show qualitatively distinct responsiveness to commensal and pathogenic bacterial species, thus illustrating the importance of the epithelial cell layer as a sensor for current environmental conditions and the instruction of adjacent DCs (Figure 8-5).

The Immunoregulatory Role of Vitamin A and Retinoic Acid in the Mucosal Immune System

Recently, it has been recognized that vitamin A and its metabolites have potent immunoregulatory activities in the mucosal immune system (Figure 8-6). Dendritic cells have been shown to produce retinoic acid, which provides yet another type of intestine-specific environmental conditioning agent for activation of T cells and B cells in the GALT and associated lymphoid tissues. Retinoic acid (**RA**), produced by gut dendritic cells or from dietary sources, not only induces addressin-associated homing receptors on T and B cells, but also provides important signals that induce differentiation and class switching of IgA-producing B cells. Retinoic acid also

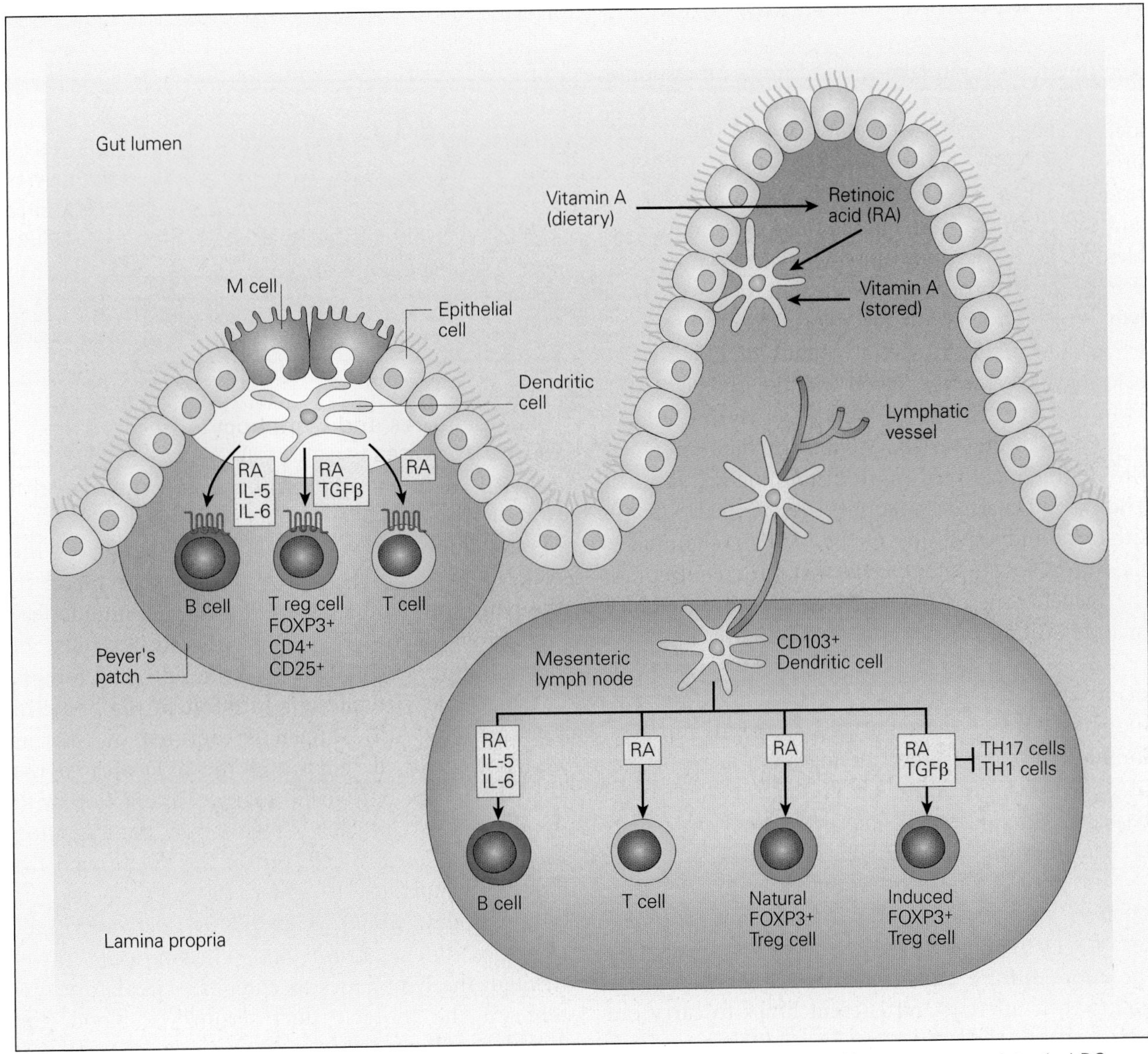

Figure 8-6. Schematic representation of the role of vitamin A and retinoic acid (RA) in the mucosal immune system. Intestinal DCs produce RA from stored or dietary sources of vitamin A and promote the expression of gut-homing addressin receptors by T and B lymphocytes, the peripheral generation of forkhead box P3 (FOXP3)+ regulatory T (Treg) cells, and class switching to IgA. RA has an important role in these three processes. Peyer's patch DCs and mesenteric lymph-node DCs that arrive from the intestine express enzymes that allow them to metabolize RA, perhaps from retinol carried in the serum or stored in the intestine. Alternatively, DCs may transport RA metabolized from dietary carotenoids or other vitamin A derivatives by intestinal epithelial cells to lymphoid tissues.

induces a subset of forkhead box P3 (**FOXP3**)+ regulatory T cells, which are important for maintaining immune tolerance in the gut (*Chapter 7*). These findings show that retinoids provide important positive and negative regulatory signals to fine-tune the mucosal immune system and suggest the potential for therapeutic manipulation of the levels of retinoic acid to not only enhance immunoregulatory pathways, but to directly inhibit the generation of inflammatory T cell populations.

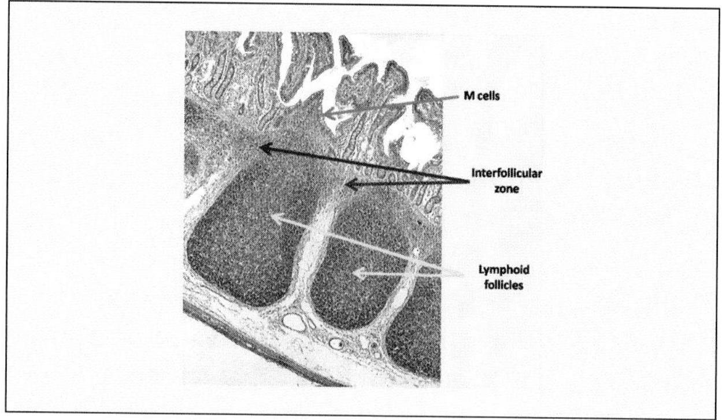

Figure 8-7. Histochemical section of Peyer's patch. The main parts of the tissue are labeled with arrows, epithelial M cells, interfollicular T zone (stained in brown), and B cell follicles. Below the epithelium and dispersed in the T zone, abundant MHC-II+ dendritic cells are localized.

The Adaptive Immune Mucosal Defense System: Inductive and Effector Sites

The initiation of antigen-specific immune responses in the mucosal immune system occurs at special locations, referred to as inductive sites. There, uptake, processing, and presentation of antigen take place, resulting in the development of a set of lymphocytes and cell products, e.g., antibody and cytokines, capable of carrying out the complex functions of immune defense and homeostasis. In the case of GALT, these lymphocytes migrate to the mesenteric lymph nodes where they undergo several rounds of cell division before they enter the blood via the thoracic duct. From the blood these lymphocytes may traffic back to epithelial sites in the vicinity of their inductive site or they may seed more distal mucosal surfaces. Their epithelial destinations are termed effector sites. The inductive sites of the MALT contain all of the immunocompetent cells that are required for the generation of an immune response, which include APCs, T cells, and B cells. Peyer's patches (Figure 8-7), in the gut, and the NALT—two of the main components of the MALT—are important inductive tissues for the generation of mucosal immunity through either the ingestion or inhalation of antigen in the intestinal and respiratory tracts, respectively, and are also sites of induction of allergic sensitization (*Chapter 18*).

The common mucosal immune system (**CMIS**) refers to an integrated pathway that allows communication between the organized inductive sites with the more diffuse effector sites of the MALT, enabling their afferent and efferent limbs to carry out host-protective immunity against pathogenic microorganisms and other potentially noxious substances. Shown in Figure 8-8 is a schematic representation of how the CMIS connects inductive sites in Peyer's patches and the NALT with effector sites such as the lamina propria of the intestinal and respiratory tracts, and glandular tissues. The homing of lymphocytes from inductive sites to distant effector sites allows for the antigen-specific T helper 2 (**Th2**) cell–dependent IgA responses, and T helper 1 (**Th1**) cell–dependent and cytotoxic T lymphocyte (**CTL**)-dependent immune responses, to be expressed throughout the entire mucosal immune system.

Inductive Sites and Lymphocyte Recirculation to Effector Sites

One of the amazing attributes of the adaptive immune system is its capacity to recirculate its lymphocytes throughout the body, referred to as the recirculating pool (*Chapter 2*), from the blood to the lymph or the lymph to blood. This unique feature provides the basis for the exquisite ability of the immune system to sense the entry of foreign substances at virtually any location in the body. In the case of GALT, antigen is captured by M cells and is transferred to DCs in the SED area of the PP where they engage in cognate interaction with T cells and B cells. This is followed by the migration of activated T and B cells out of the PP through the efferent lymphatics to enter the local mesenteric lymph nodes (**MLN**) (Figure 8-9). Activated cells undergo differentiation and effector cells travel through the lymphatics to enter the circulatory system via the thoracic duct. From the blood, the T and B cells seed the lamina propria of the ileum and, amazingly enough, the lamina propria of remote mucosae. For example, effector cells induced at the PP arrive at (or migrate to) the intestinal lamina propria (**LP**). In nursing mothers,

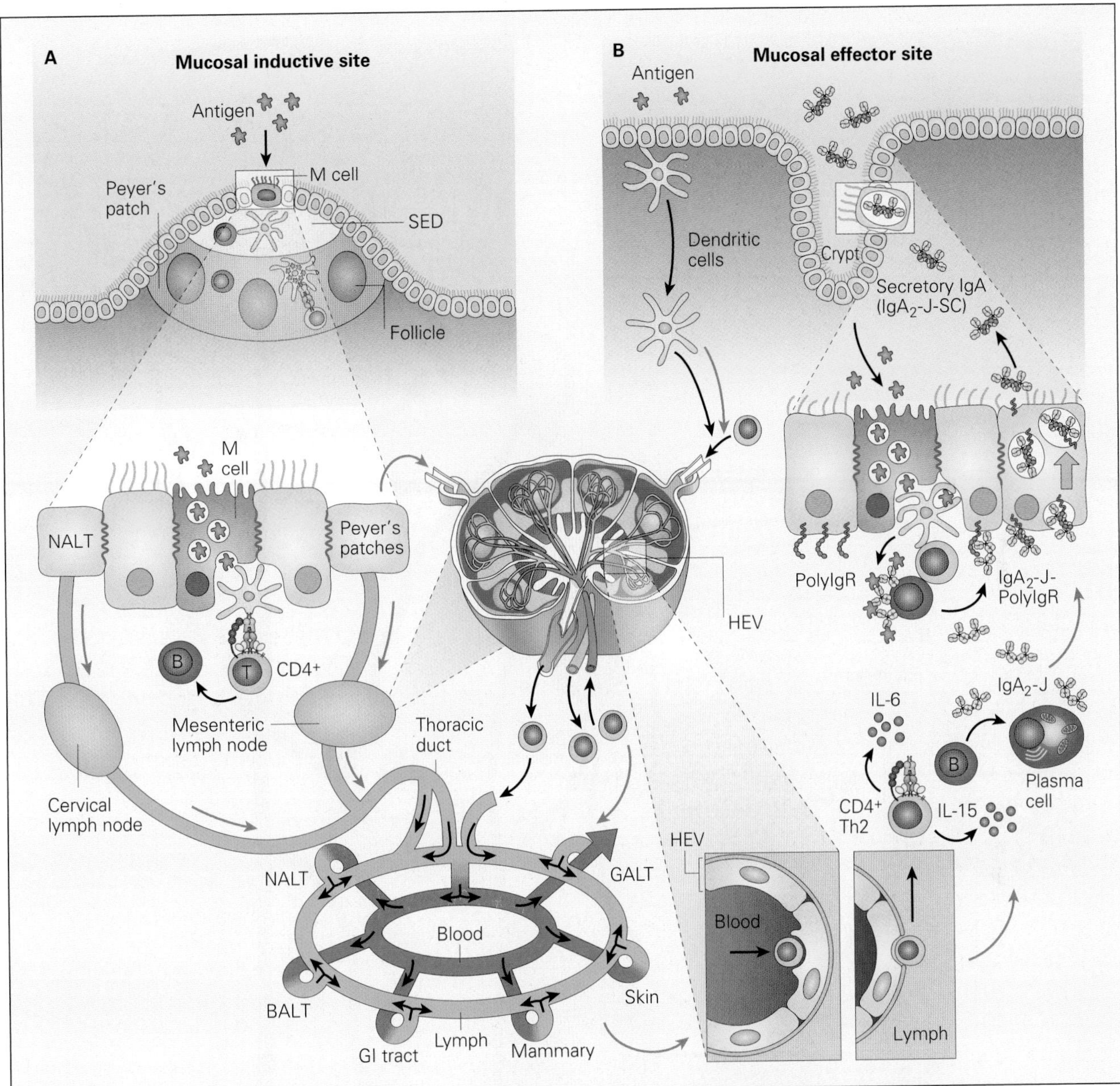

Figure 8-8. Schematic representation of the CMIS illustrating the transport of luminal antigens from the NALT and Peyer's patches through M cells that are present in the epithelium overlying the NALT and Peyer's patch follicles, respectively. Dendritic cells process and present antigens to T cells in these lymphoid tissues, which are referred to as inductive sites. CD4+ T cells that are stimulated by dendritic cells then preferentially induce IgA-committed B cell development in the germinal center of the lymphoid follicle. After IgA class switching and affinity maturation, B cells rapidly migrate from the NALT and Peyer's patches to the regional cervical lymph nodes and mesenteric lymph nodes, respectively, through the efferent lymphatics. Antigen-specific CD4+ T cells and IgA+ B cells migrate to effector sites (such as the nasal passage and intestinal lamina propria) through the thoracic duct and blood circulation. IgA+ B cells and plasmablasts then differentiate into IgA-producing plasma cells in the presence of cytokines such as interleukin-5 (IL-5) and IL-6 that are produced by T helper 2 (Th2) cells, and they subsequently produce dimeric (or polymeric) forms of IgA. These dimeric forms of IgA then become secretory IgA by binding to polymeric Ig receptors (which become the secretory component in the process of secretory IgA formation) that are displayed on the monolayer of epithelial cells lining the mucosa. Secretory IgA is then released into the nasal passage and intestinal tract.

it has been shown that many of these intestinal effector B and T cells specifically migrate to the mammary gland, releasing their products, i.e., cytokines and antimicrobial SIgA antibodies, into the colostrum and breast milk, to passively protect the newborn through a remarkable maternal-infant biologic relationship referred to as the *enteromammary circulation* (Box 8-1 and Figure 8-10).

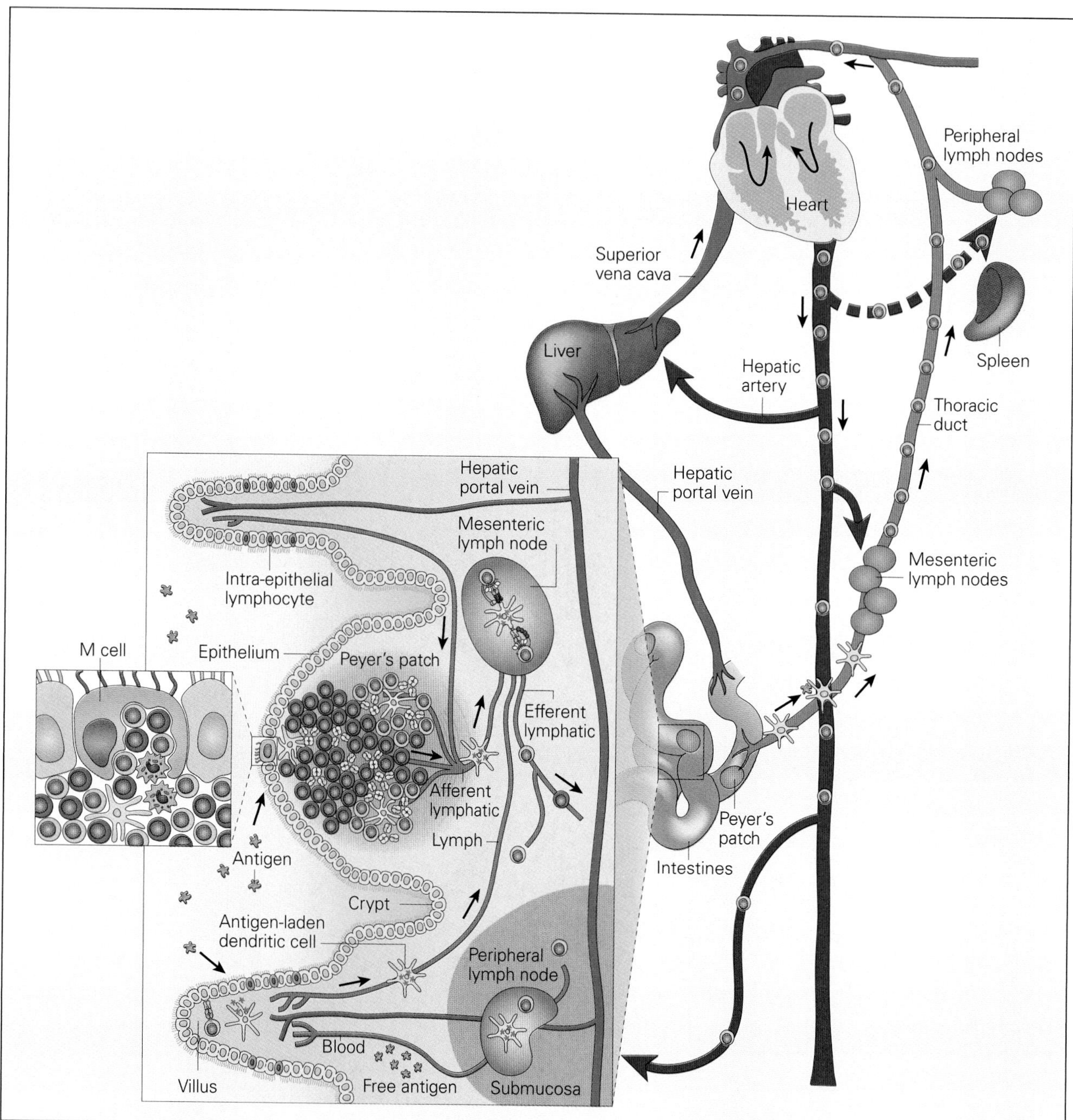

Figure 8-9. Schematic representation of the recirculating pool of lymphocytes sensitized in an inductive site in the Peyer's patch of the small intestine. In the case of GALT, antigen is captured by M cells and is transferred to DCs in the SED area of the Peyer's patch (PP) where they engage in cognate interaction with T cells and B cells. This is followed by the migration of these cells out of the PP through the efferent lymphatics to enter the local mesenteric lymph nodes (MLN). Activated cells undergo differentiation, and effector cells travel through lymphatics to enter the circulatory system through the thoracic duct. From the blood, the T and B cells seed the lamina propria of the small intestine and mucosae of other remote effector sites.

Lymphocyte Homing into Mucosal Compartments: The Role of Adhesion Molecules

The selective migration of lymphocytes into the mucosal tissues is carried out through specific homing molecules consisting of adhesion molecules and ligands, i.e., integrins and ICAMs (*Chapter 5*) expressed on the membrane of the migrating lymphocytes and specific ligands on the vascular endothelium in the mucosal tissue (Figure 8-11). Thus, effector sites receive activated effector and memory cells, which will populate the extensive areas of the

Box 8-1

The Enteromammary Circulation

Lactating mammary glands are another part of the mucosal immune system and in the human participate in a set of remarkable immunologic events that link the inductive sites of the GALT, BALT, and MALT of the mother with the effector sites of the gut and the upper airways of the breast-fed infant (Figure 8-10).

After initial sensitization to food antigens or microflora found in the GALT and BALT of the mother, primed B and T lymphocytes from Peyer's patches or peribronchial lymphoid tissues leave these sites via lymph and peripheral blood and home to the lactating mammary gland, where local production of secretory antibodies (sIgA and sIgM) specific for these antigens occurs. Breast milk, therefore, contains a boutique of specialized antibodies resulting from antigenic stimulation in the inductive sites of the MALT both in the gut and the airways of the mother. This has been documented by showing that sIgA from breast milk exhibits antibody specificity for a wide range of common intestinal as well as respiratory pathogens. The secretory antibodies are thus highly targeted against infectious agents in the mother's environment, which are those likely to be encountered by the infant during its first weeks of life. In addition to its role in infectious disease, the benefits of breast-feeding in prevention of allergic disease in the infant are well documented. Thus, breast-feeding represents a unique immunological integration of the mucosal immunologic systems of the mother and child that has biologic significance both in the protection afforded the breast-fed infant against infectious disease as well as in the prevention of allergic disease (*Chapter 18*).

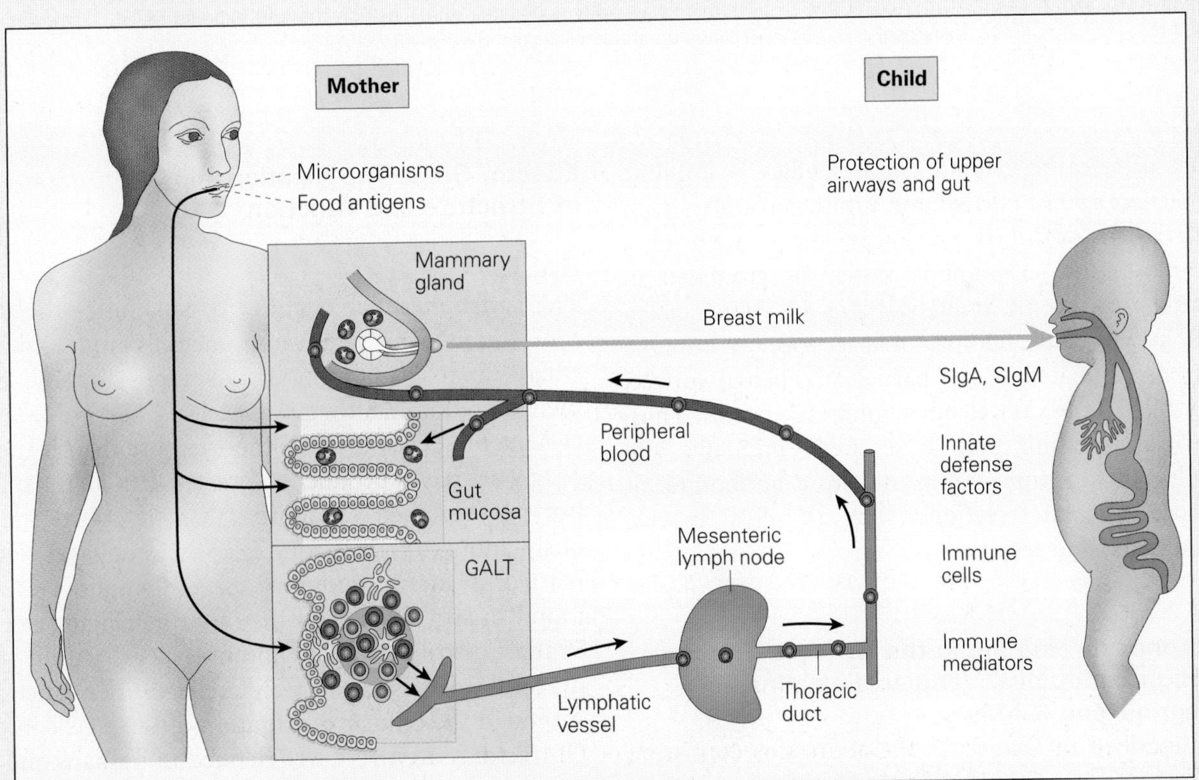

Figure 8-10. Integration of mucosal immunity between the mother and the newborn, showing the linkage of the mucosal immunologic systems of the mother and child. After initial sensitization to the food antigens and microflora found in the GI tract of the mother, primed B and T lymphocytes from Peyer's patches leave via lymph and peripheral blood to the lactating mammary gland, where local production of secretory antibodies (sIgA and sIgM) specific for enteric antigens (microorganisms and food proteins) occurs. By this mechanism, the breast-fed infant receives relevant secretory antibodies directed against the antigens found in the maternal GI tract reflecting her intestinal microenvironment, and hence the infant is better protected both in the gut and in the upper airways in the same way as the mother's gut mucosa is protected by similar antibodies. (Adapted with permission from Brandtzaeg P. Mucosal immunity: integration between mother and the breast-fed infant. *Vaccine.* 2003; 21:3382–8.)

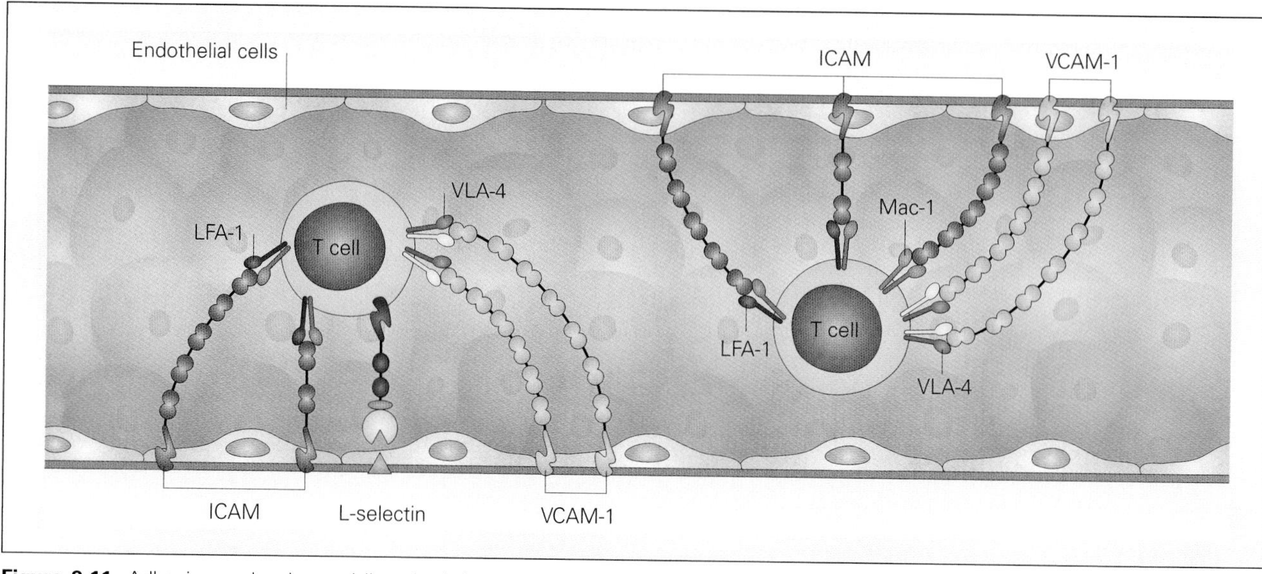

Figure 8-11. Adhesion molecules and ligands. It is possible to differentiate two migration patterns of mucosal and systemic activated cells. Mucosal activated lymphocytes (the T cell on the right) migrate to the regional lymph nodes after activation and then return to mucosal sites directed by adhesion molecules (LFA-1, αEβ7, and VLA-4) on their surface that recognize ligands on mucosal endothelial cells (ICAM-1 and 2, MAdCAM-1, and VCAM-1). Systemic activated lymphocytes (the T cell on the left) express LFA-1, L-selectin, and VLA-4 that recognize ICAM, mannose, and VCAM-1 ligands on endothelial cells. See Box 8.2.

mucosae, releasing cytokines or antibodies for immune protection against current and future encounters with antigen. As described previously, the concept of a common mucosal immune system is grounded in observations of the traffic patterns of Peyer's patch lymphocytes and findings that a specific immune response, initiated at one particular mucosal surface, may offer protection at other mucosal surfaces. Thus, mucosal immunization at a single inductive site results in the appearance of SIgA antibodies at remote mucosal secretions, such as saliva, mucus, milk, tears, and feces.

Lymphocyte Homing in the GI Tract: The Role of High Endothelial Venules, Selectins, Integrins, and ICAMs

As described in *Chapter 5*, the addressins consisting of selectins, integrins, and ICAMs play an important role in the migration of leukocytes from blood vessels into tissues during inflammation. They also play a role in the homing of lymphocytes from inductive sites to effector sites through structures called high endothelial venules (**HEV**), described in *Chapter 2*. Shown in Box 8-2 and Figure 8-11 are the lymphocyte receptors and addressin ligands involved in homing into mucosal effector sites of the GI tract.

Effector Sites: The Relationship of Structure and Function

GALT

The gastrointestinal tract is, perhaps, after the thymus, the site where most immune cells are found and where up to 70 percent of the total lymphoid elements, predominantly plasma cells (**PCs**), are located (*Chapter 6*). These PCs synthesize more than 3 grams of IgA per day, a production greater than all the other isotypes together. In addition, as described previously, numerous accessory cells (macrophages, DCs, mast cells, and eosinophils) and T lymphocytes are found in specific sites of the intestine (Figure 8-12). Spatial distribution of immune cells within the mucosal tissues is closely related to function. Although the cellular distribution of these cells in the GI tract has been very well defined in humans and in several animal models, there still exists a paucity of information concerning similar distributions in other regions of the mucosal immune system, such as the respiratory and genitourinary tracts.

In the adult human GI tract, a full array of immune cells is found. As shown in Figure 8-12, there are three main compartments in the small intestine where specific cell subpopulations preferentially lodge, which include the epithelium, lamina propria, and submucosa. Within the epithelium, a vast number of

Box 8-2

Lymphocyte Homing in the GI Tract

Naïve lymphocytes enter mucosal or systemic lymphoid tissues from the blood through specialized HEV that consist of cuboidal endothelial cells. In the GALT, HEV are present in the interfollicular zones, which are rich in T cells. In effector sites such as the lamina propria of the GI tract, the endothelial venules are less pronounced and tend to occur near villus crypt regions. Mucosal addressin cell adhesion molecule-1 (MAdCAM-1) is the most important addressin expressed by PP HEV or lamina propria venules (LPV) (*Chapter 5*). Peripheral lymph node addressin (PNAd) and vascular cell adhesion molecule (VCAM-1) are the principal addressins expressed by peripheral lymph node and skin HEV, respectively.

The major homing receptors expressed by lymphocytes are the integrins, a large class of molecules characterized by a heterodimeric structure of α and β chains (*Chapter 5*). In general, the type of homing receptor is determined by the integrin expressed with the α_4 chain; the β_1-integrin characterizes the homing receptor for the skin, whereas the β_7-integrin characterizes the receptor for the gut. The pairing of α_4 with β_7 is thus responsible for lymphocyte binding to the MAdCAM-1 that is expressed on HEVs in PPs and GI tract LPVs.

The C-type lectins L-, E-, and P-selectin (*Chapter 5*) also serve as homing receptors. L-selectin has a high affinity for carbohydrate-decorated PNAd, which is of central importance in peripheral lymph node homing of B and T cells. L-selectin can also bind to carbohydrate-decorated MAdCAM-1 and is an important initial receptor for homing into GALT HEVs.

Chemokines are also involved in lymphocyte homing, with different chemokine-receptor pairs controlling migration into different lymphoid tissues (*Chapter 9*). For example, the loss of secondary lymphoid tissue chemokine (SLC) results in a lack of naïve T-cell or dendritic-cell migration into the spleen or PPs. CCR4, which responds to the thymus activation-regulated chemokine (TARC) and macrophage-derived chemokine (MDC), mediates the arrest of skin-homing T cells but does not affect $\alpha_4\beta_7$hi T-cell migration in the GI tract. Conversely, memory $\alpha_4\beta_7$hi T cells that express the receptor for thymus-expressed chemokine (TECK), CC9, migrate into the lamina propria of the GI tract. Both human $\alpha_E\beta_7$+ and $\alpha_4\beta_7$hi CD8 T cells express CCR9, suggesting that TECK-CCR9 is also involved in lymphocyte homing and the arrest of IELs in the GI tract epithelium.

lymphoid cells can be found as IELs. These cells are heterogeneous in nature, but many CD2+CD4–CD8– cells (presumably NK cells) may be found there, as well as numerous TCR2 CD8+ T lymphocytes and a prominent TCR1 T lymphocyte population expressing the gamma/delta TCR. The importance of the epithelial location is evident, since in the small and large intestines, more than 50 percent of the total lymphoid cells localize there.

The LP of the intestine may be subdivided into villus LP and crypt LP. The villus LP is considered the absorptive area of the small intestine, whereas the crypt LP is the secretory area. In the villus LP, CD4+ and CD8+ T lymphocytes, NK cells, mast cells, eosinophils, and MHC-II+ DCs are abundant. DCs are localized just beneath the epithelial basement membrane (**BM**), and some of their dendrites may be found between the enterocytes, sampling antigens from the intestinal lumen. Close to these DCs, CD8+ T lymphocytes are localized in significant numbers by the BM, and many CD4+ T lymphocytes are found around the lacteal vessel of the villus. Also, NK, mast cells, and eosinophils are randomly distributed in the LP. In this way, the absorptive zone (villi) is populated with APCs and lymphocytes at the very entrance of foreign antigen, ready to induce an immune response or tolerance. Although significant numbers of NK cells and T lymphocytes are found in the crypt LP, the secretory zone of the intestine, the main populations at that site are intra-epithelial lymphocytes, macrophages, mast cells, and eosinophils. Effector sIgA-producing PCs at that site synthesize significant amounts of antibodies that are readily secreted into the gut lumen. Additionally, MHC-II-negative macrophages may function as scavenger cells, removing apoptotic PCs at the site.

Finally, the intestinal submucosa is populated with significant numbers of MHC-II+ DCs and mast cells, in close vicinity to neural terminals and blood vessels. Their function has not yet been elucidated, but it may relate to the modulation and amplification of the immune response through common neural mediators, like nitric oxide (**NO**) and serotonin, thus playing a role in the neuroimmune axis with the central nervous system.

Innate Immune Lymphoid Cells

IELs are interspersed between the columnar epithelial cells of the villi in the small and large intestines and constitute the first immune cell line of defense

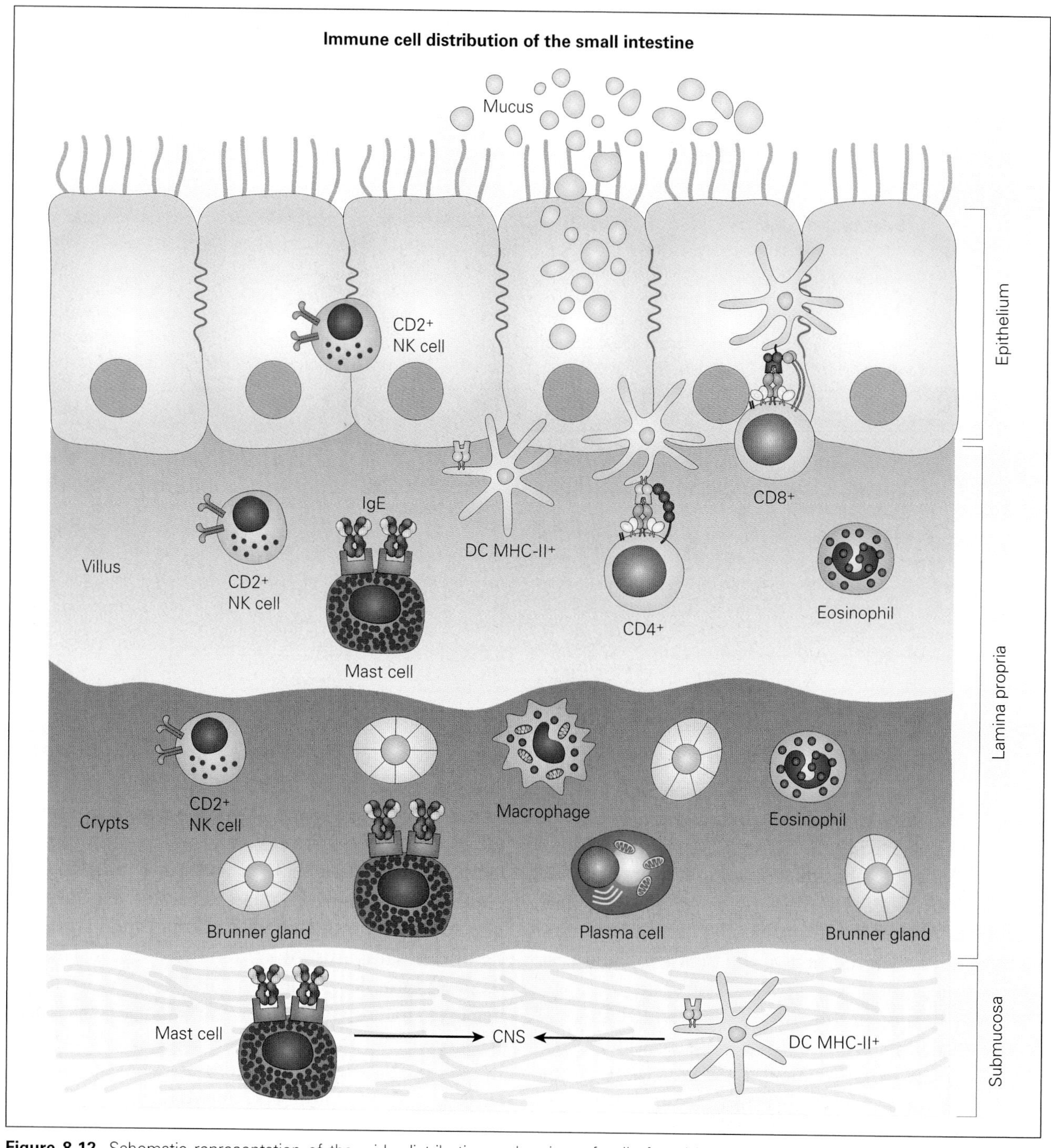

Figure 8-12. Schematic representation of the wide distribution and variety of cells found in the small intestine. In the adult human GI tract, a full array of immune cells is found. There are three main compartments in the small intestine where specific cell subpopulations preferentially lodge: (1) the epithelium; (2) the lamina propria; and (3) the submucosa. CD2+ = NK lymphocyte, CD4+ = T helper lymphocyte, CD8+ = cytotoxic T lymphocyte, CNS = central nervous system, DC = dendritic cell, and MHC-II = class II major histocompatibility complex antigens.

at those sites. IELs are a heterogeneous collection of lymphoid cells, and at least two types of T cells may be identified there on the basis of their T cell antigen receptor and phylogenetic appearance: TCR1 (TCRγδ) and TCR2 (TCRαβ) IEL cells (*Chapters 2* and *7*).

As described in Chapter 7, the T cell receptor has two forms based on different polypeptide chains. The most common T cell receptor (TCRαβ) is made up of alpha (α) and beta (β) chains and is found on about 95 percent of circulating T cells. A second type of TCR (TCRγδ) has gamma (γ) and delta (δ) chains and is found on about 5 percent of circulating T cells, but is the predominate cell type in the MALT found within the population of lymphocytes known as IELs. The γδ T cells are peculiar in that they do not seem to require antigen processing and MHC presentation of peptide epitopes for activation, although some recognize MHC-IB molecules. Furthermore, γδ T cells are believed to have a prominent role in the recognition of lipid antigens.

Because the γδ T cells do not need antigen processing and the presentation of peptides via the APC/MHC system required by the more abundant αβ T cells, they are ready to function immediately at mucosal surfaces with properties similar to the innate immune system believed to function as a first line of defense. Therefore, many consider these cells as a bridge between innate and adaptive immunity, similar to other unconventional T cell subsets bearing invariant TCRs, such as the natural killer T (**NKT**) cells (*Chapter 3*). Like these NKT cells, γδ T cells exhibit several characteristics that place them at the border between the more evolutionarily primitive innate immune system that permits a rapid beneficial response to a variety of foreign agents, and the adaptive immune system, where B and T cells coordinate a slower but highly antigen-specific immune response, leading to long-lasting memory against subsequent challenges by the same antigen.

B1 lymphocytes are a thymic-independent CD5+ subpopulation of B cells that provide an appreciable proportion of natural IgM with highly cross-reactive specificities (*Chapter 6*). In mice, it has been demonstrated that B1 cells can populate the gut lamina propria with IgA-producing plasma cells. This may account for an early, functionally important contribution to the development of thymic-independent natural IgA in the neonatal gut. However, the anatomic localization of B1 lymphocytes and their maturational development with age have not been studied in detail in the human.

Although several animal models have been used to study mucosal immune development, few human studies have been conducted. The distribution of lymphoid cells that populate the three major mucosal compartments do not vary importantly across species but may differ with maturational age. Although lymphoid cells are found most abundantly in the GALT, their spatial distribution in the human GI tract is attained later in life (Figure 8-12). In pigs, CD2+ lymphoid cells are found in low numbers in the epithelium and lamina propria at birth; no CD4+ or CD8+ T cells are present at that time. Later colonization of the mucosae with commensal bacteria stimulates the arrival of lymphoid cells to these tissues, and by the third week of life, significant numbers of CD4+ T cells can be identified in the lamina propria, whereas CD8+ T cells arrive later and are localized at the epithelial basement membrane interface. At weaning, these numbers increase significantly; however, adult numbers and spatial localization within these tissues are achieved only after three months of age.

The NALT and BALT

Little is known about lymphocyte populations in the human respiratory tract. The NALT and BALT are very well defined in rodents, but in humans, their presence is not necessarily constitutive, although antigenic exposure may induce their formation. As described previously, in the human pharynx, a set of lymphoid organs surrounds the nasal and oral passages, termed Waldeyer's ring, which includes the adenoids, tonsils, and other lymphoid structures. In rodents, the NALT is formed by lymphoid aggregates in the nasal cavity at the entrance to the pharyngeal duct. The many lymphocytes found in and below the epithelium lining the nasal passages into the pharynx are known as diffuse NALT. Similar to Peyer's patches, M cells covering lymphoid aggregates, such as tonsils, can be found, playing presumably the same function. Particulate antigens are taken up by M cells, whereas soluble antigens can pass directly through the nasal epithelium into the submucosal lymph nodes. In mice, NALT lymphocytes are mainly B cells outnumbering T cells by 2:1. CD4+ T cells are the predominant T cell subpopulation. The NALT is an important inductive site of immune responses after nasal immunization, and activated lymphocytes reach the cervical lymph nodes through afferent lymphatics. Also, the NALT is an inductive site for IgA class switching, and IgA blasts migrate from the NALT to effector sites, such as the nasal passages. Active T cell-mediated suppression and tolerance are also induced via the nasal mucosa down-regulating IgE and delayed-type hypersensitivity (**DTH**) responses, thereby lowering the impact of developing allergic disease and autoimmune disorders. In mice, this activity resides in the organized lymphoid tissue of the lymph nodes that drain the nose, suggesting that Treg cells may be one mechanism of tolerance induction.

BALTs ensure the sterility of the gas exchange apparatus while avoiding sensitization by inhaled antigens. BALT refers to the bronchial lymphoid aggregates and the less-organized lymphoid tissue in humans and other species. About 10 to 20 percent of the interstitial lymphocyte pool is composed of T cells. There is a priority to avoid inflammation within the bronchial lumen or mucosa. To achieve this, mechanisms of downregulation restrict cell activation and recruitment of nonspecific inflammatory cells to sites of tissue injury and regional lymph nodes that are primary sites for antigen handling and the induction of immune responses rather than the mucosal lymphoid tissues. TCR1 T cells promote tolerance to inhaled antigens, and also alveolar macrophages exert an antiproliferative effect on T cells, preventing antigen presentation at the mucosal surface. These observations are finding clinical application in the human in the form of new uses of mucosal delivery of antigen (allergen), such as sublingual immunotherapy (**SLIT**) as described below and in Chapter 18.

The Development of the BALT

There are relatively fewer BALT structures in the human in contrast to rodents, where the BALT develops in early postnatal life and contains a full set of T cell phenotypes by the fourth day after birth. In humans, lymphoreticular aggregates appear at one week of age. In rodents and chickens, the BALT can be identified in the bifurcations of major bronchial divisions where M cells are found in the epithelium of structures similar to PPs heavily infiltrated with lymphocytes and resident APCs. Plasma cells are found only around the BALT periphery. In rats and rabbits, the cell population associated with the HEV of the BALT is composed of 55 percent of T cells, 2 percent of surface IgG (**sIgG**), 28 percent of sIgM, and 27 percent of SIgA-expressing B cells. The BALT is also an early site for antigen uptake since epithelial cells can present soluble antigen to MHC-II+ DCs found beneath the respiratory epithelium.

T lymphoblasts circulate from mediastinal lymph nodes via the thoracic duct in the recirculating pool to mucosal surfaces, where they play a role in the downregulation of mucosal immune responses in the BALT after antigen inhalation. Respiratory tract immunization has little influence on the intestinal immune response. However, the regional lymph nodes that allow a connection between the generalized immune response and the lung provide a vehicle for systemic sensitization. Regional distribution of nerve fibers in the BALT suggests the existence of important neuroimmunological control mechanisms in the bronchial mucosa, similar to those found at the intestinal submucosa, with possible implications in clinical conditions such as asthma.

The Synthesis and Transport of IgA into External Secretions

As described previously, activated B cells in the inductive sites migrate to effector sites, where they differentiate into IgA plasma cells under the influence of Th2-type cytokines, mainly IL-4, IL-6, and TGF-β. Most of the PCs at the mucosal tissues simultaneously synthesize IgA and J chain (joining chain), allowing the assembly of dimeric SIgA (trimeric and tetrameric forms can also be found) that is able to attach to the polymeric immunoglobulin receptor (**pIgR**), expressed at the basolateral surface of epithelial cells (*Chapter 6*). Following receptor-mediated endocytosis, the pIgR-SIgA complex is transported in intracellular vesicles, within which neutralization of intracellular pathogens, such as viruses, and antigens can take place. At the apical surface of the epithelial cell, the pIgR is cleaved to give rise to the secretory component (**SC**) that now forms part of the SIgA molecule, providing additional resistance to proteolysis (Figure 8-13). SC expression in the salivary glands and the intestinal epithelium increases soon after birth, and levels similar to those in adults are expressed in intestinal crypts. SC is essential for the transport of polymeric immunoglobulins (**Igs**), being a prerequisite for the development of effective mucosal defense.

The Maturation of sIgA Production

Two subclasses of IgA are found in humans (*Chapter 6*). More than 95 percent of plasma IgA belongs to the IgA1 subclass, whereas almost equal proportions of IgA1 and IgA2 are found in external secretions. Because IgA in plasma is produced by plasma cells in peripheral lymphoid tissues, whereas sIgA is produced by plasma cells in the mucosal LP, the rates of maturation differ, probably due to the immediate challenge by the endogenous microbiota

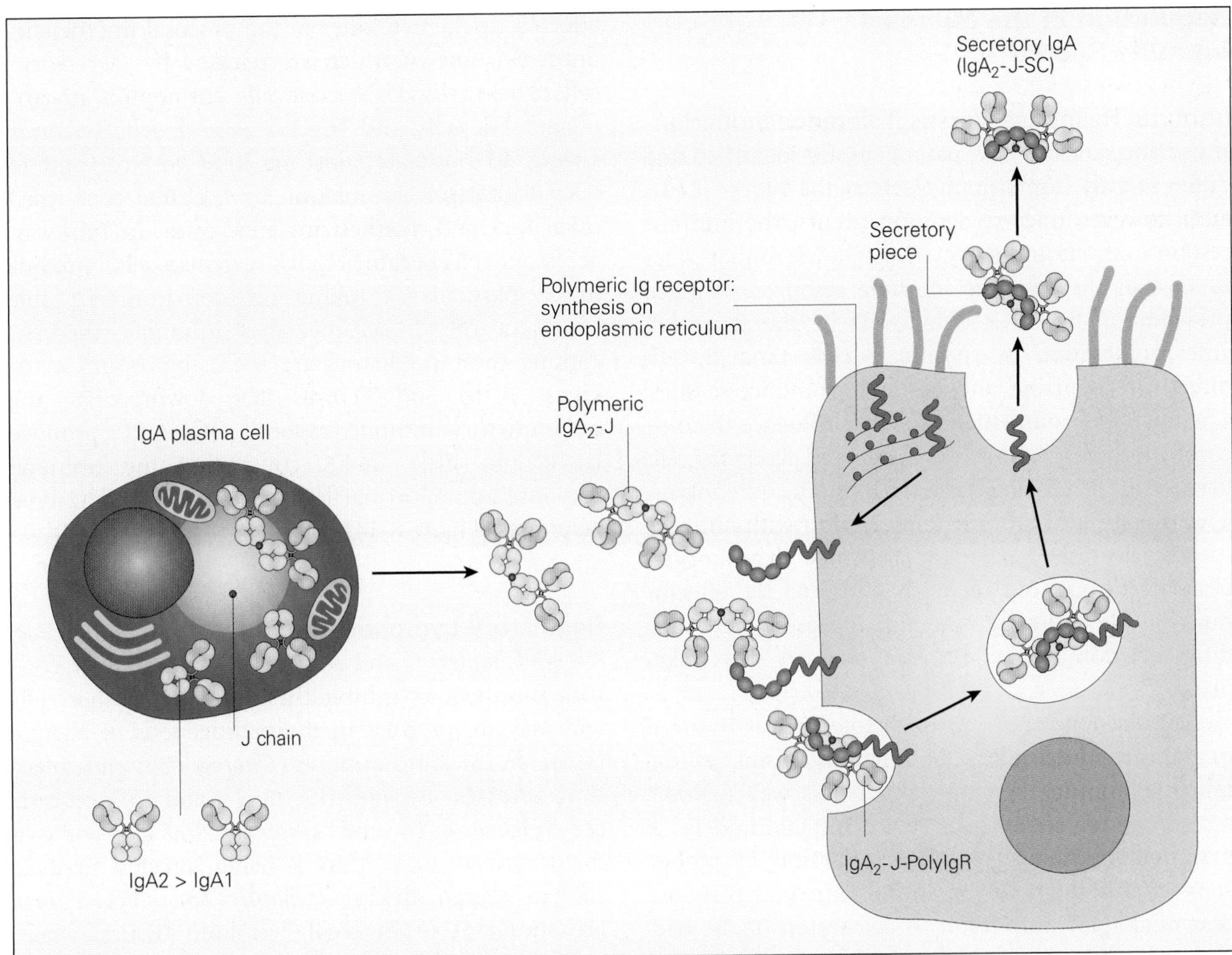

Figure 8-13. Secretory IgA is produced by plasma cells at the LP of mucosal tissues. J chain links two monomeric IgA and binds to the pIgR expressed at the basolateral surface of the epithelial cell. The complex pIgR-IgA is then endocytosed and transported to the apical surface of the cell. During this travel, IgA may bind to intracellular antigens. At the apical surface, the pIgR undergoes proteolytic cleavage and is released in the mucosal surface as the secretory component (SC) bound to SIgA. There are relatively greater amounts of IGA2 than IgA1 in external secretions than in serum.

colonizing mucosal surfaces immediately postpartum. SIgA is detected in mucosal secretions between one week and two months of age. Salivary levels of IgA peak by six weeks of age and remain consistent until exposure to increased antigen load, when they rise significantly. Adult levels of IgA are reached in external secretions as early as seven years of age, whereas adult levels in blood plasma are not reached until adolescence.

The Function of SIgA in Immune Exclusion

SIgA may capture antigens in the external secretions, at the epithelial surface, or attach to antigen located within the mucosal LP. In the latter case, bound antigen is then transported to the mucosal lumen by the epithelial pIgR system, eliminating (i.e., excluding) foreign antigen from the body. At the mucosal surfaces, immune exclusion is accomplished by SIgA neutralizing, aggregating, agglutinating, and allowing physical and chemical mechanisms to eliminate antigens before they are able to enter the body. The fact that IgA does not fix complement under physiological conditions and that external secretions inhibit complement activation (*Chapter 4*) allows IgA to dispose of antigen in a noninflammatory manner. In addition to binding antigen via its paratopes, SIgA interacts with lectins on the surface of microorganisms via its hinge region carbohydrates, resulting in aggregation and clearance. IgA may also participate in antibody-dependent cell cytotoxicity (**ADCC**) through binding to IgAα receptors. IgAα receptors are found on monocytes, PMNs, and eosinophils.

Regulation in the Mucosal Immune System

Immune Response Versus Tolerance Induction

It remains unclear how pathogens are identified and differentiated from commensals at the mucosal surface; however, once recognition occurs, the immune response at the inductive sites follows similar steps to that of the systemic immune response. Antigen presentation by APCs is followed by the activation and proliferation of specific T cells (and B cells directly recognizing antigen) at the inductive sites. The microenvironmental cytokines influence the outcome of the response, where APCs and accessory cells drive Th0 T cells toward a Th1 or Th2 phenotype. T cells engage in a cognate interaction with antigen-specific B cells, and then activated lymphocytes circulate throughout the body and seed the effector mucosal site and/or remote mucosal sites where final differentiation into effector or memory cells takes place.

The mechanism(s) by which tolerance is induced to harmless molecules and microorganisms by the mucosal immune system is much less well defined, but there are some clues from animal models. A principal mechanism is the elimination of pathogens without engendering an inflammatory response that might not only result in disruption of the barrier epithelium, but also provide cytokine signals and upregulation of costimulatory molecules to activate the immune system. Several levels of control of the immune response can be identified. The nature of the antigen is the first level of control. Microorganisms contain PAMPs, which engage PRRs on APCs of the innate immune system, bringing about upregulation of MHC-I and MHC-II and costimulatory molecules. Replicating microorganisms are much more likely to induce productive immune responses than nonreplicating, inactivated organisms—presumably related to their ability to react with immunoreactive APCs. Soluble antigens, in contrast, are handled differently by pathways that stimulate immune tolerance, e.g., Treg cells. This may explain, in part, the failure to induce immunity by oral and nasal immunization using soluble antigens. A second level of control is at the level of the APCs, since immature DCs or nonprofessional APCs (epithelial cells) lack costimulatory molecules needed for proper T cell activation. The final outcome may be anergy, unresponsiveness (*Chapters 7* and *19*), or apoptosis (*Chapter 9*) of T cells. Another level of control is affected by the cytokines in the mucosal microenvironment, some of which are released by "accessory" cells. These cells (DCs, mast cells, eosinophils, macrophages, NK cells, and TCR1 T gamma/delta cells) are known to populate most mucosal surfaces and to react to antigen stimulation by releasing preformed mediators and synthesizing new ones. In this way, accessory cells became "quick response cells," providing a particular cytokine microenvironment able to direct the T cell-mediated immune response. Among these mediators are the "suppressor" cytokines, IL-10 and TGF-β, that downregulate the inflammatory immune response. DCs in PPs produce IL-10 and little IL-12, controlling the immune response and allowing the development of Th2-type responses (Figure 8-14).

Regulatory Lymphocytes

Tregs (*Chapters 5* and *9*) are cells that actively control, suppress, or inhibit the function of other cells and play major roles in the pathogenesis of allergic (*Chapter 18*), autoimmune (*Chapter 19*), and infectious diseases (*Chapters 12, 13, 14,* and *15*) and cancer (Figure 8–14 and *Chapter 20*). Currently, a major investigative effort is being directed to their role in allergic disease (*Chapter 18*). CD4+ Tregs are abundant in mucosal lymphoid tissues, where they downregulate Th1 and Th2 responses. These cells are characterized by CD25 expression, CTLA-4 binding, and by the production of regulatory cytokines (IL-10 and TGF-β). Expression of CD25 on T cells is associated with natural regulatory function; CD25 is the α-chain of the IL-2 receptor and is also a marker of T cell activation. FOXP3 is the key regulatory gene in the development of CD25+ Tregs, which can be induced in the periphery, and their conversion into Tregs is dependent on TGF-β. Tr1 cells are a subtype of Tregs found in both humans and mice that are characterized by their low proliferative capacity, their production of high levels of IL-10, their production of low levels of IFN-γ, and their failure to produce IL-4. Another subset of Tregs, termed Th3, which produces high levels of TGF-β, plays an important role in the induction of oral tolerance. Tr1 cells seem to exert their suppressive activity due to their ability to produce high levels of IL-10 and TGF-β, whereas Th3 cells may act solely through the production of TGF-β, which has been claimed also to induce IgA class switching *in vitro*. The generation of active suppression or

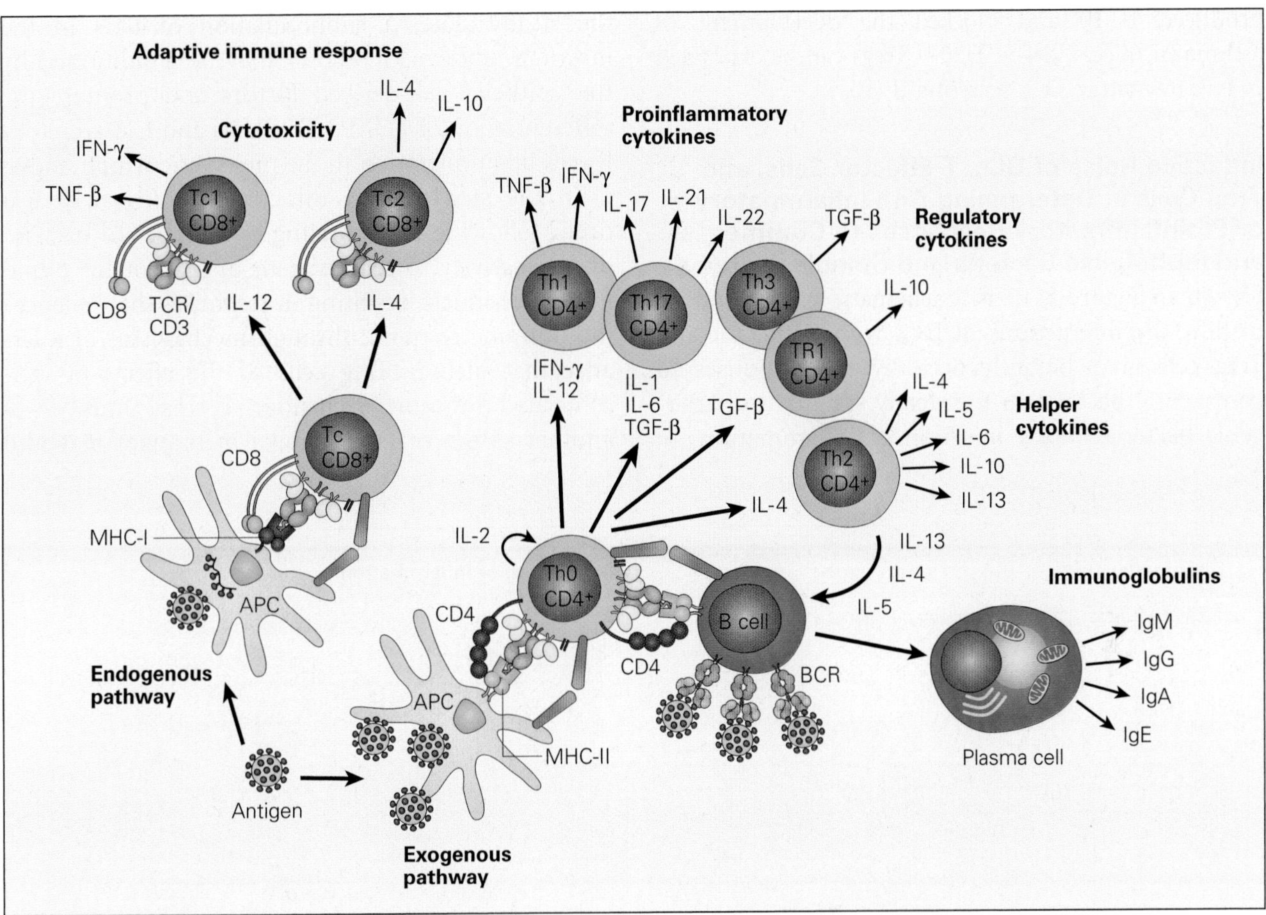

Figure 8-14. Immune regulation in mucosal surfaces is a complex interplay between innate and adaptive immune mechanisms. Antigen presentation by DCs and microenvironmental cytokines released by quick response cells like intraepithelial lymphocytes (IEL), mast cells (MCs), and macrophages, have a profound impact in the outcome of the immune response, either inducing cell-mediated immunity (CMI) with Th1 cells, antibody-mediated immunity through Th2 cells, or immune regulation and tolerance with T regulatory cells (Tregs). Activated macrophages are able to break tolerance by releasing IL-12 and IFN-γ.

clonal anergy and/or deletion is due to the induction of TGF-β-producing Th3 cells that downregulate host responses.

T-cell anergy is a state of unresponsiveness characterized by a lack of proliferation and IL-2 synthesis (*Chapter 19*). Oral tolerance may be achieved by anergized CD4+ T cells. It is thought that anergic T cells may retain some functional activity and are able to upregulate IL-10 and TGF-β production, downregulating DC expression of CD80/86 (*Chapter 9*). Therefore, anergic T cells could also function as regulatory cells by releasing TGF-β resembling Treg cells that suppress immune responses. In the scenario, where Th1 or Th2 cells become anergic, subsets of these cells may switch to become Treg cells producing IL-10 and/or TGF-β. Oral and nasal tolerance also have been shown to block mast cell function in animal models and may be a route for the control of allergies and inflammatory responses in the human.

Furthermore, antigen presentation by DCs regulates tolerance by the deletion of self-reactive T cells, the induction of nonresponsiveness by immature DCs expressing low levels of costimulatory molecules, and the expansion of Tregs. In humans, two major subpopulations of DCs have been described: $CD11c^{hi}$ (myeloid DCs) and $CD11c^{lo}$ (plasmacytoid or lymphoid DCs). In the mouse, three major functionally distinct types exist: plasmacytoid DCs (B220+, Gr1+, and IFN-α production), myeloid DCs (CD11b+CD8α−), and lymphoid DCs (CD8α+). Activated DCs influence the generation of polarized IL-12 (Th1) and IL-4 (Th2) lymphocytes. Tregs may be stimulated *in vivo* by specific subsets of IL-10-producing DCs. Two different pulmonary subsets of DCs exhibiting plasmacytoid morphology induce Tr1-type Tregs *in vitro* and *in vivo.* Th1-type Tregs are induced by pulmonary CD8α+ DCs, and Th2-type Tregs are induced by pulmonary CD8α− DCs secreting IL-10. These Tregs produced IL-10 and blocked the development of asthma in mice. CD4+CD25+ Tregs can be expanded *in vivo* by mature DCs secreting IL-10.

Inductive Roles of DCs, T Effector Cells, and Treg Cells in Determining Anti-Inflammatory or Proinflammatory Responses to Commensal and Pathogenic Bacteria and Soluble Proteins

Shown in Figure 8-15 is a schematic representation of how the interactions of DCs with T effector and Treg cells may be influenced by the responses to commensal bacteria in the steady state or to pathogenic bacteria during infection or inflammation. In the steady state, a subpopulation of DCs in the intestine (shown in yellow) may be conditioned by the epithelial-cell-derived factors and promote the differentiation of FOXP3 Treg cells and IgA-secretory B cells upon migration to the mesenteric lymph nodes.

In the steady state, this conditioning may also occur following the sampling of commensal bacteria or alternatively to self antigens or to proteins found in food products, resulting in responses that "silence" the immune response through mechanisms of tolerance that include Treg cells or the effects of IgA-associated immune exclusion. A small number of another subset of DCs (shown in orange) may also

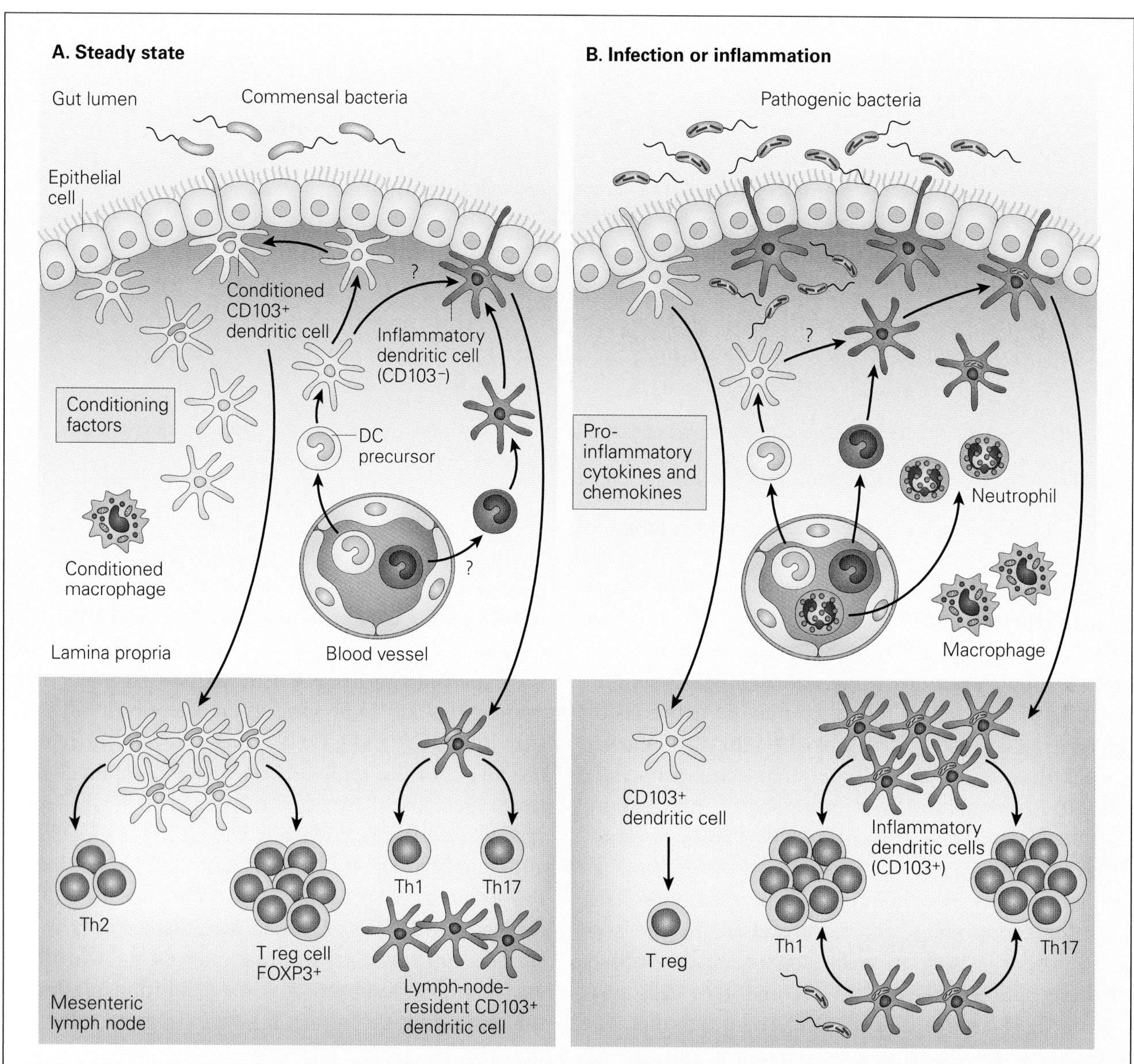

Figure 8-15. Panel A: Schematic representation of the interactions of DCs with T effector and Treg cell responses to commensal bacteria in the steady state. Panel B: The anti-inflammatory or proinflammatory responses in the steady state or during infection or inflammation.

be recruited to mesenteric lymph nodes in the steady state that may have escaped conditioning and drive T helper populations toward Th1 or Th17 profiles. Since these cells exist in small numbers, they will not give rise to disease in the steady state, but could act as sentinels when pathogenic bacteria are encountered or produced in excess, as in the case where aberrant responses to soluble proteins give rise to disease symptoms, as in the case of food allergy (*Chapter 18*).

In contrast to the responses seen with commensal bacteria, some pathogenic bacteria possess sufficient virulence factors that allow them to invade the intestinal epithelium and to subvert the immune response and enhance their replication (Figure 8-15B). This would then result in the activation of the cytosolic- or cell membrane–associated activation of PRRs and the enhanced production of proinflammatory cytokines, e.g., TNF-α, and chemokines that would then promote the recruitment and influx of neutrophils, monocytes/macrophages, and DC precursors derived from the vascular compartment (Figure 8-15B). These newly arrived DCs have not undergone sampling of the luminal contents with conditioning; this sampling results in the production of Treg cells and IgA-associated immune exclusion, which then induce a cascading set of cellular responses brought about by proinflammatory Th1 and Th17 responses.

Clinical Relevance of the Mucosal Immune System

Mucosal Immunization

The majority of disease-causing human pathogens, primarily viruses and bacteria, invade the body via the mucosal membranes, predominately the respiratory and gastrointestinal tracts. Although antibiotic treatment and conventional immunization programs have greatly reduced the burden of infectious diseases caused by these pathogens, there still remains the need for a better means of protective immunity. Currently, the vast majority of available vaccines is administered by the parenteral route and induces excellent systemic immunity that only blocks disease development once the pathogen has crossed the mucosal or skin barriers into the normally sterile systemic environment (*Chapter 23*). However, the mucosal surfaces remain susceptible to infection. The goal of mucosal immunization is to prevent the initial stages of infection (the adherence and colonization of pathogens) by providing protection at the portal of entry of the infecting pathogen, thereby blocking disease development.

Mucosal immunization offers several advantages over traditional vaccines administered via the parenteral route (Table 8-2). It is a cost-effective, safe, and noninvasive method of immunization suitable for mass immunization, and because of its needle-free application, the risk of needle stick injury or cross-contamination with blood-borne transmission of viral agents (e.g., hepatitis B or C or HIV) is reduced. The oral or nasal route of vaccine administration, the two applications in common use, is more acceptable to recipients than injections, and mucosal vaccines are simpler to administer and distribute. Mucosal immunization stimulates both local (sIgA and CMI) and systemic immunity (IgG and CMI). One of the interesting observations made by Dr. Albert B. Sabin in studies of infants with a measles vaccine delivered by aerosol was that infants as young as four to six months could be effectively immunized without the inhibitory effect of maternal measles-neutralizing serum antibody seen in infants immunized by the parenteral route. Mucosal immunization can be accomplished using either recombinant-attenuated viruses or bacteria or inactivated microbes expressing relevant antigens from the pathogen that prime and induce memory in the immune system. Several attenuated viral vaccines have been licensed for routine immunization via the mucosal route, e.g., live oral poliovirus (**OPV**) vaccine, oral rotavirus vaccine, and love attenuated influenza vaccine (administered via the nasal route) (*Chapter 23*). Another possibility is the creation of mucosal vaccines in the form of edible transgenic plants expressing relevant antigens of the pathogen, such as hepatitis B and rotavirus. However, to date, the level of protein expressed in plants is variable

Table 8-2. Advantages of mucosal immunization over immunization via the parenteral route

Advantages of mucosal immunization
A cost-effective, safe, and noninvasive method
A "needle-less" method, with an ease and efficiency of vaccination to a large population by nonmedical staff
Elimination of blood-borne transmission of viral agents (e.g., hepatitis and HIV)
Mucosal immunization stimulates both "local" (SIgA and CMI) and "systemic" immunity (IgG and CMI)
Allows immunization of younger infants, e.g., four to six months; no inhibitory effect of maternal antibody

and often too low for effective immunization and may even induce tolerance. For those reasons, most of the mucosal immunization protocols use high amounts of antigen, microbial-derived adjuvants (mainly the cell-binding component of toxins), and numerous immunizations in order to induce an effective mucosal immune response. None of these approaches to date have had practical application to human and animal medicine. Therefore, new strategies for mucosal immunization are needed and will require a deeper understanding of the regulatory mechanisms of the mucosal immune response to shed light on a more effective way of manipulating it for clinical use. The following section describes some results of animal studies that have explored alternative routes of immunization, adjuvants, and delivery systems with the potential for mucosal immunization in the human.

Routes of Immunization

Several routes of immunization have been explored in both the experimental animal and the human, utilizing various common portals of entry. Shown in Table 8-3 are some of the routes of mucosal immunization that have been explored together with the relative immunogenic effectiveness of each. Single and even repeated immunization at the same mucosal site is not effective at inducing vigorous immune responses even if high doses of antigen are utilized. A combination of systemic priming and mucosal boosting appear to be more effective at inducing mucosal immunity than with single immunization. Systemic immunization may be of considerable importance in the induction of protective responses in genital secretions. Rectal immunization of humans induced specific antibodies at the site of immunization, in saliva, and in other remote secretions. Rectal lymphoid tissues may be an important source of IgA precursor cells destined for the genital tract. Mucosal and systemic immunity can also be achieved by transdermal scarification, such as used in smallpox vaccination, and by topical application of an antigen to intact skin, and as described below, with the use of an appropriate adjuvant. The mechanisms underlying the induction of mucosal immunity by transcutaneous vaccines remain elusive. Nasal immunization with mucosal adjuvants induces superior immune responses in external secretions such as saliva and, surprisingly, in female genital secretions of rodents, rhesus monkeys, chimpanzees, and humans.

Although mucosal immunization relies heavily on the concept of a common mucosal immune system that allows the stimulation of immune responses at effector sites of the mucosal surfaces distant from the initial inductive site of mucosal immunization, new evidence suggests a certain degree of compartmentalization of the local immune response (Table 8-3). Cell trafficking among the various compartments is facilitated by a complex network of interactions mediated by mucosal addressins, integrins, and chemokines, allowing the tissue-specific migration (homing) of immune cells from the inductive to the effector sites. Consequently, certain routes are more favorable for inducing immunity at the desired effector site. This knowledge should be taken into consideration in the design of every novel type of vaccine that is contemplated to be used for mucosal immunization.

Mucosal Adjuvants

Mucosal vaccines containing adjuvants may be used both to prevent mucosal infections through the activation of antimicrobial immunity and to treat systemic inflammatory diseases through the induction of antigen-specific mucosal tolerance (*Chapter 11*). Several mucosal adjuvants have been developed for

Table 8-3. Compartmentalization of the mucosal immune system in mice and humans

Route	Effective response	Noneffective response
Oral	Small intestine (proximal), ascending colon, and mammary and salivary glands	Distal large intestine, genital mucosa, and tonsils
Rectal	Rectum	Small intestine and proximal colon
Nasal or tonsilar	Upper airway, regional secretions, and genital mucosa	Gut
Vaginal	Genital mucosa	
Skin	Gut (?)	

(Adapted from Gerdts V, Mutwiri GK, Tikoo SK, et al. Mucosal delivery of vaccines in domestic animals. Vet Res. 2006;37:487–510.)

human use, including among others cholera toxin, cholera toxin B subunit, *E. coli* heat-labile enterotoxin, synthetic cytidine-phosphate-guanosine (**CpG**) and CPG oligodeoxynucleotides (**CpG ODN**), and cytokines and chemokines, with the aim of improving the induction of mucosal Th1 and Th2 responses. Mucosal delivery systems, in particular virus-like particles, have also been shown to enhance the binding, uptake, and half-life of the antigens, as well as to target the vaccine to mucosal surfaces. DNA vaccines are currently being developed for administration at mucosal surfaces. However, there have also been failures, such as the withdrawal of an oral rotavirus vaccine and a nasal influenza vaccine, because of their potential side effects (Box 8-3). These experiences illustrate that in developing new strategies for mucosal immunization to improve immunogenicity, safety must always be a prime concern.

Mucosal adjuvants can act through TLRs on epithelial cells, improving antigen delivery to mucosal inductive sites by increasing the permeability of the epithelial layer or by targeting M cells. Adjuvants including enterotoxins and cytokines upregulate costimulatory and MHC-II molecule expression in APCs and stimulate their maturation, favoring their interaction with B and T cells. Also, they can stimulate maturation and differentiation of effector B cells and trigger B cell switching for production of IgA antibodies. Mucosal adjuvants play a major role in the differentiation of CD4+ T cells and subsequent Th1- or Th2-type responses for protection against intracellular pathogens or toxins.

The use of cytokines and chemokines as adjuvants is an attractive strategy as they act through specific receptors and influence the development of Th1- or Th2-type immune responses (*Chapter 9*). Mucosal delivery of cytokines avoids the toxicity often found in parenteral administration. IL-1 enhances mucosal Th2-type immune responses, and IL-12 induces antibodies to nasally co-administered antigens in both systemic and mucosal compartments. Lymphotactin (Lptn) is a C chemokine produced predominantly by NK and CD8+ T cells, including TCR1 T IELs. Nasal co-administration of antigen and Lptn enhanced antibody responses both in plasma and in mucosal secretions. RANTES (defined in Chapter 9) also displays mucosal adjuvant activity for nasally co-administered protein antigens and supports Th1-associated plasma IgG subclass responses. Nasally delivered MIP-1α promotes strong plasma IgG antibodies as well as mucosal and systemic CMI responses to co-administered antigen. In contrast, MIP-1β supports higher levels of mucosal SIgA. Also, chemokines are directly involved in mucosal homing of effector B and T cells. A major role for IL-5 and IL-6 is the induction of sIgA+ B cells to differentiate into IgA-producing PCs in both mice and humans. Therefore, their use could boost mucosal immunity.

Bacterial DNA contains immunostimulatory sequences recognized by nonspecific immune mechanisms. These sequences consist of short palindromic nucleotides around a CpG dinucleotide core. CpG motifs induce B cell proliferation and Ig synthesis as well as secretion of Th1-type cytokines by a variety of immune cells. CpG motifs enhance systemic and mucosal immune responses when given to mice by the nasal or oral route. Two of the innate molecules induced by CpG (IL-12 and RANTES) link the mucosal innate and adaptive immune systems. QS-21 is a highly purified complex triterpene glycoside that promotes both humoral and CMI responses when added to systemic and nasal vaccines. Low oral doses of QS-21 promote mucosal sIgA responses, while stronger Th1-type responses are seen after immunization with high oral doses. The enhancement of the

Box 8-3

Nasal Vaccination, *Escherichia coli* Enterotoxin, and Bell's Palsy

An inactivated influenza vaccine that had been originally developed by the Swiss for parenteral administration consisting of the hemagglutinin and neuraminidase surface antigens of influenza virus incorporated into liposomes was subsequently used in the formulation of an influenza virus vaccine for intranasal administration. To optimize both mucosal and systemic immune responses to the nasal vaccine, heat-labile *Escherichia coli* enterotoxin, a powerful mucosal adjuvant, was included in the formulation. The initial clinical studies showed that significant nasopharyngeal and serum antibody responses to influenza virus were elicited by this vaccine and that the vaccine was protective against influenza in both adults and children. Approval of the vaccine for distribution and use in Switzerland followed. However, after its clinical use, Bell's palsy was identified in some recipients of this intranasal vaccine attributable to the immunization, and the product was withdrawn from the market.

immune response may be due to the improvement of antigen uptake.

Mucosal immunization may be used both to prevent mucosal infections through the activation of antimicrobial immunity and to treat selected autoimmune, allergic, or infectious-immunopathological disorders through the induction of antigen-specific tolerance. The development of mucosal vaccines, whether for prevention of infectious diseases or for immunotherapy, requires antigen delivery and adjuvant systems that can efficiently help to present vaccine or immunotherapy antigens to the mucosal immune system. Promising advances have recently been made in the design of more efficient mucosal adjuvants based on detoxified bacterial toxin derivatives or CpG motif-containing DNA, and even more striking progress has been made in the use of virus-like particles as mucosal delivery systems for vaccines and of cholera toxin B subunit as an antigen vector for immunotherapeutic tolerance induction. However, two recently developed mucosal vaccines for human use against rotavirus diarrhea and influenza were withdrawn after a short period on the market because of adverse reactions among the vaccinees, thus emphasizing the difficult and challenging task also for mucosal immunization of combining vaccine and adjuvant efficacy with safety and acceptability.

Delivery Systems

In order to avoid antigen degradation and the use of high doses of antigen, delivery systems targeting mucosal inductive sites have been devised for mucosal immunization. Among them, viral envelope proteins of reoviruses have been used because of their specificity to bind to M cells in Peyer's patches. However, for human mucosal immunization, it is necessary to determine the specific serotype with affinity for human M cells. Also, antigens incorporated in nontoxic and nonimmunogenic vehicles, like carboxymethyl cellulose, are used for oral, nasal, and vaginal immunization, promoting local and systemic immune responses. Immunostimulating complexes (**ISCOMs**) made of a mixture of cholesterol and Quil A are effective oral delivery systems that promote mucosal and systemic immunity. Finally, bacterial and viral vectors have been used with variable results in experimental models. One disadvantage of this approach is that the elicited immune response also recognizes the vector hampering repeated use of it. Recently approved live influenza vaccine for nasal administration in humans represents a significant advance in mucosal vaccines.

Mucosal AIDS Vaccine

HIV infection has become one of the largest pandemics in history (*Chapter 13*). Since 70 to 80 percent of people contract the disease through mucosal contact, and the intestine is recognized as a virus reservoir, mucosal immunization seems to be a practical approach to control the disease. High levels of HIV-neutralizing IgA and HIV-reactive T cells in the genitourinary tract confer resistance to infection in about 30 percent of patients. Experimental vaccination in rhesus macaques, designed to mimic the mucosal immunity seen in these patients, showed promising results, but failed to prevent infection, stressing the importance of dissecting in more detail the mechanisms underlying mucosal immunity before attempting immunization.

Immunocontraceptives

Control of fertility through the immune response is an old idea based on the evidence that up to 30 percent of human infertility is associated with antisperm antibodies and T cells. Since this immune-mediated infertility apparently causes no other health problems, mucosal immunity against sperm antigens may be an approach to control conception. Male immunization would render sperm nonviable, while female immunization would result in sperm motility reduction or impaired sperm penetration into the oocyte. Another approach is to target reproductive hormones to interfere with their function and reduce fertility. In order to use these alternatives, effective mucosal immunization protocols must be designed, although lack of knowledge of the mucosal immune system of the genitourinary tract still impairs progress in this area.

Immunopathologic Conditions Associated with the Mucosal Immune System

The etiology of most systemic and mucosal immunopathologic disorders is unknown. Many are multifactorial, have a genetic basis, and are possibly triggered by microbial agents and environmental pollutants emanating from the ever-increasing technologic complexity of the industrialized world. Although there has been considerable progress in understanding the physiology of the mucosal immune system, it is not known with certainty how the local immune system targets a harmful molecule or recognizes a harmless particle. These inadequacies make an accurate diagnosis difficult, and most treatments are focused on alleviating symptoms rather than on attacking the cause of the problem. Deeper knowledge about the etiology of the issue, the mucosal physiology, and the nature of the antigen challenge is needed to enable a more rational manipulation of the mucosal immune response to alleviate and prevent these problems. The following sections emphasize the possible mucosal immune involvement in immunopathologic conditions affecting the mucosal immune system, rather than on symptoms and treatment, which are dealt with below.

Inflammatory Bowel Diseases

The two major inflammatory bowel diseases (**IBD**) in the human, regional ileitis (Crohn's disease) and ulcerative colitis, are characterized by abdominal pain, diarrhea, bloody stools, weight loss, and intestinal inflammation, and represent chronic, relapsing, inflammatory, and tissue-destructive diseases of the gastrointestinal tract. Although the etiologies remain unknown, there is evidence for a failure of the mucosal immune system to appropriately sense luminal antigens, leading to a breakdown in tolerance to the endogenous microbiota. IBD may result from an initial insult followed by an inappropriate and sustained immunologic response to normal microbiota. Altered regulatory T cell-mediated mechanisms and an imbalance of regulatory cytokines have been demonstrated in experimental models, especially excessive production of Th1-cell IFN-γ in response to auto-antigens and intestinal microbiota. In murine IBD, an exacerbated Th2-biased response is elicited after luminal antigen presentation by DCs to naïve T cells. IL-4 and IL-13 generated by these activated Th2 cells promote IgE production by B cells that sensitizes mast cells in the mucosa. A subsequent challenge with antigen triggering an IgE-mediated inflammatory response and further release of Th2 cytokines by T cells may offer yet another pathogenetic event contributing to the chronic intestinal inflammation seen in many immunologically altered conditions.

In contrast to these proinflammatory models, production of the immunoregulatory cytokines IL-10 and TGF-β by Treg cells may also be involved in colitis prevention. Mucosal tolerance is one of the major immunoregulatory mechanisms for the maintenance of host homeostasis (*Chapter 11*). In addition to the involvement of Th1 and Th2-type CD4+ T cells in the induction and regulation of oral and mucosal tolerance, IL-10 and/or TGF-β from Th3 or Treg CD4+ T cells are essential cytokines that not only induce oral tolerance and downregulate mucosal inflammation, autoimmune, and hyperimmune responses, but also maintain homeostasis. In this way, the involvement of at least two separate sets of CD4+ T cells have been defined, i.e., the Th1 and Th2 cell set that upregulates and the Th3 and Treg cell set that downregulates immune responses. In addition, recent reports have described an altered balance between Th17 and Th1 cells at mucosal sites and an important role of IL-23 and Th17 cytokines in intestinal homeostasis (*Chapter 9*). The possible CD4+ T cell modulation of the GALT of HIV-infected patients that has been associated with enhanced Th17 cell and polyfunctional HIV-specific T cell responses represents new research challenges for the future, which should reap a harvest of improved management of those who suffer from IBD and other immunologically mediated disorders affecting the mucosal immune system.

Over the last few years, significant progress has been made in our understanding of the role of defective innate immune mechanisms in the pathogenesis of IBD and other autoinflammatory diseases (*Chapter 19*). Variations in nucleotide oligomerization domain (**NOD**)2/caspase recruitment domain (**CARD**)15 have been identified as risk factors contributing to the genetic susceptibility to Crohn's disease. These data suggest that NOD2/CARD15 and NF-κB activation may play critical roles in the induction of intestinal mucosal inflammation and may represent the initial response of the GALT innate immune system necessary for the maintenance of gut homeostasis. Crohn's disease is now being considered as an impaired and inadequate innate immune reaction and no longer solely as a hyper-responsiveness of the adaptive mucosal immune system. Studies of defective NOD2/CARD15 expression suggest that macrophages and epithelial cells could be the locus of the primary pathophysiological event and that T cell activation might be a secondary effect inducing the chronicity of the inflammation, perhaps as a compensatory mechanism to inadequate innate immunity. In addition to NOD2/CARD15, there are other innate pathways, e.g., TLRs, defensins that can be blocked by commensal and pathogenic bacteria, allowing them to become more invasive and pathogenic. More research in this area will undoubtedly shed more important insights on the pathogenesis of IBD that should translate into improved diagnostic and therapeutic procedures for patients with IBD.

Asthma

Allergic diseases such as asthma are caused by exaggerated Th2-biased immune responses in genetically susceptible individuals (*Chapter 18*). Allergic hyperreactivity is defined as an exaggerated immune response, typically IgE, toward harmless antigenic stimuli. Immune regulation can be achieved by Th1 responses that counterregulate Th2 reactivity, or through regulatory T cells, which can suppress both Th1 and Th2 cells through the secretion of IL-10 and TGF-β. CD4+CD25+ Tregs suppress antigen-induced airway eosinophilia via their influence on the development of the Th2 phenotype. In children, tolerance to cow's milk proteins correlates with the presence of circulating CD4+CD25+ Tregs capable of suppressing potential effector cells. IL-10-secreting Tr1 cells also have been shown to prevent the induction of allergic diseases. Th1-like Tregs producing both IFN-γ and IL-10 express FOXP3 in conjunction with T-bet, a marker of the Th1 cell subset of Tregs. The factors driving the acquisition of regulatory activity in the periphery are not yet understood, but CD4+CD25+ Tregs may educate CD4+CD25− T cells to become suppressor cells via cell-cell contact. Th1-like, Th2-like, and Tr1 Tregs all suppress the proliferation and differentiation of both Th1- and Th2-type effector cells through the production of suppressive cytokines.

Another possibility for the emergence of allergic diseases and asthma is a deficiency in the suppressive activity of CD4+CD25+ T cells rather than insufficient numbers of Tregs in atopic individuals. In this sense, impaired expansion of natural and/or adaptive Tregs may lead to the development of allergy and asthma, and treatment to induce allergen-specific Tregs could provide curative therapies for these problems. Immunotherapies that enhance the development of allergen-specific Tregs may provide safe, specific, and long-lasting control of allergic diseases and asthma. Further understanding of the mechanisms involved in inducing these cells is necessary to utilize them more efficiently in therapeutic strategies.

Food Allergy

The term food allergy, synonymous with food hypersensitivity and food intolerance, is a general term describing abnormal responses to ingested food (*Chapter 18*). Food-induced allergic disorders are reported in up to 8 percent of children less than three years of age and in approximately 2 percent of the adult population. These food hypersensitivities are IgE-mediated, and the exaggerated immune response (also non-IgE-mediated) is directed toward harmless antigenic stimuli. This IgE overproduction in the mucosa sensitizes mast cells (abundant in these tissues) with a high proportion of specific antibody in the alimentary tract. Upon ingestion, the food antigens cross-link mast cell-bound and basophil-bound IgE located in mucosal tissues, inducing the release of chemical mediators of inflammation.

Infant susceptibility to food-allergic reactions may be the result of immaturity of the gastrointestinal barrier and of the immune system. Some studies suggest that breast-feeding promotes oral tolerance, preventing food allergy and atopic dermatitis in young children.

Tolerance Induction and Transplantation as Treatment for Disease

The induction of tolerance for the treatment of hypersensitivities and autoimmunity through mucosal administration of allergens or autoantigens is a therapeutic possibility intensely studied by clinicians. Autoimmunity toward self components of the body may occur through several mechanisms described elsewhere in this book (*Chapter 19*), but the reasons for their occurrence remain elusive. Symptoms of autoimmune diseases such as multiple sclerosis, rheumatoid arthritis, lupus, and type I diabetes may be diminished or reversed by induction of mucosal tolerance. Oral or nasal administration of the initiating self antigens could induce mucosal tolerance, lowering the harmful systemic immune response. MS patients suffer a slow degradation of neural myelin by the immune response, resulting in the loss of nerve function. Similar symptoms develop in mice suffering from experimental autoimmune encephalomyelitis (**EAE**). It has been demonstrated that the administration of high doses of myelin basic protein to animals undergoing EAE by oral or nasal routes suppressed myelin deterioration in these mice. Similarly, oral administration of protein antigens in human clinical trials has inhibited some forms of autoimmune diseases, such as multiple sclerosis, rheumatoid arthritis, uveitis, and diabetes. The induction of tolerance through mucosal immunization may theoretically provide a novel means to facilitate organ transplantation by tolerizing the immune system of a potential organ recipient, e.g., to a relevant donor MHC antigen.

Sublingual Immunotherapy

Over the past ten years, several immunotherapies for allergen desensitization have been developed, especially for inhaled antigens (*Chapter 18*). There is now emerging evidence that the administration of small but gradually increasing amounts of allergen to patients with allergic disease by the sublingual route, at regular intervals, can increase tolerance to the allergen. It is claimed that the advantages of this immunotherapy include avoiding injections, fewer doctor visits, and lower side effects. However, the therapy requires four to five months to yield results. Apparently, SLIT is safe and effective, but perhaps less effective than injection immunotherapy, since it needs up to 300× higher allergen doses, and its long-term efficacy is unclear.

Several recent studies have suggested that sublingual immunization with allergens can achieve a reduction in allergic disease manifestations, utilization of anti-allergic medications, and possibly a safer, more cost-effective method of immunotherapy than the more traditional, subcutaneous route of immunization (*Chapter 18*). Although the protective mechanism of immunotherapy for allergic disease was thought traditionally to be related to the production of IgG antibodies that could exert a blocking effect by the binding of specific antibodies of a class other than IgE to the allergen, thereby reducing IgE activity, recognition of the role of Treg cells in modulating the allergic response and their stimulation by immunotherapy suggest that this mechanism may be more central to the development of tolerance by both the subcutaneous as well as the sublingual routes of immunotherapy for allergic disease. However, because of wide differences in the types of allergens, and their doses and frequency of administration in published studies of SLIT, it is difficult to compare the results of different trials. Strict standardization of the procedure by additional studies will be required for a critical evaluation of the results and a general acceptance of this procedure.

IgA Deficiency

A selective deficiency in IgA is the most common primary immunodeficiency in humans and occurs at a frequency between 1:300 and 1:500 persons (*Chapter 16*). Despite the fact that more IgA is synthesized daily than all of the other immunoglobulin isotypes combined, the vast majority of individuals with a selective deficiency of IgA are asymptomatic, apparently because increased IgM production serves as a compensatory mechanism for IgA deficiency. However, there are individuals with selective IgA deficiency who have significant allergic diseases and autoimmune disorders. Why this disparity exists remains unclear but may be related to the fact that a subset of those with a selective deficiency of IgA is also deficient in IgG2 and in a variety of T cell functions. Common infections observed in symptomatic patients with selective IgA deficiency are recurrent ear infections, sinusitis, bronchitis, and pneumonia. People with selective IgA deficiency may be more susceptible to allergic diseases such as asthma and food allergies. The spectrum of autoimmune disorders seen in individuals with selective IgA deficiency include rheumatoid arthritis, systemic lupus erythematosus, and immune thrombocytopenic purpura. As the case study described in this chapter demonstrates, patients with IgA deficiency are more susceptible to the development of anti-IgA-related anaphylactoid reactions to blood transfusions, immunoglobulin replacement therapy, and the administration of other plasma products containing small amounts of IgA.

Case Study: Clinical Relevance

Let us now return to the case study of IgA deficiency presented earlier and review some of the major points of the clinical presentation to see how they relate to the mucosal immune system.

- The mucosal immune system is found at the interface of the internal environment of the host and the external environment that comes into contact with the mucosal surfaces of respiratory, gastrointestinal, genitourinary, and mammary systems.
- The bulk of serum IgA is produced in mucosal tissues where the dimeric form of the molecule is found with a secretory component that protects the molecule at certain sites (e.g., the gastrointestinal tract) from degradation by proteolytic enzymes.

Case Study: Clinical Relevance (continued)

- At these locations, the mucosal immune system contains all the elements of the innate and adaptive immune systems that respond to foreign substances, including infectious agents and nonreplicating substances such as allergens.
- The patient's prior history of multiple episodes of bronchitis and otitis media in childhood is consistent with the loss of one of the major antimicrobial protective components of the mucosal immune system, i.e., secretory IgA.
- The association of a wide variety of other immune-mediated disorders seen in those with IgA deficiency, e.g., celiac disease, is also related to the loss of the normal protective mechanisms directed at other foreign substances in certain foods, e.g., gliadin fraction of glutens found in wheat, barley, and oats, which gives rise to the clinical manifestations of malabsorption, diarrhea, and weight loss seen in these patients.
- In those deficient in IgA, such as the patient described in this case, the development of serum IgG-associated anti-IgA antibodies occurs, which is responsible for the anaphylactoid hypersensitivity reactions seen in patients following the administration of blood, intravenous gamma globulin (which invariably contains small amounts of IgA), or other blood products.
- Intravenous gamma globulin should not be administered to IgA-deficient patients, and if blood transfusions are required, these patients should receive saline-washed packed red blood cells, which will eliminate exposure to IgA either in whole blood or in packed (non-washed) red blood cells.

Key Points

- The MALT is located where antigen most often enters the body and produces a large percentage of the body's activated memory lymphocytes and antibody molecules (IgA).
- Lymphocytes activated within the MALT tend to recirculate to mucosal immune tissues, including some distant from the site of their activation. This is a particularly important mechanism for lactating women to pass antibodies specific for their intestinal flora to their infants.
- M cells in the intestinal and respiratory tract epithelium transport antigen to the underlying immune tissues for lymphocyte activation.
- Mucosal immune responses have the complete range of effector functions found in the peripheral immune system. In addition, they have higher numbers of gamma-delta T cells and B1 B cells, whose antigen receptors are less diverse but are especially adapted to respond to mucosal pathogen antigens.
- Regulatory T cells are especially important in the mucosal immune system, where tolerance to food antigens and commensal organisms is needed and inflammation must be avoided.
- Mucosal immunization offers some advantages and some challenges compared with conventional immunizations.
- Mucosal pathologies are well documented, but their underlying mechanisms are not well understood.

Study Questions/Critical Thinking

1. How do SIgA molecules reach the respiratory epithelial surface and what are their effector functions there?
2. IgA does not activate complement; is this an advantage or a disadvantage? Explain your answer.
3. Compare how dendritic cells acquire antigen for processing and presentation in the skin and in Peyer's patches.
4. Compare the immune response to commensal bacteria and pathogenic bacteria in the MALT. What regulates these two kinds of responses?
5. Describe the roles of intraepithelial lymphocytes, gamma-delta T cells, and B1 B cells in the mucosal immune system.

Suggested Reading

Bellanti JA. Biological significace of the secretory A immunoglobulins. Pediatrics. 1971; 48: 715–29.

Bellanti JA, Zeligs BJ, Mendez-Inocencio J, et al. Immunologic studies of specific mucosal and systemic immune responses in Mexican school children after booster aerosol or subcutaneous immunization with measles vaccine. Vaccine. 2004; 22: 1214–20.

Belyakov IM, Hel Z, Kelsall B, et al. Mucosal AIDS vaccine reduces disease and viral load in gut reservoir and blood after mucosal infection of macaques. Nature Med. 2001; 7: 1320–6.

Bienenstock J, Clancy RL. Bronchus-associated lymphoid tissues. In J. Mestecky, J. Bienenstock, M.E. Lamm, et al. Mucosal Immunology. 3rd ed. Maryland Heights (MO): Elsevier Academic Press; 2005.

Cebra JJ, Jiang HQ, Sterzl J, et al. The role of mucosal microbiota in the development of and maintenance of the mucosal immune system. In P.L. Ogra, J. Mestecky, M.E. Lamm, et al. Mucosal Immunology. 2nd ed. San Diego: Academic Press; 1999.

Chehade M, Mayer L. Oral tolerance and its relation to food hypersensitivities. J Allergy Clin Immunol. 2005; 115; 3–12.

Cripps AW, Gleeson M. Ontogeny of mucosal immunity and aging. In P.L. Ogra, J. Mestecky, M.E. Lamm, et al. Mucosal Immunology. 2nd ed. San Diego: Academic Press; 1999.

Delves PJ, Lund T, Roitt IM. Antifertility vaccines. Trends Immunol. 2004; 23: 213–9.

Devereux G. The increase in the prevalence of asthma and allergy: food for thought. Nat Rev Immunol. 2006; 6: 869–74.

Elson CO, Cong Y, McCracken VJ, et al. Experimental models of inflammatory bowel disease reveal innate, adaptive and regulatory mechanisms of host dialogue with the microbiota. Immunol Rev. 2005; 206; 260–76.

Faria AM, Weiner HL. Oral tolerance. Immunol Rev. 2005; 206: 232–59.

Fujihashi K, McGhee JR. Thl/Th2/Th3 cells for regulation of mucosal immunity, tolerance and inflammation. In J. Mestecky, J. Bienenstock, M.E. Lamm, et al. Mucosal Immunology. 3rd ed. Maryland Heights (MO): Elsevier Academic Press; 2005.

Fukaura H, Kent SC, Pietrusewicz MJ, et al. Induction of circulating myelin basic protein and proteolipid protein-specific transforming growth factor-beta1-secreting Th3 T cells by oral administration of myelin in multiple sclerosis patients. J Clin Invest. 1996; 98: 70–7.

Gerdts V, Mutwiri GK, Tikoo SK, et al. Mucosal delivery of vaccines in domestic animals. Vet Res. 2006; 37: 487–510.

Harrison LC. Vaccination against self to prevent autoimmune disease: the type 1 diabetes model. Immunol Cell Biol. 2008; 86: 139–45.

Kaetzel CS. The polymeric immunoglobulin receptor: bridging innate and adaptive immune responses at mucosal surfaces. Immunol Rev. 2005; 206: 83–99.

Kaul R, Plummer FA, Kimani J, et al. HIV-1-specific mucosal CD8+ lymphocyte responses in the cervix of HIV-1-resistant prostitutes in Nairobi. J Immunol. 2000; 164: 1602–11.

Kraal G. Nasal-associated lymphoid tissue. In J. Mestecky, J. Bienenstock, M.E. Lamm, et al. Mucosal Immunology. 3rd ed. Maryland Heights (MO): Elsevier Academic Press; 2005.

Kutteh WH. Mucosal immunity in the human female reproductive tract. In P.L. Ogra, J. Mestecky, M.E. Lamm, et al. Mucosal Immunology. 2nd ed. San Diego: Academic Press; 1999.

Larche M, Akdis CA, Valenta R. Immunological mechanisms of allergen-specific immunotherapy. Nat Rev Immunol. 2006; 6: 761–71.

Latiff AH, Kerr MA. The clinical significance of immunoglobulin A deficiency. Ann Clin Biochem 2007; 44: 131–9.

Lefrancois L, Puddington L. Basic aspects of intraepithelial lymphocyte immunobiology. In P.L. Ogra, J. Mestecky, M.E. Lamm, et al. Mucosal Immunology. 2nd ed. San Diego: Academic Press; 1999.

Lefrancois L, Puddington L. Intestinal and pulmonary mucosal T cells: local heroes fight to maintain the status quo. Ann Rev Immunol. 2006; 24: 681–704.

Lin TJ, Befus D. Mast cells and eosinophils in mucosal defenses and pathogenesis. In P.L. Ogra, J. Mestecky, M.E. Lamm, et al. Mucosal Immunology. 2nd ed. San Diego: Academic Press; 1999.

Medina E, Guzman CA. Modulation of immune responses following antigen administration by mucosal route. FEMS Immunol Med Mic. 2000; 27: 305–11.

Mowat AW, Weiner HL. Oral Tolerance. Physiological basis and clinical applications. In P.L. Ogra, J. Mestecky, M.E. Lamm, et al. Mucosal Immunology. 2nd ed. San Diego: Academic Press; 1999.

Round JL, Mazmanian SK. The gut microbiota shapes intestinal immune responses during health and disease. Nat Rev Immunol. 2009; 9: 313–23.

Sabin AB, Flores Arechiga A, Fernandez de Castro J, et al. Successful immunization of children with and without maternal antibody by aerosolized measles vaccine: I. Different results with undiluted human diploid cell and chick embryo fibroblast vaccines. J Am Med Assoc. 1983; 249: 2651–62.

Savage DC. Mucosal microbiota. In P.L. Ogra, J. Mestecky, M.E. Lamm, et al. Mucosal Immunology. 2nd ed. San Diego: Academic Press; 1999.

Snoeck V, Peters IR, Cox E. The IgA system: a comparison of structure and function in different species. Vet Res. 2006; 37: 455–67.

Stiehm RE. The four most common pediatric immunodeficiencies. Adv Exp Med Biol. 2007; 601: 15-26.

Stumbles PA, McWilliam AS, Holt PG. Dendritic cells and mucosal macrophages. In P.L. Ogra, J. Mestecky, M.E. Lamm, et al. Mucosal Immunology. 2nd ed. San Diego: Academic Press; 1999.

Umetsu DT, DeKruyff RH. A role for natural killer T cells in asthma. Nat Rev Immunol. 2006; 6: 953–8.

Vassallo RR. Review: IgA anaphylactic transfusion reactions: part I; Laboratory diagnosis, incidence, and supply of IgA-deficient products. Immunohematology. 2004; 20: 226–33.

Vega-Lopez MA, Telemo E, Bailey M, et al. Immune cell distribution in the small intestine of the pig: immunohistological evidence for an organized compartmentalization in the lamina propria. Vet Immunol Immunop. 1993; 37: 49–60.

Vega-Lopez MA, Arenas-Contreras G, Bailey M, et al. Development of intraepithelial cells in the porcine small intestine. Dev Immunol. 2001; 8: 147–58.

World Health Organization. The World Health Report 2004. Geneva: World Health Organization, 2004.

Yoshikawa T, Gon Y, Matsui M, et al. IgE-mediated allergic responses in the mucosal immune system. In P.L. Ogra, J. Mestecky, M.E. Lamm, et al. Mucosal Immunology. 2nd ed. San Diego: Academic Press; 1999.

Chapter 9

Cytokines, Chemokines, and the Immune System

Joseph A. Bellanti, MD
Alejandro Escobar-Gutiérrez, PhD
Joost J. Oppenheim, MD

LEARNING OBJECTIVES

When you have completed this chapter, you should be able to:

- Describe the characteristics of a cytokine
- Understand the general classification of cytokines and their subfamilies
- Understand the various roles of individual interleukin molecules
- Describe the interactions between cytokines and their receptors
- Understand how cytokines can have both pro-inflammatory and anti-inflammatory properties
- Explain the contributions of cytokines to innate and adaptive immunity
- Understand the extrinsic and intrinsic pathways of apoptosis
- Have a general understanding of growth factors and their role in normal development and malignancy
- Explain how chemokines differ from other cytokines
- Understand the basics of cytokine signaling, including the JAK/STAT pathway
- Describe a few examples of how cytokines and their antagonists are used clinically to treat immunologically mediated diseases
- Summarize the role of cytokines in health and disease

Case Study

A previously healthy thirty-three-year-old woman was seen in the emergency room with a two-day history of lethargy and malaise. During the past three days she experienced three episodes of vomiting, diarrhea, and flu-like symptoms. Over the past twenty-four hours she developed severe continuous pain in the right upper arm associated with severe weakness for which acetaminophen was prescribed by her family physician. Also at this time she had noticed that her lips and tongue were swollen and she felt short of breath. Due to suspicion of impending laryngeal edema, she was given intramuscular epinephrine and was transferred to the acute medical intensive care unit for further evaluation and management.

On admission she was agitated, restless, and incontinent and had a pulse rate of 110/min, respiratory rate of 22/min, blood pressure of 60/40 mm, and a temperature of 38.9° C. Three hours later she started to develop swelling of the face with no erythema or other skin lesions. Examination of the oral cavity revealed an edematous tongue, pharynx, and buccal mucosa with no detectable lymphadenopathy. Lungs auscultation revealed diffusely scattered rhonchi, and cardiovascular examination was normal. Abdominal examination revealed localized tenderness in the left lower quadrant. The laboratory parameters following admission showed an elevated leukocyte count of 21,000/mm^3 with 70 percent neutrophils and 15 percent band forms. The C-reactive protein (CRP), urea, and creatinine were elevated. A provisional diagnosis of meningococcal septicemia was made and treatment was initiated with a third-generation cephalosporin. Intravenous fluids and oxygen therapy by mask were administered and intake and output was strictly maintained.

Over the next eighteen hours a non-blanching erythematous rash appeared over the right upper arm; it progressed rapidly to peeling over the medial aspect of the arm with gross swelling (Figure 9-1). A diagnosis of necrotizing fasciitis was considered (Box 9-1). X-rays of the arm revealed no bony injury and no crepitus was evident in the subcutaneous tissues. The patient continued to be clinically unstable due to hypotension and required constant monitoring. Repeat blood samples continued to reveal an elevated white cell count and CRP, but with

Case Studies (continued)

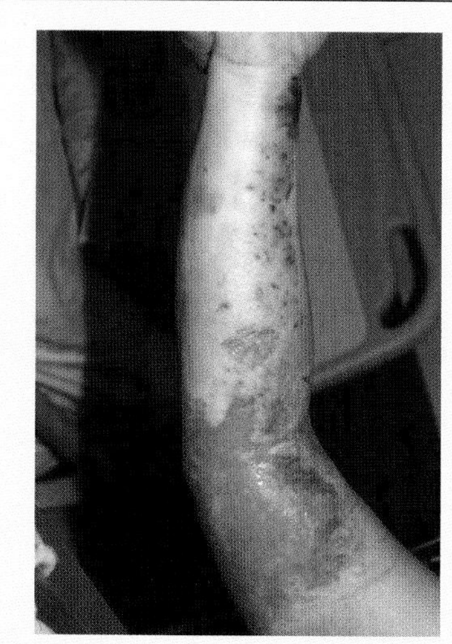

Figure 9-1. Photograph of the right upper limb of the patient showing diffuse swelling of the skin and subcutaneous tissues as well as early signs of desquamation (peeling of the skin). (Courtesy of Madhusudhan TR, Sambamurthy S, Williams E, et al. Surviving streptococcal toxic shock syndrome: a case report. J Med Case Reports. 2007;1:118.)

normal coagulation parameters. Creatine kinase levels, however, were elevated and reached values as high as 9,367U/liter on the fifth hospital day. Although initial blood cultures were negative, a repeat blood culture at forty-eight hours following admission was positive for *alpha hemolytic (viridans) Streptococcus mitis.* Emergency surgery was considered, including the option of an amputation or a disarticulation.

Based on the positive blood culture, antibiotic therapy was changed to imipenem to cover both staphylococcal and streptococcal infection; clindamycin was also given for its improved soft tissue penetration and ability to halt toxin production. The patient gradually improved over the next twenty hours and after twenty-four hours was transferred to the medical ward for further management. Oral clindamycin was continued for an additional two weeks until her blood parameters were normalized. The skin lesions disappeared over the next three weeks with full recovery of her upper limb function.

Introduction

Cytokines are a group of protein and peptide molecules that comprise the intercellular communication network of every cell system of the body, including the immune system. They function as signaling molecules to regulate the growth, differentiation, activation, and inhibition of all cellular aspects of

Box 9-1

Toxic Shock Syndrome and Necrotizing Fasciitis

Toxic shock syndrome (TSS) is an illness of acute onset characterized by fever, rash, and hypotension that can lead to multiple organ failure and lethal shock, as well as desquamation in patients who recover. Although TSS was originally linked to the use of tampons, it is now known to result from wounds or surgical incisions where bacteria can enter the body and cause infection or following the use of contraceptive sponges and diaphragm birth control methods. The toxin-producing causative agent is primarily *Staphylococcus aureus* although a similar condition, called toxic shock-like syndrome (TSLS), results from *Streptococcus pyogenes* infection. Both diseases are caused by bacterial superantigens (SAGs) secreted from either *Staphylococcus aureus* or group A streptococci (GAS) that bypass normal antigen presentation by binding to class II major histocompatibility complex molecules on antigen-presenting cells and to specific variable regions on the β-chain of the T cell antigen receptor (*Chapter 7*). Such superantigens bind to MHC-II molecules on APCs outside the peptide-binding groove and to the TCR variable chains on the T cell. Through this interaction, SAGs activate T cells at orders of magnitude above antigen-specific activation, resulting in massive cytokine release. This massive cytokine release, sometimes referred to as a "cytokine storm," is believed to be responsible for the most severe features of TSS. Soft-tissue infections such as necrotizing fasciitis and myonecrosis are common complications of invasive GAS infections, although these sequelae are not necessary for the development of streptococcal TSLS. Necrotizing fasciitis or fasciitis necroticans, commonly known as "flesh-eating bacteria," is a rare infection of the deeper layers of skin and subcutaneous tissues, easily spreading across the fascial planes within the subcutaneous tissues. Many types of bacteria can cause necrotizing fasciitis (e.g., group A streptococcus, *Vibrio vulnificus, Clostridium perfringens*, and *Bacteroides fragilis*), but group A streptococcus (also known as *Streptococcus pyogenes*) is the most common cause.

Table 9-1. Comparison of cytokines and hormones

Property	Cytokines	Hormones
Pleiomorphism	Produced by and affects many cell types	Produced by single cells
Redundancy	Very high	More restricted
Synergism	Very high	Relatively low
Autocrine, paracrine, or endocrine	Generally localized to tissues	Present in plasma

both the innate and adaptive immune responses. Although cytokines manifest these global effects on virtually all somatic cells, this chapter will focus on their interactive roles with immune cells. The term "immune response" will therefore be used broadly, as introduced in Chapter 1, to denote cells and tissues engaged in host defense, homeostasis, and surveillance, and includes not only the roles of cells of the innate and adaptive immune systems but also those of the hematopoietic, endothelial, mesenchymal, and epithelial cells. Chemokines are a specialized subset of cytokines that function to induce directed cell movement, i.e., chemotaxis, in nearby responsive cells; they are chemotactic cytokines, hence the name "chemokines". **Chemokines** recruit leukocytes to sites of inflammation and play an important role in lymphocyte trafficking (*Chapter 2*). Cytokines and chemokines are involved in every aspect of cellular pathophysiology and, within the immune system, play a central role in cell development and differentiation, as well as inflammatory and immune responses from the initial induction of the **innate immune response** (*Chapter 3*), progressing to the vast array of feedback signals and the DNA recombinatorial and mutational events involved in the **adaptive immune system** (*Chapters 6* and *7*). This chapter will describe how cytokines and chemokines are involved in maintaining balanced homeostasis of the innate immune system (*Chapter 3*) and the adaptive immune system (*Chapters 6* and *7*) in health and how they play critical roles in the pathogenesis of infectious diseases, the allergic and autoimmune disorders, and in cancer.

Cytokines are signaling molecules similar to hormones and neurotransmitters that enable one cell to communicate with another. Cytokines differ, however, from conventional hormones in several important ways (Table 9-1). For example, unlike hormones, which are produced as single cell products of the endocrine system, are present in plasma, and affect specific target cells, cytokines show **pleiomorphism**, i.e., they are produced as multiple products by a variety of cells, are more localized to tissues, and affect a larger number of cells of the immune system. Secondly, cytokines show a high degree of **redundancy** in their biologic function, and different cytokines may have similar effects in contrast to hormones whose effects are more restricted. Cytokines also display a relatively higher degree of **synergism** than hormones so that their combined effects are greater than the sum of their individual effects.

Despite their differences, cytokines are similar to hormones in their modes of action, including the following:

- ***autocrine***, if the cytokine acts on the cell that secretes it,
- ***paracrine***, if the action is restricted to the immediate vicinity of a cytokine's secretion, and
- ***endocrine***, if the cytokine diffuses to distant regions of the body (carried by blood or plasma) to affect different tissues (Table 9-1 and Figure 9-2).

Cytokines are uniquely involved in several cascading events—they affect immune responses and participate in the development of stem cells into

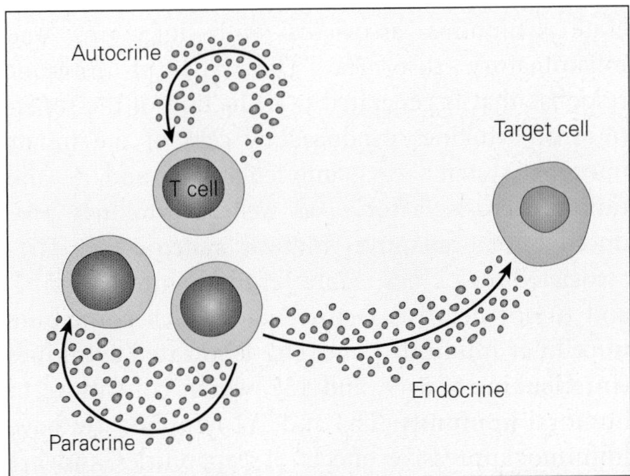

Figure 9-2. Schematic representation of the various effects of cytokines: autocrine, paracrine, and endocrine effects.

immune cells, direct cell trafficking and their location in lymphoid tissues and organs, and mediate the nature and magnitude of their response after activation of the innate or adaptive immune systems by stimulation by pathogen-associated molecular patterns (**PAMPs**) (*Chapter 3*) or antigens (*Chapters 6* and *7*), respectively (Figure 9-3). Due to their pivotal role in both innate and adaptive immune responses, cytokines are also involved in the pathogenesis and symptomatology of a wide variety of immunologically mediated diseases, including infectious diseases (*Chapters 12, 13, 14,* and *15*), autoimmune disorders (*Chapter 19*), allergic diseases (*Chapter 18*), and malignancies (*Chapter 20*). However, the functions of cytokines are not limited to the immune system alone; they also are involved in several developmental and homeostatic processes affecting other organ systems, such as the neurologic and the endocrine systems, and play critical roles in hematopoiesis, angiogenesis, bone turnover, inflammation, and tissue healing. Shown in Figure 9-3 is a schematic overview representation of the panoply of cytokines produced by cells of the innate and adaptive immune systems as well as by epithelial and vascular endothelial cells in response to PAMPs and antigens (*Chapters 1* and *3*). The complexity of the interactions of the cytokines is illustrated not only by their multiple cellular sources of production but also by their cascading modes of action on subsequent cells once produced.

Cytokines derived predominantly from cells of the innate immune system are uniquely important in initial response to foreign configurations as well as subsequent adaptive immune responses (Figure 9-3). They initiate both immune responses and generate symptoms associated with infections and inflammatory disorders. The type of immune response that is generated is a function of the repertoire of cytokines produced by cells of the innate immune system, e.g., interleukins 1 and 6 and tumor necrosis factor α, as well as cytokines produced by the adaptive immune system, e.g., Th1-associated cytokines, (interferon γ, interleukin 2, and tumor necrosis factor beta), which contribute to cellular immunity, and Th2-associated cytokines (interleukins 4, 5, 9, and 13), which contribute to humoral immunity. Th3 and Tr1 lymphocytes have immunosuppressive effects or capabilities and are characterized by their production of transforming growth factor β and interleukin 10, respectively and, when reduced in quantity, contribute to the development of allergic and autoimmune diseases. T helper type 17 cells (**Th17**) are likewise triggered by several cytokines, e.g., interleukins 6 and 23, and when fully activated produce interleukin 17A, 17F, and 22. The production of proinflammatory cytokines, e.g., interleukin 1 and tumor necrosis factor α, contributes to inflammatory diseases characterized by systemic symptoms, e.g., fever, through their effects on the central nervous system and other tissues.

Overstimulation of cytokine production can trigger a dangerous syndrome known as a **cytokine storm**. This is seen in a variety of clinical conditions, including overwhelming sepsis caused by gram-negative bacterial organisms and by toxic shock syndrome, primarily caused by toxic shock syndrome toxin-1 produced by staphylococci (Box 9-1). This syndrome results from the stimulation by superantigens produced by certain bacterial components, e.g., staphylococci, which bind directly to the variable regions of β chains of T cell receptors, causing them to be cross-linked with major histocompatibility complex (**MHC**) molecules of antigen-presenting cells (**APCs**), usually outside the normal antigen-binding groove, resulting in toxicity from massive cytokine release (*Chapters 10* and *12*).

Cytokine Classification

Cytokine Nomenclature

Cytokines have been traditionally named according to their cell of origin or to their specific functions. This early method of nomenclature posed several problems not only because of its imprecise and sometimes mysterious descriptive nature but also because it was soon realized that each cytokine had overlapping properties with other cytokines owing to structural homologies of the cytokines themselves or to the specific receptors to which they bind. This problem is being resolved in recent years as cytokines and their receptors are being better understood based on their precise molecular structures or genomic origins. For ease of discussion, however, in this chapter the cytokines will be presented first in the more traditional functional format, followed by more recent molecular descriptions of their overlapping functions based on molecular structures.

Shown in Table 9-2 is a classification of cytokines based on their functional properties. They are

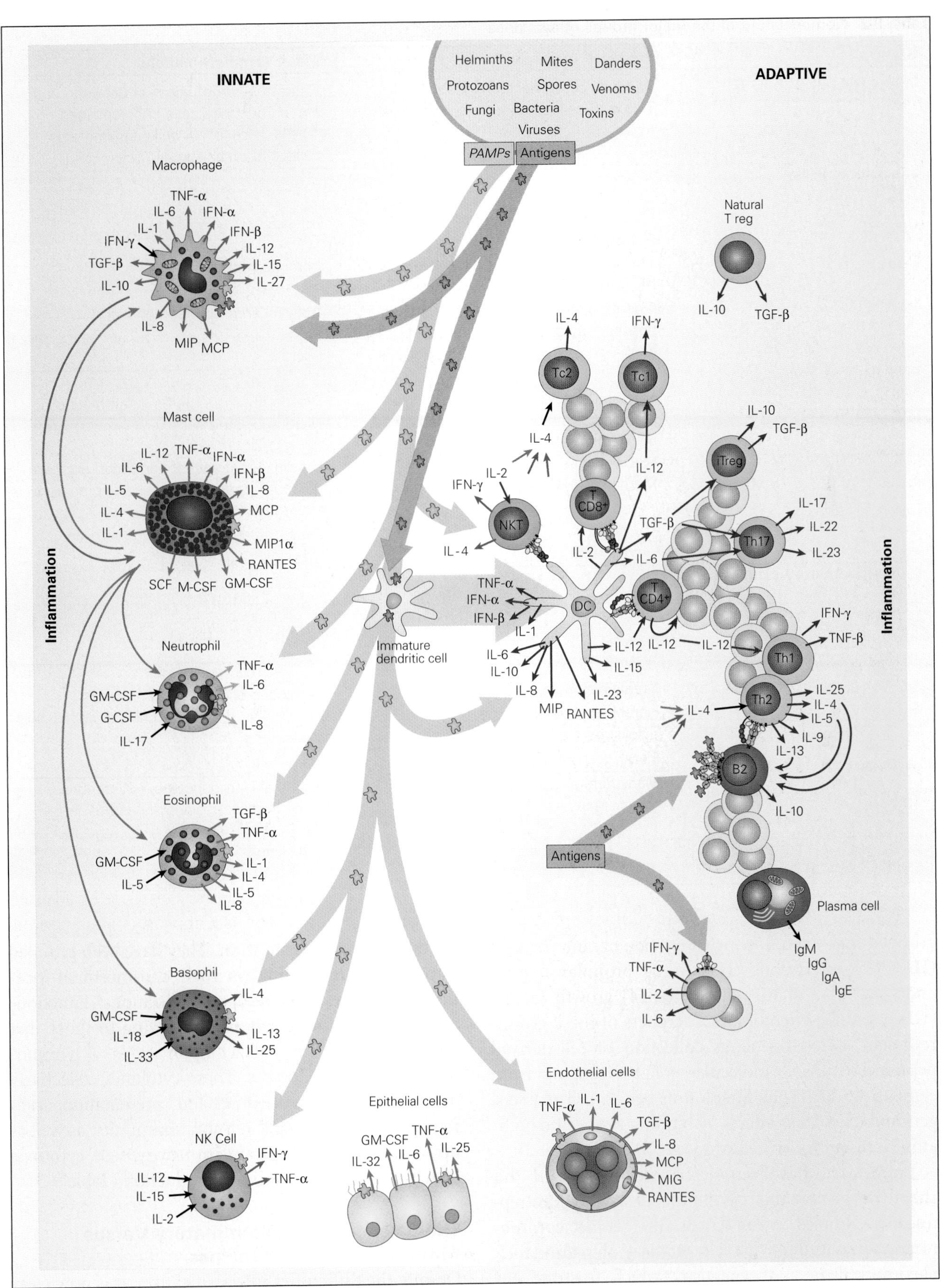

Figure 9-3. Schematic representation of the production and actions of cytokines and chemokines by cells of the innate and adaptive immune systems as well as by epithelial and vascular endothelial cells in response to stimulation by PAMPs and antigens.

Table 9-2. Nomenclature of the major groups of cytokines

Group	Produced mainly by	Major targets/functions
Interleukins (IL-1 to IL-37)	Dendritic cells, macrophages, NK cells, T cells, B cells, and other somatic cell types	Regulates communication between and among dendritic cells, macrophages, T cells, B cells, NK cells, inflammatory cells, and other somatic cells
Interferons (IFNs)		
Type I		
IFN-α	Plasmacytoid dendritic cells, macrophages	Antiviral
IFN-β	Fibroblasts	
Type II (IFN-γ)	Th1 and Tc1 cells, Tγδ cells, NKT cells, NK cells	Immune regulation
Type III (IFN-λ)	T and B lymphocytes, NK cells, macrophages, fibroblasts, endothelial cells, epithelial cells, osteoblasts, and others	Antiviral and immunomodulatory
Proinflammatory cytokines		
TNF-α	Macrophages, mast cells	Proapoptotic, promotes inflammation
IL-1	Macrophages, keratinocytes, and other nucleated cells	Most nucleated cells
IL-6	Macrophages, lymphoid cells	B cells, hepatocytes, hematopoietic cells
IL-17	Memory T cells, Th17 cells, NK cells	APCs, DCs, and stromal cells; promotes autoimmunity
TNF-β/lymphotoxin	Th1 cells	Proapoptotic, promotes inflammation, lymphoid organogenesis
Anti-inflammatory cytokines		
IL-10	Tr1	Dampens inflammation, immunosupressive
TGF-β	Th 3	
	IL-35?	
Growth factors		
G-CSF	Fibroblasts, macrophages	Hematopoietic cells, granulocytes
GM-CSF	Fibroblasts, macrophages	Monocytes, progenitor cells, dendritic cells
M-CSF	T cells, others	Monocytes
TGF-β	Platelets, nucleated cells	Many cells
Chemokines CL CCL CXCL CX_3CL	Many different cell types	Neutrophils, monocytes, NK, dendritic, T and B cells, eosinophils and basophils, mast cells, endothelial cells; regulates cell trafficking

grouped into the following categories: (1) interleukins (**ILs**); (2) interferons (**IFNs**); (3) proinflammatory and anti-inflammatory cytokines; (4) growth factors (**GFs**); and (5) chemokines. Members of these groups represent a heterogeneous collection of cell-derived peptides with low molecular weights ranging from eight to 45 kDa that function as cell-to-cell messengers and exert their effects by binding to specific high-affinity receptors on cell surfaces.

From what has been described thus far in this chapter, it is clear that cytokines and chemokines represent a complex set of structurally distinct communication molecules with a great deal of redundancy, pleiomorphism, and synergism, which frustrate any attempt at classification. Several criteria have been used for the cytokine classification. They have been grouped into families depending on their chromosomal locations, structures, and receptor utilizations. Functionally, they can also be grouped according to those that are produced by or that act upon APCs, T lymphocytes, and B lymphocytes. These cytokines collectively mediate antigen processing and presentation, cell-mediated immunity, and humoral immunity, as well as immunosuppression, proinflammatory, and cytotoxic activity and immunoglobulin production (Table 9-3).

The Balance of Proinflammatory Versus Anti-inflammatory Cytokines

Despite the difficulties in classification, it is now clear that cytokines can exert opposing (**antagonistic**)

Table 9-3. Functional classification of cytokines

Cytokines produced by or acting upon:	Example of cell type	Example of cytokine	Function
Antigen-presenting cells	Dendritic cells, macrophages	IL-12	Antigen processing and presentation; T cell differentiation
T lymphocyte	**CD4**		
	Th1	IFN-γ	Cell-mediated immunity
	Th2	IL-4, IL-5, IL-9, IL-13	Humoral immunity
	Th17	IL-17, IL-22	Proinflammatory
	Treg[a]	(IL-35)	Immunosuppression
	Tr1	IL-10	Immunoregulatory
	Th3	TGF-β	Immunosuppression
	CD8	TRAIL/Fas-2	Cytotoxic activity
B lymphocyte	Th2-B cell interaction	Produced by Th2 cells IL-4 IL-5 IL-9 IL-13	Immunoglobulin production

a. The classical Treg activity (both nTreg and iTreg effects) are considered cell contact–dependent and do not synthesize cytokines. IL-35 has not get been confirmed.

functions and represent the molecules par excellence that maintain the immunologic balance between the external and internal environments described in Chapter 1. Cytokines accomplish these antagonistic effects by either promoting or inhibiting inflammation (*Chapter 5* and Figure 9-4).

Thus, cytokines are reactive molecules that can both promote and counteract inflammation; this is accomplished because the same molecules are able to react with receptors that share homologies and that can be activated or turned off depending on the nature of the foreign insult and the resulting inflammatory response. Shown in Figure 9-5 is a schematic representation of the overlapping nature of the major groups of cytokines (interleukins, interferons, growth factors, and chemokines). The resulting proinflammatory/anti-inflammatory paradigm is superimposed on this overlapping and cascading set of responses and is responsible for the clinical expressions of cytokine production in health and disease.

Cytokines and Cellular Immunity

Cellular immunity may be defined as any manifestation of the adaptive immune response in which antigen-specific T cells play a pivotal role (*Chapters 1* and *7*). These immune responses are characterized by the clonal selection and development of antigen-specific T lymphocytes through their T cell receptors (**TCRs**). Upon expansion, these T cells not only serve as effector cells for the recognition and elimination of pathogens and other foreign configurations, but also generate memory cells for long-term resistance to disease. The understanding of T cell

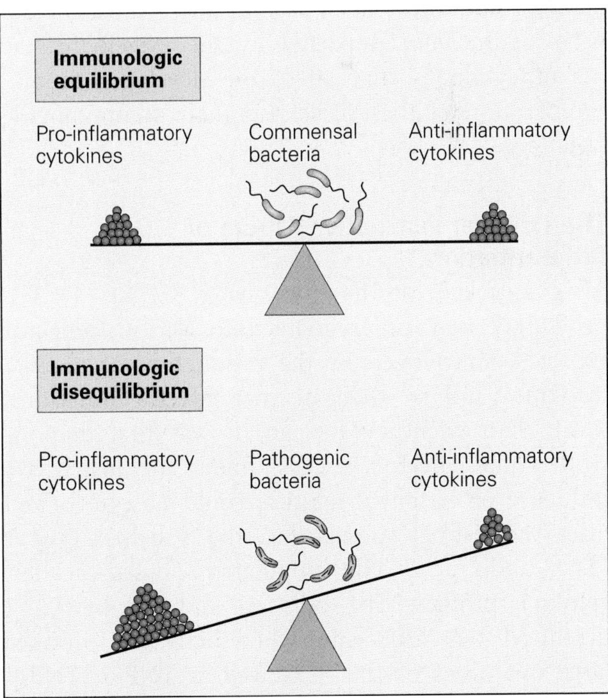

Figure 9-4. Schematic representation of the opposing proinflammatory and anti-inflammatory functions of cytokines in maintaining immunologic equilibrium. The balanced production of pro-inflammatory and anti-inflammatory cytokines in response to commensal bacteria in the gastrointestinal tract resulting in immunologic equilibrium (upper panel) is contrasted to the immunologic disequilibrium seen when pathogenic bacteria are introduced (lower panel).

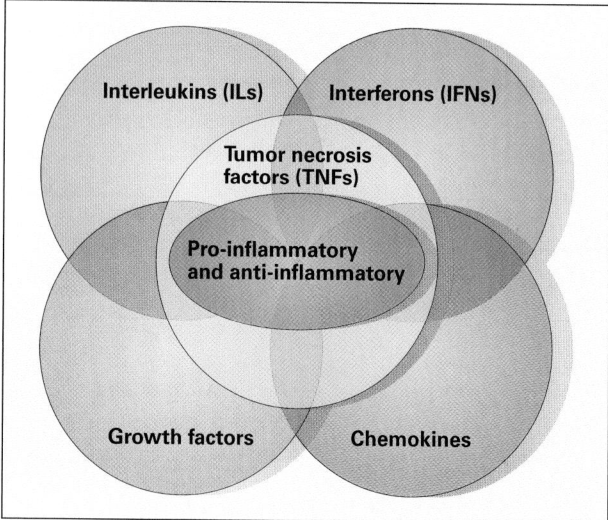

Figure 9-5. Schematic representation of the overlapping nature of the five major groups of cytokines (interleukins [ILs], interferons [IFNs], tumor necrosis factors [TNFs], growth factors, and chemokines), and superimposed on this overlapping and cascading set of responses is the pro-inflammatory/anti-inflammatory paradigm.

differentiation has undergone considerable expansion from what was originally demonstrated. The division of lymphocytes into CD4+ and CD8+ populations and the elucidation of their subsets have been significantly impacted by the ever-increasing list of cytokines that affect the development and proliferation of these cells and their accompanying functions.

The Original Instructive Model of T Cell Differentiation

After antigenic stimulation, naïve CD4+ T cells proliferate and differentiate into various effector subsets characterized by the production of distinct cytokines and by their distinct effector functions. More than twenty years ago, it was first demonstrated that effector T cells, under the instructive influence of certain cytokines, could be categorized into two distinct subsets, i.e., the T helper type 1 (**Th1**) and type 2 (**Th2**) populations, based on their cytokine profiles. Th1 cells are induced by IL-12 produced by APCs and when activated produce large quantities of IFN-γ as well as TNF-α, TNF-β (also called lymphotoxin [**LT**]), and IL-10 can cause self-destructive inflammation (*Chapter 19*). In contrast, Th2 cells are induced by IL-4 and when activated produce predominantly IL-4, as well as IL-5, IL-9, IL-10, IL-13, IL-21, and IL-31 and can diminish cellular inflammation (Figure 9-6). Th1 cells elicit delayed-type hypersensitivity responses, activate macrophages, and are highly effective in clearing intracellular pathogens. Th2 cells, in contrast, are particularly important for the production of immunoglobulins (**Igs**), e.g., IgG and IgE, through their collaboration with B cells and play major roles in host defense against parasites and in allergic disease. As will be described later, other newly discovered T cell subsets, e.g., T regulatory (**Treg**), Th3, Tr1, and Th17 cells, are now known to play critical roles in silencing or enhancing the proinflammatory responses of the immune system, respectively. This knowledge is assuming considerable clinical importance and is providing the tools with which to better diagnose and treat a wide variety of allergic and autoimmune diseases, as well as enhancing the treatment of patients receiving transplanted organs or with malignancy.

The process by which an uncommitted Th cell develops into a mature Th1 or Th2 cell has provided a useful model for an understanding of developmentally regulated gene expression (Figure 9-6). There is good evidence to indicate that this differentiation process is highly plastic. Many factors influence the decision of a T cell to become a Th1 or Th2 cell that expresses T-bet or GATA3, respectively (Box 9-2). The cytokines IL-12 and IL-4, acting through the signal transducer and activator of transcription (**STAT**) 4 and STAT6, respectively, are key determinants of the outcome. It has been proposed also that antigen dose, co-stimulators, genetic modifiers, and other non-cytokine factors have crucial roles in determining the dominance of a particular Th cell response. How each signal influences the differentiation process is an area of active investigation and, often, lively controversy.

For almost two decades, the Th1/Th2 paradigm has offered a productive conceptual framework for both the study of T cell differentiation as well as a basis for an understanding the pathogenesis of a variety of autoimmune and allergic disorders. However, the discovery of new T cell subsets and cytokines has required a revision of the Th1/Th2 paradigm in the context of new T cell subsets and their signature cytokines. The discovery of Treg cells and the identification of a novel effector T cell population referred to as Th17 cells has opened new diagnostic and therapeutic applications for a wide variey of infectious, allergic, and autoimmune diseases and cancer.

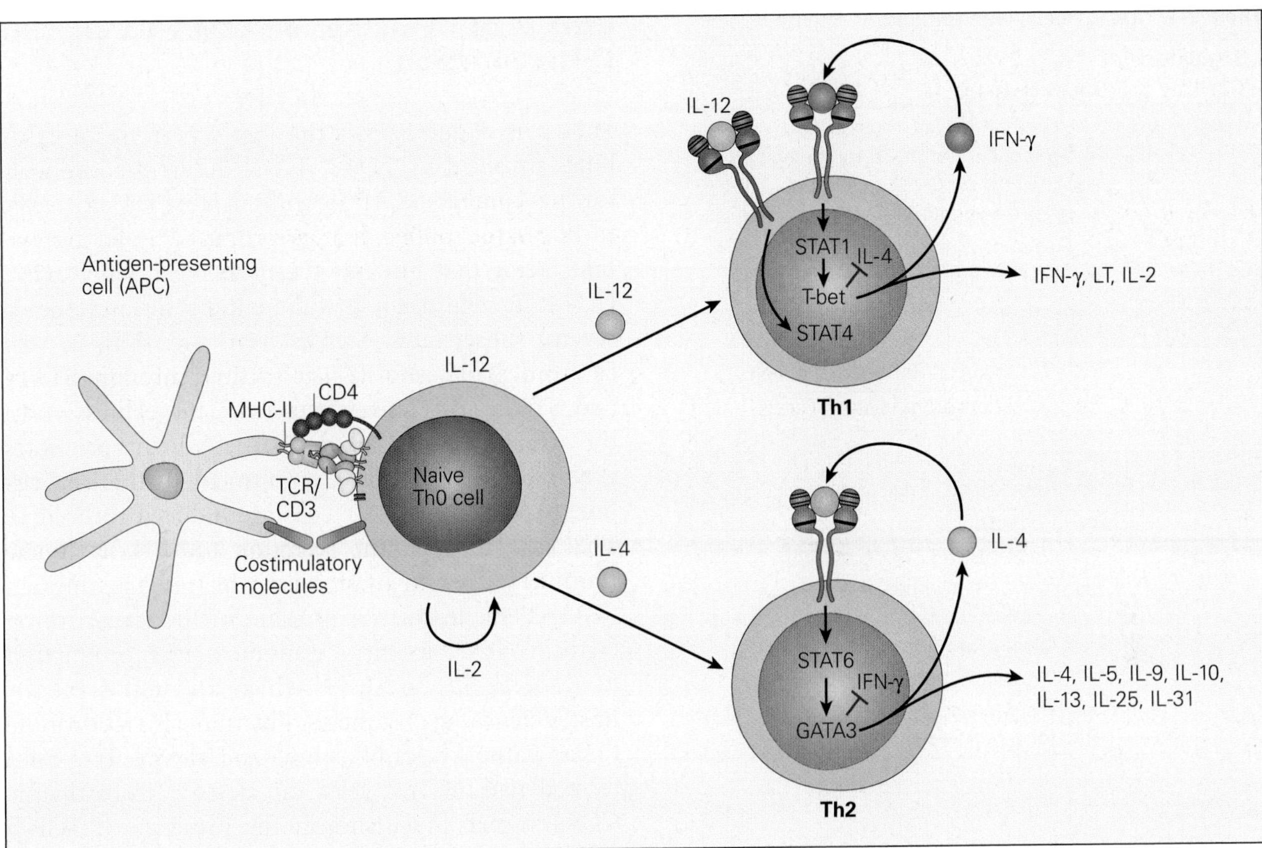

Figure 9-6. The original instructive model of helper T cell differentiation. Following antigen processing and presentation of peptides to an uncommitted, naïve helper T (Th0) cell precursor, it can become activated to differentiate into either a Th1 or Th2 cell under the instructive influence of interleukin-12 (IL-12) or IL-4, respectively. Th1 cells express T-bet and secrete their signature cytokine interferon-γ (IFN-γ) and others. Th2 cells express GATA-3 and secrete their signature cytokine IL-4 as well as other cytokines.

T Regulatory Cells

Several subsets of reg (Treg cells) capable of controlling effector T cell responses have also been described in Chapter 7; these include both naturally occurring Treg (nTreg) and induced Treg (iTreg) cells (Table 9-4). Although naturally occurring Treg cells originate directly from thymic precursors, induced Treg cells, Tr1 cells, and Th3 regulatory T cells differentiate from peripheral T helper cell precursors through the actions of different cytokines.

> **Box 9-2**
>
> ### T-bet and GATA3 Transcription Factors
>
> Two important transcription factors:
>
> - T-bet is a member of the T box family of transcription factors. It is a master switch in the development of T helper 1 (Th1) cell responses through its ability to regulate expression of the IL-12 receptor, inhibit signals that promote Th2 cell development, and promote the production of IFN-γ.
> - GATA3 is a 444-amino transcription factor that binds with high affinity to related consensus DNA sites (GATA, GATTA, and GATCT) and that is important in regulating Th2 cell differentiation.

The Two Major Pathways of T Cell Differentiation: The CD4+ T Helper and the CD8+ T Cytotoxic Populations and Their Subsets

Shown in Figure 9-7 is a schematic representation of the two major arms of the T cell system that include the CD4+ T helper (**Th**) and the CD8+ T cytotoxic (**Tc**) populations. The CD4+ Th cell population is made up of several effector subsets that include the Th1, Th2, Th17, and Treg populations. The CD4+ Th cells and their subsets are the

Table 9-4. CD4+ T cells with regulatory activity

Regulatory T cell	Characteristic
nTreg	CD25+ FOXP3+ thymus-derived Not dependent on IL-10 for biologic activity Mediates self-tolerance/prevents autoimmune disease
iTreg	Peripheral-derived Treg cells Dependent on CTLA-4 for suppressive activity FOXP3+ CD25+ TGF-β responsible for their induction
Th3	Peripheral-derived regulatory T cells FOXP3− Characterized by TGF-β production Mediates mucosal tolerance/antigen-specific IgA production
Tr1	Peripheral-derived Treg cells FOXP3− or + at times Characterized by IL-10 production Possibly derived from Th1-like/Th2-like lymphocytes or naïve T cells ±CD25 expression (reflecting their effector function-activation)

key orchestrators of adaptive immune responses in mammalian hosts and each of their effector subsets mobilizes a distinct module of antimicrobial immunity. Th1 cells direct the elimination of intracellular microbial pathogens, viruses, and tumors; Th2 cells induce the expulsion of intestinal helminths; and Th17 cells promote resistance to extracellular bacteria and fungi. Treg cells suppress immune and inflammatory reactions and ensure that the host's intrinsically self-recognizing repertoire of lymphocytes does not mount a response against its own tissues or innocuous environmental antigens (*Chapters 7* and *19*).

The CD8+ Tc population is similarly comprised of subpopulations that include Tc1 and Tc2 subsets. Tc1 cells are active in the destruction of virally infected or malignant cells. During their ontogeny in the thymus and their subsequent differentiation in secondary lymphoid tissues, CD4+ T cells and CD8+ T cells undergo a sequence of complex and mechanistically distinct processes that result in the acquisition of helper or regulatory repertoire as well as cytotoxic activity, respectively (*Chapters 2* and *7*).

Effects of Cytokines on CD4+ T Cell Differentiation

Shown in Figure 9-8 is the vast repertoire of cytokines involved in CD4+ T cell differentiation. Following contact of APCs with naïve CD4+ T cells, the cytokine milieu that is produced is an important factor that initiates the process by which naïve CD4+ T cells begin to differentiate toward one of several subset fates. Signals from the TCR, as well as from IL-12 and IFN-γ (acting through STAT4 and STAT1, respectively), increase the expression of the transcription factor T-bet, which promotes IFN-γ production and commitment to the Th1 cell lineage. Naïve CD4+ T cells are induced to become Th2 cells through the secretion of IL-4 by innate immune cells and mast cells, which signal through STAT6. This leads to expression of the transcription factor GATA3, in turn resulting in the production of IL-4, IL-5, and IL-13, which are important for host defense against helminths and also contribute to the pathogenesis of asthma and allergy. Treg cells, termed natural Treg cells, can develop from thymic CD4+ T cell precursors in the presence of TGF-β and IL-2. In the periphery, naïve CD4+ T cells can also be converted to become inducible T reg cells by signaling through STAT5 in the presence of TGF-β, which results in upregulation of the transcription factor forkhead box P3 (**FOXP3**). Treg cells produce high levels of IL-35, CTLA-4, and TGF-β. Retinoic acids, which are abundant in the liver and intestine, increase FOXP3 expression. In the presence of commensal bacteria, dendritic cells synthesize retinoic acid from vitamin A, which not only upregulates the FOXP3 transcription factor, but also downregulates the expression of the retinoic acid-related orphan receptors (**RORγt** and **RORα**), thereby inhibiting the activation of naïve T cell precursors into Th17 cells. Treg cells, therefore, have an important role in peripheral self-tolerance and immune suppression (*Chapter 8*). Th17 cells develop from naïve CD4+ T cells in response to IL-6, IL-1β, IL-23, and TGF-β. IL-1β, IL-6, and IL-23 activate STAT3, which increases the expression of the transcription factors RORγt and RORα, which in turn promote the expression of IL-17A, IL-17F, IL-21, and IL-22. IL-23 seems to stabilize and increase the pathogenicity of Th17 cells. Th17 cells are important for host defense against extracellular bacteria (*Chapter 12*) and are involved in mediating autoimmune

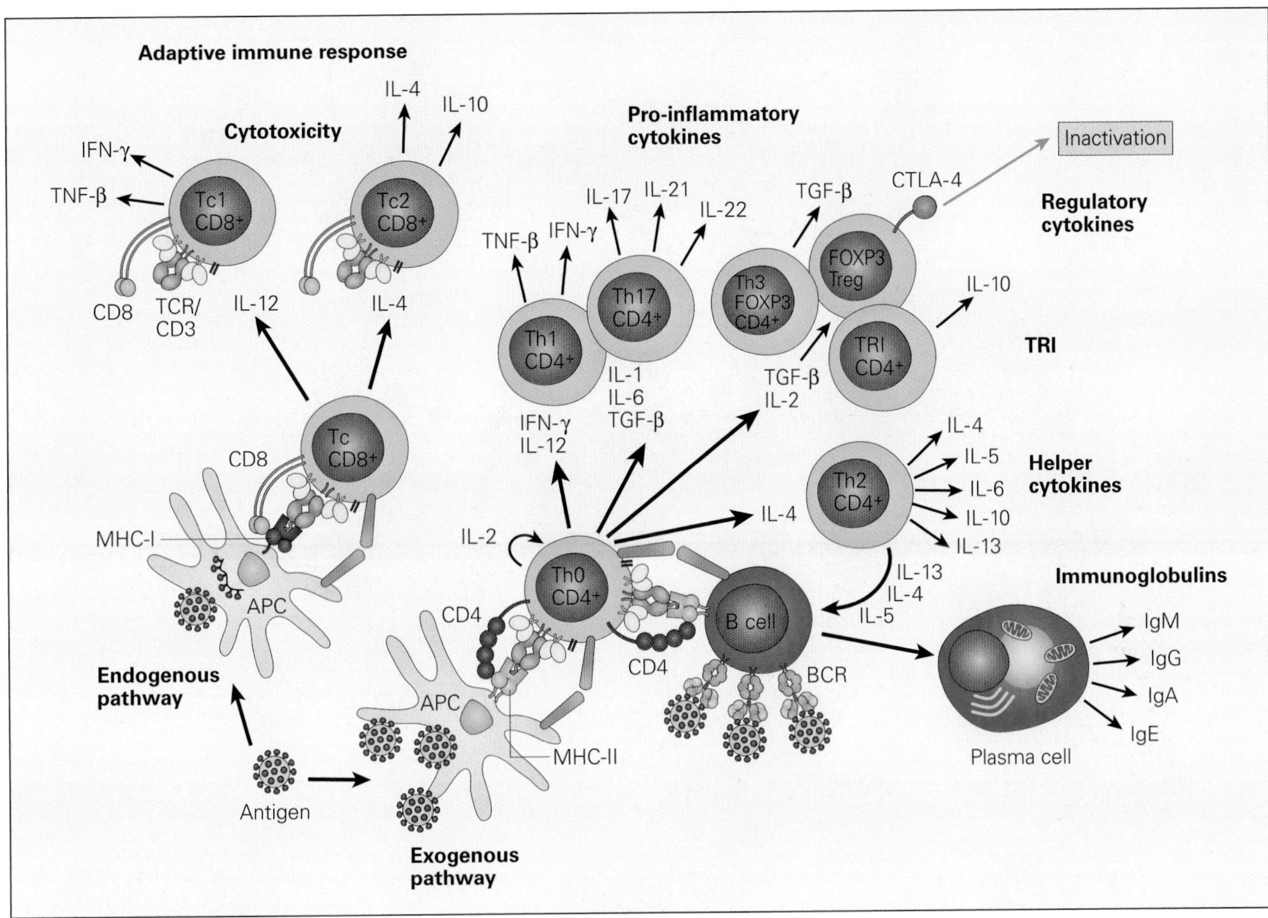

Figure 9-7. Schematic representation of the two major pathways of T cell differentiation: the CD4+ T helper (Th) and the CD8+ T cytotoxic (Tc) populations and their subsets. Following uptake and processing of an antigen by an APC shown in the figure as a dendritic cell, peptide is presented either to the CD8 population in the context of MHC-I or to the CD4 subpopulation in the context of MHC-II following which a cascading set of cellular lymphoproliferative and differentiative steps are initiated under the inductive influence of cytokines that ultimately determine their effector functions.

disease (*Chapter 19*). IL-22 tempers the inflammatory effects of IL-17A and IL-17D.

Subset Flexibility and Plasticity

One of the major hallmark properties of Th differentiation is the amazing capacity of subset flexibility and plasticity rendered by cytokines (Figure 9-8). At present, lineage commitment is defined by the signature cytokines that differentiated cells secrete (i.e., IFN-γ, IL-4, and IL-17, for Th1, Th2, and Th17 cells, respectively). However, additional complexity is becoming evident. For example, although Treg cells are sometimes immunosuppressive and produce IL-10, all CD4+ T cell subsets can produce the immunoregulatory cytokine IL-10, which is crucial for dampening immune responses. Furthermore, Th17 cells can, at times, also produce IFN-γ, and so the relationship between Th1 cells and Th17 cells is currently being intensively scrutinized. Similarly, although Th17 cells produce IL-21 and IL-22, it also seems that under some circumstances, T cells can produce IL-21 or IL-22 without producing IL-17 (*Chapter 12*). Another limitation adding to the complexity of cytokine secretion by T cell subsets is that proposed models that involve the selective expression of master regulators might not be appropriate. For example, FOXP3 and RORγt can be co-expressed and can interact. Moreover, some Treg cells can be induced to become Th17 cells (Figure 9-8). Therefore, Th1 and Th2 CD4+ T cell subsets should be viewed as terminally differentiated lineages, but the Th17 and Treg subsets retain some flexibility and plasticity. The extent to which some aspects of T cell subsets are firmly fixed and others remain plastic is the subject of current intense investigation.

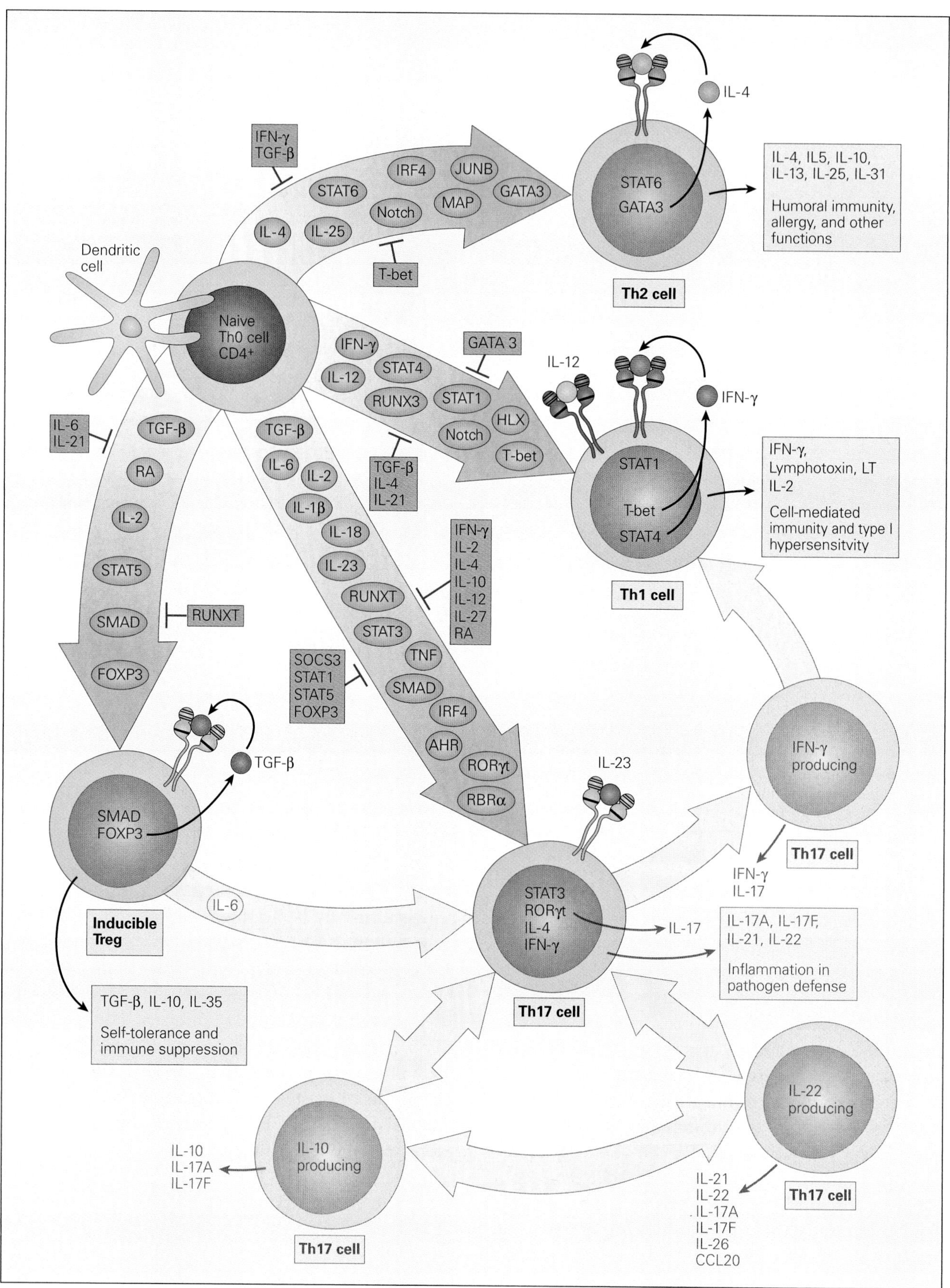

Figure 9-8. Schematic representation of the effects of the vast repertoire of cytokines involved in the inductive phases of CD4 T cell differentiation from naïve Th0 precursors and their subsequent terminal development into four major effector T helper subsets, the Th2, Th1, Th17, and Treg cells and their signature cytokines, i.e., IL-4, IFN-γ, IL-17, and TGF-β, IL-10, and IL-35, respectively. The four major pathways of differentiation are indicated by the heavier arrows that are intersected by T bar located cytokines designating their inhibitory functions. Shown in ghosted arrows and cells is the great plasticity that these terminally differentiated Th17 and Treg cells display in transitioning from one to another.

Cytokine Receptors and Signaling Pathways

Before the properties and functions of individual cytokines are described, it is important to review the characteristics of the cytokine receptors to which the cytokines bind and the subsequent signaling pathways that result following this initial binding. Cytokines are proteins and key mediators of cellular proliferation, differentiation, and apoptotic cell death and play a central role in both the activation and effector phases of innate and adaptive immune responses. All cytokine receptors consist of proteins found at the surface of cells that are composed of three components: (1) an **extracellular portion**, (2) a **transmembrane portion**, and (3) an **intracytoplasmic portion**. The cytokine first binds to the extracellular portion of the receptor, following which a signal is generated through a series of conformational changes of the cytokine receptor and a cascading set of biochemical reactions (involving primarily the addition of phosphate groups to substrates, i.e., phosphorylation, through the action of a variety of kinases), during which the signal is transmitted through the cytosolic and nuclear regions of the cell, leading to the ultimate construction of a biologically functional product, e.g., antibody, cytokine.

For ease of discussion, these cascading steps have been used throughout this book and may be described in their simplest format as the "three Ts": transduction→transcription→translation (Box 9-3 and Figure 9-9). These signaling pathways are usually activated by ligand-induced receptor clustering, bringing together the cytoplasmic portions of two or more receptor molecules in a process analogous to signaling described for B and T cell receptors for antigens (*Chapters 6* and *7*). These signaling pathways involve several substrates, including janus kinases (**JAKs**) and signal transducers and activators of transcription (**STATs**), and will be described in greater detail in a separate section of this chapter (Table 9-5).

Box 9-3

The Signaling Pathways of Cytokines with Their Receptors: Transduction→Transcription→Translation (the "Three Ts")

All cellular activity involved in maintenance of balance between the external and internal environments is dependent on the initiation of extracellular signals that are received by cells at their membranes and then transmitted to the nuclear DNA and then to cytoplasmic RNA with the ultimate production of a protein which performs any of a number of functions. This set of cascading events, shown in Figure 9-9, is at the heart of cellular and molecular biology and involves the "three Ts," a triad of **transduction→transcription→translation** that will be repeated time and time again in various derivative forms throughout this book. Therefore, it is crucial for the student to have a fundamental understanding of these molecular events in order to not only comprehend the cacophony of acronyms that derive from them and that comprise their infrastructure but also to understand the clinical applications of molecular biology in the diagnosis, treatment, and prevention of immunologically mediated disorders.

Transduction

Following the initial binding of a cytokine with the extracellular portion of its receptor and clustering of one or more of various portions of the ligand-receptor complex, a signal is transmitted across the cell membrane to the cytosol by the first "T" of the process, referred to as "transduction" (from the Latin, denotes leading across). The signal is generated at this step of the process by a series of biochemical reactions involving kinases that are enzymes that phosphorylate cytoplasmic substrates that are then activated and can phosphorylate other substrates, leading eventually to a final product called a transcription factor, which initiates the second "T" of the process, referred to as "transcription."

Transcription

Once the transcription factor enters the nucleus and lodges on a region of the DNA molecule referred to as the promoter region, a portion of the gene is expressed with the formation of a messenger RNA (mRNA) by the process of transcription (from the Latin, denotes writing across). The mRNA leaves the nucleus to be situated on the ribosomes of the endoplasmic reticulum. The mRNA provides a molecule that contains the antisense nucleotide sequence necessary to initiate the third "T" of the process, referred to as "translation."

Translation

Following its placement on the surface of a ribosome in the endoplasmic reticulum, the mRNA serves as a template for the ligation of specific amino acid-transfer RNAs, following which the amino acids are fastened together into protein molecules by translation (from the Latin, denotes carrying across).

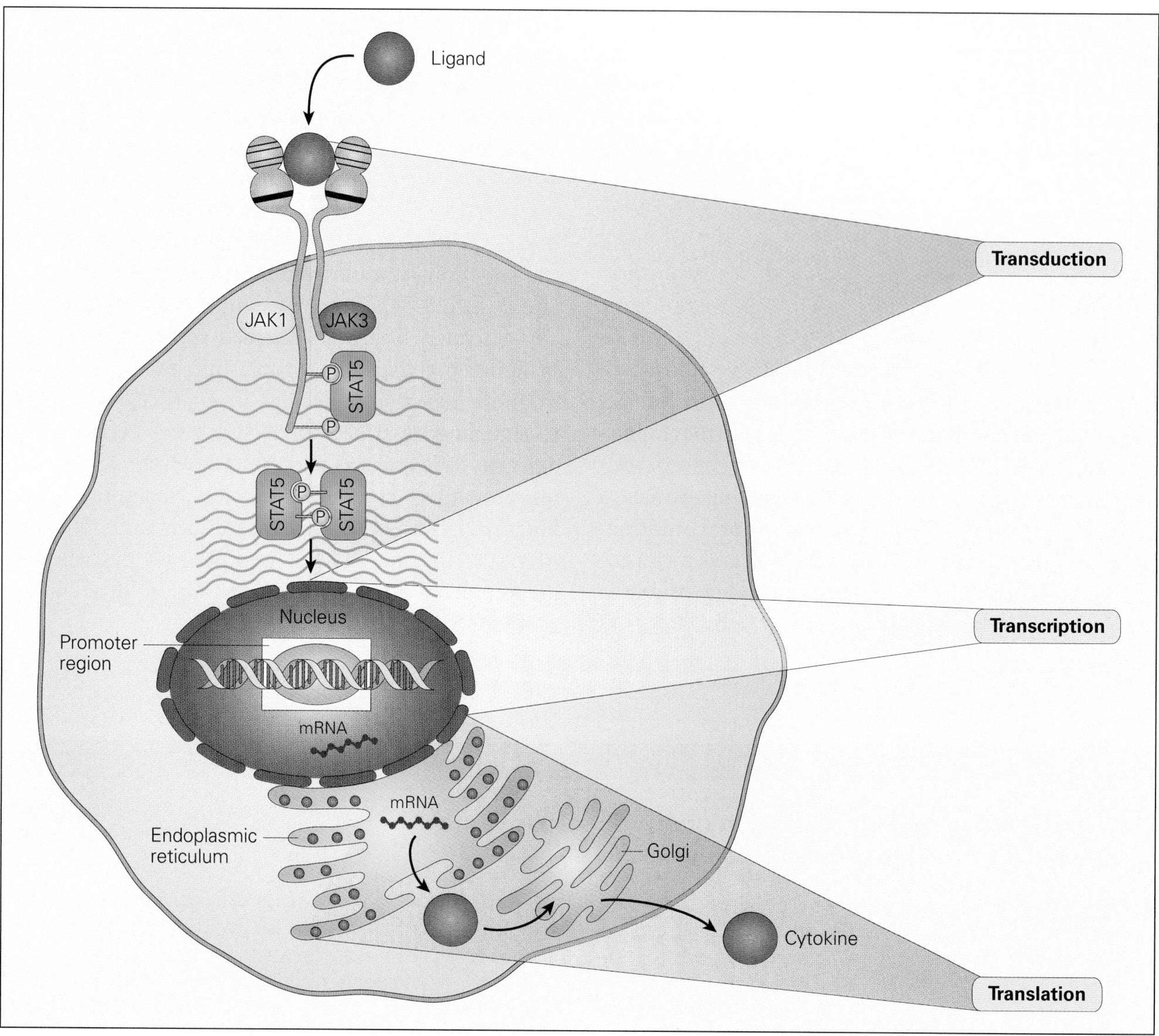

Figure 9-9. Transduction→Transcription→Translation (the "three Ts.")

The Molecular Basis for Cytokine and Cytokine Receptor Pleiotropy and Redundancy

Pleiotropy and redundancy have now become better understood as a result of recent advances in the understanding of the molecular structures of cytokines and their cytokine receptors as well as the signaling pathways that are activated following their interaction. Cytokines and cytokine receptors consist of various protein moieties that are shared respectively with one another. As will be described in detail below, the pleiotropic properties of a cytokine are related to its ability to bind to receptors that are found on multiple cellular lineages or by its ability to activate multiple signaling pathways that differentially contribute to different functions. Overlapping actions or redundancy are related to the finding that different cytokines can bind to the same or to a variety of receptors that share the same or similar molecular motifs.

The function of a cytokine is determined both by molecular signals resulting from binding to its cognate receptor as well as the receptor structure itself, which collectively predict its signaling function. For this reason, cytokines have been divided into a limited number of families based primarily on structural features of their receptors. Cytokines and chemokines bind to cell surface receptors that belong to the eight families shown in Table 9-5 and in Figure 9-10A and B.

Table 9-5. Cytokine receptor families and subfamilies

Cytokine receptor family	Subfamily	Cytokine	Signaling
Class I (hematopoietin)		IL-2	JAK1, JAK3, STAT5
	γc-utilizing	IL-4	JAK1, JAK3, STAT6
	(common γc chain)	IL-7	JAK1, JAK3, STAT5
		IL-9	JAK1, JAK3, STAT5
		IL-15	JAK1, JAK3, STAT5
		IL-21	JAK1, JAK3, STAT3
	βc-utilizing	GM-CSF	JAK1, STAT3
	(GM-CSF common β chain)	IL-3	JAK2, STAT5
		IL-5	JAK2, STAT5
	gp130-utilizing	IL-6	JAK1, STAT3
	(IL-6 receptor common gp130)	IL-11	JAK1, STAT3
		IL-27	JAK1, STAT1, STAT3, STAT4, STAT5
		IL-31	JAK1, STAT3, STAT5
		LIF	JAK1, STAT3
		OSM	JAK1, STAT3
		CNTF	JAK1, STAT3
		CT-1	JAK1, STAT3
		CLC	JAK1, STAT3
Class II (interferon)[a]	IFNAR1, IFNAR2	IFN-α, IFN-β	JAK1, TYK2, STAT1, STAT2
	IFNGR1, IFNGR2	IFN-γ	JAK1, JAK2, STAT1
	IL-10R	IL-10	JAK1, TYK2, STAT3
	IL-20R1, IL-20R2, IL-22R	IL-19, IL-20, IL-22, IL-24, IL-26	STAT1, STAT3
	IL-28R	IL-28, IL-29, IL-30	STAT1, STAT2, STAT3, STAT4, STAT5
Tumor necrosis factor (TNF) family receptors	TNFR1, BAFFR, TNFR2, TACI, CD40, BCMA, OX40. CD27, HVEM, DcR3, LTβR, 41B3, Fas, GITR, CD30, DR1-4, RANK, TL1A, TWEAKR, EDAR	TNF-α, LTα, LTβ, FasL, CD40L, OX-40L, 4-1BBL, TRAIL, BlyS, CD27L, CD30L, APRIL, GITRL, CD30L, BTLA, RANKL, TWEAK, EDA	NF-κB, TRAF6, MyD88, IRAK, IRAK4
IL-1/TLR	IL-R1	IL-1α/β	IRAK, MyD88, TRAF6, NF-κB, TIR
	IL-1R2	IL-1F, IL-1G	
	IL-18R	IL-18	
	ST-2	IL-33, IL-36α,β,γ, IL-36Ra, IL-37,	
	IL-Rrp2	(IL-38)	
Th17 receptors	IL-17RA	IL-17A	TRAF6, JNK, Erk1/2, p38, AP-1, NF-κB
	IL-17RB	IL-17B, IL-17C, IL17-D	
	IL-17RC	IL-17E (IL-25)	
	IL-17RD	IL-17F	
	IL-17RE (IL-17RA + IL-17RB)		
TGF-β receptor serine kinase family	TGFBR1	TGF-β1	SMADs
	TGFBR2	TGF-β2	
		TGF-β3	
Tyrosine kinase receptors		Stem cell factor	Ras/Raf/MAPK Stromal cell
	CSF-1R/c-Fms	CSF-1(M-CSF)	Ras/Raf/MAPK
		Flt-3 ligand	Ras/Raf/MAPK
	?	IL-32	NF-κB, p38 MAPK
	CD-4	IL-16	
	CSF-1R	IL-34	Erk
Chemokine receptors	CXC receptors	CXC ligand	MAP kinase pathway
	CC receptors	CC ligand	
	C receptors	C ligand	
	CX_3C receptors	CX_3C ligand	

a. Class II (interferon) in this table refers to all classes of interferons.

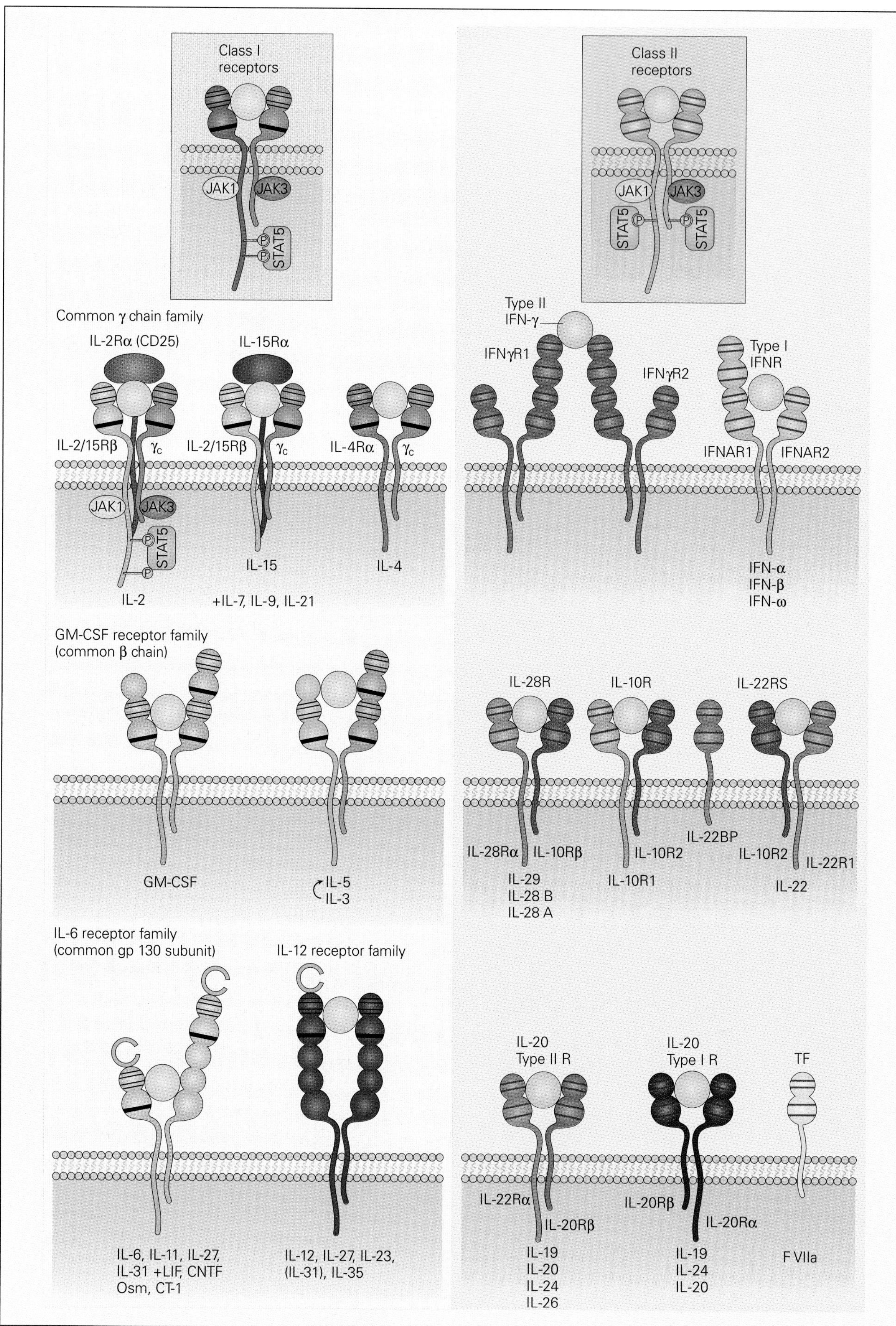

Figure 9-10A. Schematic representation of the class I and class II cytokine receptor families and subfamilies.

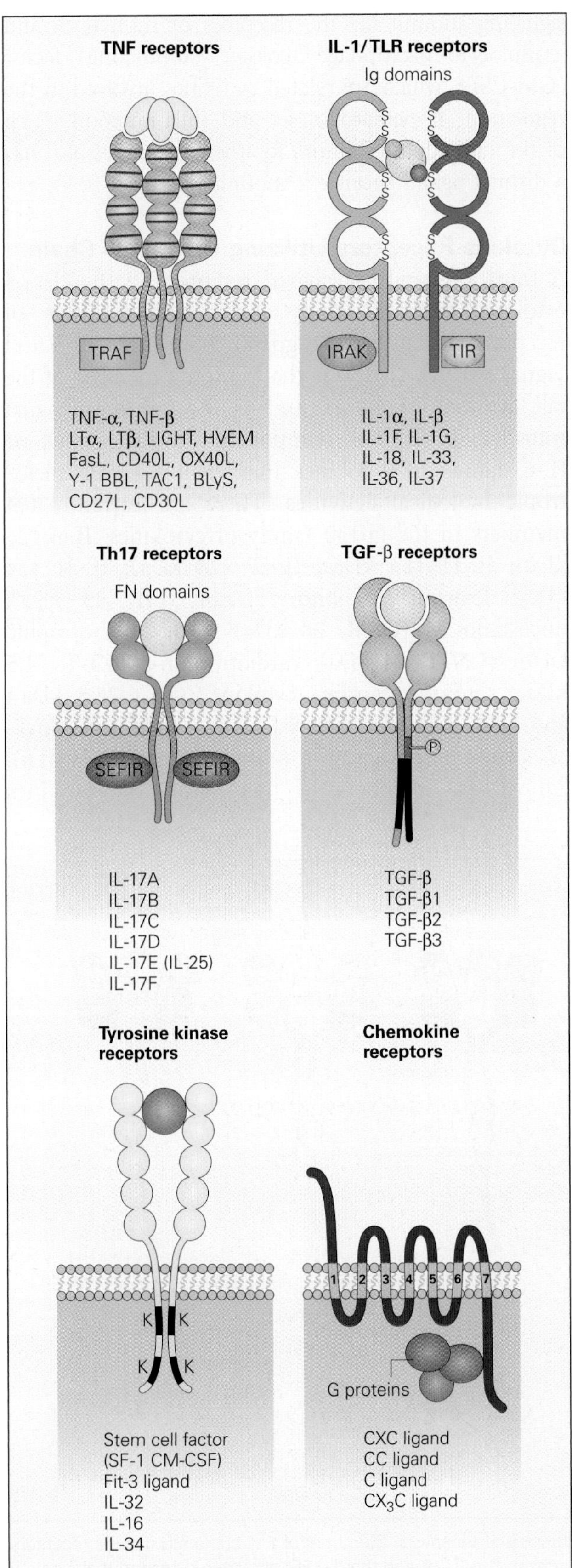

Figure 9-10B. Schematic representation of the tumor necrosis factor (TNF), IL-1/TLR, Th17, TGF-β serine kinase, tyrosine kinase, and chemokine receptor families.

Cytokine Receptor Families and Subfamilies

Class I cytokine receptors, also called hemopoietin receptors, include many interleukins and constitute the largest group among the cytokine receptor family (Table 9-5 and Figure 9-10A). As will be described in greater detail below, the class I family is divided into three subfamilies: (1) the **γc-utilizing** (common γc chain), (2) the **βc-utilizing** (GM-CSF common β chain), and (3) the **gp130-utilizing** (IL-6 receptor common gp130) subfamilies. A cardinal feature of cytokines that bind to the type 1 cytokine receptors is their similarity in a basic structure, each containing four anti-parallel α helices with two long and one short loop connection arranged in an up-up-down-down configuration (Figure 9-10A). Because of this structure, these cytokines have also been referred to as the α-helical bundle cytokine family. They contain one or more copies of a domain with two conserved pairs of cysteine residues and a membrane-proximal sequence of tryptophan (W)-serine-X-tryptophan (W)-serine (**WSXWS**), where X is any amino acid. The conserved features of the receptors form structures that bind the four α-helical cytokines, but the specificity for individual cytokines is determined by amino acid residues that vary from one receptor to another. These receptors consist of unique ligand-binding chains and one or more signal-transducing chains that are often shared by receptors for different cytokines. All the class I cytokine receptors engage JAK-STAT signaling pathways that induce new gene transcription (Table 9-5).

Subfamilies of Class I Cytokine Receptor Family: The γc Chain, the βc Chain, and gp130 Chain

A significant feature of the class I cytokine receptors is their use of a common, shared receptor subunit as a signal-transducing chain together with other cytokine-specific chains. When subgrouped by shared receptors, there are three major subfamilies of receptors in the class I cytokine receptor family: (1) those that use the γc chain, (2) others that use the βc chain, and (3) still others that use the gp130 chain (Table 9-5 and Figure 9-10A). In this respect, the shared receptors have not only taught us much about the basic structural and chemical mechanisms of protein-protein cross-reactivity in general but also have provided a better understanding of the pleomorphism and redundancy that characterize the cytokines.

Cytokine Receptors Utilizing the γc Chain

The cytokines IL-2, IL-4, IL-7, IL-9, IL-15, and IL-21 all bind to receptors that share a common γc receptor subunit (Figure 9-10A and Figure 9-11). The γc common subunit and the ligand-specific subunits are expressed predominantly on lymphocytes, although they can be found on other hematopoietic cells as well. Therefore, these cytokines are critically important for the development and function of lymphoid cells. The classic clinical consequence of this shared receptor chain is seen in the mutation of the γc gene responsible for X-linked severe combined immunodeficiency (**SCID**), which is characterized by a lack of T cells and NK cells and poorly functioning B cells (*Chapter 16*). This disorder, which has proved to be the most common form of SCID in humans, is thus designated as a T-B+ SCID. Although the lack of γc abrogates signaling by all of the cytokines that utilize this subunit (i.e., IL-2, IL-4, IL-7, IL-9, IL-15, and IL-21), the lack of IL-7 signaling is predominantly responsible for the SCID phenotype.

Cytokine Receptors Utilizing the βc Chain

A second class I cytokine receptor subfamily utilizes the βc membrane protein that serves as a shared signaling subunit for the receptors of IL-3, IL-5, and granulocyte-macrophage colony stimulating factor (**GM-CSF**), which are related cytokines involved in the regulation of hematopoiesis and inflammation. Each of the individual receptors for these cytokines also has a distinct ligand-specific α subunit (Figure 9-10A).

Cytokine Receptors Utilizing the gp130 Chain

A third subfamily of shared receptors in the class I cytokine receptor family includes the cluster of receptors that utilize the gp130 chain (Table 9-5 and Figure 9-10A). Gp130 is the founding member of the tall cytokine receptors and is the common signal transducing receptor component for the gp130, or IL-6, family of cytokines that exhibit highly pleiotropic biological activities. There are currently ten members in the gp130 family of cytokines: IL-6 (26 kDa); IL-11 (23 kDa); IL-27 (28 kDa); IL-31 (24 kDa); leukemia inhibitory factor (**LIF**, 23 kDa); oncostatin M (**OSM**, 28 kDa); ciliary neurotrophic factor (**CNTF**, 24 kDa); cardiotrophin-1 (**CT-1**, 21.5 kDa); cardiotrophin-like cytokine (**CLC**, 22.5 kDa); and an IL-6 mimic referred to as Kaposi's sarcoma–associated herpes virus IL-6-like protein (**KSHV-IL6**). All of the members of this family of cytokines

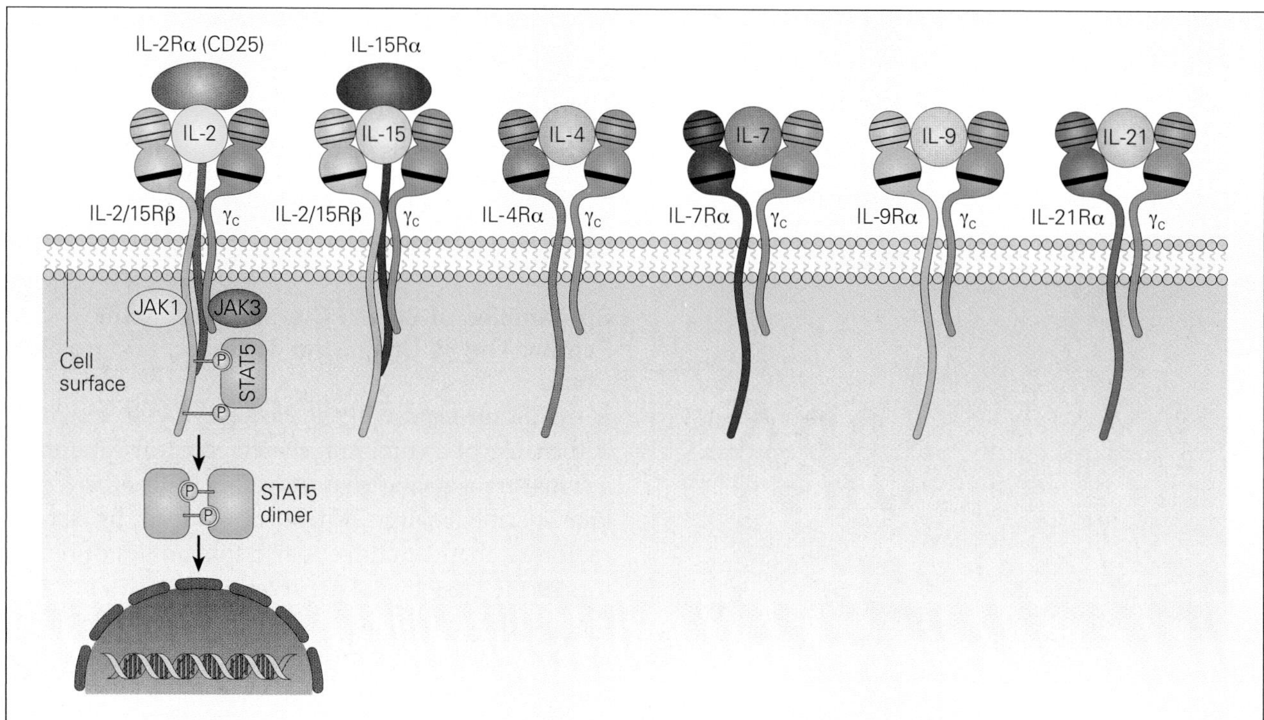

Figure 9-11. The structure of the common cytokine-receptor γ-chain subfamily of receptors. Members of this subfamily include receptors for IL-2, IL-4, IL-7, IL-9, IL-15, and IL-21, which all contain a common γc chain. The IL-2R and the IL-15R also have a second β chain IL-2/15Rβ subunit in common, but differ from each other by the presence of a unique third subunit, i.e., IL-2Rα or IL-15Rα, respectively. IL-4, IL-7, IL-9, and IL-21, in addition to having a common γc chain, each have a distinctive IL-4α, IL-7α, IL-9α, or IL-21 α chain, respectively.

signal through the common membrane receptor subunit gp130. A major distinguishing feature of gp130 cytokines is that they possess the unique site III receptor-binding site at the tip of the cytokine that is necessary for gp130 activation. In contrast, the IL-12 subfamily members (IL-12, IL-23, IL-27, IL-31 and IL-35) share either a p35 or p40 ligand chain.

Class II Cytokine Receptors

The class II cytokine receptors constitute a second major group of receptors that includes IFN-α/β, IFN-γ, IL-10, IL-19, 20, 22, 24, 26, IL-28, 29, and 30 (Figure 9-10A). These receptors are similar to type I receptors by virtue of two extracellular domains with conserved cysteines, but type II receptors do not contain the WSXWS motif (Table 9-5 and Figure 9-10A). They consist of one ligand-binding polypeptide chain and one signal-transducing chain. For example, the interferon receptors for IFN type I (IFN-α and IFN-β) and IFN type II (IFN-γ) consist of IFNAR1 and IFNAR2 and IFNGR1 and IFNGR2, respectively. In each case, the cytokine binding chains are IFNAR1 for IFN-α and IFNGR1 for IFN-γ, while the signal-transducing chain for IFN-α is the IFNAR2 and for IFN-γ is IFNGR2. All type II cytokine receptors engage JAK-STAT signaling pathways. With the exceptions of IL-22 binding protein (**IL-22BP**) and tissue factor (**TF**), receptor complexes are formed by two chains, one chain with a relatively short cytoplasmic domain (e.g., IL-10 receptor β [IL-10Rβ]) and one chain with a longer cytoplasmic domain (for example, IL-10Rα). The characteristics of this family are that since one chain is found in several receptor complexes, not only can one cytokine ligand bind to several different receptors, but also several cytokine ligands can bind to the same receptor.

TNF Family Receptors

TNF receptors belong to a large family of proteins (some are not cytokine receptors) with conserved trimeric, cysteine-rich extracellular domains, and shared intracellular signaling mechanisms that induce apoptosis and/or stimulate gene expression (Box 9-4, Table 9-1, Figure 9-10B, and Figure 9-12).

Box 9-4

TNF Cell Signaling

As will be described later in this chapter, the TNF receptor superfamily can be divided into three subfamilies on the basis of the types of intracellular signaling molecules recruited, e.g., FADD, TRADD, or TRAF. The cytoplasmic domains of several receptors, including TNFR1, Fas, DR3, DR4, and DR5, contain a conserved ~80 amino acid motif termed the death domain (DD). This element is required for recruitment of DD-containing adaptor molecules that are involved in the initiation of apoptotic cell death (see below). For this reason, these receptors have been termed "death receptors." The function of a number of death receptors may be down-regulated by decoy receptors, cell surface molecules that bind ligand but lack functional intracellular domains. Other TNF receptor superfamily receptors that lack death domains (e.g., CD27, CD30, CD40, HVEM, TNFR2, LT-βR, OX40, and 4-1BB) associate with different types of adapter molecules, most importantly members of the TRAF (TNFR-associated factor) family, as described below. Two receptors, TNFR1 (TNF receptor type 1; CD120a; p55/60) and TNFR2 (TNF receptor type 2; CD120b; p75/80), bind to TNF-α. TNFR1 is expressed in most tissues and can be fully activated by both the membrane-bound and soluble trimeric forms of TNF, whereas TNFR2 is found only in cells of the immune system and responds to the membrane-bound form of the TNF homotrimer. Although most information regarding TNF signaling is derived from TNFR1, TNFR2 is most highly expressed by Treg cells and down-regulates the pro-inflammatory TNF-TNFR1 effects.

The signaling pathway of TNFR1 is shown in Figure 9-12. Upon contact with their ligand, TNF receptors form trimers, their tips fitting into the grooves formed between TNF monomers. This binding causes a conformational change to occur in the receptor, leading to the dissociation of the inhibitory protein SODD from the intracellular death domain. This dissociation enables the adaptor protein TRADD to bind to the death domain, serving as a platform for subsequent protein binding. Following TRADD binding, three pathways can be initiated.

- **Activation of NF-κB:** TRADD recruits TRAF2 and RIP. TRAF2 in turn recruits the multicomponent protein kinase IKK, enabling the serine-threonine kinase RIP to activate it. An inhibitory protein, IκBα, that normally binds to NF-κB and inhibits its translocation, is phosphorylated by IKK and subsequently degraded, releasing NF-κB. NF-κB is a heterodimeric transcription factor that translocates to the nucleus and mediates the transcription of a vast array of proteins involved in cell survival and proliferation, inflammatory response, and anti-apoptotic factors.
- **Activation of the MAPK pathways:** Of the three major MAPK cascades, TNF is a potent activator of the stress-

(continued)

Box 9-4 (continued)

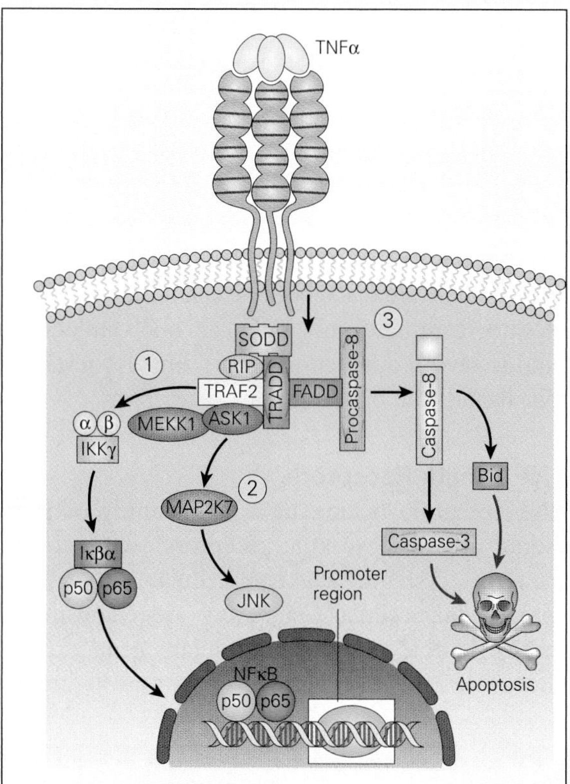

Figure 9-12. Signaling pathways of TNFR1. Step 1: Signaling adapter molecule activates the IKK complex of NF-κB to the nucleus that triggers the translation. Step 2: The activation of MAP2K7. Step 3: Activation of Caspase-8, which triggers apoptosis through the activation of Caspase-3.

related JNK group, evokes moderate response of the p38-MAPK, and is responsible for minimal activation of the classical ERKs. TRAF2 activates the JNK-inducing upstream kinases of MEKK1 and ASK1 (either directly or through GCKs and Trx, respectively), and these two kinases phosphorylate MAP2K7, which then activates JNK. JNK translocates to the nucleus and activates transcription factors such as c-Jun and ATF2. The JNK pathway is involved in cell differentiation and proliferation and is generally pro-apoptotic.

- **Induction of death signaling:** Like all death-domain-containing members of the TNFR superfamily, TNF-R1 is involved in death signaling. However, TNF-induced cell death plays only a minor role compared to its overwhelming functions in the inflammatory process. Its death-inducing capability is weak compared to other family members (such as Fas) and is often masked by the anti-apoptotic effects of NF-κB. Nevertheless, TRADD binds FADD, which then recruits the cysteine protease caspase-8. A high concentration of caspase-8 induces its autoproteolytic activation and subsequent cleaving of effector caspases, leading to cell apoptosis.

The myriad and often-conflicting effects mediated by the above pathways indicate the existence of extensive crosstalk. For instance, NF-κB enhances the transcription of C-FLIP, BCL-2, and cIAP, inhibitory proteins that interfere with death signaling. On the other hand, activated caspases cleave several components of the NF-κB pathway, including RIP, IKK, and the subunits of NF-κB itself. Other factors, such as cell type, concurrent stimulation of other cytokines, or the amount of reactive oxygen species (ROS) can shift the balance in favor of one pathway or another. Such complicated signaling ensures that whenever TNF is released, various cells with vastly diverse functions and conditions can all respond appropriately in inflammation.

As described in greater detail below, TNF is the principal mediator of the acute inflammatory response to Gram-negative bacteria and other infectious microbes and is responsible for many of the systemic complications of severe infections. The name of this cytokine derives from its original identification as a serum factor that caused necrosis of tumors. TNF is also called TNF-α to distinguish it from the closely related TNF-β (also called LT).

The TNF receptors are members of a large family of more than twenty proteins, many involved in immune and inflammatory responses. These receptors exist as trimers in the plasma membrane, even before binding of TNF (Figure 9-12). Of these receptors, the most clinically important include TNFRI, TNFRII, and CD40. There are two distinct TNF receptors: TNFRI (55 kD), expressed by most cell types; and TNFRII (75 kD), restricted to lymphoid cells. CD40 is constitutively expressed on B cells and CD40L on activated T cells, and these are important in isotype switching (*Chapter 6*).

The binding of TNF with TNFRI, TNFRII, and CD40 leads to the recruitment of proteins, called TNF receptor-associated factors (**TRAFs**) with gene expression and the production of other inflammatory mediators (Figure 9-12). As will be described later in this chapter, the binding of TNF to TNFRI also leads to another signaling pathway with recruitment of an adapter protein that activates caspases and triggers apoptosis and programmed cell death.

Clinical Relevance of TNF and TNF Receptors

Many studies have implicated TNF in the pathogenesis of the chronic inflammatory diseases rheumatoid arthritis (**RA**) and Crohn's disease (**CD**). Levels of TNF are highly elevated in the synovial fluid and the serum of patients with RA, as well as in the gut mucosa of patients with CD. This suggests that the pro-inflammatory effects of TNF might underpin the severe inflammatory symptoms observed in these diseases. Of particular relevance to RA, TNF inhibits the synthesis of proteoglycan and bone formation and stimulates resorption of proteoglycan and bone, contributing to the devastating osseous clinical manifestations of patients with severe RA. In addition, TNF-overexpressing transgenic mice develop chronic inflammatory polyarthritic disease. These findings have prompted the development of specific TNF inhibitors, which are demonstrating great benefit in the treatment of RA and CD. The two best-characterized of these inhibitors are monoclonal anti-TNF antibodies (infliximab and adalimumab) and chimeric TNFRII-Fc fusion proteins (etanercept and lenercept). Clinical studies of these compounds have demonstrated that they can induce striking improvement in RA patients (*Chapters 11* and *19*). Side effects of TNF-antagonism include increased incidence of infection, particularly with *Mycobacterium tuberculosis*, and an increased incidence of cancer. Because of this susceptibility to mycobacterial infection associated with the use of these agents, careful evaluation of patients should be performed prior to initiation of this type of therapy.

Mutations of TNFRI are associated with autosomal dominant periodic fever syndromes (*Chapters 16* and *19*). These patients have missense mutations in exons encoding the extracellular regions of TNFRI that are thought to affect normal TNFRI function, prompting the designation TNFRI-associated periodic syndromes (**TRAPS**). Humans with heterozygous mutations in the fragment apoptosis stimulating (**Fas**) receptor have also been identified with lymphadenopathy and splenomegaly due to the accumulation of unusual CD4–CD8 T cells, as well as the production of autoantibodies. In this disease, called autoimmune lymphoproliferative syndrome or ALPS, the Fas mutations act as dominant negative inhibitors of intracellular signaling, causing defective apoptosis in all carriers of Fas mutations and overt disease in a variable percentage of family members (*Chapter 16*).

The gene encoding CD40 ligand is defective in X-linked Hyper IgM syndrome (**X-HIM**), a rare inherited disorder in which affected male children generate only IgM antibodies, many of which are autoantibodies (*Chapters 6* and *16*). Patients with X-HIM frequently suffer opportunistic infections, usually bacterial, and have an increased susceptibility to cancer. In humans, mutations of transmembrane activator and calcium-modulator and cyclophilin-ligand interactor (**TACI**), a member of the TNF-receptor superfamily, and mutations of BLymphocyte stimulator (**BLyS**), also known as B cell activating factor (**BAFF**), have been found in patients with common variable immunodeficiency affecting B cell numbers and function (*Chapter 16*).

IL-1/TLR Family

The IL-1/TLR family of receptors comprises at least eleven members capable of binding IL-1, IL-18, and IL-1F5-10, IL-33 (IL-1F11) (Table 9-5 and Figure 9-10B). IL-1 mediates its biologic effects through a membrane receptor called the type I IL-1 receptor, which engages signal transduction pathways that activate NF-κB and AP-1 transcription factors. There are three members of the IL-1 gene family: two antagonists, IL-1α and IL-1β, and one IL-1 receptor antagonist (IL-1Ra). IL-1α is usually active in a membrane-associated form, while IL-1β functions as a soluble cytokine. The type I IL-1 receptor is a member of a family of integral membrane proteins that contain an extracellular ligand-binding Ig domain and a Toll-IL-1 receptor (**TIR**) signaling domain in the cytoplasmic region. The TIR domain was described in reference to TLRs in Chapter 3. The signaling events that occur when IL-1 binds to the type I IL-1 receptor are similar to those associated with TLRs.

The biologic effects of IL-1 are similar to those of TNF and appear to be dose-dependent. When secreted at low concentrations, IL-1 functions as a mediator of local inflammation acting on endothelial cells to increase expression of surface molecules that mediate leukocyte adhesion, such as ligands for integrins (*Chapter 5*). When secreted in larger quantities, IL-1 enters the bloodstream and exerts systemic endocrine effects, including fever (this is why IL-1 was sometimes called endogenous pyrogen), synthesis of acute-phase plasma proteins by the liver, and neutrophil and platelet production by the bone marrow. The biologic similarities between IL-1 and TNF end there.

Because the cytokines and their receptors are structurally different, there are several differences between the function of the two cytokines, e.g., IL-1 does not induce apoptotic death of cells. However, administration of IL-1 to cancer patients was shown to result in severe hypotension and shock.

IL-1/TLR Signaling

There are two cell surface receptors for IL-1: type I (**IL-1RI**) and type II (**IL-1RII**). Both of these bind ligand (Figure 9-13), but only IL-1RI transduces signal. Ligand binding to IL-1R, IL-18R, and TLRs results in NF-κB activation. These receptors all associate with the adapter protein MyD88. Notably, MyD88 has a C-terminal TIR domain and an N-terminal death domain. MyD88 allows the recruitment of IL-1 receptor-associated kinase (**IRAK**), which also has an N-terminal death domain. IRAK, in turn, permits the recruitment and activation of a member of the TRAF family, TRAF6. This leads to the activation of other kinases, including the phophosphorylation of IκB, which leads to its degradation within proteosomes, freeing bound NF-κB for nuclear translocation. The IL-RII captures IL-1 with high affinity and prevents it from activating IL-RI. It has therefore been called a decoy receptor (Figure 9-13) and is used as an IL-1 antagonist.

Clinical Relevance of IL-1 and IL-1/TLR Receptors

Because of the importance of IL-1 in the pathogenesis of fever, it logically follows that agents that inhibit IL-1 would be therapeutically useful. Indeed, IL-1Ra, the naturally produced antagonist, has been studied in a variety of settings. The IL-1Ra drug, anakinra, has been found to be efficacious in the treatment of rheumatoid arthritis as well as other autoinflammatory disorders, including Muckle-Wells disease, neonatal multisystem inflammatory disease, and Still's disease. Recently, the human monoclonal antibody, canakinumab, which targets IL-1β, was approved by the FDA for the treatment of cryopyrin-associated periodic syndromes (**CAPS**), specifically familial cold autoinflammatory syndrome (**FCAS**) and Muckle-Wells syndrome (**MWS**) (*Chapters 11* and *19*).

Th17 Receptors

For more than twenty years, the dominant paradigm in T cell-mediated disease, whether infectious or autoimmune, stated that immune responses are controlled by Th1 or Th2 cells. Th1 cells secrete IFN-γ and are induced to differentiate by cues from IL-12, whereas Th2 cells secrete IL-4, IL-5, and IL-13, and are triggered to develop by IL-4. Development of each T-helper lineage is self-reinforcing and mutually antagonistic, and all immunologically mediated diseases have traditionally been viewed in the confines of this model. A major evolution in T cell biology occurred with the discovery of a new subset of CD4+T cells, termed Th17 after their signature cytokine, IL-17 (Table 9-5, Figure 9-10B, and *Chapter 7*). The implications for understanding—and ultimately treating—autoimmunity are profound. For years, it was considered that Th1 cells were the major mediators of inflammation in autoimmune syndromes, particularly in rheumatoid arthritis, Crohn's disease, and multiple sclerosis, but it is now evident that Th17 cells are the primary drivers of these autoimmune diseases. This discovery emerged from reports comparing IL-12 and IL-23, the heterodimeric cytokines that share a common subunit, IL-12p40 (Figure 9-10A).

In addition to secreting IL-17, Th17 cells produce other pro-inflammatory cytokines, including IL-6, IL-11, IL-17F, IL-22, IL-26, IL-1β, TNF-α, GM-CSF, and various chemokines (Figure 9-14). Collectively, these factors induce expression of classic inflammatory effectors, including IL-6, CXC chemokines, and acute-phase proteins. IL-17A and its close homolog IL-17F are co-expressed in Th17 cells and share a chromatin locus that undergoes remodeling.

As described previously, there exists an important inverse relationship between Th17 and Treg cells with reference to their role in mucosal immunity. Dendritic cells favor the development of FOXP3+ Treg cells in response to commensal bacteria by the conversion of vitamin A to retinoic acid, which in turn down-regulates the production of Th17 cells through inhibition of RORγt. Failure of vitamin A conversion following exposure of dendritic cells to pathogenic bacteria, on the other hand, will lead to the inhibition of Treg development and will upregulate the production of Th17 cells through activation of RORγt by IL-6 and IL-23.

TGF-β Receptor Serine Kinase Family

The TGF-β serine kinase family are a family of more than forty cytokines that inhibit cellular proliferation and can induce apoptosis of a variety of cell types. TGF-βs are involved in a number of biological processes, including tissue remodeling, wound repair,

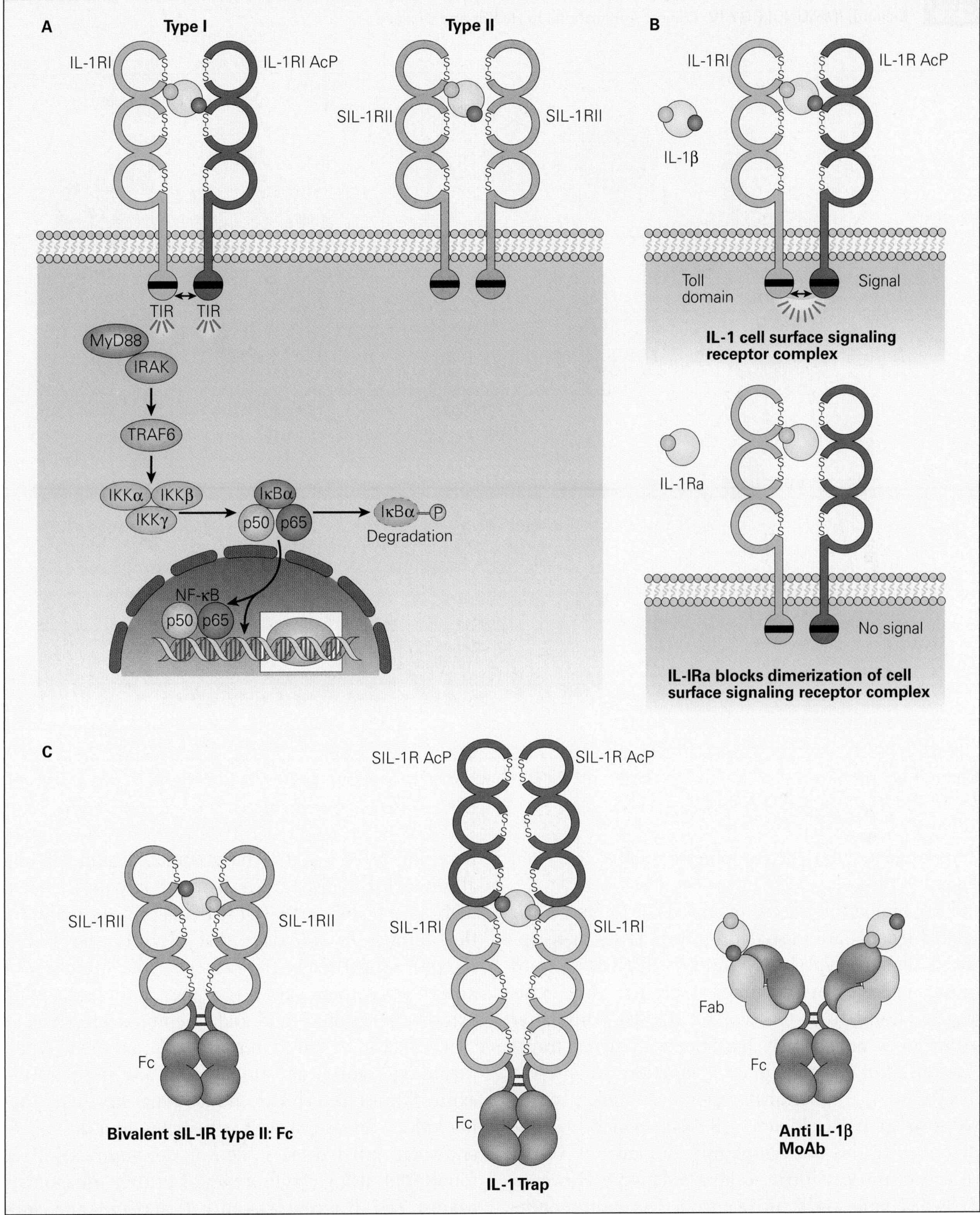

Figure 9-13. Mechanisms of signal transduction by IL-1 receptor (IL-1R) and related receptors. Panel A: The cytokine IL-1β has two different receptor binding sites (IL-1RI [green]) and IL-1 receptor accessory protein (IL-1R AcP) [blue]). The IL-1 receptor type I (IL-1RI) binds one site of IL-1β (green) and IL-1R AcP engages the second site (blue). The resulting complex activates the cell. The IL-1 receptor type II (SIL-1RII) consists of two identical SIL-1RII chains, and since IL-1β can bind only one of these chains, signaling does not occur, and it functions only as a decoy receptor. Panel B: The naturally occurring IL-1 receptor antagonist (IL-1Ra) possesses only IL-1RI binding site and, therefore, following binding of the IL-1Ra antagonist with the type I IL-1 receptor, it prevents bona fide IL-1β from binding to its receptor. This forms the basis of the clinical use of a commercially available biologic immune modifier (anakinra). Panel C: The soluble IL-1 receptor type 2 (SIL-1RII) is shown as a bivalent construction of the extracellular domains of the receptor; two identical chains are linked by the Fc segment of IgG1. The IL-1 trap contains the extracellular segment of both IL-1 receptor chains fused into a dimeric molecule using the complement domain of IgG1. The IL-1 trap allows high-affinity IL-1β binding similar to that on the cell surface. Monoclonal antibodies that can bind and neutralize two IL-1β molecules (canakinumab) cytokine traps (Rilonacept) may present some advantages over other cytokine-targeting agents. (Adapted from Dinarello CA. Setting the cytokine trap for autoimmunity. Nat Med. 2003;9:20–2.)

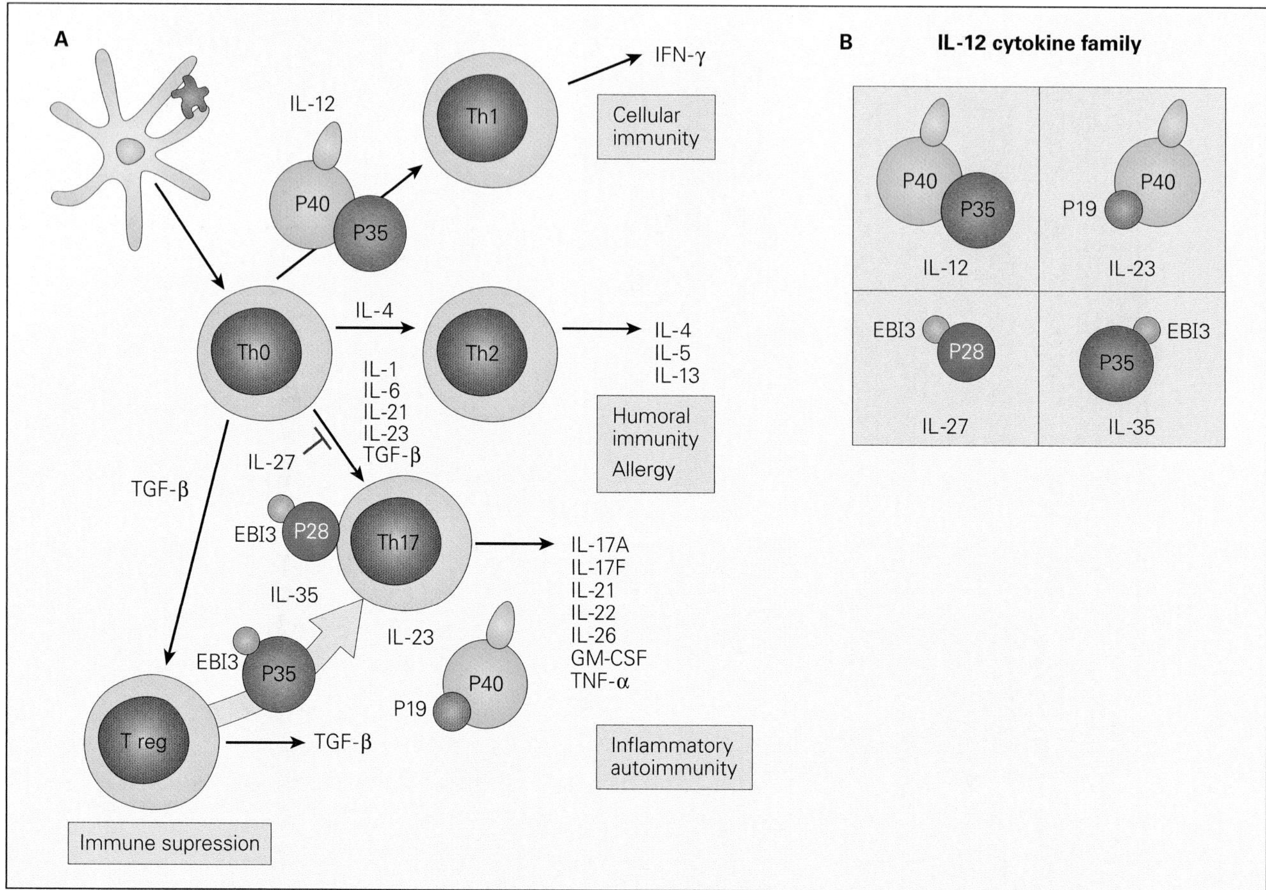

Figure 9-14. Mechanism of signal transduction by Th17 and related receptors showing the inverse relationship between Treg and Th17 cells.

development, and hematopoiesis (Table 9-5 and Figure 9-10B).

The biological effects of the TGF-βs and their related ligands are mediated by two classes of receptor, designated type I (RI) and type II (RII). A third group of receptors, denoted type III, also exists (e.g., TGF-βRIII in the case of TGF-β). This latter group does not actively participate in signal transduction, but is thought to function to present ligands to the functional receptors. Similar to the receptor tyrosine kinases (**RTKs**), which will be described below, the cytoplasmic domains of TGF-β receptors possess intrinsic kinase activity. However, TGF-βRI and TGF-βRII encode serine/threonine kinases. The signaling cascade appears to be initiated by the binding of TGF-β to the type II receptor, inducing the assembly of a ternary complex containing TGF-β, TGF-βRII, and TGF-βRI.

TGF-β receptors are serine/threonine kinase receptors that exist in several different forms. There are three TGF-β receptor types that are distinguished by their structural and functional properties. Receptor types I and II have similar ligand binding affinities for TGF-β1; TGF-β receptor type III has a high affinity for both TGF-β1 and -β2. In addition, the number of cytokines that bind to the TGF-β receptor superfamily far exceeds the number of known receptors, suggesting the promiscuity that exists between the ligand and receptor interactions.

TGF-β can be found in many different tissue types, including brain, heart, kidney, liver and testes. Overexpression of TGF-β can induce renal fibrosis, causing kidney disease, as well as diabetes, and ultimately end-stage renal disease. Recent developments have found that, using certain types of protein antagonists against TGF-β receptors can halt and in some cases reverse the effects of renal fibrosis.

Signaling

Ligand binding of TGF-β first occurs to the type II receptor, which then allows the recruitment of the type I receptor (Figure 9-15). The type II receptor is

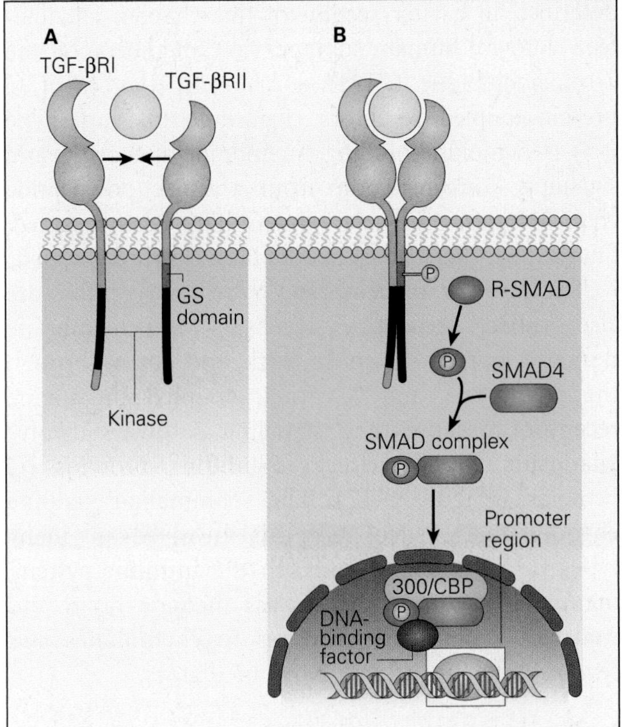

Figure 9-15. Schematic representation of TGF-β signaling pathways. Panel A: TGF-β first binds to TGF-βRII, which then recruits TGF-βRI. Panel B: Following the joining of the two receptor chains, the constitutively active kinase found on TGF-βRII then phosphorylates the GS domain of TGF-βRI. The phosphorylated GS domain is responsible for phosphorylating other key signaling intermediates, referred to as SMADs, a class of proteins that modulate the activity of TGF-β ligands. They form complexes, often with other SMADs, enter the nucleus, serve as transcription factors, and regulate transcription of specific target genes.

thought to have a constitutively active kinase that phosphorylates the type I receptor. The type I receptor is structurally distinct from the type II receptor in having a juxtamembrane domain that precedes the kinase domain, which is referred to as the GS domain. It is this site that is phosphorylated by the type II receptor following which the phosphorylated GS is responsible for phosphorylating other key signaling intermediates referred to as SMADs, a class of proteins that modulate the activity of transforming growth factor beta ligands. They form complexes, often with other SMADs, enter the nucleus, serve as transcription factors, and regulate transcription of specific target genes. It is not clear whether activation of the type I receptor is due to enhancement of its kinase activity, to the appearance of substrate-binding sites, or to a combination of the two.

Receptor Tyrosine Kinases

Receptor tyrosine kinases (**RTKs**) are the high-affinity cell surface receptors for many polypeptide growth factors, e.g., epidermal growth factor (**EGF**), cytokines, and hormones, e.g., insulin (Table 9-5 and Figure 9-10B). These receptors have been shown to be not only key regulators of normal cellular processes but also to play a critical role in the development and progression of many types of cancer. Many new therapeutic agents for neoplastic disease have shown efficacy by inhibiting these tyrosine kinase-signaling pathways.

Although most of the RTKs not typically classified as receptors for cytokines, some are. These include receptors for colony-stimulating factor-1 (**CSF-1**), stem cell factor (**SCF**, **c-KIT ligand**, or **Steel factor**), platelet-derived growth factor (**PDGF**), and FMS-like tyrosine kinase 3 ligand (**FLT3-L**). All of these have important hematological effects and tend to be included in discussions of cytokines. The structure of SCF and CSF-1 is similar to that of the cytokines that bind class I receptors, as they too form four α-helical bundles, even though their receptors are entirely distinct. The similarities in the three-dimensional structure point to a common evolutionary ancestor. It is therefore reasonable to define these factors as cytokines. The receptors in this subfamily typically have five immunoglobulin-like loops in their ligand-binding extracellular domains. The cytoplasmic domain contains a tyrosine kinase catalytic domain interrupted by an "insert region" that does not share homology with other tyrosine kinases. This segment is used to recruit various signaling molecules.

Family Members and Actions of RTKs

Bone marrow stromal cells can synthesize SCF as either a secreted or a transmembrane protein. SCF is required to make stem cells responsive to other CSFs. SCF is widely expressed during embryogenesis and is also detectable in the circulation of normal adults. It has effects on germ cells, melanocytes, and hematopoietic precursors, as well as important effects on the differentiation of mast cells. Naturally occurring mouse mutations of SCF (Steel) or its receptor (W) have been recognized for many years. These mice have defects in hematopoiesis and fertility, lack mast cells, and have absent coat pigmentation.

CSF-1, also known as monocyte-macrophage-CSF or macrophage-CSF (**M-CSF**), is a hematopoietic growth factor that supports the survival and differentiation of monocytic cells. It is produced by a wide variety of cells, including monocytes, smooth muscle cells, endothelial cells, and fibroblasts. M-CSF-deficient mice manifest monocytopenia and osteopetrosis. IL-34 is a new cytokine that binds to the CSF-1 receptor. FLT3-L synergizes with other cytokines, including SCF, in inducing proliferation of hematopoietic precursors. FLT3-L is also an important regulator of dendritic cells.

Tyrosine Kinase Signaling

The first step in signaling by the RTKs is ligand-induced receptor dimerization (Figure 9-16). Dimerization brings the two kinase domains into proximity and results in the activation of phosphotransferase activity. This leads to autophosphorylation of the receptor subunits on the tyrosine residues, which are then bound by a variety of signaling molecules, initiating signal transduction. During this important step, the signaling and adapter molecules recognize phosphotyrosine residues on the RTKs by virtue of either their src homology 2 (**SH2**) domains or their phosphotyrosine-binding (**PTB**) domains.

Chemokine Receptors

Chemokine receptors activate directional cellular migration upon binding chemokines. As will be described in a later section of this chapter, all nineteen known human subtypes are members of the 7-transmembrane (**7TM**) domain superfamily of G protein-coupled receptors (Figure 9-10B and Table 9-5). Chemokine-binding, membrane-anchoring and signaling domains come from a single polypeptide chain. Homo- and heterodimers have been reported, but the physiologic form has not been clearly delineated.

The seven-transmembrane α-helical receptors are also called serpentine receptors transmembrane domains appear to snake back and forth through the membrane, and G protein-coupled chemokine receptors, because their signaling pathways involve guanosine triphosphate GTP-binding proteins (G proteins) (Figure 9-17). The mammalian genome encodes many such receptors involved in many types of sensory responses. In the immune system, members of this receptor class mediate rapid and transient mobilizing responses to chemokines and several different inflammatory mediators.

The Interleukins

The interleukins (ILs) are cytokines that regulate the communication and crosstalk between and among the many cells that comprise the innate and adaptive immune systems as well as with other non-immune target cells and tissues such as endothelial and epithelial cells. Shown in Table 9-6 is a list of the major interleukins that have been identified together with their targets and some examples of their mechanisms of action.

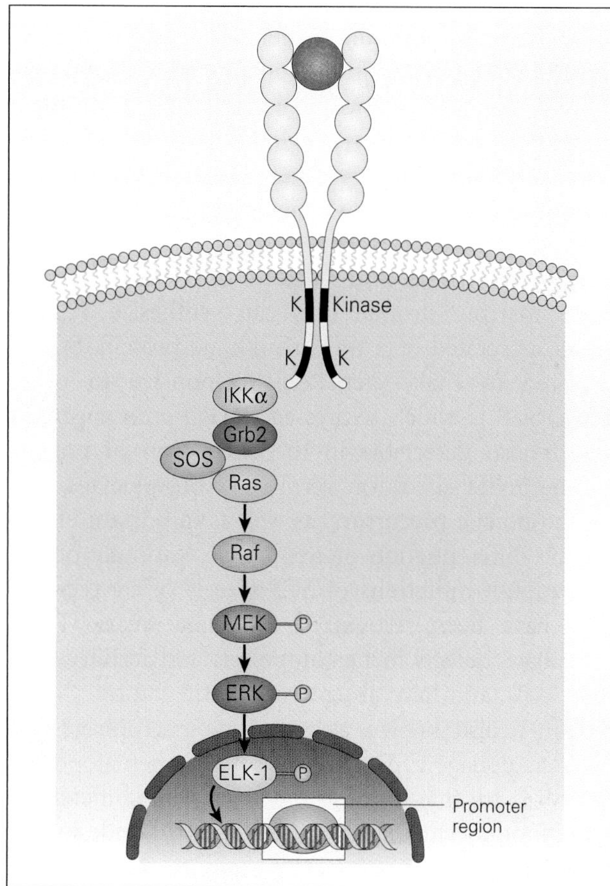

Figure 9-16. Mechanism of signal transduction by receptor tyrosine kinases.

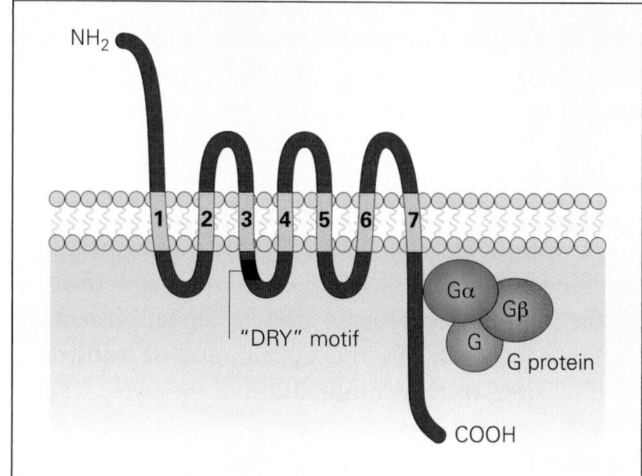

Figure 9-17. The seven-transmembrane α-helix structure of a G-protein-coupled chemokine receptor.

Interleukin-1

Interleukin-1 (IL-1), one of the first cytokines to be identified, was originally described functionally as a factor that could promote inflammation and fever, activate thymocytes and lymphocytes, increase the number of bone marrow cells, and cause degeneration of bone joints by stimulating osteoclasts to resorb bone. IL-1 has two distinct forms, IL-1α and IL-1β; these two forms are 26 percent homologous at the amino acid level and belong to a family of cytokines known as the IL-1 superfamily (Table 9-7). IL-1α usually acts locally as a membrane-associated cytokine, while IL-1β acts systemically as a soluble cytokine. One of the functions of IL-1 is to enhance the activation of T cells in response to antigen. The activation of T cells by IL-1 leads to increased T cell production of IL-2 and of the IL-2 receptor, which in turn augments the activation of the T cells in an autocrine loop. IL-1 also induces expression of IFN-γ by T cells. This effect of T cell activation by IL-1 is mimicked by other pro-inflammatory cytokines such as IL-6 and TNF-α. In addition to its effects on T cells, IL-1 can induce proliferation in non-lymphoid cells. Both IL-1α and IL-1β form an important part of the inflammatory response of the body against infection and in the regulation of hematopoiesis. Both forms of IL-1 can increase the expression of adhesion factors on endothelial cells, enhancing the transmigration of leukocytes from the vascular compartment to tissue sites of infection and can also reset the hypothalamus thermoregulatory center, leading to an increased body temperature. IL-1 was originally referred to as endogenous pyrogen and is an important component of the inflammatory response that helps the body's immune system to fight infection (*Chapter 5*).

The IL-1s are secreted primarily by dendritic cells and macrophages but also from neutrophils, endothelial cells, smooth muscle cells, glial cells, astrocytes, B and T cells, fibroblasts, and keratinocytes (Table 9-6). Production of IL-1 by these different cell types occurs only in response to cellular stimulation, specifically in response to PAMPs, which bind to detection molecules of the innate immune system, called pattern-recognition receptors (**PRRs**), e.g., TLRs, and by stimulants of the inflammasome pathway, as will be described below. TLRs are not only present on cell surface membranes but also within cytoplasmic membrane-bound vesicles and induce intracellular signaling cascades that give rise to the production of IL-1 and other inflammatory cytokines (*Chapter 3*). As described previously, there are two forms of IL-1 receptors, IL-1RI and IL-RII. Both forms of IL-1 bind to IL-1RI, which is composed of two related (but not identical) subunits, i.e., IL-1RI and IL-1RI AcP that transmit intracellular signals via a common pathway that is shared with certain other receptors, including the Toll family of innate immune detectors and the receptors for IL-18 and IL-33. IL-1RII, in contrast, binds IL-1α and IL-1β, but does not transduce signals. IL-1RII, therefore, acts as a decoy receptor that can sequester IL-1 and prevent it from activating IL-1RI (Figure 9-13).

The Interleukin-1 Superfamily

Shown in Table 9-7 are other members of the interleukin-1 superfamily in addition to IL-1α and IL-1β. IL-1 receptor antagonist (**IL-1Ra**) is a cytokine that competes for receptor binding with IL-1α and IL-1β, blocking their role in immune activation. Two other cytokines, IL-18 and IL-33, have structural homologies with IL-1 and signal via IL-18R and ST2 to produce Th1 or Th2 cytokines, respectively.

Inflammasomes, the Innate Immune System, and IL-1

As previously described in Chapter 3, the innate immune system provides a critical protective function during the initial phase of microbial invasion as well as a homeostatic safeguard for the removal of worn out or effete cellular components during the healthy physiologic state using germline-encoded PRRs that not only detect danger signals generated by microbes but also by endogenous products of injured tissues that also can initiate inflammatory responses. In this respect, a major pathway utilized by the innate immune system to carry out these functions relies on the production of potent pro-inflammatory cytokines, most notably IL-1β, through specialized cytoplasmic multimeric protein structures called **inflammasomes** found within phagocytic cells of the innate immune system, particularly dendritic cells and macrophages. The inflammasome (from the Latin word *inflammare*, which means to set on fire; from the Greek word *soma*, which means body) is a danger-sensing complex that triggers innate immunity-linked inflammatory processes by induction of pyroptosis, a process of programmed cell death distinct from apoptosis (*Chapter 5*). In the detection of external and internal pathogenic signals, the innate immune system utilizes five types of PRRs: (1) TLRs, (2) C-type lectin receptors (**CLRs**), (3) nucleotide-binding oligomerization domanis (**NOD**)-like

Table 9-6. The major interleukins: Sites of production, targets, and actions

Interleukin	Produced mainly by	Major targets	Examples of actions
IL-1	Macrophages, monocytes, dendritic cells, neutrophils, endothelial cells, smooth muscle cells, glial cells, astrocytes, T cells, fibroblasts, keratinocytes, and synovial cells	Endothelial cells, adhesion factors, hypothalamus, leukocytes, hepatocytes, thymocytes, and lymphocytes	Co-stimulation of APCs and T cells, promotes inflammation and fever, acute phase response, hematopoiesis
IL-2	Th1 cells, NK cells	Th0 cells, CD8 cytotoxic cells, Treg cells, B cells	Activation and proliferation of T cells, enhancement of NK functions, Treg cell survival; apoptosis of lymphocytes
IL-3	T cells	Hematopoietic stem cells, bone marrow stromal cells, dendritic cells	Growth of hematopoietic progenitor cells, stimulates granulocyte production
IL-4	Th2 cells, mast cells, eosinophils, NKT cells, $\gamma\delta$ T cells	T cells, B cells, macrophages	Th2 cell differentiation and humoral immunity, B cell proliferation, IgE and MHC-II expression on B cells, eosinophil and mast cell growth and function, inhibition of IFN-γ production
IL-5	Th2 cells, mast cells, NK cells	Eosinophils, B cells, T cells	Stimulates production and function of eosinophils
IL-6	T cells, macrophages	B cells, T cells, hepatocytes, megakaryocytes, macrophages, endothelial cells, and fibroblasts	Mediator of inflammation, acute phase response, fever, B cell proliferation, thrombopoiesis, synergistic with IL-1 and TNF on T cells and with TGF-β in the differentiation of Th17 cells
IL-7	Stromal cells	Immature and mature T and B lymphocytes	Development of T, B, and NK cells and homeostasis
IL-8 (CXCL8)	Macrophages, epithelial cells, endothelial cells, keratinocytes, synovial cells, hepatocytes	Neutrophils, CD8 cells, endothelial cells	A chemokine; chemoattractant properties for neutrophils and CD8 T cells; proangiogenic
IL-9	Th2 cells	Th2 cells, mast cells; switch to IgE	Promotes allergic inflammation; antiparasitic
IL-10	Th2 cells, macrophages, tumor cells, B cells, Tr1 cells	Th1 cells, B cells, DCs	Inhibits cytokine production, suppresses cellular immunity, promotes B cell proliferation and antibody production, mast cell growth
IL-11	Bone marrow stroma	B cells, myeloid progenitor cells, megakaryocytes, hepatocytes	Lymphopoietic/hematopoietic and osteotrophic properties; acute phase response
IL-12	Myeloid dendritic cells, macrophages, blastoid B cells	Th1 cells, NK cells	Differentiation and proliferation of Th1 cells and NK cells, IFN-γ production, suppresses Th2 responses
IL-13	Th2 cells, mast cells, eosinophils	B cells; activation of monocytes, mast cells and eosinophils	IL-4-like activities, important mediator of allergic inflammation and disease; Th2 polarization
IL-14	This cytokine has not been identified at the gene level		
IL-15	Macrophages, epithelial cells, EC, NK cells, T cells, non-T cells, muscle cells, fibroblasts	NK cells, T cells	Lymphocyte effects and activation of NK cells, lymphoproliferative

Table 9-6. The major interleukins: Sites of production, targets, and actions (continued)

Interleukin	Produced mainly by	Major targets	Examples of actions
IL-16	Lymphocytes, epithelial cells	CD4+ T cells, eosinophils, macrophages, DCs, mast cells	Chemotactic for monocytes, eosinophils, dendritic cells and CD4+ T cells
IL-17 Family	CD4+ and CD8+ T cells, Th17 cells, NK cells	T cells, fibroblasts, APCs, neutrophils	Drives acute inflammatory responses and promotes autoimmune diseases
IL-18	Macrophages, keratinocytes, astrocytes, DCs, osteoblasts	Th1 cells, NK cells	Together with IL-12 induces Th1 cell-mediated immunity by stimulating NK cells and T cells with release of IFN-γ
IL-19	B cells, monocytes, and nonimmune epithelial tissues	Monocytes, T cells, keratinocytes	Inflammatory responses, wound healing, re-epithelialization
IL-20	Skin, synovial fibroblasts, macrophages, endothelial cells, epithelial cells	Keratinocytes, fibroblasts	Regulates proliferation and differentiation of keratinocytes during inflammation, particularly inflammation associated with the skin, e.g., psoriasis
IL-21	Activated CD4+ T cells and NKT cells	CD4+ and CD8+ T cells, B cells, NK cells	Important in destruction of virally infected or cancerous cells
IL-22	Th22 CD4+ T lymphocytes, Th17, NK cells, macrophages, fibroblasts	Hepatocytes, fibroblasts, keratinocytes, mesangial cells, epithelial cells	IL-22 suppresses inflammation, acute phase response, and autoimmune diseases; promotes wound repair and epithelial barrier function
IL-23	Antigen presenting cells, dendritic cells, synovial fibroblasts, macrophages	Th17 memory cells	Stimulates Th17 cells to produce cytokines known to drive inflammatory responses, including TNF, IL-6, IL-17, GM-CSF, CXCL1, and CCL20
IL-24	Monocytes, macrophages and T cells, keratinocytes, melanocytes	Skin, lung, reproductive tissues, and tumor cells	Promotes wound healing, psoriasis, and tumor cell apoptosis
IL-25 (IL-17E)	Th2 cells, mast cells, eosinophils, basophils, epithelial cells	Th2 cells, switch to IgE	Induces Th2 responses, suppresses IL-17, regulates immunity of the gut, and is implicated in chronic inflammation of the gastrointestinal tract
IL-26	Memory T cells, mast cells	Epithelial cells	Proinflammatory effects; induces the transcription factors STAT1 and STAT3, which enhance IL-10 and IL-8 secretion and expression of the CD54 molecule on the surface of epithelial cells
IL-27	Macrophages, dendritic cells, and epithelial cells	Th1 cells; suppresses Th17 precursors and induces IL-10	Acts in synergy with IL-12 in the induction of Th1 cells, induces production of IFN-γ, MHC-I expression, anti-angiogenic effects, inhibits differentiation of Th17 cells

(continued)

Table 9-6. The major interleukins: Sites of production, targets, and actions (continued)

Interleukin	Produced mainly by	Major targets	Examples of actions
IL-28/IFN-λ2, 3 IL-29/IFN-λ1	Virus-infected cells, myeloid DCs	Virus-infected cells	Antiviral effects; IL-28 has two isoforms, IL-28A (IFNλ2) and IL-28B (IFNλ3); together with IL-29 (IFNλ3) belongs to the IFN-λ family. Like other IFNs, IL-28 and IL-29 play a role in immune defense against viruses. IFN-λ molecules signal through a receptor formed by an interferon receptor subunit, IL-28RA, and the IL-10R, common to several members of the IL-10 family.
IL-30	IL-30 and EBI3 form the IL-27 heterodimer expressed by antigen-presenting cells, i.e., dendritic cells	Naïve CD4+ cells	Promotes polarization toward a Th1 phenotype with expression of γ-interferon and IL-10 induction
IL-31	Th2 cells	Monocytes, epithelial cells, keratinocytes, eosinophils	Plays a role in cell-mediated immunity and inflammatory skin diseases
IL-32	T cells, monocytes, fibroblasts, epithelial cells and NK cells	T cells and monocytes	Induces proinflammatory cytokines, TNF-α, IL-1β, IL-6 and CXC chemokine family members and stimulates the release of prostaglandins from monocytes
IL-33	Endothelial cells, epithelial cells, fibroblasts, smooth muscle cells, dendritic cells, activated macrophages, and Th2 cells	Th2 cells	IL-1 family member, induces Th2 cells to produce type 2 cytokines
IL-34	Many tissues and spleen	Macrophage progenitors and CSF-1R+ monocytes	Generates myeloid progenitors and activates monocytes
IL-35 (mouse)	Treg cells	CD25+ lymphocytes, suppresses Th17 cells	Inhibits CD4+CD25$^-$ and Th17 cells, suppresses autoimmune disease
IL-36 α,β,γ IL-1 F6, F8, F9 (IL-1Rrp2 & AcP)	Skin and monocytes	Macrophages, DCs	Elevated in skin inflammation
IL-36Ra IL-1 F5 (IL-1Rrp2 & AcP)	Monocytes, B cells, DCs/Langerhans cells, keratinocytes, and gastric fundus parietal and chief cells	Macrophages, DCs	Antagonist of IL-36
IL-37 IL-1 F7	Monocytes, DCs, epithelial cells, tumor cells	Inhibits DCs and macrophages	Anti-inflammatory by suppressing IL-12, IL-3, IL-6, TNF and chemokines; synergizes with TGF-β

receptors (**NLRs**), (4) RIG-like helicases (**RLHs**), and (5) DNA sensors absent in melanoma 2 (**AIM2**) and (DNA-dependent activator of IFN (**DAI**)-regulatory factors) (Table 9-8). These receptors recognize conserved molecular moieites found on a wide variety of microbes (**"nonself"**) as well as those present in disorganized or modified self-structural proteins (**"modified self"**). Collectively, these danger-detecting PRRs recognize innate-stimulating triggers known as PAMPs or danger-associated molecular patterns (**DAMPs**) or alarmins, respectively (*Chapter 3*).

Location of PRRs

Generally, PRRs are found in two forms in the cell, either as (1) **membrane-associated PRRs**, located on the surface membranes of cells or as intra-cytosolic membrane-structured vesicles; and (2) **nonmembrane-associated PRRs**, found only in the cytosol as free structures (Table 9-8 and Figure 9-18). For example, the C-type lectin receptors and some of the TLRs that predominantly sense bacterial moieties, i.e., TLR-1, 2, 4, 5, 6, and 10, are found on the cell surface, while those TLRs

Table 9-7. The interleukin-1 superfamily

Member	Other names	Structural characteristics	Function
IL-1F1 IL-1F2 IL-1F3 IL-1F4 IL-1F5/IL-36Ra IL-1F6/IL-36α IL-1F7/IL-37 IL-1F8/IL-36β IL-1F9/IL-36γ IL-1F10 (IL-38) IL-1F11	IL-1α IL-1β IL-1Ra IL-18, IFN-γ-inducing factor IL-36Ra IL-36α, IL-1Rrp2 IL-37 IL-36β, IL-1Rrp2 IL-36γ, IL-1Rrp2 IL-1H IL-1ε, IL-1Hy2, IL-33	Components of the IL-1 cytokine	Pro-inflammatory cytokines; wide range of autoimmune and febrile; Autoinflammatory diseases, e.g., RA, IBD, psoriasis, FMF, gout, type II diabetes
IL-1 Receptor Antagonist (IL-1Ra)	IL-36Ra IL-1F7 IL-1F10	Heterodimer	Blocks effects of IL-1; Wide range of autoimmune and inflammatory diseases, RA, IBD, psoriasis
IL-18 IL-33	IL-1F4 IL-1F11	Structural homology Structural homology	IL-1-like cytokines that signal via IL-18R or the ST-2 receptor and induce Th1 or Th2 cytokines, respectively

that sense nucleic acids, such as ss RNA, ds RNA and CpGDNA, i.e., TLR3, 7, 8, and 9, respectively, are found within cytosolic double-membraned vesicles (*Chapter 3*). The NLRs, the RLHs, and the DNA sensors (i.e., AIM2 and DAI), on the other hand, are examples of free cytosolic PRR structures.

The PRRs were initially shown to discriminate self from nonself, recognizing microbial products or PAMPs to stimulate innate immunity to fight infections. More recently, this distinction is proving to be more complex and it is now well-recognized that endogenous ligands, released from dying or damaged cells, or metabolic products, e.g., uric acid, can also provide danger signals or alarmins that trigger these PRRs. The sensing of these exogenous and endogenous danger signals is rapidly being recognized in the etiology of a wide array of diseases ranging from autoimmunity to cancer.

Structure and Function of the PRRs

The basic structure of the PRRs involves the scaffolding of various protein domains with one another into critical locations within cells. Components and specific structures of individual PRRs are shown in Table 9-8 and Figure 9-18 and are described in Box 9-5.

The basic function of innate immunity is to control infection and eliminate pathogens as well as to marshal the T and B cell responses of adaptive

Table 9-8. PRRs of the innate immune system and their danger-inducing ligands

Pattern-recognition receptors (PRRs)	Danger-inducing ligands (PAMPs and DAMPs)	Function
Membrane-associated PRRs		
Toll-like receptors (TLRs)	Molecular moieties found on bacteria and viruses and from damaged and necrotic cells	Initiate signaling pathways, e.g., NF-κB, to modulate gene expression; indirectly activates the inflammasome
C-type lectin receptors (CLRs)	Carbohydrate moieties on microbes or cell surfaces	Serve as antigen receptors on APCs but also regulate the migration of dendritic cells and their interaction with lymphocytes
Nonmembrane-associated PRRs		
NOD-like receptors (NLRs)	Intracellular bacterial or viral components	Discriminate between pathogenic and commensal bacteria; directly activates the inflammasome
RIG-like helicases (RLHs)	Viral RNA	Promote type 1 interferon synthesis in cells infected by viruses to control the infection
DNA sensors (AIM2 and DAI)	Double-stranded DNA	Direct binding to double-stranded cytosolic DNA and activate inflammasome

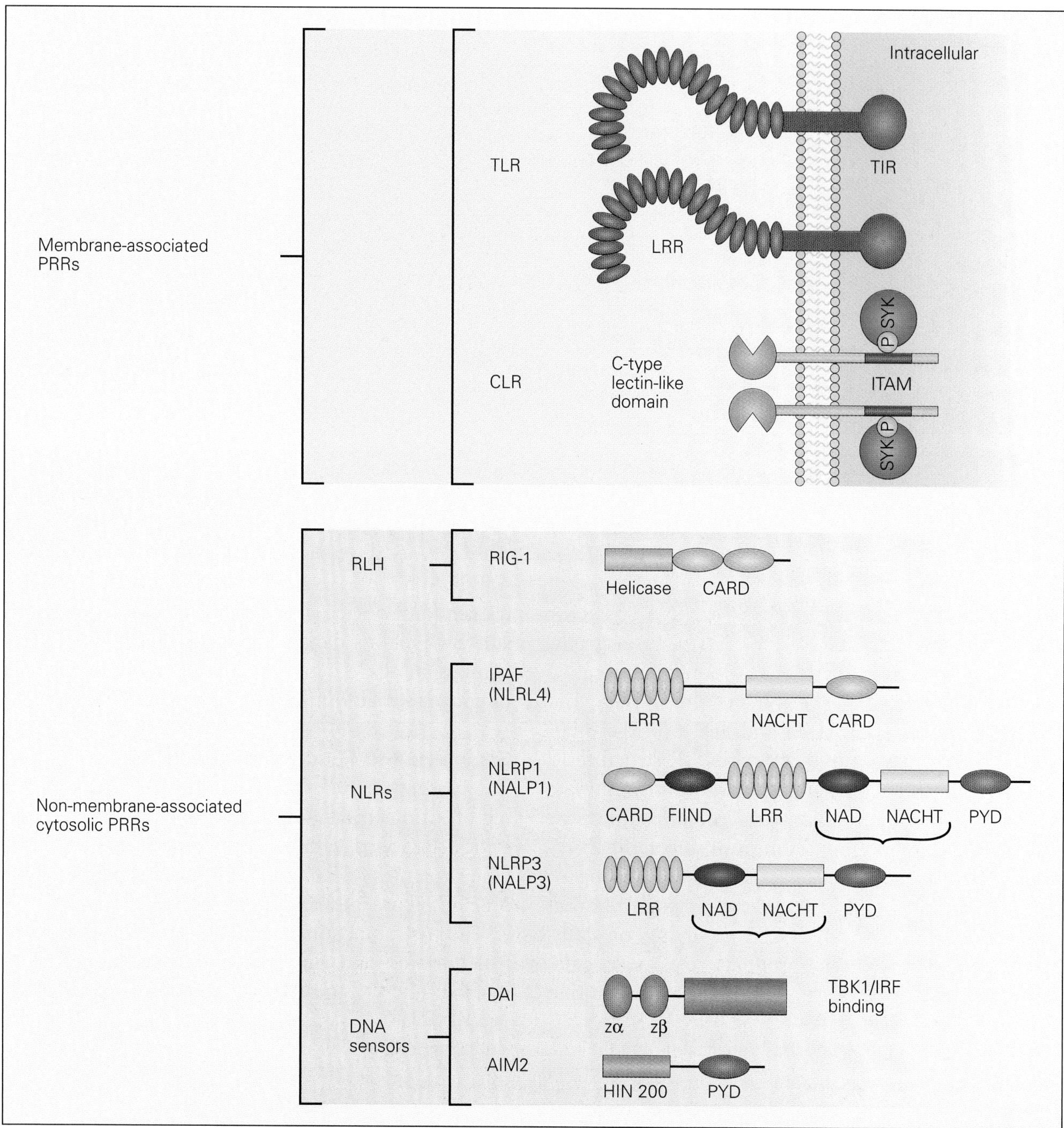

Figure 9-18. Schematic representation of the structural differences between the various families of membrane-associated and nonmembrane-associated PRRs.

immunity (*Chapter 3*). The PRRs are the sentinel recognition molecules to accomplish these functions. In the control of infection, innate immune cells often are themselves killed in the microbicidal killing process and utilize two of the four known host cell-killing mechanisms (*Chapter 5*): (1) autophagy, wherein damaged or infected organelles are sequestrated into autophagic compartments, i.e., autophagosomes, that eventually fuse with lysosomes and recycle their cellular contents, and (2) pyroptosis, or cell death associated with inflammasome-related inflammatory cytokine synthesis. In contrast to autophagy, wherein caspase is inhibited, pyroptosis is associated with caspase 1 activation (Box 9-6).

Inflammasome Structure and Function

Following the binding of a foreign danger-inducing stimulus with any of the innate immune receptors, a

Box 9-5

Structure of Individual PRRs

The basic structure of the PRRs involves the scaffolding of various protein domains with one another (Figure 9-18). The TLRs are made up of two domains, the ligand-sensing Leucine-Rich Repeats (LRRs) and a cytoplasmic signaling domain that triggers the final common pathway of IL-1 activation for every TLR, called the Toll/IL-1 Receptor (TIR) domain. The C-type Lectin Receptor (CLR) is composed of a CLR domain and a cytoplasmic Immunoreceptor Tyrosine-based Activation Motif (ITAM). The NOD-Like Receptors (NLRs) are made up of three domains that are (1) LRRs, (2) a Nucleotide Oligomerization Domain (NOD), and (3) an adapter domain (described in greater detail below) and are found in all of the NLR families. As will be described in greater detail below, specialized NLRs participate in the formation of several types of inflammasomes, the best characterized of which is the NLRP3 inflammasome. The RIG-Like Helicases (RLHs) are composed of three domains, one helicase domain, and two CARDs. The newly discovered DNA sensors each contain two domains; the DNA-dependent Activator of IFN regulatory factors (DAI) (also referred to as DLM-1/ZBP1) is made up of two Z-DNA binding domains (Zα and Zβ) and the Absent In Melanoma-2 (AIM2), composed of a pyrine domain (PYD) and a Hemopoietic IFN-inducible Nuclear protein of a 200-amino acid motif (HIN-200) domain.

Box 9-6

Apoptosis, Autophagy, Oncosis, and Pyroptosis

Cell death can occur by at least four different processes: apoptosis, autophagy, oncosis, and pyroptosis (*Chapter 5*). Apoptosis and autophagy are mechanisms that maintain normal intracellular homeostasis and do not lead to inflammation, in contrast to oncosis and pyroptosis, which are associated with the release of intracellular contents, necrosis, and inflammation. Pyroptosis is a pathway morphologically and mechanistically distinct from the other forms of cell death in which caspase 1 dependence is a defining feature. Unlike apoptosis, which involves caspase 3, caspase 6, and caspase 8, in pyroptosis, caspase 1 is the enzyme that mediates this process of cell death. Furthermore, loss of mitochondrial integrity and release of cytochrome *c*, which can activate apoptotic caspases, do not occur during pyroptosis. Furthermore, loss of mitochondrial integrity and release of cytochrome *c*, which can activate apoptotic caspases, do not occur during pyroptosis.

series of signaling pathways are activated through the "the three Ts" of transduction, transcription, and translation described previously. A key structure involved in these processes is the inflammasome, which serves as a tri-molecular platform for the subsequent generation of IL-1β and other related cytokines of the IL-1 family, i.e., IL-18 and IL-33 through a series of caspase-linked reactions. There are several families of inflammasomes but only four have been studied in great detail (Table 9-9).

The basic structure of the inflammasome in each of the inflammasome families is similar and consists of three major components: (1) an NLR, (2) an adapter protein, and (3) a caspase (Table 9-10). The nomenclature of the inflammasome takes its name from the NLR embedded in this tri-molecular structure (Table 9-9). Although many inflammasomes are being described, the most extensively studied inflammasome is the NLRP3 inflammasome, and most of the currently recognized monogenic clinical disorders involve disruption of this pathway (*Chapter 19*). Shown in Figure 9-19 is a schematic representation of the tripartite structure of the NLRP3 inflammasome.

The Components of the Inflammasome

NOD-like Receptors

In humans, the twenty-three members of the NLR family have similar structural components, although there are minor differences in each of the members. Their basic structure is composed of three differentiable parts: (1) an N-terminal end, also called the effector domain, which could be either a PYrine domain (**PYD**), a caspase recruitment domain (**CARD**), or a baculovirus inhibitor of apoptosis repeat domain (**BID**) molecule; (2) a central nucleotide and oligomerization binding domain, usually called a NACHT domain; and (3) a C-terminal domain made of leucine-rich repeats (**LRR**s) that under normal conditions maintains the receptor in an inhibited state and essentially has a similar structure and function as the ligand-sensing LRRs found in the TLRs (*Chapter 3*) (Figure 9-19).

The earliest described receptors, NOD1 and NOD2, are involved in the generation of signals that activate gene expression of unknown molecules through an NF-κB/MAPK-dependent pathway. However, the

Table 9-9. Four of the best-studied inflammasomes

Family	Components: NLR	Components: Adapter protein	Components: Caspase	Activation signals	Examples of clinical significance
IPAF (now called NLRC4)	IPAF	ASC	Caspase-1	Many flagelllin containing bacteria (flagellin dependent), *Legionella pneumophila* (flagellin independent)	Triggering inflammatory responses following infection with selected bacteria
NALP1 inflammasome	NALP1	ASC	Caspase-1 and 5	*Bacillus anthracis* lethal toxin (LT)	Triggering inflammatory response to *Bacillus anthracis* LT
Cryopyrin/NALP3 (NLRP3) inflammasome	NALP3 (or NLRP3) Cryopyrin	ASC and Cardinal	Caspase-1	Asbestosis, silica, aluminum adjuvants, uric acid, cholesterol	Monogenic cryopyrinopathies; autoinflammatory diseases; inflammatory response and adaptive immune enhancement of adjuvants; detrimental inflammatory response of gout
AIM2 inflammasome (*Francisella*-sensing inflammasome)	DNA sensor	None	Caspase-1	Viral, host, and bacterial ds DNA	Triggering inflammatory responses following infection with *Francisella*; Ds DNA vaccinia

principal role of the majority of them is the discrimination between pathogenic or commensal bacteria. Of clinical importance is the recent identification of mutations of NOD2/CARD15 in patients with Crohn's disease and NOD1 in patients with vitiligo. Apart from the detection of bacterial components that are common to both pathogenic and nonpathogenic bacteria, NLRs appear to identify the formation of pores produced by bacterial secretion systems in the cellular membrane to allow the entrance of the pathogen (intracellular bacteria) or the delivery of bacterial products inside of the host cell, events that contribute to the evasion strategies of bacteria that contribute to their virulence (*Chapter 12*).

Adapter Proteins

The second component of the inflammasome is the adapter protein that bridges the interaction between the NLR with the caspases and contains two protein interaction domains (either CARD or PYD), one that binds to the NLR and the other that binds to the caspase (Figure 9-19). So far, two different molecules have been described as adapter proteins: (1) the apoptosis-associated speck-like

Table 9-10. Structural components of an inflammasome

Component	Substructure	Function
Nod like receptor (NLR)	**Effector domain:** The N-terminal (PYD, CARD, or BID)	Recruits the caspase 1 via the multimerization of the adapter protein(s)
	Central domain: A (NOD) central domain	Provides an energy source for inflammasome activation
	Sensor domain: The C-terminal LRRs	Ligand-sensing and autoregulation portion of the inflammasome
Adapter protein	Bridging protein interaction domains (either CARD or PYD)	Recruitment of the procaspase subunits p10 and p20
Caspase	Inflammatory caspases (cysteine-aspartate proteases) caspases-1, -4, -5, -11, and -12	Function to cleave procaspases into active caspases and cleavage proinflammatory zymogen precursors into their active inflammatory cytokines, e.g., pro IL-1$\beta \rightarrow$IL-1β

protein containing a CARD (**ASC**) and (2) the Cardinal molecule.

Caspase

The third component of the inflammasome is the caspase that cleaves the zymogens into smaller active cytokines, e.g., pro-IL-1β to active IL-1β (Figure 9-19 step 9). Originally, caspases were linked to the induction of apoptosis, but this enzyme subset generates inflammatory cytokines and comprises caspases 1, 4, 5, 11, and 12. They are therefore termed as inflammatory caspases.

The Two Steps of IL-1β Synthesis

It is now generally recognized that the synthesis of IL-1β takes place in two steps (Figure 9-20). The first phase (Figure 9-20A) requires a microbial stimulus that is detected by a PRR, such as a TLR-4, that induces the synthesis of pro-IL-1β through the NF-κB and MAPK signaling pathways. This is followed by a second phase (Figure 9-20B) that requires the cleavage of pro-IL-1β to its active IL-1β form. This is accomplished through the assembly and activation of the inflammasome platform with the production of a heterotetrameric caspase-1 complex triggered by a wide variety of danger-inducing stimuli. These stimuli can include microbial PAMPs as well as other DAMPs such as monosodium urate (**MSU**) crystals, ATP, silica, asbestos, β amyloid, cholesterol and alum (Figure 9-20B). The molecular events of the activation of the inflammasome and production of IL-1β and other pro-inflammatory cytokines are described in Box 9-7.

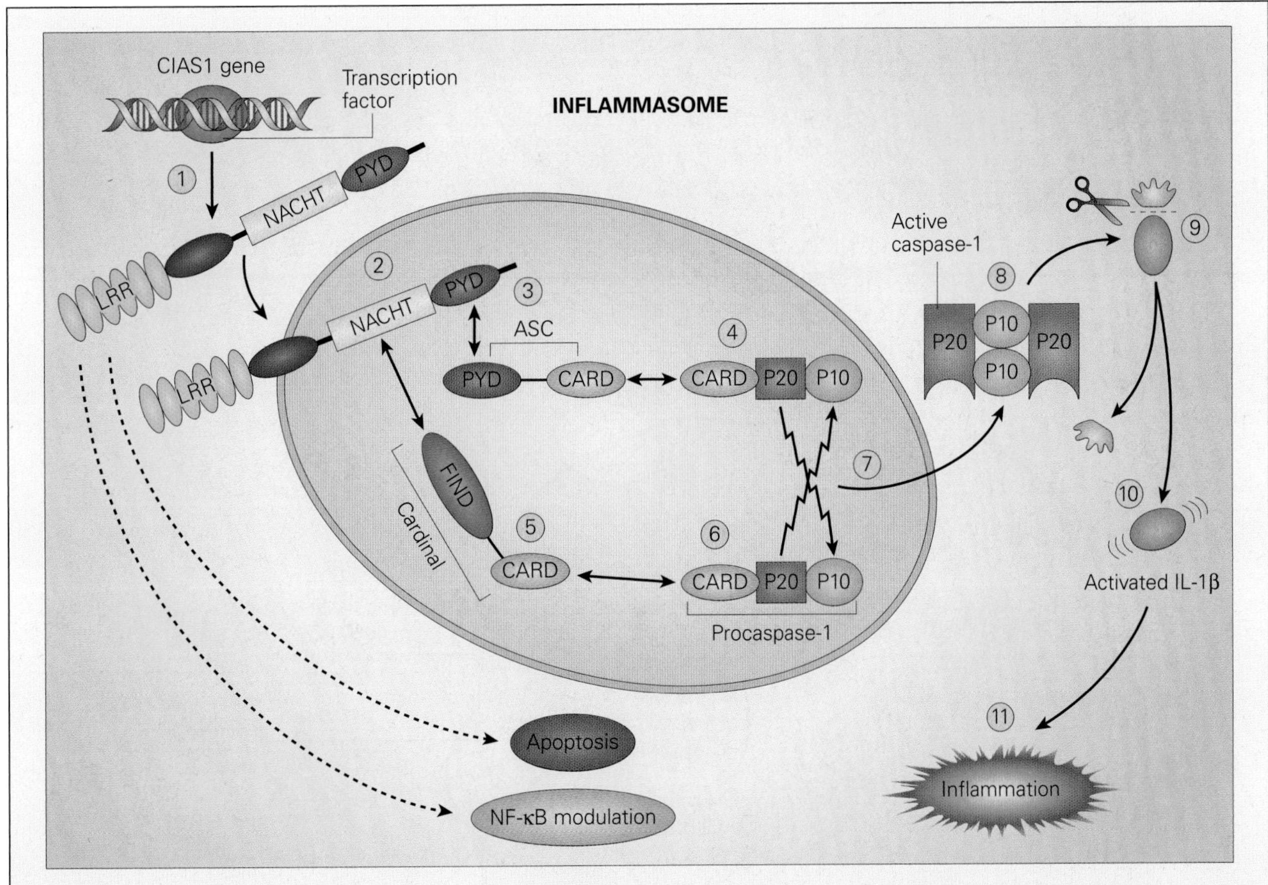

Figure 9-19. Schematic representation of the tripartite structure and assembly of the NLRP3 (cryopyrin) inflammasome. The structure consists of: (1) NLRP3 (made up of LRR, NACHT, and PYD); (2) adapter proteins ASC and Cardinal (made up of PYD and CARD and FIIND and CARD, respectively); and (3) the procaspase-1. The numbers in the figure refer to the sequential components involved in the assembly and activation of the inflammasome. Step (1) involves the initial transcription of the CIAS1 gene and translation of its product, NLRP3. After activation, the NLRP3 recruits other components of the inflammasome (2), which include either the ASC (3) and the procaspase-1 (CARD-P20-P10) (4) or the Cardinal (5) and another procaspase-1 (6). Following dimerization of the two procaspase-1 components (7) the production of an active caspase-1 (8) cleaves the pro-IL-1β (9) into an activated IL-1β (10), resulting in inflammation (11). CIAS1 gene = the gene that encodes NLRP3; named after cold-induced autoinflammatory syndrome (CIAIS) 1, the condition in which this gene is mutated in the cold-associated periodic syndromes (CAPS). (Adapted with permission from Goldbach-Mansky R, Dailey NJ, Canna SW, et al. Neonatal-onset multisystem inflammatory disease responsive to interleukin-1β inhibition. N Engl J Med (Suppl) 2006;355:581–92.)

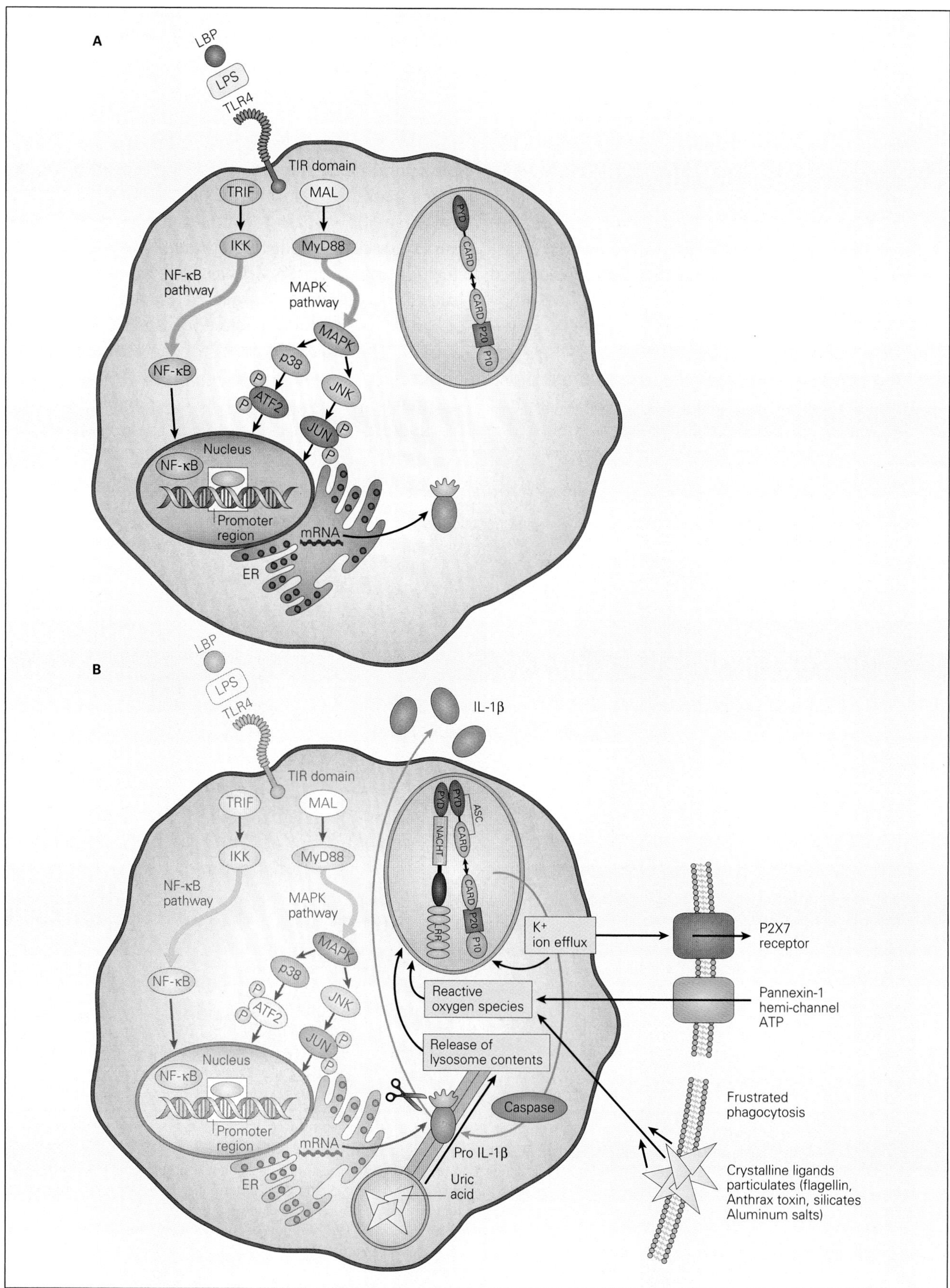

Figure 9-20. Schematic representation of the two phases regulating IL-1β production. Panel A: Phase 1 requires the generation of intracellular stores of pro-IL-1β following a priming signal, often from PRRs such as TLRs that activate NF-κB and MAPK signaling pathways. Panel B: The pro-IL-1β is then cleaved in the second phase into the active cytokine IL-1β by the newly assembled caspase-1 complex.

Box 9-7

Molecular Events Associated with Inflammasome Activation and IL-β Release

Current evidence concerning the formation of the inflammasome suggests at least a two-phase process. The first is related to the activation of the cell through stimulation of various PRR sensors (e.g., TLRs, NLRs), leading to the synthesis of pro-IL-1β (Figure 9-20A) The second event is the activation of a NLR by the presence of various secretion systems and by potassium efflux and generation of reactive oxygen species (Figure 9-20B). This disruption of the cellular membrane works as a signature for the presence of pathogenic bacteria in the cell and allows the completion of any of two events that trigger the final signal to initiate the activation of the inflammasome: (1) the secretion of ATP that is linked to changes in the electrolyte composition of the cytoplasm due to the formation of bacterial-induced pores, i.e., the efflux of potassium outside of the cell that contributes to the activation of the NALP3 inflammasome, or (2) the formation of reactive oxygen species (ROS) that are attributed to the stimulation of NADPH oxidase pathway that is related to frustrated phagocytosis of large particles, e.g., silica, alum, and uric acid that are unable to be taken up by the macrophages, i.e., uric acid crystals. These molecular events are finding clinical application and are providing a basis for a better understanding of the role of the immune system in health, e.g., the use of alum adjuvants in vaccines, as well as in disease, e.g., gout, diabetes, and sarcoidosis.

Inflammasome Mechanism of Action

Activation of the inflammasome has been linked to two critical intracellular events, either of which must occur in order for the complex to proceed to its completion. These include (1) pore formation in the cellular membrane that can be induced by pore-forming microbes, which is required for the efflux of potassium and ATP generation; and (2) the generation of ROS, an essential mechanistic step of inflammasome activity. Shown in Figure 9-20B is a schematic representation of these two critical steps involved in inflammasome activation.

Autoinflammatory Diseases

Recent data support the important role of IL-1β in the inflammatory processes associated with many autoinflammatory diseases of complex origin, e.g., silicosis, asbestosis, and gout (*Chapter 19 Annex*). In addition to these disorders, many rare monogenic and polygenic diseases are thought to be involved in defects of the pathway synthesis of IL-1β, resulting in its overproduction and the consequent pathogenic chronic or periodic inflammatory attacks. For this reason, they have been called autoinflammatory diseases, and one group involves mutations in the genes encoding different components of the inflammasomes. Thus, they have been classified according to the inflammasome affected and the product that is overproduced. In this functional classification, the first type correspond to defects found in the NLRP3 inflammasome and for this reason they have been termed cryoparinopathies or cryopyrin-associated periodic syndromes (**CAPS**), resulting in periodic episodes of inflammation due to the overproduction of IL-1β after innocuous stimulation from cold, i.e., familial cold autoimmune syndrome (**FCAS**) or others, for reasons still not understood completely, i.e., neonatal onset multisystem inflammatory disease (**NOMID**) (*Chapter 19 Annex*).

Clinical Applications of the IL-1 Superfamily

Knowledge of these molecular discoveries is now assuming clinical significance. The IL-1Ra is a cytokine that is now available clinically in the form of human recombinant form of IL-1Ra, commercially known as anakinra, used in the treatment of rheumatoid arthritis and a number of less common autoinflammatory diseases, such as familial Mediterranean fever and gout (*Chapter 11*). As a result of its ability to bind to the same IL-1RI receptor on the cell surface as IL-1β, IL-1Ra prevents signal transduction and subsequent proinflammatory effects that, if excessive, may be detrimental. Anakinra is proving to be effective in the treatment of several autoinflammatory conditions (*Chapter 19 Annex*).

Interleukin-2

Interleukin-2 (IL-2) is another key interleukin that was first discovered as a lymphocyte mitogenic factor (**LMF**) and later described as T cell growth factor (**TCGF**). Subsequently, TCGF was designated IL-2 because, in addition to T cells, LMF also activated B cells, NK cells, and monocytes. IL-2 is produced primarily by CD4+ T helper cells as a result of antigen-driven, autocrine T cell activation and is the major interleukin responsible for clonal T cell proliferation. This property of IL-2 to produce long-term cultures of T cells made possible the cultivation and discovery of the human immunodeficiency virus (**HIV**) (Box 9-8).

Box 9-8

IL-2 and the Discovery of HIV as the Causative Agent of AIDS

Working with human retroviruses in the early 1970s, Dr. Robert Gallo and his colleagues at the National Institutes of Health recognized that to detect reverse transcriptase-producing human retroviruses, there was a need to culture human blood cells for long periods and in greater numbers than possible with systems of colony growth on agar available at that that time. Analyzing conditioned media from various cell types, including activated T cells, this group was the first to find a growth factor that promoted long-term lymphoid cell growth, which they called T cell growth (mitogenic) factor. This finding enabled the group to isolate the first human retrovirus, human T cell leukemia virus-1 (HTLV-1), in 1979 and later the human immunodeficiency virus (HIV) in 1983 (*Chapter 19*).

IL-2 is also necessary for the maturation of a unique subset of T cells in the thymus and the periphery that are termed T regulatory (Treg) cells (*Chapters 2* and *7*). After exiting the thymus, Treg cells function to prevent other T cells from reacting against "self-antigens," which could result in autoimmunity (*Chapter 7*). Treg cells accomplish this by inhibiting the maturation of antigen-presenting dendritic cells. Thus, IL-2 is required to discriminate between self and nonself, one of the unique characteristics of the immune system. The stimulatory effect of IL-2 on Tregs is deficient in mice with IL-2 gene deletion. This accounts for the unexpected finding that such mice often develop hyperproliferative lymphadenopathy and autoimmune hemolytic anemia.

IL-2 has been found to be similar to IL-15 in terms of function. Both cytokines are able to facilitate production of immunoglobulins made by B cells and induce the differentiation and proliferation of natural killer cells. The primary differences between IL-2 and IL-15 are found in their cell sources and adaptive immune responses. For example, T lymphocyte-derived IL-2 participates in the maintenance of Treg cells and suppresses self-reactive T cells. On the other hand, IL-15 is derived from non-lymphocytic cells and is necessary for maintaining highly specific cytotoxic T cell responses by supporting survival of CD8 memory T cells and proliferation of NK cells. IL-15 supports Treg cells less well. The differences in function in these two cytokines stem from the use of differing receptors with distinct signal transduction pathways, which are described in an earlier section.

Interleukin-2 belongs to a group of cytokines, which includes IL-4, IL-7, IL-9, IL-15, and IL-21; this group recognizes cell receptors belonging to the common cytokine-receptor γ-chain family of receptors (Figure 9-11). IL-2R consists of three components:

1. IL-2 receptor alpha (IL-2Rα), also called CD25 and T cell activation antigen (Tac), which is specific only for IL-2;
2. IL-2 receptor beta (IL-2Rβ) or CD122, which is shared by IL-2 and IL-15; and
3. a common gamma chain (CD132), which is shared by all members of this cytokine family.

Knowledge of these molecules finds clinical application in the primary immunodeficiencies, as deficiencies of these various molecules are associated with susceptibility to infection as described below and in Chapter 16. The IL-2 receptor is not expressed on the surface of resting T cells and is present only transiently on the surface of activated T cells; it disappears within six to ten days of antigen presentation. It is noteworthy that the CD25 chain is constitutively expressed in the "natural" Treg cells of thymic origin, and this characteristic is used for the identification of these cells. In contrast to T helper cells, NK cells constitutively express IL-2 receptors and will secrete TNF-α, IFN-γ, and GM-CSF in response to IL-2, which in turn activates macrophages.

The IL-2 receptor uses a signaling pathway that involves Janus kinase-1 (**JAK1**), JAK3, and STAT5, which are described elsewhere in this chapter. The IL-2/IL-2R interaction stimulates the growth, differentiation, and survival of antigen-selected CD4+ helper cells as well as CD8+ cytotoxic T cells via the activation of specific genes. As such, IL-2 is necessary for the development of T cell immunologic memory, a unique characteristic of the immune system that depends upon the expansion of the number and function of antigen-selected T cell clones.

Clinical Applications of IL-2 and IL-2R

There are several clinical applications that emanate from this knowledge of IL-2 structure, function, and genomic origins. One of the serious immune deficiency disorders of infants, X-linked SCID, involves dysfunction of the common gamma chain of the IL-2R (*Chapter 16*, Box 9-9). Other clinical applications of IL-2 and its receptor include the

Box 9-9

Common Gamma Chain Dysfunction and X-Linked Severe Combined Immunodeficiency

Most cases of SCID are due to mutations in the gene encoding the common gamma chain (γc), a protein that is shared by the receptors for interleukins IL-2, IL-4, IL-7, IL-9, IL-15, and IL-21. In SCID, γc is expressed, but its binding to JAK3 is reduced (*Chapter 16*). Since these interleukins and their receptors are involved in the development and differentiation of T and B cells and because the common gamma chain is shared by many interleukin receptors, mutations that result in a non-functional common gamma chain cause widespread defects in interleukin signaling. The result is a near-complete failure of the immune system to develop and function, with low or absent T cells and NK cells as well as non-functional B cells. These abnormalities explain the unusually severe and widespread spectrum of infections seen in children afflicted with this disorder (*Chapter 16*).

The common gamma chain is encoded by the IL-2 receptor gamma gene, or IL-2Rγ, which is located on the X-chromosome. Therefore, immunodeficiency caused by mutations in IL-2Rγ is known as X-linked severe combined immunodeficiency and the condition is inherited in an X-linked recessive pattern. All males with the defective X-linked allele will have the clinical disease. Females with one defective and one normal allele will be healthy carriers. Half of their male children will have X-linked SCID, and their female children will have a 50 percent chance of being carriers.

availability of biotechnically engineered products for the treatment of patients with a variety of autoimmune diseases and malignancy (*Chapter 11*).

A recombinant form of IL-2 is now available as aldesleukin. It has been approved by the U.S. Food and Drug Administration (FDA) for the treatment of specific cancers (malignant melanoma, renal cell cancer), and is in clinical trials for the treatment of chronic viral infections and for use as a booster (adjuvant) for vaccines (*Chapter 11*). The role of IL-2 in HIV therapy remains to be fully determined.

Many of the immunosuppressive drugs used in the treatment of autoimmune diseases (e.g., corticosteroids) and organ transplant rejection (e.g., cyclosporine, tacrolimus) work by inhibiting the production of IL-2 by antigen-activated T cells. Others, such as sirolimus (also known as rapamycin) like corticosteroids, block IL-2R signaling and expand Treg cells, thereby preventing the clonal expansion and function of antigen-selected T cells (*Chapter 11*). Sirolimus is a relatively new immunosuppressant drug used to prevent rejection in organ transplantation, and is especially useful in kidney transplants (*Chapter 22*).

Anti-IL-2 Receptor Antibodies

As described previously, IL-2 is an important immune system regulator necessary for the clonal expansion and survival of activated T lymphocytes. The IL-2Rα (CD25, Tac) is expressed only by the already activated T lymphocytes and resting Treg cells. Therefore, an intensive research effort has been directed toward the development of effective and safe anti-IL-2 antibodies. By the use of recombinant gene technology, mouse anti-Tac antibodies have been modified (humanized), leading to the development of two chimeric mouse/human anti-Tac antibodies, basiliximab (Simulect) and daclizumab (Zenapax). These drugs act by binding the IL-2Rα chain, preventing the IL-2-induced clonal expansion of activated lymphocytes and shortening their survival. They are used in the prophylaxis of acute organ rejection after bilateral kidney transplantation, and both have been shown to be effective and with few side effects (*Chapters 11* and *22*).

Interleukin-3

Interleukin-3 (IL-3) stimulates the proliferation of hematopoietic pluripotent progenitor cells, such as those responsible for granulocyte production (Figure 9-21 and Table 9-6). It is secreted by activated T cells to support growth and differentiation of myeloid precursor cells from the bone marrow. The human IL-3 gene encodes a protein 152 amino acids in length, and the naturally occurring IL-3 is glycosylated. The human IL-3 gene is located on chromosome 5, only nine kilobases from the GM-CSF gene, and its function is quite similar to GM-CSF.

Interleukin-4

Interleukin-4 (IL-4) is a cytokine secreted mainly by Th2 cells but also by mast cells and eosinophils (Table 9-6 and Figure 9-22). It has many biological roles, including the stimulation of B cell– and T cell–proliferation, and the differentiation of CD4+ T cells into Th2 cells. IL-4 is a key regulator of the humoral arm of adaptive immunity, induces B cell class switching to IgE production, and upregulates MHC-II production. This cytokine also activates mast cells by binding to IL-4 receptors on their cell surfaces.

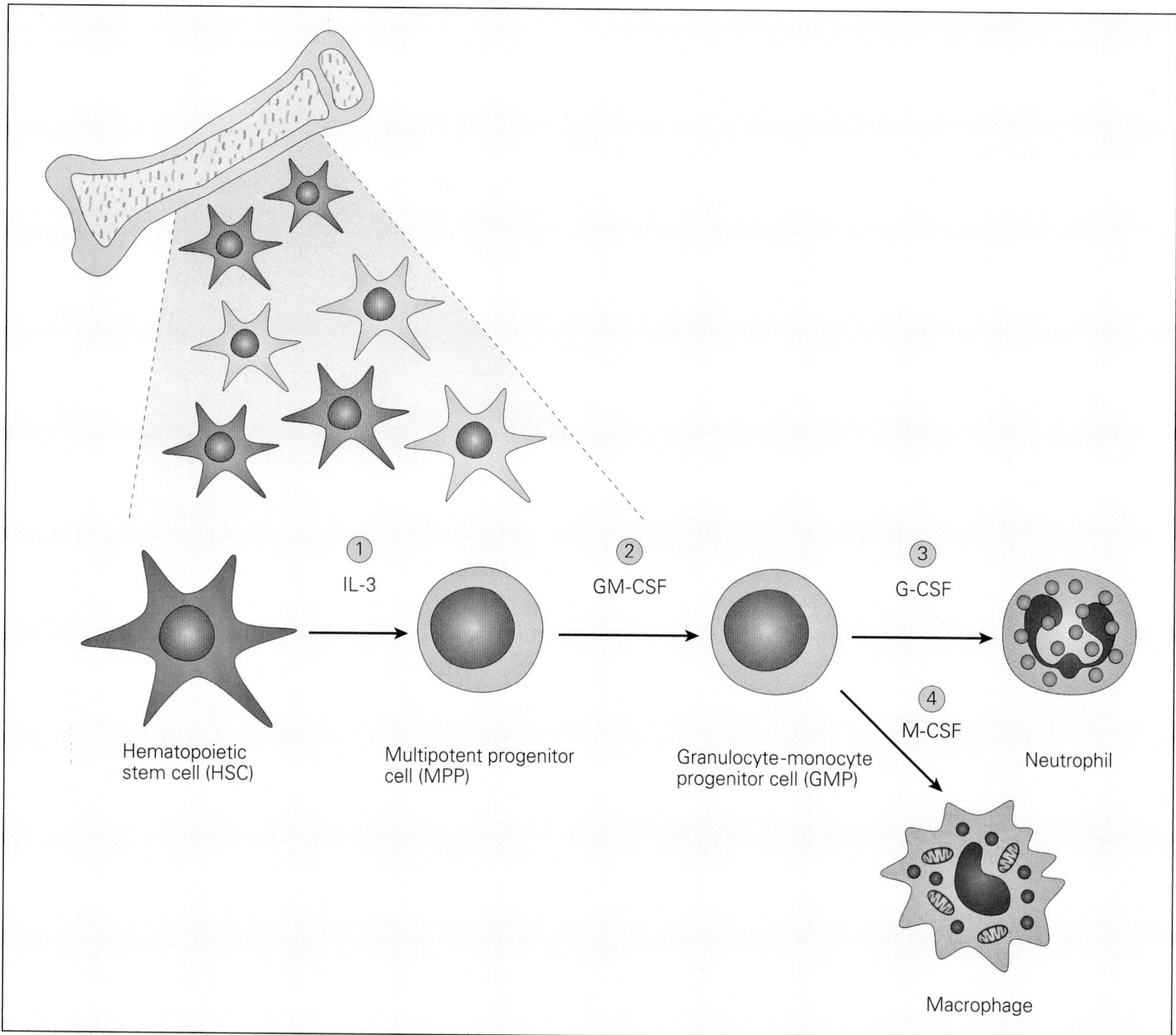

Figure 9-21. Schematic representation of the effects of IL-3 and other growth factors on granulocyte and macrophage production from hematopoietic stem cell (HSC) precursors.

IL-4 and Allergic Diseases

Dysregulation of IL-4 expression often leads to the production of immunoglobulin E and Th2 cytokine-mediated allergic inflammation, including allergen-induced asthma, rhinitis, and anaphylaxis (Figure 9-23 and *Chapter 18*). More than 25 percent of the population in industrialized countries suffers from IgE-mediated allergies. IL-4 and IL-13 are important inducers of B cell isotype switching and IgE production. IgE is involved in the development of immediate allergic reactions that are mediated by IgE-dependent mast cells (Figure 9-23). In addition, IL-4 and IL-13 also promote expression of endothelial adhesion molecules and production of chemokines, many of which are also importantly involved in allergic asthmatic inflammation. As will be described below, IL-5 produced by Th2 cells actively promotes the production and survival of eosinophils and airway hyperactivity.

Interleukin-5

Interleukin-5 (IL-5) is produced by Th2 cells and mast cells (Figure 9-22 and Figure 9-23). Its functions are to stimulate B cell growth and increase immunoglobulin secretion. It is also a key mediator in eosinophil development and activation. IL-5 is a 115-amino acid Th2 cytokine that is part of the hematopoietic family. Unlike other members of this cytokine subfamily (namely IL-3 and GM-CSF), this glycoprotein is a homodimer in its active form.

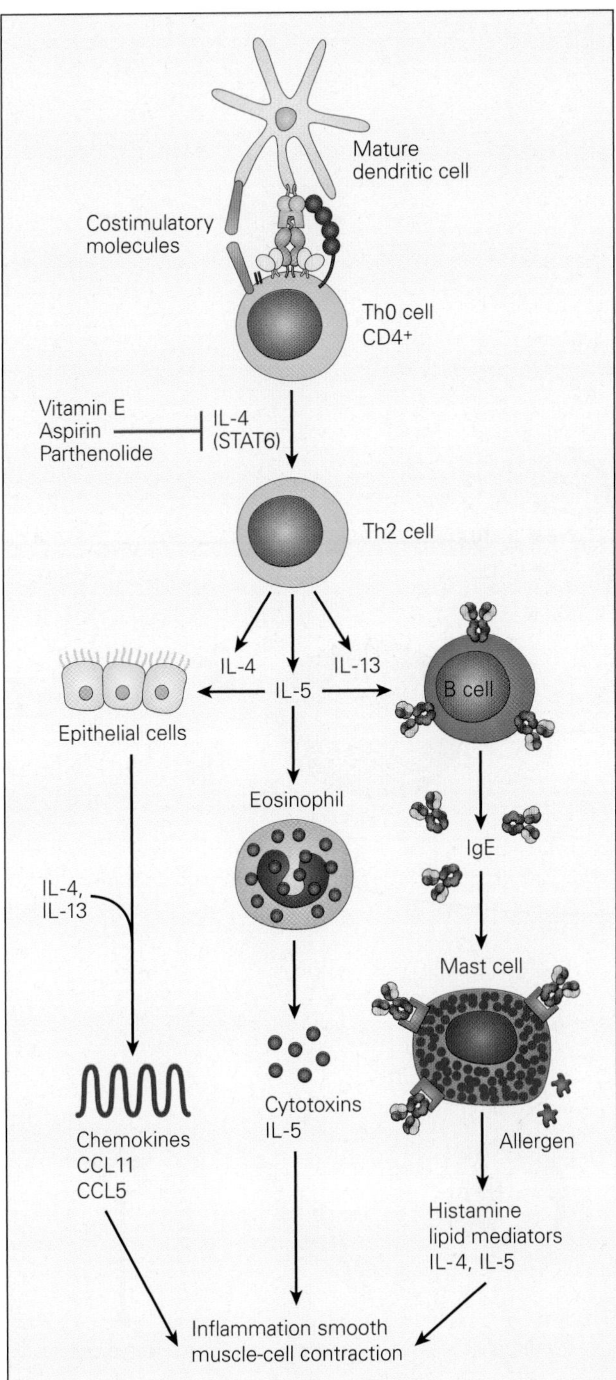

Figure 9-22. Schematic representation of the many roles of IL-4 and other cytokines on multiple immune stem and epithelial cells. IL-4 not only participates in the polarization of naïve CD4+ T helper (Th0) cells toward the Th2 subset and together with IL-5 activates epithelial cells to produce chemokines, but also is produced by mast cells to promote inflammation. Vitamin E, aspirin, and parthenolide have been shown to inhibit the expression of IL-4, whereas they have no effects on the production of Th1 cytokines.

The IL-5 gene is located on chromosome 5 in humans and chromosome 11 in the mouse. This gene is in close proximity to genes encoding IL-3, IL-4, and GM-CSF, which are often co-expressed in Th2 cells. Interleukin-5 is also expressed by eosinophils and has been observed in the mast cells of asthmatic airways by immunohistochemistry. IL-5 expression is regulated by several transcription factors, including GATA-3. Interleukin-5 has long been associated with several allergic diseases, including allergic rhinitis and asthma; in these conditions, an increased number of eosinophils has been observed in the circulation, airway tissues, and induced sputum. A major location of eosinophils is the gastrointestinal tract, where recently they have been implicated in several pathologic conditions affecting all segments of this system, including eosinophilic esophagitis, grastroenteritis, and colitis (*Chapter 18*). Eosinophils clearly have an important role in the pathology of these diseases.

The IL-5 Receptor

The IL-5 receptor (IL-5R) belongs to the class I cytokine receptor family and is a heterodimer composed of two polypeptide chains, one α subunit that binds IL-5 and confers upon the receptor cytokine specificity, and one β subunit that contains the signal transduction domains (Figure 9-10A).

α Chain

The IL-5Rα chain is exclusively expressed by eosinophils, some basophils, and murine B1 cells or B cell precursors. Like many other cytokine receptors, alternative splicing of the α chain gene results in expression of either a membrane-bound or soluble form of the α chain. The soluble form does not lead to signal transduction and therefore has an antagonistic effect on IL-5 signaling. Both monomeric forms of IL-5Rα are low-affinity receptors, while dimerization with the β chain produces a high-affinity receptor. In either case, the α chain exclusively binds IL-5 and the intracellular portion of IL-5Rα is associated with JAK2, a protein tyrosine-kinase essential in IL-5 signal transduction.

β Chain

The β subunit of the IL-5 receptor is responsible for signal transduction and contains several intracellular signaling domains. Unlike the α chain, the β chain does not bind IL-5, is not specific for this cytokine, and is expressed on practically all leukocytes. In fact, the β subunit of the IL-5 receptor is also found in

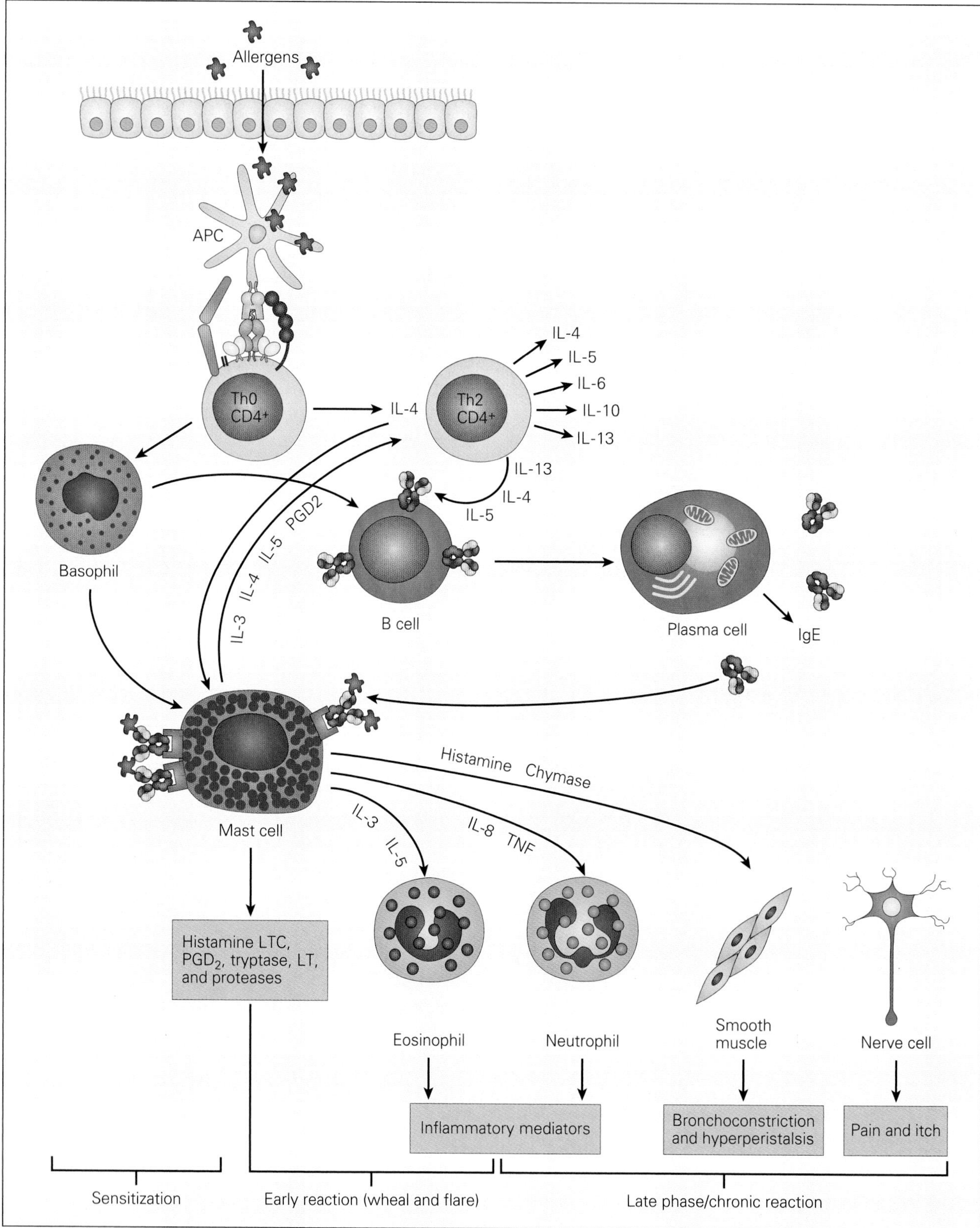

Figure 9-23. Immune pathways of allergic disease. IL-4 is a key player in the pathogenesis of allergic (atopic) disorders. In addition to its role in promoting the polarization of naïve Th0 CD4+ T helper cells toward the Th2 subset, IL-4 subsequently promotes allergic disease by many mechanisms including B cell isotype switching and immunoglobulin E production, mast cell activation leading to the release of other cytokines, and mediators contributing to inflammation, bronchoconstriction, and pain and itching characteristic of many allergic diseases and asthma. These effects are seen in all phases of allergic disease pathogenesis, including sensitization and progressing to the early and late phases of these disorders.

IL-3 and GM-CSF receptors, where it is associated with the IL-3Rα and GM-CSFRα subunits, respectively (Figure 9-10A). Therefore, it is known as the common β receptor or βc. Like the IL-5Rα subunit, the β subunit's cytoplasmic domain is constitutively associated with JAK2, as well as Lyn, another tyrosine kinase, both of which are essential for IL-5 signal transduction.

Effect of IL-5 on Eosinophils

Eosinophils are terminally differentiated granulocytes found in most mammals. In a healthy host, the principal role of these cells is the elimination of antibody-bound parasites through the release of cytotoxic granule proteins. Given that eosinophils are the primary IL-5Rα-expressing cells, it is not surprising that this cell type responds to IL-5. In fact, IL-5 was originally discovered as an eosinophil colony-stimulating factor; it is a major regulator of eosinophil accumulation in tissues and can modulate eosinophil behavior at every stage from maturation to survival. Shown in Figure 9-22 and Figure 9-23 are schematic representations of the central role of mast cells under normal conditions and in allergic inflammation. This figure illustrates the pleiomorphic roles of IL-4 and IL-5 on many cells of the immune system, including Th2 cells, B cells, mast cells, and eosinophils.

Interleukin-6

Interleukin-6 (IL-6) is produced by macrophages, fibroblasts, endothelial cells, and activated T helper cells (Table 9-6). IL-6 acts in synergy with IL-1 and TNF-α in innate immune responses and in T cell activation. IL-6 has also been called a myokine since it is a cytokine produced from muscle and is elevated in response to muscle contraction. Additionally, IL-6 stimulates osteoclast formation, which leads to bone resorption and remodelling.

IL-6 is one of the most important mediators of fever and of the acute phase response in the liver. IL-6 also enhances the differentiation of B cells and their consequent production of immunoglobulin. Chronic inflammation resulting in persistent IL-6 production has led to the development of B cell lymphomas and myelomas (*Chapter 21*). Glucocorticoid synthesis is also enhanced by IL-6. An additional effect of IL-6 is to stimulate increased energy mobilization in muscle and adipose tissue, leading to increased body temperature. Unlike IL-1, IL-2, and TNF-α, IL-6 does not induce cytokine expression; its main effect, therefore, is augmentation of the responses of immune cells to other cytokines. Inhibitors of IL-6 (including estrogen) are used in the treatment of postmenopausal osteoporosis. As will be described below, IL-6 together with TGF-β induces the Th17 pathway. Furthermore, IL-6 is one of the important pro-inflammatory cytokines produced by the Th17 lymphocyte.

The IL-6 Receptor

IL-6 signals through a cell-surface class I cytokine receptor complex consisting of the ligand-binding IL-6Rα chain (CD126) and the signal-transducing component gp130 (CD130). CD130 is a common signal transducer for a subfamily of IL-6-related cytokines and is almost ubiquitously expressed in most tissues, in contrast to CD126, which is restricted to certain tissues. As IL-6 interacts with IL-6Rα, it triggers the gp130 and IL-6R proteins to form a complex and thus activates gp130. These complexes of IL-6 and IL-6Rα bring together the intracellular regions of gp130 to initiate a signal transduction cascade through the JAK and STAT transcription factors.

IL-6 is probably the best studied of the cytokines that use gp130 in their signaling complexes. Other cytokines that signal through receptors containing gp130 are IL-11, IL-27, IL-31, ciliary neurotrophic factor (**CNTF**), cardiotrophin-1 (**CT-1**), cardiotrophin-like cytokine (**CLC**), leukemia inhibitory factor (**LIF**), oncostatin M (OSM), and an IL-6 mimic referred to as Kaposi's sarcoma-associated herpes virus IL-6-like protein (**KSHV-IL-6**). These cytokines are commonly referred to as the IL-6-like or gp130-utilizing cytokines (Figure 9-10A).

In addition to the membrane-bound receptor, a soluble form of IL-6R (sIL-6R) has been purified from human serum and urine. Many neuronal cells are unresponsive to stimulation by IL-6 alone, but differentiation and survival of neuronal cells can be mediated through the action of IL-6 bound to sIL-6R. The sIL-6R/IL-6 complex can stimulate neuronal outgrowth and promote survival of neurons and, hence, may be important in nerve regeneration through remyelination. Neutralizing antibody to IL-6 is proving to be effective in the treatment of inflammatory diseases such as juvenile idiopathic arthritis (**JIA**), RA, and Castleman's disease, a rare form of IL-6-dependent plasma cell leukemia.

Box 9-10

Homeostasis and T- and B-Cell Development

Homeostasis of T cells can be defined as the ability of the immune system to maintain normal T cell counts and to restore T cell numbers following T cell depletion or expansion. These processes are governed by extrinsic signals, most notably cytokines. Two members of the common γ-chain family of cytokines, IL-7 and IL-15, are central to homeostatic proliferation and survival of mature CD4+ and CD8+ T cells. Recent evidence suggests that other cytokines, including IL-2, IL-10, IL-12, interferons, and TGF-β, all play important but different roles at distinct stages of T cell homeostasis. Likewise, in the bone marrow, B cell specification and commitment is driven by the concerted action of transcription factors and IL-7 signaling.

Interleukin-7

Interleukin-7 (IL-7), a homeostatic lymphocyte growth factor secreted by the stromal cells of the bone marrow and thymus, is capable of stimulating the proliferation of immature lymphoid progenitors and mature lymphocytes (Table 9-6). During certain stages of B cell maturation and lymphoid proliferation, IL-7 is crucial for T and NK cell survival, development, and homeostasis of peripheral lymphocytes (Box 9-10, *Chapter 2*, and *Chapter 6*). B and T cells can originate via different pathways that appear to be used with varying frequencies in the animal host. IL-7 appears to play a crucial role in the maturation of both T and B cells and the survival of mature CD4+ and CD8+ T cells. Thymic stromal-derived lymphopoietin (**TSLP**) and IL-7 share a common receptor chain, IL-7Rγ (also called γc chain of the IL-2 family) (Figure 9-10A, Figure 9-11, and Figure 9-24). IL-7 is involved in T cell homeostasis, while TSLP favors Th2 responses and induces production of pro-allergic cytokines.

Interleukin-8

Interleukin-8 (IL-8) is a chemokine produced by macrophages, monocytes, neutrophils, NK cells, and other cells, such as epithelial and endothelial cells. IL-8 was renamed CXCL8 by the Chemokine Nomenclature Subcommittee, although its approved gene symbol remains IL-8. Macrophages are the primary cells that phagocytose and process an antigen

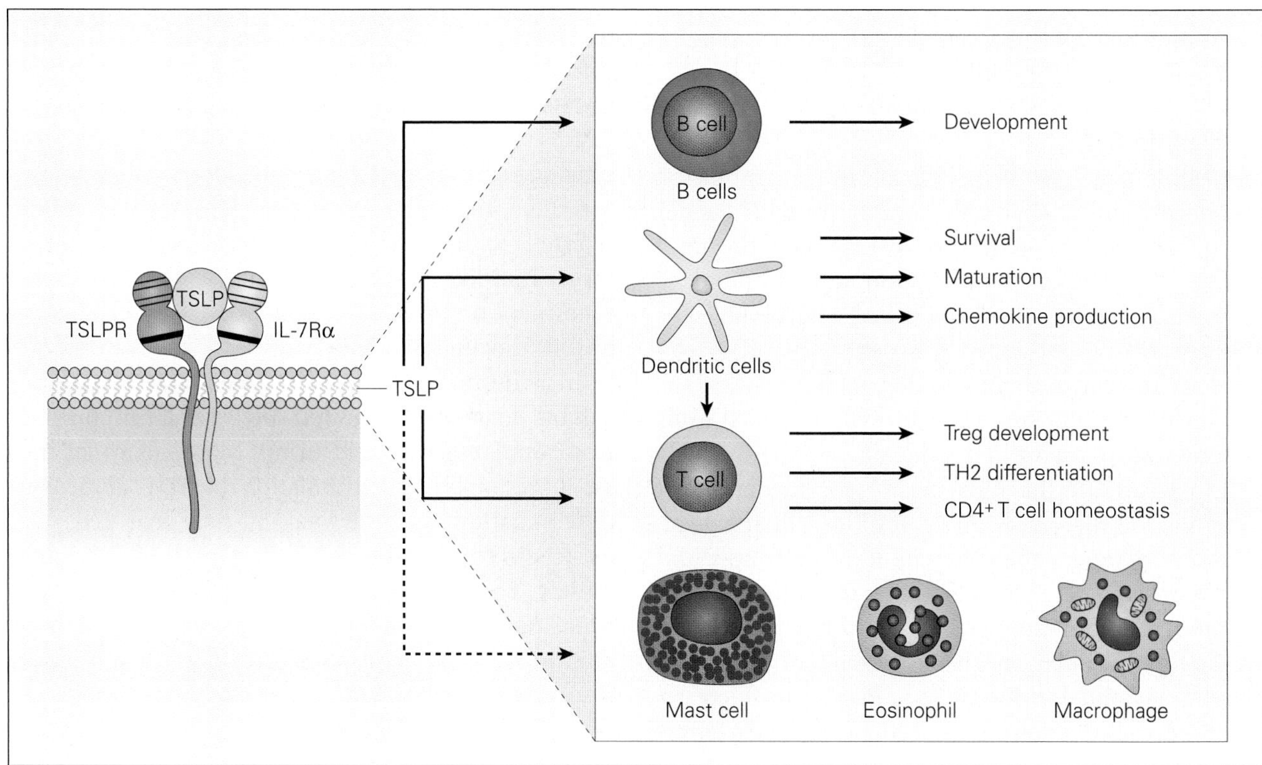

Figure 9-24. Biological function of thymic stromal-derived lymphopoietin (TSLP). Left panel: The TSLP receptor complex consists of a heterodimer of TSLPR (homologous to the γc chain of the IL-2 family) and IL-7Rα. Right panel, inset: TSLP stimulation of its receptor induces the activation and phosphorylation of STAT5 (P-STAT5), as well as activation of other as-yet-unidentified pathways that affect many cell lineages, including B cells, DCs, and T cells. Mast cells, eosinophils, and macrophages may also respond to TSLP.

on initial encounter. Upon processing, they release cytokines to signal other immune cells to come into the site of inflammation. IL-8 is one such chemokine that serves as an intercellular signal that attracts neutrophils and some CD8+ T cells to the site of inflammation (Table 9-6). IL-8 is often associated with acute inflammation and has potent angiogenic protumor growth effects based upon its chemotactic stimulating effects on endothelial cells.

Interleukin-9

Interleukin-9 (IL-9) is a cytokine produced by CD4+ helper cells and specifically by Th2 polarized cells (Table 9-6). IL-9 elicits many effects on lymphoid cells and mast cell lineages. Interestingly, the gene encoding this cytokine has been thought to have a role in asthma. Genetic studies on a mouse model of asthma demonstrated that this cytokine is a determining factor in the pathogenesis of bronchial hyperresponsiveness (*Chapter 18*).

Interleukin-10

Interleukin-10 (IL-10) functions mostly as an anti-inflammatory cytokine, capable of inhibiting synthesis of many pro-inflammatory cytokines like interferon-gamma, IL-2, IL-3, TNF-α, and GM-CSF. The IL-10 protein is a homodimer of 178 amino-acid-long subunits made by numerous cells, including Th1 and Th2 lymphocytes, cytotoxic T cells, B lymphocytes, mast cells, mononuclear phagocytic cells, and dendritic cells (Table 9-6). Monocytes and B cells are the major sources of IL-10 in humans; however, the primary T cell source for IL-10 is a subset of regulatory T lymphocytes named Tr1 antigen-induced cells, as described below and shown in Table 9-4. IL-10 is primarily responsible for inhibiting production of a wide variety of cytokines, including the following:

- inhibition of IFN-γ and IL-2 production by Th1 lymphocytes;
- inhibition of IL-4 and IL-5 production by Th2 lymphocytes;
- inhibition of IL-1β, IL-6, IL-8 (CXCL8), IL-12, and TNF-α production by mononuclear phagocytes; and
- inhibition of IFN-γ and TNF-α production by NK cells.

In addition, IL-10 inhibits MHC-II, CD23, intercellular adhesion molecule 1 (**ICAM-1**), and CD80/CD86 expression by dendritic cells and other APCs, eliminating the ability of the APC to provide the accessory signals necessary for T helper activation. IL-10 is also released by cytotoxic T cells and inhibits the action of NK cells during the immune response to viral infection (*Chapter 13*). Paradoxically, IL-10 is also stimulatory towards certain T cells, mast cells and B cells and thus can promote antibody production.

Other cytokines that are structurally and functionally related to IL-10 include IL-19, IL-20, IL-22, IL-24, and IL-26; it is likely that IL-28 and IL-29 also belong to the same class II subfamily since they all utilize members of the IFN family of receptors (Figure 9-10A).

These latter two cytokines and their receptors loosely share homologies with IFN and IFN receptors and display antiviral activity. In contrast to IL-10, none of these cytokines significantly inhibits cytokine synthesis, an activity that remains unique for IL-10 and IL-37 family members.

Interleukin-11

Interleukin-11 (IL-11) is a cytokine that originates from bone marrow stroma and megakaryocytes and is known to activate B cells (Table 9-6). It belongs to the IL-6 superfamily and is also known as adipogenesis inhibitory factor (AGIF) and oprelvekin. IL-11 has been demonstrated to improve platelet recovery after chemotherapy-induced thrombocytopenia, induce acute phase proteins, modulate antigen-antibody responses, and participate in the regulation of bone cell proliferation and differentiation. Due to this property, IL-11 may prove useful as a therapeutic for osteoporosis. Besides its lymphopoietic/hematopoietic and osteotrophic properties, it also functions in many other tissues, such as brain, gut, and testis. IL-11 stimulates the growth of certain lymphocytes and, in the murine model, stimulates an increase in the cortical thickness and strength of long bones.

Interleukin-12

Interleukin-12 (IL-12) is a cytokine that induces the differentiation of naïve T cells into Th1 cells (Figure 9-25). IL-12 is produced by myeloid dendritic cells and macrophages in response to antigenic stimulation and is composed of a bundle of four alpha helices encoded by two separate genes, IL-12A (P35) and IL-12B (P40) (Table 9-6 and Figure 9-25). IL-12 stimulates the production of IFN-γ and TNF-α from T and NK cells and suppresses IL-4 production and other Th2 cytokines. T cells that produce IL-12 have

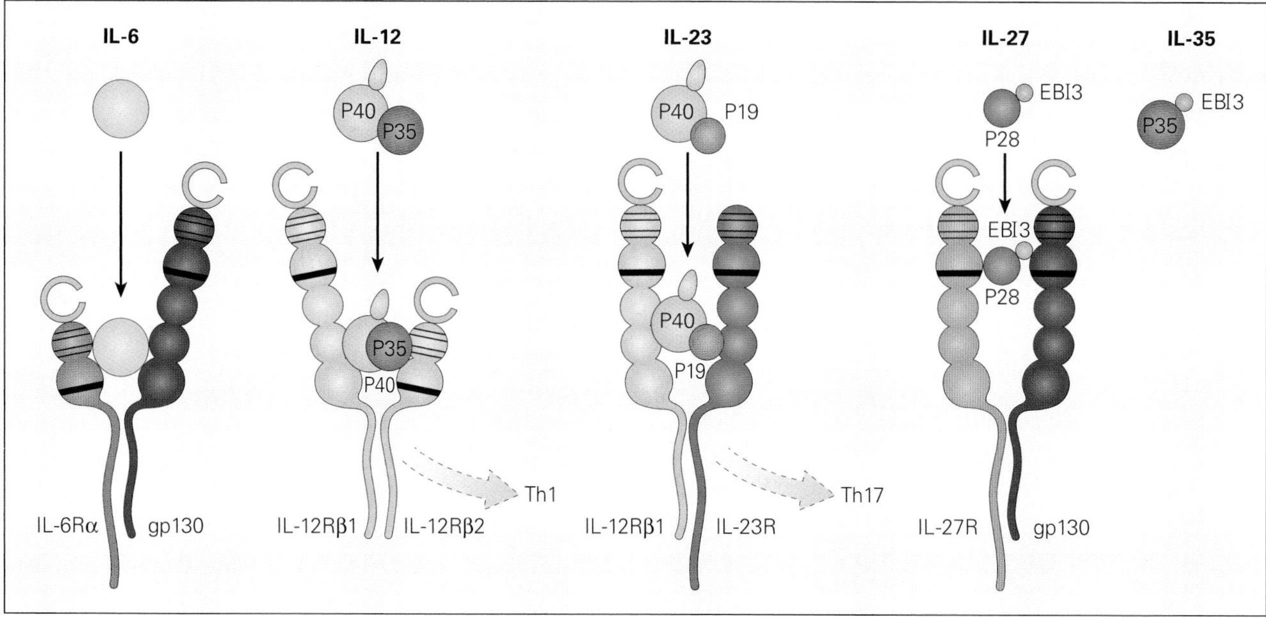

Figure 9-25. The IL-6 and IL-12 cytokine family: structural and biological characteristics. IL-12R and IL-23R share a common IL-12Rβ1 chain. IL-12 and IL-23 share a common P40 subunit that binds to the common IL-12Rβ1 receptor chain. The binding of cytokine IL-12 to the common IL-12R chain promotes Th1 cell development, and the binding of cytokine IL-23 to the IL-23R favors Th17 development. The gp130 chain of the IL-6R is common to the IL-27R.

a coreceptor, CD30, which is associated with IL-12 activity.

IL-12 is part of the IL-12 family that is composed of IL-12, IL-23, IL-27, and the newly identified IL-35. The IL-12-related cytokines are heterodimeric proteins comprised of an α chain (P19, P28, or P35) and a β chain (P40 or EBI3) (Figure 9-25). IL-12 binds to the IL-12 receptor, which is a heterodimeric receptor formed by IL-12Rβ1 and IL-12Rβ2. IL-12Rβ2 is considered to play a key role in IL-12 function, since it is found on activated T cells; it is stimulated by cytokines that promote Th1 cell development and inhibited by those that promote Th2 cell development. Upon binding, IL-12Rβ2 becomes tyrosine phosphorylated and provides binding sites for kinases, TYK2, and JAK2. These kinases are important in activating critical transcription factor proteins such as STAT4 that are implicated in IL-12 signaling in T cells and natural killer (**NK**) cells. This pathway is known as the JAK-STAT pathway.

IL-12 plays an important role in the activities of natural killer cells and T lymphocytes. IL-12 enhances the cytotoxic activity of NK cells and CD8+ cytotoxic T lymphocytes in part through the production of IFN-γ. There also seems to be a link between IL-2 and the signal transduction of IL-12 in NK cells. IL-2 stimulates the expression of the two IL-12 receptors maintaining the expression of a critical protein involved in IL-12 signaling in NK cells. Enhanced functional responses to IL-2 and IL-12 were demonstrated by IFN-γ production and enhanced killing of target cells. Patients with defects in IL-12 P40 and IL-12R comprise part of a spectrum of several molecular defects affecting the IL-12/IFN-γ axis (*Chapter 12*). Patients affected by these IL-12 mutations have been identified by their extreme susceptibility to infections caused by non-tuberculosis mycobacteria and BCG vaccine (*Mycobacterium bovis*, Calmette-Guérin strain).

IL-12 also plays a role in autoimmunity. Administration of IL-12 to people suffering from autoimmune diseases, for example, was shown to worsen the autoimmune phenomena. This is believed to be due to its key role in induction of Th1 immune responses. In contrast, in a mouse model of autoimmunity, IL-12 gene knockout in mice or treatment of mice with IL-12-specific antibodies ameliorated the disease. IL-12 also has been shown to have anti-angiogenic activity and to block the formation of new blood vessels. This effect is related to an increased production of interferon gamma, which in turn increases the production of a chemokine such as inducible protein-10 (IP-10 or CXCL10), which is directly responsible for this anti-angiogenic effect. Because of its ability to induce immune responses and its anti-angiogenic activity, there has been a growing interest in testing IL-12 as a possible anti-cancer drug. Although it has not been shown to have substantial anti-tumor activity to date, it may prove to be useful as a vaccine adjuvant (*Chapter 23*). Recent studies suggest that blockage of IL-12 may also be useful in the treatment of diseases such as psoriasis and inflammatory bowel disease.

Interleukin-13

Interleukin-13 (IL-13) is a cytokine secreted by many cell types and is an important mediator of allergic inflammation and disease (Table 9-6). IL-13 has effects on immune cells similar to the closely related cytokine IL-4; but, more importantly, it has been implicated as a central mediator of the pathologic changes induced by allergic inflammation in many tissues (Figure 9-23, and *Chapter 18*). IL-13 induces its effects through a multi-subunit receptor that includes the alpha chain of the IL-4 receptor (IL-4Rα), which is also a component of the IL-4 receptor, and at least one of two known IL-13-specific binding chains (Figure 9-10A). Most of the biological effects of IL-13, like those of IL-4, are linked to STAT6.

The functions of IL-13 overlap considerably with those of IL-4, especially with regard to changes induced on hematopoietic cells, but these effects are probably less important given the more potent role of IL-4. Thus, although IL-13 can induce immunoglobulin E (**IgE**) secretion from activated human B cells, deletion of IL-13 from mice does not markedly affect either Th2 cell development or antigen-specific IgE responses induced by potent allergens. In contrast, deletion of IL-4 abrogates these responses. Thus, rather than being a lymphoid cytokine, IL-13 acts more prominently as a molecular bridge linking allergic inflammatory cells to the nonimmune cells in contact with them, thereby altering physiological function.

IL-13 specifically induces pathophysiological changes in parasitized organs that are required to expel the offending organisms or their products (*Chapter 15*). For example, expulsion from the gut of a variety of mouse helminths requires IL-13 secreted by Th2 cells. IL-13 induces several changes in the gut that create an environment hostile to the parasite, including enhanced contractions and glycoprotein hypersecretion from gut epithelial cells that ultimately lead to detachment of the organism from the gut wall and its removal.

The eggs of the parasite *Schistosoma mansoni* may lodge in a variety of organs, including the gut wall, liver, lung, and even central nervous system, inducing the formation of granulomas under the control of IL-13. Here, however, the eventual result is organ damage, and often profound or even fatal disease, not resolution of the infection. An emerging concept is that IL-13 may antagonize Th1 responses that are required to resolve intracellular infections. In this immune-dysregulated context, marked by the recruitment of aberrantly large numbers of Th2 cells, IL-13 inhibits the ability of host immune cells to destroy intracellular pathogens.

IL-13 induces many features of allergic lung disease, including airway hyperresponsiveness, goblet cell metaplasia, and glycoprotein hypersecretion, which all contribute to airway obstruction (*Chapter 18*). IL-4 also contributes to these physiologic changes but appears to be less important than IL-13. IL-13 also induces secretion of chemokines that are required for recruitment of allergic effector cells to the lungs. Studies of STAT6 transgenic mice suggest the interesting possibility that IL-13 signaling occurring only through the airway epithelium is required for most of these effects. While no studies have yet directly implicated IL-13 in the control of human diseases, many polymorphisms in the IL-13 gene have been shown to confer an enhanced risk of atopic respiratory diseases such as asthma.

Although IL-13 is associated primarily with the induction of airway disease, it also has anti-inflammatory properties. Airway matrix metalloproteinases (**MMPs**), which are protein-degrading enzymes, are required to induce egression of effete parenchymal inflammatory cells into the airway lumen, where they are then cleared. Among other factors, IL-13 induces these MMPs as part of a mechanism that protects against excessive allergic inflammation and asphyxiation.

Interleukin-14

Although several studies have reported a number of biologic properties of a cytokine that has been dubbed interleukin-14 (IL-14), these have neither been confirmed nor has the putative molecule been cloned. Thus, considerable doubt has been raised as to the actual existence of this cytokine.

Interleukin-15

Interleukin-15 (IL-15) is a cytokine with structural similarity to IL-2 that is secreted by mononuclear phagocytes and some other nonlymphoid cells following infection by viruses (Table 9-6 and Figure 9-10A). This cytokine is most potent in inducing proliferation of natural killer (NK) cells, i.e., cells of the innate immune system whose principal role is to kill virally infected cells. Maintenance of memory cells does not appear to require persistence of the original antigen; instead, survival signals for memory lymphocytes are provided by cytokines such as IL-15. Since IL-15 is less active in stimulating Treg cells than IL-2, it may prove to be a better immune adjuvant for supplementing vaccines and for treatment of immunosuppressed patients,

Interleukin-16

Interleukin-16 (IL-16) is released by a variety of cells (including lymphocytes and some epithelial cells) and has been characterized as a chemoattractant for certain immune cells expressing the cell surface molecule CD4 (Table 9-6). IL-16 was originally described as a cytokine that could attract activated T cells in humans and was previously called lymphocyte chemoattractant factor (**LCF**). Since then, this interleukin has been shown to recruit and activate many other cells expressing the CD4 molecule, including monocytes, eosinophils, dendritic cells, and CD4+ T cells. IL-16 is produced as a precursor peptide (pro-IL-16) that requires processing by an enzyme called caspase-3 to become active.

Interleukin-17

Interleukin-17 (IL-17 or IL-17A) is the founding member of a group of cytokines called the IL-17 family. IL-17 is produced by cells belonging to a CD4+ subpopulation, different from Th1 or Th2, designated as Th17 cells characterized by the production of IL-17A and IL-17F cytokines (Table 9-6). However, dual producers of IL-17A and IFN-γ have also been detected. Differentiation of Th17 cells is initiated by a combination of the cytokines transforming growth factor-beta 1 (TGF-β1) and IL-6 or IL-1, and maintained by IL-23 secreted from APCs (Figure 9-25 and *Chapter 12*). Th17 cells are a distinct lineage of T cells that produce IL-17, IL-17F, IL-21, and IL-22 and have not only been shown to play critical roles in autoimmunity and tissue inflammation but also to be critical regulators of host immunity against bacterial, fungal, and viral infections at mucosal surfaces (*Chapter 8*). In addition, Th17 cells produce a range of other factors known to drive inflammatory responses, including TNF-β, IL-6, GM-CSF, CXCL1, and CCL20. The key contribution of the Th17 cell subset to normal immune responses remains undefined, but it has been shown that they can play a role in the clearance of certain infectious agents and in exacerbating autoimmune diseases. Unlike Th1 and Th2 cells, Th17 cell production of IL-17A and F is not stable, but these cells can revert to Th1 or Th2 cell types (Figure 9-8).

IL-17 Family

In addition to IL-17A, members of the IL-17 family include IL-17B, IL-17C, IL-17D, IL-17E (also called IL-25), and IL-17F (Figure 9-10B and Figure 9-14). All have a similar protein structure, with four highly conserved cysteine residues critical to their three-dimensional shape, yet they have no sequence similarity to any other known cytokines.

IL-17 is produced mainly by CD4+ Th17 cells and memory cells and acts upon T cells, fibroblasts, and APCs (Table 9-6). Numerous immune regulatory functions have been reported for the IL-17 family of cytokines, presumably due to their induction of many immune-signaling molecules. Most notably, IL-17 is involved in inducing and mediating pro-inflammatory responses. IL-17 is commonly associated with allergic responses. In fact, IL-17 actually has suppressive effects on IFN-γ and the Th1 pathway and induces the production of many other cytokines (i.e., IL-6, G-CSF, GM-CSF, IL-1β, TGF-β, and TNF-α), chemokines (including IL-8, GRO-α, and MCP-1), and prostaglandins (e.g., PGE2) from many cell types (fibroblasts, endothelial cells, epithelial cells, keratinocytes, and macrophages). The release of cytokines causes many functions, such as airway remodeling, a characteristic of IL-17 responses. The increased expression of chemokines attracts other cells, including neutrophils but not eosinophils. As a result of these roles, the IL-17 family, and in particular IL-17A and IL-17F, is pro-inflammatory and has been linked to many immune/autoimmune-related diseases, including rheumatoid arthritis, asthma, lupus, allograft rejection, and anti-tumor immunity. IL-17 levels are not only elevated in patients with these autoimmune diseases but also are decreased following clinical improvement.

Regulation of IL-17 Expression

Much progress has been made in the understanding of the regulation of IL-17. Production of IL-17 is now demonstrated to be dependent on IL-23, and STAT3 and NF-κB signaling pathways are required for this IL-23-mediated IL-17 production (Figure 9-14). Another molecule, suppressors of cytokine-signaling3 (**SOCS3**), plays an important role in suppressing IL-17 production (Box 9-11, Figure 9-26).

In the absence of SOCS3, IL-23-induced STAT3 phosphorylation is enhanced, and phosphorylated STAT3 binds to the promoter regions of both IL-17A and IL-17F, increasing their gene activity (Figure 9-26). As described previously, the interplay of IL-1/IL-6/IL-23/TGF-β is crucial for Th17 development, while IL-27 appears to exert an inhibitory effect on its development (Figure 9-14). Several groups have now identified ways to induce IL-17 production both *in vitro* and *in vivo* by the combination of TGF-β and IL-6 without the need for IL-23. Although IL-23 is not required for initiating IL-17 expression, IL-23 does play a role in promoting survival and/or proliferation of the IL-17-producing T cells.

IL-17 Receptor Family Distribution and Signaling

The IL-17 receptor family consists of five broadly distributed receptors that present with individual ligand specificities. Within this family of receptors, IL-17R is the best described. IL-17R binds both IL-17A and IL-17F and is expressed in multiple tissues: vascular endothelial cells, peripheral T cells, B cell lineages, fibroblasts, lung cells, myelomonocytic cells, and marrow stromal cells (Figure 9-14). Another member of this receptor family, IL-17RB, is expressed in the kidney, pancreas, liver, brain, and intestine; it binds both IL-17B and IL-17E. IL-17RC is expressed by the prostate, cartilage, kidney, liver, heart, and muscle, and its gene may undergo alternate splicing to produce a soluble receptor in addition to its cell membrane-bound form. Similarly, the gene for IL-17RD may undergo alternative splicing to yield a soluble receptor. This feature may allow these receptors to inhibit the stimulatory effects of their as-yet-undefined ligands. The least described of these receptors, IL-17RE, is known to be expressed in the pancreas, brain, and prostate. Signal transduction by these receptors is as diverse as their distribution. Similar to the IL-17 ligands, their receptors are not similar to other cytokine receptors.

Box 9-11

Suppressors of Cytokine Signaling

Suppressors Of Cytokine Signaling (SOCS) are a family of intracellular proteins, several of which have emerged as key physiological regulators of cytokine responses, including those that regulate the immune system. SOCS proteins seem to regulate signal transduction by combining direct inhibitory interactions with cytokine receptors and signaling proteins with a generic mechanism of targeting associated proteins for degradation. Evidence is emerging for the involvement of SOCS proteins in diseases of the human immune system, which raises the possibility that therapeutic strategies based on the manipulation of SOCS activity might be of clinical benefit, e.g., neuro-inflammatory diseases and malignancy.

Interleukin-18

Interleukin-18 (IL-18) is a cytokine produced by macrophages that belongs to the IL-1 superfamily and, together with IL-12, collaborates to induce cell-mediated immunity following infection with microbial products like LPS (Table 9-6). It is one of the pro-inflammatory cytokines produced by the inflammasome described previously. After stimulation by IL-18, NK cells and certain T cells release the pivotal Th1 cytokine, IFN-γ, which plays an important role in activating macrophages, T lymphocytes, and other cells.

Interleukin-19

Interleukin-19 (IL-19) is a cytokine that belongs to the IL-10 family of cytokines, which include IL-10, IL-20, IL-22, IL-24, IL-26, and several virus-encoded cytokine mimics. It signals through the same cell surface receptor (IL-20R) that is used by IL-20 and IL-24 (Figure 9-10A). The IL-19 gene is expressed in resting monocytes, B cells, and nonimmune cells. Its expression by monocytes is induced by LPS (Table 9-6). IL-19 activates monocytes to secrete IL-6 and TNF-α and produce reactive oxygen species. It is upregulated by IL-4 and GM-CSF and downregulated by IFN-γ. Consistent with a positive-feedback loop, in the presence of IL-19, increased numbers of IL-4 and fewer IFN-γ-producing cells are observed, thus promoting Th2 immune deviation.

Interleukin-20

Interleukin-20 (IL-20) is another member of the IL-10 family of cytokines and is produced by skin, synovial fibroblasts, and macrophages and acts upon activated keratinocytes and fibroblasts; it

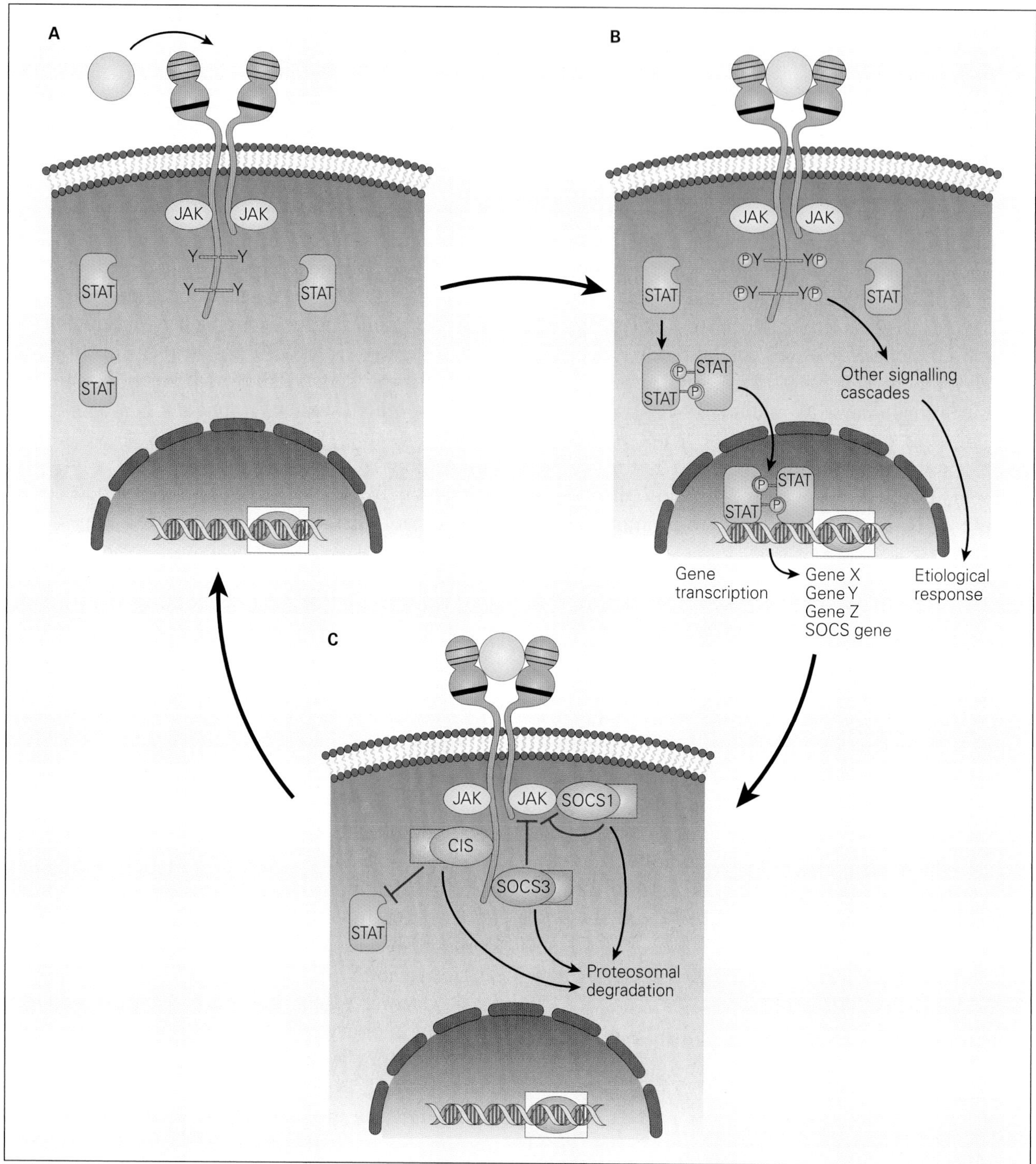

Figure 9-26. SOCS proteins are negative-feedback inhibitors of cytokine signal transduction. Panel A: In unstimulated cells, signaling molecules, such as the JAKs and STATs, are inactive and, typically, SOCS genes are not expressed. Panel B: After binding of cytokines, receptor aggregation occurs; receptor-associated JAKs are brought together, which allows cross-phosphorylation (P) and activation. The active JAKs tyrosine (Y) phosphorylate and activate several signaling proteins, including the cytokine receptors. Panel C: The SOCS proteins act in a negative-feedback loop to quench signal transduction by interacting directly with JAKs (SOCS1) and inhibiting their catalytic activity; CIS is thought to bind receptor sites, which blocks the recruitment and activation of STATs; and SOCS3 seems to inhibit JAKs after gaining access by receptor binding.

transmits an intracellular signal through two distinct cell-surface receptor chains on keratinocytes and other epithelial cells (Figure 9-10A and Table 9-6). IL-20 regulates proliferation and differentiation of keratinocytes during inflammation, particularly inflammation of the skin, e.g., psoriasis. In addition, IL-20 causes proliferative expansion of multipotential hematopoietic progenitor cells.

Interleukin-21

Interleukin-21 (IL-21) is a newly described cytokine produced by activated CD4+ T cells and NKT cells (Table 9-6). It has been the object of intensive research because of its homology to IL-2, IL-4, and IL-15, and its ability to promote both innate and adaptive immune responses. IL-21 augments the proliferation of CD4+ and CD8+ T lymphocytes and regulates the profile of cytokines secreted by these cells, drives the differentiation of B cells into memory cells and terminally differentiated plasma cells, and enhances the activity of NK cells. It is a cytokine that has potent upregulatory effects on cells of the immune system, including NK cells and cytotoxic T cells that can destroy virally infected or cancerous cells. This cytokine induces cell division/proliferation of its target cells. IL-21 elicits its effects on immune cells by interacting with a cell surface receptor known as the IL-21 receptor, IL-21R, that is expressed on bone marrow cells and on various lymphocytes, including Th17 cells.

Interleukin-22

Interleukin-22 (IL-22) is a member of the IL-10 family and functions to promote innate immunity of tissues against infection (*Chapter 3*). IL-22 is produced by Th17 cells, mast cells, and macrophages and fibroblasts (Table 9-6). There are potent interactions of IL-22 and IL-17 signal pathways in tissue inflammation and autoimmune diseases. Initiation of the JAK1/TYK2/signal transducer and activator STAT3 pathway appears to be the major mode of IL-22 signal transduction, through activation of STAT1, mitogen-activated protein (**MAP**) kinases, and NF-κB, activator, among others. IL-22 signaling is established by binding of the cytokine to its heterodimeric receptor complex consisting of the interferon receptor-related proteins IL-22R1 and IL-10R2 (Figure 9-10A). Since IL-10R2 is an ubiquitous protein, cellular IL-22 responsiveness is mainly determined by expression of the IL-22R1 receptor chain. Interestingly, IL-22R1 expression is restricted to non-leukocytic cells. Therefore, IL-22 appears to be unique among cytokines in that this protein is incapable of mediating functions between leukocytes, but is rather specialized to transmit information between leukocytes and the non-leukocytic cells, such as hepatocytes, pancreatic acinar cells, colonic myofibroblasts, synoviocytes, and cells of epithelial origin, such as keratinocytes, lung, and colon carcinoma cells. IL-22 promotes the barrier functions of epithelial lining cells and the production of antimicrobial proteins (*Chapters 1, 8,* and *12*). IL-22 and IL-17 were found to be coordinately induced by TGF-β and IL-6 during Th17 differentiation. However, IL-22 knockout mice exhibit greater inflammatory reactions, suggesting that IL-22 actually downregulates IL-17 inflammatory responses.

Interleukin-23

Recent studies have provided evidence for a third effector of the CD4+ Th17 pathway, interleukin-23 (IL-23). The differentiation and expansion of this pathway is initiated and maintained by a combination of the cytokines TGF-β1 and IL-6 or IL-1, together with IL-23 secreted from APCs. These T cells, as described above, have been designated Th17 based on their production of IL-17A and IL-17F—cytokines not produced by either Th1 or Th2 CD4+ T cells. In addition to IL-17, Th17 cells produce a range of other cytokines known to regulate inflammatory responses, including TNF, IL-6, GM-CSF, IL-22, and some chemokines (Table 9-6).

IL-23 is a heterodimeric cytokine consisting of two subunits; one is called p40, which is shared with the cytokine IL-12, and the other is called p19 (the IL-23 alpha subunit) (Figure 9-25). IL-23 is an important participant in the inflammatory response against infection. It upregulates the matrix metalloprotease MMP9, increases angiogenesis, and reduces CD8+ T cell infiltration. Recently, IL-23 has been implicated in the growth of malignant tumors.

Knockout mice deficient in either p40 or p19 or in either subunit of the IL-23 receptor (IL-23R and IL12R-β1) develop less severe symptoms of multiple sclerosis and inflammatory bowel disease (Figure 9-25), highlighting the importance of IL-23 in promulgating IL-17-dependent autoimmune and autoinflammatory diseases (*Chapter 19*).

Interleukin-24

Interleukin-24 (IL-24) is a cytokine belonging to the IL-10 family of cytokines that signals through two heterodimeric receptors, IL-20R1/IL-20R2 and IL-22R1/IL-20R2 (Figure 9-27). This interleukin is also known as melanoma differentiation-associated 7 (**mda-7**) due to its discovery as a tumor-suppressing protein. IL-24 appears to promote cell survival and proliferation by inducing rapid activation of the transcription factors STAT1 and STAT3. This cytokine is predominantly released by activated monocytes,

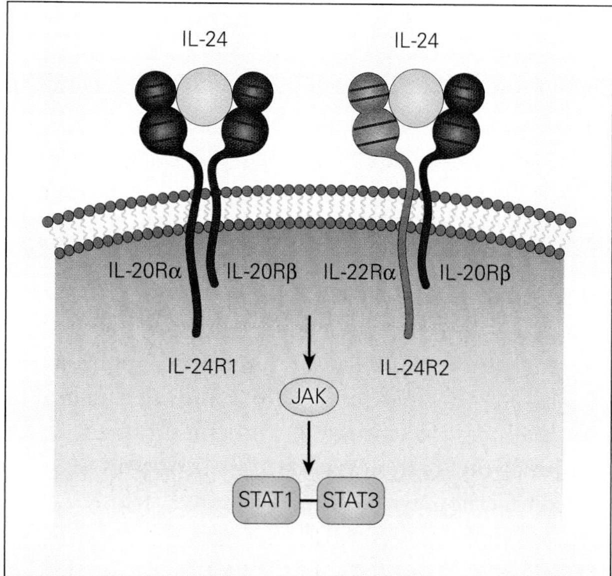

Figure 9-27. Schematic representation of the two types of IL-24 receptors. IL-24R1 consists of IL-20Rα/IL-20Rβ and IL-24R2 consists of IL-22Rα/IL-20Rβ.

macrophages, Th2 cells, melanocytes, and keratinocytes and acts on non-hematopoietic tissues such as skin, lung, and reproductive tissues (Table 9-6). IL-24 performs important roles in wound healing, psoriasis, and cancer. Several studies have shown that apoptotic cell death occurs in cancer cells/cell lines following exposure to IL-24. The gene for IL-24 is located on chromosome 1 in humans.

Interleukin-25

Interleukin-25 (IL-25) is a cytokine that belongs to the IL-17 cytokine family and is secreted by Th2 cells and mast cells (Table 9-6). It is also known as IL-17E. IL-25 induces Th2 polarization by producing other cytokines, including IL-4, IL-5, and IL-13 in multiple tissues, which in turn stimulates the expansion of eosinophils. This cytokine is an important molecule controlling immunity of the gut and has been implicated in chronic inflammation associated with the gastrointestinal tract. Further, the IL-25 gene has been identified in a chromosomal region associated with autoimmune diseases of the gut, such as inflammatory bowel disease (**IBD**), although no direct evidence suggests that IL-25 plays any role in this disease.

Interleukin-26

Interleukin-26 (IL-26) is a 171-amino acid protein, which is similar in amino acid sequence to interleukin-10. IL-26 is produced by memory T cells and mast cells and has pro-inflammatory effects (Table 9-6). It was originally called AK155 and is composed of a signal sequence, six helices, and four conserved cysteine residues. IL-26 is expressed in certain herpes virus-transformed T cells but not in primary stimulated T cells. IL-26 signals through a receptor complex comprised of two distinct proteins called IL-20R1 and IL-10R2 (Figure 9-10A). By signaling through this receptor complex, IL-26 induces rapid phosphorylation of the transcription factors STAT1 and STAT3, which enhance IL-10 and IL-8 (CXCL8) secretion and CD54 (ICAM-1) expression on epithelial cell surfaces.

Interleukin-27

Interleukin-27 (IL-27) is a heterodimeric cytokine belonging to the IL-12 family of ligands that is composed of two subunits, Epstein-Barr virus (**EBV**)-induced gene 3 (**EBI3**) (also known as IL-27B) and IL27-p28 (also called IL-30) (Figure 9-25). IL-27 plays an important function in regulating the activity of B and T lymphocytes. IL-27 is produced by macrophages and dendritic cells and induces Th1 cytokines such as IFN-γ with consequent antiangiogenic and antitumor effects (Table 9-6). IL-27 inhibits the differentiation of Th17 cells (Figure 9-14). The effects of IL-27 are elicited by its interaction with a specific cell surface receptor complex composed of two proteins known as IL-27R and gp130 (Figure 9-25). Consequently, IL-27 is also a member of the IL-6 subfamily that uses gp130.

Interleukin-28 and Interleukin-29

Interleukin-28 (IL-28A and IL-28B) and interleukin-29 (IL-29) belong to the group of type III interferons known as interferon lambda (IFN-λ) (Figure 9-10A). Both IL-28 and IL-29 are produced by virus-infected cells and play a role in immune defense against viruses (Table 9-6). Similar to other IFNs, both interleukins play a significant role in immune defense against viruses (*Chapter 13*), as well as in some malignancies (*Chapter 20*). This family of molecules signals through a receptor formed by an interferon receptor subunit, IL-28R (also called IFN-γR1 or CRF2-12) and IL-10R2, common to several members of the IL-10 family (Figure 9-10A). IL-28 and IL-29 genes are found on human chromosome 19. This is described in greater detail below in the IFN section.

Interleukin-30

Interleukin-30 (IL-30) is produced by dendritic cells and activates naïve CD4+ T cells (Table 9-6) and is a protein with a molecular weight of twenty-eight kilodaltons, which is identical to the p28 component of IL-27 and therefore IL-30 is sometimes called IL27-p28. The other chain of IL-27 is EBI3. IL-30 is a member of the long-chain, four-helix bundle family of cytokines, making it structurally similar to IL-6. Shown in Figure 9-25 is a schematic representation of some of the structural molecules that explains the overlapping complexity of these cytokines. Since IL-30 is a component part of IL-27, the IL-30 expressed by antigen-presenting cells triggers expansion of antigen-specific naïve CD4+ T cells and promotes polarization toward a Th1 phenotype with expression of gamma-interferon (Table 9-6).

Interleukin-31

Interleukin-31 (IL-31) is a cytokine with a four-helix bundle structure, which is preferentially produced by Th2 cells (Table 9-6). The structure of IL-31 places it in the IL-6 family of cytokines (Figure 9-10A). IL-31 signals via a receptor complex that is composed of IL-31 receptor A (IL-31RA) and oncostatin M receptor subunits. These receptor subunits are expressed in activated monocytes and in unstimulated epithelial cells. IL-31 is believed to play a role in inflammation of the skin.

Interleukin-32

Interleukin-32 (IL-32) is a cytokine produced by T cells, monocytes, fibroblasts, epithelial cells, and NK cells and acts as a proinflammatory stimulant on T cells and monocytes (Table 9-6). IL-32 can induce monocytes and macrophages to secrete TNF-α, IL-1β, IL-6, and two CXC chemokine family members involved in several autoimmune diseases, i.e., IL-8 and MIP-2/CXCL2. IL-32 (previously termed NK transcript 4) is an inflammatory cytokine produced by mitogen-activated lymphocytes, IFN-γ activated epithelial cells, and IL-12-, IL-18-, and IL-32-activated NK cells. In addition, IL-32 activates arachidonic acid metabolism in peripheral blood mononuclear cells by stimulating the release of prostaglandins. IL-32 is produced by T cells, monocytes, fibroblasts, epithelial cells, and NK cells and acts as a pro-inflammatory stimulant on T cells and monocytes.

Interleukin-33

Interleukin-33 (IL-33) is structurally related to IL-1 and induces helper T cells to produce type 2 cytokines. This cytokine was previously called NF-HEV because it appeared to play a role as a nuclear factor (**NF**) in high endothelial venules (**HEVs**) (*Chapter 2*). IL-33 is produced by T cells and most nonimmune cell types and its mRNA is broadly expressed in various organs (Table 9-6). Expression within these organs is restricted to a few cell types, such as epithelial cells from the bronchus or the small airways, fibroblasts, and smooth muscle cells. Some expression of mouse IL-33 mRNA has been seen in dendritic cells, activated macrophages, and Th2 cells, but in general, levels are low.

IL-33 mediates its biological effects by interacting with the orphan IL-1 receptor, ST2, activating intracellular molecules in the NF-κB and MAP kinase-signaling pathways that drive production of type 2 cytokines (e.g. IL-4, IL-5, and IL-13) from polarized Th2 cells. The induction of these type 2 cytokines by IL-33 *in vivo* is attributed to severe pathological changes observed in mucosal organs. *In vivo*, IL-33 induces the expression of IL-4, IL-5, and IL-13 and leads to severe pathological changes in mucosal organs.

Interleukin-34

Interleukin-34 (IL-34) is composed of a homodimer of 241 amino acids produced by many tissues, including the spleen, thymus, liver, small intestine, and colon and promotes the growth and survival of macrophage progenitors and interacts with the CSF1R of monocytes (Table 9-6).

Interleukin-35

Interleukin-35 (IL-35) is a heterodimeric protein consisting of IL-12α (p35) and IL-27β chains that are encoded by separate genes called IL-12A and EBI3, respectively. IL-35 is a member of the IL-12 family (Figure 9-25) and is a homologue of IL-27 and is produced by Treg cells (Table 9-6). It produces its suppressive effects by inducing proliferation of CD25+ Treg cells and reducing the activity of Th17 cells.

Interferons

A second major group of cytokines are the **interferons** (IFNs) (Tables 9-2 and 9-7), a family of pleiotropic cytokine proteins produced by the cells of the immune system and other cell types of most vertebrates in response to challenges by foreign agents, such as viruses, bacteria, fungi, parasites, and tumor cells (*Chapter 13*). Although the interferons were originally described as major antiviral proteins, they also exhibit downregulatory effects on the growth of normal and malignant hematopoietic cells *in vitro* and *in vivo*. There are three major different classes of IFNs:

1. Type I, alpha and beta (IFN-α, IFN-β),
2. Type II, gamma (IFN-γ),
3. Type III, lambda (IFN-λ).

These IFN classes differ in their cells of origin and properties, but all IFNs exert their biologic effects by binding and signaling through specific cell receptors (Tables 9-2 and 9-5).

In the majority of cases, the production of interferons is induced in response to viruses and bacteria and/or their products (e.g., viral glycoproteins, viral RNA, bacterial endotoxin, bacterial flagella, and CpG DNA). They can also be induced by polyclonal mitogens and other cytokines, e.g., IL-1, IL-2, IL-6, IL-10, IL-12, TNF, and CSFs. Type I and type III IFNs are produced by many cell types; type II IFN is made by a more restricted family of cells of the immune system consisting of CD4+ and CD8+ T cells, Tγδ, NKT, and NK cells (Table 9-11). Type I IFNs are particularly produced in great abundance by plasmacytoid dendritic cells (**pDCs**); Type II IFN-γ has relatively weak antiviral activity and is more effective as an immunostimulatory molecule that promotes Th1 responses. All IFNs have multiple functions (i.e., are pleiotropic) and are host species-specific rather than virus-specific. Upon release by virus-infected cells, IFNs bind to specific receptors on other cells and trigger synthesis of antiviral proteins that inhibit viral replication by several mechanisms (*Chapter 13*). Interferons are induced immediately after viral infection but disappear rapidly. Their metabolism and excretion take place mainly in the liver and kidneys.

Other effects common to all IFNs include anti-oncogenic properties, macrophage and natural killer

Table 9-11. Properties of the major interferons: Type I, type II, and type III

Class	Interferon type	Properties					
		Acid and heat lability	Cell of origin	Species specificity	Biological activity	Subtypes	Receptor
Type I	IFN-α	Stable	All somatic nucleated cells; plasmacytoid dendritic cells (pDCs) are major producers	Yes	Antiviral effects; induction of MHC-I on all somatic cells; activation of NK cells and macrophages	Several (see Box 9–12)	IFNAR1 and IFNAR2
	IFN-β		Usually made by many cell types; fibroblasts are major producers	Yes		Two major types: IFN-β1, IFN-β3 IFN-β2 is IL-6	IFNR1 and IFNR2
Type II	IFN-γ	Labile	NK, NKT, Tγδ, Th1 CD4+ and Tc1 CD8+ cells.	Yes	Induction of MHC-I on all somatic cells and of MHC-II on APCs and somatic cells; activation of macrophages, neutrophils, NK, and APC cells; promotion of Th1 cell-mediated immunity; low antiviral effects; suppression of Th2 cells; anti-angiogenic effects	One type	IFNGR1 and IFNGR2
Type III	IFN-λ	Stable	All nucleated cell types	Yes	Antiviral and immunomodulatory	IFN-λ1, IFN-λ2, and IFN-λ3 (also called IL29, IL28A, and IL28B, respectively)	IL10R2 (CRF2-4) and IFNLR1 (CRF2-12)

Box 9-12

Human Type I Interferons

Human type I IFNs comprise a vast and growing group of IFN proteins, designated IFN-α (alpha), IFN-β (beta), IFN-κ (kappa), IFN-δ (delta), IFN-ε (epsilon), IFN-τ (tau), IFN-ω (omega), and IFN-ζ (zeta, also known as limitin). There are thirteen subtypes of IFN-α proteins that are called IFNA1, IFNA2, IFNA4, IFNA5, IFNA6, IFNA7, IFNA8, IFNA10, IFNA13, IFNA14, IFNA16, IFNA17, and IFNA21. The IFN-α molecules are encoded by genes found together in a cluster on chromosome 9. Two types of IFN-β have been described, IFN-β1 (IFNB1) and IFN-β3 (IFNB3) (a gene designated IFN-β2 actually produces IL-6).

lymphocyte activation, and enhancement of the expression of major histocompatibility complex glycoprotein classes I and II (*Chapter 10*). Thus, the IFNs promote the presentation of foreign peptides to T cells.

Type I IFNs: IFN-α and IFN-β

Type I interferons contain at least thirteen IFN-α and IFN-β members in humans (Box 9-12). They are expressed as a first line of defense against viruses and are known to play a critical role in the antiviral response (*Chapter 13*). Type I IFNs combat viruses both directly by inhibiting virus replication within cells and indirectly by stimulating the innate and adaptive antiviral immune responses. Type I IFNs modulate the adaptive immune response by increasing MHC-I expression to promote antigen presentation, enhance T cell survival, and stimulate dendritic cell maturation. As will be described in greater detail below, certain type I IFNs have been approved for use in clinical conditions, including multiple sclerosis, chronic hepatitis B and C, and malignant diseases such as hairy cell leukemia, malignant melanoma, and AIDS-related Kaposi's sarcoma.

In order for interferons to exert their biological effects, binding to their respective cognate receptors is required. Both IFN-α and IFN-β bind to the same receptor, known as type I IFN receptor (IFNR), which consists of two distinct components: (1) IFNAR1 (previously called α subunit) and(2) IFNAR2 (previously called β subunit) chains (Table 9-11, and Figures 9-10A and 9-28).

Type II IFN: IFN-γ

IFN-γ (gamma) is the only member of the type II IFNs and is produced by T cells (Th1, Tc1, Tγδ, and NKT) and NK cells and perhaps by dendritic cells (Table 9-11). This cytokine has a role in many different types of immune reponses, such as cell-mediated immunity, inflammation, antibody production, and viral infection. Although the antiviral activity of IFN-γ is low, it plays a major role in Th1 cell-mediated immune reactions activating macrophages and increasing the expression of MHC-II on APCs. IFN-γ-stimulated macrophages display increased phagocytic properties and have a greater capacity to kill intracellular pathogens, to upregulate the synthesis of other cytokines, and to enhance their ability to present antigen. IFN-γ secreted by Th1 cells also exerts a suppressive effect on Th2 cells, promotes IL-12 production by dendritic cells and macrophages, and induces an isotype class switch from IgM to IgG (*Chapter 6*). IFN-γ and TNF-α are the major cytokines involved in mediating the macrophage infiltration and granuloma formation seen in tuberculosis and other chronic infections (*Chapter 12*).

In contrast to IFN-α and IFN-β, IFN-γ binds to another receptor on a target cell called the IFN-γ receptor (**IFNGR**), following which a signal is elicited within the cell. The IFNGR is made up of two subunits designated IFNGR1, associated with JAK1, and IFNGR2, associated with JAK2. The major ligand-binding subunit is the 90 kDa IFNGR1, to which IFN-γ binds. IFNGR2 is a 62 kDa protein that plays a minimal role in ligand binding, but its signaling function is critical in the generation of IFN-γ signals (Figures 9-10A and 9-28).

Type III IFN: IFN-γ

The recently identified type III IFN group consists of three IFN-λ (lambda) molecules called IFN-λ1, IFN-λ2, and IFN-λ3 (also called IL-29, IL-28A, and IL-28B, respectively) (Table 9-11). As described previously, these IFNs signal through a receptor complex consisting of IL-10R2 (also called CRF2-4) and IL-28R (also called IFN-γR1 or CRF2-12). The heterodimeric receptor mediates JAK1 activation and tyrosine phosphorylation of STAT factors, leading to biological responses similar to those mediated by type I IFNs. The IFN-λs have been demonstrated to be induced after stimulation with several single-stranded RNA (ssRNA) viruses, whereas the inducibility with other viruses and other genomes (DNA and double-stranded RNA [dsRNA]) is not clear. In contrast to IFN-α and IFN-β, which exert their effects by both directly inhibiting virus replication in the cells and indirectly by stimulating the innate and

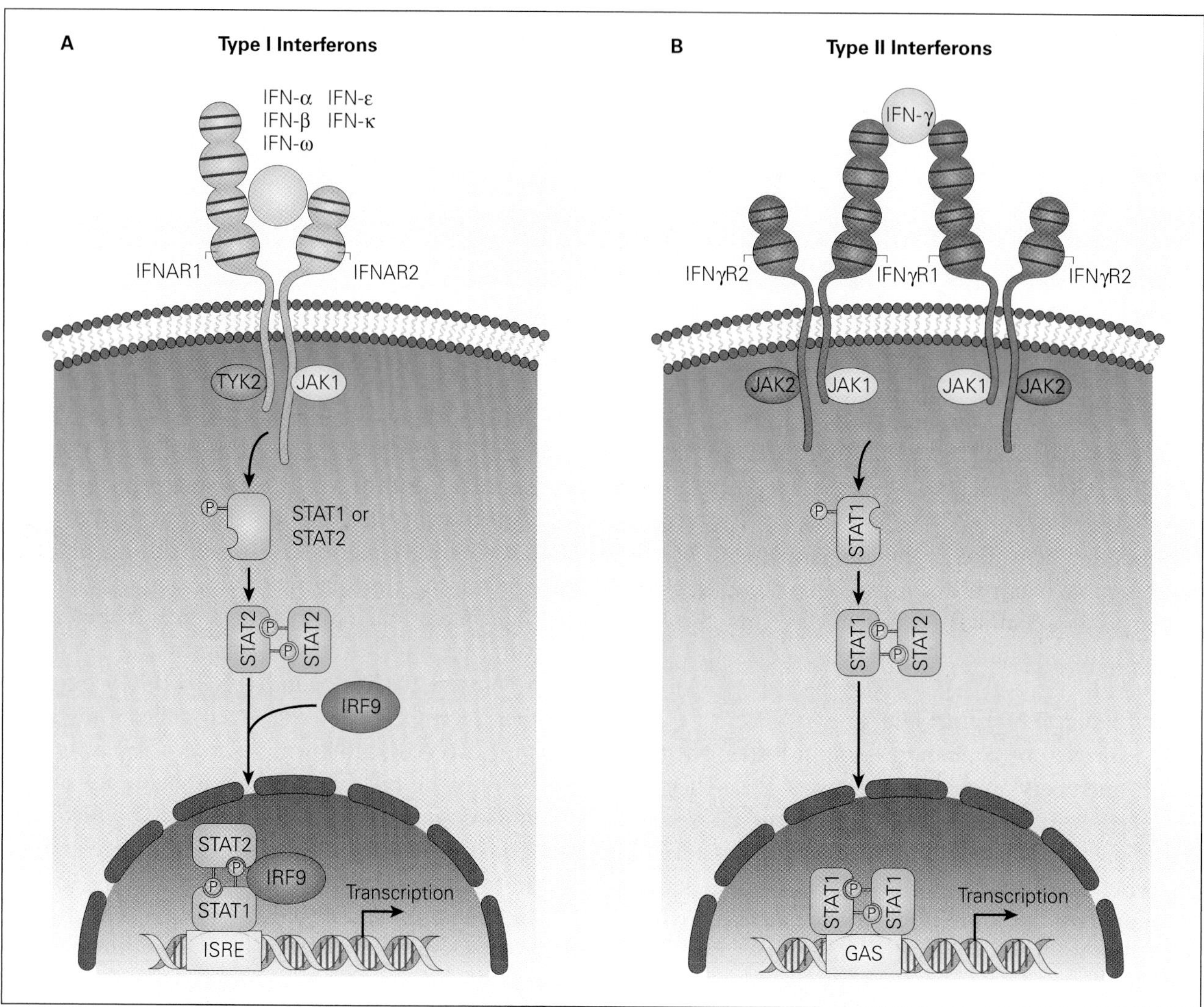

Figure 9-28. Signaling pathways of type I and type II interferons. Panel A: All type I interferons bind to the type I IFN receptor, which is composed of two subunits, IFNAR1 and IFNAR2, which are associated with tyrosine kinase 2 (TYK2) and JAK1, respectively. Following phosphorylation and dimerization of STAT1 and STAT2 they form a complex together with IRF9 (IFN-regulatory factor 9) that translocates to the nucleus either as a STAT1/STAT2/IRF9 heterodimer complex or a STAT1/STAT1/IRF9 homodimer complex, either of which can bind to the IFN-stimulated response elements (ISREs) in DNA to initiate gene transcription. In the figure, only the STAT1/STAT2/IRF9 heterodimer complex is shown. Panel B: IFN-γ binds to the type II IFN receptor composed of IFNGR1 and IFNGR2 chains which are associated with JAK1 and JAK2, respectively. They promote the phosphorylation and dimerization of STAT1 and STAT2 to form either a STAT1-STAT2 heterodimer or a STAT1-STAT1 homodimer complex, either of which can translocate to the nucleus and bind to GAS (IFN-gamma-activated site) elements that are present in the promoter region of certain ISGs, thereby initiating the transcription of these genes. In the figure, only the STAT1-STAT1 homodimer is shown.

adaptive immune responses, IFN-λ exerts a significant portion of its antiviral activity *in vivo* via stimulation of the immune system rather than through induction of the antiviral state.

Clinical Uses of the Interferons

Shown in Table 9-12 are the clinically approved uses of the three major types of interferons, IFN-α, IFN-β, and IFN-γ. Although all have overlapping properties, their distinct biologic activities have provided the basis for their effective use in a variety of clinical entities. The major side effects of interferon therapy consist of localized injection site reactions (e.g., pain and inflammation) and systemic flu-like symptoms (e.g., muscle pain, fatigue, and fever).

Alpha interferon. Various subtypes of IFN-α, e.g., alpha 2B, are indicated for the treatment of chronic hepatitis C virus (**HCV**) infection in patients eighteen years of age or older with compensated liver disease who have anti-HCV serum antibodies and/or the presence of HCV RNA. Not all strains of HCV are sensitive to interferon. Other

Table 9-12. Examples of the clinical uses of the three major classes of interferons

Interferon type	Target	Clinical use
IFN-α	Liver	Chronic HCV infection
	Malignant cell	Kidney cancer, malignant melanoma, multiple myeloma, carcinoid tumors, and hairy cell leukemia
IFN-β	CNS	Multiple sclerosis
IFN-γ	Phagocytic cell	Chronic granulomatous disease (CGD)

causes of hepatitis, such as viral hepatitis B or autoimmune hepatitis, should be ruled out prior to initiation of therapy since the use of alpha interferon has not been shown to be effective with these entities. In some patients with chronic HCV infection, IFN-α normalizes serum ALT concentrations, reduces serum HCV RNA concentrations to undetectable quantities (<100 copies/mL), and improves liver histology. IFN-α is also used in the treatment of certain malignancies, e.g., kidney, malignant melanoma, multiple myeloma, carcinoid tumors, and hairy cell leukemia (Table 9-12). The mechanism by which IFN-α exerts antitumor or antiviral activity is not clearly understood. However, it is believed that direct antiproliferative action against tumor cells, inhibition of virus replication, and modulation of the host immune response play important roles in antitumor and antiviral activity.

Beta interferon. IFN-β-1b has been shown to possess both antiviral and immunoregulatory activities and is indicated for use in ambulatory patients with relapsing-remitting multiple sclerosis (**MS**) and to reduce the frequency of clinical exacerbations (Table 9-12). Administration of IFN-γ promotes exacerbations of MS, whereas recombinant IFN-β has been shown, in controlled clinical trials, to suppress disease manifestations. Although the mechanism(s) by which IFN-β exerts its actions in MS are not clearly understood, its beneficial effects on the disease probably result from different mechanisms of action, such as modulation of IgG synthesis in plasma cells, stimulation of IL-1 receptor antagonist production, inhibition of proliferation of leukocytes, or inhibition of IL-1β and TNF-α. IFN-β also increases IL-10 levels, decreases antigen presentation in microglia, reduces T cell migration into the brain by inhibition of the activity of T cell matrix metalloproteinases, and downregulates expression of adhesion molecules.

Gamma interferon. Gamma interferon is used to reduce the frequency and severity of serious bacterial infections occurring in patients with the genetic phagocytic cell immune deficiency disorder, chronic granulomatous disease (**CGD**) (*Chapter 16*). It is often used together with antibiotics to help prevent the serious bacterial infections associated with the disorder (Table 9-12). This medication is also used to slow down the progress of the genetic bone disease malignant osteopetrosis.

ProInflammatory/ Anti-Inflammatory Cytokines

From what has been described thus far, several of the cytokines exert either pro-inflammatory or anti-inflammatory effects (Table 9-2). Although these are molecules with overlapping functions classified in other groupings, it is useful to refer to them as either pro-inflammatory or anti-inflammatory cytokines. It should be pointed out, however, that the classification of cytokines as either pro-inflammatory or anti-inflammatory is somewhat arbitrary since, because of their overlapping molecular structures and functions, a given cytokine can be pro-inflammatory in one circumstance and anti-inflammatory in another. However, this arbitrary classification may be useful not only because of the increasing clinical importance of the cytokines in the pathogenesis of many disease processes (*Chapter 5*) but also because of the ever-increasing number of biologic response modifiers now becoming available for the treatment of these diseases (*Chapter 11*).

Tumor Necrosis Factors

Prominent among the pro-inflammatory cytokines is the tumor necrosis factor (TNF) family, which includes two homologous proteins primarily derived from mononuclear phagocytes and other cells (e.g., TNF-α, also called cachexin or cachectin) and lymphocytes (e.g., TNF-β, usually called LT) (Table 9-2). The most potent inducer of TNF-α by monocytes is lipopolysaccharide (**LPS**), acting through TLR4 (*Chapter 3*). Since LPS is often contaminated with lipoproteins and lipid A, its action is dependent on its purity. LPS free of lipoprotein and lipid A only

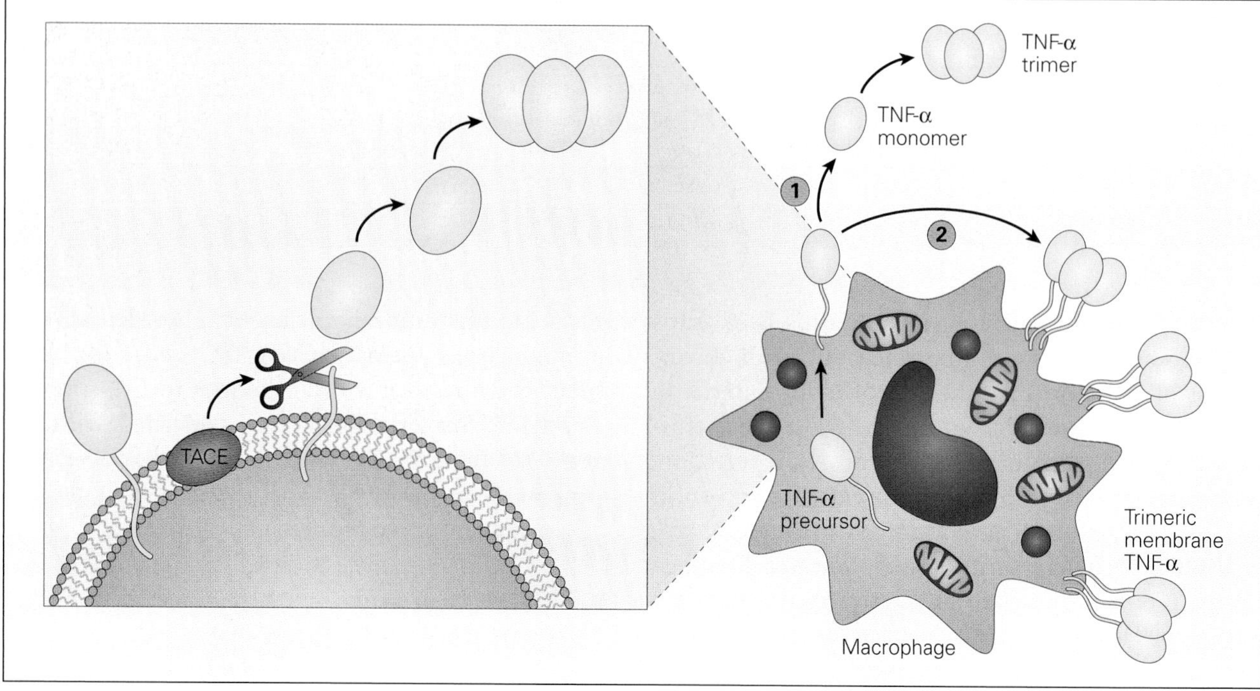

Figure 9-29. Extracellular and membrane forms of TNF-α. Left panel: TNF-α is initially synthesized as a precursor TNF-α monomer that inserts into the cell membrane and is cleaved by TACE; the TNF-α monomer is then released from the cell and spontaneously forms a trimer. Inset (1) shows the release of the TNF-α monomer and its extracellular trimerization; (2) alternatively, trimerization of the TNF-α monomer may also occur at the membrane.

act on TLR4; the lipoprotein and lipid A contaminants act on TLR-2. The active form of TNF-α is a homotrimer (Figure 9-29) that exerts a number of pro-inflammatory actions similar to those of IL-1β and IL-6 on various organ systems, by any of the following possible mechanisms:

- On the hypothalamus: It stimulates the hypothalamic-pituitary-adrenal axis by stimulating the release of corticotropin releasing hormone (CRH). TNF-α can also suppress appetite and participates in the induction of fever.
- On the liver: It initiates the acute phase response, leading to an increase in the synthesis of C-reactive protein (**CRP**) and a number of other acute-phase proteins. It also induces insulin resistance by promoting serine-phosphorylation of insulin receptor substrate-1 (**IRS-1**), which impairs insulin signaling.
- On endothelial cells: It interacts with endothelial cells to induce adhesion molecules such as intercellular adhesion molecule-1 (**ICAM-1**), vascular cell adhesion molecule-1 (**VCAM-1**), and E-selectin, thus facilitating the egress of granulocytes, lymphocytes, and monocytes into inflammatory loci (*Chapter 5*).
- On neutrophils: It activates neutrophils to adhere to endothelial cells for interepithelial transmigration into tissues.
- On macrophages: It stimulates phagocytosis and production of IL-1β, reactive oxygen species (**ROS**), nitric oxide (**NO**), and the inflammatory lipid prostaglandin E2 (**PGE2**).
- It is also responsible for the cardinal signs of inflammation: calor (heat), dolor (pain), rubor (redness), and edema (swelling) (*Chapter 5*).
- Whereas high concentrations of TNF-α induce shock-like symptoms, prolonged exposure to low concentrations can result in cachexia, a wasting syndrome. This consequence can be observed, for example, in patients with malignancy, tuberculosis, or advanced HIV infection (AIDS) and who can present with clinical cachexia.
- TNF-α also causes apoptotic cell death, cellular proliferation, differentiation, inflammation, tumorigenesis, and viral replication.
- Dysregulation and in particular overproduction of TNF-α have been implicated in a variety of human autoimmune disorders, e.g., rheumatoid arthritis, psoriasis, and Crohn's disease (*Chapter 19*). Conversely, inhibition of TNF-α activity has been implicated in cancer (*Chapter 20*).
- Surprisingly, TNF-α stimulates TNFR2 leading to lymphocyte proliferation and expansion; TNFR2, on the other hand, is expressed predominantly by Treg cells and when this pathway is activated by TNF-α has a negative feedback anti-inflammatory effect.

TNF-α is initially synthesized as a precursor TNF-α monomer which inserts into the cell membrane and is cleaved by the TNF-alpha converting enzyme (**TACE**), a membrane-associated metalloprotease (Figure 9-29). The TNF-α monomer is then released from the cell and spontaneously forms a trimer (the active form of TNF-α). Alternatively, some cells without an active TACE mechanism do not cleave the membrane-inserted TNF-α and there is spontaneous trimerization of the TNF-α in the membrane. This membrane TNF-α trimer is biologically active. Although all TNF-α producing cells express biologically active TNF-α trimer, macrophages have an active TACE and secrete the cytokine, whereas T cells primarily express the membrane TNF-α trimer.

The other tumor necrosis factor, TNF-β or LT-α produced in lymphocytes, can be synthesized and processed as a typical secretory protein but is usually linked to the cell membrane by forming heterotrimers with a third membrane-associated member of this family, lymphotoxin-beta (**LT-β**), which bind, and the resultant heterotrimer is responsible for peripheral lymphoid organ development through the production of chemokines.

TNF Receptors

As described previously, there are two distinct receptors for TNF-α, TNF receptor 1 (TNFR1[p55], CD120a) and TNF receptor 2 (TNFR2[p75], CD120b). TNF-α and TNF-β bind to these two distinct cell surface receptors with similar affinities and produce non-identical effects (Table 9-5 and Figure 9-12). TNFR1 is widely expressed on many cells and contains a death domain that can mediate cytotoxic effects, whereas TNFR2 expression is limited to T lymphocytes and signals proliferative responses. TNFs induce antitumor immunity through direct cytotoxic effects on cancerous cells and by stimulating antitumor immune responses. TNF-α is a potent activator of neutrophils and promotes adherence, degranulation, and the respiratory burst. It also mediates chemotaxis by inducing chemokines, induces vascular leakage, has negative inotropic effects, and is the primary endogenous mediator of toxic shock and sepsis (*Chapter 3*). Elevated serum concentrations of both shed forms of TNFR1 (p55) and TNFR2 (p75) have been found in systemic lupus erythematosus and rheumatoid arthritis as well as in certain forms of cancer.

Clinical Implications of TNF

TNF promotes the inflammatory response, which in turn causes many of the clinical problems associated with autoimmune disorders such as rheumatoid arthritis, ankylosing spondylitis, Crohn's disease, and psoriasis. Elevated levels of TNF-α have also been found in a subset of patients with refractory asthma and with chronic viral infections, e.g., HIV infection. These disorders are sometimes treated by TNF antagonist preparations that inhibit TNF. These TNF inhibitors include monoclonal antibody preparations such as infliximab (Remicade) or adalimumab (Humira), or consists of a circulating receptor fusion protein such as etanercept (Enbrel) (*Chapter 11*). Shown in Figure 9-30 is a schematic representation of the role of TNF-α and other mediators in the pathogenesis of RA showing the different mechanisms of action of anti-TNF-α monoclonal antibodies and fusion proteins

Because of the importance of TNF-α in antibacterial defense by granuloma formation (*Chapter 12*), one of the major adverse effects of treating patients with anti-TNF preparations is infection. Active tuberculosis may develop soon after the initiation of treatment with the TNF antagonists. Before prescribing the drug, physicians should therefore screen patients for latent tuberculosis infection or disease. The anti-TNF monoclonal antibody antagonists infliximab and adalimumab and the fusion protein etanercept have label warnings stating that patients should be evaluated for latent tuberculosis infection and treatment should be initiated prior to starting therapy with these medications.

TNF-β

TNF-β (usually called LT-α) is characterized by its ability to kill a number of different cell types *in vitro*, as well its ability to induce terminal differentiation in others. Like TNF-α, TNF-β is involved in the regulation of various biological processes, including cell proliferation, differentiation, apoptosis, lipid metabolism, coagulation, and neurotransmission. One significant non-proliferative response to TNF-β is an inhibition of lipoprotein lipase present on the surface of vascular endothelial cells. In general, TNF-α and TNF-β display similar biological activities in *in vitro* systems, although the latter is often less potent or displays apparent partial activities. TNF-β can be synthesized by antigen or mitogen-stimulated T cells (Th1 and Tc1 cells), mast cells, fibroblasts, endothelial cells, and epithelial cells. It is processed as a typical secretory protein but is usually linked to the cell surface by forming heterotrimers with a third, membrane-associated member of this family, LT-β.

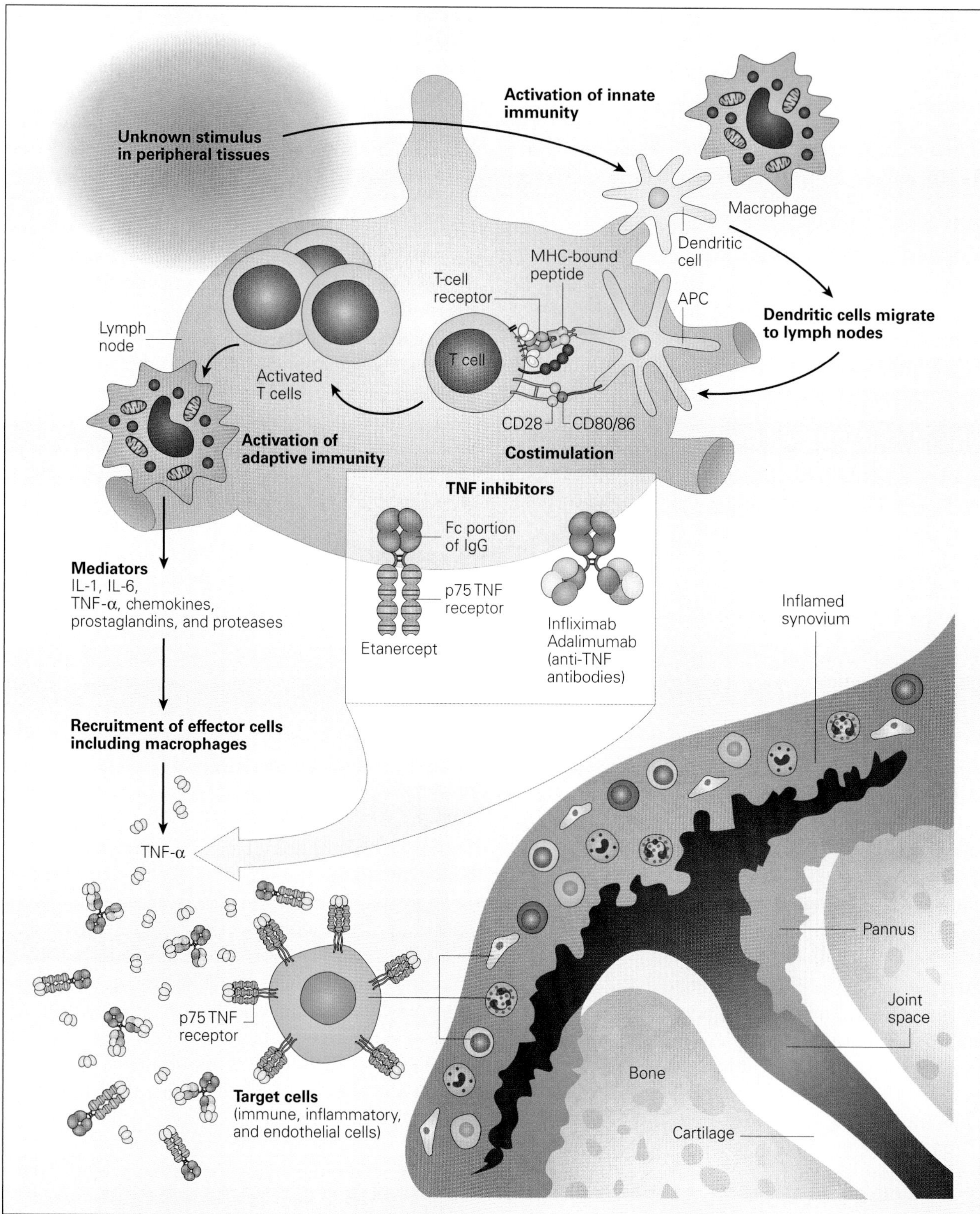

Figure 9-30. Schematic representation of the role of TNF-α and other mediators in the pathogenesis of RA showing the different mechanisms of action of anti-TNF-α monoclonal antibodies and fusion proteins. The pathogenesis of RA is thought to be initiated by an infective agent or some other stimulus that binds to dendritic cell receptors, leading to innate immune system activation. Activated DCs migrate into lymph nodes, presenting antigen to T cells utilizing a set of TCR/CD28 dual activation signals. Activated T cells not only proliferate and stimulate macrophages but also migrate into the synovial tissues of joints, producing TNF-α and other pro-inflammatory cytokines and mediators that stimulate macrophages and fibroblasts as well as chondrocytes, osteoclasts, and B cells. TNF-α, thus, serves as a central focalizing component in the cascade of cytokines and mediators which promote inflammation. Infliximab and adalimumab are monoclonal anti-TNF-α antibodies that bind to TNF-α with high affinity and prevent it from binding to its receptors. Etanercept is a fusion protein consisting of two p75 TNF receptors that are linked to the Fc portion of human IgG1, which also binds to TNF-α and prevents it from interacting with its receptors on cell surfaces.

Surprisingly, unlike TNF-α knockout mice, which have normal lymphoid development, LT-α (TNF-β) knockout mice exhibit a major defect in secondary lymphoid organ development and lack normal lymph nodes and Peyer's patches. Although the humoral immune responses of these mice are impaired, their cell-mediated immune responses are intact. Thus, the interaction of LT-α with one of its other receptors (LT-βR) accounts for the normal development of lymphoid organs.

The Anti-inflammatory Cytokines: IL-10 and TGF-β

As will be described below in the section on growth factors, there are a number of cytokines with anti-inflammatory activities. These are primarily associated with the Treg cells, and the most significant of these cytokines are IL-10 and TGF-β.

Apoptosis or Programmed Cell Death

Some cytokines, including a number of TNF family members, such as TNF-α, TNF-Related Apoptosis Inducing Ligand (**TRAIL**), and Fas, have the capacity to kill cells, while others promote their survival; this section will describe the role of cytokines in apoptosis. Apoptosis (Greek, *apo*, from; *ptosis*, falling), or programmed cell death, is a process conducted in multicellular organisms by which cells that are old, surplus, damaged, or abnormal and would otherwise interfere with normal cellular functions are promptly removed from the body. It represents a component of normal development during the ontogeny of the immune system in which autoreactive cells are removed in the thymus, for example, as well as a system of removal of abnormal cells, e.g., viral infected or malignant cells. In contrast to necrosis, which is a form of uncontrolled cell death that results from acute cellular injury due to a variety of stimuli and results in inflammation, apoptosis involves the death of cells in a controlled, regulated fashion and does not result in inflammation (*Chapter 5*). This makes apoptosis distinct from necrotic forms of cell death in which uncontrolled cell death not only leads to lysis of cells and inflammatory responses to released intracellular components but also to potentially serious health problems. Apoptosis, by contrast, is a process in which cells play an active role in their own death (which is why apoptosis is often referred to as cell suicide), and the cell debris is usually rapidly removed by phagocytosis.

Upon receiving specific signals instructing a cell to undergo apoptosis, a number of distinctive biochemical and morphological changes occur in it. Apoptosis is characterized by membrane blebbing, translocation of phosphatidylserine from the inner leaflet of the cell membrane to the outer surface, nuclear fragmentation, and activation of a number of suicide proteases called cysteine-aspartate proteases (**CASPASES**). These caspases breakdown or cleave key cellular substrates that are required for normal cellular function, including structural proteins in the cytoskeleton, mitochondria, and DNA, and nuclear proteins such as DNA repair enzymes. Some of these changes are illustrated in Figure 9-31, which shows a cell undergoing apoptosis with shrinkage, the formation of membrane blebs, and apoptotic bodies being phagocytosed by a macrophage.

Induction of Apoptosis

There are two major pathways of apoptosis: (1) the extrinsic pathway and (2) the intrinsic pathway (Figure 9-32).

In the extrinsic pathway, certain specific cytokine ligands bind to cell surface receptors, can be either soluble factors, referred to as death receptors, following which apoptosis signals are stimulated that lead to the development of a Death-Inducing Signaling Complex (**DISC**). Death receptors belong to the TNF gene superfamily and can activate a caspase cascade within seconds of ligand binding and play an important role in apoptosis. Induction of apoptosis via this mechanism is therefore very rapid. Death receptors belong to the TNF gene superfamily and generally can have several functions other than initiating apoptosis. The best characterized of the death receptors are CD95 (or Fas), TNFR1, and the TRAIL receptors, DR4 and DR5.

The ligands that bind to the death receptors can be either soluble factors, such as TNF-α, or can be expressed on the surface of cells, such as cytotoxic T lymphocytes. Cytotoxic T lymphocytes can also kill cells by directly inducing apoptosis by opening up perforin pores in the target cell membrane and releasing granzymes, which bypass the normal apoptotic pathway (*Chapter 1*). The latter occurs when T cells recognize damaged or virus-infected cells and initiate apoptosis in order to prevent damaged cells from becoming neoplastic (cancerous) or virus-infected cells from spreading the infection. The pores are created by the action of secreted

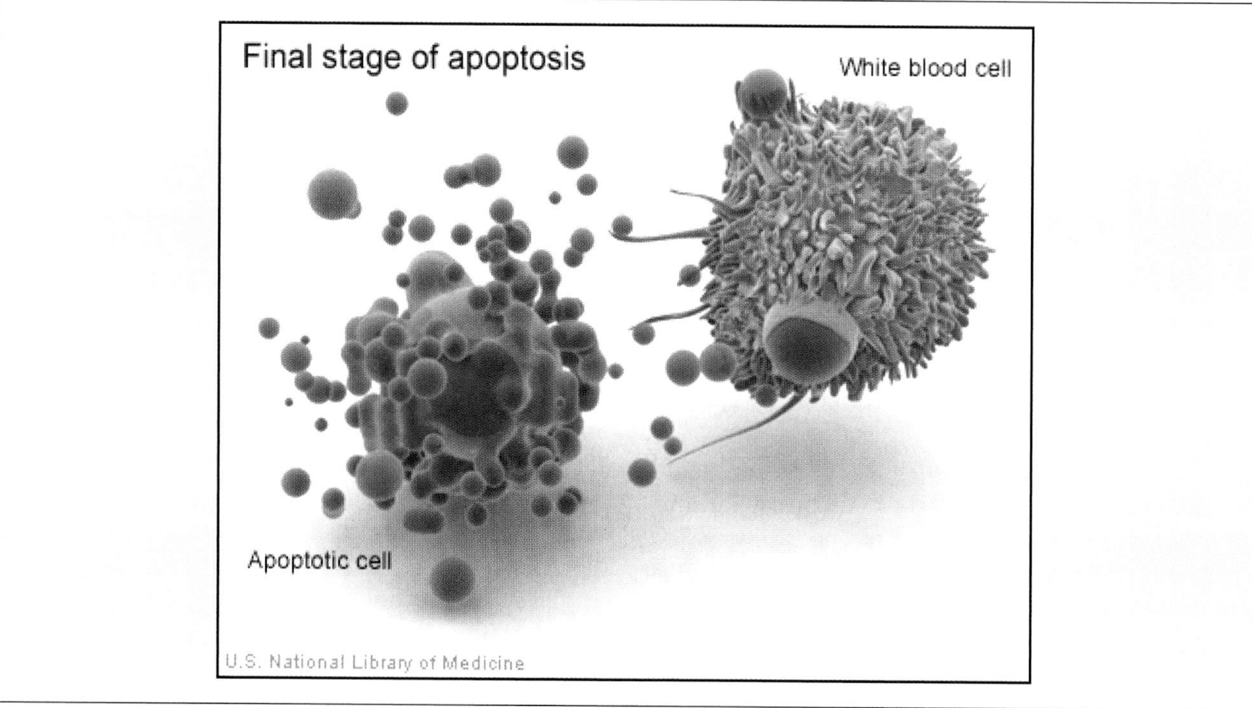

Figure 9-31. An illustration of a cell undergoing apoptosis showing shrinkage, the formation of membrane blebs, and apoptotic bodies being phagocytosed by a white blood cell, i.e., a macrophage that is consuming cell debris. (Courtesy of the National Library of Medicine.)

perforin, and the granules contain granzyme B, a serine protease which activates a variety of caspases by cleaving aspartate residues. The second way cytotoxic cells can kill a target cell is by binding to the Fc portion of an IgG antibody attached to a target cell in the antibody-dependent cellular cytotoxicity (**ADCC**) reaction; this is also the mechanism of cytotoxicity exhibited by natural killer (NK) cells (*Chapter 1*). The sensitivity of cells to any of these stimuli can vary depending on a number of factors such as the expression of pro- and anti-apoptotic proteins, e.g., the BCL-2 (B Cell Lymphoma 2) proteins or the inhibitor of apoptosis proteins (**IAP**), the severity of the stimulus, and the stage of the cell cycle. Some of the major stimuli that can induce apoptosis are outlined in Figure 9-32.

In other cases, apoptosis can be initiated following intrinsic signals that are produced after cellular stress. Cellular stress may occur from exposure to radiation or chemicals or to viral infection. It might also be a consequence of growth factor deprivation or oxidative stress caused by free radicals. In general, intrinsic signals initiate apoptosis via the involvement of the mitochondria with the release of cytochrome C. The relative ratios of the various BCL-2 proteins can often determine how much cellular stress is necessary to induce apoptosis (Box 9-13).

Signaling by TNFR1

Binding of TNF-α to TNFR1 results in receptor trimerisation and clustering of intracellular death domains (Figure 9-32). This allows binding of an intracellular adapter molecule called TNFR-associated death domain (**TRADD**) via interactions between death domains. TRADD has the ability to recruit a number of different proteins to the activated receptor. Recruitment of TNF-associated factor 2 (**TRAF2**) leads to activation of NF-κB and the JNK/Ap-1 pathway. TRADD can also associate with an adaptor protein called Fas-associated death domain (**FADD**), which leads to the induction of apoptosis via the recruitment and cleavage of procaspase-8 (Figure 9-32).

Signaling by CD95/Fas

The ligand for CD95 (CD95L or FasL) is also thought to be a trimer that on association with the receptor promotes receptor trimerization, which results in intracellular clustering of parts of the receptor called death domains. This allows the adapter protein FADD to be associated with the receptor through an interaction between homologous death domains on the receptor and on FADD. The CD95-FADD complex recruits procaspase-8 to form DISC, which activates caspase-8 to execute apoptosis.

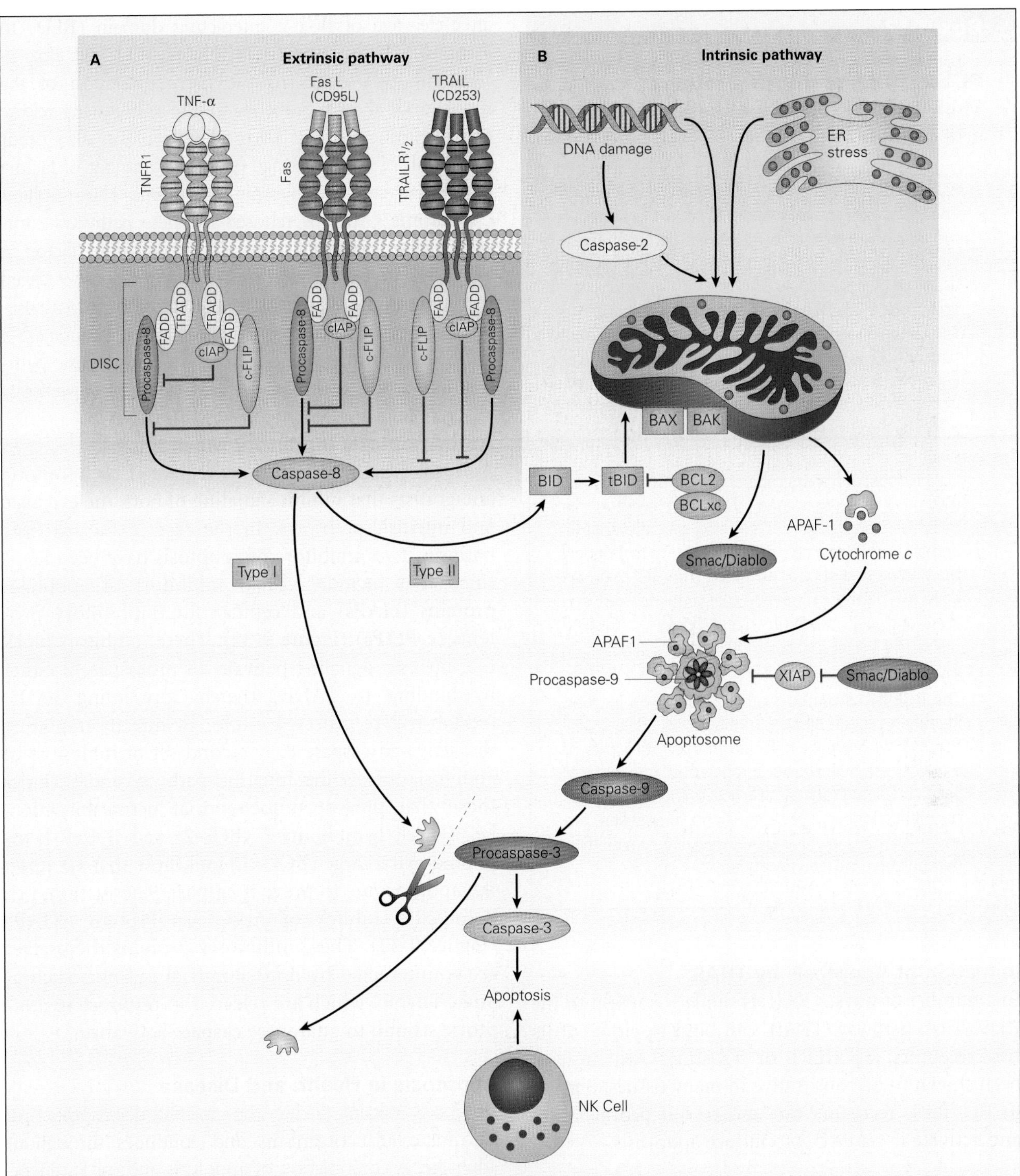

Figure 9-32. Schematic representations of the two major pathways of apoptosis. Panel A: The extrinsic pathway. The extrinsic pathway depicted on the left is characterized by death-inducing signaling complexes involving the TNFR1/TNF-α, Fas/FasL, and TRAILR1 or TRAILR2. Encountering its ligand (TNF-α), TNFR1 recruits two adaptor proteins, TRADD and FADD, via homotypic interactions between death domains of both, followed by recruitment of procaspase-8 monomers and activation to caspase-8. Similar interactions occur between FasL and TRAIL with their respective receptors with the exception that TRADD is not recruited in these two pathways. In the type I pathway, activated caspase-8 cleaves procaspase-3 into its active caspase-3 form, which then triggers apoptosis. In the type II pathway, caspase-8 cleaves BID into a cleavage product, tBID, which then promotes the release of cytochrome C from the mitochondrion, and subsequent events join with those of the intrinsic pathway. Panel B: The intrinsic pathway. Following DNA damage or any of a number of stresses affecting the endoplasmic reticulum (ER) or from the tBID generated from the extrinsic pathway, cytochrome C is released from the mitochondrion. Following the combination of the released cytochrome C with APAF-1, they form a complex with procaspase-9 called the apoptosome that leads to the activation of caspase-9. The activated caspase-9 then cleaves procaspase-3 and joins with the type I pathway of the extrinsic pathway into a final common pathway leading to apoptosis. Also shown is apoptotic induction by a natural killer (NK) cell. Also shown in red are molecules that inhibit apopotosis in the intrinsic pathway, referred to as cIAPs and c-FLIP. Similarly, there are inhibitors of tBID-induced cytochrome C release and mitochondrial permeability shown in red which include BCL-2 and BCL-xL.

Box 9-13

BCL-2, BAD, and BAX Proteins: Their Clinical Significance in Health and Cancer

1. BCL-2
   The BCL-2 proteins are a family of proteins involved in the intrinsic response to apoptosis. Some of these proteins (such as BCL-2 and BCL-XL) are anti-apoptotic, while others (such as BAD or BAX) are pro-apoptotic (Figure 9-32). The sensitivity of cells to apoptotic stimuli can depend on the balance of pro- and anti-apoptotic BCL-2 proteins. When there is an excess of pro-apoptotic proteins, the cells are more sensitive to apoptosis; when there is an excess of anti-apoptotic proteins, the cells will tend to be more resistant.
2. BAD
   Unlike most other members of the BCL-2 family, (BCL-xL/BCL-2-Associated Death promoter), a death enhancer, has no C-terminal transmembrane-domain for targeting to the outer mitochondrial membrane and nuclear envelope. The BCL-2 genes encode a family of proteins that regulates cell survival and cell death in many tissues, including mammary tissue and breast cancer.
3. BAX
   The BCL-2-Associated X protein gene was the first identified pro-apoptotic member of the BCL-2 protein family. They are believed to exert their pro- or anti-cell death activities through the transport of salts and biological materials across the membranes of mitochondria. These transport processes are essential for maintaining cell viability, while their deregulation can lead to cancer.

Induction of Apoptosis by TRAIL

In a number of ways, TRAIL is similar in action to the CD95/FasL pathway. TRAIL can bind to either of its two receptors, TRAILR1 or TRAILR2, which have been shown to be constitutive in many tissues. Similar to Fas, these receptors can also recruit procaspase-8 and activate it via FADD to induce apoptosis.

DISC Formation and the Common Pathway

Binding of death-inducing ligands such as TNF-α, FasL, and TRAIL to their receptors results in the formation of a multiprotein complex called the death-inducing signaling complex, or DISC, which is formed by (1) the receptor, (2) the adaptor protein, and (3) the procaspase-8. The DISC activates caspase-8, which can directly cleave procaspase-3 and execute apoptosis (type I pathway) or indirectly can enter the intrinsic pathway after cleavage of BCL-2 interacting domain (**BLD**) to form tBID (truncated BID) (Figure 9-32 and Box 9-13). The tBID leads to the permeabilization of the mitochondrial membrane, with the subsequent release of cyochrome C. This permeabilzation can also occur as a result of DNA damage or after a number of factors that stress the endoplasmic reticulum. The resultant cytochrome C that is released by these pathways combines with apoptotic peptidase activating factor 1 (**APAF-1**) to form a complex with procaspase-9 called the apoptosome that leads to the activation of caspase-9. The activated caspase-9 then cleaves procaspase-3 and joins with the type I pathway of the extrinsic pathway into a final common pathway leading to apoptosis.

Anti-Apoptotic Inhibitory Mechanisms

Apoptotic pathways are also regulated by apoptotic antagonists that inhibit signaling of both the extrinsic and intrinsic pathways. In the case of the extrinsic pathway, two inhibitors of apoptosis have been identified that include cellular inhibitors of apoptosis proteins (**cIAPs**) and cellular flICE-inhibitory proteins (**c-FLIPs**) (Figure 9-32). These inhibitors block the intrinsic signaling pathway of procaspase-8 either by binding to FADD, thereby preventing FADD recruitment of procaspase-8, or by directly inhibiting the activated caspase-8. A second set of inhibitors of apoptosis affects the intrinsic pathway and includes those that prevent mitochondrial permeabilization, i.e., B Cell Lymphoma-2 (**BCL-2**) and B Cell Lymphoma-extra Large (**BCL-xL**) and those that act upon the apoptosome to prevent caspase-9 activation, i.e., X-linked Inhibitor of Apoptosis Protein (**XIAP**) (Figure 9-32). These inhibitory proteins themselves are counteracted by mitochondrial proteins such as Smac/Diablo, which are released in response to apoptotic stimuli to guarantee caspase activation.

Apoptosis in Health and Disease

Apoptosis occurs during the normal development of all multicellular organisms and continues throughout adult life. A combination of apoptosis and cell proliferation is responsible for sculpting tissues and organs in developing embryos. Apoptosis is also an important part of the regulation of the immune system. T lymphocytes mature in the thymus, but before they can enter the bloodstream, they are tested to ensure that they are effective against foreign antigens and are not reactive against normal, healthy cells (*Chapters 2* and *7*). The induction of apoptosis is the process by which any ineffective or self-reactive T cells are removed.

Problems with the regulation of apoptosis have been implicated in a number of diseases. Cancer is a disease that is often characterized by too little apoptosis. Cancer cells typically possess a number of mutations that have allowed them to ignore normal cellular signals regulating their growth; they therefore become more proliferative than normal. In the case of cancer, mutations may occur that prevent cells from being able to undergo apoptosis. In these cases, there is no check on the cellular proliferation of these mutated cells; their progressive accumulation results in the formation of tumors, e.g., B cell lymphoma and BCL-2 (Box 9-13). In many cases, these tumors can be difficult to kill; many cancer treatments rely on damaging the cells with radiation or chemicals, and mutations in the apoptotic pathway often produce cells that are resistant to this type of attack. Another group of conditions characterized by too little apoptosis can be seen within the autoimmune lymphoproliferative syndrome (**ALPS**) (*Chapter 16*). These include a group of clinical disorders caused by mutations of any number of components of the apoptotic pathway, e.g., defective CD95, CD95L, caspase 8, or caspase 10, which manifest with findings of lymphoproliferation and autoimmunity. Understanding how apoptosis is regulated in these conditions is therefore an area of current major interest for the development of treatments.

There are also diseases in which too much apoptosis is thought to be part of the problem, e.g., neurodegenerative diseases, such as Parkinson's disease, Alzheimer's disease, and preeclampsia. Apoptosis is also thought to play a role in the progression of many autoimmune diseases (*Chapter 19*). For example, excessive proliferation of synovial cells in rheumatoid arthritis is thought to be due in part to the resistance of these cells to apoptotic stimuli. In other cases, poor regulation of apoptosis in T lymphocytes can result in autoreactive T cells entering the circulation and contributing to the onset of autoimmune diseases.

In conclusion, it is clear that the elimination of cells by apoptotic death is essential for the maintenance of homeostatic well-being in both health and disease. This is achieved by a number of precisely regulated pathways in which cytokines and intracellular enzymes play crucial roles.

Growth Factors

Growth factors (GFs) and colony-stimulating factors (CSFs) include another group of cytokines that stimulate the proliferation of specific pluripotent stem cells of the bone marrow (Table 9-2 and Table 9-13). These factors are proteins that bind to receptors on cell surfaces, with the primary result of activating cellular proliferation and/or differentiation. Many of these cytokines are quite pleiotropic and stimulate cellular division in numerous different cell types, while others are specific to a particular cell type.

Hematopoietic Growth Factors: Colony-Stimulating Factors

Both red and white blood cell production is regulated with great precision in healthy humans, and the production of granulocytes is rapidly increased during infection (*Chapter 2*). The proliferation and self-renewal of red and white blood cells depends on glycoprotein growth factors called stem cell factors (**SCFs**) which regulate the proliferation and maturation of descendent cells that enter the blood from the marrow. In the case of red cells, the SCF is erythropoietin (**EPO**). EPO is synthesized primarily by the kidney and is the primary regulator of erythropoiesis. EPO stimulates the proliferation and differentiation of immature erythrocytes; it also stimulates the growth of erythoid progenitor cells (e.g., erythrocyte burst-forming and colony-forming units) and induces the differentiation of erythrocyte colony-forming units into proerythroblasts (Table 9-13). When patients suffering from anemia from a variety of causes (e.g., infection and/or kidney failure) are given EPO, the result is a rapid and significant increase in red blood cell count. EPO is also produced by neural cells, and its use may prevent the severity and chronic effects of strokes.

CSFs stimulate the production of committed myeloid-monocytic stem cells and include Granulocyte-Macrophage CSF (**GM-CSF**), Granulocyte CSF (**G-CSF**), and Macrophage CSF (**M-CSF**) (Table 9-13). They are active on progenitor cells and/or differentiated end-product cells (Figure 9-21).

Thrombopoietin is a growth factor responsible for the differentiation of myeloid progenitor cells to megakaryocytes, the precursor cells that ultimately produce platelets (Table 9-13).

Therapeutic Uses of Hematopoietic Growth Factors

Hematopoietic growth factors are used therapeutically in several clinical situations in which stimulation of the production of red or white blood cells is required (Table 9-14). EPO has been found to be useful in the treatment of patients with aplastic anemia and Myeloidysplastic SynDrome (**MSD**) by augmenting

Table 9-13. Growth factors

Factor	Principal source	Primary activity	Comments
Granulocyte colony-stimulating factor (G-CSF, CSF 3)	Endothelium, macrophages, fibroblasts	Promotes proliferation of granulocyte precursors	G-CSF exists in two forms, a 174- and 180-amino-acid-long protein of molecular weight 19,600. The 174-amino acid form is produced by recombinant DNA (rDNA) technology and is available as filgastrim
Granulocyte-macrophage-CSF (GM-CSF, CSF 2)	Endothelium, macrophages, fibroblasts, T cells	Promotes proliferation of precursors for granulocytes, macrophages, and dendritic cells	Activation of mature monocytes
Macrophage-colony-stimulating factor (M-CSF, CSF 1)	Endothelium, macrophages, fibroblasts	Promotes proliferation of monocyte/macrophage precursors	M-CSF enhances the production of interferons, prostaglandin E, IL-1, G-CSF, and TNF-α in mature monocytes
Platelet-derived growth factor (PDGF)	Platelets, endothelial cells, placenta	Promotes proliferation of fibroblasts, glial, and smooth muscle cells	Composed of two polypeptide chains, A and B, that form homodimers (AA or BB) or heterodimers (AB)
Epidermal growth factor (EGF)	Submaxillary gland, Brunner's gland, kidney, mammary gland, and tumor cells	Promotes proliferation of mesenchymal, glial, and epithelial cells	Promotes angiogenesis and wound healing, mammary tissue development and homeostasis, and acts as an oncogene
Transforming growth factor (TGF-α)	Macrophages, brain cells, keratinocytes, and tumor cells	Stimulates neural cell proliferation in the adult injured brain and heals wounds	Upregulated oncogene in some human cancers and aids mammary gland development
Transforming growth factor (TGF-β)	Tumor cells, T reg, and Th3 cells and platelets	Anti-proliferative effects on endothelial cells, macrophages, and T and B cells; suppression of hematopoiesis, myogenesis, adipogenesis, and adrenal steroidogenesis; induction of IgA responses in gut-associated lymphoid tissues (GALT)	Induces Treg cells, promotes wound healing, and acts as an oncogene; an immunosuppressive agent and macrophage chemoattractant
Fibroblast growth factors (FGFs)	Wide range of cells	Promotes proliferation of many cells; inhibits some stem cells; induces mesoderm to form in early embryos	Promotion of endothelial cell proliferation, angiogenesis, and wound healing
Nerve growth factor (NGF)	Nerve cells	Essential for neuronal survival and differentiation	Several related proteins first identified as proto-oncogenes
Erythropoietin (EPO)	Kidney and neural cell types	Promotes proliferation and differentiation of erythrocyte precursors	Useful in treatment of a variety of anemias and in prevention of chronic effects of strokes
Insulin-like growth factor-I (IGF-I)	Primarily liver	Promotes proliferation of many cell types	Related to IGF-II and proinsulin, also called somatomedin C

Table 9-13. Growth factors (continued)

Factor	Principal source	Primary activity	Comments
Insulin-like growth factor-II (IGF-II)	Variety of cells	Promotes proliferation of many cell types, primarily of fetal origin	Related to IGF-I and proinsulin
Vascular endothelial growth factor (VEGF)	Most tissues and most tumors	Stimulates endothelial cells, hematopoiesis, and bone formation	Suppresses dendritic cell maturation; promotes tumor growth and angiogenesis

erythrocyte production. G-CSF and GM-CSF have been found useful in hematopoietic stem cell transplantation, not only by increasing leukocyte production in bone marrow recipients, but also in enriching the number of harvested hematopoietic stem cells obtained from pretreated donors prior to leukapheresis. Chemotherapy can cause myelosuppression and unacceptably low levels of white blood cells, making patients prone to infections and sepsis (*Chapter 16*). In oncology, a recombinant form of G-CSF, e.g., filgastrim, is used in the treatment of certain cancer patients to accelerate recovery from neutropenia after chemotherapy, allowing higher-intensity treatment regimens. GM-CSF also has been used to augment dendritic cell function in cancer patients.

The recombinant human G-CSF synthesized in an *E. coli* expression system is called filgrastim. Filgrastim (Neupogen) and PEG-filgrastim (Neulasta) are two commercially available forms of recombinant human G-CSF (**rhG-CSF**). The structure of filgrastim differs slightly from the structure of the natural glycoprotein. The polyethylene glycol (**PEG**) form has a much longer half-life, reducing the necessity of daily injections. Another form of recombinant human G-CSF, called lenograstim, is synthesised in chinese hamster ovary cells (CHO cells).

Table 9-13 also includes several other growth factors, most of which are not directly involved in immune responses. These are briefly described below, with the notable exception of the TGFs, which are described more completely because of their increasing immunologic importance, particularly in immune regulation.

Platelet-Derived Growth Factor

Platelet-derived growth factor (PDGF) is composed of two distinct polypeptide chains, A and B, that form homodimers (AA or BB) or heterodimers (AB) (Table 9-13). The c-Sis proto-oncogene has been shown to be homologous to the PDGF A chain. Only the dimeric forms of PDGF interact with the PDGF receptor. Like the EGF receptor, the PDGF receptors have intrinsic tyrosine kinase activity. Following autophosphorylation of the PDGF receptor, numerous signal-transducing proteins associate with the receptor and are subsequently tyrosine phosphorylated.

Proliferative responses to PDGF action are exerted on many mesenchymal cell types. Other growth-related responses to PDGF include cytoskeletal rearrangement and increased polyphosphoinositol turnover. Again, like EGF, PDGF induces the expression of a number of nuclear localized proto-oncogenes, such as Fos, Myc, and Jun. One of the primary effects of TGF-α is to enhance PDGF expression.

Table 9-14. Clinical uses of hematopoietic growth factors

Disease	Modality	Effects
Aplastic anemia	Erythropoietin (EPO)	Increases red blood cells
Myelodysplastic syndrome (MDS)		
Neutropenia	G-CSF	Increases neutrophils in clinical situations involving decreased production, e.g., post-chemotherapy
Bone marrow transplantation	G-CSF, GM-CSF	Increase leukocytes
Leukemias (acute myelogenous leukemia)	G-CSF, GM-CSF	Priming regimen in induction therapy
Augment antitumor immunity	GM-CSF	Augments dendritic cell function

Epidermal Growth Factor

Epidermal growth factor (EGF) is a growth factor that plays an important role in the regulation of cell growth, as well as proliferation and differentiation of epidermal cells (Table 9-13). Like all growth factors, EGF binds to specific high-affinity, low-capacity receptors on the surface of responsive cells. Intrinsic to the EGF receptor is tyrosine kinase activity, which is activated in response to EGF binding. The kinase domain of the EGF receptor phosphorylates the EGF receptor itself (autophosphorylation) as well as other proteins in signal-transduction cascades that associate with the receptor following activation. Experimental evidence has shown that the neu proto-oncogene is a homologue of the EGF receptor.

EGF has proliferative effects on cells of both mesodermal and ectodermal origin, particularly keratinocytes and fibroblasts. EGF, for example, exhibits growth effects on certain tumors as well as hair follicle cells and also has the effect of decreasing gastric acid secretion. Because of its known tumor growth effects, antibodies to receptors for EGF are being used to reduce tumor growth in patients with breast cancer, e.g., anti-human epidermal growth factor receptor (**anti-HER**) (*Chapter 11*).

Transforming Growth Factors

Transforming growth factors (TGFs) include TGF-α and TGF-β molecules (Table 9-13). Although these proteins were originally identified by their capacity to induce oncogenic transformation in rat kidney fibroblasts, the name "transforming growth factor" is somewhat arbitrary; the two classes of TGFs are not structurally or genetically related to one another, and they also act through different receptor mechanisms. Furthermore, they do not actually induce cellular transformation, but are growth factors that promote the growth of transformed cells.

TGF-α, produced in macrophages, brain cells, and keratinocytes, induces epithelial development and is upregulated in some human cancers, especially carcinomas. It is closely related to EGF and can also bind to the EGF receptor with similar effects. TGF-β, a prototypical member of the TGF-β family, is comprised of three known subtypes in humans, TGF-β1, TGF-β2, and TGF-β3. These regulate a broad range of cellular responses, including cell proliferation, differentiation, adhesion, migration, and apoptosis. Another molecule, activin bA, shares with TGF-β similar structure and functions in suppressing inflammatory reactions, and promoting tissue repair. This group of cytokines are produced by macrophages, T cells, natural killer cells, epithelial cells, and glial cells. TGF-β1 is a potent, suppressive cytokine critically involved in the induction of tolerance and the regulation of immune responses. This cytokine is produced by natural CD4+CD25+ Tregs which represent 5–10 percent of peripheral CD4+ T cells and are released by the thymus in the first days after birth (*Chapter 2*). Natural CD4+CD25+ Tregs mediate their regulatory function, in part, (CTLA4 is also crucial) by the expression of TGF-β1 (*Chapter 7*). After antigen challenge, another TGF-β1 producing-Treg subpopulation, the Tr1 cells, is induced in peripheral lymphoid tissues. The mechanism through which TGF-β1 mediates its tolerogenic functions is not completely understood. Membrane-bound TGF-β might be one of the major cytokines responsible for immunosuppression of CD4+CD25+ Treg cells and dendritic cells. Furthermore, TGF-β1 is also involved in the development, differentiation, expansion, or suppressive mechanism of both natural Treg cells as well as the induction of Treg cells from naive T cells, although the underlying molecular mechanisms remain elusive.

TGF-β1 is now considered an important cytokine in the immune suppression of different models of autoimmunity and allergy; its presence has the following effects: (1) it suppresses antigen-specific Th1 and Th2 cells, as well as allergen-specific IgE synthesis; (2) it down-regulates FcγRI expression on Langerhans cells; (3) it blocks the maturation of immature dendritic cells; and (4) it promotes the switch to IgA production. Shown in Box 9-14 are the many pleiotropic effects of TGF-β.

Fibroblast Growth Factors

Fibroblast growth factors (**FGFs**), are a family of growth factors involved in wound healing and embryonic development (Table 9-13). The FGFs are heparin-binding proteins and interactions with cell-surface associated heparan sulfate proteoglycans have been shown to be essential for FGF signal transduction. There are twenty-two members of the FGF family which have been identified in the human, all of which are structurally related signaling molecules.

One of the most important functions of bFGF (FGF2), like vascular endothelial growth factor (**VEGF**), is the promotion of endothelial cell proliferation and the physical organization of endothelial cells into tube-like structures. It thus promotes

Box 9-14

Pleiotropic Effects of TGF-β

TGF-β and related factors exhibit their pleiotropic effects through binding to transmembrane serine-threonine kinase receptors type I (TβRI) and type II (TβRII). The TGF-β family of receptors has intrinsic serine/threonine kinase activity and therefore induces distinct cascades of signal transduction. Upon ligand-induced heteromeric complex formation between TβRI and TβRII, TβRI is phosphorylated and activated by TβRII kinase and mediates specific intracellular signaling through phosphorylation of receptor-regulated Smads (R-Smads). Phosphorylated R-Smads interact with co-Smad (Smad4) and translocate into the nucleus, where they regulate transcription of target genes in cooperation with various transcription factors and transcriptional coactivators or corepressors.

TGF-β has potent anti-proliferative effects on a wide variety of cells, including epithelial cells, endothelial cells, and hematopoietic cells, although under certain conditions, it promotes the proliferation of mesenchymal cells, including fibroblasts, chondrocytes, and osteoblasts. TGF-β also induces the deposition of extracellular matrix proteins. TGF-β and its close family member activin βA are known to induce expression of collagen and other extracellular matrix components. Since deposition of matrix is required for tissue repair, the proliferative effects of TGF-β may be harmful. The inflammatory effects of tissue repair represent a major complication in life-threatening conditions, particularly asthma and nephritis, wherein the thickened basal membranes diminish gas or ion exchange, i.e., lung remodeling and chronic kidney disease, respectively. Antagonists of TGF-β are being developed to overcome these detrimental effects.

angiogenesis, the growth of new blood vessels from the preexisting vasculature. The bFGF is as potent an angiogenic factor as VEGF, and to a lesser extent, PDGF. As well as stimulating blood vessel growth, bFGF is an important player in wound healing. It stimulates the proliferation of fibroblasts that give rise to granulation tissue, which fills up a wound space/cavity early in the wound-healing process.

Vascular Endothelial Growth Factor

VEGFs are a family of proteins that include VEGF-A, VEGF-B, VEGF-C, VEGF-D, and the placental growth factor (**PLGF**). These proteins engage the VEGF tyrosine-kinase receptors, VEGFR1, VEGFR2, and VEGFR3, and the neuropilins, NP-1 and NP-2. Initially thought to mediate only endothelial-cell function, the VEGFs have been shown to mediate many functions of the immunologic, hematologic, and neurologic systems, as well as the promotion of bone formation. They also suppress dendritic cell maturation and promote tumor growth and angiogenesis.

Clinical Significance of VEGF

VEGF has been implicated in breast cancer patients with poor prognosis, rheumatoid arthritis, diabetic retinopathy, and wet-form, age-related macular degeneration (**AMD**), which is the leading cause of blindness of the elderly in the industrialized world. Anti-VEGF therapies are now available and have become important in the treatment of certain cancers and in age-related macular degeneration (*Chapter 11*). They include a wide variety of monoclonal antibodies such as bevacizumab (Avastin), antibody derivatives such as ranibizumab (Lucentis), or orally available small molecules that inhibit the tyrosine kinases stimulated by VEGF: lapatinib (Tykerb), sunitinib (Sutent), sorafenib (Nexavar), axitinib, and pazopanib.

Nerve Growth Factor

Nerve growth factor (**NGF**) is a small secreted protein which induces the differentiation and survival of particular target neurons (Table 9-13). It is perhaps the prototypical growth factor, and was the first to be described by Rita Levi-Montalcini and Stanley Cohen, who were rewarded with the 1986 Nobel Prize for Physiology and Medicine.

NGF is critical for the survival and maintenance of sympathetic and sensory neurons. After release from the neural cells, NGF binds to and activates its high-affinity receptor (TrkA) and is internalized by the responsive neuron. NGF binding and activation of TrkA is required for NGF-mediated neuronal survival and differentiation.

Insulin-Like Growth Factors

IGF-I (originally called somatomedin C) is a growth factor structurally related to insulin (Table 9-13). IGF-1 is mainly secreted by the liver in response to stimulation by growth hormone (**GH**) and is important in normal physiologic cell function as well as in number of pathological states, including cancer. IGF-II (also referred to as somatomedin A and insulin-like growth factor) is almost exclusively expressed in embryonic and neonatal tissues. Following birth, the levels of detectable IGF-II protein fall significantly (Table 9-13). For this reason, IGF-II is thought to be a fetal growth factor. The IGF-II receptor is identical to the mannose-6-phosphate receptor and is thought to be responsible for the delivery of lysosomal enzymes to the lysosomes.

Chemokines

Introduction

Chemokines are a family of small polypeptide cytokines that function as chemoattractants that induce directed cell migration, e.g., chemotaxis (*Chapter 5*). Their name is derived from their two properties, i.e., they are chemotactic cytokines. Chemokines are produced by many different cell types and serve to mobilize cells involved in a variety of immune responses, both innate and adaptive. Chemokines consist of a family of mediators that share structural and functional features and are characterized by their small size (i.e., approximately eight to fourteen kilodaltons) and the presence of two to six cysteine residues; these residues are important because they make up one to three internal disulfide loops in conserved locations that are key to forming their three-dimensional shape (Figure 9-33A). Chemokines bind to characteristic cell membrane receptors composed of seven transmembrane regions, which are members of the family of G-protein coupled receptors (**GPCR**). Originally chemokines were given specific names such as macrophage inflammatory protein (**MIP**), macrophage-derived chemokine (**MDC**), thymus-expressed chemokine (**TECK**), regulated upon activation normal T cell expressed and secreted (**RANTES**), lymphotactin, and eotaxin. More recently, an official nomenclature was developed taking into consideration the structural characteristics of the molecules.

The chemokine family of mediators is classified into four groups (C, CC, CXC, and CX_3C) according number and location of the first two conserved cysteine (C) residues in the molecule (Figure 9-33B). Each group contains a number of individual family members that are designated by the name of the group to which it belongs, followed by an L referring to the ligand and its number (Tables 9-15, 9-16, and 9-17).

Chemokine Receptors

The biological effects of the chemokines are mediated by chemokine receptors that are G-protein-linked seven-transmembrane receptors expressed on the surfaces of certain cells (Figure 9-33). Following interaction with their specific ligands, chemokine receptors trigger a flux of intracellular calcium (Ca^{++}) ions (calcium signaling) and another signal cascade that generates the chemotactic response of

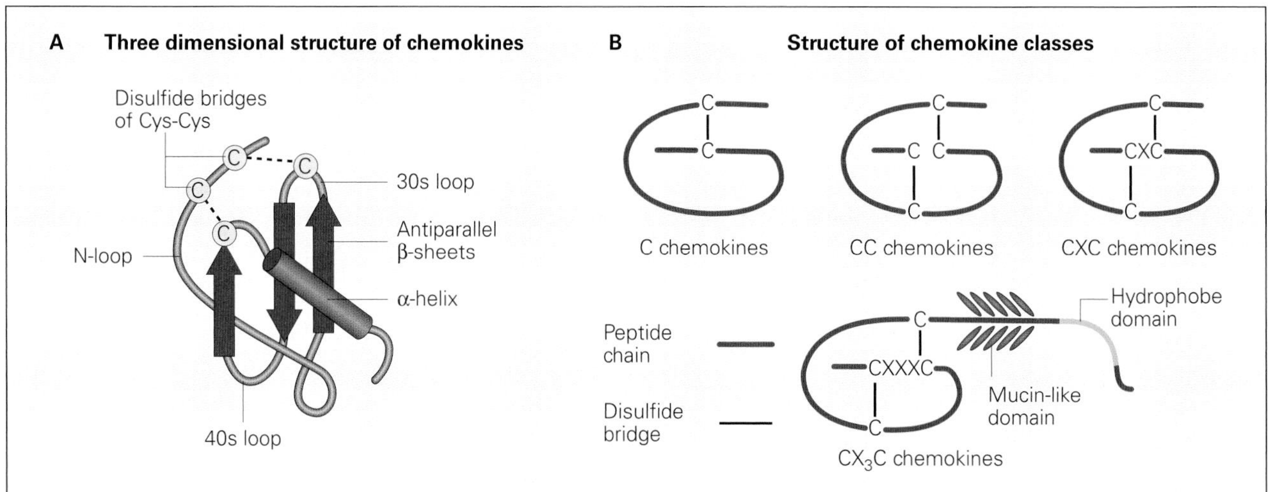

Figure 9-33. Chemokine structure. Panel A: Schematic representation of the three-dimensional structure of a chemokine showing the four cysteine residues that make up the two internal disulfide cys-cys bridges of the molecule. Panel B: The spatial relationship of the two cys-cys bridges gives rise to the nomenclature of the chemokines.

that cell, thus trafficking the cell to a desired location within the organism. These chemokine receptors are divided into different families according to the family of chemokines they bind (C, CC, CXC, or CX_3C):

- CXC chemokine receptors (seven members)
- CC chemokine receptor (ten/eleven members)
- C chemokine receptor (one member, XCR1)
- CX_3C chemokine receptor (one member, CX_3CR1)

Table 9-15. The two members of the C chemokines group

Member		Function
XCL1 XCL2	Lymphotactin	Attracts T cell (CD4+) and precursors

C Chemokines

The chemokines known as C chemokines are unlike all other chemokines in that they contain only one

Table 9-16. List of various members of the CC chemokines and CXC chemokines groups

Member	CC Chemokines Function	Member	CXC Chemokines Function
CCL1 (I-309)	Monocytes, Tregs, Th2>Th1 cells	CXCL1 (Groα) CXCL2 (Groβ) CXCL3 (Groγ)	Effects mainly on neutrophils and to a lesser extent on monocytes, lymphocytes, EC, basophils, eosinophils, and melanocytes. Angiogenic
CCL2 (MCP-1) CCL3 (MIP-1α) CCL4 (MIP-1β) CCL5 (RANTES)	Induce the migration of monocytes and other cell types such as NK cells, dendritic cells, T and B cells, eosinophils, and basophils and in the case of RANTES and MIP-1α and MIP-1β, can suppress HIV infection		
CCL6 (MRP-1)	T, B lymphocytes, macrophages, NK cells	CXCL4 (PF4)	Inhibits PMN adherence to EC. Anti-angiogenic
CCL7 (MCP-3) CCL8 (MCP-2)	Monocytes, T, NK cells, eosinophils, basophils, DC cells	CXCL5 (ENA78) CXCL6 (GCP2)	PMN, EC. Angiogenic PMN, EC. Angiogenic
CCL9/CCL10 (MRP-2)	Monocytes, PMNs, T cells	CXCL7 (NAP2)	PMN, EC, mast cell. Angiogenic
CCL11 (Eotaxin)	Th2 T cells, eosinophils, basophils		
CCL12 (MCP-5)	Monocytes, T and B cells, eosinophils		
CCL13 (MCP-4)	Monocytes, T cells, basophils, eosinophils, DC cells	CXCL8 (IL-8)	PMN, basophil, CD8 T cell, EC (macrophage adhesion). Angiogenic
CCL14a (HCC-1)	Monocytes, T cells, eosinophils		
CCL14b (HCC-3)	Unknown		
CCL15 (HCC-2)	Monocytes, T cells, eosinophils, DC cells	CXCL9 (MIG) CXCL10 (IP10) CXCL11 (I-TAC)	Anti-angiogenic T cells, NK cells (inhibits EC)
CCL16 (HCC-4)	Monocytes and T cells		
CCL17 (TARC)	Th2 cells and Treg cells		
CCL18 (PARC)	B cells and naïve T cells		
CCL19 (ELC)	T and B cells, NK cells, and mature DC cells		
CCL20 (LARC)	Immature DC cells and some T cells		
CCL21 (SLC)	T and B cells, NK cells, and mature DC cells		
CCL22 (MDC)	Th2 cells and Treg cells	CXCL12 (SDF-1)	Inhibits HIV-1, most leukocytes, T and B lymphocytes, bone marrow progenitor cells, EC, cerebellar cells Angiogenic Binds to CXCR4 mutated in WHIM (Chapter 16)
CCL23 (MPIF-1)	PMNs, macrophages, T cells		
CCL24 (Eotaxin 2)	T cells, eosinophils, basophils, monocytes		
CCL25 (TECK)	Thymocytes, T cells, and monocytes		
CCL26 (Eotaxin 3)	Eosinophils, basophils		
CCL27 (CTACK)	CLA+ memory T cells		
CCL28 (MEC)	Naïve T cells	CXCL13 (BCA-1)	B cells and some T cells
		CXCL14 (BRAK)	Monocytes
		CXCL15 (Lungkine)	Neutrophils
		CXCL16	NKT cells, T cells

Note: EC = epithelial cells.

disulfide bridge connecting two cysteine residues (Figure 9-33A, Table 9-15). Two chemokines have been described for this group: XCL1 (lymphotactin-α) and XCL2 (lymphotactin-β). Although it is known that lymphotactins attract T cells, their other effects remain unclear.

CC Chemokines

The CC chemokines have two adjacent disulfide bridges near their amino terminus (Figure 9-33B and Table 9-16). In mammals, there have been at least twenty-eight distinct members of this group, which includes CC chemokine ligands (**CCL**)-1 to -28, with CCL9 and CCL10 now identified as the same molecule but two distinct CCL14 molecules (Table 9-16). CC chemokines induce the migration of monocytes and other cell types such as T cells, epithelial cells (**ECs**), NK cells, eosinophils, mast cells, and dendritic cells. The CC chemokines induce cellular migration by binding to and activating CC chemokine receptors, ten of which have been discovered to date and are called CCR1-10. These receptors are expressed on the surface of different cell types, allowing their specific attraction by the chemokines. For example, the CC chemokine that attracts naïve T lymphocytes is CCL28, which expresses the chemokine receptor CCR10. The CCL11 (Eotaxin) chemokine can attract eosinophils that express CCR3. The CCL5 (or RANTES) chemokine attracts cells such as T cells, eosinophils, and basophils that express the receptor CCR5. In a similar fashion as cytokines, ligand-receptor interaction in the chemokine family shows not only redundancy but also binding promiscuity; that is, a single chemokine may bind to several receptors and a single chemokine receptor may react to several chemokines. For example, CCL5 (RANTES) binds CCR1 and CCR5. Also, CCR3 recognize CCL11 (eotaxin), CCL13 (monocyte chemoattractant protein-3 [**MCP-3**]) and CCL28 (mammary-enriched chemokine [**MEC**]). Interestingly, receptors for some of the chemokines, namely CCR5 and CXCR4, also act as co-receptors along with CD4 for the entry of HIV-1 into human T cells and monocytes (*Chapter 13*). Furthermore, β defensins also are chemotactic by interacting with CCR2 and/or CCR6. Consequently, chemokines frequently exhibit considerable overlapping effects (i.e., redundancies).

CXC Chemokines

The CXC chemokine group has the two adjacent disulfide bridges separated by an amino acid (X) between these residues and is comprised of sixteen members with effects mainly on neutrophils and endothelial cells and, to a lesser extent, on lymphocytes (Figure 9-33B, Table 9-16). One of the interleukins is now recognized as a CXC chemokine. For example, IL-8 induces neutrophils to leave the bloodstream and enter into the surrounding tissue and now is identified as CXCL8 (Table 9-16). CXC chemokines bind to CXC chemokine receptors, of which seven have been discovered to date, designated CXCR1-7.

CX_3C Chemokines

A fourth group of chemokines has also been discovered and members have three amino acids between the two cysteines (Figure 9-33B, Table 9-17) and are named CX_3C chemokines (or δ chemokines). The only CX_3C chemokine discovered to date is called fractalkine (or CX_3CL1). It is both secreted and tethered to the surface of the cell that expresses it, thereby serving as both a chemoattractant and as an adhesion molecule. This chemokine binds to its corresponding receptor, CX_3CR.

Function of Chemokines

Chemokines released by infected or damaged cells form a concentration gradient ranging from the lowest to a highest chemokine concentration (Figure 9-34). Attracted cells move through the gradient toward the higher concentration of chemokine.

The major role of chemokines is to guide the migration of cells. Cells that are attracted by chemokines follow a signal of increasing chemokine concentration toward the source of the chemokine. Some chemokines control cells of the immune system during processes of immune surveillance, such as directing lymphocytes to the lymph nodes so that they can screen for invasion of pathogens by interacting with antigen-presenting cells residing in these tissues. These are known as homeostatic chemokines and are produced and secreted without any need to stimulate their cell source. Some chemokines have roles in development; they promote angiogenesis (i.e., the growth of new blood vessels), promote lymphoid tissue organogenesis, or guide

Table 9-17. CX_3C chemokines

Member	Function
CX_3CL1 (fractalkine)	Acts on monocytes, NK, and T cells neuronal cells; adherence to EC

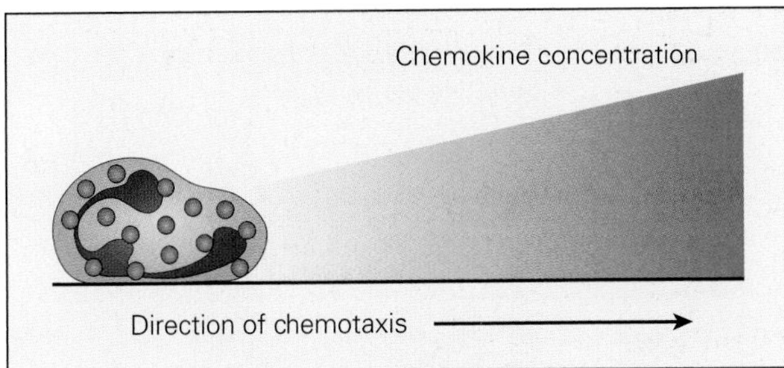

Figure 9-34. Schematic representation of the attraction of cells by chemokines toward the higher concentration of chemokine.

cells to tissues that provide specific signals that are critical for cellular maturation. Other chemokines are inflammatory chemokines that are released from a wide variety of cells in response to bacterial or viral infection and agents that cause physical damage, such as silica or the urate crystals associated with gout. Their release can also be stimulated by pro-inflammatory cytokines such as IL-1β. Inflammatory chemokines function mainly as chemoattractants for leukocytes, recruiting monocytes, neutrophils, and other effector cells from the blood to sites of infection or tissue damage. Certain inflammatory chemokines can also activate cells to initiate an immune response or can promote wound healing. They can be released by many different cell types and serve to guide cells of both the innate immune system and adaptive immune system.

Cytokines and Signaling Pathways

As described throughout this book, the basic function of the immune system is to maintain a homeostatic balance between the external and internal environments of the host. This is accomplished through a variety of receptors and their signaling pathways that are available in all cells of the body and that transmit molecular signals from a cell's exterior in the form of a variety of ligands (e.g., hormones and/or cytokines) to its interior. Cytokines carry out their many functions through signaling pathways, the two most important of which are the JAK-STAT and the NF-κB pathways. The knowledge of the molecular components of these pathways forms the basis for diagnosis and treatment of a number of clinical entities, including autoimmune disorders (*Chapter 19*), immune deficiency disorders (*Chapter 16*), allergic diseases (*Chapter 18*), and malignancies (*Chapters 20* and *21*).

Each cytokine binds to a specific cell-surface receptor followed by a cascade of intracellular-signaling events that results in altered cell functions. This may include either the upregulation or downregulation of numerous genes and their transcription factors, in turn resulting in the production of other cytokines, an increase in the number of surface receptors for other molecules, and/or the suppression of their own effect by feedback inhibition.

The JAK-STAT Pathway

Of particular importance in cell signaling associated with cytokines is the JAK-STAT signaling pathway, which is involved with regulation of cellular responses to cytokines, e.g., interferons, interleukins, and growth factors. Employing JAKs and STATs, the pathway transduces the signal carried by these intracellular polypeptides to the cell nucleus, where activated STAT proteins modify gene expression. Although STATs were originally discovered as targets of Janus kinases, it has now become apparent that certain stimuli can activate them independent of JAKs. The pathway plays a central role in principal cell fate decisions, regulating the processes of cell proliferation, differentiation and apoptosis. It is particularly important in hematopoiesis, the production of blood cells.

The NF-κB Signaling Pathway

Another essential signaling pathway important in cytokine synthesis and regulation is the NF-κB pathway (Figure 9-35). This pathway, which involves NF-κB, an inducible transcription factor of the Rel family (Box 9-15), is unique in terms of its duality of function and represents an example of a family of transcription factors that can either promote harmful inflammation or guide the beneficial aspects of tissue regeneration required for repair of inflamed tissues. NF-κB can exist in several dimeric forms, but the p50/p65 heterodimer is the predominant one. The NF-κB pathway plays a key role in programmed cell death, e.g., apoptosis. This duality of function is exemplified by many of the cytokines, chemokines, and their respective receptors, which utilize this pathway. As described previously, TNF-α, for example, can activate NF-κB and is also endowed with this same dual capacity to either harm or heal by triggering inflammation or regeneration.

There are two pathways of NF-κB activity: (1) the NF-κB1 canonical pathway, which is the prime

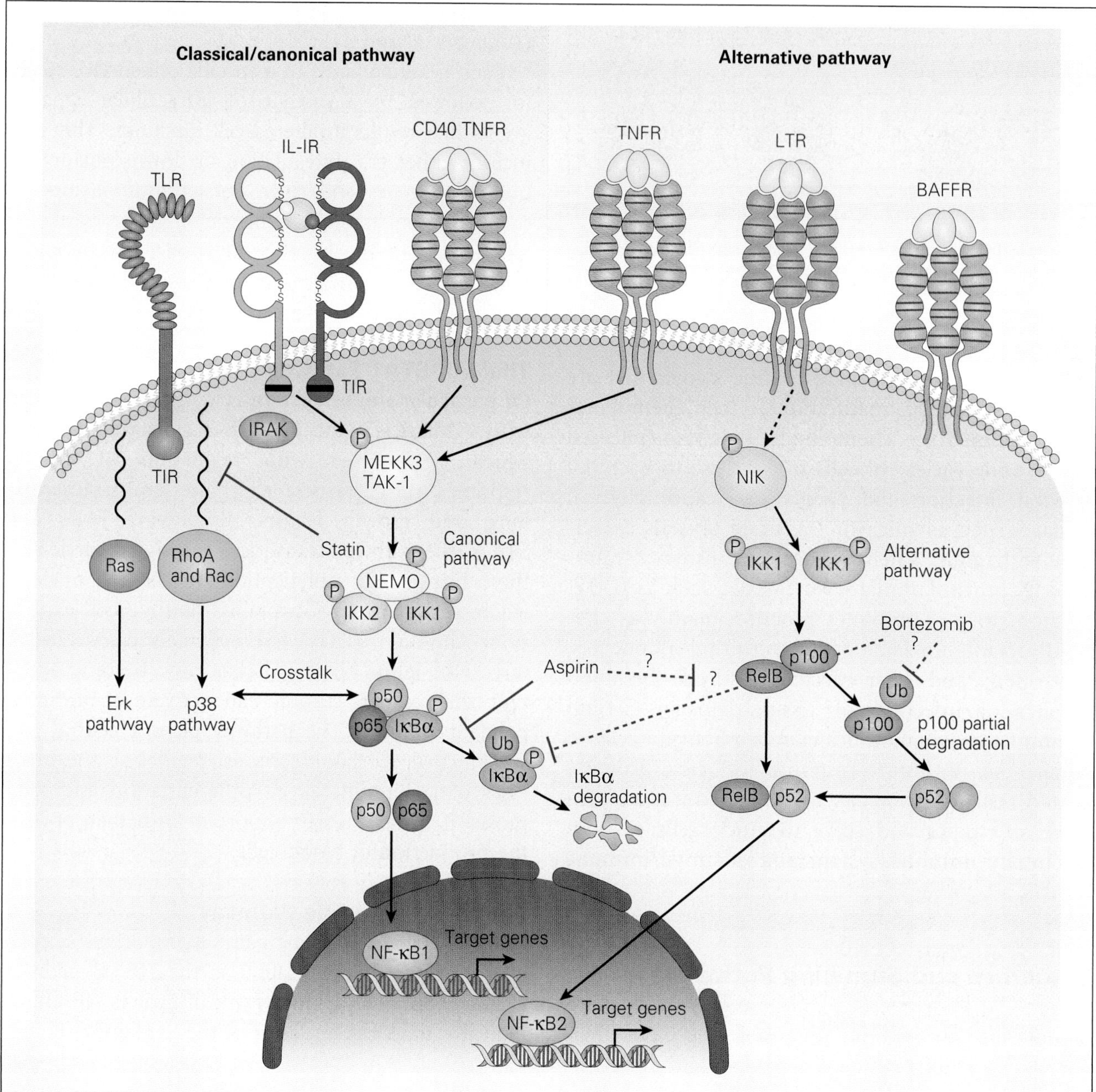

Figure 9-35. Schematic representation of NF-κB signaling pathways showing the two pathways of NF-κB activity: (1) the NF-κB1 "canonical" pathway, which is the prime pathway of the innate immune system, and (2) the NF-κB2 "alternative" pathway, which is used by the adaptive immune system.

pathway of the innate immune system, and (2) the NF-κB2 alternative pathway, which is used by the adaptive immune system (Figure 9-35). The canonical pathway is activated by any of several ligands, such as those that activate the TLRs, IL-1R, or CD40/TNFR, resulting in translocation of the NF/κB1 (p50/p65) dimer to the promoter region of genes involved in activation of inflammatory and cell survival responses. The alternative pathway is activated by ligands that bind to tumor necrosis factor-α receptors (TNFR); LT-α receptor (LTR); or BAFF receptor (**BAFFR**), which release the active NF-κB2 (p52-RelB) heterodimer into the nucleus (Figure 9-35). This alternative pathway is involved in the development of secondary lymphoid organs, B cell maturation, and the adaptive immune response (*Chapter 2*).

Box 9-15

Components of the NF-κB System

The NF-κB family consists of the following five subunits:

- Rel-A
- RelB
- c-Rel
- p50
- p52

(Rel-A, RelB, c-Rel: p65 — larger members containing transactivating factors)

NF-κB1 (p50/p65) and NF-κB2 (p52/RelB) are key transcription factors synthesized as large precursor molecules of 105 kilodaltons (p105) and 100 kilodaltons (p100), respectively, and are partially proteolyzed by the 26S proteasome, resulting in the mature active transactivating complexes. The NF-κB1 and NF-κB2 heterodimers are then translocated into the nucleus to activate target genes (Figure 9-35).

Mode of Action of the NF-κB Factors

The classical or canonical pathway is triggered by bacterial and viral infections, as well as by pro-inflammatory cytokines. The complex that mediates this pathway is a trimolecular complex called inhibitor of NF-κB kinase (**IKK**). This complex is composed of two catalytic subunits, IKK1 (also known as IKKα) and IKK2 (also known as IKKβ), and a regulatory subunit, NF-κB essential modulator (**NEMO**) (also known as IKK-γ) (Figure 9-35). This trimolecular IKK complex phosphorylates NF-κB-bound IκBs, thereby targeting them for proteasomal degradation and liberating NF-κB dimers made up of the p65 and p50 subunits to enter the nucleus and activate the transcription of target genes.

This reaction mostly depends on the catalytic subunit IKK2, which carries out the phosphorylation of IκB. Interestingly, in the canonical pathway especially in the macrophages, the IKK1 subunit has a negative-regulatory role by phosphorylation of the NF-κB subunits p65 (RelA) and c-Rel on sites that accelerate their nuclear turnover, thereby contributing to the termination of the NF-κB mediated gene-induction response. Thus, the hallmark event that characterizes the activity of the NF-κB pathway is the generation of its activity through the release of an inhibitory factor that normally keeps the transcription factor in an inhibited state. In the canonical pathway, one key regulatory mechanism is the sequestration of NF-κB complexes in the cytoplasm by interaction with the inhibitory IκB protein. NF-κB complexes are rapidly activated by means of an "upstream" Janus kinase that phosphorylates and thereby releases the inhibitory subunit, which is degraded in the 26S proteasome. In the canonical pathway, phosphorylation of IκB is critical for activation of the NF-κB1 complex. That activity is orchestrated by a cascade of kinases, including a complex consisting of IKK1, IKK2, and the other regulatory factor NEMO.

In the alternative pathway, the slower *de novo* synthesis of NF-κB-inducing kinase (**NIK**), the first kinase in the cascade is the rate-limiting step in the activation. NIK then activates the IKK1–IKK1 homodimeric complex that in turn phosphorylates and partially degrades the p100-RelB (NF-κB2) complex into active p52-RelB (NF-κB2) (Figure 9-35).

Clinical Significance of the NF-κB Signaling Pathway

The NF-κB signaling pathway is a multi-component pathway that regulates the expression of hundreds of genes that are involved in diverse and key cellular and host processes, including cell proliferation, cell survival, the cellular stress response, innate immunity, and inflammation. Dysregulation or malfunctioning of the NF-κB pathway, either by mutation or epigenetic mechanisms, is involved in many human and animal diseases, especially those associated with chronic inflammation, immunodeficiency, or cancer. Shown in Table 9-18 is a list of inherited human genetic diseases associated with mutations in the NF-κB signaling pathway.

The activation of NF-κB depends on many post-translational modifications in key molecules, which either directly influence the cascade or indirectly modulate the cascade through the regulation of intersecting pathways. These post-translational modifications include isoprenylation (Box 9-16) of the GTPases Ras and Rho, whose well-described pathways impinge on NF-κB, and the ubiquitination of IKK2, which directly modulates NF-κB (Figure 9-35). There is considerable crosstalk between cyclooxygenase-mediated prostaglandin metabolism and NF-κB. Aspirin blocks IκB phosphorylation, whereas statins inhibit the canonical NF-κB pathway, resulting in the attenuation of experimental autoimmune encephalitis and other autoimmune diseases. Regulation of NF-κB therefore can be achieved to a certain extent by means of widely used drugs, including statins, aspirin, and glucocorticoids. The development

Table 9-18. Inherited human genetic diseases with mutations in the NF-κB signaling pathway

Pathology	Phenotype	Gene/chromosome	Mutations
Incontinentia pigmenti	Skin inflammation Missing/deformed teeth Retinal vessel detachment CNS dysfunctions	NEMO (Chr. X)	Genomic rearrangement (70–80%) Stop or frameshift mutations generating large NEMO deletions Rare missense mutations
EDA-ID	Recurring infections Impaired development of skin adnexes	NEMO (Chr. X)	Short truncations affecting the ZF; Missense mutations in various domains of NEMO
OL-EDA-ID	Same as EDA-ID plus Increased bone mass Impaired function of lymphatic vessels	NEMO (Chr. X)	Addition of 27 aa at the C-ter of NEMO
Immunodeficiency (without EDA)	Recurring infections	NEMO (Chr. X)	Missense mutations; short truncation of the N-ter of NEMO
EDA-ID(T)	Same as EDA-ID plus impaired T cell proliferation	IκBα (Chr. 14)	Heterozygous missense mutation abolishing IκBα phosphorylation by IKK
Immunodeficiency	Recurring infections	IRAK-4 (Chr. 12)	Missense/nonsense mutations and microdeletions (1–2 nuc) affecting the kinase domain
Cylindromatosis/MFT	Tumors developing at skin adnexes	CYLD (Chr. 16)	Stop or frameshift mutations deleting the catalytic domain Rare missense mutations

of drugs targeting the ubiquitin system and the proteasome should increase the repertoire of classes of therapeutics that influence NF-κB. The conundrum, however, for transcription factors such as NF-κB is that, although they are pathogenic in inflammation, they may be necessary for regeneration and for the termination of autoimmunity through the apoptotic elimination of self-reactive T cells. Whether targeting NF-κB directly will tip this balance to physiological amounts remains a challenge.

Summary

Once the field that dealt exclusively with the study of mechanisms of resistance to infectious diseases, immunology has evolved into a clinical discipline in which it now plays a significant role in diagnosis, treatment, and prevention of a myriad of diseases that were previously diagnostic and therapeutic orphans. As the field of clinical immunology has progressed from an observation-based entity to an interventional-clinical discipline, it has placed into the hands of the health care provider the necessary tools to diagnose and treat patients suffering from such diseases as rheumatoid arthritis, diabetes mellitus type 1, multiple sclerosis, asthma and allergy, transplant-related disorders, and chronic viral infections, including HIV/AIDS, immune deficiencies, and cancer. Central to this supernova expansion in the field of immunology is the rapidly growing knowledge of cytokines, chemokines, and their effects on the immune system. These achievements in clinical care have been made possible by seminal discoveries of basic and clinical scientists that have led to new research strategies resulting in the approval of flagship therapies targeting TNF for rheumatoid arthritis and that are now paving the way for new cytokine-targeted treatments for numerous other immunologically mediated diseases as described in detail in Chapter 11.

Box 9-16

Prenylation or isoprenylation or lipidation is the addition of hydrophobic molecules to a protein. It is usually assumed that prenyl (3-methyl-2-buten-1-yl) groups facilitate attachment to cell membranes, similar to lipid anchors like the GPI anchor, though direct evidence is missing. Prenyl groups have been shown to be important for protein-protein binding through specialized prenyl-binding domains.

Because of the continuing discoveries of the cytokines, chemokines, and the receptors to which they bind, it is difficult to predict the infinite number of products that will emerge as a result of this ever-expanding list of pro-inflammatory and anti-inflammatory molecules. But we can be certain of one thing: they will continue to provide the tools for better diagnosis and treatment of a multitude of diseases that were once relegated to chapters of medical textbooks as diseases of unknown etiology treated empirically with agents whose mechanisms of action were unknown. The future of cytokines is here, and for patients with immunologically mediated diseases, the future will be brighter and more hopeful.

Case Study: Clinical Relevance

Let us now return to the case study of the streptococcal toxic shock syndrome presented earlier and review some of the major points of the clinical presentation and how they relate to the immune system:

- Toxic shock syndrome (TSS) is an acute-onset illness characterized by fever, rash, and hypotension that can lead to multiple organ failure and lethal shock, as well as desquamation in patients who recover. The disease is caused by bacterial superantigens (SAGs) secreted from Staphylococcus aureus or group A streptococci that bypass normal antigen presentation by binding to class II major histocompatibility complex molecules on antigen-presenting cells and to specific variable regions on the β chain of the T cell antigen receptor.
- Shown in Table 9-19 is a comparison of the diagnostic criteria by which staphylococcal and streptococcal TSS are currently defined.
- Through this interaction, SAGs activate T cells at orders of magnitude above antigen-specific activation, resulting in massive cytokine release that is believed to be responsible for the most severe features of TSS and which is referred to as "cytokine storm."
- The profound clinical consequences of Gram-positive toxic shock associated with "cytokine storm" are hypothesized to stem from excessive Th1 responses to superantigens that results in a systemic release of pro-inflammatory cytokines, including IL-1, TNF-α, and IFN-γ.
- The evidence supporting the importance of T cells in toxic shock led to the expectation that T cell-derived cytokines would play a key role in the pathogenesis of toxic shock. The pathogenetic role of IFN-γ, the hallmark cytokine of Th1 activation, has been validated by the finding that IFN-γR knockout mice are resistant to endotoxin or staphylococcal enterotoxin B (SEB)-induced shock. However, in other studies, treatment with anti-IFN-γ Abs appears only partially protective.
- Recent studies of experimental mouse models of toxic shock suggest that the release of cytokines, including TNF-α, occurs in a biphasic manner; an "early" release of cytokines at two hours, and a "delayed" release before death at seven hours. Mortality and cytokine release at both time points were dependent on TCRαβ T cells. Anti-TNF-α pretreatment inhibited the early TNF-α response and was protective against shock, but delayed anti-TNF-α treatments were not. These results demonstrate that TCRαβ T cells are critical for lethality in toxic shock, but it is the early TNF-α response and not the later cytokine surge that mediates lethal shock.

Table 9-19. Diagnostic criteria for staphylococcal and streptococcal toxic shock syndrome

Staphylococcal toxic shock syndrome	Streptococcal toxic shock syndrome
1. Fever 2. Hypotension 3. Diffuse macular rash with subsequent desquamation 4. Three of the following organ systems involved: • Liver • Blood • Renal • Mucous membranes • Gastrointestinal • Muscular • Central nervous system 5. Negative serologies for measles, leptospirosis, and Rocky Mountain spotted fever, as well as negative blood or cerebral spinal fluid cultures for organisms other than *S. aureus*	1. Isolation of group A streptococci from • A sterile site for a definite case • A nonsterile site for a probable case 2. Hypotension 3. Two of the following symptoms: • Renal dysfunction • Liver involvement • Erythematous macular rash • Coagulopathy • Soft-tissue necrosis • Adult respiratory distress syndrome

Key Points

- Cytokines are small proteins that function as intercellular communication molecules. They may act on the producing cell (autocrine), an adjacent cell (paracrine), or a distant organ (endocrine). They may also act redundantly, synergistically, or antagonistically.
- Cytokines bind to specific membrane receptors, activating intracellular signaling pathways that modify cell function.
- Cytokines are classified by their functions into six major groups: interleukins, interferons, pro-inflammatory cytokines, anti-inflammatory cytokines, growth factors, and chemokines.
- There are thirty-seven presently known interleukin molecules that regulate communication between and among the many cells that comprise the innate and adaptive immune systems.
- Interferons are cytokines, which in addition to their classical antiviral functions, exhibit downregulatory effects on the growth of normal and malignant hematopoietic cells *in vitro* and *in vivo*; there are three different classes: type I (IFN-α, IFN-β), type II(IFN-γ), and type III (IFN-λ).
- Apoptosis is a complex process that occurs via both extrinsic and intrinsic pathways and is regulated by a variety of cytokines.
- Growth factors (GFs) and colony-stimulating factors (CSFs) induce growth by stimulating the proliferation of specific pluripotent stem cells of the bone marrow.
- Chemokines are a family of small polypeptide cytokines that function as chemoattractants that induce directed cell migration, e.g., chemotaxis.
- Cytokine activity occurs through a variety of complex signaling processes, including the JAK-STAT and the NF-κB signaling pathways.
- Cytokines are demonstrating ever-increasing clinical significance as knowledge of their roles and signaling mechanisms continues to provide tools for better diagnosis and treatment of a multitude of immune-mediated diseases.

Study Questions/Critical Thinking

Pick the one BEST answer for each question by picking the letter of the correct choice.

1. Cytokines may exhibit __________ action, signaling the cells that produce them.
   a. antagonistic
   b. autocrine
   c. endocrine
   d. paracrine
   e. synergistic
2. Cytokines are NOT
   a. antigen-specific
   b. capable of activating more than one cell type
   c. made by lymphocytes
   d. small protein molecules
   e. synthesized *de novo* in response to antigen or other cytokines
3. Several cytokines may have the same effect on the cells they bind. This is an example of
   a. a cascade
   b. antagonism
   c. pleiotropism
   d. redundancy
   e. synergy
4. Characterization of cytokine activities is NOT made more difficult by their
   a. gene structure
   b. pleiotropism
   c. redundancy
   d. secretion close to target cell membranes
   e. short half-lives
5. Interferons
   a. activate B cells to make virus-specific antibodies
   b. are Th2 cytokines
   c. are virus proteins that interfere with activation of cytotoxic T cells
   d. block virus infection of host cells
   e. inhibit virus replication by infected cells
6. A cytokine can do all of the following EXCEPT
   a. bind to receptors that do not share cytokine-binding subunits
   b. bind to its specific receptor on the same cell that produced it
   c. bind to receptor antagonists produced by pathogenic viruses
   d. compete with other cytokines whose receptors share signal-transducing subunits
   e. upregulate (increase) synthesis of high-affinity subunits for its receptor
7. Members of a cytokine receptor family
   a. all bind the same cytokines
   b. are grouped together because they share antigen specificity

c. are often found on the same cells
d. are similar in protein structure and sometimes in regions of amino acid sequence
e. are specific for cytokines produced by a single cell type

8. The ability of a cytokine to change gene expression in the target cell is influenced by all of the following EXCEPT

a. presence of high-affinity receptors on the target cell
b. presence of soluble cytokine receptors
c. proximity of the producing and target cells
d. rate of transport of cytokine-receptor complexes into the cytoplasm
e. simultaneous production of another cytokine whose receptor uses the same signal-transducing subunit

9. Cytokines are NOT

a. able to inhibit the function of other cytokines
b. able to stimulate the synthesis of other cytokines
c. produced by more than one cell type
d. small protein molecules
e. stored in the cell for quick release

10. The IL-2R subfamily consists of receptors for IL-2, IL-4, IL-7, IL-9, and IL-15. This group of cytokine receptors

a. binds all five cytokines to promote synergistic action on target cells
b. binds cytokines that are produced by the same cell
c. each has a unique high-affinity cytokine-specific α chain
d. shifts the immune response toward cellular immunity
e. each has a unique signal-transducing γ chain

11. An antagonist for cytokine X may NOT be

a. cytokine A, competing for a shared receptor subunit
b. cytokine B, which acts synergistically with cytokine X
c. cytokine C, which inhibits the activation of the cell that produces cytokine X
d. made by microorganisms
e. soluble cytokine X receptors

12. A knockout mouse for a particular cytokine allows immunologists to characterize cytokine function

a. by doing a dose-response study with competing cytokines
b. in the absence of all other cytokines
c. on all cell types simultaneously
d. under controlled conditions of local cytokine concentrations
e. with defined cell populations

13. Activated Tc can regulate immune responses by signaling activated lymphocytes to undergo

a. apoptosis
b. clonal deletion
c. clonal proliferation
d. cytotoxicity
e. somatic hypermutation

Suggested Reading

Ahmed CM, Johnson HM. IFN-gamma and its receptor subunit IFNGR1 are recruited to the IFN-gamma-activated sequence element at the promotor site fo the IFN-gamma-activated genes: evidence of transactivational activity in IFNGR1. J Immunol. 2006; 177: 315–21.

Artis D, Kane CM, Fiore J, et al. Dendritic cell-intrinsic expression of NF-kappa B1 is required to promote optimal Th2 cell differentiation. J Immunol. 2005; 1174: 7154–9.

Brennan F, Beech J. Update on cytokines in rheumatoid arthritis. Curr Opin Rheumatol. 2007; 19: 296–301.

Bueno C, Criado G, McCormick JK, et al. T cell signaling induced by bacterial superantigens. Chem Immunol Allergy. 2007; 93: 161–80.

Clerico M, Contessa G, Durelli L. Interferon-beta1a for the treatment of multiple sclerosis. Expert Opin Biol Ther. 2007; 7: 535–42.

Conti P, Youinou P, Theoharides TC. Modulation of autoimmunity by the latest interleukins (with special emphasis on IL-32). Autoimmun Rev. 2007; 6: 131–7.

Deb DK, Sassano A, Lekmine F, et al. Activation of protein kinase C delta by IFN-gamma. J Immunol. 2003; 171: 267–73.

De Togni P, Goellner J, Ruddle NH, et al. Abnormal development of peripheral lymphoid organs in mice deficient in lymphotoxin. Science. 1994; 264: 703–7.

Dunn GP, Koebel CM, Schreiber RD. Interferons, immunity, and cancer immunoediting. Nat Rev Immunol. 2006; 6: 836–48.

Dupuis S, Jouanguy E, Al-Hajjar S, et al. Impaired response to interferon-alpha/beta and lethal viral disease in human STAT1 deficiency. Nat Genet. 2003; 33: 388–91.

Edwards CK, Bendele AM, Reznikov LI, et al. Soluble human p55 and p75 tumor necrosis factor receptors reverse spontaneous arthritis in transgenic mice expressing transmembrane tumor necrosis factor alpha. Arthritis Rheum. 2006; 54: 2872–85.

Faulkner L, Cooper A, Fantino C, et al. The mechanism of superantigen-mediated toxic shock: not a simple Th1 cytokine storm. J Immunol. 2005; 175: 6870–7.

Fina D, Fantini MC, Pallone F, et al. Role of interleukin-21 in inflammation and allergy. Curr Drug Targets Inflamm Allergy. 2007; 6: 63–8.

Hotchkiss RS, Nicholson DW. Apoptosis and caspases regualate death and inflammation in sepsis. Nat Rev immunol. 2006; 6: 813–22.

Hotchkiss RS, Strasser A, McDunn JE, et al. Cell death. New Engl J Med. 2009; 361: 1570–83.

Kaminska J, Kowalska M, Kotowicz B, et al. Pretreatment serum levels of cytokines and cytokine receptors in patients with non-small cell lung cancer, and correlations with clinicopathological prognostic factor. Oncology. 2006; 70: 115–25.

Kilani RT, Mackova M, Davidge ST, et al. Endogenous tumor necrosis factor alpha mediates enhanced apoptosis of cultured villous trophoblasts from intrauterine growth-restricted placentae. Reproduction. 2007; 133: 257–64.

Krammer PH, Arnold R, Lavrik IN. Life and death in peripheral T cells. Nat Rev Immunol. 2007; 7: 532–42.

Lachmann HJ, Kone-Paut I, Kuemmerle-Deschner JB, et al. Canakinumab in CAPS study group: use of canakinumab in the cryopyrin-associated periodic syndrome. 2009; 360: 2416–25.

Leung S, Qureshi SA, Kerr IM, et al. Role of STAT2 in the alpha interferon signaling pathway. Mol Cell Biol. 1995; 15: 1312–7.

Lundberg P, Welander PV, Edwards CK, et al. Tumor necrosis factor (TNF) protects resistant C57BL/6 mice against herpes simplex virus-induced encephalitis independently of signaling via TNF receptor 1 or 2. J Virol. 2007; 81: 1451–60.

Madhusudhan TR, Sambamurthy S, Williams E, et al. Surviving streptococcal toxic shock syndrome: a case report. J Med Case Reports. 2007; 1: 118.

Marchetti M, Monier MN, Fradagrada A, et al. Stat-mediated signaling induced by type I and type II interferons (IFNs) is differentially controlled through lipid microdomain association and clathrin-dependent endocytosis of IFN receptors. Mol Biol Cell. 2006; 17: 2896–909.

Markowitz CE. Interferon-beta: mechanism of action and dosing issues. Neurology. 2007; 68 Suppl 4: S8–11.

McCormick JK, Yarwood JM, Schlievert PM. Toxic shock syndrome and bacterial superantigens: an update. Ann Rev Microbiol. 2001; 55: 77–104.

Platanias LC. Mechanisms of type-I- and type-II-interferon-mediated signaling. Nat Rev Immunol. 2005; 5: 375–86.

Platanias LC, Fish EN. Signaling pathways activated by interferons. Exp Hematol. 1999; 27: 1583–92.

Sakamoto E, Hato F, Kato T, et al. Type I and type II interferons delay human neutrophil apoptosis via activation of STAT3 and up-regulation of cellular inhibitor of apoptosis. J Leuk Biol. 2005; 78: 301–9.

Salem HA, Eissa LA, Rabbie AM, et al. Evaluation of some biochemical markers as prognostic factors in malignant lymphomas. Pak J Pharm Sci. 2006; 19: 219–30.

Scheller C, Sopper S, Ehrhardt C, et al. Caspase inhibitors induce a switch from apoptotic to pro-inflammatory signaling in CD95-stimulated T lymphocytes. Eur J Immunol. 2002; 32: 2471–80.

Schrader JW. Interleukin is as interleukin does. J Immunol Methods. 2003; 276: 1–3.

Schutze S, Tchikov V, Schreider-Brachert W. Regulation of TNFR1 and CD95 signaling by receptor compartmentalization. Nat Rev Mol Cell Biol. 2008; 9: 655–62.

Shuai K, Ziemiecki A, Wilks AF, et al. Polypeptide signaling to the nucleus through tyrosine phosphorylation of the JAK and STAT proteins. Nature. 1993; 366: 580–3.

Sims JE, Nicklin MJ, Bazan JF, et al. A new nomenclature for the IL-1 family genes. Trends Immunol. 2001; 22: 536–7.

Tamai M, Kawamaki A, Tanaka F, et al. Significant inhibition of TRAIL-mediated fibroblast-like synovial cell apoptosis by IFN-gamma through JAK/STAT pathway by translation regulation. J Lab Clin Med. 2006; 147: 182–90.

Toh ML, Miossec P. The role of T cells in rheumatoid arthritis: new subsets and new targets. Curr Opin Rheumatol. 2007; 19: 284–8.

Weaver CT, Hatton RD. Interplay between the TH17 and T reg cell lineages: a co-evolutionary perspective. Nat Rev Immunol. 2009; 9: 883–9.

Wu T, Xie C, Bhaskarabhatla M, et al. Excreted urinary mediators in an animal model of experimental immune nephritis with potential pathogenic significance. Arthritis Rheum. 2007; 56: 949–59.

Youssef S, Steinman L. At once harmful and beneficial: the dual properties of NF-κB. Nat Immunol. 2006; 7: 901–2.

Chapter 10

Immunogenetics

Kathleen E. Sullivan, MD, PhD
Eleni E. Magira, MD

Case Studies

Case Study 1

A six-month-old boy was evaluated for recurrent infections. He has had two ear infections that resolved promptly with antibiotics, as well as recurrent candida and thrush. Topical treatment of the candidal infections was not effective. At the age of four months, he developed a cytomegalovirus pneumonitis, which has persisted. IgG, IgA, and IgM levels were slightly low for his age. His total T cell count as determined by CD3 expression was normal at 1,800 cells/mm^3. His CD4 T cell count was low at 325 cells/mm^3 and his CD8 T cell count was normal at 1,200 cells/mm^3. Lymphocyte proliferation responses to mitogens were approximately 50 percent of the control. The diminished CD4 T cell level was suggestive of MHC-II deficiency; MHC-II expression was directly measured by flow cytometry and was found to be absent on B cells and stimulated T cells.

Case Study 2

A twenty-year-old man with a one-year history of back pain was seen by an orthopedic surgeon. His back pain began acutely with a presumed viral infection but never completely resolved. X-rays showed sacroileitis and early vertebral squaring, establishing the diagnosis of ankylosing spondylitis. At the age of twenty-four, he started nonsteroidal anti-inflammatory medications, which allowed him to continue his usual activities. He developed recurring episodes of iridocyclitis after age thirty and also developed enthesitis (an inflammation of the entheses, the location where a bone has an insertion to a tendon or a ligament; from the Greek *enthetos*, implanted, and *-itis*, inflammation), costosternal tendonitis, sternoclavicular arthritis, and hip arthritis. His symptoms typically worsened with infection and although he has had considerable progression since age thirty, he has maintained an active lifestyle through the use of nonsteroidal medications and acupuncture. He is considering the use of TNF-α inhibitor therapy.

Case Study 3

A twenty-five-year-old woman presented to the emergency department with vomiting. She had a three-month history of progressive fatigue and

LEARNING OBJECTIVES

When you have completed this chapter, you should be able to:

- Understand the structure and function of MHC molecules
- Describe the differences between MHC-I and MHC-II expression
- Understand associations between specific MHC molecules and diseases such as rheumatoid arthritis and ankylosing spondylitis
- Understand the role of immunogenetics in transplantation
- Explain the differences between hyperacute, acute, and chronic rejection
- Understand graft-versus-host disease and the various preventative measures currently employed
- Recognize the importance of immunogenetics in health and disease

Case Studies (continued)

shortness of breath. Recently she had developed bruising with minimal trauma. In the emergency department, she was found to have a hemoglobin level of 2.9 gm/dl, a white count of 700 cells/mm^3, and a platelet count of 3,000/mm^3. After multiple transfusions, a bone marrow biopsy and aspirate were performed that demonstrated cellularity of <10 percent. A chromosomal breakage analysis ruled out Fanconi's anemia and a karyotype analysis on the marrow cells was normal. She was treated with cyclosporine and cyclophosphamide. All three hematopoietic lineages rose modestly, but the effect was not sustained. She then received a course of anti-lymphocyte globulin with no effect. A decision was made to perform a bone marrow stem cell transplant. The patient had no siblings and a search for a donor was made through the National Marrow Donor Program where a match was found and recruited. The patient received conditioning and an unrelated stem cell transplant from that donor. She later developed acute grade III graft-versus-host disease, which was treated with steroids. Once the graft-versus-host disease resolved, the patient was discharged and has continued on multiple immunosuppressive medications but with normal hematologic parameters.

Introduction

Immunogenetics has classically referred to the study of major histocompatibility complex (**MHC**) genes and their relation to disease. The term has been broadened in recent years, however, to encompass all aspects of genetic influences on host immune responses. The study of immunogenetics has been greatly enhanced by the availability of an increasing number of emerging techniques of modern molecular biology such as the use of microarrays, which have clearly had profound effects in the delineation of genetic controls affecting all aspects of the innate and adaptive immune responses (*Chapter 25*). These include a wide array of individual differences ranging from those affecting innate immune response molecular recognition, e.g., toll-like receptor (**TLR**) expression, cytokine production, adhesion molecule expression, and molecular signaling pathways of adaptive immunity, to those that affect the clinical expression of specific infection, allergic disease, autoimmune disorders, and malignancy. Since these topics will be covered in other sections in the book, this chapter will confine itself to the structure and function of MHC molecules and their clinical application in health and disease.

Physiology: The Major Histocompatibility Complex

Background

The MHC molecules are glycoproteins encoded in a large cluster of genes located on chromosome 6. They were first identified by their potent effect on the immune response to transplanted tissue (*Chapter 22*). For that reason, the gene complex was termed the "major histocompatibility complex." MHC genes (called the H-2 complex in mice) were first recognized in 1937 as a barrier to transplantation in mice. In humans, these genes are often called human leukocyte antigens (**HLA**), as they were first discovered through antigenic differences between white blood cells from different individuals. MHC is the term for the region located on the short arm of chromosome 6p21.31 in humans and chromosome 17 in mice. In humans, it contains more than 200 genes (Figure 10-1).

The principal function of the MHC is to present antigen to T cells to discriminate between self (our cells and tissues) and nonself (the invaders or modified self). Two main characteristics of the MHC make it difficult for pathogens to evade immune responses. First, the MHC is polygenic. It contains several different MHC-I and MHC-II genes so that every individual possesses a set of MHC molecules with different ranges of peptide-binding specificities. Second, the MHC is extremely polymorphic. The MHC genes display the greatest degree of polymorphism in the human genome. There are multiple variants of each gene within the population as a whole. The different variants that are inherited by an individual from a parent are known as *alleles*. The numbers of alleles recognized at the classical loci are presented in Table 10-1. Polymorphic sites are found predominantly in specific regions of the MHC-I and MHC-II molecules called domains, which will be described in greater detail below. Although each HLA molecule shows slight differences in its amino acid sequence from one another, causing a slightly altered three-dimensional structure in the peptide-binding cleft, the basic structures of MHC-I and MHC-II molecules are very similar (Figure 10-2). The charge characteristics of the groove determine which peptides can be presented. Since different antigenic peptides have different shapes and charge characteristics, it is important that the human population overall has a large array of different HLA

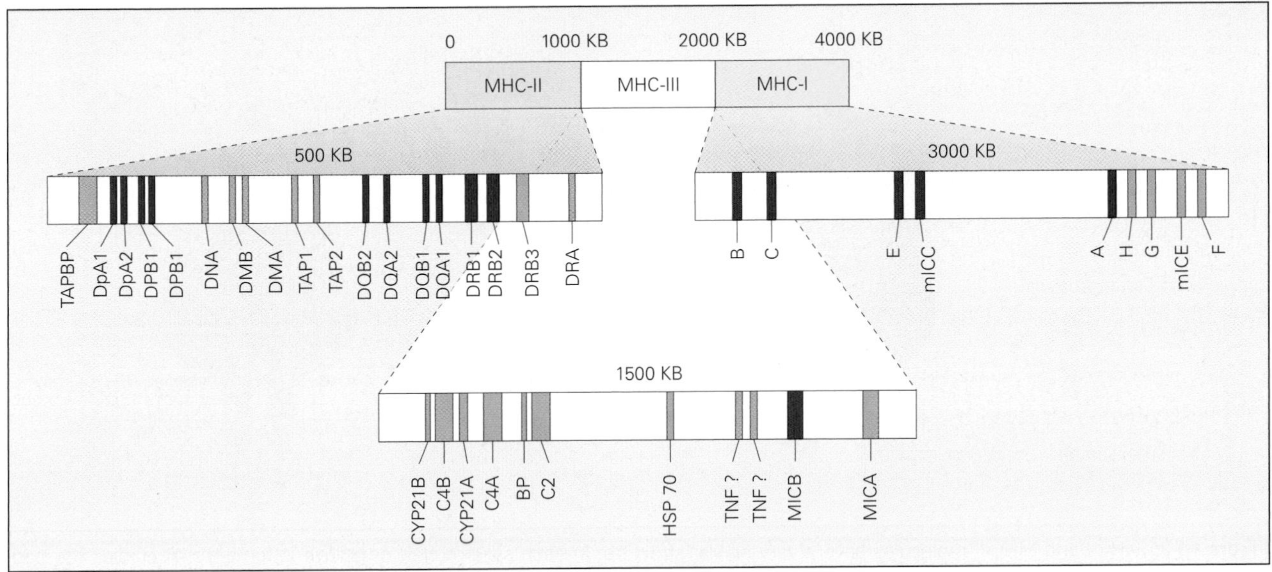

Figure 10-1. Genetic map of the MHC regions. This map has been simplified to demonstrate organizational themes within the MHC. There are more than 200 genes within these regions.

molecules, each with different shaped peptide-binding areas (clefts) to cope with the multitude of self and nonself peptides presented.

MHC Structure and Function

The MHC has three regions: MHC-I, MHC-II, and MHC-III (Figure 10-1). The classical HLA antigens encoded in each region include HLA-A, -B, and -C in the MHC-I region, and HLA-DR, -DQ, and -DP in the MHC-II region. The MHC-III region includes several genes involved in the complement cascade (C4A, C4B, C2, and FB) (*Chapter 4*), the TNF-α and TNF-β (LTα) genes, the CYP21 gene that encodes an enzyme in steroid metabolism, the HSP70 gene that encodes a

Table 10-1. The number of alleles within each HLA locus

	Number of antigens defined by serologic methods	Number of alleles defined by DNA methods
MHC-I loci		
HLA-A	28	545
HLA-B	61	894
HLA-Cw	10	307
MHC-II loci		
HLA-DRB1	24	494
HLA-DQB1	9	83
HLA-DQA1	0	34
HLA-DPB1	6	126
HLA-DPA1	0	23

(As of April 2007.)

chaperone, and many other genes of unknown immunological function. In general, when we refer to MHC, we are referring to either MHC-I or MHC-II molecules.

Shown in Figure 10-3 is a schematic representation of the chromosomal locations and genetic loci responsible for MHC-I and MHC-II synthesis. MHC-I molecules consist of two polypeptide chains, a larger α chain encoded on chromosome 6 in the MHC region and a smaller β2 microglobulin encoded on chromosome 15 (Figures 10-2 and 10-3). The class I α chains consist of a single polypeptide composed of three extracellular domains named α_1, α_2, and α_3, a transmembrane region that anchors it in the plasma membrane, and a short intracytoplasmic tail (Figure 10-2). The β_2 microglobulin consists of a single non-polymorphic molecule noncovalently bound to the alpha chain and is encoded on chromosome 15 (Figure 10-2 and Figure 10-3). The α_1 and α_2 domains fold together into a single structure consisting of two segmented α helices lying on a sheet of eight antiparallel β strands. The folding of the α_1 and α_2 domains creates a long cleft or groove that is the site at which peptide antigens bind to the MHC-I molecule and are presented to the CD8 lymphocyte.

MHC-II molecules consist of two polypeptide chains, α and β, both encoded in the MHC-II region on chromosome 6 and noncovalently linked to one another (Figure 10-2 and Figure 10-3). The α and β chains each consist of two extracellular domains referred to as α_1 and α_2 and β_1 and β_2,

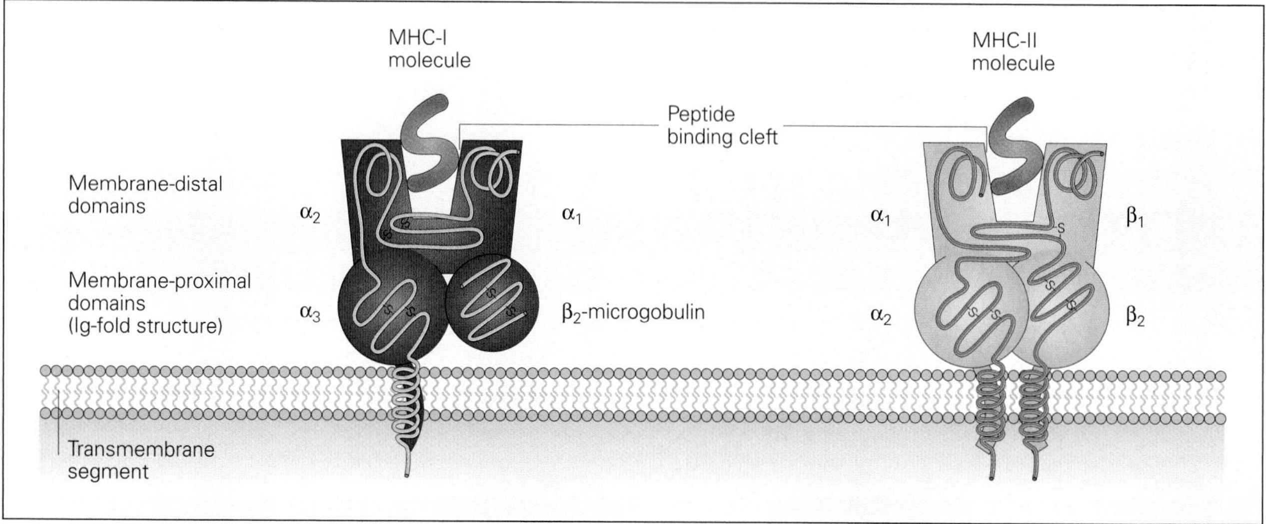

Figure 10-2. MHC-I and MHC-II molecules have a very similar structure. In each case, a cleft or groove is formed that cradles the peptide. The charge characteristics of the groove determine which peptides can be presented.

respectively, and, similar to the MHC-I α chain, the α and β chains of the MHC-II molecule also consist of a transmembrane segment and a cytoplasmic tail (Figure 10-2). The extracellular membrane-proximal α_2 and β_2 domains are homologous to immunoglobulin-constant domains (*Chapter 6*).

The crystallographic structure of the MHC-II molecule shows that it is folded very much like the MHC-I molecule (Figure 10-4). The major differences between the two molecules lie at the ends of their peptide-binding clefts, which are more open in MHC-II molecules compared with MHC-I molecules. The MHC-II molecule cleft is made up of a noncovalent association between the α_1 and β_1 domains and that binds the peptide through multiple van der Waals forces and hydrogen bonds (Figure 10-5). The main consequence of this difference is that the ends of a peptide bound to an MHC-I molecule are buried within the molecule whereas the ends of peptides bound to MHC-II molecules are not. This allows more flexibility in the length and types of peptides that MHC-II molecules can bind. Peptides that bind a specific class II molecule will share the same middle anchor residues but may vary in length and sequence of other residues.

Expression of MHC Molecules

MHC-I proteins are expressed on all nucleated cells, in contrast to MHC-II molecules, which are restricted to antigen-presenting cells (**APCs**) (Table 10-2). Lymphocytes, macrophages, dendritic cells, Langherans cells, and some endothelial cells are the predominant cells that express MHC-II. Nonnucleated cells such as mammalian red blood cells express little or no MHC-I and thus, pathogens within red blood cells can go undetected by cytotoxic T cells, e.g., malaria. The expression of both MHC-I and MHC-II molecules is regulated by cytokines (*Chapter 9*). Interferon-γ (**INF-γ**) increases the expression of MHC-I or MHC-II molecules and can induce the expression of MHC-II molecules on certain cell types that do not normally express them. This may be very important both in normal immunologic function and in autoimmunity. The level of MHC molecule expression plays an important role in T cell activation and therefore differences in levels of expression are significant (*Chapter 7*). Shown in Table 10-3 is a comparison of the principal differences between MHC-I and MHC-II molecules.

Antigen Presentation

T cells recognize foreign antigens in the form of short peptides that have been processed and displayed on the cell surface bound to MHC-I or MHC-II molecules (Figure 10-5). The MHC-peptide complex is as critical to adaptive immunity as the T cell receptor (**TCR**) (*Chapter 7*). Antigens are often categorized according to whether they are derived from (1) viruses, intracellular bacteria, or protozoan parasites (endogenous pathogens); or (2) exogenous pathogens that replicate outside of the cell (*Chapter 1*). Intracellular antigens are presented to T cells by any nucleated cell because MHC-I expression is ubiquitous. In contrast, exogenous antigens are taken up by professional APCs, which process the antigens

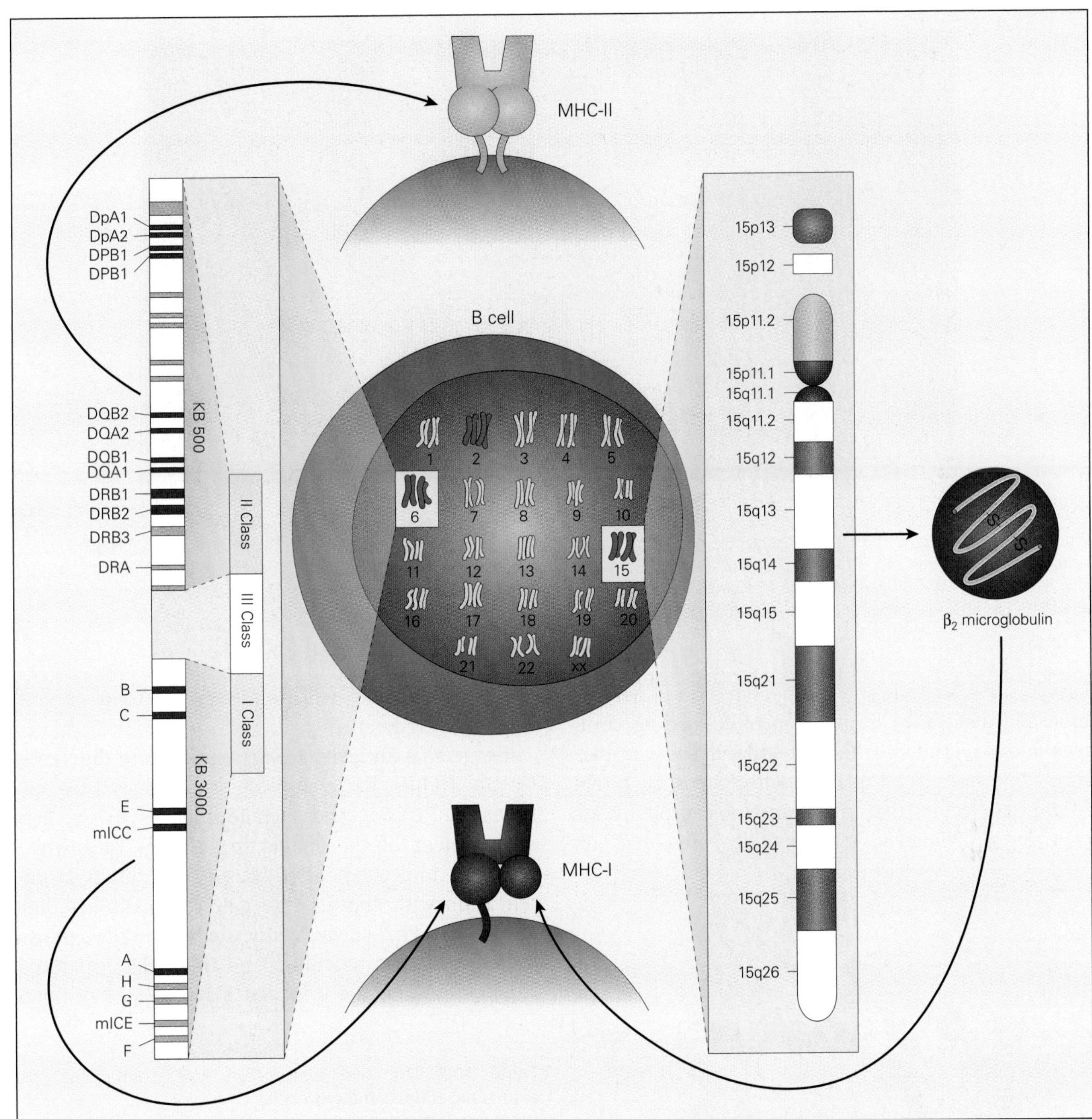

Figure 10-3. Schematic representation of the chromosomal location and genetic loci responsible for MHC-I and MHC-II synthesis.

and present them in the context of MHC-II. An important function of a professional APC, e.g., dendritic cell (**DC**), is to deliver a second signal (costimulation) to the T cell to alert it to the presence of infection (*Chapter 7*).

Endogenous antigens, including misfolded proteins and pathogen-derived peptides, are processed by the proteasome (Figure 10-6A). This complex of proteases typically generates peptides of four to twenty amino acids with a hydrophobic carboxy terminus. After trimming of the peptide by cytosolic proteases, the antigenic peptides are translocated to the endoplasmic reticulum by the transporters associated with antigen processing (**TAP1** and **TAP2** molecule). Meanwhile, a new MHC-I molecule is being synthesized in the endoplasmic reticulum. As it folds, it is bound by calnexin, which is then replaced by calreticulin and β_2 microglobulin. The new MHC-I molecule associates with the MHC-I peptide loading complex. Tapasin physically links the MHC-I molecules and the TAP transporters. As the peptide enters from the cytosol, the cleft of the class

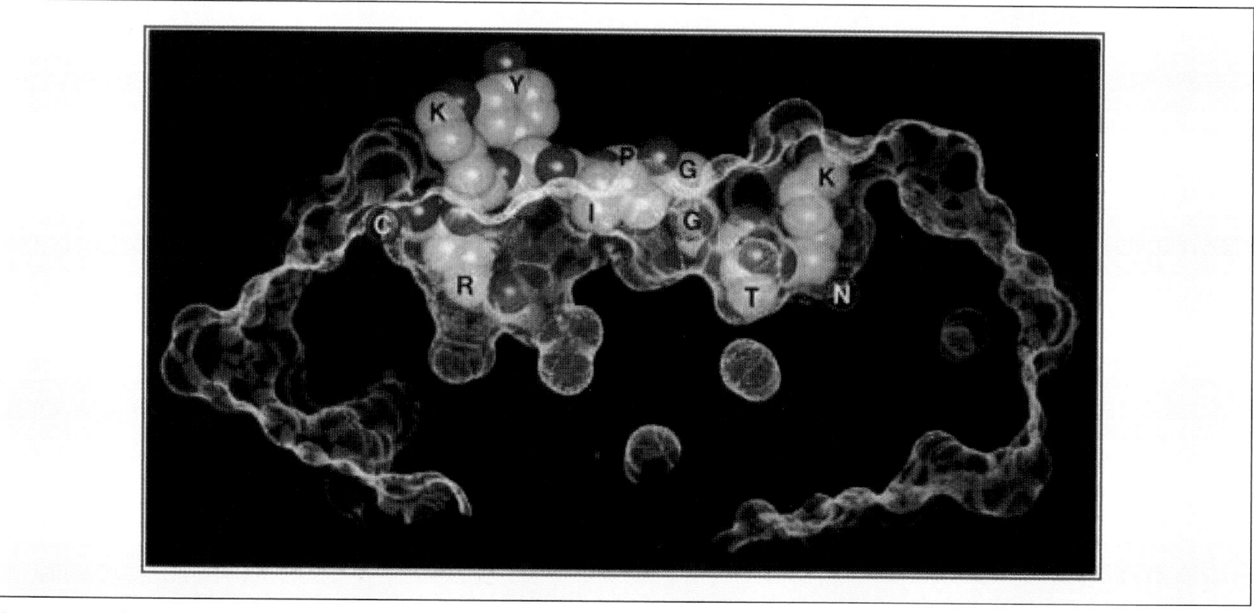

Figure 10-4. Structure of an HLA-DQ molecule. An influenza virus nucleoprotein peptide (KTGGPIYKR) bound to HLA-A*6801, shows insertion of Thr (T) and Arg (R) buried in specificity pockets of the HLA molecule. (Reproduced with permission from Guo HC, Madden DR, Silver ML, et al. Comparison of the P2 specificity pocket in three human histocompatibility antigens: HLA-A*6801, HLA-A*0201, and HLA-B*2705. Proc Natl Acad Sci USA. 1993;90:8053–7.)

I molecule receives it and the peptide-bound MHC-I molecule dissociates from the peptide-loading complex and is recruited to the cell surface. This complex machinery has several quality-control steps, such that MHC-I molecules that fail to assemble properly are degraded. Ultimately, the peptide presented on MHC-I molecule will stimulate a CD8 T cell response (Figure 10-7).

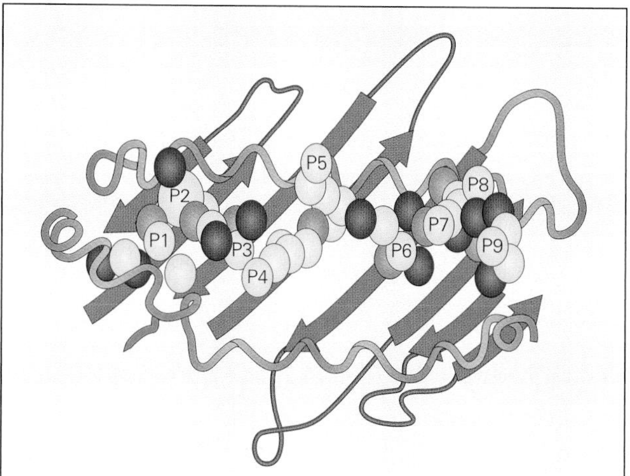

Figure 10-5. An example of a peptide held within an MHC-II groove. The fit of the peptide within the groove is very specific. The MHC-II molecule cleft is made up of a noncovalent association between the α_1 and β_1 domains that bind the peptide through multiple van der Waals forces and hydrogen bonds. The α_1 and β_1 domains are shown lying on a sheet of eight antiparallel β strands. The folding of the α_1 and β_1 domains creates a long cleft or groove that is the site at which peptide antigens bind to the MHC-II molecule and are presented to the CD4 lymphocyte.

Exogenous antigens are processed quite differently (Figure 10-6B). Bacterial proteins are cleaved by proteases, cathepsins, and metalloproteases in the acid environment of the endocytic pathway. Meanwhile, MHC-II molecules assemble in the endoplasmic reticulum with another molecule called the invariant chain (**li**). The newly synthesized molecules transit the endoplasmic reticulum and the Golgi apparatus. After passage of the li-loaded MHC-II-DM complex

Table 10-2. The two classes of MHC molecules are expressed differentially on cells

Human tissue	MHC-I	MHC-II
T cells	+++	+ (activated T cells)
B cells	+++	+++
Macrophages	+++	++
Other antigen-presenting cells (APCs) (e.g., Langerhans)	+++	+++
Epithelial cell of the thymus	+	+++
Neutrophils	+++	–
Hepatocytes	+	–
Kidney	+	–
Brain	+	–
Red blood cells	–	–

Note: + = degree of expression; – = lack of expression.

Table 10-3. Features of MHC-I and MHC-II molecules

Feature	MHC-I	MHC-II
Polypeptide chains	A single α chain (44–47 kD) noncovalently linked to the β_2-microglobulin chain (12 kD)	A single α chain (32–34 kD) noncovalently linked to a single β chain (29–32 kD)
Distribution	All nucleated cells	Antigen-presenting cells
Composition of antigen-binding clefts	α_1 and α_2 domains	α_1 and β_1 domains
Binding site for T cell co-receptor	CD8 binds to the α_3 region	CD4 binds to the β_2 region
Size of peptide-binding cleft	Accommodates peptides of 8–11 residues	Accommodates peptides of 10–30 residues or more
Nomenclature in the human	HLA-A, HLA-B, HLA-C	HLA-DR, HLA-DQ, HLA-DP

through the Golgi into the late endosomes, the invariant chain is cleaved by acid proteases, leaving a residual peptide referred to as the CLass II-associated Invariant chain Peptide (**CLIP**) in the MHC-II cleft. CLIP occludes the MHC-II cleft and prevents peptides from loading until the molecule is in the lysosomal or late endosomal compartment containing the peptides. At that point, HLA-DM molecules remove CLIP from the cleft and stabilize the molecule while the peptide is loaded into the cleft. HLA-DO molecules can also facilitate this process in some settings. The fully assembled and loaded MHC-II molecule is recruited to the surface and serves to stimulate predominantly CD4 positive T cells (Figure 10-6B and Figure 10-7).

The segregation of antigens as either MHC-I-presented or MHC-II-presented has important functional consequences. Intracellular organisms such as viruses are largely inaccessible to antibodies, thus the need for the recruitment and presentation of antigen to CD8 T cells that can kill the host cell harboring the virus (*Chapter 13*).

Extracellular pathogens generally require opsonization and phagocytosis for clearance (*Chapter 12*). Opsonization with antibody improves phagocytosis and presentation of extracellular pathogen-derived peptides to CD4 T cells via MHC-II, which allows the CD4 T cells to direct an antibody response by B cells.

Nomenclature of HLA

The HLA nomenclature has developed historically from the original serological designations. Polymorphisms in proteins were originally defined by antibody reaction patterns. Modern definitions utilize DNA sequences to define alleles. The current nomenclature was recommended during the Tenth International Histocompatibility Workshop in 1987, with minor modifications added in 1990. The rules governing nomenclature are shown in Box 10-1.

Each chromosome is found twice (diploid) in each individual, and therefore a normal tissue type of an individual will involve twelve HLA antigens (three HLA class I loci [A, B, and C] from each parent and three class II loci [DR, DQ, and DP] from each parent). HLA-DM and HLA-DO are not highly polymorphic and are not typed. These twelve antigens are inherited co-dominantly. The MHC phenotype of a person describes which alleles the person carries without reference to inheritance. For example, someone might be typed as HLA-A1, -A3; B7, B8; Cw2, Cw4; DR15, DR4, DQ3, DQ6, DP4, DP4. A haplotype is the set of HLA antigens inherited from one parent. For example, the mother of the person whose HLA type is given above might have HLA-A3, -A69; B7, B45; Cw4, Cw9; DR15, DR17, DQ6, DQ2, DP2, DP4. Therefore, the A3, B7, Cw4, DR15, DQ6, and DP4 were all passed on from the mother to the child above. This group of antigens is a haplotype. Siblings have a one-in-four probability of inheriting identical haplotypes from parents and are likely to provide the best match for transplantation (*Chapter 22*).

Despite the enormous number of alleles at each expressed locus, the number of haplotypes observed in the population is much smaller than theoretical expectations. This is because certain alleles tend to occur together on the same haplotype rather than segregating randomly. This is called linkage disequilibrium.

Linkage Disequilibrium

Linkage disequilibrium is a genetic phenomenon in which two alleles are found together with a higher

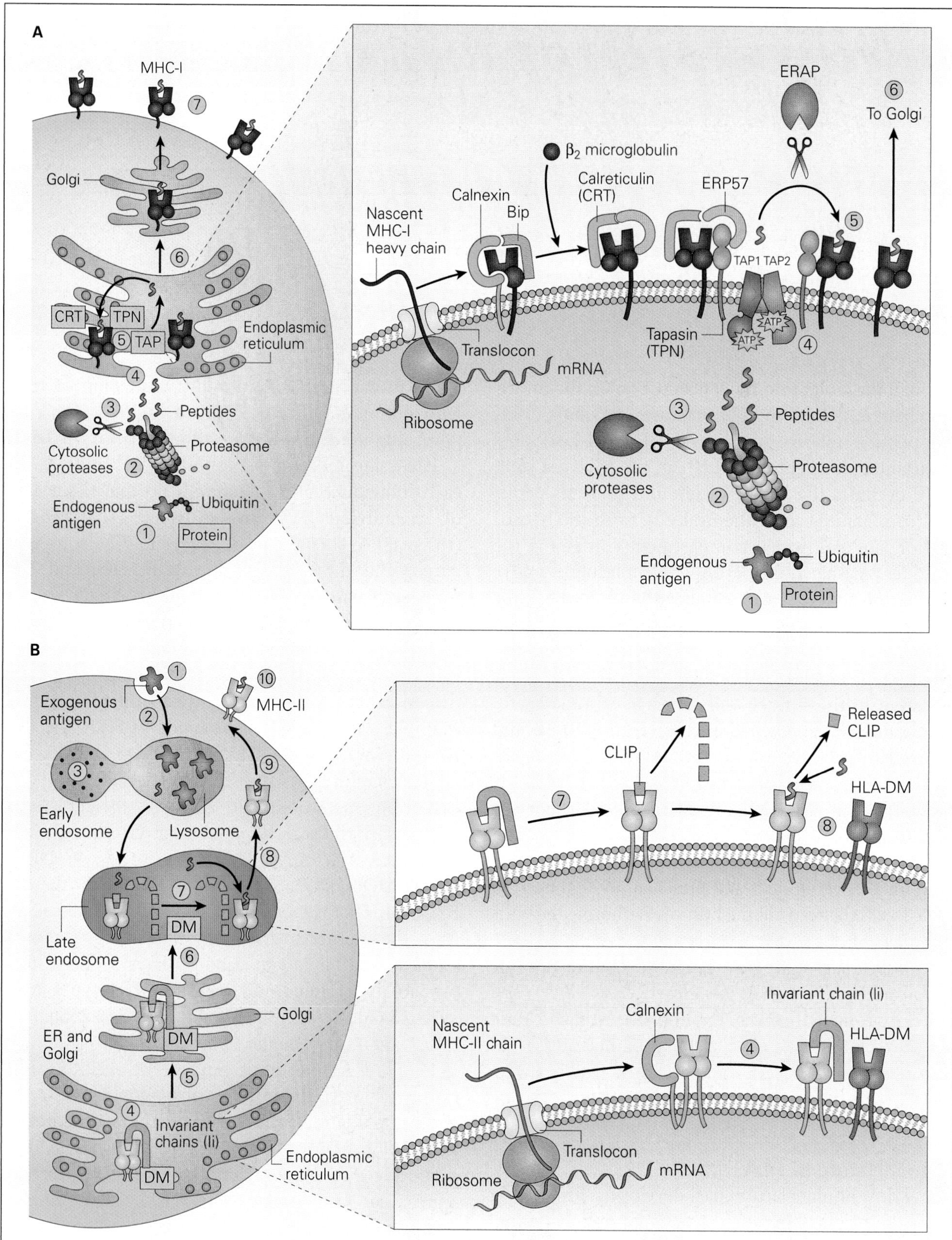

Figure 10-6. Peptide loading of MHC-I and MHC-II molecules. Panel A: shows the synthesis and peptide loading of MHC-I through the endogenous pathway. Endogenous proteins (e.g., a self-protein or a viral protein) synthesized in the cytoplasm are modified initially by ubiquitin (1), following which they are processed by the proteasomes (2). After trimming by cytosolic proteases (3), the peptides enter the endoplasmic reticulum via the TAP 1 and TAP 2 transporters (4). The MHC-I alpha chain, which is initially formed as a linear peptide in the ER, is then folded with the help of several chaperones (calnexin, calreticulin [CRT]). Binding immunoglobulin protein (BiP) and endoplasmic

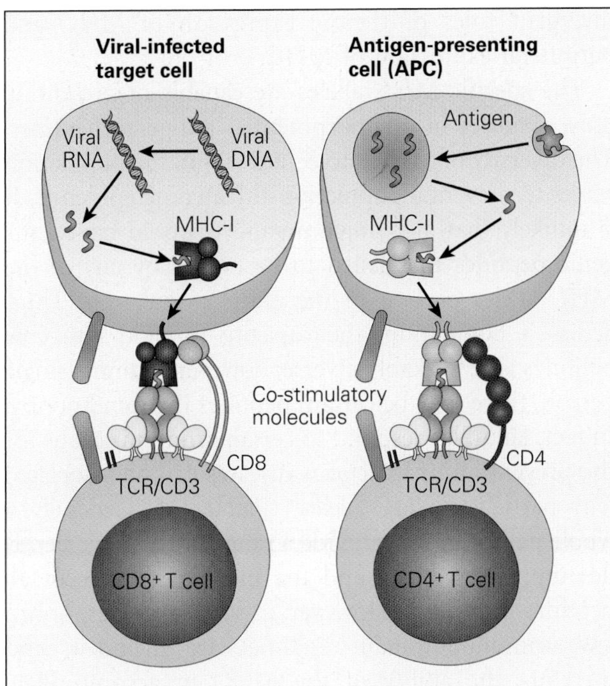

Figure 10-7. Endogenous antigens are generally presented to CD8+ T cells (left panel), and exogenous antigens are generally presented to CD4+ T cells (right panel).

> **Box 10-1**
>
> **Nomenclature of HLA**
>
> The following are the rules that dictate the nomenclature of HLA:
>
> - The prefix HLA precedes all antigens or alleles.
> - A capital letter indicates a specific locus (A, B, C, or D). All genes in the region D are prefixed by the letter D followed by a second letter indicating the subregion of D (DR, DQ, DP, DM, or DO).
> - Loci coding for the specific class II peptide chains are next identified (A1, A2, B1, and B2). Greek letters are used for protein designations, whereas Latin capital letters are used for gene/allele designations, i.e., DRβ1 versus DRB1.
> - Specific alleles are designated by an "*" followed by a two-digit number indicating the most closely associated serologic specificity, followed by a two-digit number that defines the unique allele. For example, the serologically defined HLA-A2 specificity actually comprises seventy-seven distinct variant alleles. These alleles are now referred to as HLA–A*0201 through *0299.
> - Some alleles have a third two-digit number (HLA-B*350101 and B*350102) which indicates that the two variants differ by a silent nucleotide substitution, but not in amino acid sequence 6. To avoid possible confusion between HLA-C locus, alleles, and complement components, C locus alleles are designated with Cw.

frequency than normally expected. It is the non-random association between alleles at different loci. For example, if 16 percent of the population has a particular HLA-A antigen (A1) and 10 percent of the population has a particular HLA-B antigen (B8), the chance of finding A1 genetically linked to B8 on the same chromosome is given by the product of their gene frequencies (16 percent × 10 percent = 1.6 percent). In practice, this does not always occur. Certain combinations of A and B specificities occur more frequently than would be expected if their association were random. The combination of A1 and B8 is found at a frequency of 8.8 percent in human populations compared to an expected frequency of 1.6 percent. Such paired specificities are said to be in linkage disequilibrium. In Caucasians, the HLA-A1, B8, DR3 (DRB1*0301), DQ2 (DQB1*0201) haplotype is highly conserved in the population. At HLA class II, this phenomenon is so pronounced that the presence of specific HLA-DR alleles can be used to predict the HLA-DQ allele with a high degree of accuracy before testing. The HLA alleles are ordered on chromosome 6 as DP-DQ-DR-B-Cw-A. Those alleles that are physically closest to each other usually have the highest linkage disequilibrium. It is possible that certain haplotypes may be advantageous in some immunological sense, so that they have a positive selective advantage.

Figure 10-6. (continued) reticulum protein 57 (ERP57), during which the β2 microglobulin is added to the alpha chain, complete the synthesis of the complete MHC-I molecule (right inset in panel A). The complex is held together by tapasin (TPN), which facilitates transfer of the peptide to the antigen-binding cleft (5). The peptide-loaded MHC-I complex is then transferred to the Golgi (6) and then transported to the surface of the cell (7). Panel B: Shows the uptake of protein and peptide loading of MHC-II through the exogenous pathway. Exogenous proteins are taken up (1) and processed in the early endosomal compartment (2) and cleaved into peptides by cathepsins and other acid proteases (3). MHC-II molecules are formed in the endoplasmic reticulum with the help of the chaperone calnexin (4) and are held ready by the invariant chain (Ii); the complex is later fused with the HLA-DM (DM) (right lower inset in panel B). After passage of the Ii-loaded MHC-II-DM complex through the Golgi (5) into the late endosomes (6), the invariant chain is cleaved by acid proteases, leaving a residual peptide referred to as the class II-associated invariant chain peptide (CLIP) (7) in the MHC-II cleft (right upper inset in panel B). The HLA-DM facilitates the insertion of the peptide in the MHC-II cleft replacing CLIP (8). The MHC molecule loaded with peptide is transported (9) and expressed on the cell surface (10).

Molding the Immune Response

The role of the MHC molecules is to present antigen in such a manner that T cells are capable of recognizing it. This occurs at two separate sites and times in the development of a host response. Maturation of T cells occurs in the thymus and relies on a sequential interaction with resident thymic cells (*Chapters 2* and *7*). Immature CD4/CD8 double-positive thymocytes interact with MHC and peptide in the cortex of the thymus. This initial step is one of positive selection for T cells expressing T cell receptors of sufficient affinity for self-MHC. In the subsequent negative selection step, immature T cells are eliminated in the medulla if their interactions with self-MHC self-peptide are too strong. This important step eliminates most of the autoreactive cells. At the end of this process, a repertoire of T cells exists with moderate affinity for self and ability to recognize a diverse array of foreign antigens.

Critical to this process is the expression of functional MHC molecules and the loading of these MHC molecules with self-antigen such that T cells bearing self-reactive T cell receptors can be eliminated. A disease of humans known colloquially as the "bare lymphocyte syndrome" and more appropriately as MHC-I or MHC-II deficiency has provided important insights into the role of MHC molecules (case 1). In this disorder, CD4 T cells develop poorly in the absence of MHC-II, and CD8 T cells develop poorly in the absence of MHC-I expression. This is believed to occur because the cells cannot be positively selected for self in the absence of the preferred type of MHC for that class of T cells. As described previously, CD4 T cells preferentially recognize antigen in the context of MHC-II, and CD8 T cells preferentially recognize antigen in the context of MHC-I. Patients with this disorder have recurrent infections with bacteria, viruses, and parasites because they are unable to present the relevant antigens to the T cells (*Chapter 16*). Even after stem cell transplantation, the T cell numbers remain diminished because they are still maturing in a thymic environment that lacks MHC expression. T cell function that relies on peripheral recognition of self-MHC, in contrast, improves after stem cell transplantation, and the infection pattern improves. This is believed to be due to the donor monocytes, macrophages, and B cells serving as antigen-presenting cells to the donor T cells. Studies of these patients and corresponding knockout mice have confirmed the important role of thymic education in the development of a host response and demonstrated the divergent roles of thymic expression of MHC and peripheral expression of MHC.

The specific MHC alleles are capable of presenting only a subset of all the potential antigenic peptides. The diversity of MHC molecules within the population serves to prevent a population-threatening epidemic. It is unlikely that any single organism would have antigenic peptides that failed to be bound by any of the MHC alleles present in the entire population. Thus, across a population, the capacity to bind antigenic peptides is remarkably diverse; however, within a single person, there may be certain peptides that bind poorly. In fact, failure to respond to certain immunizations for the prevention of infectious diseases can be associated with particular MHC alleles (*Chapter 23*). Generally, a whole pathogen will provide a range of antigenic peptides for presentation, and the inability to present all peptides is unlikely. However, in some vaccines, only a few immunodominant epitopes are included, and therefore the ability of the MHC to accommodate those antigenic peptides becomes more important.

Pathophysiology

MHC Associations with Disease

Thus far, the importance of the MHC in molding the immune response to infectious threats has been emphasized. Individual HLA alleles dictate the specificity of T cell interactions and guide antigen-specific immune events. Polymorphisms are therefore implicated in disease pathogenesis when specific HLA genes are associated with diseases. The majority of associations between HLA and diseases are with class II alleles. Table 10-4 presents some of the better-known disease associations. In most cases, bearers of a particular HLA molecule are more susceptible to a disease, but there are also examples wherein a particular allele confers protection from disease. In addition to classical allele-specific disease associations, there are also examples of structural elements (MHC epitopes) being associated with disease. Alleles may possess unique epitopes that potentially play a critical role in peptide binding and TCR recognition. Table 10-5 refers to residues on the HLA-DQβ1 and DRβ1 molecules that have been demonstrated to have an important role. For example, the DQβ R55 L56 D57/E70 D71 epitope is positively associated with acute inflammatory demyelinating polyneuropathy (i.e., the susceptible element), whereas the R55 P56 D57 epitope is negatively associated (i.e., the protective element).

Table 10-4. Disease associations with MHC antigens

Disease	Allele(s) associated with susceptibility	Relative Risk
Addison's disease	DR3	6
Ankylosing spondylitis	B27	70–100
Behcet's syndrome	B51	3–6
Celiac disease	DR3, DQA1*0501, DQβ1*0201	> 200
Congenital adrenal hyperplasia	B47	15
Dermatitis herpetiformis	DR3	15–18
Goodpasture syndrome	DR2	16–20
Graves' disease	DR3	4
Hashimoto's disease	DR11	3
Hereditary hemochromatosis	A3/B14	90
Insulin-dependent diabetes mellitus	B35, Cw04	1–3
Idiopathic membranous glomerulonephritis	DR3	12
Multiple sclerosis	DR2, DQ6	5–12
Myasthenia gravis	DR3	10
Narcolepsy	DR2, DQβ1*0602	130
Psoriasis vulgaris	Cw6	13
Pemphigus vulgaris	DRβ1*0402-DQβ1*0302 DRβ1*1401-DQβ1*0503	14–21
Rheumatoid arthritis	DR4	4–10
Systemic lupus erythematosus	DR3	3–6
Sarcoidosis	DRβ1*1101	1.5–3.6

Note: Relative risk is calculated by dividing the frequency of the HLA allele in the patient population by the frequency in the general population. A positive association is indicated by a relative risk of more than 1.0, and a negative association by a relative risk of less than 1.0.

MHC Associations with Autoimmune Diseases

Although the association of MHC alleles with autoimmune diseases has been recognized for many years, the specific mechanism underlying the association is still not fully understood (*Chapter 19*). There are several hypotheses regarding the role of specific MHC molecules in the predisposition to autoimmune disease, and there is experimental evidence to support each hypothesis.

In the first hypothesis, a specific MHC molecule presents the self-protein less effectively than non-disease-related MHC. This may seem counterintuitive,

Table 10-5. Susceptibility and resistance to disease mediated by specific epitopes

Disease	Positional residues associated with susceptibility	Positional residues associated with resistance
Insulin-dependent diabetes mellitus	DQβ1 57, DQα1 52	
Rheumatoid arthritis	DRβ1 67, 70, 71, 74	
Tuberculoid leprosy	DRβ1 13, 70, 71	
Beryllium hypersensitivity	DPβ1 55, 69 (DRβ1 57, 71)	
Acute inflammatory demyelinating polyneuropathy	DQβ1 55, 56, 57/70,71	DQβ1 55, 56, 57
Epithelial ovarian carcinoma	DQα1 11, 55(p1); 66, 69(p6); 52	DRβ1 67, 70, 71
Pulmonary tuberculosis	DRβ 37, 71	

but inefficient presentation of self-peptides could lead to failure of negative selection in the thymus and escape from autoreactive T cells to the periphery. Insulin-dependent diabetes mellitus is known to be associated with DRβ1*0302, DQβ1*0401 (in Caucasians), and DRβ1*0405, DQβ1*0401 or DRβ1*0901, DQβ1*0303 (in Japanese). These human MHC-II alleles and a murine MHC molecule called I-A^{g7}, which is found in a spontaneously diabetic mouse model, are all very unstable MHC molecules. These unstable molecules are capable of presenting very few peptides, and this is also associated with escape of autoreactive T cell clones into the periphery.

A second hypothesis comes directly from observations of patients with rheumatoid arthritis. Most Caucasian patients with rheumatoid arthritis have HLA-DRβ1*0401. In other ethnicities, other DR types predominate. When compared, all the rheumatoid arthritis-associated DR types have a conserved amino acid sequence, although there are differences in the specific binding pockets of the different DR molecules. The conserved amino acid sequence, or shared epitope, is LLEQ(K/R)RAA at position 67–74 of the DRβ1 chain. The hypothesis is that these DR types with a shared epitope select for a very specific population of T cells that are able to present the autoantigen. In the case of rheumatoid arthritis, as is true for most autoimmune diseases, the specific autoantigen remains unknown.

Each of these hypotheses is supported by direct experimental evidence in one or more models. There are also hypotheses that implicate the MHC without invoking its role as an antigen-presenting molecule. There are stretches of chromosome 6 across which recombination is suppressed, punctuated by regions of high recombinational activity leading to linkage disequilibrium. Therefore, while the description of specific diseases being associated with DR alleles is common, it may be that adjacent genes that were co-inherited on the haplotype are actually driving the disease association. Genes which are in linkage disequilibrium with DR include DQ and DP; the gene for the pro-inflammatory cytokine TNF-α; the MHC genes encoding peptide-loading proteins (HLA-DM and TAP); MICA/MICB, which encode stress-induced proteins that interact with natural killer cells and Tγδ cells; and the nonclassical MHC-I gene, HFE, which is the gene defective in hereditary hemochromatosis. There is modest evidence for each of these genes contributing to the susceptibility to autoimmune diseases in humans.

The concept of molecular mimicry also has been invoked to understand the close relationship between ankylosing spondylitis and HLA-B27 (case 2). About 90 percent of patients with ankylosing spondylitis carry HLA-B27, yet only a small fraction of people carrying HLA-B27 develop ankylosing spondylitis. The most obvious explanation is that exposure to an uncommon organism is required to trigger the inflammation in HLA-B27-positive individuals. Indeed, ankylosing spondylitis has been known to occur subsequent to infection with *Salmonella, Shigella, Chlamydia,* and other organisms associated with reactive arthritis or Reiter's disease. Nevertheless, experimental evidence to date does not provide strong support for that model.

The leading hypothesis for the association of ankylosing spondylitis with HLA-B27 relates to its unique biochemical characteristics. Mice and rats expressing human HLA-B27 consistently develop colitis that is dependent on colonization with gut flora. Immunization with HLA-B27 results in a more robust response to *Chlamydia*, suggesting that the HLA-B27 itself can alter immune responses to infections independently of antigen presentation. This may relate to the high rate of protein misfolding that occurs with HLA-B27, which could allow the B27 itself to be an antigen or to bind peptides aberrantly.

Transplantation

The MHC is best known as a barrier to transplantation (*Chapter 22*). Solid organs and hematopoietic stem cells are usually at least partially matched to the recipient. The graft is likely to be rejected as foreign if the recipient has competent T cells, and conversely, the graft can reject the recipient if the graft contains competent T cells and the recipient does not, in a condition called graft-versus-host disease (**GVHD**).

As described previously, the MHC region contains three genes encoding MHC-I molecules (i.e., HLA-A, HLA-B, and HLA-C) and three genes encoding MHC-II molecules (i.e., HLA-DR, HLA-DQ, and HLA-DP). In principle, a fully matched donor-recipient pair would have the same alleles at all twelve loci (six are maternally inherited and six are paternally inherited). In practice, it is infrequent that all six loci of the donor would be fully cross-matched with those of the recipient. It is not clear, however, which HLA loci are most important for optimal matching. The traditional gold standard for serologic matching employed hyperimmune sera from multiparous women isoimmunized during pregnancy by fetal cells containing their husband's MHC. It is not yet clear, however, whether matching on a DNA level using more current PCR methodology will markedly improve graft survival, although it is a general truth that the better the match, the longer the survival (*Chapter 22*).

There are two potential mechanisms by which a solid organ is rejected as a result of alloreactivity, i.e., immunogically mediated response to antigens that are distinct between members of the same species (Figure 10-8). The first mechanism of graft rejection occurs by direct recognition of the graft. This takes place when MHC molecules shed from the graft on recipient antigen-presenting cells are recognized by recipient T cells in regional lymphoid tissue (Figure 10-8A). This occurs without respect to any donor peptide that may be in the cleft of the donor MHC but requires both the presence of APCs in the graft as well as adequate lymphatic drainage to regional lymph nodes. Presentation of the foreign MHC and generation of an appropriate co-stimulatory signal results in activation of the recipient T cells with rejection of the graft (Figure 10-8A). A second mechanism of graft rejection occurs by indirect recognition of the graft. Trauma from the transplant itself can occur during the procedure, with release of foreign proteins from the graft that are taken up and processed by recipient APCs resulting from the pro-inflammatory environment. Following peptide presentation and appropriate co-stimulatory signals, the recipient T cells are activated with rejection of the graft (Figure 10-8B). Approximately 1 to 7 percent of naïve T cells are capable of responding to alloantigens by either mechanism.

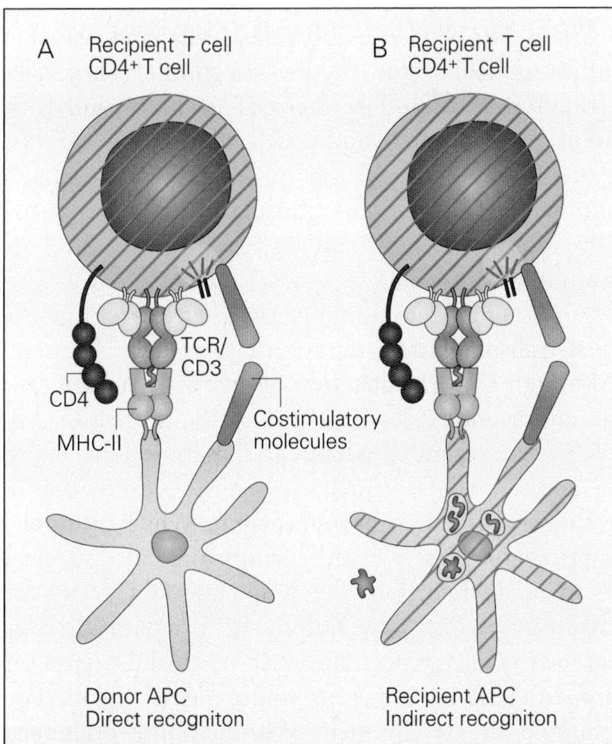

Figure 10-8. Alloreactivity: direct and indirect responses to alloantigen. Panel A: Direct alloresponses rely on the T cell receptor on recipient T cells recognizing the MHC of donor antigen-presenting cells (APCs) as foreign. This occurs without respect to the peptide in the cleft. Following migration of donor APCs to regional lymphoid tissue of the recipient, the foreign MHC is recognized by the TCR of the recipient's T cells with subsequent T cell activation and graft rejection. Panel B: In indirect alloresponses following trauma, foreign antigens are released from the graft and are processed by recipient APCs and the resultant peptides are presented to recipient T cells with subsequent T cell activation and graft rejection. In both cases, co-stimulation is required.

Clinical Manifestations and Treatment

Solid Organ Transplantation

Immunosuppressive medications have revolutionized the field of transplantation (*Chapters 11* and *22*). Generally, these drugs either globally suppress T cell reactivity or lead to the death of reactive T cells. These agents are required for any form of transplantation across MHC barriers. In the case of solid organ transplantation, organs are fully (living donor) or partially (living donor or cadaveric donor) HLA matched for the recipient. For kidney transplants, the overall rate of graft failure in the first year is 10 percent, and the overall rate of graft failure at five years is 35 percent (*Chapter 22*). The likelihood of graft rejection is increased with increasing MHC disparity. In addition to MHC matching, there are two additional compatibility tests that are performed for renal-transplant recipients. Kidneys are also matched for ABO blood group antigens. When kidneys are transplanted into ABO-incompatible recipients, only 50 percent of the kidneys function at one year post-transplant. The last level of matching that is performed is called cross-matching (Table 10-6). This assay determines whether there is preexisting antibody in the recipient to donor histocompatibility antigens. The determination of antibody to ABO blood groups or

Table 10-6. Implications of transplant cross-match testing

Type of test	Implications
Antibodies to HLA-A, B, and C	Positive antibodies are an absolute contraindication to transplant
Antibodies to HLA-DR, DQ	High titer antibodies are a relative contraindication
Autoantibody cross-reacting with donor	Does not affect transplant unless directed at organ

donor MHC antigens is important for preventing graft rejection, as will be described below. This is generally a problem with patients who have received more than one graft, but also can be seen in patients receiving their first graft. In the past, liver transplants were matched only for ABO and by cross-matching. The short half-life of the liver once removed from the body made it difficult to do any additional MHC matching. Recently, it has been shown that partial matching for MHC antigens improves survival, and technical advances now allow more rapid MHC typing.

Cadaveric kidneys are usually MHC-typed for HLA-A, HLA-B, and HLA-DR. This information along with the age of the donor and his or her medical history is matched to the best available patient within the distribution area. Until quite recently, the MHC typing done in this setting was performed using serologic methods because of the necessity of speed. PCR has replaced serologic typing at most facilities (*Chapter 22*). Sibling-matched renal transplants have the best outcome, with cadaveric 6/6 and 5/6 matches having the next-best outcomes.

Hyperacute, Acute, and Chronic Graft Rejection

Graft rejection can occur with any graft other than an autotransplant. Even fully matched sibling donor grafts can be rejected due to incompatibility at minor histocompatibility loci. These minor loci are not well understood and represent a variety of genes that are not accessible to typing methods but can still influence alloreactivity. Rejection of grafts is traditionally divided into three phases: hyperacute, acute, and chronic (*Chapter 22*). **Hyperacute rejection** is due to preformed antibodies to ABO or MHC antigens on the graft. Hyperacute rejection due to antibodies and complement activation has been one of the major obstacles to using xenotransplants therapeutically. In hyperacute rejection, the graft rapidly becomes tender and swollen. Arterioles may also show necrosis or thrombosis. The goal of the pretransplant cross-matching is to avoid this type of rejection and has been responsible for making this complication rather rare. Patients with multiple anti-MHC antibodies who are typically cross-match positive have been unable to safely receive transplants in the past. Recent work using plasmapheresis of the recipient prior to transplant and intravenous gammaglobulin, however, has allowed some patients with multiple anti-MHC antibodies to safely receive a kidney transplant (*Chapter 11*).

Acute rejection is a second type of graft rejection that has become exceedingly common in transplant recipients; most patients will have at least one episode of rejection in the first three months post-transplant. Rejection is accompanied by signs of inflammation and organ dysfunction. Biopsy findings of acute rejection usually demonstrate a mixed cellular infiltrate. The vasculature is normally marked by swollen endothelial cells and variable adherent leukocytes. Acute rejection is normally treated with high-dose steroids or, if severe, with addition of immunosuppressive drugs (*Chapter 11*). Patients are generally on a cocktail of immunosuppressive drugs post-transplant and they usually require a significant increase in the level of immunosuppression.

Once graft rejection occurs after three months post-transplantation, rejection is considered chronic. Although this classification seems at first artificial, its importance is documented by the diverse quality of the rejection process. The rejection is more insidious and is usually progressive and poorly responsive to immunosuppression. While immunosuppression has markedly improved the survival from acute rejection, the frequency and effects of chronic rejection have not altered dramatically over the last twenty years. The rates of chronic rejection are different for different transplanted organs. For example, the development of bronchiolitis obliterans after two or three years in most patients receiving lung transplants has significantly limited the use of this type of transplant. Conversely, cardiac transplant recipients have fairly low rates of chronic rejection. Rejection of renal transplants is moderately frequent with the expected half-life for unrelated kidney transplants being seventeen years. Chronic rejection is primarily due to slow cumulative damage from infiltrating cells and vascular compromise.

Bone Marrow Transplantation

Bone marrow transplantation in humans was first performed on twins after pioneering work in mice demonstrated its feasibility. Following the discovery of the MHC in 1968, the entire field of transplantation evolved dramatically. Bone marrow or stem cell transplantation is substantially different than solid organ transplantation (*Chapter 22*). Immunocompetent cells in both the recipient and donor can reject each other. Donor rejection of the recipient is termed GVHD and will be described below. Rejection of the graft by the recipient is a significant problem in all cases except patients with severe combined immunodeficiency (*Chapter 16*). Bone marrow recipients who do not have severe combined immunodeficiency are typically treated with some combination of radiation and myelosuppressive drugs to facilitate engraftment (*Chapter 11*).

Stem cell transplantation can be categorized in a variety of ways. Stem cells can be obtained from bone marrow, umbilical cord, or peripheral blood-harvesting techniques. The donor can be the patient, a sibling, an unrelated partially matched donor, or a parent. Finally, the transplant can be described in terms of the recipient/stem cell preparation. The source of stem cells appears to make little difference, although there is some evidence suggesting that cord blood transplants may be associated with lower rates of GVHD. The type of donor represents the single most important variable in determining outcome. Autologous transplants are performed for certain malignancies and autoimmune diseases and carry a very low rate of GVHD. Surprisingly, the risk is not zero, possibly because the cells that normally regulate self-responses are impaired in this setting. Sibling-matched transplants are the next most successful type of stem cell transplant. In this situation, not only is GVHD infrequent and often of low grade intensity, but also the graft is infrequently rejected. Unrelated matched donors can be either marrow donors or cord blood donors.

Cord blood does not contain sufficient stem cells to repopulate an adult and is reserved for pediatric transplants. When cord blood is stored or someone enrolls in the National Marrow Donor Program, low-resolution typing results are recorded. A search using the patient's typing data is performed using a computer algorithm, and matches are confirmed prior to transplant using high-resolution typing to ensure the best possible match. An appropriate cord blood match simply requires shipping to the institution performing the transplant. When a match is identified through the National Marrow Donor Program, the stem cell donor needs to be recruited and scheduled for either a peripheral harvest or a marrow harvest.

Since marrow harvesting is painful, a better option for most donors is to undergo induction of stem cell release following administration of hematopoietic growth factors and harvesting of peripheral blood (*Chapter 9*). Unrelated stem cell transplants that match at least five of six loci (HLA-A, HLA-B, and HLA-DR are usually typed) have been shown to be as statistically successful as six-of-six matches. Unfortunately, unrelated donor transplants that appear to be fully matched are not as successful as sibling matches because of minor differences within the MHC and at minor histocompatibility loci. The greater the degree of disparity, the more morbidity and mortality is seen. Haploidentical transplants (from a parent) have the highest morbidity and mortality. These are typically performed only on patients with severe combined immunodeficiency where time is of the essence and there is no opportunity to wait for a better match (*Chapter 16*).

The final variables relate to the preparation of the patient and the stem cells. For stem cell transplants that are not fully matched, the T cells in the donor marrow or blood must be removed so they will not cause GVHD. There are a number of methods for purifying the stem cells away from the undesired T cells. The goal is not to completely eliminate T cells, but to reduce their number to the point where alloreactive T cells are unlikely to be a part of the graft.

Today, stem cell transplantation is most often performed for malignancies (*Chapter 21*); however, significant numbers of patients with immunodeficiencies, congenital hematologic disorders, and inborn errors of metabolism receive stem cell transplants. In situations where it is important to eliminate abnormal cells (malignant or nonfunctional), the conditioning procedures can be quite rigorous. This conditioning is referred to as myeloablative, which implies that the patient would die without the stem cell "rescue." In this sense, it is similar to stem cell transplants performed for fatal radiation injury. In truth, the conditioning is often not fully myeloablative. Certain resistant cells survive, and the stromal cells required for stem cell development are preserved as well. Nevertheless, the conditioning procedure is associated with significant morbidity and mortality. One of the greatest predictors of mortality is the time to emergence of neutrophils. To address this, patients are sometimes supported with the use of myeloid growth factors to induce more rapid neutrophil recovery (*Chapter 9*). The return of lymphoid cells varies widely.

When the donor and recipient are matched, the stem cells are not purified, and mature T cells are infused with the stem cells. In these cases, lymphoid reconstitution is rapid. When the stem cells are depleted of T cells, as would be the case for a non-fully matched transplant, lymphoid recovery can take several months; this delay also poses a significant risk of infection. When the immune system is normal prior to transplantation, recovery is quicker. In contrast, when lymphocytes have to completely redevelop, such as in severe combined immunodeficiency, recovery is much slower. T cell depleted transplants for severe combined immunodeficiency often lead to T cell recovery in approximately three months, while B cell recovery can take years (*Chapter 16*).

Although infection remains the most significant complication of stem cell transplantation, recipients can also develop anemia and thrombocytopenia as the marrow recovers, as well as a peculiar liver disease known as veno-occlusive disease, which is thought to be caused by endothelial cell damage. Long-term issues include endocrine abnormalities, poor growth, secondary malignancies, and incomplete immunologic function. Most of these are independent of the MHC; however, GVHD is the most feared long-term management issue for caregivers.

Graft-Versus-Host Disease

Graft-versus-host disease (GVHD) is categorized as **acute** when it occurs within the first 100 days after transplantation and **chronic** if it occurs more than 100 days after the transplantation. The pathogenesis of acute GVHD is due to a combination of tissue damage from the conditioning, donor T cell recognition of the host, antigen-presenting cells, and cytokines (IL-2, IFN-γ, and TNF-α). Risk factors for GVHD are shown in Box 10-2. The earliest sign of acute GVHD is usually a skin eruption that appears on the hands, feet, and face. The rash may spread into generalized erythroderma. A skin biopsy can confirm the diagnosis, but is often unnecessary. The second tissue that is typically involved in GVHD is the bowel. Diarrhea and abdominal cramps occur when the epithelial necrosis of the gut is extensive. In the liver, biliary epithelial cells (but not hepatocytes) are involved, and the patient develops jaundice. Although the level of immunocompromise may not be clinically apparent, it is invariably present and quite severe.

Box 10-2

Developing GVHD

These are the risk factors for developing GVHD:

- HLA mismatch
- Donor/recipient gender mismatch
- High numbers of T cells transfused from donor
- Host exposure to previous blood product transfusions
- Older age of donor or host

Organ fibrosis with collagen deposition and atrophy are the hallmarks of chronic GVHD and resemble some spontaneously occurring autoimmune disorders such as systemic lupus erythematosus (**SLE**) or scleroderma. The diagnosis may be made clinically or by biopsy. Although a dry, itchy rash is one of the most common manifestations, dry eyes and dry mouth (sicca syndrome) are nearly as common. The skin may become thickened and features of hypopigmentation and hyperpigmentation may also occur. Chronic GVHD may also involve the lungs and produce obliteration of small airways. When severe, chronic GVHD can be fatal. The incidence of chronic GVHD varies according to many of the same factors affecting acute GVHD. Additionally, CMV infection in the host or donor and previous acute GVHD are associated with an increased incidence of chronic GVHD.

The current approaches for the prevention of GVHD are:

1. **Elimination of the donor T cells:** This can be accomplished by *in vitro* manipulation of the donor's cells. Some residual T cells are needed to ensure engraftment.
2. **Immunosuppressive therapy:** This therapy consists of combined regimens of methotrexate (MTX), cyclosporin (CsA), tacrolimus (FK 506), and/or a corticosteroid. These immunosuppressive agents used to prevent GVHD also may be used to treat established GVHD (*Chapter 11*).

Autoimmune Disease

Autoimmune diseases affect approximately 4 percent of the population in industrialized countries

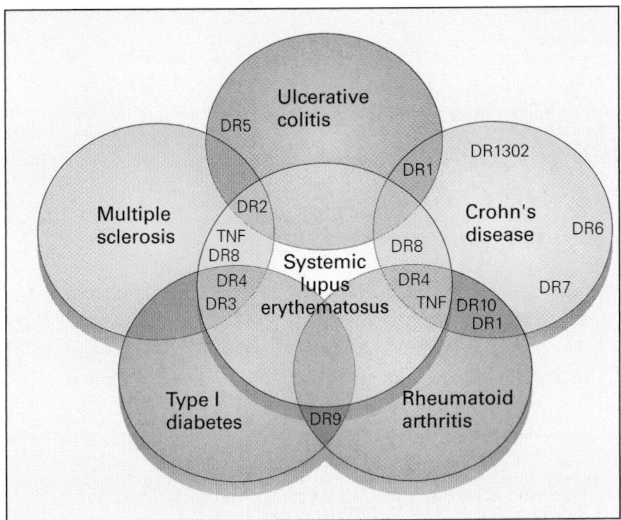

Figure 10-9. Schematic representation of the principal shared and distinct MHC haplotype associations in six immune-mediated diseases. (Adapted from Fernando MM, Stevens CR, Walsh EC, et al. Defining the role of the MHC in autoimmunity: a review and pooled analysis. PLoS Genet. 2008;4:e1000024.)

and are characterized by an immune-mediated destruction of autologous cells and/or tissues (*Chapter 19*). As described previously (Table 10-4), several autoimmune diseases such as multiple sclerosis, type 1 diabetes, systemic lupus erythematosus, ulcerative colitis, Crohn's disease, and rheumatoid arthritis are strongly associated with certain classical HLA class II and/or class I genes. Shown in Figure 10-9 is a schematic representation of the principal shared and distinct MHC haplotype associations in six of these autoimmune diseases.

The primary pathogenetic mechanisms of tissue injury in the autoimmune diseases are generally thought to be due to aberrant T cell or B cell recognition of self-antigens as foreign (*Chapter 19*). Although the mechanisms of recognition of antigen presented by the MHC to T cells are well-recognized (*Chapter 7*), the specific antigen(s) responsible for initiating the destructive immune reaction is unknown in most cases. Generally, autoimmune diseases are associated with organ dysfunction. For example, thyroiditis is associated with a pleomorphic cellular infiltrate, destruction of the organ, and either hypothyroidism or hyperthyroidism. Insulin-dependent diabetes mellitus is similarly characterized by infiltrates of CD4+ and CD8+ T cells in the pancreatic islands of Langerhans. In these cases, the inflammation causes endocrine dysfunction that leads to the diagnosis and appropriate replacement therapy. Other autoimmune diseases require therapy more specifically directed at the inflammatory aspect of the disease. For example, Crohn's disease can be treated with topical anti-inflammatory agents, but the most common strategy is to treat it with systemic steroids or a TNF-α inhibitor (*Chapter 11*). Interestingly, this same strategy is very effective for rheumatoid arthritis, and there is a growing realization that while the triggers and specific manifestations of different autoimmune diseases may be distinct, the final inflammatory pathways may be quite similar.

Therapy for autoimmune diseases has not progressed dramatically in the last few decades. Newer immunosuppressive medications such as FK506, cyclosporine, and rapamycin have been beneficial in both the transplant setting and in the treatment of autoimmune diseases (*Chapters 11* and *22*). Conceptually, however, this represents more aggressive immunosuppression as opposed to a different type of therapy. Current research strategies are now being directed to the induction of tolerance to self-antigens (*Chapter 19*). Tolerance in animal models is often induced by exposing the animal to antigen administered via a mucous membrane prior to a challenge (*Chapter 8*). A similar phenomenon probably exists in humans, but lack of knowledge of the relevant antigens and the ineffectiveness of this method in established disease has limited its usefulness in humans. A more direct approach has been tested in animal models; it utilizes dendritic cells pulsed with antigen and then reinfused into the animal. The pulsed dendritic cells act to induce tolerance in the T cell compartment. These tolerizing strategies hold promise for the treatment of autoimmune disease and offer the theoretical advantage of eliminating one specific pathologic response and yet retaining host responses that are necessary for host defense.

All of these tolerizing strategies require identification of the antigen; this has been a significant hurdle for clinical immunologists. One approach has been to liberate peptides from MHC molecules and sequence the released peptides for identification. While this is simple in concept, in reality, since many hundreds of peptides may be present at any given time, those peptides present at the highest frequency may not necessarily be those with pathogenic potential. Additional research may allow identification of the pathologic self-peptides and facilitate specific immunotherapy for autoimmune diseases.

Case Studies: Clinical Relevance

Let us now return to the case studies of MHC-II deficiency, ankylosing spondylitis, and aplastic anemia presented earlier and review some of the major points of the clinical presentation and how they relate to the immune system:

Case Study 1: MHC-II Deficiency (Bare Lymphocyte Syndrome)

In this case, the diagnosis of MHC-II deficiency (aka, bare lymphocyte syndrome) was made after flow cytometry indicated MHC-II expression to be absent on B cells and stimulated T cells (*Chapter 24*). A sibling-matched bone marrow transplant was performed that was unsuccessful. The patient was retransplanted using the same donor and very high levels of stem cells. This second transplant was successful.

There are four known genetic types of MHC-II deficiency (CIITA, RFXANK, RFX5, and RFXAP; see Figure 10-10). Each of the genetic types affects transcription of all of the MHC-II genes, i.e., DR, DQ, and DP expression are deficient in each type. In some cases, transcription of MHC-I genes is partially affected. Most cases of isolated MHC-I deficiency are due to TAP1 or TAP2 defects. These molecules oversee peptide loading onto MHC-I molecules in the endoplasmic reticulum (Figure 10-11).

- One of the consequences of MHC-II deficiency is impaired positive selection of CD4 T cells (*Chapter 7*). This is felt to be the explanation for the characteristic CD4 T cell lymphopenia. The CD4 T cells that do develop in the thymus and exit to the periphery are competent to deliver CD40L signals to B cells, and patients do produce some immunoglobulin (*Chapter 6*). However, CD4 T cells do not recognize antigen in the absence of MHC-II and do not secrete a typical array of cytokines (*Chapter 9*). Thus, antibody production is not normal, and CD4 T cell function is compromised with respect to antigen-specific responses.

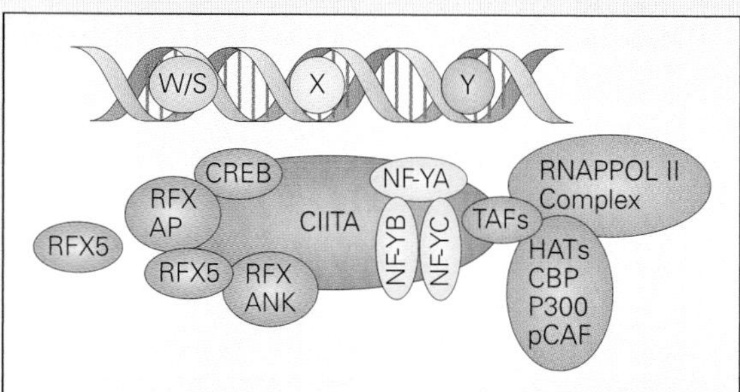

Figure 10-10. Genetic bases for MHC-II deficiency. CIITA, RFXANK, RFX5, and RFXAP mutations are associated with MHC-II deficiency. Each of the pink and yellow ovals represent transcription factors that attach to various promoter regions W/S, X, and Y involved in the transcriptional regulation of MHC-II. The purple shapes represent proteins that are not gene-specific and that do not bind to the promoter regions. The complexity of the transcriptional regulation likely reflects the need for tight control of antigen presentation.

- Patients with MHC-II deficiency are prone to infections with bacteria, fungi, viruses, and protozoa (*Chapters 12-15*). Death is common between six months to five years in the absence of successful stem cell transplantation. The infections can involve any organ, but the respiratory tract and the gastrointestinal tract are the two most common sites. Patients with MHC-II deficiency do not have severe combined immunodeficiency because they often produce immunoglobulin and their T cells are capable of sustaining proliferation after stimulation with mitogens. In spite of this, their infection pattern resembles that seen in patients with severe combined immunodeficiency. This is because they have significant compromise in both functional immunoglobulin production and functional T cell responses. While the T cells can proliferate to nonspecific signals, they can seldom respond to specific antigens because the antigens have no mechanism for presentation to the T cells. Similarly, B cells are able to produce antibody, but infrequently make specific antibody to antigens or immunizations because the T cell help for immunoglobulin production is severely compromised.
- As is true for many patients with immunodeficiencies, patients with MHC-II deficiency develop autoimmune disease more frequently than others (*Chapters 16* and *19*). Sclerosing cholangitis is the most common of the autoimmune diseases, and nonspecific colitis with villous atrophy is seen nearly as frequently.
- The outlook for patients with MHC-II deficiency is quite poor in the absence of stem cell transplantation. On the other hand, patients with MHC-I deficiency are often treated with supportive care. Their immunodeficiency is much milder, and sinopulmonary infections are the dominant feature. This may be because the MHC-II molecules can present intracellular antigens that have been shed into the extracellular space or because the MHC-I deficiency is generally leaky with a low level of MHC-I expression detectable.
- Stem cell transplantation for patients with MHC-II deficiency has been disappointing to date. In the early 1990s, less than 50 percent of patients receiving transplants survived. Nearly all the successful transplants were from HLA-identical donors; this is believed to be due to the lack of rejection of the donor marrow when HLA-matched and because matched transplants contain potential antigen-presenting cells. In the case of a transplant from a parent, the donor cells would be only half-matched. The recipient's CD8 T cells are capable of recognizing the mismatched HLA alleles as foreign, and the graft is rejected. In addition, the donor stem cells are more highly purified in the case of a mismatched

Case Studies: Clinical Relevance (continued)

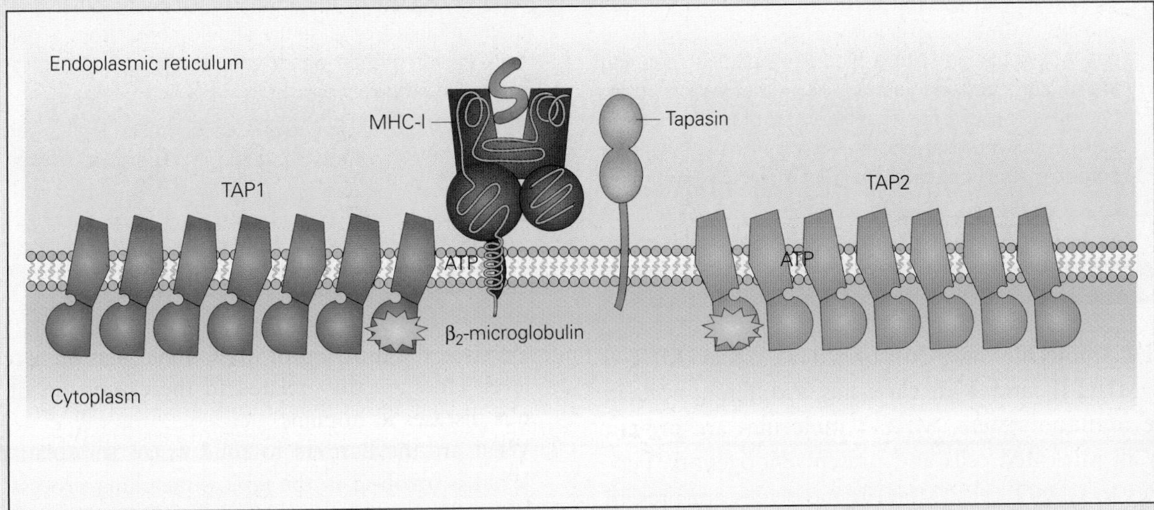

Figure 10-11. Genetic bases for MHC-I deficiency. TAP1 and TAP2 mutations are associated with MHC-I deficiency.

transplant, and engraftment of antigen-presenting cells is delayed compared to matched transplants. Increased conditioning prior to the transplant has improved the rate of graft rejection, but haploidentical stem cell transplantation is still much less successful in patients with MHC-II deficiency than in other forms of immunodeficiency or for malignancy.

Case Study 2: Ankylosing Spondylitis

- The relationship between HLA B27 and infection with enteric pathogens and arthritis is poorly understood. More than 90 percent of Caucasians with ankylosing spondylitis carry HLA B27 while it is found in only 5 to 14 percent of the general population. There are other related MHC-I alleles that are associated with ankylosing spondylitis in other ethnicities. In some cases, ankylosing spondylitis follows an infection with *Salmonella, Shigella, Yersinia*, or *Chlamydia*, suggesting infection can trigger the process in genetically susceptible individuals. Patients with inflammatory bowel disease develop a similar spondyloarthropathy, and those with ankylosing spondylitis have been found to have subclinical colonic ulcers. Thus, one hypothesis is that exposure to enteric bacteria is part of the pathophysiologic process involved in autoinflammatory diseases (*Annex, Chapter 19*).
- TNF-α is a pro-inflammatory cytokine expressed by cells infiltrating the joints of patients with ankylosing spondylitis. While nonsteroidal anti-inflammatory agents provide pain relief and limited anti-inflammatory effects, they do not alter the progressive course of the disease. Only TNF-α inhibitors have been shown to limit disease progression (*Chapters 9* and *11*).

Case Study 3: Aplastic Anemia

- Aplastic anemia can have multiple causes. In some cases, aplastic anemia follows exposure to certain drugs, environmental toxins, or radiation. Roughly 25 percent of cases of aplastic anemia have been attributed to drug exposure; the strongest association has been found with nonsteroidal anti-inflammatory drugs, anti-thyroid drugs, allopurinol, sulfonamides, gold, furosemide, corticosteroids, and phenothiazines. A genetic predisposition is thought to underlie certain idiosyncratic responses, and the MHC region has been specifically implicated as sensitive to clozapine. Idiopathic aplastic anemia is strongly associated with HLA-DR2. MHC-I alleles have also been implicated in some studies with HLA-B14 and HLA-B7 overrepresented in patients with aplastic anemia.
- In aplastic anemia, the stem cells in the bone marrow are reduced in number and are hyporesponsive to hematopoietic growth factors. T cells over-produce the inhibitory factors interferon-γ and TNF-α. These two cytokines suppress proliferation and induce apoptosis of hematopoietic progenitors (*Chapter 9*). Initial treatment of aplastic anemia, once the patient is stabilized, is directed at the abnormal T cells. Cyclosporine, cyclophosphamide, anti-thymocyte globulin, antilymphocyte globulin, and corticosteroids have all been used successfully and intensive immunosuppression for 6 months results in a response in approximately 70 percent of the patients (*Chapter 11*). Relapse, the emergence of a clonal disease, and myelodysplasia, however, can occur.

Case Studies: Clinical Relevance (continued)

- Transfusion is required at some point for nearly all patients with aplastic anemia. This is an issue for a patient population with a high likelihood of requiring stem cell transplantation. Alloimmunization from transfusions increases the likelihood of graft rejection and overall morbidity from a stem cell transplant. A potential stem cell donor should never be used as a red cell or platelet donor and transfusions other than those required emergently should come from a partially HLA matched donor or a single donor to minimize alloimmunization.
- Refer to the chapter above for a complete discussion of bone marrow transplantation and graft-versus-host disease.

Key Points

- MHC molecules are categorized as either MHC-I or MHC-II, and each class has a different role in the immune system. MHC-I molecules are present on all nucleated cells and present endogenous peptides to CD8 T cells; MHC-II molecules are present only on cells of the immune system and present exogenous peptides to CD4 T cells.
- Many human diseases are associated with the inheritance of specific HLA alleles, including ankylosing spondylitis, rheumatoid arthritis, and type I diabetes mellitus.
- Transplant rejection can be either direct or indirect. Direct alloresponses rely on the T cell receptor recognizing the donor antigen-presenting cells (APCs) as foreign. This occurs without respect to the peptide in the cleft. In indirect allo-responses, the foreign cell antigens are processed and the resultant peptides are presented by host APCs to host T cells resulting in T cell activation and graft rejection.
- Rejection of a graft can occur with anything other than an autotransplant. Even fully matched sibling donor grafts can be rejected due to incompatibility at minor histocompatibility loci.
- With bone marrow transplantation, immunocompetent cells in both the recipient and donor can reject each other. Donor rejection of the recipient is termed graft-versus-host disease (GVHD).
- Stem cell transplantation is most often performed for malignancies; however, significant numbers of patients with immunodeficiencies, congenital hematologic disorders, and inborn errors of metabolism receive stem cell transplants as well.
- The field of immunogenetics is expanding rapidly, and new immunosuppressive therapies for autoimmune diseases and transplant recipients are on the horizon.

Study Questions/Critical Thinking

1. Describe the function of MHC molecules on a cellular level. How are they related to the expression of various diseases in humans?
2. What are the barriers to solid organ transplantation? What is involved in the typical matching process?
3. What are the differences between hyperacute, acute, and chronic rejection? Explain their timing and reversibility.
4. What are the risk factors for developing graft-versus-host disease, and what are the current approaches to prevent this from occurring?
5. Describe the role of immunosuppressive medications in the treatment of autoimmune diseases. Name a few specific diseases being treated with immunosuppressive therapy.

Suggested Reading

Fernando MM, Stevens CR, Walsh EC, et al. Defining the role of the MHC in autoimmunity: a review and pooled analysis. PLoS Genet. 2008; 4: e1000024.

Klein J, Sato A. The HLA system: first of two parts. N Eng J Med. 2000; 343: 702–9.

Klein J, Sato A. The HLA system: second of two parts. N Eng J Med. 2000; 343: 782–6.

Lennon-Dumenil AM, Bakker AH, Wolf-Bryant P, et al. A closer look at proteolysis and MHC-class-II-restricted antigen presentation. Curr Opin Immunol. 2002; 14: 15–21.

Lie BA, Thorsby E. Several genes in the extended human MHC contribute to predisposition to autoimmune disease. Curr Opin Immunol. 2005; 17: 526–31.

Oldstone MBA. Molecular mimicry and immune-mediated diseases. FASEB J. 1998; 12: 1255–65.

Petersdorf E, Anasetti C, Martin P, et al. Genomics of unrelated-donor hematopoietic cell transplantation. Curr Opin Immunol. 2001; 13: 582–9.

Thorsby E. Invited anniversary review: HLA associated diseases. Hum Immunol. 1997; 53: 1–11.

Van Kaer L. Major histocompatibility complex class I-restricted antigen processing and presentation. Tissue Antigens. 2002; 60: 1–9.

Section Two

MECHANISMS OF RESPONSE

Chapter 11

Advances in Clinical Immunomodulation

Robert P. Nelson, Jr., MD
Mark Ballow, MD
Joseph A. Bellanti, MD

LEARNING OBJECTIVES

When you have completed this chapter, you should be able to:

- Define immunomodulation broadly to include immunopotentiation, immunosuppression, or induction of immunologic tolerance
- Describe the important role of immunomodulatory therapies in the treatment of many diseases. You should also be able to give a few specific examples of treatments with immunomodulatory agents, including their targets and modes of action
- Understand the system of nomenclature for monoclonal antibodies
- Explain the proposed mechanisms of IVIG immunoregulatory activity and name a few different diseases for which it is a successful treatment
- Appreciate the variety of therapeutic immunoglobulins that have been developed, including monoclonal and polyclonal immunoglobulins directed against microbes and cells
- Understand the extracorporeal therapy, plasmapheresis, and its indications
- Describe the basic mechanisms of action of glucocorticosteroids and some of their common side effects
- Understand the differences between monoclonal antibodies, therapeutic fusion proteins, recombinant cytokines, and soluble receptor constructs and their different modes of action as immunomodulators
- Gain an appreciation of the exciting future of immunomodulatory treatments in health and disease

Case Study

A two-year-old boy presents to his pediatrician with a nine-day history of daily fevers > 39°C, irritability, a polymorphous rash on the trunk (Figure 11-1A) and extremities most prominent in the diaper area (Figure 11-1B), bilateral nonexudative bulbar conjunctivitis (Figure 11-1C), cracked lips, and strawberry tongue (Figure 11-1D), as well as edema and erythema on his hands and feet (Figure 11-1E and Figure 11-1F). The child was well prior to the onset of the present illness and there was no history of a preceding sore throat or other infection. Laboratory tests showed an elevated white cell count of 15,900/mm^3 with 80 percent neutrophils and 10 percent band forms and an elevated erythrocyte sedimentation rate of 45 mm/hr. Based on the history and physical findings, a diagnosis of Kawasaki disease was made.

Kawasaki disease is an acute febrile illness of unknown etiology that primarily affects infants and children. The disease was recognized and first reported as a separate entity by Dr. Tomisaku Kawasaki in 1967 and was later reported in the English-language literature in 1974. The histopathological changes of Kawasaki disease are consistent with a systemic vasculitis with multiorgan involvement similar to those seen in periarteritis nodosa (PAN), differing, however, by the involvement of medium- and smaller-sized arteries. The clinician should consider Kawasaki disease as a possible cause of this boy's rash after excluding several other diseases of childhood that enter into the differential diagnosis (Table 11-1).

Diagnosis of Kawasaki Disease

At the present time, the diagnosis of Kawasaki disease is based on characteristic features of the history and physical findings that were developed by the Japan Kawasaki Disease Research Committee and subsequently adopted by the American Heart Association (Box 11-1).

Treatment of Kawasaki Disease

In the absence of a known etiologic agent, initial therapy for Kawasaki disease is directed at reducing fever and other inflammatory features with

Case Study (continued)

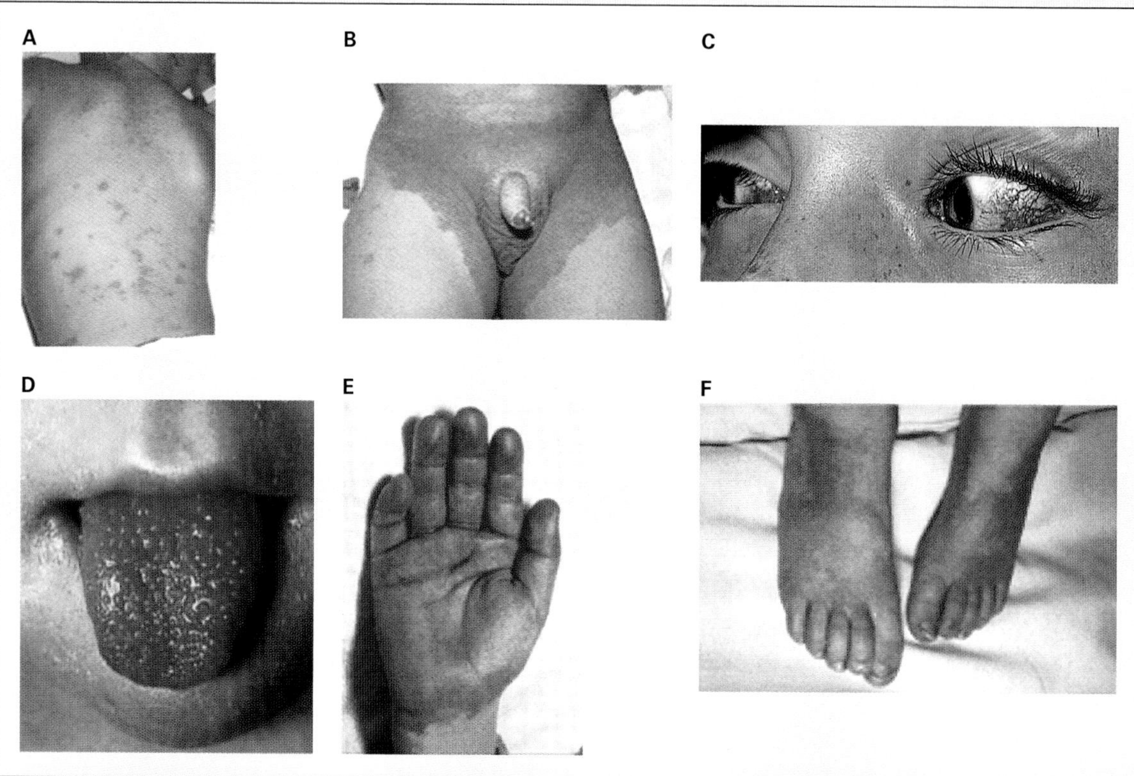

Figure 11-1. Erythema and edema in a patient with Kawasaki's disease. Panel A: Erythematous maculopapular rash on the skin of the back; Panel B: diffuse, confluent erythematous rash in the diaper area; Panel C: bilateral nonexudative bulbar conjunctivitis; Panel D: strawberry tongue; Panels E and F: edema and erythema on the hand and feet, respectively. Photos A, B, E, and F reproduced with permission from Trager JD. Images in clinical medicine. Kawasaki's disease. N Engl J Med. 1995;333:1391; Photos C and D, courtesy of Dr. Charlotte Barbey-Morel and Dr. Thomas Rubio.

the ultimate aim of preventing the development of coronary artery abnormalities, i.e., aneurysms, and subsequent myocardial ischemic injury. Long-term therapy is targeted at avoiding coronary thrombosis by preventing platelet aggregation.

Current recommendations for initial therapy (preferably given within the first ten days of the onset of illness) include intravenous immunoglobulin (IVIG) administered as a single bolus of 2 g/kg to help prevent coronary artery abnormalities and the oral administration of acetylsalicylic acid (i.e., aspirin) in high dosages to hasten resolution of the acute inflammatory manifestations of Kawasaki disease, especially fever. When the treatment is initiated within ten days of the onset of symptoms, the prevalence of aneurysms is reduced from 20–25 percent to less than 5 percent at six to eight weeks after initiation of therapy. Aspirin is continued until the ESR, CRP, and platelet counts return to normal, which typically occurs within four to six weeks.

Table 11-1. Diseases that should be included in the differential diagnosis of Kawasaki disease

Measles
Scarlet fever
Drug reactions
Stevens-Johnson syndrome
Other febrile viral exanthems
Toxic shock syndrome
Rocky Mountain spotted fever
Staphylococcal scalded skin syndrome
Juvenile idiopathic arthritis (JIA)
Leptospirosis
Mercury poisoning

Box 11-1

Kawasaki Disease

Criteria Required to Diagnose Kawasaki Disease

- A fever that lasts for a minimum of five days.
- Presence of four of the following five conditions:
  1. Bilateral conjunctival injection.
  2. Changes of the mucosa of the oropharynx, including an injected pharynx, erythematous and/or dry and cracked lips, and a strawberry tongue.
  3. Edema and/or erythema of hands and/or feet. Desquamation (usually beginning periungually) in the convalescent phase.
  4. Rash (primarily truncal), polymorphous usually non-vesicular, sometimes only present in the perineum.
  5. Cervical lymphadenopathy.
- Illness not explained by other known disease processes.

Additional Findings Not Included in the Major Diagnostic Criteria But Often Present in Patients with Kawasaki Disease

- Cardiovascular manifestations, the leading cause of morbidity and mortality, include coronary aneurysms, which are reported in 20–25 percent of children with Kawasaki disease, pancarditis, myocarditis, and pericarditis with pericardial effusion. Involvement of the left coronary artery is more common than involvement of the right coronary artery.
- Patients with giant aneurysms (internal diameter of at least 8 mm) have the worst prognosis and are at the greatest risk of developing thrombosis, stenosis, and myocardial infarction. Long-term follow-up studies demonstrate the resolution of coronary aneurysms within 5–18 months in approximately 50 percent of patients.
- During the acute phase, children may develop aseptic meningitis, pneumonitis, arthritis and arthralgia, uveitis, gastrointestinal symptoms such as diarrhea, vomiting, and abdominal pain, and hydrops of the gallbladder.
- Laboratory findings include leukocytosis with left shift in the acute phase along with elevated erythrocyte sedimentation rate (ESR) and C-reactive protein (CRP). Elevated liver transaminase levels and sterile pyuria are also seen. An increased number of circulating platelets (thrombocytosis) is typically present in the second week of the illness.

Introduction

One of the greatest contributions of immunology to medicine in recent years has been the translation of basic complex cellular and molecular workings of the immune system into new procedures and products that not only promote health and well-being in the healthy host, but also provide novel therapies for patients suffering from diseases for which no effective treatment modalities have been available. These advances were made possible not only by the landmark contributions of pioneering immunologists and clinicians of the past two centuries interested in the treatment of infectious diseases with hyperimmune serum or gamma globulin, but also as a result of the remarkable progress in biotechnology and molecular biology in more recent years, which has provided new modalities to enhance the reactivity of the immune system when it is functioning suboptimally, as in the case of immunodeficient states (*Chapter 16*), or to diminish immune reactivity when it is hyperreacting, as in the case of the allergic (*Chapter 18*) or autoimmune diseases (*Chapter 19*). Collectively, these activities are referred to as immunomodulation, and the procedures or substances, e.g., drugs, used to accomplish them are called immunomodulators.

Immunomodulation may be defined as the process by which the immune response is adjusted or changed to another desired level utilizing three interventive strategies of **immunopotentiation**, **immunosuppression**, or induction of **immunologic tolerance**. Shown in Table 11-2 is a broad classification of immunomodulators together with their mechanisms of action and some examples of their applications in health and disease based on this paradigm. For ease of discussion, the immunomodulators may be arbitrarily divided into three major groups based on whether the direction of immunomodulation is upward, i.e., increased immune reactivity, or downward, i.e., decreased immune reactivity: (1) **group 1** agents, commonly referred to as immunopotentiators, include those

Table 11-2. Classification of three groups of immunomodulatory (IM) agents, with mechanisms of action, examples, and potential recipients of each

Group	Direction of IM effect	Mechanism of action	Example of IM agents	Healthy or diseased subjects who receive immunomodulators
Group 1				
Immunopotentiators Subgroup 1a nonspecific	↑	No requirement for antigenic specificity	Adjuvants, hormones (e.g., vitamin D)	Healthy subjects receiving vaccines for prevention of infectious diseases
Subgroup 1b specific		Require antigenic specificity	Vaccines, polyclonal antibodies, monoclonal antibodies	Antibody replacement therapy for patients with humoral immunodeficiency
Group 2				
Immunosuppressants Subgroup 2a nonspecific	↓	Produce broad-based immunosuppression at multiple sites	Irradiation, cytotoxic drugs, glucocorticoids, immunophilins (e.g., cyclosporine), intravenous immunoglobulin (IVIG)	Subjects with autoimmune disorders, allergic diseases, and cancer
Subgroup 2b specific		Target specific cells, cytokines, or receptors	Therapeutic polyclonal and monoclonal antibodies (e.g., anti-TNF agents), therapeutic fusion proteins (e.g., etanercept), soluble receptor constructs (e.g., anakinra), cytokines (e.g., interferons)	
Group 3				
Tolerance-inducing agents or procedures	↓	Directed at provoking immune tolerance by involvement of Treg cells, immunosuppressive cytokines (e.g., TGF-β, IL-10), or other mechanisms	Allergy immunotherapy (SCIT and SLIT)	Subjects with allergic disease

Note: SCIT = subcutaneous immunotherapy; SLIT = sublingual immunotherapy.

that enhance immune reactivity, and these can be further subdivided into nonspecific (**subgroup 1a**) and specific modalities (**subgroup 1b**); (2) **group 2** agents, commonly referred to as immunosuppressants, are those that diminish immune reactivity and include agents that exert their effects by either broadly depressing immune function at multiple sites of the immune system (**subgroup 2a**) or those targeting specific cells, cytokines, or cytokine receptors at specific sites (**subgroup 2b**); and, (3) **group 3** agents are those that exert their effects by diminishing immune responsiveness by induction of immune tolerance.

It is important for the clinician and all health care providers who treat or care for patients receiving immunomodulators to understand that their use carries with it both beneficial as well as detrimental aspects. Immunomodulatory agents that induce broad-based immunosuppressive effects, e.g., corticosteroids, or targeted effects, e.g., anti-TNF-α agents, for example, can benefit patients with autoimmune disease, e.g., rheumatoid arthritis, but are known to also predispose them to frequent and morbid infections, e.g., tuberculosis, as well as to autoimmune disease and cancer. Similarly, agents that provide physiological or supraphysiological levels of cytokine activity, e.g., interferon alpha, for the treatment of chronic hepatitis B or C infection can cause or exacerbate autoimmune disease in patients receiving them. Other agents, such as the growth factors that stimulate hematopoiesis, e.g., erythropoietin or granulocyte colony-stimulating factor (**G-CSF**) (*Chapter 9*) can also lead to myelodysplastic syndrome, leukemia, or other forms of lymphoproliferative disease (*Chapter 21*). These recently approved immunomodulators are rapidly becoming primary or adjunctive treatments for patients treated by clinical immunologists/allergists, rheumatologists, and other specialists. This chapter will describe the major immunomodulatory agents and some of their current clinical indications as well as their potential adverse effects.

Group 1 Immunopotentiators

This group of immunomodulators includes those modalities that enhance immune reactivity and are generally referred to as immunopotentiators (Table 11-2). They consist of adjuvants, vaccines, and immune globulin used in the prevention or treatment of infectious diseases. These can be further subdivided into nonspecific (subgroup 1a) and specific modalities (subgroup 1b).

Subgroup 1a Nonspecific Immunopotentiators

This subgroup of immunopotentiators achieves enhancement of immune reactivity nonspecifically primarily by activation of antigen-presenting cells (**APCs**) of the innate immune system, most notably dendritic cells and macrophages (*Chapter 3*). These agents do not require antigen specificity and include exogenous agents such as inorganic salts, e.g., aluminum salts, and organic substances, e.g., squalene, commonly used as adjuvants in vaccines (*Chapter 23*) as well as endogenous substances, e.g., hormones such as estrogens, which also enhance immune reactivity nonspecifically. Although adjuvants primarily activate cells of the innate immune system, when used in combination with specific vaccine antigens, they activate the adaptive immune system and accelerate, prolong, or enhance antigen-specific adaptive immune responses. Activation of cells of the innate immune system by adjuvants occurs by their interactions with pattern-recognition receptors (**PRRs**), specifically Toll-like receptors (**TLRs**) located on or within these cells (*Chapter 3*). Recent evidence suggests that the molecular mechanism of activation of macrophages by alum is mediated by activation of the NALP3 inflammasome, release of inflammatory cytokines (interleukins [**IL**]) IL-1β, IL-18, and IL-33, and potassium efflux, events similar to that seen following natural infection (Figure 11-2 and *Chapters 3* and *9*).

Subgroup 1b Specific Immunopotentiators

In contrast to the nonspecific subgroup 1a immunopotentiators, a second subgroup of agents, **subgroup 1b specific immunopotentiators,** exerts its immunopotentiating effects by antigen-specific modalities of adaptive immune responses through immunization with antigen-specific vaccines (**active immunization**) or by the administration of preformed polyclonal antibodies (**passive immunization**) (Table 11-2). The antigen-specific vaccines are used primarily for the prevention or treatment of infectious diseases and will be described in greater detail in *Chapter 23.* This section will describe the historical landmarks of serum therapy, the later applications of pooled gamma globulin and hyperimmune preparations containing elevated levels of antibody to specific microbial agents as replacement therapy for patients with humoral immune deficiencies as well as their use as immunosuppressant modalities in autoimmune and inflammatory diseases.

Historical Landmarks of Serum Therapy

The history of antibody therapy as an immunopotentiating modality began in the late 1800s with the work of von Behring and Kitasato, who discovered that patients suffering from diphtheria when treated with serum from horses immunized with diphtheria toxin recovered from this previously almost universally fatal disease (Figure 11-3). This form of treatment was called serum therapy or passive immunization because whole serum from the blood of immunized animals was used. Although antibodies were not recognized or characterized until decades later, von Behring specifically used the term antibodies in his writings. For his role in the discovery and development of serum therapy for diphtheria, he was awarded the first Nobel Prize in Medicine in 1901. Following these initial successes, serum therapy of other infectious diseases continued and was widely used for prophylaxis and treatment of several viral and bacterial diseases during the early 1900s using sera obtained from convalescent patients or from horses immunized with specific bacteria or toxins. However, when antibiotics became widely available in the 1940s, serum therapy of most bacterial infections was less frequently used.

The next major landmark of serum therapy occurred in the 1940s during World War II when Cohn, working on techniques for the fractionation of plasma proteins for the production of serum albumin as a plasma expander for wounded soldiers, developed

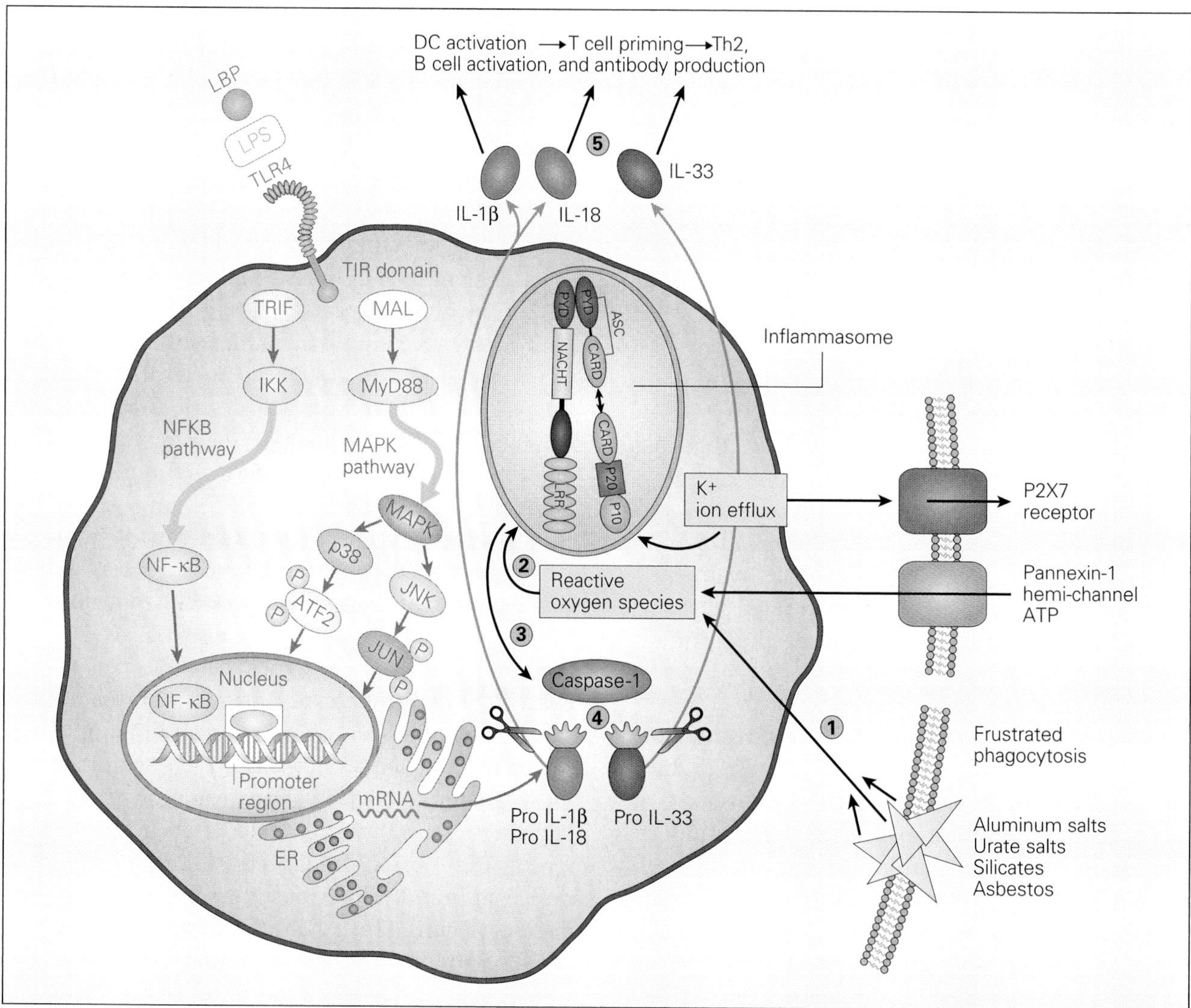

Figure 11-2. Schematic representation of the proposed adjuvant mechanism of action of alum in innate immunity showing the critical roles of the NALP3 inflammasome and potassium efflux leading to the secretion of pro-inflammatory cytokines as well its collaborative role in adaptive immunity through Th2/B cell activation and antibody production. The uptake of alum salts induces the synthesis of reactive oxygen species (1) which in turn stimulates the activation of the NALP3 inflammasome (2) which generates an active caspase-1 (3) that mediates the cleavage of pro-IL-1β, pro-IL-18, and pro-IL-33 to the synthesis (4) and release (5) of active IL-1β, IL-18, and IL-33, respectively. IL-1β and IL-18 are believed to be involved in dendritic cell (DC) activation and T cell priming to a Th2 phenotype that is favored by IL-33 to promote B cell activation and antibody production. Also shown in the figure are the roles of potassium efflux and ATP entry through the Pannexin-1 hemi-channel events, which are important in the activation of the inflammasome.

the cold ethanol process of plasma fractionation. The basis for the Cohn procedure was to use varying concentrations of ethanol at low temperatures coupled with reduced pH and lowered ionic strength. This discovery led to the fractionation of human plasma into several useful plasma components other than albumin, including gamma globulin. These early gamma globulin products were used in subsequent years for the prevention of measles, poliomyelitis, mumps, pertussis, and hepatitis A, but were gradually replaced with the vaccines for these diseases that were developed in subsequent years. The Cohn process still serves as a major foundation for the production of all gamma globulin products by the blood industry.

In 1952, the discovery by Colonel Bruton of agammaglobulinemia in an eight-year-old boy demonstrated the effective subcutaneous use of pooled human gamma globulin in preventing infection in this patient (Figure 11-3 and *Chapter 16*). This discovery by an astute clinician not only provided the basis for replacement therapy for antibody-related immune deficiencies by gamma globulin, but also paved the way for subsequent development of clinical immunology made by countless basic and

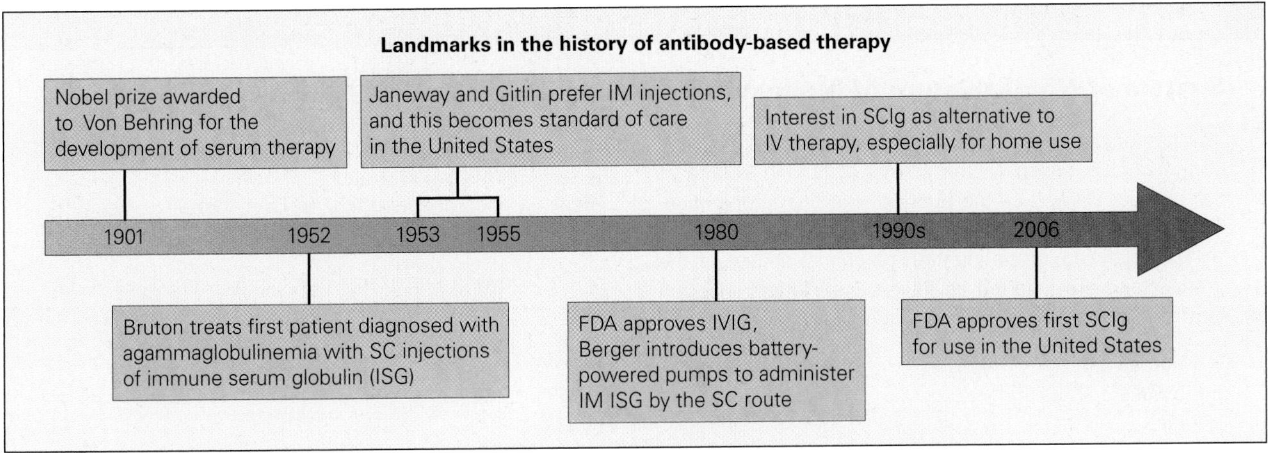

Figure 11-3. Schematic representation of some of the historic landmarks of antibody-based serum therapy.

clinical immunologists in subsequent years. In the 1950s, the intramuscular use of gamma globulin was favored by Janeway and Gitlin over the subcutaneous route. Still later, as will be described below, preparations of gamma globulin suitable for intravenous delivery became available and more recently immunoglobulin replacement by slow subcutaneous infusion was introduced (Figure 11-3).

Although serum polyclonal antibody preparations and pooled gamma globulin continued to be used for the prevention of several viral infectious diseases, e.g., hepatitis A, and for replacement therapy of patients with agammaglobulinemia, problems related to allergic reactions including a risk for anaphylactoid reactions, lot-to-lot variation, and uncertain dosing limited the continued use of these preparations. In addition, the active antigen-specific antibodies in a polyclonal preparation typically represented only a relatively small portion of the total antibodies (1 percent); the rest of the antibodies were not only ineffective, but could at times contribute to adverse effects. It was not possible to produce large amounts of antibodies with the desired specificity until the 1970s, when another extraordinary discovery was made.

The Discovery of Hybridoma Technology for the Production of Monoclonal Antibodies

In 1975, Kohler and Milstein made the remarkable discovery that the progeny of fusion between a normal antibody-secreting B cell (i.e., plasma cell) and a myeloma cell of animal or human origin, referred to as a hybridoma, was capable of producing large quantities of homogenous antibody to a single antigenic specificity, i.e., monoclonal antibody (**mAb**) (Figure 11-3 and *Chapter 6*). For this outstanding contribution, Köhler and Milstein together with Jerne received the Nobel Prize in Physiology or Medicine in 1984 for their work in this field. This discovery initiated a paradigm shift for the *in vitro* production of therapeutic monoclonal antibodies (e.g., anti-TNF agents), therapeutic fusion proteins (e.g., etanercept), soluble receptor constructs (e.g., anakinra), and cytokines (e.g., interferons) that has continued to the present and that has revolutionized the field of medical diagnostics and therapeutics for infectious diseases, allergic diseases, autoimmune disorders, and cancer (Table 11-2). Since monoclonal antibodies contained varying quantities of foreign mouse protein, however, a major limitation of the hybridoma technology was an inability to produce a completely human monoclonal antibody preparation for human use since administration of these murine mAbs in humans could result in adverse immune responses against the foreign proteins with the generation of human anti-mouse antibodies (**HAMAs**). However, with the advent of a number of molecular biologic techniques, i.e., recombinant DNA technology, and an increased understanding of antibody structure and function, chimeric and humanized mAbs could now be developed. Finally, phage-display techniques and other molecular biology techniques, including the generation of transgenic animals, allowed the development of fully human antibodies (*Chapter 25*). During a period of three to four decades beginning in the 1970s and continuing to the present, we are witnessing the fruits of this paradigm shift that have resulted in a number of useful therapeutic antibodies approved for clinical use, which will be described below. Shown in Box 11-2

Box 11-2

System of Nomenclature of Monoclonal Antibodies and Fusion Proteins

The nomenclature of various classes of monoclonal antibody (mAb) is based on the animal or human source of the product as well as the purity of the final preparation. All mAbs end in the suffix -mab.

The following letters identify the animal source of the product and are inserted as infixes (i.e., letters inserted into a word) preceding the -mab stem:

u – human
o – mouse
a – rat
e – hamster
i – primate
xi – chimera

The suffix of the product name denotes its class and is based on purity and the degree of residual foreign protein in the preparation:

-umab = human monoclonal antibody (100 percent human and contains no mouse protein)
-omab = mouse protein (100 percent mouse protein)
-zumab = humanized monoclonal antibody (contains < 5 percent mouse protein)
-ximab = chimeric monoclonal antibody (contains > 5 percent mouse protein)
-cept = receptor-antibody fusion protein (receptor attached to Fc of IgG1)

The following are examples of infixes for disease, target class, or tumor:

viral – vir-
bacterial – bac-
immune – lim-
cardiovascular – cir-
colon tumor – col-
ovary tumor – gov-

The starting prefix is a distinct syllable that creates a unique mAb name; a consonant is often dropped to make the name more pronounceable, e.g., the "m" in "lim." Examples:

oma li(m) zu mab = omalizumab
ritu xi mab = rituximab
dac li(m) zu mab = daclizumab

and Figure 11-4 is the nomenclature used to describe mAbs and fusion proteins.

Intravenous Immunoglobulin

Immunoglobulin was introduced as an intravenously administered product in 1981, and this mode of therapy has essentially replaced the use of intramuscular preparations for the treatment of immunodeficiency diseases (Figure 11-3). All intravenous immunoglobulin (**IVIG**) products are prepared initially by the Cohn method of cold ethanol fractionation of plasma derived from multiple donors (10,000 to 60,000). Ethanol fractionation is followed by processes that remove antibody aggregates and inactivate viral pathogens. Preparations are usually supplied as 5 percent, 10 percent, or 12 percent protein solutions. A 20-percent preparation is also available for subcutaneous (**SC**) use. Ninety-five to 99 percent of the IVIG is IgG (with trace amounts of IgA and IgM), and IgG subclass distribution of approved products is similar to that of normal human serum. Some products contain extremely low quantities of IgA, which may be useful for patients with antibody deficiency and low IgA and who would be capable of producing IgE-associated anti-IgA antibodies when given products with higher IgA content. The use of a low IgA-containing product in selected individuals minimizes the risk of IgA sensitization and possible anaphylactic reactions. However, patients with a isolated IgA deficiency should not receive IVIG, even those with low IgA-containing products. All currently available preparations are otherwise equivalent; therefore, products

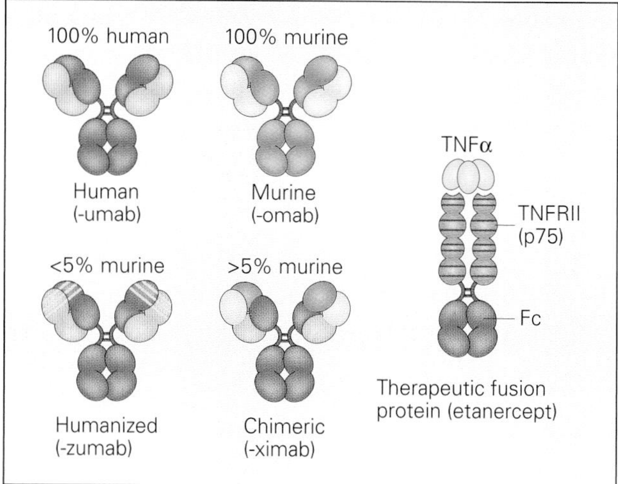

Figure 11-4. Schematic representation of various mAbs and fusion proteins.

may be chosen on the basis of cost, availability, and/or convenience and formulation (e.g., a lyophilized versus a liquid form).

Indications for Replacement Therapy with IVIG

IVIG is indicated as replacement therapy for patients with primary immunodeficiency diseases who are incapable of normal antibody production (*Chapter 16*). Because of the twenty to thirty day half-life of IgG (*Chapter 6*), infusions are given every three to four weeks at a dose of 400–600 mg/kg to achieve a trough IgG level greater than 500 mg/dl, a level correlated with a decreased frequency of infections. The number of infections, days missed from school or work, or days hospitalized may not be sufficient indicators of adequate treatment, and improvement or maintenance of pulmonary function may be a more important measure of successful therapy.

Quartier and associates studied the clinical features and outcomes of 31 patients with X-linked agammaglobulinemia who received IVIG replacement therapy between 1982 and 1997. Although early treatment with IVIG and the achievement of a trough serum IgG level of > 500 mg/dl was effective in preventing severe acute bacterial infections, pulmonary disease and sinusitis still occurred. This may have reflected the greater advantage of parenterally administered IgG in providing resistance to systemic infection but its relatively lesser effectiveness in providing local defense at mucosal surfaces, sites where secretory IgA plays a greater protective role (*Chapter 8*). The authors suggested that maintaining a higher serum IgG level (e.g., > 800 mg/dl) might delay or prevent the decline in pulmonary function observed in some patients. A period of approximately three to six months following initiation of monthly infusions or changing the dosage is required to reach equilibration, i.e., the steady state. For patients who catabolize infused IgG relatively rapidly, more frequent infusions, e.g., smaller doses given every two to three weeks, may maintain the serum level in the normal range. The rate of elimination of IgG may also be higher during a period of active infection, at which time more frequent serum IgG determinations and adjustments to higher dosages or shorter intervals may be required.

Adverse Reactions Associated with IVIG

Adverse effects are generally associated with the presence of infections and are presumably mediated by the formation/degradation of immune complexes. Risks of these adverse reactions are relatively high during the initial treatment, and actively infected patients should initially receive half the maintenance dose, i.e., 200 mg/kg, followed two weeks later by the remaining half to achieve a full dose. Treatment should not be discontinued due to active infection and adverse reactions are uncommon after normal serum IgG levels are reached.

The most common side effects include flushing, headache, nausea, vomiting, and myalgias that are often infusion-rate dependent. Severe anaphylactic episodes occur rarely in patients who have IgE antibodies directed toward IgA. Aseptic meningitis is a rare complication, especially following large doses (1–2 gm/kg), rapid infusions, and the treatment of patients with autoimmune disorders or inflammatory disease. Pretreatment with aspirin (15 mg/kg/dose), acetaminophen (15 mg/kg/dose), diphenhydramine (1 mg/kg/dose), and/or hydrocortisone (6 mg/kg/dose, maximum 100 mg) one hour prior to the infusion may prevent adverse reactions. Acute renal failure is a rare but serious complication of IVIG treatment and occurs primarily in patients with autoimmune disease who are receiving large doses and in those with preexisting renal insufficiency. IVIG that contains sucrose as a stabilizer may confer greater risk of renal failure. It may be necessary, therefore, to monitor blood urea nitrogen and creatinine before and periodically thereafter in patients at risk, including those with preexisting renal insufficiency, diabetes mellitus, dehydration, sepsis, paraproteinemia, concomitant use of nephrotoxic agents, and those over 65 years of age.

One preparation of IVIG used previously was taken off the market in 1994 following a series of occurrences of hepatitis C infection. Routine screening for hepatitis C RNA by reverse transcriptase PCR and the addition of viral inactivation processes in the final manufacturing step (e.g., treatment with solvent/detergent, pasteurization, and/or nanofiltration) have significantly reduced the risk of viral transmission. There have been no reports of human immunodeficiency virus transmission or prion-associated Creutzfeldt-Jakob disease in recipients of IVIG.

Hyperimmune Globulin Preparations for the Treatment and Prevention of Infection

In contrast to polyclonal preparations of pooled gamma globulin obtained randomly from large groups of donors, hyperimmune globulin preparations are obtained from plasma of multiple donors with high titers of specific IgG antibody, which may be elevated as a consequence of natural infection or exposure or after purposeful immunization. A number of preparations are available that are usually administered via the intramuscular route, although some are available as intravenous products (Table 11-3). Since these products contain higher levels of antibody directed to specific disease-causing microbes than polyclonal preparations, they therefore provide greater protection.

Hepatitis B hyperimmune globulin is derived from the plasma of multiple donors with high antibody titers to the hepatitis B surface antigen, which passively immunizes people exposed to hepatitis B. Similar products are available for the prevention of rabies and tetanus. These preparations are given intramuscularly and adverse effects may include local pain and redness at the sight of injection, occasional urticaria/angioedema, and rare systemic anaphylactoid reactions.

Cytomegalovirus (CMV) immune globulin, an intravenous preparation containing relatively high levels of anti-CMV antibodies, is effective at reducing the incidence or attenuating the severity of CMV disease, providing prophylaxis for patients at risk to CMV infection, e.g., renal transplant recipients at risk for primary CMV disease. Side effects are similar to those seen with routine IVIG infusions.

Respiratory syncytial virus (RSV) immune globulin is available for prevention of serious lower respiratory disease in patients at high risk for RSV disease and together with a monoclonal preparation, described in the next section, have appeared to have significantly diminished the incidence of RSV-related hospitalizations, severity of illness, and cost of RSV-related care of infants at risk for significant RSV disease, although a relatively high cost-to-benefit ratio exists.

Shown in the Annex to this chapter are several groups of biologic response modifiers that have become available as a result of technologic advances. These modifiers have shown great promise in the treatment of a wide variety of immunologically mediated disease.

Table 11-3. Hyperimmune globulin preparations for the treatment and prevention of infection

Tetanus
Rabies
Hepatitis B
Cytomegalovirus (CMV)
Respiratory syncytial virus (RSV) (also available as a monoclonal antibody preparation)
Varicella/zoster

Monoclonal Antibody Preparations Directed Against Microbial Pathogens

There has been limited experience with monoclonal antibody preparations for treatment or prevention of infectious disease agents, with the notable exception of products targeted to the prevention of RSV infection. **Palivizumab** (Table 11A-1 in the Annex) is an intramuscularly administered anti-RSV monoclonal antibody preparation that reduces the risk of hospitalization attributable to RSV infections in high-risk pediatric patients, including those infants delivered between 32 and 35 weeks of gestation. Studies have shown that infants and children with chronic lung disease (**CLD**), formerly designated bronchopulmonary dysplasia (**BPD**), as well as prematurely born infants without CLD, were hospitalized less frequently while receiving palivizumab; this treatment may be preferable to **RSV hyperimmune globulin** because it is not only easier to administer (intramuscular), but also does not interfere with measles-mumps-rubella and varicella vaccination responses known to occur with the hyperimmune polyclonal preparation. However, since RSV-IGIV provides additional protection against other respiratory viral illnesses, it may be preferred for selected high-risk children, including those with underlying primary immunodeficiency or human immunodeficiency virus infection who may benefit from the broader coverage of RSV-IGIV infused prior to hospital discharge during the RSV season. RSV-IGIV is contra-indicated, and palivizumab is not recommended for children with cyanotic congenital heart disease. Additional information regarding guidelines and indications for RSV prophylaxis are provided by the American Academy of Pediatrics.

Group 2 Immunosuppressants

This group of immunomodulators diminish immune reactivity and include agents that exert their immunosuppressant effects by either broadly depressing immune function at multiple sites of the immune system (subgroup 2a) or those targeting specific cells, cytokines, or cytokine receptors at specific sites (subgroup 2b) (Table 11-2).

Subgroup 2a Nonspecific Immunosuppressants

The subgroup 2a agents comprise a group of nonspecific modalities including irradiation, the cytotoxic drugs, glucocorticoids, immunophilins (e.g., cyclosporine), IVIG, and plasmapheresis (Table 11-2).

The Major Immunosuppressive Agents Used Clinically Today: Irradiation and Drugs

Irradiation and chemotherapeutic cytotoxic pharmaceuticals possess potent immunosuppressive activities that are useful for the treatment of diseases characterized by disordered immunological function or patients undergoing transplantation (*Chapter 22*). Irradiation (total body or localized), azathioprine, methotrexate, and cyclophosphamide are the predominant modalities commonly used at this time for a variety of immunomodulating purposes. Mycophenolate mofetil is a recent addition to this group of drugs.

Irradiation

High dose, total body irradiation (**TBI**) has profound immunosuppressive effects and is useful for preparing patients for human stem cell transplantation (**HSCT**) (*Chapter 22*). Following TBI, 80 percent of lymphocytes undergo prompt intermitotic death (i.e., killing of the cells between two successive mitoses during the cell cycle). Some lymphocytes survive, but high rates of sustained allogeneic engraftment occur when TBI is combined with an alkylating agent. B lymphocytes undergo interphase and mitotic death; precursors to all T cell subpopulations are sensitive, and the homing activity of cells is affected. TBI prevents primary immune responses to neoantigens more effectively than modifying responses to recall antigens. Irradiation of lymph tissues, known as total lymph node irradiation, is effective for the treatment of Hodgkin's disease, solid organ graft rejection, and severe rheumatoid arthritis, and as a component of conditioning prior to HSCT. Local irradiation, including regional lymph node irradiation, produces lymphopenia and decreased delayed hypersensitivity responses but does not appear to increase susceptibility to infection.

Azathioprine

Azathioprine is a member of a group of immunosuppressive agents referred to as purine antagonists. Following oral administration, azathioprine is metabolized in the liver to the purine analogue 6-mercaptopurine, which integrates into DNA and causes death of rapidly dividing precursor cells of the bone marrow and intestine. It prevents or minimizes immune-mediated rejection of transplanted organs and modulates autoimmune diseases, including rheumatoid arthritis, Crohn's disease, ulcerative colitis, and chronic graft-versus-host disease (**GVHD**) following HSCT (*Chapters 10* and *22*). Therapeutic immunosuppression occurs at doses of 1.5 mg/kg, a dose not often profoundly myelosuppressive. As in many forms of primary and secondary immunodeficiency, long-term therapy is associated with an increased risk of squamous cell carcinoma and lymphoreticular malignancies.

Methotrexate

Methotrexate is a folic acid antagonist that inhibits dihydrofolate reductase, leading to an accumulation of inactive oxidized folates and cessation of nucleotide synthesis, resulting in the death of cells that are in the process of synthesizing DNA (S-phase). Nonproliferating cells are resistant to the drug. The reduced folate leucovorin reverses the drug's physiological effects and is used to treat clinical methotrexate toxicity and is referred to as "leucovorin rescue." Methotrexate also inhibits macrophage activation, as demonstrated in an animal model of adjuvant arthritis. It is given to humans to prevent GVHD following HSCT and for the treatment of rheumatoid arthritis and psoriasis. Given as a weekly oral dose, methotrexate has a steroid-sparing effect in severe asthmatics; however, the potency of this effect remains controversial. Methotrexate has proven short-term efficacy for the treatment of juvenile rheumatoid arthritis (**JRA**), now referred to as juvenile idiopathic arthritis (**JIA**). There are several risk factors that contribute to enhanced hematologic toxicity of methotrexate, including renal insufficiency, concomitant nonsteroidal anti-inflammatory and trimethoprim-sulfamethoxazole administration, intravascular volume depletion, and folate deficiency. Chronic use of the drug is associated with hepatic fibrosis, which leads to cirrhosis in some patients, a complication that is not uniformly predicted by hepatocellular enzyme elevation. Periodic liver biopsy should therefore be considered for long-term recipients of the drug. Methotrexate is teratogenic and its use should be avoided, if possible, in pregnant women. It does not appear to be carcinogenic.

Cyclophosphamide

Cyclophosphamide is an alkylating agent that forms covalent bonds with DNA leading to mutations, DNA fragmentation, and cell death. It suppresses cellular immunity, inhibits antibody (and autoantibody production), and is primarily used as conditioning therapy prior to HSCT and for the treatment of autoimmune diseases and vasculitis. It is given as a single daily oral dose for the treatment of Wegener's granulomatosis or as monthly intravenous "pulse" therapy, usually in combination with maintenance oral prednisone, for the treatment of lupus erythematosus. Adverse effects include leukopenia, sterility, hemorrhagic cystitis, and malignancy, including leukemias and transitional cell carcinoma. A thorough review of these potential effects should be undertaken with the patient and documented in the medical record prior to treatment.

Mycophenolate Mofetil

Mycophenolate mofetil (**MMF**) is an ester of mycophenolic acid that inhibits the enzyme inosine monophosphate dehydrogenase (without incorporation into DNA), interrupting the *de novo* pathway of guanosine nucleotide synthesis. T and B lymphocytes are critically dependent on *de novo* purine synthesis for DNA replication, whereas other cell types rely on nucleoside salvage pathways. Therefore, MMF inhibits T cell proliferation following mitogen and alloantigen stimulation, inhibits antibody production by B lymphocytes, and prevents glycosylation of adhesion proteins. The latter effect inhibits recruitment of lymphocytes to inflammatory foci. The administration of MMF helps prevent the rejection of renal, cardiac, and hepatic allografts and is commonly used in conjunction with glucocorticosteroids and cyclosporine. It is also being investigated for the treatment of several autoimmune diseases.

Glucocorticosteroids

Glucocorticosteroids (**GCs**) are potent catabolic hormones that have both anti-inflammatory and immunosuppressive properties. In general, the therapeutic uses of GCs are based primarily on their anti-inflammatory properties; at higher doses, however, they may exert immunosuppressive effects.

The anti-inflammatory effects of GCs include the reduction of tissue destruction, vasodilatation, vascular permeability, and acute phase reactivity. GCs alter the circulating number and function of neutrophils, eosinophils, macrophages, and lymphocytes. Following their administration, they induce redistribution of lymphocytes and cause an increase in neutrophils and a rapid and transient decrease in circulating lymphocytes. It is noteworthy that the lymphocytopenia is selective; i.e., T lymphocytes are depleted from the circulation to a greater extent than are B lymphocytes. One of the reasons for the paradoxical increase in neutrophil count in the circulation and reduction at sites of inflammation is related to glucocorticoid-mediated downregulation of endothelial adhesion molecules ICAM and ELAM-1 (*Chapter 5*). Although neutrophils are increased in number in the circulation their function is repressed, in part, by glucocorticoid-mediated IL-8 inhibition. Eosinophil adherence and degranulation are also inhibited. The well-recognized corticosteroid-induced neutrophilia is therefore the result of increased release from bone marrow progenitors, increase in neutrophil circulating half-life and prevention of adherence to vascular endothelium and migration into inflammatory sites. The striking degree of eosinopenia following corticosteroid administration is also felt to be due to a redistribution of circulating eosinophils from the vascular space into other body compartments.

Monocyte-mediated effects of GCs are inhibited by interference with recruitment, Fc-receptor function, antigen processing, and MHC-II and IL-1 production. GCs reroute the trafficking of lymphocytes from recirculating to nonrecirculating pools in lymph nodes and bone marrow. Immature lymphocytes and thymocytes are susceptible to glucocorticoid-induced apoptosis, while T cell proliferation to soluble and cellular antigens and production of IL-2 is inhibited. B cells are likewise redistributed, although immunoglobulin production is not directly inhibited. Nonetheless, serum IgG levels may be lower in subjects treated with GCs, secondary to cytokine-mediated pathways or increased immunoglobulin metabolism. Thus, it is important to recognize that steroid-dependent asthmatics may have low total IgG levels secondary to increased catabolism rather than decreased production, which makes immunoglobulin replacement therapy unnecessary and generally ineffective for the treatment of severe asthma.

Molecular Mechanisms of Action of Corticosteroids

The anti-inflammatory and immunosuppressive effects of corticosteroids are now better recognized by a greater understanding of the molecular mechanisms involved in gene transcription affecting both innate and adaptive immune responses. The molecular signaling events occurring after interaction of a cytokine, e.g., IL-2, with its receptor are shown in Figure 11-5A. In the inactive state, NF-κB is part of a trimolecular complex consisting of a heterodimer of p65 and p50 (the NF-κB) anchored in the cytoplasm by IκBα; above this complex, there exists a trimolecular complex called inhibitor of NF-κB kinase (**IKK**) composed of IKK1 (also known as IKKα), IKK2 (also known as IKKβ), and the NF-κB essential modulator (NEMO, also called IKKγ), which regulate the activation of the NF-κB. Following binding of a cytokine, e.g., IL-2 to its cell surface receptor, signals are generated, resulting in the activation of IKK1 (also called the IκB kinase), which results in the phosphorylation and proteolytic degradation of IκBα (Figure 11-5A). This then releases activated NF-κB (composed of the p50/p65 heterodimer), which then translocates into the nucleus where it attaches to the glucocorticoid regulatory element (**GRE**) in the promoter regions of inflammatory mediator genes in the DNA. Together with the participation of a transcriptional complex consisting of RNA polymerase II (Pol II), transcription factors II (**TFIIs**), and other transcription-associated factors (**TAFs**), transcriptional and translational events occur with gene expression and synthesis of pro-inflammatory cytokines, i.e., IL-1, IL-2, IL-6, IL-8, interferon gamma (**IFN-γ**), and tumor necrosis factor alpha (**TNF-α**).

A schematic representation of the molecular events associated with the anti-inflammatory effects of GCs is shown in Figure 11-5B. GCs initially interact with the intracytoplasmic glucocorticoid receptor (**GR**), which exists in an inactive form until it binds a GC. Binding of GC with its GR forms a complex consisting of four components: (1) GC, (2) GR and two chaperone heat shock proteins, (3) HSP-70, and (4) HSP-90. These binding events then lead to conformational changes in the GR resulting in the release of the two HSP chaperone molecules and the unmasking of a DNA-binding region of the activated GR/GC, causing it to bind to the GRE. Although glucose metabolism is controlled by either enhancement or inhibition of gene transcription, the anti-inflammatory effects result predominately from transcription inhibition and blockage of synthesis of inflammatory mediators by direct GRE-DNA binding or by the production of inhibitory proteins.

The GR/GC complex is thought to block NF-κB activity by either of two possible mechanisms: (1) inhibition through protein-protein interactions between the ligand-activated GR and NF-κB or (2) increased expression of IκBα through IκBα gene upregulation, thereby curtailing the activation of NF-κB and preventing subsequent transcriptional and translational events with blockage of inflammatory cytokine synthesis and induction of apoptosis in activated cells (Figure 11-5B). Thus, T cells are prevented from proliferating and being activated, cytotoxic T lymphocyte (**CTL**) activation is inhibited, and neutrophils and monocytes display poor chemotactic responses.

Another anti-inflammatory effect of GCs results from the upregulation of ANXA1 gene and its product, lipocortin (Annexin A1). Lipocortin blocks arachidonic acid degradation at the membrane level by inhibition of phospholipase A2, resulting in a broad and potent reduction in leukotriene synthesis, mediating their partial anti-asthmatic activity. Moreover, GCs limit the production of prostaglandins by inhibiting the gene transcription of COX-2, the rate-limiting enzyme for prostaglandin synthesis. A counterbalancing mechanism of the anti-inflammatory effects of glucocorticoids is mediated by IL-1, which opposes their action. Collagenase, a proteolytic enzyme active at the inflammatory sites, is also inhibited at the transcriptional level by the GCs. The GR complex formed by GCs binds to the protein c-JUN, one of the constituents of the activating protein-1 transcription factor complex (**AP-1**) that acts as an early response transcription factor, inducing the synthesis of collagenase. AP-1 induced transcription is then downregulated by GCs, preventing collagenase synthesis and further degradation of tissue at the inflammatory site. Finally, GCs inhibit nitric oxide synthetase, which decreases production of nitric oxide, a potent vasodilator and mediator of inflammation (*Chapter 5*).

The Clinical Significance of Glucocorticoid Therapy

The diverse anti-inflammatory and immunosuppressive activities of GCs have great clinical significance for the treatment of allergic, dermatological, and the autoimmune and autoinflammatory diseases. GCs are used to prevent GVHD and solid organ graft rejection. Patients receiving transplants usually receive combination immunosuppressive therapy, which increases the risk of bacterial, viral, and fungal infections. GCs are used also as an antimicrobial adjunct for the treatment of *Pneumocystis jirovecii* pneumonia by improving oxygenation and decreasing clinical progression to ventilator dependence, while the antifungal medication kills the organism. Multiple systemic GCs are available for clinical use, and a large variety of agents may be topically applied to the skin, conjunctiva, nasal mucosa, rectal mucosa, or delivered to pulmonary tissue by inhalation.

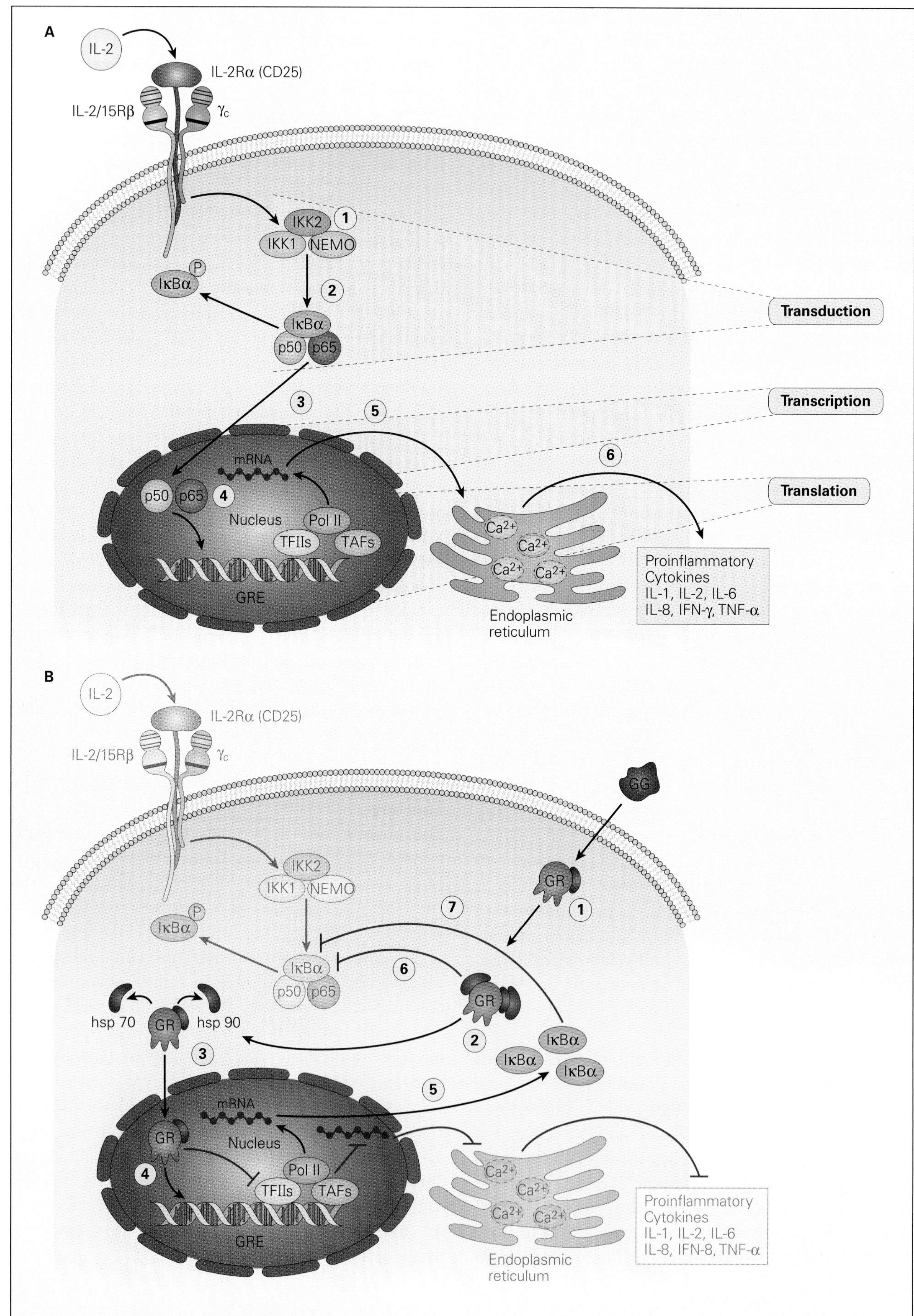
A
IL-2
IL-2Rα (CD25)
IL-2/15Rβ
γc
IKK2
1
IKK1
NEMO
P
IκBα
2
IκBα
p50
p65
Transduction
3
5
Transcription
mRNA
6
p50
p65
4
Translation
Nucleus
Pol II
TFIIs
TAFs
Ca2+
Ca2+
Ca2+
Ca2+
Proinflammatory
Cytokines
IL-1, IL-2, IL-6
IL-8, IFN-γ, TNF-α
GRE
Endoplasmic
reticulum
B
IL-2
IL-2Rα (CD25)
IL-2/15Rβ
γc
GG
IKK2
IKK1
NEMO
GR
P
IκBα
7
1
IκBα
6
p50
p65
GR
hsp 70
GR
hsp 90
2
IκBα
3
IκBα
IκBα
5
mRNA
GR
Nucleus
4
Pol II
TFIIs
TAFs
Ca2+
Ca2+
Ca2+
Ca2+
Proinflammatory
Cytokines
IL-1, IL-2, IL-6
IL-8, IFN-8, TNF-α
GRE
Endoplasmic
reticulum

Pharmacologic Properties and Potencies of Various Glucocorticoid Preparations

Shown in Table 11-4 are relative pharmacologic properties and potencies of various glucocorticosteroid preparations. GCs can be divided into three groups based on their plasma and biologic half-lives: short-acting, intermediate-acting, and long-acting drugs. Hydrocortisone is a short-acting GC that is assigned an anti-inflammatory and endocrine potency of "1" and a sodium-retaining potency of "2." The sodium-retaining potency of intermediate-acting drugs, which include prednisone, prednisolone, and methylprednisolone, is less than that of hydrocortisone. The long-acting preparations are virtually devoid of sodium-retaining activity and include dexamethasone, triamcinolone acetonide, fluticasone propionate, budesonide, and betamethasone dipropionate (Table 11-4). The administration of GCs in multiple doses daily, such as every six to eight hours, maximizes both their anti-inflammatory effects and adverse side effects, including hypothalamic-pituitary suppression. Less effective (and less toxic) regimens include single daily morning administration and alternate-morning dosing.

The glucocorticoid potency of cortisol is dependent upon its 11-betahydroxyl group; 11-keto compounds (cortisone and prednisone) must be converted to the corresponding 11-betahydroxyl compound to be active. Prednisolone or methylprednisolone, 11-betahydroxyl compounds, may be preferred for patients with impaired liver function or congestive heart failure. The administration of a large bolus or "pulse" dose (i.e., methylprednisolone, 15–30 mg/kg) daily for one to three days may be used at monthly intervals to achieve potent anti-inflammatory activity while limiting daily chronic exposure. The efficacy of such treatment has been demonstrated in controlled studies of patients with rheumatoid arthritis, lupus nephritis, and interstitial lung disease. General guidelines for clinicians treating allergic, inflammatory, and autoimmune conditions stress the importance of not only utilizing sufficient quantities to control the disease, but also the necessity to then taper the dose to the lowest quantity necessary to maintain disease remission while limiting side effects. Adverse effects are minimized by alternate-day oral administration, pulse therapy, the use of topical preparations, and the incorporation of adjunctive inflammatory/immunosuppressive medications. These strategies may permit the avoidance of toxicities that universally occur eventually in patients given supraphysiological doses.

Potentially serious side effects in adults include the development of hypertension, gastritis, cataracts, glucose intolerance, weight gain, and osteoporosis; occasionally, aseptic necrosis of the large joints, psychogenic effects, and increased susceptibility to viral, fungal, and mycobacterial infections may also occur. It is important to recognize that long-term use of GCs can result in hypothalamic pituitary axis suppression. Since fatal Addisonian crises have been known to occur following general surgical procedures during steroid withdrawal, patients receiving long-term GC administration should be treated with higher dosages (i.e., two to three times maintenance) prior to major surgical procedures to avoid this complication. Growth failure complicates GC use in children. The probability that most patients will experience iatrogenic complications with extended use underscores the clinicians' responsibility to inform patients of these potential adverse outcomes. Although many physicians request that patients provide signed informed consent documenting that these issues have been discussed prior to initiating therapy, this practice is not universally performed.

Immunophilin Ligands

Cyclosporine, tacrolimus, and sirolimus are potent immunosuppressant drugs that function as ligands of

◀**Figure 11-5.** Panel A: Schematic representation of the IL-2 signaling pathway. Binding of IL-2 to its receptor transduces a signal and activates the IKK complex (1). This then leads to subsequent phosphorylation of IκBα (2), releasing NF-κB (p50p65) (3) that then translocates to the nucleus and binds to a promoter region called the glucocorticoid regulatory element (GRE) (4). This promotes the activation of the RNA polymerase II (Pol II) with the collaboration of initiation factors (TFIIs and TAFs) that leads to the transcription of mRNA and its translocation to the endoplasmic reticulum (5), thus initiating the translational synthesis of pro-inflammatory cytokines IL-1, IL-2, IL-6, IL-8, IFN-γ, and TNF-α (6). Panel B: Schematic representation of the mechanism of glucocorticoid (GC) action through its inhibitory repression of NF-κB activity. After GC binding to its intracytoplasmic receptor (GR) to form the GR/GC complex (1), the two chaperone molecules that are initially added to the complex (2) lead to conformational changes of the GR are then dissociated (3) and permit activation of the GR/GC complex, which translocates to the nucleus (4). The GR/GC complex not only inhibits the initiation complex at the GRE promoter region, but also activates the transcription of other mRNAs that encode the synthesis of blocking molecules, such as IκBα (5). It has been proposed that NF-κB can be inhibited either by the GR/GC/chaperone complex (6) or alternatively by the newly synthesized IκBα (7), leading ultimately to the inhibition of the synthesis of pro-inflammatory cytokines.

Table 11-4. Relative pharmacologic potencies, equivalent dosage, and biologic and plasma half-life (t1/2) of glucocorticosteroid preparations

Preparation	Anti-inflammatory potency[a] dose (mg)	Equivalent pharmacologic potency[b]	Mineralocorticoid activity[a]	Plasma activity t1/2 (hr)	Biologic activity t1/2 (hr)	HPA axis suppression (mg)[c]
Cortisone	0.8	25	2.0	1.5	8–12	20–35
Prednisone	2.7	5.0	1.0	2.7	12–36	7.5
Prednisolone	4.0	5.0	1.0	2.75	12–26	7.5
Methylprednisolone	5.0	4.0	0	3.0	12–26	7.5
Triamcinolone	5.0	4.0	0	4.2	24–48	5–7.5
Dexamethasone	30	0.75	0	5.0	36–54	1–1.5

a. Relative to hydrocortisone, which is assigned a value of 1.
b. Range, 0–4.
c. Daily dose that usually leads to hypothalamic-pituitary (HPA) suppression.

immunophilins, i.e., members of a family of highly conserved proteins found mainly within the cytoplasm of cells that function as cis-trans peptidylprolyl isomerases (peptidylprolyl isomerases). These immunophilin ligands are derived from fungi that inhibit T cell activation through a series of calcium-dependent signaling events involved in cytokine gene transcription. They not only play especially important roles in suppression of solid organ allograft rejection, but are also the mainstays of GVHD prevention following HSCT (*Chapter 22*) and are increasingly becoming useful for the treatment of autoimmune conditions (*Chapter 19*). Cyclosporine (CsA) is a cyclic hexapeptide that blocks the calcium-dependent signal-transduction pathway emanating from the T cell receptor, thereby inhibiting the activation of helper CD4+ T cells. Tacrolimus (FK506) differs structurally from CsA but also interferes with T cell receptor-dependent cell activation (Figure 11-6).

Shown in Figure 11-7 is a schematic representation of the cellular sites of action of tacrolimus and cyclosporine at critical points in the signaling pathway following cytokine-mediated activation. Shown in Figure 11-7A are the normal signaling events that occur following IL-2 activation. Following binding of a cytokine to its receptor, e.g., IL-2, the increase in cytoplasmic calcium concentration within and released from the endoplasmic reticulum activates calmodulin, which in turn initiates a cascade of events involving increased phosphatase activity of calcineurin, leading to the dephosphorylation of the nuclear factor of activated T cells (**NFAT**) and its translocation to the nucleus, where it initiates gene transcription.

The effects of CsA and tacrolimus antagonize these cytokine-mediated pathways (Figure 11-7B). Upon entry into the cells, these compounds form tight complexes with two different immunophilins; cyclosporine binds to cyclophilin and tacrolimus to the FK506 binding protein (**FKBP**)-12. The resulting complexes subsequently bind to calcineurin, and after binding, either complex exerts its effects through a common final metabolic pathway that involves inhibition of phosphatase activity of calcineurin and prevention of NFAT dephosphorylation, the previously described critical steps in the induction of gene transcription. This action not only prevents the nuclear translocation of NFAT, but also renders it incompetent. CsA and tacrolimus inhibit IL-2, IL-3, IL-4, IFN-γ, GM-CSF, and TNF-α and mRNA expression. In addition to NFAT, other transcriptional factors including NF-κB and the Spi-1/PU.1 consensus motif known as PU box are also inhibited. Additionally, T cell receptor–mediated apoptosis of lymphocytes and thymocytes is augmented by tacrolimus but not by CsA, providing yet another mechanism by which graft rejection is inhibited.

Clinical Uses of the Calcineurin Inhibitors

CsA is used clinically to prevent GVHD following HSCT and graft rejection of solid organ transplants. It is also effective in the treatment of many diseases, including psoriasis, ocular disease associated with Behcet's disease, endogenous uveitis, atopic dermatitis, rheumatoid arthritis, Crohn's disease, nephritic syndrome, aplastic anemia, pure red cell aplasia, polymyositis/dermatomyositis, pyoderma gangrenosum, and severe asthma. Tacrolimus helps

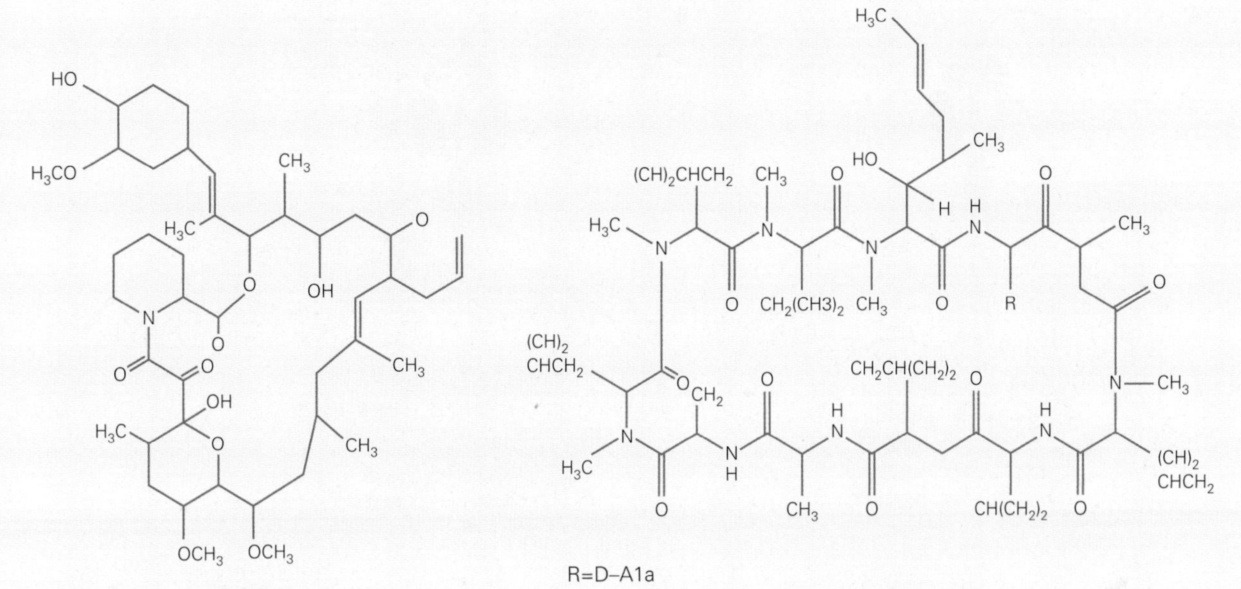

Tacrolimus

Molecular formula $C_{44}H_{69}NO_{12}$–H_2O
Molecular weight 822.03

Cyclosporine

Molecular formula $C_{62}H_{111}N_{11}O_{12}$
Molecular weight 1202.61

Figure 11-6. Comparison of chemical structures of tacrolimus and cyclosporine.

prevent solid organ rejection and GVHD. The use of CsA and tacrolimus is somewhat complex and requires close monitoring of blood levels because of their erratic absorption and also because elevated blood levels resulting from administration of multiple drugs metabolized by the hepatic p450 cytochrome system can lead to major clinical toxicities. Adverse effects include nephropathy, hypertension, diabetes mellitus, susceptibility to infection, development of malignancies, and post-transplant lymphoproliferative disorders. Tacrolimus is associated with less hypertension and less concomitant glucocorticosteroid requirement in renal transplant recipients, but a higher frequency of moderate-to-severe neurotoxicity in liver transplant patients with hepatitis C.

Sirolimus (rapamycin) is another immunosuppressive drug that has recently become available. It is a macrocyclic lactone produced by *Streptomyces hygroscopicus* that specifically inhibits T lymphocyte activation and proliferation in response to antigenic and cytokine stimulation. Unlike the similarly named tacrolimus, sirolimus is not a calcineurin inhibitor. The mechanism of action of sirolimus is distinct from that of cyclosporine and tacrolimus. However, it has a similar suppressive effect on the immune system. In contrast to tacrolimus, which inhibits the production of IL-2, sirolimus inhibits the response to IL-2 and thereby blocks activation of T and B cells. Although sirolimus initially binds intracellularly to the same immunophilin FKBP-12 as tacrolimus, after producing the immunosuppressive sirolimus-FKBP-12 complex, it subsequently binds to and inhibits the activation of a regulatory kinase, known as the mammalian target of rapamycin (**mTOR**). This inhibition suppresses cytokine-driven T cell proliferation, inhibiting the progression from the G1 to the S phases of the cell cycle. Sirolimus is indicated for the prophylaxis of organ rejection in patients receiving renal transplants not only since it has less renal toxicity than the calcineurin inhibitors, but also because of its possible additional advantage as a treatment for steroid-refractory acute GVHD therapy.

Immunosuppressant Applications of Polyclonal IVIG in the Immunomodulation of Autoimmune, Allergic, and Inflammatory Disorders

Mechanisms of Action of IVIG

During the course of its successful utilization in replacement therapy in patients with antibody

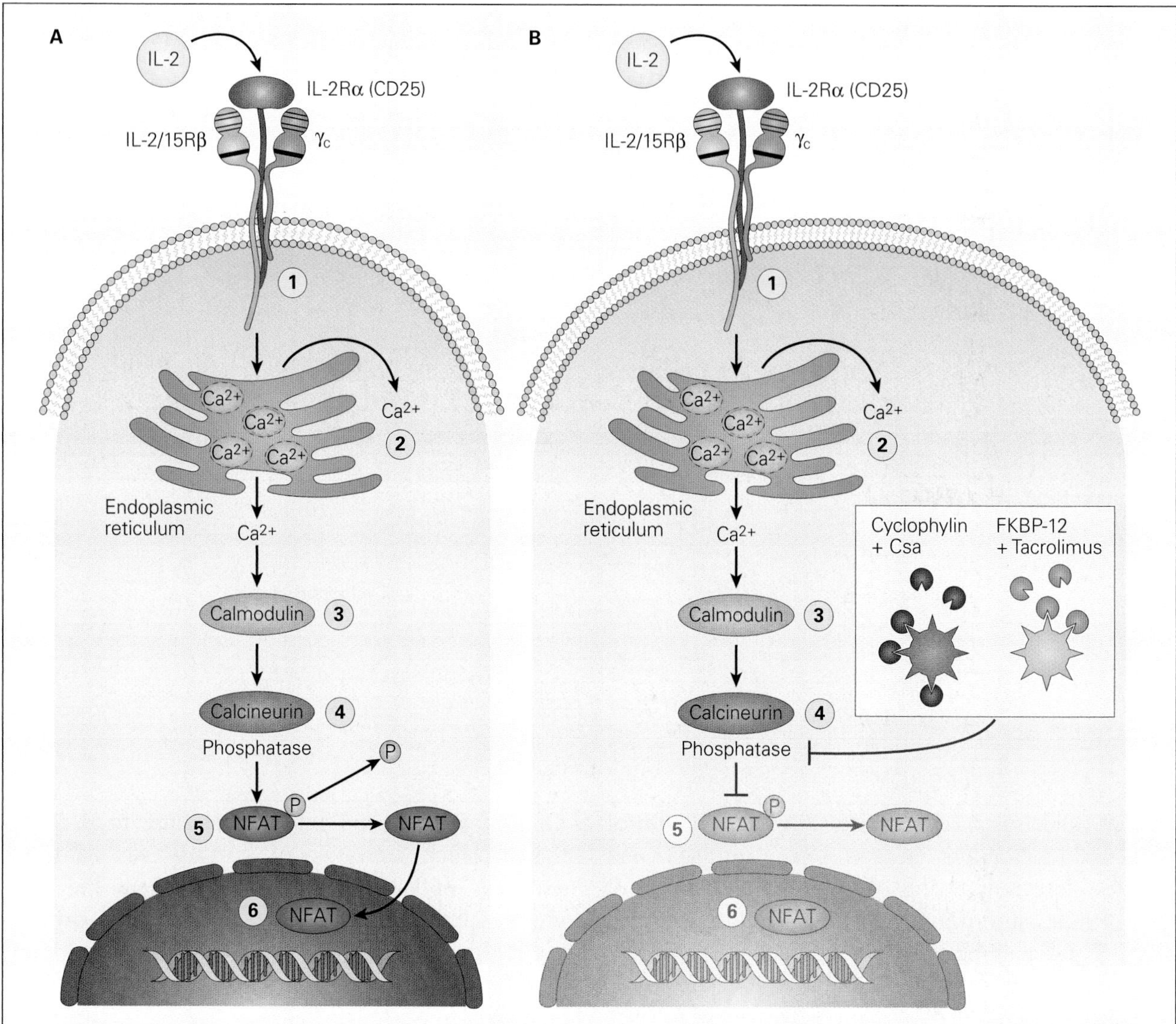

Figure 11-7. Schematic representation of the sites of action of two calcineurin inhibitors, cyclosporine (CsA) and tacrolimus. Panel A: Schematic representation of the normal signaling events that occur following binding of a cytokine, e.g., IL-2, to its receptor. Following cytokine binding, a signal is transduced (1), leading to increased calcium concentration within and released from the endoplasmic reticulum (2). This then leads to activation of calmodulin (3), which in turn activates increased phosphatase activity of calcineurin (4), leading to the dephosphorylation of NFAT (5) and the translocation of the activated NFAT to the nucleus (6), where it initiates gene transcription and subsequent translational events, leading to the synthesis of pro-inflammatory cytokines. Panel B: Schematic representation of the mechanism of sites of action of CsA and tacrolimus through their inhibitory repression of calcineurin activity. Following the same cytokine-induced signaling pathways described in A (1–3), entry of CsA and tacrolimus into the cells leads to the formation of tight complexes with two different immunophilins; CsA binds to cyclophilin (red) and tacrolimus to FKBP-12 (green). The binding of either complex to calcineurin leads to inhibition of its phosphatase activity (4) and prevention of NFAT dephosphorylation (5). This action not only prevents the nuclear translocation of NFAT, but also inhibits mRNA expression and subsequent synthesis of IL-2, IL-3, IL-4, IFN-γ, GM-CSF, and TNF-α.

deficiency, intramuscular IgG or IVIG was also found to be effective in the treatment of a number of diseases characterized by hyperactive immune responses, autoimmunity, or chronic inflammation, e.g., idiopathic thrombocytopenic purpura (**ITP**), neutropenia, alopecia, skin lesions, arthritis, reactive airway disease, and diarrhea. Often, these effects occurred rapidly following immunoglobulin replacement therapy, and the benefits appeared to wane as trough levels of IgG were reestablished. Shown in Table 11-5 are several mechanisms of action of IVIG that have been proposed to explain its immunosuppressant action.

The Use of IVIG in ITP

Imbach and his coworkers initially reported the efficacy of IVIG for the treatment of immune thrombocytopenia in children, introducing a new era of immunoglobulin therapy for inflammatory and autoimmune disease. The proposed mechanism of action in immune thrombocytopenia is phagocytic cell Fc receptor blockade in reticuloendothelial tissues of the spleen and liver. Purified Fcγ fragments prepared from IVIG also were shown to result in the elevation of platelet counts in children with immune-mediated thrombocytopenia. Autoantibody-coated platelets survive, and the tempo of this response makes IVIG treatment attractive when platelet recovery is required immediately.

The Use of IVIG in Kawasaki Disease and Autoimmune Disease

One of the best demonstrated anti-inflammatory effects of IVIG is exemplified in the treatment of Kawasaki syndrome as described above in the case presentation. In addition to a high content of antibodies to a number of cytokines, receptors, and membrane molecules potentially important in immune regulation, IVIG also contains antibodies to a broad range of staphylococcal and streptococcal enterotoxins

Table 11-5. Proposed mechanisms of immunosuppressant action of IVIG

✓ **Fc receptor blockade or modulation** Fc receptor blockade of reticuloendothelial cell system and mononuclear phagocytes Competitive interaction of IVIG with circulating IgG-sensitized platelets for Fc receptors on macrophages Soluble Fcγ receptors compete with membrane Fc receptors (RES) for circulating IgG-sensitized platelets
✓ **Immunomodulation (either immunopotentiation or immunosuppression)** Enhancement of T cell regulatory function Inhibition of B cell function and/or antigen-processing cells via FcγRIIB– receptor
✓ Neutralization or binding of autoimmune antibodies by anti-idiotypic antibodies in the IVIG, leading to restoration of idiotype-anti-idiotypic network
✓ Inhibition of complement uptake on target tissues; prevent complement-dependent immune damage to tissues and cells
✓ Inhibition of cytokine/interleukin production/action
✓ Neutralization of bacterial enterotoxin superantigens
✓ Saturation of the FcRn receptor to accelerate the catabolism of autoantibodies
✓ Inhibition of Fas-mediated cell death by Fas-blocking antibodies in the IVIG

that function as T cell superantigens. Kawasaki disease, the prototypical superantigen-mediated condition, responds favorably to neutralization of bacterial superantigen enterotoxins that cause vascular endothelial inflammation and damage. IVIG is also efficacious for the treatment of toxic shock syndrome, especially when employed during the early phases of the disease (*Chapter 9*). Studies in animals and humans have demonstrated that IVIG inhibits the binding of activated fragments of C3 and C4 to target cells, a mechanism that has been invoked to explain the reversal of complement-mediated endomysial capillary damage in patients with dermatomyositis.

Abnormalities in the idiotype network are also important in the pathogenesis of a number of autoimmune diseases (*Chapter 6*). The presence of anti-idiotypic antibodies in IVIG was first suggested by the response to IVIG therapy of a patient with autoimmunity to Factor VIII. F(ab′)2 fragments from commercial sources of IVIG are capable of binding and neutralizing autoantibodies to Factor VIII, thyroglobulin, DNA, intrinsic factor, and neutrophil cytoplasmic proteins. This mechanism may also explain the beneficial effects of IVIG therapy for the treatment of patients with vasculitides associated with anti-neutrophil cytoplasm antibody (**ANCA**), i.e., ANCA-positive vasculitis, who are refractory to other forms of conventional immunosuppressive therapy. In toxic epidermal necrolysis (**TEN** or Lyell's syndrome), a condition characterized by severe drug-induced bullous skin lesions with a mortality rate of up to 30 percent, apoptosis of keratinocytes is seen, resulting in large areas of dermo-epidermal junction detachment, giving the appearance of scalded skin. In this condition, IVIG blocks the effects of FasL on the Fas receptor on keratinocytes, prevents apoptosis, and is associated with disease arrest followed by rapid healing and favorable outcomes in affected patients. These findings suggest that IVIG may be useful in other Fas--mediated inflammatory or autoimmune diseases (*Chapter 9*).

IgE production by B cells is inhibited *in vitro* by IVIG, an effect that is accompanied by a decrease in mRNA Cε transcripts. *In vitro* lymphocyte proliferative responses to a variety of T cell mitogens are suppressed, an effect that requires the Fc portion of the molecule, given that the F(ab′)2 fragments of IgG have no effect. The synthesis of various cytokines from monocytes is also suppressed, an effect mediated through the Fcγ receptor on mononuclear cells and T lymphocytes.

B cells and a subpopulation of T cells express a low-affinity Fcγ receptor (FcγRIIB), a receptor subtype that provides an inhibitory signal via an immunoregulatory tyrosine-based inhibition motif (**ITIM**) (*Chapters 6* and *7*). Coligation of the B cell receptor and FcγRIIB appears to be induced by the binding of IVIG through the Fc moiety of the IgG to the FcγRIIB receptor, and the anti-idiotypic specificity of the IgG molecule to the B cell receptor. Inhibitory Fcγ receptors are also present on basophils and mast cells. Samuelsson et al. investigated a murine model of immune thrombocytopenia and found that the protective effects of IVIG required the FcγRIIB, since either disruption of the receptor or blockade with a monoclonal antibody reversed the therapeutic effects. Thus, modulation of B cell immunoglobulin synthesis and effector responses of other cell types, including macrophages and mast cells, is through the FcγRIIB receptor and its negative regulatory signaling motifs (*Chapter 6*).

Another mechanism proposed to explain the immunomodulating effects of IVIG on serum autoantibody levels in patients is the saturation of the FcRn receptor (Table 11-5). The FcRn receptor (neonatal Fc receptor) appears to protect immunoglobulin molecules from catabolism in the endocytotic vesicles of endosomes, thus prolonging the half-lives of these plasma proteins. By saturating protective receptors in proportion to the concentration of exogenous immunoglobulin, catabolism of IgG autoantibodies appears to be accelerated (*Chapter 6*). Hansen and Balthasar demonstrated this in a rat model of immune thrombocytopenia; IVIG enhanced the clearance of anti-platelet antibodies by saturating the FcRn receptor in a dose-dependent fashion.

No single mechanism can account for the immunoregulatory activities of IVIG; perhaps the immunomodulatory effects of IVIG are best explained by a summation of multiple influences exerted by these and still other yet to be determined mechanisms on various pathways of inflammatory and immune effector responses.

Plasmapheresis

Plasmapheresis is a particular type of extracorporeal procedure, i.e., apheresis, in which the blood of a donor or patient is passed through an apparatus that removes selected plasma proteins from the intravascular compartment and returns the cellular remainder to the circulation. The technique is usually given as a series of treatments over a period of several weeks or months. Since plasmapheresis removes IgM and IgG and immune complexes, the procedure is clinically useful for the emergent treatment of thrombotic thrombocytopenic purpura, myasthenia gravis, Goodpasture's syndrome, and hyperviscosity secondary to Waldenström's macroglobulinemia. Although plasmapheresis is transiently effective for the treatment of diseases characterized by autoantibodies and/or immune complexes, such as systemic lupus erythematosus and cryoglobulinemia, the pathogenic antibody or complex production unfortunately recurs following cessation of treatment. Therefore, in formulating more protracted treatment regimens for these chronic diseases, plasmapheresis is usually combined with other immunosuppressive therapies (e.g., cyclophosphamide and/or glucocorticosteroids). Also available are semi-selective apheresis techniques that employ affinity separation methods that permit the removal of specific blood components. One example is *Staphylococcus aureus* Cowan strain I-derived protein A column, which binds the Fc portion of IgG and has been used for the treatment of idiopathic thrombocytopenic purpura.

Subgroup 2b Specific Immunosuppressants

The subgroup 2b agents include a variety of agents that target specific cells, cytokines, or receptors. These include therapeutic polyclonal and monoclonal antibodies, therapeutic fusion proteins (e.g., etanercept), soluble receptor constructs (e.g., anakinra), and cytokines (e.g., interferons) (Table 11-2). A partial list of the polyclonal and monoclonal immunomodulator antibody therapies that have had greater than five years clinical use in humans is shown in Table 11-6. A more complete listing of monoclonal antibody preparations, fusion proteins, recombinant cytokines, monoclonal antibodies used for *in vivo* imaging, and soluble receptor constructs are shown in the Annex to this chapter, Tables 11A-1–11A-6.

Polyclonal Antibody Directed Against Cells: The Conquest of Erythroblastosis Fetalis by Rh (D) Immune Globulin

One of the most successful immunological clinical interventions ever developed in humans has been the use of Rh (D) immune globulin, an enriched fraction of antibodies directed against the D blood group antigen, for the prevention of rhesus D alloimmunization in pregnancy (*Chapter 23*). Erythroblastosis

Table 11-6. Immunomodulator antibody therapies with greater than five years clinical use in humans

Therapeutic antibodies	Target	Major indications	Adverse effects
Polyclonal			
Rh (D) immune globulin	D antigen	Rh-negative mothers	Anaphylactoid reactions
Antithymocyte globulin	Thymocytes	Aplastic anemia, organ rejection	Serum sickness, opportunistic infections
Intravenous immunoglobulin	Multiple organisms	Immunodeficiencies post-hematopoietic cell transplant	Anaphylactoid reactions
	Fc receptors	Chronic lymphocytic leukemia	
	Idiotypes	Pediatric AIDS, immune-mediated thrombocytopenia, Kawasaki disease	
Monoclonal			
Muromonab-CD3	CD3+ T cells	Organ rejection	Opportunistic infections
Infliximab	TNF-α	Rheumatoid arthritis, regional ileitis (Crohn's disease)	Reactivation of tuberculosis
Alemtuzumab	CD52+ cells	Refractory chronic lymphatic leukemia	Opportunistic infections
Rituximab	CD20+ B cells	Non-Hodgkin's lymphoma, autoimmune diseases (e.g., SLE)	Opportunistic infections
Ibritumomab tiuxetan	CD20+ B cells	Refractory non-Hodgkin's lymphoma (NHL)	Opportunistic infections

fetalis, the severe anemia of the fetus and newborn resulting from a blood group incompatibility between the fetus and its mother, caused primarily by antibodies to the fetal D antigen, is now a rarity (Table 11-6). The condition has been successfully prevented in literally thousands of newborns by administering Rh (D) immune globulin to Rh-negative mothers within 72 hours of the birth of Rh-positive babies. This passively blocks sensitization of mothers, whose next offspring then escapes the risk of hemolysis.

Antithymocyte globulin (**ATG**), an example of an isotypic antibody product (*Chapter 6*) prepared by immunizing mammals (e.g., horses, rabbits, sheep, or goats) with human thymic lymphocytes, binds to surfaces of circulating T lymphocytes and leads to their elimination; this results in profound suppression of cellular immune responses (Table 11-6). It is used for the treatment of idiopathic aplastic anemia, the prevention of rejection of allogeneic tissues, and the acute rejection of solid organ renal and cardiac transplants. The half-life is between three and nine days. ATG may cause thrombocytopenia, and patients receiving it for the treatment of aplastic anemia may require prophylactic platelet transfusions during the course of treatment. Other serious toxicities include serum sickness and nephritis (*Chapter 17*).

Monoclonal Antibody Directed Against Cells

Muromonab-CD3 is a biologically purified murine IgG2a monoclonal antibody directed against the CD3 antigen, a glycoprotein that is present on the surface of the human T cell receptor (**TCR**) and whose functional presence is required for normal signal transduction (*Chapter 7* and Table 11-6). *In vivo* administration of muromonab-CD3 results in a rapid decrease in circulating CD3+CD8+ and CD3+CD4+ cells, which remain undetectable in the peripheral blood from two and seven days following infusion. Since muromonab is comprised entirely of mouse protein, it provokes the production of neutralizing heterologous antibodies with repeated treatments, which may not only abrogate some of its activity, but also may contribute to hypersensitivity reactions (*Chapter 17*). It is approved for the treatment of acute allograft rejection in renal transplant recipients and for glucocorticosteroid-resistant acute allograft rejection of heart and liver transplants (*Chapter 22*). Most patients experience an acute clinical syndrome called cytokine release syndrome associated with the initial dose, manifestations of which range from a flu-like illness to capillary leak, hypotension, and multiorgan failure.

Alemtuzumab is a recombinant DNA-derived humanized monoclonal antibody that is directed against CD52, a 21–28 kDa cell surface protein expressed on normal and malignant B and T lymphocytes, NK cells, monocytes, macrophages, and tissues of the male reproductive system (Table 11-6). Alemtuzumab is an approved therapy for B cell chronic lymphocytic leukemia (**B-CLL**) in patients who fail initial therapy. The broad array of immune cells that carry the CD52 receptor predict that the immunosuppressive properties in patients are more profound than those observed with monoclonal therapies directed at more selective receptors. Profound lymphopenia can therefore occur, sometimes accompanied by opportunistic infections. Antimicrobial prophylaxis is recommended following the last dose until the patient's absolute CD4+ cell count is greater than 200 cells/mm^3, the median time to which is two months. Although CD52 is not present on erythrocytes or hematopoietic stem cells, life-threatening bone marrow aplasia has resulted from exposure to recommended dosages. Clinical trials seeking to determine its graft-versus-host preventive potential are in progress. This treatment may prove to be useful as conditioning prior to hematopoietic cell transplantation and for the treatment of immune-mediated severe aplastic anemia.

Ibritumomab, the parent compound of **rituximab,** is a chimeric murine/human monoclonal antibody directed against CD20 that is present on B lymphocytes (Table 11-6). It is produced by mammalian cell (Chinese hamster ovary) suspension culture and purified by affinity and ion exchange chromatography that includes a viral inactivation step. Rituximab was the first antibody to be licensed for the treatment of human malignancies and is widely used for the treatment of non-Hodgkin's lymphoma (**NHL**) (*Chapter 21*). CD20, a 33–37 kDa phosphoprotein expressed on both normal and most malignant B lymphocytes, functions as a calcium channel subunit that regulates cell cycle progression by inhibiting transition from G_1 to S phase. The Fab domain of rituximab binds to CD20 and recruits effector cells that mediate B cell destruction. Mechanisms that may explain rituximab-mediated B cell lysis include complement-dependent cytotoxicity, antibody-dependent cellular cytotoxicity (**ADCC**), apoptosis induction, and the modulation of regulatory T cells. Rituximab is a highly efficient agent, and intravenous administration in humans results in the disappearance of B cells from the circulation for weeks to months, depending on the dosing schedule. CD20 is expressed on >90 percent of non-Hodgkin's lymphomas and mature normal B cells but not hematopoietic cells, pro-B cells, normal plasma cells, or other normal tissues. It is approved for the treatment of patients with relapsed or refractory, low-grade or follicular, CD20-positive, B cell NHL (*Chapter 21*). It is also being evaluated for the treatment of several autoimmune conditions (*Chapter 19*).

By linking ibritumomab to a radioactive atom of the isotope yttrium-90 using tiuxetan (a chelating agent), the first radioimmunotherapy to gain FDA sanction was produced. It is useful for the treatment of follicular or transformed B cell NHL that has recurred after standard therapy. The addition of the radioactive atom appears to boost response rates by combining the specificity of the antibody with the cytotoxic impact of molecular radiotherapy, and in one multicenter study, an impressive 80 percent response was seen.

Monoclonal Antibody Directed Against Pathogenic Antibody

Omalizumab is a recombinant humanized monoclonal anti-IgE antibody that binds to the Cε3 domain located on the Fc portion of an IgE molecule, the same domain that attaches to the FcεR1 (*Chapter 18*). This action decreases the antigen-specific binding of IgE to tissue mast cells and basophils, effectively inhibiting the elicitation process and the subsequent release of mediators responsible for Type I-mediated allergic diseases (*Chapter 18*). Although omalizumab reduces the amount of free IgE, it does not bind to IgE already bound to effector cells. This monoclonal antibody preparation contains 5 percent murine sequences (needed for the IgE-binding portion) and 95 percent human residues from a human IgG1 kappa framework and is therefore considered as a humanized monoclonal antibody (Figure 11-4). The effect of omalizumab is to provide incremental improvement in symptoms of atopic patients, i.e., asthma, who are already being managed with pharmacological therapy, and represents a new approach of "short-circuiting" another critical step in the pathogenesis of allergic diseases. The subcutaneous injection is administered every two to four weeks in a dose that is based not only on body weight, but also on the level of total serum IgE in the patient. Its use is currently limited to patients with moderate-to-severe persistent allergic asthma and who have inadequately responded to the usually effective armamentarium of less costly standard pharmacologic and immunotherapeutic therapies, in which case its addition has been shown to reduce the frequency of asthma exacerbations, inhaled glucocorticosteroid requirements, and rescue medication use. A schematic representation of the mode of action and points of interaction within the immune response of several monoclonal antibody and fusion protein preparations is shown in Figure 11-8.

Recombinant Interferons

Interferons are recombinant DNA products obtained from the bacterial fermentation of *Escherichia coli* that bear genetically engineered plasmids containing an interferon alpha or interferon gamma gene (*Chapter 25*). These soluble proteins are available for intramuscular, subcutaneous, intralesional, or intravenous injection and mimic naturally occurring endogenous interferons. This family of interferon molecules was named for its capacity to "interfere" with *in vitro* infectivity of virions into mammalian cells. This occurs by the binding of interferon to a specific Type 1 or Type 2 receptor on the cell membrane and initiation of a complex sequence of intracellular events that results in decreased cell proliferation, enhancement of phagocytosis by monocytes/macrophages, and augmentation of the cytotoxicity of specific lymphocytes. (*Chapters 9* and *13*). Although these *in vitro* effects do not precisely correlate with clinical results they do suggest that these compounds might be capable of modulating the clinical expression of a wide array of immunologically mediated diseases.

Interferon alpha-2B, **interferon beta**, and **interferon gamma** are FDA-approved for a number of malignant conditions and viral infections, as shown in Table 11-7. The administration of specific preparations is rarely associated with hypersensitivity reactions (e.g., urticaria, angioedema, bronchoconstriction, and anaphylaxis). Other common side effects include fever, transient skin rashes, flu-like symptoms, and bone marrow suppression. Thirty percent of patients experience neuropsychiatric symptoms, most commonly depression, and some, on rare occasion, experience autoimmune disorders, e.g., disease exacerbation in patients with psoriasis, ischemic events, and infections. Interferon alpha may also substantially increase serum theophylline levels.

Interleukin-2

Interleukin-2 (IL-2), described as a T cell growth factor in 1976, stimulates growth of T lymphocytes from normal human marrow (*Chapters 7* and *9*). Discovery of the IL-2 gene in 1983 made it possible for large-scale production by gene expression of a product that is biologically and functionally similar to natural IL-2. The administration of IL-2 leads to measurable changes in the function of a wide variety of immune cells and serves as one of the most important key pivotal cytokines of the immune system (*Chapter 9*). IL-2 is FDA-approved and considered standard therapy for metastatic renal cell carcinoma; approximately 15–20 percent of patients experience an objective response with therapy, although the complete response (CR) rate is 5–7 percent (*Chapter 20*). Nonetheless, 80 percent of complete responders experience a response duration of greater than two years. Although treatment-related mortality of systemic IL-2 therapy is less than 1 percent, toxicities are significant and include hypotension requiring pressors, major organ failure, myocardial infarction, and potentially fatal systemic capillary leak. Fisher reported a long-term median response duration of 16.3 months, with 10–20 percent estimated to be alive at five to ten years post-treatment.

TNF Inhibitors

Tumor necrosis factor-alpha (TNF-α) is a pro-inflammatory cytokine produced mainly by monocytes and macrophages (*Chapter 9*). It mediates its inflammatory action by increasing the transport of white blood cells to sites of inflammation, and through additional molecular mechanisms initiates and amplifies inflammation. TNF-α specifically induces IL-1 and IL-6, promotes leukocyte migration, activates neutrophils and eosinophils, and induces acute phase-reactant production and tissue-degrading enzymes. Tumor necrosis factor inhibitors bind to TNF and block its action, thereby reducing the inflammatory response, which is especially useful for treating autoimmune diseases.

There are several licensed tumor necrosis factor inhibitors currently available that include one therapeutic fusion protein, i.e, etanercept, and three monoclonal preparations, i.e., infliximab, adalimumab, and certolizumab pegol (Table 11-8). Although these four agents are all biologic anti-TNF therapeutics, their methods of administration, dosing, and side effect profiles are somewhat different. These differences may be accounted for by fundamental differences in their biologic structure, which affects their mechanisms of action.

Mechanism of Action of the Various TNF Inhibitors

There are two forms of TNF-α, the soluble and membrane-bound varieties (*Chapter 9*). Some of the TNF inhibitors target only the soluble, while others

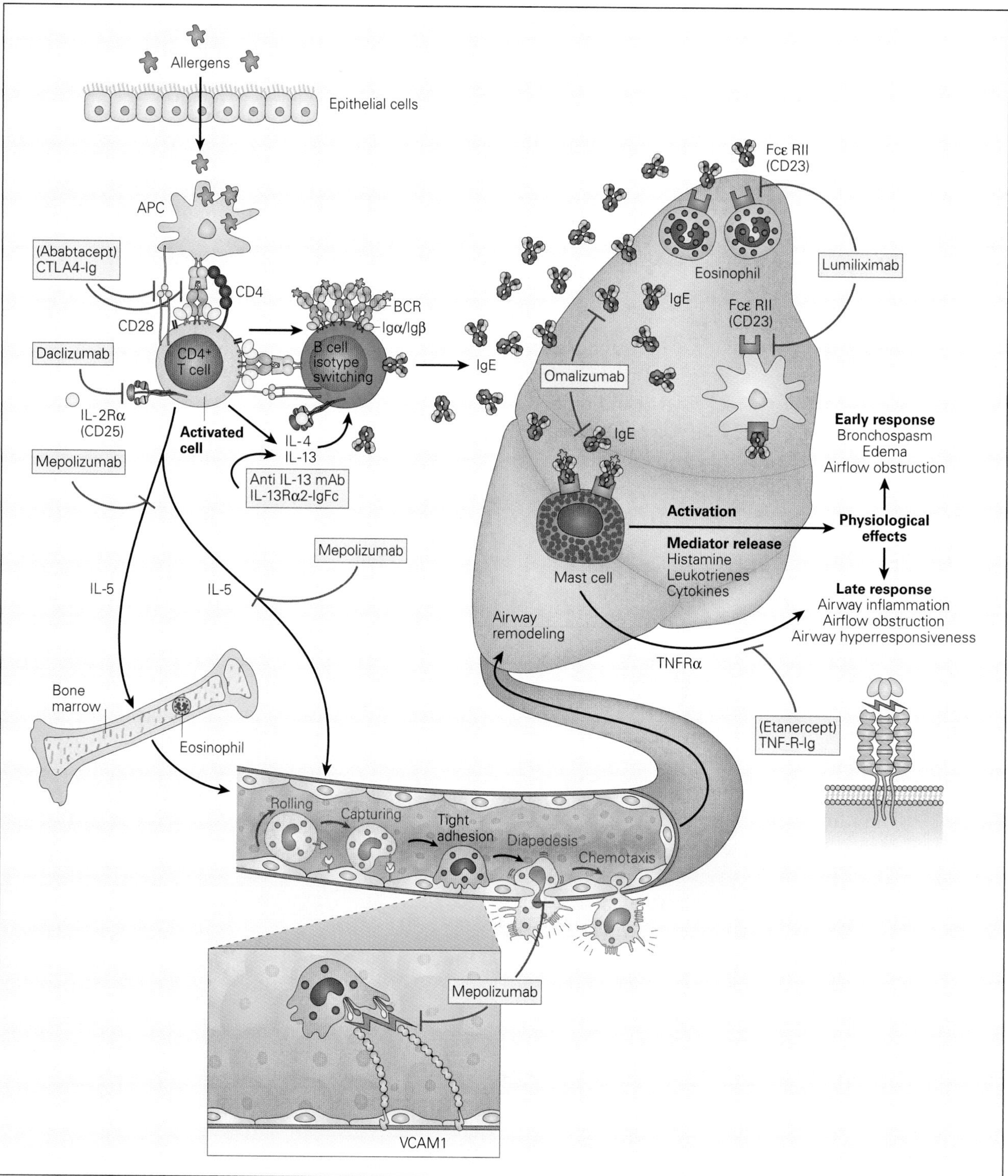

Figure 11-8. A schematic representation of the mode of action and points of interaction within the immune response of several monoclonal antibody and fusion protein preparations. (Adapted from Ballow M. Biologic immune modifiers: trails and tribulations—are we there yet? J. Allergy Clin Immunol 2006; 118; 1209–15.)

target both the soluble and the membrane-associated forms of the cytokine. Shown in Figure 11-9 is a schematic representation of the differences in mechanism of action between monoclonal antibody and therapeutic fusion protein preparations that target these forms. Both infliximab and adalimumab target both soluble and membrane-associated TNF and are therefore more potent than etanercept, which

Table 11-7. Clinical indications for the use of recombinant interferon in human illness

Interferon-alpha-2a	Interferon-alpha-2b	Interferon-alpha-n
Malignant melanoma	Malignant melanoma	
Condylomata	Follicular lymphoma	Follicular lymphoma
AIDS-related Kaposi's sarcoma	AIDS-related Kaposi's sarcoma	
Condyloma acuminata	Condyloma acuminata	
Chronic hepatitis C	Chronic hepatitis B	
Chronic myelogenous leukemia	Chronic hepatitis C	
Interferon-beta-1b		
Relapsing-remitting multiple sclerosis (ambulatory patients)		
Interferon-gamma		
Chronic granulomatous disease		
Idiopathic pulmonary fibrosis		

targets only mainly soluble TNF. These monoclonal antibodies also fix complement and have the ability to lyse cells, in contrast to etanercept, which does not fix complement and has no cytolytic effects. While potentially contributing to their therapeutic efficacy in disorders such as Crohn's disease (for which both of these monoclonal antibodies are now FDA-approved), these mAbs also carry black-box

Table 11-8. List of TNF inhibitors

Product	Brand name	Type	Target	Molecular structure	Clinical indication(s)
Therapeutic Fusion Protein					
Etanercept	Enbrel	Receptor-antibody fusion protein (receptor attached to Fc of IgG1)	TNF-α and TNF-β	TNFR-IgG1 Fc fusion protein	Rheumatoid arthritis; juvenile idiopathic arthritis; psoriatic arthritis; ankylosing spondylitis; plaque psoriasis
Monoclonal Antibody or Fab′ Fragment Preparations					
Infliximab	Remicade	-ximab	TNF-α	Chimeric IgG1κ anti-TNF-α recombinant monoclonal antibody to TNF-α	Rheumatoid arthritis; ankylosing spondylitis; psoriatic arthritis; chronic severe plaque psoriasis; Crohn's disease; ulcerative colitis
Adalimumab	Humira, Trudexa	-umab	TNF-α	Human IgG1κ anti-TNF-α recombinant antibody to TNF-α	Rheumatoid arthritis; juvenile idiopathic arthritis; psoriatic arthritis; ankylosing spondylitis; Crohn's disease; plaque psoriasis
Certolizumab pegol	Cimzia	-zumab	TNF-α	Humanized, recombinant Fab′ anti-TNF-α antibody fragment conjugated to polyethylene glycol	Crohn's disease

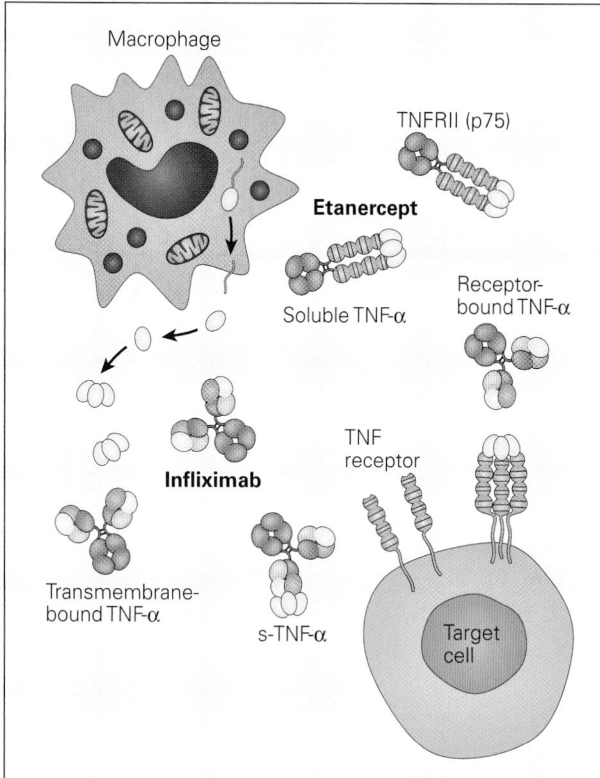

Figure 11-9. Schematic representation of the differences in mechanism of action between monoclonal antibody and therapeutic fusion protein anti-TNF-α preparations that target soluble TNF-α (s-TNF-α) and membrane-associated forms of TNF-α. Etanercept targets primarily the s-TNF-α, in contrast to infliximab, which targets both forms.

warnings. In addition, infliximab has a higher propensity for the development of anaphylaxis, perhaps as a result both of its chimeric structure and its intravenous route of administration.

Etanercept is a therapeutic fusion protein made from the combination of two naturally occurring soluble human 75-kilodalton TNF receptors linked to an Fc portion of an IgG1. Etanercept is capable of reducing the signs and symptoms of patients with rheumatoid arthritis who have inadequate responses to disease-modifying anti-rheumatic drugs (**DMARDs**).

There are two types of TNF receptors: (1) those found on the surface of virtually all nucleated cells that respond to TNF by releasing other cytokines, and (2) soluble TNF receptors, which are used to deactivate TNF and blunt the immune response (*Chapter 9*). Etanercept mimics the inhibitory effects of naturally occurring soluble TNF receptors, the difference being that etanercept, because it is a fusion protein rather than a simple TNF receptor, has a greatly extended half-life in the bloodstream, and therefore a more profound and long-lasting biologic effect than a naturally occurring soluble TNF receptor. Since the mechanism of TNF inhibition by etanercept involves receptor binding rather than an antibody-mediated monoclonal action, it targets mainly the soluble form of TNF and not the membrane-associated TNF, with no complement activation and no cell lysis. Etanercept is currently licensed in the United States for treatment of rheumatoid arthritis, polyarticular juvenile idiopathic arthritis, psoriatic arthritis, and ankylosing spondylitis.

Infliximab is an IgG1 kappa chimeric monoclonal antibody that binds specifically and with high affinity to TNF-α. Infliximab is active for patients with rheumatoid arthritis, particularly when used with methotrexate. It is also indicated for patients with Crohn's disease who experience an inadequate response to conventional therapy. Side effects include autoantibody production and a lupus-like syndrome, acute infusion reactions, infections, and possible increased incidence of malignancy. The discordant responses in Crohn's between infliximab and etanercept are noteworthy and may be due in part to diverse effects on T lymphocytes.

Adalimumab, a fully human-derived recombinant monoclonal antibody against TNF- α, is effective for the treatment of patients with moderately to severely active rheumatoid arthritis, long-standing recalcitrant psoriasis, and psoriatic arthritis.

Certolizumab pegol is a humanized, recombinant Fab′ fragment with high affinity for TNF-α that has been conjugated to polyethylene glycol (approximately 40kDa) as a means of prolonging elimination half-life. This antibody is reported to target both the soluble and membrane-bound forms of TNF-α. In contrast to etanercept and adalimumab, owing to the absence of the Fc moiety in the preparation, certolizumab pegol shows no complement fixation, antibody-dependent cell-mediated toxicity, induction of neutrophil degranulation, and no apoptosis induction in human peripheral blood monocytes or lymphocytes. Certolizumab pegol was approved for treatment of Crohn's disease in the United States in April 2008. Pre-licensing studies of certolizumab pegol for treatment of moderate-to-severe Crohn's disease have shown some improvement of disease manifestations.

Side Effects of the TNF Inhibitors

A large group of side effects has been reported in association with TNF inhibitor therapy, including infections, malignancies, demyelinating conditions, and lupus-like conditions. Treatment with TNF inhibitors predisposes patients to *Mycobacterium tuberculosis* infections and reactivation, which may occur within weeks after initiation of treatment, with atypical presentations including disseminated and extrapulmonary disease. PPD testing is recommended for all patients who are considered candidates for tumor necrosis inhibitor therapy, together with the more specific interferon-gamma release assays (**IGRAs**). The full measure of adverse effects may take years to assess, as has been the case with other broad immunosuppressives such as glucocorticosteroids. At present, combination therapy with a TNF inhibitor and rituximab is not recommended, as administration of rituximab results in B cell depletion that may last for more than six months, and the safety of TNF inhibition in patients who have received rituximab has not been established.

Clinical Impact of the TNF Inhibitors

With the advent of mass-marketing directly to patients, there has been relatively broad acceptance of these potent immunosuppressive medications for the treatment of chronic inflammatory conditions that often require more than one agent or the sequential administration of medications of incremental potency. At the time of this publication, we are experiencing a major shift in treatment algorithms made possible by these new agents. It is important to recognize that although these inhibitors of tumor necrosis factor have provided immense clinical value for a number of immunologically mediated diseases for which no effective therapy was available, their long-term safety has yet to be defined, and a number of safety issues make the prescribing of these medications a task that is at present complicated and that should receive careful and continual scrutiny.

IL-1 Receptor Inhibitors

Anakinra is an interleukin-1 receptor antagonist (IL-1Ra) that blocks IL-1, a protein involved in the inflammation and joint destruction associated with rheumatoid arthritis (*Chapter 9*). Methods for monitoring side effects are currently being developed and may soon be available.

IL-2 Receptor Inhibitors

The interleukin-2 receptor (IL-2R) is comprised of at least three genetically distinct subunits termed alpha, beta, and gamma (*Chapter 9*). The cluster of differentiation (**CD**) cell surface marker for the alpha subunit of the high-affinity IL-2 receptor is CD25. Humanized or chimeric monoclonal antibodies directed against CD25 are promising immunosuppressive agents due to improved pharmacokinetic profiles and less toxicity. Three monoclonal antibodies that target the IL-2 receptor are currently approved for human use, including daclizumab, denileukin diftitox, and basiliximab. Daclizumab and basiliximab have proven effective for the prevention and/or treatment of solid organ transplantation rejection, which suggests that they may be useful for the prevention/treatment of GVHD after HSCT. Denileukin diftitox, otherwise known as Ontak, is an antineoplastic agent, an engineered DNA recombinant protein combining interleukin-2 and diphtheria toxin fragments A and B that can bind to IL-2 receptors and introduce the diphtheria toxin into cells that express those receptors, killing the cells (*Chapter 20*). The drug has been effective in some malignancies, i.e., cutaneous T cell lymphoma, whose malignant cells express the CD25 component of the IL-2 receptor and has some efficacy in the treatment of glucocorticosteroid-refractory GVHD after allogeneic bone marrow transplantation.

Basiliximab is a chimeric (murine/human) monoclonal antibody that inhibits the generation of antigen-specific cytotoxic T lymphocytes but has little effect on the cytolytic activity of established antigen-specific T cell clones. This makes anti-CD25 antibodies particularly potent when combined with CsA.

Daclizumab is a humanized monoclonal antibody that targets primarily human T lymphocytes expressing the high-affinity IL-2R. It directly and specifically interferes with IL-2 signaling at the receptor level by inhibiting the association and subsequent phosphorylation of the IL-2R beta and gamma chains. It rapidly saturates IL-2R alpha (CD25) on lymph node lymphocytes. It is useful for the prevention of solid organ graft rejection and for the treatment of steroid-refractory GVHD. One advantage of relatively specific (anti-CD25) immunosuppressive therapy is the low incidence of infusion-related reactions; few serious side effects are seen, especially with daclizumab and basiliximab.

Abatacept (CTLA-4Ig) is a recombinant fusion protein comprising the extracellular domain of human CTLA-4 and an Fc domain of human IgG1 that has been modified to prevent complement fixation. Abatacept competitively binds with high avidity to CD80/CD86, preventing these molecules from engaging CD28 on T cells, and thereby preventing full T cell activation. Abatacept has been approved by the FDA for use in adult patients with moderate-to-severe rheumatoid arthritis who have not responded adequately to medications such as methotrexate or TNF antagonists.

The development programs for several of the newer immunological therapies, including abatacept, has often assessed patients taking another concomitant anti-inflammatory medication or disease-remitting agent such as methotrexate. With other biological agents, combination therapy with standard immunosuppressives has afforded synergistic clinical efficacy, and in some cases, beneficial pharmacokinetic interactions. The degree of synergistic effectiveness with newer biologic agents remains to be fully defined, as does the extent to which adverse effects may be additive or "synergistic."

Group 3 Tolerance-Inducing Agents or Procedures

Group 3 agents or procedures represent a group of emerging modalities that exert their effects by diminishing immune responsiveness by induction of immune tolerance in clinical conditions where the loss of tolerance is considered to be the central importance in the pathogenesis of such disorders as allergy, asthma, (*Chapter 18*) and autoimmune diseases (*Chapter 19*). This represents the newest of modalities that achieve immunomodulation and represents the most specific and potentially safest means of averting or treating allergic diseases and autoimmune disorders. Although the strategy of vaccination with self-antigen to promote self-antigen-specific tolerance for autoimmune diseases is therapeutically effective in inbred rodent models, its translation in humans has met with lesser success. Recent trials of nasal insulin vaccine in humans at risk of type 1 diabetes, however, have provided some evidence of tolerance induction as a basis for continued exploration of this form of immunomodulation. More clinically promising are studies of oral tolerance to food and inhalant antigens for the treatment of allergic disease in the human (*Chapter 18*). The field of allergen-specific immunotherapy is experiencing exciting and novel developments for the treatment of allergic diseases not only by the more traditional subcutaneous immunotherapy (**SCIT**), but more recently in the form of oral and sublingual immunotherapy (**SLIT**), in which allergen is administered either subcutaneously or orally or sublingually in gradually increasing doses, respectively. The recent explosive expansion of knowledge of T cell function and cytokine physiology and their reciprocal regulation and counterbalance between different T cell subsets is anticipated to facilitate new strategies for immunologic intervention and new forms of prevention and therapy for these conditions utilizing such tolerance-inducing agents or procedures (*Chapters 7* and *9*).

Conclusions

The human immune response has permitted the survival of our species for countless millennia despite its exposure to an ever-changing and hostile external environment. The impact of medical therapies that have been derived from an understanding of the functioning of the immune system is enormous. Jenner's seminal discovery in 1796 that cowpox inoculation of humans could provide solid protective immunity to smallpox not only laid the groundwork for modern-day discoveries in vaccine development, but also gave birth to a period of medical inquiry that has led to the development of interventions that have prevented or eradicated human diseases through immunization and other innovative immune therapies (*Chapter 23*). Nonetheless, many other diseases have not been successfully addressed, and new pathogens continue to emerge.

Although we are endowed from birth with a great diversity of potential immunological responses, the immune system usually requires the continual postnatal fine regulation and tuning to maintain a homeostatic balance between our internal bodily environment and the multiple foreign agents in the external environment that give rise to human disease. For the most part, the challenge has been met successfully, but, on rare occasion, aberrant imbalances result either from genetically determined failure of proper immune recognition of foreignness or from the evasive capacity of the foreign agent to elude immune recognition, resulting in a variety diseases that take the form of chronic infectious diseases, allergic diseases, autoimmune disorders, and malignancy. Presently, although progress has been made to address some of the challenges posed by the persistent plague of malignant diseases and diseases of organ dysfunction through immunomodulation and transplantation, answers to a number of other therapeutic questions are inadequate and remain unanswered. These health issues have prompted the immunological community to seek a greater understanding of the immunopathophysiology of human illness through scientific inquiry, from which a whole new group of available immodulatory therapies has sprung forth. We are now challenged scientifically to discover new insights and, clinically, to continue to learn how to administer novel medicines safely. It is sobering to contemplate perhaps an even greater challenge—that of developing creative ways to distribute these technology-driven resources to a greater segment of the population in need.

Case Study: Clinical Relevance

Let us now return to the case study of Kawasaki disease presented earlier and review some of the major points of the clinical presentation and how they relate to the immune system:

- Kawasaki disease (KD) is an acute childhood illness manifested by high spiking fever and skin rash that usually affects previously healthy infants and children.
- Although the precise etiology of KD is unknown, the disease and the diagnosis is established by the presence four of five classical features: rash; red eyes; red lips and mouth; swollen and red hands and feet; and swollen lymph nodes in the neck.
- These symptoms resolve spontaneously within one to three weeks, or sooner after treatment with intravenous gamma globulin and aspirin. However, inflammation of medium-sized arteries throughout the body, particularly of the coronary arteries, can occur during the acute illness and result in coronary artery aneurysms in 25 to 30 percent of untreated patients.
- In severe cases, KD leads to myocardial infarction, and EKG changes are seen consistent with those in adults with the same condition; coronary artery aneurysm rupture may lead to sudden death.
- Although treatment with intravenous gamma globulin is an effective therapy for KD, its mechanism of action is unknown, and not all children respond with the same degree of clinical improvement.
- Several clinical features of KD support an infectious etiology that includes abrupt onset of symptoms that are compatible with infection, and resolution of the illness in one to three weeks, even without treatment and usually without recurrence. The young age group that is affected, the winter-spring predominance of cases in non-tropical climates, and the existence of epidemics or clusters of cases that spread in a wave-like manner throughout a community also suggest an infectious cause. In the 40 years since Tomisaku Kawasaki initially described the clinical features of KD, many possible etiological agents have been suggested, but none have been confirmed by subsequent studies.
- Recent studies examining tissues from fatal cases of KD revealed that oligoclonal IgA plasma cells infiltrate inflamed tissues, including coronary arteries, suggesting that these cells are producing IgA antibody specific for a putative antigen.
- The prominence of IgA plasma cells in the vascular infiltrate in the early, acute, and subacute stages of KD suggests an antigen-driven immune response to an etiologic agent (such as a virus), with a respiratory or gastrointestinal portal of entry. It has been speculated that this unusual immune response is integral to the pathogenesis of the illness.

A

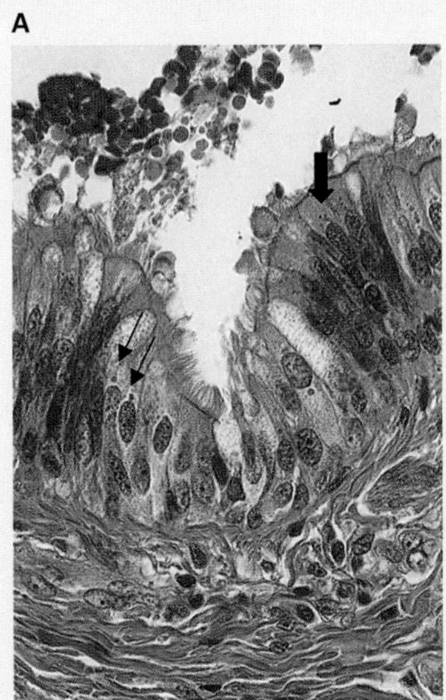

B

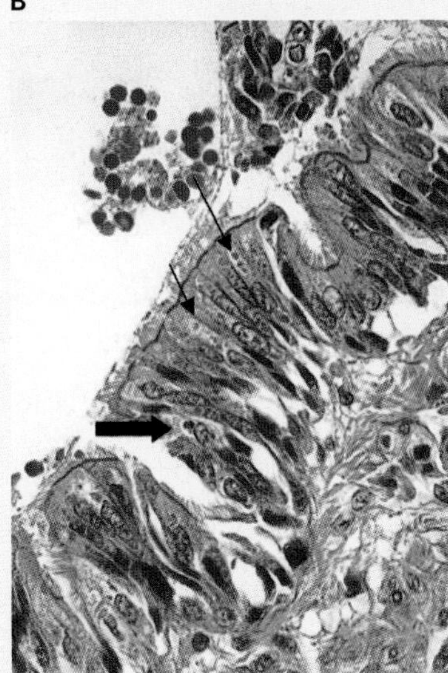

Figure 11-10. Both panels show cytoplasmic inclusion bodies are visible in ciliated bronchial epithelium by light microscopy in acute KD. Hematoxylin-eosin-stained sections show amphophilic spheroidal cytoplasmic inclusion bodies (thin arrows) and irregular, golden yellow, granular, supranuclear pigment resembling classic lipofuscin (thick arrows). Original magnifications × 640 for both panels. (Reproduced with permission from Rowley AH, Baker SC, Shulman ST, et al. Cytoplasmic inclusion bodies are detected by synthetic antibody in ciliated bronchial epithelium during acute Kawasaki disease. J Infect Dis. 2005;192:1757–66.)

Case Study: Clinical Relevance (continued)

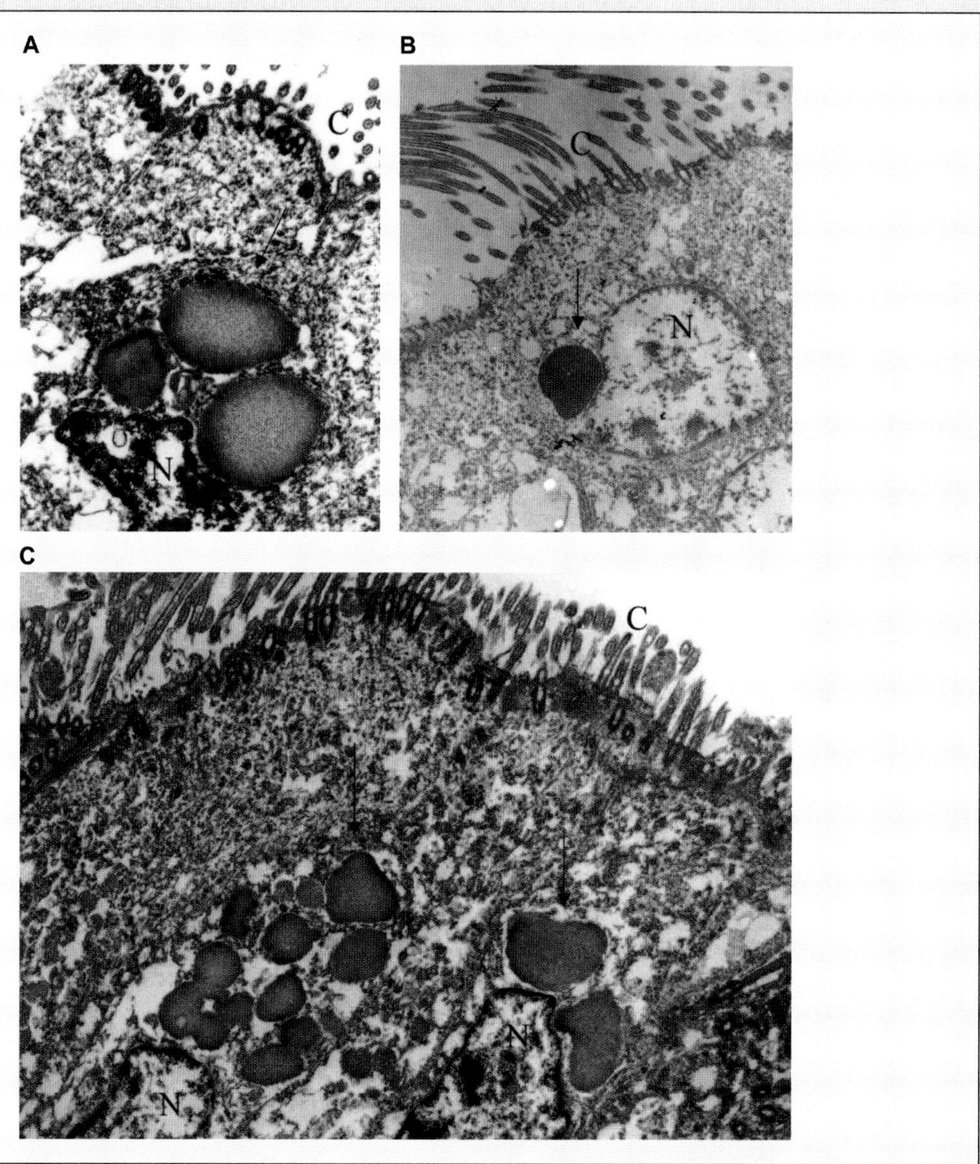

Figure 11-11. Homogeneous cytoplasmic perinuclear inclusion bodies observed by transmission electron microscopy in patients with acute KD. Panel A: Three regular, homogeneous perinuclear inclusion bodies (arrow) are observed in a ciliated bronchial epithelial cell from patient 3. Panel B: A single homogeneous spheroidal inclusion body (arrow) is observed indenting the nucleus of a ciliated bronchial epithelial cell from patient 2. Panel C: Multiple homogeneous bodies (arrows) are observed in ciliated bronchial epithelial cells from patient 4. Original magnifications × 17,000 for panel A and × 14,000 for panels B and C. C = cilia; N = nucleus. (Reproduced with permission from Rowley AH, Baker SC, Shulman ST, et al. Cytoplasmic inclusion bodies are detected by synthetic antibody in ciliated bronchial epithelium during acute Kawasaki disease. J Infect Dis. 2005;192:1757–66.)

- Using synthetic versions of these oligoclonal KD antibodies produced by these cells, an antigen has been found in acute-KD-inflamed ciliated bronchial epithelium light (Figure 11-10). Electron microscopy (Figure 11-11) studies have demonstrated that the antigen is localized to cytoplasmic inclusion bodies in tissues inflamed by acute KD.

Key Points

- IVIG has a wide range of proposed immunomodulatory activities and is indicated as replacement therapy for patients with primary immunodeficiency diseases, as well as treatment for immune thrombocytopenia, Kawasaki disease, and toxic shock syndrome.
- Hyperimmune globulin is used for prevention of various diseases; examples include prevention of hepatitis B, RSV, and CMV.
- Recombinant monoclonal and polyclonal antibodies have been developed as effective treatments for various diseases; these therapeutic antibodies target specific cell markers on T cells, B cells, and IgE.
- Plasmapheresis is an effective method of removing plasma proteins. IgM and IgG are effectively reduced, and the procedure is clinically useful for the emergent treatment of thrombotic thrombocytopenic purpura, myasthenia gravis, Goodpasture's syndrome, and hyperviscosity secondary to Waldenström's macroglobulinemia.
- Irradiation (total body or localized) and drugs such as azathioprine, methotrexate, and cyclophosphamide are the predominate modalities commonly used at this time for a variety of immunomodulating purposes. Mycophenolate mofetil is a recent addition to this group of drugs.
- Glucocorticosteroids are potent catabolic anti-inflammatory and immunosuppressive hormones. They exert their effects through gene transcription modulation, causing inhibition of pro-inflammatory cytokines IL-1, IL-2, IL-6, IL-8, IFN-γ, and TNF-α.
- The immunophilin ligands cyclosporine, tacrolimus, and sirolimus are important immunosuppressive medications that inhibit T cell activation. These compounds play important roles in the suppression of solid organ allograft rejection and are the mainstays of GVHD prevention following HSCT.
- Recombinant hematopoietic growth factors, recombinant interferons, TNF inhibitors, and IL receptor antagonists are also important emerging immunomodulatory treatments.

Study Questions/Critical Thinking

1. When should IVIG treatment be considered? List a few possible side effects.
2. What types of immunomodulatory therapies are available for the prevention of RSV infection, and how do they work?
3. How do monoclonal and polyclonal antibody treatments differ? Name a few examples in each category.
4. How does plasmapheresis work? With what conditions is it useful?
5. Explain the mechanism of glucocorticosteriods. What are some common side effects?
6. What are some of the clinical indications for immunophilin ligands such as cyclosporine, tacrolimus, and sirolimus?

Suggested Reading

Akdis M, Akdis CA. Therapeutic manipulation of immune tolerance in allergic disease. Nat Rev Drug Discov. 2009; 8: 645–60.

American Academy of Pediatrics Committee on Infectious Diseases and Committee of Fetus and Newborn. Prevention of respiratory syncytial virus infections: indications for the use palivizumab and update on the use of RSV-IGIV. Pediatrics. 1998; 102: 1211–6.

Anderson RE, Warner NL. Ionizing radiation and the immune response. Adv Immunol. 1976; 24: 215–335.

Ballow M. Biologic immune modifiers: trials and tribulations—are we there yet? J Allergy Clin Immunol. 2006; 118: 1209–15.

Ballow M. Mechanisms of action of intravenous immune serum globulin in autoimmune and inflammatory diseases. J Allergy Clin Immunol. 1997; 100: 151–7.

Ballow M. The IgG molecule as a biological immune response modifer: mechanics of action of intravenous immune serum globulin in autoimmune and inflammatory disorders. J Allergy Clin Immunol. 2011; 127: 315–23.

Basta M, Dalakas MC. High-dose intravenous immunoglobulin exerts its beneficial effect in patients with dermatomyositis by blocking endomysial deposition of activated complement fragments. J Clin Invest. 1994; 94: 1729–35.

Berger M, Pinciaro PJ, Althaus A, et al. Efficacy, pharmacokinetics, safety, and tolerability of flebogamma® 10% DIF, a high-purity human intravenous immunoglobulin, in primary immunodeficiency. J Clin Immunol. 2010; 32: 321–9.

Bernard A, Boumsell L. Human leukocyte differentiation antigens. Presse Med. 1984; 13: 2311–6.

Bonaros N, Mayer B, Schachner T, et al. CMV-hyperimmune globulin for preventing cytomegalovirus infection and disease in solid organ transplant recipients: a meta-analysis. Clin Transplant. 2008; 22: 89–97.

Borin G, Pezzoli A, Marchiori F, et al. Synthetic and binding studies on the calcium binding site I of bovine brain calmodulin: II: Synthesis and CD studies on the cyclic 20-31 sequence. J Peptide Protein Res. 1985; 26: 528–38.

Boumpas DT, Austin HA, Fessler BJ, et al. Systemic lupus erythematosus: emerging concepts: part I: renal, neuropsychiatric, cardiovascular, pulmonary, and hematologic disease. Ann Intern Med. 1995; 122: 940–50.

Brandt SJ, Peters WP, Atwater SK, et al. Effect of recombinant human granulocyte-macrophage colony-stimulating factor on hematopoietic reconstitution after high-dose chemotherapy and autologous bone marrow transplantation. N Eng J Med. 1988; 318: 869–76.

Brazelton TR, Morris RE. Molecular mechanisms of action of new xenobiotic immunosuppressive drugs: tacrolimus (FK506), sirolimus (rapamycin), mycophenolate mofetil and leflunomide. Curr Opin Immunol. 1996; 8: 710–20.

Bresnihan B. Anankinra as a new therapeutic option in rheumatoid arthritis: clinical results and perspectives. Clin Exp Rheumatol. 2002; 20: S32–4.

Bresnihan B. Effects of anankinra on clinical and radiological outcomes in rheumatoid arthritis. Ann Rheum Dis. 2002; 61 Suppl 2: ii74–7.

Broide DH. Immunomodulation of allergic disease. Annu Rev Med. 2009; 60: 279–91.

Burk ML, Matuszewski KA. Muromonab-CD3 and antithymocyte globulin in renal transplantation. Ann Pharmacother. 1997; 31: 1370–7.

Burks AW, Sampson HA, Buckley RH. Anaphylactic reactions after gamma globulin administration in patients with hypogammaglobulinemia: detection of IgE antibodies to IgA. N Eng J Med. 1986; 314: 560–4.

Burnstein KL, Cidlowski JA. Regulation of gene expression by glucocortisoids. Annu Rev Physiol. 1989; 51: 683–99.

Busse W, Corren J, Lanier BQ, et al. Omalizumab, anti-IgE recombinant humanized monoclonal antibody, for the treatment fo severe allergic asthma. J Allergy Clin Immunol. 2001; 108: 184–90.

Centers for Disease Control and Prevention. Outbreak of hepatitis C associated with intravenous immunoglobulin administration—United States, October 1993-June 1994. J Am Med Assoc. 1994; 272: 424–5.

Champlin R, Ho W, Gale RP. Antithymocyte globulin treatment in patients with aplastic anemia: a prospective randomized trial. N Eng J Med. 1983; 308: 113–8.

Chew AL, Bennet A, Smith CH, et al. Successful treatment of severe psoriasis and psoriatic arthritis with adalimumab. Br J Dermatol. 2004; 151: 492–6.

Chen Y, Bond E, Tompkins E, et al. Asymptomatic reaction of JC virus in patients treated with natalizumab. N Engl J Med. 2009; 361: 1067–74.

Contreras M, de Silva M. The prevention and management of haemolytic disease of the newborn. J R Soc Med. 1994; 87: 256–8.

Dahl MG, Gregory MM, Scheuer PJ. Liver damage due to methotrexate in patients with psoriasis. Br J Med. 1971; 1: 625–30.

Debre M, Bonnet MC, Fridman WH, et al. Infusion of Fc gamma fragments for treatment of children with acute immune thrombocytopenic purpura. Lancet. 1993; 342: 945–9.

Deresinski SC. Hyperimmune products in the prevention and therapy of infectious disease: a report of a hyperimmune products expert advisory panel. BioDrugs. 2000; 14: 147–58.

Dijkmans BA, Jansen G. Antimetabolites in the treatment of arthritis: current status of the use of antimetabolites. Nucleos Nucleot Nucl. 2004; 23: 1083–8.

Dumont FJ. Alemtuzumab (millennium/ILEX). Curr Opin Invest Drugs. 2001; 2: 139–60.

Duvic M, Cather J, Maize J, et al. DAB389IL2 diphtheria fusion toxin produces clinical responses in tumor stage cutaneous T cell lymphoma. Am J Hematol. 1998; 58: 87–90.

Eibl MM. History of Immunologlobulin replacement. Immunol Allergy Clin. 2008: 28: 737–64.

Eisenbeis CF, Caligiuri MA, Byrd JC. Rituximab: converging mechanisms of action in non-Hodgkins lymphoma? Clin Cancer Res. 2003: 9: 5810–2.

Ensley RD, Bristow MR, Olsen SL, et al. The use of mycophenolate Mofetil (RS-61443) in human heart transplant recipients. Transplantation. 1993: 56: 75–82.

No author listed. Etanercept: soluble tumour necrosis factor receptor, TNF receptor fusion protein, TNFR-Fc, TNR 001, enbrel. Drugs R D. 1999; 1: 75–7.

Fauci AS, Haynes BF, Katz P, et al. Wegener's granulomatosis: prospective clinical and therapeutic experience with 85 patients for 21 years. Ann Intern Med. 1983; 98: 76–85.

Fauci AS, Murakami T, Brandon DD, et al. Mechanisms of corticosteroid action on lymphocyte subpopulations: VI: lack of correlation between glucocorticosteroid receptors and the differential effects of glucocorticosteroids on T-cell subpopulations. Cell Immunol. 1980; 49: 43–50.

Fischl M, Galpin JE, Levine JD, et al. Recombinant human erythropoietin for patients with AIDS treated with zidovudine. N Eng J Med. 1990: 322: 1488–93.

Fisher RI, Rosenberg SA, Fyfe G. Long-term survival update for high-dose recombinant interleukin-2 in patients with renal carcinoma. Cancer Journal from Scientific American. 2000; 6 Suppl 1: S55–7.

Foss FM. Interleukin-2 fusion toxin: targeted therapy for cutaneous T cell lymphoma. Ann N Y Acad Sci. 2001; 941: 166–76.

Garces K. Anankinra: interleukin-1 receptor antagonist therapy for rheumatoid arthritis. Issues in Emerging Health Technologies. 2001; 101: 1–4.

Hammond WP, Price TH, Souza LM, et al. Treatment of cyclic neutropenia with granulocyte colony-stimulating factor. N Eng J Med. 1989; 320: 1306–11.

Hansen RJ, Balthasar SP. Effects of intravenous immunoglobulin on platelet count and antiplatelet disposition in a rat model of immune thrombocytopenia. Blood. 2002; 100: 2087–93.

Hartung HP, Mouthon L, Ahmed R, et al. Clinical application of intravenous immunoglobulins (ivig)—beyond immunodeficiencies and neurology. Clin Exp Immunol. 2009; 158 Suppl 1: 23–33.

Imbach P, Barandun S, Baumgartner C, et al. High-dose intravenous gammaglobulin therapy of refractory, in particular idiopathic thrombocytopenia in childhood. Helv Paediatr Acta. 1981; 36: 81–6.

The Impact-RSV study Group. Palivizumab, a humanized respiratory syncytial virus monoclonal antibody, reduces hospitalization from respiratory syncytial virus infection in high-risk infants. Pediatrics. 1998; 102: 531–7.

Kazatchkine MD. Anti-idiotypic suppression of autoantibodies with high dose intravenous immunoglobulins. Prog Clin Biol Res. 1990; 337: 411–4.

Kinder AJ, Hassell AB, Brand J, et al. The treatment of inflammatory arthritis with methotrexate in clinical practice: treatment duration and incidence of adverse drug reactions. Rheumatology. 2005; 44: 61–6.

Kircher B, Latzer K, Gastl G, et al. Comparative in vitro study of the immunomodulatory activity of humanized and chimeric anti-CD25 monoclonal antibodies. Clin Exp Immunol. 2003; 134: 426–30.

Kishiyama JL, Valacer D, Cunningham-Rundles C, et al. A multicenter, randomized, double-blind, placebo-controlled trial of high-dose intravenous immunoglobulin for oral corticosteroid-dependent asthma. Clin Immunol. 1999; 19: 126–33.

Kressebuch H, Schaad UB, Hirt A, et al. Cerebrospinal fluid inflammation induced by intravenous immunoglobulins. Ped Infect Dis J. 1992; 11: 894–5.

Lederman HM, Roifman CM, Lavi S, et al. Corticosteroids for prevention of adverse reactions to intravenous immune serum globulin infusions in hypogammaglobulinemic patients. Am J Med. 1986; 81: 443–6.

Leung DY. Kawasaki syndrome: immunomodulatory benefit and potential toxin neutralization by intravenous immune globulin. Clin Exp Immnol. 1996; 104 Suppl 1: 49–54.

Macris MP, Frazier OH, Lammermeier D, et al. Clinical experience with muromonab-CD3 monoclonal antibody (OKT3) in heart transplantation. J Heart Transplant. 1989; 8: 281–7.

Maloney DG, Liles TM, Czerwinski DK, et al. Phase I clinical trial using escalating single-dose infusion of chimeric anti-CD20 monoclonal antibody (IDEC-C2B8) in patients with recurrent B-cell lymphoma. Blood. 1994; 84: 2457–66.

Mattila PS. The action of cyclosporine A and FK506 on T-lymphocyte activation. Biochem Soc Trans. 1996; 24: 45–9.

Newburger JW, Fulton DR. Kawasaki disease. Curr Opin Pediatr. 2004: 16: 508–14.

Newcombe C, Newcombe AR. Antibody production: polyclonal-derived biotherapeutics. J Chromatogr B. 2007; 848: 2–7.

Nousari HC, Sragovich A, Kimyadi-Asadi A, et al. Mycophenolate mofetil in autoimmune and inflammatory skin disorders. J Am Acad Dermatol. 1999; 40: 265–8.

Present DH, Korelitz BI, Wisch N, et al. Treatment of Crohn's disease with 6-mercaptopurine: a long-term, randomized, double-blind study. N Eng J Med. 1980; 302: 981–7.

Quartier P, Debre M, De Blic J, et al. Early and prolonged intravenous immunoglobulin replacement therapy in childhood agammaglobulinemia: a retrospective survey of 31 patients. J Pediatr. 1999; 134: 589–96.

Roenigk HH Jr, Auerbach R, Maibach HI, et al. Methotrexate in psoriasis: revised guideline. J Am Acad Dermatol. 1988; 19: 145–56.

Rowley AH, Baker SC, Shulman ST, et al. Cytoplasmic inclusion bodies are detected by synthetic antibody in ciliated bronchial epithelium during acute Kawasaki Disease. J Infect Dis. 2005; 192: 1757–66.

Samuelsson A, Towers TL, Ravetch JV. Anti-inflammatory activity of IVIG mediated through the inhibitory Fc receptor. Science. 2001; 291: 484–6.

Sandborn WJ, Hanauer SB, Katz S, et al. Etanercept for active Crohn's disease: a randomized, double-blind, placebo-controlled trial. Gastroenterology. 2001; 121: 1088–94.

Sehgal SN. Ragamune® (RAPA, rapamycin, sirolimus): mechanism of action immunosuppressive effect results from blockade of signal transduction and inhibition of cell cycle progession. Clin Biochem. 1998; 31: 335–40.

Siddiqui MA, Scott LJ. Infliximab: a review of its use in Crohn's disease and rheumatoid arthritis. Drugs. 2005; 65: 2179–208.

Sieper J, Van den Brande J. Diverse effects of infliximab and etanercept on T lymphocytes. Sem Arthritis Rheum. 2005; 34: 23–7.

Stewart GE, Diaz JD, Lockey RF, et al. Comparison of oral pulse methotrexate with placebo in the treatment of severe glucocorticosteroid-dependent asthma. J Allergy Clin Immunol. 1994; 94: 482–9.

Sultan Y, Rossi F, Kazatchkine MD. Recovery from anti-VIII:C (antihemophilic factor) autoimmune disease is dependent on generation of antiidiotypes against anti-VIII:C autantibodies. Proc Nat Acad Sci USA. 1987; 86: 828–31.

Thyer J, Unal A, Thomas P, et al. Prion-removal capacity of chromatographic and ethanol precipitation steps used in the production of albumin and immunoglobulins. Vox Sanguinis. 2006; 91: 292–300.

van der Spek J, Hemard A, Dautry-Varsat A, et al. Epitope tagging of DAB389IL-2: new insights into C-domain delivery to the cytosol of target cells. Leukemia. 1994; 8 Suppl 1: S144–8.

Voso MT, Pantel G, Rutella S, et al. Rituximab reduces the number of peripheral blood b cells in vitro mainly by effector cell-mediated mechanisms. Haematologica. 2002; 87: 918–25.

Waldmann TA, Levy R, Coller BS. Emerging therapies: spectrum of applications of monoclonal antibody therapy. Hematology American Society of Hematology Education Program. 2000; 394–408.

Weinblatt ME, Kremer JM, Bankhurst AD, et al. A trial of etanercept, a recombinant tumor necrosis factor recipient: Fc fusion protein, in patients with rheumatoid arthritis receiving methotrexate. N Eng J Med. 1999; 340: 253–9.

Weisman MH, Moreland LW, Furst DE, et al. Efficacy, pharmacokinetic, and safety assessment of adalimumab, a fully human anti-tumor necrosis factor-alpha monoclonal antibody, in adults with rheumatoid arthritis receiving concomitant methotrexate: a pilot study. Clin Therapeutics. 2003; 25: 1700–21.

Wiseman GA, Witzig TE. Yttrium-90 ((90)Y) Ibritumomab Tiuxetan (Zevalin®)) induces long-term durable responses in patients with relapsed or refractory B-cell non-Hodgkin's lymphoma. Cancer Biother and Radio. 2005; 20: 185–8.

Yazici Y, Erkan D, Paget SA. Monitoring by rheumatologists for methotrexate-, etanercept-, infliximab-, and anankinra-associated adverse events. Arthritis Rheum. 2003; 48: 2769–72.

Yu Z, Lennon VA. Mechanism of intravenous immune globulin therapy in antibody-mediated automimmune diseases. N Eng J Med. 1999; 340: 227–8.

Biologic Response Modifiers

The ***Biologic Response Modifiers*** listed in the following tables represent the currently available FDA-approved products as of the publication of this textbook edition. For the most recently FDA-approved products, the reader is referred to the following Drugs@FDA website which is updated on a timely basis, which can be accessed at http://www.accessdata.fda.gov/scripts/cder/drugsatfda/ or by the QR code shown above.

Table 11A-1. Therapeutic monoclonal antibodies to a variety of cellular and molecular targets

Product	Brand name	Type	Target	Molecular structure	Clinical indication(s)
Abciximab	ReoPro c7E3 Fab	-ximab	Glycoprotein (GP) IIb/IIIa receptor of human platelets	Chimeric human monoclonal antibody; Fab portion	Patients undergoing coronary intervention for prevention of cardiac ischemic complications
Alemtuzumab	Campath, Campath-1H, Mabcampath	-zumab	CD52 (cell surface glycoprotein)	Humanized IgG1κ recombinant monoclonal antibody to CD52	Chronic B lymphocyte leukemia (B-CLL)
Basiliximab	Simulect	-ximab	CD25 (IL-2Rα)	Chimeric IgG1κ, recombinant antibody to CD25	Prophylaxis of acute organ rejection in adults following cadaveric or living-donor renal transplantation
Belimumab	Benlysta	umab	BlyS, also referred to as BAFF and TNFSF13B	Human IgG1λ monoclonal anti-BLyS	Treatment of adult patients with active, autoantibody-positive, systemic lupus erythematosus (SLE)
Bevacizumab	Avastin rhuMAb VEGF	-zumab	VEGF (vascular endothelial growth factor)	Humanized monoclonal antibody to VEGF	Metastatic colorectal cancer; unresectable, locally advanced, recurrent, or metastatic non-small cell lung cancer, metastatic breast cancer, glioblastoma renal carcinoma
Canakinumab	Ilaris	umab	IL-1β	Human IgG1κ monoclonal anti-IL-1β	Cryopyrin-Associated Periodic Syndromes (CAPS), in adults and children ≥4 years of age, i.e., FCAS and MWS

(Continued)

Table 11A-1. Therapeutic monoclonal antibodies to a variety of cellular and molecular targets (continued)

Product	Brand name	Type	Target	Molecular structure	Clinical indication(s)
Cetuximab	Erbitux	-ximab	EGF (epidermal growth factor) receptor	Chimeric monoclonal antibody to EGF	Metastatic colorectal cancer, head and neck cancer, metastatic breast cancer, glioblastoma renal carcinoma
Daclizumab	Zenapax	-zumab	CD25 (IL-2Rα)	Humanized IgG1 monoclonal antibody	Renal allograft rejection
Denosumab	Xgeva	umab	RANKL	Human IgG2 monoclonal antibody that binds to human RANKL	Prevention of skeletal-related events in patients with bone metastases from solid tumors
	Prolia	umab	RANKL	RANKL	Treatment of postmenopausal women with osteoporosis at high risk for fracture
Eculizumab	Soliris, 5G1.1	-zumab	Complement protein C5 thereby inhibiting its cleavage to C5a and C5b and prevention of generation of the terminal C5–9 lytic membrane attack complex (MAC)	Humanized IgG2/4κ monoclonal antibody to C5	Paroxysmal nocturnal hemoglobinuria
Efalizumab (has been withdrawn from the market after report of progressive multifocal leukencephalopathy)	Raptiva, Xanelin, hu 1124	-zumab	CD11a (α-subunit of leukocyte function antigen-1 [LFA-1])	Humanized IgG1κ recombinant monoclonal anti-CD11a antibody to α-chain of LFA-1	Chronic, moderate-to-severe plaque psoriasis
Gemtuzumab ozogamicin	Mylotarg, hP67.6	-zumab	CD33	Humanized IgG4κ monoclonal antibody to CD33 conjugated with the toxin calicheamicin	CD33 positive acute myeloid leukemia
Ibritumomab tiuxetan	Zevalin	Murine	CD20	Murine IgG1κ monoclonal antibody to CD20, conjugated to a chelator (tiuxetan), to which a radioactive isotope (either yttrium-90 or indium-111) is added	Non-Hodgkin's lymphoma (CD20-positive, low-grade, or follicular) which is relapsed or refractory to rituximab, in combination with rituximab
Ipilimumab	Yervoy	umab	CTLA-4	Human IgG1κ monoclonal anti-CTLA-4	Treatment of unresectable or metastatic melanoma
Muromonab-CD3	Orthoclone OKT3	Murine	CD3	Murine IgG2a monoclonal antibody to CD3	Renal, cardiac, hepatic allograft rejection

Table 11A-1. Therapeutic monoclonal antibodies to a variety of cellular and molecular targets (continued)

Product	Brand name	Type	Target	Molecular structure	Clinical indication(s)
Natalizumab	Tysabri	-zumab	α4-subunit of α4β1 and α4β7 integrins; blocks binding of VLA4 to VCAM-1 and binding of α4-β7 to MAdCAM-1	Humanized IgG4κ monoclonal antibody to a4-integrins	Relapsing forms of multiple sclerosis and Crohn's disease
Ofatumumab	Arzerra	umab	CD20	IgG1κ human monoclonal anti-CD20 antibody	Treatment of patients with chronic lymphocytic leukemia (CLL) refractory to fludarabine and alemtuzumab
Omalizumab	Xolair	-zumab	IgE; leads to reduction of mediator release from and presence of IgEεRI receptors on basophils and mast cells	Humanized IgG1κ recombinant monoclonal antibody to IgE	Moderate-to-severe IgE-mediated, persistent asthma (US) or severe asthma (EU), in adults and children over 12 years old, inadequately controlled by inhaled corticosteroid treatment
Palivizumab	Synagis, MEDI-493	-zumab	RSV F (fusion) protein	Humanized IgG1κ recombinant monoclonal antibody to RSV F protein	Prevention of serious lower respiratory tract disease caused by respiratory syncytial virus (RSV) in pediatric patients at high risk of RSV disease
Panitumumab	Vectibix, ABX-EGF	Murine	Human EGFR (Epidermal Growth Factor Receptor)	Murine recombinant human IgG2 monoclonal antibody to EGFR	Treatment of EGFR-expressing, metastatic colorectal carcinoma with disease progression on or following fluoropyrimidine-, oxaliplatin-, and irinotecan- containing chemotherapy regimens
Ranibizumab	Lucentis rhuFab V2; IgG1k (derived from Avastin (bevacizumab)	-zumab	VEGF-A	Humanized IgG1 Fab fragment antibody to VEGF-A	Neovascular (wet) age-related macular degeneration. Metastic cancer of colon or rectum, non-small cell lung cancer, breast cancer, glioblastoma multiforme, renal cell carcinoma
Rituximab	Rituxan, Mabthera	-ximab	CD20	Chimeric IgG1 recombinant monoclonal antibody to CD20	Rheumatoid arthritis; B cell non-Hodgkin's lymphoma; chronic lymphocytic leukemia (CLL)

(*Continued*)

Table 11A-1. Therapeutic monoclonal antibodies to a variety of cellular and molecular targets (continued)

Product	Brand name	Type	Target	Molecular structure	Clinical indication(s)
Tocilizumab	Actemra, MRA	-zumab	IL-6 receptor (IL-6R)	Humanized, recombinant monoclonal antibody to IL-6R	Rheumatoid arthritis (Japan), systemic-onset juvenile idiopathic arthritis (Japan)
Tositumomab I131	Bexxar	Murine	CD20	Murine, IgG2a monoclonal recombinant antibody to CD20 covalently bound to Iodine-131	Non-Hodgkin's lymphoma (CD20 positive, follicular), which is refractory to rituximab and relapsed following chemotherapy
Trastuzumab	Herceptin	-zumab	c-erbB2/HER2	Humanized recombinant anti-HER2 receptor antibody that kills HER2 expressing cancer cells	HER2 overexpressing breast cancer, HER2 overexpressing metastatic gastric or gastroespheogeal junction adenocarcinoma
Ustekinumab	Stelara	umab	p40 subunit common to both IL-12 and IL-23	Human IgG1α monoclonal anti-p40 subunit common to IL-12 and IL-23 cytokines	Treatment of adult patients (≥18 years) with moderate to severe plaque psoriasis who are candidates for phototherapy or systemic therapy

Annex 11A-2. Therapeutic monoclonal antibodies to TNF-α

Product	Brand name	Type	Target	Molecular structure	Clinical indication(s)
Adalimumab	Humira, Trudexa	-umab	TNF-α	Human IgG1κ anti-TNF-α recombinant antibody to TNF-α	Rheumatoid arthritis; juvenile idiopathic arthritis; psoriatic arthritis; ankylosing spondylitis; Crohn's disease; plaque psoriasis
Infliximab	Remicade	-ximab	TNF-α	Chimeric IgG1κ anti-TNF-α recombinant monoclonal antibody to TNF-α	Rheumatoid arthritis; ankylosing spondylitis; psoriatic arthritis; chronic severe plaque psoriasis; Crohn's disease; ulcerative colitis
Certolizumab pegol	Cimzia	-zumab	TNF-α	Humanized, recombinant Fab′ anti-TNF-α antibody fragment conjugated to polyethylene glycol	Crohn's disease, active rheumatoid urthritis
Golimumab	Simponi	-vmab	TNF-α	Human IgG1κ anti-TNF-α monoclonal antibody	Rheumatoid arthritis; Psoriatic arthritis; ankylosing spondylitis

Annex 11A-3. Therapeutic Fusion Proteins

Product	Brand name	Type	Target	Molecular structure	Clinical indication(s)
Abatacept	Orencia, CTLA4Ig, BMS-188667	Receptor-antibody fusion protein (receptor attached to Fc of IgG1)	B7-1 (CD80), B7-2 (CD86)	CTLA-4-Human IgG1 fusion protein	Rheumatoid arthritis, juvenile idiopathic arthritis
Alefacept	Amevive, BG 9273	Receptor-antibody fusion protein (receptor attached to Fc of IgG1)	CD2	LFA-3-IgG1 Fc fusion protein	Moderate-to-severe chronic plaque psoriasis
Denileukin diftitox	ONTAK	Receptor antibody fusion protein (receptor attached to Fc of IgG1)	IL-2 Receptor	Recombinant fusion protein expressing amino acid residues of diphtheria toxin fragment A and B, followed by the sequence for IL-2	Recurrent CD25 positive, cutaneous T cell lymphoma
Etanercept	Enbrel	Receptor-antibody fusion protein (receptor attached to Fc of IgG1)	TNF-α and TNF-β	TNFR-IgG1 Fc fusion protein	Rheumatoid arthritis; juvenile idiopathic arthritis; psoriatic arthritis; ankylosing spondylitis; plaque psoriasis
Rilonacept	Arcalyst	Receptor-antibody fusion protein (IL-1R1 and IL-IRAcP fusel to Fc of IgG1)	IL-1	IL-1 TRap	Cryopyrin-Associated Periodic Syndromes (CAPS), including FCAS and MWS

Annex 11A-4. Monoclonal Antibodies Used for *In Vivo* Imaging

Product	Brand name	Type	Target	Molecular structure	Clinical indication(s)
Arcitumomab	CEA-SCAN	Murine	CEA	Murine monoclonal IgG1, ^{99m}Tc-labeled	Diagnostic imaging of CEA+ colorectal cancers
Capromab pendetide	Prostascint, 7E11-C5.3	Murine	Prostate Specific Membrane Antigen (PSMA)	Murine monoclonal IgG1κ, ^{111}In labeled	Diagnostic imaging of metastatic prostate cancer in newly diagnosed, high risk patients
Technetium (^{99m}Tc) nofetumomab merpentan	Verluma	Murine	40 kDA carcinoma-associated antigen	Murine monoclonal Fab' fragment attached to the chelator merpentan for conjugation with ^{99m}Tc	Diagnostic imaging of lung cancer, GI, breast, ovary, pancreas, kidney, cervix, and bladder carcinoma
Sulesomab Fab' fragment	Leukoscan, IMMU-MN3	Murine	CEA carcinoembryonic antigen); NCA-90 (surface granulocyte nonspecific cross-reacting antigen) on neutrophils	Murine monoclonal Fab'-SH fragments for conjugation with ^{99m}Tc	Diagnostic imaging of infection/inflammation in bone (suspected osteomyelitis); marketed/approved in European Union

Annex 11A-5. Recombinant Cytokines

Product	Brand name	Type	Target	Clinical indication(s)
Interferon alpha-2a	Roferon-A, IFN-α2A	Recombinant, human	IFN type I R	Hairy cell leukemia; chronic hepatitis C; chronic myelogenous leukemia (Philadelphia chromosome positive, minimally pretreated)
Interferon alpha-2b	Intron A, IFN-α2B	Recombinant, human	IFN type I R	Hairy cell leukemia; malignant melanoma; follicular lymphoma; condylomata acuminata; AIDS-related Kaposi's sarcoma; chronic hepatitis B; chronic hepatitis C
Interferon beta-1a	Rebif	Recombinant, human, glycosylated	IFN type I R	Relapsing forms of multiple sclerosis
Interferon beta-1b	Betaseron	Recombinant, human	IFN type I R	Relapsing forms of multiple sclerosis
Interferon gamma	Actimmune	Recombinant, human	IFN type II R	Chronic granulomatous disease; severe, malignant osteopetrosis
Oprelvekin	Neumega, IL-11, rhIL-11	Recombinant, human IL-11	IL-11 R	Risk of, or preexisting, severe thrombocytopenia and/or need for platelet transfusions following myelosuppressive chemotherapy in patients with nonmyeloid malignancies
Denileukin (diftitox)	Ontak	Recombinant DNA-derived cytotoxic protein composed of diptheria toxin fragments A and B and sequences for IL-2	IL-2R	Treatment of patients with persistent or recurrent cutaneous T-cell lymphoma whose malignant cells express the CD25 component of the IL-2 receptor

Annex 11A-6. Soluble Receptor Constructs

Product	Brand name	Type	Target	Molecular structure	Clinical indication(s)
Anakinra	Kineret	Decoy antagonist	IL-1 type I receptor (IL-1RI)	Recombinant, nonglycosylated form of the human IL-1 receptor antagonist (IL-1Ra)	Moderately to severely active rheumatoid arthritis, in patients 18 years of age or older who have failed one or more disease-modifying antirheumatic drugs
Rilonacept	Arcalyst, IL-1 trap, IL-1 blocker	IL-1 trap fusion protein	IL-1 beta (IL-1β)	Dimeric fusion protein; ligand-binding domains of IL-1 receptor (IL-1R) and IL-1 receptor accessory protein (IL-1RAcP) linked to human IgG1	Cryopyrin-associated periodic fever syndromes (CAPS), including Muckle-Wells syndrome (MWS) and familial cold autoinflammatory syndrome (FCAS) in children 12 years and older

Chapter 12

Immunity to Bacteria

Steven M. Holland, MD
Alexandra Freeman, MD
Joseph A. Bellanti, MD

Case Study

A 14-year-old male was in his usual state of good health when he developed a fever of 103° F, chills, and mild right hip pain while attending summer camp. He was active in sports and attributed the pain to trauma while playing hockey earlier in the year. The hip pain and fever persisted, and 10 days later, because of radiation of the pain to the right lower abdomen, he was evaluated at an emergency department for suspected appendicitis. It was ruled out because of normal findings on physical examination as well as a normal WBC count, and he was discharged on symptomatic treatment. Because of persistence of fever and worsening of the right hip pain, he was taken two days later to another emergency department, where a blood culture was obtained and intravenous ceftriaxone was started empirically at a dose of 2 grams daily. The culture subsequently revealed methicillin-sensitive *Staphylococcus aureus*, following which he was hospitalized and his treatment was changed to intravenous nafcillin at a dose of 200 mg/kg/day in 6 divided doses. Initial X-rays of the hips and femurs showed no evidence of trauma or other pathologic changes (Figure 12-1). A subsequent MRI study with contrast, however, revealed the presence of an effusion in the right hip and edema of the head of the right femur, and he was immediately taken to surgery, where drainage of the hip was performed. Laboratory tests on admission revealed a WBC of 8,300/mm^3 (normal, 4,800–10,800/mm^3), with 65 percent neutrophils, 22 percent lymphocytes, and 13 percent monocytes; however, an erythrocyte sedimentation rate of 70 mm/hr (normal 0–12 mm/hr) and a C-reactive protein (CRP) of 20 (normal up to 0.9) were found.

Despite several days of continuous antibiotic therapy, the fever and right hip pain persisted and a repeat MRI study revealed that pockets of pus had developed in the soft tissues in the proximity of the right femoral head together with a focus of pyomyositis in the right gluteus medius muscle. Subsequently, the patient underwent several surgical procedures to drain these abscesses and for removal of inflammatory and necrotic tissue from the right hip joint. His clinical course was further complicated by the development of an allergic rash to nafcillin requiring a change to cefazolin at a dose of 2 grams every 8 hours and the addition of ciprofloxacin for treatment of *Pseudomonas aeruginosa*, which was isolated from cultures obtained at surgery.

LEARNING OBJECTIVES

When you have completed this chapter, you should be able to:

- Understand the array of biochemical, functional, and anatomical features that bacteria possess to evade the immune system and successfully infect its host
- Appreciate the variety of immunological mechanisms within the innate and adaptive immune systems that have evolved to destroy different groups of bacteria
- Describe the three different relationships between the host and bacteria: symbiosis, commensalism, and pathogenicity
- Understand the differences between acute and chronic bacterial infection and the immune mechanisms involved in each
- Explain the differences between a host's immune response to primary and secondary exposure to a particular bacterium
- Understand how excessive immune reactivity can lead to autoimmunity, and give a few examples of such autoimmune conditions
- Utilize this knowledge for the prevention of bacterial infection in the healthy host and for the management of bacterial infection in disease states

Case Study (continued)

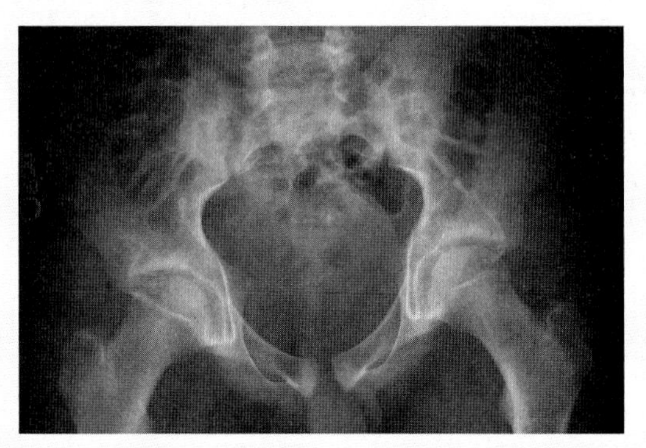

Figure 12-1. Initial X-ray of the hips and femoral heads of a patient on admission showing no abnormalities. (Courtesy of Georgetown University Hospital.)

He was treated with antibiotics for a total of eight weeks (six weeks intravenously and two weeks with oral linezolid), following which he appeared clinically improved. One week after discontinuation of antibiotic therapy, however, he again developed fever and was readmitted to the hospital for further evaluation and reinitiation of intravenous antibiotic therapy. An MRI revealed an enhanced signal within the right femoral head, and further surgical drainage of the right hip was performed. Cultures from the drainage site again revealed methicillin-sensitive *Staphylococcus aureus*. A week later, because of severe hip pain, another MRI study showed dislocation of the femoral head. The proximal end of the right femoral head was resected and histopathologic examination revealed a heavy inflammatory infiltration characterized predominantly by neutrophils (Figure 12-2).

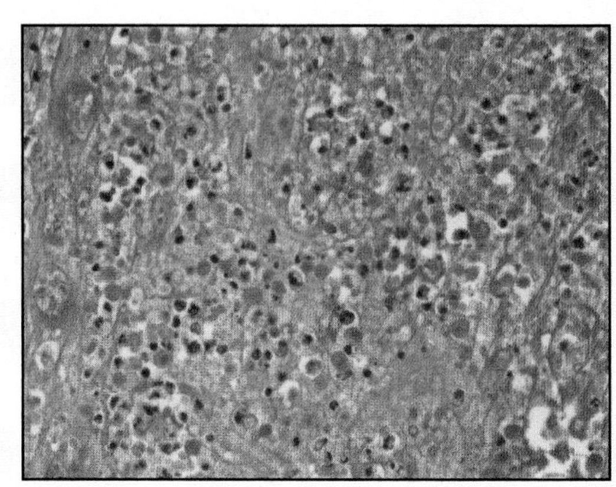

Figure 12-2. Photomicrograph of an H & E section of excised inflammatory tissue from the right femoral head of the patient showing a dense neutrophilic infiltrate associated with hemorrhage (×4,000). Note that many of the cells are ghost cells (necrotic PMNs). (Courtesy of Dr. Pedro de Brito.)

Following this procedure, the patient's clinical status improved markedly. He remained afebrile, the pain subsided, and he was discharged from the hospital on long-term antibiotic treatment, physical therapy, and rehabilitation.

Introduction

The world is awash in bacteria, from soil to water to air. Deep seas and high peaks have niches that are harsh yet permissive for unique bacterial species and strains that have long adapted to and exploited their surroundings, not by overwhelming them but by profiting from them and by yielding profit in return. Plants and animals, humans among them, have had to cope with bacteria from the beginning stages of multicellular evolution due to the simple fact that the bacteria were here first (*Chapter 2*). Therefore, it makes sense that mammalian immunity is deeply informed by the presence, or possible presence, of bacteria.

Despite the extraordinary toll that bacterial infections have traditionally taken on human life, it is important to keep in mind that the overall number of discrete bacteria globally is extraordinarily large, while the total number of species and strains that infect humans is really quite small. The mere fact that we can divide the bacterial world into pathogens (the subject of medical microbiology) and nonpathogens (the bulk of the biota) indicates that there may be something important about the few organisms that we do care about in our daily encounters. Added to this complex milieu is the fact that bacteria have impressive mutational capacity and have evolved ways to readily exchange DNA, allowing for rapid bulk changes as opposed to slow and incremental ones that the human immune system employs. Fortunately for us, most bacteria have no interest in becoming human pathogens and do not exert themselves to target humans. However, those few bacteria (and viruses) that almost exclusively come to fruition in humans, such as *M. tuberculosis*, are living blueprints of the gaps or potential gaps in the human immune armor.

The principles of immunology were initially defined in cell cultures, mouse colonies, and basic science laboratories. However, it was only in the clinic that the true mechanisms of human bacterial immunity were determined by the recognition of humans with defects in discrete pathways of their immune system (*Chapter 16*). These defects can be as extensive as neutropenia, with its broad susceptibility to bacterial and fungal infections, or as narrow as X-linked chronic granulomatous disease (**CGD**), with its susceptibility to only a few bacteria and fungi.

It has long been apparent that there are several different aspects of the human immune response; the two main categories of these responses are humoral and cellular (*Chapter 1*). Among the humoral components are all things soluble, including complement, mannose binding lectin, and antibody. Among the cellular factors are neutrophils, eosinophils, basophils, monocytes, and lymphocytes. However, it is now appreciated that another pervasive distinction cuts through these broad categories—the division into innate and adaptive immunity. Innate responses are preformed, unaltered over time, and have stereotypic binding sites, reactions, and capabilities. This innate response is highly efficient and has been highly conserved throughout evolution (*Chapter 2*). Therefore, complement, mannose binding lectin, and phagocytes all fall into the innate category, since they are preformed and largely unaltered by their interaction with their targets (*Chapter 3*).

In contrast, the adaptive immune responses involve mature antibody production and result from a bewildering array of feedback signals, DNA recombination, mutation, refinement, and splicing; this process results in maturation of immature B cells to mature plasma cells (*Chapter 6*) and development of a similarly complex T cell system, with many opportunities for perfection, perversion, or destruction along the way (*Chapter 7*). Over the last few years, the molecular and mechanistic explosion of information about these areas has led to novel and exciting insights into the nature and development of immunity. Nowhere have these developments found greater clinical application than in the host responses to bacterial infection.

The Bacterial-Host Cell Interaction

The outcome of the interaction between a bacterial organism and the host that it encounters is determined both by the properties of the infecting microorganism as well as the host's total immunologic response to the infecting agent. Therefore, any discussion of the immune mechanisms to bacterial infection must of necessity take into account properties of both the bacterium as well as the immune defenses summoned by the host in response to the strategies of the invading organisms. As with other infectious diseases caused by viruses, fungi, and parasites, successful infection by a bacterium is dependent largely on the ability of the organism to evade the defenses of innate and adaptive immunity as well as the transmissibility of the organism. As will be described in greater detail below, the effectiveness of the immune response to the bacteria is further modified by the status of the host immune arsenal, which in turn is influenced by a number of factors, including age, nutritional status, and comorbid illness. This chapter will first describe some of the bacterial properties that allow infections to occur, followed by the immune responses directed by the host to contain these infections.

Bacteria

Bacterial Cell Structure: Cell Wall Structure, PAMPs, Capsules, and Secretory Systems

Bacteria are prokaryotes lacking well-defined nuclei and membrane-bound organelles and with chromosomes composed of a single, continuous strand of DNA arranged in a closed DNA circle localized to a region of the cell called the nucleoid (Figure 12-3). The space between the inner and outer cell membrane in Gram-negative bacteria is referred to as the periplasmic space or periplasm. All the other cellular components, including the ribosomes, are scattered throughout the cytoplasm. The ribosomes are the protein-synthesizing factories found in all cells, including bacteria, involved in the translation of the genetic code from the molecular language of their DNA nucleic acid structure to that of amino acids and then to the synthesis of proteins (*Chapter 25*). However, there are structural differences between bacterial and eukaryotic ribosomes. Some antibiotics, for example, will selectively inhibit the functions of bacterial ribosomes, but not those of the eukaryote. This permits the antibiotic to kill the bacteria but not the eukaryotic organisms they are infecting.

Some bacteria contain surface projections, including the whip-like flagella, that provide a means of locomotion and the hair-like pili that assist the bacteria in attaching to other cells and surfaces as well as for conjugation, during which two bacteria exchange fragments of plasmid DNA. The flagella and pili can

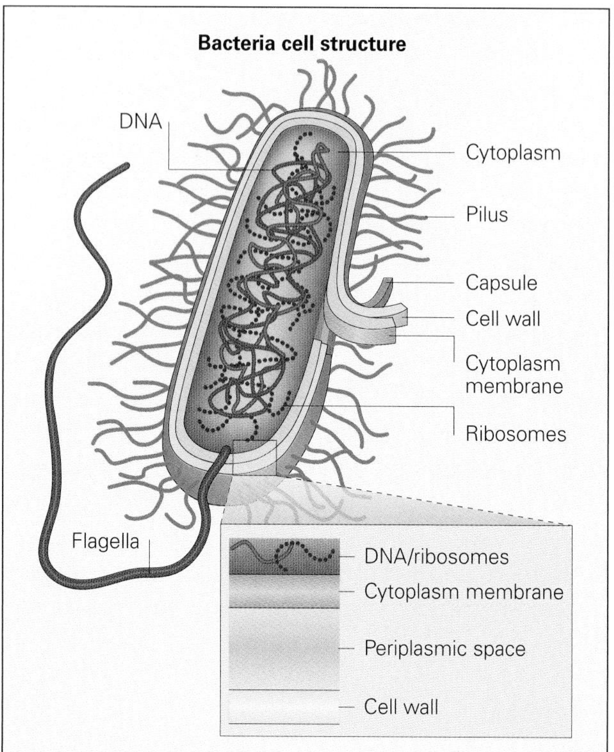

Figure 12-3. Schematic representation of the general structure of a bacterial cell showing key structures, which are both critical to the survival of the bacteria as well as those which may be targeted by the host immune response.

be targeted by antibody production, which is a beneficial protective immune response used by the host in countering the bacterial pathogen.

Bacterial Cell Wall Structures Targeted by the Immune system

Shown in Figure 12-4 is a schematic representation of bacterial cell wall structures found on Gram-negative and Gram-positive bacteria compared to a mycobacterium; it demonstrates how these components may be targeted by various elements of the immune system. All bacteria are protected by a covering layer on its outer surface referred to as the cell envelope, which consists of a thin cytoplasmic lipoprotein cell membrane surrounded by a more rigid peptidoglycan cell wall that is thicker in Gram-positive bacteria than in Gram-negative. In addition, Gram-negative bacteria also have an outer lipid bilayer cell membrane in which the lipopolysaccharide (**LPS**) is embedded. Lysosomal enzymes and lysozymes are active against the peptidoglycan layer, whereas cationic proteins and complement are effective against the outer lipid bilayer of the Gram-negative bacteria. The cell wall of mycobacteria is abundant in lipid, particularly mycolic acid and glycolipids such as lipoarabinomannan. The compound cell wall of mycobacteria is extremely resistant to breakdown, and explains why this organism can persist in macrophages for long periods of time. Some species of bacteria have a third protective covering, a capsule made up of polysaccharides. Capsules play a number of roles, but the most important is to protect the bacteria from being phagocytosed (engulfed) by phagocytic cells of the innate immune system. As will be described in greater detail below, the capsule is a major virulence factor in many disease-causing bacteria, such as *Escherichia coli* and *Streptococcus pneumoniae.* Many of these bacterial cell wall structures function as pathogen-associated molecular patterns (**PAMP**) that provide "danger signals" that bind to pattern-recognition receptors (**PRRs**) that alert the innate immune system into action (*Chapter 3*).

Modes of Bacterial Immunopathogenicity

Bacteria generally exert their pathogenic effects through two mechanisms: (1) bacterial replication and invasiveness and (2) elaboration of toxins (Figure 12-5). Most bacteria are intermediate between these two extremes, having some properties of invasiveness associated with the production of locally acting toxins and spreading factors (tissue-degrading enzymes), such as the case with *Staphylococcus aureus.*

Bacteria produce two major types of toxic substances: (1) **exotoxins**, which are proteins released extracellularly into the medium or at local sites in which it grows; and (2) **endotoxins**, which consist of lipid and polysaccharide moieties that form part of the bacterial cell wall, i.e., LPS. Exotoxins account for some of the consequences of classic infectious diseases. Anthrax, for example, produces a potent toxin that can cause lethal hemorrhage and necrosis not by bacterial replication but by the elaboration of its exotoxin. Similarly, diarrhea in cholera is due to elaboration of an exotoxin by *Vibrio cholera* within the gastrointestinal tract, as the organism is not invasive. *Clostridium difficile* is another gastrointestinal infection commonly seen in patients receiving antibiotic therapy that induces its deleterious effect solely through its toxin production.

Certain strains of bacteria produce many exotoxins that, in turn, are associated with specific clinical entities. For example, staphylococcus produces a variety of exotoxins (A, B, C, D, E, F) that are

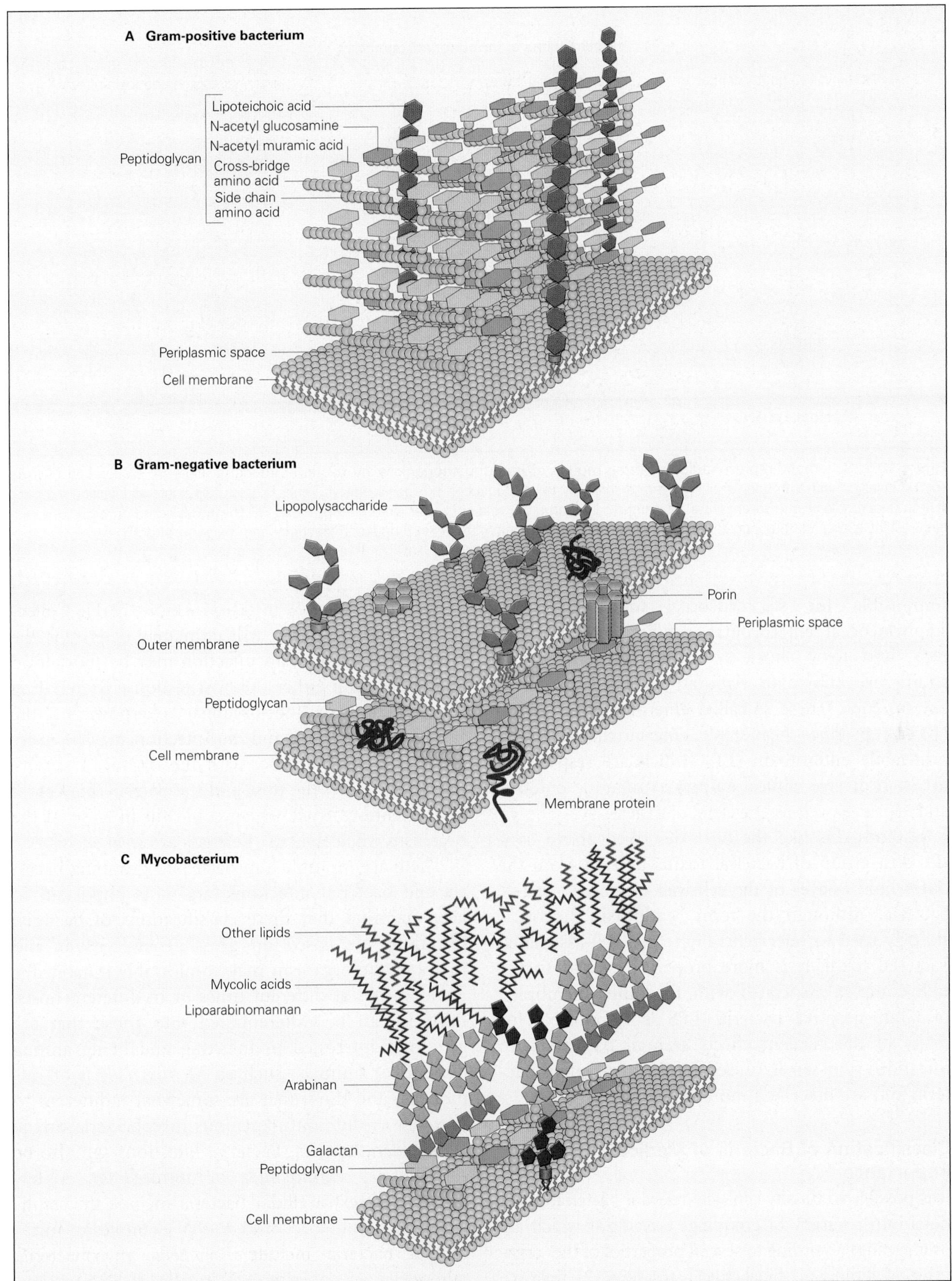

Figure 12-4. Schematic representation of different bacterial cell wall structures. Panel A: All bacteria have an inner lipoprotein cell membrane and a peptidoglycan wall. Panel B: Gram-negative bacteria also have an outer lipid bilayer in which lipopolysaccharide (LPS) is embedded. Panel C: Mycobacteria are abundant in lipid, particularly mycolic acid and glycolipids such as lipoarabinomannan.

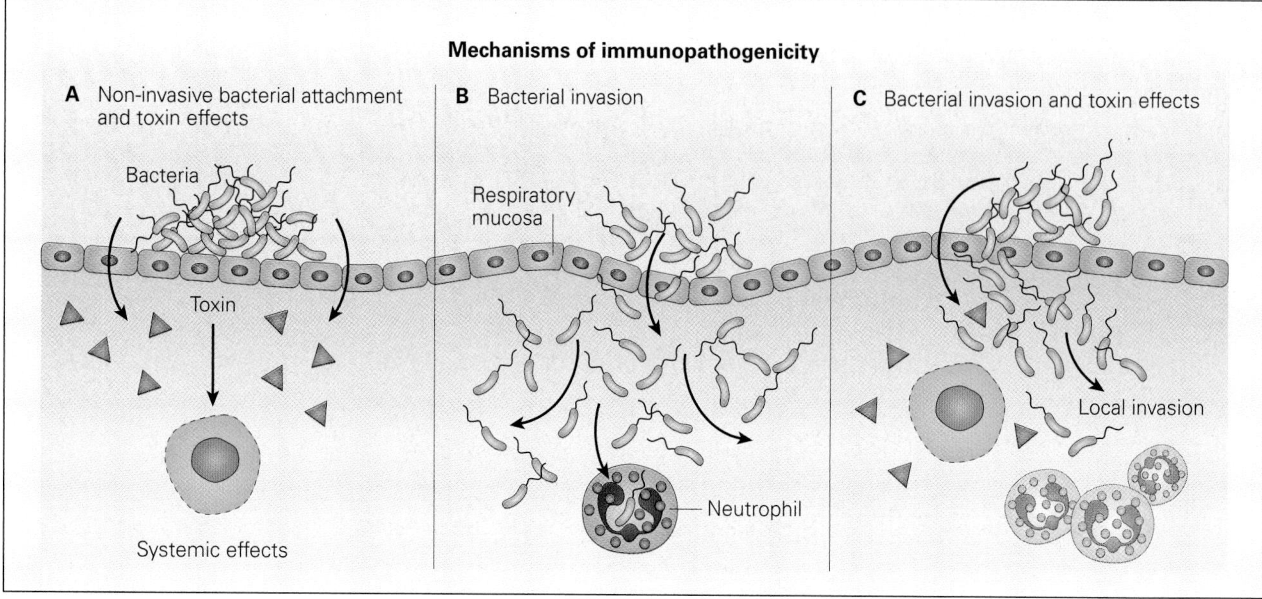

Figure 12-5. Schematic representation of three modes of immunpathogenicity by bacterial infection: Panel A: Elaboration of toxin and no invasion with immunopathology exerted solely by toxin production (toxigenic effect). Panel B: Exclusive bacterial invasion resulting in immunopathology due to an acute neutrophilic inflammatory response (bacterial effect). Panel C: The most common situation, with bacterial invasion and immunopathology resulting from inflammation and toxin production (bacterial and toxigenic effect).

responsible for staphylococcal food poisoning, staphylococcal enterocolitis, exfoliative skin disorders, and toxic shock syndrome. *Escherichia coli* strains are known to elaborate different classes of enterotoxins. These so-called enterotoxigenic *E. coli* (**ETEC**) produce heat-stable enterotoxin (**ST**) and heat-labile enterotoxin (**LT**), which are responsible for such diverse clinical entities as infantile enteritis and sepsis as well as travelers' diarrhea.

Enterotoxins like the ones described above consist of a group of bacterial toxins derived from the outer lipid bilayer of the cell wall of Gram-negative bacteria. Although the term "endotoxin" is occasionally used to refer generally to any cell-associated bacterial toxin, it is more properly reserved to the LPS complex associated with the outer membrane of Gram-negative bacteria. LPS is responsible for many of the virulent effects seen in patients with infections and sepsis caused by Gram-negative bacteria and are described more fully below.

Classification of Bacteria of Medical Importance

It is possible to classify clinically relevant bacterial infections into a variety of groupings (several of which are overlapping) according to several properties of the organism, including: (1) biochemical structure, (2) invasive properties (i.e., virulence), and (3) intracellular or extracellular sites of infection (Table 12-1). Collectively, these properties will ultimately determine the fate of an infection; an infection may be short-lived and acute, with either the host response terminating the infection or the organism overpowering the host. On the other hand, an infection may be more protracted and chronic, with the organism surviving. In this case, the host and the parasite may enter into a tenuous truce which could tilt in favor of the organism when the host defenses are weakened.

There are multiple approaches to grouping bacteria and bacterial infections, and it is important to keep in mind that these classifications of bacterial infections are based on gross generalizations and that any one organism may comfortably inhabit different camps at different times or in different hosts. Bacteria can be differentiated into those that are genuinely interested in infecting and living among humans or animals, such as *M. tuberculosis* or salmonella, and those that are somewhat indifferent to us, such as the nontuberculous mycobacteria or the *Burkholderia* species. Bacterial infections can also be classified as *extracellular* or *intracellular.* A few examples of extracellular bacteria include the staphylococci, streptococci, and *E. coli*; examples of intracellular bacteria include *Legionella*, mycobacteria, salmonella, mycoplasma, chlamydia, rickettsiae, spirochetes, and actinomycetes. Bacteria can also be

Table 12-1. Possible classifications of bacterial infections

Property	Example	Immunological mechanism
Biochemical	Cell wall structure	
	Lipoprotein cell membrane	Cationic proteins and complement
	Peptidoglycan cell wall	Lysosomal enzymes, lysozymes
	Capsule	Antibody and phagocytosis
Functional	Bacterial virulence (adhesins, hemolysins, proteases, toxins)	Antibody
Anatomic	Extracellular versus intracellular sites of infection	Antibody and phagocytosis Opsonic uptake (antibody and complement)

characterized according to their ability to cause acute infection, chronic infection, or toxin-associated infection (Table 12-2). Some of these categories can overlap, depending on the clinical and host situations. Toxins can be transferred among organisms, so that an organism (e.g., *S. aureus*) can be toxin negative at one point and then acquire toxin-production capacity at another point and cause toxic shock syndrome (*Chapter 3*). The knowledge of these various biochemical, structural, and physiologic properties of bacteria that lead to these classifications is crucial for an understanding of the various host immunological mechanisms that have evolved to destroy the different groups of bacteria (Table 12-2).

Host-Bacterial Relationships: Symbiosis, Commensalism, and Pathogenicity

To further expand on the classification of bacteria and the concept of pathogenicity, one needs to understand the development of the continuum of relationships between the host and parasite, which include symbiosis, commensalism, and pathogenicity (Figure 12-6). Symbiosis and commensalism are usually grouped under the general heading of mutualism. Opportunism is a collective term that refers to the balanced relationship between the microbe and its host. In this relationship the organism can sustain itself, invade the host, and cause infection but only cause disease when the defenses of the host immune system are diminished. An "opportunistic" infection is a clinical term that refers to those infections to which immunocompromised individuals (such as those with HIV/AIDS) are susceptible.

Symbiosis refers to the relationship between two different species where at least one partner benefits without harming the other. The production of vitamin K by *E. coli* in the gastrointestinal tract of the human is one example of symbiosis. The term "commensal" is derived from the medieval Latin term "commensalis," meaning "at table together,"

Table 12-2. Classification of bacterial diseases according to characteristics of the bacteria and host immune responses

Characteristics of the bacteria			Host immunity mechanisms				
			Innate immunity		Adaptive immunity		
					Antibody		
Type	Examples	Histopathology	Phagocytosis	Inflammatory response	Serum	Mucosal	CMI
Acute							
Localized	*S. aureus*	PMNs ("abscess")	+	+	+	?	?
	S. pyogenes						
Generalized	*N meningitidis*	Varied	+	+	+	+	?
Chronic	TB, leprosy, brucellosis	Macrophages (*"granuloma"*)	+ (NK cells)	+	−	−	++
Toxigenic	Diphtheria, tetanus, cholera	None (exotoxin)	−	−	+	+	−
	E. coli	Varied (exotoxin)	?	−/+	?	?	−

Note: The + and − denote the degree of involvement.

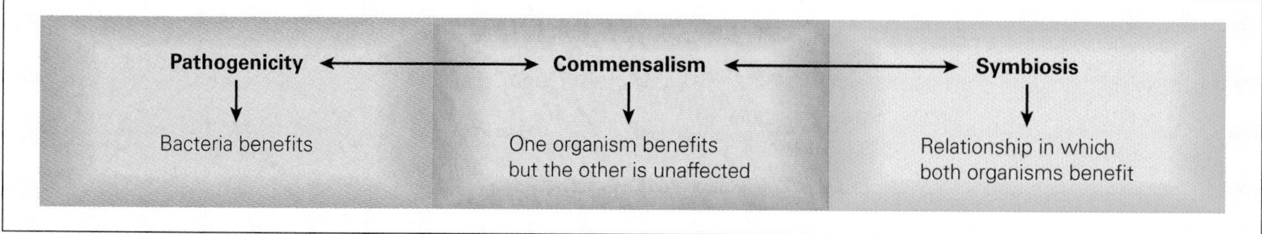

Figure 12-6. A schematic representation of the continuum between pathogenicity, commensalism, and symbiosis distinguished by the identification of specific benefits derived by one or both members of a host-bacterial partnership. Commensalism or symbiosis is a potential but not inevitable outcome of the dynamic coevolution of host-bacterial relationships.

and generally refers to partners that coexist without detriment but without obvious benefit to one another. Most of our bacterial symbionts and commensals reside in our gastrointestinal tract, where they play a key role in both the development and maintenance of the immune system. These bacteria are also involved in maintaining the homeostatic balance of the gastrointestinal mucosal immune system important in distinguishing harmful foreign invaders from more beneficial luminal inhabitants, i.e., commensal bacteria and food antigens required for nutrition (*Chapter 8*).

At the other end of the host-parasite continuum is a pathogenic relationship carried out by more virulent organisms that results in damage to the host where only the bacteria benefit (Figure 12-6). Symbiosis and commensalism have been viewed as potential outcomes of a dynamic "arms race" initiated when a pathogen encounters a vulnerable host. In this race, a change in one combatant is matched by an adaptive response in the other. In some settings, the arms race evolves toward attenuation of virulence of the organism and peaceful coexistence, with or without frank codependence (symbiosis) or commensalism. In other circumstances, the pathogenic relationship is sustained by the development of effective countermeasures of the bacteria that bypass the host's innate or adaptive defenses.

Commensal bacteria play an important role in providing the normal flora of the gastrointestinal tract. There is mounting evidence that commensals acquired during the early postnatal period are required for the development of tolerance, not only to themselves, but also to other luminal antigens, e.g., food antigens (*Chapter 8*). Commensal bacteria may directly influence the intestinal epithelium to limit immune activation. The mammalian gut must be sufficiently permeable to support efficient absorption of nutrients; at the same time, it must avoid potentially damaging immune responses to dietary proteins and pathogenic organisms. A breakdown of this delicate balance has been implicated in the development of allergic disease and autoimmune disorders in humans, e.g., Crohn's disease. Innate defenses, such as epithelial production of beta-defensins and mucins, also help prevent bacteria from crossing the mucosal barrier. Commensals can also limit pathogen invasion through the production of antibacterial proteins termed colicins. Additional protection is afforded by products of the adaptive immune system. Secretory immunoglobulin A (**sIgA**) directed against commensal antigens is specifically induced in the intestinal mucosa. In contrast to sIgA production by B cells in response to pathogen-derived epitopes, which requires costimulation by antigen-specific T cells, induction of sIgA against commensal antigens is T cell independent in mice (*Chapter 8*). This allows the host to respond to shifts in the commensal flora without eliciting a deleterious immune response.

Commensals may therefore occupy an ecological niche that would otherwise be occupied by organisms with more adverse outcomes. When the normal commensal flora is disturbed, as occurs with prolonged antibiotic usage, the overgrowth of other pathogenic organisms can take place, such as *Clostridium difficile*, a major cause of antibiotic-induced pseudomembranous colitis and diarrhea. Several studies suggest that the administration of nonpathogenic "probiotic" organisms such as lactobacilli can be useful in the management of this condition as well as in the treatment of some allergic conditions (*Chapter 18*).

Opportunistic microorganisms include bacteria, viruses or fungi that take advantage of certain opportunities, such as weakened host defense, to cause disease. These microorganisms often can lie dormant in body tissues for many years, such as the human herpes viruses (*Chapter 13*), or bacteria, fungi, or parasitic agents that are extremely common but typically nonpathogenic in the healthy host. When the immune system cannot respond adequately, these microorganisms can multiply and cause disease, e.g., HIV infection.

Virulence and Immune Response Evasion Factors of Bacteria: Adhesins, Anti-Phagocytic Factors, Toxins, Invasins, and Host Cell Alteration Factors

Bacterial pathogens have evolved complex and effective methods to overcome innate and adaptive immune mechanisms, which the host employs in bacterial defense and which will be described in greater detail below. The mechanisms used by the pathogen to evade the host's immune response include a number of strategies and specific bacterial factors that are shown in Table 12-3. Ironically, these mechanisms at times can achieve their evasion by interfering or blocking the host's immune responses while at other times attaining their survival advantage by co-opting, enhancing, or directing the defense mechanisms against the host. Although the various virulence strategies used by viral and bacterial pathogens are numerous, there are several general mechanisms that are used to subvert and exploit immune systems that are shared between these diverse microbial pathogens. The success of each pathogen is directly dependent on its ability to mount an effective anti-immune response within the infected host, which can ultimately result in acute disease, chronic infection, or pathogen clearance.

Mechanisms Used by the Pathogen to Evade the Host's Immune System

One of the principal ways that bacteria can evade the host immune response is by the secretion of modulators or toxins (Table 12-3). Many bacteria secrete toxins that can alter host cells and lead to disease manifestations. For instance, some bacteria secrete hemolysins that can lyse red blood cells, leading to anemia. Other bacteria produce proteases that through their proteolytic effects achieve a wide range of evasion strategies, such as cleavage of important host immune components, e.g., complement components and antibody. Although sIgA protects the mucosal surfaces against inhaled and ingested bacterial pathogens (*Chapter 8*), many pathogenic bacteria, such as *Haemophilus influenzae* and *Neisseria gonorrhoeae,* produce proteases that cleave IgA, making the molecule ineffective. The ability to drive bacterial molecules directly into host cells is another strategy used by several bacterial pathogens to subvert and overcome host defenses. *Mycobacterium tuberculosis,* for example, has developed a specialized secretion system that is needed to deliver major T cell antigens (ESAT-6 and CFP-10) into macrophages and presumably other proteins that are needed for bacterial replication inside these cells.

Since recognition of the exposed surfaces of bacteria provides the key interface between the bacterial pathogen and the immune system for initiation of microbial clearance, constitutively expressed bacterial surface structures or those modified by the bacteria through mutation represent yet another set of important mechanisms of immune subversion utilized by the bacteria. Examples of these include carbohydrate capsules, adhesins (fimbriae and pili), LPS with lengthy chain structures, hypervariability of O antigen of LPS, bacterial secretion systems, and enzymes that can modify antigenic expression of bacterial cell wall structures (Table 12-3). Another set of mechanisms used by bacteria to undermine immune clearance once the bacteria have breached these initial barriers is by subversion of the phagocytic pathways. This may occur either by avoidance of internalization or by interference of phagocyte killing by prevention of phagolysosome fusion (*Chapter 5*). This failure of phagosolysosome fusion has been shown to be particularly important for survival of the tubercle bacillus within infected macrophages. *M. tuberculosis* glycolipids can interfere with phagosome/lysosome fusion through blockage of a normal host-trafficking event that is regulated by phosphatidylinositol 3-phosphate (**PI3P**), a host-membrane component that is essential for phagolysosome biosynthesis. PI3P is believed to present a docking site for several proteins involved in the maturation of phagosomes into lysosomes. In uninfected cells, the generation of PI3P regulates the delivery of phagocytosed cargo to lysosomes. *M. tuberculosis* interferes with this trafficking event by actively preventing PI3P accumulation on phagosomal membranes and therefore thwarts the formation of the phagolysosome and assures its survival within infected macrophages.

The innate immune response may also be compromised by bacteria-blocking innate immune receptors as shown by Yersinia or Salmonella, or as in the case of *S. aureus* and *Shigella* with the blockage of cytokine activity resulting from the interference of binding of cytokines to their receptors. Bacterial pathogens have developed ways to avoid peptidoglycan processing and

Table 12-3. Anti-immune strategies of bacteria

Strategy	Factor	Mechanism
Secreted modulators or toxins	Many toxins	Host cells cytotoxicity
	Proteases	Degradation of complement or antibody by proteases (sIgA)
	ESAT6 and CFP10	T cell antigens injected into macrophages needed for intracellular replication
Bacterial molecular surface structures that prevent immune recognition	Carbohydrate capsules	Hides complex proteins and carbohydrates from immune recognition
	Adhesins (fimbriae and pili)	Enable bacterial invasion, preventing bacterial wall exposure to TLRs and other sensors
	Hypervariability of O antigen of LPS	Enables reinfection of the host by different strains of the same species
	Long chain LPS	Prevents complement deposition and MAC insertion into the bacterial membrane
	Bacterial secretion systems (T3SS and T4SS in Gram-negative and secretion systems of M. TB and pores formed by Gram-positives)	Export virulence factors into the environment or intracellular into the host cells, e.g., transport of substances to avoid phagolysosomal fusion
	PagL or 3-O-deacylase and PagP or palmitoyl-transferase of Salmonella	Lipid A modifiers
	Peptidoglycan hydrolases of Listeria	Cleavage of peptidoglycan from bacterial surfaces promoting NOD2 sensing to promote bacterial pathogenesis
Bacterial subversion of phagocytes	Yersinia proteins Yop H, E, O, and T	Avoidance of internalization during phagocytosis
	Shigella and Listeria lysins to escape from phagosome	Interference of phagocyte killing
	M. tuberculosis glycolipidis and carbohydrates to prevent phagolysosome fusion	Interference of phagocyte killing
	SifA effectors for Salmonella to alter Salmonella-containing vacuole composition	Interference of phagocyte killing
	IpaB and SipB of Shigella and Salmonella	Activate caspase-1 and increase inflammation, resulting in the spread of infection by infected phagocytes
	Lethal toxin of *B* anthracis	Cleaves MAPKK and blocks NF-κB activation in the phagocyte
Blockage of innate immune receptors	Virulence antigen of Yersinia (LCrV)	TLR2 and CD14 agonist that increases !L-10 and decreases inflammation
	PgtE protease of Salmonella	Cleaves defensins and cathelicidins (cationic peptides)
	Sap A-F of Salmonella	Removal of surface cationic peptides
	Spi2 in Salmonella-containing vacuole (SCV)	Inhibition of NADPH oxidative killing
Competitive inhibition of cytokines by bacteria	S aureus protein A	Activation of TNFR1
	OspG (type III secretion system) of Shigella	Inhibition of ubiquitin-conjugated enzymes leading to decreased degradation of IκB
Blockage of adaptive immunity	*H. pylori* LPS binding to C type lectin	Blocks Th1 development
	Binding of Vac A of *H. pylori* to IL-2R	Decreases NFAT and T cell activation
	Binding of Opa protein of *N. gonorrhea* to CEACAM1	Decreases CD4 T cell proliferation

Table 12-3. Anti-immune strategies of bacteria (continued)

Strategy	Factor	Mechanism
Manipulation of apoptotic cell death by bacteria	Production of T3SS of Chlamydia	Decrease apoptosis
	SopB/SigD of Salmonella	Inhibition of AKt/protein kinase with resultant decreased apoptosis
	SipB of Salmonella	Activation of caspase-1

recognition by NOD-like receptors (**NLRs**) using virulence strategies that block genes involved in peptidoglycan synthesis, turnover, and recycling. As described in *Chapter 9*, NOD1 and NOD2 are leucine-rich repeat (**LRR**) intracellular proteins that function analogously to TLRs to detect peptidoglycan inside host cells. Human NOD1 detects N-acetylglucosamine-N-acetylmuramic acid, a tripeptide motif characteristic of Gram-negative organisms, while NOD2 detects a N-acetylglucosamine-N-acetylmuramic acid dipeptide. Activation of either nucleotide-binding oligomerization domains (**NOD**) leads to NF-κB activation and inflammatory responses. Surface-located and secreted peptidoglycan hydrolases have also been identified that also function as virulence factors. These findings suggest that blockage of synthesis or cleavage of peptidoglycans represent bacterial virulence mechanisms that exploit NOD2 and the innate inflammatory response to promote bacterial pathogenesis.

The adaptive immune system can likewise be circumvented by blockage of Th1 development, diminution of nuclear factor of activated Tcells (**NFAT**) and T cell activation, and by inhibition of CD4 T cell proliferation by bacteria such as *H. pylori* or *N. gonorrhea*. One of the ultimate mechanisms of immune evasion by bacteria is their ability to manipulate apoptotic cell death by the inhibition of protein kinases or by activation of caspase-1 activity, as in the case of Salmonella (Table 12-3).

The Host Response to Bacterial Infection

Anatomic and Physiologic Barriers of the Innate Immune Response: Skin, Mucosa, and Secretions

As described in Chapter 1, even before the components of innate and adaptive immunity are summoned in response to an invading bacterium, anatomic and physiologic barriers are available to prevent the entry of the organism and establishment of infection (Figure 12-7). Mucosal and epithelial surfaces provide mechanical barriers against invasion by bacteria and other pathogens. In modern medicine, the majority of severe infection-predisposing conditions are iatrogenic, due to disruptions of these barriers through surgery, indwelling catheters, intubation, and associated alteration of the normal host flora brought about by antibiotic therapy. Additionally, fatty acids produced by the sebum in the skin are toxic to many bacterial organisms. Breaks in skin integrity, following burns for instance, allow local penetration of resident flora, such as *Staphylococcus aureus* or *Pseudomonas aeruginosa*, with establishment of severe infection. The oral mucositis that follows chemotherapy or radiotherapy similarly allows for local penetration of resident oral flora, leading to inflammation and pain. Although most of these oral organisms are not intrinsic pathogens, in the setting of a weakened host response, e.g., neutropenia, more severe disease may occur. Line infections are a common complication of long-term intravenous therapy, leading to bacteremia often caused by skin flora such as *Staphylococcus epidermidis*. These examples of breaks in epithelial integrity confirm the critical role that mechanical barriers play in protection.

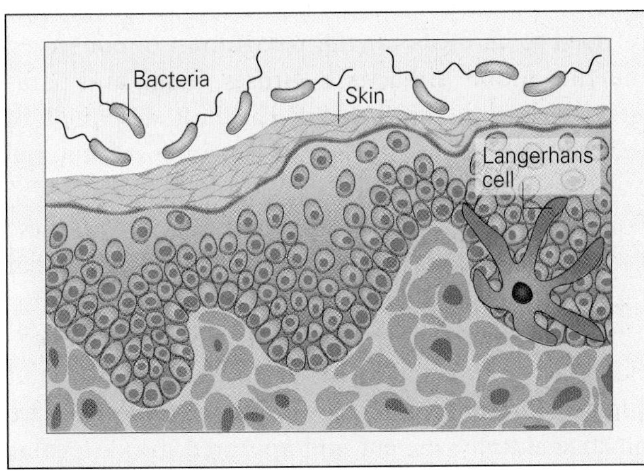

Figure 12-7. Schematic representation of the anatomic barrier to penetration by bacteria provided by the skin.

Mucosal surfaces such as those lining the respiratory passages are cleansed by the ciliary action of respiratory epithelia in the trachea or bronchi; when these functions are ablated, as in cystic fibrosis or ciliary immotile syndrome, conditions for bacterial infection are established. The gastric mucosa utilizes acid pH to inhibit bacterial growth. Conditions in which gastric acidity is ablated clearly predispose to increased rates of bacterial pneumonia in hospitalized patients, and increased rates of tuberculosis in countries where the disease is endemic. Skin cells also produce antibacterial peptides in high quantity, such as beta-defensins, as do bronchial epithelial cells. Tears and saliva contain lactoferrin, an iron-binding protein that inhibits bacterial growth by chelating iron, an essential growth factor for nearly all bacteria. Lactoferrin also plays an important intracellular antibacterial role within neutrophils (*Chapter 5*).

Innate Immune Factors

If bacteria overcome the mechanical barriers provided by the skin and mucous membranes, innate immune responses are activated next; these include **complement opsonization, phagocytosis** (*Chapter 4*), and the **inflammatory response** (*Chapter 5*). Bacterial products, the products of complement-mediated opsonization, and tissue activation lead to elaboration of chemokines and cytokines that attract neutrophils and macrophages to infected tissue sites from the circulation through the process of chemotaxis and diapedesis (*Chapter 1*). One of the most significant developments in immunology has been the definition of how the innate immune system functions at a molecular level. As described in Chapter 3, during the course of evolution, the innate immune system has developed receptors referred to as PRRs for the recognition of conserved moieties found in bacteria, viruses, fungi, and parasites referred to as PAMPs. The best described of the PAMPs are those associated with bacterial cell wall structures described previously (Figure 12-8). Following recognition of bacterial PAMPs by these PRRs, several signaling pathways are activated that result in the production of a wide variety of cytokines that contribute to both the protective beneficial and detrimental manifestations of innate and adaptive immune responses. These responses are phylogenetically ancient and appeared during evolution prior to the appearance of T and B lymphocyte components of the adaptive immune system (*Chapter 2*) and are found both on cells as well as in soluble proteins found in tissues and serum (Table 12-4).

Among the most important and best-studied PRRs are the Toll-like receptors (**TLRs**), which are a set of primary transmembrane proteins found on immune cells that serve as a key part of the innate immune recognition system (*Chapter 3*). TLRs are preferentially expressed on phagocytes, dendritic cells, and epithelial cells at critical sites of bacterial entry into the host. Each cell type can express a different combination of receptors, and this repertoire can be altered by inflammatory stimuli, allowing the greatest possible recognition coverage to a diverse range of pathogens (Figure 12-8). Shown in Box 12-1 are some of the historical milestones that led to the discovery of the TLRs. The better characterized bacterial cell wall structures and TLRs to which these bacterial ligands bind are summarized in Table 12-5. Their activation not only stimulates innate immune responses to these threats, but also leads to activation of the adaptive immune system, linking innate and acquired immune responses.

Evidence is mounting that TLRs are fundamental if not essential to an effective host response to microbial infection affecting both the innate and the adaptive immune systems. Moreover, the linkage between the innate and adaptive immune system is bidirectional. Not only does the innate immune system regulate the subsequent development of the adaptive immune system, but there is evidence in humans that the adaptive immune system can regulate the efficiency of the innate immune system. Cytokines secreted by T helper type 1 and 2 cells regulate the expression and function of TLRs on monocytes and dendritic cells, thereby affecting the clinical manifestations of disease (*Chapter 9*).

Since the success of vaccines depends on appropriate innate immune TLR activation, TLR ligands are sometimes used as adjuvants to improve the immunogenicity of vaccines (*Chapter 23*). Although TLR activation is likely to be essential for effective host defense against infectious pathogens, this activation may paradoxically contribute to the pathophysiologic manifestations of disease, including apoptosis-induced tissue injury, the manifestations of septic shock, and autoimmune disease (*Chapters 3* and *19*). Another recent application of the use of TLR ligands in boosting vaccine effectiveness has

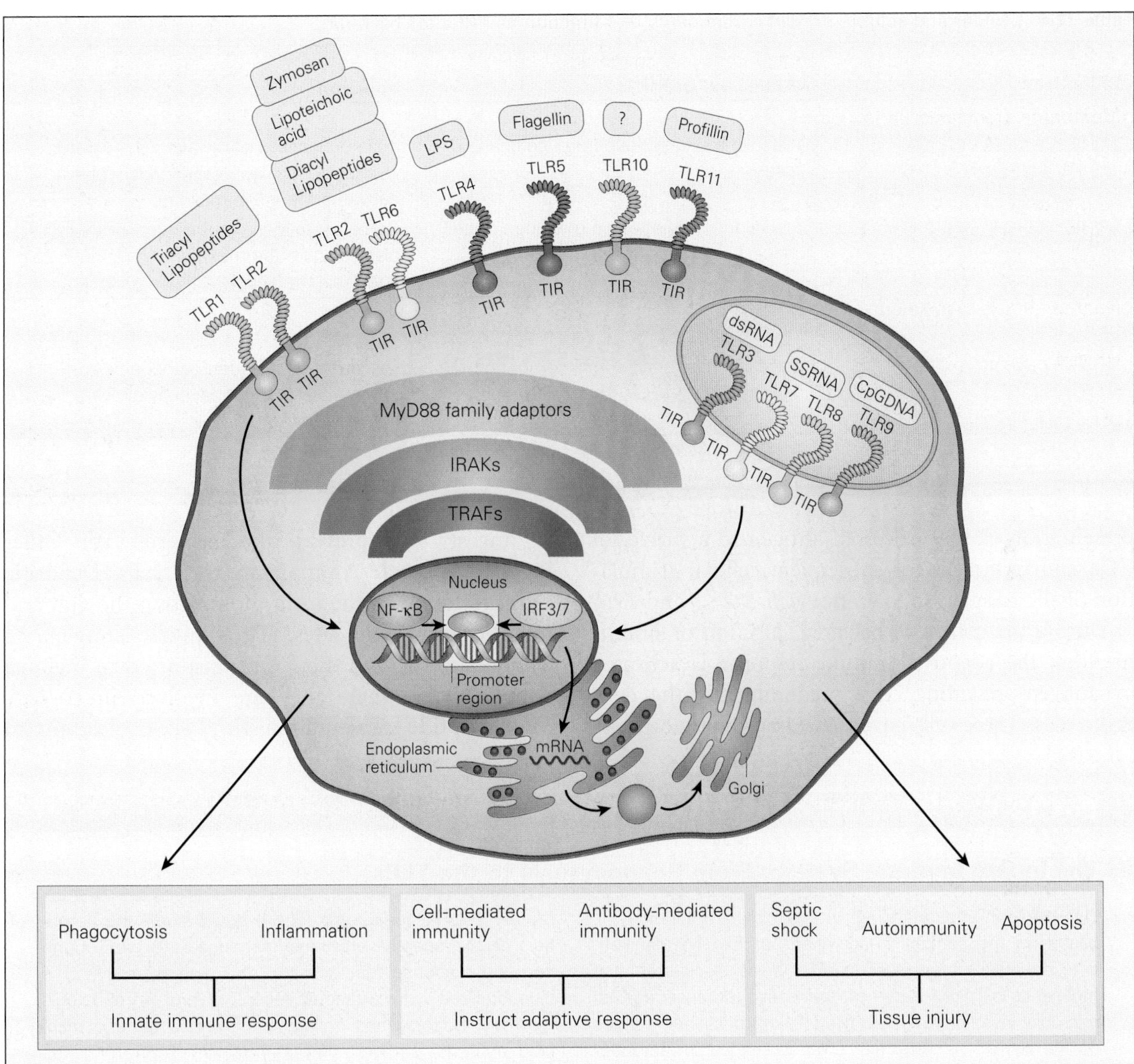

Figure 12-8. **Schematic representation of TLRs and their respective PAMPs.** Upon recognition of PAMPs by their extracellular, leucine-rich repeat domains, TLRs transduce signals by recruitment of MyD88 family members that help the recruitment of interleukin-1 receptor–associated kinases (IRAKs) and tumor necrosis factor receptor-associated factors (TRAFs) to form the initial signaling complexes. Different PAMPs associated with a variety of bacteria can induce these pathways with induction involved in specific beneficial biological functions in innate and adaptive immune responses as well as those that are detrimental and contribute to tissue injury.

been directed to their use in allergy immunotherapy (*Chapter 18*). A ragweed-pollen antigen vaccine conjugated to an immunostimulatory sequence of DNA containing a CpG motif that binds to TLR9 was shown to offer long-term clinical efficacy in the treatment of patients with ragweed-allergic rhinitis.

Adaptive Immune Factors

Following the activation of the innate immune system, the stage is now set for the mobilization of components of the adaptive immune system in the bacterial host cell interaction. Shown in Table 12-6 are the major lymphocyte domains of adaptive immunity, including the CD4 and CD8 populations together with their subpopulations of cells and functions. As described in Chapter 1 and in a subsequent segment of this chapter, these various cell components and cell products (i.e., cytokines) collaborate in a highly intricate network of responses beginning with the processing of antigens by antigen-presenting cells (predominantly dendritic cells) and subsequent

Table 12-4. Cellular and soluble protein components that function as PRRs for bacteria

PRRs	Danger-inducing ligands (PAMPs and DAMPS)	Function
Membrane associated PRRs		
Toll-like receptors (TLRs)	Molecular moieties found on bacteria and viruses	Initiate signaling pathways, e.g., NF-κB, to modulate gene expression; indirectly activates the inflammasome
C-type lectin receptors (CLRs)	Carbohydrate moieties on microbes or cell surfaces	Serve as antigen receptors on APCs but also regulate the migration of dendritic cells and their interaction with lymphocytes
Nonmembrane associated PRRs		
NOD-like receptors (NLRs)	Intracellular bacterial or viral components	Discriminate between pathogenic and commensal bacteria; directly activate the inflammasome

presentation of the processed antigen to a variety of CD4 and CD8 cells for subsequent cellular stimulation or silencing, as in tolerance (*Chapters 9* and *19*).

During the course of bacterial infection or immunization, the adaptive immune response is activated by antigen-presenting cells, predominantly the dendritic cells. These cells have the extraordinary capacity to ingest and present the bacterial (or other ingested) peptide components to T cells. Dendritic cells are found in the skin, the mucosa, the gut, and most other tissue sites. They ingest antigen, or whole bacteria, and then are transported to regional lymph nodes where they are involved in cognate MHC-peptide presentation to T cells, leading to

Box 12-1

The Innate Immune System: From Phagocytosis to the TLRs

Our present understanding of microbial immunology is based on the seminal observations of Elie Metchnikoff, who during his studies of starfish larvae discovered that mobile cells might serve in the host's defense against microbial invaders. In 1884, Metchnikoff published studies on the planktonic water flea *Daphnia magna* and its interaction with a yeast-like fungus. He found that cells of the water flea, which he termed phagocytes, were attracted to and engulfed the foreign spores. "The spores that reached the body cavity are attacked by blood cells and—probably through some sort of secretion—are killed and destroyed," he wrote. For this work, Metchnikoff received the 1908 Nobel Prize in Medicine.

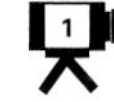

It took immunologists more than 100 years to work out the mechanism by which cells of the innate immune system rapidly recognize microbial invaders. In the mid-1990s, two key discoveries propelled our understanding of the mammalian innate immune system. The first came from the study of the genetic control of early embryonic development in *Drosophila* by Christiane Nusslein-Volhard, for which she received the 1995 Nobel Prize in Medicine. The second came from Medzhitov, Janeway, and colleagues who implicated the Toll protein in recognition of foreign microbes and in activation of host defense. They showed that a human homolog of the *Drosophila* Toll protein Toll-like receptor 4 (TLR4) could signal the activation of the adaptive immune response, the part of the immune response that consists of T and B cells and is characterized by rearranged receptors and immunologic memory. Poltorak and colleagues, using a genetic mapping analysis, showed that mammalian TLR4 mediates the recognition of LPS, a cell envelope component of Gram-negative bacteria.

These discoveries led immunologists to search for other ligands recognized by TLRs (Figure 12-8). Initial studies of TLR2 led to the finding that microbial lipoproteins trigger host responses through TLR2. TLR2/6 heterodimers mediate the response to diacylated lipoproteins, whereas TLR2/1 heterodimers recognize triacylated lipoproteins. Later studies showed that TLR9 is activated by unmethylated DNA sequences (CpG dinucleotides) found in bacterial DNA and that TLR5 is activated by bacterial flagellin. Specific TLRs are also involved in viral recognition (*Chapter 13*). TLR3 is activated by virus-derived double-stranded RNA and TLR7 and TLR8 by virus-derived single-stranded RNA. The finding that different TLRs have distinct patterns of expression, particularly on monocytes, macrophages, dendritic cells, B cells, endothelia, and epithelia, suggests that each TLR could trigger a specific host response.

Table 12-5. Summary of human TLRs

Receptor	Ligand(s)	Pathogen
TLR 1	Triacyl lipoproteins	Gram-negative bacteria, mycobacteria
TLR 2	Lipoproteins Lipoteichoic acids Lipoarabinomannan	All bacteria Gram-positive bacteria Mycobacteria
TLR 4	Lipopolysaccharides Lipopeptides	Gram-negative bacteria Gram-negative bacteria
TLR 5	Flagellin	Bacteria
TLR 6	Diacyl lipoproteins	Mycobacteria
TLR 9	Unmethylated CpG DNA	Bacteria

activation of B and T cell components of the adaptive immune response. Certain Gram-negative enteric bacteria stimulate antibody that is primarily of the IgM class. Furthermore, in certain localized infections (particularly those of the respiratory and gastrointestinal tracts), local IgA antibody synthesis occurs and is important for local bacterial defense (*Chapter 8*).

The host response to infection by bacteria or to immunization with bacterial antigens leads to a sequential appearance of specific antibodies. The antibody appearing initially is usually of the IgM variety and is followed by IgG, IgA, and IgE production. These differences, in order of appearance, reflect isotype switching of antibody from early IgM to later forms of isotypes with greater affinity (*Chapter 6*). On a molecular basis, IgM antibodies have greater relative opsonizing, bactericidal, and agglutinating capacities than IgG; the IgG antibodies, on the other hand, possess greater relative precipitating and neutralizing capacities (*Chapter 6*). The IgM formed early in the immune response appears to function best as an opsonin, facilitating and cooperating with the phagocytic events. IgM can immobilize bacteria by agglutination or, in the case of some Gram-negative bacteria, lyse cell walls with complement (*Chapter 4*). Since IgM is confined largely to the vascular compartment, it seems to be uniquely well suited to perform its function within the bloodstream. IgG antibody, on the other hand, can diffuse quite readily between vascular and extravascular compartments. IgG shows good precipitating capacity and is effective in neutralizing toxins.

Table 12-6. Components and functions of the adaptive immune system involved in the bacterial host cell interaction

Domain	Major components	Functions
CD4	Th1	Cell-mediated immunity
	Th2	Help B cells make antibody
	Th17	Promotes both mucosal beneficial antimicrobial peptide synthesis as well as detrimental inflammatory responses
	Th3 (Treg)	Downregulate excessive responses by IL-10 and TGF-β
CD8	T cytotoxic cells (Tc)	Destroy target cells, including infected macrophages

IgA in secretions appears to have a number of novel features that make it well suited to function at body surfaces (*Chapter 8*). Secretory IgA, in its dimeric form with an additional secretory component, is endowed with a unique stability and resistance to proteolytic cleavage, allowing it to function within the milieu in which other immunoglobulins would be degraded, such as in the gastrointestinal tract (*Chapter 8*). Some bacteria, such as *Neisseria gonorrhea*, are capable of degrading IgA. Upon subsequent encounter between a B cell and its cognate bacterial pathogen, there occurs a secondary or "rapid recall" that results in the elaboration of greater quantities of high titer IgG antibody, the so-called "booster" or secondary anamestic response (*Chapter 6*).

Certain bacterial infections induce immune responses carried out by several members of the CD4 helper and CD8 cytotoxic subpopulations (*Chapter 7*). These subpopulations, e.g., Th1, contribute to bacterial clearance, the promotion of inflammation, e.g., Th17, or the suppression of an overactive T cell response, e.g., Treg cells (Table 12-6). These T cell responses are seen most prominently in intracellular chronic infections such as tuberculosis.

Collaboration of Innate and Adaptive Immune Responses

The wide variety of pathogenic infections caused by bacteria is countered by an equally diverse set of innate and adaptive immune responses of the host. Successful immunity must be a concerted effort between the various immune responses, working in stepwise fashion to address, contain, or kill bacterial invaders. The contribution of the various components of the innate and adaptive immune responses will vary during the course of acute, chronic, and toxigenic bacterial infections, as described below.

If a bacterium breaks through the host's anatomic and physiologic barriers, it will first encounter tissue macrophages and dendritic cells that are not particularly well suited for initial clearance of bacteria. The most effective response to an acute bacterial infection is triggered by neutrophils (i.e., polymorphonuclear leukocytes [**PMNs**]) that are summoned by bacterial factors such as formyl methionyl-leucyl-phenylalanine (**fMet-Leu-Phe**), complement components (C3a and C5a), and chemokines that promote their emigration from the vascular compartment into tissues (Figure 12-9).

When neutrophils encounter the bacteria, they usually ingest it into a phagolysosome and degrade the microbe (*Chapter 5*). This process is typically effective and leads to the cardinal signs of inflammation, i.e., *calor* (heat), *dolor* (pain), *rubor* (erythema), and *tumor* (swelling). Some encapsulated bacteria, such as pneumococcus, however, are capable of resistance to efficient phagocytosis by virtue of their capsules, and this may contribute to their increased pathogenicity; however, with the subsequent development of antibody (an effective opsonin) and opsonic complement component C3b, the pneumococci are opsonized and phagocytosis is then facilitated (Figure 12-10).

If the bacteria are not successfully killed at local sites, they may continue to replicate locally or further invade the host by way of the lymphatics to the regional lymph nodes or the bloodstream to the spleen (Figure 12-11).

The well-known red streaks that extend up the arm (lymphangitis) with enlarged regional (e.g., epitrochlear or axillary) lymph nodes or an enlarged spleen (splenomegaly) are examples of regional and systemic spread of the invading bacteria into

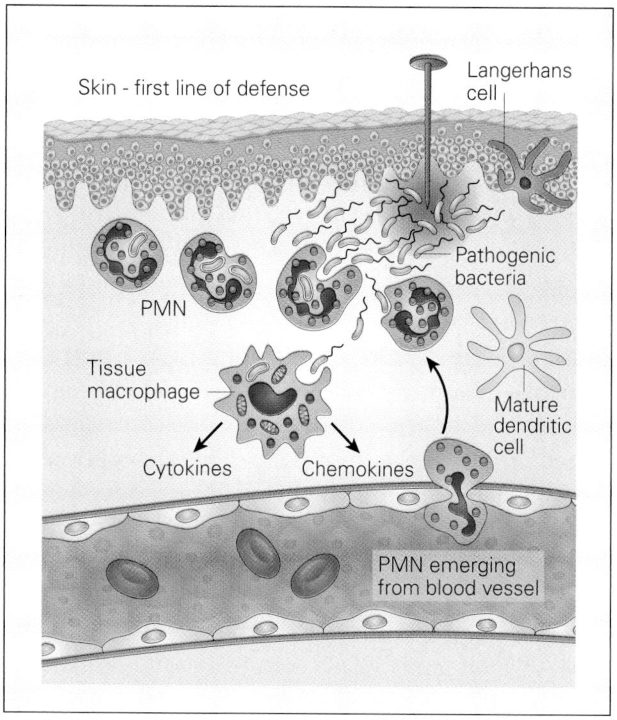

Figure 12-9. Schematic representation of phagocytosis by polymorphonuclear leukocytes (PMNs) and tissue macrophages following penetration of the skin and introduction of pathogenic bacteria into deeper tissues. The PMNs are more efficient in phagocytosis than are the macrophages. Note that the PMNs are mobilized into tissues from blood vessels during the inflammatory response.

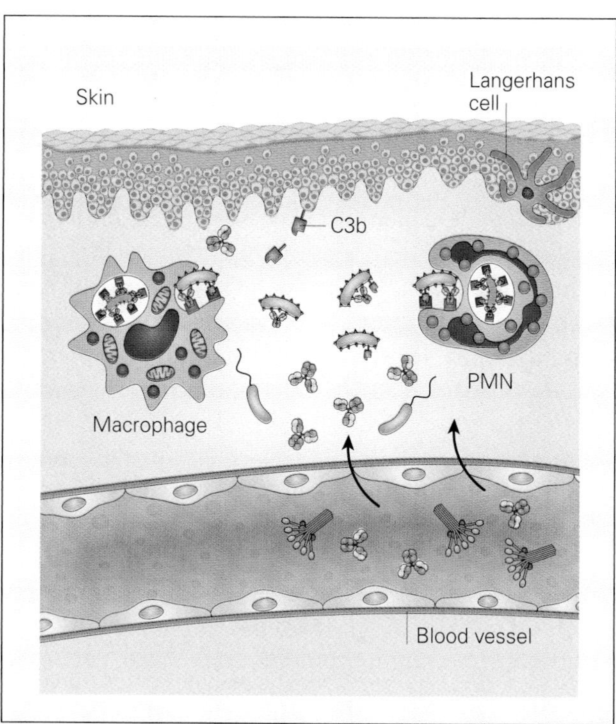

Figure 12-10. Schematic representation of the enhancement of phagocytosis occurring with the development of specific antibody together with the participation of complement (C3b) as opsonins. IgG and intact complement are shown as opsonins in the blood; in tissue, C3b can be generated from the innate response (lectin and/or alternative pathways) or from the adaptive (IgM and/or IgG-activated classical pathway).

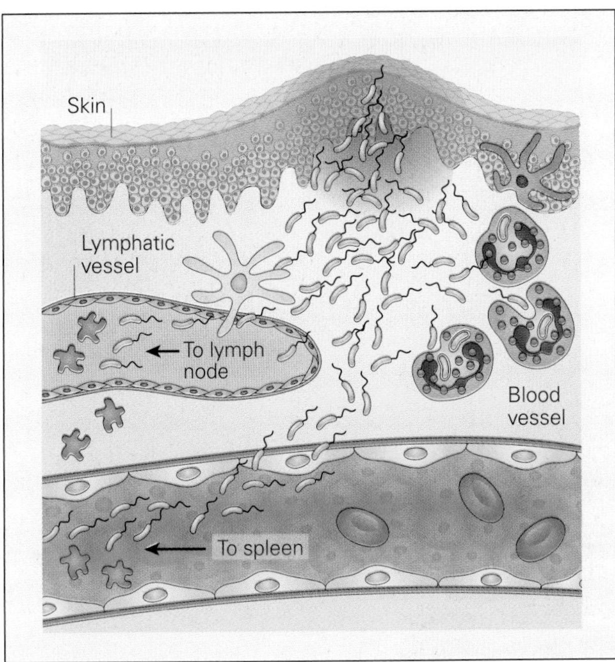

Figure 12-11. Schematic representation of the cellular events occurring if the PMN leukocytes are unsuccessful in killing the bacteria. The organisms are shown replicating in the tissues and entering a lymphatic channel and blood vessel.

lymphatic vessels or bloodstream, respectively. When bacteria or bacterial products enter lymph nodes via the lymphatics or the bloodstream, they encounter macrophages and dendritic cells that will attempt again to ingest, degrade, and present peptide fragments to naive Th0 lymphocytes by cognate interactions, and after their activation into various T helper subsets, initiate the development of subsequent humoral and cell-mediated adaptive immune responses (Figure 12-12).

The Interactive Antibacterial Protective Mechanisms in Acute, Chronic, and Toxigenic Bacterial Infections

The compartments of the immunologic system work in concert so that, when the innate immune defense mechanisms of the host have been surmounted and specific adaptive immunologic responses have been engaged, the products of the latter enhance the former. These mechanisms vary according to the previously described patterns seen in acute, chronic, or toxigenic bacterial infections.

Acute Bacterial Infections

Acute bacterial infections can be produced by many bacteria, but classic examples include the staphylococci and streptococci, bacteria that cause infections globally and with high frequency (Table 12-2). These Gram-positive bacteria display a propensity for attachment to skin and mucous membranes, making possible their transfer between and their long-term domicile in humans. Staphylococci often cause skin infections, typically initiated by a break in the epithelium, leading to local bacterial replication. As described previously, the release of bacterial protein products (fMet-Leu-Phe) together with host chemotactic factors, i.e., C3a, C5a, and chemokines, leads to the chemotaxis of host neutrophils with resultant inflammation (*Chapter 5*).

Shown in Figure 12-13 are two types of mechanisms of bacterial clearance by phagocytes that are related to the virulence of an invading extracellular acute disease-producing bacterium. Nonencapsulated organisms are readily phagocytosed by neutrophils in an opsonin-unenhanced fashion and are readily killed. In contrast, encapsulated organisms are often poorly ingested by neutrophils alone; however, with the production of antibody and complement opsonization, phagocytosis by neutrophils is greatly enhanced and subsequent killing is permitted. Although T cell-mediated immune mechanisms can enhance phagocytosis by macrophages, since such organisms are not regularly phagocytosed by macrophages, this scheme normally appears to be of relatively lesser importance (Figure 12-13). If the inflammation progresses, it creates a lake of dead neutrophils (pus) with surrounding wall formation, i.e., an abscess, and with the persistence of sequestered bacteria, the inflammation can progress to chronicity with the clinically perplexing sequelae of tissue injury and necrosis, as seen in the case presentation. As described previously, bacteria are made more attractive for neutrophils by host components called opsonins that allow for easier neutrophil attachment to and ingestion by these cells. Some of these opsonins are preformed, such as complement or mannose-binding lectin (*Chapter 4*). Other opsonins include antibodies that are derived from previous experience with the organism; these provide a unique and highly efficient set of molecules that make subsequent encounters with bacteria more efficient as a result of the enhanced quantity and affinity of the antibody produced during the secondary immune response (*Chapters 1* and *6*). Although the early phases of the encounter of bacteria determine whether the infection is contained to the skin and superficial tissues (as is almost always the case), the

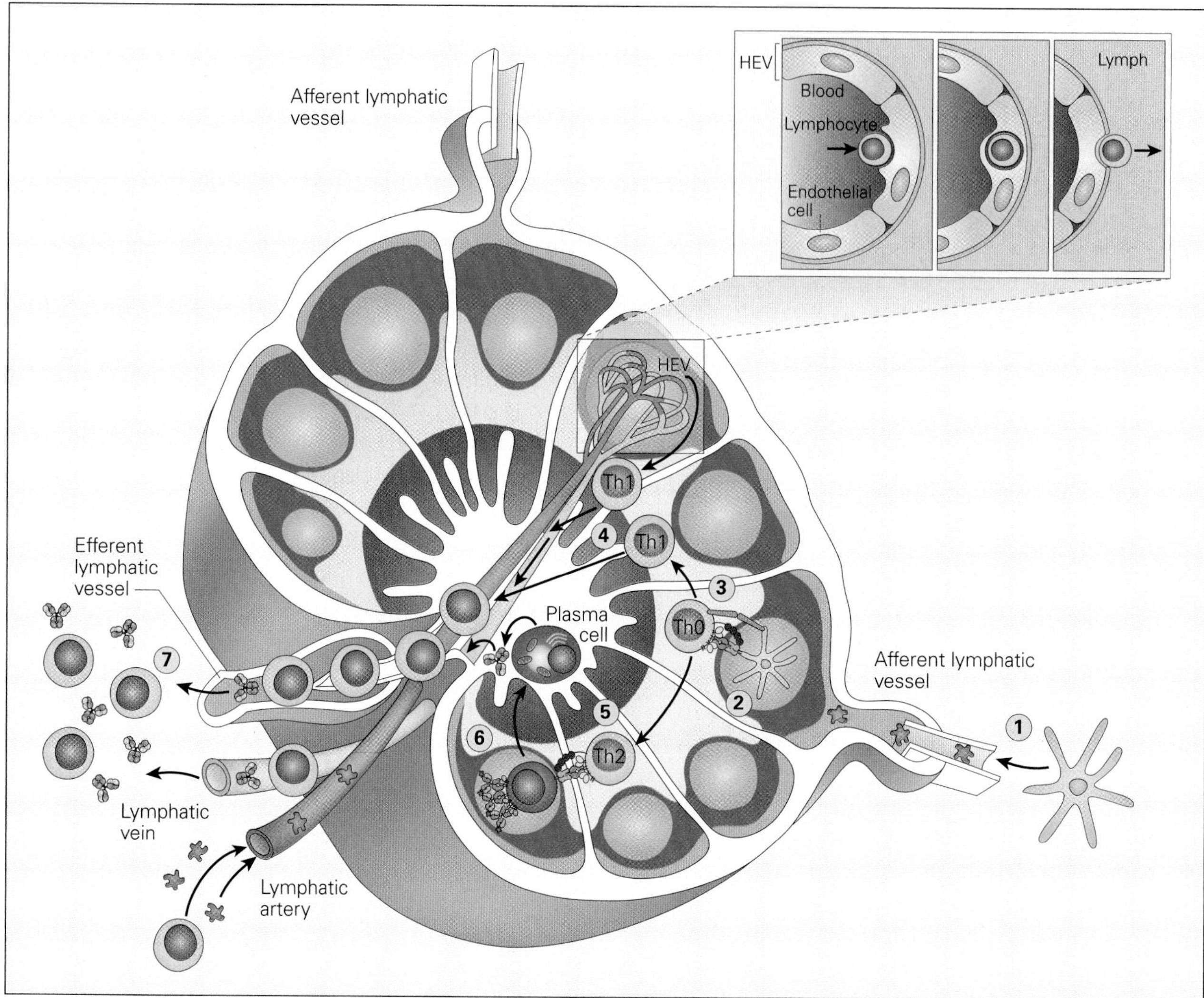

Figure 12-12. Schematic representation of induction of the adaptive immune responses in a lymph node with elaboration of cell-mediated immune responses and antibody. After bacteria or bacterial products enter lymph nodes via the lymphatics (1) or the bloodstream (2), they encounter macrophages and dendritic cells that will attempt again to ingest, degrade, and present peptide fragments to naive Th0 lymphocytes by cognate interactions (3), and after their activation into various T helper subsets, initiate the development of subsequent Th2/B cell-interactive humoral (4). Th1 cell-mediated adaptive immune responses are also generated from Th0 precursors or may enter from the blood into lymph via the post-capillary high endothelial venules (HEV) (5). Antibody subsequently produced by plasma cells as well as activated Th1 lymphocytes leave the lymph node through the efferent lymphatic vessels (7).

infection will be capable of spreading locally or systemically. If this happens, the organism triggers a complex set of responses that are sometimes called the systemic inflammatory response syndrome (**SIRS**) (*Chapter 3*).

Chronic Bacterial Infections

Protracted or chronic bacterial infections are often caused by organisms that have an intracellular phase; this requires that they are adept at the penetration, evasion, and exploitation of the host immune responses. The classic example of a chronic bacterial infection is seen with *Mycobacterium tuberculosis*, the causative organism of tuberculosis. These bacteria invade the host and set up a long-standing relationship by killing some cells and chronically infecting others, eliciting an unstable detente with host immunity that is typically detected only indirectly by demonstration of an antigen-specific tuberculin skin test (**TST**) in response to antigens derived from *M. tuberculosis*, known as purified protein derivative (**PPD**) (*Chapter 7*). Shown in Figure 12-14 is a schematic representation of three outcomes of the interaction of a

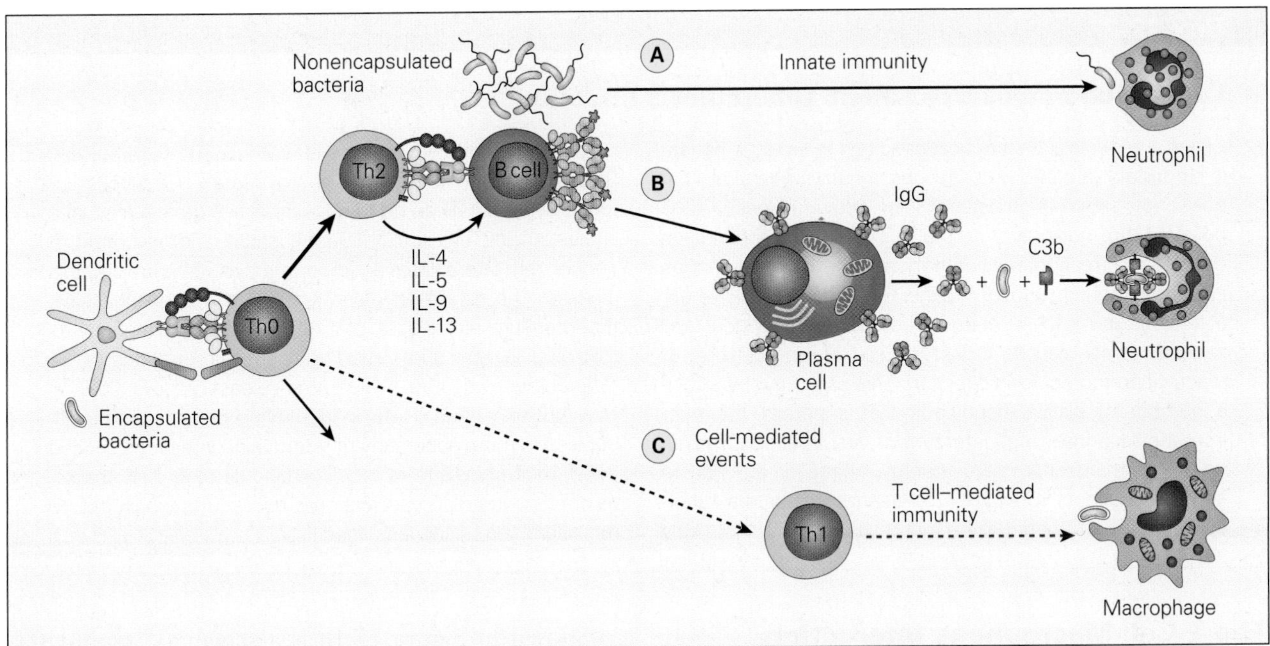

Figure 12-13. Schematic representation of relative roles of antibody and cell-mediated events in the enhancement of phagocytosis in acute bacterial infections. Panel A: Phagocytosis of an unencapsulated organism through an unenhanced process. Panel B: The enhanced process of phagocytosis through antibody and complement. Panel C: The relatively lesser important role of cell-mediated immune (CMI) events during acute infection. Note the interrelationship of antibody and phagocytosis by PMNs and its relatively greater importance than CMI events during acute bacterial infections.

mycobacterium and a macrophage, illustrating either killing of the organism by the macrophage (Figure 12-14A), killing of the macrophage by the organism (Figure 12-14B), or survival of both the organism and the cell, as seen in chronic infection (Figure 12-14C). This third interaction between the host and the tubercle bacillus is thought to be the basis for latent tuberculosis infection (**LTBI**), which establishes an armistice between the host and the bacterium that can be broken, as seen by reactivation of the active infection at a later point in life, when the balance is tipped in favor of the bacterium (Figure 12-3 and Box 12-2).

Shown in Figure 12-15 are two types of mechanisms of bacterial clearance by phagocytes that are related to the virulence of an invading intracellular chronic disease-producing bacterium, such as the tubercle bacillus. In contract to the scenario seen with acute infections described above, these organisms are not readily phagocytosed by opsonin-dependent uptake by neutrophils, but because of their intracellular location within macrophages, T cell-mediated immune mechanisms that enhance phagocytosis and intracellular killing by macrophages are of crucial importance. This pathway is of greater importance than the opsonin-mediated pathway in these types of chronic bacterial infections.

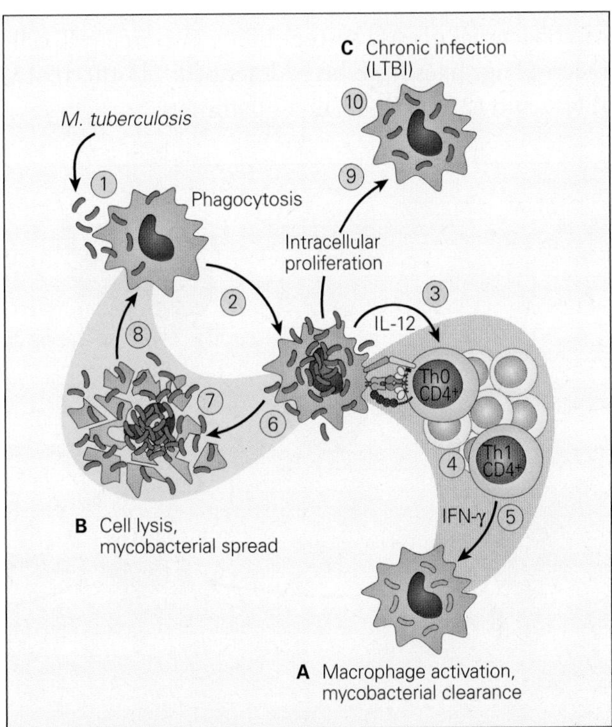

Figure 12-14. Schematic representation of three modes of interaction of the tubercle bacillus with a macrophage. Panel A: The macrophage kills the organism. Panel B: The organism kills the macrophage. Panel C: The organism takes up residence in the macrophage and establishes chronic infection, where both the tubercle bacillus and macrophage can survive together in a tenuous chronic infection.

Box 12-2

Latent Tuberculosis or Latent Tuberculosis Infection

Latent tuberculosis is a clinical condition in which a patient is chronically infected with *Mycobacterium tuberculosis* but does not show manifestations of active disease. It is believed (but not proven in the human) that the condition develops from an interaction between the tubercle bacillus and a macrophage shown in panel C of Figure 12-14, where a tenuous armistice is established between the host and parasite, which can be broken in later life in the form of reactivation tuberculosis infection. This can occur by any of a number of clinical conditions that suppress the host immune response, e.g., intercurrent viral infection, malnutrition, immunosuppressive therapy, aging, or the use of anti-TNF-α agents (*Chapter 11*). Patients with latent tuberculosis are not thought to be infectious, and it is not likely to contract TB from someone with latent tuberculosis. Since the main risk is that approximately 10 percent of these patients will go on to develop active tuberculosis at a later stage of their life, the identification and treatment of people with latent TB is an important part of controlling this disease. The recent development of highly specific assays that measure the release of IFN-γ from blood lymphocytes following *in vitro* stimulation with specific peptides of *M. tuberculosis*, i.e., the IFN-gamma release assays (IGRAs) have not only been useful in identifying patients with LTBI, but also in more accurately differentiating infections caused by *M. tuberculosis* from those caused by other mycobacteria or following BCG vaccination (*Chapter 23*), which can be misdiagnosed by the less specific TST.

The T Cell-Macrophage Interaction

Having presented the importance of the T cell-macrophage interaction in chronic bacterial infection, it may now be possible to describe some of the important recent genetic and molecular discoveries that have contributed to a better understanding of human mycobacterial disease susceptibility. Two major T cell-macrophage axes have been described: (1) the IL-12/IFN-γ and (2) the IL-23/IL-17 pathways.

Shown in Figure 12-16 is a schematic representation of the IL-12/IFN-γ axis. As can be seen, there are many T cell-macrophage-interactive cytokine pathways involved in chronic bacterial microbicidal activity. Deficiencies in any of these cytokine pathways have been described that contribute to increased mycobacterial disease susceptibility. Disruptions of the IL-12/IFN-γ pathway, such as mutations of the IFN-γ receptor, IL-12 receptor b1 (IL-12Rb1), and IL-12 p40 genes have been recognized (*Chapter 9*).

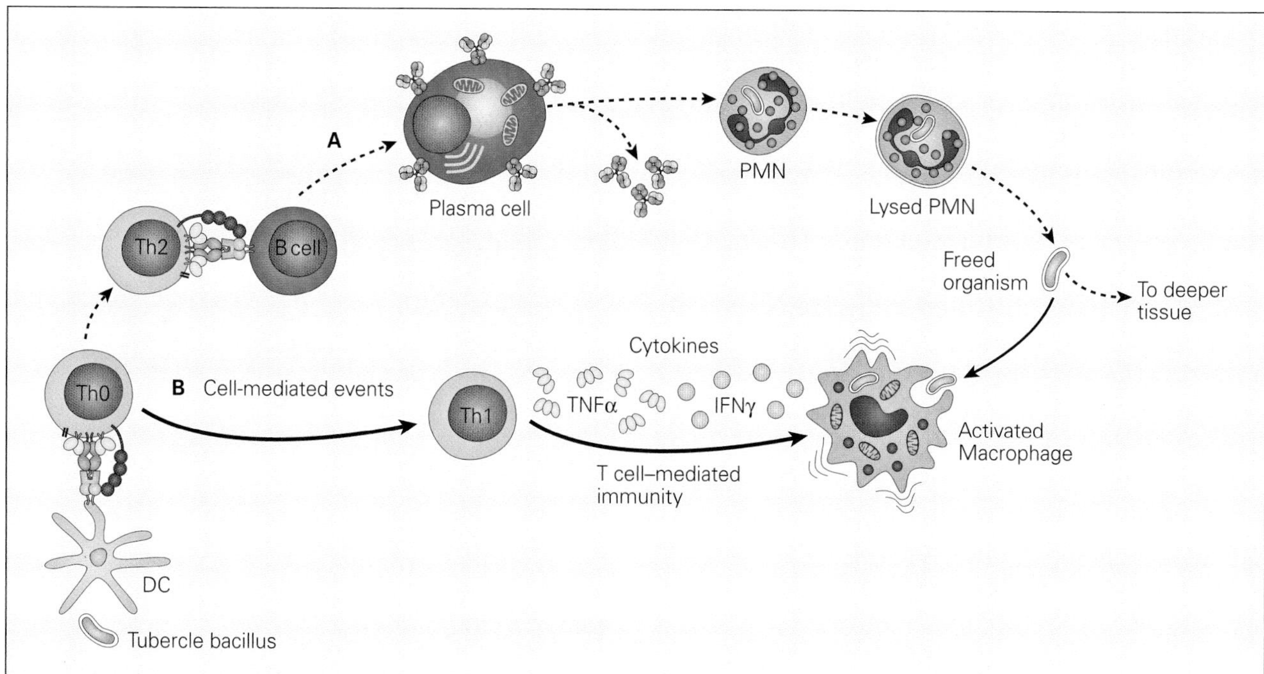

Figure 12-15. Schematic representation of the relative roles of antibody and cell-mediated events in the enhancement of phagocytosis during *chronic* bacterial infections. Panel A: PMNs show limited microbicidal activity. Panel B: The major cellular response in chronic infection is carried out through cytokine-induced stimulation of macrophages by TNF-α and IFN-γ.

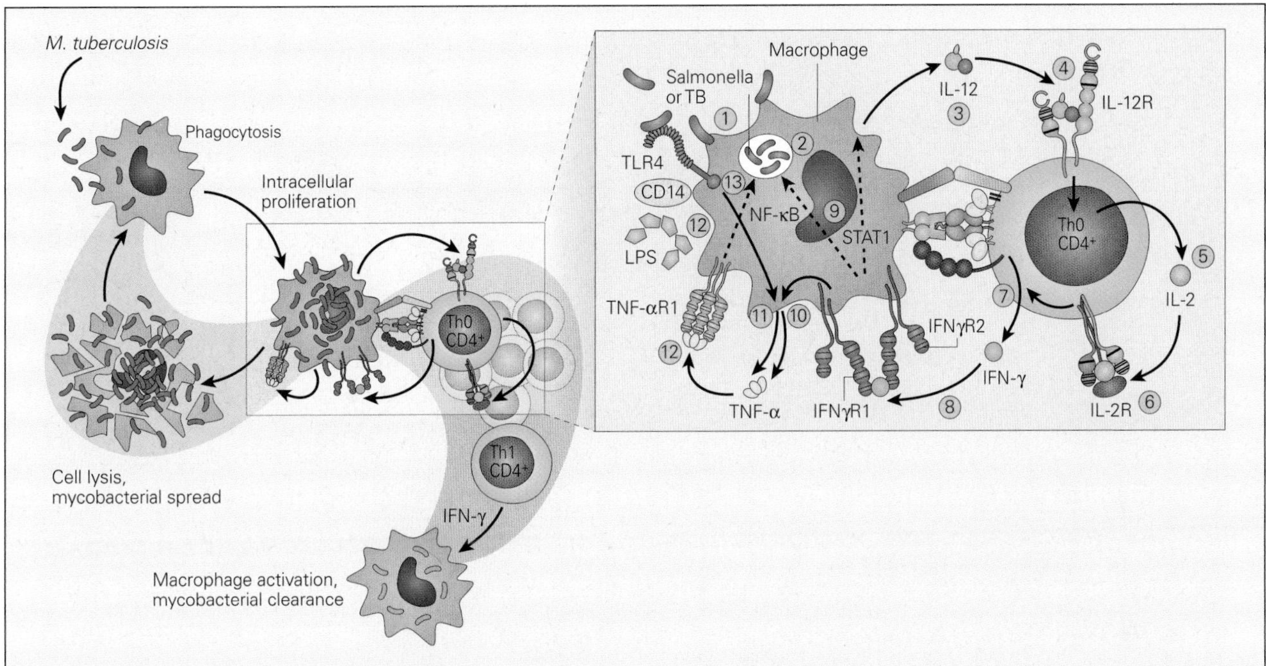

Figure 12-16. Schematic representation of the IL-12/IFN-γ pathway illustrating various activation pathways associated with the killing of intracellular bacterial organisms such as *M. tuberculosis* (TB) and *Salmonella*. Following the uptake of the TB by the macrophage (1) into a phagosome (2), the macrophage is stimulated to produce IL-12 (3). The binding of IL-12 to its IL-12R on a Th CD4+ cell (4) induces the synthesis of IL-2 (5), and after autocrine binding of IL-2 to its IL-2R (6) leads to the synthesis of IFN-γ (7). The binding of IFN-γ to its receptor (8) activates both the STAT1 and NF-κB pathways (9) to kill the TB and to further enhance IL-12 production; the IFN-γ-activated macrophage (10) and TLR4 activation by the TB (11) induce TNF-α production that, after binding to its receptor (12), leads to further enhancement of intracellular killing of the TB (13).

These mutations are associated with heightened susceptibility to disease caused by intracellular pathogens, including nontuberculous mycobacteria, vaccine-associated Bacille Calmette Guerin (**BCG**), Salmonella species, and some viruses. Shown in Figure 12-17 is a photograph of an infant with complete IFN-γR1 deficiency vaccinated with BCG who developed dissemination of the BCG (i.e., BCGosis) as a result of this deficiency.

The second T cell-macrophage axis important for the maintenance of normal bacterial clearance is the IL-23/IL-17 pathway shown in Figure 12-18. This pathway is particularly important at mucosal surfaces. IL-23 exerts its effects by activation of Th17 cells. The subsequent production of cytokines by these cells has opposing beneficial and detrimental effects; the production of IL-22 and IL-17 leads to the generation of antimicrobial peptides by epithelial cells, while IL-17 can also increase granulocyte production and influx, promoting inflammation. The IL-23/17 axis appears to not only play an important protective role in antibacterial and antifungal immunity (*Chapter 14*), but also is an important regulator of immune responsiveness in various inflammatory diseases, e.g., Crohn's disease, arthritis, and allergic airway inflammatory disease.

Granuloma Formation

The T cell-macrophage balance is further maintained by the creation of a structure referred to as a

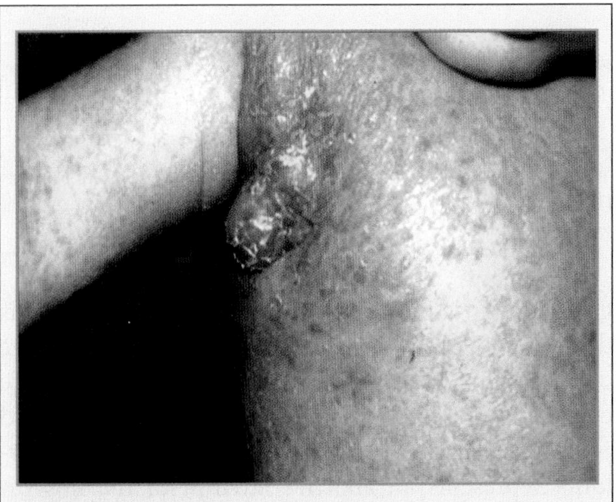

Figure 12-17. Photograph of an infant with complete IFN-γR1 deficiency who was vaccinated with BCG and who developed dissemination of the BGC (BCGosis) as a result of a defect of the IL-12/IFN-γ pathway. The deficiency permitted the spread of the BCG infection to a regional lymph node with suppurative inflammation swelling and erythema in the right axilla. (Courtesy of Dr. Sergio Rosenzweig.)

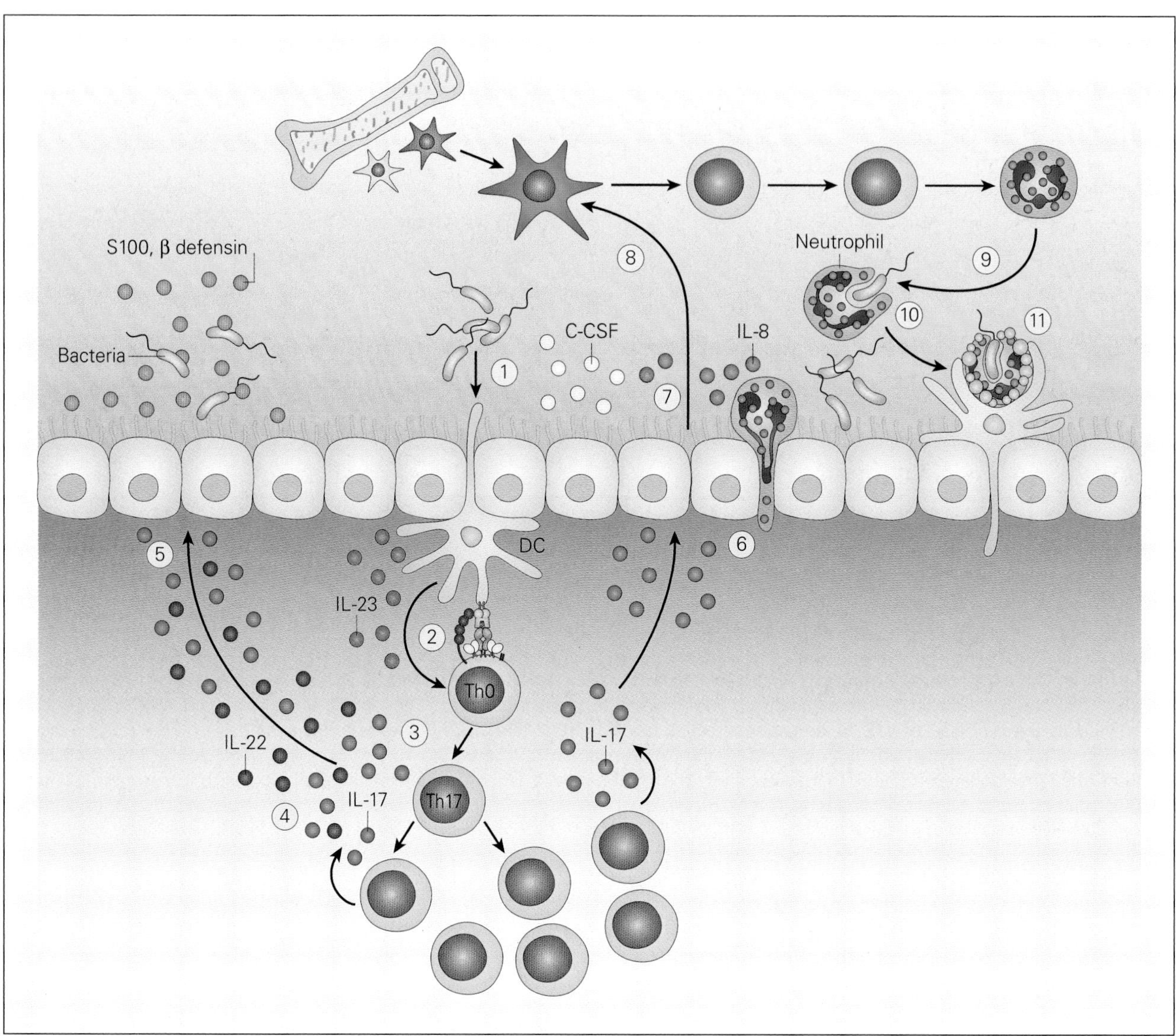

Figure 12-18. Schematic representation of the IL-23/17 axis involved in host antibacterial defense at a mucosal surface. Mucosal dendritic cells activated by bacterial pathogen (1) produce IL-23 (2), which then activates the production of resident memory Th17 cells from naive Th0 cells (3) to produce IL-17 and IL-22 (4), which then induce epithelial cells to secrete antimicrobial peptides, e.g., β-defensins and S-100 proteins (5). IL-17 also induces epithelial cells (6) to produce granulopoietic and chemotactic factors, e.g., G-CSF, IL-8 (7), which then leads to bone marrow granulocyte production (8). The granulocytes then home to the mucosal surface (9), where they phagocytose bacteria (10) and following their apoptotic cell death, their resultant apoptotic fragments are phagocytosed by dendritic cells (11).

granuloma (*Chapter 5*). The term "granuloma" is derived from the anatomical "granular" appearance of the lesions on gross examination and is a structure consisting mainly of epithelioid macrophages and other inflammatory and immune cells. The granuloma represents an abortive attempt of the host to wall off a foreign substance that can neither be killed nor completely eliminated. The formation of a granuloma is highly dependent on pro-inflammatory cytokines, e.g., TNF-α and IFN-γ (Figure 12-19). However, when the T cell-macrophage balance of the granuloma is disturbed by immune suppression, illness, malnutrition, or old age, organisms emerge and enter a replicative stage, resulting in reactivation of chronic infection, e.g., reactivation tuberculosis. A specialized form of immunosuppression has recently been recognized with the current availability and usage of biologic immunomodulators such as anti-cytokine preparations (*Chapter 11*). The increasing use of anti TNF-α preparations, for example, for the treatment of rheumatoid arthritis and other inflammatory conditions has unfortunately led to reactivation of chronic infections such as tuberculosis and fungal infections (Figure 12-20).

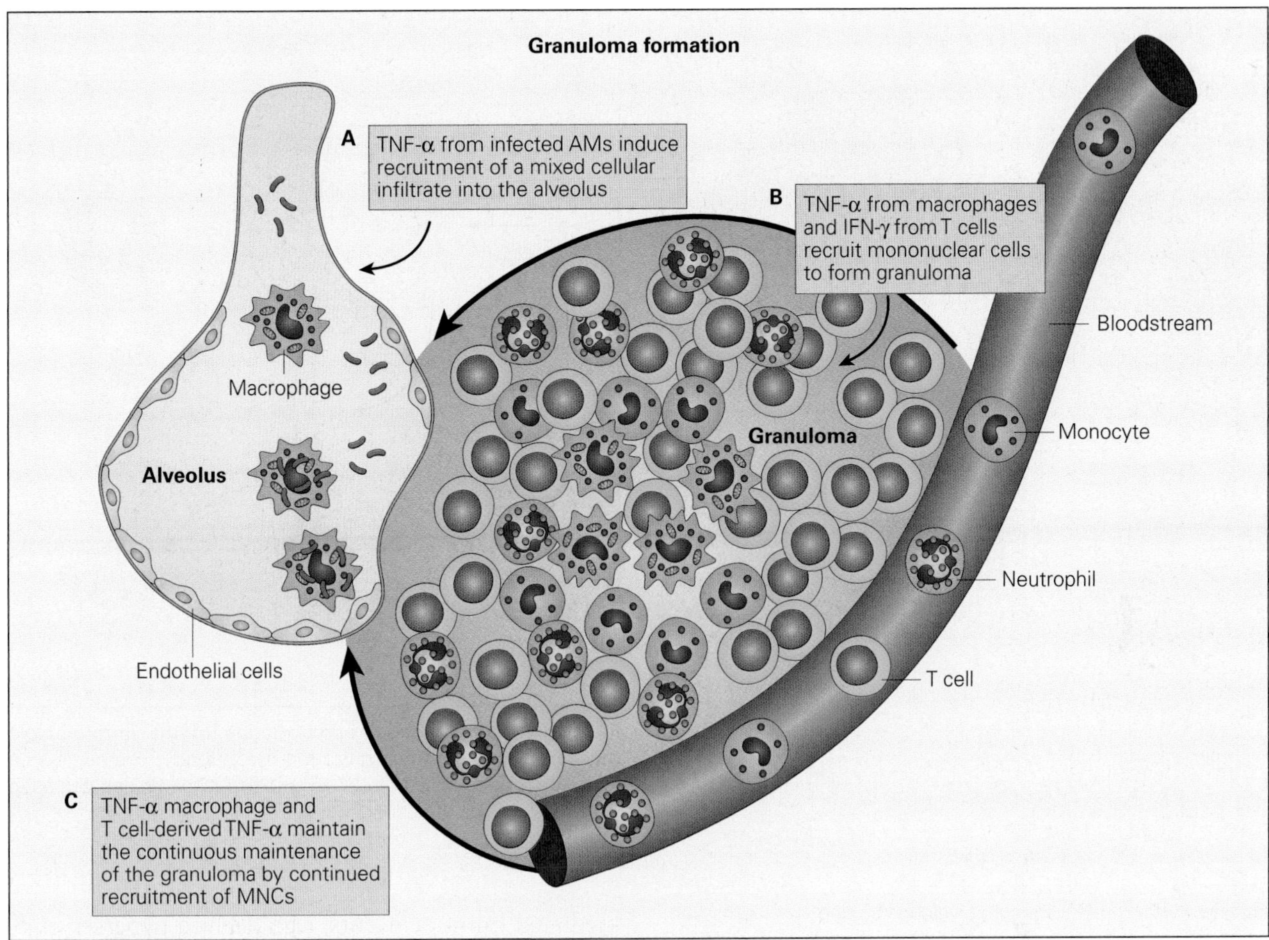

Figure 12-19. TNF acts at multiple steps in protective granuloma formation in response to *M. tuberculosis* infection. Panel A: TNF-α derived from infected alveolar macrophages initially induces recruitment of a mixed cellular alveolar and interstitial infiltrate. Panel B: Under the influence of TNF-α and T cell-derived IFN-γ, mononuclear cells accumulate to form a highly structured granuloma. Here, TNF-α and IFN-γ activate mycobactericidal pathways within macrophages and regulate excessive inflammation by inducing apoptosis of T cells. Panel C: Macrophage and T cell-derived TNF-α is necessary to continuously orchestrate the recruitment of mononuclear cells into granulomas in order to maintain effective containment of mycobacterial foci of infection. (Adapted from Ehlers S. Why does tumor necrosis factor targeted therapy reactivate tuberculosis? J Rheumatol Suppl. 2005;74:35–9.)

Toxigenic Infection

A third pattern of antibacterial protective mechanisms is directed against the exotoxins produced by pathogenic bacteria. Exotoxins are extracellular products that may be produced even after minimal infection of the host or may be produced outside the host and enter via ingestion, e.g., botulism. The prime defense of the host against these toxins is through neutralization by the production or administration of specific antibody (antitoxin). This detoxification process leads to the production of toxin-antitoxin complexes that are usually removed by phagocytic degradation (Figure 12-21).

A Summary of Innate and Adaptive Immune Responses of a Nonimmune and Susceptible Host to an Acute Bacterial Pathogen: Primary Encounter

Following exposure of a nonimmune and susceptible host to an acute bacterial pathogen, there is a period of time referred to as the incubation period or prodromal period, when bacterial replication takes place and there are no clinical symptoms (Figure 12-22). During this period, elements of the innate immune system begin to be stimulated with uptake and degradation of bacteria by macrophages (and dendritic cells), with the beginning of antigen presentation to

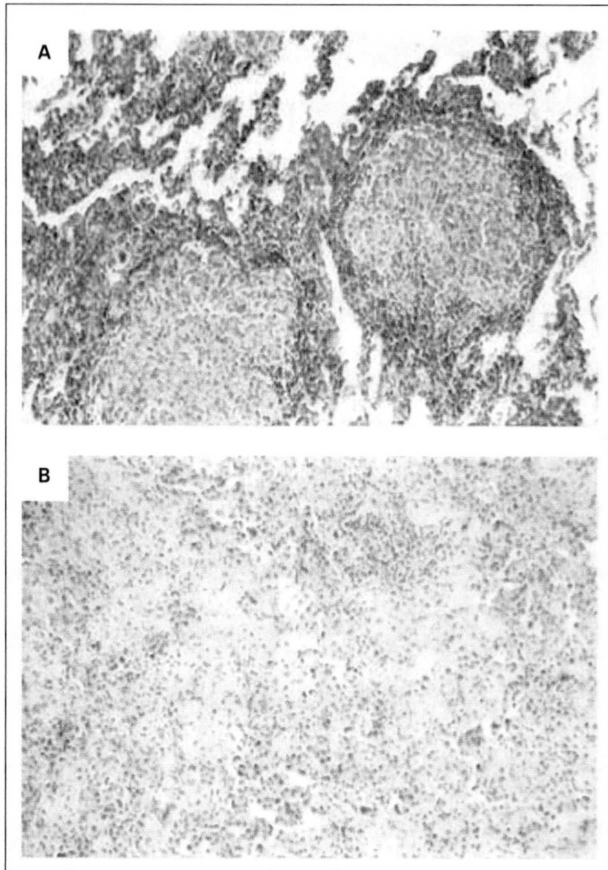

Figure 12-20. Panel A: Photomicrographs of lung specimens from a patient with tuberculosis and granuloma formation who did not receive infliximab. Panel B: A patient with tuberculosis with a breakdown of granuloma formation who received infliximab. The specimen from the patient who did not receive infliximab shows well-formed granulomas with negligible overt necrosis (panel A). The specimen of lung parenchyma from the patient who received infliximab shows prominent interstitial fibrosis and lymphoid inflammation without granulomas (panel B). (Reproduced with permission from Keane J, Gershon S, Wise RP, et al. Tuberculosis associated with infliximab, a tumor necrosis factor alpha-neutralizing agent. N Engl J Med. 2001;345:1098–104.)

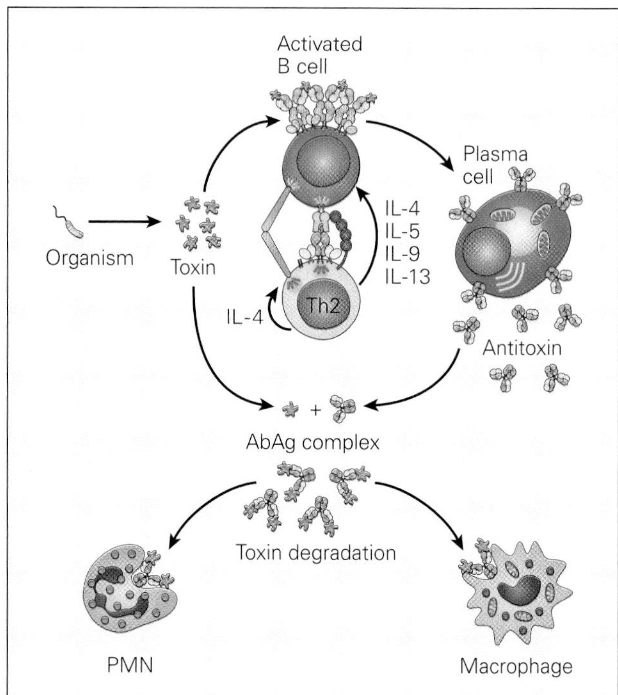

Figure 12-21. Schematic representation of the immunologic mechanism of toxin neutralization by antibody. The neutralized toxin-antitoxin complexes are shown being taken up and degraded within both types of phagocytic cells.

T cells and the interaction of B cells for induction of CMI and the subsequent production of antibody, respectively. During this phase, the production of pro-inflammatory cytokines contributes to the onset of symptoms, e.g., IL-1 with fever and TNF-α with malaise and myalgia. This occurs as a consequence of the increased quantities of pathogen and a corresponding innate response above a clinical threshold.

This stage is followed shortly by the initiation of the adaptive immune response, first with the stimulation of the CD8 population of T cells and then by the emergence of CD4 T cells. The Th1 subpopulation of the CD4 cells is involved in the development of cell-mediated immune events, e.g., delayed hypersensitivity, and the Th2 with the interaction with B cells for the sequential production of specific immunoglobulin-associated antibodies directed against various components of the bacterial cell wall or structures (Figure 12-22). A robust IgM antibody response is seen initially, followed within the first 7 to 10 days by IgG and later IgA antibodies in serum and in external secretions in the form of sIgA antibodies. Collectively, these immune reactions usually lead to the clearance of the bacterial pathogen and to a stage of convalescence with full recovery from this initial infection and resistance to subsequent infection with the same organism.

A Summary of Innate and Adaptive Immune Responses Following a Subsequent Encounter of an Immune Host with an Acute Bacterial Pathogen: Secondary Encounter

Having described the immunologic events occurring with bacterial infection during a primary encounter with an acute bacterial pathogen, it may now be

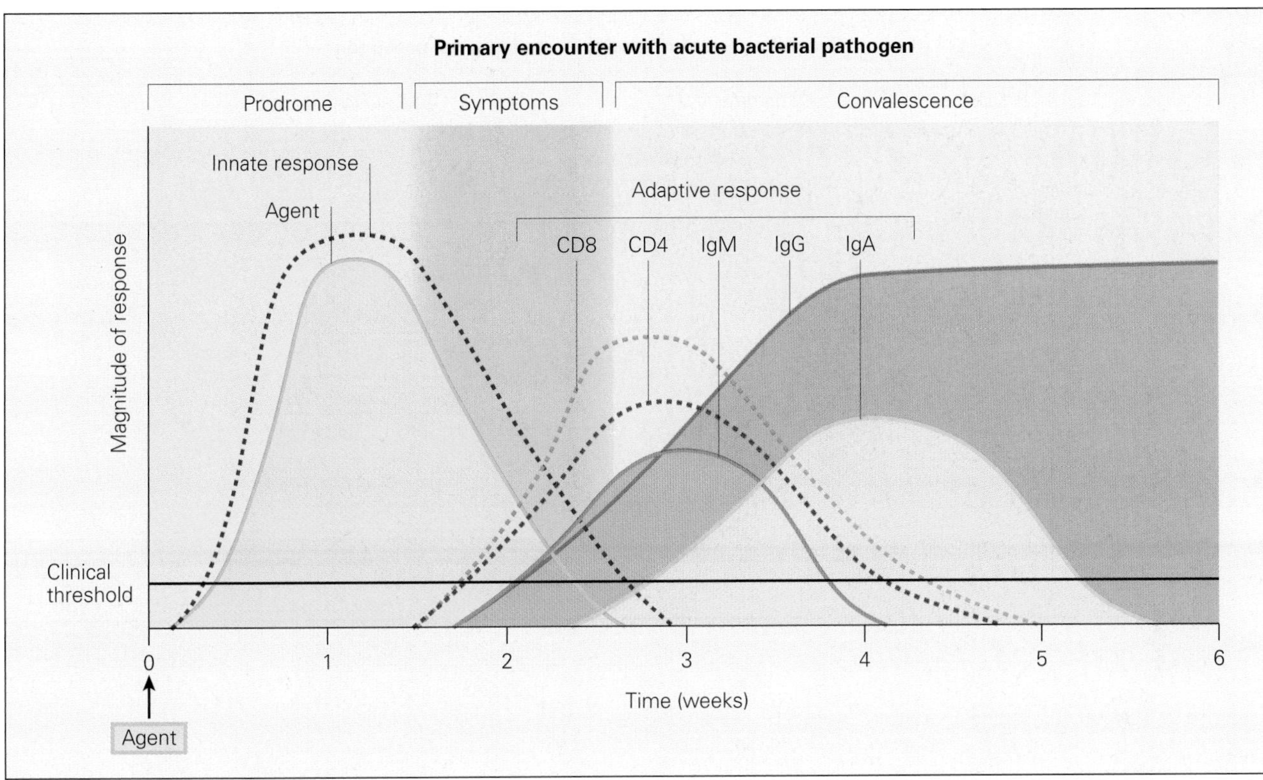

Figure 12-22. Schematic representation of the innate and adaptive immune responses following encounter of a nonimmune and susceptible host with an acute bacterial pathogen.

possible to describe innate and adaptive immune responses occurring during a subsequent encounter with the same bacterial pathogen (Figure 12-23).

In contrast to events seen during a bacterial infection following the initial encounter of a nonimmune host with an acute bacterial pathogen, the innate and adaptive immune responses following an encounter with the same pathogen are quite different (Figure 12-23). In this scenario, following processing and presentation of antigen by the innate immune system to a bank of presensitized memory T and B lymphocytes, there is expansion of these cells and a rapid control of the infection by the adaptive immune response. Because of the limited replication of the bacterial pathogen and subliminal innate immune stimulation below a clinical threshold, there are few pro-inflammatory cytokines produced, and therefore minimal clinical manifestations seen. Moreover, because of the presence of memory cells, the subsequent appearance of CD8, CD4 cells, and specific immunoglobulin isotypes occurs much earlier, and the levels of IgM are much lower and those of IgG and IgA are much higher than those seen during first encounter, events characteristic of the anamnestic or booster response (*Chapter 6*). Collectively, these immune reactions usually lead to minimal or no replication of a bacterial pathogen with few or no clinical manifestations and maintenance of health and freedom from disease.

A Summary of Innate and Adaptive Immune Responses Following an Encounter of a Nonimmune Host with a Chronic Bacterial Pathogen: Evasion of the Immune Response and Persistence of the Bacterial Pathogen with Immunopathology

The initial innate and adaptive immune response events occurring following the encounter of a nonimmune host with a chronic bacterial pathogen are similar to those seen in the primary encounter of a host with an acute bacterial pathogen with the same sequential appearance of CD8, CD4, and immunoglobulin isotypes (Figure 12-24). However, in contrast to the primary encounter, in this scenario the bacterial pathogen evades the host immune response and persists in the host for extended periods of time. The continued presence of bacterial antigen resulting from the persistent infection drives

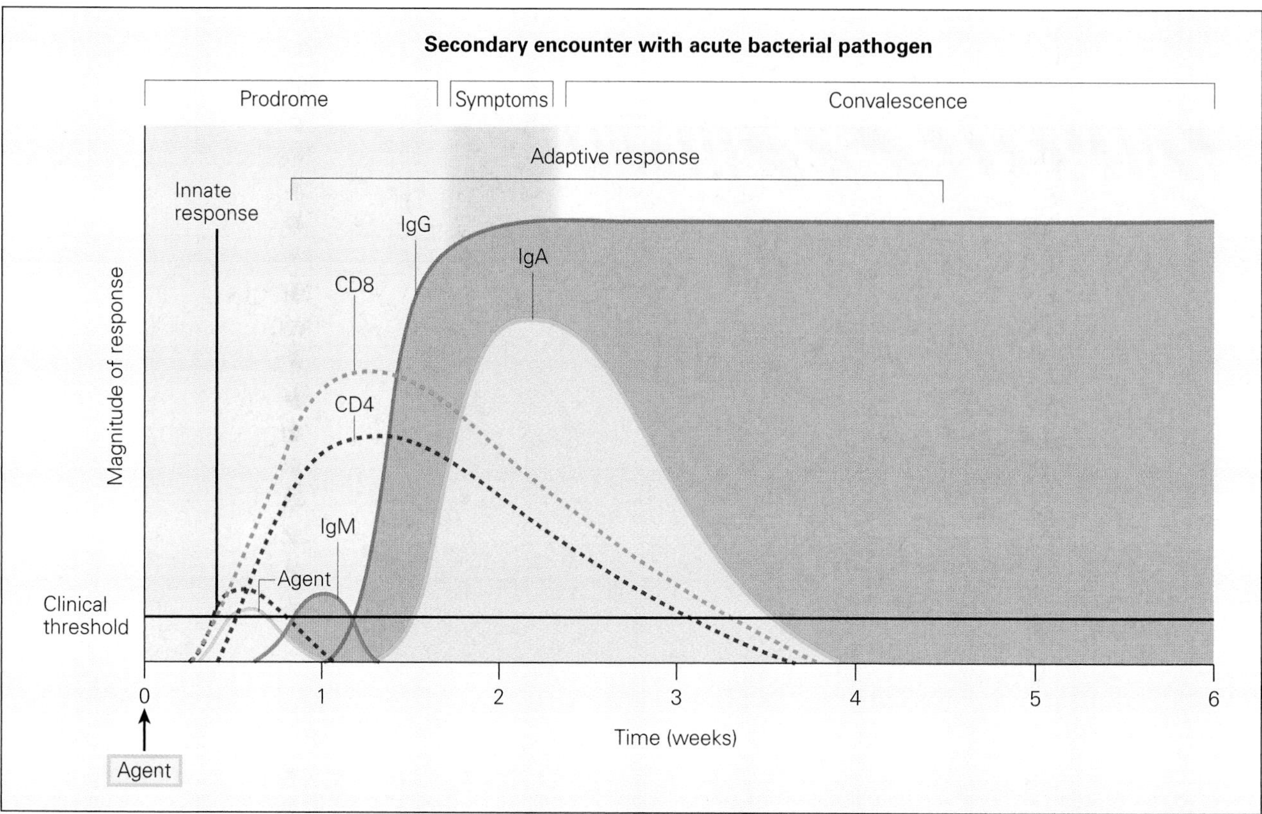

Figure 12-23. Schematic representation of the innate and adaptive immune responses following a subsequent encounter of an immune host with the same acute bacterial pathogen.

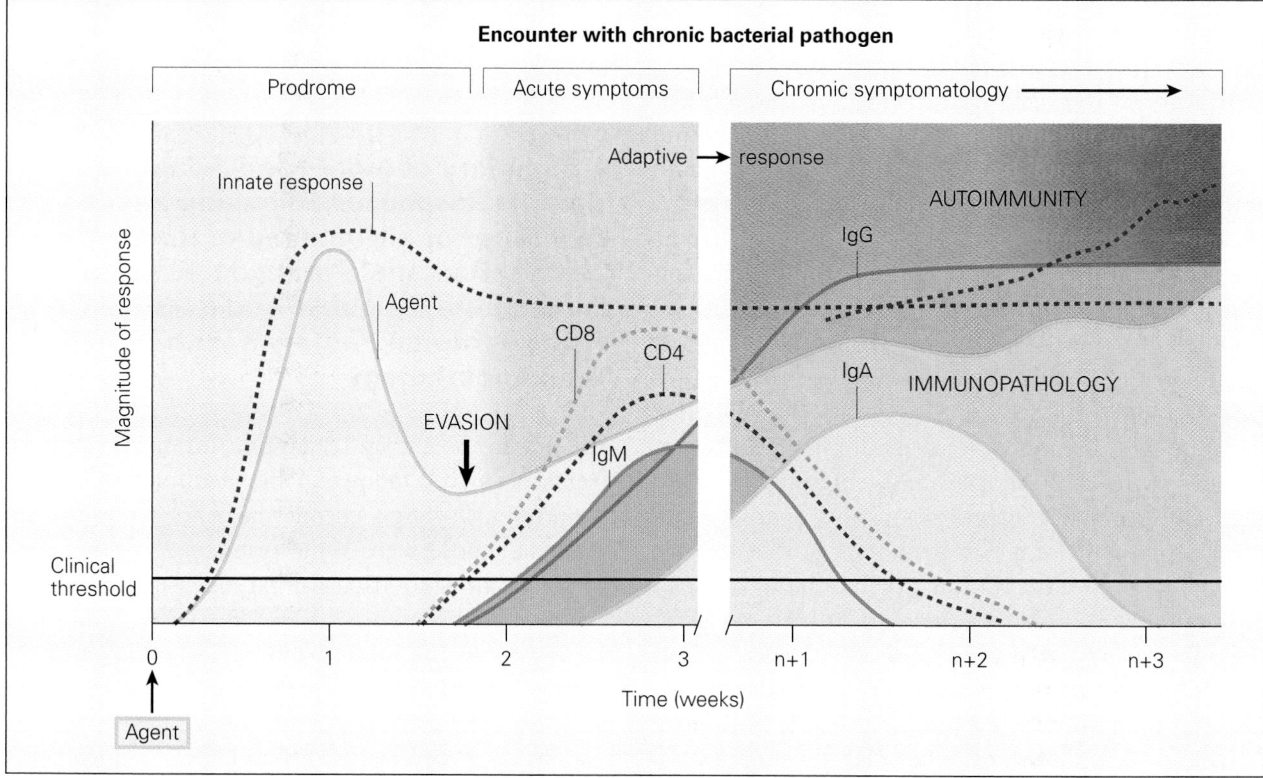

Figure 12-24. Schematic representation of the innate and adaptive immune responses following the encounter of a nonimmune host with a chronic bacterial pathogen: evasion of the immune response and the persistence of the bacterial pathogen with immunopathology.

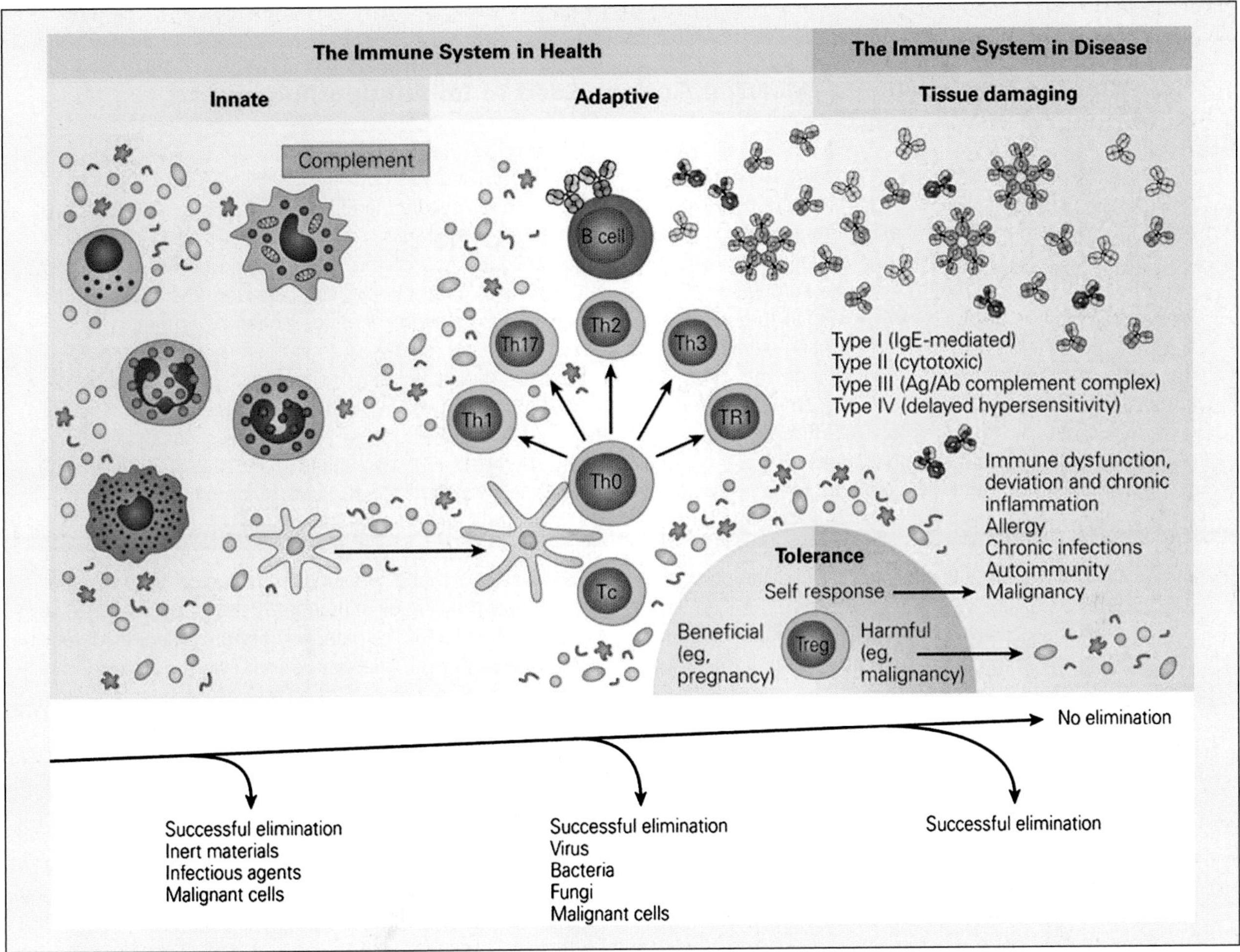

Figure 12-25. Schematic representation of the total immunologic capability of the host based on the efficiency of the elimination of foreign matter.

continued stimulation of both the innate and adaptive immune systems, resulting in the deleterious expressions of the immune response (*Chapter 1* and *Chapter 17*) with resultant immunopathology and frequently the expressions of autoimmunity or autoinflammatory disease (Figures 12-24 and 12-25 and Box 12-3).

Immunologic Injury Secondary to Bacterial Infection

Having presented the basis for immunologic injury resulting from the persistence of bacterial antigen, it is now possible to cite examples of some of the many presumed immune-mediated sequelae of chronic bacterial infection. Group A beta-hemolytic streptococcal infection leads to post-streptococcal glomerulonephritis in what has been shown to involve immune complex (Type III) injury; this process is mediated by the formation of streptococcal antigen, antibody, and complement complexes that deposit in renal glomeruli with resultant inflammation and immunologic injury. Rheumatic heart disease results from the production of anti-streptococcal antibodies that cross-react with cardiac tissue and central nervous tissue (i.e., Sydenham's chorea) in a Type II reaction. Pediatric autoimmune neuropsychiatric disorders associated with streptococcal infection (**PANDAS**) is a syndrome in which tics (motor and/or vocal) and/or obsessive-compulsive disorder are thought to be exacerbated in temporal correlation to a group A beta-hemolytic streptococcal infection. It is important to be aware of these complex subsequent interactions of the immune response with bacterial infection that may be responsible for these and other immunologically mediated disorders.

Box 12-3

How Can the Persistence of Bacterial Antigen Lead to Immunopathology and Autoimmune Phenomena?

As described in Chapter 1, the immune system is clearly a physiologic system of cells and cell products designed to recognize and remove foreignness and a system in which the body attempts to maintain homeostasis between the internal and external environments. The summation of the total immunologic capability of the host to all foreign matter is shown schematically in Figure 12-25 and is based upon the following assumptions concerning the immune response: (1) the foreign substance, e.g., immunogen (antigen) drives the system, i.e., active immune responses occur only as long as the foreign substance is present and will cease after it is removed; (2) there are three phases through which all foreign substances are removed; and (3) the extent of the progression through these three phases will be determined by the efficiency of elimination of the foreign substance.

The first phase involves the *innate* immune response and consists of those ancient responses to a first encounter with a foreign configuration—*phagocytosis* and the *inflammatory response.* In the case of an encounter with a bacterium, the processing by APCs and cognate presentation of peptide to the T cell repertoire leads to the initiation of the *adaptive immune* responses, which consist of two basic effector systems: (1) B lymphocyte-mediated humoral immunity with the elaboration of antibody associated with five major classes of immunoglobulin (IgM, IgD IgG, IgA, and IgE) and (2) T lymphocyte-mediated antigen elimination, including both the CD4 and CD8 universes of cells. A sophisticated addition to these systems is the capacity to enhance these immunologic responses through the action of the *biologic amplification system(s)* of cytokines, chemokines, complement, and the coagulation cascade (*Chapter 4*) and a bank of "memory cells" that can expand rapidly when antigen is re-encountered. If antigen is successfully eliminated at these two phases of innate and adaptive immunity, the immunologic response terminates. Normally, most bacteria are successfully eliminated in these first two stages, and this beneficial outcome characterizes "the immune system in health."

If bacteria cannot be eliminated at these first two stages, persistence of antigen can lead to the development of the *tissue-damaging responses* (*Chapter 17*). Bacterial persistence may result either from the adapted state of bacterial virulence of the pathogen or from a genetic defect in the interactive innate/adaptive immune responses of the host, resulting in bacterial evasion of the host immune responses and the emergence of the deleterious manifestations of tissue injury. Following antigen persistence resulting from either of these possibilities, four types of immunopathologic interactions of the Gell and Coombs classification can be elicited: Types I, II, III, and IV (*Chapter 17*). These responses are no longer beneficial to the host and are manifested as the immunologically mediated diseases that represent "the immune system in disease."

Case Study: Clinical Relevance

Let us now return to the case study of chronic osteomyelitis presented earlier and review some of the major points of the clinical presentation and how they relate to the immune system:

- Chronic osteomyelitis is an example of a chronic bacterial infection usually caused by *Staphylococcus aureus* that manifests with systemic symptoms of fever, loss of function, and bone pain. Although typical laboratory findings include leukocytosis and elevated sedimentation rate, these hallmark acute phase markers were not initially present and the absence of these contributed to the delay in diagnosis.
- The diagnosis was finally made by isolation of the causative organism from blood culture, and although intensive antibiotic therapy was initiated, the infection persisted.
- This case presentation illustrates how an acute infectious disease can evade the immune responses and lead to sequestration of the bacteria in sites not accessible to antibiotic therapy; the acute infection then progressed to a chronic infection characterized by chronic inflammation in which the production of pro-inflammatory cytokines, e.g., TNF-α, led to bone destruction.
- The resolution of the infection was achieved only with surgical curettage of the sequestered infected tissue and additional antibiotic treatment.
- This case presentation not only illustrates the principles and mechanisms of acute and chronic inflammatory responses to bacterial infection, but also the practical importance of early diagnosis and prompt treatment of these infections.

Summary

The immune mechanisms displayed by the host in bacterial defense are best viewed according to the type of host-bacterium interaction, intracellular or extracellular, with broad overlap in the categories of acute, chronic, or toxigenic infections. Bacterial pathogens evoke many immune effector mechanisms. The interwoven participation of both innate and adaptive immune mechanisms occurs in all successfully handled bacterial infections; the relative roles of each, however, vary with the type of infection. At times, the products of the immune response can be harmful and are manifested as immune-mediated diseases.

Key Points

- Bacteria generally exert their pathogenic effects through two mechanisms: (1) bacterial replication and invasiveness without toxicity and (2) toxicity as a result of elaboration of toxins without invasiveness.
- Host-bacterial relationships can take on three different forms: symbiosis, commensalism, or pathogenicity. Symbiosis and commensalisms are grouped together in the category of mutualism.
- Depending on the host's immune response, bacterial infection can result in either acute or chronic disease.
- The persistence of bacterial antigen can lead to immunopathology and autoimmune sequelae, such as post-streptococcal glomerulonephritis and rheumatic heart disease.

Study Questions/Critical Thinking

1. Name a few biochemical, anatomical, and functional properties that bacteria developed to evade the immune system.
2. What are the primary differences between acute and chronic bacterial infections? Give an example of each.
3. Describe the difference between and exotoxin and an endotoxin and give an example of each type of toxin and the organism that produces it.
4. Once a bacterium penetrates the host's anatomical barriers of mucosal and epithelial surfaces, what immune cells does it encounter first? How are the innate and adaptive immune responses stimulated?
5. How does the immune system respond differently during a secondary encounter with the same pathogen?

Suggested Reading

Ehlers S. Why does tumor necrosis factor targeted therapy reactivate tuberculosis. J Rheumatol Suppl. 2005; 74: 35–9.

Finlay BB, McFadden G. Anti-immunology: evasion of the host immune system by bacterial and viral pathogens. Cell. 2006; 124: 767–82.

Foster TJ. Immune evasion by staphylococci. Nat Rev Microbiol. 2005; 3: 948–58.

Gan YH. Interaction between Burkholderia pseudomallei and the host immune response: sleeping with the enemy? J Infect Dis. 2005; 192: 1845–50.

Hoesel LM, Gao H, Ward PA. New insights into cellular mechanisms during sepsis. Immunol Res. 2006; 34: 133–41.

Holland SM. Interferon gamma, IL-12, IL-12R and STAT-1 immunodeficiency diseases: disorders of the interface of innate and adaptive immunity. Immunol Res. 2007; 38: 342–6.

Hooper LV, Gordon JI. Commensal host-bacterial relationships in the gut. Science. 2001; 292: 1315–8.

Iwatsuki K, Yamasaki O, Morizane S, et al. Staphylococcal cutaneous infections: invasion, evasion and aggression. J Dermatol Sci. 2006; 42: 203–14.

Keane J, Gershon S, Wise RP, et al. Tuberculosis associated with infliximab, a tumor necrosis factor alpha-neutralizing agent. N Engl J Med. 2001; 345: 1098–104.

Mahenthiralingam W, Urban TA, Goldberg JB. The multifarious, multireplicon Burkholderia cepacia complex. Nat Rev Microbiol. 2005; 3: 144–56.

Mayer-Scholl A, Averhoff P, Zychlinsky A. How do neutrophils and pathogens interact? Curr Opin Microbiol. 2004; 7: 62–6.

Otto M. Bacterial evasion of antimicrobial peptides by biofilm formation. Curr Top Microbiol Immunol. 2006; 306: 251–8.

Quinn MT, Ammons MC, Deleo FR. The expanding role of NADPH oxidases in health and disease: no longer just agents of death and destruction. Clin Sci (Lond). 2006; 131: 1–20.

Salgame P. Host innate and Th1 responses and bacterial factors that control Mycobacterium tuberculosis infection. Curr Opin Immunol. 2005; 17: 374–80.

Sansonetti PJ. The bacterial weaponry: lessons from Shigella. Ann NY Acad Sci. 2006; 1072: 307–12.

Voyich JM, Musser JM, DeLeo FR. Streptococcus pyogenes and human neutrophils: a paradigm for evasion of innate host defense by bacterial pathogens. Microbes Infect. 2004; 6: 1317–23.

Zabel BA, Zuniga L, Ohyama T, et al. Chemoattractants, extracellular proteases, and the integrated host defense response. Exp Hematol. 2006; 34: 1021–32.

Chapter 13

Mechanisms of Immunity to Viral Disease

Joseph A. Bellanti, MD
Barry T. Rouse, DVM, PhD, DSc

Case Study

An eight-year-old male was taken to an emergency department by his mother for evaluation of a small cluster of vesicular lesions on the left upper lip. Prior to this episode, the child had an intercurrent URI characterized by nasal discharge and sore throat. The child was irritable and complained of pain and stated that he "does not want to go to school with this terrible thing on my lip". His mother explained that the child gets the sores on his lip approximately every other month during the winter months, with each episode lasting one to two weeks. The mother stated that she applies ice to the child's lip for a few minutes when the outbreaks occur to relieve the pain but had used no other specific therapy. The episodes of recurrent lesions were usually associated with intercurrent colds or stressful situations and they healed spontaneously within several days without any specific therapy. One year prior to the onset of these recurrent lesions, the child had a more extensive outbreak of oral lesions, which were characterized by widespread, small, superficial ulcers of the oral

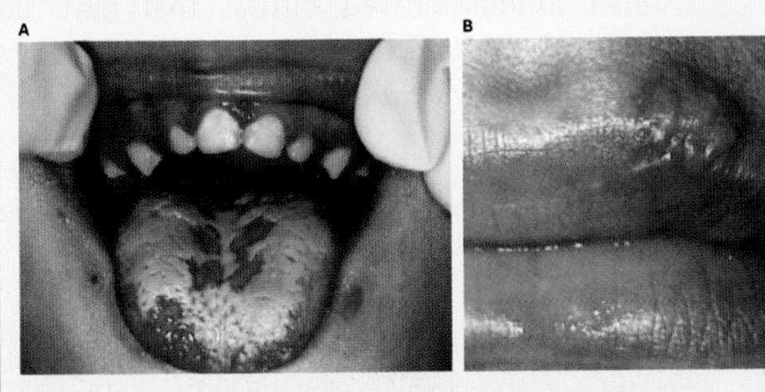

Figure 13-1. Panel A: An extensive outbreak of oral lesions in the patient in the preceding year, which were characterized by widespread, small, superficial ulcers of the oral mucosa and tongue with swollen and ulcerated gingivae. Panel B: A more recent cluster of confluent raised vesicular lesions on the vermillion border of the left upper lip, surrounded by an erythematous border. (Reproduced with permission from Leão JC, Gomes VB, Porter S. Ulcerative lesions of the mouth: an update for the general medical practitioner. Clinics (Sao Paulo). 2007;62:769–80.)

LEARNING OBJECTIVES

When you have completed this chapter, you should be able to:

- Understand that viruses can cause acute and chronic infection in the human host and give a few examples of each
- Appreciate the concept of "tropism" and the mechanisms by which viruses attach to and enter host cells
- Explain the differences between latent, persistent, and chronic viral infection
- Understand the structure, life cycle, and pathogenicity of HIV and the categories of antiretroviral therapies that have been developed thus far
- Distinguish the various categories of viral infections: localized, generalized, inapparent, and latent infection
- Describe the various components of the innate and adaptive immune response to viral infection
- Describe prions and their relationship to viral infection
- Summarize the clinical relevance of mechanisms of viral immunity in health and disease

Case Study (continued)

mucosa and tongue with swollen, ulcerated, and hemorrhagic gingivae (Figure 13-1A). His mother stated that the child was otherwise healthy and had no underlying conditions and was not receiving any medication.

Physical examination revealed the presence of a cluster of confluent, raised vesicular lesions on the vermillion border of the left upper lip surrounded by an erythematous border (Figure 13-1B). Herpes simplex type 1 was recovered from a needle aspirate of one of the vesicles. This case report illustrates a classic primary oral infection with Herpes simplex type 1 consisting of an extensive gingivostomatitis occurring during the previous year, which then cleared and resulted in a latent infection that was periodically exacerbated during stressful situations with the subsequent occurrence of recurrent periodic localized herpes labialis.

Introduction

Viruses are infectious agents that are obligate intracellular parasites. A complete viral particle, or virion, may be regarded as a basic block of genetic material, consisting of either a DNA or RNA genome and surrounded by a protective coat of protein, i.e., capsid, which may also serve as a vehicle for its transmission from one host cell to another. In addition, many viruses are surrounded by a viral envelope, which consists of a lipid bilayer membrane containing viral glycoproteins that may protrude as spikes. There also may be a layer between the viral nucleoprotein and the envelope referred to as the tegument that generally contains proteins that aid in viral DNA/RNA replication and evasion of the immune response (Figure 13-2).

Several viral agents that were once major human pathogens have been successfully controlled, either by the widespread use of effective vaccines (*Chapter 23*) or by other eradication schemes such as improved sanitation and the control of mosquito vectors. Thus, smallpox has been eradicated, poliomyelitis is close to being eliminated, and other formerly common viral infectious diseases such as measles, mumps, and rubella are no longer significant pathogens in the Western world. However, many other viruses remain important causes of disease, perhaps because they possess a wide range of strategies that help bypass or evade immune defenses. Effective vaccines directed at these agents still need to be developed. Moreover, some new viral agents arising from animal sources have become significant pathogens when transmitted to the human (Table 13-1). Most notable among these is the lentivirus, now called human immunodeficiency virus (**HIV**), the causative agent of the acquired immunodeficiency syndrome (**AIDS**); this human virus presumably arose from a natural viral infection of chimpanzees. In 2007, more than 25 years after its jump to humans, global HIV/AIDS estimates indicate that more than 25 million persons had died from and 33 million people were living with HIV with no prospect for a cure (Table 13-2). Currently, we do not have effective HIV vaccines that either prevent infection or minimize disease severity, although some recent trials with developing vaccines have shown some glimmer of promise.

Other animal-derived viruses that have become human pathogens include those responsible for severe acute respiratory syndrome (**SARS**) (caused by a

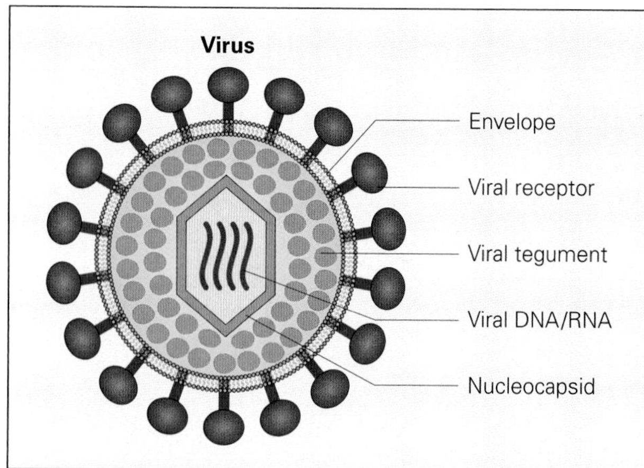

Figure 13-2. Schematic representation of a viral particle.

Table 13-1. High frequency of animal sources of emerging human pathogens

HIV
Avian (H5N1) and swine influenza (H1N1)
Human monkeypox in the United States
Nipah virus
BSE and vCJD
SARS
Ebola

Note: BSE = bovine spongiform encephalopathy, also known as mad cow disease; vCJD = variant Creutzfeldt-Jakob disease, a rare and fatal human neurodegenerative condition; SARS = severe acute respiratory syndrome, a respiratory disease in humans caused by SARS coronavirus (SARS-Cov).

Table 13-2. Global HIV/AIDS estimates, 2009

People living with HIV, 2009	33.3 million
New HIV infections in 2009	2.6 million
Deaths due to AIDS in 2009	1.8 million
Cumulative HIV-related deaths	> 30 million

Source: The 2010 UNAIDS *Report on the Global AIDS epidemic.*

SARS coronavirus), avian (H5N1) and swine H1N1 influenza. Animal influenza viruses are known to occasionally jump to humans, which can lead to devastating worldwide pandemics. The most dramatic example of this occurred with the pandemic of influenza of 1918, of possible avian and swine origin which caused an estimated worldwide mortality of 20 to 50 million deaths (Figure 13-3).

Other recent events that highlight the importance of understanding antiviral immune responses include the prospect that viral pathogens such as the now-extinct smallpox virus could be used as an agent of bioterrorism. Furthermore, viruses are suspected of contributing to the development of certain chronic human diseases, including malignancies, autoimmune diseases, and perhaps some neuroinflammatory diseases. Some have suggested that chronic fatigue syndrome may also have a viral etiology, and recently a xenotropic murine leukemia virus–related virus (**XMRV**) has been isolated from the blood cells of patients with this disorder. A further justification of the need to understand how viruses can either cause disease or how they are restrained from doing so by the immune system is substantiated by recent developments in cellular and molecular biology (*Chapter 25*). These advances have also generated several novel therapeutic modalities (*Chapter 11*) that can either prevent viral-induced clinical disease or minimize its consequences once infection has occurred.

During the past 50 years, the increased awareness of the escalating prevalence of viruses as etiologic agents of human infectious diseases has stimulated widespread interest in their pathogenicity and immunogenicity. Three major events have given great impetus to increase our knowledge and understanding of both the protective immune responses to viruses as well as their role in immunopathology. These include the following: (1) the devastating effects of HIV infection and AIDS; (2) the possibility that exotic viral pathogens, such as smallpox virus, can be used as weapons of bioterrorism; and (3) the natural emergence of new viral pathogens, e.g., swine H1N1 influenza, with potential to cause global pandemics.

The spectrum of diseases produced by viruses ranges from **acute** to **chronic** forms of viral infections. Acute viral infections are characterized by

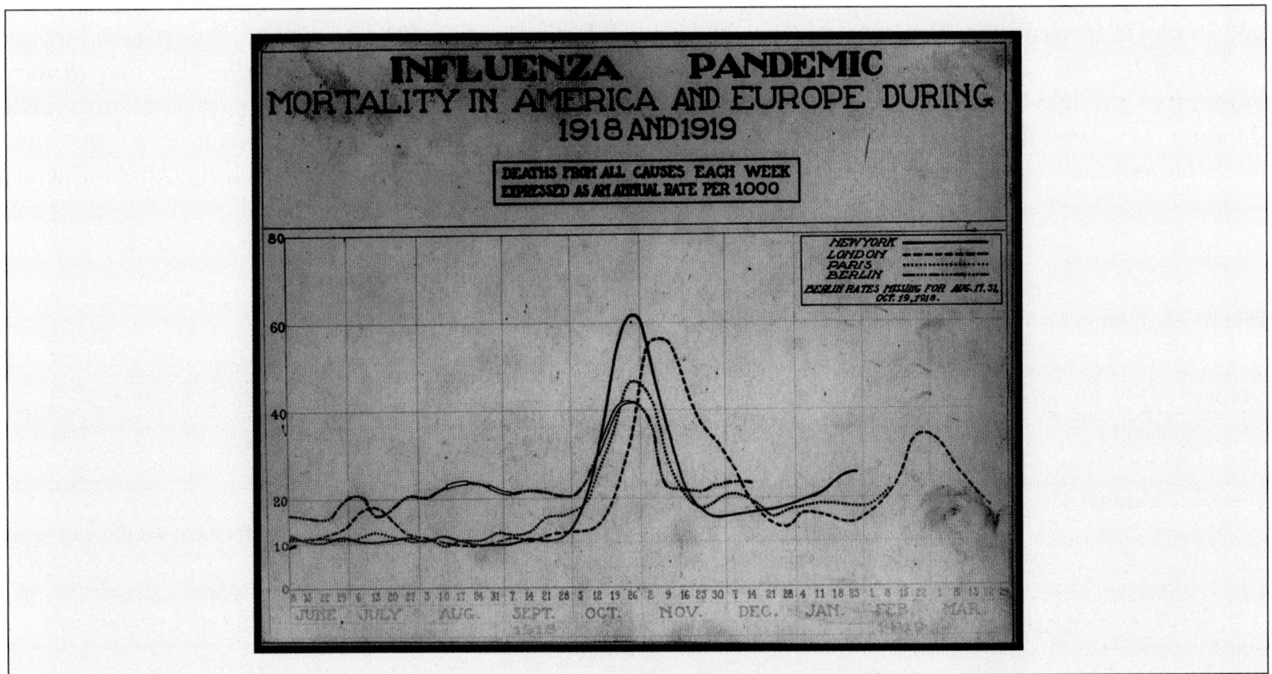

Figure 13-3. Mortality rates in the United States and Europe during the 1918–19 influenza epidemic. (Courtesy of Dr. Jeffrey K. Taubenberger.)

rapid viral clearing or widespread dissemination, infection, or death. Chronic viral infections, on the other hand, are characterized by prolonged viral replication and the capability of the virus to persist and to evade the host's immune response, with the possible consequences of tissue injury. In some cases, this could result not only in autoimmune disease (*Chapter 19*), but also in malignancy (*Chapter 20*). The recent discoveries of an association between viruses and human cancer has initiated areas of intense research that have found clinical application in the form of new vaccines for the prevention of human cancer, e.g., hepatitis B virus (**HBV**) and human papilloma virus (**HPV**) vaccines, which have been shown to prevent the subsequent development of hepatocellular carcinoma and some types of cervical cancers, respectively (*Chapter 23*).

New products to modulate the immunologic system (up- or downregulation) are becoming increasingly available through rapid advances in molecular biotechnology (*Chapter 11*). These products, collectively known as biologic response modifiers, are applicable to the prevention, diagnosis, and treatment of viral infections, tumors, and autoimmune diseases. These new modalities include interferons, interleukins, viral receptor inhibitors, and a host of monoclonal antibodies and fusion protein molecules directed against receptors and their ligands (*Chapters 9* and *11*). Thus, it is important for the student of all ages to have a fundamental grasp of immunologic mechanisms. Not only do these mechanisms drive the normal processes of antiviral immunity, but they also provide a clearer understanding of atypical responses seen during viral infection and their clinical sequelae.

Classification of Viral Infections

All viruses that infect humans represent foreign genetic material that will sound an alarm, i.e., a "danger signal," and alert a wide range of host immune reactions in an attempt to identify and eliminate the virus and minimize the consequences of its infection. The outcome of this encounter will depend on multiple factors, including (1) the primary properties of the virus itself; (2) the circumstances of exposure, such as the route and dose of the infecting viral agent; and (3) the degree of susceptibility of the host, which includes genetic factors, age, and numerous physiologic variables. Accordingly, viruses can infect and cause disease only if sufficient numbers of target cells in the host can be successfully infected, damaged, or destroyed by the virus. As previously described, the outcome of some viral infections can be decided quickly and are referred to as acute viral infections (Table 13-3). Alternatively, the viral-host interaction may be more prolonged and lead to chronic viral infections, which occur when viruses are not successfully controlled by the host and persist for prolonged and sometimes indefinite periods of time. Examples of these chronic viral infections are well illustrated by all members of the herpes virus family as well as HIV-1 (Table 13-3 and Figure 13-4).

Chronic infections may include (1) **latent infections**, which are characterized by an initial (episomal) acute infection that progresses to a dormant infection; and (2) **persistent infections**, which involve continuous viral replication that may or may not impair cell function. The essential features of a persistent infection include integration of the viral genome into the host DNA with chronic and low levels

Table 13-3. Examples of virus-target cell interactions and clinical sequelae

		Clinical manifestations	
Type	**Virus**	**Early**	**Late**
Acute infection	Poliovirus, smallpox, rhinovirus, rubeola, rubella, mumps, rotavirus	Paralysis, rash, common cold, parotitis, diarrhea	? sequelae
Chronic infection			
Latent	Herpes simplex virus (HSV-1, HSV-2)	Gingivostomatitis, genital herpes	Recurrent herpetic infection
	Varicella-zoster virus (VZV)	Varicella	Herpes zoster (shingles)
Persistent, some viral replication	HIV	AIDS (infectious mono-like picture)	Infections and malignancies
	Human papilloma virus (HPV)	Warts	Cervical cancer
	Hepatitis B virus (HBV)	Acute hepatitis	Hepatic adenocarcinoma

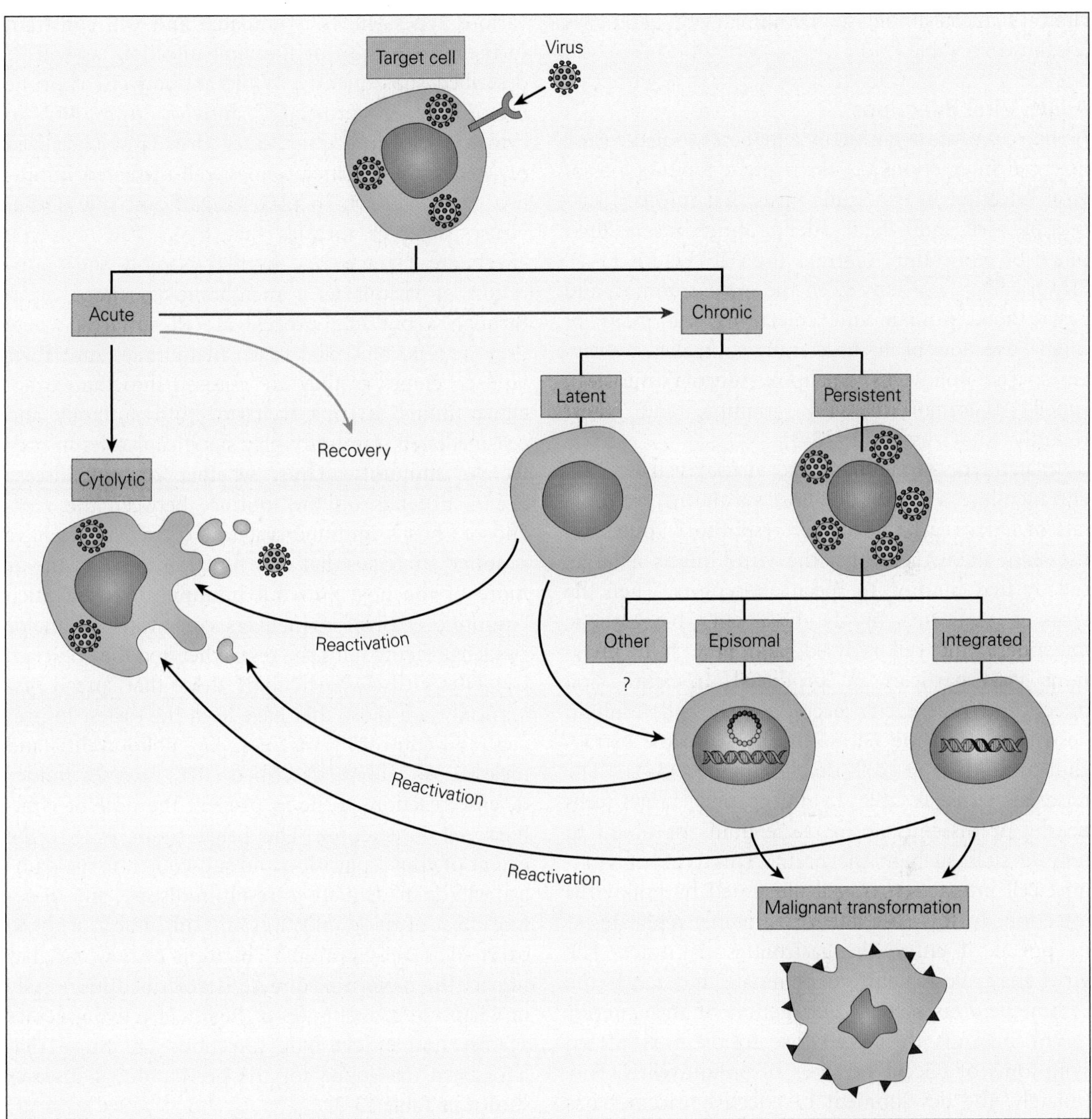

Figure 13-4. Schematic representation of acute and chronic virus-target cell interactions. In acute (cytolytic) viral infections, viruses infect a target cell by first binding to specific receptors then replicate by the host cell's biosynthetic machinery following which the cell is lysed and new fully infectious viral particles are produced. The host undergoing an acute viral infection may recover with termination of the infection or may proceed to a chronic viral infection, where the virus persists in either a latent or persistent infection in which the virus exists in an episomal form or may be integrated within the DNA of the cell. These persistently infected cells may be reactivated to a cytolytic infection with cell destruction and release of fully infectious virus or at times may undergo malignant transformation.

of virus replication in tissues that are constantly regenerated, e.g., HPV in warts. A late sequela of persistent HPV infection is cervical cancer. In the case of latent infections, the viral genome is ensconced in the absence of viral production and is placed securely within the cell, hidden from the arsenal of the immune system. Latency is seen primarily with the herpes family of viruses, including herpes simplex virus type 1 and 2 (**HSV-1** and **HSV-2**), varicella-zoster virus (**VZV**), Epstein-Barr virus (**EBV**), cytomegalovirus (**CMV**), roseola virus (**HHV-6**), and human herpes virus 8 (**HHV8**) (Kaposi's sarcoma-associated herpes virus). Episodic reactivation of the virus is a hallmark of latent infections, as seen with recurrent "cold" sores (HSV-1) or shingles (VZV). Multiple examples of the three types of the viral-host cell interaction and clinical sequelae among several human viral pathogens are shown in Table 13-3.

Acute Viral Infections

Perhaps the most common and best-studied virus-host cell interactions are the acute cytolytic types of viral infection in which the virus first infects a susceptible cell and then, after a brief intracellular phase of replication, destroys the cell (Figure 13-4). Historically, these have been the most common and best-studied human viral infections and many of them have now been successfully controlled by vaccines, e.g., poliovirus, smallpox, rubeola (measles), rubella (German measles), mumps, and, most recently, rotavirus (Table 13-3).

In cytolytic viral infections, viruses usually gain entrance into a susceptible host via the natural portals of entry, e.g., the oral or respiratory route and the skin, following which the virus infects a target cell by first binding to specific receptors. Then the virus is replicated by the host cell's biosynthetic machinery, the cell is lysed, and new, fully infectious viral particles are produced. In acute viral infections, these events occur quickly and result in destruction and the release of virus into the extracellular fluid after cell death (Figure 13-4). The released virus is able to infect new target cells nearby or disseminate in tissue fluids or blood to remote sites such as the brain. This type of viral-host cell interaction is well-illustrated by poliovirus infection. In this case, the virus mainly replicates at its portal of entry, the gastrointestinal tract. The virus may subsequently disseminate and target the central nervous system; destruction of the anterior motor neurons then gives rise to the well-known symptoms of flaccid paralysis of poliomyelitis. Fortunately, the development of effective vaccines has resulted in almost worldwide eradication of this disease (*Chapter 23*).

For cytolytic viruses to cause disease, there needs to be sufficient host cell destruction either at the site of initial infection or in distal organs to which the virus has disseminated. If damage is restricted to the portal of entry, localized symptoms are seen, such as with common upper respiratory tract infections, e.g., the common cold caused by rhinoviruses. On the other hand, if virus is disseminated and damage is more widespread, the symptoms of disease are of a more generalized nature, e.g., poliomyelitis. Invariably, the released virus will be recognized by the immune system and host defenses of various types will be stimulated and will constrain further progression of the viral infection, as will be described subsequently. While antibody is of prime importance in protective antiviral immunity to cytolytic viral infections, since virus is not localized or shed from cell membranes, cell-mediated immunity is not known to play a significant role. Other viruses such as measles that have acute cytolytic effects are characterized by the assembly and maturation of virions as a membrane-associated event through a budding process at cell surfaces, where they incorporate cell surface membranes into their viral envelopes as they are released into the extracellular fluids. In this scenario, both antibody and cell-mediated immunity play significant roles in protective immunity. Thus, whether or not disease occurs depends on the footrace between the virus and the host's immune system. Several viruses have acquired strategies that may function to blunt one or more of the host antiviral immune defenses. Such "immune evasive" maneuvers constitute the major challenge facing both the researcher and the clinician. Cytolytic viruses, particularly those that spread systemically, are those that have been the easiest to prevent and control by vaccines, e.g., poliomyelitis and measles. As will be described later, vaccines induce defense reactions to be in place at the time of viral-host cell interaction. The usual result is that the extent of viral replication and subsequent tissue damage will be inadequate to result in disease, and therefore most of these infections are subclinical, with no overt signs or symptoms. The topic of how vaccines impact the pattern of disease is described more fully in Chapter 23. Examples of highly effective vaccines against human cytolytic infections are those that have been developed for the prevention of diseases shown in Table 13-3.

Chronic Viral Infections

In contrast to the acute cytolytic viral infections, chronic viral infections are caused by viruses that infect and often replicate more slowly within host cells and may not cause rapid cell destruction and disease (Table 13-3 and Figure 13-4). These chronic infections can be further subdivided into latent and persistent chronic viral infections. Viruses that cause persistent infection are those that continue to replicate after an initial infection, producing infectious virus with or without cell death. Examples are HIV, HPV, and HBV. Some viruses persist but may take on an alternative form of replication referred to as "latency". This is what typically occurs with herpes virus infections. Latency is usually not a permanent situation and can be reactivated by a variety of clinical conditions, such as stress, intercurrent viral infection, and the use of steroids or immunosuppressive medications. Examples include recurrent cold sores or genital lesions, as occurs with herpes simplex virus or shingles in the case of VZV disease.

Latent Chronic Viral Infections

The first type of chronic viral infection is latency, where the virus persists in a more hidden fashion (Table 13-3 and Figure 13-4). Infections of the human with any of the members of the herpes virus family are examples of latent chronic viral infections with varying capacities to either remain latent or be reactivated with active production of infectious virions. These viruses all share the ability to remain potentially infectious, but dormant, in the body for life. In contrast to persistent chronic viral infection, where the viral genome is integrated into host DNA, latent viruses occur as found in an epigenetic or episomal location within the nucleus (Figure 13-4). Of all the human herpes viruses known to date, CMV is arguably the one whose infection causes the most morbidity and mortality. Although primary infection with this agent generally does not produce symptoms in healthy adults, several high-risk groups (e.g., the fetus and immunocompromised patients, including individuals infected with HIV) are at risk of developing life-threatening (i.e., pneumonia) and sight-threatening (i.e., chorioretinitis) CMV disease. CMV has emerged in recent years as the most important cause of congenital infection in the developed world, often leading to hearing dysfunction and less commonly to mental retardation and developmental disability. Two other viruses of this group, human herpes virus (HHV-1 and HHV-2) and VZV, may remain latent in the nerve cells of sensory ganglia for months or years, and when reactivated can cause symptoms such as recurrent oral, e.g., HHV-1 or genital lesions in the case of HHV-2 and herpes zoster with VZV.

Although the mechanism(s) by which reactivation occurs is poorly understood, it seems to be related to conditions that depress cell-mediated immune function, such as stress or excessive exposure to sunlight, as well as underlying diseases, such as lymphoreticular malignancies, e.g., lymphoma (Figure 13-5) (*Chapter 21*). Herpes zoster infections are believed to represent a reactivation of a latent varicella viral infection that has occurred previously and remained dormant in sensory ganglia throughout life. In the modern world, HIV infection is a common cause of reactivation of clinical disease caused by these chronic latent viral infections, e.g., recurrent HSV or herpes zoster lesions. Zoster is usually a onetime event that commonly occurs in the elderly because of a progressive decline in cell-mediated immunity to VZV with aging (*Chapter 2*) and this is the basis for current recommendations for zoster vaccine in individuals older than 60 years (*Chapter 23*). Similar to the decreased prevalence of varicella following the introduction of the varicella vaccine, herpes zoster may soon become less common owing to the recent availability of the new herpes zoster vaccine (*Chapter 23*).

Persistent Chronic Viral Infections

In the persistent form of chronic viral infection, the virus has acquired a sophisticated means to evade the immune response by assimilation of its genome into the host's genetic apparatus either by direct incorporation of its viral nucleic acid into the host DNA or by epigenetic (episomal) mechanisms that involve differences in DNA methylation, as well as differences in chromatin structure involving histone modifications (Table 13-3 and Figure 13-4). In this scenario of integrated infection, the virally infected cell may or may not express viral antigens on its cell membrane (Figure 13-4). In either case, the virus has effectively evaded the host immune response by either downregulation of MHC-I expression (in the case of integrated infections that express viral antigen) or by lack of immune recognition in the case of those integrated infections not expressing viral antigens on cell membranes of the infected target cell.

Until recently, most integrated infections were observed only with DNA viruses and in experimental animal systems and under specialized circumstances, e.g., inoculation of virus into a host at birth or shortly thereafter. It is now known that integrated infections can be seen with both DNA and RNA viruses and represent an important part of human viral infection; they are important in the development of human cancer (*Chapter 20*) and possibly in the immunopathology associated with autoimmune diseases (*Chapter 19*). HPV, a DNA virus, is associated with human vulvar cancer. HPV-16 and HPV-18 DNA integration into the host cell

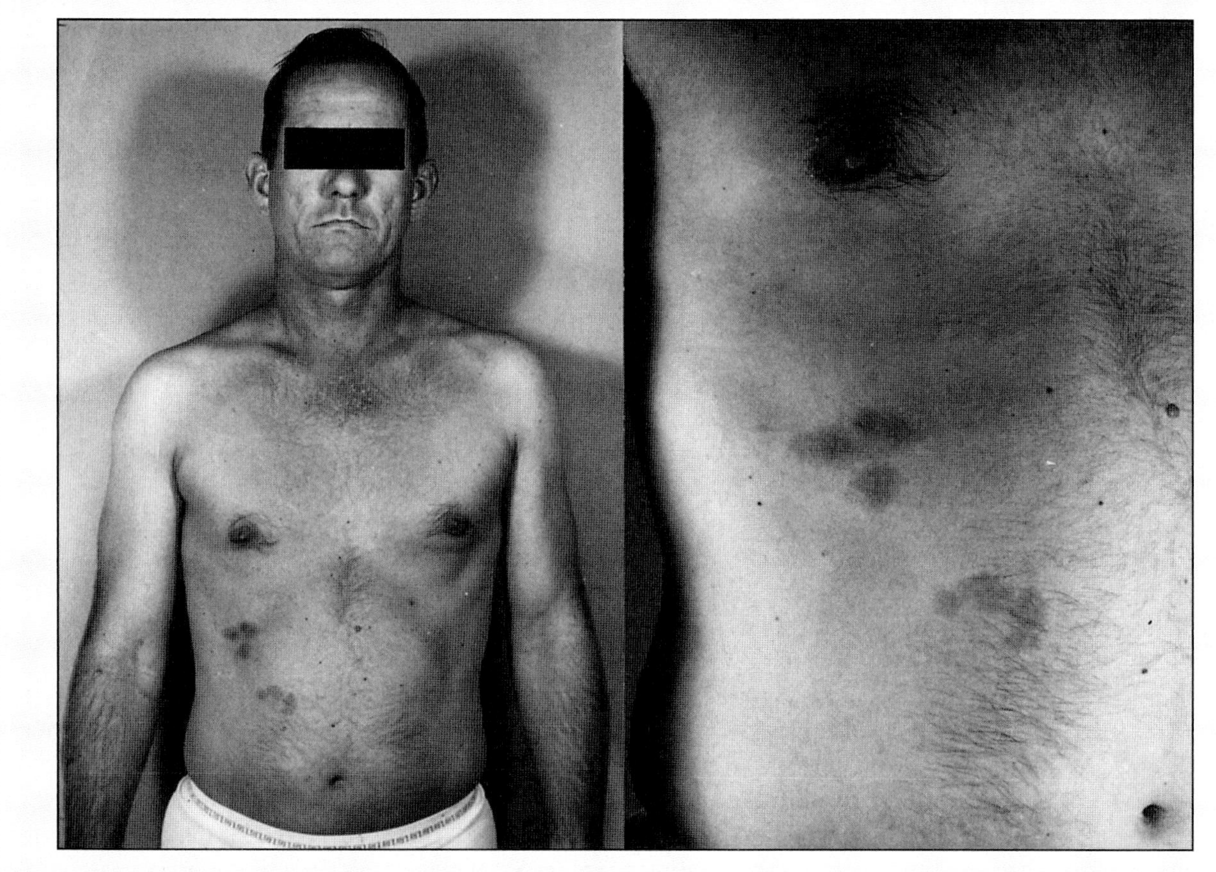

Figure 13-5. Lesions of herpes zoster in a patient with lymphoma. (Courtesy of Dr. S. Gerald Sandler.)

genome seems to be related to the stage of progression of epithelial cell dysplasia in tissues of the human female genital tract and, therefore, may be responsible for the development of HPV-associated invasive cervical and vulvar carcinoma in women. A quadrivalent human papilloma virus vaccine containing types 6, 11, 16, and 18 is now available for immunization of girls and women 9 to 26 years of age for the prevention of cervical cancer, precancerous or dysplastic lesions, and genital warts and for boys and men ages 9 to 26 for the prevention of genital warts. A recently approved bivalent HPV vaccine containing types 16 and 18 is indicated for the prevention of cervical cancer in girls and women ages 9 to 26 (*Chapter 23*).

Integration into host DNA is not limited to DNA viruses but is also seen with RNA viruses such as the primate lentiviruses, e.g., human immunodeficiency virus type 1 (**HIV-1**). These viruses through the retrograde production of viral complementary DNA (**cDNA**) by reverse transcriptase traverse the nuclear envelope and are integrated within host DNA. The most clinically important of these lentiviruses is the HIV-1, the causative agent of HIV infection and AIDS in the human. Another agent is the human T cell lentivirus, human T cell leukemia virus type 1 (**HTLV-1**), the causative agent of one form of human leukemia (Box 13-1). Recently, a related and possibly contagious rodent retrovirus, XMRV, has been isolated from the blood cells of patients with the chronic fatigue syndrome (**CFS**) as well as from patients with an aggressive form of prostate cancer, suggesting a retroviral link between the two disorders.

The outcome of this persistent viral-host infection is highly variable and is dependent not only on continued presence of viral genome, but also on the type of changes induced by the virus on the infected host cell. The infected cell may continuously release virus to the extracellular fluids without cell destruction, as in the case of the spread of rubella virus to daughter cells during intrauterine

Box 13-1

Viruses as Causative Agents in Leukemia and Lymphoma

Viruses of the retrovirus and herpes virus families are etiological agents of human leukemias and lymphomas. The human T-cell leukemia virus type 1 (HTLV-1) causes one form of adult T-cell leukemia. Epstein-Barr virus (EBV) is associated with Burkitt's lymphoma, Hodgkin's lymphoma, and other lymphomas in immunosuppressed individuals. The discovery of human herpes virus type 8 (HHV-8) has led to the identification of a rare and unusual form of virus-associated malignancy, e.g., Kaposi's sarcoma. Individuals infected with the human immunodeficiency virus type 1 (HIV-1) are at greatly increased risk of developing lymphoma, but the mechanism of lymphomagenesis is indirect. Recent data suggest that hepatitis C virus infection is also associated with an increased incidence of lymphoma.

infection. In some instances, lysis of the infected cell occurs, with the spread of virus to adjacent neighboring cells (Figure 13-4). Cells that are persistently infected with these viruses may escape rapid removal by the host immune response by virtue of their intracellular domicile. A critical feature of this mode of infection determines which arm of the adaptive immune system is stimulated during recovery and resistance. If virus is released extracellularly, antibody is of primary importance; if virus is localized on cell membranes, cell-mediated immunity appears to assume greater importance. This will be described in greater detail below.

Given these various modes of viral infection, it will become apparent that the corresponding immunologic responses of the host, i.e., innate and adaptive immune responses, will be determined by the nature of these viral host cell interactions and the degree to which the virus can evade recognition by the immune system and persist.

Patterns of Disease: Localized, Generalized, Inapparent, and Latent Infections

Biologic classification systems allow us to arbitrarily divide the types of viral infection according to their clinical appearance into the following classes: **localized**, **generalized**, **inapparent**, and **latent**.

Localized infections are those in which viral multiplication and cell damage remain at the portal of entry. The virus may first infect and then spread from cell to cell either directly (in the case of cytolytic viruses) or by contiguity (as with chronic persistent viral infections). The virus may then exert its effect by forming a single lesion or a group of lesions at the portal of entry. For example, warts represent a type of localized infection of the skin caused by HPV, and the common cold is a type of localized infection of the respiratory tract caused by rhinoviruses (Table 13-3). These infections induce hardly any viremia in the infected host.

In the setting of **generalized infection**, on the other hand, viruses undergo a progression through a number of steps, including the following: (1) primary multiplication at the portal of entry and spread to regional lymph nodes; (2) spread of progeny virus through blood to internal organs (viremia); (3) replication at an internal site; and (4) secondary viremia with spread to target organs, causing cell damage, pathologic lesions, and clinical disease. Shown in Figure 13-6A is a schematic representation of the various portals of entry of different viruses, which include: (1) the respiratory route, e.g., rhinovirus, influenza, and respiratory syncytial virus (**RSV**); (2) the gastrointestinal tract, e.g., rotavirus, poliovirus, and hepatitis A; (3) the skin, through the bite of an arthropod vector, e.g., dengue virus, yellow fever virus, or through the use of a syringe, e.g., HIV, HBV, and HCV; and (4) the genitourinary tract, e.g., HIV and HPV. Replication of virus at these portals of entry can give rise to localized inflammatory responses responsible both for localized symptoms as well as the induction of immune protective responses. Shown in Figure 13-6B is a schematic representation of those viruses that gain entry into the systemic vascular or lymphatic compartments that contribute to more systemic symptoms of generalized infection. Protective immune responses initiated at mucosal sites of the mucosa-associated lymphoid tissues (**MALT**) can also gain widespread distribution to other sites of the immune system through the recirculating pool (*Chapters 2 and 8*).

Generalized infection may be seen either with the cytolytic infections, e.g., poliovirus infection, or with the acute infection of VZV. In the case of the cytolytic viruses, the effects of disease appear to be caused by the direct spread of virus and cell death. In the case of the membrane-associated persistent viruses, the

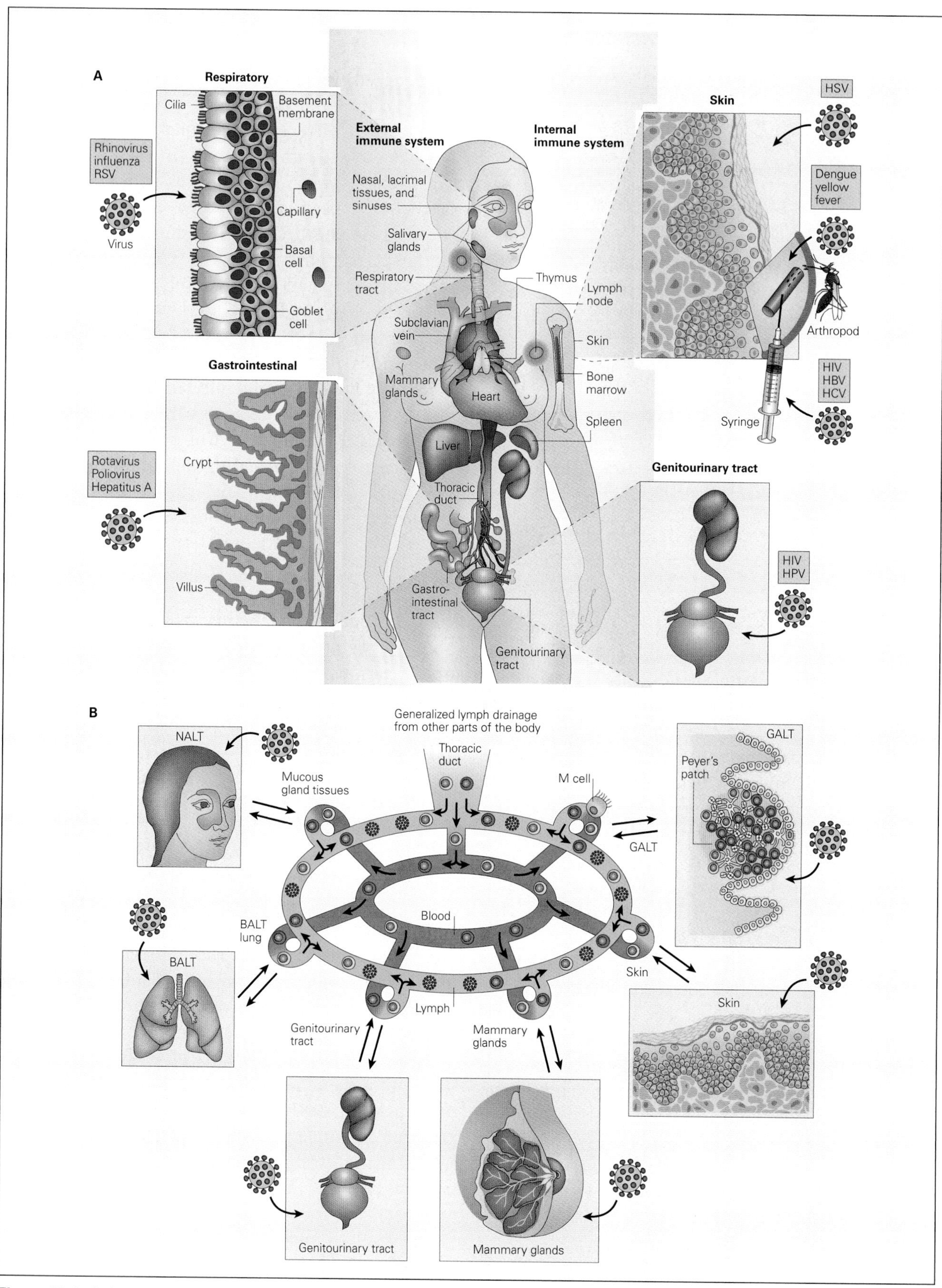

Figure 13-6. **Schematic representation of the portals of entry and sequential steps of viral replication involved the in pathogenesis of localized and generalized types of viral infections.** Panel A: Shows various portals of entry of different viruses that include the respiratory tract; the gastrointestinal tract; the skin, through the bite of an arthropod vector or through the use of a syringe; and the genitourinary tract. Panel B: Shows how viruses can replicate locally with localized infections or gain entry into the systemic vascular or lymphatic compartments that contribute to more systemic symptoms of generalized infection. Protective immune responses initiated at these mucosal sites of the mucosa-associated lymphoid tissues can also gain widespread distribution to other sites of the immune system through the recirculating pool.

disease pattern appears not only to be related to the spread of virus and cell death, but additionally, some of the manifestations may be due to hypersensitivity, e.g., the rash of measles. Still other manifestations of disease may be mediated by the effects of humoral antibody, e.g., renal injury, e.g., glomerulonephritis mediated by viral-antiviral complexes, e.g., hepatitis B virus, or by the effects of cell-mediated immunity or meningeal infiltration, e.g., HSV-1. These will be described below in greater detail.

Many infections of both acute and chronic varieties may occur without clinical symptoms of disease; these are known as **inapparent viral infections.** These appear to be of great importance in medicine because they confer immunity without overt clinical disease. This may be due to the nature of the virus or the status of host immunity. Failure of the virus to reach the target organ may be another cause of inapparent infection. In some cases of poliomyelitis, for example, in which limited replication of virus occurs in the gastrointestinal tract, the infection may not spread to the central nervous system. Instead, a localized infection may occur within the gastrointestinal tract that may be abortive or productive of few signs and symptoms within the infected host and yet capable of transmission to another susceptible individual with the production of overt paralytic disease. The use of live attenuated viral vaccines may be considered as a special case of inapparent infection, in which a purposeful attempt is made to produce a subclinical infection with resultant protective immunity without disease. Because of the uncommon but serious complication of vaccine-associated paralysis that rarely occurs following administration of the live oral poliovirus vaccine (**OPV**), the inactivated poliovirus vaccine (**IPV**) in developed countries is now used for routine immunization of infants, children, and adults (*Chapter 23*).

Immune Responses to Viral Infection Based on Viral Pathogenesis

Having described the various forms of acute and chronic viral-host cell interactions, it may now be possible to construct a central unifying description of how the immune responses may be involved in these relationships. Immunity to viruses depends upon the coordinated, interrelated, and interactive functions of numerous cell types and their products that comprise both the innate and adaptive immune systems (Table 13-4). Moreover, the immune responses to viruses are best understood in the context of viral pathogenesis with a delineation of components of the various phases of viral infection. The following components will be addressed: the environment, target cells, recovery and resistance mechanisms, innate and adaptive immune responses to viral infection, and a concept of immunologic balance based upon the model of efficiency of elimination of foreignness presented in Chapter 1.

Table 13-4. Components of the innate and adaptive immune responses

The environment
Target cells
Classification of immune responses to viral infection: recovery and resistance mechanisms
Innate immune responses to viral infection
Macrophages and dendritic cells
Interferons
NK cells
Complement
Adaptive immune responses to viral infection
B cells
T cells
CD4+ T cells (Th1, Th2, Th17, Tr1, and Th3)
CD8+ T cells (T cytotoxic [Tc])
Cytokines
Concept of immunologic balance (efficiency of elimination of foreignness)

The Environment

Viruses are found in the external environment as obligate intracellular parasites and require host cells to survive, replicate, and eventually infect another host. In order to do so, the virus must breach the natural anatomic barriers of the skin or mucous membranes of a vulnerable host and gain access to its susceptible target cells through one of the natural portals of entry, i.e., the respiratory, gastrointestinal, and genitourinary systems (Figure 13-7). In addition to these points of entry, some viruses are transmitted from the environment by biting insects that may deliver virus directly into the blood, bypassing the anatomic and physiologic barriers of innate defense. In the modern world, "artificial insects" (syringes) achieve the same purpose as exemplified by the transmission of HIV and hepatitis B and C by intravenous drug users and recipients of blood products. Viruses are extremely diverse in their capacity to infect, persist, and initiate disease in the targeted host; they utilize a variety of

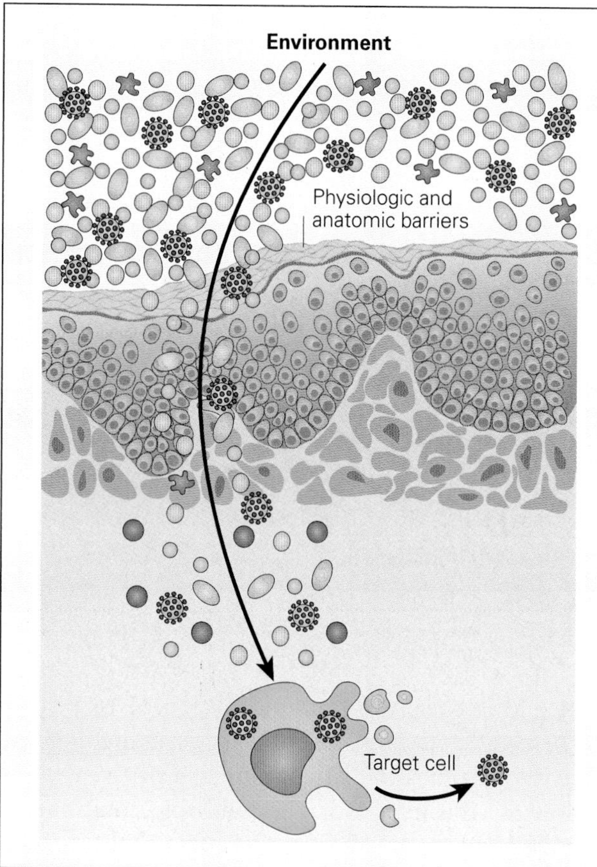

Figure 13-7. Schematic representation of the entry of infectious virus particles from the external environment and infection of a target cell of a susceptible host. This occurs only after the natural physiologic and anatomic barriers of the skin and mucosal tissues are breached.

entry strategies, including transmission via infectious respiratory secretions, fecal-oral spread, sexual contact, and bloodborne entry.

Target Cells

Following entry, viruses are not able to infect all cells indiscriminately, but bind to selected host cells via specific receptors located on target cells of the susceptible host. This selective property of viruses to infect particular target cells is referred to as "tropism" (Figure 13-8). Shown in Table 13-5 are some examples of viral tropism for various target cells, together with associated specific receptors on selected target cells to which virus binds. The selective capacity for a target cell to either manifest susceptibility for or a resistance to infection by a given virus appears to have a genetic basis. This concept is exemplified by the resistance to HIV-1 transmission of certain populations of individuals mediated by certain chemokine receptors, i.e., CXCR4 and CCR5, as described below.

Following attachment of the virus to a target cell, it penetrates and then uncoats its protein capsid, releases its nucleic acid into the cytoplasm, and begins the process of transcription followed by the production of viral proteins essential for viral replication (Figure 13-9A). As a general rule, DNA viruses replicate in the nucleus and RNA viruses in the cytoplasm (notable exceptions are influenza virus, which has a nuclear phase, and the pox viruses, which replicate in the cytoplasm). Some viruses can incorporate their nucleic acid into the cellular DNA of the nucleus. As will be described below, HIV does so through the elaboration of a cDNA through its reverse transcriptase. The viral genome is then replicated and assembled with other key components of the virus to form new "progeny" viral particles (virions) that are then released extracellularly to infect neighboring cells and tissues (Figure 13-9A).

Shown in Table 13-6 are the various pattern-recognition receptors (**PRRs**) of the innate immune system involved in viral genome recognition (*Chapters 3* and *9*).

Mitochondrial antiviral signaling (**MAVS**) is a protein that activates NF-κB and IRF 3; for RIGI, the intermediary protein is mitochondria-bound IPS1.

Classification of Immune Responses to Viral Infection

Immunity has been classically defined as encompassing all those mechanisms that are concerned with the recognition of foreignness or in response to danger signals. These immune mechanisms include both the primary encounter of a host who is susceptible and nonimmune, as well as the subsequent encounters of a host who manifests protective immunity as a result of prior exposure. Those immune mechanisms the host employs upon initial encounter with a virus are the **resistance mechanisms**, which include both natural anatomic and physiologic factors as well several components of the **innate immune system**. Those mechanisms that are employed by the host upon all subsequent encounters with the same or a similar virus are termed the **recovery mechanisms** that consist of those associated with the **adaptive immune system**. Shown in Table 13-7 is a summary of the major resistance and recovery mechanisms of viral immunity.

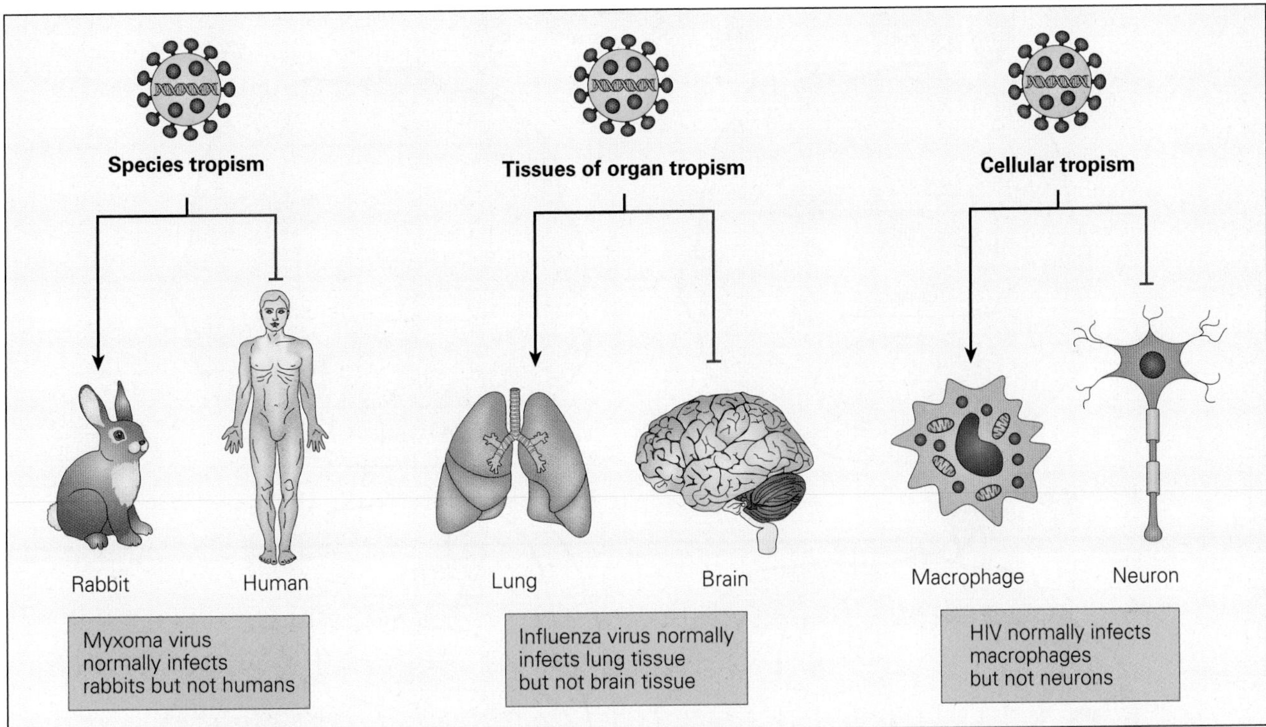

Figure 13-8. Levels of viral tropism. Viral tropism can be divided into three distinct categories depending on the physiological level at which it is measured. Tropism in which the virus replicates in one host species but not another is known as host tropism; tropism in which the virus replicates in a particular tissue or organ but not another is known as tissue tropism; and tropism in which the virus replicates in one cell type but not another is known as cellular tropism.

The Innate Immune Responses to Viral Infection

The innate immune system plays a key role in the host's initial encounter with viruses that have successfully overcome the initial barricades provided by the anatomic and physiologic components of host defense. Prominent among these are the macrophages and dendritic cells and their associated PRRs, the interferons, the natural killer (**NK**) cells, and complement (Table 13-7). These components function both as part of innate immunity and in collaboration with components of adaptive immunity.

Following replication and release of virions from infected cells, they are taken up by macrophages and dendritic cells in the extracellular tissues; here, they are degraded and processed for eventual presentation to the T cells of the adaptive immune system (Figure 13-10). Recently, Toll-like receptors (**TLRs**) and other PRRs on the surface of these cells have been recognized to serve as

Table 13-5. Examples of viral tropism for various target cells and associated specific receptors

Target cell	Virus	Specific receptor
T helper lymphocyte	Human immunodeficiency virus type 1 (HIV-1)	CD4 and co-receptors CCR5, CXCR4
B lymphocyte	Epstein-Barr virus (EBV)	Complement receptor type 2 (CR2), also called CD21
Neurons	Poliovirus	Poliovirus receptor
	Rabies	Acetylcholine receptor
Respiratory mucosal cell	Rhinovirus	CD54 (intercellular adhesion molecule 1 [ICAM-1])
	SARS	Angiotensin-converting enzyme 2 (ACE2)
Basal mucosal and epithelial cells	Human papilloma virus (HPV)	?

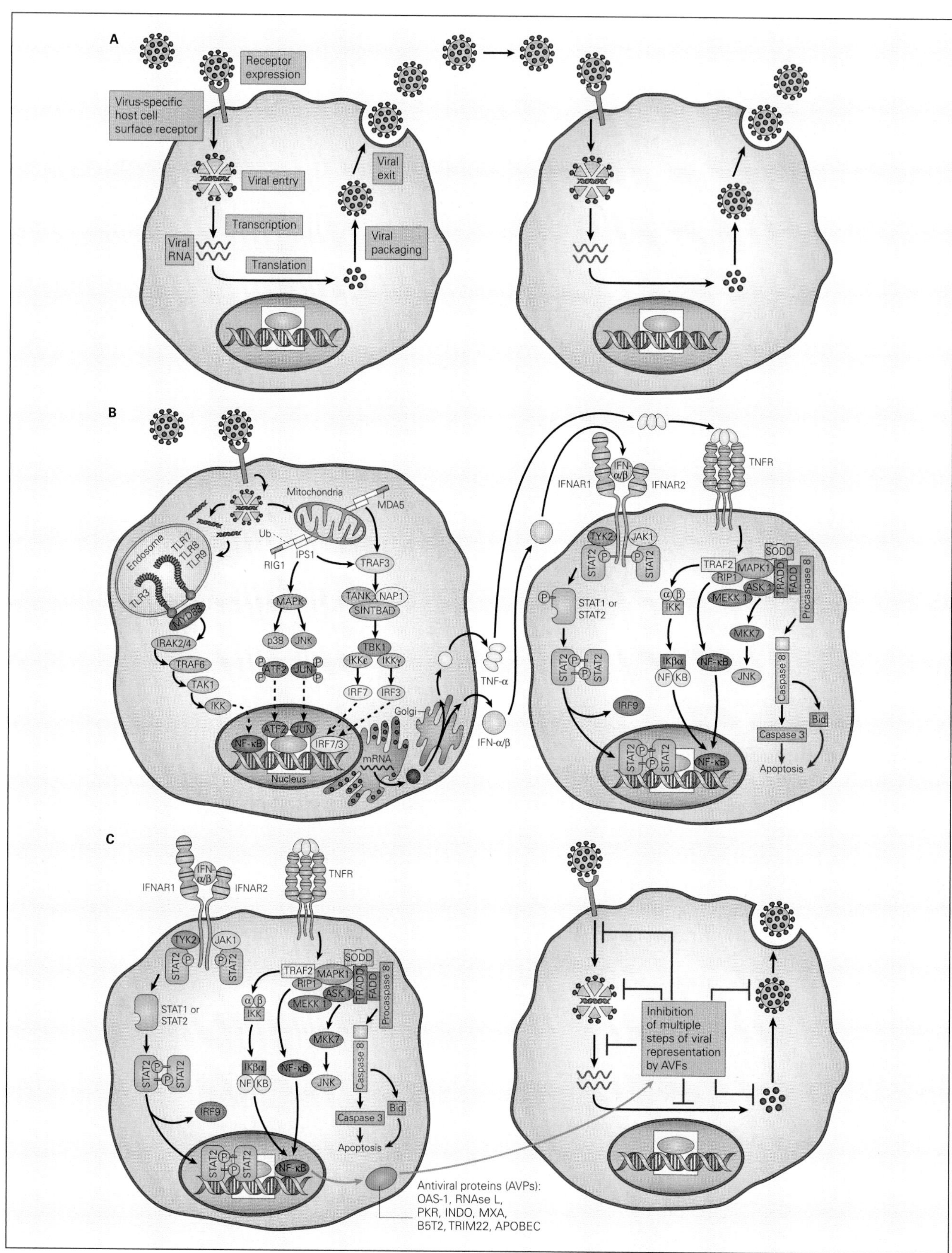

Figure 13-9. **Schematic representation of the viral-host cell interactions.** Panel A: Shows a simplified viral cycle with viral entry and replication in a target cell and transmission of the newly assembled viral particles to another susceptible cell. Panel B: Shows the PRR pathways involved in the production of antiviral cytokines, e.g., TNF-α and Type I interferon (IFN-α) after the viral molecules are recognized by intracellular sensors of the innate immune system (left cell), as well as the cytokine pathways stimulated by these antiviral cytokines in healthy target cells (right cell). Panel C: Following the binding of TNF-α and Type I interferon to their respective receptors, a number of antiviral proteins are produced that block the synthesis of infectious virus at multiple steps.

Table 13-6. Pattern-recognition receptors of the innate immune system involved in viral genome recognition

Pattern-recognition receptors	Function
Toll-like receptors (TLRs)	Initiate signaling pathways, e.g., MyD88 or TRIF, to modulate gene expression of antiviral cytokines, e.g., interferons, TNF-α
NOD-like receptors (NLRs)	NOD2 has also been shown to bind to MAVS (IPS1) in response to ssRNA or viral RNA treatment and activates the IFN response
RIG-like helicases (RLH)	RIG-1 binds to MAVS to promote Type 1 interferon synthesis in cells infected by viruses to control the infection
DNA sensors (DAI)	DAI (DNA-dependent activator of IFN-regulatory factors)

important sensing molecules to perform these functions (*Chapter 9*).

Mammalian hosts have evolved a variety of membrane-associated PRRs (e.g., TLRs) and non-membrane-associated PRRs, e.g., NOD-like receptors (**NLRs**), RIG-like helicases (**RLH**), and DNA sensors (AIM2 and DAI) for sensing a wide range of pathogens (primarily bacterial but also viral) (*Chapters 3* and *9*). These innate immune mechanisms have been recognized as crucial players in the host immune response to microbial invaders. Many innate receptors are expressed on cell surfaces, while others are found intracellularly on endocytic vesicle membranes or other intracellular organelles. The defining characteristic of these receptors is their location on cells that carry out a sentinel function in sensing foreignness at sites where early detection and responsiveness is critical. Thus, TLRs are not only expressed on circulating cells and tissue immune cells, such as monocytes, macrophages, dendritic cells, and granulocytes; they are also present in airway epithelium, skin, gastrointestinal tract, and other important target sites of host-pathogen interaction.

The TLR family is composed of membrane proteins with domains designed to sample the environment for pathogen-associated molecular patterns (**PAMPs**) (Box 13-2). Shown in Table 13-8 is a summary of the properties of the known human TLRs. TLRs become activated and transmit signals through their cytoplasmic Toll/interleukin-1 receptor (**TIR**) domains, resulting in the transcriptional induction of multiple genes involved in innate and adaptive immunity, including the type 1 interferons, interferon alpha (**IFN-α**) and interferon beta (**IFN-β**) (Box 13-3). Different TLR molecules recognize specific PAMPs; among these, TLR3, TLR7, TLR8, and TLR9 appear to play important roles in identifying viral products. TLR7 and TLR8 become activated by recognition of single-stranded RNA, whereas DNA activates TLR9. Specifically, TLR9 becomes activated in response to infection with DNA viruses, such as herpes viruses, and TLR7 and TLR8 respond to RNA viruses, such as influenza viruses and HIV. In

Table 13-7. Major resistance and resolution mechanisms of viral immunity

Type of encounter	Immunity mechanisms	Characteristics	Examples
Initial	Innate	Resistance	Skin, mucous membranes, fever, secretions, interferon Innate immunity Macrophages and DCs Pattern recognition receptors Interferons Mast cells and basophils NK cells Complement
Subsequent	Adaptive	Recovery	Adaptive immunity B cells T cells (Th [Th1, Th2, and Th3], Tc) Cytokines and chemokines

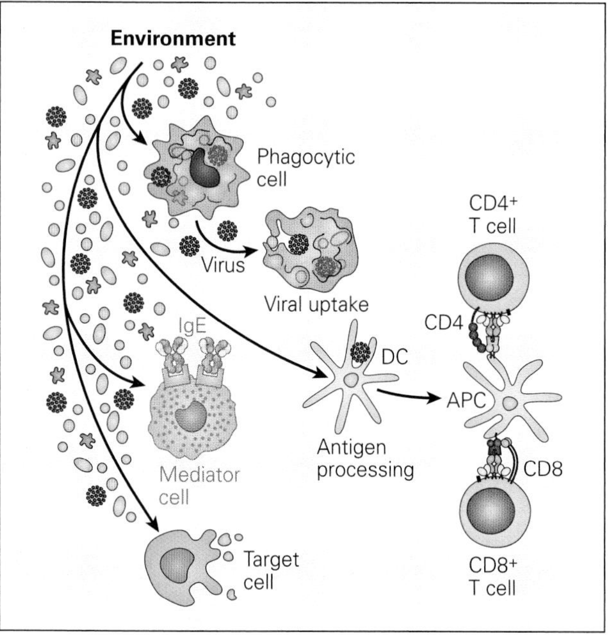

Figure 13-10. Schematic representation of the uptake of viruses by phagocytic cells (macrophages) and dendritic cells and their presentation to T cells.

contrast, TLR3 appears to represent a more general sensor of viral infection through detection of double-stranded RNA (dsRNA), a byproduct of viral replication and transcription for both RNA and DNA viruses. These four TLR molecules are localized mainly in endosomal compartments of the cell.

The interaction with their ligands leads to activation of a number of molecular events associated with innate immunity, such as enhanced antigen presentation and increased cytokine production (Table 13-8). In the case of TLR7/8/9, this involves endosome-mediated internalization of viruses; with TLR3, the ligands include products of viral replication from lysed and/or apoptotic virus-infected cells. In order to achieve optimal contact of the viral genome with its corresponding TLR, this most likely involves the critical importance of degradation of a subset of virus particles in the endosome. In addition, some cell surface-expressed TLRs, such as TLR4, have been shown to bind to specific viral glycoproteins and induce IFN production in a different range of cells.

Box 13-2

Toll-Like Receptors

It has been estimated that most mammalian species have between 10 and 15 types of Toll-like receptors. Ten TLRs have been identified in humans, (TLR1 to TLR9 and TLR11) and equivalent forms of many of these have been found in other mammalian species (*Chapter 3*). The function of TLRs in all organisms appears to be similar enough to use a single model of action. Each Toll-like receptor forms either a homodimer or heterodimer in the recognition of a specific or set of specific molecular determinants present on microorganisms.

Because the specificity of Toll-like receptors (and other innate immune receptors) cannot be changed, these receptors must recognize patterns that are constantly present as threats, not subject to mutation, and highly specific to threats (i.e., not normally found in the host where the TLR is present). Patterns that meet this requirement are usually critical to the pathogen's function and cannot be eliminated or changed through mutation; they are said to be evolutionarily conserved. Well-conserved features in pathogens include bacterial cell-surface lipopolysaccharides (LPS), lipoproteins, lipopeptides, and lipoarabinomannan; proteins such as flagellin from bacterial flagella; double-stranded RNA of viruses or the unmethylated CpG islands of bacterial and viral DNA; and certain other RNA and DNA (*Chapter 3*). Shown in Table 13-8 is a summary of the properties of the known human TLRs that are activated by viruses.

Table 13-8. Summary of known human Toll-like receptors reactive with viruses

Receptor	Ligand PAMP(s)	Activation cascade(s)
TLR 3	double-stranded RNA (as found in certain viruses), poly I:C	TRIF/TICAM (MyD88 independent)
TLR 4	lipopolysaccharide; viral glycoproteins	MyD88 dependent TIRAP; MyD88 independent TRIF/TICAM/TRAM
TLR 7	small synthetic compounds; single-stranded RNA	MyD88 dependent IRAK
TLR 8	small synthetic compounds; single-stranded RNA	MyD88 dependent IRAK
TLR 9	unmethylated CpG DNA	MyD88 dependent IRAK

Box 13-3

The Interferons

Interferons (IFNs) are a family of cytokines produced by white blood cells, fibroblasts, or T cells as part of an immune response to a viral infection or other immune triggers (*Chapter 9*). Four classes of interferons have been identified: interferon-alpha (IFN-α), interferon-beta (IFN-β), interferon-gamma (IFN-γ), and interferon-lamda (IFN-λ). IFN-α and IFN-β are known as Type I IFNs since they share the same receptor for binding to cells (*Chapter 9*). IFN-γ is referred to as Type II interferon and binds to a distinct receptor different from that used by Type I IFNs. A Type III interferon has been identified, called IFN-λ, which binds to a heterodimeric receptor made up of one chain similar to the IL-10 receptor (IL-10R) and the other chain representing a totally new and novel IFN receptor (*Chapter 9*). Deficient induction of IFN-λ has recently been observed in a subset of patients with asthma triggered by rhinovirus infection. Each class displays different effects, although their activities overlap. IFN-α and IFN-β are grouped together as type I interferons; IFN-α is produced by white blood cells and IFN-β by fibroblasts; and IFN-γ is produced by Th1 cells and cells of the innate immune system, such as NK cells, NK T cells, macrophages, and some subtypes of dendritic cells.

Cytokines and the Interferons Involved with Viral Infection

Infection by viruses results in the induction of cytokines from a variety of cell sources. These participate in numerous phases of the host response to viruses. They include the acute inflammatory response, the induction of an antiviral state that principally involves interferons (Box 13-3), as well as cytokines that regulate the nature of the ensuing adaptive immune response. In fact, cytokines constitute a major means of communication between the innate and adaptive aspects of the immune response to viruses. As described previously in Chapter 9, cytokines are also critical participants in the adaptive immune defenses.

The initial cytokines emanate mainly from infected cells or cells directly contacted by virions. The first cytokines produced consist primarily of IFN-α and IFN-β (Box 13-3), along with tumor necrosis factor alpha (**TNF-α**), IL-6, IL-14, and interferon gamma (**IFN-γ**). Some of these help orchestrate an anti-inflammatory reaction that contributes to immunity. Some viruses may themselves encode molecules that mimic cytokines or cytokine receptors, and these may interfere with the function of their normal counterparts. These so-called virokines and viroreceptors may help the virus sidestep control by the host.

Perhaps the most critical cytokines produced that contribute to the early control of virus infections are the interferons (Box 13-3). These can be produced by infected cells themselves or nearby cells exposed to products released from the infected cells. The products so far identified include interferon itself, some other cytokines, viral nucleic acids, and other TLR ligands, as well as stress proteins such as heat shock proteins. An additional major source of IFN-α that is abundantly produced upon viral infection derives from plasmacytoid dendritic cells (**PDC**). These cells have stores of the cytokine that are rapidly released when viruses contact their cell membrane. PDC are found in some tissue entry sites but also in the blood. Rapid interferon release in the blood by PDC may account for many of the acute symptoms of viral infections, such as chills, fever, nausea, and general malaise. While we know various means by which viruses cause cells to synthesize and/or release interferons, we have minimal understanding of the molecular pathways that control these events. One molecular inducer already identified is double-stranded RNA (**dsRNA**). Such molecules are produced as replication intermediates by most DNA and RNA virus infections.

The interferon response is quite short-lived and functions only when the interferons bind to specific receptors located at cell surfaces (Figure 13-11). Receptors for α/β (Type I) and γ interferons (Type II) are distinct and their binding transduces disparate signals to cells (*Chapter 9*). The outcome of receptor binding is that cells undergo a marked change in gene expression with up to 300 new cellular proteins being synthesized. One major consequence of this event is that the cell develops an antiviral state that can inhibit a wide range of viruses. Understanding this antiviral state at a molecular level is in its infancy, but several clues have emerged. For example, interferon can increase the production of an inactive cellular protein kinase RNA-dependent (**PKR**). If the cell is then infected by a virus, the dsRNA made

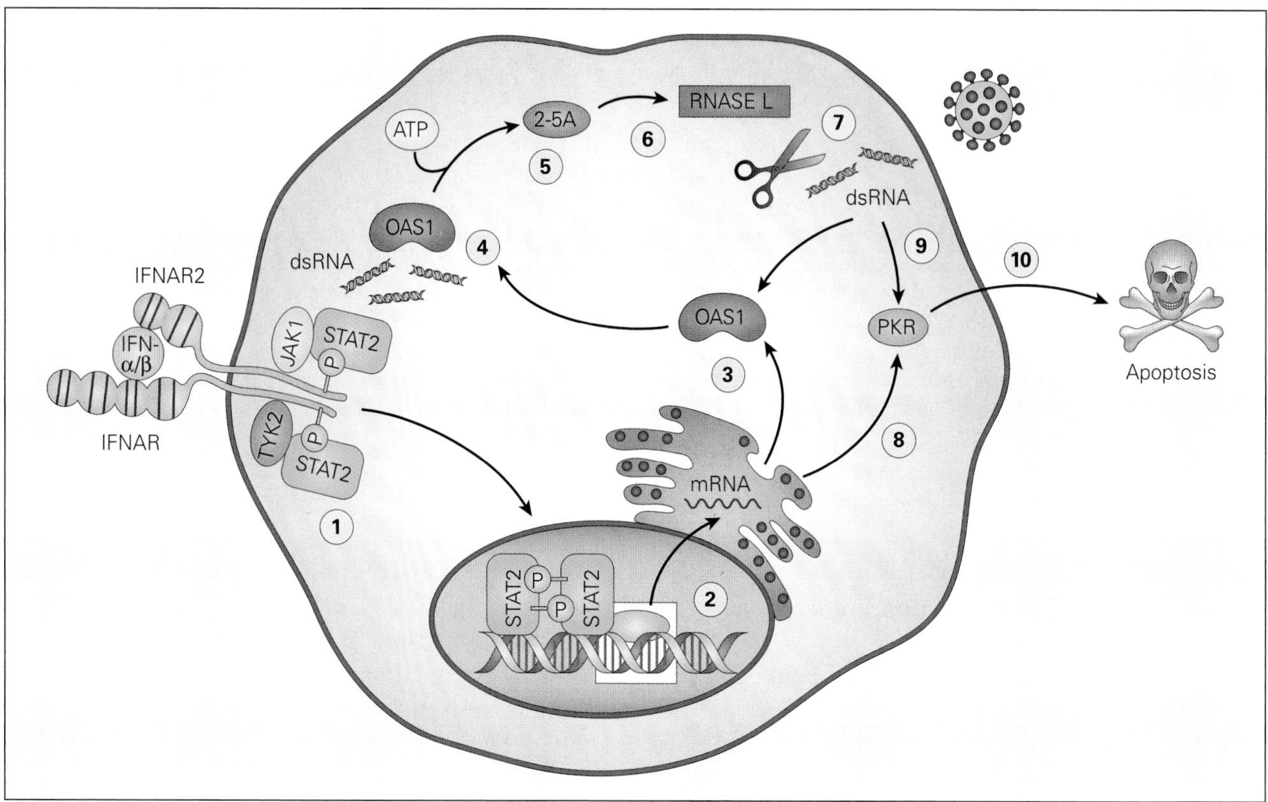

Figure 13-11. Schematic representation of antiviral action of interferon (IFN) mediated through the production and activation of 2′-5′ oligosynthetase. The binding of the IFN to its receptor activates the JAK/STAT pathway, (1) leading to the translocation of the STAT2 homodimer to the promoter region of the nuclear DNA and to the transcription of mRNA (2). This then leads to the translational synthesis of 2′-5′ oligosynthetase (OAS1) (3). The newly formed OAS1/dsRNA complex (4) leads to the production of 2′-5′ adenosine (2-5A) from its ATP precursor (5), which activates the RNAse L (6) to cleave viral dsRNA (7), which has been generated from the entry of the virion shown on the right upper side of the cell. The translational synthesis of the protein kinase RNA-dependent (PKR) (8) resulting from IFN stimulation is also activated by dsRNA (9) resulting from viral entry and will lead to apoptosis (10).

during its replication activates the PKR, which halts both viral and cellular protein synthesis and induces apoptosis (Figure 13-11).

Interferons also induce the enzymes RNase and 2′-5′ oligosynthetase. The latter is activated by dsRNA and in turn activates the RNase to degrade all viral and host mRNA. One of the possible interesting applications of this action of interferon is its effects on depleting cellular sources of ATP in CFS, which is thought by some to be caused by chronic viral infection, most recently by a xenotropic murine leukemia virus-related virus (**XMRV**). This depletion of cellular ATP caused by a persistent viral infection may be one the major causes of the inexorable fatigue that patients with disorder suffer from.

Additional antiviral mechanisms induced by interferons include the GTPase MX, which is antiviral to negative strand RNA viruses such as influenza. Others include interferon regulatory proteins, nitric oxide synthase (**NOS**) made by interferon gamma, activated antiviral NK cells, and the ubiquitin proteasome components that are involved in protein degradation. Many more antiviral mechanisms will almost certainly be discovered, and understanding how they function at a molecular level should lead to the design of novel therapeutics that will permit us to contain infection. Viruses of course do not stand by idle, but have evolved their own defenses against host protection. Some of these viral strategies are discussed subsequently.

During the early stages of viral replication associated with the intracytoplasmic release of the viral nucleic acid, the infected cell is stimulated to produce alpha and beta interferons (Figure 13-9B). These interferons can provide a signal to neighboring cells to directly inhibit viral metabolism. They do this by binding to IFN receptors on neighboring cells, where the production of antiviral proteins (**AVPs**) is stimulated. The AVPs can switch the cell from a viral-sensitive to a viral-resistant state, thus protecting them from being infected. IFN-γ produced by activated T cells, as described below, also

Table 13-9. Representation of the participation of various CD4 and CD8 T cell subsets in several antiviral defense functions

T cell	T cell subset	Antiviral function	Mechanism
CD4+	Th1	Variety of CMI events (e.g., inflammation)	Release of pro-inflammatory cytokines (e.g., IL-2, IFN-γ, and TNF-α)
	Th2	Involvement in antibody production	Th2 B cell collaboration
	Th17	?	
	Tr1, Th3 reg cells	Immunoregulation	Elaboration of immunosuppressive cytokines (e.g., IL-10 and TGF-β)
CD8+	T cytotoxic cells (Tc1 and Tc2 cells)	Lysis of viral-infected target cells	Apoptosis

induces the synthesis of the major histocompatibility complex (**MHC-I**) molecule, which makes the cell more readily recognized by cytotoxic T cells. The prevention of viral infection of neighboring cells by AVPs gives the immune system time to mobilize the T cell responses of adaptive immunity.

Adaptive Immune Responses to Viral Infection

At this point in the struggle between the virus and the host, the T cell plays a pivotal role in bridging the antiviral defense systems of innate and adaptive immunity. Shown in Table 13-9 and Figure 13-12 is a representation of how the various CD4 and CD8 T cell subsets participate in several intricate, interdependent, and interrelated antiviral defense systems. The CD4 lymphocyte population consists of at least four major subsets: (1) the Th1 cells, which are involved in many of the cell-mediated immune functions associated with viral immunity through the production of pro-inflammatory cytokines; (2) the Th2 cells, which through their collaboration with B cells help induce antiviral antibody; (3) the Th17, whose antiviral role has not yet been established; and (4) the Th3 and Tr1 Treg cells, which are critically involved in the immunoregulation of many components of adaptive immunity and which may be the ultimate arbiters of whether a viral infection is cleared or whether it may go onto chronicity.

Shown in Figure 13-13 is a schematic representation of how a virus-infected target cell can be killed by antibody, NK cells, or T cytotoxic (**Tc**) CD8+ cells. As will be described in greater detail below, a viral-infected target cell may be killed by the cytolytic action of antibody-mediated complement activity through the classical complement pathway (Figure 13-13A and *Chapter 4*). Alternatively, the killing can also occur by a CD8+ T cytotoxic cell facilitated by the prior elaboration of interferons, as described previously (Figure 13-13A). One of the consequences of interferon signaling is an increased expression of the major histocompatibility molecules, particularly MHC-I, by the target cell. These MHC-I molecules are synthesized within the endoplasmic reticulum as part of the endocytic pathway of antigen processing (*Chapter 10*), where the MHC-I comes in contact with viral peptide fragments and the complex is then carried to the cell

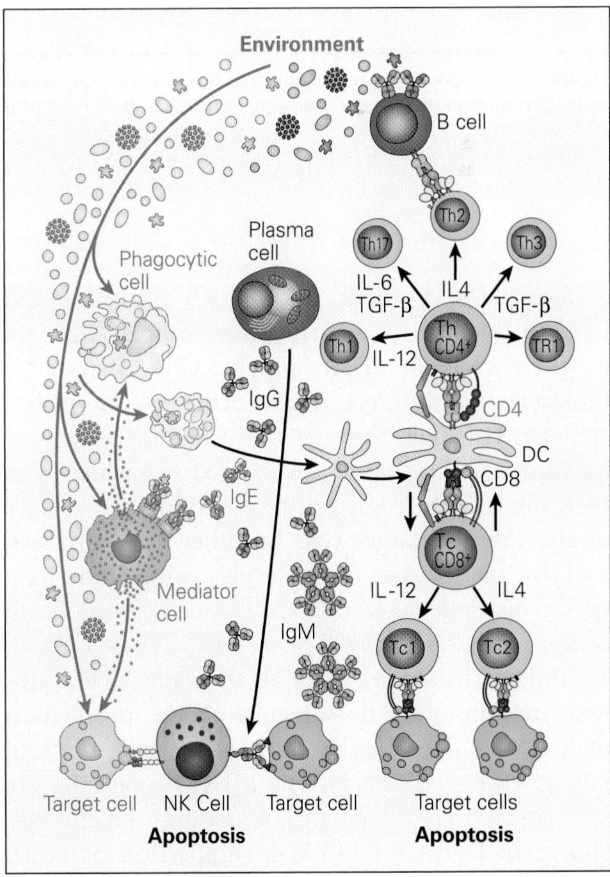

Figure 13-12. Schematic representation of the role of CD4 and CD8 T cell subsets in antiviral immunity.

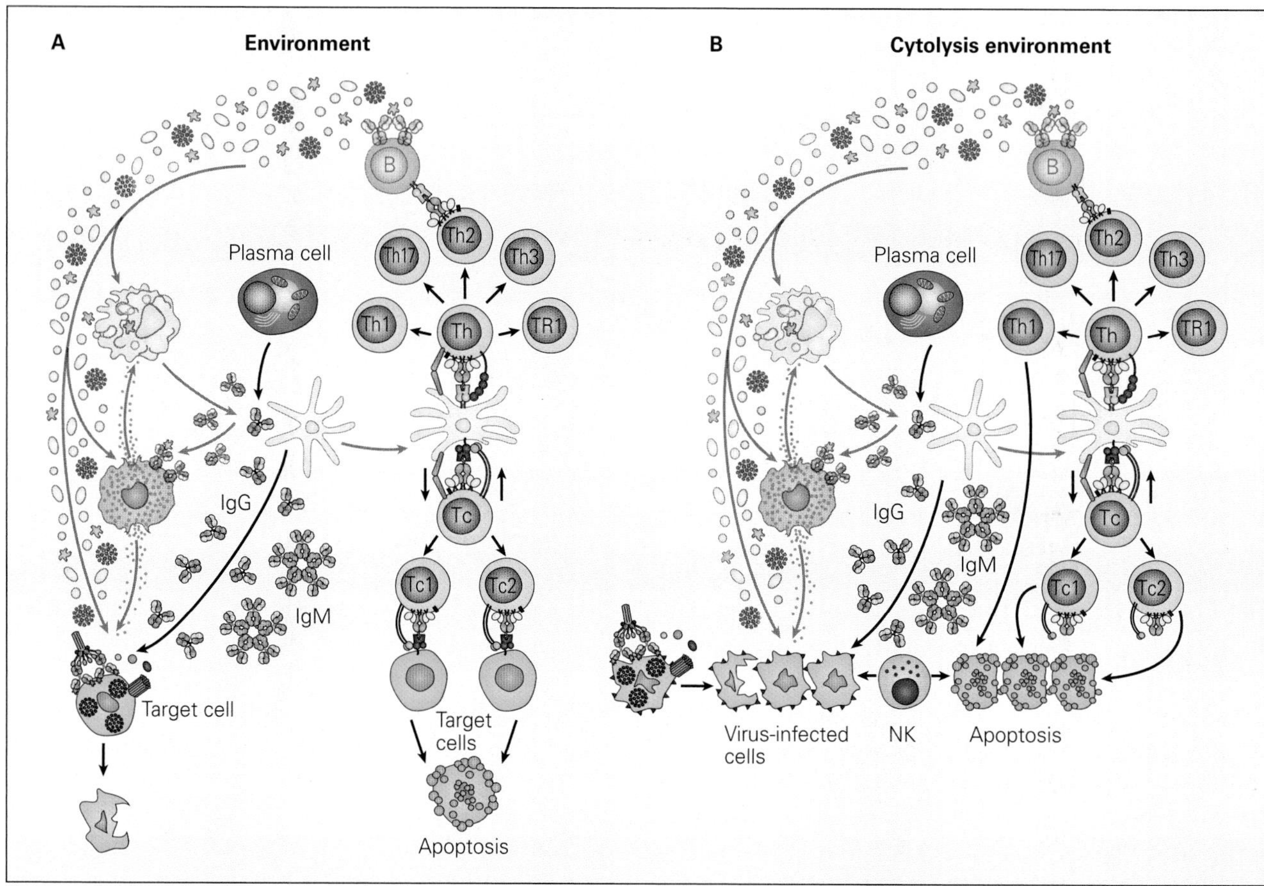

Figure 13-13. **Schematic representation of the killing of virus-infected target cells by antibody, NK cells, or T cytotoxic (Tc) CD8+ cells.** Comparison of the beneficial and detrimental outcomes of the killing of target cells by antibody, NK cells, or cytotoxic T cells. Panel A: Shows the killing of viral-infected target cells by the cytolytic action of antibody-mediated complement activity through the classical complement pathway or by CD8+ T cytotoxic cells. Panel B: Shows the killing of infected target cells by NK cells, which is particularly important when the killing by CD8+ T cells is evaded by the downregulation of target cell MHC-I production.

surface. CD8 cytotoxic T cells will recognize and bind to this MHC-I viral peptide complex through its T cell receptor (**TCR**) and the CD8 co-receptor molecule. An indirect signal may also be generated by Th1 cells through the elaboration of proinflammatory cytokines, e.g., TNF-α, which can then bind to their specific receptors on the surface of the infected target cell. In either case, this will lead to the release of molecules within the cell, which disrupts nuclear DNA and causes cell death by apoptosis (*Chapter 9*).

Some viruses may attempt to evade CD8 cytotoxic responses by downregulating the production of the MHC-I molecules essential for this mode of killing. However, cells lacking MHC-I molecules are still susceptible to killing by natural killer cells. Shown in Figure 13-13B is a comparison of target cell killing utilizing the CD8 cytotoxic subset and MHC-I with natural killer/target cell killing.

As stated previously, immunity to viruses depends on the coordinated functions of numerous cell types and their products. Most recently, these have included the subset of T cells, called Treg cells, that regulate several important components of the immune system through the elaboration of immunosuppressive cytokines, particularly interleukin 10 (**IL-10**) and TGF-β (*Chapters 7* and *9*). There has been considerable interest in the Treg cell regarding its specific role in protective as well as tissue-damaging T cell responses to several classes of microbes, particularly viruses. These relationships range from situations in which the Treg response seems to contribute to the manifestations of several diseases by helping to minimize tissue damage by counteracting the activity of immunoinflammatory T cell reactions to those in which major immune dysfunction leads to serious immunopathology caused by enhancement of immunoinflammatory T cell reactions.

Table 13-10. Some of the currently recognized mechanisms used by viruses to evade host immune responses and countermeasures used by the host

Host component targeted by the virus	Example of evasion mechanism used by the virus	Countermeasures used by the host
MHC products	Inhibition of MHC-I and MHC-II molecules at many levels of transcription, protein synthesis, accelerated destruction, intracellular retention, and increased clearance from the cell surface	Acquisition of other mechanisms of cytotoxic activity, e.g., antibody-complement-mediated killing and NK activity
CD4 helper T cell function	Paramount destruction by HIV, leading to inhibition of all CD4+ subsets	Counter by augmenting other components of the innate and adaptive immune responses' regulatory measures?
CD8+ T cell cytotoxicity	Blockage of cytotoxicity by loss of MHC-I	Use of NK cell-mediated cytotoxicity
Apoptosis	Blockage by synthesis of anti-apoptotic proteins	?
Cytokines	Interference with cytokine production	Utilization of new cytokine pathways and redundancy in cytokine functions
Humoral responses	Interference with Fc and complement components	Utilization of alternate complement pathways

In several parasitic infections, for example, Treg cells maintain equilibrium to ensure parasite persistence, minimal tissue damage, and immunity to reinfection (*Chapter 15*). In contrast, accumulating evidence suggests that the inability to clear viral infections with persistence of viral antigen plays a pathogenetic role in the immunopathology of allergic and autoimmune diseases, as well as in the evasion of protective immune responses responsible for the progression of cancer (*Chapter 18*). Although there are several unresolved questions about the role of Treg cells in microbial infections, learning how to successfully manipulate Treg responses holds great promise in the control of these diseases through the use of immunomodulators and the development of more effective vaccines (*Chapters 11* and *23*). Most recently, the T helper CD4+ type 17 (Th17) cells have been identified as a distinct lineage of T cells that produce the effector molecules IL-17, IL-17F, IL-21, and IL-22 (*Chapters 7* and *9*). Although the role of Th17 cells in autoimmunity is well documented, there is growing evidence that the Th17 lineage and other interleukin IL-17-producing cells are critical for host defense against bacterial and fungal and possibly viral infections at mucosal surfaces. These recent studies suggest that the function of IL-17-producing cells is to serve as a bridge between innate and adaptive immunity against infectious diseases at mucosal sites.

Antibody and complement also play key roles in the body's major antiviral defense mechanisms. Both infected target cells and extracellular free viruses express viral antigens on their surfaces, to which antiviral antibody can bind (Figure 13-13A). Following the binding of antibody to viral antigens on membrane surfaces, complement may be activated with generation of membrane-attack complexes, resulting in target cell lysis with loss of intracellular contents (*Chapter 4*). Similarly, viruses can be inactivated directly by complement in the presence or absence of antibody. For most viruses, inactivation requires only the early components of the complement cascade (C1, C4, and C2), while other membrane-associated viruses require inactivation by later components of the MAC-mediated pathway. The binding of antibody or antibody complement on the surface of a viral particle destroys the infectivity of the virus and prevents it from infecting another uninfected target cell.

Antibody also plays a role in antiviral immunity through the mechanism of antibody-dependent cellular cytotoxicity (**ADCC**) by NK cells; antibody bridges the Fc receptor on the NK cell and attaches to viral antigen on the cell membrane of the virus-infected target cell. IgG antibodies provide a major barrier to spread between cells and tissues and are particularly effective in the blood and interstitial fluids. The production of secretory IgA antibody has been shown to be effective at mucosal surfaces and serves to provide a first line of protective immunity at these surfaces (*Chapter 8*). Vaccines that stimulate these mucosal antibodies have been found to be effective in preventing initial and subsequent infections. New strategies are being increasingly directed at the development of viral vaccines that stimulate these antibodies at mucosal surfaces, e.g., intranasal influenza vaccines and orally administered rotavirus vaccines (*Chapter 23*).

Following immunization or infection with viruses, there is a sequential appearance of the molecular varieties of antibody (*Chapter 6*). Initial antibody in serum is usually associated with the IgM class and is followed later by IgG antibody. The precise timing of the IgA antibody is unknown, but it appears within a few days or several weeks after the appearance of IgM and IgG antibody. Since IgM production is more pronounced in the fetus or newborn than in the adult, the measurement of elevated total levels of IgM or more importantly IgM-specific antibodies seen in intrauterine infections, such as those caused by the toxoplasma, rubella, cytomegalovirus, and herpes viruses, (**TORCH**) syndrome, and HIV infection has been found to be useful in diagnosing these infections in early life.

Mechanisms Used by the Virus to Evade Immune Responses

Throughout the course of evolution, there has been a continuous set of interactions between host and pathogens, each attempting to assert its survival advantage over the other. As described in *Chapter 2*, the development of the immune system in the species, i.e., phylogeny, may be considered as a series of genetically determined cellular adaptations that occurred in response to an ever-changing and potentially hostile environment. In each of these situations, the best-adapted form that survived in each new environment was the one best selected for its continued existence. Thus, the development of all innate and adaptive immune responses to viral infection occurred as a continuing set of adaptive responses to a changing environment. Viruses likewise have exhibited many genetically determined adaptive transformations to counter and evade host defenses. Shown in Table 13-10 are some of the currently recognized mechanisms used by viruses to evade host immune responses.

Concept of Immunologic Balance

Throughout this book, the concept of immunologic balance has been stressed as a central unifying theme for an understanding of the clinical applications of immunology in health and disease (Figure 13-14). This model presents the responses of the immune system in three progressive phases, each based on the efficiency of elimination of foreign substances, i.e., phase 1, **innate immunity**; phase 2, **adaptive immunity**; and phase 3, **the tissue-damaging effects**. Most foreign configurations are eliminated efficiently during the first two phases of innate immunity and adaptive, which, when efficiently eliminated, characterize the **immune system in health**. If foreignness cannot be eliminated efficiently in the first two phases and persists or is continually reintroduced, the third phase, the most harmful, emerges and contributes to the pathogenesis of immunologically mediated disorders. It represents the **immune system in disease** in the form of allergic disease, autoimmunity, or malignancy. Chronic viral infection represents the example *par excellence* of persistence of antigen wreaking immunologic havoc by contributing to the pathogenesis of these disorders. This model is built on the premise that the immune system is a physiologic system of cells and cell products that respond to danger signals and that recognize and remove foreign configurations with or without detriment to its own tissues. In performing these functions, the immunologic system attempts to maintain a balance between the internal and external environments, and the efficiency with which foreignness is eliminated will determine whether the outcome of this struggle will be beneficial or harmful. Nowhere is this concept of immunologic balance better exemplified than with the host immune response to viral invaders, particularly those that persist.

Human Immunodeficiency Virus: Epidemiology

This section will be devoted to a description of the antiviral mechanisms of immunity that are seen in the devastating disease caused by HIV-1 infection. Because of its worldwide prevalence and lethality, accompanied by its sophisticated viral-host cell interaction, it not only represents the greatest example of how a virus can subvert, evade, and ultimately destroy the immune system, but also presents the ultimate challenge for the clinical management of the most devastating and evasive infectious disease of our time.

The origins of HIV in the human are believed to have arisen in Africa (Box 13-4). The first cases of AIDS were reported in the United States during the

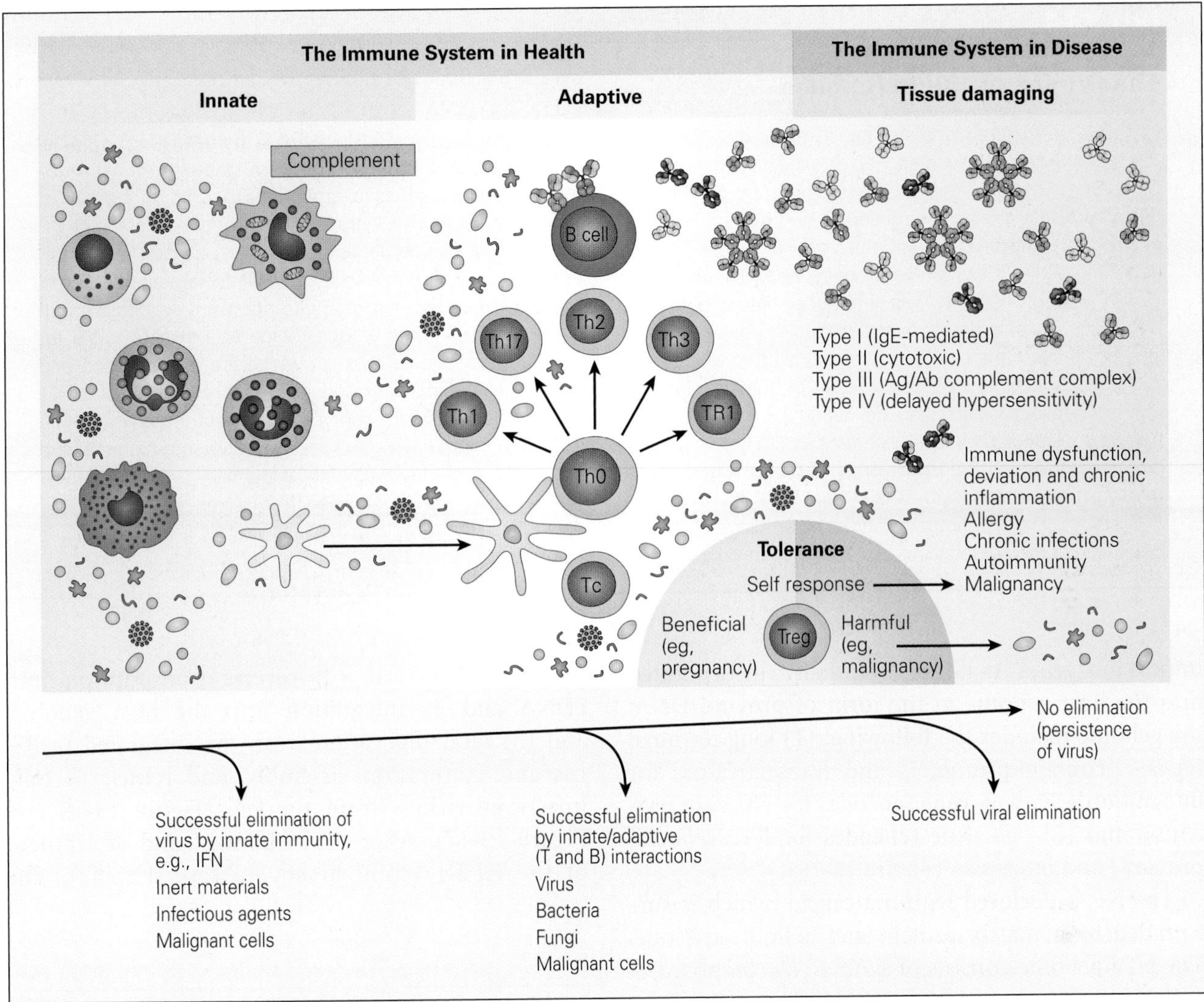

Figure 13-14. Schematic representation of responses of the immune system in three progressive phases, each based on the efficiency of elimination of foreign substances, i.e., phase 1, innate immunity; phase 2, adaptive immunity; and phase 3, the tissue-damaging effects. Chronic viral infections comprise a major source of persistent antigen and etiologic agent for immunologically mediated disorders.

summer of 1981 in five young men, all active homosexuals, who were treated for biopsy-confirmed *Pneumocystis carinii* pneumonia, and in a group of Haitian patients with opportunistic infections and Kaposi's sarcoma (Figure 13-15). As described previously, since then, the number of infections with HIV throughout the world has grown to pandemic proportions, resulting in an estimated 65 million infections and 25 million deaths. HIV continues to disproportionately affect certain geographic regions (e.g., sub-Saharan Africa and the Caribbean) and subpopulations (e.g., women in sub-Saharan Africa, men who have sex with men, injection-drug users, and sex workers). Effective prevention and treatment of HIV infection with antiretroviral therapy (**ART**) is now available, even in countries with limited resources. Nonetheless, comprehensive programs are needed to reach all persons who require treatment and to prevent transmission of new infections.

Human Immunodeficiency Virus: Structure and Pathogenicity

Human immunodeficiency virus is a member of the *Retroviridae* family, subfamily *Lentivirinae,* and consists of a spherical virion 80–100 nm in diameter and with a unique three-layer structure (Figure 13-16). The innermost layer is the genome-nucleoprotein (**NP**) complex with reverse transcriptase (**RT**), integrase, and protease. The HIV genome contains

Box 13-4

The Origins of HIV in Humans

HIV-1 was first introduced into the human population from the chimpanzee subspecies *Pan troglodytes* in southern Cameroon. Chimpanzees in this region carry SIV strains (SIVcpzptt) that are closely related to two distinct lineages of HIV-1, i.e., the main (M) and the new (N) groups. The origin of the outlier (O) group might be related to a jump from *Gorilla gorilla.* SIVcpzptt was introduced into the human population multiple times, over decades to possibly centuries, but these transfer events probably started to increase in the 1920s to the 1950s as a result of human migration into this dense tropical region. Following this founder event, human population density and contact had to be sufficiently high for subsequent transmission and spread. It is possible that a single transmission of HIV-1 group M spawned the > 60–80 million infections that have taken place since the beginning of the epidemic.

By contrast, HIV-2 originated in humans from a cross-species transmission from sooty mangabeys in West Africa (near or in Guinea-Bissau) around 1930–1955. In the 1980s, the incidence of HIV-1 group M in central Africa and HIV-2 in west Africa expanded exponentially, but clearly at different rates, as the prevalence of HIV-1 M infections (28 million) far exceeded that of HIV-2 infections (< 1 million). In stark contrast, HIV-1 groups O and N are responsible for < 25,000 infections, most of which are in Cameroon and Gabon. The expansion and divergent evolution of HIV-1 group M into diverse subtypes has been dated to 1956–1976 and might have coincided with human emigration and the seeding of new regional epidemics in central Africa. (Reproduced with permission from Ariën KK, Vanham G, Arts EJ. Is HIV-1 evolving to a less virulent form in humans? Nat Rev Microbiol. 2007;5:141–51.)

important genes that are eventually incorporated into the host genome in the form of proviral DNA; the genome includes the following: (1) long terminal repeats (contain promoters and transactivators for integration); (2) *gag*- gene (encodes for NC core proteins); and (3) *pol*- gene (encodes for RT, RNaseH, protease, and integrase) (Figure 13-16).

The NP is enclosed within a capsid, which is surrounded by a matrix protein and a lipid envelope. The HIV genome consists of a 70S RNA composed of two 35S RNA subunits and a tRNA. The surface glycoproteins (**GP**) include gp120, crucial for attachment of the virion to a CD4 receptor on a T cell, and a gp41, important for fusion of the viral envelope with the cel membrane, allowing the viral nucleic acid to enter the cell. The HIV envelope glycoproteins (Env) are organized on virions as trimeric spikes of noncovalently associated heterodimers of gp120 and gp41. Gp120 contains highly conserved binding sites for the co-receptor CD4 and the two chemokine receptors CCR5 and CXCR4. In addition, gp120 contains externally oriented variable loops (V1, V2, V3, and V4) that by their variability protect underlying gp120 core domain (Figure 13-16). It is this variability that has thwarted all attempts at developing a gp120-based HIV vaccine.

Human Immunodeficiency Virus: HIV-1 Life Cycle and Viral Integration

The life cycle of HIV can be divided into several phases: (1) attachment, fusion, and entry of the virus into the cell; (2) reverse transcription into cDNA and its integration into the host genome; and (3) viral replication from the integrated provirus and maturation, assembly, and release of fully infectious virions from the cell (Figure 13-16 and Figure 13-17). After initial contact and attachment of the HIV-1 virion to any of several cells of the

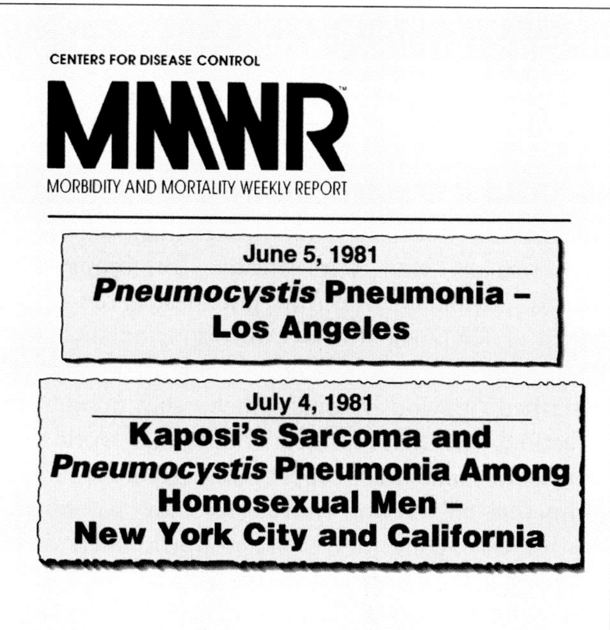

Figure 13-15. First reported U.S. cases of opportunistic infections and Kaposi's sarcoma reported by the CDC in 1981 that were later identified as HIV-1 infections.

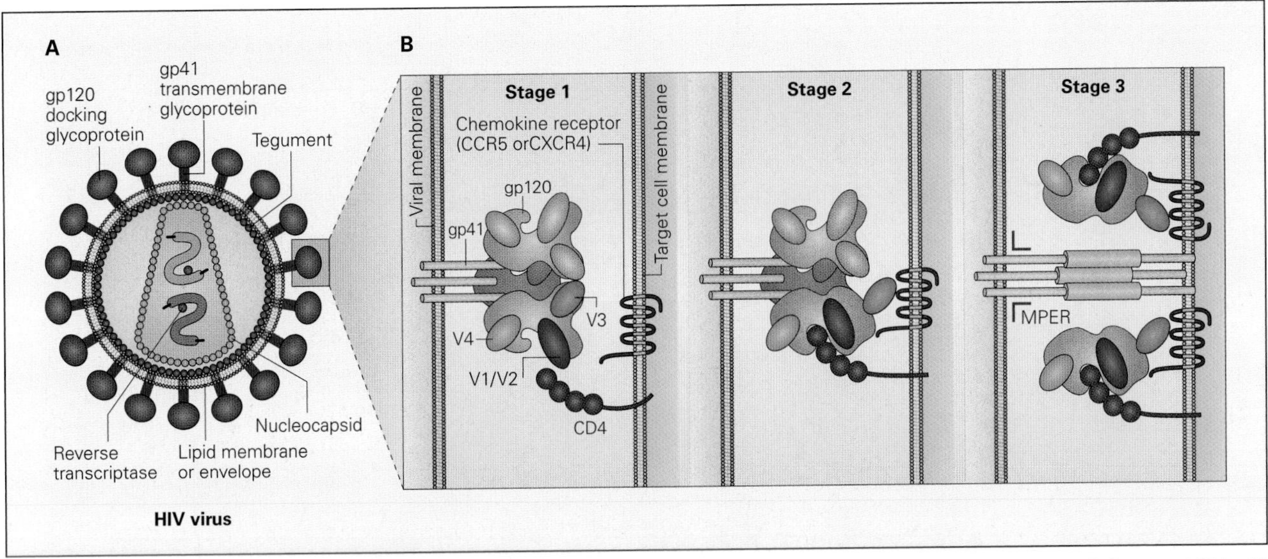

Figure 13-16. Panel A: Schematic representation of the structure of the HIV-1 virion showing the trimeric spikes of three gp120/gp41 heterodimers on the viral envelope. Panel B: Stage 1, structure of the gp120/gp41 heterodimer on the viral envelope showing the externally oriented variable loops V1/V2, V3, and V4 on the gp120 and the CD4 and CCR5 and CXCR4 chemokine receptors located on the surface of a CD4+ T cell. Stage 2 shows the insertion of the CD4 into a binding pocket located between V1/V2 and V4 loops and the attachment of V3 to either of the two chemokine receptors. Stage 3 shows the separation of the gp120 from the gp41 components, which in turn fuse with the cellular membrane, allowing the entry of the viral genome into the cell.

immune system (e.g., lymphocytes or monocytes), there is a cascade of intracellular events, the end result of which is the production of massive numbers of new viral particles, death of the infected cells, and ultimate devastation of the immune system. Figure 13-17 is a schematic representation of the various steps involved in the HIV-1 life cycle, from the initial attachment of the HIV-1 viral particle to a CD4+ T cell through the budding of new viruses from that cell.

Attachment, Fusion, and Entry of the Virus into the Cell

The first phase begins with the binding of the glycoprotein gp120 to the CD4 co-receptor of a helper T cell as well as to CC chemokine receptor type 5 (**CCR5**) or CXC chemokine receptor type 4 (**CXCR4**) (Figure 13-16). The binding of the CD4 occurs in a pocket between V1/V2 and V4, while the binding of the chemokine receptor to the trimeric gp120/gp41 heterodimers occurs through V3. The binding of the three gp120/gp41 heterodimers to these co-receptors facilitates the splitting of the gp120 from the three gp41 components, which in turn are free to fuse with the cellular membrane and ultimately allow the entry of the viral genome into the cell (Figure 13-16, Stage 3).

Reverse Transcription Into CDNA and Its Integration into the Host Genome

Following entry into the cell, the viral RNA is retrotranscribed into double-stranded, complementary DNA (**dscDNA**) in the cytoplasm by its reverse transcriptase, following which it enters the nucleus through a nuclear pore (Figure 13-17). The dscDNA either circularizes as circular non-integrated DNA or is integrated as a provirus into the host cell genome. After integration, the provirus remains quiescent, existing in a permanent post-integration latent state until its activation.

Activation of the HIV Provirus, Assembly, and Release of Infectious Virions

Activation of the HIV provirus occurs concurrently with the activation of the infected CD4+ T cell (Figure 13-17). On activation, the viral genome is transcribed into mRNA by the synergic interaction of three cellular transcription factors: (1) nuclear factor-κB (**NF-κB**), (2) nuclear factor of activated T cells (**NFAT**), and (3) specificity protein 1 (**SP1**) with the elongation factor, i.e., the viral transactivator (**Tat**). The regulator of virion (**Rev**), an HIV viral protein, regulates the splicing and cytosolic transport of some of the viral mRNAs to the cytoplasm, where they are translated into regulatory and structural viral proteins that are cleaved by viral proteases

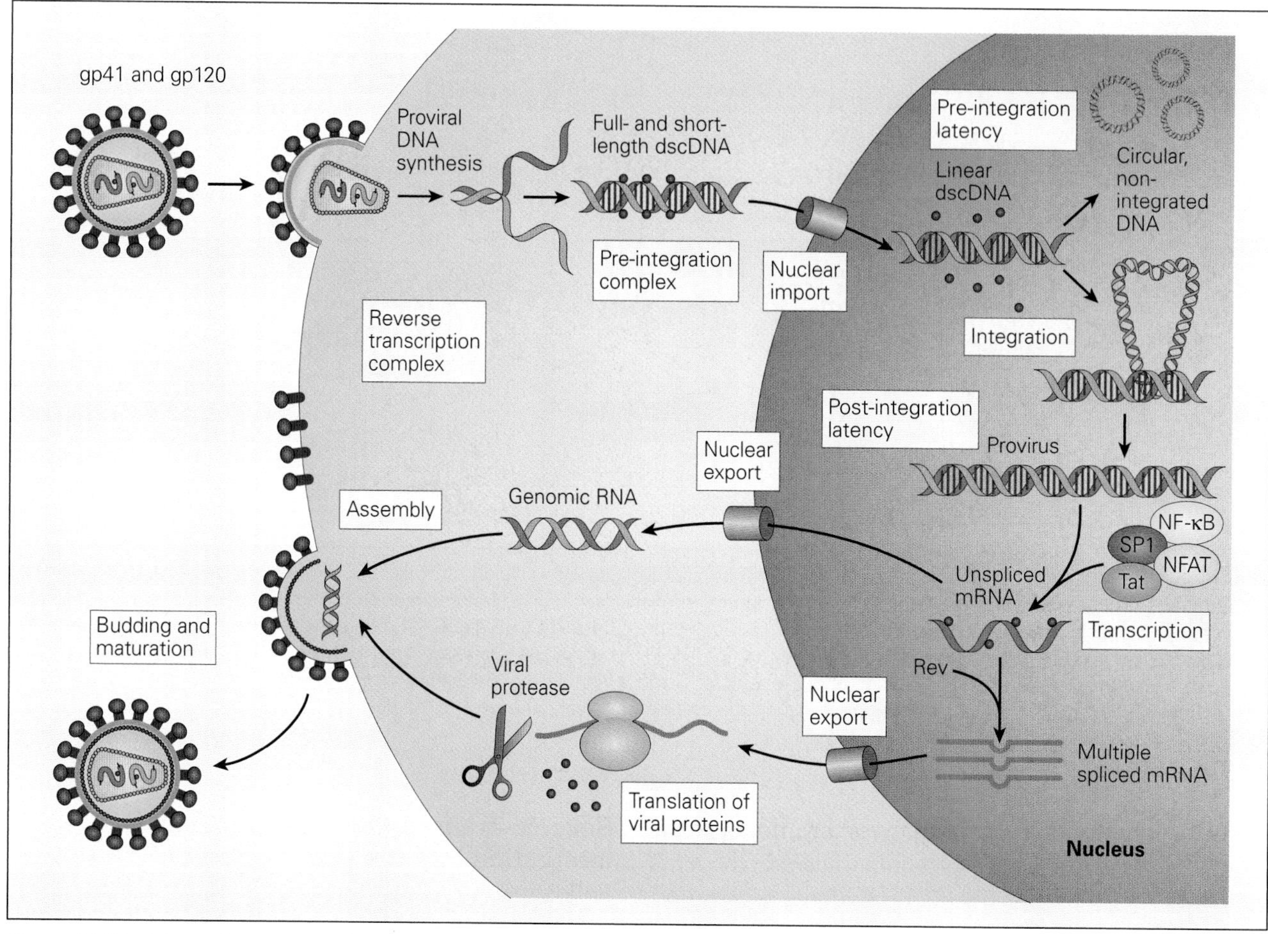

Figure 13-17. Schematic representation of the various steps involved in the HIV-1 life cycle, from initial attachment of the HIV-1 viral particle to a CD4+ T cell, fusion, and entry of the virus into the cell, conversion of the viral RNA by reverse transcription into cDNA, its integration into the host genome and activation of the HIV provirus, and its assembly and release of infectious virions through budding of new viruses from the infected cell. (Adapted with permission from Coiras M, López-Huertas MR, Pérez-Olmeda M, et al. Understanding HIV-1 latency provides clues for the eradication of long-term reservoirs. Nat Rev Microbiol. 2009;7:798-812.)

(Figure 13-17). New virions assemble and bud through the cell membrane, maturing through the activity of the viral protease.

HIV-1 Tropism

As described previously, HIV-1 manifests a tropism for many key cells of the immune system and infects predominantly CD4 cells, dendritic cells, and macrophages. HIV enters a cell by means of the binding of the two non-covalently associated viral glycoproteins (gp120 and gp41) located in the viral envelope (Figure 13-17). Although the gp120 binds to CD4, which is expressed in varying concentrations in various target cells, since the highest concentration of this co-receptor is found on activated T helper CD4+ cells, they constitute the principal target of infection and a reservoir for latency. Moreover, the infected macrophages and dendritic cells that are less accessible to antiviral treatment also serve as secondary reservoirs and represent a major obstacle for therapeutic eradication strategies.

A fascinating example of natural resistance to HIV infection is seen in individuals with a rare hereditary mutation of the chemokine receptor targets of HIV. Tropism of HIV-1 has been found to be restricted in individuals lacking CCR5 who are unusually resistant to HIV infection (Box 13-5). The HIV that causes primary infection uses CCR5 as a co-receptor and requires only a relatively low level of CD4 on the surface of the cell it infects. This virus that utilizes this chemokine receptor selectively infects dendritic cells, macrophages, and T cells *in vivo* and is referred to as a macrophage-tropic or R5 virus. In contrast, lymphocytotropic variants that infect only CD4 cells and use the CXCR4 as a coreceptor are referred to as X4 viruses. R5 variants are the most frequent isolates.

The multi-stratified mucosal epithelia found in the vagina, penis, cervix, and anus serve as targets of

Box 13-5

Genetic Alleles with Associated Decreased Susceptibility to HIV-1 Infection

Studies of exposed seronegative individuals in Gambia with persistent high-risk sexual behavior have suggested these individuals to be less susceptible to human immunodeficiency virus type 1 (HIV-1) infection because they carry the chemokine receptor (CR) gene alleles CCR5 open reading frame (ORF) Delta32, CCR5 promoter 2459G, or CCR2 ORF 64I (CCR2-64I). All three of these alleles have been found to diminish HIV-1 infectivity and/or disease progression. The results of these studies suggest that the CCR5 ORF Delta32/wt-CCR5-2459 A/G genotype combination offers an advantage in resisting sexual HIV-1 transmission and that this effect is mediated by a relative paucity of CCR5 on potential target cells of HIV-1. Conversely, the risk for HIV-1 infection associated with a common CXCL14 (SDF1) polymorphism, and CXCR4 variation varies in an African population.

viral attachment and portals of entry of HIV-1. The dendritic cells found in these areas become the adventitious targets for HIV and initiate infection by gp120 attaching to a cell surface adhesion molecule named dendritic cell-specific intercellular adhesion molecule-3 grabbing non-integrin (**DC-SIGN**), also known as CD209. A second type of mucosa found in the intestine, rectum, and endocervix consists of a single layer of epithelial cells. These cells carry CCR5 and other HIV-binding molecules (glycosphingolipid galactosyl ceramide) that serve as points of HIV-1 attachment and entry.

Treatment of HIV: The Development of Antiretroviral Agents

The development of antiviral agents was made possible as a result of the intensive research and increased understanding of the HIV-1 genome and the specific molecular pathways associated with its replication in infected host cells. The products of the polymerase (*pol*- gene) not only serve important functions in viral replication, but also act as targets for a variety of antiviral agents that have been developed for the treatment of HIV infection and are referred to as antiretroviral drugs. When several of these agents, typically three or four, are taken in combination, the approach is known as highly active antiretroviral therapy, or (**HAART**). The American National Institutes of Health and other organizations recommend offering antiretroviral treatment to all patients with AIDS.

Shown in Figure 13-18 is a schematic representation demonstrating the various points at which the products of the HIV-1 genome are targeted by the various classes of antiretroviral drugs. These medications have been classified according to the various points that they target in the replication cycle of HIV-1 and are shown in Table 13-11 together with their mechanisms of action. They include the following:

- Nucleoside/nucleotide reverse transcriptase inhibitors (**nRTI**) inhibit reverse transcription by being incorporated into the newly synthesized viral DNA and preventing its further elongation.
- Non-nucleoside reverse transcriptase inhibitors (**NNRTI**) inhibit reverse transcriptase directly by binding to the enzyme and interfering with its function.
- Maraviroc and Enfuvirtide are the two currently available agents in this class.
- Protease inhibitors (**PIs**) target viral assembly by inhibiting the activity of protease, an enzyme used by HIV to cleave nascent proteins for final assembly of new virions.
- Integrase strand transfer inhibitors inhibit the enzyme integrase, which is responsible for integration of viral DNA into the DNA of the infected cell. There are several integrase inhibitors currently under clinical trial, and Raltegravir became the first to receive FDA approval in October 2007.
- Fusion/entry inhibitors interfere with binding, fusion, and entry of HIV-1 to the host cell by blocking one of several targets.
- Maturation inhibitors inhibit the last step in gag processing in which the viral capsid polyprotein is cleaved, thereby blocking the conversion of the polyprotein into the mature capsid protein (p24). Because viral particles resulting from treatment with these agents have a defective core, the virions released consist mainly of noninfectious particles. There are no drugs in this class currently available, although two are under investigation, Bevirimat and Vivecon.

The Prion Diseases

Previously, a group of fatal neurodegenerative diseases in both animals and the human were thought to be caused by viral agents with long incubation periods and a slow pathogenesis and were therefore

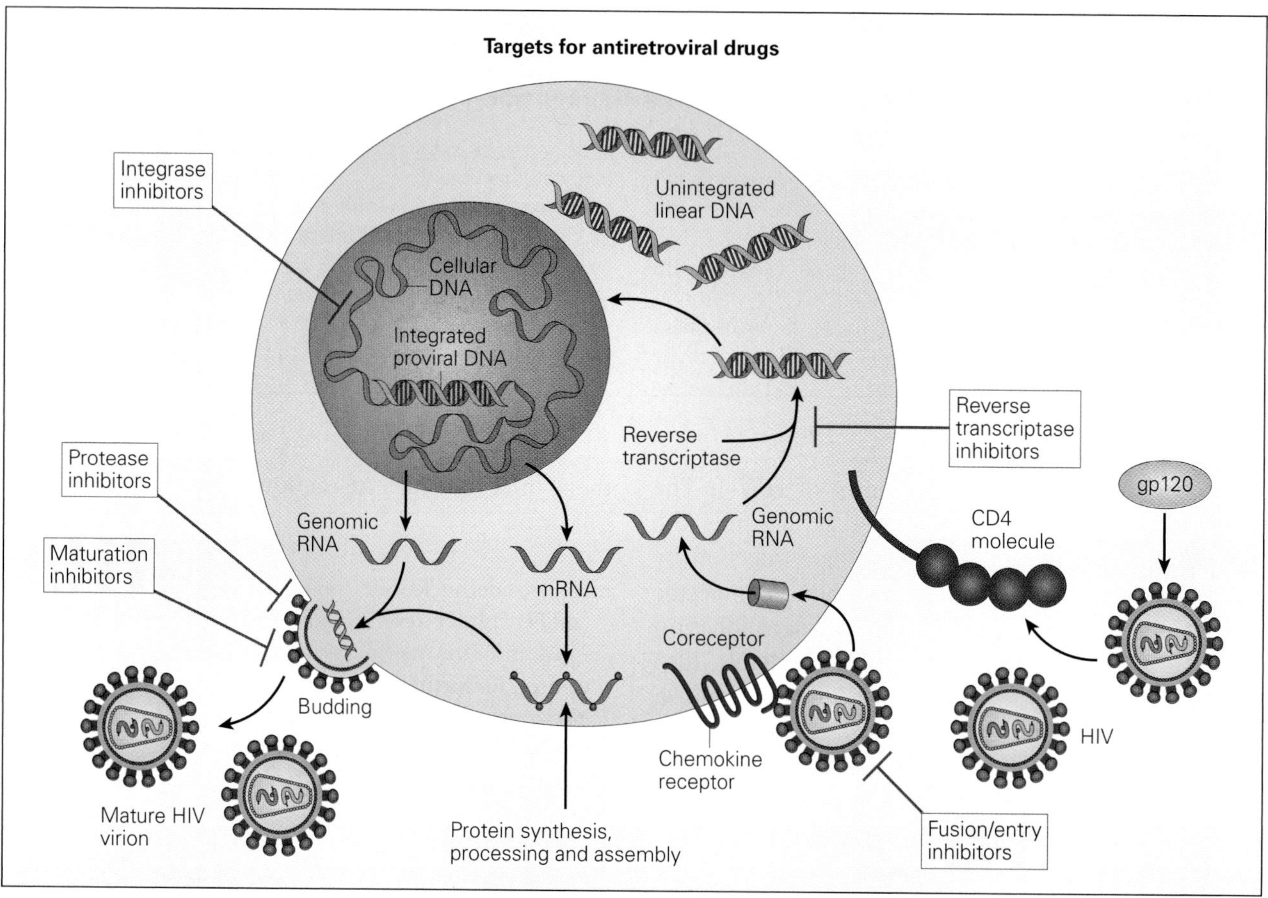

Figure 13-18. Various products of the HIV-1 genome and the points at which they serve as targets for antiviral drugs.

called "slow viral infections." Despite their suspected viral etiology, attempts at viral isolation from affected tissues were uniformly unsuccessful. These diseases are now considered to be caused by proteins, which, despite the fact that they lack a nucleic acid genome, have the unusual capacity to serve as infectious transmittable agents and are called prions. Prion diseases are often called spongiform encephalopathies because of the post mortem appearance of the brains of affected animals or humans that contain large vacuoles in neurons of the cortex and cerebellum, resembling a sponge-like structure. Many of these diseases are known to be transmissible and are referred to as transmissible spongiform encephalopathies (**TSEs**). Their pathogenesis is based on the self-propagating amyloid form of the protein PrP. PrPcs is the normal form of Prp found on the membranes of cells. Upon acquisition of the infectious isoform of PrP, known as PrPSc, the PrPc proteins are converted into the infectious prion isoform by conformational changes. Shown in Table 13-12 are examples of the spongiform encephalopathies in animals and the human.

Although most mammalian species develop these diseases, the greatest knowledge of the pathogenesis of the spongiform encephalopathies came from studies of the strange neurodegenerative disease of kuru seen in the aborigines of New Guinea. The aborigines practiced a primitive ritualistic form of cannibalism consisting of eating human brain tissues obtained from deceased members of a tribe. Since in general, women ate brain tissue rather than the men, it was more frequently the women and children who died relatively rapidly of the disease after consuming infected brain tissue. The other more recent observations that demonstrated a chain of transmission of the spongiform encephalopathies from animals to the human were made in the so-called "mad cow disease" or bovine spongiform encephalopathy (**BSE**), resulting from the ingestion by cattle of feed prepared from the remains of scrapie-infected sheep and cattle. Following

Table 13-11. Various antiretroviral drugs used for the treatment of HIV, together with their mechanisms of action

Drug class	Brand name	Generic name	Mechanism of action
Nucleoside/nucleotide reverse transcriptase inhibitors (NRTIs)	Combivir	Lamivudine/ Zidovudine (AZT)	An activated nucleotide triphosphate that has greater affinity for reverse transcriptase than for human DNA polymerase; causes chain termination during DNA synthesis.
	Truvada	Tenofovir/ Emtricitabine	
	Zerit	Stavudine	
	Ziagen	Abacavir	
	Viread	Tenofovir	
Non-nucleoside reverse transcriptase inhibitors (NNRTIs)	Atripla	Efavirenz/ Tenofovir[a]/ Emtricitabine[a]	Noncompetitive inhibitors of reverse transcriptase that do not require phosphorylation; bind at sites distinct from nucleosides.
	Viramune	Nevirapine	
	Sustiva	Efavirenz	
	Intelence	Etravirine	
	Rescriptor	Delavirdine	
Fusion/entry inhibitors	Fuzeon	Enfuvirtide	Prevents fusion of virus with cell membrane; binds gp41 (envelope protein) and prevents conformational change that allows virus to fuse.
	Selzentry	Maraviroc	Blocks cell entry by preventing the interaction between human CCR5 and HIV-1 gp120.
Protease inhibitors (PIs)	Kaletra	Lopinavir/ Ritonavir	Inhibits HIV protease; prevents cleavage of viral polyproteins that are necessary for maturation of infectious virus.
	Crixivan	Indinavir	
	Reyataz	Atazanavir	
	Aptivus	Tipranavir	
	Prezista	Darunavir	
	Lexiva	Fosamprenavir	
Integrase strand transfer inhibitors	Isentress	Raltegravir	Inhibits catalytic activity of HIV-1 integrase; prevents covalent insertion of linear HIV-1 DNA into host genome, causing a rapid drop in viral load.
Maturation inhibitors	Currently not FDA approved.	Bevirimat Vivecon	Inhibits viral maturation by blocking cleavage of the Gag capsid precursor, capsid-SP1; results in non-functional capsid proteins and non-infectious HIV particles.

a. Tenofovir and Emtricitabine are nucleoside reverse transcriptase inhibitors (NRTIs).

ingestion, it takes approximately four to seven years for cattle to show symptoms of the disease; however, once symptoms become evident, the cattle die within weeks. In March 1996, the British government announced a possible link between BSE and Creutzfeldt-Jacob disease (**CJD**), a sporadic and rare but fatal human disease that usually strikes people over 65 and that occurs on a worldwide basis at an estimated annual rate of one case per one million population. Although the cases in humans were suspected to result from the ingestion of beef from affected cattle, about 10 to 15 percent of CJD cases are inherited.

Table 13-12. Examples of the spongiform encephalopathies in animals and humans

ANIMALS
Scrapie: sheep
TME (transmissible mink encephalopathy): mink
CWD (chronic wasting disease): mule deer, elk
BSE (bovine spongiform encephalopathy): cows
HUMANS
CJD: Creutzfeld-Jacob disease
GSS: Gerstmann-Straussler-Scheinker syndrome
FFI: Fatal familial insomnia
Kuru
Alpers syndrome

CJD variant CJD (**vCJD**), Gerstmann-Straussler Scheinker disease (**GSS**), kuru, and other diseases caused by prions are fatal illnesses characterized by a rapidly progressive dementia, myoclonus, psychiatric changes, often-typical EEG changes, and spongiform neuropathologic changes. The infection is not associated with any obvious inflammatory or immunologic response in the host, and the disease is invariably fatal. Prions are resistant to a number of standard sterilization and disinfection procedures. Most cases are sporadic (about 90 percent), and most of the rest are inherited. However, in a small number of cases, iatrogenic transmission of CJD has been associated with percutaneous exposure to medical instruments, such as brain electrodes contaminated with prion/CNS (central nervous system) tissue residues. Possible iatrogenic transmission has also been associated with transplantation of CNS and corneal tissues and recipients of human growth hormone and gonadotropin derived from cadaveric material. A case of vCJD has been associated with a blood transfusion. Although the occurrence of CJD has been associated with the unusual feeding practice of animal husbandry described above, there have been no documented cases of person-to-person transmission.

Summary: Immune Responses to Acute and Chronic Viral Infection

It may now be possible to construct a central unifying hypothesis that summarizes interactions of the various components of innate and adaptive immunity that participate in the host-parasite defense against viral agents. For ease of discussion, viral infections may be divided into acute and chronic viral infections.

For a nonimmune and susceptible host, primary encounter with certain viruses, e.g., cytolytic viruses, leads to acute viral infections where viral replication is rapid and is countered quickly by components of the innate and adaptive immune responses. In this scenario, the duration of the illness is short and the illness terminates quickly (Figure 13-19). The infection is countered by a robust initial innate immune response characterized by extensive viral replication and release of an array of pro-inflammatory cytokines responsible for many of the associated symptoms (e.g., myalgia or fever). This is followed within one to two weeks with a brisk adaptive immune response with stimulation of both components of CMI and humoral immunity and recovery. If the virus is subsequently re-encountered, the extent of viral replication and stimulation of the innate immune response is minimal, and therefore associated clinical symptoms are limited. The magnitude of the adaptive immune response, however, is quite expansive owing to the booster stimulation of pre-sensitized memory cells, and recovery is complete (Figure 13-19).

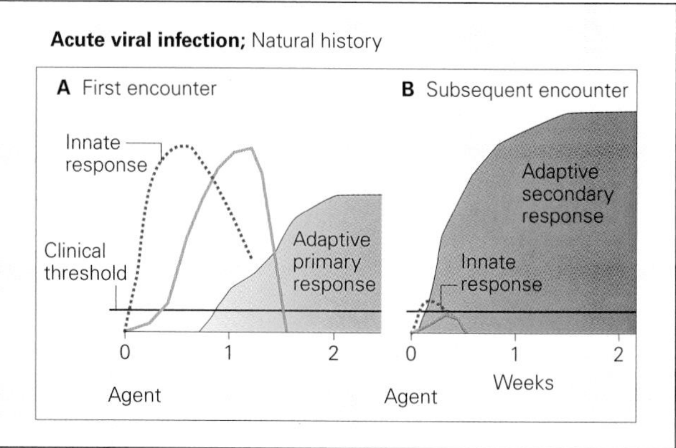

Figure 13-19. Schematic representation of immunologic responses seen during acute viral infections, upon initial encounter (A) and subsequent encounter (B).

A second category of viral infection includes the chronic viral infections where the same initial phases of viral entry and stimulation of both innate and adaptive immune responses are seen (Figure 13-20). These infections are caused primarily by viruses that enter into a latent or persistent state and endure within cells, often during the entire lifespan of the individual. In contrast to the clearing and resolution of illness associated with acute viral infections, these viruses have learned how to evade the immune responses and persist. The best studied

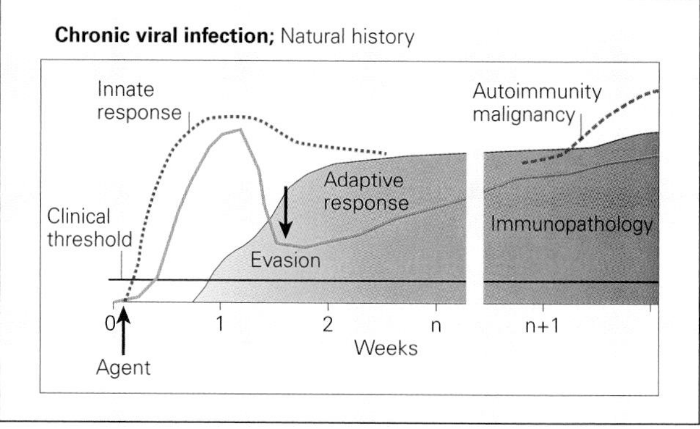

Figure 13-20. Schematic representation of immunologic responses seen during chronic viral infections showing evasion of immune responses with persistent viral antigen and resultant immunopathology in the form of chronic infection, autoimmunity, and malignancy.

Table 13-13. Schematic representation of acute and chronic viral infections and types of protective and tissue-damaging immune responses stimulated by them

Category of viral infection	Functional type of viral infection	Examples of viruses	Innate immunity	Adaptive immunity		Tissue-damaging (tertiary) immune responses
				CMI	Humoral	
Acute	Cytolytic	Poliovirus measles, influenza	+	–	4+	–
			+	2+	4+	+
Chronic	Persistent and latent	HIV, herpes, hepatitis, HPV	+	4+	1+	4+

Note: The plus signs show the degree of involvement.

of these are the herpes viruses, all of which display alternative forms of gene expression, i.e., latency or integration, during their continued existence. Some persist in a latent form that at times may become fully productive, e.g., herpes simplex and varicella-zoster viruses. In either event, because of the persistence of viral antigen, these chronic viral infections enter into the tertiary deleterious phase of immunity described previously that often results in immunopathology with clinical expressions of autoimmunity or cancer (Figure 13-20). Many of the perplexing problems encountered in medicine today result from those viruses that have acquired the most sophisticated evasion mechanisms and present with varied expressions of chronic viral infection. These are seen in patients whose immune systems have been immunosuppressed as a result of chronic viral infection, e.g., HIV infection, transplantation, or malignancy, as well as the immunosuppressive agents that are used for their treatment or management.

Shown in Table 13-13 are some examples of the various types of viruses that cause acute and chronic viral infections together with the relative roles of the three phases of the immune response: innate immunity, adaptive immunity, and the tertiary immune responses to these agents.

Case Study: Clinical Relevance

Let us now return to the case study of recurrent herpes labialis presented earlier and review some of the major points of the clinical presentation and how they relate to the immune system:

- Recurrent herpes labialis is an example of a chronic viral infection usually caused by herpes simplex type 1 that manifests with recurrent episodes of reactivation of the latent virus, which usually resides in dorsal root ganglia.
- Shown in Figure 13-21 is a schematic representation of the host-parasite relationship of infection caused by herpes simplex in the human; following infection of susceptible hosts, < 1 percent present with clinically discernible disease as exemplified by the primary herpetic gingivostomatitis seen in the clinical case (Figure 13-1A); > 99 percent of infected hosts present with clinically inapparent or subclinical infection
- Following primary infection with herpes simplex, the majority of patients (70–90 percent) enter into a chronic infection characterized by latent infection where the viral genome resides within the nucleus as an episome; the manifestations of recurrent herpes labialis represent the reactivation of the latent infection, which can be triggered by any of a number of stressful conditions, e.g., intercurrent respiratory infections in the case presented.
- During reactivation, the latent virus enters into an active cytolytic phase with the release of fully infectious virions that can now infect another susceptible host. In contrast to acute cytolytic infections caused by poliovirus, for example, which are addressed mostly by antibody-mediated immunity and not by T cell immunity, membrane-associated viruses such as herpes simplex require both antibody and cell-mediated immunity for maintenance of protective immunity.
- In one study evaluating specific cell-mediated immunity to HSV type 1 (HSV-1) in patients with recurrent herpes labialis (Figure 13-22), specific reduction of cell-mediated immunity to HSV-1 was demonstrated during the quiescent period between recurrences. This may in part account for the propensity of these individuals to develop recurrent herpetic infections during periods of recrudescence.

Case Studies: Clinical Relevance (continued)

Virus

Susceptible host

Gingivostomatitis

Herpes labialis

<1%

>99%

Primary infection

Clinical disease

Gingivostomatitis
Vulvovaginitis
Eczema herpecticum
Traumatic herpes
Keratoconjunctivitis
Meningoencephalitis
Visceral herpes

Inapparent infection

Recurrent manifestations

Herpes labialis
Herpes genitalis
Herpetic stromal keratitis
Localized encephalitis

Excitants

Fever
Sunshine
Trauma
Menstruation
Gastrointestinal upsets
Psychic upsets

Carriers (70%–90% of population)
(antibodies and virus persist)

Reactivation of latent herpetic infection

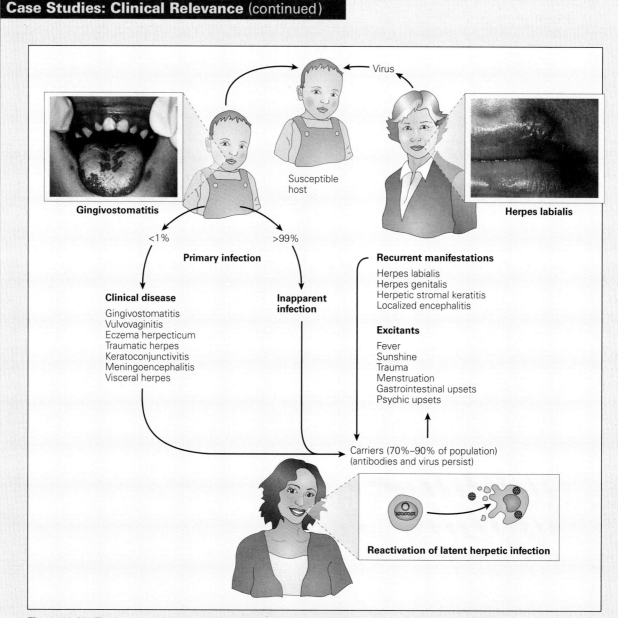

Figure 13-21. The host-parasite relationship of infection caused by herpes simplex infection in the human.

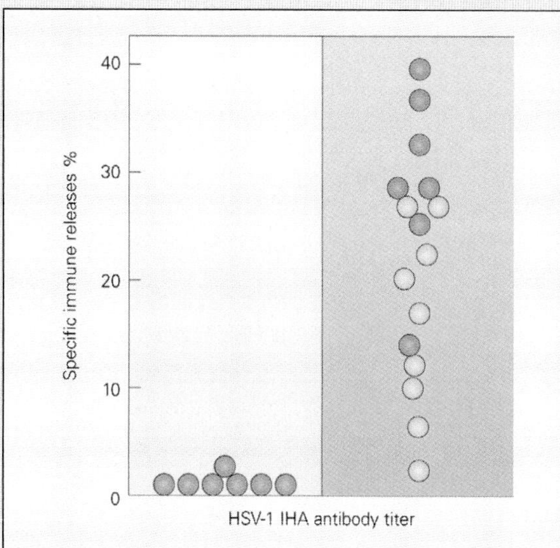

Figure 13-22. Schematic representation of decreased levels of cell-mediated immunity to HSV-1 in asymptomatic subjects with recurrent herpes labialis (turquoise dots) compared to healthy controls without HSV-1 recurrence (orange dots) as determined by a Cr51-specific immune release using a lymphocyte interaction with a target cell consisting of a MA-160 human prostatic adenoma cell line persistently infected with HSV-1. (Adapted from Thong YH, Vincent MM, Hensen SA, et al. Depressed specific cell-mediated immunity to Herpes simplex virus type 1 in patients with recurrent herpes labialis. Infect Immun. 1975;12:76–80.)

Key Points

- Viral infections can be classified as acute or chronic; within the category of chronic infection, viruses can cause persistent infection or latent infection.
- Immunity to viruses depends upon the coordinated functions of numerous cell types and their products, including both the innate and adaptive immune response.
- HIV/AIDS is an example of the vast impact that viral infection can have on society; numerous antiretroviral therapies have been developed to target different aspects of this RNA virus' pathogenicity, but we have a great deal to learn about the disease.
- Viruses have many mechanisms to evade host immune responses, and host cells often respond by developing countermeasures; the host-viral relationship is constantly evolving in this manner.

Study Questions/Critical Thinking

1. Give a few examples of viruses that cause persistent and latent chronic infections.
2. What is necessary for cytolytic viruses to cause disease?
3. Which viruses are suspected to be related to the development of leukemia and lymphoma?
4. How does HIV replicate within host cells and what particular proteins are targeted with current antiretroviral therapy?
5. How are Toll-like receptors involved in the immune response to viral infection?
6. What is the role of interferons in fighting viral infection? What about antibodies and complement?

Suggested Reading

Bergman IM. Toll-like receptors (TLRs) and mannan-binding (MBL): on constant alert in a hostile environment. Ups J Med Sci. 2011; 116: 90–9.

Brandenburg B, Zhuang X. Virus trafficking: learning from single-virus tracking. Nat Rev Microbiol. 2007; 5: 197–208.

Carson KR, Evens AM, Richey EA, et al. Progressive multifocal leukoencephalopahty after rituximab therapy in HIV-negative patients: a report of 57 cases from the research on adverse drug events and reports projects. Blood. 2009; 113: 4834–40.

Carson KR, Focosi D, Major EO, et al. Monoclonal antibody-associated progressive multifocal leucoencephalopathy inpatients treated with rituximab, natalizumab and efalizumab: a review from the research on adverse drug events and reports (RADAR) project. Lancet Oncol. 2009; 10: 816–24.

Centers for Disease Control and Prevention. The global HIV/AIDS pandemic, 2006.

———. Morbidity and Mortality Weekly Report 11 55 2006; 31: 841–4.

———. Erratum in Morbidity and Mortality Weekly Report 55 2006. page 881.

Chang MH, You SL, Chen CJ, et al. Taiwan hepatoma study groups: decreased incidence of hepatocellular carcinoma in hepatitis B vaccines: a 20-year follow-up study. J Nat Cancer Inst. 2009; 101: 1348–55.

Coiras M, Lopez-Huertas MR, et al. Understanding HIV-1 latency provides clues for the eradication of long-term reservoirs. Nat Rev Microbiol. 2009; 7: 798–812.

Contoli M, Message SD, Laza-Stanca V, et al. Role of deficient type III interferon-lambda production in asthma exacerbations. Nature Med. 2006: 12: 1023–6.

Day CL, Kaufmann DE, Kiepiela P, et al. PD-1 expression on HIV-specific T cells is associated with T-cell exhaustion and disease progression. Nature. 2006; 443: 350–4.

Drugge JM, Allen PJ. A nurse practitioner's guide to the management of herpes simplex virus-1 in children. Pediatr Nurs. 2008; 24: 310–8.

Garcia-Sastre A, Biron CA. Type 1 interferons and the virus-host relationship: a lesson in détente. Science. 2006; 314: 879–82.

Gennery AR, Cant AJ. Advances in hematopoetic stem cell transplantion for primary immunodeficiency. Immunol Allergy Clin North Am. 2008; 28: 439–56.

Hladik F, Liu H, Speelmon E, et al. Combined effect of CCR5-Delta32 heterozygosity and the CCR5 promoter polymorphism -2459 A/G on CCR5 expression and resistance to human immunodeficiency virus type 1 transmission. J Virol. 2005; 79: 11677–84.

Jarrett RF. Viruses and lymphoma/leukaemia. J Pathol. 2006; 208: 176–86.

Kawai T, Akira S. Innate immune recognition of viral infection. Nat Immunol. 2006; 7: 131–7.

Khader SA, Gaffen SL, Kolls JK. Th17 cells at the crossroads of innate and adaptive immunity against infectious diseases at the mucosa. Mucosal Immunol. 2009; 2: 403–11.

Krugman S, Ward R, Katz S. Infectious diseases of children. St. Louis: Mosby; 1977.

Lindå H, von Heijne A, Major EO, et al. Progressive multifocal leukoencephalopathy after natalizumab monotherapy. N Eng J Med. 2009: 361: 1081–7.

Lombardi VC, Ruscetti FW, Das Gupta J, et al. Detection of an infectious retrovirus, XMRV, in blood cells of patients with chronic fatigue syndrome. Science. 2009; 326: 585–9.

Major EO. Progressive multifocal leukoencephalopathy in patients on immunomodulatory therapies. Ann Rev Med. 2010; 61: 35–47.

Major EO. Reemergence of PML in natalizumab-treated patients—new cases, same concerns. N Eng J Med. 2009: 36: 1041–3.

McFadden G, Mohamed MR, Rahman MM, et al. Cytokine determinants of viral tropism. Nat Rev Immunol. 2009; 8: 645–55.

Pantaleo G, Harari A. Functional signatures in antiviral T-cell immunity for monitoring virus-associated diseases. Nat Rev Immunol. 2006; 6: 417–23.

Petersen DC, Glashoff RH, Shrestha S, et al. Risk for HIV-1 infection associated with a common CXCL14 (SDF1) polymorphism and CXCR4 variation in an African population. J Acquir Immune Defic Syndr. 2005; 40: 521–6.

Rouse BT, Suvas S. Regulatory cells and infectious agents: détentes cordiale and contraire. J Immunol. 2004: 173: 2211–5.

Rowland-Jones S, Dong T. HIV: tired T cells turn around. Nature. 2006; 443: 282–3.

Sapp M, Day PM. Structure, attachment and entry of polyoma- and papillomoviruses. Virology. 2009; 384: 400–9.

Suvas S, Kumaraguru U, Pack CD, et al. CD4+CD25+ T cells regulate virus-specific primary and memory CD8+ T cell responses. J Exp Med. 2003: 198: 889–901.

Suvas S, Rouse BT. Regulation of microbial immunity: the suppressor cell renaissance. Viral Immunol. 2005; 18: 411–8.

Suvas S, Rouse BT. Treg control of antimicrobial T cell responses. Curr Opin Immunol. 2006; 18: 344–8.

Thong YH, Vincent MM, Hensen SA, et al. Depressed specific cell-mediated immunity to herpes simplex virus type 1 in patients with recurrent herpes labialis. Infect Immun. 1975; 12: 76–80.

Tortorella D, Gewurz BE, Furman MH, et al. Viral subversion of the immune system. Ann Rev Immunol. 2000; 18: 861–926.

Van Kaer L, Joyce S. Viral evasion of antigen presentation: not just for peptides anymore. Nat Immunol. 2006; 7: 795–7.

Wang Z, Choi MK, Ban T, et al. Regulation of innate immune responses by DAI (DLM-1/ZBP1) and other DNA-sensing molecules. Proc Nat Acad Sci USA. 2008; 15: 5477–82.

Watts JC, Balachandran A, Westaway D. The expanding universe of prion diseases. PLoS Pathog. 2006; 2: 152–63.

Yuan W, Dasgupta A, Cresswell P. Herpes simplex virus evades natural killer T cell recognition by suppressing CD1d recycling. Nat Immunol. 2006; 7: 835–42.

Chapter 14

Mechanisms of Fungal Immunity

Luigina Romani, MD, PhD
Joseph A. Bellanti, MD

Case Study

A 19-year old man presented with oral candidiasis (thrush) since the age of three years. *C. albicans* infection was proven by culture and he was treated with the prophylactic use of ketoconazole. The patient had one brother and two sisters. His brother had intermittent thrush and seizures since childhood and developed hydrocephalus when he was 18 years old, following which he died one year later from candidal meningitis. His mother gave a history of vaginal candidiasis for the past eight years concurrent with a five-year history of dermatophytosis involving the skin of her hands and neck. A history of oral and vaginal candidiasis was also obtained from a maternal aunt since early childhood. In addition, a maternal uncle had a history of dermatophytosis since childhood, and both of his daughters died of invasive candidal infection.

Complete blood counts performed on the patient, his mother, maternal aunt, and maternal uncle were within the normal range. The total counts of CD3+ T cells, CD4+ T cells, CD8+ T cells, memory T cells, follicular helper T cells, effector memory T cells, regulatory T cells, B cells, and natural killer T cells were within normal limits, as were the basal levels of immunoglobulins. In the patient, delayed-type hypersensitivity skin tests were negative for tuberculin but positive for *Candida*. Autoimmune regulator (AIRE) gene analysis revealed a wild type sequence. The fatal illness caused by *Candida* infection within several male and female members of this kindred without any other associated factors suggested a hereditary form of chronic mucocutaneous candidiasis.

LEARNING OBJECTIVES

When you have completed this chapter, you should be able to:

- Describe the differences between acute and chronic fungal infection
- Classify the five categories of fungal infections: opportunistic, superficial, cutaneous, subcutaneous, and systemic
- Explain the basic role of Toll-like receptors (TLR) as activators of innate and adaptive immunity to fungi
- Understand how Th17 and Treg cells contribute to the fine-tuning of immune responses to fungi
- Gain an appreciation for the future of fungal immunology research and its importance for the development of therapies and immunization
- Utilize this knowledge for a better understanding of antifungal immunity in the normal host as well as in individuals with genetic defects of fungal immunity

Introduction

Fungi are a class of infectious agents that were previously classified as "plantlike" in their structure and organization. A more recent classification system suggested by genomic analysis places the fungi within a separate kingdom of the eukaryotes, the fungi; this classification is unlike most other microorganisms, which are part of the prokaryotes. One of the outstanding characteristics of fungi, unlike the prokaryotic organisms, is their ability to commonly exist in nature in two different forms, a property known as dimorphism. These include: (1) a filamentous branching form, referred to as the vegetative or hyphal form, and (2) an oval or spherical form, referred to as the yeast phase. Although both forms are important for infection, the filamentous hyphal form is more invasive than the yeast form.

The effects of fungi on the human host are both **beneficial** (e.g., production of vitamins, antibiotics, fermentation reactions, and maintenance of the geochemical structure of the earth's soil) and **detrimental** (e.g., a major source of opportunistic infections in immunocompromised hosts). While the other classes of pathogenic microorganisms have been largely controlled through chemotherapy, immunization, and public health measures, there is a notable lack of success in the control of fungi and their pathogenic effects. Ironically, with the advent of new antibiotics for the treatment of bacterial infections and the introduction of potent corticosteroid and immunosuppressive agents for allergic and autoimmune diseases (*Chapter 11*), there has been an increased upsurge of fungal infections resulting from a changed flora and fungal overgrowth following the use of these agents.

The fungi have presented two additional problems for health care providers in recent years. The first is seen in the form of hypersensitivity reactions that are known to be caused by immunologic reactions to the organisms brought about by the increased use of immunosuppressive agents. The second challenge is a series of perceived illnesses described predominantly in the lay literature, such as "yeast connection" and "sick building syndrome." These conditions have no known immunologic basis and have not been validated by evidence-based biomedical research, yet they are believed to be related to fungal infection. This chapter will focus primarily on mechanisms of protective immunity to fungi and pathogenesis of diseases that result from either infection or hypersensitivity reactions to these fungal agents. The chapter will also include a description of how the fungi evade the immune response by using some of the host's immunologic machinery against itself.

Pathogenesis of Fungal Diseases

In order to understand the mechanisms of immunity involved in fungal diseases, it may be helpful to first describe the various types of interaction that a fungus can have with a host. The eventual outcome of such an interaction will depend upon (1) the properties of the fungus and (2) the status of the host in which the interaction occurs.

The properties of a potentially pathogenic fungus include its ability to establish either a *localized* infection at the portal of entry or its capacity to become *invasive* and establish deeper infections in tissues or at times generalized infection. Examples of localized infections include those fugal infections restricted to body surfaces, such as those caused by *Candida* or the dermatophytes. Fungal infections of a more generalized nature include histoplasmosis, coccidiomycosis, and blastomycosis. Certain fungi have a polysaccharide capsule that may be of importance in resisting phagocytosis in a manner similar to that described for the encapsulated bacteria (*Chapter 12*).

Acute Versus Chronic Fungal Infections

A second important consideration in the pathogenesis of fungal infections is whether a disease is *acute* or *chronic.* The chronicity reflects adaptation of the fungus to its host. Those fungal infections that are characterized by the initiation of an acute inflammatory component of the innate immune system have been most responsive to disposal by subsequent activation of the host's adaptive immune mechanisms and also to treatment; those fungi that evade the initial recognition by the host's innate immune system and establish quiet residence with minimal tissue damage are most apt to continue their parasitic domicile within the host as chronic infections by not invoking a robust adaptive immune response. In general, if the defense mechanisms of the host are adequate to resist the initial attack by fungus, the disease will be acute and self-limiting. If, on the other hand, the nature of the virulence factors of the organism or the size of the initial inoculum overwhelm the host defense factors, or if the defense mechanisms are incompletely developed (as in the newborn host) or suppressed (as with patients receiving immunosuppressive therapy), the eventual outcome will be unfavorable for the host and will lead to chronic systemic and sometimes fatal infection. With the development of chronic infection in an otherwise immunocompetent host, there may be the development of a prominent delayed hypersensitivity (cell-mediated immune response) with subsequent granuloma formation (*Chapter 7*).

Environmental Factors

Environmental factors affect the host-fungus relationship. For example, the arid climate of the western

United States is associated with a high incidence of fungal disease such as coccidiomycosis (San Joaquin Valley Fever). It seems that the immune system of otherwise normal individuals is ineffective under these environmental conditions. This may be related to either a high concentration of infecting inoculum of the pathogen in these areas or diminished efficiency of the innate immune responses in the host. A pathogen in high enough concentration can overwhelm the defense mechanisms of the normal host. Other types of fungal infections are more commonly seen with different environmental conditions, such as occupations in which the skin is subjected to immersion in water, predisposing the host to superficial infections of the skin.

Classification of Fungal Diseases

Fungal diseases are commonly classified according to their site of infection, depth of penetration of human tissue, and the susceptibility of the immunocompromised host. Fungal infection classification includes the following categories: (1) opportunistic infections; (2) superficial mycoses; (3) cutaneous mycoses; (4) subcutaneous mycoses and (5) systemic mycoses (Table 14-1). All five categories are described in greater detail below.

Opportunistic Fungal Infections

Perhaps the most common of the human diseases caused by fungi are the so-called opportunistic fungal infections (Table 14-1). These fungi include *Candida albicans*, Aspergillus spp, and *Phycomycetes* (*Mucor, Rhizopus*); these are normally nonpathogenic in humans but may behave as virulent organisms in individuals with depressed immune function, e.g., the newborn infant, patients with HIV infection/AIDS, lymphoreticular malignancy, and those receiving immunosuppressive therapy or excessive use of broad spectrum antibiotics. Patients with certain metabolic diseases such as diabetes mellitus are also more susceptible to infections caused by these organisms (Table 14-2). Under circumstances in which either innate or adaptive immune responses are depressed, the fungi may establish a variety of localized or generalized, acute, or chronic opportunistic fungal infections (Figure 14-1).

Table 14-2. Clinical conditions that predispose to opportunistic fungal infection

Newborn infant
HIV infection/AIDS
Lymphoreticular malignancy
Patients receiving immunosuppressive therapy or antibiotic therapy
Diabetes mellitus

Of the opportunistic fungi, Candida is the most common and the most important in humans. This microorganism inhabits the normal mucous membranes of the mouth, vagina, and gastrointestinal tract. Thrush and vulvovaginitis are examples of infection of the mucous membranes caused by Candida. Thrush, a localized infection of the mucous membranes of the mouth and pharynx, consists of discrete whitish patches; it is commonly seen during the early newborn period and in young infants and is presumably acquired through passage through the birth canal and related to the immaturity of the T cell immune system seen during early infancy (*Chapter 2*). Secondary skin infection in the diaper

Table 14-1. Examples of types of fungal disease

Type of infection	Example of disease	Etiologic agent	Clinical presentation
Opportunistic	Thrush vulvovaginitis pneumonitis	*Candida albicans*, Aspergillus spp, *Phycomycetes (Mucor, Rhizopus)*	Whitish plaques and radiographic lung densities
Superficial	Pityriasis versicolor	*Malassezia furfur*	Hypopigmented macules
Cutaneous	Tinea capitis Tinea corporis Onychomycosis	*Microsporum audouini* *Trichphyton rubrum* *Epidermophyton*	Ringworm lesion of scalp Infection of the skin Infection of nails
Subcutaneous	Sporotrichosis	*Sporothrix schenckii*	Budding yeast in tissue exudate
Systemic	Blastomycosis Coccidioidomycosis Histoplasmosis Cryptococcosis	*Blastomyces dermatitidis, Coccidioides immitis, Histoplasma capsulatum, Cryptococcus neoformans*	Radiographic lung densities or meningitis

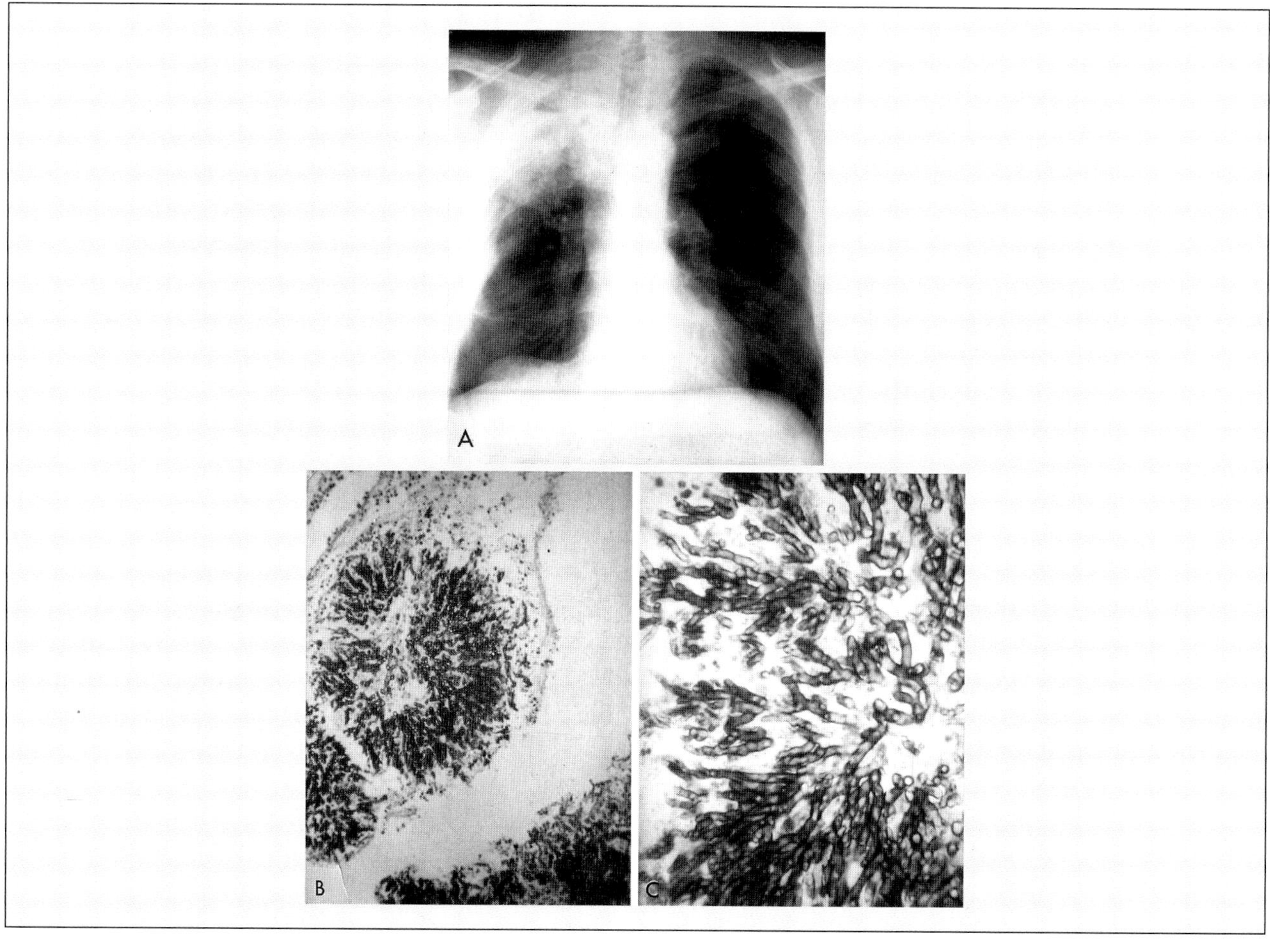

Figure 14-1. Aspergillus infection in a 57-year-old male with bronchogenic carcinoma. Panel A: Chest x-ray showing area of increased density in the right upper lobe. Panel B: Photomicrograph of section of lung showing hyphae of *Aspergillus fumigatus* in the wall of a pulmonary abscess (hematoxylin and eosin stain × 100). Panel C: Photomicrograph of same section of lung as shown in Panel B, under increased magnification, hematoxylin and eosin stain × 600. (Courtesy of Dr. John Guerrant).

area is also seen during this period, causing a beefy red erythematous lesion.

Candidal infection is also seen in individuals receiving broad-spectrum antibiotics or with depressed adaptive immunity, such as patients receiving immunosuppressive therapy. These opportunistic fungal infections may be acute and self-limiting or chronic; occasionally, the infection becomes disseminated, particularly in very immature infants or individuals with severely depressed immune functions. The opportunistic fungi may become invasive and involve virtually every tissue of the body. A particularly severe chronic form of mucocutaneous candidiasis that is often serious and life-threatening is seen in children with severe T cell immune deficiency (*Chapter 16*). The condition involves mucous membranes of the mouth, the respiratory and gastrointestinal tracts, the skin, and the nails. This presenting clinical picture is so common that if candidiasis is seen beyond the newborn period in individuals not receiving antibiotics, a diligent search should be made for diseases with deficient T cell immunity (e.g., AIDS).

Another type of involvement with these opportunistic fungi is seen in clinical situations, in which prosthetic valves or devices are used, e.g., the use of indwelling catheters or valves used for the treatment of cardiac disease or hydrocephalus. These prostheses act as foci and, since they are avascular, are not accessible to the normal clearing mechanisms of the host's immune system.

Superficial, Cutaneous, and Subcutaneous Fungal Infections

In addition to their propensity to cause opportunistic infections in immunocompromised hosts, fungi can also be responsible for superficial infections of the upper layers of the skin and deeper cutaneous and subcutaneous infections once they breach the integrity of the integument or mucous membranes in an otherwise immunologically normal host (Table 14-1). Pityriasis versicolor is an example of a superficial fungal infection of the skin caused by *Malassezia furfur* and is characterized by hypopigmented macules. Other types of fungi affecting upper layers of the skin and its appendages, i.e., hair and nails, are referred to as the dermatophytes. Included in this group are members of the following genera: Microsporum, Trichophyton, and Epidermophyton. These organisms all have a predilection for keratin-rich tissues such as the skin, hair, and nails, as they appear to have the capacity to degrade keratin and utilize its breakdown products as a nutritional source. These fungi can produce infection of the scalp (tinea capitis), the skin (tinea corporis), or the nails (onychomycosis) (Table 14-1).

Some fungi also have the capability to invade deeper subcutaneous tissues. One example is *Sporothrix schenckii,* which causes sporotrichosis (Table 14-1). This organism is found in soil and on plants and is introduced into the body by penetration of the skin with contaminated splinters, thorns, and soil. Once established, infection tends to be localized in subcutaneous tissues and become associated with draining ulcerated lesions. There also may be involvement of the lymphatics with lymphadenopathy and occasionally systemic spread.

The mechanisms of immunity responsible for the susceptibility to or protection from these fungal infections are not known, but T cell immunity appears to be an important immune mechanism during the course of these fungal infections. Since antibody has been found in individuals with and without infection, antibody determinations offer little diagnostic or prognostic value. Certain localized manifestations of the skin occur during the course of these fungal infections and are referred to as "Id" reactions. Although the mechanism of these reactions is one of delayed hypersensitivity, their role in immunity remains unclear.

Systemic Fungal Infections

Systemic mycoses represent the most serious of all fungal infections (Table 14-1). Fungal infections of this type include blastomycosis, coccidioidomycosis, histoplasmosis, and cryptococcosis. Adaptive immune responses are stimulated during these infections and appear to be important mechanisms of protective immunity. Thus, the development of serum antibody, including precipitins, agglutinins, and complement-fixing antibodies, offers both diagnostic and prognostic value. The pathogenesis of these infections usually invokes the introduction of the organism through a break in the skin or entry into the respiratory tract by inhalation (Figure 14-2). Following limited replication at the entry point, the organism may be cleared by the innate immune response (phagocytosis by macrophages). Following infection, an inflammatory response characterized by granuloma formation is commonly seen (*Chapter 7*). In many infections, such as histoplasmosis, caseous necrosis may also develop, and recovery from the illness may occur with microangiographic evidence of calcification, similar to that seen in tuberculosis.

In addition, cell-mediated immunity, i.e., delayed hypersensitivity, may develop during the course of these systemic mycoses. Until the 1970s blastomycin, coccidioidin, and histoplasmin were available for use in delayed hypersensitivity testing, which offered some aid in the diagnosis of these systemic mycoses. More recently, other fungal antigens have been identified for use in in-vitro tests of cellular immunity that show comparable results to skin testing.

The Immune Response to Fungi: From Microbe Sensing to Host Defensing

Most pathogenic fungi need a stable host-parasite interaction characterized by an immune response robust enough to allow host survival but not so strong as to eliminate the pathogen, thereby allowing the establishment of commensalism and latency (*Chapter 12*). Therefore, the balance of pro-inflammatory and anti-inflammatory signaling is a prerequisite for a successful host/fungal interaction.

The host defense mechanisms against fungi are numerous and range from protective mechanisms that appeared early in the evolution of multicellular organisms (*Chapter 2*) (collectively referred to as "innate immunity"), to sophisticated attuned mechanisms that are specifically induced during infection and disease ("adaptive immunity"). The two systems are intimately linked and controlled by sets of molecules and receptors that act to generate a highly coordinated and integrated process for protection against fungal pathogens. Traditionally considered only as a first line of defense, innate immunity has recently received renewed attention because it discriminates between pathogens and self through a set of pattern-recognition receptors (**PRRs**), which activate adaptive immune mechanisms by provision of specific signals (*Chapters 3* and *9*). Dendritic cells (**DCs**) are uniquely

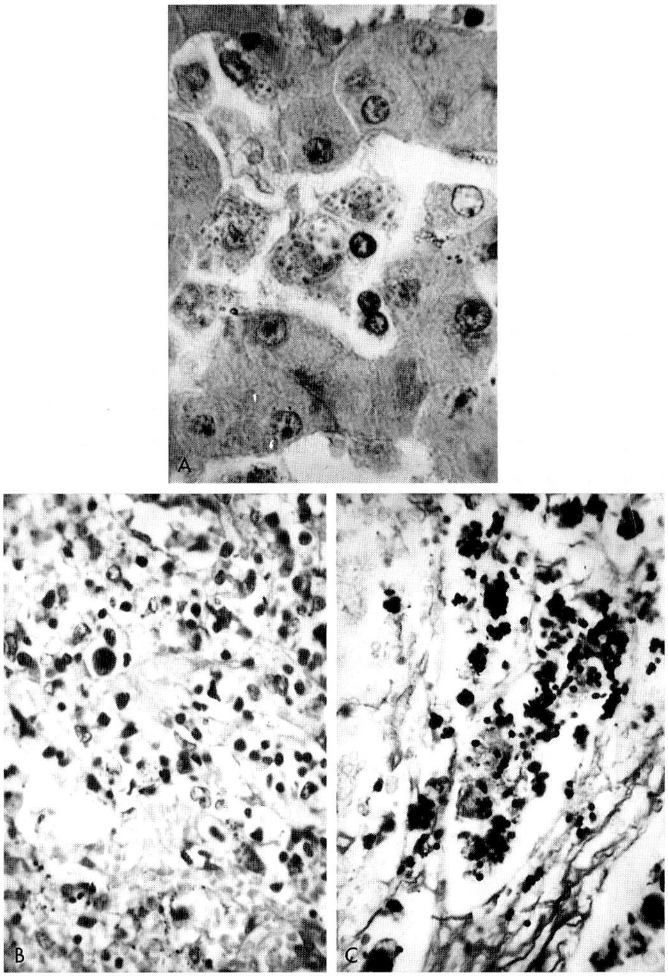

Figure 14-2. Panel A: Photomicograph of a liver section from a 60-year-old man who died of myeloid metaplasia complicated by systemic histoplasmosis showing *Histoplasma capsulatum* organisms within Kupffer cells (hematoxylin and eosin stain × 600). Panel B: Section of spleen showing *Histoplasma capsulatum* organisms within macrophages (hematoxylin and eosin stain × 100). Panel C: Section of a lymph node showing *Histoplasma capsulatum* organisms in tissue (silver methemamine stain × 100). (Courtesy of Dr. Daniel Mohler.)

proficient at uptake of extracellular foreign substances, including fungus-associated material, which after processing, present resulting peptide fragments to specific populations of T helper (**Th**) effector and T regulatory cells (**Tregs**) for subsequent induction of a balanced adaptive immune response. This dichotomous Th cell model of adaptive immunity has proven to be a useful construct that illustrates the general principle that diverse effector functions are required for eradication of different fungal infections. This paradigm has not only contributed to a better understanding of basic host immune responses to fungi, but has also provided a conceptual clinical framework to better examine new strategies of immune interventions. The development of a dominant Th1 response driven by inteleukin 12 (**IL-12**) is required for the ultimate expression of protective immunity to fungi. The optimal activation of phagocytes at sites of infection is facilitated not only by the production of the signature cytokine interferon gamma (**IFN-γ**) by Th1 cells, but also through the phagocytosis-enhancing effects of opsonizing antibody. The newly described Th17 developmental pathway may play an important inflammatory role previously attributed to uncontrolled Th1 responses and serves to accommodate the seemingly paradoxical association of chronic inflammatory responses with fungal persistence in the face of an ongoing inflammation (*Chapter 9*). In addition to efficient control of pathogens, tightly regulated mechanisms are required to balance protective immunity and immunopathology. A number of protective mechanisms, including the generation of Tregs

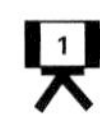

and the secretion of anti-inflammatory cytokines, such as IL-10, are key in maintaining a healthy balance between protection and immunopathology (Figure 14-3).

Inflammation and Immunity: From Protection to Disease Promotion

Inflammation is a key feature of fungal infection and disease. The inflammatory response may not only serve to limit infection, but an overzealous or heightened inflammatory response can, at times, also contribute significantly to fungal pathogenicity and disease accentuation, as illustrated by the occurrence of severe fungal infections in patients with the immune reconstitution inflammatory syndrome (**IRIS**) (Box 14-1). These patients may experience intractable fungal infections despite recovery from immunosuppression and the return of pathogen-specific immunity.

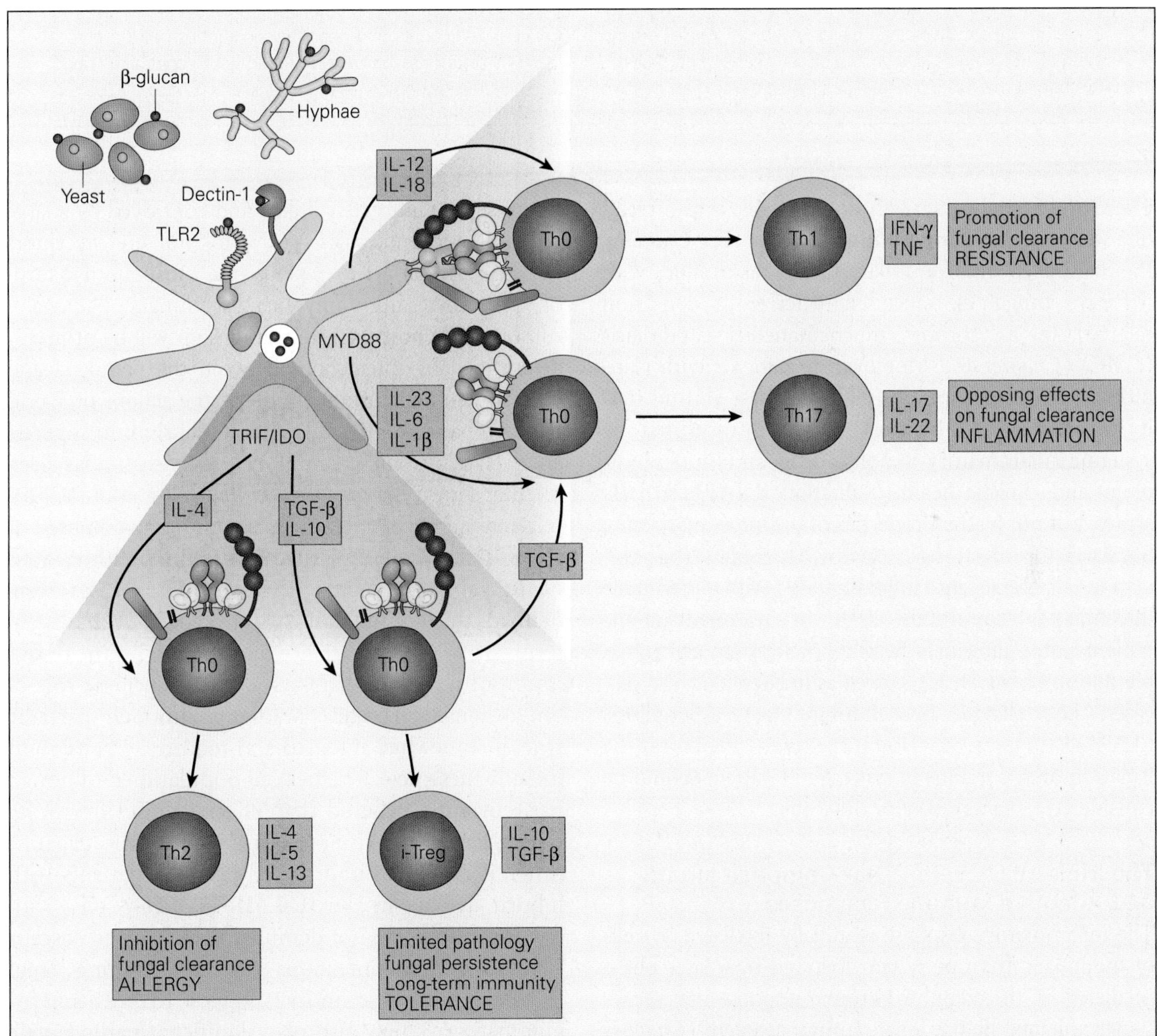

Figure 14-3. Protective immunity against fungal pathogens is achieved by the integration of two distinct arms of the immune system, the innate and adaptive responses. Innate and adaptive immune responses are intimately linked and controlled by sets of molecules and receptors that act to generate the most effective form of immunity for protection against fungal pathogens. Although Th1 responses driven by the IL-12 /IFN-γ axis are central to protection against fungi, other cytokines and T cell-dependent pathways have come of age. The newly described Th17 developmental pathway may also play an important inflammatory role previously attributed to uncontrolled Th1 responses. Regulatory T cells in their capacity to inhibit aspects of innate and adaptive antifungal immunity have become an integral component of immune resistance to fungi and provide the host with immune defense mechanisms adequate for protection, without necessarily eliminating fungal pathogens, which would impair immune memory or cause an unacceptable level of tissue damage. Th2 lymphocytes driven by IL-4 may contribute to the inhibition of fungal clearance as well as the development of allergy. The enzyme indoleamine 2,3-dioxygenase (IDO) contributes to immune homeostasis by inducing Tregs and taming overzealous or heightened inflammatory responses.

Box 14-1

The Immune Reconstitution Inflammatory Syndrome (IRIS)

Soon after the advent of potent highly active antiretroviral therapy (HAART), successful immune restoration in HIV-infected patients became associated with an exuberant inflammatory response and the worsening of clinical manifestations characterized by a recrudescence of opportunistic infections. This entity, known as immune reconstitution inflammatory syndrome (IRIS), is seen not only in other immunocompromised patients, but also in immunocompetent individuals. The syndrome IRIS is best characterized as a collection of localized and systemic inflammatory responses of varying degrees that displays both beneficial and deleterious features during an invasive opportunistic infection. Infections most commonly associated with IRIS include cytomegalovirus, herpes zoster, Mycobacterium avium complex (MAC), Pneumocystis *jiroveccii* (the causative agent of pneumocystic pneumonia), and Mycobacterium tuberculosis and a variety of mycoses. AIDS patients are more at risk for IRIS if HAART is initiated for the first time or if they have recently been treated for an opportunistic infection. It is generally advised, therefore, that when patients have low initial CD4+ T cell counts and opportunistic infection at the time of their HIV diagnosis, they receive treatment to control the opportunistic infections before HAART is initiated (*Chapter 13*).

Therefore, fungal outgrowth does not occur as a result of a weak or inefficient immune response. For *Candida*, the failure to resolve inflammation associated with defective fungal clearance characterizes a condition referred to as chronic mucocutaneous candidiasis (**CMC**) (*Chapter 16*). Moreover, in patients with Candida systemic infection, the clinical course and mortality were predicted by host responses measured by systemic inflammatory response (**SIR**) and acute physiology and chronic health evaluation II (**APACHE II**) scores, but not by the properties of the infecting species. Similarly, for infections caused by Aspergillus, the association of persistent inflammation with intractable infection is commonly seen in non-neutropenic patients after allogeneic hematopoietic stem cell transplantation (*Chapter 22*), as well as in allergic fungal diseases, i.e., allergic bronchopulmonary aspergillosis (**ABPA**) (*Chapter 18*). Not surprisingly, therefore, the isolation of Aspergillus in critically ill patients could be considered a marker of poor outcome.

The Molecular Events That Comprise Innate and Adaptive Immune Responses

The inflammatory response is initially mediated by cells of the innate immune system followed by a later phase mediated by the adaptive immune response that senses signals initiated by the innate immune system (*Chapters 3* and *5*). Most of the innate mechanisms are inducible upon infection and their activation requires contact with invariant evolutionarily conserved molecular structures shared by large groups of pathogens, i.e., pathogen-associated molecular pattern (**PAMPs**), which are recognized by a set of PRRs, including Toll-like receptors (**TLRs**) and C-type lectins, which are described in greater detail below (*Chapters 3* and *9*). Innate and adaptive immune responses are intimately linked and controlled by a large repertoire of molecules, i.e., cytokines and receptors (*Chapter 9*) that act to generate the most effective form of protective immunity against fungal pathogens. Although the host-parasite relationship will be primarily determined by interactions between the pathogen and cells of the innate immune system, the actions of T cells will feed back into this dynamic equilibrium to suppress an overzealous innate immune response. It has been recently shown that conventional adaptive immune Treg cells may suppress the early innate immune responses.

As described previously, the immunopathogenesis of fungal infections and associated diseases were defined during the last two decades, primarily in terms of a Th1/Th2 balance. However, with the recognition of new T cell subsets, the pathogenetic role of the original Th1/Th2 paradigm, although partially true, is somewhat outdated and requires expansion to include these new T helper cell populations. Although it is currently believed that Th1 responses driven by the IL-12/IFN-γ axis are central to protection against fungi, it is also an undisputed fact that patients with inborn deficits in the IL-12/IL-23-IFN-γ axis, with few exceptions, do not demonstrate increased susceptibility to most infectious agents, including fungi (*Chapter 12*). These findings suggest that other cytokine pathways may also play significant pathogenetic roles in antifungal immunity. The participation of both the Th17 pathway, playing a crucial inflammatory role previously attributed to uncontrolled Th1 cell reactivity, together with the Treg cells, responsible for fine-tuning the delicate balance between protective and deleterious aspects of antifungal immunity, have now become the hallmark component of the immune response to opportunistic fungi.

The Innate Antifungal Immune Response: Its Role in Pathogen Sensing and Shaping of the Adaptive Immune Response

The bulwark of the mammalian innate antifungal defense system is built upon effector mechanisms mediated by cells, cellular receptors, and a number of humoral factors (*Chapter 3*). Pathogenic fungi first interact with a variety of host cells during the initiation of disease. The environmental milieu then has a profound impact on the capacity of cells to optimally phagocytose fungi in the natural environment where a pathogen is encountered. This may explain why "delocalized," i.e., systemic fungal infections are less controllable diseases and why fungi have exploited a variety of mechanisms or putative virulence factors to evade phagocytosis, escape destruction, and survive within macrophages. Humoral factors and antibodies not only contribute to and enhance the innate cellular defense mechanisms, but also have been shown to play an important immunoregulatory role.

The constitutive mechanisms of innate immune defense are present at sites of continuous interaction of fungi with immune components found at body surfaces (*Chapter 8*). These include not only the barrier function provided by mucosal epithelial surfaces of the respiratory, gastrointestinal, and genitourinary tracts, but also by the microbial antagonism offered by the commensal microbiota, e.g., lactobacilli and bifidobacteria, that have shown clinical efficacy in the biotherapy of candidiasis, i.e., probiotics. Together with defensins and collectins, these components collectively comprise the major constitutive mechanisms of fungal immunity. Most of the host defense mechanisms, however, are inducible upon infection and, therefore, their activation requires that PAMPs be recognized by a set of PRRs, including TLRs and other moieties, as will be described below.

Antigen-independent recognition of fungi by the PRRs of the innate immune system leads to the immediate mobilization of immune effector and regulatory mechanisms of the adaptive immune system that provide the host with three crucial survival advantages: (1) rapid initiation of both innate and adaptive immune responses and creation of the inflammatory and co-stimulatory milieu for antigen recognition; (2) the establishment of a first line of defense, which holds the pathogen in check during the maturation of the adaptive immune response; and (3) steering of the adaptive immune response toward the cellular or humoral elements most appropriate for protective immunity against the specific pathogen. Therefore, in order to achieve optimal activation of antigen-specific adaptive immunity, it is first necessary to activate the pathogen-detection mechanisms of the innate immune response.

The structural composition of the mammalian innate antifungal defense system is built upon effector mechanisms mediated by cells, cellular receptors, and a number of humoral factors (*Chapter 3*). The professional phagocytes, consisting of polymorphonuclear leukocytes (neutrophils), mononuclear leukocytes (monocytes and macrophages), and dendritic cells, play essential roles. The antifungal effector functions of phagocytes include fungicidal and growth-inhibiting mechanisms as well as processes that resist fungal infectivity, including inhibitory effects on dimorphism and the promotion of phenotypic switching. The optimal restriction of fungal growth occurs via a combination of oxidative and complementary nonoxidative mechanisms, the latter consisting of intracellular or extracellular release of effector molecules, defensins, neutrophil cationic peptides, and iron sequestration (*Chapter 5*). Enzymes such as nicotinamide adenine dinucleotide phosphate (**NADPH**) oxidase and inducible nitric oxide synthase (**iNOS**) initiate the oxidative pathways known as the respiratory burst (*Chapter 5*). Myeloperoxidase, a lysosomal hemoprotein found in azurophilic granules of neutrophils and monocytes, but not in macrophages, is also a mediator in the oxygen-dependent killing of fungi. The clinical significance of these molecular events is seen in patients with inherited X-linked chronic granulomatous disease (**CGD**) resulting from a deficiency in the formation of activated oxygen radicals due to an NADPH-oxidase deficiency who demonstrate an increased susceptibility to aspergillosis (*Chapter 16*). The successful transplantation of bone marrow cells transfected with the NADPH oxidase gene has recently been shown to restore fungicidal activity of CGD patients. Myeloperoxidase deficiency predisposes to pulmonary candidiasis and aspergillosis, although it has not been shown to play an isolated role in fungal host defense in the absence of the NADPH oxidase complex.

The fact that both quantitative and qualitative defects of neutrophils are associated with an undue susceptibility to major disseminated fungal infections supports the important role of neutrophils in the protective immunity to fungal diseases. Their functions may well go beyond microbicidal activity and also include an immunoregulatory role in adaptive immunity. Myeloid suppressor cells have been shown recently to be responsible for immunosuppression observed in a variety of clinical conditions that include tumor growth (*Chapter 20*), overwhelming infections, graft-versus-host disease, and pregnancy. Moreover, the reciprocal relationship of neutrophils and T lymphocytes further illustrates the highly coordinated and unified processes that comprise immune resistance to fungi. Collectively, this new knowledge makes the traditional dogma of a dichotomy between neutropenia and T cell-specific defects less tenable and somewhat obsolete.

Evasion Mechanisms Utilized by Fungi

Macrophages are a heterogeneous population of tissue resident cells possessing the machinery for antigen presentation; however, their main contribution to antifungal defense is mediated through phagocytosis and killing of fungi. Not surprisingly, therefore, fungi have exploited a variety of mechanisms or putative virulence factors to evade phagocytosis, escape destruction, and survive within macrophages. Moreover, macrophages paradoxically provide a mechanism of fungal dissemination by providing a protected environment in which the dimorphic fungi multiply and disseminate from their initial portals of entry, e.g., the lung, to other tissues and organs. *H. capsulatum* represents an example of how a successful intracellular pathogen can utilize mammalian macrophages as a vehicle of transmission from initial entry in the lung to other tissue sites.

Humoral factors such as complement and antibodies also contribute to and enhance the innate defense mechanisms. Complement, a group of bioamplification proteins activated in cascading fashion (*Chapter 4*), antibodies, mannose-binding protein (**MBP**), and collectins promote binding of the fungal organism to the phagocyte surface with subsequent opsonization and represent a recognition mechanism carried out by a variety of receptors and PRRs that have a hierarchical organization. The specific biological activities of the complement system and antibodies that contribute to host resistance are multifaceted and interdependent. For example, antibodies greatly contribute to the activation of the complement system by fungi, and complement is essential for antibody-mediated protection. Each receptor on phagocytes not only mediates distinct downstream intracellular events related to clearance, but also participates in complex and disparate functions related to immunomodulation and activation of immunity, depending on the cell type. Engagement of CR3, also known as CD11b/CD18, not only represents one of the most efficient means of engulfing opsonized fungi, but also displays the remarkable characteristic of a broad recognition capacity for a diversity of fungal ligands. Moreover, the multiplicity of binding sites and the existence of different activation states of phagocytes enable CR3 to engage in dissimilar positive and negative effector activities against fungi. Since signaling through CR3 may not consistently lead to phagocyte activation without the concomitant engagement of receptors for the Fc portion of immunoglobulins, i.e., FcRs (*Chapter 6*), this may contribute to its role in intracellular fungal parasitism. Of interest are the contrasting findings that when *H. capsulatum* uses the CR3 receptor for entry into macrophages, it survives, but when taken up by DCs, it is rapidly degraded. Candida also exploits entry through CR3 to assure its survival within DCs. On the other hand, ligation of the antibody-coated fungi to the FcRs is usually sufficient to trigger phagocytosis, a vigorous oxidative burst, and the generation of pro-inflammatory signals. Ultimately, recognition of antibody-opsonized fungi represents either a beneficial outcome for the host or a high-level threat for the pathogen.

The lack of susceptibility to fungal infections seen in antibody-deficient patients as well as the presence of normal levels of specific antifungal antibodies found in patients with progressive fungal infections have been the main arguments against a protective role of antibodies in fungal infections. Recent advances have perhaps rendered these arguments less relevant by the demonstration of both the protective and non-protective properties of anti-fungal antibodies as well as the variable amounts and composition of antibodies seen in patients with fungal infections. Moreover, the tenuous role of antibody is not only supported by the finding of antibodies to heat shock protein 90 (**HSP90**) in patients recovering from *C. albicans* infections that correlate with protection against disseminated disease, but also by the identification of anti-HSP90 antibodies that synergize with antifungal chemotherapy in patients with AIDS. Complement, antibodies, and collectins not only fulfill the requirement of a first line of defense against fungi, but have also an impact on the inflammatory and adaptive immune responses through several mechanisms, including regulation of cytokine secretion by and co-stimulatory molecule expression on phagocytes. The local release of these effector molecules regulates cell trafficking in various types of leukocytes, thus initiating an inflammatory response, activating phagocytic cells to a microbicidal state, and directing Th/Treg development.

Sensing Fungi: The TLR and Non-TLR Pathogen-Detection Systems

A number of cell wall components of fungi may act through several distinct PRRs, each activating specific antifungal programs on phagocytes and DCs (*Chapters 3* and *9*) (Figure 14-4). However, another function of innate immunity that is being recognized is its role in promoting sterile inflammation—that is, inflammation caused by endogenous TLR ligands. In this regard, TLR activation itself is a double-edged sword. Thus, members of the TLR family are involved in the pathogenesis of a number of autoimmune diseases, as well as chronic inflammatory disorders such as asthma, rheumatoid arthritis, and infectious diseases. TLRs might also promote the pathogenesis of infections through hyperinduction of pro-inflammatory cytokines or by facilitating tissue damage or impairing protective immunity. Not surprisingly, therefore, the exploitation of PRRs may also provide a mechanism to divert and subvert host immune responses by fungi.

The different impact of TLRs on the expressions of innate and adaptive Th immune reactivity to fungi is related to the ability of individual TLRs to activate specialized antifungal effector pathways on phagocytes and DCs. TLRs influence specific antifungal programs of phagocytes, such as the respiratory burst, degranulation, and production of chemokines and cytokines. The recognition that both the quantity and specificity of toxic neutrophil products generated during inflammation ultimately determines whether the relative outcome leads to beneficial fungicidal activity versus deleterious inflammatory cytotoxicity to host cells underscores the critical pivotal role that TLRs play in antifungal immunity.

C-type lectin receptors (i.e., dectin-1 and 2, DC-SIGN, mannose receptor [**MR**]) and the galectin family are major mammalian PRRs for several fungal components and are the prototype molecules of the innate non-TLR signaling pathway for innate antifungal sensing (*Chapter 9*). The findings that N-linked mannosyl residues on fungal cells bind to MR, O-linked mannosyl residues bind to TLR4, and the critical role of mannosylation for optimal T cell activation to fungal antigens collectively provide mechanistic insights into the cooperative signaling between TLRs and non-TLRs for full immune cell activation. Dectin-1 is a myeloid-expressed transmembrane receptor possessing a single extracellular non-classical C-type-lectin-like domain that specifically recognizes the cell wall carbohydrate β1, 3 glucans of many fungi (Figure 14-4). As for TLRs, avoiding dectin-1 recognition could be a counter-strategy of fungi for immune evasion. The cytoplasmic tail of the receptor contains an immunoreceptor tyrosine-based activation-like motif (**ITAM**) related to those of adaptive antigen receptors that can mediate myeloid cell activation, cytokine production, and a variety of anti-fungal responses through the tyrosine kinase Syk/cytoplasmic caspase-recruiting domain (**CARD**) 9-dependent pathways.

Tuning the Adaptive Immune Responses: The Instructive Role of DCs

DCs are bone marrow–derived cells of both lymphoid, i.e., plasmacytoid DCs (pDCs) and myeloid stem cell origins, i.e., myeloid DCs (mDCs), that populate all lymphoid and nearly all nonlymphoid tissues and organs (*Chapter 3*). The dual activation/tolerization function of these DCs is mediated by their capacity to change the context of antigen presentation and to communicate to T cells the nature of the antigens they are presenting. DCs are uniquely adept at decoding fungus-associated information and translating it in qualitatively different adaptive T cell immune responses. A number of PRRs determine the functional plasticity of DCs in response to fungi and contribute to the discriminative recognition of the different fungal morphotypes. This process exemplifies the importance of PRRs not only in directing early immune responses, but also in orchestrating many aspects of adaptive immunity. The ability of a given DC subset to respond with flexible activating programs to different stimuli as well as the ability of different T cell subsets to convert into each other confers unexpected plasticity to the DC system.

DCs (both human and murine) are now known to recognize and internalize a number of fungi, including *A. fumigatus*, *C. albicans*, *C. neoformans*, *H. capsulatum*, and *Malassezia furfur*. DCs are capable of internalizing different fungal morphotypes through different receptors by phagocytosis. These events are consistent with the view that fungi have exploited common pathways for entry into DCs, which may include a lectin-like pathway for

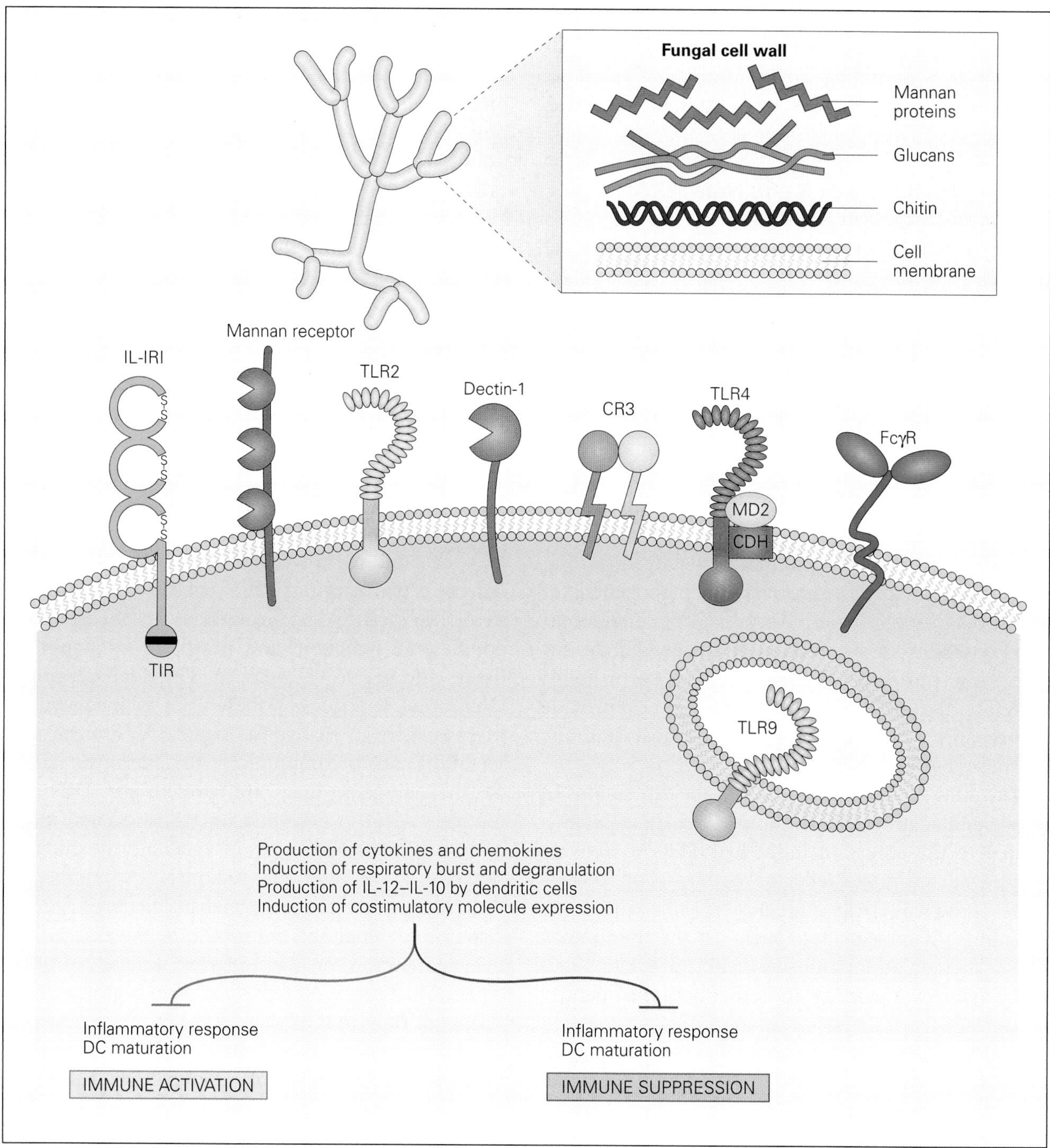

Figure 14-4. Role of Toll-like receptors (TLR) as activators of innate and adaptive immunity to fungi. Recognition of fungi and fungal PAMPs (pathogen-associated molecular patterns), mainly associated with fungal cell walls (top right schematic inset), leads to activation of specialized antifungal effector functions in neutrophils, such as the respiratory burst and degranulation and the production of directive cytokines by dendritic cells (see text). This translates into inflammatory responses and immune activation as well as inhibition of one or both. Blue and red lines refer to positive and negative signals, respectively.

unicellular yeast forms and opsono-dependent pathways for filamentous hyphal forms (Figure 14-4). As previously described, PRRs provide a pivotal contribution to fungal recognition and activation by DCs. Recent research findings have highlighted the involvement of both the TLR/Drosophila myeloid differentiation primary response gene 88 (**MyD88**)/Toll/IL-1 receptor domain-containing adaptor protein-inducing IFN (**TRIF**) and dectin-1-Syk-CARD9 signaling pathway in DC maturation and secretion of cytokines in response to fungi (*Chapter 9*). The engagement of distinct receptors by different fungal morphotypes translates into downstream signaling events, ultimately regulating cytokine production and co-stimulation, events greatly influenced by fungal opsonins, such as the mannose-binding lectins (**MBL**). This may explain the increased susceptibility to fungal infections in patients with defective MBL or MBL gene polymorphisms (*Chapter 16*).

Fungus-pulsed DCs *in vitro* and *in vivo* translate fungus-associated information to Th1, Th2, Th17, and Treg subsets. *In vivo*, the balance between the two DC subsets can determine whether protective or non-protective antifungal cell-mediated immune responses develop. Fungus-pulsed DCs have also been shown to activate different CD4+ Th cells upon adoptive transfer in a murine model of allogeneic bone marrow transplantation. More recent data have shown that the infusion of different DC subsets activates different immune responses. For example, the infusion of pDCs in bone marrow-transplanted mice has been shown to result in a concomitant Th1/Treg cell priming, eventually leading to fungal growth restriction, limited inflammatory pathology, and, interestingly, transplantation tolerance. These results, together with the finding that fungus-pulsed DCs could reverse T cell anergy in patients with fungal diseases, may suggest the utility of DCs for fungal vaccines and vaccination (*Chapter 23*).

A remarkable and important feature of DCs is their capacity to produce IL-10 in response to fungi. These IL-10-producing DCs activate CD4+CD25+ Treg cells that are essential components of antifungal resistance (*Chapter 9*). Thus, by subverting the DC morphotype-specific program of activation, the activity of opsonins, antibodies, and other environmental factors may subsequently modify DC functioning and Th/Treg selection *in vivo*, ultimately impacting fungal virulence. In this scenario, the qualitative development of a given Th subset response to a fungus may not depend exclusively on the nature of the fungal form being phagocytosed and presented. Rather, the nature of the cell response is determined by the type of cell signaling initiated by the ligand receptor interaction in DCs. For Candida, for example, which is sensed by dectin-1 receptor, the paradigm would predict that dimorphism per se can no longer be considered the single most important factor in determining commensalism versus infection, nor can specific forms of the fungus be regarded as absolutely indicative of saprophytism or infection at a given site. The selective exploitation of receptor-mediated entry of fungi into DCs could therefore explain the full range of host immune-parasite relationships, including saprophytism and infection. Importantly, as both fungal morphotypes, but particularly the hyphal forms, activate gut DCs for the local induction of Treg cells and because the morphogenesis of *C. albicans* is activated *in vivo* by a wide range of signals, it appears that the discriminative response toward Treg cell function is of potential teleological significance. This dichotomy in morphotype sensing could indeed permit fungal persistence in the absence of pathological consequences of an exaggerated immunity and possible autoimmunity, conditions that determine the very basis of fungal commensalisms. Therefore, in addition to the induction of phase-specific products enhancing fungal survival within the host, transition from the yeast to the hyphal phase of the fungus will favor fungal commensalism resulting from the participation of immunoregulatory events that will benefit the host.

The Adaptive Immune Response to Fungi: Th1/Th2/Th17 Cells

Generation of a dominant Th1 response driven by IL-12 is essentially required for the expression of protective immunity to fungi (Figure 14-3). Through the production of the signature cytokine IFN-γ and help provided by opsonizing antibodies, the activation of Th1 cells is instrumental in the optimal activation of phagocytes at sites of infection. Therefore, the failure to deliver activating signals to effector phagocytes may predispose patients to overwhelming infections, limit the therapeutic efficacy of antifungals and antibodies, and favor persistency and/or commensalisms. Immunological studies in patients with polar forms of paracoccidioidomycosis (Box 14-2) demonstrate an association between Th1-biased reactivity and the asymptomatic and mild forms of the infection, as

Box 14-2

Paracoccidioidomycosis (also known as Brazilian blastomycosis, South American blastomycosis, Lutz-Splendore-de Almeida disease, and Paracoccidioidal granuloma) is a mycosis caused by the fungus *Paracoccidioides brasiliensis*. Sometimes called South American blastomycosis, paracoccidioidomycosis is caused by a different fungus than that which causes blastomycosis, *Blastomyces dermatitidis*.

opposed to the positive correlation of Th2 responses with the severity of the disease and poor prognosis. Patients with inborn errors of the IL-12/IL-23/IFNγ-mediated axis of immunity are susceptible to disseminated paracoccidioidomycosis (*Chapter 16*).

IL-4 acts as the most potent proximal signal for commitment to Th2 reactivity that dampens protective Th1 responses and favors fungal allergy (Figure 14-3). IL-4 may both deactivate and activate phagocytes and DCs for certain specialized functions; for example, it may inhibit the antifungal effector activities of phagocytes, yet may promote IL-12 production by DCs. Thus, the most important mechanism underlying the inhibitory activity of IL-4 in fungal infections relies on its ability to act as the most potent proximal signal for commitment to Th2 reactivity that dampens protective Th1 responses and favors fungal allergy. In atopic subjects and neonates, the suppressed DTH response to fungi is associated with elevated levels of antifungal IgE, IgA, and IgG (*Chapter 18*). However, susceptibility to fungal infections may not always be associated with an overt production of IL-4.

IL-12, by initiating and maintaining Th1 responses, was thought to be responsible for hyperreactive immune and autoimmune disorders. This was also the case in fungal infections where immunoregulation proved to be essential in regulating inflammation and uncontrolled Th1/Th2 antifungal reactivity. Over the past several years, however, the demise of the Th1/Th2 dichotomy paradigm has been accompanied by a renaissance in probing the basic tenets of CD4+ T cell biology (*Chapter 9*). As a result, instead of only two distinct "fates" for developing T cells, research has identified alternative fates and more flexibility in the T cell cytokine repertoire than previously envisioned.

Th17 cells are now thought to be a separate lineage of effector Th cells contributing to immune pathogenesis previously attributed to the Th1 lineage (Figure 14-3 and *Chapter 9*). They produce unique cytokines (IL-17, IL-17F, IL-21, and IL-22) and express transcription factors distinct from Th1 and Th2 cells. Naive mouse and human CD4+ T cells activated in the presence of TGFβ and IL-6 express the transcription factor, retinoid-related orphan receptor gamma t (**RORγt**), and become Th17 cells that are stabilized by DC-derived IL-23 and amplified by IL-1 and IL-21. IL-6, IL-21, and IL-23 all induce phosphorylation of signal transducer and activator of transcription 3 (**STAT-3**) that has multiple binding sites on the IL-17A promoter. In contrast, TGFβ with IL-2 upregulates expression of the transcription factor, forkhead box P3 (**FOXP3**), and activate "inducible" Tregs that suppress immune responses. Several lines of evidence further support the notion of a reciprocal relationship between FOXP3+ Tregs and Th17 cells: IL-2 inhibits differentiation of Th17 cells; retinoic acid, a Vitamin A metabolite produced by CD103+ DCs in the gut, enhances Tregs but inhibits Th17 cell differentiation, and the transcription factors that differentiate Tregs and Th17 cells physically associate with each other (*Chapter 9*). In addition, since TGFβ can induce both RORγt and FOXP3, it is interesting that the level of TGFβ and the presence of cytokines such as IL-6 and IL-21 dictate whether expression of RORγt/RORα or FOXP3 predominate and, depending on the level of free transcription factors, determine whether T cells will differentiate into the Treg or Th17 phenotype. These transitional cellular forms once again illustrate the great plasticity of the T helper cell repertoire (*Chapter 9*).

Emerging data on the mechanism by which Th17 cells induce tissue inflammation suggest that IL-17/Th17 cells first infiltrate the site of tissue inflammation and then recruit other pro-inflammatory effector T cells (including Th1 cells) and innate cells (including neutrophils) to sites of tissue inflammation. These various cell types coordinately mediate inflammation, host defense, and tissue damage. Additionally, since IL-17 receptors are widely expressed on parenchymal/tissue cells and IL-17 induces production of IL-1, IL-6, TNF-α, matrix metalloproteinases, IL-8, and chemokines, these mediators coordinate infiltration of other cell types to the site of inflammation and generate massive tissue inflammation at the site where IL-17 is abundantly produced.

Th17 cells are induced in fungal infections through TLR- and non-TLR-dependent signaling pathways. Th17 lymphocytes are an important component of the human T cell memory repertoire to *C. albicans* and *A. fumigatus*, and defective Th17 cell differentiation has been linked to mucocutaneous candidiasis in patients with primary immunodeficiencies (*Chapter 16*). However, both positive and negative effects on immune resistance have been attributed to Th17 and IL-17 receptor (IL-17R) signaling in experimental fungal infections. Thus, the role of IL-17 and Th17 cells in immunity versus pathology in fungal infections and diseases remains controversial. It has been proposed that the protective versus disease-promoting effect of the IL-17/Th17 pathway may depend on the stage and site of infection; in an early stage of infection, for example, IL-17 may be able to exert some forms of antifungal resistance via defensins and neutrophils, while in a later phase of infection, the failure to downregulate microbe-induced expression of IL-17 could eventually lead to infection with chronic inflammation.

The mechanisms that link inflammation to chronic infection have been attributed to the detrimental potential of IL-17A that, although promoting neutrophil recruitment, can impede the timely restriction of neutrophil inflammatory potential, thus preventing optimal protection. IL-17A also is known to activate the inflammatory program of neutrophils by counteracting IFN-γ-dependent activation of the enzyme indoleamine 2,3-dioxygenase (**IDO**) and, as will be further described below, is known to limit the inflammatory status of neutrophils by inducing the release of metalloproteinases and oxidants. Collectively, these events likely account for the high inflammatory pathology and tissue destruction associated with Th17 cell activation (Figure 14-3).

The association between unrestricted inflammation and impairment in antifungal immunity has provided new strategies for the development of novel forms of immune therapy for fungal infections that are directed to restrict inflammation in order to stimulate an effective immune response. Thus, the Th17 pathway could be involved in the immunopathogenesis of chronic fungal diseases where persistent fungal antigens may maintain aberrant immune reactivity. Additionally, Th17 activation could account for the exacerbation of autoimmunity induced by fungal β-glucans. In experimental models, neutralization of IL-17 has been shown to increase fungal clearance, ameliorate inflammatory pathology, and restore protective Th1 antifungal resistance, findings that support the potential therapeutic utility of immunomodulatory strategies directed at reducing Th17-driven hyper-inflammation in fungal infections.

Collectively, these new findings may also find application in the restoration of immune homeostasis from its dysregulated state by the control of the fungal microbiota, including both those found within an individual host as commensals as well as those encountered ubiquitously in nature. Since the inflammatory response resulting from the activation of the IL-23/IL-17 axis leads to immune dysregulation, the potential for activation of Tregs that are the integral and essential components of protective immunity to fungi presents itself as a means to prevent dysregulated immunity.

Despite the strong evidence supporting the role of the IL-23/IL-17 axis in antifungal immunity, there are a number of other immunologic components that need to be considered. These include the dependency of Th17 cells on the plasticity of the complex human CD4+ T cell repertoire as well as the relative contributions of various populations of IL-17-producing cells to the pathogenesis of infections and diseases caused by the different fungi. Th17 cells, for example, also produce IL-22, a member of the IL-10 family of cytokines, which has been shown to play a more important role than IL-17 in host defense in the lung and gastrointestinal tract (*Chapter 8*). Recent findings in animal models of candidiasis and aspergillosis suggest that the IL-23/IL-22/defensin pathway is also crucially involved in the control of fungal growth at mucosal and non-mucosal sites, particularly under conditions of Th1 deficiency. Although some studies have suggested that the Th17 cells may exert their protective role in fungal infections through production of IL-22, IL-22-producing Th17 cells, however, failed to confer the same level of resistance to reinfection and to inflammatory pathology conferred by the Th1/Treg axis. Thus, in the relative absence of protective Th1/Treg cells, the IL-22+/Th17 cells may fulfill the role of an "emergency" protective response that exploits primitive anti-fungal effector defense mechanisms. This finding suggests that functionally distinct "modules" of immunity evolved to provide resistance, i.e., the ability to limit fungal burden, or tolerance, i.e., the ability to limit the host damage in response to fungi.

The IFN-γ/IDO Axis and Its Role in Fungal Immunity

The IDO pathway and its downstream enzymes comprise a metabolic axis involved in the degradation of tryptophan to a variety of kynurenine metabolites (Figure 14-5). Found in innate immune cells, including macrophages, polymorphonuclear neutrophils (**PMN**), and epithelial cells, IDO is a key player in the suppression of acute and chronic inflammatory responses. Through local tryptophan starvation, IDO can stimulate a Gcn2-induced stress-signaling pathway that upregulates translation of the NF-IL6/CEBPβ transcription factor isoform LIP, which alters immune-related gene expression, including the key immune modulatory factors IL-6, TGFβ, and IL-10.

The role of IDO in mammalian cells was generally unclear before the seminal studies that correlated IDO activity with T cell suppression. In addition to directly suppressing T cell activation, IDO+ pDCs have also been reported to induce a population of Tregs by inducing naïve CD4+ T cells to differentiate to FOXP3+ Tregs, as well as by activating resting natural Tregs to become potently suppressive. Interestingly, Tregs have been shown to induce IDO in DCs through CTLA-4-mediated reverse signaling. Therefore, it has been suggested that communication between IDO+ pDCs and Tregs may result in a positive feedback loop of immunosuppression. Shown in Figure 14-5 is a schematic representation of the metabolic events involved in the activation of IDO in pDCs by a variety of activators, including IFN-γ, following which the IDO-activated pDC displays a dual role in both augmenting the suppression of an immune response first by the induction of naive Th0 cells into Treg cells through a CTLA-4/B7.1 interaction and second by the down-regulation of T effector cells following tryptophan degradation.

Naturally occurring IL-22+Th17 cells are highly enriched at mucosal sites, where continuous exposure to ubiquitous fungi occurs either through inhalation or via commensalism in the respiratory and gastrointestinal tracts, respectively (*Chapter 8*). This requires a sophisticated degree of host-parasite adaptation to which a number of complex integrated innate and adaptive immune responses contribute (Figure 14-5). In this scenario, the IFN-γ/IDO axis, leading to sequential Th1/Treg activation upon exposure to fungi at mucosal sites, may have evolved to accommodate fungal persistence, i.e., commensalism, in an inflammatory environment rich in IFN-γ. In contrast, the occurrence of IL-22+Th17 cells employing ancient effector mechanisms of immunity may represent a primitive mechanism of resistance against the fungus under conditions of limited inflammation. Thus, the exploitation of the IFN-γ/IDO axis for functional specialization of antifungal effector and regulatory mechanisms may have allowed commensal or ubiquitous fungi to co-evolve with the mammalian immune system to survive in conditions of high-threat inflammation.

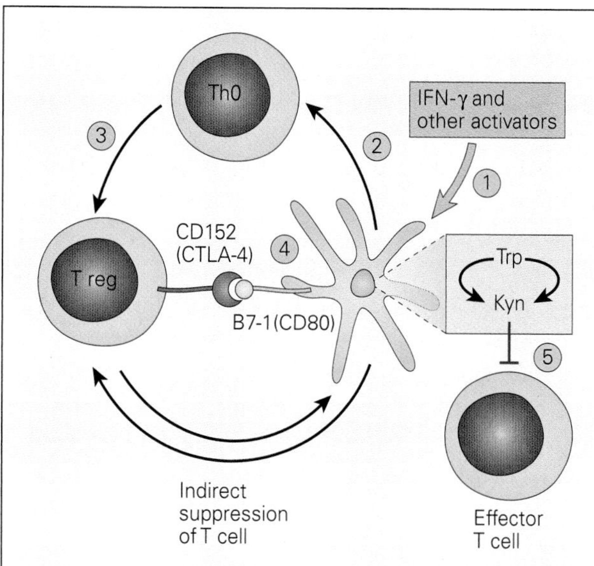

Figure 14-5 Schematic representation of the central role of IDO in the metabolic events involved in the activation pDCs. Following activation of the DC by a variety of activators including IFN-γ, (1) IDO-activated DC displays a dual role in both augmenting the suppression of an immune response by the induction of naïve Th0 cells (2) into Treg cells (3) through a CTLA-4/B7.1 interaction (4) as well as the down-regulation of T effector cells following tryptophan degradation (5).

Dampening Inflammation and Allergy to Fungi: A Task for Treg Cells

As described previously, the inflammatory response to fungi may serve to limit infection but may also contribute to pathogenicity, as documented by the occurrence of severe fungal infections in patients with IRIS. These patients may experience intractable fungal infections despite recovery from neutropenia with the occurrence of adaptive immune responses. The above considerations suggest that in fungal diseases, a series of complex induced immunoregulatory elements are essential and may contribute to the fine-tuning of inflammation and Th reactivity to fungi. In this regard, CD4+ T cells are known to be comprised of a series of induced Treg cells that, in contrast to the natural T cells produced in the thymus, are primed locally (*Chapter 9*). These induced Treg cells include (1) Tr1 cells producing IL-10 and (2) Th3 cells producing transforming growth factor TGFβ. These locally induced Treg cells contribute to the immunomodulation of antimicrobial immune responses by fine-tuning and balancing the other effector axis, minimizing harmful inflammatory consequences. The final outcome of this dynamic equilibrium will not only be determined by interactions between pathogens and cells of the innate immune system, but also by the actions of these induced Tregs on the adaptive immune function. Conceptually, in a similar fashion to their effects on immunity against pathogens, Treg cells can also impede effective immunosurveillance of tumors (*Chapter 20*). At the present time, the concept of aberrant numbers and/or functions of Treg cells has been incorporated within the global view of counter-regulatory elements affecting self versus nonself discrimination. The Treg cell population is recognized as having great clinical applications in the outcome of infection, autoimmunity, transplantation, cancer, and allergic disease.

Clinical Consequences of Immune Dysregulation

A number of clinical observations suggest an inverse relationship between IFN-γ and IL-10 production in patients with fungal infections. High levels of IL-10, negatively affecting IFN-γ production, are detected in chronic candidal diseases, in the severe form of endemic mycoses, and in neutropenic patients with aspergillosis (*Chapter 16*). Fungal polysaccharides are known to negatively modulate cell-mediated immunity (**CMI**) through the production of IL-10, a finding suggesting that IL-10 production may be a consequence of infection. However, tolerance to fungi can also be achieved through the induction of Treg cells capable of finely tuning antifungal Th reactivity. Naturally occurring Treg cells operating in the respiratory or the gastrointestinal mucosa account for the lack of pathology associated with fungal clearance in mice with fungal pneumonia or mucosal candidiasis. Distinct Treg populations capable of mediating anti-inflammatory or tolerogenic effects are coordinately induced after exposure to *Aspergillus conidia*. Ultimately, the inherent resistance to Aspergillus diseases suggests the existence of regulatory mechanisms that provide the host with protection from infection and tolerance to allergy. It has been demonstrated that a division of labor occurs between functionally distinct Treg cells that are coordinately activated after exposure of mice to resting *Aspergillus conidia*. Early in infection, inflammation is controlled by the expansion, activation, and local recruitment of Treg cells suppressing neutrophils through the combined actions of IL-10 and cytotoxic T lymphocyte antigen (**CTLA**)-4 on IDO, as described previously (Figure 14-5). Late in infection, and similarly in allergy, tolerogenic Treg cells that produce IL-10 and TGFβ inhibit Th2 cells and prevent allergy to the fungus.

The Molecular Bases of Chronic Mucocutaneous Candidiasis

It has long been recognized that the ability of *C. albicans* to establish an infection involves multiple components of the fungus, but its ability to persist in host tissue might involve primarily the immunosuppressive property of a major cell wall glycoprotein, mannan. Although epitopes of mannan exist endowed with the ability to induce protective antibodies to the fungus, mannan and oligosaccharide fragments could also function as potent inhibitors of CMI and appear to contribute to the immune deficit of patients with CMC (*Chapter 16*). Although encompassing a variety of clinical entities, CMC has also been associated with autoimmune polyendocrinopathy-candidiasis-ectodermal dystrophy (**APECED**), an entity in which the AIRE gene (a gene thought to be normally involved in the ontogeny of CD25+ Treg cells) is mutated. In CMC, both anergy and active lymphoproliferation and variable DTH reactivity to the fungus are indeed observed. As described previously, this has been associated with a defective type 1 cytokine production without obvious increase in type 2 cytokine production (namely IL-4 or IL-5). However, both elevated and diminished levels of IL-10 have also been observed in patients with CMC, a finding suggestive of an inherent defect in receptor-mediated signaling to fungal polysaccharide that may predispose affected patients to a dysfunctional induction of Treg cells that in turn may lead to an impaired capacity of Th1-dependent clearance of the fungus without the activation of Th2 cells.

Collectively, these observations suggest that the capacity of Treg cells to inhibit aspects of innate and adaptive immunity may be central to their regulatory activity in fungal infections. This may result in the generation of immune responses vigorous enough to provide adequate host defense, without necessarily eliminating the pathogen (which could limit immune memory) or causing an unacceptable level of host damage. Although the immunopathogenesis of fungal infections and associated diseases have been previously attributed to a Th1/Th2 imbalance, a more contemporary explanation should include the pivotal role of the various types of Treg cells and their immunoregulatory controls over the Th1, Th2, and Th17 inflammatory responses.

The Central Role of the Tryptophan Metabolic Pathway in Tolerance and Immunity to Fungi: Implications for Fungal Disease and Commensalism

As described previously, the inflammatory/anti-inflammatory state of DCs is strictly controlled by the IFN-γ/IDO metabolic pathway involved in tryptophan catabolism and mediated by the enzyme IDO (Figure 14-5). The IFN-γ/IDO axis plays an important immunoregulatory role in infection, pregnancy, autoimmunity, transplantation, and neoplasia. IDO-expressing DCs are regarded as regulatory DCs specialized to cause antigen-specific immune suppression, e.g., tolerance or otherwise negatively regulating responding T cells. In experimental fungal infections, IDO blockade has been shown to greatly exacerbate infections, aggravate the associated inflammatory pathology, and abolish resistance to reinfection. These events are caused by the dysregulation of innate and adaptive immune responses resulting from the IDO-blocked DCs that fail to induce the suppressive activity of suppressor CD4+CD25+ Treg cells producing IL-10. These findings provide novel mechanistic insights into the complex events occurring at the fungus/pathogen interface that relate to the dynamics of host adaptation by fungi. Thus, the production of IFN-γ may be squarely placed at this interface, where IDO activation likely exerts a fine control over both inflammatory and adaptive antifungal responses.

It may now be possible to construct a central unifying hypothesis to explain several unexplained findings of candidiasis focusing on the pivotal role of IDO in immunoregulation. Shown in Figure 14-6 are two possible molecular mechanisms by which depressed immune function may be involved in the persistence of *C. albicans* as a chronic infection. In the first of these, since *C. albicans* is a commensal of the human gastrointestinal and genitourinary tracts and IFN-γ is an important mediator of protective immunity to the fungus, the IFN-γ/IDO axis may accommodate fungal persistence in a host environment rich in IFN-γ by upregulation of IDO in DCs. This, in turn, leads to an increase in Treg cells and a decrease in effector cells. In its ability to downregulate antifungal Th1 responses in the gastrointestinal tract, IDO behaves in a fashion similar to that described in mice with colitis where IDO expression correlates with the occurrence of local tolerogenic responses. An alternative possibility invokes the high levels of IL-10 production, such as those seen in patients with CMC, which may be a consequence of IDO activation by the fungus, impairing antifungal Th1 immunity and thus favoring persistent infection.

In aspergillosis, the level of inflammation and IFN-γ in the early stage sets the subsequent adaptive stage by conditioning the IDO-dependent tolerogenic program of DCs and the subsequent activation and

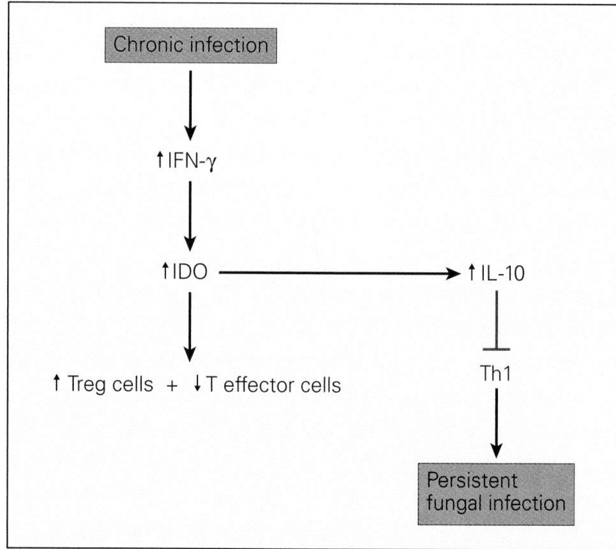

Figure 14-6 Schematic representation of two possible molecular mechanisms by which depressed immune function may be involved in the persistence of *C. albicans* as a chronic infection. In the pathway shown on the left, the IFN-γ/IDO axis may accommodate fungal persistence in a host environment by increased IDO resulting from a host environment rich in IFN-γ, leading to an increase in Treg cells and a decrease in T effector cells. In the pathway shown on the right, the high levels of IL-10 production may be a consequence of IDO activation by the fungus, impairing antifungal Th1 immunity and thus favoring persistent infection.

expansion of tolerogenic Tregs preventing allergy to the fungus. Therefore, regulatory mechanisms operating in the control of inflammation and allergy to the fungus are different but interdependent, as the level of the inflammatory response early in infection may impact on susceptibility to allergy in conditions of continuous exposure to the fungus. Early Treg cells, by affecting Th1-induced IFN-γ-production, indirectly can exert a fine control over the induction of late tolerogenic Tregs. Thus, a unifying mechanism linking natural Tregs to tolerogenic respiratory Tregs in response to the fungus is consistent with the revisited "hygiene hypothesis" of allergy in infections and may provide mechanistic explanations for the significance of the variable level of IFN-γ seen in allergic diseases and asthma and for the paradoxical worsening effect on allergy of Th1 cells. IDO has a unique and central role in this process as it may participate in the effector and inductive phases of anti-inflammatory and tolerogenic Tregs.

Working Hypothesis of the Pathogenesis of Diseases That Result From Hypersensitivity Reactions to Fungal Agents

There are three probable outcomes that could result from the interaction between the host immune response and a fungal agent that determine whether the outcome will result in protective immunity or a hypersensitivity reaction. This working hypothesis is based on the concept of immunologic balance and the efficiency of antigen elimination described in Chapter 1 and Figure 14-7. The degree to which fungal antigen persists, is reintroduced, or is eliminated will determine the expression of the host reaction.

If fungal antigen is successfully eliminated either by the components of phagocytosis and inflammation of the first phase of innate immunity, or by development of antibody and cell-mediated immunity of adaptive immunity, no further host interaction is seen. If, on the other hand, the fungus is not successfully eliminated or is reintroduced in either a live or inactivated form, the persistence of fungal antigen and interaction with components of either antibody or cell-mediated immune responses may lead to further host interaction with the development of immunologically mediated injury of the lung, as described in Chapter 18. For example, if IgE antibody is stimulated, particularly in an atopic patient, that individual could express symptoms of asthma mediated by a Type I reaction. If precipitating antibody is stimulated and fungal antigen persists or is reintroduced via the respiratory tract, an immune-complex (Type III) reaction might result in conjunction with a cell-mediated (Type IV) component to result in a mixed-type hypersensitivity reaction characteristic of extrinsic allergic alveolitis (Farmer's lung disease). Similarly, the combination of a Type I IgE-mediated reaction to *Aspergillus* antigen, for example, in an atopic patient together with an immune-complex (Type III) reaction could result in another type of mixed type hypersensitivity reaction

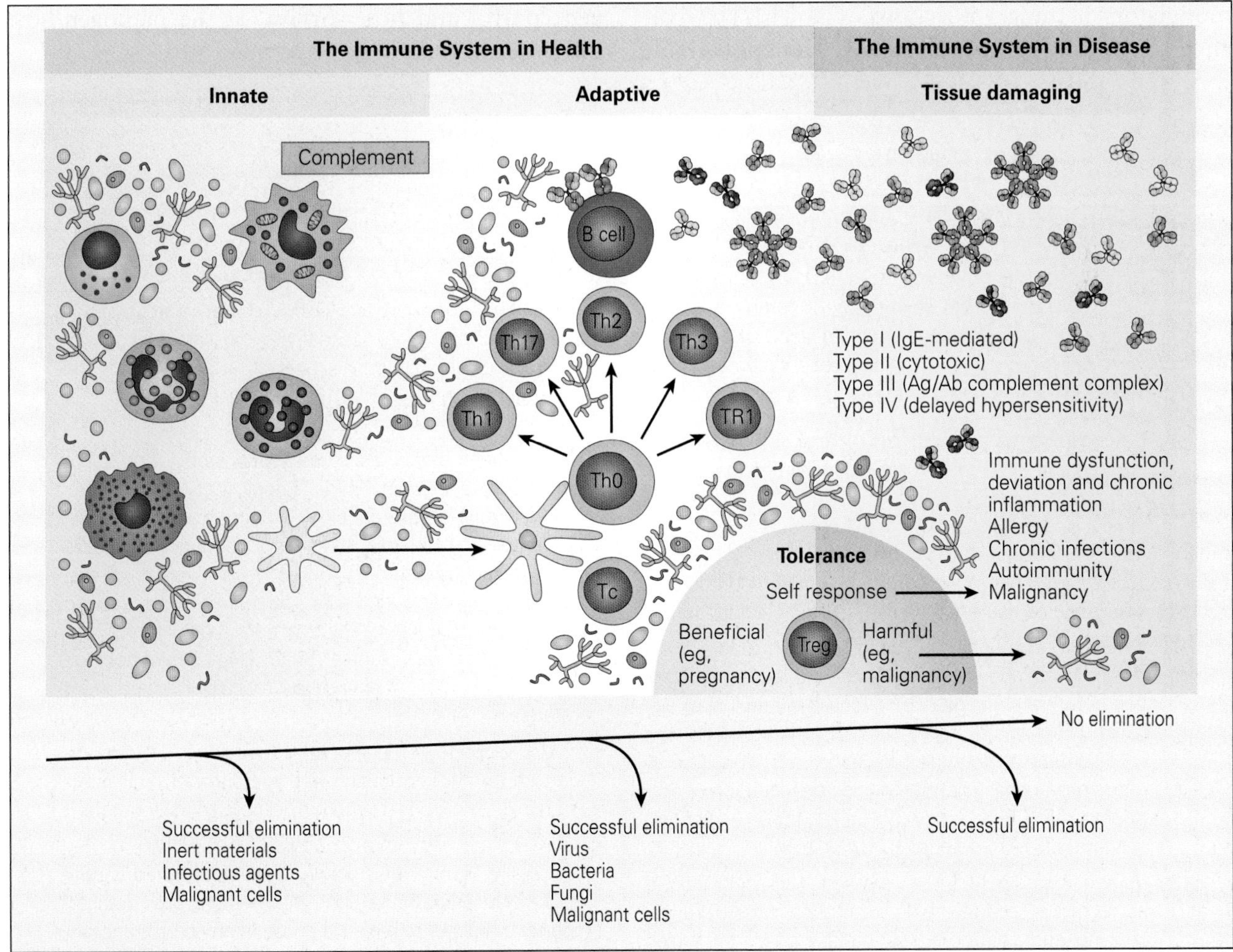

Figure 14-7 Schematic representation of the total immunologic capability of the host, based on the efficient elimination of foreign matter. Fungi persist because of a variety of inherited immunosuppressure conditions affecting immunologic recognition of fungal antigens or signaling mechanisms or metabolic defects (e.g., diabetes).

characteristic of allergic bronchopulmonary aspergillosis (**ABPA**) (*Chapter 18*).

Conclusions

A finely orchestrated balance between activating and inhibitory signals is fundamental for the ability of the immune system to effectively attack and eliminate pathogenic fungi and/or coexist with commensals without reacting against self-antigens. Derangements of this balance may underlie the pathogenesis of chronic infections and autoimmune inflammatory diseases. New discoveries in the field of fungal immunology have offered grounds for a better comprehension of cells and immune pathways that are amenable to manipulation in patients with or at risk of fungal infections. Preclinical studies have shown the potential therapeutic role of a variety of cytokines, growth factors, and immunomodulators in fungal infections. The Th1/Th2 balance itself can be the target of immunotherapy. However, the new findings provide the basis for novel immunomodulatory therapies that are strictly required to limit inflammation in order to stimulate an effective immune response. Despite the redundancy and overlapping repertoire of antifungal effector mechanisms, the pivotal role of different types of Tregs in the control of Th1/Th2 inflammatory responses as well as in Th17 antagonism suggests that manipulation of Tregs could be a promising therapeutic approach devoid of risks associated with interference with homeostatic mechanisms of the immune system. In this regard, the potential of the anti-TNF antibody, e.g., Infliximab, to induce anti-inflammatory cytokines IL-10 or TGFβ via retrograde signaling or through induction of a certain subset of Tregs is of interest. Likewise, tryptophan metabolites and Th17 inhibitors are likely candidates as potent regulators in a reciprocal two-edged sword interaction capable of taming overzealous or heightened inflammatory host responses to the benefit of pathogen control and host survival at the pathogen/host interface.

Case Studies: Clinical Relevance

Let us now return to the case study of chronic mucocutaneous candidiasis presented earlier and review some of the major points of the clinical presentation and how they relate to the immune system:

- Mucocutaneous candidiasis, vaginal candidiasis, thrush, and onychomycosis (fungal infection of the nail) occur in several clinical conditions, ranging from infection, e.g., HIV and metabolic defects (e.g., diabetes) that promote the growth of the organism as well as a variety of immune defects of innate and adaptive immunity, particularly those affecting T cell function.
- Inherited immunologic conditions include some recently described genetic disorders affecting recognition of fungal antigens, e.g., dectin-1 mutations, or signaling mechanisms, e.g., CARD9 mutations, as well as disorders of immune regulation, e.g., the autoimmune polyendocrinopathy–candidiasis–ectodermal dystrophy (APECED) syndrome, and Job's (hyper-IgE) syndrome (STAT3 defects) (*Chapter 16*).
- Shown in Figure 14-8 is a schematic representation of some of the recently identified mechanisms of fungal sensing and control illustrating the points at which mutations of key sensing and signaling molecules occur lead to defective antifungal responses.
- The finding of a positive *Candida*-delayed hypersensitivity skin test suggests that the Th1 limb of T helper CD4+ cellular function is normal, indicating that the adaptive immune system is functioning and that the defect lies elsewhere.
- The patient described in the case study represents an example of dectin-1 deficiency that led to defective sensing of the candidal β-glucan by the dectin-1 receptor on epithelial cells and phagocytes (Figure 14-8). This resulted in defective activation of the CARD9 signaling complex, which, in turn, led to defective production of IL-6 and IL-23, which are cytokines needed to help drive CD4+ T lymphocytes toward the Th17 phenotype, a STAT3-dependent process.
- Th17 lymphocytes elaborate interleukin-17 (augmenting neutrophil production and recruitment) and interleukin-22, which are synergic in the STAT3-dependent production of antimicrobial peptides by epithelial cells.
- A family history elucidating several affected family members together with the results of detailed genetic studies revealed the condition to be transmitted in an autosomal recessive mode of inheritance (Figure 14-9).

Case Studies: Clinical Relevance (continued)

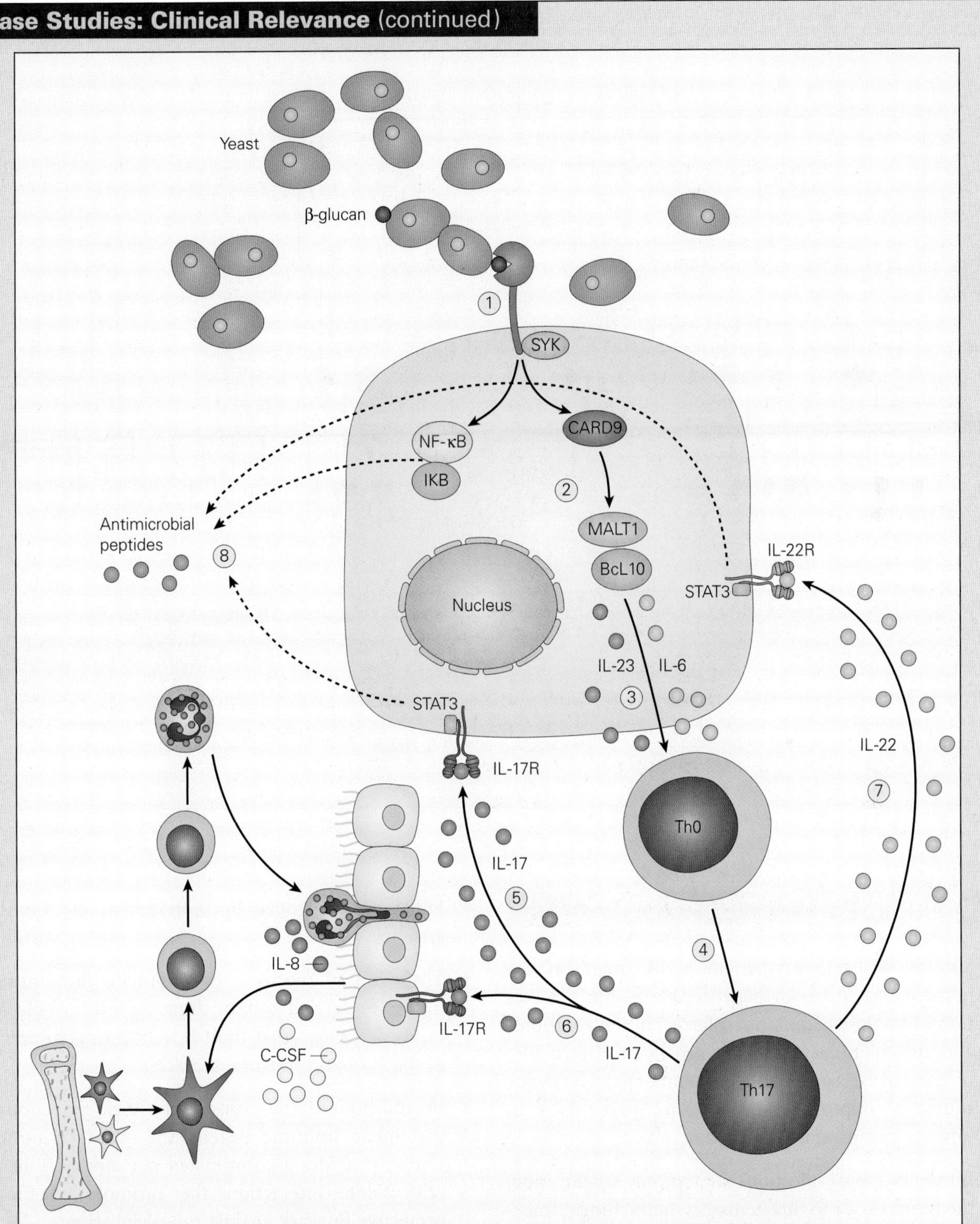

Figure 14-8 Schematic representation of some of the recently identified mechanisms of fungal sensing and control, illustrating the points at which mutations of key sensing and signaling molecules occur that lead to defective antifungal responses. The β-glucan on the budding yeast forms of Candida binds to dectin-1 on epithelial cells and phagocytes (1), leading to activation of the CARD9 (2) signaling complex (along with MALT1/Bcl-10). This in turn produces IL-6 and IL-23 (3), cytokines that help drive CD4+ T lymphocytes toward the Th17 phenotype (4), a STAT3-dependent process. Mutations in CARD9, detin-1 and STAT3 have been associated with defective antifungal responses. Th17 lymphocytes elaborate interleukin-17 (augmenting neutrophil production and recruitment) (5) and interleukin-22 (6), which are synergic in the STAT3-dependent production of antimicrobial peptides by epithelial cells (7 and 8).

Case Studies: Clinical Relevance (continued)

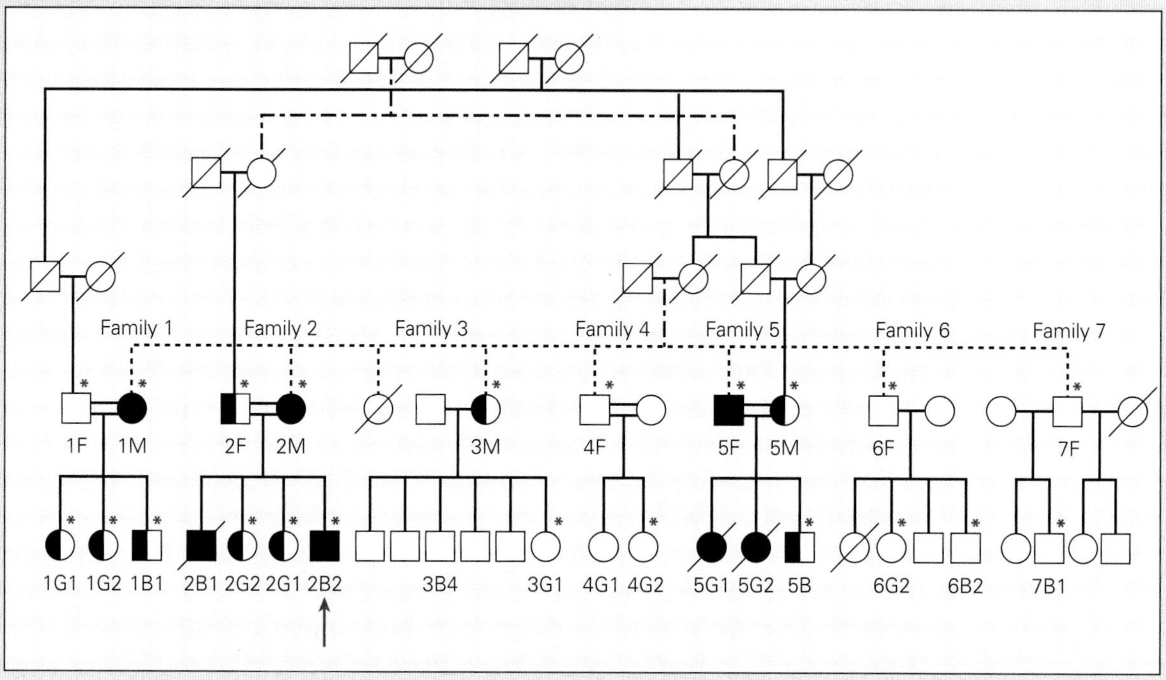

Figure 14-9 Pedigree of an Iranian family with chronic mucocutaneous candidiasis. The patient (2B2) described in the case presentation is indicated by the red arrow. A slash denotes a deceased family member. Circles denote female family members; squares are male family members; solid circles and squares are patients with chronic mucocutaneous candidiasis who were homozygous for point mutation in CARD9; half-solid circles and squares represent members who were heterozygous for this mutation; open circles and squares represent healthy members with wild-type CARD9, and double horizontal lines indicate consanguinity in a married couple. Asterisks indicate family members whose samples were submitted to DNA sequencing. (Reproduced with permission from Glocker EO, Hennigs A, Nabavi M, et al. A homozygous CARD9 mutation in a family with susceptibility to fungal infections. N Engl J Med. 2009;361:1727–35.)

Key Points

- Similar to bacteria, the effects of fungi on the human host are both beneficial (e.g., the production of vitamins, antibiotics, fermentation reactions, and the maintenance of the geochemical structure of the earth's soil) and detrimental (e.g., a major source of opportunistic infections, particularly in immunocompromised hosts).
- Although fungal infections are typically self-limiting, the number of life-threatening systemic fungal infections has risen steadily over the past three decades.
- The increased prevalence of fungi as agents of disseminated infection has been seen, particularly in patients undergoing surgical or chemotherapeutic interventions and/or with underlying immunological deficiencies that allow fungi to overwhelm the protective antifungal host defense mechanisms.
- Fungi are controlled by both innate and immune systems.
- The primary mechanisms of innate immunity to fungi are carried out by fungal sensing molecules on macrophages that limit infection to colonization of the skin and mucosal surfaces.
- In addition to the control of fungal infection by the innate immune system, the adaptive immune system provides a coordinated network of T helper cell/cytokine interactions that promote an efficient protective bulwark against fungal invasion.
- Although Th1 responses driven by the IL-12 /IFN-γ axis are central to protection against fungi, other cytokines and T cell-dependent antifungal mechanisms of immunity have been recognized.
- The newly described Th17 developmental pathway has been shown to play an inflammatory role

previously attributed solely to uncontrolled Th1 responses and serves to accommodate the seemingly paradoxical association of chronic inflammatory responses with fungal persistence in the face of an ongoing inflammation.

- Regulatory T cells (Tregs) in their capacity to inhibit aspects of innate and adaptive antifungal immunity have become an integral component of immune resistance to fungi and provide an effective mechanism to counterbalance and limit the degree of inflammatory responses that would otherwise be detrimental to host defense.
- Molecular defects in specific aspects of these innate and adaptive protective mechanisms have recently been identified and provide new opportunities for novel and interventive therapeutic and preventive modalities.

Study Questions/Critical Thinking

1. Each of the following clinical conditions have been associated with an increased prevalence of fungal infections EXCEPT:

   a) HIV/AIDS
   b) Diabetes
   c) Chronic granulomatous disease (CGD)
   d) X-linked agammaglobulinemia (X-LA)

2. Patients with CGD frequently manifest infection with which fungal organism?

   a) Aspergillus
   b) Candida
   c) Histoplasma
   d) Coccioimycoccosis

3. Each of the following molecular defects predispose patients with candidal infection EXCEPT:

   a) STAT3
   b) Dectin-1
   c) CARD9
   d) BTK

4. A 23-year-pld patient presenting with SOB, cough, and a golden sputum with no known infectious disease contact whose laboratory tests show an elevated IgE and eosinophilia should raise the most likely possibility of which of the following entities:

   a) Asthma
   b) Wegener's syndrome
   c) Bronchopulmonary aspergillosis (BPA)
   d) Extrinsic allergic alveoltis

Acknowledgment

We thank Cristina Massi Benedetti for dedicated editorial assistance. This study was supported by the Specific Targeted Research Project "ALLFUN" (FP7–Health–2010–single–stage, contract number 260338) and by the Italian projects AIDS RF-PGN-2009-1302800.

Suggested Reading

Brown GD. Dectin-1: a signaling non-TLR pattern recognition receptor. Nat Rev Immunol. 2006; 6: 33–43.

Ferwerda B, Ferwerda G, Plantinga TS, et al. Human decetin-1 deficiency and mucocutaneous fungal infections. N Eng J Med. 2009; 361: 1760–7.

Glocker EO, Hennigs A, Nabavi M, et al. A homozygous CARD9 mutation in a family with susceptibility to fungal infections. N Eng J Med. 2009; 36: 1727–35.

Heitman J, Filler SG, Edwards JE Jr, et al., eds. Molecular principles of fungal pathogensis. Washington, DC: ASM Press; 2006.

Holland S. Yeast infections—human genetics on the rise. N Eng J Med. 2009; 361: 1798–801.

Netea MG, Brown GD, Kullberg BJ, et al. An integrated model of the recognition of *Candida albicans* by the innate immune system. Nat Rev Microbiol. 2008; 6: 67–78.

Predergast GC, Metz R, Muller AJ. Towards a genetic definition of cancer-associated inflammation: role of the IDO pathway. Am J Pathol. 2010; 176: 2082–7.

Romani J, Puccetti P. Protective tolerance to fungi: the role of IL-10 and tryptophan catabolism. Trends Microbiol. 2006; 14: 183–89.

Romani L, Puccetti P. Controlling pathogenic inflammation to fungi. Expert Rev Anti Infect Ther. 2007; 5: 1007–17.

Romani L, Puccetti P. Dendritic cells in immunity and vaccination against fungi. In Handbook of dendritic cells: biology, diseases, and therapies, 2nd vol. Lutz MB, Steinkasserer A, eds. Weinheim, Germany: Wiley-VCH Verlag GmbH & Co; 2006.

Romani L. Cell-mediated immunity to fungi: a reassessment. Med Mycol. 2008: 1–15.

Romani L. Immunity to fungal infection. Nat Rev Immunol. 2004; 4: 1–23.

Segal BS, Kwon-Chung J, Walsh TJ, et al. Immunotherapy for fungal infections. Clin Infect Dis. 2006; 42: 507–15.

Singh N, Perfect JR. Immune reconstitution syndrome associated with opportunistic mycoses. Lancet Infect Dis. 2007: 7: 395–401.

Zelante T, Fallarino F, Bistoni F, et al. Indoleamine2,3-dioxygenase in infection: the paradox of an evasive strategy that benefits the host. Microbes Infect. 2009; 11: 133–41.

Chapter 15

Clinical Immunology of Parasitic Diseases

Susana Mendez, DVM, PhD
Ricardo T. Fujiwara, PhD

Case Studies

Case Study 1

A well-developed, well-nourished 18-old-year male from Patna (Bihar, India) was hospitalized with a chief complaint of fever of 10 days duration, cough, fatigue, chills, abdominal pain, and weight loss. The present illness began about one month before, when he developed generalized weakness, fatigue, fever, and weight loss. He was not receiving medications and there was no history of exposure to animals or other people with similar symptoms. There was a history of kala-azar in several of his brothers and sisters.

Physical examination revealed a thin male with pale conjunctivae, no icterus or rash, normal jugular venous pressure (JVP), and no lymphadenopathy. Examination of the chest revealed decreased breath sounds at the right lung base but no rales or wheezes. The cardiac examination was normal. The abdominal examination revealed a large palpable liver 4 cm below the right costal margin with a liver span of 13 cm and a greatly enlarged spleen palpable 9 cm below the left costal margin. The extremities showed a moderate degree of muscle wasting and the neurologic examination was normal.

Laboratory tests showed a hemoglobin level of 8.8 g/dl, a hematocrit of 21 percent, and a total white blood count (WBC) of 2,000/mm^3, with 65 percent neutrophils, 14 percent lymphocytes, 20 percent monocytes, and 1 percent eosinophils. The platelet count was 106,000/mm^3 and the A/G ratio was 0.45 (normal is 1.5) with a total globulin of 9.1 g/dl (normal is 2.3–3.5). A pleural effusion was detected by CT scan and a pleural tap was performed that revealed a transudate with a total WBC count of 330/mm^3 with 23 percent neutrophils, 67 percent lymphocytes, 10 percent monocytes, total protein of 1.7 g/dl, glucose of 133 mg/dl, and LDH of 62 u/l. Culture of the pleural fluid was negative. Abdominal sonography revealed an enlarged liver with a heterogeneous echo pattern, a dilated portal vein, and a hugely enlarged spleen with a normal homogenous echo pattern. Bone marrow biopsy revealed the presence of multiple intracellular oval bodies measuring 2–3 μ in diameter within monocytes and macrophages.

LEARNING OBJECTIVES

When you have completed this chapter, you should be able to:

- Understand that infections caused by protozoan, helminthic, or arthropod parasites are referred to as parasitic diseases
- Appreciate that parasites are classified as protozoans (single-cell parasites) or metazoans (multicellular parasites)
- Explain the various targets of parasitic infections to include the gastrointestinal tract, lungs, bloodstream, or solid organs
- Know that metazoans are also called helminths (worms)
- Classify the helminths into the flatworms (Platyhelminthes) and the roundworms (nematodes [Nemathelminthes])
- Describe the innate and adaptive immune responses to parasitic infections
- Recognize that elevated IgE levels and eosinophilia occur in several helminthic infections
- Appreciate that the medically important flatworms are further divided into the flukes (Trematoda) and tapeworms (Cestoda)
- Recognize that tapeworms live in the gut but also can infect solid organs
- Know that flukes can live in blood vessels, lungs, or liver
- Provide examples of the clinical consequences of parasitism, which include anemia, development of space-occupying lesions or granulomas in solid organs, allergic reactions, obstruction of blood vessels or lymphatics, induction of cancer, blindness, and diarrhea
- Describe the role of immunity to parasites in health and disease

Case Studies (continued)

Case Study 2

An 18-month-old male was seen by his primary care physician for a very pruritic rash on his feet and buttocks of several months duration. Because initial treatment with a topical steroid ointment offered no relief, the child was subsequently started on topical clotrimazole with no improvement. After two weeks, the mother became increasingly concerned as her son was unable to sleep at night and began losing weight due to poor appetite, and he was taken to an emergency room.

Physical examination revealed an irritable child with an erythematous, raised, serpiginous rash on the right buttock measuring 2–3 mm in width and 5 cm in length that tunneled beneath the skin in a burrowing track. A more obviously undulating and serpiginous track-like skin lesion was present along the lateral aspect of the right side of the neck. Scattered erythematous papules studded the skin of the right calf. The remainder of the physical examination was unremarkable.

Laboratory tests showed a hemoglobin concentration of 13.6 g/dl, a hematocrit of 36 percent, a total WBC count of 12,000/mm^3 with 32 percent neutrophils, 31 percent lymphocytes, 12 percent monocytes, and 25 percent eosinophils, and a platelet count of 300,000/mm^3. A skin biopsy specimen taken from the leading edge of the tract on the buttock revealed chronic inflammatory changes compatible with nonspecific dermatitis.

Case Study 3

A 50-year-old white male presented with upper abdominal pain and tenderness in the epigastric region that began one month before accompanied by diarrhea, weight loss, and episodes of nausea and vomiting. The patient had received a liver transplant eight months earlier and had been treated with continuous dexamethasone therapy since then. In addition to the worsening of his abdominal pain, he developed increasing nausea and vomiting and mild constipation. He was admitted for further evaluation and treatment. The patient resided in Africa and denied a history of alcohol intake or smoking.

Physical examination revealed a thin, somewhat malnourished male in no distress with a blood pressure of 97/58 mm Hg, a heart rate of 100/min, a respiratory rate of 16/min, and an oral temperature of 98.6° F. Examination of the skin and bulbar conjunctivae revealed no evidence of icterus or rash, and the remainder of the physical exam was within normal limits. Abdominal ultrasound and a computerized tomogram of the abdomen were normal.

Laboratory tests showed a hemoglobin of 8.6 g/dl, a hematocrit of 25 percent, a total WBC count of 7,300/mm^3 with 43 percent neutrophils, 26 percent lymphocytes, 10 percent monocytes, and 21 percent eosinophils, and a platelet count of 350,000/mm^3. Stool culture revealed no bacterial pathogens, and a stool examination for ova and parasites was negative for helminths and protozoa. A biopsy of the small intestine revealed sections of a small helminth and helminth larvae within the mucosa; several subsequent serial stool examinations continued to show small larvae.

Introduction

Infections caused by protozoan, helminthic, or arthropod parasites are referred to as parasitic diseases. Shown in Table 15-1 are some examples of parasitic diseases commonly occurring in humans together with their clinical manifestations. Parasites are eukaryotic organisms that obtain food and shelter by living on or within other organisms and derive all benefits from their association with the host, who may either be unharmed or may suffer from the consequences of this encounter. The parasitic diseases continue to result in large-scale morbidity, mortality, and economic loss to humans and their domestic animals in both industrialized and developing countries.

The immunologic responses of the host to parasitic infections are essentially the same as those that govern responses to other infectious agents such as bacteria (*Chapter 12*) or viruses (*Chapter 13*), but they involve more complex host-parasite interactions. As described in Chapter 1, immunology was founded by the study of the body's protective defense response to infectious microorganisms, and yet, microbial prokaryotes only tell half the story of the immune response to the universe of microbial agents, i.e., the microbiota that confront the host's immune system. Eukaryotic pathogens—the protozoa, helminths, fungi and ectoparasites—have all been powerful selective forces for evolution of the immune system. Often, as with lethal intracellular protozoan parasites, the focus has been on acute

Table 15-1. Examples of parasitic diseases and their clinical manifestations

Phylum	Representative parasites	Disease produced and symptoms
Protozoa		
Sarcomastigophora		
Trichomonadida	*Trichomonas vaginalis*	Trichomoniasis (STD)
Diplomonadida	*Giardia lamblia*	Giardiasis (diarrhea)
Kinetoplastida	Leishmania spp	Cutaneous, visceral, mucocutaneous leishmaniasis
	Trypanosoma spp	African trypanosomiasis, "sleeping sickness" (meningoencephalytis)
	Trypanosoma cruzi	Chagas' disease (acute, illness and death; chronic heart, intestinal, and oesophageal damage and progressive weakness)
Amoebida	*Entamoeba histolytica*	Amebiasis (dysentery, liver abscesses)
Apicomplexa	Plasmodium spp	Malaria
	Toxoplasma gondii	Toxoplasmosis (damage to the brain, eyes, or other organs if immunocompromised)
Helminths		
Nematodes	Hookworms (Ancylostoma spp and *Necator americanus*)	Hookworm disease (anemia) and cutaneous larva migrans
	Ascaris lumbricoides	Ascariasis (cough, wheezing, abdominal distention, and obstruction)
	Trichuris trichiura	Trichuriasis (bloody diarrhea)
	Strongyloides stercoralis	Mild abdominal tenderness, urticaria, hyperinfection syndrome
	Wuchereria bancrofti, Brugia malayi	Lymphatic filariasis (elephantiasis)
	Loa Loa	Loiasis (eye worm)
	Onchocerca volvulus	Onchocerciasis (river blindness)
Platyhelminthes		
Trematodes (flukes)	Schistosoma spp	Schistosomiasis (acute hepatosplenomegaly, urticaria; chronic abdominal tenderness, bloody diarrhea, and right heart failure)
Cestodes	Taenia spp	Intestinal discomfort, neurocysticercosis
Arthropoda		
	Pulex irritans	Flea bites
	Tunga penetrans	Burrowing flea, pain, and infection
	Pediculus humanus capitis, corporis	Head louse, body louse
	Phthirus pubis	Pubic louse
	Sarcoptes scabiei	Scabies
	Ticks (*Riphicephalus, Ixodes, Argus,* etc.)	Tick bites: injury, tissue damage, and tick paralysis

infections and the inflammatory responses they evoke. Long-lived parasites such as the helminths, however, are more remarkable for their ability to persist and to downregulate host immunity, protecting them from elimination.

Although strong immune responses may be generated during parasitic infections, they do not always lead to protection, and as is often the case with infectious disease, the immune response to parasites can even produce more serious harmful effects than those produced by the organism itself. Some examples of harmful adverse effects of parasitic infection include the hepatic granulomas of schistosomiasis, the glomerulonephritis seen in certain forms of malaria, and antibody-mediated anaphylactic shock resulting from a ruptured hydatid cyst or the release of parasitic fragments following the excessively rapid killing of filarial worms by drugs. During parasitic infections, the interactions of the host and the parasite provide a fascinating example of an evolutionary struggle between two combatants in which each attempts to maintain a survival advantage over the other and in which the immune system plays a key role in determining the victor. As with other infectious diseases, an understanding of the basic mechanisms of pathogenesis and host protection to parasitic infection is of paramount importance in mounting effective preventive and therapeutic measures for the control of these diseases. Moreover, this knowledge is equally important for understanding the harmful expressions of the immune response to parasitic infection in the form of hypersensitivity reactions that often contribute to immunologically mediated diseases.

Hallmarks of the Immune Response to Parasitic Infections

The Innate Immune Response to Parasites

It is now well established that the innate immune response is the single most critical event in the host defense to virtually every known category of microbial pathogen (*Chapter 3*). During the early stages of infection, the host innate immune system rapidly detects and responds to parasitic infection through a set of innate immune receptors referred to as pattern recognition receptors (**PRRs**), the most extensively studied of which are the Toll-like receptors (**TLRs**) (*Chapters 3* and *9*). This initial encounter of the innate immune response and PRRs with the pathogen not only begins the process of recognition and elimination of the organism through its primordial mechanisms, but also orchestrates the subsequent development of the adaptive immune response, which is necessary for the ultimate removal of the organism and protection of the host against reinfection. Therefore, in the absence of recognition by innate immune receptors, the host may quickly become overwhelmed by the parasitic pathogen, resulting in disease and possibly death. Conversely, if activation of innate immune receptors is excessive, high levels of pro-inflammatory mediators such as interleukin-12 (**IL-12**), tumor necrosis factor (**TNF-α**), reactive nitrogen intermediates (**RNIs**), and reactive oxygen species (**ROS**) can be detrimental to the host. Therefore, how the innate immune system detects and responds to invading parasites in this initial encounter is crucial to understanding how infection is controlled, as well as how excessive immune responses are avoided.

In mammalian cells, TLRs are crucial for many aspects of microbial elimination, including recruitment of phagocytes to infected tissue and subsequent microbial killing. TLRs expressed by immune cells, mostly macrophages and dendritic cells (**DCs**), also have a role in shaping long-term adaptive immunity (*Chapter 3*). However, when activated to excess, TLRs mediate pathology, as in the case of septic shock induced by infection with Gram-negative bacteria and lipopolysaccharide (**LPS**). Although the importance of innate immunity in resistance to parasitic infections is well established, the molecular mechanisms underlying recognition of parasitic agents by innate immune cells are only now beginning to be understood. Major advances have identified bacterial and viral molecules that act as TLR agonists (i.e., PAMPs) and have identified how these pathogens can manipulate TLR-induced signaling cascades to prolong their own survival (*Chapters 12* and *13*). Now this area, of research is emerging with new and exciting insights into how the TLR signaling system responds to infection by protozoa, including *Trypanosoma cruzi*, *Trypanosoma brucei*, Leishmania, Plasmodium spp, and *Toxoplasma gondii*—pathogens that every year account for immense human suffering and death worldwide. Shown in Figure 15-1 is a schematic representation of the molecular events associated with activation of Toll-like receptors by protozoan pathogen-associated molecular patterns (**PAMPs**).

Several studies have shown that the glycosylphosphatidylinositol (**GPI**) molecule is abundantly expressed by many protozoan parasites and functions to anchor proteins to the surface of eukaryotic cells such as lymphoid and myeloid lineages and to activate them. The GPIs for *Trypanosoma cruzi*, *Trypanosoma brucei*, Leishmania spp, or *P. falciparum* thus represent PAMPS for these parasites and consist of a variety of different molecular forms composed of differing chemical structures (Figure 15-1). TLR activation by these different parasite molecules triggers nuclear factor-κB (**NF-κB**) and mitogen-activated protein kinase (**MAPK**) signaling pathways to induce the expression of proinflammatory cytokine genes that directly control parasite replication. At the same time, genes that encode anti-inflammatory cytokines are induced. These counteract and control an excessive and therefore deleterious immune response (*Chapter 9*). An appropriate balance therefore exists between the proinflammatory and anti-inflammatory response, which facilitates host parasitism, and persistent

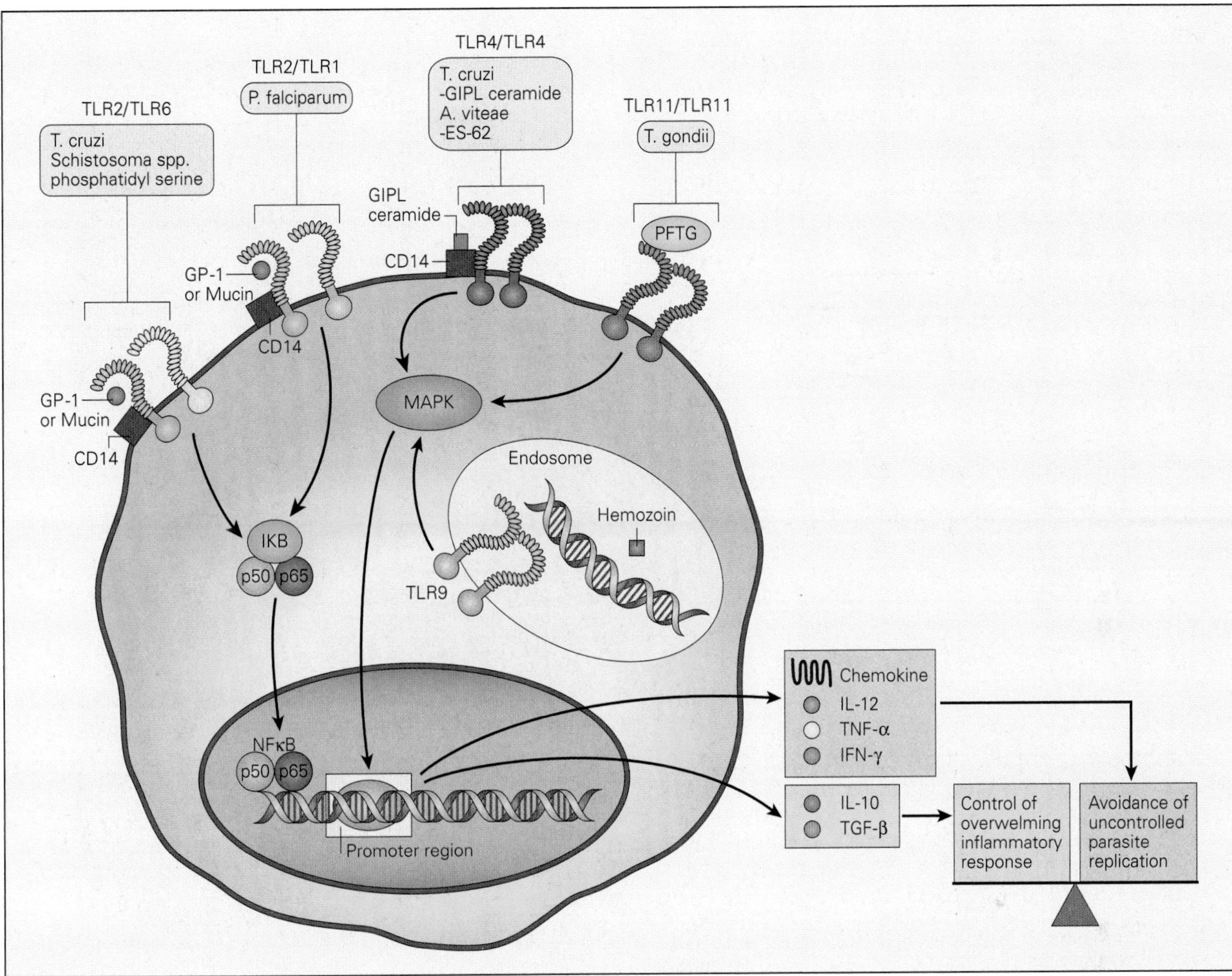

Figure 15-1. Schematic representation of the molecular events associated with activation of Toll-like receptors by PAMPs of parasites. The engagement of TLRs by parasitic PAMPs induces the activation of both NF-κB and the MAPK pathways that induce the expression of pro-inflammatory cytokines like IL-12, TNF-α, and IFN-γ, as well as anti-inflammatory cytokines like IL-10 and TGF-β. The production of these pro-inflammatory and anti-inflammatory cytokines contributes to a balanced host-parasite interaction. (Adapted from Gazzinelli RT, Denkers EY. Protozoan encounters with Toll-like receptor signalling pathways: implications for host parasitism. Nat Rev Immunol. 2006;6:895-906.)

infection, sometimes necessary to maintain protection (i.e., premonition, as will be described later).

In recent years, worm-derived molecules have also been proven to interact with TLRs. The interactions of parasites with TLRs is not only restricted to protozoa; metazoan helminths also possess molecules that can interact with the receptors. The following examples illustrate some of the known interactions of parasite-related PAMPs with TLRs. The schistosome-derived lyso-phosphatidylserine facilitates the interaction of IL-10 with the development of T regulatory (**Treg**) cells following TLR2 engagement. Schistosome double-stranded RNA (**dsRNA**) interacts with the DCs TLR3. The filarial glycoprotein ES-62 (from the rodent filaria *Acanthocheilonema viteae*) drives the differentiation of DCs to a DC2 phenotype, which initiates the T helper 2 (**Th2**) responses). It also suppresses LPS-mediated induction of the Th1-inducing cytokine IL-12 by macrophages; TLR4 is required for this molecule's effects on macrophages and dendritic cells.

Th1/Th2 Polarization

As described previously, the innate immune response sets the stage for the subsequent adaptive immune response that, depending upon the molecular structures of the PAMPs associated with the parasite, induces a balanced set of pro-inflammatory and anti-inflammatory cytokines associated with Th1 and Th2 profiles (Figure 15-2). In general, parasitic infections

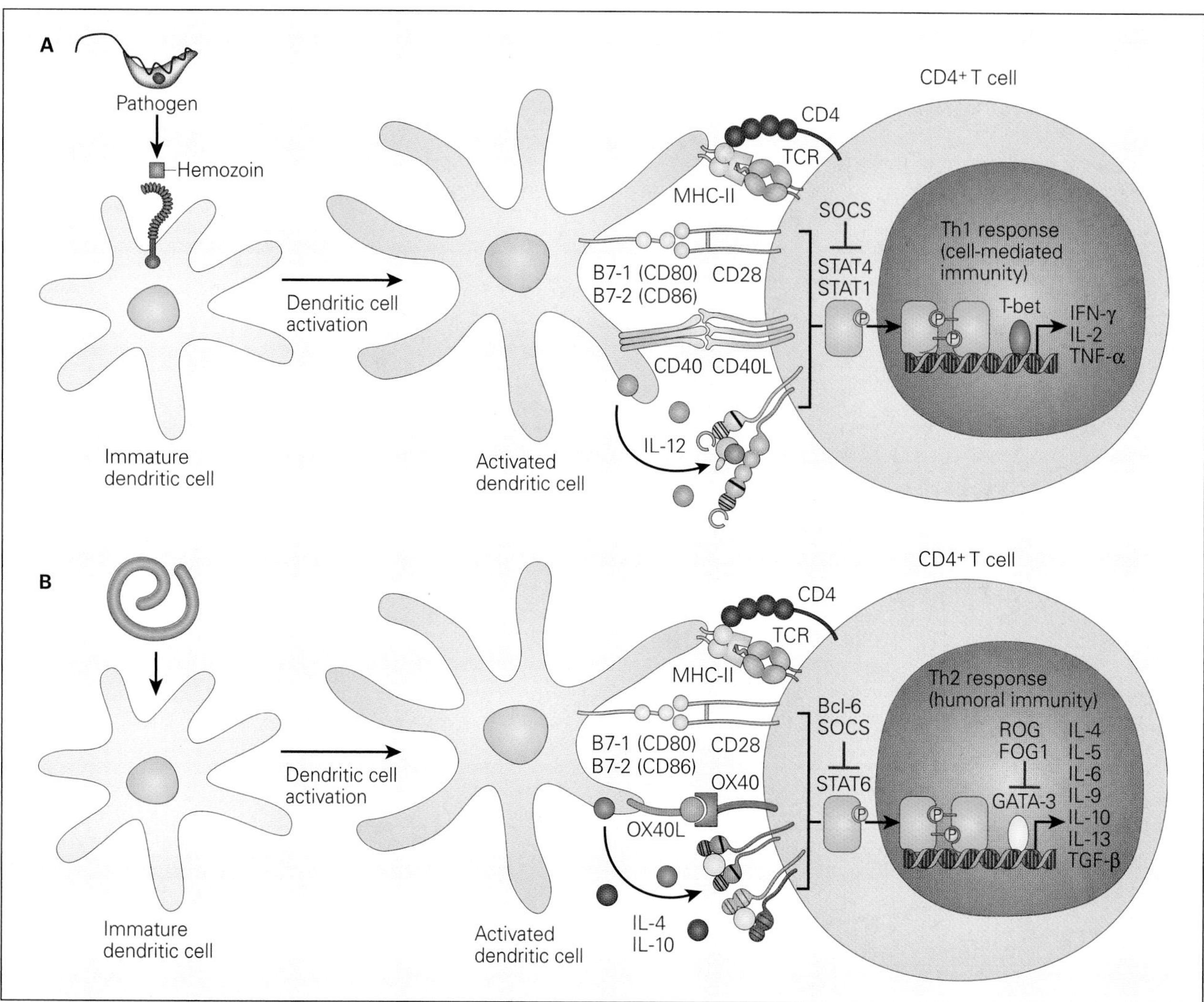

Figure 15-2. Model of Th1 /Th2 cell development. For both T helper 1 (Th1) and Th2 cell differentiation, antigens are presented to naive CD4+ T cells by dendritic cells (DCs). The interaction of co-stimulatory molecules (CD40–CD40L, OX40–OX40L, and/or CD80–CTLA4/CD28) with their respective ligands together with the local cytokine environment promotes the differentiation of naive T cells into interferon-γ (IFN-γ)-secreting Th1 cells or interleukin-4 (IL-4)-secreting Th2 cells. Panel A: In Th1 cell development, certain pathogens or PAMPs trigger antigen-presenting cells through TLRs to secrete IL-12, which promotes the differentiation of naive T cells into IFN-γ-secreting Th1 cells. Panel B: In Th2 cell development, the inability of antigen to activate DCs to produce IL-12 results in a default pathway of naive T cell differentiation into IL-4-secreting Th2 cells. (Adapted from Sacks D, Noben-Trauth N. The immunology of susceptibility and resistance to Leishmania major in mice. Nat Rev Immunol. 2002;2:845-58.)

often induce CD4+ T cell responses that are highly polarized in terms of cytokine production. This phenomenon is striking in helminthic infections that, in contrast to the majority of pathogenic organisms, routinely trigger strong Th2 responses, i.e., IL-4, eosinophilia, IgE, and mastocytosis. Conversely, many other parasitic protozoa induce CD4+ T cell responses with a Th1 cytokine profile. This striking difference represents a vivid example of immunologic class selection. Sometimes a switch in the immunological profile occurs during the same parasitic infection. Leishmania is an intracellular protozoan that elicits a Th1 response from the host. However, the immune response in advanced cases of American mucocutaneous and diffuse forms of leishmaniasis is skewed toward a Th2 response. Similarly, as will be described below, the cellular profile of hepatic granulomas caused by Schistosoma spp changes from Th1 to Th2 when they become chronic, favoring the development of fibrosis and other clinical complications associated with the granulomas. Although this description focuses mainly on role of the classic Th1/Th2 paradigm in parasitic immunity, recent studies with Leishmania have suggested an important role of

IL-27 and other subpopulations of CD4+ T cells such as Th17 that may also participate in the balance between immunity and pathology (*Chapter 9*).

Premunition or Concomitant Immunity

Most parasites are able to survive the immune response and produce long-lasting infections directed to ensure their subsequent transmission to other susceptible non-immune hosts. In the case of protozoan infections caused by Toxoplasma or Leishmania, chronicity is characterized by a state of latency in which replication of the parasite is minimal and the infection is subclinical and asymptomatic. The presence of the parasite in low numbers, paradoxically, is responsible for a relative immunity to severe infection by the same pathogen (i.e., premunition or concomitant immunity) (Box 15-1). Ironically, complete eradication of the infectious process in the infected host eliminates premunition and leaves the host susceptible to reinfection.

Most helminth infections also induce different levels of concomitant immunity, often developing with age (*Chapter 2*). As an example, immunoepidemiological studies of humans living in endemic areas where Schistosoma spp is prevalent have revealed that individuals who have passed their teen years generally have significantly less intense infections than younger children despite similar levels of exposure to infectious parasites. Following treatment, the older individuals are resistant to reinfection whereas younger children exposed to the same degree of infectious challenge become as heavily infected as they were prior to treatment. Acquisition of immunity with age is also typical of most soil-transmitted helminth infections (i.e., Ascaris, Trichuris). The development of concomitant immunity depends not only on the ability of the parasite to escape protective immune responses, but also on the generation of specific mechanisms of immunoregulation, i.e., Treg cells, that serve both to prevent parasite elimination and suppress immunopathology. This will be described in greater detail below.

Box 15-1

Premunition or concomitant immunity refers to the relative immunity to severe infection by a particular pathogen as a result of a chronic low-grade infection by the same pathogen (from the Latin word *praemunitio*, which means fortification beforehand, and from *praemunitus*, which is the past participle of *praemunire*, which means to fortify in advance).

Evasion Mechanisms and Immunomodulation

Another fascinating aspect of parasitic infections is the variety of mechanisms by which parasites evade the immune response. The parasite can hide within the host cells (i.e., Leishmania), produce waves of progeny with different surface antigens (i.e., African trypanosomiasis), or incorporate host antigens (i.e., Schistosoma) on the cell surface of the parasite thereby subverting the immune system's recognition of foreignness. Nonspecific immunosuppression is characteristic of a number of parasitic infections. There has been a resurgence of interest in helminth immunology with a particular emphasis on the induction of immunoregulatory mechanisms in the parasitized host (*Chapters 7* and *9*). These regulatory mechanisms facilitate chronic persistence of the worms while at the same time limiting the immunopathology likely to arise from persistent antigenic stimulation. This appears to have a major impact on ongoing immune responses to autoantigens, allergens, co-infections, and vaccines. In some instances, they may also provide a beneficial outcome (i.e., reducing autoimmune responses and allergic reactions); in others, however, the result may be detrimental (i.e., downmodulating protective responses to ongoing infections or vaccines). The immunomodulatory properties of helminth infections are starting to be exploited for therapeutic purposes in situations where an exacerbated immune response is present (i.e., asthma, autoimmune disease).

Protozoa

Protozoan Infections

Infections with protozoa may be classified into four general groups according to the location of the parasite within the infected host which include the following sites: (1) intracellular, (2) blood and intracellular, (3) blood, and (4) intestinal. The most important protozoan diseases and their immunological features are highlighted and summarized in Table 15-2.

Intracellular Protozoan Infection

This group of parasites is characterized by their intracellular localization in the vertebrate host (Table 15-2). The manifestations of each protozoan infection vary depending on the site and extent of

Table 15-2. Immunologic characteristics of protozoan infections in the human

	Immune mechanisms		
		Adaptive	
Type of infection	**Innate**	**Cellular**	**Humoral**
Intracellular			
Leishmania spp			
Cutaneous	Phagocytosis, complement macrophage activation, NK cells, TLR2	Th1 CD4, CD8, IFN-γ (in mucocutaneous leishmaniasis, a Th2 response is also elicited)	–
Mucocutaneous			+ (not protective)
Visceral			++ (not protective)
Toxoplasma gondii			++ (secretory)
Plasmodium spp			++ (neutralizing)
Blood and intracellular			
Trypanosoma cruzi	Phagocytosis, complement macrophage activation, NK cells, TLR2	CD4, CD8, IFN-γ	+
Blood			
Trypanosoma gambiense	TLR2, complement	IFN-γ, TNF-α	++ (neutralizing)
Trypanosoma rhodesiense			++ (neutralizing)
Intestinal			
Entamoeba histolytica	ADCC, complement, eosinophils, mast cells, macrophage activation, TLR4	Th1, CD4	++ (secretory)
Giardia intestinalis			++ (secretory)

Note: The plus signs present the degree of reactivity.

tissue involvement within the body and are reflected in the immune response that is elicited.

Leishmania Infections

As examples of infection with intracellular protozoa, those caused by Leishmania spp vary from localized cutaneous lesions (cutaneous Leishmaniasis caused by *L. major*), to the more extensive metastatic lesions of the skin, mouth, and pharynx (mucocutaneous Leishmaniasis caused by *L. braziliensis*), to the systemic involvement seen in visceral leishmaniasis (kala-azar, caused by *L. donovani*) (Table 15-2). Figure 15-3 illustrates the wide clinical spectrum of Leishmaniasis. Although circulating antibody has not been demonstrated in the cutaneous form, it is present in the mucocutaneous and visceral forms. However, protective immunity has not been correlated with the presence of antibody; conversely, antibody actually contributes to the immunopathology associated with the disease. Cellular mechanisms (i.e., macrophage and neutrophil activation, CD4+ and CD8+ T cells) appear to be responsible for protective immunity in leishmaniasis.

Toxoplasmosis

Another example of intracellular parasitism is toxoplasmosis. Human infection with *Toxoplasma gondii* can either be congenital or acquired (Table 15-2). When acquired, it is among the most common opportunistic infections in HIV-infected individuals. Congenital

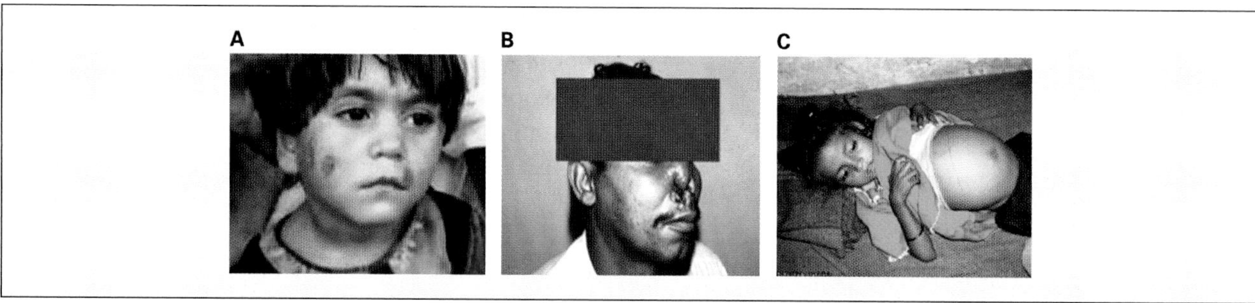

Figure 15-3. Clinical spectrum of various manifestations of human leishmaniasis. Panel A: Cutaneous leishmaniasis lesions in a Pakistani child. (Reproduced with permission from Khan SJ, Muneeb S. Cutaneous leishmaniasis in Pakistan. Dermatol Online J. 2005;11:4.) Panel B: Mucocutaneous leishmaniasis (espundia). Panel C: Five-year-old girl with advanced kala-azar.

infection occurs as a result of maternal infection and transmission to the fetus and may be reflective of developmental immaturity of the fetal immune system and greater susceptibility to infection (*Chapter 2*).

T. gondii is transmitted to humans by three principal routes (Figure 15-4). First, humans can acquire *T. gondii* by eating raw or inadequately cooked infected meat, especially pork, mutton, and wild

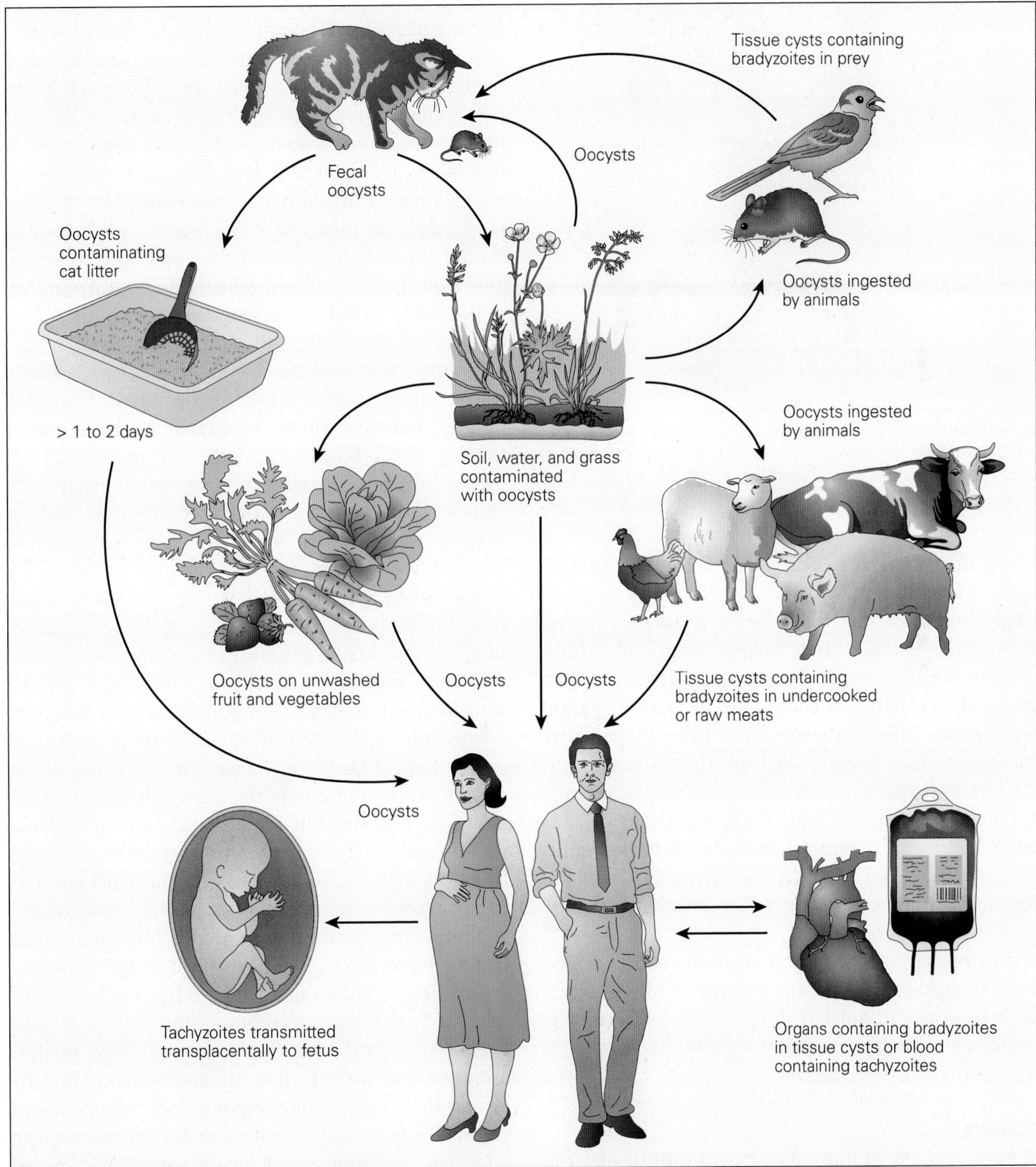

Figure 15-4. Schematic representation of the three principal routes of transmission of *T. gondii* to humans. The feline intestinal tract is the only source for the production of *T. gondii* oocysts, which can be transmitted to humans through the ingestion of tissue cysts in undercooked meat, animal contaminated sources (e.g., soil, cat litter, garden vegetables, and water) or transplacental transmission from an infected pregnant mother to her unborn fetus. Transmission can also occur from donor-related tissues, e.g., blood or organ transplants.

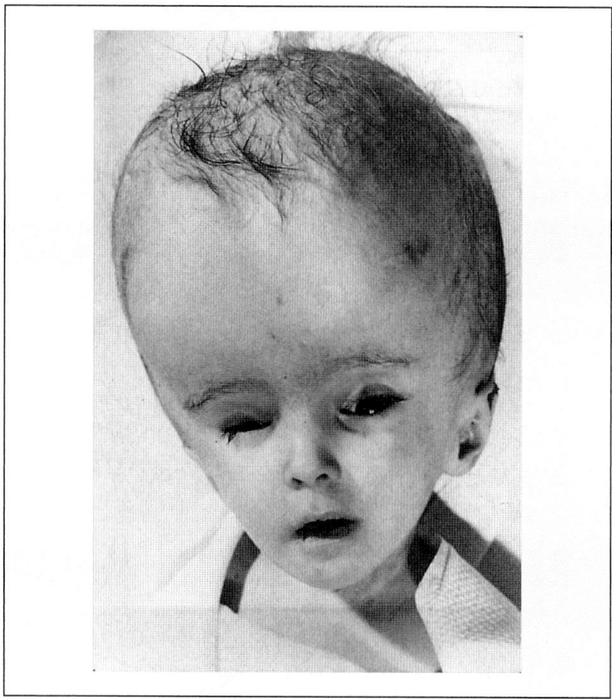

Figure 15-5. Photograph of an infant with congenital toxoplasmosis and extreme hydrocephalus resulting from congenital infection with *T. gondii* toxoplasmosis. (Courtesy of Dr. Leon Jacobs.)

game, or uncooked foods that have come in contact with infected meat. Second, humans can inadvertently ingest oocysts that cats have passed in their feces, either from a litter box or from soil. Third, women can transmit the infection transplacentally to their unborn fetus. In adults, the incubation period for *T. gondii* infection ranges from 10 to 23 days after the ingestion of undercooked meat and from five to 20 days after the ingestion of oocysts from cat feces.

The most frequent clinical manifestations of congenital infection are calcification, hydrocephalus (Figure 15-5), and microcephaly that lead to neurologic disturbances, muscle tone disturbances, seizures, and chorioretinitis.

In nonimmunocompromised individuals infected with Toxoplasma, both humoral and cellular immune responses are stimulated, but cellular immunity is protective while the humoral response appears to be only of diagnostic value.

Malaria

A third example of intracellular parasitism is malaria, which is of widespread importance in the world (Table 15-2 and Figure 15-6).

When an infected Anopheles mosquito bites a human, it injects sporozoites into the small blood vessels. Sporozoites migrate to the liver where they infect hepatocytes, after which the parasite develops into a multinucleate liver stage (schizont) that contains merozoites (Figure 15-6). This stage is referred to as exoerythrocytic schizogony and may occur with a single infecting parasite (e.g., *P. falciparum*) or with multiple organisms (e.g., *P. vivax*, *P. ovale*). The mature schizonts eventually rupture, releasing thousands of uninucleate merozoites into the bloodstream, each of which can infect a red blood cell. Within the red blood cell, the merozoite develops to form either an erythrocytic stage (blood stage) schizont or a spherical or banana-shaped uninucleate gametocyte. The gametocyte, which is the sexual stage of the parasite, is infectious for mosquitoes that ingest it while feeding. Within the mosquito, gametocytes develop into female and male gametes (macrogametes and microgametes, respectively), which undergo fertilization and then develop into sporozoites that can infect humans.

Symptoms of malaria include fever, chills, arthralgia, vomiting, anemia caused by hemolysis, hemoglobinuria, and convulsions. There may be the feeling of tingling in the skin, particularly with malaria caused by *P. falciparum*. The classical symptom of malaria is a cyclical fever pattern occurring every two days in *P. falciparum*, *P. vivax*, and *P. ovale* infections (tertian fever). Severe malaria is almost exclusively caused by *P. falciparum* infection and is associated with coma and death if untreated. Splenomegaly, severe headache, cerebral ischemia, hepatomegaly, and hemoglobinuria with renal failure, i.e., black water fever, may also be seen in severe malaria. Young children and pregnant women are especially vulnerable. Chronic malaria is seen in both *P. vivax* and *P. ovale* infections, but not in *P. falciparum*, where only the acute fulminating form is usually observed. In the chronic form of malaria, the disease can relapse months or years after initial infection, with recurrent waves of parasitemia emanating from the persistence of latent parasites in the liver.

Protective immunity can occur following initial infection and render the host shielded against subsequent disease. Individuals who are repeatedly exposed to malaria develop antibodies against the sporozoite, liver-stage, blood-stage, and/or sexual-stage malaria antigens. It is thought that antibodies acting directly against these antigens are responsible for the decreased susceptibility to malaria infection and disease seen in adults in malaria-infested areas. Antibodies directed against the sexual stages of plasmodia may also reduce malaria transmission. Additional components of naturally acquired immunity include the release of cytokines that act against all stages of the parasite and also

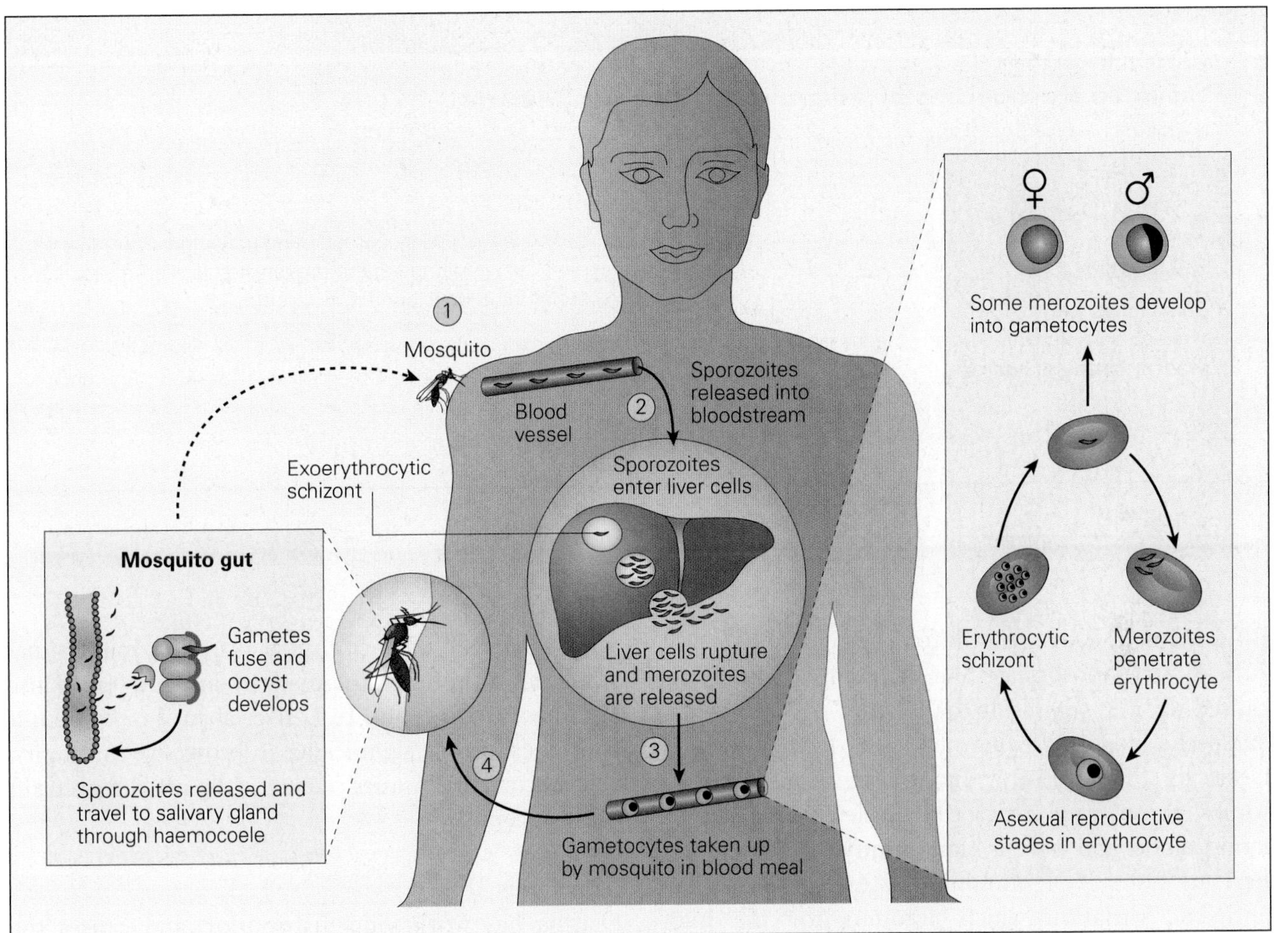

Figure 15-6. The life cycle of *Plasmodium falciparum* in the human host and mosquito vector. The mosquito injects sporozoites into the host (1), which are carried through the blood to the liver (2), where they invade hepatocytes and undergo a process of asexual (mitotic) replication to give rise to an exoerythrocytic schizont. Up to this point, the infection is nonpathogenic and clinically silent. After about seven days, the liver schizonts rupture to release many thousands of merozoites into the blood (3). Each merozoite invades an erythrocyte and divides mitotically to form an erythrocytic schizont containing up to 20 daughter merozoites (right, inset). These merozoites can reinfect fresh erythrocytes, giving rise to a cyclical blood-stage infection with a periodicity of 48 to 72 hours, depending on the *Plasmodium* species. As-yet-unknown factors trigger a subset of developing merozoites to differentiate into male and female gametocytes, which, when taken up by a feeding mosquito, give rise to extracellular gametes (4). In the mosquito mid-gut, the gametes fuse to form a motile zygote (ookinete), which penetrates the mid-gut wall and forms an oocyst, within which meiosis takes place and haploid sporozoites develop (left, inset). (Reproduced with permission from Stevenson MM, Riley EM. Innate immunity to malaria. Nat Rev Immunol. 2004;4:169-80.)

a cytotoxic T cell response directed at liver stages of the parasite. Shown in Box 15-2 are some of the presumed mechanisms of adaptive immunity to malaria.

Other immunologically mediated features of clinical importance associated with malarial infection include glomerulonephritis and hemolytic anemia caused by immune complex (Type III) injury and autoantibody production, respectively (*Chapter 17*). These will be described in greater detail below.

Blood and Intracellular Protozoan Infections

Trypanosomiasis is an example of both blood and intracellular (*Trypanosoma cruzi*) and blood-borne (*Trypanosoma gambiense, Trypanosoma rhodesiense*) parasitism (Table 15-2). These two major trypanosome infections of the human are found in widely separated geographic areas of the world and have equally divergent clinical expressions. American trypanosomiasis (Chagas disease) is caused by *T. cruzi*, which reproduces intracellularly with relatively few trypanosome forms found in the bloodstream. Following inoculation from infected reduviid bugs, an acute local inflammatory reaction occurs (e.g., periorbital edema, Romaña's sign, or chagoma), and the parasite rapidly becomes intracellular in cells of the reticuloendothelial system. The localization in cardiac muscle accounts for the manifestations or cardiomyopathy in Chagas disease. Recently, the recognition of antimyocardial antibodies has led to the suggestion that these may be involved in an autoimmune process.

Box 15-2

Presumed Mechanisms of Adaptive Immunity to Malaria

- Antibodies block invasion of sporozoites into liver cells.
- IFN-γ and CD8 T cells inhibit parasite development in hepatocytes.
- Antibodies block invasion of merozoites into erythrocytes.
- Antibodies prevent sequestration of infected erythrocytes by preventing binding to adhesion molecules on the vascular endothelium.
- IFN-γ and CD4+ T cells activate macrophages to phagocytose intra-erythrocytic parasites and free merozoites.
- Antibodies neutralize parasite glycosylphosphatidylinositol and inhibit induction of the inflammatory cytokine cascade.
- Antibodies mediate complement-mediated cytolysis of extracellular gametes and prevent fertilization of gametes and the development of zygotes.

Reproduced with permission from Stevenson MM, Riley EM. Innate immunity to malaria. Nat Rev Immunol. 2004;4:169-80.

Blood-Borne Protozoan Infections

African trypanosomiasis or sleeping sickness is caused by *T. gambiense* or *T. rhodesiense*, which enter the host following the bite of the infected tsetse fly (Table 15-2). Unlike American trypanosomes, those from Africa can be detected in circulating blood and have a high affinity for the central nervous system. Of immunologic importance is the antigenic variation which accounts for the high degree of reinfections, i.e., relapses, and the lack of durable immunity in the disease. Another striking feature of sleeping sickness is the marked increase of IgM in serum and cerebrospinal fluid. Although these blood-borne parasites can be neutralized by circulating antibody, owing to its extreme antigenic variation, the parasite is protected and is permitted to establish new generations of parasites that are antigenically different from the original strain.

Intestinal Protozoan Infections

Amebiasis

Another type of protozoan infection is that caused by *Entamoeba histolytica,* the only known intestinal amoeba that is pathogenic for the human (Table 15-2). Although the infection may be asymptomatic, occasionally the parasite becomes infective, penetrates tissue, and gives rise to symptomatic disease. Symptomatic infections are commonly divided into those with manifestations restricted to the gastrointestinal tract (i.e., intestinal amebiasis) and those whose expressions are more generalized (i.e., extraintestinal amebiasis). The most frequent presentation of the symptomatic infections is intestinal amebiasis, while hepatic amebiasis is the most common form of extraintestinal amebiasis. Although there is an antibody response after invasive infection (e.g., liver abscess or colitis), it is of questionable significance in protective immunity, since recurrent episodes of enteric disease can occur in these patients.

Giardiasis

Giardia has worldwide distribution and causes the most frequent protozoan intestinal infection in the United States (Table 15-2). It is the most commonly identified cause of water-borne disease associated with breakdown of water purification systems, drinking from contaminated streams, travel to endemic areas (e.g., Russia, India, the Rocky Mountains, etc.), and day care centers. There is evidence that mucosal immunity plays a significant protective role in Giardia infection, and mouse studies have also suggested a role for cellular immune response (i.e., neutrophils, CD4, and CD8 T cells) (*Chapter 8*). A definitive study of the human immune response to the parasite has not been possible since most cases of *Giardia* infection occurs in immunodeficient patients, particularly those with an IgA deficiency (*Chapter 16*). Other intestinal parasites (Cryptosporidium, Microspora) common among the immunocompromised are described below.

Immunity against Protozoa

Protozoa are a highly diverse group of parasites that constitute an important cause of morbidity and mortality worldwide. There are more than 50,000 species of protozoa, of which one-fifth are capable of causing parasitic diseases. Parasitic protozoa are, in general, minute organisms that have short generation times and high rates of reproduction. As described previously, they can either have an intracellular domicile or can exist as extracellular forms, sometimes depending on the life cycle phase. Parasitic protozoa frequently include complex life cycles and manifest specialized ways of entering and maintaining themselves within their hosts.

Nonimmunologic Host Defense

In addition to the immune mechanisms of host protection to parasitic infection, there are a number of non-immunologic means by which the host can nonspecifically counteract parasites. These nonspecific mechanisms are dictated by the presence or absence of a variety of serum components that result in impairment in development or even death of the parasite. The best-studied non-specific protective mechanism is perhaps the differential resistance of red blood cells (containing genetic variants of hemoglobin) to invasion and growth of Plasmodium spp, the causative agents of the different forms of malaria. Individuals with sickle cell trait (heterozygous for sickle cell hemoglobin), for example, are significantly more resistant to *Plasmodium falciparum* infection. Similarly, red blood cells lacking the Duffy antigen are not susceptible to *P. vivax* infection. These two mutations have possibly emerged in malaria-endemic populations as a result of the selective pressures exerted by the disease. Although non-specific factors can play a key role in resistance, they usually work in conjunction with the host's immune system.

Innate Immune Host Defense

Complement and Other Soluble Factors

The most important humoral component of the innate immune response is the C3 component of complement (*Chapter 4*). Complement activation provides a first line of defense against parasites that are extracellular. Normally this reactive molecule is short-lived but it can covalently attach to proteins (i.e., via the alternative pathway), carbohydrates (i.e., mannose residues via the lectin pathway), or antibodies (i.e., via the classical pathway) in the cell surface, recruit the serum factor b, and generate the active C3 convertase (C4b-C2a). If it binds to a host cell, regulators of the complement system rapidly inactivate it. However, parasites lack the host regulatory proteins, and thus the C3 convertase rapidly amplifies itself. The resulting activation of the complement cascade leads to formation of the lytic membrane attack complex (**MAC**), as well as the opsonic C3b recognized by C3b receptors on phagocytes. Complement also serves to activate the acute inflammatory response by generation of the C5a fragment, which not only is a potent chemoattractant for neutrophils, but can also activate the vascular endothelium directly. Through its anaphylatoxin activity, C5a also amplifies the inflammatory signals by activating mast cells to release their preformed vasoactive mediators through a non-IgE-mediated mechanism (*Chapter 17*). This mechanism is particularly important to combat intestinal extracellular parasitic infections by purging the worms from the intestinal tract.

In addition to complement, other soluble mediators provide a barrier to parasitic infection. Best studied in the human is a trypanolytic factor that confers resistance against *Trypanosoma brucei rhodesiense*, one of the causative agents of African trypanosomiasis (sleeping sickness) by directly lysing the parasite. A similar serum factor may be responsible for resistance to Mediterranean leishmaniasis manifested by adults or to pediatric kala-azar, a visceral form of leishmaniasis that primarily affects children between one and five years of age. However, it is not clear whether these *in vitro* findings have any resistance-conferring effects during natural infection in the human. Other non-immune factors, such as fever and host gender, may also play a role in the host's resistance to various protozoan parasites.

Natural Antibody

Even when parasites infect a host for the first time there may be some naturally occurring IgM "natural" antibody which may bind to their surface structures and provide some degree of protective immunity. The basis for the development of this normal serum antibody without known exposure to the specific antigen is not clear but is generally thought to result from exposure to naturally occurring cross-reacting antigens, i.e., molecular mimicry (*Chapter 19*). However, it is known that even very low affinity IgM can participate in the destruction of parasites through activation of the classical complement pathway and formation of the lytic MAC.

Antigen-Presenting Cells and Innate Recognition

As described previously, innate recognition plays a critical role in the triggering of adaptive immunity. Antigen-presenting cells (**APCs**) discriminate pathogens by PRRs that recognize PAMPs shared by different groups of microbes (*Chapter 3*). TLR ligation with the PAMPs triggers the initiation of the innate immune response, which includes upregulation of iNOS and increased production of cytokines such as TNF-α, IL-1, and IL-12. Although it is not clear to what extent TLRs serve as PRRs, parasites such as *T. brucei, Leishmania* spp, and *P. falciparum* express GPI lipid anchors on their surface, which are an important set of PAMPs (Figure 15-1). TLR2 is the PPR that can recognize these GPI structures on *T. cruzi* gycoconjugates. As another example, a lipopeptidophosphoglycan present on the surface of *Entamoeba histolytica*, appears to be able to elicit an innate immune response via TLR2 and TLR4.

Cells Involved in Innate Immune Cellular Mechanisms

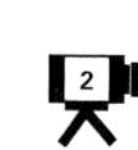

Phagocytosis represents an innate first line of defense against protozoan pathogens (Table 15-2). Although macrophages are resident in almost all tissues and are found in particularly large numbers in mucosal tissues, neutrophils, normally present in very large numbers only in the blood, can be recruited rapidly to tissues at any site where the complement cascade has been activated (*Chapter 4*). Both cell types possess receptors for C3b, which is one of the major opsonic factors promoting phagocytosis. Phagocytosis by neutrophils and monocytes and their secreted products (lysozyme, ß-glucuronidase, ROIs, cytokines, and chemokines) has been shown to play significant roles in protection against both intracellular and intestinal parasites. Evasion of the phagocytic mechanisms achieved by Leishmania, trypanosomes, and Toxoplasma is a critical adaptation of the mammalian host.

Most innate cellular defenses do not eliminate parasites directly, but they trigger other effector cells. In the case of intracellular protozoa, the cellular innate immune response is primarily mediated by natural killer (**NK**) and mononuclear cells. When the immune cells encounter the pathogen, a cytokine loop is activated that results in macrophage activation (Figure 15-7A). Macrophages (in toxoplasmosis and trypanosomiasis) and dendritic cells (in leishmaniasis) produce IL-12, which activates NK cells. Unlike T and B lymphocytes, NK cells can be activated almost immediately by type 1 interferons or IL-12. As a result, NK cells enter tissues and rapidly attack infected cells long before antigen-specific T or B cells are generated. In responses to parasitic infection, NK cells produce interferon γ (**IFN-γ**) that enhances NK activity by promoting the rapid differentiation of pre-NK cells. It also activates more macrophages so that production of TNF-α is augmented by IFN-γ. The combination of IFN-γ and TNF-α further activates macrophages and is thought to play an important role in granuloma formation (*Chapter 5*), as will be described below. This activation not only limits parasite proliferation by its direct or indirect cytotoxic action, but also has been shown to trigger a specific immune response by enhancing antigen presentation. The inhibition of parasite replication or its destruction is the result of various effector mechanisms: (1) ROIs, primary H_2O_2, and (2) RNIs, represented mainly by the production of nitric oxide (NO). TNF-α also "primes" neutrophils, causing them to activate oxygen-dependent intracellular killing mechanisms and making them more effective.

In the case of extracellular parasites, opsonization by complement or antibodies may trigger antibody-dependent cellular cytotoxicity (**ADCC**) and recruitment of NK cells, neutrophils, and eosinophils; the latter will degranulate, contributing to the creation of a toxic environment around the parasite.

Other populations that may provide a rapid cytokine response to intracellular parasites are gamma delta T (**Tγδ**) cells (*Chapter 7*). These lymphocyte populations express T cell receptors chains of limited diversity, which may have been designed for innate recognition of microbial structures or self-components expressed in infections of host cells particularly at mucosal sites. In humans. Tγδ cells represent a very small percentage of lymphocytes in the periphery (5–10 percent), but they are abundant in the epithelium and mucosae (*Chapter 8*). Moreover, their numbers increase in peripheral blood in response to protozoan infections (Toxoplasma and malaria). Therefore, it is likely that Tγδ cells help to restrict the parasite growth prior to the development of the adaptive immune response exerted by αβ T cells.

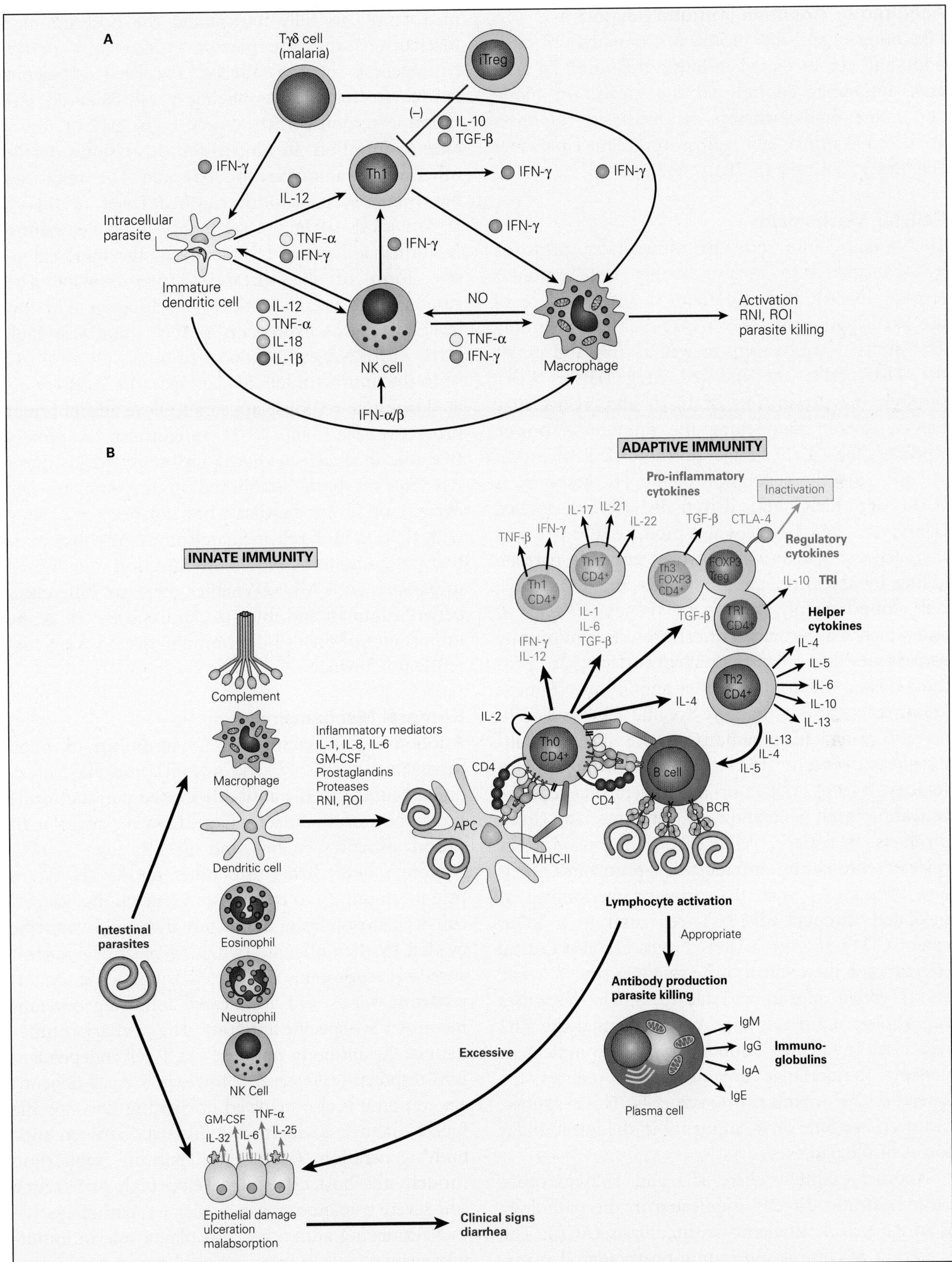

Figure 15-7. Regulation of the immune response to protozoan infections by cell-mediated immune responses. Panel A: Regulation of the immune response in intracellular protozoan infections by cell-mediated immune responses (CMI). Panel B: Regulation of the immune response in extracellular protozoan infections by antibody-mediated immune responses.

Acquired or Adaptive Immune Response

Like other organisms, protozoa stimulate both antibody and cell-mediated immune responses. In general, antibodies control parasite growth in blood and tissue fluids, whereas cell-mediated responses are directed principally against intracellular parasites (Figures 15-7A and 15-7B).

Cellular Mechanisms

Traditionally, immunity to intracellular protozoa was considered to involve mainly Th1 responses (Figure 15-7A). Recently, there is also evidence of the participation of other CD4+ subsets, including Th2-directed mechanisms as well as Treg and possibly Th17 cells; the induced Treg (**iTreg**) cells, through the production of IL-10 and TGFβ, may play a role in dampening the immune response, whereas the Th17 may promote inflammation (*Chapter 9*). The generation of the Th1 response is IL-12 dependent and driven by NK-cell-derived IFN-γ; activated Th1 cells also produce IFN-γ to further activate macrophages, which enhance parasite killing by the production of RNIs and ROIs. Tγδ cells, found mainly in mucosal tissues (*Chapter 8*) and which may provide critical protective immunity to parasites that infect at mucosal surfaces, also produce IFN-γ, which may further amplify macrophage killing of parasites. Parasite-specific CD8+ T cells are also generated in response to the infection, killing the parasites by IFN-γ production, direct cytotoxicity (CD8+ cells), or subsequent macrophage activation and generation of cytokines and toxic products. In malaria, cellular immunity plays a key role in eliminating intrahepatic sporozoites. It is now recognized that the primary mechanism is mediated through CD8+ T cells and to a lesser extent CD4+ T cells. CD8+ T cells are also critical effectors for the control of Leishmania spp, *T. cruzi*, and *T. gondii* infections (Table 15-2). Th2 responses can also occur in response to Toxoplasma; the Th2 response involving antibodies and complement destroys extracellular organisms and reduces the spread of the organism between cells. This response, however, has little or no influence in the intracellular forms of the parasite.

Another example where Th1 and Th2 responses are mixed and directly implicated in the pathology is in American cutaneous leishmaniasis (**ACL**). The spectrum of clinical and immunopathological manifestations of ACL (localized, mucocutaneous, and diffuse) has been the subject of many investigations in attempts to fully understand the host immune mechanisms that are playing crucial roles in the pathogenesis of the disease. Localized cutaneous lesions are regarded as having a well-balanced Th1 immune response with a very high level of resistance to infection. In mucocutaneous lesions, on the other hand, a mixture of Th1 and Th2 responses has been observed, with elevated levels of IFN-γ, IL-4, and IL-10 in the secondary, mucosal lesions. In diffuse cutaneous leishmaniasis, the most extensive form of the disease, a predominant Th2 response has been identified, resulting in very low levels of mRNA expression of IFN-γ and very high levels of mRNA expression of IL-4.

In the murine model of giardiasis, the T cell-mediated immune response appears to have an important protective role (Table 15-2). In contrast, the protective role of T cell-mediated immunity to giardiasis has not yet been established in the human, e.g., chronic or severe giardiasis has not been associated with defects in T cell-mediated immunity, but antibody response to *G. intestinalis* infection is depressed in patients with AIDS. Whether there are differences between human and murine giardiasis as well as the importance of the cellular immune response are currently unknown.

Humoral Mechanisms

Antibodies can contribute to immunity through three mechanisms: (1) via opsonization and subsequent binding of the antibody-coated parasite to the Fc receptor on the macrophage, (2) via classical activation of complement, and (3) through ADCC. Although neutralizing antibodies appear to play a role in immunity to trypanosome infections, in African trypanosomiasis, the humoral response may be evaded by the antigenic switching of critical variant surface glycoproteins (**VSG**). Parasitemia manifest as recurring waves and are cleared following development of VSG-specific antibody. The primary component of the antibody response is a T cell-independent IgM response (*Chapter 6*). However, a T cell-dependent response is also involved in eliciting VSG-specific IgG. Nonetheless, due to the disparity between antibody generation (days) and parasite replication (hours), the host can still develop high parasitemia and severe trypanosomiasis-associated pathology.

Neutralizing antibodies also play a role in immunity against malaria infection, and for several years, a major effort has been directed to the development of vaccines that are targeted to the generation of malaria-specific, neutralizing antibodies that could potentially avoid the invasion of hepatocytes or erythrocytes by the parasite. In humans living in endemic areas for *P. falciparum*, there is evidence for an antibody-mediated development of immunity. This form of immunity is directed against asexual blood stages, and although its mechanisms of action are not entirely clear, it probably involves agglutination of parasitized erythrocytes, inhibition of cytoadherence to small blood vessels, and/or blocking of red blood cell invasion by free merozoites. Naturally acquired humoral immunity against invasive stages of parasites is generally inefficient and in most circumstances must work concomitantly with cell-mediated immunity to confer complete protection.

Secretory antibodies (sIgA) seem to play a role in protection against *T. gondii* cysts and enteric protozoan infections such as *Entamoeba histolytica* and *Giardia intestinalis* (*Chapter 8* and Table 15-2). In genital infections of humans due to *Trichomonas vaginalis*, a local IgE response is stimulated. The allergic reaction provokes intense discomfort, and by increasing vascular permeability, this reaction permits IgG antibodies to reach this site of infection and immobilize and eliminate these organisms. Although the role of antibodies in resistance to most intracellular protozoa is limited, there is evidence that they may still play a role in protection. As an example, antibody production generated as a consequence of a Th2 cell response (directed to extracellular parasites) seems to be required for survival of mice to toxoplasmosis in a toxoplasma challenge murine model. In most cases, however, intracellular protozoa induce polyclonal activation of B cells that, in turn, generates hypergammaglobulinemia. Although this antibody response is useful for diagnostic purposes, systemic antibodies seem to play no role in protection and may be responsible for certain immunopathologic syndromes (e.g., hyperviscosity and type II and III hypersensitivity, as described below in the immunopathology section) (*Chapter 17*).

Immunopathology Associated with Protozoan Infections

Protozoan infection frequently results in tissue damage leading to disease, which is often chronic, lasting months or years, and associated with an immune response directed at parasitic antigens and changes in cytokine profiles (*Chapter 17*). Alternatively, disease manifestations may be due to toxic protozoan products and/or to mechanical damage. This type of chronic infection is likely to frequently result in immunopathology.

Hyperviscosity Syndrome

Hyperviscosity syndrome occurs when plasma proteins increase serum viscosity, leading to vascular stasis, infarction, thrombosis, tissue injury, and rupture of small blood vessels. Increases in blood viscosity most often occur secondary to increases in circulating macromolecules such as immunoglobulin (i.e., hypergammaglobulinemia) or fibrinogen. The clinical hallmarks of hyperviscosity syndrome include the presence of bleeding secondary to paraproteins covering the platelet surface, visual disturbances due to retinal vein distension, retinal hemorrhage or thrombosis, and central nervous system (**CNS**) impairment such as dizziness, somnolence, or stupor. Other clinical manifestations include peripheral neuropathy, weakness, fatigue, renal failure, and congestive heart failure due to increased plasma volume. It has been suggested that this phenomenon is responsible for various clinical syndromes in trypanosomiasis (i.e., increase in circulating IgM), visceral leishmaniasis (i.e., polyclonal activation of B cells), and other protozoan infections where hypergammaglobulinemia is present.

Autoimmunity (Type II Hypersensitivity)

Autoantibodies directed to a number of different host antigens (e.g., red blood cells, laminin, collagen, or DNA) have been demonstrated during the course of several protozoan infections in a type II Gel and Coombs type of immune injury (*Chapter 17*). These autoantibodies may induce a direct cytotoxic effect on host cells (e.g., autoantibodies coat red blood cells with resultant hemolytic anemia). Alternatively, autoantibodies may be pathogenic through a buildup of antigen-antibody-complement immune complexes in tissues such as the kidneys, leading to glomerulonephritis through type III (as described below), as well as type II hypersensitivity reactions or other forms of chronic host inflammatory response.

A particularly good example of a protozoan infection in which autoimmunity appears to be an important contributor to pathogenesis is Chagas disease. Chagas heart disease develops in approximately one-third of individuals infected with the protozoan parasite *Trypanosoma cruzi.* Antibodies and cytotoxic lymphocytes appear in the muscle of infected animals that cause cytopathologic changes in the absence of parasites. This type of experimental data, combined with the fact that the parasite itself seems not to cause the tissue pathology, leads one to conclude that autoimmunity may play a key role in the pathogenesis of these disorders.

Another example is malaria. Experimental findings have revealed that infected animals may produce antibodies to certain molecules that could react to epitopes present in erythrocytes and leukocytes. In humans, anti alpha-galactosyl antibodies and anti-band-3 antibodies (molecules present in the surface of the erythrocyte) have been shown in patients infected with *P. falciparum*.

In another study involving patients suffering visceral leishmaniasis or kala-azar, most individuals were found to display polyclonal activation (with increases of IgG and IgM) and anti-immunoglobulin antibodies. Anti-smooth muscle antibodies were also observed. Although glomerulonephritis is not a common feature of human visceral leishmaniasis, it may occur in some cases, although its association with autoantibodies is unclear.

Immune Complex Disease (Type III Hypersensitivity)

In type III hypersensitivity, soluble immune complexes composed of aggregates of antigens, IgG and IgM antibodies, and complement form in the blood and are deposited in various tissues (typically the skin, kidney, and joints) (*Chapter 17*). This type of hypersensitivity reaction develops as a result of systemic exposure to an antigen and is dependent on the type of antigen and antibody and the size of the resulting complex. More specifically, complexes that are too small remain in circulation; complexes that are too large are removed by the glomerulus; and intermediate complexes, particularly those in slight antigen excess (*Chapter 17*), may become lodged in the tissues leading to tissue damage. Immune complexes have been found circulating in serum and deposited in the kidneys and other tissues of humans with visceral leishmaniasis, quartan malaria, toxoplasmosis, trypanosomiasis, and *Encephalitozoon* infections.

The most severe clinical manifestation caused by immune complex is their deposition in the kidneys, which may lead to glomerulonephritis. Immune complex deposition in the glomerulus results in activation of the complement cascade, which may involve either the classic or alternative pathway (*Chapter 4*). The immune complexes may activate endogenous glomerular cells. The production of chemotactic factors results in the accumulation of leukocytes and platelets within the glomerulus and, consequently, the promotion of an inflammatory response. Presentation may vary from asymptomatic hematuria to a full-blown acute nephritic syndrome consisting of proteinuria, edema, hypertension, and renal failure.

Cellular Hypersensitivity/Immune Mediators (Type IV Hypersensitivity)

Cellular hypersensitivity has also been observed in protozoan diseases (*Chapter 17*). For example, in cutaneous leishmaniasis, cell-mediated immune responses to leishmanial antigen produce lesions that display many of the characteristics of granulomas observed in tuberculosis. In these lesions, an ongoing immune response to the parasites causes a continuous influx of inflammatory cells, leading to sustained reactions and chronic pathologic changes at the sites of infection. During a parasitic infection, cytokines and other secreted products are released from activated immune cells. These mediators, in turn, influence the action of other cells and may be directly involved in pathogenesis. An example is TNF-α, which is released by different subsets of lymphocytes and, especially, macrophages. TNF-α may be involved in the muscle wasting observed in chronic stages of African trypanosomiasis. Similarly, TNF-α has also been implicated in the cachexia and wasting seen in *L. donovani* infection, cerebral malaria in *P. falciparum* in children, and decreased survival of *T. cruzi*-infected mice. Therefore, there appears to be a delicate balance between the factors involved in resistance to infectious agents and those that ultimately produce pathology and manifestations of clinical disease. Although low TNF-α levels in mice infected with malaria have been associated with protective immunity, there is evidence that when levels of the cytokine increase beyond certain critical levels, there may be pathological damage.

Helminths

Helminthic Infections

Helminths may be grouped according to their major site of infection: intestinal, intestinal and tissue, and tissue. Examples of helminths that cause human infection and their main immunological features are summarized in Table 15-3.

Intestinal Helminths

Adult tapeworms (*Taenia saginata, Diphilobotrium-latum*), pinworms (*Enterobius vermicularis*), and whipworms (*Trichuris trichiura*) live exclusively in the intestine. Their interaction with the host is limited. Humoral responses are particularly elevated, and IgE can be detected in serum. Intestinal infections can also elicit cellular immune responses that are responsible for worm expulsion. However, reinfections can occur, and chemotherapy is usually required to eliminate the worms.

Intestinal and Tissue Helminths

The second group of helminths of importance in human infection is characterized by more complex life cycles, in which the parasites are found as adults in the intestinal tract and as migratory larvae in tissues. Ascarids, hookworms (e.g., *Necator americanus*), and Trichinella illustrate this type of parasitic infection. Active infection with *Ascaris*, in which eggs are ingested, and hookworm, in which larvae penetrate the skin, elicits similar immunological responses from the host. Following entry, the larvae migrate through the tissues and reach the lungs, develop and migrate up the trachea, are swallowed, and enter the intestine. During the migration, the larvae cause a prominent granulocytic response in tissues characterized by eosinophils, which become activated in the presence of antibody (i.e., IgE). Larvae of the related dog and cat ascarids (*Toxocara canis* and *T. cati*) and the dog hookworm (*Ancylostoma caninum*) migrate through tissues but do not develop into adult worms. The eggs of the *Toxocara* spp are ingested and the larvae freed; hookworm larvae penetrate the skin and migrate through various tissues of the body. They induce an intense inflammatory reaction characterized by the migration of mononuclear leukocytes and eosinophils from the vascular compartment into tissues. When the larvae stop migrating, a granulomatous reaction develops with a thick fibrous capsule, within which the larvae may survive for years. In addition to the cellular response, migrating helminths induce antibody production in the host. Unlike Ascaris and hookworms, *Trichinella spiralis* develops in the intestinal mucosa. Within seven days, larvae are shed by the female worms into the circulation, are carried throughout the body, and invade into skeletal muscle. In the intestine, an acute inflammatory reaction is also initiated associated with antibody production. Adult worms are

Table 15-3. Immunologic characteristics of helminthic infections in the human

	Immune mechanisms			
		Humoral		
Type of infection	Cellular	IgE	Other Ig	DTH[2]
Intestinal				
Taenia saginata *Enterobius vermicularis* *Trichuris trichiura*	Th2: eosinophils, Th2 cytokines, ADCC (worm expulsion)	+	IgG, sIgA	−
Intestinal and tissue				
Ascaris lumbricoides Human hookworm	Th2: eosinophils, Th2 cytokines, ADCC (worm expulsion)	++	IgG sIgA (stimulated by adult forms in the intestine only)	+
Canine hookworm Toxocara spp Echinococcus spp *Taenia solium* (larvae)	Th2: eosinophils, ADCC	+++	IgG	++ (granulomas encapsulating worms)
Tissue				
Schistosoma spp	Th1–Th2 switch	++	IgG	+++ (granulomas encapsulating eggs)

Note: The plus signs denote the degree of involvement.

eliminated from the intestinal tract in two to three weeks, but the larvae, which have become encysted, evoke an intense inflammatory response in the musculature, accounting for the symptoms of the disease (e.g., myalgia).

The most serious human cestode infections are caused by the larvae of Echinococcus spp and *Taenia solium* (described below under "Accidental Parasitism in Humans"). The larval form of these tapeworms hatches from the egg in the intestine of the intermediate host (human), migrate though the body, and form cysts in various tissues. These cysts are very immunogenic and induce a strong response detectable as serum antibody (i.e., IgE and other immunoglobulins). If a cyst containing larvae of *Echinococcus* is ruptured, a life-threatening anaphylactic reaction may occur.

Tissue Helminths

Following penetration of the skin by cercariae of *Schistosoma mansoni, S. hematobium,* or *S. japonicum,* the schistosomules migrate first to the lung and finally to the venules of the pelvic or mesenteric veins. In the venules, they mature to adult worms and the female deposits eggs, most of which are passed in urine or in feces. Some of the eggs, however, are carried to the liver, where they elicit an intense cellular response characteristic of the disease (i.e., granuloma). Thus, the damage seen in schistosomiasis is primary the result of the cellular reaction elicited by the eggs. This early phase of hepatic schistosomiasis is characterized by an infiltration of inflammatory cells. When production and destruction of eggs reach equilibrium, fibrosis occurs and the infection enters a chronic phase, which may last many years and in which the host is relatively resistant to reinfection. Although disease in schistosomiasis is apparently associated with the tissue response to the eggs, host protection to reinfection is apparently based on continuous presence of the adult worm. The immunobiology of schistosomiasis is described in greater detail below.

Immunity Against Helminths

Nonimmunological Factors

Genetics and Human Behavior

Epidemiologic studies in areas where helminth infections are present have revealed differences in susceptibility to infection among affected individuals. Genetic loci for susceptibility to schistosomiasis and ascariasis have been mapped, and there is evidence for genetic control of filarial infections. In addition to genetic factors, human behavior, particularly with regard to hygiene and food, is a major factor influencing susceptibility. Helminths do not replicate within the host; the number of worms present at any one time represents a dynamic balance between the rate of infection and the efficiency of the host's defense. This balance is affected by individual susceptibility as well as by changes in host's behavior or ability to express forms of nonspecific or specific defense. Age, diet, hormonal changes, and immune suppression may enhance susceptibility to helminthic infections.

Surface and Chemical Barriers

For parasites that are ingested orally, stomach acidity and other protective physiologic factors of the bowel may eliminate opportunistic parasites that are not adapted to these adverse conditions. Worms entering through the skin must survive physical barriers such as the intact epidermis and secretions (i.e., sweat and sebum) and, if they breach these barriers, must also avoid other inflammatory responses in the dermis. In the tissues, worms need the correct sequence of environmental signals to mature. Lack of appropriate signals represents a form of nonspecific resistance that may prevent further parasite development.

Immunological Factors

The parasite may not die as a result of the nonimmune host response. Prolonged survival may result in pathology from the continuing inflammatory response. Examples of this are seen in human eosinophilic enteritis caused by *Ancylostoma caninum*, cutaneous larva migrans caused by Ancylostoma spp, and visceral larva migrans caused by Toxocara spp.

All helminths stimulate strong immune responses in the host that often do not appear to be protective. The high prevalence of helminth infection in endemic areas (up to 100 percent), the abundance of chronic infections, and the elevated rates of reinfection after treatment suggest that protective immunity against helminths is weak or perhaps absent altogether in humans. Some degree of concomitant immunity, however, seems to develop upon infection as evidenced by a number of factors, including (1) a decreased prevalence of most helminthic infections with age, (2) an increased prevalence in endemic areas of non-parasitized individuals suspected to be immune, (3) an enhanced susceptibility in immunosuppressed individuals, and (4) the development of acquired immunity in laboratory animal models.

Since helminths are extracellular organisms too large to be phagocytosed, they invoke protective immediate-type hypersensitivity reactions, characterized by IgE production, local and peripheral eosinophilia, basophil and mast cell involvement (histamine release), and Type 2 cytokines (IL-4, IL-5, IL-6, IL-13, and IL-10) produced by CD4+ Th2 cells. Paradoxically, although this type of immune response is normally associated with detrimental pathological reactions (i.e., pruritus, anaphylaxis), in the case of helminthic infection, it appears to serve a more beneficial protective function by providing a means of worm expulsion and larval killing.

As humans age, they eventually develop immunity to most helminths. Hookworm infections, however, appear to be the exception, with adults harboring greater parasite numbers than children. This observation has suggested that hookworms may have unique mechanisms to evade or suppress the host's immune response. Although these mechanisms are not completely understood, they appear to involve the capacity to release a number of specific parasite-derived molecules that allow the worms to modulate or evade the host immune response in several ways including skewing of cytokine production and the induction of T regulatory cells and their immunoregulatory products (*e.g.* IL-10, TGFß, and PGE2).

Humoral Responses: IgE and IgA Antibodies

Antibodies that bind to surface antigens may attract complement- or cell-mediated effectors that can damage the worm (e.g., ADCC). Neutrophils, eosinophils, phagocytes, and NK cells all mediate ADCC. Ligation of the low affinity IgG FcγRIII receptor (CD16, expressed in neutrophils, NK cells, and macrophages) activates several cytolytic pathways (*Chapter 6*). Ligation of both the low affinity IgE receptor FcεRII (CD23, expressed in eosinophils), as well as the high affinity FcεRI (expressed mainly by basophils and mast cells, but also by eosinophils), for example, have been specifically involved in eosinophil-mediated cytotoxicity against schistosome larvae (*Chapter 18*). Encapsulation of trapped worms by inflammatory cells may also result in killing the worm, although this is not always the case. Specific antibodies may also block enzymes released by the worm, thus interfering with its ability to penetrate tissues or to feed.

IgE Antibody

IgE antibodies produced in response to parasitic infection react only with certain helminth antigens. Following the binding of these antigens with membrane-bound IgE antibody on mast cells, eosinophils, and basophils, the release of pharmacologically active mediators from these cells causes two major effects: (1) local inflammation that augments the ability of the immune system to damage the helminth and (2) smooth muscle relaxation that aids in expulsion of parasites from the gastrointestinal tract (*Chapter 18*). An exacerbated IgE production, however, can also cause a local allergic reaction or even anaphylaxis, as described below. The increase in IgE is mainly induced by IL-4 produced by mast cells as well as by CD4+ Th2 cells. However, most of the IgE produced is not antigen-specific. It has been proposed that such polyclonal IgE responses may represent a mechanism to saturate cellular IgE receptors, rendering them refractory to specific stimulation by parasite antigens.

IgA Antibody

IgA is the signature immunoglobulin found in the external secretions of the mucosa-associated lymphoid tissues (**MALT**) (*Chapter 8*), including the gastrointestinal, respiratory, and urogenital tracts. It provides protective immunity against a wide variety of microbes, e.g., viruses and bacteria. Although the role of IgA antibodies in anti-parasitic immunity is less well understood, their production has been observed in intestinal infections caused by *Ascaris* and *Trichuris* spp, where they have been shown to bind to eosinophils and induce their degranulation. Despite the abundance of IgA antibodies in the intestinal lumen, however, little is known about their specific role in protection against other human helminthic infections.

Cellular Responses

Eosinophils

Eosinophilia is a characteristic response in helminthic infections. Eosinophils are attracted to sites of helminth invasion by chemotactic molecules released by degranulating mast cells (Figure 15-8). Recruitment of eosinophils is regulated by CD4+ Th2 cells and driven by IL-5, possibly in synergy with IL-13 and granulocyte-macrophage colony-stimulating factor (**GM-CSF**) (*Chapter 9*). The effector functions of eosinophils are mediated by stimuli that induce degranulation. Activated eosinophils migrate to

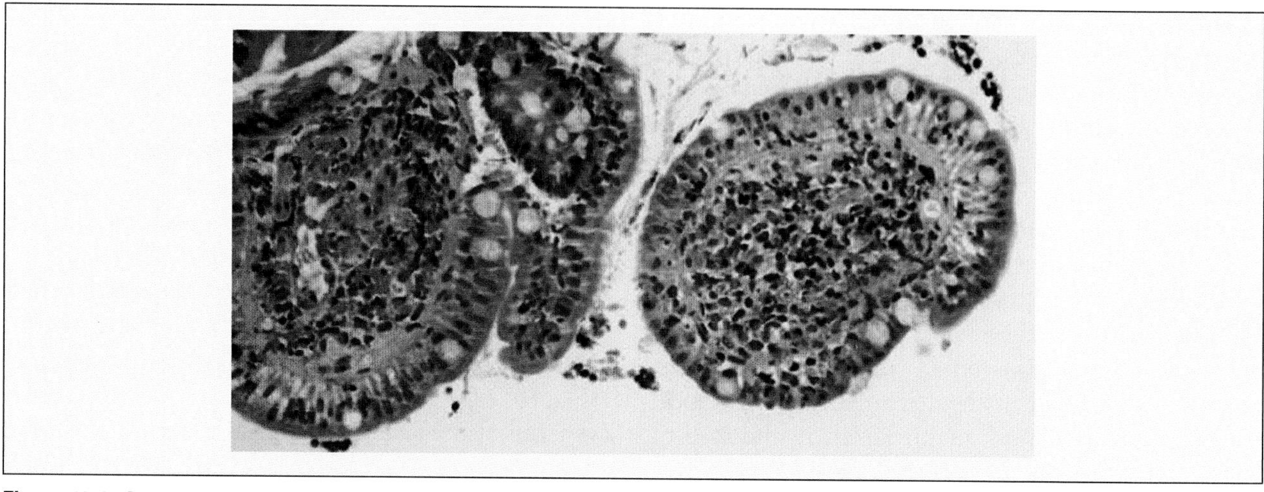

Figure 15-8. Duodenal biopsy showing a profuse eosinophilic infiltrate in the submucosal areas (in pink). (Reproduced with permission from Ralph A, O'Sullivan MV, Sangster NC, et al. Abdominal pain and eosinophilia in suburban goat keepers–trichostrongylosis. Med J Aust. 2006;184:467-9.)

infected tissue sites and attach to the parasite surface coated by immunoglobulins or complement factors such as C3b, where they degranulate, releasing oxidants, nitric oxide, lytic enzymes, and pro-inflammatory eicosanoids that are toxic, causing small perforations in the tegument of the helminth. Eosinophil degranulation can be regulated by multiple components, including those that primarily stimulate these cells (e.g., immunoglobulins and lipid mediators), priming antigens, chemokines, and cytokines. Given the diversity of parasitic worms, it is important to point out that eosinophilic responses may not be universally effective against all parasites.

Mast Cells and Basophils

Mast cells are stimulated following the binding of antigen with IgE attached to their membrane-associated FcεRI receptors to synthesize another group of mediators, which cause prolonged symptoms (i.e., the late-phase response) several hours after initial antigen binding (*Chapter 17*). These mediators include (1) chemokines and platelet-activating factors that attract leukocytes; (2) cytokines (including IL-4) that activate eosinophils and stimulate their synthesis in the bone marrow; and (3) leukotrienes that promote increased blood flow, smooth muscle constriction, and mucus secretion. Basophils also constitute a major source of Th2-polarizing cytokines IL-4 and IL-13 in response to antigen or IgE-FcεRI cross-linking. Therefore, it is possible that basophils and mast cells constitute a constant source or Th2 cytokines in the presence of circulating helminth antigens that provide a local environment for the induction of subsequent adaptive immunologic events.

T Cells

Although the Th1 cells of the T cell repertoire comprise the classic cellular response in helminth infections, they may individually be of limited protective benefit. More recent knowledge involving the participation of other T cell subsets is beginning to offer a more complete picture of T cell-related antiparasitic protective immunity (*Chapter 7*). Sensitized T cells may assault helminths by two mechanisms. First, cytotoxic CD8+ T cells may attack helminths that are deeply embedded in the intestinal mucosa or are undergoing tissue migration, although this mechanism is more likely to be efficient in killing larvae. Second, the development of delayed type hypersensitivity (**DTH**) by Th1 cells that attract lymphocytes and monocytes to produce granulomas may create an environment unsuitable for the parasite. The immunological events associated with granuloma formation are described more fully below in the immunopathology section.

More is known concerning the protective role of Th2 cells in helminthic infection. Worm antigens preferentially stimulate Th2 responses (Figure 15-9). 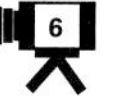 They produce cytokines such as IL-4, IL-5, IL-6, and IL-13 that promote antibody production. Collectively, these cytokines enable B lymphocytes to proliferate and synthesize and secrete antibodies and enable antibody-producing cells to switch the class of antibodies being produced (*Chapter 6*). Another major function of the cytokines produced by Th2 cells is to enable B lymphocytes to produce

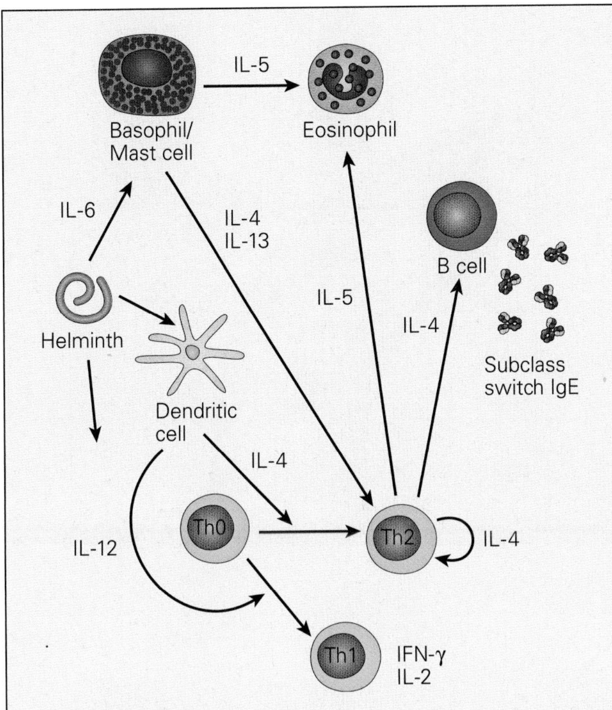

Figure 15-9. Schematic representation of the pivotal role of the Th2 cell in cytokine production and IgE synthesis in the immune response to helminth infection.

IgE that will lead to eosinophil activation and parasite killing.

The Biology of Schistosomes

Shown in Figure 15-10 is the life cycle of *Schistosoma mansoni.* Infection is initiated by cercariae, which burrow into the skin, transform into schistosomula, and then enter the vasculature and migrate to the portal system, where they mature into adult worms. Within the vasculature, eggs released by female parasites cross the endothelium and basement membrane of veins and traverse the intervening tissue, basement membrane, and epithelium of the intestine (*S. mansoni* and *Schistosoma japonicum*) or bladder (*S. haematobium*) en route to the exterior. An adult female can produce approximately 300 eggs/day. However, 50 percent of the eggs do not leave the body but are trapped within the tissues, where they induce immunopathologic responses, e.g., granuloma formation. During the course of infection, mediators are released from cells of the immune system as well as from the parasite, and mediator receptors are induced on the surface of the adult worms.

Immunology of Human Infection with Schistosoma

Shown in Figure 15-11 are three broad categories of specific immune responses that result from infection with two helminthic agents, *Schistosoma mansoni* and *Brugia malayi.* One group of individuals has immunological responses described as modified Th2 cell responses. They have relatively higher levels of Th2 cells, with lower Th1 cell responses, and express high levels of IL-10, which suggests a strong regulatory Treg cell activity. The Th2-type antibody profiles are dominated by the IgG4 isotype with relatively little IgE. These individuals often have clinically silent infections and are the main reservoir for subsequent transmission. A second group of individuals is relatively resistant to infections and shows well-balanced immune responses characterized by the presence of equal numbers of Th1, Th2, and Treg cells. Although the Th1 and Th2 cell responses are balanced, they are of sufficient magnitude to kill the invading helminths. This is also reflected in a less skewed distribution of IgG4 and IgE isotypes in the Th2-type antibody profile. At the other extreme, some individuals develop uncontrolled inflammatory (Th1) disease. In this stage of schistosomiasis, strong immune responses can be mounted against eggs that are trapped in tissues, such as the liver or the bladder wall, leading to the formation of granulomas. Uncontrolled inflammatory responses, often characterized by type 1 responses in peripheral blood, are associated with hepatosplenic disease and show low levels of IgG4 but prominent IgE responses. In filariasis, strong type 1 immune responses are associated with lymphatic inflammation. This leads to pathological outcomes, such as elephantiasis, which is caused by the failure of lymphatic drainage and opportunistic secondary infection. In such cases, it would be expected that a low activity of regulatory T cells occurred.

Development of the Immune Response to Schistosoma during Infection

Shown in Figure 15-12 are the immune responses that occur during the course of a typical Schistosomal infection that progresses through at least three phases. In the first phase occurring during the first three to five weeks of acute infection, the host is exposed to migrating immature parasites during which time the dominant response is Th1-like. As the parasites mature, mate, and begin to produce eggs at five to six weeks, a second phase emerges where the response is markedly altered and is characterized by a decreasing

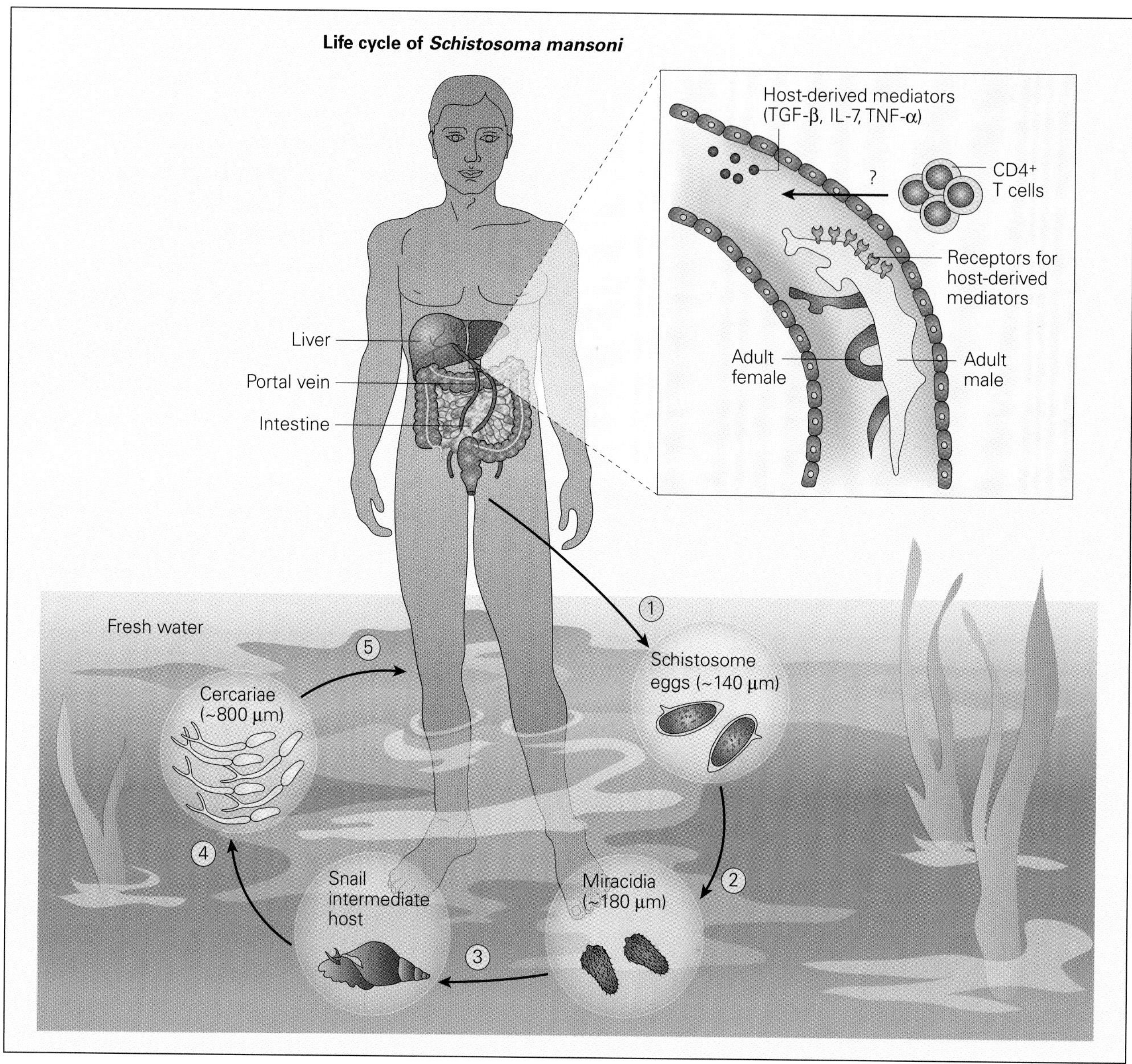

Figure 15-10. Schematic representation of the life cycle of Schistosoma mansoni. (1) After the eggs of the intestine-dwelling adult parasite are emitted in the feces and into the water; (2) the ripe miracidia hatch out of the eggs; (3) the miracidia search for a suitable freshwater snail that acts as an intermediate host following which they undergo development through a series of sporocyst steps; (4) the sporocysts progress to the generation of cercaria that emerge from the snail into the water; (5) the cercaria propel themselves in the water seeking and finally penetrating the skin of their final host; the cercariae, burrow into the skin, transform into schistosomula, and then after a series of migratory steps through the lung and liver, enter the vasculature and migrate to the portal system, where they mature into adult worms. The inset at the top right shows that after pairing with the adult male worm in the mesenteric venules, the female worm begins production of eggs that are released into the external environment with the feces. (Adapted with permission from Pearce EJ, MacDonald AS. The immunobiology of schistosomiasis. Nat Rev Immunol. 2002;2:499-511.)

Th1 component with the emergence of a strong Th2 response. The third phase of infection, occurring after six weeks, is characterized by a chronic stage of infection during which infections are long-lived and worms continue to produce eggs—300 per day in the case of each *Schistosoma mansoni* female. In this third phase, after an initial increase, the Th2 response is downmodulated and the granulomas that now form around newly deposited eggs are smaller in size than at earlier times during infection. From studies performed in a mouse model, there appears to be a correlation between the inability to form granulomas or the development and persistence of a highly pro-inflammatory Th1-like response beyond the acute phase, with the development of hepatotoxic disease. In contrast, Th2 cell-mediated granulomas seem to protect

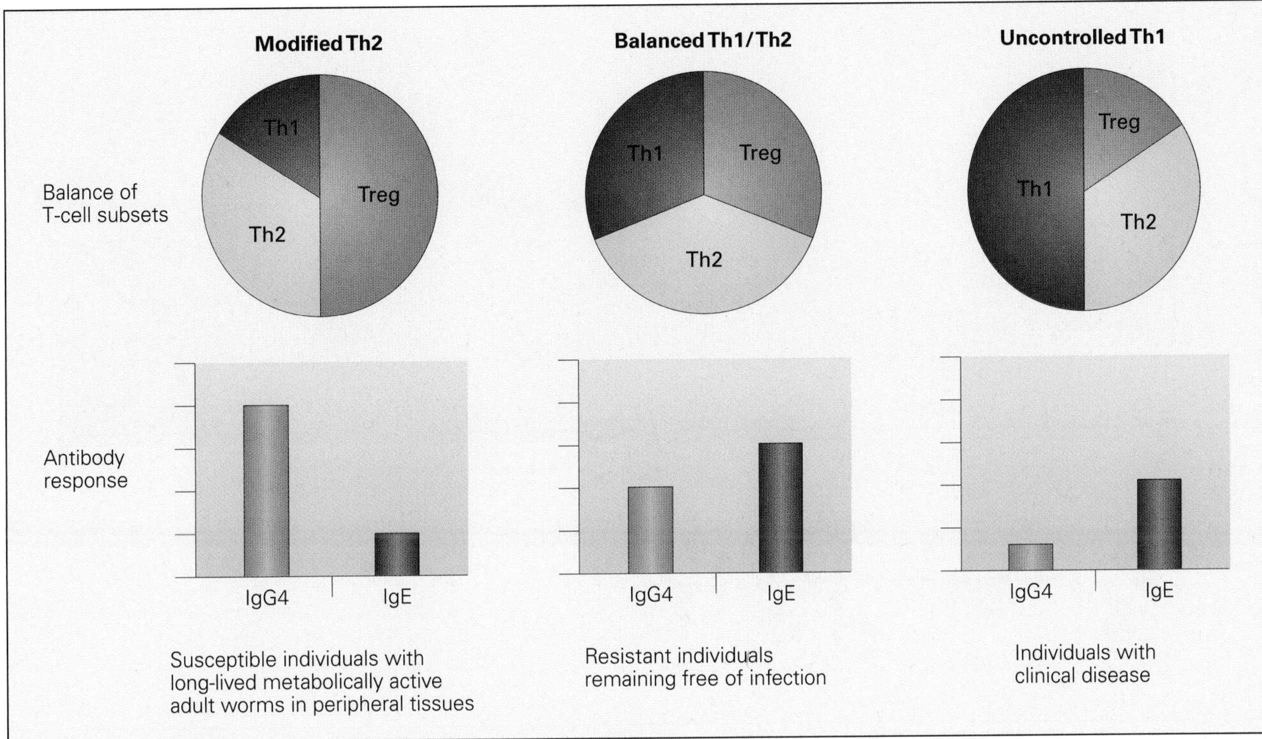

Figure 15-11. Schematic representation of three broad categories of specific adaptive immune responses that result from infection with two helminthic agents, *Schistosoma mansoni* and *Brugia malayi.* Patients in the modified Th2 category (left panel) show a predominant Treg, high Th2, low Th1; high Ig4 low IgE; and have silent infections and serve as reservoirs; patients in the balanced Th1/Th2 category (center panel) have equal Th1, Th2, and Treg, less skewed IgG4 and IgE, and are relatively resistant to infection; patients in the uncontrolled Th1 category (right panel) have a predominant Th1, a relatively low Treg that favors a greater IgE response and show clinical disease. Immunology of human infections with *Schistosoma mansoni* and *Brugia malayi.* (Adapted from and reproduced with permission from Maizels RM, Yazdanbakhsh M. Immune regulation by helminth parasites: cellular and molecular mechanisms. Nat Rev Immunol. 2003;3:733-44.)

hepatocytes but are associated with the development of fibrosis. Although the occurrence of severe fibrosis in human schistosomiasis is clear, there is debate over the existence of the hepatotoxic form of the disease. Th2 responses are also strongly implicated in naturally acquired resistance to reinfection with schistosomes.

Immunopathology Associated with Helminthic Infections

Intestinal worms cause a variety of pathologic changes in the host, some reflecting physical damage to the tissues, others resulting from the immune response against the parasite.

Physical Factors

The most obvious forms of direct damage are those resulting from the blockage of internal organs of the infected host or from the effects of pressure exerted by parasites that include the following changes:

- Large worms can physically block the intestine, and this may occur after some forms of chemotherapy.
- Granulomas that form around schistosome eggs retained in the portal circulation of the liver may block hepatic blood flow that may lead to pathological changes in the liver as well as other organs (e.g., congestive heart failure) (Figure 15-13). In later stages of the disease, as the eggs die and the granulomas resolve, fibrosis can develop. This can lead to increased portal hypertension and the development of esophageal varices. Bleeding from these varices is the most common cause of death due to schistosomiasis.
- Filarial parasites cause significant pathology either through obstruction and damage of the lymphatic system by adult parasites, as is the case with *Brugia* spp and *Wuchereria bancrofti*, or through cutaneous and ocular irritation by larval transmission stages (microfilariae) of *Onchocerca volvulus.*
- Pressure atrophy is also characteristic of the growth of larval tapeworm cysts; the hydatid cyst, the larva of *Echinococcus granulosus*, can be found in the liver, brain, lungs, or body cavity. The larvae of *Taenia solium* frequently develop in the central nervous system and eyes. Some of the neurological symptoms of the resulting condition are caused by the pressure exerted by the cysts.

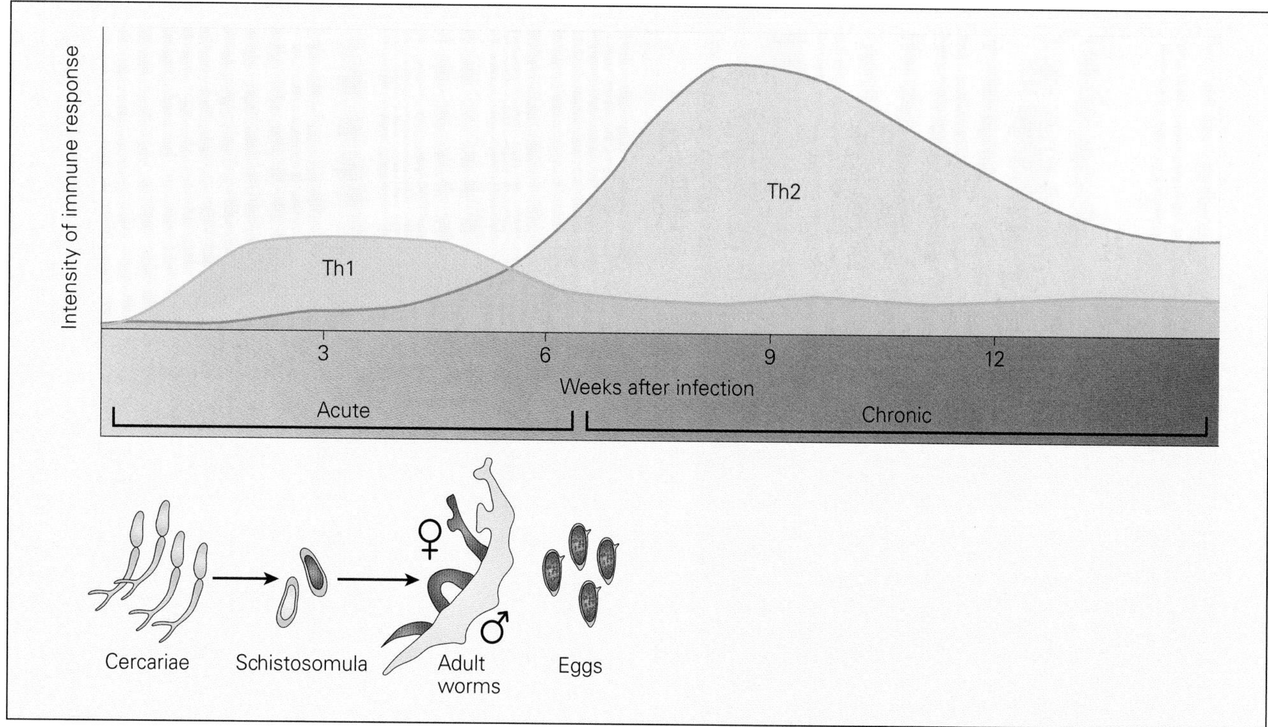

Figure 15-12. Schematic representation of the three phases of the development of the immune response occurring during *Schistosoma* infection. The first phase is characterized by a predominant Th1 response. The second phase is the Th2 predominant phase where a decreasing Th1 component is seen with the emergence of a strong Th2 response and which correlates with increased egg production and granuloma formation. The third phase is the chronic phase characterized by continued egg production, decreased Th2 response, and granuloma shrinkage. (Adapted with permission from Pearce EJ, MacDonald AS. The immunobiology of schistosomiasis. Nat Rev Immunol. 2002;2:499-511.)

In infection with any schistosome species, chronic disease is the result of the ongoing host response to accumulating tissue-trapped eggs (Figure 15-13). In *Schistosoma mansoni* and *Schistosoma japonicum* infections, the liver is the principal site that is affected because many of the eggs are carried by the blood into this organ, the sinusoids of which are too small for the eggs to traverse. Thus, the liver becomes a dead-end organ for the eggs, which eventually die within the hepatic tissues. Intestinal damage by traversing eggs can also be problematic. During *Schistosoma haematobium* infection, the passage of eggs across the urinary bladder wall causes damage to this organ, with resultant hematuria. The CD4+ T cell response that is induced by egg antigens orchestrates the development of granulomatous lesions—which are composed of collagen fibers and cells, including macrophages, eosinophils, and CD4+ T cells—around the individual eggs (Figure 15-13). A central role for TNF-α in the development of the granuloma has also been proposed (*Chapter 12*). As the eggs die, the granulomas resolve, leaving fibrotic plaques. Severe consequences of infection with *S. mansoni* and

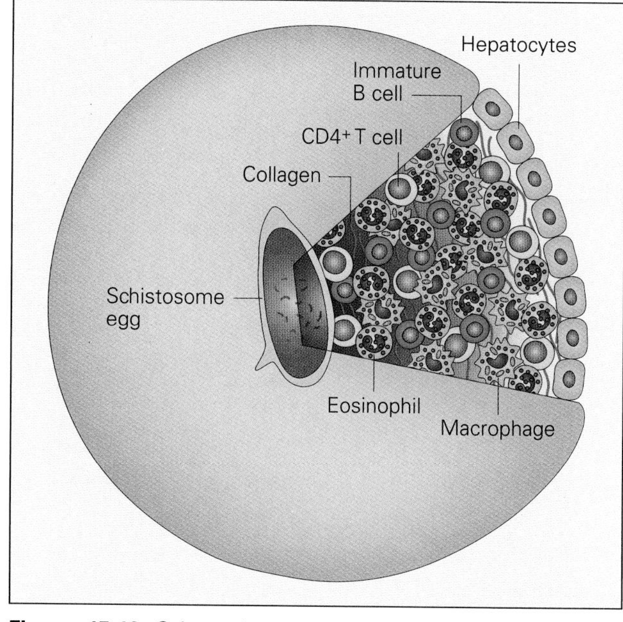

Figure 15-13. Schematic representation of a schistosomal granuloma in the liver showing the pleomorphic infiltration of macrophages, eosinophils, and CD4+ cells together with collagen deposition following schistosoma egg deposition and persistence. (Adapted with permission from Pearce EJ, MacDonald AS. The immunobiology of schistosomiasis. Nat Rev Immunol. 2002;2:499-511.)

S. japonicum are the result of an increase in portal blood pressure as the liver becomes fibrotic, congested, and harder to perfuse. Under these conditions, the diameter of the portal vein increases and the wall of the portal vein becomes fibrotic. Associated with these changes is the development of ascites (i.e., the accumulation of serous fluid in the peritoneal cavity) and portal-systemic venous shunts (i.e., new blood vessels that bypass the liver), which can rupture, leading to life-threatening bleeding. The most serious effects of infection with *S. haematobium* are bladder cancer and genital schistosomiasis, a condition in which eggs pass through the cervix in women or into the testes in men.

Immediate Hypersensitivity (Type I)

Type 1 hypersensitivity or immediate hypersensitivity is an IgE-mediated allergic reaction provoked by re-exposure to specific antigens (*Chapter 17*). It is generated following contact of antigen with pre-existing IgE antibody attached to the high-affinity FcεRI receptors found on mast cells and basophils. These cells are activated by the cross-linking of the FcεRI receptors via antigen binding to the bound IgE molecules. Such cross-linking leads to rapid degranulation (i.e., within minutes) of the mast cells with the release of primary mediators (histamine, serotonin, and others) stored in the granules. These mediators cause all the normal consequences of an acute inflammatory reaction—increased vascular permeability, smooth muscle contraction, granulocyte chemotaxis, and extravasation. Mast cell activation via FcεRI also leads to the active production of two other types of mediators called secondary mediators. These secondary mediators, unlike the stored granule contents, must be newly synthesized *de novo* and comprise arachidonic acid metabolites (i.e., prostaglandins and leukotrienes) and proteins (i.e., cytokines and enzymes). The most dramatic effects of these secondary mediators include the contraction of intestinal and bronchial smooth muscles as well as increased vascular permeability and mucus secretion. In addition, a variety of cytokines are released by mast cells (IL-4, IL-5, and IL-6), some of which have profound modulatory effects on the immune response and recruitment of leukocyte populations, e.g., chemokines, while others may contribute to the pathology, e.g., TNF-α. Allergens, and in particular helminth antigens, have an innate preference for the induction of IgE antibodies that can prime mast cells for this immediate type of anaphylactic response. In addition to these antigens, cross-linking of FcεRI receptors can also be achieved by carbohydrate-binding lectins. Galectin-3, associated with mast cell granules, for example, can bind to oligosaccharides attached to both IgE and its IgE receptor and induce degranulation. In this respect, it is of interest that galectins identified in the parasitic nematodes *Onchocerca volvulus* and *Teladorsagia circumcincta* have been shown to bind IgE.

Type I hypersensitivity reactions may be either local or systemic. Symptoms vary from mild irritation to sudden death from anaphylactic shock. Immediate hypersensitivity reactions such as urticaria and angioedema are found in the acute stages of many helminthic infections (e.g ascaridiasis, ancylostomiasis, and Strongyloides infections). Rupture of hydatid cysts (*Echinococcus granulosus*) may cause a systemic reaction and anaphylactic shock.

Immune Complex-Mediated Hypersensitivity (Type III)

As described in *Chapter 17*, the reaction of an excess of soluble antigen with circulating antibody results in the formation of complexes in the zone of antigen excess, which can induce activation of the classical complement pathway with a resultant inflammatory response. In contrast to immune complexes formed within the infected tissue that cause localized inflammatory reactions (i.e., rashes) (Type IIIA), immune complexes formed within the bloodstream or lymphatics can form more serious systemic inflammatory reactions at sites where they deposit (Type IIIB). In patients with chronic schistosomal infections, deposition of immune complexes on blood vessel walls can also cause complement-dependent aggregation of platelets and the release of clotting factors, leading to the formation of microthrombi, while complexes deposited in the kidney can cause glomerulonephritis and progressive kidney damage, resulting in nephropathy.

Delayed Hypersensitivity (DTH Type IVA)

Perhaps the most classic example of DTH Type IVA reactions (*Chapter 17*) in helminth infections is the granuloma formation in schistosomiasis. The mechanisms of granuloma formation, modulation, and subsequent fibrosis are complex. DTH reactions require the involvement of sensitized T cells, which upon renewed antigen encounter, release cytokines resulting in the recruitment and activation of effector cells that can mediate tissue damage (*Chapter 7*). Due to the time required for antigen processing and presentation to T cells, cytokine release, and cell recruitment, DTH reactions take two to three days to fully develop. DTH Type I reactions are characterized by a predominant Th1 response, with cells secreting IL-2, IFN-γ, and TNF-α. In mice, a predominantly Th1 reaction in the early stages of schistosomal infection shifts to an egg-induced Th2-biased profile. Similar mechanisms involving Th1 cell-induced helminthic pathology could also be operative in the human.

DTH Type IVA is the most common cause of pathology observed during helminth infections and is associated with the production by CD4+ T cells of the Th2 cytokines IL-4 and IL-5 and the subsequent recruitment of eosinophils (Figure 15-9). Chronic stimulation with parasite antigens results in granuloma formation, with the presence eosinophils and their products as the most characteristic features. The formation of eosinophilic abscesses and granulomas caused by human enteric infection with the canine hookworm *A. caninum* is probably one of the more common underlying causes of eosinophilic enteritis in humans. Similarly, eosinophilic granulomas largely account for the pathology caused by the migration of the dog ascarid larvae in the skin, liver, lung, and eyes of their natural or accidental hosts (i.e., visceral larva migrans).

A third pathological consequence of T cell-mediated immunity is the excessive collagen deposition and fibrosis, seen especially in the liver and lung, following inflammation and tissue damage caused by the host's hypereactivity to parasitic antigens. The formation of fibrotic tissue probably occurs as a host-protective effect in an attempt to wall off an invading parasite. Collagen deposition during liver fluke infection, for example, protects the host from damage caused by the flukes, and fibrosis usually resolves after early elimination of schistosomal infections. It is only after chronic stimulation by parasitic infestation that the pathologic sequelae of parasitic disease are seen. As described previously, this has been best studied in Schistosoma infections, where hepatic fibrosis rather than egg-induced granuloma formation itself, is the main cause of severe disease and death in humans infected with *Schistosoma mansoni* and *S. japonicum*. In schistosomiasis, fibrosis leads to progressive occlusion of the portal veins, portal hypertension, splenomegaly, collateral venous circulation, portocaval shunting, and gastrointestinal varices. Transforming growth factor β (TGFβ) is the key cytokine involved in the fibrogenic process, causing both fibroblast proliferation and upregulation of collagen synthesis; its expression is under the control of the Th2 cytokines IL-4 and IL-13.

Evasion of Immunity by Parasites

As with bacterial and viral infections, parasites that cause persistent or chronic infection have learned how to evade the immune response (*Chapters 12* and *13*). In general, when assaulted by a new foreign invader, the host's immune system reacts with three basic outcomes: early and complete expulsion of the foreign agent; overwhelming infection with failure of control; or persistence of the pathogen with potential long-term carriage or induction of disease. This last scenario is the most frequently seen with parasitic infections in the human and represents the classic example of persistence of foreignness and induction of immunologically mediated disease described in Chapter 1 and in Chapter 17. The complexity of the life cycles of parasites reflects their exquisite ability to adapt to a variety of hostile environments both in the vector as well as in the host. In this way, many parasites escape immune recognition and maximize the probability of being transmitted to another uninfected host. Their success as parasites, in fact, depends on a series of intricate and highly evolved host adaptations that enable them to successfully evade destruction by the immune system and to survive. Some of the mechanisms used by parasites to evade a host's immune responses are shown in Table 15-4.

Resistance to Macrophage Killing of Intracellular Parasites

The antimicrobial mechanisms that can be induced in phagocytic and even non-phagocytic host cells after contact with intracellular parasitic protozoa represent the main defensive machinery of many nucleated cells (Table 15-4). The acidified hydrolytic environment of host cell lysosomes, for example, is lethal for acid-protease-sensitive parasites that are not able to avoid or modify this compartment (*Chapter 5*). *Toxoplasma gondii* resides in a phagosome that restricts its fusion with endosomes and lysosomes. This parasite actively penetrates host cells by an actin-myosin-dependent gliding motility. In the process, it establishes

Table 15-4. Mechanisms of evasion used by parasites

General mechanism	Parasites	Specific mechanism and molecules
Resistance to macrophage killing	Trypanosoma spp	Escape of phagolysosome via Tc-TOX
		LPG inhibits phagosome maturation
	Leishmania spp	Amastigote hydrolases make them resistant to the acidic environment of the phagolysosome
	Toxoplasma gondii	Avert phagolysosome formation
Resistance to complement	*Trypanosoma cruzi*	gp160
	Trypanosoma brucei	gp63
	Leishmania spp	Lipophosphoglycan (LPG), gp63
	Entamoeba histolytica	Galactose residues (Gal/GalNac)
	Trichomonas vaginalis	Cysteine proteinases, adhesions
	Schistosoma mansoni	Glycocalyx coat shedding
	Schistosomula	Complement inhibitors (proteases)
	Adult *Fasciola hepatica*	Glycocalyx coat shedding
Molecular mimicry	Plasmodium spp	MSP, 1-thymosine-like
	Trichomonas vaginalis	Adhesins
	Helminths	Cytokine-like genes
Antigenic variation	*Trypanosoma brucei*	Changes in VSG expression
	Plasmodium spp	Stage-specific proteins
	Trichomonas vaginalis	P270, adhesins
	Giardia intestinalis	Changes is VSP expression
Antigen modulation and disguise	*Trypanosoma cruzi*	Elimination of immune membrane complex
	Leishmania spp	Antibody capping
	Entamoeba hystolitica	Antibody capping
	Trichomonas vaginalis	Coating with host plasma proteins
	Schistosoma mansoni	Coating with cell surface molecules
Suppression or modulation of host immunity	*Trypanosoma cruzi*	Decrease in IL-2, increase in PGE2 and TGFβ
	Trypanosoma brucei	Decrease of MHC-II and antigen presentation
	Leishmania spp	Overeactive macrophages, decrease in IL-2
		gp63 cleaves CD4 molecules
	Toxoplasma gondii	GPI motifs decrease MHC-I and MHC-II expression
	Plasmodium falciparum	Decrease in IL-12, increase in PGE2 and TGFβ
	Helminths	Cystatin-like molecules, protease inhibitors, prostanoids
	Filaria, Ascaris	Increase in IL-10 and TGFβ
	Ancylostoma spp	CSP variation reduces efficacy of T cell response
	Schistosoma mansoni	Decrease of T cell proliferation
		Enzymes disrupt antigen presentation pathway
		Secreted products interact with immune function
		Serine proteinase decreases elastase function

a compartment called a parasitophorous vacuole (**PV**) that lacks integral membrane proteins of host cell origin and is modified by secreted parasite proteins. In this way, the PV does not fuse with host cell lysosomes and, therefore, with inhibition of PV acidification, *T. gondii* is protected and can resume its life cycle inside the host. Dead or opsonized parasites are internalized via classical receptor-mediated phagocytosis and are killed by the internal fusion of endosome with lysosome (*Chapter 5*).

T. cruzi trypomastigotes actively invade the host cell by a Ca2+ regulated lysosomal exocytic pathway. The membrane of the PV that contains the parasite inside the cell host is derived from lysosomes; the vacuole itself remains acidic and potentially fusigenic with other lysosomes (Figure 15-14). After cell invasion, *T. cruzi* escapes to the cytosol to survive and continue its growth and development. Exit from the vacuole is mediated by a parasite-secreted protein (Tc-TOX), which has membrane pore-forming activity at acidic pH (Table 15-4).

Leishmania promastigotes are internalized by macrophages via conventional receptor-mediated phagocytosis. The parasites do not seem to remodel the phagosome in a major way because it rapidly fuses with late endosomes or lysosomes, generating a PV that maintains an acidic pH and hydrolytic activity. The LPG present in the membrane of Leishmania can inhibit phagosome maturation. The amastigotes are resistant to low pH environment and acid hydrolases, presumably by producing an abundance of cell surface and secreted glycoconjugates and metalloproteinases

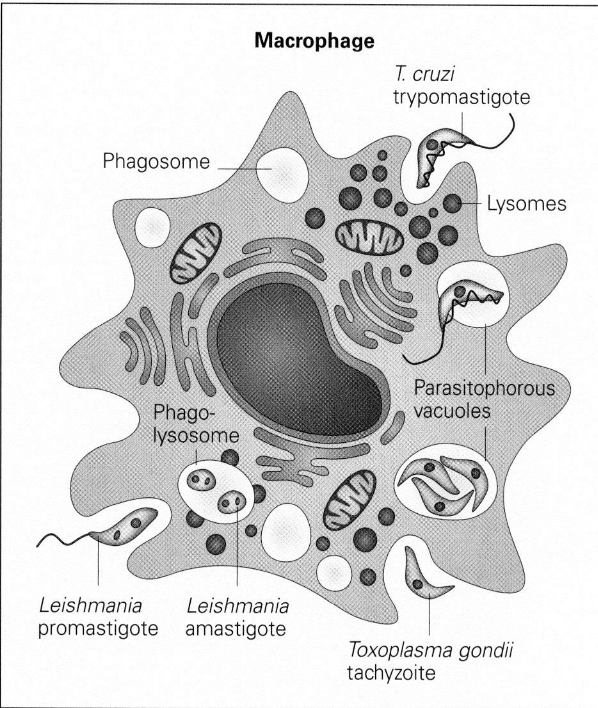

Figure 15-14. Schematic representation of evasion of macrophage uptake and killing of various parasitic protozoa. The formation of parasitophorous vacuoles that lack integral membrane proteins of host cell origin prevents the fusion of the phagosome with host cell lysosomes. This leads to the subsequent inhibition of PV acidification following which the parasite is protected from the microbicidal action of the macrophage and can resume its life cycle inside the host.

(i.e., gp63) that protect the cell from proteolytic damage, and by the presence of large amounts of catalase and superoxide dismutase, which degrade the oxygen intermediates produced by the macrophage.

Resistance to Complement-Mediated Lysis

The complement system provides an important host-protective mechanism against microbial infections (*Chapter 4*). To counter the host's complement defenses and to assure their survival, parasites have developed novel ways to avoid the complement activity and allow them to survive in the host (Table 15-4). The alternative pathway of complement activation provides a first line of defense against extracellular parasites that must be subverted for infection to proceed. Some parasites are resistant to complement-mediated lysis. For example, the infective metacyclic and bloodstream trypomastigotes of *T. cruzi* express a 160-kD glycoprotein (gp160) that can bind to C3b and C4b and inhibit the uptake of subsequent components of the complement cascade, thus preventing convertase formation. In the case of *Leishmania*, when the promastigotes develop into infective metacyclic forms, their membrane is altered, with expression of a modified surface lipophosphoglycan (**LPG**) that is approximately twice as long as the form of non-infective promastigotes and may act as a barrier for insertion of the lytic C5b-C9 MAC. In addition, during transformation into the infective stage, Leishmania promastigotes enhance synthesis of the surface proteinase gp63, which can cleave C3b to the inactive iC3b form, thus preventing deposition of the MAC. Some African trypanosomes (*T. brucei gambiense* and *T. brucei rhodesiese*) that can cause sleeping sickness have several homologous genes encoding gp63-like proteins, similar to those from *Leishmania. Entamoeba histolytica* resist complement-mediated lysis by proteolytic degradation of C3 and C5 and by the presence of galactose- and N-acetyl-D-galactose (**Gal/GalNAc**)-containing cell surface receptors, which bind to C8 and C9, preventing assembly of the MAC and further lysis. The same degradation of complement component C3 appears to contribute to the resistance of *Trichomonas vaginalis* due the trichomonal adhesins and cysteine proteases present in the parasite's surface.

Among helminths, the parasitic worm *Schistosoma mansoni* undergoes a stage-specific transformation that permits it to resist complement-mediated damage. The free-swimming cercaria shed by the snail vector activates complement very efficiently while the schistosomula released after skin penetration is much less sensitive to lysis by complement. One of the first steps the infecting parasite takes is shedding of the coat, which is a strong direct activator of the alternative pathway of complement. The release of the glycocalyx coat may consume complement thus reducing the effective complement concentration around the penetrating larvae (Table 15-4). Similar shedding of glycocalyx has been reported in *Fasciola hepatica. S. mansoni* also avoid the complement effect by the presence of two complement inhibitors in the surface of adult worms. Another protective mechanism employed by schistosomulae of *S. mansoni* to avoid complement killing is the proteolytic degradation of complement proteins such as C3, C3b, iC3b, and C9 by a membrane-secreted protease.

Molecular Mimicry

The original concept of molecular mimicry was based upon the expression of host protein homologues by the parasite, which would result in poor immunogenicity of the parasite, resulting in a passive evasive tactic to escape from or reduce the immune detection of the parasite through the possession of shared host-parasite epitopes (*Chapter 19*). This original concept of molecular mimicry was subsequently expanded to include escape through a more aggressive form or mimicry by participation of host immunoregulatory molecules, e.g., TGFβ, IL-10, or receptors (*Chapter 9*). The aggressive response against foreign molecules similar to the host's is a significant concept not only important in the immunity against parasites, but also in the pathogenesis of autoimmunity (*Chapter 19*). Molecular mimicry is common in human malaria and can modulate the cellular immune response and the release of cytokines. For example, the GPI moiety that anchors a range of merozoite surface proteins (**MSPs**) appears to have a marked insulin-mimetic effect, increasing the synthesis of TNF-α and IL-1β in macrophages; this is responsible for the typical malarial fevers and the production of acute-phase proteins (Table 15-4). Similarly, sequences homologous to 1-thymosin (a thymic hormone that modulates the differentiation of T cells) have been identified in two *P. falciparum* proteins. Like the human hormone, synthetic peptides from those sequences showed a similar effect on T cell maturation, suggesting that it might interfere with the development of effective cellular immunity against this parasite. The same adhesin proteins of *Trichomonas vaginalis* described previously as an important antigenic variation factor are also an example of molecular mimicry. These proteins appear to mimic the structure of malic enzyme, which may account for their poor immunogenicity.

In helminths, cytokine-like molecules of parasite origin, including homologues of IFN-γ, TGF-ß, and macrophage inhibitory factor (**MIF**), have been identified in several helminth species. Although their impact on host immunity is as yet not clear, these cytokines may be able to interfere with the regulation of the host immune response and potentiate parasite survival.

Antigenic Variation

Another mechanism of immune evasion used by protozoan parasites is exemplified by infections caused by species of Plasmodium spp, *Trypanosoma brucei* complex, *Giardia intestinalis*, and *Trichomonas vaginalis* (Table 15-4). These infections are characterized by a prolonged course with fluctuating numbers of and an undulating periodic pattern of appearance of parasites that demonstrate different surface antigens. The first mechanism of immune evasion described for a parasite was the antigenic variation in African trypanosomes, the *Trypanosoma brucei* complex. These organisms have the ability to shift their antigenicity due to the acquisition of the so-called VSG coat, whose molecular identity periodically changes, permitting a portion of the parasite population to avoid antibody-mediated killing throughout an infection. In consequence, this repeated antigenic change of VSG in trypanosomes allows them to evade the antibody response, resulting in the successive surges of parasitemia, a situation similar to being infected successively by related, but not identical, pathogens.

Antigenic variation has also been described in Plasmodium spp. Once the *Plasmodium* parasite is established in the host, it evades the immune response by changing its surface antigens as it passes through the various stages of its life cycle. In this way, each phase of the cellular cycle is associated with the expression of stage and species-specific proteins, many of which are inserted into the membrane surface of the parasite or the red blood cells they invade. Again, this diversity results in antibody responses that confer only variant-specific protection.

In *Giardia intestinalis*, antigenic variation is caused by an exchange of the parasite's variant surface protein (**VSP**) coat. Immune evasion has been commonly attributed to antigenic variation, and both immunological and non-immunological host mechanisms are known to act as selection factors mediating which VSPs are expressed. The biological role of these proteins in the evasion of the immune responses, however, is still unclear.

Like the other protozoan parasites, *Trichomonas vaginalis* also displays antigenic variation as a mechanism of immune evasion. The alternate expression of highly immunogenic glycoproteins (mostly P270) and adhesins indicates the resistance to antibody response. Only the organisms that are P270-negative can parasitize host cells and are resistant against antibody-mediated complement lysis *in vitro.*

Antigenic Modulation and Antigenic Disguise

Other mechanisms of host immune evasion are associated with the ability of the parasite to modulate its surface constituents (i.e., antigenic modulation) or to coat itself with host proteins (i.e., antigenic disguise) (Table 15-4). The concept of antigenic modulation differs from antigenic variation since it involves mechanical changes of membrane composition by the parasite rather than alterations of genetic expressions of surface molecules. To circumvent the antibody response and the antibody-dependent lytic effect mediated by complement, Leishmania and *E. histolytica* concentrate antibodies that have been deposited on its surface toward a specific region, i.e., polarize the antibodies, where they are spontaneously eliminated as molecular aggregates (i.e., capping). *T. cruzi* eliminates the immune membrane complexes by surface molecular turnover through the endocytic pathway (*Chapters 1* and *10*). One example of antigenic disguise in protozoan parasites has been described for *Trichomonas vaginalis*, which can coat itself with host plasma proteins. This coating camouflage impedes host immune system recognition of the parasite as foreign.

The existence of shared antigens between schistosomes and their hosts has also been described. The parasite adsorbs host molecules onto their tegument, including MHC antigens, immunoglobulins, blood group antigens, C1q receptors, contrapsin (an antithrombotic serum serine protease inhibitor), and low-density lipoproteins (possibly causing the progressive loss of antibody-binding sites with maturation). This antigenic disguise or camouflage might protect the worm against antibodies and cells that could otherwise lead to its elimination. Schistosomulae of *S. mansoni* have also the capacity to absorb complement inhibitors from a host's tissues.

Suppression or Modulation of Host Immunity

In a general way, protozoan parasitic infections lead to inhibition of host immunity as an adaptive mechanism for survival. This restraint is commonly attributed but not limited to (1) the proliferation of suppressor T cells and/or macrophages that inhibit the immune system by secretion of regulatory cytokines (immunomodulation); (2) the production of specific immune suppressor substances by the parasite, which could either inhibit the cellular immune response or degrade immunoglobulins directed against the parasite (immunosuppression); and (3) non-specific stimulation of antibody-producing B cells (polyclonal activation), rather than stimulation of specific anti-parasite B cells.

During infection with *P. falciparum*, circulating T cells are reduced in number, accompanied by a decrease in lymphoproliferative responses and cytokine release by peripheral blood mononuclear cells when stimulated by malarial antigens (Table 15-4). Although some malarial antigens have been reported to directly induce immunosuppression, prostaglandin secreted by activated macrophages might also be responsible for the low cellular response. The circumsporozoite surface protein (**CSP**) has been shown to be an antigen crucially implicated in protective immunity to Plasmodium infection and formed the basis for the first *P. falciparum* subunit vaccine. Recent analysis of the immune response against malarial CSP suggest that some *P. falciparum* strains contain CSP variants with T cell epitopes that would prevent the binding of the original T cell epitopes to the major histocompatibility complex (**MHC**) molecule, thereby altering memory T cell effector functions. Polyclonal B cell activation is also reported to be implicated in Immunosuppression in human malaria.

In African trypanosomiasis, parasitic products activate macrophages and CD8+ T cells, causing changes in the pattern of cytokines that are released from these cells. Among these, the GPI moiety of the VSG coat appears to overactivate macrophages to produce TNF-α and induce CD8+ T cells to secrete high levels of IFN-γ. In turn, the high levels of IFN-γ result in the decrease of IL-2 receptor expression and IL-2 synthesis, which impair the proliferative T cell response to avoid parasite elimination.

Similar to the African trypanosomiasis, infection by *T. cruzi* induces a T cell immunomodulation by a decrease in the expression and synthesis of IL-2. In addition, other mechanisms may contribute to this negative immunomodulation, including (1) downregulation of components of the T cell receptor complex; (2) T cell receptor dysfunction; (3) defects in the processing and MHC-II antigen presentation; (4) T cell and macrophage suppressor activity; and (5) prostaglandin E2 production. *Trypanosoma cruzi* also induces polyclonal B cell activation with subsequent overproduction of IgM antibodies, which bind to the trypomastigote surface and interfere with the binding of IgG inhibitory antibodies and further elimination of parasite.

In Leishmania infections, some components from the parasite including GPIs can inhibit the expression of the MHC-I and MHC-II molecules on macrophages (Table 15-4). It has also been shown that gp63 from *L. major* and *L. donovani* cleave CD4 molecules on T cells, interfering with the interaction between antigen-presenting cells and T helper cells. Leishmania spp and *E. histolytica* induce the release of prostaglandin E2 and TGF-ß, resulting in the blockage of macrophage function. In addition, Leishmania can modulate IL-12 production by suppression of transcription of its gene and increase IL-10 production by infected macrophages and regulatory T cells.

The TGF-ß production and reduction of MHC-II presented by *T. cruzi* and Leishmania is also the mechanism of modulation observed in *T. gondii* infection. In addition, these parasites can induce the production of other regulatory cytokines such as IL-10 by endogenous regulatory T cells, which along with TGF-ß may inhibit the Th1 cytokine synthesis and macrophage activation, which could be characterized as an i-Treg type of immune response (Figure 15-7A). Finally, extracellular protozoa such as *G. intestinalis, E. histolytica*, and *Trichomonas vaginalis* can evade the humoral immune response by production of enzymes that degrades antibodies, most of them effective against the parasite.

Despite their extracellular localization, it has been demonstrated for some helminthic infections that macrophages are incompetent antigen presenters. Possibly the quantity of polysaccharides and glycoconjugates produced may interfere with antigen processing. In addition, some filarial worms can release cystatin-like molecules that may block the antigen-processing pathway, whereas antigen processing in B cells can be blocked by an aspartic protease inhibitor from *Ascaris lumbricoides*.

In a general way, helminthic chronic infection leads to an impairment of the T cell proliferation, which is caused mostly by secreted parasite products. This could be observed in patients infected with filarias (*Wuchereria bancrofti* and *Brugia malayi*), *S. mansoni*, Taenia, and hookworms. Filarial and teniaed parasites use endogenous and exogenous arachidonic acid to produce and release prostanoids (prostacyclin and prostaglandin E2), which in addition to their anti-inflammatory properties may also inhibit T cell proliferation. The suppression of T cell proliferation in *S. mansoni* and hookworm infection is associated with excrete or secrete (**ES**) products released by the parasite. Secreted products from the helminths can also modulate granulocyte functions. In this context, an immunoreactive neutrophil inhibitor factor (**NIF**) and a NIF-like activity are detectable in the ES products of *Ancylostoma ceylanicum*. In addition, Ancylostoma hookworms were shown previously to release a tissue inhibitor of metalloproteases (**TIMP**) in abundance. Mammalian TIMPs were show previously to stimulate host cell production of IL-10. Therefore, the possibility remains that adult hookworms directly stimulate host IL-10 production, which in turn suppresses proliferative responses. A serine protease inhibitor was identified in tegumental detergent extracts from adult worms of *S. mansoni*, which can block the activity of neutrophil elastase.

Accidental Parasitism in Humans

Even in industrialized urban environments, humans are exposed to a number of zoonotic animal parasites unexpectedly and unintentionally that result in what is commonly referred to as accidental parasitism. There are many reports in the literature describing various accidental parasitoses in humans; the most prevalent types are briefly summarized in Table 15-5.

These accidental parasitoses very often result in symptoms mimicking allergic or hypersensitivity diseases and must be included in the differential diagnosis of the allergic diseases (*Chapter 17*). These include the cutaneous and visceral forms of larval migrans that result from ingestion of nematode larvae of dogs or cats by small children with resultant hypersensitivity manifestations mimicking allergy, the more serious sequelae of echinococcal disease resulting from ingestion of tapeworm larvae of various species of echinococcus with resultant cyst formation in various organs, the neurological manifestations of neurocysticercosis following ingestion

Table 15-5. Examples of various types of accidental parasitoses in humans

Parasite	Disease	Reservoir	Target Organ	Clinical Presentation
Ancylostoma braziliense, Ancylostoma caninum	Larva migrans Cutaneous	Dog, cat	Skin	Pruritic lesions with red tracks and vesicles
Toxocara canis, Toxocara cati	Visceral	Dog, cat	Gastrointestinal tract, liver, lungs, eye	Fever, malaise, wheezing, hepatomegaly, leukocytosis, eosinophilia, elevated IgE, hypergammaglobulinemia, vision loss
Echinococcus granulosus	Echinococcosis	Dog, sheep, fox	Liver, lungs, kidney and spleen; cystic hydatid disease	Generalized malaise, palpable or X-ray identified lung or abdominal mass, hypersensitivity (anaphylaxis)
Echinococcus multilocularis			Alveolar hydatid disease	
Taenia solium	Neurocysticercosis	Pig, human	Skeletal muscle, brain	Myopathy, neurologic symptoms, seizures
Anisakis simplex, Pseudoterranova decipiens	Anisakiasis	Fish	Gastrointestinal tract	Acute abdominal pain, nausea, and vomiting, severe eosinophilic granulomatous response; can mimic allergic response to fish ingestion

Table 15-6. Opportunistic parasitic infections seen in immunocompromised hosts

Parasite	Disease	Classification	Clinical presentation	Target organ	Susceptible host
Microsporidia	Microsporidiosis	Now considered fungi	Diarrhea	Gastrointestinal tract	Immunocompromised patients AIDS
Cyclospora cayetanensis	Cyclosporiasis	Protozoa	Diarrhea	Gastrointestinal tract	Immunocompromised patients AIDS
Cryptosporidium parvum	Cryptosporidiosis	Protozoa	Diarrhea	Gastrointestinal tract	Immunocompromised patients AIDS
Strongyloides stercoralis	Strongyloidiasis	Nematode	Abdominal pain, distension, shock, pulmonary and neurologic complications and septicemia	Gastrointestinal tract	Immunocompromised patients AIDS
Pneumocystis carinii	*Pneumocystis carinii* pneumonia PCP)		Pneumonia	Lungs	Immunocompromised patients AIDS
Toxoplasma gondii	Toxoplasmosis	Protozoa	Cerebral toxoplasmosis	CNS	Immunocompromised patients AIDS
			Congenital toxoplasmosis	CNS, liver, lymphoid tissues	Fetuses
Sarcoptes scabiei	Scabies	Ectoparasites	Skin infection	Skin	Normal hosts and immunocompromised patients

Table 15-7. Anti-parasitic vaccines currently under investigation

Infection	Leader candidate vaccine	Status
Hookworm infections	Larval antigen Na-ASP-2 (larval secreted antigen)	Clinical trials (Brazil)
Schistosomiasis	Sh28 GST (*S. haematobium* 28 kDa Glutathione-S- Transferase)	Clinical trials (Africa)
Trichomoniasis	SolcoTrichovac[a]	Licensed
Cutaneous leishmaniasis	Leishmanization (live parasites) Leish-111F (multicomponent)	Discontinued Clinical trials (South America)
Malaria	Pre-erythrocytic stages RTS,S/ASO2 Blood-stage malaria MSP-1 (merozoite surface protein) AMA-1 (apical merozoite antigen-1) Transmission blocking TBV25-28	Clinical trials (Africa) Clinical trials, possibly in combination with RTS, S In development

a. Licensed in Russia

of *Taenia solium*, and the acute early and late manifestations of anisakiasis following the ingestion of larvae of the nematodes *Anisakis simplex* and *Pseudoterranova decipiens* in raw or uncooked fish.

Parasitic Infections in Immunosuppressed Individuals

A wide variety of infectious agents, including viruses and bacteria but also parasites, although not infectious for normal hosts are known to be predominantly transmittable to immunosuppressed individuals who show a particular susceptibility to these agents, i.e., opportunistic infectious agents (*Chapter 12*). Parasites that show this propensity for selective infectivity are referred to as opportunistic parasites and give rise to opportunistic parasitic infections associated with severe morbidity and mortality (Table 15-6). These include microsporidiosis, cyclosporiasis, and cryptosporidiosis, responsible for a protracted and debilitating illness with diarrhea. Strongyloidiasis, often asymptomatic in immune, normal individuals, can become disseminated when patients with chronic strongyloidiasis become immunosuppressed. It presents with abdominal pain, distension, shock, pulmonary and neurologic complications, and septicemia, and is potentially fatal. Eosinophilia is often present but is sometimes absent. *Pneumocystis carinii* pneumonia (PCP) and cerebral toxoplasmosis are commonly seen in immunocompromised individuals and patients with AIDS. Finally, ectoparasitic infections such as scabies and demodectic mange, uncommon in immunocompetent individuals, can be present in immunocompromised patients and need to be taken into consideration when dermatological lesions are present.

Anti-Parasitic Vaccines

Vaccine development is widely recognized as one of the most cost-effective modalities to improve public health and to protect humans against infectious diseases (*Chapter 23*). Although vaccines are well accepted and employed for the prevention of many viral and bacterial diseases, the use of vaccination to control parasitic diseases is still investigational. Although there are no commercially available anti-parasitic vaccines currently on the market, some for protozoan and helminthic diseases currently undergoing clinical trials are shown in Table 15-7.

Case Studies: Clinical Relevance

Let us now return to the case studies presented earlier and review some of the major points of the clinical presentation and how they relate to the immune system:

Case Study 1: Visceral Leishmaniasis or Kala-Azar

- Visceral leishmaniasis is a protozoan disease caused by Leishmania donovani, which is transmitted to humans by the bite of a suitable sand fly vector of the Phlebotomus species in endemic areas of the

(continued)

Case Studies: Clinical Relevance (continued)

world that include the Indian subcontinent, northern and eastern China, the Middle East, the Mediterranean basin, and eastern Africa.

- In the case report, the patient lived in an endemic area of India and reported a strong family history of kala-azar in his brothers and sisters and presented with the classical nonspecific features of the disease including fever, chills, abdominal pain, fatigue, and weight loss.
- The onset of symptoms over a one-month period was consistent with the typical pattern of an insidious subacute form of the disease, with fever, weakness, loss of appetite, pallor, and weight loss. However, the most significant clinical finding was the abdominal enlargement due to hepatosplenomegaly; as time progressed, the spleen became massively enlarged.
- The laboratory findings of anemia, leukopenia, and thrombocytopenia were consistent with parasitic invasion of the bone marrow with a myelophthisic replacement of normal blood-forming elements; the abnormal A/G ratio with 9 gm/dl of globulin documented the significant hypergammaglobulinemia that accompanies kala-azar; and the leukopenia may have contributed to a secondary pulmonary infection and pleural effusion.
- The diagnosis was established by bone marrow biopsy that revealed the presence of the typical morphology of the L. donovani organism within monocytes and macrophages.
- Injectable antimony-containing compounds are the principal medications used to treat leishmaniasis. These include meglumine antimoniate (Glucantime) and sodium stibogluconate (Pentostam). Other drugs that may be used when there is lack of response to these compounds include pentamidine and amphotericin B.
- A new oral treatment (Miltefosine) has been employed in India with promising results.

Case Study 2: Cutaneous Larva Migrans due to Ancylostoma Spp

- Cutaneous larva migrans is a distinctive serpiginous cutaneous eruption caused by a wide variety of canine and feline hookworms for which humans are accidental hosts.
- Although larva migrans is often thought of as a tropical infection, an increasing number of cases have been reported in cooler northern climates.
- In the United States, cutaneous larva migrans is most often caused by the larvae of the nematodes Ancylostoma braziliense and Ancylostoma caninum, the hookworms of wild and domestic dogs and cats. Because the larvae are located 1–2 cm ahead of the advancing edge of the lesion, biopsies rarely reveal an organism; the clinical signs are crucial for its correct diagnosis.
- Typically, humans become infected when they have prolonged contact with warm, sandy, shady areas frequented by dogs and cats. In children, as with the more systemic visceral larva migrans, exposure commonly occurs in play areas such as sandboxes where contamination with canine or feline stool is found.
- The clinical syndrome begins when larvae penetrate the skin and migrate in the epidermis. This migration is marked by tortuous, intensely pruritic, thin, elevated, erythematous tracts, 2–3 mm wide, containing serous fluid.
- The finding of a marked eosinophilia together with a typical history of a migratory intensely pruritic skin eruption suggest the diagnosis (Figure 15-15).
- A number of treatments are curative, including oral thiabendazole, topical thiabendazole, and oral ivermectin. Topical thiabendazole is an effective treatment without the side effects of oral thiabendazole.

Case Study 3: Hyperinfection by Strongyloides in an Immunocompromised Patient

- As a result of a previous liver transplant and the requirement for continuous high-dose corticosteroid immunosuppressive therapy, this immunocompromised patient developed a parasitic infection caused by Strongyloides stercoralis following cutaneous penetration by larvae of the nematode.
- This infection is potentially lethal because of its capacity to cause an overwhelming autoinfection, particularly in the immunosuppressed host.
- The organism is widely distributed in the tropics. Adult parasites reside in the gastrointestinal mucosa and produce eggs, which after hatching release rhabditiform larvae. Subsequent autoinfection occurs when a subset of these larvae convert to filariform larvae that can penetrate mucosa into the vasculature or skin. This conversion from rhabditiform to filariform larvae is enhanced in immunocompromised individuals.
- Most people are asymptomatic at the time of cutaneous penetration by larvae, although some develop a mild rash or urticaria. Eosinophilia is common. The pulmonary phase can be associated with cough, shortness of breath, wheezing, fever, and transient pulmonary infiltrates. Once the parasite reaches the

Case Studies: Clinical Relevance (continued)

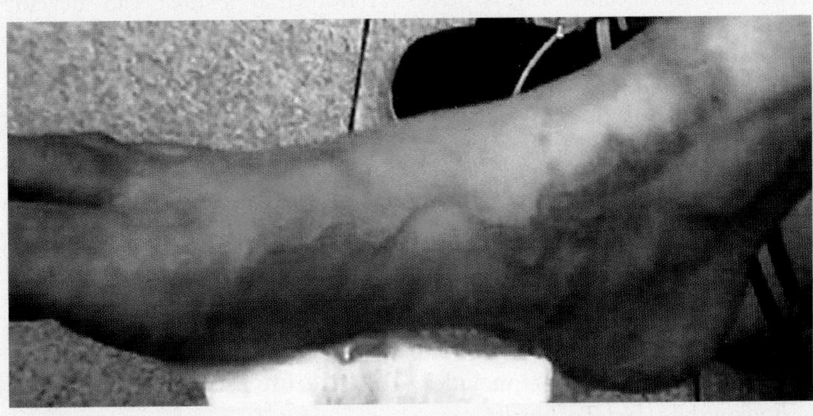

Figure 15-15. A typical cutaneous serpentine-like track (measuring approximately 12 cm) characteristic of cutaneous larva migrans on the dorsal aspect of the right foot of another patient. (Reproduced with permission from Hamat RA, Rahman AA, Osman M, et al. Cutaneous larva migrans: a neglected disease and possible association with the use of long socks. Trans R Soc Trop Med Hyg. 2010;104:170-2.)

gut, it can produce epigastric or diffuse abdominal pain, anorexia, and nausea with or without diarrhea. Alternatively, the adult worm can reside in the mucosa for years, causing no symptoms or only occasional mild gastrointestinal symptoms. Eosinophilic granulomatous enterocolitis and inflammatory mass lesions have been reported.

- The hyperinfection syndrome can occur when an infected individual becomes immunocompromised. Some patients present with predominant pulmonary symptoms and can progress to the acute respiratory distress syndrome (ARDS). Others may present with intestinal symptoms.
- Concurrent polymicrobial bacterial infections often occur as a result of concomitant invasion of bacteria attached to the surface of the filariform larvae. This facilitates entry of bacterial intestinal organisms and is a major cause of sepsis; multiorgan failure, meningitis, peritonitis, and endocarditis have been reported and are associated with a high rate of mortality.
- Unlike other nematodes, eggs are not detected in stool, and the diagnosis requires detection of larvae in stool. However, since 25 percent of patients do not have larvae in random stool samples, multiple stool specimens should be obtained.
- The diagnosis was established by a biopsy of the small intestine that demonstrated sections of a small helminth and helminth larvae within the mucosa and the presence of small larvae in several subsequent stool examinations.
- Complete eradication is necessary to eliminate the potential risk for reactivation. Recent studies using a single dose of oral Ivermectin (200 μg/kg) have shown that this regimen is the best treatment for uncomplicated or chronic strongyloidiasis. Ivermectin, however, is active against the intestinal worms only.
- Since recurrent infection from migrating larvae can also develop, a second dose of Ivermectin is recommended after two weeks of initial treatment. Fulminant disseminated disease requires repeated doses on days 2, 15, and 16. Alternatively, two to three courses of thiabendazole can be used as a second choice for the treatment of the hyperinfection syndrome. Mortality rates nonetheless remain high.

Key Points

- Parasites that infect the human are generally classified as unicellular protozoans and multicellular metazoans (helminths).
- These two major groups of parasites are generally responsible for a heterogeneous collection of chronic infections in the host, which are countered by an equally heterogeneous variety of immunologic responses involving the innate and adaptive immune systems.
- To address infections caused by parasites, certain components of either the innate or adaptive immune responses target various phases of the parasite during its life cycle.

- Protozoans can be further classified according to the location of the infection into (1) intracellular protozoans, (2) blood and intracellular forms, (3) blood borne, and (4) intestinal protozoans.
- Protozoans such as *Plasmodium*, *Leishmania*, and *Trypanosoma* produce infections in the human after their transmission from a variety of vectors, or following their ingestion, as in the case of *Toxoplasma*, *Giardia*, and *Entamoeba*.
- Helminths have been divided into two groups: (1) flatworms, which comprise both flukes (trematoda, e.g., *Schistosoma*) and tapeworms (cestoda like taenias), and (2) roundworms (nematodes) that include ascarids, pinworms, hookworms, and *Trichinella*.
- Infections caused by helminths found in the intestine, in tissues, or at both sites are associated with a prominent adaptive immune response characterized by elevated serum IgE levels and eosinophilia.
- Innate immunity plays an important role in parasitic infections through the presence of phagocyte sensors like PRRs that react with conserved moieties, i.e., pathogen-associated molecular patterns in the parasites.
- The PAMPs can trigger dichotomous responses (i.e., tolerance or inflammation) depending on the particular PRR that the parasite engages.
- Phagocytosis can be potentiated by the effect of both antibody and complement-associated opsonins as well as by adaptive immune cytokine systems that promote cytolysis of the parasite, as in the case of intracellular parasitic infections.
- Although humoral immunity generally protects the host against extracellular parasitic forms and cellular immunity against intracellular stages, there is considerable overlap in the immune response(s) directed against a single parasite; the host immune anti-parasitic protective mechanisms are therefore heterogeneous and depend on many factors, including the stage of the parasite, the genetic susceptibility of the host, the age of first host exposure, and a variety of mechanisms of immunologic evasion employed by the parasite.
- The mechanisms of immunologic evasion include antigenic variation of the parasite, resistance to phagocytic uptake and lysis, intracellular immune modulation, and molecular mimicry.
- One hallmark of the immune response against parasitic infections is the phenomenon called premunition. This event implies the relative immunity against further colonization and severe infection that a host can develop when maintaining small number of parasites in the intestinal mucosa.
- Chronic parasitic infections potentiate the occurrence of different immunologic complications in the host, including hypersensitivity reactions, as well as other adverse responses, including hyperviscosity syndrome, obstruction of blood and lymphatic vessels, cancer, and blindness.

Study Questions/Critical Thinking

1. During persistent parasitic infections, the process that benefits the host from further parasitism by its capacity to express a low quantity of pro-inflammatory and anti-inflammatory cytokines is called:
   1. Immune tolerance
   2. Immunomodulation
   3. Premunition
   4. Antigenic variation
   5. Evasion
2. Each of the following are protozoan infections that can be eliminated by humoral immunity, EXCEPT:
   1. Malaria
   2. Trypanosomiasis
   3. Visceral Leishmaniasis
   4. Amebiasis
   5. Giardiasis
3. The most common complications of congenital toxoplasmosis are listed below, EXCEPT:
   1. Chorioretinitis
   2. Hydrocephalus
   3. Microcephaly
   4. Intracranial calcification
   5. Cyclical fever pattern
4. Each of the following are TRUE statements concerning mechanisms of immunity against malaria, EXCEPT:
   1. Antibodies block invasion of sporozoites into liver cells
   2. IFN-γ and CD8 T cells inhibit parasite development in hepatocytes
   3. Protective antibodies prevent sequestration of infected erythrocytes by preventing binding to adhesion molecules on the vascular endothelium
   4. IFN-γ activates macrophages to enhance phagocytoses of intra-erythrocyte located parasites and free merozoites

5. Antibody neutralization of glycosylphosphatidylinositol promotes induction of the inflammatory cytokine cascade

5. Each of the following are mechanisms by which parasites evade phagocytosis by macrophages, EXCEPT:

   1. Formation of a parasitophorous vacuole
   2. Glycocalyx coat shedding
   3. Synthesis of cysteine proteinases
   4. Presence of gp60 and 63 proteins
   5. Production of complement proteases

Suggested Reading

Anderson CF, Stumholfer JS, Hunter CA, et al. IL-27 regulates IL-10 and IL-17 from CD4+ cells in nonhealing leishmania major infection. J Immunol. 2009; 183: 4619–27.

Barbieri CL. Immunology of canine leishmaniasis. Parasite Immunol. 2006; 28: 329–37.

Barry JD, McCulloch R. Antigenic variation in trypanosomes: enhanced phenotypic variation in a eukaryotic parasite. Adv Parasitol. 2001; 49: 1–70.

Borkow G, Bentwich Z. HIV and helminth co-infection: is deworming necessary? Parasite Immunol. 2006; 28: 605–12.

Brodskyn C, de Oliveira CI, Barral A, et al. Vaccines in leishmaniasis: advances in th last five years. Expert Rev Vaccines. 2003; 2: 705–17.

Brooker S, Bethony J, Hotez PJ. Human hookworm infection in the 21st century. Adv Parasitol. 2004; 58: 197–288.

Carvallho EM, Bastos LS, Araujo MI. Worms and allergy. Parasite Immunol. 2006; 28: 525–34.

de Spilva NR, et al. Soil-transmitted helminth infections: updating the global picture. Trends Parasitol. 2003; 19: 547–51.

Eckmann L. Mucosal defences against giardia. Parasite Immunol. 2003; 25: 259–70.

Eisenberg JN, Lei X, Hubbard AH, et al. the role of disease transmission and conferred immunity in outbreaks: analysis of the 1993 cryptosporidium outbreak in Milwaukee, Wisconsin. Am J Epidemiol. 2005; 161: 62–72.

Garside P, Kennedy MW, Wakelin D, et al. Immunopathology of intestinal helminth infection. Parasite Immunol. 2000; 22: 605–12.

Gazzinelli RT, Denkers EY. Protozoan encounters with Toll-like receptor signaling pathways: implications for host parasitism. Nat Rev Immunol. 2006; 6: 895–906.

Ghosh M, Bandyopadhyay S Present status of anti-leishmanial vaccines. Mol Cell Biochem. 2003; 253: 199–205.

Girard MP, Reed ZH, Friede M, et al. A review of human vaccine research and development: malaria. Vaccine. 2007; 25: 1567–80.

Gramicca M, Gradoni L. The current status of zoonotic leishmaniasis and approaches to disease control. Int J Parasitol. 2005; 35: 1169–80.

Hamat RA, Rahman AA, Osman M, et al. Cutaneous larva migrans: a neglected disease and possible association with the use of long socks. T Roy Soc Trop Med H. 2010; 104: 170–2.

Harnett W, Harnett MM. Molecular basis of worm-induced immunomodulation. Parasite Immunol. 2006; 28: 535–43.

Hodgkin J. Dissecting worm immunity. Nat Immunol. 2004; 5: 471–2.

Hokke CH, Deelder AM. Schistosome glycoconjugates in host-parasite interplay. Glycoconjugate J. 2001; 18: 573–87.

Holland MJ, Harcus YM, Balic A, et al. Th2 induction by nippostrongylus secreted antigens in mice deficient in B cells, eosinophils or MHC class I-related receptors. Immunol Lett. 2005; 96: 93–101.

Hotez PJ, Bethony J, Bottazzi ME, et al. New technologies for the control of human hookworm infection. Trends Parasitol. 2006; 22: 327–31.

Hotez PJ, Brooker S, Bethony JM, et al. Hookworm infection. N Eng J Med. 2004; 351: 799–807.

Jones J, Lopez A, Wilson M. Congenital toxoplasmosis. Am Fam Physician. 2003; 15: 2131–8.

Kariuki TM, Farah IO. Resistance to re-infection after exposure to normal and attenuated schistosome parasites in the baboon model. Parasite Immunol. 2005; 27: 281–8.

Khamesipour A, Rafati S, Davoudi N, et al. Leishmaniasis vaccine candidates for development: a global overview. Indian J Med Res. 2006; 123: 423–38.

Maizels RM, Balic A, Gomez-Escobar N, et al. Helminth parasites—masters of regulation. Immunol Rev. 2004; 201: 89–116.

Maizels RM, Yazdanbakhsh M. Immune regulation by helminth parasites: cellular and molecular mechanisms. Nat Rev Immunol. 2003; 3: 733–44.

Mansfield JM, Paulnock DM. Regulation of innate and acquired immunity in African trypanosomiasis. Parasite Immunol. 2005; 27: 361–71.

Matuschewski K. Vaccine development against malaria. Curr Opin Immunol. 2006; 18: 449–57.

Mauel J. Vaccination against leishmania infections. Curr Drug Targets Immune Endocri Metabol Disord. 2002; 2: 201–26.

Meeusen EN. Immunology of helminth infections, with special reference to immunopathology. Vet Parasitol. 1999; 84: 259–73.

Melby PC. Recent developments in leishmaniasis. Curr Opin Infect Dis. 2002; 15: 485–90.

Mountford AP. Immunological aspects of schistosmiasis. Parasite Immunol. 2005; 27: 243–6.

Pearce EJ, MacDonald AS. The immunobiology of schistosomiasis. Nat Rev Immunol. 2002; 2: 499–511.

Pepin J, Meda HA. The epidemiology and control of human African trypanosomiasis. Adv in Parasitol. 2001; 49: 71–132.

Reed SG, Campos-Neto A. Vaccines for parasitic and bacterial diseases. Curr Opin Immunol. 2003; 15: 456–60.

Reed ZH, Friede M, Kieny MP. Malaria vaccine development: progress and challenges. Curr Mol Med. 2006; 6: 231–45.

Sacks D, Noben-Trauth N. The immunology of susceptibility and resistance to leishmania major in mice. Nat Rev Immunol. 2002; 2: 845–58.

Sacks D, Sher A. Evasion of innate immunity by parasitic protozoa. Nat Rev Immunol. 2002; 3: 104–1047.

Sacks D, Sher A. Evasion of innate immunity by parasitic protozoa. Nat Immunol. 2002; 3: 1041–7.

Shinkai K, Mohrs M, Locksley RM. Helper T cells regulate type-2 innate immunity in vivo. Nature. 2002; 420: 825–9.

Soulsby EH. The evasion of the immune response and immunological unresponsiveness: parasitic helminth infections. Immunol Lett. 1987; 16: 315–20.

Spiegelberg HL. Structure and function of Fc receptors for IgE on lymphocytes, monocytes, and macrophages. Adv Immunol. 1984; 25: 61–88.

Stevenson MM, Riley EM. Innate immunity to malaria. Nat Rev Immunol. 2004; 4: 169–80.

Taylor MD, LeGoff L, Harris A, et al. Removal of regulatory T cell activity reverses hyporesponsiveness and leads to filarial parasite clearance in vivo. J Immunol. 2005; 174: 4924–33.

Section Three

CLINICAL APPLICATIONS OF IMMUNOLOGY

Chapter 16

Immune Deficiency Disorders

Steven M. Holland, MD
Joseph A. Bellanti, MD

LEARNING OBJECTIVES

When you have completed this chapter, you should be able to:

- Recognize the differences between the primary immunodeficiencies and those secondary to other diseases
- Identify general features of the molecular and phenotypic characteristics of the primary immunodeficiencies
- Classify the key molecular defects responsible for immunodeficiency disorders affecting various components of the innate and adaptive immune systems
- Utilize the Online Mendelian Inheritance in Man (OMIM®) knowledge base of human genes and genetic disorders for more detailed genetic and clinical information concerning the primary immunodeficiencies
- Explain how the molecular defects seen in the primary immunodeficiencies contribute to the clinical manifestations of the disorders
- Correlate the molecular basis of these disorders with the most current forms of therapy
- Utilize the knowledge you have gained not only for the recognition of these rare disorders, but also for the management of more commonly encountered diseases that present with recurrent infection, autoimmunity, or malignancy

Case Study

An eight-year-old boy was well until the age of four years, when he developed pneumonia secondary to rubeola. The birth, developmental, and family histories were normal and his only male sibling was well. At four and a half years, the patient experienced chills, fever, and pain in the left knee. Physical examination was unremarkable except for a few scattered petechiae on both arms and tenderness of the left knee. The white blood cell (WBC) count was 16,400/mm^3 with 88 percent neutrophils; blood culture findings were normal. The pain and fever disappeared with administration of penicillin.

Two weeks later, fever recurred. Pneumonia was diagnosed and sulfadiazine was administered. Four days later, mumps and gastroenteritis developed and the boy was admitted to Walter Reed Hospital under the care of Colonel Ogden C. Bruton (Figure 16-1). The patient experienced a prolonged febrile course complicated by recurrent otitis media (OM). The throat, blood, and ear cultures were positive for type 14 pneumococcus (*S. pneumoniae*).

The child improved after 10 days of treatment with penicillin. Another episode of OM developed two months later. Two days afterward, fever and left shoulder pain developed. The WBC count was 25,000/mm^3 with 91 percent neutrophils. Antibiotics were again administered, and six months later fever recurred and type 33 pneumococci were recovered from the bloodstream.

After convalescence, a tonsillectomy and adenoidectomy were performed in the hope of decreasing the number of infections. During the next four years, however, the patient experienced 15 episodes of high fever resulting from sepsis which yielded pneumococci from culture on seven occasions. He also experienced two episodes of pneumonia, three episodes of OM, two episodes of mumps ("epidemic parotitis"), and a single episode of "herpes zoster" (Figure 16-2). Prophylactic sulfadiazine and pneumococcal vaccine were ineffective in controlling infection. Entirely unusual, however, was the striking occurrence of the same pneumococcal serotype during subsequent bouts of infection, i.e., type 33, type 6 (Figure 16-2).

Case Study (continued)

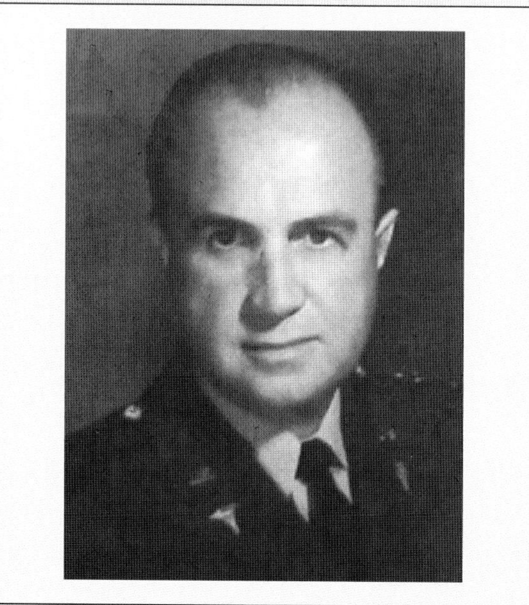

Figure 16-1. Colonel Ogden C. Bruton (1925–1994).

At the time of hospitalization at Walter Reed Army Hospital in 1946, the hospital had recently acquired a then-newly developed instrument for the free boundary electrophoretic measurement of serum proteins by the Tiselius method (*Chapter 6*). Using this methodology, analysis of a serum specimen from the patient was found to be completely lacking in the gamma globulin peak. Based upon this finding, Colonel Bruton initiated replacement therapy with monthly subcutaneous injections of gamma globulin (Cohn Fraction II) following which the child improved dramatically with cessation of his recurrent infections (*Chapter 11*).

This is the first recorded case of X-linked agammaglobulinemia (XLA) or Bruton's agammaglobulinemia described by an astute clinician and which demonstrates many of the major characteristics of this disorder, including male sex, early onset, recurrent high grade pyogenic infections, ineffectiveness of most forms of conventional therapy, and the favorable response to injected gamma globulin.

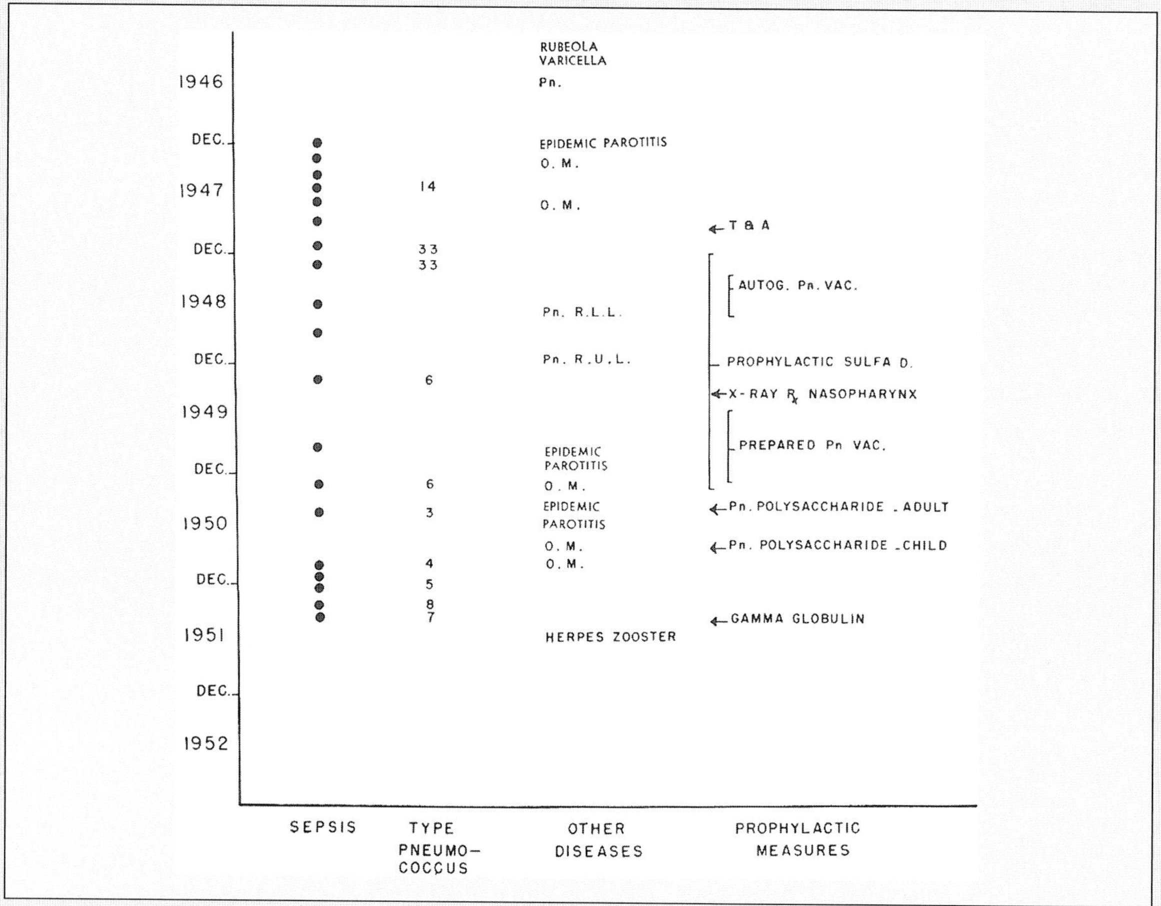

Figure 16-2. Chart published by Bruton showing his original observations of recurrent infection due to the same type of pneumococcus in his patient with agammaglobulinemia. (Reproduced with permission from Bruton, OC, Agammaglobulinemia. Pediatrics 1952;9:722.)

Throughout the text of this chapter, references are made to the Online Mendelian Inheritance in Man (OMIM®), a comprehensive, timely, and authoritative knowledge base of human genes and genetic disorders. Created by Dr. Victor McKusick in the 1960s and published as Mendelian Inheritance in Man in 12 editions, the final published in 1998, OMIM is available online at ***http://www.omim.org/*** or can be accessed by the following quick response (QR) code:

It is continuously updated, derived from the published biomedical literature, and is written and edited by staff and faculty at Johns Hopkins University with input from scientists and clinicians around the world. As of January 19, 2011, OMIM comprised 20,306 entries describing more than 13,600 genes and about 7,000 disorders or traits. OMIM is written as free-text descriptions of genes and disorders, but its structured entries have numerous organized links to genomic, genetic, clinical, and animal model resources. OMIM citations are listed in this chapter with each of the primary immune deficiency disorders to provide the reader with the most current tools to access additional information on these complex disorders.

Introduction to Immune Deficiency Disorders

The immune deficiency conditions are a group of disorders that result from one or more abnormalities of the immune system and that manifest clinically as an increased susceptibility to infection. This group of human diseases was ushered in by a single seminal observation made by a clinician who carefully studied a child with recurrent respiratory infections and who later documented the first immune deficiency disorder in the human. In 1952, Colonel Ogden Bruton (Figure 16-1), while searching for the reasons why a young child hospitalized at Walter Reed Army Hospital in Washington, DC, was suffering from repeated and life-threatening infections, found that the child was unable to synthesize specific antibodies and, later, that the child's serum lacked gamma globulin. Further, the child's susceptibility to infection was reversed by the administration of serum gamma globulin. This landmark discovery represents a consummate example of clinical research that led not only to the current explosive molecular and phenotypic dissection of the immunodeficiencies that are described in this chapter, but that also set the stage for the subsequent development of clinical immunology as we know it today.

General Considerations

X-linked agammaglobulinemia (**XLA**) represents the first of over 150 entities that have come to be known as the primary immunodeficiency disorders, which will be described in greater detail in this chapter. Although these are rare, they have been useful in unraveling many of the molecular pathways that govern both the innate and the adaptive immune systems and that have provided new diagnostic and therapeutic modalities for the treatment of a wide variety of allergic (*Chapter 18*), autoimmune disorders (*Chapter 19*), and malignant diseases (*Chapters 20* and *21*).

In addition to the primary immunodeficiencies, which have been observed mainly in children, there exist a more frequently encountered group of secondary immunodeficiencies that occur both in children and adults and that are the consequence of another disorder or underlying condition, infectious disease, genetic disorder or chromosomal abnormality, age, surgery or trauma, lymphoproliferative malignancies, or treatment with immunosuppressive agents that also result in an increased susceptibility to infection. Shown in Table 16-1 is a list of some of the more frequently encountered secondary causes of immunodeficiency.

Developmental Background

Because most of the primary immunodeficiencies result from abnormalities in cellular maturation emanating from known molecular lesions in signaling pathways, transcription molecules, or cytokine systems, it may be useful to frame these defects according to the normal ontogenetic development of the immune system described in Chapter 2 and that are shown schematically in Figure 16-3. The fetal bone marrow provides stem cells that have the potential to progressively differentiate into: (1) a hematopoietic lineage that contains individual precursor cells that

Table 16-1. Some of the more frequently encountered secondary causes of immunodeficiency

Cause	Example
Another disease or underlying condition	Uremia Diabetes mellitus Malnutrition and vitamin and mineral deficiencies Protein-losing enteropathies Nephrotic syndrome Myotonic syndrome Sickle cell disease Allergic diseases and asthma Autoimmune diseases Stress Pregnancy
Infectious diseases	HIV infection/AIDS Viral exanthema (measles, varicella) Cytomegalovirus infection Epstein-Barr virus (EBV) infection Congenital rubella Bacterial infection Mycobacterial, fungal, or parasitic disease
Genetic disorder or chromosomal abnormality	Cystic fibrosis Down syndrome
Age	Premature and newborn Elderly
Surgery or trauma	Splenectomy Burns Anesthesia
Lymphoproliferative malignancies	Leukemias Lymphomas Multiple myeloma
Treatment with immunosuppressive agents	Radiation therapy Immunosuppressive drugs Corticosteroids Antilymphocyte or antithymocyte globulin Biologic response modifiers (anticytokine monoclonal antibodies or receptor binding agents)

give rise to the erythrocytes, granulocytes, monocytes, and platelets; and (2) a lymphopoietic lineage that contains precursor cells that give rise to T lymphocytes, B lymphocytes, and natural killer (**NK**) cells.

Mononuclear cells (monocytes) migrate to the lung, liver, spleen, brain, and peripheral lymph nodes where they differentiate into specialized macrophages (e.g., alveolar cells, Kupffer cells, and microglial cells) capable of antigen uptake, processing, and antigen presentation to T lymphocytes (*Chapter 7*). Lymphoid precursors are influenced by cytokines as well as a variety of hormonal factors that cause them to differentiate into mature T lymphocytes (e.g., thymic hormones) or B lymphocytes. Although the hormonal source of B cell maturation in the chicken is known to be derived from the bursa of Fabricius, the source of only some of the factors in the bone marrow responsible for B cell differentiation is known in the human (*Chapter 6*).

T cells may be recognized by the presence of the T cell receptor (**TCR**) as well as specific membrane proteins referred to as cluster of differentiation (**CD**) molecules recognized by specific monoclonal antibodies which differentiate lymphocytes into two major families, CD4+ T helper and CD8+ T cytotoxic cells (*Chapters 1* and *7*). These CD surface proteins on T cells change during maturation. For example, they appear and then disappear as the cell matures from a stem cell to a fully developed T lymphocyte, e.g., double negative CD4−/CD8−, to a double positive CD4+/CD8+, to a specialized mature T cell bearing a single marker, i.e., CD4+ or CD8+ single positive T cells, which emigrate from the thymus into the peripheral tissues (*Chapters 2* and *7*). B cell differentiation shows similar changes of cell surface proteins with maturation (*Chapter 2* and *6*). Pre-B cells have no surface immunoglobulin but later develop surface IgM and IgD immunoglobulins and then lose these as the cell differentiates into fully developed B cells bearing IgM, IgG, IgA, or IgE.

In animal systems, removal of the thymus (e.g., in the mouse) or bursa (e.g., in the chicken) during the earliest stages of development produces characteristic immunologic defects, i.e., profound deficiencies of cell-mediated immunity or in antibody production, respectively. If both organs are removed, a combined immune deficiency results. These experimental studies in the animal have served as important models for counterpart primary immunodeficiencies in the human.

Until recently, it has been difficult to place the developmental origin of the NK cell in the developmental scheme of monocytes, myeloid cells, T cells, or B cells. NK cells share some surface membrane characteristics of both T lymphocytes and monocytes. It is now recognized that there exists a "natural" population of NK cells and an induced population of NK cells bearing an invariant T cell receptor that are referred to as iNKT cells (*Chapter 3*). These cells also play an important role in killing of cancer cells (*Chapter 20*) and viral-infected cells (*Chapter 13*).

The Primary Immunodeficiencies

The in-depth study of the primary immunodeficiencies is of extraordinary importance not only because

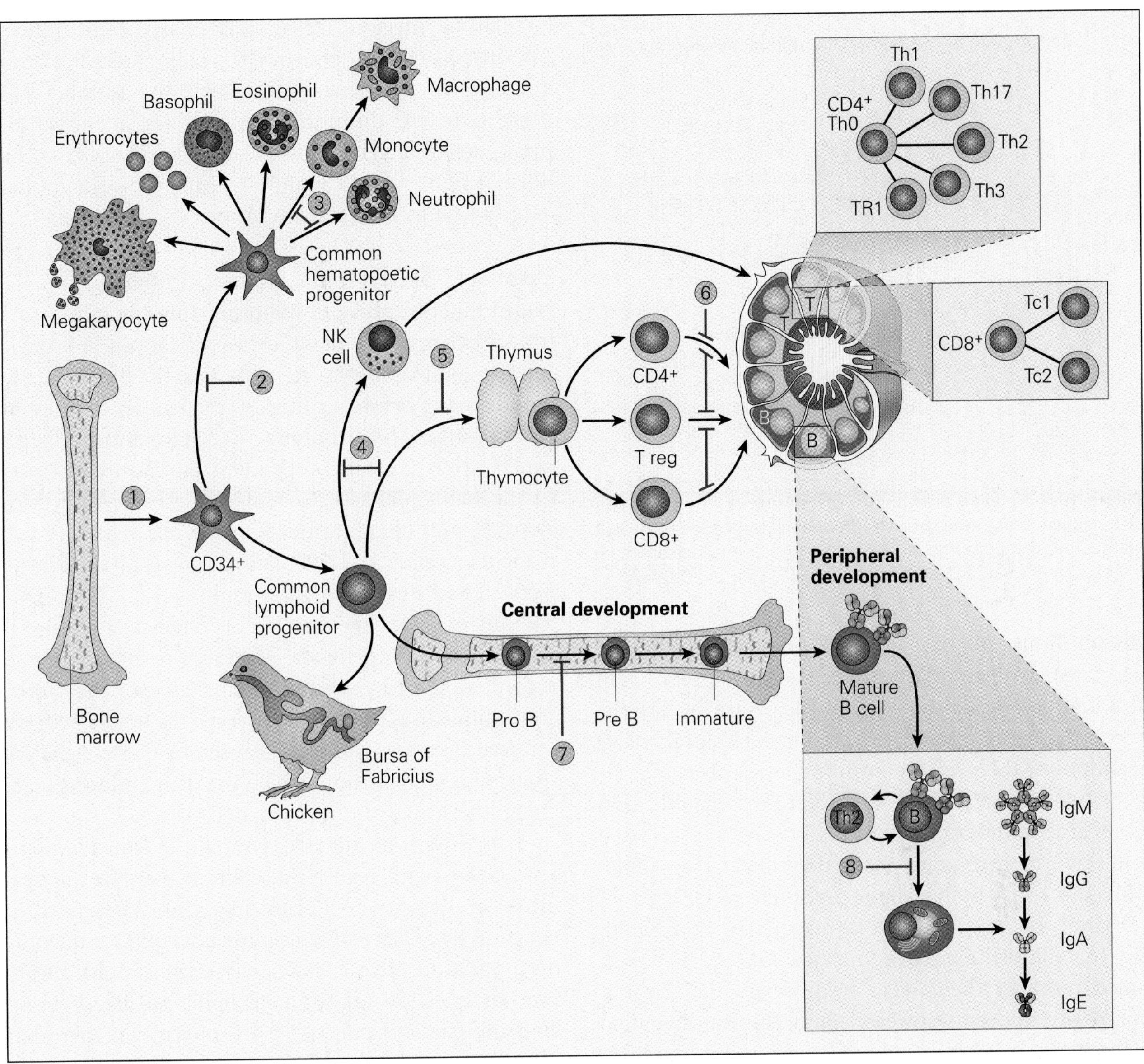

Figure 16-3. **Schematic representation of points in immunologic development at which dysfunction or deficiency can occur in the various primary immunodeficiencies.** 1. Reticular dysgenesis; 2. Aplastic anemia; 3. Chronic granulomatous disease; 4. Severe combined immune deficiency (SCID); 5. DiGeorge syndrome; 6. Coronin-1 A deficiency; 7. X-linked agammaglobulinemia (XLA); 8. Common variable immunodeficiency (CVID).

affected patients need care, but also because the infections seen in these patients are not quite like those in normal subjects. Moreover, the molecular and phenotypic dissection of immunodeficiencies shows genes and pathways critical in the control of environmental exposures that have been important drivers of evolution. Scientifically, fundamental mechanisms of action are most clearly defined in genetic immunodeficiencies, but difficult to sort out in otherwise healthy people. Since research in the field of the primary immunodeficiencies is moving extremely rapidly, this chapter includes areas that are inherently dynamic and, therefore, should be regarded as a set of signposts, not petrified truths.

White blood cells (**WBCs**) come in two main types, lymphoid (T, B, and NK) and myeloid (neutrophils, eosinophils, basophils, and monocytes/macrophages), each with their respective host defenses, and relatively specific and reproducible patterns of susceptibility to infection. Therefore, the study of genetic immunodeficiencies is fundamentally about understanding the mechanisms of resistance to infection (*Chapters 12–15*). The immunodeficiencies have been classically divided into: (1) the phagocytic cell deficiencies, (2) the complement deficiencies, (3) the antibody deficiencies, (4) the cell-mediated deficiencies, and (5) the combined cellular and antibody deficiencies. Shown in Figure 16-4 are the relative frequency

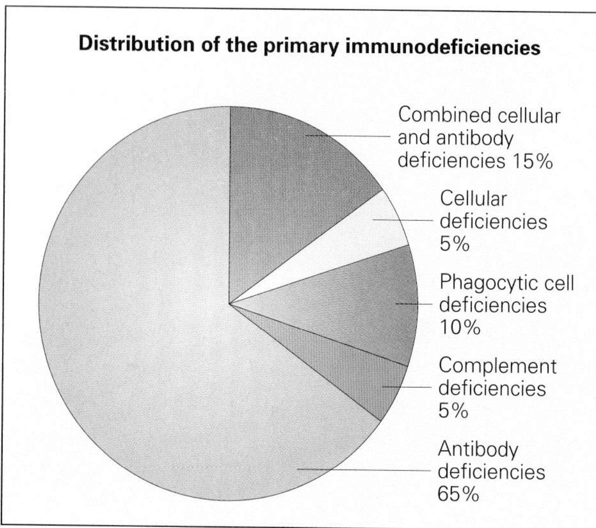

Figure 16-4. Relative distribution of the primary immunodeficiencies according to a more traditional classification. (Adapted with permission from Stiehm ER, editor. Immunologic disorders in infants and children. 5th ed. Philadelphia: Elsevier, Inc.; 2004.)

distributions of the primary immunodeficiencies according to this classification. As can be seen from this figure, the antibody deficiencies are by far the most frequently diagnosed. From a comprehensive standpoint, the primary immunodeficiencies may be classified using a more contemporary classification according to the component cell type or transcription molecule or cytokine system they affect (see Tables 16A-1 to 16A-8 in the Annex to this chapter).

Clinically, immune defects have been thought to be the almost exclusive purview of pediatricians, since most of these were traditionally first recognized in children. However, with the improvement and greater availability of easily administered antibiotics and antifungal agents, many of the milder cases are being surreptitiously, unknowingly, but successfully treated in the outpatient setting, only to present later in life, even into adulthood, with slightly different clinical manifestations than those classically described. Therefore, immunodeficiency is no longer the isolated province of the pediatric immunologist, but must be considered in many of the presentations of infection and inflammatory complications encountered in adults.

Abnormalities of Number and/or Function of Phagocytic Cells

Cells of the phagocytic cell system include circulating monocytes and tissue macrophages as well as circulating myeloid cells, particularly neutrophils. Abnormalities of phagocytic cells include both quantitative deficiencies in which the numbers of these cells are diminished as well as a variety of functional deficiencies where the numbers may be normal but they manifest intrinsic functional defects (Table 16A-1 in the Annex).

Disorders of Myeloid Cells and Defects

Mature neutrophils develop in the bone marrow from the myeloid stem cell over about 14 days. Mature neutrophils spend only 6 to 10 hours in the bloodstream before exiting by diapedesis to sites of inflammation. Neutrophilia (> 7,500 neutrophils/μL in adults) is typically dependent on causes extrinsic to the neutrophils (e.g., acute or chronic infection, steroids, and epinephrine). On the other hand, neutropenia (mild: < 1,500 neutrophils/μL, moderate: 1,500–1,000 neutrophils/μL, and severe: < 500 neutrophils/μL) can be intrinsic or extrinsic to neutrophils or their progenitors. Although neutropenia can accompany many immunodeficiencies, the most common causes include infections, particularly those induced by viruses, or those caused by Gram-negative bacteria as well as those which are drug induced (e.g., chemotherapy, immune mediated).

A myeloid immune defect should be considered in any patient with recurrent, severe bacterial or fungal infection. Unusual organisms (e.g., *Burkholderia cepacia* complex, *Chromobacterium violaceum*) or uncommon locations (e.g., visceral abscess) should always prompt questions about neutrophil integrity. Severe viral and parasitic infections are not typically increased in patients with phagocytic cell defects, and should prompt interest in disorders involving lymphocytes.

The structural and molecular composition of normal neutrophils contains many morphologic and biochemical components involved in the uptake and digestion of foreign substances (*Chapter 5*). Shown in Figure 16-5 is a schematic representation of the normal intracellular primary and secondary granule contents involved in microbicidal activity.

Severe Congenital Neutropenia (MIM ID #202700)

Severe congenital neutropenia (**SCN**) comprises a heterogeneous group of disorders with variable inheritance patterns that share bone marrow maturation arrest at the promyelocyte or myelocyte stage and severe chronic neutropenia (< 200 neutrophils/μL) (Table 16A-1 in the Annex). Some are associated with

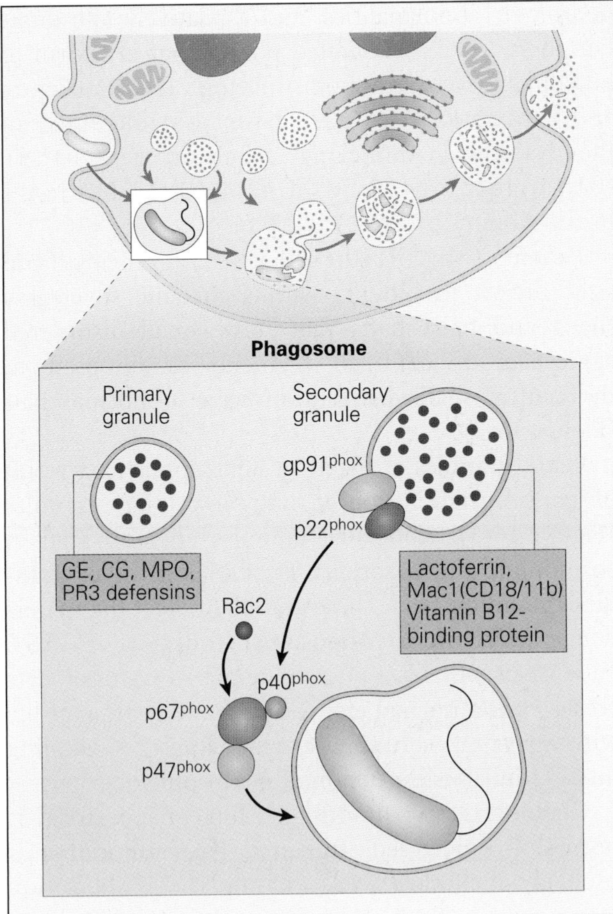

Figure 16-5. Schematic representation of a normal neutrophil. Primary granules arise early in neutrophil ontogeny in the bone marrow and contain numerous enzymes, including neutrophil or granulocyte elastase (GE) and cathepsin G (CG), embedded in a glycocalyx, as well as proteinase 3 (PR3), myeloperoxidase (MPO), and defensins. Secondary granules arise later in bone marrow development and contain lactoferrin and vitamin B12 binding protein, as well as membrane-bound proteins such as Mac-1 (CD18/CD11b) and the cytochrome b complex (gp91^{phox} and p22^{phox}). P47^{phox} and p67^{phox} are joined together in the cytoplasm but not phosphorylated. Neutrophils typically ingest bacteria, fungi, and complex particles into a phagosome, which then serves as the main locus for granule discharge, keeping the concentration of discharged proteins high and exposure of the cell to toxic degradation products minimal.

an increased susceptibility to acute myeloid leukemia. Approximately 30 percent of cases of severe congenital neutropenia have dominant mutations in neutrophil elastase (ELA2, 19p13.3). Surprisingly, mutations in this same gene also cause cyclic neutropenia. The clinical manifestations of SCN appear promptly after birth: 50 percent are symptomatic in the first month, and 90 percent within six months. Omphalitis, upper and lower respiratory tract infections, and skin and liver abscesses are common. Treatment with subcutaneous granulocyte colony-stimulating factor (**G-CSF**) (5 μg/kg/d; range 1–120 μg/kg) has dramatically reduced infections and hospitalizations and increased survival (*Chapter 9*). Somatic mutations in the G-CSF receptor occur in patients with ELA2 mutations and are associated with myeloid leukemias. An elastase-interacting protein, growth factor independent-1 (GFI-1, MIM #600871), acts as a repressor of elastase production and so also can cause SCN. Dominant GFI-1 mutations that blocked elastase repression have been associated with neutropenia and abnormal lymphocyte function. An X-linked form of severe congenital neutropenia (**XLN**) is due to discrete mutations in the Wiskott-Aldrich syndrome protein (**WASP**).

Cyclic Neutropenia/Cyclic Hematopoiesis (MIM ID #162800)

Cyclic neutropenia is an autosomal dominant disease characterized by regular cyclic fluctuations in all hematopoietic lineages, but symptoms are only due to decreased numbers of neutrophils. In affected patients, neutrophil counts cycle about every 21 days (ranging from 14 to 36 days); severe neutropenia (< 200/μL) usually lasts 3–10 days. Most patients become symptomatic in early childhood and present with aphthous oral ulcers, gingivitis, lymphadenopathy, pharyngitis, tonsillitis, or skin lesions. Permanent teeth may be lost due to chronic gingivitis and periapical abscess. Bone marrow aspirates during neutropenia show maturation arrest at the myelocyte stage, or, less frequently, bone marrow hypoplasia. Administration of G-CSF elevates neutrophil counts in cyclic neutropenia and dramatically improves quality of life and survival. Interestingly, the frequency of infections and hospitalizations appears to diminish with age.

Kostmann's Syndrome (MIM ID #610738)

In 1956, Kostmann described a Swedish kindred with severe congenital neutropenia inherited in an autosomal recessive pattern. The absolute neutrophil count (**ANC**) in affected patients is characteristically less than 200/mm^3, which results in an increased susceptibility to frequent bacterial infections. A subset of patients with Kostmann's syndrome has been identified whose symptoms result from deficiency of elastase (Table 16A-1 in the Annex). Mutations in the granulocyte colony-stimulating factor receptor (CSF3R) gene have been identified in patients with Kostmann's syndrome, but these are thought to be acquired defects. Recently, the genetic basis for Kostmann's syndrome has been identified in the original family and in a large Kurdish cohort as a recessive mutation in the HAX-1 (1q21.3) gene, a genetic locus that encodes a protein with anti-apoptotic function.

P14 Deficiency (MIM ID #610389)

Another form of congenital neutropenia seen in patients with p14 deficiency is an autosomal recessive disorder with ANCs below 500/μL, partial albinism, short stature, and B cell and cytotoxic T cell deficiency. Protein p14 is required for the proper biogenesis of endosomes and the subcellular relocation of mitogen-activated protein kinase (**MAPK**) signaling to late endosomes.

Some Additional Rare Conditions Affecting Myeloid Cells

There are a few rare genetic conditions affecting myeloid cells, which include patients with metabolic defects affecting either the enzyme glucose-6-phospatase or the Wiskott-Aldrich syndrome (**WAS**) gene (Table 16A-1 in the Annex). The first two conditions are inherited in an AR fashion and affect either the synthesis of the glucose-6-phospatase or its transporter, i.e., (1) patients with neutropenia with cardiac and urogenital malformations caused by an AR mutation affecting the gene G6PC3 and its product glucose-6-phospatase and enhances apoptosis, and (2) patients with glycogen storage disease type 1b caused by a mutation of the transporter 1 of glucose-6-phospatase, which results in the same phenotype, respectively. A third group of defects of myeloid cells referred to as X-linked neutropenia/myelodysplasia is caused by X-linked inherited gain-of-function mutation of the WAS gene, a regulator of actin cytoskeleton, resulting in loss of autoinhibition and neutropenia and monocytopenia. Another rare inherited myeloid cell defect affecting patients' mental retardation and short stature is the AD condition, β-actin deficiency, in which the ACTB gene is mutated, resulting in deficiency of motility.

Defects of Granule Formation and Content

Chediak-Higashi Syndrome (MIM ID #214500)

The Chediak-Higashi syndrome (**CHS**) is a rare multisystem autosomal recessive disease with oculocutaneous albinism, frequent bacterial infections, neurologic abnormalities, and a relatively late onset lymphoma-like "accelerated phase" that is a form of hemophagocytic lymphohistiocytosis (**HLH**) (Figure 16-6). Mutations for CHS have been identified in the lysosomal trafficking regulator gene, LYST (CHS1; 1q42.1-q42.2; MIM #214500) (Table 16A-1 in the Annex).

Patients with CHS have hair color ranging from light brown to blonde, with a metallic silver-gray sheen and hair shafts that show small disordered aggregates of clumped pigment, as opposed to the central shaft distribution seen in normal hair (Figure 16-7).

Giant granules are seen in neutrophils as a result of inappropriate fusion of multiple primary granules (Figure 16-8). Abnormal granules are also seen in eosinophils and basophils, as well as in other granule-containing cells. These granules reflect the underlying defect in the lysosomal transporter, LYST. Patients usually have poor bone marrow granulocyte release, but a normal circulating granulocyte half-life with elevated serum lysozyme levels, suggesting intramedullary destruction of neutrophils.

Chemotaxis is diminished, but phagocytosis is normal or increased. Impaired bacterial killing is probably due to low levels and impaired mobilization

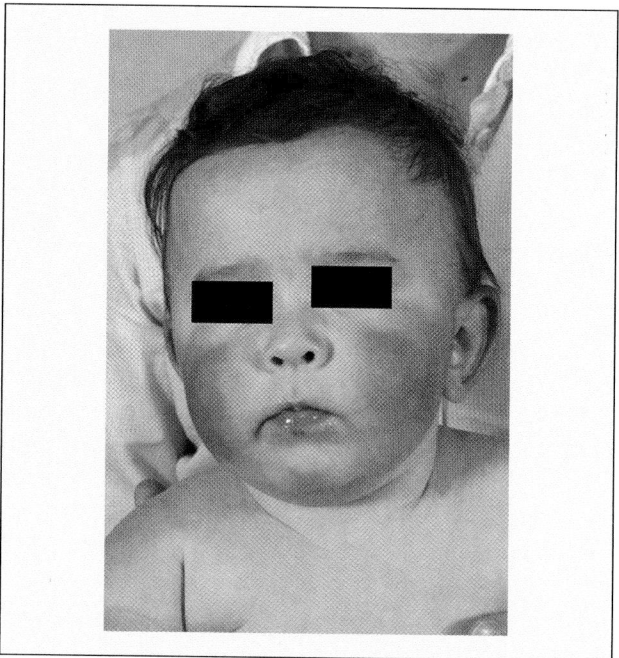

Figure 16-6. Child with the Chediak-Higashi syndrome (CHS) showing the typical light brown hair with a metallic silver-gray sheen. (Reproduced with permission from Zarzour W, Kleta R, Frangoul H, et al. Two novel CHS1 (LYST) mutations: clinical correlations in an infant with Chediak-Higashi syndrome. Mol Genet Metab. 2005;85:125–32.)

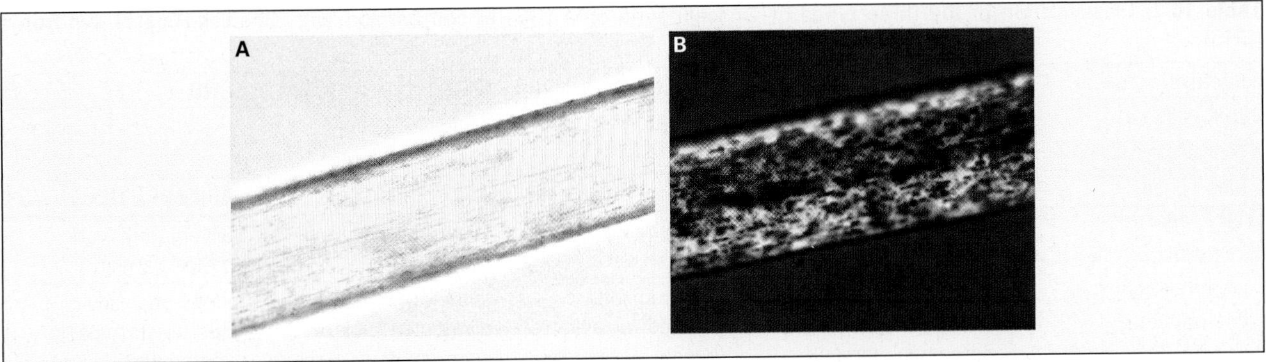

Figure 16-7. Panel A: Normal. Panel B: Chediak-Higashi syndrome patient hair shafts. Note evenly distributed pigment in the normal hair compared with clumped pigment in the patient's hair. (Reproduced with permission from Zarzour W, Kleta R, Frangoul H, et al. Two novel CHS1 (LYST) mutations: clinical correlations in an infant with Chediak-Higashi syndrome. Mol Genet Metab. 2005;85:125–32.)

of primary and secondary granule enzymes. NK cell cytotoxicity is diminished, but antibody-dependent cell-mediated cytotoxicity (**ADCC**) is intact. B cell function appears intact.

The accelerated phase of CHS is similar to other hemophagocytic syndromes, characterized by fever, hepatosplenomegaly, lymphadenopathy, cytopenias, hypertriglyceridemia, hypofibrinogenemia, hemophagocytosis, and tissue lymphohistiocytic infiltration. Etoposide (VP16), steroids, and intrathecal methotrexate (when the CNS is involved) have been successful. However, without successful bone marrow transplantation, the accelerated phase usually recurs and is fatal. Bone marrow transplantation cures the immune defect in CHS and the accelerated phase, but it does not prevent the central or peripheral neurologic problems.

Griscelli Syndrome (GS) Type 2 (MIM ID #607624)

In 1978, Griscelli and coworkers first reported a syndrome associating partial albinism with immunodeficiency in two patients with silvery gray hair and frequent pyogenic infections that clinically resembled CHS (Table 16A-1 in the Annex). However, these cases differed from CHS by the absence of characteristic giant granules in granulocytes, by differences in the hair and skin revealed by light and electron microscopy, and by the presence of defects in cellular and humoral immunity. Since then, a little more than 60 cases of GS have been reported in the literature in association with primary neurologic manifestations, with immunologic abnormalities or with silvery gray hair and hypopigmented skin as the sole abnormality.

GS is now classified into three types on the basis of clinical, genetic, and molecular features. Shown in Table 16-2 is a comparison of the three types of

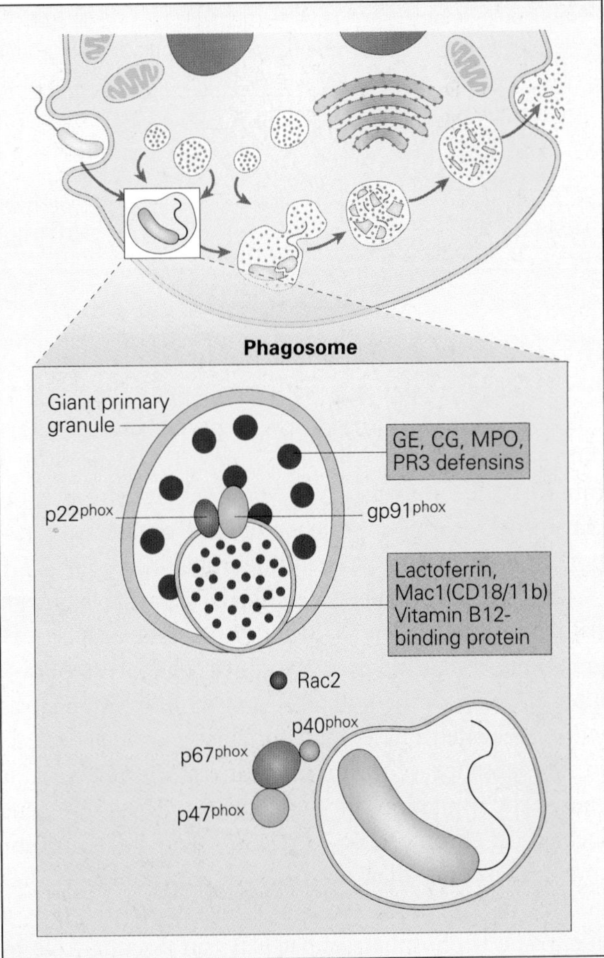

Figure 16-8. Schematic representation of a neutrophil from a patient with Chediak-Higashi syndrome showing giant primary granules caused by fusion of many smaller primary granules and secondary granules. The condition is caused by a mutation in the lysosome trafficking gene LYST (CHS1) that results in impairment in the ability of the primary and secondary granules to fuse with the phagosome. Although the initial dimer gp91^{phox} and p22^{phox} is formed, note the failure of the later addition of p47^{phox} and p67^{phox}. These abnormal granules not only impair the ability of neutrophils to traverse endothelium by virtue of their size, but also impair neutrophil killing of bacteria by failure of complete assembly of the NADPH oxidase complex.

Table 16-2. Classification of the three types of Griscelli syndrome (GS) in comparison with Chediak-Higashi syndrome (CHS)

Feature	GS1	GS2	GS3	CHS
Gene involved	Myosin Va on Ch 15q21	Rab27a on Ch 15q21	MLPH on Ch 2q37.3, F-exon of Myosin Va	LYST on Ch 1q42-43
Inheritance	Autosomal recessive	Autosomal recessive	Autosomal recessive	Autosomal recessive
Hair color	Silvery gray with metallic sheen	Silvery gray with metallic sheen	Silvery gray with metallic sheen	Silvery gray with metallic sheen
Light microscopy of hair structure	Large, irregularly distributed melanin aggregates, primarily in medulla	Large, irregularly distributed melanin aggregates, primarily in medulla	Large, irregularly distributed melanin aggregates, primarily in medulla	Small, regularly distributed melanin aggregates
Light microscopy of skin	Increased pigment in melanocytes with sparse pigment in keratinocytes	Increased pigment in melanocytes with sparse pigment in keratinocytes	Increased pigment in melanocytes with sparse pigment in keratinocytes	Decreased pigment in both melanocytes and keratinocytes
Neurologic defects	Severe (mental retardation, hypotonia, seizures)	May be seen (due to lymphohistiocytic infiltration), less severe	Absent	Common (seizures and progressive neurologic deficit)
Immune defects	Absent	Hypogammaglobulinemia, NK cell defects, suppressed delayed type hypersensitivity (DTH)	Absent	Defective chemotaxis, NK cell defects

Griscelli syndrome in comparison with the CHS. GS type 1 includes patients with silvery gray hair, light-colored skin, early-onset severe psychomotor retardation, and normal immune status. It is caused by a mutation in the myosin Va (**MYO5A**) gene located on chromosome 15q21, which regulates organelle transport in both melanocytes and neuronal cells.

GS type 2 (originally described as partial albinism with immunodeficiency) includes patients with silvery gray hair, frequent pyogenic infections of skin and internal organs, hemophagocytic lymphohistiocytosis with accelerated phases, and variable neurologic defects in the absence of primary neurologic disease. It is caused by mutation in the Rab27a (**RAB27A**) gene located on chromosome 15q21, less than 1.6 cm (antimorgan, a unit that describes a recombination frequency of 1%) from the MYO5A gene. RAB27A is a guanosine triphosphatase that plays an essential role in peripheral transport of melanosomes to the neighboring cells such as keratinocytes and granule exocytosis in cytotoxic T lymphocytes. A mutation in the RAB27A gene results in partial albinism of the skin and hair and uncontrolled T lymphocyte and macrophage hyperactivation, resulting in the hemophagocytic syndrome. Hemophagocytic syndrome is characterized by infiltration of lymph nodes and other organs (including the brain) by polyclonal, activated T cells, mostly of the CD8 subset, and by activated macrophages that phagocytized blood cells.

GS type 3 represents the restricted expression of the disease and is characterized by hypopigmentation in the hair and skin. No abnormalities of the nervous and immune systems are seen. Two cases of this type have been reported. In the first case, a mutation was found in the gene located on chromosome 2q37.3 that encodes melanophilin, which is a member of the Rab effector family. The second case was caused by an F-exon deletion in the MYO5A gene. Melanophilin helps in the capture and local movement of melanosomes in the actin-rich cell periphery of melanocytes by forming a protein complex with Rab27a and MyoVa. The different expressions of the same disease reflect the complex molecular pathways that are required for the exocytosis of secretory granules by melanocytes, neurons, and immune cells.

Neutrophil-Specific Granule Deficiency (MIM ID #245480)

Neutrophil-specific granule deficiency is a rare, heterogeneous, autosomal recessive disease characterized by profound reduction or absence of neutrophil-specific granules and their contents, as well as the primary granule product, defensins (Tables 16A-1 to 16A-8 in the Annex).

Mutations in [CAAT enhancer binding protein epsilon gene (**C/EBPE**) 14q11.2] have been found in several cases. The product of the mutated gene is C/EBPE, one of the transcription factors that play critical roles in myelopoiesis and cellular differentiation (Figure 16-9). Recurrent pyogenic infections of the skin, ears, lungs, and lymph nodes are the rule. Neutrophil morphology is abnormal, with bilobed neutrophil nuclei (pseudo-Pelger-Huët anomaly); electron microscopy shows absent secondary granules in some patients and empty granules in others. Staphylococcidal activity may be reduced, but candidacidal activity and superoxide production are normal. Bleeding due to abnormalities of platelet-associated high molecular weight von Willebrand factor and platelet fibrinogen and fibronectin has also been reported.

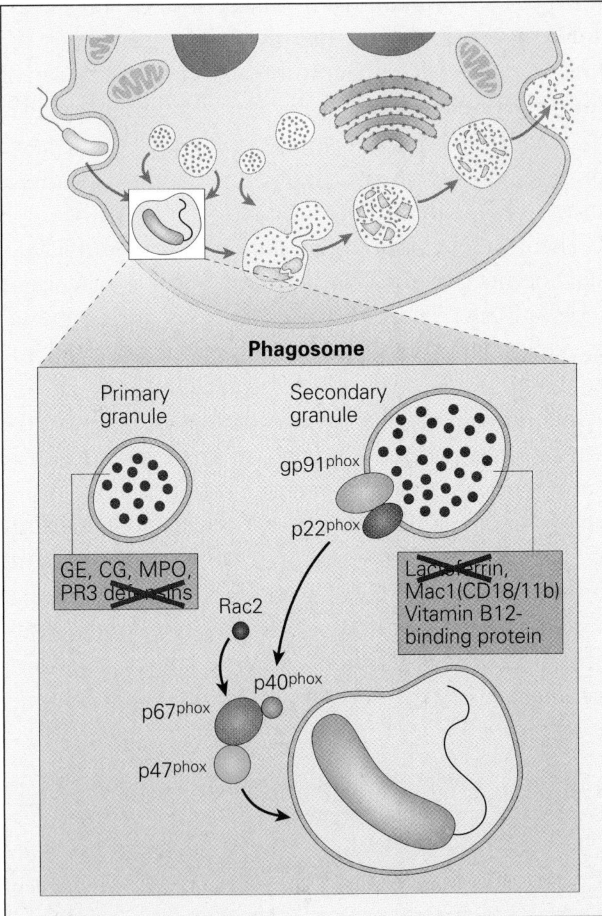

Figure 16-9. Schematic representation of a neutrophil in neutrophil-specific granule deficiency due to mutation of C/EBPE. Note the absence of lactoferrin and secondary granules, but also the absence of defensins, since these primary granule products are transcriptionally controlled by the same gene that regulates secondary granule products like lactoferrin.

Specific granule deficiency can be diagnosed on peripheral smear by finding that neutrophils are slightly larger and paler than normal, along with abnormal neutrophil nuclear morphology. Eosinophils may not be detectable on routine smears. Immunoblotting or ELISA shows absence of neutrophil lactoferrin and defensins. The inflammatory response is poor; Gram-positive coccus infections are common and require prolonged and intensive antibiotic therapy.

Hermansky-Pudlak Syndrome Type II (HPSII) (MIM ID #608233)

Hermansky-Pudlak syndrome type II (**HPSII**) is an autosomal recessive disease that is caused by disruption of the adaptor protein-3 complex (Table 16A-1 in the Annex). The adaptor protein (**AP**) complex plays a fundamental role in vesicle formation and in cargo selection in the vesicular trafficking system of the cell. Patients with HPSII present with mutations in the gene encoding for the beta subunit of the AP-3 complex. Clinically, the syndrome is characterized by oculocutaneous albinism and platelet defects due to absence of platelet dense bodies. Disruption of the AP-3 complex differentially affects vesicular trafficking in melanocytes, platelets, cytotoxic T lymphocytes, and NK cells. Neutropenia, often severe, is associated with diminished amounts of neutrophil elastase.

Defects of Oxidative Metabolism

Chronic Granulomatous Disease (CGD) (MIM ID #306400)

This disorder is the most common of the syndromes associated with defective oxidative metabolism resulting in diminished bactericidal activity (Table 16A-1 in the Annex). In most cases, it is inherited as an X-linked trait, although autosomal recessive forms are known. The underlying defect is impaired generation of activated forms of oxygen, i.e., superoxide (O_2^-) and hydrogen peroxide (H_2O_2) due to a variety of enzymatic defects involving the nicotinamide adenine dinucleotide phosphate (**NADPH**) oxidase system (*Chapter 5*).

The NADPH oxidase is a multicomponent enzyme complex required for the generation of superoxide and its metabolites hydrogen peroxide and bleach (Figure 16-10). The structural components are referred to as phox (phagocyte oxidase) proteins. At rest, the complex exists as separate components: the cytochrome b558 is comprised of gp91^{phox}, the 91kd beta chain, and p22^{phox} the 22kd alpha chain. Together they form a complex that binds heme and flavin, embedded in the walls of secondary granules. In the cytosol are the structural proteins p47^{phox} and p67^{phox}, and the regulatory components p40^{phox} and RAC. p47^{phox} and p67^{phox} are phosphorylated and bind tightly together on neutrophil activation. In association with p40^{phox} and RAC, they join to the complex of gp91^{phox} and p22^{phox} to form the intact NADPH oxidase. This complex harvests an electron from NADPH and donates it to molecular oxygen, creating superoxide (O_2^-). Superoxide dismutase (**SOD**) converts O_2^- to H_2O_2. Myeloperoxidase converts H_2O_2 to bleach by combination with chlorine. Phagocyte production of O_2^- facilitates activation of certain proteins inside the phagosome.

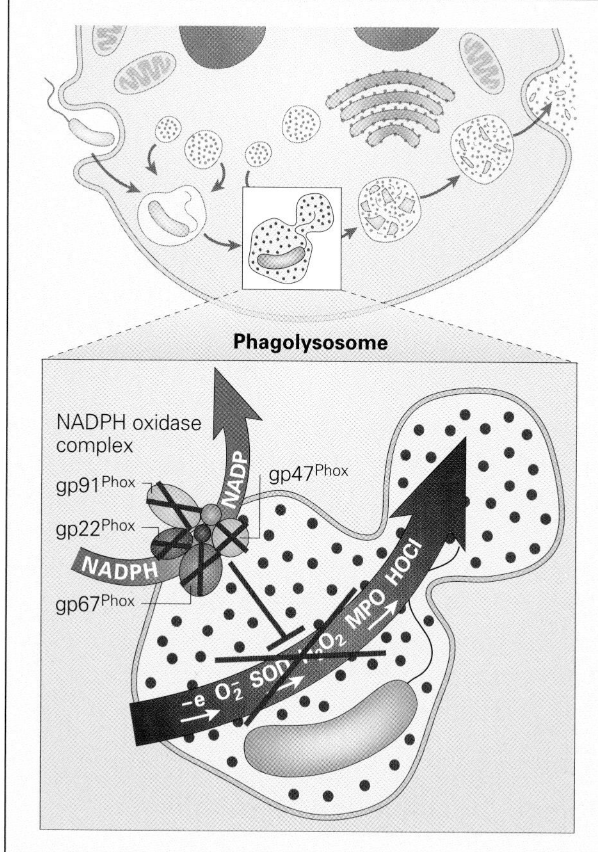

Figure 16-10. Schematic representation of a neutrophil in chronic granulomatous disease (CGD). The NADPH oxidase is assembled on either the wall of the phagolysosome, or the plasma membrane, depending on whether the invader has been engulfed or is too large to be ingested. After cellular activation the secondary granule fuses with the phagolysosome, embedding the cytochrome components in the wall of the vesicle. p47^{phox} and p67^{phox} become phosphorylated and tightly associated in the cytosol, followed by transit to the transmembrane cytochrome complex. When p40^{phox} and RAC join the complex, the mature NADPH oxidase is formed, and is capable of harvesting an electron from NADPH, oxidizing it to NADP+, and delivers that electron to molecular oxygen in the phagosome, generating superoxide (O_2^-). Superoxide is converted to hydrogen peroxide (H_2O_2) by superoxide dismutase (SOD); this in turn is converted to hypohalous acid (HOCl or bleach) by myeloperoxidase (MPO). Mutations in the four structural genes of the NADPH oxidase (gp91^{phox}, p22^{phox}, p47^{phox}, and p67^{phox}) cause CGD. Gp91^{phox} is X-linked recessive, while the others are autosomal recessive.

Mutations in gp91^{phox}, p22^{phox}, p47^{phox}, and p67^{phox} cause chronic granulomatous disease (**CGD**), characterized by recurrent life-threatening infections due to catalase-positive bacteria and fungi and granulomatous complications (MIM #306400, 233690, 233700, and 233710). Shown in Figure 16-10 and Table 16-3 are the NADPH oxidase mutations that give rise to CGD together with their inheritance patterns, chromosomal locations, and relative frequencies. The gp91^{phox} variant is X-linked, located on Xp21, and accounts for about two-thirds of cases; the other three variants have an autosomal recessive pattern of transmission, and p47^{phox}, located on chromosome 7, accounts for about 25 percent, with p22^{phox}, located on chromosome 16, and p67^{phox}, located on chromosome 1q42, accounting for the rest.

There are no autosomal dominant cases of CGD. CGD occurs in 1/200,000 live births, but this may be an underestimate. The majority of patients are diagnosed as toddlers and young children; infections or granulomatous lesions are usually the first manifestations.

Symptoms usually begin during the first few years of life, with the advent of recurrent disseminated abscesses or pneumonias. The lung, skin, lymph nodes, and liver are the most frequent sites of infection in patients in North America and Western Europe (Figure 16-11A and Figure 16-11B).

The characteristic suppurative granulomas scattered throughout the body at these sites gave rise to the name of the entity. Individual granulomas

Table 16-3. NADPH oxidase mutations associated with diverse CGD variants together with chromosomal locations and frequencies

CGD variant	Mendelian inheritance	Chromosomal location	Frequency (%)
gp91^{phox}	XL	Xp21	65
p47^{phox}	AR	7	25
p22^{phox}	AR	16	<5
p67^{phox}	AR	1q42	<5

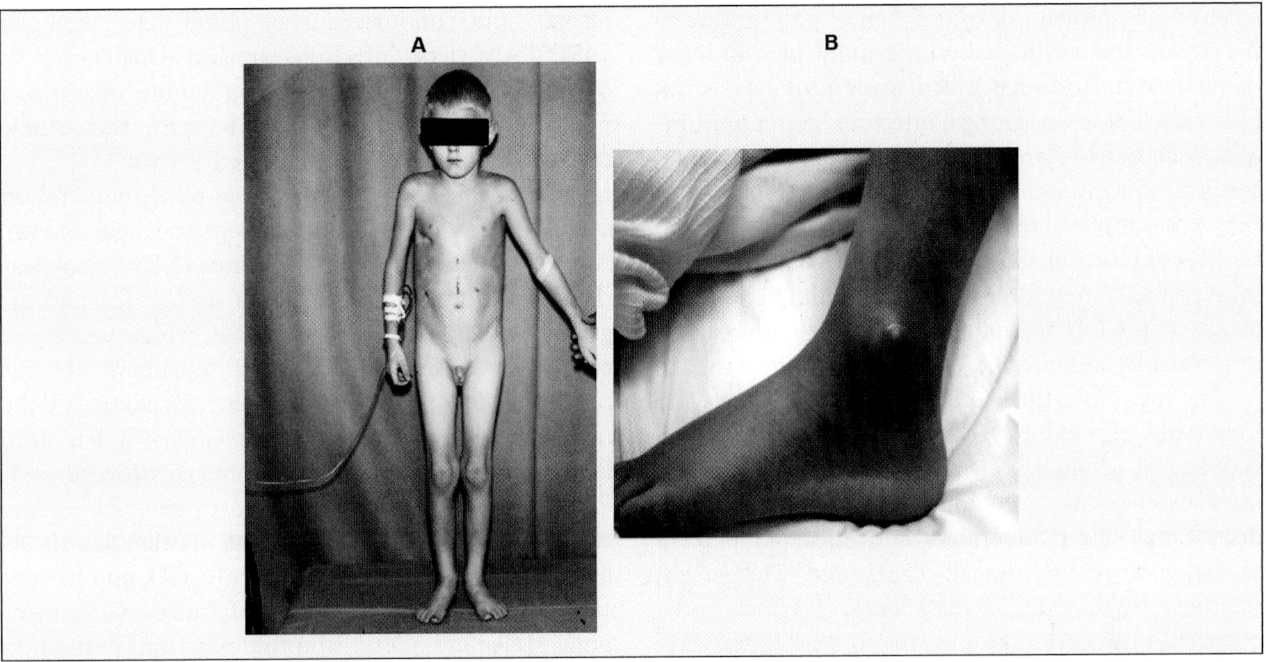

Figure 16-11. Panel A: Photograph of a nine-year-old boy with chronic granulomatous disease. Note thoracotomy and right upper abdominal laparotomy scars at sites of prior therapeutic procedures to drain abscesses of the lung and liver. Panel B: Staphylococcal osteomyelitis in a patient with X-linked CGD. Note the impending rupture of the infection through the lateral malleolus. Osteomyelitis in CGD is typically staphylococcal or caused by *Serratia marcescens*.

consist of peripheral collections of lymphocytes and macrophages surrounding a central necrotic core, superficially resembling the granulomas seen in tuberculosis (Figure 16-12 and *Chapter 13*).

The epidemiology of CGD infections in less developed countries is not as well defined, but it differs slightly from North America and Europe. In countries where BCG vaccination is still administered, local BCG lymphadenitis is common. In North America, the overwhelming majority of infections in CGD are due to only five organisms: *S. aureus*, *Burkholderia cepacia* complex, *Serratia marcescens*, *Nocardia*, and *Aspergillus*. In contrast to other primary immunodeficiencies, the infectious agents found in CGD are of low virulence in normal individuals and are characteristically catalase-positive. Certain catalase-negative organisms, such as *Streptococcus pneumoniae* and *Streptococcus pyogenes*, which also produce hydrogen peroxide, do not often infect these patients. It has been postulated that the alternative source of hydrogen peroxide produced by these organisms partially corrects the intracellular short supply found in CGD cells and therefore is given as an explanation of why patients with CGD are not susceptible to this class of bacteria. However, this explanation is unlikely since most bacteria and all fungi are catalase and hydrogen peroxide producing, indicating that there must be other factors that regulate the specific virulence of the infecting organisms for CGD patients.

Trimethoprim/sulfamethoxazole (**TMP/SMX**) prophylaxis has reduced the frequency of bacterial infections markedly. In patients receiving TMP/SMX prophylaxis, staphylococcal infections are essentially confined to the liver and cervical lymph nodes. In

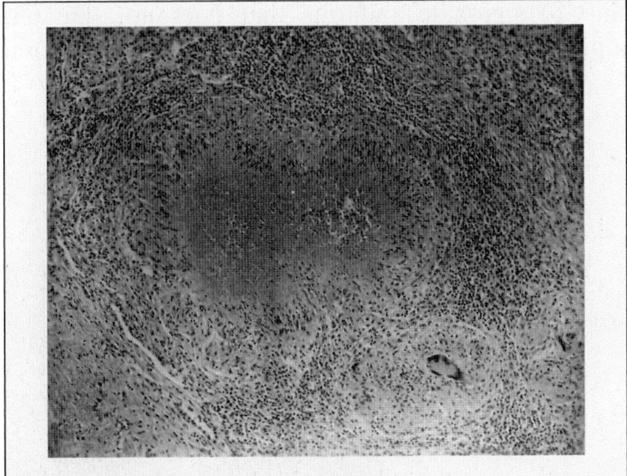

Figure 16-12. Photomicrograph of a typical granuloma seen in chronic granulomatous disease. Note the central area of necrosis surrounded by a rim of chronic inflammatory cells consisting of lymphocytes and macrophages and a multinucleated Langerhans giant cell in the lower right. Hematoxylin and eosin stain, x 120.

recent years, fungal infections, typically those due to *Aspergillus* species, have become more predominant (*Chapter 14*). Although itraconazole prophylaxis has been shown to reduce fungal infection, newer antifungals, such as voriconazole and posaconazole, should further reduce fungal mortality in CGD. The use of IFN-γ has been shown to reduce the number and severity of infections in CGD by 70 percent compared to placebos. Therefore, current recommended prophylaxis in CGD is trimethoprim/sulfamethoxazole, itraconazole, and interferon gamma.

The gastrointestinal and genitourinary tracts are frequently affected by granulomata (Figure 16-13). Esophageal, jejunal, ileal, cecal, rectal, and perirectal involvement with granulomata mimicking Crohn's disease have been described, and affect 43 percent of patients with X-linked CGD and 11 percent of those with p47^{phox} deficiency. Gastric outlet obstruction is common and may be the initial presentation of CGD. Bladder granulomata and ureteral obstruction are common in patients with defects in gp91^{phox} and p22^{phox} and readily relieved with steroids. Prednisone 1 mg/kg for a brief initial period then tapered to a low dose on alternate days is usually successful. However, relapse or recurrence of gastrointestinal granulomatous disease is common, requiring the frequent use of prolonged low-dose steroid therapy. The use of infliximab increases the rates of fungal and bacterial infection in CGD, just as it does in normal individuals (*Chapter 12*).

The X-linked gp91^{phox} carrier females typically have two populations of phagocytes: one that produces superoxide and one that does not. Discoid lupus erythematosus-like lesions, aphthous oral ulcers, and photosensitive rashes are seen in gp91^{phox} carriers. Infections are not usually seen in female carriers unless the population of normal neutrophils is below 5 to 10 percent; then, these carriers are at risk for CGD type infections.

The diagnosis of CGD is made by demonstration of reduced or absent superoxide generation. Although the nitroblue-tetrazolium (**NBT**) assay was the most widely known diagnostic test for chronic granulomatous disease in the past, which was based on the direct reduction of NBT by superoxide free radical to form an insoluble blue formazan in the normal and its absence in the patient, it has been largely replaced by the flow cytometric dihydrorhodamine (**DHR**) assay, which is now preferred because of its speed, ease of use, ability to distinguish X-linked from autosomal patterns of CGD, and its sensitivity to very low numbers of functional neutrophils (*Chapter 24*). Immunoblot and mutation analysis has also been used to identify specific proteins and mutations. The precise gene defect should be determined when possible, as it is critical for genetic counseling and is prognostically significant. p47^{phox} deficiency has a significantly better prognosis than X-linked disease: mortality for the X-linked form has been shown to be about 5 percent per year, compared to 2 percent per year for the autosomal recessive varieties.

Bone marrow transplantation leading to stable chimerism has been successfully performed in patients with CGD, including for refractory infection, predominantly from *Aspergillus*. In some studies using reduced-intensity non-ablative bone marrow transplantation from HLA-identical siblings into CGD patients, success was greater in children

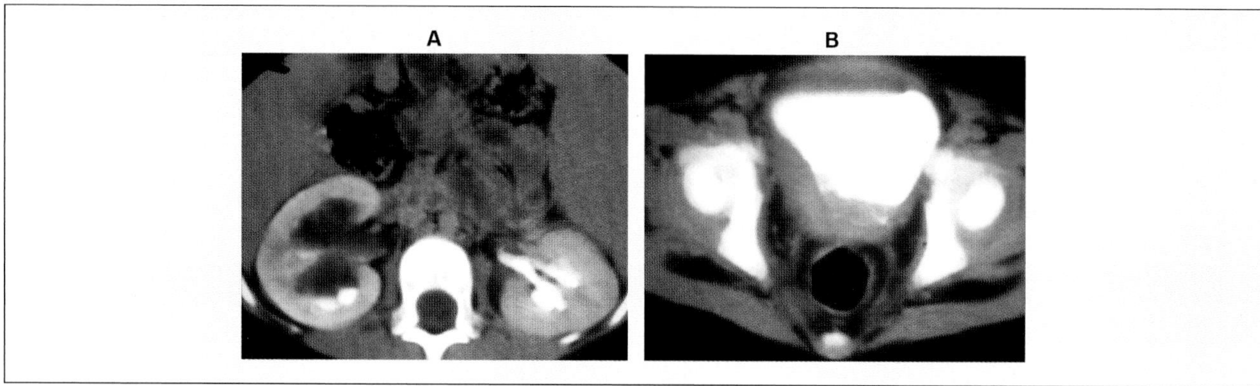

Figure 16-13. The granulomatous complications of CGD can affect the hollow viscera, as well as the lung, skin, and retina. Bowel, bladder, and ureter granulomata are especially difficult to treat, but are highly steroid-responsive. Panel A: Shown is a CT scan of the kidneys. Panel B: Pelvis (B) in a three-year-old boy with X-linked CGD who presented with dysuria. Note the right hydronephrosis (A) due to the extensive right posterior bladder granuloma formation (B). This process was rapidly steroid responsive and completely resolved within days of steroid therapy.

than adults, but transplant-related toxicities, such as graft versus host disease, remained problematic. Gene therapy for p47^{phox} and gp91^{phox} deficiencies have been successful, but not durable.

RAC2 Deficiency (MIM ID #602049)

RAC2 is a hematopoietic-specific Rho-GTPase that plays a stimulus-specific role in regulating reduced NADPH oxidase activation and other functional responses in neutrophils, such as the regulation of the actin cytoskeleton. An autosomal dominant mutation in the Rho GTPase RAC2 (RAC2, 22q12.13-q13.2), a member of the Rho family of GTPases needed for connection of the actin cytoskeleton and superoxide production, caused severe immune deficiency in a boy (Table 16A-1 in the Annex). He had delayed umbilical cord separation, perirectal abscesses, and impaired wound healing without pus, despite neutrophilia. Chemotaxis, superoxide production, azurophilic granule release, and phagocytosis were impaired. Bone marrow transplantation was curative.

The rationale for bone marrow transplantation in RAC2 deficiency is based on the ability of hematopoietic stem cell and progenitor (**HSC/P**) precursors after intravenous administration to lodge in the medullary cavity and be retained in the appropriate marrow space, a process referred to as homing (*Chapter 2*), a multistep process encompassing a sequence of highly regulated events that mimic the migration of leukocytes to inflammatory sites (*Chapter 5*). This process includes an initial phase of tethering and rolling of cells to the endothelium via E- and P-selectins, firm adhesion to the vessel wall via integrins that appear to be activated in an "inside-out" fashion, transendothelial migration, and chemotaxis through the extracellular matrix (**ECM**) to the inflammatory nidus (*Chapter 5*).

Myeloperoxidase Deficiency (MIM ID #254600)

Myeloperoxidase (**MPO**; 16q23) is an enzyme synthesized in neutrophils and monocytes, packaged into azurophilic granules, and released either into the phagosome or the extracellular space, where it catalyses the conversion of H_2O_2 to hypohalous acid (in neutrophils, the halide is Cl^- and the acid is bleach). Myeloperoxidase deficiency is an autosomal recessive disease with variable expressivity. It is the most common primary phagocytic cell disorder, occurring in 1/4,000 individuals with complete MPO deficiency and in 1/2,000 with partial defects. Although in vitro MPO deficient neutrophils are markedly deficient in killing *C. albicans* and hyphal forms of *A. fumigates* (*Chapter 14*), clinical infection in MPO deficiency is rare. Mucocutaneous, meningeal, bone, and disseminated candidiasis have been described, but diabetes mellitus appears to be a critical cofactor for these infections in the context of MPO deficiency. Diagnosis is established by performance of neutrophil or monocyte peroxidase histochemical staining or by direct MPO measurement. There is no specific treatment for MPO deficiency.

The Leukocyte Adhesion Deficiencies

Over the years, a number of defects of leukocyte movement from the blood into tissues has been identified which predispose patients to recurrent infection. These include a group of molecular defects that come under the general heading of leukocyte adhesion deficiency (**LAD**). These molecular lesions are responsible for the clinical manifestations resulting from an impaired step in the inflammatory process, namely, the emigration of leukocytes from the blood vessels to sites of infection, which requires adhesion of leukocytes to the endothelium (*Chapter 5*). Leukocyte adhesion to each other, endothelium, and to bacteria is required for travel, communication, and inflammation to fight infection. The leukocyte adhesion molecules, predominantly the integrins and selectins, mediate these processes. Leukocyte β2 integrins are heterodimeric molecules on neutrophils, monocytes, and lymphocytes that attach to intercellular adhesion molecules (**ICAMs**) on the endothelium in order to exit the circulation (Figure 16-14). ICAMs are also expressed on other leukocytes, mediating some forms of cell-cell adhesion. Certain β2 integrins bind directly to pathogens or to a complement. The integrins are composed of an α chain (CD11a, CD11b, or CD11c) noncovalently linked to a common β2 subunit, CD18. The αβ heterodimers of the β2 integrin family are CD11a/CD18 (lymphocyte-function-associated antigen-1, [**LFA-1**]), CD11b/CD18 (macrophage antigen-1, [**Maca-1**]; complement receptor-3, [**CR3**]), and CD11c/CD18 (p150,95; complement receptor-4, [**CR4**]). Since CD18 is required for normal expression of the αβ heterodimers, mutations that eliminate or impair CD18 lead to either very low or no expression of CD11a, CD11b, and/or CD11c. These mutations lead to inability of leukocytes to bind to

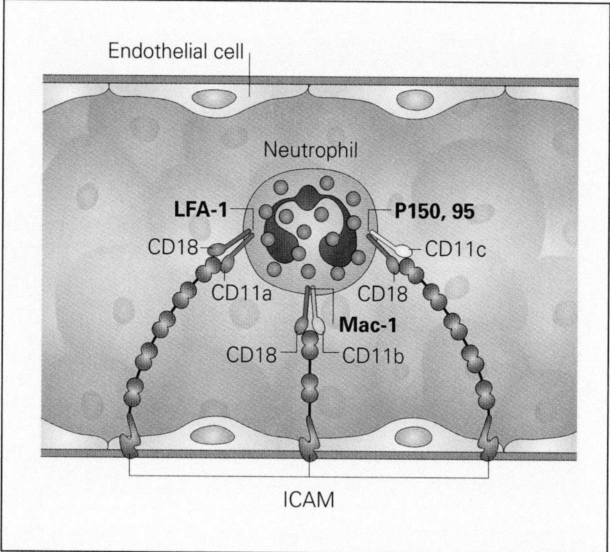

Figure 16-14. Leukocyte adhesion via integrins. Neutrophils attach to endothelium via PMN-surface receptors composed of heterodimeric CD18 molecules with their partners, CD11a, CD11b, and CD11c. These in turn bind to cell surface molecules on the endothelium, composed of the intercellular adhesion molecules (ICAM) 1 and 2. Mutation of CD18 leads to loss or impairment of all the heterodimers, disabling tight adhesion and vascular exit of neutrophils. Therefore, CD18 deficiency leads to leukocyte adhesion deficiency type I (LAD I).

endothelium, with each other, to certain pathogens, or to complement opsonized particles, thereby causing leukocyte adhesion deficiency type I (ITGB2, 21q22.3; MIM #116920).

Over the past 20 years, in addition to LAD I, two additional defects of the leukocyte adhesion cascade have been described, referred to as LAD II and LAD III, involving several precise ordered steps such as rolling, integrin activation, and firm adhesion of the leukocytes.

LAD I Deficiency (MIM ID #116920)

Leukocyte adhesion deficiency type I (**LAD I**) is an autosomal recessive disease due to mutations in CD18 (*INTG2;* 21q22.3) (Table 16A-1 in the Annex). The prominent clinical feature of these patients is recurrent bacterial infections, primarily localized to skin and mucosal surfaces. The severity of clinical infectious complications among patients with LAD I appears to be directly related to the degree of CD18 deficiency. Two phenotypes, designated as severe deficiency and moderate deficiency, have been defined. Patients with severe LAD I have < 1 percent normal expression of CD18, while patients with the moderate phenotype can show from 1 to 30 percent of normal values. Patients with severe deficiency of CD18 surface expression exhibit a more relentless form of disease, with earlier, more frequent, and more serious episodes of infection, often leading to death in infancy. Patients with a lesser amount of surface expression of CD18 (2.5 to 10 percent) who manifest the moderate-to-mild phenotype exhibit fewer serious infectious episodes and may survive into adulthood. Rarely, CD18 may be present on the leukocyte surface, but it will be non-functional due to the mutation.

In the severe form of LAD I deficiency, infections are usually apparent from birth onward, and common clinical findings include omphalitis with delayed separation of the umbilical cord, persistent leukocytosis (> 15,000/μL) in the absence of obvious active infection, and severe gingivitis and periodontitis with associated loss of dentition and alveolar bone. Recurrent infections of the skin, lung, bowel, and perirectal area are usually due to Gram-positive cocci or Gram-negative bacilli. Wounds characteristically show necrotic ulceration without pus or neutrophil invasion and leave dystrophic "cigarette-paper" scars (Figure 16-15A and Figure 16-15B). Moderate phenotype patients have normal umbilical stump separation, fewer life-threatening infections, milder leukocytosis, and tend to be diagnosed later in life. However, periodontal disease and delayed wound healing are still common. Neutrophil transfusions may be helpful in severe acute infections, but their use is anecdotal. Bone marrow transplantation is the only definitive corrective treatment. Although gene therapy is attractive and has been shown to be successful in mice and dogs, its use in the human has not been demonstrated. The absence of pus formation at the sites of infection is one of the hallmarks of LAD I. Severe gingivitis and periodontitis are major features among all patients who survive infancy. Impaired healing of traumatic or surgical wounds is also characteristic of this syndrome

LAD II Deficiency (MIM ID #266265)

Leukocyte adhesion deficiency type II (**LAD II**), also known as congenital disorder of glycosylation type IIc (CDG-IIc), is a very rare autosomal recessive disease due to mutations in the GDP-fucose transporter, FUCT1 (11p11.2). Patients with LAD II have defective fucosylation of many molecules, including the neutrophil selectin ligand sialyl-Lewis^{X} as well as blood group antigens, leading to the Bombay (hh) blood type. Selectins mediate the

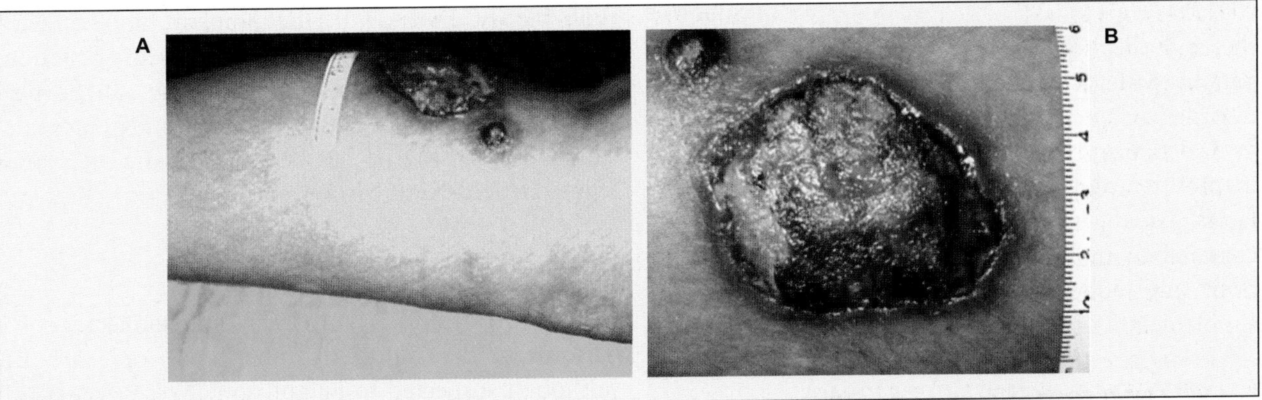

Figure 16-15. Panel A: Characteristic skin ulcerations of LAD I showing the ulcerative lesions with minimal inflammation. Panel B: Note the extensive scab overlying the wound with no pus formation. Biopsy showed no neutrophil exudation.

loose, rolling adhesion of neutrophils along post-capillary venules (*Chapter 5* and Figure 16-16). In contrast to the tight adhesion mediated by CD18 and exemplified in LAD I, the loose adhesion that allows neutrophil rolling and sampling of the endothelium is mediated by PMN CD15s and endothelial selectins. Mutations in the fucosyl transferase that are required for proper glycosylation of

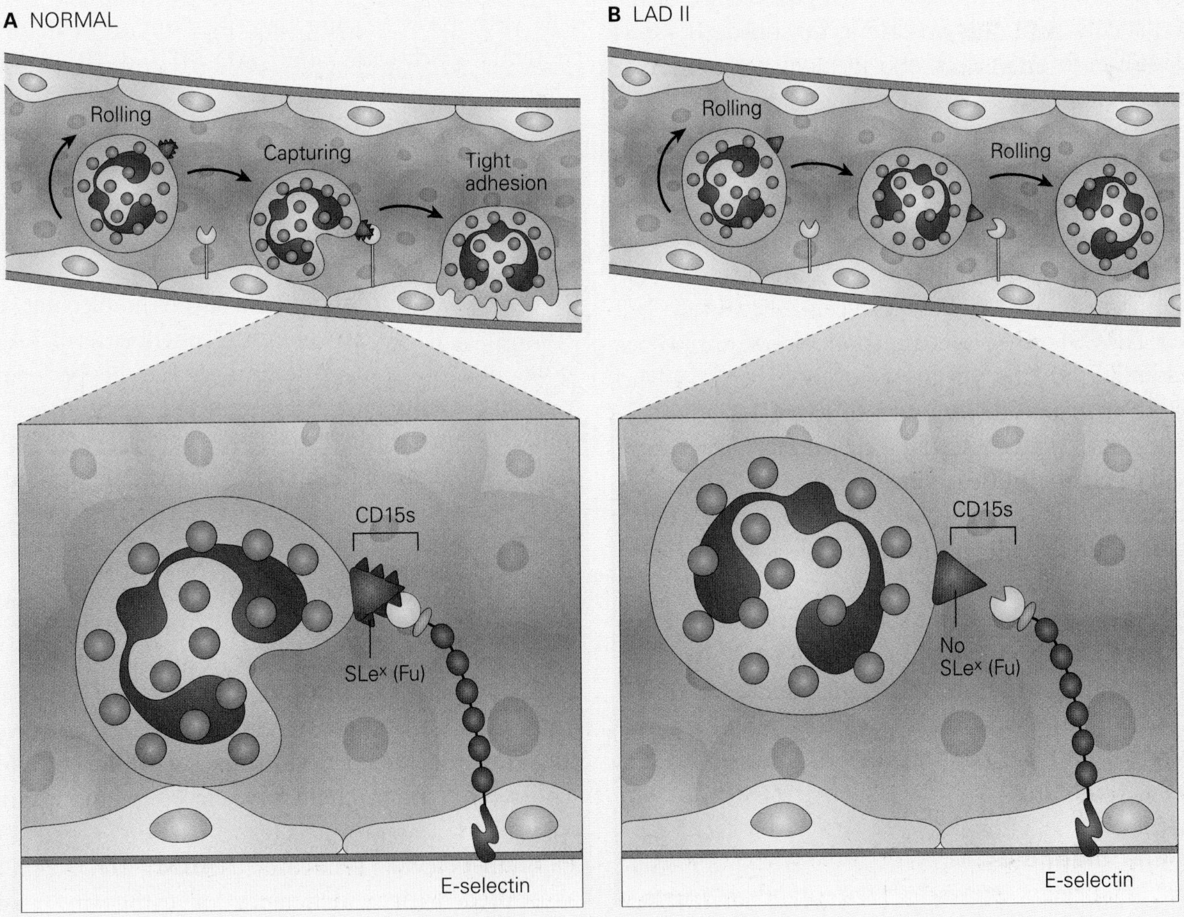

Figure 16-16. **Schematic representation of the loose adhesion that allows neutrophil rolling and sampling of the endothelium mediated by PMN CD15s and endothelial selectins.** Panel A: Shows healthy adhesion. Panel B: Mutations in the fucosyl transferase required for proper glycosylation (or addition of the tetrasaccharide SLe^X) of CD15s (FUCT1) lead to defects in proper adhesion to the endothelium and recurrent infections seen in LAD II.

CD15s (FUCT1) lead to defects in proper adhesion to the endothelium and recurrent infections seen in patients with LAD II deficiency. Typical features of the disorder include infections of the skin, lung, and gingivae, leukocytosis and poor pus formation, as well as mental retardation, short stature, and distinctive facies. Leukocytes from patients with LAD II deficiency show impaired neutrophil migration, aggregation, and adherence to endothelial cells. Fucose supplementation has been helpful in some cases.

LAD III Deficiency (MIM ID #612840)

Leukocyte adhesion deficiency type III (**LAD III**) is an autosomal recessive disease due to mutations in Cal DAG-GEF1 due to defective Rap 1-mediated activation of β1, β2, and β3 integrin subunits. Mutation in the KIND LIN3 (FERMT3) gene is the cause of LAD-III in patients from the Middle East, Malta, and Turkey. It seems that this rare syndrome may be due to several defects in molecules involved in integrin activation (Table 16A-1 in the Annex). The clinical picture of the four patients with this syndrome described so far is very similar to LAD I but also includes defects in platelet activation and a severe bleeding tendency.

Diagnostic Methods

A simple complete blood count (**CBC**) test revealing a profound neutrophilia is the most important diagnostic test. Quantitative measurement of the mutant proteins by a fluorescence-activated cell sorter (**FACS**) using specific monoclonal antibodies is essential for the diagnosis of both LAD I and LAD II (*Chapter 24*). A rare form of LAD I deficiency exists where CD18 cell surface expression may be normal but where functional activity is diminished due to missense mutations that abrogate specific binding sites. Functional assays must also be performed if the clinical suspicion of LAD I is high. Adhesion assays are not performed in most laboratories and should be carried out only in those that are specialized in the performance of these assays. Mutation analysis of patients' DNA should be carried out to confirm the diagnosis and for genetic counseling.

Prenatal Diagnosis

Since leukocytes express CD18 on their surface from 20 weeks of gestation, cordocentesis can establish the diagnosis. In families in whom the precise molecular defect has been previously identified, an earlier prenatal diagnosis is possible by chorionic villi biopsy. In LAD II, the Bombay blood phenotype can be checked at 20 weeks of gestation. Genetic analysis of the defective gene can be performed at 10–11 weeks of gestation. No prenatal diagnosis of LAD III has been reported so far, since the genetic defect(s) is/are not known yet.

Management and Treatment

While LAD I and II are clearly autosomal recessive disorders, the mode of inheritance of LAD III, although suspected to be autosomal recessive, is still not clear. LAD I is due to structural defects in the integrin molecule, preventing a firm adhesion to occur. In LAD II, the primary genetic defect is in a specific Golgi GDP-fucose transporter that leads to absence of the selectin ligand on the leukocyte and a defective rolling. LAD III or LAD I/variant, which was last described, is due to defects in the integrin activation process. All three syndromes are very rare, LAD I being more frequent than LAD II and III, with LAD I being described in more than 300 patients worldwide and LAD II and III in fewer than 10 children each.

The most important focus should be to control infections. Treatment includes antibiotics and in some cases bone marrow transplantation. Granulocyte transfusion should be restricted to life-threatening situations when all other measures have failed. Blood transfusion should be given in bleeding episodes in LAD III. In the severe phenotype of LAD I, bone marrow transplantation should be performed; excellent results have been reported. Gene therapy is still experimental in LAD I. In two cases of LAD II, fucose supplementation showed encouraging results.

Other Primary Immune Deficiencies Associated with Defects in Chemotaxis

Shown in Table 16A-1 in the Annex are three other rare AR primary immunodeficiencies associated with mutations affecting chemotaxis. These include localized juvenile periodontitis (**MIM ID #170650**) associated with a chemokine receptor mutation in the formyl peptide receptor 1 (**FPR1**) gene, the Papillon-Lefévre syndrome (**MIM ID #245000**) associated with a deficiency of cathepsin C, and the Shwachman-Diamond syndrome (**MIM ID #260400**) associated with a mutation in the Shwachman-Bodian-Diamond syndrome (**SBDS**) gene. The first condition is associated with periodontitis only, the second with periodontitis and palmoplantar hyperkeratosis, and the third with pancytopenia, exocrine pancreatic insufficiency, and chondrodysplasia.

Defects of Cytokine-Signaling Pathways

Interferon-γ/IL-12 Pathway Defects

The mononuclear phagocyte mediates antigen presentation, lymphocyte stimulation and proliferation, cytokine production and response through an axis referred to as the interferon-γ/IL-12 pathway (*Chapter 12*). Following infection with a variety of intracellular microbes, e.g., mycobacteria, salmonella, and certain viruses, macrophages produce interleukin-12 (**IL-12**), which in turn stimulates T cells and NK cells to produce interferon-γ (**IFN-γ**) (Figure 16-17). IFN-γ increases production of tumor necrosis factor-α (**TNF-α**), IL-12, and other cytokines that mediate mycobacterial killing through unknown mechanisms. Although IFN-α activates both the STAT1 and NEMO pathways, IFN-α signaling depends on the signal transducer and activator of transcription 1 (**STAT1**), while TNF-α signaling depends on the NF-κB essential modulator (**NEMO**) (*Chapter 9*). Defects in signaling by IFN-γ, IL-12, TNF-α, and their respective receptors are clearly identified functionally and genetically as being responsible for infections with mycobacteria, salmonella, and certain viruses.

The interferon gamma receptor is composed of a heterodimeric pair of ligand binding (IFN-γR1) and signal transducing (IFN-γR2) chains (Figure 16-18 and *Chapters 9* and *12*). As described previously, stimulation of these receptors leads to activation of STAT1 and upregulation of interferon gamma responsive genes.

Autosomal recessive mutations in either IFN-γ receptor chain lead to abolition of IFN-γ signaling associated with severe infections predominantly with mycobacteria (Figure 16-18 and Table 16A-1 in the Annex). Patients with complete receptor defects tend to present early in life, especially if

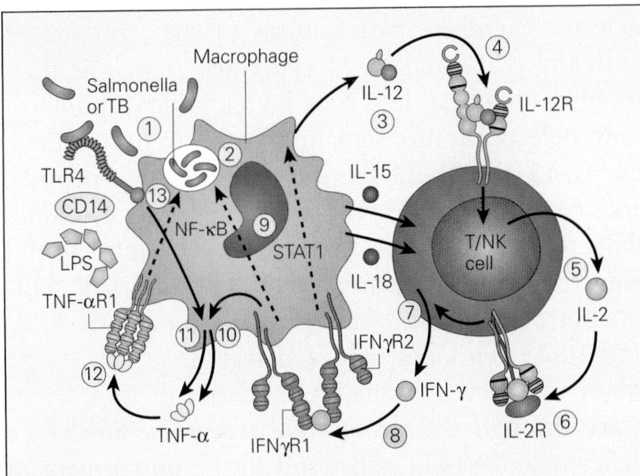

Figure 16-17. Schematic representation of the interferon-γ/IL-12 axis showing the interrelationships of the cytokine cascade for microbicidal killing of intracellular microbes, e.g., mycobacteria, salmonella, and certain viruses. Following infection with a variety of intracellular microbes, e.g., mycobacteria, salmonella, and certain viruses (#1), macrophages produce IL-12 (#3), which in turn acts on its receptor on T and NK cells (#4) to stimulate IL-2 production (#5) that binds to its IL-2R receptor (#6) to produce interferon gamma (IFN-γ) (#7). The binding of IFN-γ to IFN-γR (#8) activates the signal transducer and activator of transcription 1 (STAT1) pathway (#9) to kill the TB; tumor necrosis factor-α (TNF-α) produced both by stimulation by IFN-γ (#10) as well as by TLR4 activation (#11) binds to its receptor TNF-αR1 (#12) and mediates mycobacterial killing through unknown mechanisms (#13). IFN-γ signaling depends on the STAT1, while TNF-α signaling depends on the NF-κB essential modulator (NEMO). Defects in IL-12p40, IL-12Rβ1, IFN-γR1, IFN-γR2, and STAT1 have all been identified in patients with disseminated nontuberculous mycobacterial infections. Autoantibodies to IFN-γ have also been identified.

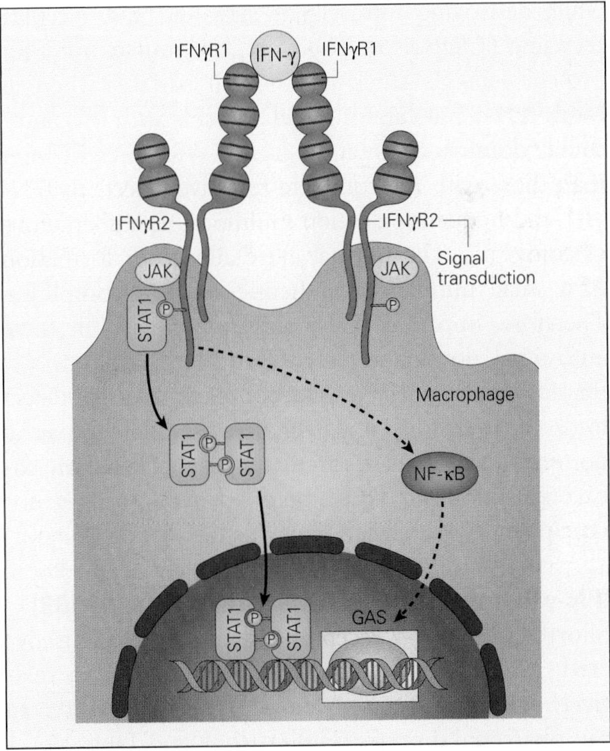

Figure 16-18. Schematic representation of the interferon gamma receptor (IFN-γR) that is composed of a heterodimeric pair of ligand-binding (IFNγR1) and signal-transducing (IFN-γR2) chains. The binding of IFN-γ with the two IFN-γR1 chains leads to the activation of the STAT1 and NF-κB signaling pathways involved in microbicidal activity shown in Figure 16-17. Mutations in either of these IFN-γR chains lead to the defective microbicidal activity and susceptibility to mycobacterial infection seen in afflicted patients.

they have received BCG vaccination (*Chapter 12*). These patients have normal tuberculin skin tests but poor or absent granuloma formation and typically develop repeated, disseminated, and life-threatening infections due to mycobacteria, salmonellae, and some viruses. Mortality is overwhelmingly due to mycobacterial disease. Bone marrow transplantation is complicated by high rates of rejection and death due to mycobacterial infection. Treatment relies entirely on antibiotic and antiviral therapy. Rare recessive mutations with partial function have intermediate phenotypes and more curable infections.

IFN-γ Receptor 1 Deficiency (MIM ID #107470)

Recessive and dominant IFNGR1 deficiencies have been described. The most common mutation of the IFN-γ/IL-12 pathway defects involves the IFN-γR1 binding chain and is due to a four-base deletion at or around base 818 (818del4), located just inside the intracellular domain of the molecule (Figure 16-18 and Table 16A-1 in the Annex). This mutation causes a truncation that preserves extracellular ligand binding while destroying intracellular signaling and receptor recycling (*Chapter 9*). Therefore, the mutant receptor protein remains stuck on the cell surface, where it binds IFN-γ but cannot signal. Patients with this autosomal dominant mutation in IFN-γR1 present later than those with the complete recessive defects in IFN-γR1 and frequently develop multifocal nontuberculous osteomyelitis. The normal allele allows for formation of a small number of authentic receptor complexes. Therefore, impaired IFN-γ signaling persists in these autosomal dominant patients, indicating that IFN-γ therapy can be effective. The complete recessive defect leads to severe disseminated disease while the partial dominant genotype leads to better-controlled mycobacterial infection. Thus, there is a very strong genotype/phenotype correlation in this IFN-γR deficiency.

IFN-γ Receptor 2 Deficiency (MIM ID #147569)

Shortly after IFN-γ receptor 1 deficiency was discovered, AR mutations were found in IFNGR2, a relatively rare molecular cause of susceptibility to mycobacterial diseases (Figure 16-18 and Table 16A-1 in the Annex). Based on the in vitro responsiveness of patients' lymphocytes to IFN-γ, the mutations can be expressed either as complete or partial. Patients with complete IFN-γR2 deficiency have either a complete absence of the receptor or the presence of a non-functional one.

The clinical presentation of complete IFN-γR2 deficiency resembles that of complete IFNGR1 deficiency and manifests early in life, with severe and often fatal infection. The most commonly encountered microbial pathogens include *Mycobacterium bovis BCG*, *Mycobacterium avium*, and *Mycobacterium fortuitum*. The only possible curative option identified to date is human stem cell transplantation (**HSCT**) (*Chapter 22*).

The IL-12/IL-23/STAT1 Signaling Pathway

In addition to the interferon-γ/IL-12 pathway, the mononuclear phagocyte/lymphocyte system utilizes a second axis, the IL-12/IL-23/STAT1 signaling pathway, to mediate antigen presentation, lymphocyte stimulation and proliferation, and cytokine production (*Chapter 12*). Shown in Figure 16-19 is a schematic representation of the IFN-γ/IL-12 axis showing the interrelationships of the cytokine cascade for microbicidal killing of intracellular microbes.

Deficiencies in this pathway can occur at several levels and lead to a susceptibility to mycobacterial infection as in the case of the IFN-γ/IL-12 pathway defects. There are two features of the structure of both the IL-12 and IL-23 cytokines as well as their receptors that can lead to a better understanding of how defects of this signaling pathway occur. First, the IL-12 and IL-23 share a common p40 peptide, and second, the receptors for these two cytokines share a common IL-12Rβ1 chain (*Chapter 9* and Figure 16-19). Therefore, a p40 deficiency will abolish both the ligand binding capacity of both IL-12 and IL-23 cytokines, and a defect in the IL-12Rβ1 chain will prevent signaling by either of these cytokines through their respective receptors. Further, a deficiency of STAT1 will result in the impairment of signaling by IFN-α/β, IFN-γ, IFN-λ, and IL-27 since they all use this common signaling molecule (Table 16A-1 in the Annex).

Mutations in IL-12p40, IL-12 receptor β1, and STAT1 are typically not as severe as complete IFN-γ receptor defects, but they also usually present with disseminated BCG, nontuberculous mycobacteria, or salmonella infections (Figure 16-19). In IL-12 receptor β1 deficiency, the infection risk for nontuberculous mycobacteria is much higher in early childhood than after age 12, and is reduced by previous BCG exposure. These patients fail to produce normal amounts of IFN-γ due to defective IL-12 signaling or IL-12 production. Because these defects

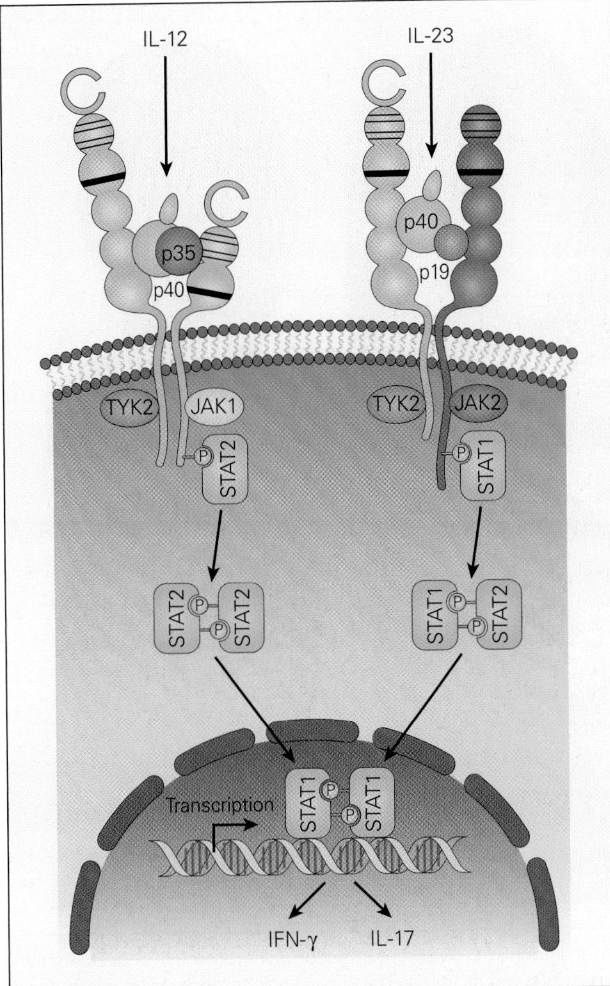

Figure 16-19. Schematic representation of the structures of IL-12 and IL-23 and binding to their specific receptors. Note that the two cytokines share a common p40 peptide and a common IL-12Rβ1 chain in their respective receptors. Binding of both IL-12 and IL-23 occurs through the common IL-12Rβ1 chain; signaling by IL-12 occurs through the binding of the p35 component of IL-12 to the IL-12Rβ2 chain, while signaling by IL-23 occurs by binding of the p19 component of the IL-23 to the IL-23R chain. After binding of IL-12 or IL-23 to their receptors and signal transduction, JAK1 or JAK2 phosphorylates IL-12Rβ2 or IL-23R, respectively, that act as docking sites for STAT2 or STAT1, resulting in their dimerization and translocation to the nucleus, where they stimulate the synthesis of IFN-γ and IL-16.

have preserved IFN-γR function, IFN-γ can be used therapeutically in addition to antimycobacterials.

Hyper-IgE and Recurrent Infection Syndrome (HIES; Job's Syndrome) (MIM ID #147060)

HIES is an immunodeficiency disorder that, in many cases, is transmitted as an autosomal dominant trait (Type 1 HIES), but that occurs sporadically in all racial and ethnic groups (Table 16A-1 in the Annex). Mutations in signal transducer and activator of transcription 3 (**STAT3**) (MIM ID #102582) have been identified as the cause of the autosomal dominant and sporadic forms of HIES. Patients with this disorder present with recurrent infections of the skin and lower respiratory system caused by *Staphylococcus aureus* (with a propensity for pulmonary abscess and pneumatoceles development), eczema, extremely elevated levels of IgE, eosinophilia, and abnormalities of the connective tissue, skeleton, and teeth (with an unusual failure/delay of shedding primary teeth) with distinctive facial features (broad nasal bridge), eczema, osteoporosis and fractures, scoliosis, hyperextensible joints, and candidiasis (Figure 16-20 and Figure 16-21). An arbitrary scoring system has been devised to aid in the formal diagnosis of HIES using both clinical and laboratory test criteria to assign a point value for each finding. IgE is greatly elevated at some point in the life of all patients with HIES, but about 20 percent drop their IgE levels below 2,000 IU/mL as they get older while retaining their susceptibility to infection (Figure 16-22).

More than one genotype may account for the HIES phenotype. An autosomal recessive variant (Type 2 HIES) has also been described with elevated IgE, severe eczema, and recurrent infections, but lacking pneumonias, pneumatoceles, and bony abnormalities (Table 16A-1 in the Annex) (MIM ID #243700). A tyrosine kinase 2 (**TYK2**) deficiency was identified in an AR-HIES patient who presented with susceptibility to intracellular bacterial and viral infections.

Peripheral blood mononuclear cells of patients with hyper-IgE syndrome have an accentuated response to lipopolysaccharide, resulting in decreased TNF-α and IFN-γ production, which could result in excessive PMN inflammatory response. At the same time, they have decreased IL-6 mediated chemokine induction, which may account for the delayed inflammatory reaction.

Eczema occurs within the first days to months of life, as do mucocutaneous candidiasis and severe diaper rash. Sinopulmonary infections, predominantly caused by *S. aureus*, *S. pneumoniae*, and *Haemophilus influenzae*, are common, as are post-inflammatory pneumatoceles. Although otitis media and externa are common, infections occur less frequently in bone and joints, and very infrequently in the liver, kidneys, and gastrointestinal tract; sepsis is rare. Infections with *Aspergillus*, *Pseudomonas*, group A streptococci, *Cryptococcus neoformans*, *Pneumocystis jiroveci*, *Histoplasma capsulatum*, and *C. albicans* are less common.

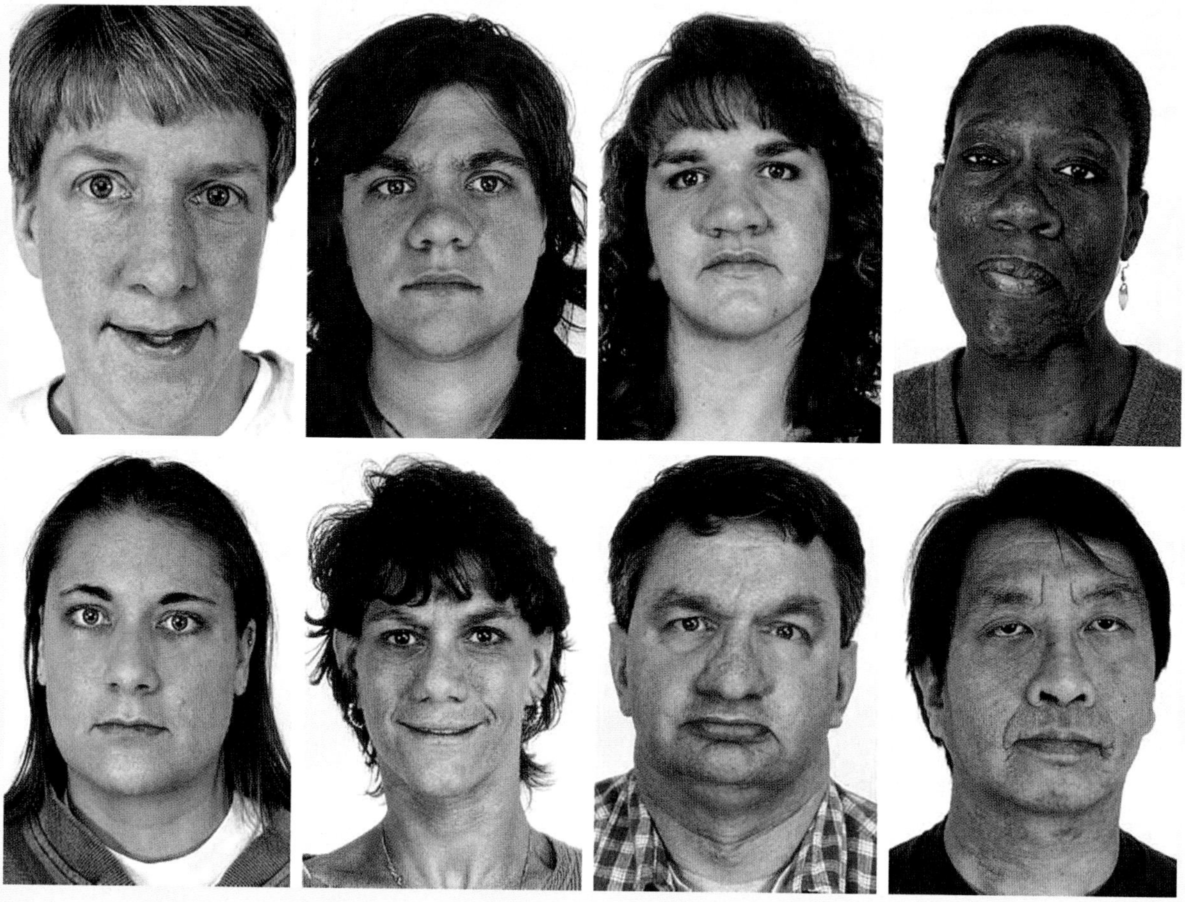

Figure 16-20. Characteristic facial appearance of patients with hyperimmunoglobulin E recurrent infection syndrome (HIES or Job's syndrome). Note that there is a characteristic facies that is apparent in both genders and all races. The facies include wide nasal width, facial asymmetry, and apparent hypertelorism. (Reproduced with permission from Grimbacher B, Holland SM, Gallin JI, et al. Hyper-IgE syndrome with recurrent infections—an autosomal dominant multisystem disorder. N Engl J Med. 1999;340:692–702.)

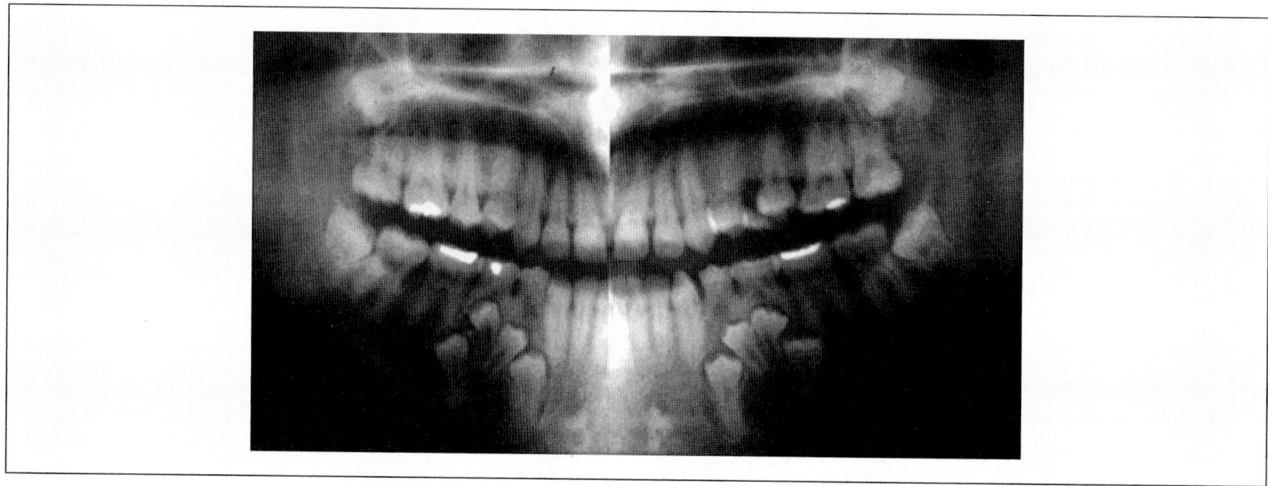

Figure 16-21. A panorex dental x-ray of both upper and lower jaws and teeth of an adult patient with HIES showing retention of primary teeth. Note the eight unerupted teeth in the lower mandible. If retained primary teeth are removed early enough, the secondary teeth erupt normally. (Reproduced with permission from Grimbacher B, Holland SM, Gallin JI, et al. Hyper-IgE syndrome with recurrent infections—an autosomal dominant multisystem disorder. N Engl J Med. 1999;340:692–702.)

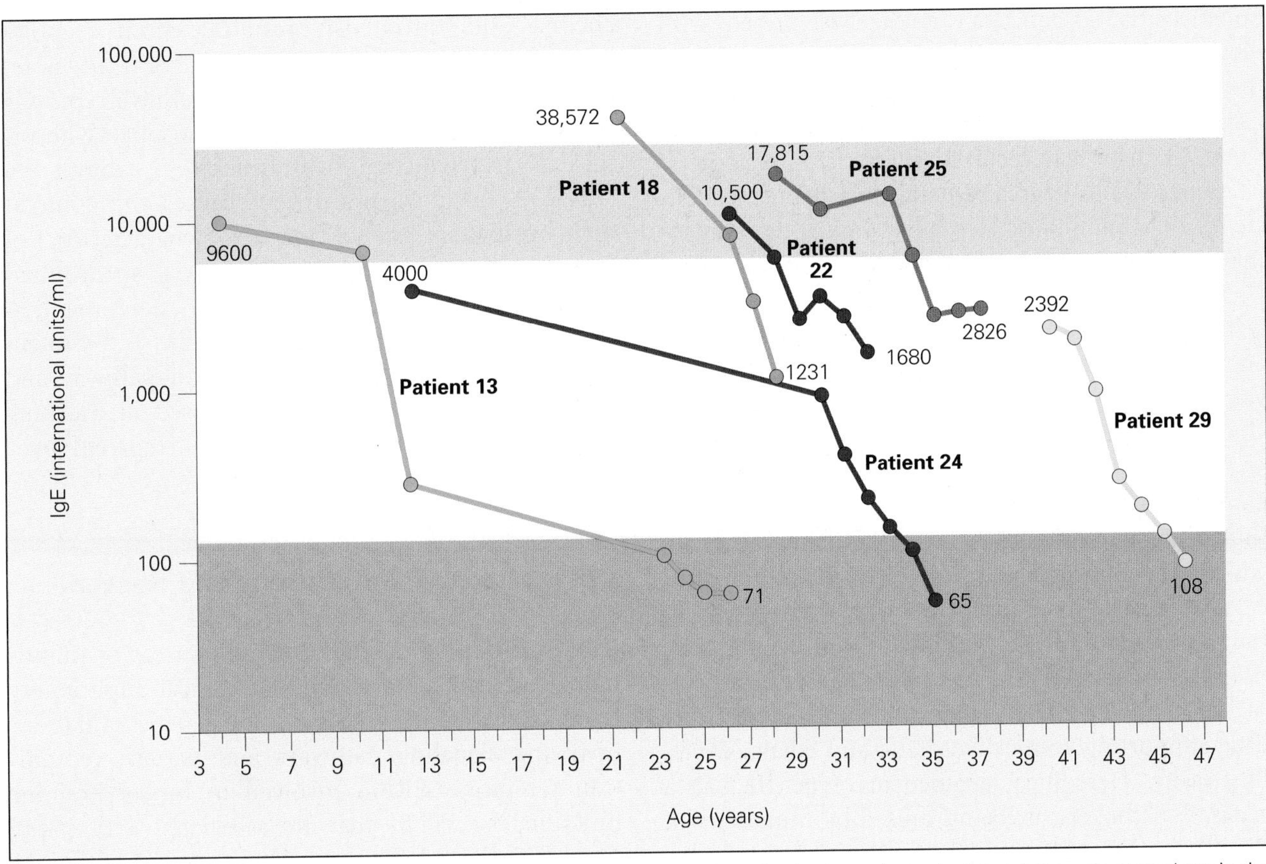

Figure 16-22. Change of IgE levels over time in selected HIES patients. Note that in the patients depicted, IgE levels started out in the extremely elevated range (upper lightly shaded bar) and fell over many years, in some cases into the normal range (lower darker shaded bar). In this study, 16 percent of patients had their IgE levels fall into the normal range over time. It remains unclear whether this change in IgE level is relevant to disease activity or for susceptibility to infection. (Reproduced wirh permission from Grimbacher B, Holland SM, Gallin JI, et al. Hyper-IgE syndrome with recurrent infections—an autosomal dominant multisystem disorder. N Engl J Med. 1999;340:692–702.)

Mucocutaneous candidiasis involving the mouth, vagina, intertriginous areas, fingernails, and toenails affects about 50 percent of HIES patients. T2 hyperintensities on MRI scanning are seen in 60 percent of adult HIES patients; carotid artery aneurysms, strokes, lymphomas, and Barrett's esophagus have also been seen. Pathologic fractures occur in the majority of patients. The use of prophylactic antibiotics (e.g., a synthetic penicillin or trimethoprim/sulfamethoxazole) directed at coverage of *S. aureus* is recommended.

Disorders of Complement

Complement Defects

Complement is an ancient bioamplification arm of the immune system developed for identifying and tagging intruders and clearing the products of immune activation (*Chapter 4*). Although considered part of the innate immune system, the complement limb can be activated through any of its three major pathways, i.e., the classical, mannose, and alternative pathways, and, as such, provides a bridge between both the innate and adaptive immune systems.

All three pathways, once activated, result in the cleavage of C3 components and utilize a final common pathway to generate important biologic products active in opsonization (C3b), anaphylatoxic activity (C3a, C5a), chemotactic activity (C5a), or in cytotoxicity MAC (5b–9) (*Chapter 4*). Defects in complement affecting each of the three pathways often can present clinically with recurrent systemic bacterial infections, autoimmunity, or both (Table 16A-2 in the Annex). Since the complement system was described in great detail in Chapter 4, this section will only briefly summarize the complement defects associated with primary immune deficiency.

As shown in Table 16A-2 in the Annex, defects in C1q, C1r, C4, and C2 deficiency can manifest not only with recurrent infection, but also with SLE-like syndrome, rheumatoid disease, infections, and in the case of C2 deficiency, with vasculitis and polymyositis. C3 deficiency can likewise present with recurrent pyogenic infections, while deficiencies of the late complement components (C5, C6, C7, C8a, C8b, and C9) as well as properdin and factor D deficiency predispose to recurrent neisserial infections.

As described in greater detail in Chapter 4, deficiency of C1 inhibitor (C1 INH) causes the autosomal dominant hereditary angioedema types I and II. In this condition, rapid swelling (edema) of the skin, mucosa, and submucosal tissues can occur in an uncontrolled fashion as "attacks" at a variety of sites, including the digestive tract, presenting with abdominal pain as well as angioedema in the skin and deeper submucosal tissues. The basis for the condition is due to a deficiency of the C1 inhibitor that normally inhibits C1, factor XII, and kallikrein, which when unregulated, can give rise to the production vasoactive substances, which gives rise to the rapid accumulation of fluid in the interstitial tissues most obvious in the face and dorsal aspects of the hands and feet, where the skin has relatively little supporting connective tissue and edema develops easily. Hereditary angioedema type III has a separate pathogenesis, being caused by mutations in the Factor XII (F12) gene, which encodes a serine protease called Factor XII.

In addition to deficiencies of the individual complement components, mutations affecting cofactors can also lead to disease manifestations. For example, mutations affecting factors H and I, which antagonize the functions of Factors B and D, can disrupt the normal control of the C3 convertase, leading to hemolytic-uremic syndrome and membranoproliferative glomerulonephritis (*Chapter 4*). Mutations can also affect components of the lectin pathway, i.e., MBP and MASP2 deficiency, leading to recurrent pyogenic infections, especially during the first years of life, and SLE syndrome in the case of deficiency of MASP2.

Deficiencies of regulatory components affecting the C3 convertase as well as factor C9 can also lead to autoimmune diseases. For example, membrane cofactor protein (CD46), which normally removes the C3 convertase from the cellular membrane, when deficient can cause glomerulonephritis and atypical hemolytic uremic syndrome by continued presence of the membrane-associated C3 convertase in patients showing an AD pattern of inheritance. Similarly, deficiency of the membrane attack complex inhibitor (CD59) that normally removes C9 from MAC has been associated with hemolytic anemia and thrombosis resulting from complement-mediated lysis of erythrocytes. A third molecule that participates in the removal of C3 convertase by anchoring CD46 is phosphatidylinositol N-acetylglucosaminyltransferase subunit a (**PIGA**), which when deficient causes the complement-mediated lysis of red cells characteristic of paroxysmal nocturnal hemoglobinuria, an acquired X-linked condition (Table 16A-2 in the Annex). A recently described mutation of ficolin 3, a protein linked to the activation of the lectin pathway and encoded by the FCN3 gene, expressed in the lung and liver, has been associated with recurrent pyogenic infections of the lung.

Defects of the Innate Immune System

One of the most rapidly developing areas of immunologic research that is finding clinical applicability is being directed to the study of genetic mutations involving signaling pathways and pattern recognition receptors (**PRRs**) involved in innate immune function, e.g., TLRs that are associated with severe innate immunodeficiency phenotypes (*Chapter 3*). These present powerful opportunities to determine the relationship between specific immunological defects and human disease processes in vivo. There are several emerging studies of human primary immunodeficiencies associated with abnormal TLR signaling that demonstrate that this pathway is critical for human defense against infection.

As described in Chapter 3 and Chapter 9, TLRs mediate recognition of microbes, regulate activation of the innate immune response, and provide a linkage with adaptive immune responses. Cellular and molecular studies over the past several years have identified a number of common TLR polymorphisms that modify the cellular immune response and production of cytokines in vitro. In addition, human genetic studies suggest that some of these polymorphisms are associated with susceptibility to a spectrum of diseases, particularly the infectious diseases.

Signaling pathways activated through receptors for IL-1β, IL-18, TNF-α, CD40, and for many of the TLRs are shared with those for ectoderm formation. These pathways converge at the activation of NF-κB, an important transcription factor dependent on the activation of the inhibitor of the NF-κB kinase (**IKK**) complex and its subsequent phosphorylation of the NF-κB inhibitor, IκB (*Chapter 9*). Defects in one of the IKK components, IKKγ, also called the NF-κB essential modulator (**NEMO**), cause ectodermal dysplasia together with a complex set of immunodeficiencies with dysfunction of the innate (Toll-like receptors, TNF-αR, and IL-1R) and adaptive (CD40 and IL-18) immune systems. These patients have a very significant susceptibility to nontuberculous mycobacterial infections, which may be mediated through IL-12 induction. They may also require prophylactic antibiotics and intravenous immunoglobulin due to ineffective immunoglobulin class switching (*Chapter 6*). Some patients respond well to IFN-γ treatment in the setting of disseminated mycobacterial infection. This syndrome is described in greater detail below together with the hyper IgM syndromes.

Shown in Table 16A-3 in the Annex are some of the major defects of the innate immune system that involve TLR signaling pathways and other transcription molecules. The genes and immunodeficiencies include those affecting IKKγ or NEMO, which causes X-linked anhydrotic ectodermal dysplasia with immunodeficiency (**XL-EDA-ID**); IKKα, which causes autosomal-dominant form of EDA-ID (**AD-EDA-ID**); IRAK4 deficiency, which is associated with susceptibility to severe bacterial invasive disease; and UNC93b and TLR3 deficiencies, which are associated with susceptibility to herpes simplex encephalitis.

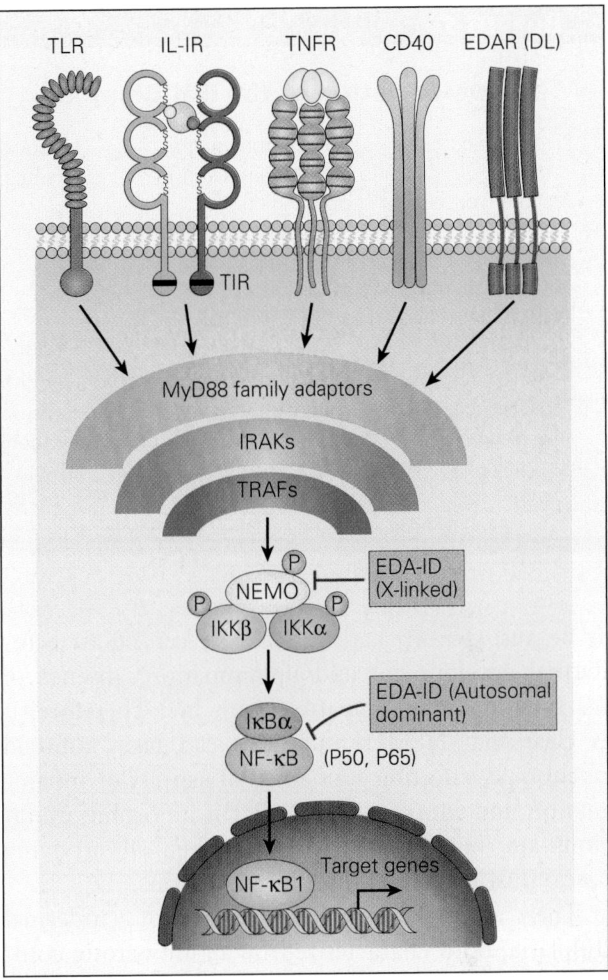

Figure 16-23. Schematic representation of NF-κB activation and NEMO deficiency. Signaling pathways, including those for ectodermal formation (EDA/DL) and inflammation (TNFR, IL1R, IL18R, CD40R, and TLR), all converge on the pathway needed to phosphorylate and ubiquitinate the inhibitor of NF-κB, i.e., IκBα. When this occurs appropriately it leads to liberation of the active p50/p65 NF-κB, which, after translocation to the nucleus, activates proinflammatory genes as well as genes responsible for skin and skeletal morphogenesis. Therefore, mutations in NEMO have the potential to impair both ectoderm formation and innate immunity. However, defective CD40 signaling also leads to impaired immunoglobulin class-switch recombination, in some cases, causing failure to switch from immunoglobulin M (IgM) to IgG, hence the occurrence of hyper IgM in some patients.

NEMO Mutations: Ectodermal Dysplasia, Anhidrotic, with Immune Deficiency (MIM ID #305100; MIM ID #300291)

Ectodermal dysplasia anhidrotic (**EDA**) with immune deficiency (**EDA-ID**) has several different inheritance patterns. Most cases are caused by mutations in the EDA gene that are inherited in an X-linked recessive pattern (EDA-ID) and are due to mutations of NEMO (IKKγ), a modulator of NF-κB activation (MIM ID #305100); less commonly, a second form of EDA-ID (MIM ID #300291) results from a gain-of-function mutation of IκBα, resulting in impaired activation of NF-κB and is inherited in an autosomal dominant pattern (Table 16A-3 in the Annex and Figure 16-23).

As described in Chapter 9, NF-κB sits at the convergence of multiple signal transduction pathways, including those for most innate immune signals (TLRs), inflammatory cytokines (IL-1β, TNF-α), IFN-γ induction by IL-18, class-switch recombination (CD40), and ectoderm formation (dysplasin) (Figure 16-23). NF-κB is an inducible transcription factor of the Rel family and is maintained normally in an inactive form in the cytoplasm by the IκBα. After activation of the IKK complex of proteins, IκBα is phosphorylated and ubiquitinated and releases the dimeric p50/p65 NF-κB to be translocated to the nucleus (Figure 16-23). The nomenclature of the IKK complex is very confusing because a variety of terms have been used to define the various components. For ease of discussion, this nomenclature is shown in Box 16-1.

Box 16-1

The Nomenclature of the IKK Complex

The IKK complex is part of the upstream NF-κB signal transduction cascade and is comprised of three subunits, each encoded by a separate gene:

-**IKK1** (also known as **IKKα**) (CHUK)
-**IKK2** (also known as **IKKβ**) (IKBKB)
-**NEMO** (also known as **IKKγ**) (IKBKG)

After binding of a ligand with a relevant receptor, the IKK is assembled and activated and can then target **IκBα** in the IκBα/NF-κB complex to affect its phosphorylation, ubiquitination, and degradation, thus releasing the active dimeric form of NF-κB consisting of p50/p65 (Figure 16-23). Because IκBα is bound to NF-κB, it maintains it in an inactive form and prevents it from translocating into the nucleus. The phosphorylation of IκBα frees the dimeric p50/65 NF-κB to move into the nucleus and subsequently promote gene transcription. NF-κB is required for the signal transduction of a number of surface and cytoplasmic receptors, including T cell receptors (TCRs), B cell receptors, IL-1 receptor and TNF receptor superfamilies, and the TLRs. The NF-κB essential modulator (NEMO) (IKKγ) serves as gatekeeper for this process. Although it has no intrinsic enzymatic activity, NEMO serves as the critical scaffolding protein for the IKK complex. NEMO is therefore an essential regulator of NF-κB signaling, and mutations have the potential to result in broad immune dysfunction as well as ectodermal and skeletal anomalies.

Because NF-κB activation is so central to ectodermal development and inflammation, absence of it's function is incompatible with life. Therefore, it is clear that NEMO mutations can have a broad phenotype, affecting fundamental aspects of inflammation and immunity, and that if amorphic mutations are incompatible with life, then all surviving cases must have hypomorphic mutations.

There are two forms of inheritance of ectodermal dysplasia, both characterized by an anhydrotic component associated with immune deficiency (EDA-ID) (Table 16A-3 in the Annex and Figure 16-23). These include (1) an X-linked form in which there is a mutation of NEMO (IKKγ) and (2) an autosomal dominant mutation that results from a gain of function mutation of IκBα. The full-blown syndrome includes pegged, gapped teeth, abnormal hair whorls and thin, sparse hair over the entire body, poor ability to sweat, and a string of infections, including those caused by *Pneumocystis*, Gram-positive, Gram-negative bacteria, viruses, and mycobacteria, but not by filamentous fungi (Figure 16-24). In the X-linked recessive form of the NEMO mutation, female carriers are mosaic with one altered and one normal copy of the gene in each cell. In about 70 percent of cases, carriers experience some features of the condition. Some of these women will have incontinentia pigmenti, somatic distributions of NEMO-deficient skin that are hypopigmented, but can also manifest erythematous skin eruptions. These signs and symptoms are usually mild and include a few missing or abnormal teeth, sparse hair, and some problems with sweat gland function. Some carriers, however, can manifest more severe features of this disorder.

Diagnosis of NEMO is difficult because the clinical presentation is rarely as clear as the full-blown cases that were described initially. Patients can have no ectodermal phenotype, can have normal antibody levels, and may have only mycobacterial infections. Even in functional studies, there are very few clear and consistent features that would allow one to either include or exclude NEMO without sequencing the gene. Therefore, in patients in whom appropriate infections have occurred and for whom no other defect is apparent, NEMO sequencing should be strongly considered (*Chapter 25*).

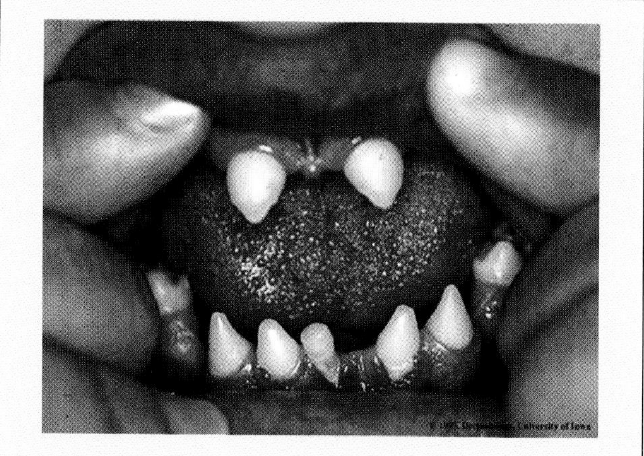

Figure 16-24. Patient with NEMO immunodeficiency showing hypodentia, cone-shaped teeth. (Reproduced with permission from the Department of Dermatology, University of Iowa.)

IRAK4 Deficiency and Gram-Positive Bacterial Infections (MIM ID #607676)

A deficiency in the interleukin-1 receptor activated kinase 4 (**IRAK-4**) has recently been associated with severe recurrent, predominantly Gram-positive bacterial infections, e.g., pneumococcal invasive disease (Table 16A-3 in the Annex). IRAK-4 is a member of the IRAK family of protein kinases involved in signaling innate immune responses from Toll-like receptors (*Chapter 9*). Clinicians treating children with recurrent invasive pneumococcal infection should therefore be aware of this novel primary immunodeficiency. IRAK-4-deficient patients predominantly suffer from recurrent infections caused by pyogenic Gram-positive bacteria, with *Streptococcus pneumoniae*, causing invasive infection in all reported cases. IRAK-4 deficiency abrogates TLR function, rendering the innate immune response to pneumococcus ineffective. IRAK-4 deficiency represents a significant diagnostic challenge as these patients generally have normal results on routine immunologic evaluation offered in most institutions because neutrophil and complement activity as well as T and B cell function are not significantly affected by IRAK-4 deficiency (*Chapter 24*). Therefore, it is conceivable that children with IRAK-4 deficiency pass unrecognized by their physicians and may be inaccurately labeled as "immunologically normal." It is recommended, therefore, that apparently healthy children who experience recurrent systemic pneumococcal disease undergo immunologic assessment of innate immunity and IRAK-4 function in addition to the routine evaluation of B cell defects that usually herald these types of infections. Early detection of IRAK-4 deficiency and related TLR signaling defects will enhance the clinical management of affected individuals by optimizing medical therapy and facilitating accurate genetic counseling for the family.

MyD88 Deficiency (MIM ID #612260), Warts, Hypogammaglobulinemia, HPV Infections, Myelokathexis Syndrome (MIM ID #193670), and Epidermodysplasia Verruciformis (MIM ID #226400)

A very rare group of innate immune system signaling defects has been described, which include (1) patients presenting with recurrent pyogenic bacterial infections with mutations in MyD88; (2) patients presenting with the constellation of warts, hypogammaglobulinemia, infections caused by HPV, and myelokathexis (**WHIM**) who have gain-of-function mutations of CXCR4, the receptor for the chemokine CXCL12; and (3) patients with epidermodysplasia verruciformis (**EV**) presenting with recurrent HPV infections and cancer of the skin with mutations of EVER1 and EVER2 of the transmembrane channel gene family, which may be involved in innate immune responses that control the clearance of EV-HPV-infected keratinocytes.

UNC93B Deficiency (MIM ID #610551), TLR-3 Deficiency (MIM ID #613002), and Susceptibility to Herpes Simplex Encephalitis

As shown in Table 16A-3 in the Annex, mutations in the signaling molecule **UNC93B** and the innate sensor TLR3 appear to be involved in selective susceptibility to recurrent viral infection. Defects in the protein UNC93B in the human predispose to susceptibility to encephalitis caused by infection with herpes simplex virus and in the mouse to cytomegalovirus (Box 16-2). The mechanism is unclear, but UNC93B1 is known to interact with the Toll-like receptors TLR3, TLR7, and TLR9, and it appears to be involved in the trafficking of these receptors within the cell (*Chapter 9*). Mutations in this gene lead to selective impairment of dsRNA-induced interferon alpha/beta and interferon 1 lambda production. Five of the 10 human Toll-like receptors (TLR3, TLR4, TLR7, TLR8, and TLR9), and four of the 12 mouse TLRs (TLR3, TLR4, TLR7, and TLR9) can trigger interferon IFN-α, IFN-β, and IFN-λ, which are critical for antiviral immunity (*Chapter 13*). On the other hand, TLR-3 participates in the innate immune response to several microbial agents and senses ds-RNA, a sign of viral infection. It acts via MYD88 and TRAF6, leading to NF-κB activation, cytokine secretion, and the inflammatory response, and deficiency of this innate immune sensor has also been shown to be associated with susceptibility to herpes simplex infection in the human.

UNC93B- and TLR3-deficient patients appear to be specifically prone to herpes simplex virus 1 (**HSV-1**) encephalitis, although clinical penetrance is incomplete, whereas IRAK-4-deficient patients appear to be normally resistant to most viruses, including HSV-1 but, as described previously, are susceptible to severe recurrent, predominantly Gram-positive bacterial infections. These experiments of nature suggest that the TLR7-, TLR8-, and TLR9-dependent induction of IFN-α, IFN-β, and IFN-λ is largely redundant in human antiviral immunity, whereas the TLR3-dependent induction of IFN-α, IFN-β, and IFN-λ is critical for primary

Box 16-2

From Worms to Mice, and Then to Children, with Herpes Simplex Virus Encephalitis

The term "UNC" derives from the UNC93 gene discovered in *Caenorhabditis elegans*, a free-living nematode (roundworm) about the size of a pinhead in studies of the regulation of muscle contraction. Mutant worms carrying semidominant gain-of-function (gf) mutations in UNC93 move sluggishly, are defective in egg-laying and defecation, and display a rubber band "uncoordinated" (UNC) response; when prodded on the head, a mutant worm contracts and then relaxes along its entire body without moving backward, in contrast to the wild-type worm, which contracts its anterior end and backs away in a more coordinated fashion.

This finding formed the basis of the discovery that a mutation in mice called the UNC93B1 mutation 3d disrupted exogenous antigen presentation and signaling via TLR 3, 7, and 9 and later to the discovery that two children with autosomal recessive deficiency in the intracellular protein UNC93B had impaired cellular interferon-α, β, and γ antiviral responses that resulted in their susceptibility to herpes simplex virus encephalitis.

Studies by Drs. Brenner, Horvitz, and Sulston using the nematode *Caenorhabditis elegans* as an experimental model system opened new understanding of pathways of cell division and differentiation from the fertilized egg to the adult, which led to the Nobel Prize in Physiology or Medicine for 2002.

immunity to HSV-1 in the central nervous system in children but redundant for immunity to most other viral infections.

Chronic Mucocutaneous Candidiasis Caused by CARD 9 Deficiency: Candidiasis, Familial, 1 (MIM ID #212050) and Candidiasis, Familial, 2 (MIM ID #114580)

Chronic mucocutaneous candidiasis (**CMC**) is a selective cellular immunodeficiency characterized by chronic infections of the skin, nails, and mucous membranes with *Candida* species, usually *C. albicans*. The clinical presentation of CMC varies and the condition is sometimes associated with endocrinopathies. Although most often occurring sporadically, autosomal recessive (Candidiasis, Familial, 1 [**CANDF1**] [MIM ID #212050]) and autosomal dominant (Candidiasis, Familial, 2; [**CANDF2**] [MIM ID #114580]) forms of the syndrome have been reported with deficiencies of CARD9 (Table 16A-3 in the Annex). Severe cases present with persistent thrush or diaper rash during the first months of life. Typically, the infection spreads from the perineal and circumoral areas over the extremities, scalp, and face, usually involving fingernails and toenails. Candidal laryngitis and esophagitis are common, yet there is little predisposition to other parenchymal involvement. *Candida* is readily cultured from infected sites. Chronic *Candida* infection may be seen in patients with more extensive immunologic compromise (Figure 16-25) and most recently in patients with HIV infection.

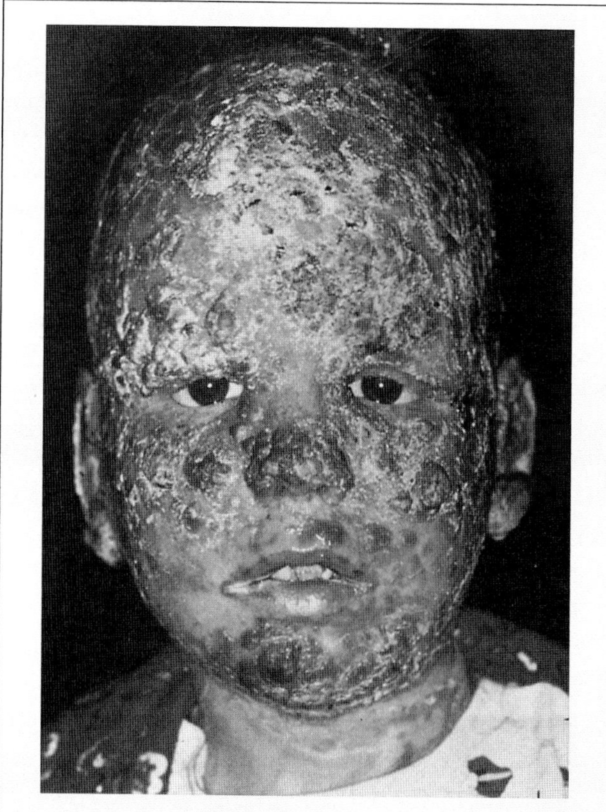

Figure 16-25. A nine-year-old boy with chronic mucocutaneous candidiasis who was found to be deficient in cell-mediated immunity. (Reproduced with permission from Schlegel RJ, Bernier GM, Bellanti JA, et al. Severe candidiasis associated with thymic dysplasia, IgA deficiency, and plasma anti lymphocyte effects. Pediatrics 1970; 45:929.)

Whereas mucocutaneous candidiasis has long been recognized as a consequence of adaptive immune deficiency caused by profound lymphocyte dysfunction, or lymphopenia, recent studies have demonstrated the important role of the innate immune system in anti-candidal protective immunity. Recognition of *C. albicans* by the innate host defense system is mediated by pattern-recognition receptors from the TLR and lectin-like-receptor families, e.g., mannans from the candida cell wall are recognized by the mannose receptor and TLR4,5 and TLR2 recognizes phospholipomannan and collaborates with the β-glucan receptor dectin-1 in the stimulation of cytokine production (*Chapter 14*). Signaling activity of dectin-1, a pattern-recognition receptor found on monocytes and dendritic cells (**DC**) able to recognize beta-1,3 and beta-1,6 glucans, has been found to be deficient in a Dutch family with recurrent candidal infection of the nails and mucosa. Another report described an extended Iranian family with predominantly mucocutaneous but also fatal candidiasis of the central nervous system caused by mutations in the critical dectin-1 signal transduction molecule, CARD9, impairing both dectin-1 signaling and Th17 production (Figure 16-26). Collectively, these studies suggest that various components of the dectin-1-CARD 9-Th17 pathways and related cytokines not only can couple the complex innate and adaptive immune responses important in anti-fungal immunity, but that defects in any of a number of these critical pathways can be responsible for the clinical spectrum of responses that characterize the heterogeneous syndrome of chronic mucocutaneous candidiasis.

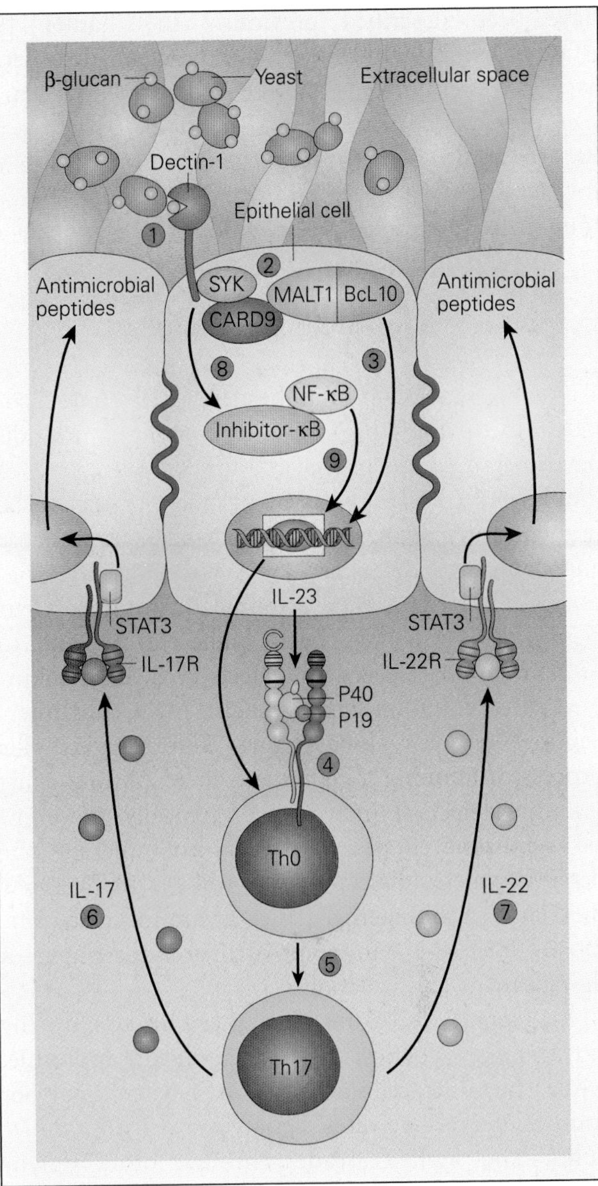

Figure 16-26. **Schematic representation of the dectin-1 signaling pathway important in fungal sensing and control.** The β-glucan on the budding yeast forms of candida bind to dectin-1 on the surface of an epithelial cell (#1) leading to activation of the CARD9 signaling complex (along with MALT1-Bcl-10) (#2). This in turn delivers a signal to the nucleus for the gene expression of IL-23 (#3) and production of IL-23 that after binding to its receptor (#4) helps drive CD4+ Th0 lymphocytes toward the Th17 phenotype, a STAT3-dependent process (#5). Th17 lymphocytes elaborate IL-17 (#6) and IL-22 (#7), which promote the synthesis of antimicrobial peptides by epithelial cells. In addition, the activation of dectin-1 also generates a signal through the NF-κB pathway (#8) that favors the gene expression and synthesis of antimicrobial peptides (#9). Molecules with identified mutations relevant to fungal susceptibility include (dectin-1, CARD9, and STAT3) have been seen in patients with chronic mucocutaneous candidiasis.

Trypanosomiasis and APOL1 Mutations (MIM ID #603743)

Protective immunity to trypanosomiasis, i.e., *Trypanosoma brucei brucei*, in the human has been associated with involvement of apolipoprotein L-I (**APOL1**), a trypanolytic component of serum (*Chapter 15*). Recently, *T. evansi* infection in a human was identified in an Indian patient whose serum was found to have no trypanolytic activity due to the lack of APOL1 (Table 16A-3 in the Annex). The defect was due to frameshift mutations in both APOL1 alleles. Trypanolytic activity was restored in vitro by the addition of recombinant APOL1. The lack of APOL1 explained the patient's infection with *T. evansi*. More recently, in African Americans, focal segmental glomerulosclerosis (**FSGS**) and hypertension-attributed end-stage kidney disease (**H-ESKD**) were found to be associated with two independent sequence variants in the APOL1 gene on chromosome 22.

Autoinflammatory Disorders

Another important group of innate immune defects are seen in the autoinflammatory disorders that have been described previously in Chapter 19 Annex. These include several monogenic disorders as well as a number of newly recognized polygenic disorders. Shown in Table 16A-4 in the Annex is a list of some of the autoinflammatory disorders together with a brief summary of their genetic mutations and clinical presentations.

Lymphocyte Immune Deficiencies

T and B lymphocyte immune deficiencies have provided the paradigms for understanding immunology, tolerance, and transplantation for over 50 years (Tables 16A-5 and 16A-6 in the Annex). The nomenclature of these immune deficiencies is dense and confusing, as diseases originally described phenotypically (e.g., severe combined immune deficiency, [**SCID**]) have been found to be due to numerous separate genetic defects (e.g., interleukin-2 receptor common gamma chain, JAK3, and interleukin-7 receptor alpha chain). Unfortunately, this process of lumping together and then splitting apart immune defects is unavoidable. Typically, the clinical syndrome is described first, followed by the detailed genetic dissection. We will try to overview this large and heterogeneous group of disorders, mostly from the standpoint of their impairment of development and function.

In general, receptors bind their ligands by the extracellular portion of the receptor molecule, while the intracellular portion engages partner molecules and activates signal transduction molecules. The signal cascades through other downstream molecules, finally governing transcription and later translation (e.g., the "3 T's"). Subsequent DNA cleavage, polymerization, and repair resulting in recombination are critical for lymphocyte diversity and antigen specificity (*Chapters* 6 and *7*). Therefore, defects that affect lymphoid ligand binding, signaling, or any of the steps of successful DNA recombination may present as defects in adaptive immunity (Tables 16A-5 and 16A-6 in the Annex).

Combined T Cell and B Cell Defects

Shown in Table 16A-5 in the Annex are the primary immunodeficiencies associated with combined defects of T cells and B cells. T lymphocytes are the pivotal cells *sine qua non* for orchestration of adaptive immunity (*Chapter 7*). They direct the killing of intracellular pathogens and the responses of B lymphocytes and antigen-presenting cells (**APCs**) in the defense against extracellular pathogens. They can also kill directly when they recognize aberrant surface molecules. Consequently, defects in T cell development and/or function invariably can also result in defects affecting B cell, NK cell, and myeloid compartments. Shown in Table 16-4 is a molecular, functional, and phenotypic classification of the combined T and B cell defects. For ease of discussion, these have been grouped both according to their functional sites of derangement, e.g., signaling, DNA rearrangement and repair or purine metabolic sites, as well as their phenotypic severity, e.g., SCID versus non-SCID. Shown in Figure 16-27 is a schematic representation of these combined T and B cell defects portrayed according to this arbitrary classification.

Severe Combined Immune Deficiencies (SCID)

Introduction

Severe combined immunodeficiency (SCID), classically referred to as the "boy in the bubble syndrome" (*Chapter 7*), is a collection of severe heritable genetic immunodeficiency disorders in which both "arms" (B cells and T cells) of the adaptive immune system may be crippled due to a defect in one of several possible genes (Table 16A-5 in the Annex, Figure 16-27 and *Chapter 7*). It is known as the "bubble boy" disease, named after David Vetter who survived isolated in a plastic bubble for 12 years because of the condition's extreme vulnerability to infectious diseases. The overall incidence is estimated to be 1 in 75,000 births, and without treatment, SCID patients usually die during infancy. Several different forms of SCID have been described based on differential involvement of T, B, and NK cell lineages. There are several types of SCID that are characterized by defective T cell function with different levels of B cell and NK cell impairment (Table 16-4 and Figure 16-27).

When considering the diagnosis of SCID, the most serious of the immune deficiency disorders, it is important to keep several things in mind. (1) SCID is a medical emergency. If the patient with SCID is to

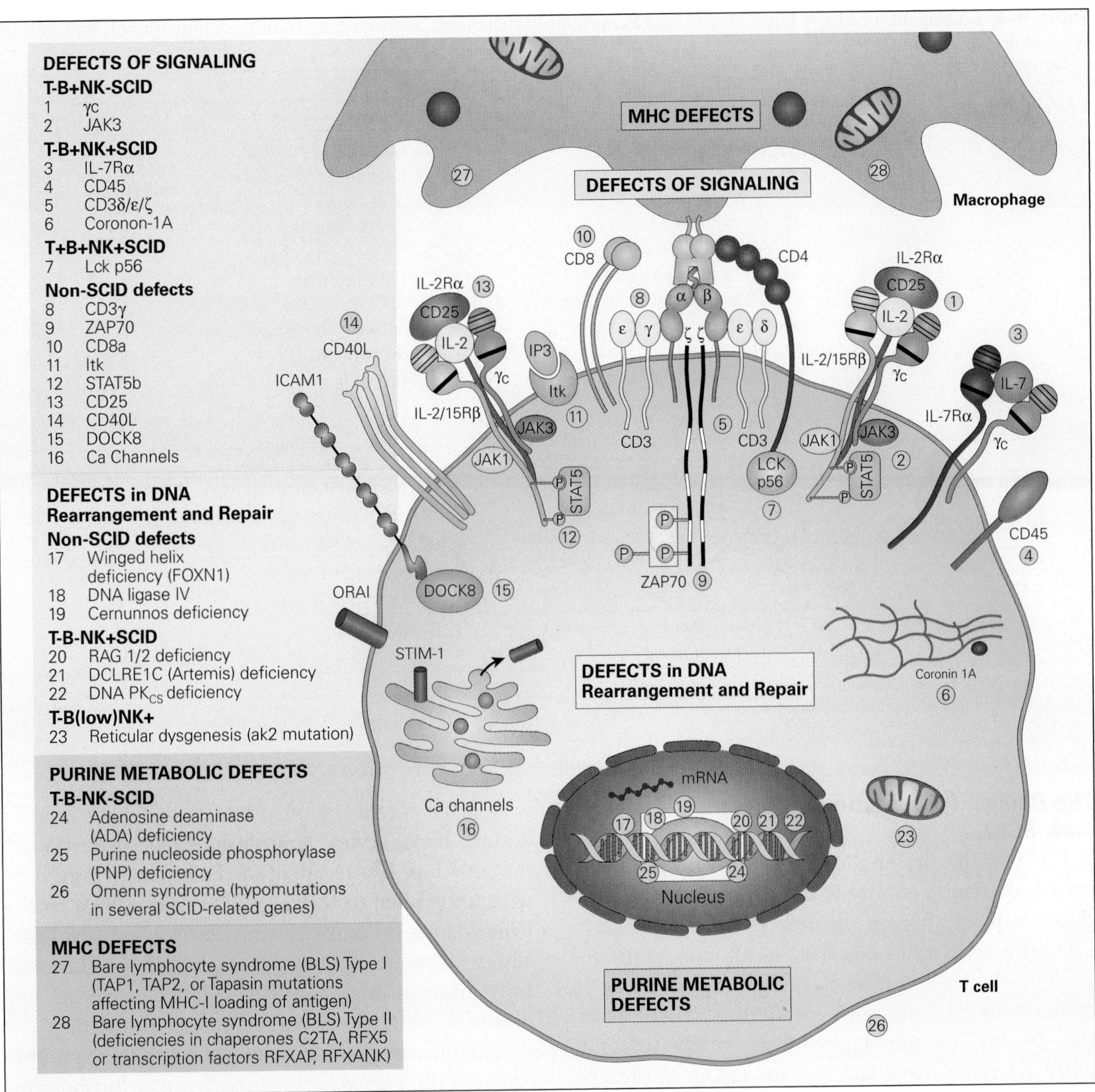

Figure 16-27. Schematic representation of the different levels at which defects of the combined T and B cell deficiencies occur divided according to the arbitrary classification shown in Table 16-4. These include defects of signaling, defects in DNA rearrangement and repair, and purine metabolic defects. Shown on the right side of the figure are molecular defects seen in conditions presenting as the SCID phenotype arranged according to various combinations of involvement of T, B, and NK phenotypes. On the left side of the figure are shown other molecular defects seen in non-SCID phenotypes.

survive transplantation, it is important to avoid community viral infections, which can be devastating; (2) persistent engraftment of maternal lymphocytes, i.e., graft-versus-host disease (**GVHD**), is both a symptom of SCID and a cause of many of the symptoms, such as failure to thrive and rash; (3) a phenotype of infections and clinical illness characterize the presentation of these patients, and the focus of laboratory testing is directed at efforts to confirm the genetic defects (*Chapter 24*); (4) since some mutations in patients with SCID are of the missense type, proteins can still be produced and detected by flow cytometry but be non-functional. Therefore, the clinical picture, typically developed out of the infection profile and the flow cytometry information, must ultimately guide decisions about which genes to sequence.

Table 16-4. Classification of the combined T and B immune deficiencies according to molecular, functional, and phenotypic characteristics

Affected function	Combined T and B immune deficiencies Non-SCID defects	 SCID defects
Defects of signaling	1. CD3γ deficiency 2. ZAP-70 deficiency 3. CD8α deficiency 4. ITK deficiency 5. STAT5b deficiency 6. CD25 deficiency 7. CD40 ligand (CD 40L) deficiency 8. CD40 deficiency 9. DOCK8 deficiency 10. Ca++ channel deficiency 11. MHC-I deficiency* 12. MHC-II deficiency*	T- B+ NK- SCID 1. γc deficiency 2. JAK3 deficiency T- B+ NK+ SCID 3. IL-7Rα deficiency 4. CD45 deficiency 5. CD3δ/CD3ε /CD3ζ deficiency 6. Coronin-1A deficiency T+ B+ NK+ SCID 7. p56Lck deficiency
Defects in DNA rearrangement and repair	1. Winged helix deficiency (FOXN1) 2. Omenn syndrome** 3. DNA ligase IV deficiency 4. Cernunnos deficiency	T- B- NK+ SCID 1. RAG 1/2 deficiency 2. DCLRE1C (Artemis) deficiency 3. DNA PKcs deficiency T- B (low) NK+ SCID 4. Reticular dysgenesis
Purine metabolic defects	1. Purine nucleoside phosphorylase (PNP) deficiency	T- B- NK- SCID 1. Adenine deaminase (ADA) deficiency

*MHC-I and MHC-II are included since they affect T cell function.
**Omenn syndrome encompasses hypomutations of many genes.

The Clinical Presentation of Patients with SCID

SCID typically presents early in life with failure to thrive, diarrhea, recurrent infections due to respiratory viruses, herpes viruses, *Pneumocystis (carinii) jiroveci*, and bacteria. Although mucosal candidiasis is common, aspergillosis is not. In contrast to patients with interferon-γ/IL-12 pathway defects, described previously, where susceptibility to both mycobacteria and BCG is present, generalized complications of BCG vaccine are common in patients with SCID when the vaccine is administered, but nontuberculous mycobacterial infections are not. The underlying defects are caused by improper lymphocyte proliferation due to failure of signal transduction (i.e., receptor defects) or toxicity (adenosine accumulation and lymphocyte death). Therefore, absolute lymphopenia is a common finding in many forms of SCID. In addition, T lymphocyte failure may facilitate persistent engraftment of maternal T lymphocytes transferred to the fetus during pregnancy, leading subsequently to the alloreactive response of the engrafted maternal T cells against the fetus referred to as GVHD, which typically presents in the neonatal infant as rash and/or diarrhea. Similarly, if children with SCID receive blood products that have residual donor lymphocytes, transfusion-associated GVHD may develop, also resulting in characteristic rash, diarrhea, and failure to thrive. SCID carries a high fatality if not diagnosed and treated as early as possible, usually with bone marrow transplantation. Therefore, early diagnosis based on a high index of clinical suspicion is essential. Treatment for all forms of SCID should include prevention of viral infection, prophylaxis against *Pneumocystis jiroveci* with trimethoprim-sulfamethoxazole, and consideration of early bone marrow transplantation or gene correction. The overall frequency of SCID is approximately 1/50,000, but the real incidence may be higher. Carrier and prenatal detection are readily accomplished once the genetic lesion is characterized (*Chapter 7*).

Unraveling the Diagnostic Dilemma of SCID

Although SCID has been classically defined by the presence or absence of T cells, B cells, and NK cells, leading to a complex nomenclature, the use of this seemingly intricate classification has the distinct advantage that with one simple flow cytometric study, one can determine which pathways are most likely to be affected (Figure 16-27,

Table 16A-5 in the Annex, and Table 16-4). Therefore, the use of specialized flow cytometry for lymphoid markers is an early step in evaluation. The reader is referred to Chapter 24 for a graphic depiction of the various combinations of surface markers for T cell, B cell, and NK cell populations determined by flow cytometry that has been found very useful in leading the clinician to the correct form of SCID. However, there is no substitute for the role of early diagnosis by the astute clinician who first suspects the condition that permits the subsequent follow-up by genetic characterization, which carries important implications for prenatal and carrier testing, transplant success, and potential genetic correction.

SCID Defects

SCID Defects of Cytokine Signaling

IL-2 Receptor Common Gamma Chain Deficiency T- B+ NK- SCID (MIM ID #300400)

The prototype for the most common form of SCID has been considered to be the X-linked **(SCID-XL)** form due to mutations in the shared IL-2 common gamma chain receptor (IL-2Rγc, Xq13) found in receptors for IL-2, IL-15, IL-4, IL-7, IL-9, and IL-21 (Figure 16-27, Table 16A-5 in the Annex, and Table 16-4). More recent data, however, indicate that JAK3 and IL7Rα deficiencies may be more common than considered previously. Shown in Figure 16-28 is the central role which the IL-2Rγc chain plays in immune responsiveness since this component is an obligatory signal transducing chain for several cytokine receptors, including IL-2R, IL-15R, IL-4R, IL-7R, IL-9R, and IL-21R (hence the designation common gamma chain) (*Chapter 9*).

Therefore, IL-2Rγc deficiency **(SCID-XL; X-linked SCID; γc deficiency; and CD132)** leads to defects in signal transduction of many cytokines simultaneously. Early lymphoid progenitors are lost because of the IL-7 defect; NK cells are lost because of the IL-15 defect. So in this form of SCID, there are few to no T cells, normal to increased numbers of B cells, and few to no NK cells; hence, it is designated as T- B+ NK- SCID (Figure 16-27, Table 16A-5 in the Annex, and Table 16-4). X-linked SCID occurs in about 1:150,000–200,000 live births and accounts for up to 50 percent of all cases of SCID. IL-2Rγc signals through JAK3, which in turn

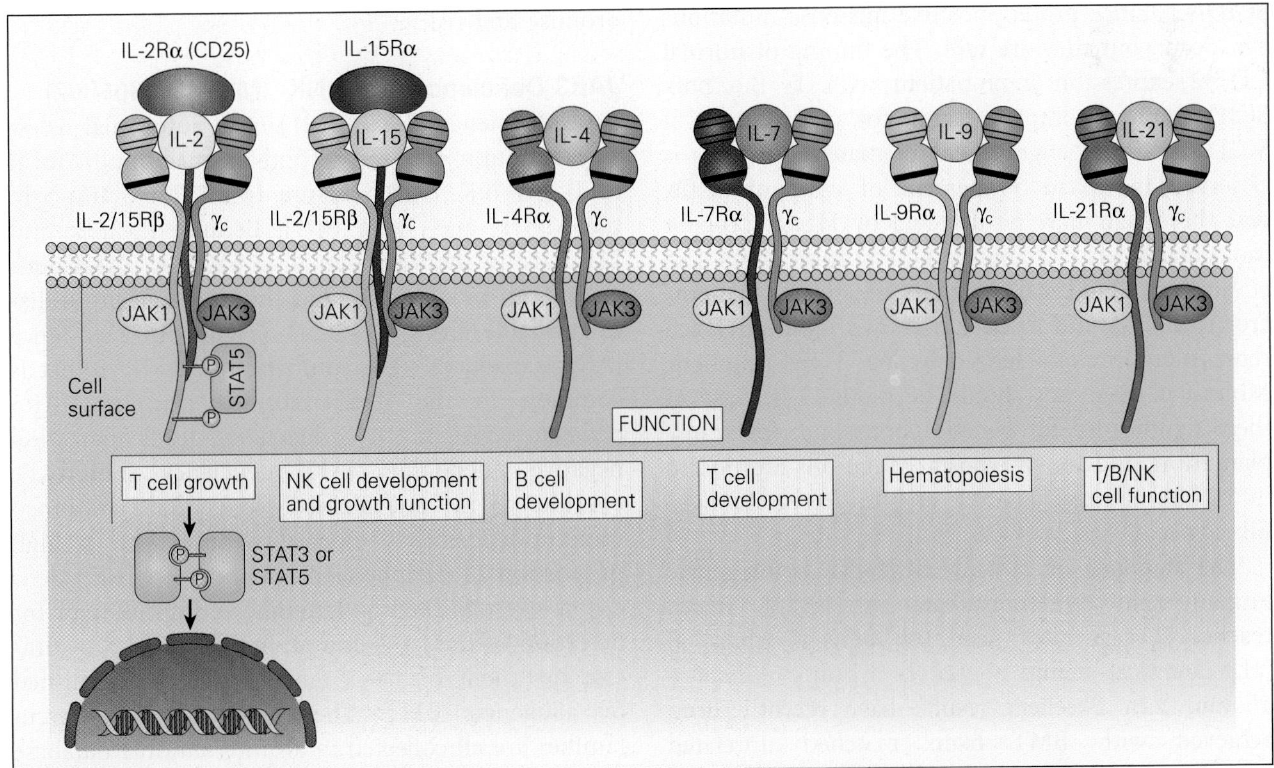

Figure 16-28. Schematic representation of the receptors that use the IL-2R common gamma chain (γc). Note that γc is linked to JAK3, and these receptors signal through STAT3 and STAT5. Therefore, mutations in γc, JAK3, and STAT5 have many overlapping features. Γc mutations exert part of their profound effect through their impact on receptors other than IL-2.

activates other JAKs and their target molecules, the signal transducers and activators of transcription, or STATs (*Chapter 9*). IL-2 signals predominantly through STAT5, which in turn translocates to the nucleus to upregulate the transcription of IL-2 activated genes.

Clinical Management of Patients with SCID

In patients with X-linked SCID, diarrhea, failure to thrive, and oropharyngeal candidiasis are common, as are recurrent pneumonias. Lymphopenia is marked, but it must be kept in mind that the average lymphocyte count for an infant is approximately 3,000/mm^3. Therefore, an absolute lymphocyte count of 1,000/mm^3 represents a significant lymphopenia. Although flow-cytometry studies in these patients show too few T and NK cells and a relative abundance of B cells, the clinical diagnosis of X-linked SCID is ultimately substantiated by flow cytometry for the IL-2Rγc chain (CD132) (*Chapter 24*). Lymphoproliferative cellular responses to mitogens are low to absent. Despite relatively normal numbers of B cells, serum immunoglobulins are very low once maternal antibody has waned, reflecting the critical loss of T cell help. Lymph nodes and lymphoid tissues are scant. Normal CD132 expression does not completely exclude a diagnosis of SCID-XL, since protein-positive missense mutations can occur, but they are rare. The finding of normal CD132 expression in a patient with T- B+ NK- SCID should prompt a search for other forms of SCID. Persistent engraftment of maternal T cells is observed in up to 50 percent of cases of SCID, and these cells may be detected by HLA-typing or molecular analysis at highly polymorphic DNA loci (*Chapters 10* and *22*). Mothers of affected patients are typically found to be carriers with skewed T cell representation characterized by low T cell numbers. Molecular diagnoses should be pursued because of their significance for genetic counseling, for transplantation, and for prognosis. Mutations are posted in an international database at http://research.nhgri.nih.gov/scid/.

The standard of care for SCID-XL is allogeneic human stem cell transplantation (BMT), which reaches success rates near 100 percent when an HLA identical sibling is used as a donor (*Chapters 10* and *22*). Excellent results have recently been achieved with BMT from matched unrelated donors. Haploidentical family (usually parental) members have been suitable donors since the 1980s, but are becoming less commonly used with the advent of comprehensive databases and molecular typing of donor and recipient. Although T cell replacement is often successful following BMT for SCID-XL, functional B cell engraftment is poor and may require replacement intravenous immune globulin (**IVIG**) therapy (*Chapter 11*). Successful in utero stem cell transplantation has been performed with good clinical and laboratory T cell reconstitution. However, this technique requires prenatal diagnosis and so is only of current value in previously diagnosed families.

XL-SCID has been the paradigm for human immunodeficiency gene therapy, since restoration of IL-2Rγc reconstitutes an effective IL-2 receptor and allows for selective growth advantage and expansion of transduced cells. This technique has been extremely successful in terms of stem cell transduction with IL-2Rγc-containing retroviruses and correction of the immune deficiency. The several unfortunate cases of lymphoproliferative disease, including leukemia, resulting from the procedure, however, have led to extensive study of the mechanics and control of retroviral integration into the newborn CD34+ stem cell. At this point, gene therapy is a research technique that has both great promise and risk.

JAK3 Deficiency T- B+ NK- (MIM ID #600802)

JAK3 deficiency (19p12-13.1) is an autosomal recessive mutation and the second most common form of T- B+ NK- SCID (Figure 16-27, Table 16A-5 in the Annex, and Table 16-4). Because IL-2Rγc and JAK3 are in the same signaling pathway, JAK3 deficiency can be clinically and immunologically indistinguishable from XL-SCID (Figure 16-27). Since JAK3 transduces signal utilizing the IL-2Rγc that is common to the IL-15 receptor complex, JAK3 deficiency, like IL-2Rγc deficiency, leads to a NK-negative phenotype. JAK3 deficiency should be considered in unexplained congenital combined immunodeficiencies, especially those with a high proportion of peripheral B-lymphocytes. JAK3 deficiency is established by lymphocyte immunoblot for detection of the JAK3 mutation (*Chapter 25*). Curative treatment of JAK3 deficiency is accomplished by allogeneic BMT. The mutations in different families are all collected in an international database available at http://bioinf.uta.fi/JAK3base/.

IL-7 Receptor Alpha Chain Deficiency (CD127) T- B+ NK+ (MIM ID #608971)

The IL-7 receptor is composed of the IL-2Rγc chain and the IL-7Rα chain (5p13), which confers specificity for IL-7 (Figure 16-27). The intact IL-7R is expressed on early lymphoid cells, including some CD34+ cells, which respond to the IL-7 produced by bone marrow stromal cells (*Chapter 6*) and in the thymus (*Chapter 7*), inducing survival and proliferation in IL-7R+ cells (*Chapter 9*). IL-7 also supports the differentiation of early thymocytes. IL-7Rα deficiency is an uncommon autosomal recessive disease causing an early block in T cell development, leading to SCID with absent T cells but normal (to elevated) B and NK cells, hence the designation T- B+ NK+ SCID, which reflects an intact IL-15 (NK cell growth) signaling (Table 16A-5 in the Annex). Clinically, these children have recurrent infections similar to those in XL-SCID and have very little lymphoid tissue. Laboratory findings include little to no proliferation to mitogens or antigens and low to absent immunoglobulins (*Chapter 24*). IL-7Rα deficiency is less common than XL-SCID and should be sought in cases of patients with SCID-like illnesses who present with normal or elevated levels of B and NK cells. The diagnosis is substantiated by flow cytometry for the IL-7Rα chain (CD127) on T, B, NK cells, or macrophages, and confirmed by mutation detection. Allogeneic stem cell transplantation is curative, but gene therapy should theoretically be effective.

CD45 Deficiency T- B+ NK- (MIM ID #608971)

CD45 is a protein tyrosine phosphatase also known as the leukocyte common antigen, since it is expressed on all nucleated hematopoietic cells and makes up to 10 percent of the cell surface area of T and B cells (*Appendix 3*). Not only does it govern signaling through the regulation of the Src family kinases p56Lck and p59fyn, it also downregulates integrin-mediated adhesion and dephosphorylates JAK kinase complexes. Two patients, one Finnish, the other Kurdish, have been reported with homozygous recessive mutations in CD45 in whom SCID occurred by six months of life. The NK numbers were low in the Finnish case and not reported in the Kurdish one. Both patients died, one of B cell lymphoma, the other of post-bone marrow transplant CMV infection (Table 16A-5 in the Annex).

CD3δ/CD3ε/CD3ξ Deficiency (MIM ID #186790/ MIM ID #186830/MIM ID #610163)

As described previously (Figure 16-27), at least four different CD3 polypeptide chains are contained within the mature TCR complex, each encompassing one (CD3γ, CD3δ, and CD3ε) or three (CD3ξ) immunoreceptor tyrosine-based activation motifs (**ITAMs**) within their cytoplasmic domains (*Chapter 7*). The CD3γ, CD3δ, and CD3ε chains are encoded within the 11q23 in contrast to the CD3ξ chain, which is found on the 1q22–q23 chromosome region. There is a growing body of evidence to suggest that a number of immunodeficiencies specifically have defects involving one or all of these polypeptide chains of the CD3 component of the TCR. Mutations affecting three of the four chains, i.e., CD3δ, CD3ε, and CD3ξ, present clinically as SCID and show a T- B+ NK+ phenotype. Mutations affecting the CD3γ chains have been reported in two brothers who did not present with the typical manifestations of increased susceptibility to infections seen in SCID, and therefore CD3γ deficiency is classified as a non-SCID defect and will be described in a later section (Table 16A-5 in the Annex and Table 16-4 and Figure 16-27).

Coronin-1A Deficiency (MIM ID #605000)

Absence of coronin-1A, a protein that antagonizes actin cytoskeleton polymerization, was reported in a girl with T- B+ NK+ SCID who suffered recurrent infections including a severe generalized varicella infection post-vaccination at the age of 13 months (Table 16A-5 in the Annex and Table 16-4). Coronins are a family of proteins that regulate the actin cytoskeleton through antagonizing actin polymerization and promoting actin severing, in contrast to the role of the Wiskott–Aldrich syndrome protein (**WASP**) that promotes actin polymerization and DOCK 8, as will be described below, that is involved in actin cytoskeleton reorganization important in the formation of the immunologic synapse (Figure 16-27). Mice with mutations in coronin-1A are T lymphocytopenic due to an inability of mature T cells to be released from the thymus into the peripheral circulation.

P56Lck Deficiency T+ B+ NK+ (MIM ID #153390)

Abnormally low expression of the cytoplasmic tyrosine kinase referred to as Lck (Table 16-4 and

Figure 16-27) that phosphorylates several of the chains of the CD3 receptor complex has been found in sporadic cases of immune deficiency and CD4 lymphocytopenia. An infant with clinical and laboratory features of SCID and selective CD4 lymphopenia and lack of CD28 expression on CD8+ T cells has been reported. T cells from this patient showed poor blastogenic responses to various mitogens and IL-2. Antibody production was variable. Bone marrow transplantation was successful in the child, and these findings suggest that a deficiency in p56Lck expression can produce a SCID phenotype in humans. The precise genetic defect responsible for the decreased expression of p56Lck in this patient was not identified but was thought to be due to aberrant alternative splicing of exon 7 of the Lck gene (Table 16-5 in the Annex).

SCID Defects in DNA Rearrangement and Repair

This next group of SCID disorders involving defects in DNA rearrangement and repair fall into the general group of defects associated with transcription (Table 16-4 and Figure 16-27). The process of successful DNA rearrangement is complex and centers around the proper handling of the recombination signal sequence (**RSS**), short DNA sequences that flank regions of the T cell receptor and immunoglobulin genes that are slated for recombination in order to generate specific lymphoid immunity (*Chapters 6* and *7*). Therefore, defects all along the recombination pathway, which includes nicking, opening, bringing together loose ends, and rejoining, result in various immune defects, ranging from forms of SCID, with profound defects in T and B cell formation, to other forms with milder defects. Some of these defects are recognized primarily as immune dysfunction (e.g., recombinase gene defects), while others may be recognized in other contexts first, and only later appreciated as having associated immune deficiencies (e.g., ataxia telangiectasia) (Figure 16-27). Since DNA breakage and repair is a complex process with many genes involved, it is not surprising, therefore, that there are many potential sites for errors leading to immune defects, radiation sensitivity, growth abnormalities, and malignancy. Shown in Table 16A-5 in the Annex, Table 16-4, and Figure 16-27 are various forms of T- B- NK+ SCID associated with defects in DNA rearrangement and repair.

RAG1/RAG2 Deficiency T- B- NK+ (MIM ID #169615/MIM ID #169616)

Recombination-activating proteins RAG1 and RAG2 regulate and mediate V(D)J recombination, the process by which genes for immunoglobulins and T cell receptors are generated (Figure 16-27, *Chapters 6* and *7*). Among these are the genes affected in severe combined immune deficiency and genes involved in ds-DNA break repair. The recombinase activating genes 1 and 2 (**RAG1** and **RAG2**) lie close together at 11p13, and this proximity is evolutionarily conserved from zebrafish onward (*Chapter 2*). Despite their physical proximity, similar names, and the coincidence of their clinical presentations, RAG1 and RAG2 are unrelated structurally, but are rather complementary proteins, both needed for successful DNA recombination. Therefore, deficiency in the capacity for DNA recombination leads to absence of both T and B cells, indicative of the critical nature of DNA recombination in their development (MIM ID #601457). The persistence of NK cells and myeloid elements in RAG deficiency confirms that NK function and myeloid function are not dependent on DNA rearrangement.

Complete autosomal recessive deficiency of either RAG1 (MIM ID #169615) or RAG2 (MIM ID #169616) is a severe and profound SCID with early presentation, severe infections, and frequent maternal engraftment (Table 16A-5 in the Annex, Table 16-4, and Figure 16-27). The predominant peripheral blood lymphocyte population virtually consists exclusively of NK cells and there is no appreciable lymphoid tissue. A diffuse erythematous rash is common and often reflects maternal engraftment with GVHD. Early bone marrow transplantation is necessary for survival.

DNA Cross-Link Repair Protein 1C (DCLRE1C) (Artemis) Deficiency T- B- NK+ SCID (MIM ID #605988)

Human Artemis deficiency results in a SCID phenotype associated with increased cellular sensitivity to DNA double-strand breaks (**DSBs**) (Table 16A-5 in the Annex). This condition represents the first human pathology associating deficient V(D)J recombination with a general DSB defect. Artemis, a protein involved in V(D)J recombination/DNA repair, located on chromosome 10p, is a DNA-joining protein that has homology to the metallo-beta-lactamase family of proteins. Autosomal recessive mutations in Artemis lead to a form of radiosensitive (RS) T- B- NK+ SCID associated with generalized radiation sensitivity demonstrated usually in dermal fibroblasts (**RS-SCID, MIM ID #602450**). Artemis deficiency is most common among those Native Americans derived from the Athabascan speaking nations, such as the Navajo, among whom the incidence is approximately 1 in 2,000 live births. Amorphic mutations lead to complete T- B- SCID. However, hypomorphic mutations have been associated with an Omenn-like phenotype and others with lymphomas.

DNA-Dependent Protein Kinase, Catalytic Subunit (DNA-PKcs) T- B- NK+ SCID (MIM ID #600899)

The DNA-dependent protein kinase is involved in the repair of double-stranded DNA breaks that occur during gene recombination essential for T and B cell development. During V(D)J recombination, the lymphoid-specific RAG1 and RAG2 proteins introduce single-stranded nicks between the coding gene segments and the flanking RSS. Recognition and repair of the DNA ends occur via the general nonhomologous end joining (**NHEJ**) pathway of DNA where DSBs are recognized by the DNA-dependent protein kinase (**DNA-PK**) complex composed of the DNA-PK catalytic subunit (**DNA-PKcs**) and the Ku70/Ku80 heterodimer (Figure 16-29).

The DNA-PK serine/threonine protein kinase activity is required for subsequent DNA end-processing and ligation. Although mutations in the DNA-PKcs gene have been predicted for a long time, spontaneous mutations have only been identified in animal models. The first human mutation in the gene encoding DNA-PKcs (PRKDC) was identified recently in a radiosensitive T- B- NK+ SCID child who presented with recurrent oral candidiasis and lower respiratory tract infections since the third month of life with progressive respiratory failure who received a successful HLA-identical bone marrow transplant. Based on the clinical presentation, a DNA-PKcs deficiency cannot be discriminated from other SCID patients. The child's fibroblasts were sensitive to ionizing radiation, indicative of a radiosensitive SCID due to a NHEJ defect. Although a DNA-PKcs mutation was identified, three other known candidate genes for radiosensitive SCID (Artemis, LIG4, and XLF (XRCC4-like factor) also know as Cernunnos) were not mutated.

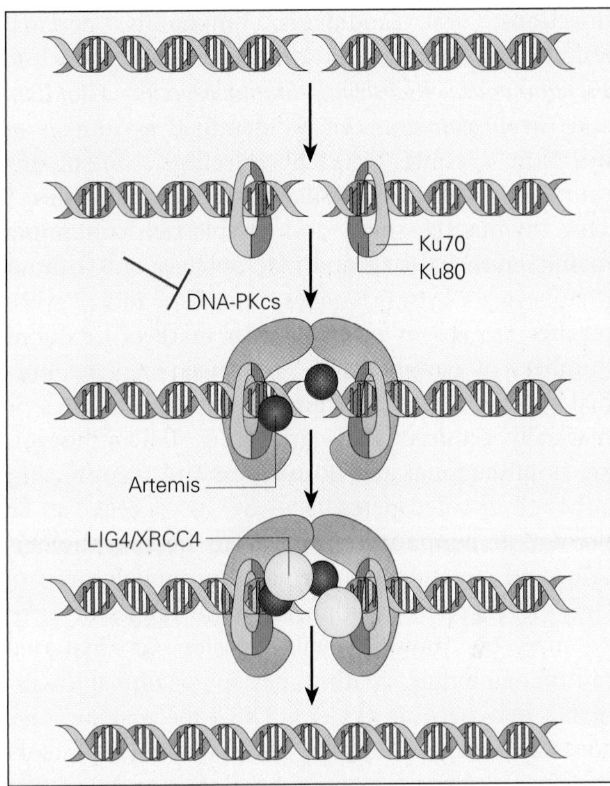

Figure 16-29. Schematic representation of the nonhomologous end-joining pathway of DNA double-strand break repair. Double-stranded DNA breaks (DSB) are recognized by the heterodimeric KU 70/80 that recruits the DNA protein kinase catalytic subunit (DNA-PKcs) necessary for the nonhomologous end joining of the DSB. A mutation of the DNA-PKcs results in a failure of DNA repair.

Reticular Dysgenesis T- B (Low) NK+ SCID (MIM ID #267500)

Reticular dysgenesis is one of the rarest and most severe forms of SCID. It is characterized by congenital agranulocytosis, lymphopenia, and lymphoid and thymic hypoplasia affecting both cellular and humoral immunity functions (Figure 16-3, Figure 16-27, Table 16A-5 in the Annex, and Table 16-4). RD is a rare and extremely serious variant of SCID. It is characterized by a congenital absence or severe depletion of T cells, neutrophils with variable (often low) numbers of B cells, and normal numbers of NK cells, platelets, and erythrocytes. Its frequency among SCIDs is believed to be 2 to 4 percent. Both males and females are affected, and consanguinity has been noted in several families. RD usually manifests early in the neonatal period with signs of sepsis, mainly caused by severe neutropenia. The affected children are usually chronically ill and anemic, fail to thrive, and have diarrhea and fevers. Recurrent infections include upper respiratory tract infections, oral candidiasis, omphalitis, perianal lesions, and abscesses. In some cases *Escherichia coli*, *Pseudomonas*, *Klebsiella*, *Staphylococcus*, *Candida*, and *Cytomegalovirus* can be identified as sources of infection. Despite recurrent infections, no significant lymphoid and tonsillar tissues can be found. The thymus is small and dysplastic, containing mainly epithelial cells and macrophages but without thymocytes. Lymph nodes, tonsils, and Peyer's patches are absent or small with markedly reduced numbers of lymphocytes. The spleen may be normal in size, but the number of lymphocytes is markedly reduced. The circulating T lymphocytes are nonfunctional and do not respond to mitogens; although elevated percentages of CD5+ cells can be present, B lymphocytes appear to be morphologically and functionally normal. Immunoglobulin G (IgG) levels can be within reference ranges at birth because of transplacental transfer of maternal immunoglobulins. With time, hypogammaglobulinemia may become evident. The bone marrow may contain normal numbers of erythroid precursors and megakaryocytes; however, other cells of the myeloid series are usually not observed. Hemoglobin values are usually within reference ranges at birth, but the patient may develop anemia secondary to sepsis and chronic illness. The underlying genetic defect for most cases of RD was recently identified in the gene encoding adenylate kinase 2 (**AK2**). However, rare patients with RD and no mutations in AK2 exist, suggesting that mutations in other genes may also cause RD. Although rare, RD has a devastating presentation involving severe neutropenia and T cell lymphopenia, in addition to non-life-threatening but still disabling sensori-neural deafness.

SCID-Related Purine Metabolic Defects

Adenosine deaminase (**ADA**) is an ubiquitously expressed enzyme that transforms adenosine into inosine and deoxyadenosine to deoxyinosine. Purine nucleoside phosphorylase (**PNP**) then converts inosine and deoxyinosine to hypoxanthine, which can either enter the purine salvage pathway or be excreted as uric acid. Since ADA and PNP work in series to handle the products of purine metabolism, it is not surprising that they have overlapping clinical and pathologic phenotypes. ADA is considered a T- B- NK- SCID in contrast to PNP deficiency, which is a milder form of non-SCID immune deficiency.

Adenosine Deaminase Deficiency T- B- NK- SCID (MIM ID #102700)

Accumulated adenosine is highly toxic, most especially to lymphocytes, and therefore levels of ADA enzyme activity are inversely correlated with disease severity (Table 16A-5 in the Annex and Table 16-4). ADA deficiency (20q13) is an autosomal recessive disorder with a highly variable disease presentation depending on the degree of residual ADA activity. Complete ADA deficiency presents early in life, with low enzyme activity, high-accumulated adenosine levels, marked panlymphopenia without significant lymphoid tissues, and only maternally transferred IgG. SCID-type infections are common. Half of cases have characteristic bony abnormalities, including flared, cupped costochondral junctions on lateral films, leading to a "rachitic rosary" (bony prominences at the costochondral junctions, reminiscent of the beads of a rosary) similar to that seen in rickets. Neurologic features are increasingly appreciated and are likely due to direct neurotoxicity of the accumulated adenosine. Partial defects in ADA activity have later and milder presentations, some in adolescence and some in adulthood. Eosinophilia, IgE elevation, and in vitro proliferation are seen in association with recurrent infections and poor autoimmunity. ADA deficiency accounts for about 20 percent of cases of SCID. ADA deficiency is one of the immune deficiencies in which somatic reversion has been best characterized and in which it is easiest to appreciate the clinical consequences of having a revertant clone.

Bone marrow transplantation is curative of the ADA deficiency but may not correct all aspects of the phenotype, including the neurocognitive defects. Pegylated bovine ADA (PEG-ADA) reduces adenosine levels and leads to marked immune improvement. Gene replacement therapy has been successful but is still experimental.

Non-SCID Defects

A number of non-SCID defects have been identified and represent the counterpoint of the combined T and B cell defects seen with the SCID defects described previously (Table 16A-5 in the Annex). For ease of discussion, these non-SCID defects can also be classified into the same three categories described for the SCID defects: (1) defects of signaling, (2) defects in DNA rearrangement and repair, and (3) purine metabolic defects (Table 16-4 and

Figure 16-27). In addition to defects affecting directly T and B lymphocytes, we include in this section a wide variety of molecular defects of major histocompatibility complex (**MHC**) I and II receptors, co-receptors, co-stimulatory molecules transcription factors, and adaptor proteins, each of which when mutated lead to defective signaling or in DNA rearrangement and repair, which can cause immune deficiency of both T and B cells.

Non-SCID Defects of Cytokine Signaling

CD3γ Chain Deficiency (MIM ID #186740)

Mutations affecting the CD3γ chains have been reported in two brothers who did not present with the typical manifestations of increased susceptibility to infections seen in SCID, and therefore CD3γ deficiency is classified as a non-SCID defect (Table 16A-5 in the Annex, Table 16-4, and Figure 16-27). One of the immunodeficient brothers was healthy at the age of 10 years, suggesting that ancillary mechanisms of T cell signaling may have compensated the genetic lesion; conversely, his brother developed an autoimmune disorder after a viral infection and died at the age of 31 months, suggesting that the CD3γ may be critical to normal T cell function and that the defect may not be entirely benign, particularly when a series of environmental insults occurs.

ZAP70 Deficiency (MIM ID #166947)

ZAP70 is a protein tyrosine kinase that associates with the CD3ζ chain and is crucial for CD8 T cell formation and function. ZAP70 becomes associated with the CD3ζ chain following receptor phosphorylation by p56Lck, a cytoplasmic tyrosine kinase (Figure 16-27). Despite the fact that ZAP70 is required for the development of single-positive CD8+ T cells in the thymus and for normal mitogen and antigen responses, ZAP70-deficient patients have normal to high lymphocyte numbers and lymphoid tissue is present. However, absolute numbers of CD8 cells are undetectable or extremely low; antibody formation is variable. Patients with ZAP70 deficiency display an autosomal recessive pattern of inheritance. The infections are consistent with SCID, including those caused by bacteria, *Pneumocystis*, and viruses, as well as oral and cutaneous candidiasis.

CD8 Deficiency (MIM ID #186910)

An autosomal recessive familial CD8 deficiency due to a single mutation in the CD8α gene has been described (Table 16A-5 in the Annex, Table 16-4, and Figure 16-27). CD8+ cells were shown to be absent in a patient with repeated bacterial infections in whom other known immunodeficiencies were ruled out. The CD8α chain was found to be completely absent in three members of this family, whereas scarce expression of CD8β chain was detected in their cytoplasm. CD8 glycoproteins are co-receptors expressed predominantly on MHC-I-restricted T cells as a disulfide-linked αβ-heterodimer, but can also be expressed as an αα-homodimer in NK cells and intraepithelial T cells. In the absence of CD8α, CD8β is retained and destroyed within the cell, whereas CD8α can be expressed at the cell surface without CD8β as CD8αα homodimers.

IL-2-inducible T Cell Kinase (ITK) Deficiency (MIM ID #186973)

Signal transduction through the T cell receptor and cytokine receptors on the surface of T lymphocytes occurs largely via tyrosine phosphorylation of intracellular substrates (*Chapters 7* and *9*). Signal transduction occurs via association of these receptors with intracellular protein tyrosine kinases. The non-receptor tyrosine kinase ITK is a member of the Tec kinase family, which also includes Bruton's tyrosine kinase (**BTK**). Two Turkish sisters, born of consanguineous parents, were reported with fatal EBV-associated lymphoproliferative syndrome and were identified to have a homozygous mutation of the ITK gene, resulting in an abnormal BG loop of the SH2 domain. Both girls developed chronic active EBV infection in early childhood that was resistant to treatment. The disorder progressed to lymphadenopathy, hepatosplenomegaly, B cell proliferation, and Hodgkin's lymphoma in one girl. There were extremely low levels of the protein in a lymph node biopsy from one of the girls. Both unaffected parents were heterozygous for the mutation.

Signal Transducer and Activator of Transcription 5B (STAT5b) Deficiency (MIM ID #245590)

STAT5b is a member of the signal transducer and activator of transcription family of proteins that regulate gene transcription in response to various cytokines and growth factors (*Chapter 9*). It plays a particularly important role in T cells, where it is a key mediator of interleukin-2-induced responses. STAT5b is present as a monomer in the cytoplasm of quiescent cells and is recruited to the activated interleukin-2 receptor (IL-2R), where it is phosphorylated by receptor-associated tyrosine kinases. The phosphorylated subunits dimerize through their SH2 domains, translocate to the nucleus, and bind DNA to regulate gene transcription. Deficiency of STAT5b causes a rare autosomal recessive disorder characterized by dwarfism associated with a normal serum growth hormone level, but very low insulin-like growth factor-1 levels (Table 16A-5 in the Annex, Table 16-4, and Figure 16-27). Other physical features include dysmorphic features, eczema, lymphocytic interstitial pneumonitis, and autoimmunity. Most patients also have a marked immunodeficiency, with recurrent varicella virus, herpes virus, and *Pneumocystis jiroveci* infections, suggesting a defect in natural killer or cytotoxic T cells. Immunophenotyping of affected patients has shown low $\gamma\delta$ T cell and natural killer cell numbers and modest T cell lymphopenia.

IL-2Rα Deficiency (CD25) (MIM ID #147730)

As described in *Chapter 9*, the IL-2R is composed of three chains (α, β, and γ) expressed on the surface of many immune cells that binds and responds to interleukin 2 (IL-2). The IL-2R plays a critical role in T cell activation, including the contribution of the IL-2Rα (also known as CD25) to the function of Treg cells. Although the defect caused by loss of IL-2Rα is relatively limited to T lymphocytes, leaving a normal number of B and NK cells, the importance of IL-2Rα deficiency is its profound effects on lymphoproliferation, lymphadenopathy, hepatosplenomegaly, autoimmunity (that may resemble IPEX syndrome), and impaired T cell proliferation (Table 16A-5 in the Annex, Table 16-4, and Figure 16-27). This also accounts for the persistent lymphadenopathy and abnormal apoptosis that are seen in this very rare autosomal recessive disorder, which has only been reported in consanguineous families.

CD40L Deficiency (MIM ID #300386) and CD40 Deficiency (MIM ID #109535)

CD40L is a T cell membrane protein that interacts with CD40, its cognate receptor, on B cells, dendritic cells, monocytes, macrophages, and activated epithelial cells. CD40L activates CD40 to drive B cell immunoglobulin class switch from IgM to IgG (class-switch recombination, CSR), as well as for subsequent maturation of antibody and formation of normal lymph node anatomy. Deficiencies of both CD40L and CD40 are described more fully below under B cell defects (Table 16A-5 in the Annex, Table 16-4, and Figure 16-27).

DOCK8 Deficiency (MIM ID #611432)

Dedicator of cytokinesis 8 (**DOCK8**), also known as Zir3, is a large (~190 kDa) protein involved in intracellular signaling networks. An autosomal recessive DOCK8 deficiency has been reported in 11 patients in association with a variant of combined immunodeficiency (Table 16A-5 in the Annex, Table 16-4, and Figure 16-27). Clinical manifestations included recurrent upper and lower respiratory and skin infections, otitis media, sinusitis, and pneumonias, recurrent *Staphylococcus aureus* skin infections with otitis externa, recurrent severe herpes simplex virus, or herpes zoster infections. An unusual hallmark susceptibility in these patients included extensive and persistent infections with molluscum contagiosum and human papillomavirus infections (Figure 16-30). Most patients had severe atopic manifestations, some with anaphylaxis, which included elevated serum IgE levels, hypereosinophilia, low numbers of T cells and B cells, low serum IgM levels, and variable IgG antibody responses. Several had squamous-cell carcinomas, and one had T cell lymphoma-leukemia. Expansion in vitro of activated CD8 T cells was impaired. Novel homozygous or compound heterozygous deletions and point mutations in the gene encoding the dedicator of cytokinesis 8 protein (DOCK8) led to the absence of DOCK8 protein in lymphocytes.

Calcium Channel Deficiency (MIM ID #610277/ORAI Calcium Release-Activated Calcium Modulator 1; ORAI1 Deficiency) (MIM ID #605921/Stromal Interaction Molecule 1; STIM1 Deficiency)

Lymphocyte activation requires Ca++ influx through specialized Ca++ channels in the plasma membrane. In T cells, the predominant Ca++ channel is the Ca++ release activated Ca++ (**CRAC**) channel encoded by the gene ORAI1. ORAI1 is activated by stromal interaction molecule 1 (**STIM1**) that is localized in the endoplasmic reticulum where it senses the concentration of stored Ca++. Following antigen binding to TCR, the endoplasmic reticulum Ca++ stores are depleted, following which STIM1 is activated and ORAI1-CRAC channel is opened, resulting in Ca++ influx and lymphocyte

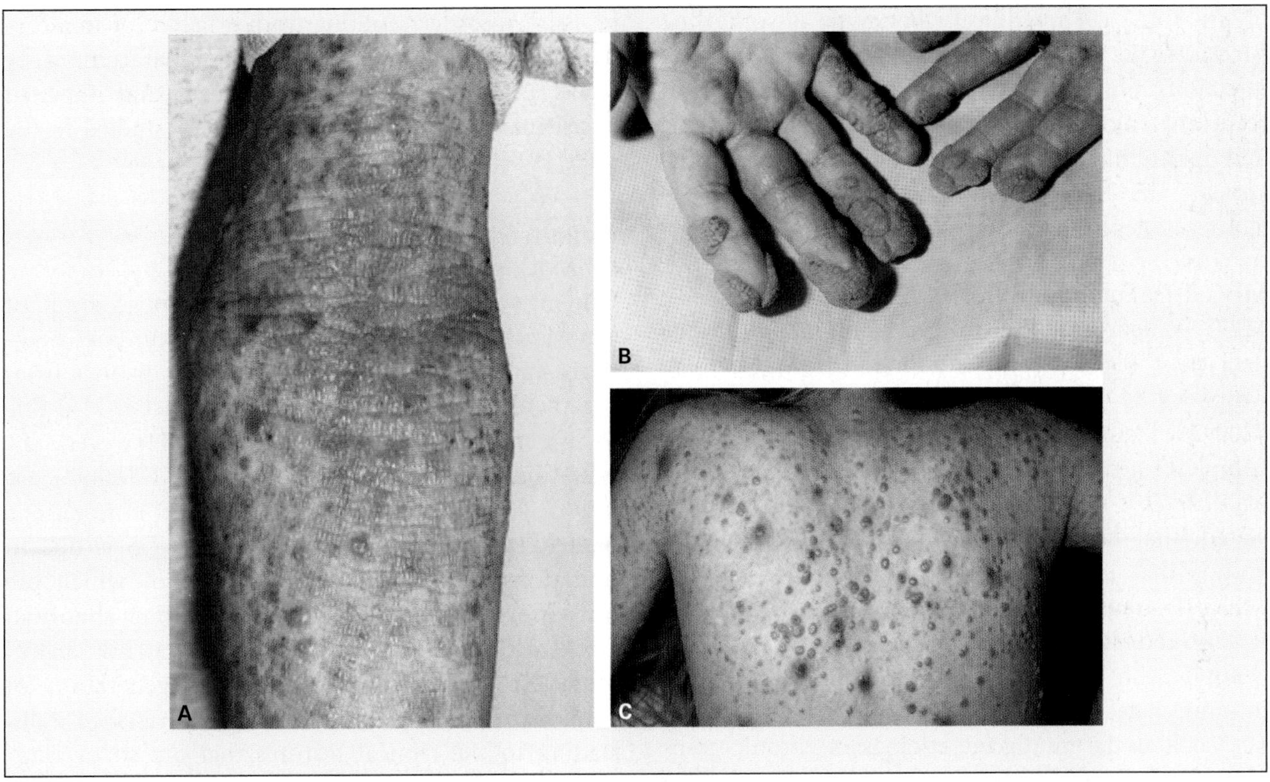

Figure 16-30. Characteristic dermatologic findings of patients with DOCK8 deficiency. Panel A: Atopic dermatitis with scattered superimposed molluscum contagiosum lesions on the inside of the arm. Panel B: Periungual and acral warts caused by the human papilloma virus (HPV). Panel C: Molluscum contagiosum on the back. (Reproduced with permission from Zhang Q, Davis JC, Lamborn IT, et al. Combined immunodeficiency associated with DOCK8 mutations. N Engl J Med. 2009;361:2046–55.)

stimulation. Mutations in either ORAI1 or STIM1 have been described as autosomal recessive disorders in patients who manifest increased susceptibility to infections similar to those seen in patients with SCID, although numbers of T cells and other lymphocytes are normal in affected individuals (Table 16A-5 in the Annex, Table 16-4, and Figure 16-27). The ORAI1 and STIM1 deficiencies, however, are not strictly T cell activation deficiencies but, rather, represent combined immune deficiencies affecting several different immune cell types.

MHC-1 and MHC-II Deficiencies

Cell surface display of antigens for adaptive immune response, whether derived from intracellular or extracellular sources, is dependent on context (*Chapter 10*). That is, appropriate recognition of antigen is contingent on appropriate binding of processed peptides to the cellular display apparatus composed of MHC proteins. This, in turn, is crucial for the stimulation of T cells and B cells for the acquisition of immunity. Therefore, in the absence of MHC molecules, immune function is impaired. Two of the classic deficiencies of TCR signaling that are indirectly responsible for T cell immune deficiencies are those that affect the MHC-I and MHC-II molecules (*Chapter 10*). These are shown in Tables 16-4 and 16A-5 in the Annex and in Figure 16-27.

MHC-I Deficiency (TAP Deficiency; Bare Lymphocyte Syndrome 1) (MIM ID #604571)

As described in *Chapter 10*, MHC-I molecules bind peptides in the endoplasmic reticulum (**ER**) that have been synthesized in the cytoplasm, such as those directed by certain viral infections or tumors. The variable portion of MHC-I joins with the MHC-I constant chain, β2 microglobulin, in the ER before being loaded with peptide by molecules of the transporter associated with antigen presentation (**TAP**) complex. TAP1, TAP2, and tapasin (TAP-binding protein), all encoded at chromosome 6p21.3, form the functional peptide transporter system that loads peptides onto the MHC-I molecule. Defects in any of the three components TAP1, TAP2, or tapasin cause reduced or absent display of MHC-I on the cell surface, resulting in bare lymphocyte syndrome type 1 (BLS1, MIM #604571,

Figure 16-27). The clinical phenotype is somewhat surprising in its mildness and lack of severe viral infections. Onset is in childhood, or even later, with recurrent sinopulmonary infections, bronchiectasis, and granulomatous skin lesions. Some of the patients have autoimmune phenomena such as glomerulonephritis and vasculitis.

MHC-II Deficiency (MIM ID #209920)

MHC-II deficiency leads to a combined immune deficiency (cellular and humoral) known as bare lymphocyte syndrome type II (BLS II, MIM #209920, Figure 16-27). It is autosomal recessive but complexly genetically heterogeneous. The expression of MHC-II is governed by an intricate transcriptional system that includes at least four complementation groups that encode necessary transcription factors: MHC-II transactivator (CIITA), RFXANK/RFX-B, RFX5, and RFXAP. The convergence of multiple genotypes on one phenotype is reminiscent of other immune defects that are dependent on a final product, such as the multigenic etiology of chronic granulomatous disease. BLS II is characterized by lack of expression of HLA DR molecules on T, B, and myeloid cells and failure to upregulate these molecules in response to interferon gamma. CD4 T lymphocyte numbers are low, but CD8 numbers are normal to high; MHC-I expression may be reduced on mononuclear cells. Immunoglobulin levels are typically low, but can be normal to high; proliferation to mitogen is normal. Allogeneic bone marrow transplantation is recommended, with earlier transplants likely to have better outcomes. Interestingly, lack of MHC-II on recipient cells has apparently not led to reduced levels of GVHD in BLS II transplants.

Non-SCID Defects in DNA Rearrangement and Repair

Winged Helix Deficiency (Nude) (MIM ID #600838)

The adaptive immune system relies on the thymic microenvironment for the production of a diverse, self-tolerant T cell receptor repertoire. The central cellular organizers of the thymic microenvironment are the thymic epithelial cells (**TECs**) that develop from endodermal precursor cells under the control of the forkhead/winged helix transcription factor (FOXN1). Defects in the forkhead box N1 transcription factor that is encoded by FOXN1 (the gene that is mutated in nude mice) is an extremely rare human autosomal recessive disorder resulting from a failure of intrathymic development of T cells and is characterized by alopecia, abnormal thymic epithelium, and impaired T cell maturation and has been widely studied in the nude FOXN1-defective mouse model.

Omenn Syndrome T+ B- NK+ (MIM ID #603554)

Omenn syndrome (**OS**) is an important example of genotype/phenotype correlation in immune function, since this syndrome is clinically distinct from complete RAG1/2 deficiency, but in fact is also due to mutations in RAG1 or RAG2. However, the mutations in OS are hypomorphic ("leaky"), as opposed to the amorphic ("complete") mutations in RAG1/2-deficient SCID. Therefore, OS is due to mutations in RAG1/2, at least one of which are missense, allowing some detectable but abnormal DNA recombination activity to persist. This "leaky" mutation is thought to allow the generation of inappropriate alloreactive clonally restricted T cells, leading to the clinical features that are so overlapping with alloreactive GVHD. The clinical hallmarks of OS are early onset generalized erythrodermia with eosinophilia and elevated IgE (Figure 16-32). Other common features are diarrhea, failure to thrive, lymphadenopathy, hepatosplenomegaly, and hypogammaglobulinemia. T cells often show activation markers, such as HLA-DR, but are poorly proliferative to antigen and sometimes to mitogen. Skin biopsies can show aggressive infiltration of the upper dermis, and diagnoses that can be entertained include histiocytosis and GVHD. Search for maternal (or transfused cell) engraftment is critical in cases of both RAG SCID and Omenn syndrome. Definitive therapy for OS is bone marrow

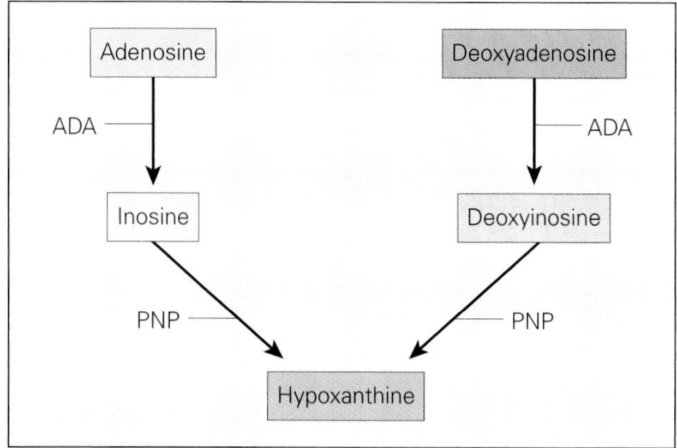

Figure 16-31. Schematic representation of purine metabolism showing the relative activities of ADA and PNP.

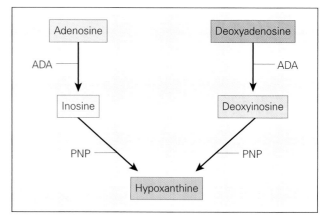

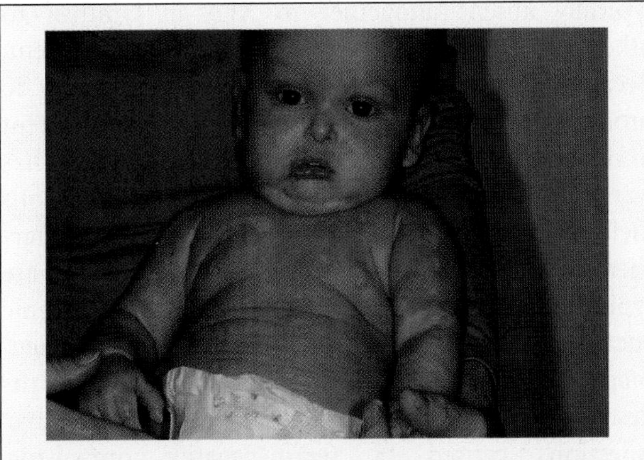

Figure 16-32. Photograph of an infant with the Omenn syndrome showing diffuse erythrodermia.

transplantation. Palliative therapies include steroids and cyclosporine to dampen the aberrant autoreactive T cell proliferation that appears to be so central to the Omenn phenotype.

DNA Ligase IV Deficiency (MIM ID #606593)

DNA ligase IV deficiency leads to defects in DNA recombination and radiation sensitivity, known as the LIG4 syndrome (Table 16A-5 in the Annex, Table 16-4, and Figure 16-27). The condition is related to defects in the general NHEJ pathway of DNA as described above for the DNA-PKcs deficiency. The genetic lesion seen in the DNA-PKcs deficiency affects a more proximal site of the NHEJ pathway than the DNA ligase IV deficiency and therefore might explain its more serious clinical SCID-like presentation than the milder non-SCID-like presentation of the LIG4 syndrome (Figure 16-29). Hypomorphic mutations in the DNA-LigIV gene have been described in patients with increased cellular sensitivity to ionizing radiation and variable immune deficiency (from no deficiency to SCID). In addition to the immune defect, most DNA-LigIV patients display developmental impairment, mainly characterized by growth retardation and microcephaly. Other features of this syndrome include developmental delay and chromosomal instability, but hypomorphic mutations can segregate these traits.

Cernunnos/XLF Deficiency (MIM ID #611290)

Cernunnos-defective patients present with a phenotype very similar to that observed in patients suffering from a DNA-LigIV deficiency (Tables 16A-5 in the Annex, Table 16-4, and Figure 16-27). The immune deficiency is mainly characterized by a profound T and B cell lymphopenia (caused by a defective V(D)J recombination) and a hyper IgM syndrome (consisting of the presence of normal or elevated amounts of serum IgM isotype contrasting with the low level of other isotypes). These immune defects result in high susceptibility to bacterial infections, and some of the patients died from septic shock. The immunodeficiency is associated with other developmental defects, mainly characterized by growth retardation and microcephaly. The increased cellular sensitivity to ionizing radiation of the primary fibroblasts from these patients is indicative of a general DNA repair defect. This diagnostic indication is strengthened by the detection of chromosomal aberrations in activated lymphocytes. The DNA repair defect has been documented by several means, including V(D)J recombination assay in fibroblasts and NHEJ assay in vitro, which pointed to a defect in one of the core NHEJ apparatus factors.

Purine Metabolic Defects

As described previously, ADA and PNP are enzymes that participate in the salvage pathway of purine metabolism involving the conversion of adenosine into inosine and deoxyadenosine to deoxyinosine by ADA and the conversion of inosine and deoxyinosine to hypoxanthine by PNP (Figure 16-31). Hypoxanthine then can either enter the purine salvage pathway or be excreted as uric acid. Since ADA affects the salvage pathway more proximally, an ADA deficiency presents with more serious clinical sequelae as a SCID phenotype owing to the accumulation of more toxic products than with a PNP deficiency.

Purine Nucleoside Phosphorylase (PNP) Deficiency (MIM ID #613179)

PNP is an enzyme downstream of ADA, where it converts inosine and deoxyinosine to hypoxanthine (Table 16A-5 in the Annex and Table 16-4). PNP is also involved in the conversion of guanosine and deoxyguanosine to guanine, which can then enter the purine salvage pathway or be excreted as uric acid. PNP deficiency (14q13, MIM #164050) is an autosomal recessive disease characterized by the accumulation of deoxyguanosine and guanosine, nucleotides that are directly toxic to lymphocytes. Accumulation of dGTP intracellularly also inhibits ribonucleotide reductase, an enzyme responsible for producing DNA precursors. PNP deficiency has a more profound effect on T than B cells. PNP-deficient patients may also have significant neurocognitive problems, including ataxia and paresis. Bone marrow transplantation is the only definitive therapy. These patients often suffer from autoimmune manifestations, especially autoimmune hemolytic anemia.

B Cell Defects

B cells begin their antigen-independent life in the bone marrow, but it is only in peripheral lymphoid tissues during the antigen-dependent phase where they encounter antigen, experience class-switch recombination (**CSR**) and expansion, and become the predominant cells in these tissues (*Chapters 2* and *6*). Their ontogeny and differentiation have been largely defined through the arduous characterization of immune defects leading to hypogammaglobulinemia, beginning with the molecular study of the flagship entity, X-linked agammaglobulinemia. The number of B cell-specific defects in antibody production is already large, and there will certainly be more causes to be found, but the major ones are now well characterized and the therapy is well developed (Table 16A-6 in the Annex and Figure 16-3). For ease of discussion, the major B cell defects can be divided into three major categories of antibody deficiencies: (1) defects in early B cell development, (2) hyper-IgM syndromes (also called class-switch recombination defects), and (3) common variable immunodeficiency (**CVID**) (Figure 16-33).

Defects in Early B Cell Development

B Cell Defects with Severe Reduction in All Serum Ig Isotypes with Absent B Cells: X-Linked Agammaglobulinemia (XLA) (MIM ID #300755)

First described in 1952 by Bruton, severe X-linked agammaglobulinemia (XLA) has been the paradigm for understanding the pure role of the B cell in immune function. The disease is now known to be due to defects in a tyrosine kinase, Bruton tyrosine kinase, BTK (MIM #300300) (Table 16A-6 in the Annex and Figure 16-33). Since BTK mutations lead to severe defects in B cell development past the pro-B cell stage (*Chapter 6*), circulating B cells are typically absent altogether in XLA in contrast to other B cell defects where these cells may be present. Because XLA affects almost exclusively the ability to produce antibody, it is not usually clinically apparent until after transplacental maternal antibody has waned after six months of age. Typical presentations include upper and lower respiratory infections, diarrhea, cellulitis, meningitis, and sepsis. Infections are typically caused by Gram-positive, highly pathogenic encapsulated organisms such as *Streptococcus pneumonia* and *Haemophilus influenzae* type b as described previously in the case presentation above. Infections caused by Gram-negative organisms, including *Campylobacter* species and *Pseudomonas* as well as other organisms such as *Pneumocystis* and herpes viruses, are not common. Although susceptibility to infection with high-grade encapsulated bacteria has been the hallmark presentation of patients with XLA, it is also known that these patients can also suffer from certain viral infections. Enterovirus infections have been especially severe in XLA, often causing a severe meningoencephalitis. The basis for this susceptibility of XLA patients to viral infection recently has been shown to be due to a special role of BTK as a key signaling molecule that interacts with and acts downstream of TLR8 and TLR9 in signal transduction, making for a unique innate defect in addition to antibody deficiency (*Chapter 9*).

XLA is easily suspected in male patients with repeated infections when flow cytometry of peripheral blood lymphocytes shows the absence of B cells, which should be readily detected in the peripheral blood of any normal boy. In any case, the finding of moderate to severe hypogammaglobulinemia with or without infections should raise a high index of suspicion for this diagnosis in a male child. Older cases have been identified, and are typically due to hypomorphic mutations. Simple demonstration of absent B cells, however, even with a positive family history of early infections and death in maternal male relatives, is not a definitive diagnosis of XLA, which requires the demonstration of absent BTK on Western blotting (which can be performed on blood monocytes) or the presence of a sequence abnormality. An extensive mutation database is available at http://www.uta.fi/laitokset/imt/bioinfo/BTKbase. Longevity and quality of life in these patients have been dramatically improved by the administration of immunoglobulin, either by the intravenous or subcutaneous routes with doses

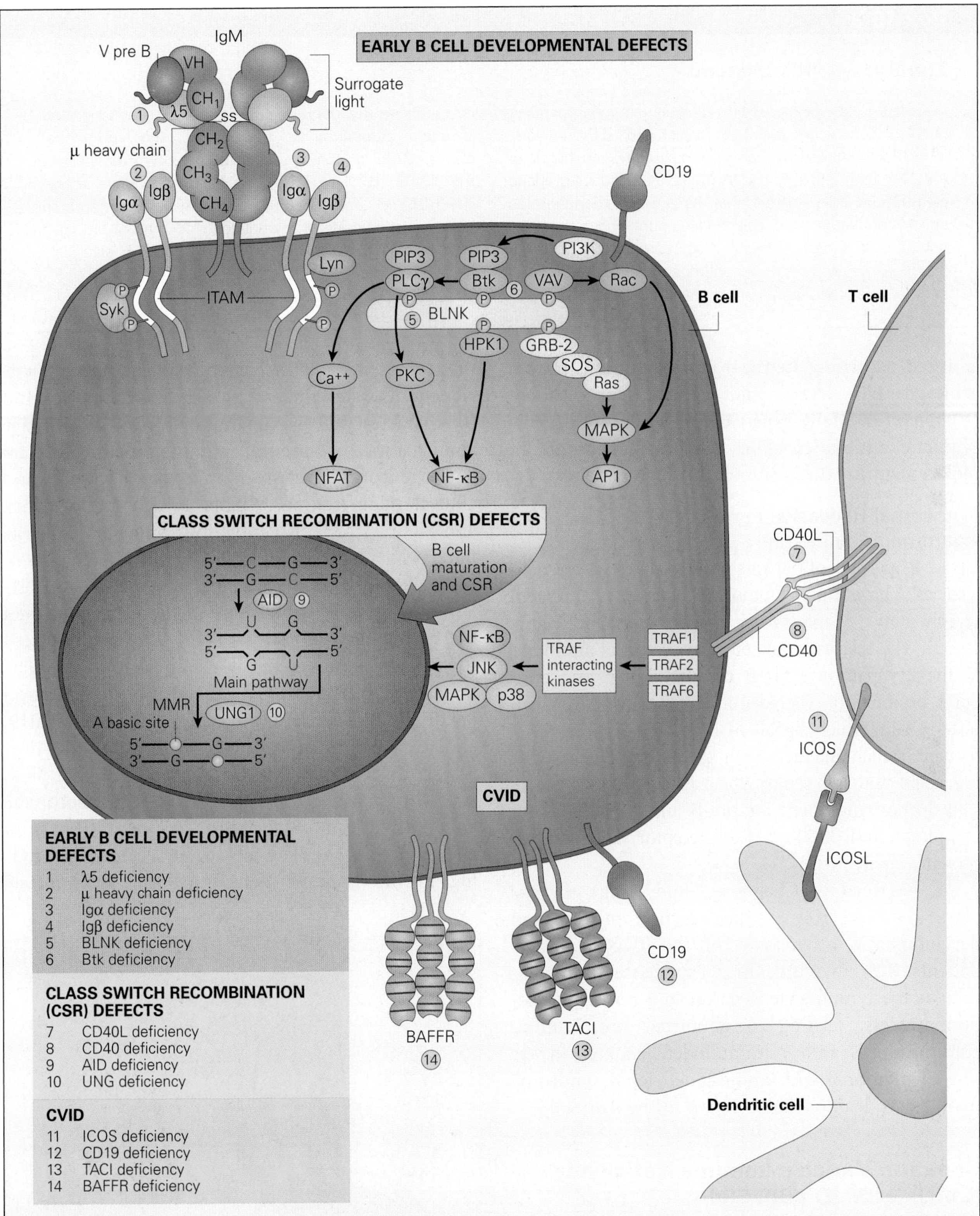

Figure 16-33. Schematic representation of the molecular events that are involved in B cell signaling. Primary B cell signaling occurs through the BCR (IgM)-associated signaling molecules Igα/β, as well as the co-stimulatory molecules CD21 and CD19. Proximal signaling occurs through Syk, BTK, BLNK, Lyn, PLCγ, and PKC. Downstream effector molecules include nuclear factor κB (NF-κB) and NFAT that translocate to the nucleus, where they affect gene transcription that controls B cell proliferation, survival, differentiation, and migration. The known human signaling defects resulting in primary immune deficiencies of B cells include (1) mutation in BTK, (2) μ heavy chain deficiency (IgM), (3) λ5 deficiency, (4) Igα deficiency, (5) Igβ deficiency, and (6) BLNK deficiency.

Box 16-3

The BAFF/APRIL System

B cells require signals from multiple sources for their development from precursor cells and differentiation into effector cells (*Chapter 6*). B cell activating factor of the TNF family (BAFF) and A proliferation-inducing ligand (APRIL) are two ligands that have been identified as critical regulators of B cell development and differentiation (Figure 16-34). Defects in the production of BAFF and/or expression of its receptors have been associated with a diverse array of human immunopathologies characterized by perturbed B cell function and behavior, including autoimmunity, malignancy, and immunodeficiency. BAFF and APRIL each bind to two receptors of the TNFR family, BCMA (B cell maturation antigen [TNFRSF 16 and CD269]) and TACI (transmembrane activator and calcium modulator and cyclophilin ligand interactor [TNFRSF 13B and CD267]). BAFF also binds selectively to the third BAFF receptor, BAFF-R (TNFRSF 13C and CD268) (Appendix 2).

adjusted according to the route of administration, achieved IgG levels, and clinical improvement (*Chapter 12*). Many experts include the use of prophylactic antibiotics along with immune globulin replacement for the treatment of these patients.

Autosomal Recessive Forms of Agammaglobulinemia

Up to 10 percent of patients with complete B cell deficiencies have an autosomal recessive pattern of inheritance (Table 16A-6 in the Annex and Figure 16-33). The relevant mutated recessive genes are found in the key pathways for B cell maturation and antibody production. The identified genes include the μ heavy chain, which signals in B cell maturation; the λ 5-chain, which interacts with the μ heavy chain; the Igα chain and Igβ chain, which provide critical signal transduction molecules for pre-B and B cell receptor complexes; and BLNK, a B cell receptor signal adapter protein (Figure 16-33).

As described in Chapters 2 and 7, the thymus plays a critical role in the selection process and developmental progression of the T cell lineage. Patients with thymoma may experience dysregulation of the lymphocyte negative and positive selection process, leading to abnormal proliferation, autoimmunity, and/or immunodeficiency as in the case of thymoma with immunodeficiency syndrome (Good's syndrome) (Table 16A-6 in the Annex).

Common Variable Immune Deficiency (CVID) (MIM ID #607594)

Severe Reduction in Serum IgG and IgA with Normal, Low, or Very Low Numbers of B Cells: The CVID Spectrum

A second major category of B cell immune deficiencies are a group of disorders referred to as CVID that represents a spectrum of primary immunodeficiency disorders that typically affects adults and is characterized by quantitative and qualitative abnormalities of humoral immune function that are heterogeneous in their immunological profile and clinical manifestations (Table 16A-6 in the Annex and Figure 16-33). Recently, four monogenic defects have been identified to result in the CVID phenotype, demonstrating that the genetic basis of CVID is highly variable. Mutations in the genes encoding the tumor necrosis factor (TNF) superfamily receptors transmembrane activator and calcium-modulating ligand interactor (**TACI**) and B cell activation factor of the TNF family receptor (**BAFF-R**), CD19, and the co-stimulatory molecule inducible co-stimulator molecule (**ICOS**) all lead to CVID and illustrate the complex interplay required to coordinate an effective humoral immune response (Box 16-3 and Figure 16-34). The molecular mechanisms leading to the immune defect are still incompletely

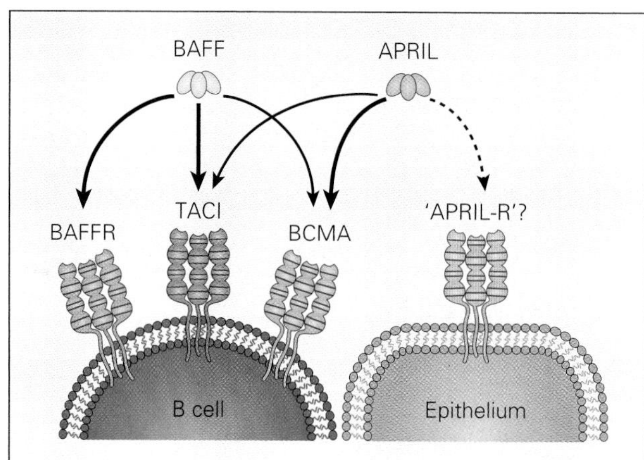

Figure 16-34. Schematic representation of BAFF/APRIL system showing the bimodal tropism of BAFF and APRIL for both the TACI and BCMA receptors and the additional selective tropism of BAFF for BAFF-R.

understood, and particularly in the case of TACI, where a number of heterozygous mutations have been found in affected individuals, the molecular pathogenesis of disease requires further elucidation. Together these defects account for perhaps 10 to 15 percent of all cases of CVID and it is highly likely that further genetic defects will be identified.

Although patients with CVID usually present with recurrent sinopulmonary infections, about 20 percent of subjects develop autoimmune complications, most often immune thrombocytopenia or hemolytic anemia (Figure 16-35). While the pathogenesis of autoreactivity is unknown for CVID subjects in general, and to a greater extent in those with autoimmunity, there is a loss of switched memory B cells. About 7 to 8 percent of CVID subjects have mutations in the transmembrane activator and TACI, a significant association with this immune defect, although the same mutations may be found in normal relatives and rarely in healthy blood donors (Figure 16-33). High numbers of IgM(+) memory B cells appear to correlate with the presence of infections, whereas decreased numbers of switched memory B cells correlate with lower serum IgG levels and increased rates of autoimmune features. Other genes that belong to the MHC-III region (*Chapter 10*) have been implicated in the pathogenesis of CVID. MSH5, a gene

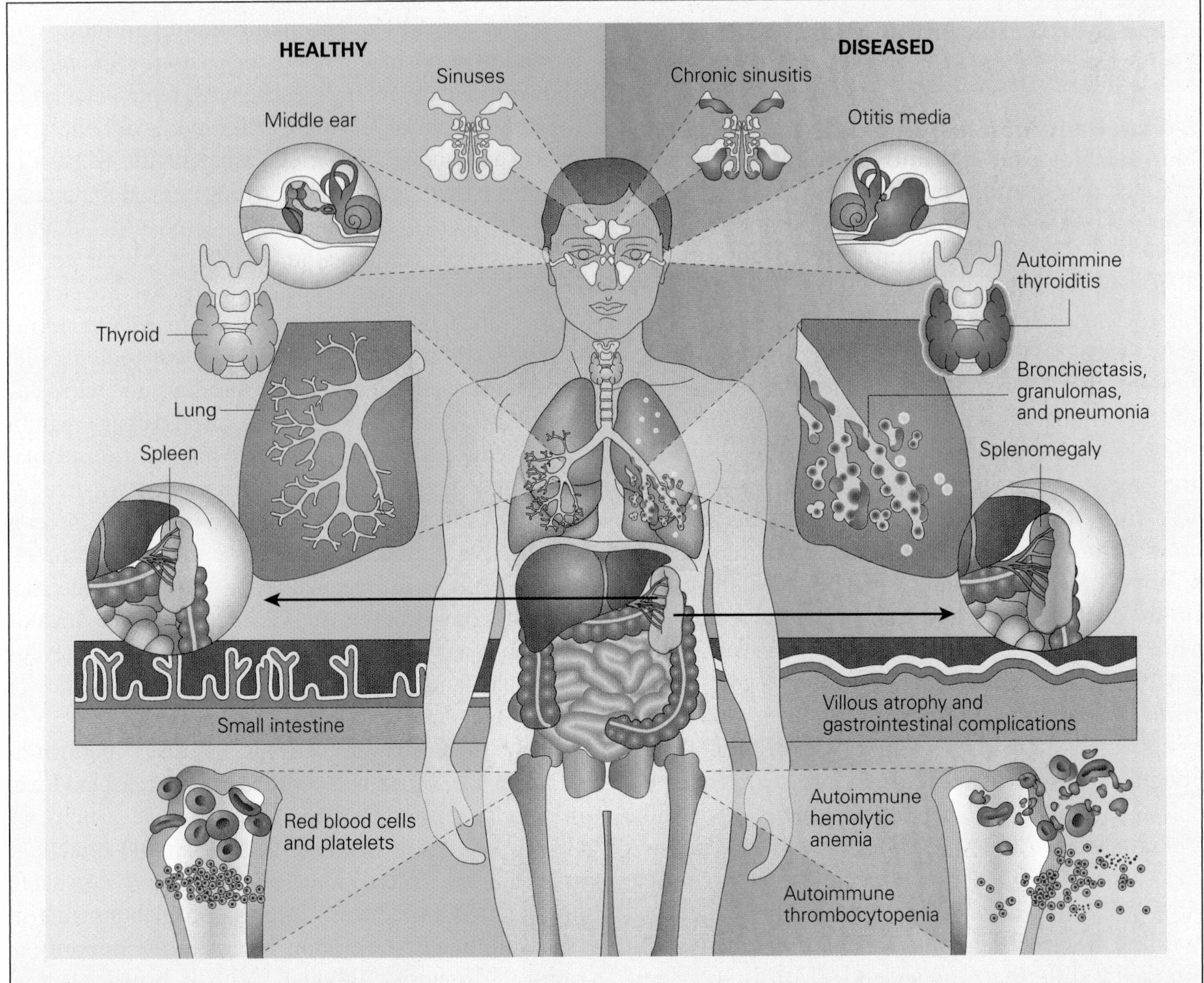

Figure 16-35. Schematic representation of infectious disease and autoimmune organ involvement in patients with CVID. Left panel shows healthy organs. Right panel shows several organ-specific infectious and autoimmune diseases, including chronic sinusitis, granulomatous lung disease, autoimmune thyroiditis, hemolytic anemia, thrombocytopenia, villous atrophy, and other gastrointestinal complications. (Adapted with permission from Park MA, Li JT, Hagan JB, Maddox DE, Abraham RS. Common variable immunodeficiency: a new look at an old disease. Lancet. 2008;372:489–502.)

encoded in the central MHC-III region, and its obligate heterodimerization partner MSH4 have a critical role in regulating meiotic homologous recombination but have not been definitively implicated in CSR.

While CVID is considered a genetic immune defect, with several of these genes having been reported as leading to the CVID phenotype, one of the most puzzling features of the disorder is the sporadic inheritance pattern and the relatively late onset. In most cases, no other family members have any immune defect. The mean age at diagnosis is between 25 and 45 years of age. These features suggest the interplay between either several or numerous genes with or without potential environmental factors.

Class-Switch Recombination (CSR) Defects

Severe Reduction in Serum IgG and IgA with Normal/Elevated IgM and Normal Numbers of B Cells: The Hyper IgM Syndromes

This is a second major class of immunodeficiencies with relatively normal numbers of hypofunctional T, B, and NK cells characterized by infections similar to those seen in patients with SCID, but typically with a more delayed and slightly milder presentation (Table 16A-6 in the Annex). Because of the fundamental T cell functional defects in these diseases, without defects in cellular survival, the suspicion of an immune deficiency may come less from the initial laboratory examination and more from careful piecing together of the clinical history, infection profile, and functional studies. Some of these cases have normal to increased IgM with low IgA and IgG and normal B cell numbers. There are four syndromes in this category recognized so far, and they are sometimes collectively grouped as the hyper IgM syndromes. These include (1) CD40 ligand (CD154) deficiency; (2) CD40 deficiency; (3) activation-induced cytidine deaminase deficiency (**AID**); and (4) uracil DNA glycosylase (**UNG**) deficiency. However, since there are several other distinct syndromes involved within the hyper IgM syndromes category, with markedly differing genetics and inconsistent elevations of IgM, it is best to refer to these syndromes as individual ones with discreet names, causes, and manifestations.

CD40 Ligand (CD154) Deficiency (MIM ID #308230)

As described previously under the combined T cell and B cell immunodeficiencies (Table 16A-5), this disease is also known as X-linked hyper IgM syndrome or XHIM or HIGM1 (Table 16A-6 in the Annex). CD40L is a member of the TNF family of ligands, so the gene is formally referred to as TNFSF5 (*Chapter 9*). CD40L is a T cell membrane protein that interacts with CD40, its cognate receptor, on B cells, dendritic cells, monocytes, macrophages, and activated epithelial cells. What was puzzling for years about this syndrome, which was first noted as yet another defect in immunoglobulin synthesis, was that the B cell phenotype was due to T cell dysfunction (*Chapter 7*). CD40L on T cells activates CD40 to drive B cell immunoglobulin class switch from IgM to IgG (class-switch recombination, CSR), as well as for subsequent maturation of antibody and formation of normal lymph node anatomy (*Chapter 6*). Shown in Figure 16-36 is a schematic representation of the critical role of CD40L/CD40 binding for the class switch and shows how a deficiency of the CD40 can lead to partial IgG/IgA/IgE hypogammaglobulinemia with normal or elevated IgM levels. In addition to directing B cell function, CD40L is critical for the control of certain intracellular parasites that are characteristic of SCID, such as *Pneumocystis jiroveci.* Other characteristic infections include *Cryptosporidium*, with eventual hepatic involvement, leading to sclerosing cholangitis, and histoplasmosis. Liver damage significantly reduces the success of bone marrow transplantation, and therefore filtered water that is free of *Cryptosporidium* is recommended once the diagnosis is suspected (this precaution may or may not be necessary, depending on regional water supplies). Other significant complications of CD40L deficiency include neutropenia, which may respond to G-CSF or IVIG, and malignancy, which may develop in adolescence or adulthood.

Flow cytometry for CD40L is easily performed (*Chapter 24*). Since it is X-linked, maternal blood can help to confirm the diagnosis if a mosaic pattern for CD40L expression is found. More than 200 mutations are cataloged (international registry: http://www.uta.fi/imt/bioinfo/CD40Lbase). Hypogammaglobulinemia is common, but IgM elevation is seen in the minority of cases at diagnosis. Although IVIG is beneficial, even with this treatment, mortality has been as high as 40 percent by 25 years as reported in European series. *Pneumocystis* prophylaxis should be instituted. BMT

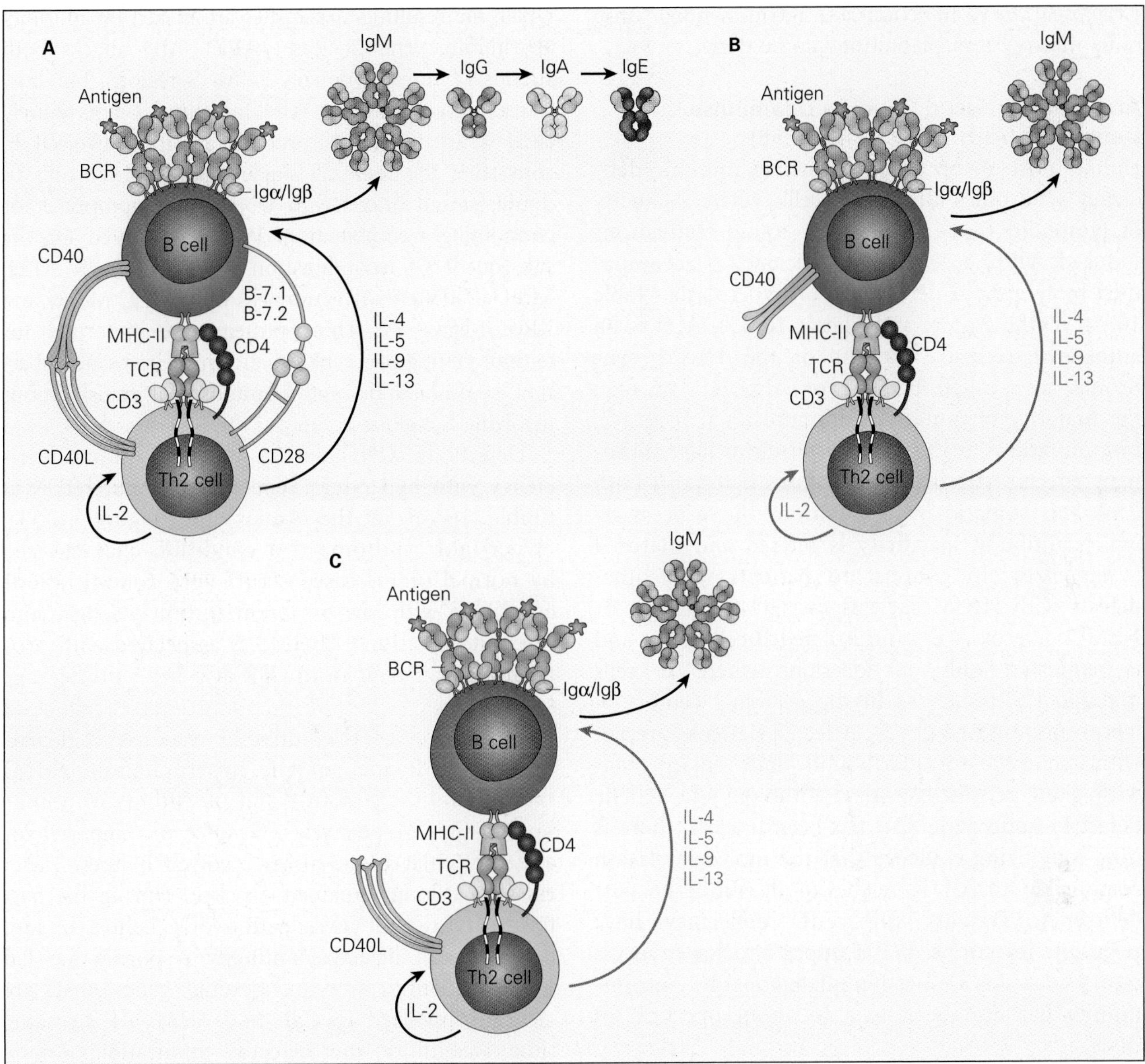

Figure 16-36. Schematic representation of the critical interaction of CD154 (CD40L) expression on the T cell with the CD40 on the B cell that is required for IgM/IgG class switching. Panel A: After cognate interaction of the MHC-II/peptide complex with the TCR of a CD4+ T cell, CD40L activates CD40 to drive B cell immunoglobulin class switch from IgM to IgG (class-switch recombination, CSR), as well as subsequent maturation of antibody from IgM→IgG→IgA→IgE. Panel B: In the absence of CD40L, there is no CD40L/CD40 interaction, no class switch, and there occurs only synthesis of IgM. Panel C: Similarly, in the absence of CD40 and lack of binding with CD40L, there is no class switch and synthesis only of IgM.

should be pursued, ideally before *Cryptosporidium* liver involvement has occurred.

CD40 Deficiency (MIM ID #109535)

Since CD40 is the cognate receptor for CD40L, it is expected that mutations in CD40 should resemble CD40L defects at both clinical and laboratory levels (HIGM3; MIM #606843) (Table 16A-6 in the Annex and Figures 16-33 and 16-36). This is indeed the case, and patients with CD40 deficiency present with hypogammaglobulinemia, impaired antibody maturation, and impaired lymphoid organ development and anatomy. The few patients identified have had *Pneumocystis*, *Pseudomonas*, and *Cryptosporidium* infections, all with clinical characteristics similar to patients with CD40L deficiency. Flow cytometry can also be used to screen for CD40 expression, but in strongly suspected cases, mutation analysis is needed (*Chapter 24*). IVIG, prophylactic antibiotics, and filtered water to prevent

Cryptosporidium infection are recommended until bone marrow transplantation can be done.

Activation-Induced Cytidine Deaminase Deficiency (AID) (MIM ID #606258)

Unlike most of the other Mendelian immune deficiency syndromes affecting B cells, where a paucity of lymphoid tissue is generally found, activation-induced cytidine deaminase deficiency is accompanied by lymphoid persistence or hyperplasia (Table 16A-6 in the Annex and Figure 16-33). AID is an autosomal recessive variant of the HIGM syndrome, also called HIGM2 or AICDA. Although the majority of mutations are autosomal recessive, rare mutations at the carboxy terminus have dominant effects. AID deficiency causes defects in both CSR and somatic hypermutation, the process by which antibody specificity is refined and matured (*Chapter 6*). In contrast to patients with other defects with HIGM such as the CD40L, CD40, or NEMO defects, AID is an isolated B cell defect and is expressed only in locations where B cells undergo CSR, such as in the germinal centers of lymph nodes (*Chapter 2*). Affected patients present with recurrent tonsillar/lymph node enlargement with giant germinal centers. Although the genetic defect(s) underlying AID has been unclear, there is now convincing evidence that the molecular lesion responsible for AID is related to an editing enzyme deficiency. Patients with AID deficiency have recurrent infections of the upper and lower respiratory tracts, as well as lymphadenopathy. Autoimmunity has also been seen in about one-fifth of cases.

Uracil DNA Glycosylase (UNG) Deficiency (MIM ID #191525)

Antibody class switching occurs in mature B cells in response to antigen stimulation and co-stimulatory signals. It occurs by a unique type of intra-chromosomal deletional recombination within special G-rich tandem-repeated DNA sequences (called switch, or S, regions located upstream of each of the heavy chain constant [CH] region genes, except Cδ [*Chapter 6*]). The recombination is initiated by the B cell-specific AID, which deaminates cytosines in both the donor and acceptor S regions. AID activity converts several deoxycytidine (dC) bases to deoxyuridine (dU) bases in each S region, and the dU bases are then excised by the UNG; the resulting abasic sites are nicked by apurinic/apyrimidinic endonuclease (**APE**). AID attacks both strands of transcriptionally active S regions, but how transcription promotes AID targeting is not entirely clear. Mismatch repair proteins are then involved in converting the resulting single-strand DNA breaks to double-strand breaks with DNA ends appropriate for end-joining recombination. Proteins required for the subsequent S-S recombination include DNA-PK, ATM, Mre11-Rad50-Nbs1, gammaH2AX, 53BP1, Mdc1, and XRCC4-ligase IV. These proteins are important for faithful joining of S regions, and in their absence, aberrant recombination and chromosomal translocations involving S regions occur.

Defects in UNG are a cause of immunodeficiency with hyper-IgM type 5 syndrome (HIGM5) (Table 16A-6 in the Annex and Figure 16-33). Hyper-IgM syndrome is a condition characterized by normal or increased serum IgM concentrations associated with low or absent serum IgG, IgA, and IgE concentrations. HIGM5 is associated with profound impairment in Ig CSR at a DNA precleavage step.

Maturation of the antibody response is dependent on CSR and somatic hypermutation (**SHM**) that modify the structure and the affinity of immunoglobulins, respectively (*Chapter 6*). The cellular and molecular mechanisms involved in these processes have long remained obscure. During the past few years, careful investigation of a cohort of rare patients with defective antibody responses has led to the identification of several genes that are critically involved in CSR and SHM. At the same time, recognition that defective maturation of antibody responses may result from different mechanisms has been essential to better define prognosis and to tailor more appropriate and specific forms of treatment.

Isotype or Light Chain Deficiencies with Normal Numbers of B Cells

There are five entities in this category recognized so far and they include: (1) Ig heavy chain mutations and deletions, (2) κ chain deficiency, (3) isolated IgG subclass deficiency, (4) IgA with IgG subclass deficiency, and (5) selective IgA deficiency.

The first two represent rare conditions with deficiencies of either IgG heavy (H) chains or IgG kappa (κ) chain deficiencies that are transmitted as autosomal recessive disorders and that are associated with recurrent bacterial infections similar to other forms of agammaglobulinemia (Table 16A-6 in the Annex).

Isolated IgG subclass deficiency is defined as a selective deficiency of one or more of the IgG subclasses with a generally accepted criterion of less than two SDs below the mean for age (*Chapter 24*). These are transmitted in a highly variable manner. Most IgG subclass-deficient patients are asymptomatic. The clinically significant IgG subclass deficiencies occur when the deficit is associated with recurrent infection and a significant defect in antibody responsiveness usually demonstrated by a failure of development of significant increases of specific antibody following immunization with protein vaccines, e.g., tetanus and diphtheria toxoids (these are associated with IgG1- and IgG3-associated antibody) or polysaccharide vaccines, e.g., pneumococcal or *H. influenzae* type B (HiB) vaccines (these are associated with IgG2- and IgG4-associated antibody) (*Chapter 24*). Subclass IgG3 deficiency is the most frequently encountered.

Some of these subclass deficiencies, e.g., IgG2, are associated with other subclass deficiencies or especially with IgA deficiency. Although previously the demonstration of diminished IgG subclasses alone was thought to be sufficient for the diagnosis of IgG subclass deficiency, it is now generally accepted that this practice is insufficient and that the diagnosis should only be made after demonstration of a failure of significant post-immunization antibody responses to the protein and/or polysaccharide vaccine antigen(s).

More commonly seen clinically is the isolated IgA deficiency that is the most frequently encountered B cell deficiency occurring in 1:400 of the population and that is transmitted in a highly variable inheritance pattern. Approximately one-third of these patients are asymptomatic, one-third present with recurrent sinopulmonary infections, and one-third with an increased frequency of autoimmune disorders such as juvenile idiopathic arthritis (**JIA**). These patients must not be treated with immunoglobulin replacement therapy because they have or will develop anti-IgA antibodies and the administration of commercial immunoglobulin products that inevitably contain small amounts of IgA may lead to nonhemolytic and sometimes-fatal anaphylactoid reactions (*Chapter 11*).

Specific Antibody Deficiency with Normal Ig Concentrations and Normal Numbers of B Cells

Perhaps the most perplexing of this class of immunodeficiency disorders is the condition referred to as specific antibody deficiency (**SAD**) with normal immunoglobulin concentrations and normal numbers of B cells (Table 16A-6 in the Annex). Several of these patients have been reported in children and adults with recurrent respiratory tract infections; however, the clinical features of SAD are not well described. The diagnosis requires a demonstration of a lack of specific antibody responsiveness following immunization as described above prior to initiation of immunoglobulin replacement therapy.

In one study by Boyle and coworkers, the clinical syndrome of SAD was evaluated by comparing the clinical features of children with SAD and those of children with recurrent infection but with normal immune function tests. SAD was defined as an adequate IgG antibody response to less than 50 percent of 12 pneumococcal serotypes tested following 23-valent unconjugated pneumococcal immunization. An adequate IgG antibody response was defined as a post-immunization titer of > 1.3 µg/mL or greater than four times the pre-immunization value. The diagnosis of SAD was made in 11 of 74 (14.9 percent) children with recurrent infection. Clinical features of the children diagnosed with SAD differed from those with normal antibody responses and included a strong history of otitis media, particularly in association with chronic otorrhea, allergic disease, particularly allergic rhinitis. The authors concluded that the diagnosis should be sought in children presenting with this distinct clinical phenotype of recurrent infection associated with chronic otorrhea and/or allergic disease.

Transient Hypogammaglobulinemia of Infancy with Normal Numbers of B Cells

Another immunoglobulin deficiency occurs as transient hypogammaglobulinemia of infancy with normal numbers of B cells, which does not have a known mode of transmission (Table 16A-6 in the Annex). This condition is thought to be due to a maturational delay in development of the adaptive immune system, and although the lowered levels of serum immunoglobulin may persist into the second year of life, the condition usually does not require treatment (*Chapter 2*).

Disorders of Immune Regulation

Introduction

As described in Chapter 1, there are three basic functions of the immune system: (1) defense, (2) homeostasis, and (3) surveillance. A decreased **defense** function is the basis for the most common manifestation of immune deficiency seen clinically as an undue susceptibility to recurrent infection. However, primary immunodeficiency disorders (**PIDs**) can also present clinically with aberrations of **homeostasis** manifested as autoimmune disease, e.g., rheumatoid arthritis (*Chapter 19*), or an impaired **surveillance** resulting in malignancy, e.g., lymphoma (*Chapter 21*). The traditional dogma that patients with PIDs are defined by their susceptibility to infections has therefore been expanded to include a new group of disorders of **immune regulation**. The immune dysregulation in these patients is expressed not only by their susceptibility to infections but also by an increased risk of allergy, autoimmunity, autoinflammatory disorders, or malignancy.

Diseases of Immune Dysregulation

Shown in Table 16A-7 in the Annex is a broad group of disorders of immune regulation that present clinically with an undue susceptibility to bacterial or viral infections, lymphoproliferative disorders, or autoimmunity. The first entity, **immunodeficiency with hypopigmentation**, has been described previously under "Abnormalities of Number and/or Function of Phagocytic Cells" (Table 16A-1 in the Annex) and includes conditions characterized by impairment in the transport, docking, or release of lytic granules for intracellular killing, e.g., phagocytic cell defects. A second group of defects of immune regulation, **familial hemophagocytic lymphohistiocytosis (FHL) syndromes**, shown in Table 16A-7 in the Annex, includes conditions with defects of cell-mediated cytotoxicity, e.g., perforin/granzyme defects, important for the clearance of viral infections or malignant cells. The third group of entities, **lymphoproliferative syndromes**, involves defects of signaling pathways responsible for defective viral clearance resulting in serious infectious mononucleosis, hemophagocytic lymphohistiocytosis secondary to viral infections, hypogammaglobulinemia, and lymphoma. The fourth collection of entities associated with disorders of immune regulation includes several clinical entities associated with **autoimmunity** resulting from defective apoptotic function and impaired Treg activity.

Shown in Table 16-5 is a more detailed summary of these four entities encompassing immune dysregulation syndromes, comparing their inheritance patterns and molecular defects with their clinical manifestations. An example of the first group of entities is Chediak-Higashi syndrome (**CHS**), which, as previously described, is an autosomal recessive disease caused by mutations of the lysosomal trafficking (**LYST**) regulator gene that impairs the intracellular transport of melanin and produces giant granules in neutrophils. This defect results in immunodeficiency with increased propensity to intracellular bacterial infections and albinism, a phenotype described similarly in Hermansky-Pudlak syndrome type 2, a condition caused by mutations in the b component of the adaptor-related protein complex 3 (**AP3**), involved in sorting of granules to the endosomal pathway (Tables 16A-1 and 16A-7 in the Annex).

The second group of diseases of immune dysregulation, the hemophagocytic lymphohistiocytosis (**HLH**) syndrome, is a collection of disorders characterized by proliferation and infiltration of hyperactive macrophages and T lymphocytes, leading to autoingestion of red blood cells by macrophages triggered by excessive lymphocyte-derived cytokine production, a phenomenon that gives this group its name. The HLH syndrome comprises both a set of genetically determined (primary) defects as well as several secondary causes of HLH that result from several other conditions including malignancy, infections (e.g., EBV and HIV), and autoimmune diseases (e.g., connective tissue diseases). The genetically determined HLH disorders are caused by mutations in several of the downstream molecules involved in the cytotoxic function of several of the cells of the immune system, e.g., macrophages, CD8+, NK, and NKT cells. Five primary disease subtypes, referred to as the FHL disorders, have been differentiated based on genetic loci that have been identified: (1) FHL1, (2) FHL2, (3) FHL3, (4) FHL4, and (5) FHL5 (Table 16-5). The primary pathogenetic mechanism underlying this immune dyregulation is a defect in cytotoxic killing of unwanted target cells due to defective perforin/granzyme activity by T and NK effector cells. This can occur by various mechanisms, including mutations of perforin, impaired transport of cytoxic granzymes, or molecules involved in maintenance of cell-to-cell contact essential for apoptosis.

As described in Chapters 1 and 7, the hallmark of cell-mediated cytotoxicity is carried out by CD8+ T cells and NK lymphocytes and depends on the coordinated assembly of perforin molecules into tubular structures forming cytolytic pores on target cells into which granzymes are introduced followed by apoptotic death of the target cells. The defective immune regulatory pathways that are found within these entities include both those that affect the assembly of perforin molecules into tubular structures as seen in FHL2, i.e., PRF1 mutations, as well as impairment in the transport and trafficking of lytic granzyme granules as seen in FHL3, i.e., UNC 13D mutation, and defective fusion between cytotoxic lymphocytes and target cells as seen in FHL4, i.e., syntaxin 11 (STX11) mutations (Table 16A-7 in the Annex and Table 16-5). In these diseases, the inability to extinguish inflammatory reactions results in sustained and excessive production of Th1 proinflammatory cytokines and IFN-γ in particular. In patients with HLH syndrome, a defect in any of the steps involving the perforin/granzyme pathway can result in a life-threatening "accelerated phase," a spectrum of manifestations consisting of susceptibility to viral infections, enhanced macrophage activity, and hemophagocytosis and is characterized by a prolonged fever and hepatosplenomegaly associated with neurologic abnormalities and cytopenias (Table 16-5).

The Lymphoproliferative Syndromes: X-Linked Lymphoproliferative Syndrome 1 (XLP1) (MIM ID #308240); X-Linked Lymphoproliferative Syndrome 2 (XLP2) (MIM ID #300635); Autosomal Lymphoproliferative Syndrome 1, EBV-Associated (ITK) (MIM ID #613011)

The third group of diseases of immune dysregulation includes the lymphoproliferative syndromes that comprise three distinct clinical presentations, each triggered by EBV infection (Table 16A-7 in the Annex and *Chapter 13*). These include two X-linked inherited disorders referred to as the X-linked lymphoproliferative (**XLP**) disorders, i.e., XLP1 and XLP2, and an autosomal recessive form ITK named after the homozygous mutation in the IL-2-inducible T cell kinase (**ITK**) gene expressed in T lymphocytes and found mutated in patients with this subtype. The genes affected in the X-linked forms are SH2D1A in XLP1, a gene encoding an adaptor protein importantly involved in intracellular signaling in T, NK, and NKT lymphocytes, and in XLP2, the BIRC4 the baculoviral IAP repeat-containing protein 4 (**BIRC4**) also called the X-linked inhibitor of apoptosis (**XIAP**) (Table 16A-7 in the Annex). Each of these three forms of lymphoproliferative diseases share a lack of NK T cells, suggesting a possible role of these rare populations of lymphocytes in controlling EBV infection (*Chapter 3*).

The X-linked lymphoproliferative syndrome 1 (XLP1), also known as Duncan's syndrome, originally described by Purtilo, is a rare, inherited immunodeficiency characterized by lymphohistiocytosis, hypogammaglobulinemia, and lymphomas, that usually develops in males in response to infection with Epstein-Barr virus (EBV) (Table 16A-7 in the Annex and Table 16-5). Mutations in the signaling lymphocyte activation molecule (**SLAM**)-associated protein (**SAP**), a signaling adaptor molecule, underlie 60 percent of cases of familial XLP. SH2D1A is the gene that encodes the SAP that is the affected moiety in XLP1. This protein serves as a negative regulator of SLAM activity, preventing cytokine activation. Mutations in SH2D1A cause a syndrome of profound susceptibility to EBV infection, manifest by the fulminant mononucleosis syndrome. The characteristic presentation was described originally in a boy with acute mononucleosis that progressed with rapid deterioration caused by hepatitis, anemia, and thrombocytopenia and culminating in the virus-associated hemophagocytic syndrome (**VAHS**). VAHS kills about 70 percent of XLP patients before the age of 10 years. However, for those who do not develop acute fulminant disease, they often develop hypogammaglobulinemia, aplastic anemia, or lymphoma. Other herpes viruses may also trigger the acute mononucleosis syndrome.

The XIAP defect seen in patients with X-linked lymphoproliferative syndrome 2 (XLP2) has been observed in three families without mutations in SAP. Apoptosis of lymphocytes from these XIAP-deficient patients is enhanced in response to various stimuli, including the T cell antigen receptor (TCR)-CD3 complex, the death receptor CD95 (also termed Fas or Apo-1), and the TNF-related apoptosis-inducing

Table 16-5. Summary of the defects of immune dysregulation comparing multiple features of genetics and inheritance patterns and molecular defects with clinical manifestations of disease susceptibility

Feature	Immunodeficiency with hypopigmentation	Hemophagocytic lymphohistiocytosis (HLH) syndromes				
Example	CHS	FHL1	FHL2	FHL3 13D	FHL4	FHL5
Gene involved	Defects in LYST	?	Defects in PRF1	Defects in UNC13D	Defects in STX11	Defects in STXBP2
Inheritance	AR	AR	AR	AR	AR	AR
Molecular defect	Impaired lysosomal trafficking; failure of lysosome/phagosome fusion	?	Defective perforin, a major cytolytic protein	Defective UNC13D required for priming vesicles for fusion	Defective syntaxin 11 required for cytotoxic/target cell contact vesicle trafficking and fusion	Defective syntaxin-binding protein
Clinical	Intracellular bacterial infections	Viral infections; enhanced macrophage activity "accelerated phase" of the disease with hemophagocytosis due to high IFN-γ production				

ligand receptor (**TRAIL-R**) (*Chapters 9* and *11*). XIAP-deficient patients, like SAP-deficient patients, also have low numbers of natural killer T lymphocytes (**NKT** cells), indicating that XIAP is required for the survival and/or differentiation of NKT cells. The observation that XIAP deficiency and SAP deficiency are both associated with a defect in NKT cells strengthens the hypothesis that NKT cells have a key role in the immune response to EBV (*Chapter 13*). Furthermore, the identification of an XLP immunodeficiency that is caused by mutations in XIAP suggests that XIAP is a potent regulator of lymphocyte homeostasis in vivo. Since some of the longer-term consequences other than acute mononucleosis occur even without EBV infection, BMT should be considered early.

Syndromes with Autoimmunity

The last group of diseases of immune dysregulation comprises several entities that are characterized by defective apoptotic killing and Treg abnormalities. These include ALPS, APECED, IPEX, and CD25 deficiency (Table 16A-7 in the Annex and Table 16-5).

Autoimmune Lymphoproliferative Syndrome (ALPS) (MIM ID #601859)

As described in Chapters 5 and 9, apoptosis is programmed cell death, without which we would readily overaccumulate cells with disastrous consequences. For lymphocytes, the critical

Lymphoproliferative disorders			**Syndromes with autoimmunity**			
XLP1	XLP2	ITK	ALPS	APECED	IPEX	CD25 deficiency
SH2D1A	XIAP	ITK	TNFRSF6 (Fas) TNFSF6 (FasL) CASP10 CASP8 NRAS	AIRE	FOXP3	IL-2Ra chain gene (IL2RA)
XL	XL	AR	AD & AR (rare) AD & AR AR AR AD	AR	XL	AR
Defective adaptor protein SAP regulating intracellular signals; required for NKT development	Defective product XIAP required for inhibition of apoptosis; required for NKT development	Defective ITK required for intracellular signaling and for NKT development	Defective apoptosis	Defective negative selection & failure of elimination of autoreactive T cells	Defective FOXP3 needed for induction of Treg cells	Defective IL-2 signaling needed for cell activation and Treg cell induction
Severe immune dysregulation in boys after primary infection with EBV, presenting as fatal mononucleosis, hemophagocytosis, hypogammaglobulinemia, and lymphoproliferation		ITK deficiency causes a fatal EBV immunodeficiency-syndrome similar to EBV-associated lymphoproliferative disorders in boys	Lymphoproliferative disease	Polyendocrinopathy autoimmune disease	Autoimmune diarrhea, early onset diabetes,thyroiditis, hemolytic anemia, thrombocytopenia, eczema	Lymphoproliferation, autoimmunity, impaired T cell proliferation

ligand-receptor interaction is between the receptor Fas (CD95) and Fas ligand (FasL, CD95L, or CD168), members of the TNF family of ligands and receptors (*Chapters 9* and *11*). Cognate interaction of Fas and FasL engages the death-inducing signaling complex (**DISC**) on the cytoplasmic side of Fas, activating caspases, leading to cell death. As a TNF receptor family member, Fas acts as a trimer (*Chapter 9*). Therefore, heterozygous mutations in Fas lead to disruption of the normal trimer oligomerization and result in deranged lymphoid apoptosis (Table 16A-7 in the Annex and Table 16-6). The consequences of this disorder of apoptosis are autoimmunity (e.g., immune thrombocytopenic purpura and hemolytic anemia) and lymphadenopathy. Infections are not part of the ALPS phenotype, unless occurring as consequences of immunosuppressive therapy or complications of splenectomy. Risks for lymphoma are greatly elevated over the general population, confirming the importance of proper regulation of cell death in lymphomagenesis (*Chapter 20*). Fas mutations have variable penetrance and expressivity. The characteristic laboratory abnormality is increased numbers of TCRαβ T cells that lack both CD4 and CD8, referred to as double-negative T (**DNT**) cells (*Chapters 2* and *7*). ALPS Ia is due to mutations in Fas, ALPS Ib is caused by mutations in FasL (TNFSF6) (Table 16A-7 in the Annex and Table 16-5). Defects in the immediate downstream caspases, i.e., caspase 8 and 10, cause ALPS II. ALPS phenotypes without genetic cause are currently called ALPS III.

The Autoimmune Polyendocrine Syndromes: Autoimmune Polyendocrine Syndrome, Type I (APS1); Autoimmune Polyendocrine Syndrome, Type 2 (APS2); Immunodysregulation, Polyendocrinopathy, and Enteropathy, X-Linked (IPEX)

The autoimmune polyendocrine syndromes (Table 16A-7 in the Annex and Table 16-6) comprise a heterogeneous group of rare diseases characterized by autoimmune activity against more than one endocrine organ, although non-endocrine organs can also be affected. There are three major "autoimmune polyendocrine syndromes" and a number of other diseases that have endocrine autoimmunity as one of their features (Table 16-6). Although the disorders may present with an extraordinary array of clinical features, they most often manifest with hypoparathyroidism, candidiasis, and adrenal insufficiency (*Chapter 14*).

Autoimmune Polyendocrine Syndrome Type I (APS1) (MIM ID #240300)

Autoimmune polyendocrine syndrome type 1, also known as the autoimmune polyendocrinopathy-candidiasis-ectodermal dystrophy (**APECED**), presents with mild immune deficiency leading to persistent mucosal and cutaneous infections with candida (candidiasis) and autoimmune dysfunction of the parathyroid gland (leading to hypocalcemia) and the adrenal glands (Addison's disease, with associated hypoglycemia and hypotension) (Table 16A-7 in the Annex and Table 16-6). In contrast to autoimmune polyendocrine syndrome type 2, which has a more complex pathogenesis and a more variable clinical presentation, the type 1 syndrome occurs is due to a monogenic defect in the autoimmune regulator (**AIRE**), a gene located on chromosome 21 (*Chapter 19*). Normal function of AIRE, a transcription factor, appears to confer immune tolerance for antigens from endocrine organs, and a deficiency of this transcription factor appears to be involved in the pathogenesis of the disorder (Figure 16-37).

Autoimmune Polyendocrine Syndrome Type II (APS1; Schmidt's Syndrome) (MIM ID #269200)

Autoimmune polyendocrine syndrome, type 2 (also known as Schmidt's syndrome) is more heterogeneous, occurs more often with an insidious onset, and has not been linked to one gene (Table 16A-7 in the Annex and Table 16-6). Rather, the condition appears to be polygenic, and although the precise mutation(s) has not been identified, patients are at a higher risk when they carry a particular HLA genotype (DQ2, DQ8, and DRB1*0404) (Figure 16-37). The features of this syndrome include Addison's disease, hypothyroidism, diabetes mellitus (type 1), and, less commonly, hypogonadism and vitiligo. Patients may also have hyperpigmentation

Table 16-6. Clinical and genetic features of the autoimmune polyendocrine syndromes.

	Autoimmune polyendocrine syndromes (APS)		
Feature	**Autoimmune polyendocrine syndrome type I (APSI) or (APECED)**	**Autoimmune polyendocrine syndrome type II (Schmidt's syndrome)**	**Immune dysregulation, polyendocrinopathy, enteropathy (X-linked) (IPEX) syndrome**
Prevalence	Rare	Common	Very rare
Time of onset	Infancy	Infancy through adulthood	Neonatal period
Gene and inheritance	AIRE (on chromosome 21, recessive)	Polygenic	FOXP3, X-linked
HLA genotype	Diabetes (risk decreased with HLA-DQ6)	HLA-DQ2 and HLA-DQ8; HLA-DRB1*0404	No association
Immunodeficiency	Asplenism, susceptibility to candidiasis	None	Overwhelming autoimmunity, loss of regulatory T cells
Association with diabetes	Yes (in 18%)	Yes (in 20%)	Yes (in majority)
Common phenotype	Candidiasis, hypoparathyroidism, Addison's disease	Addison's disease, type 1A, diabetes, chronic thyroiditis	Neonatal diabetes, malabsorption

Adapted with permission from Eisenbarth GS, Gottlieb PA. Autoimmune polyendocrine syndromes. N Engl J Med. 2004;350:2068–79.

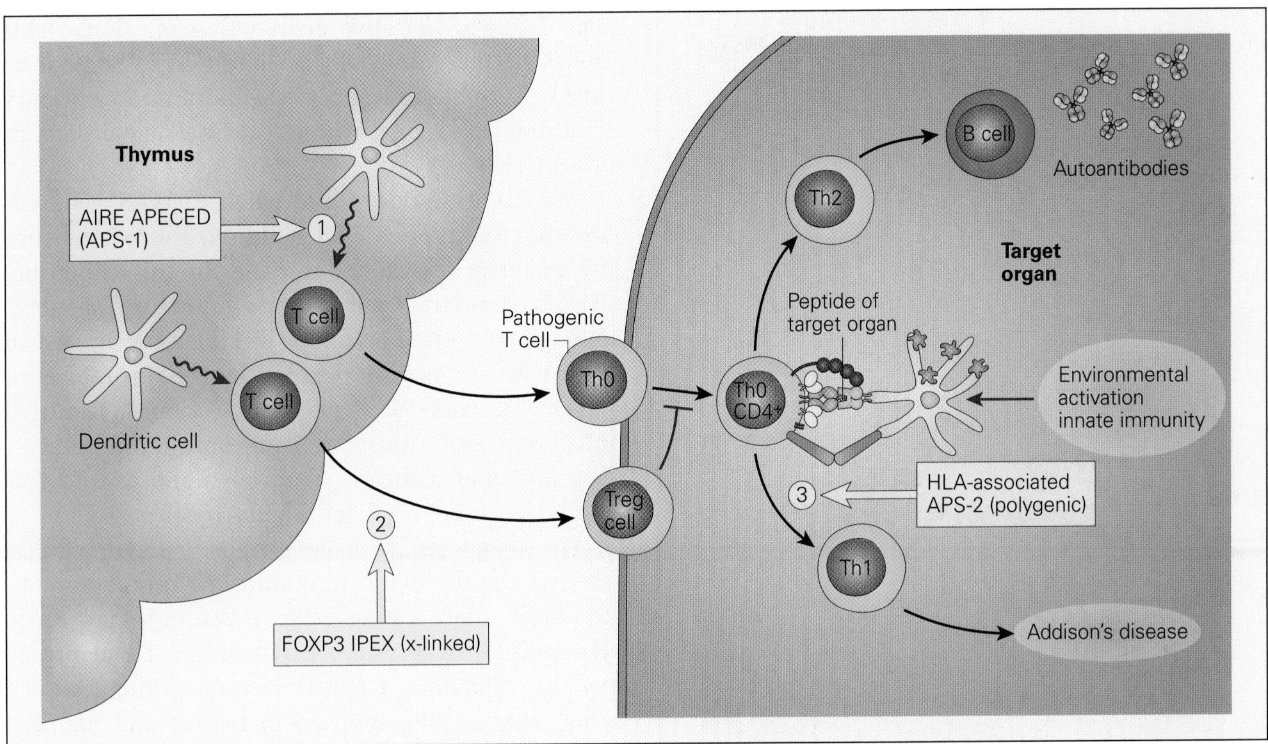

Figure 16-37. **Schematic representation of the molecular defects associated with the autoimmune polyendocrine syndromes.** Deficiency of AIRE in the thymic epithelial or DC favors the release of autoreactive pathogenic T cells to the periphery, resulting in APECED (#1); mutations in FOXP3 on T cells impair the development of Treg cells, leading to the IPEX syndrome (#2); APS-2 is a polygenic defect and has been associated with certain HLA phenotypes (#3). (Adapted with permission from Eisenbarth GS, Gottlieb PA. Autoimmune polyendocrine syndromes. N Engl J Med. 2004;350:2068–79.)

and vitiligo as well as a several-year history of intermittent, severe hypoglycemia and intermittent, severe fatigue.

Immune Dysregulation, Polyendocrinopathy, and Enteropathy (X-Linked) (IPEX) Syndrome (MIM ID #304790)

Underlying the ability to correctly activate the immune response must be the ability to correctly inactivate it. Therefore, with every antigen encounter, we undergo a phase of lymphoid expansion followed by a phase of lymphoid involution; otherwise, we would be awash in innumerable committed, expanding lymphocytes. The control of excessive responses falls to regulatory T cells, identified by the expression of FOXP3 (*Chapters 7* and *9*). Absence of regulatory T cells occurs in FOXP3 deficiency, a disease linked to the mutation and dysfunction of the transcriptional activator FOXP3 gene on the X chromosome that leads to a condition referred to as immune dysregulation, polyendocrinopathy, enteropathy, X-linked, or **IPEX** (MIM ID #304930, #304790) (Figure 16-38 and Table 16A-7 in the Annex). This is the most serious but most rare form of the autoimmune polyendocrine syndromes, and most cases present early in life with diabetes, autoimmune thyroiditis, hemolytic anemia, eczema, diarrhea, and failure to thrive. Some cases present later. About one-third of clinical IPEX cases do not have mutations in FOXP3. While males are primarily affected, female carriers might also suffer mild disease. Laboratory studies show poor ability of cells to regulate cytokine production. Infections occur in IPEX, but immune suppression is the critical therapeutic maneuver using T cell immunodulating agents such as cyclosporine (*Chapter 12*). The role of bone marrow transplantation is still evolving.

Other Well-Defined Immunodeficiencies

There are a number of primary immune deficiencies that were initially well defined by phenotypic characteristics and that do not fall into any of the previously described categories. Although mutations have been identified in many of these syndromes, the precise relationship of these genetic lesions with the

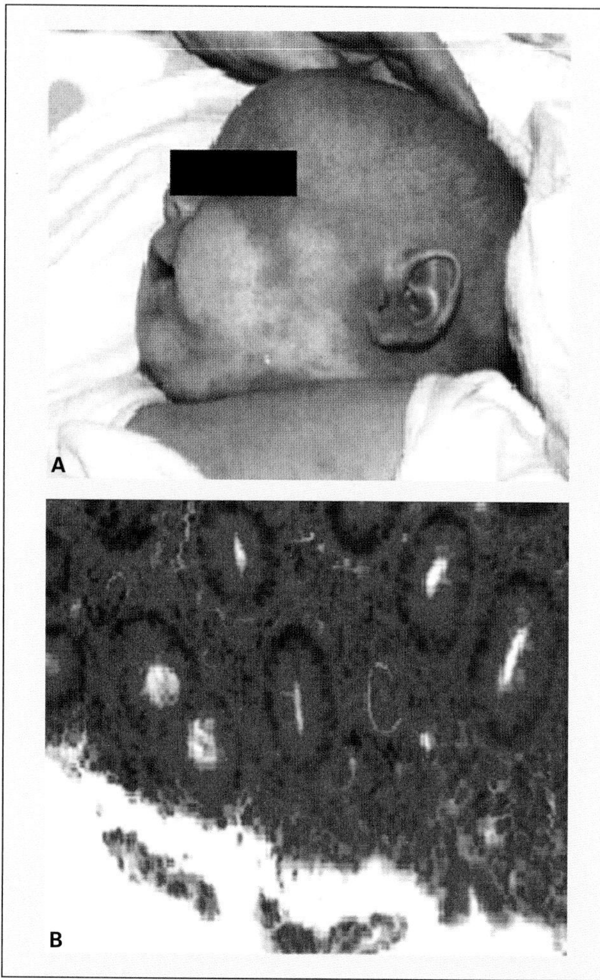

Figure 16-38. Disease manifestations of FOXP3 deficiency in a child with IPEX syndrome. Panel A: Eczema-like skin lesions on the face. Panel B: Enteritis-like picture in IPEX. Biopsy specimen of the sigmoid colon in a child with IPEX showing a colitis-like picture with infiltration by a mixed cellular infiltrate (hematoxylin and eosin staining). (Reproduced with permission from Foley SC, Préfontaine D, D'Antoni M, et al. Images in allergy and immunology: regulatory T cells in allergic disease. J Allergy Clin Immunol. 2007;120:482–6.)

morphologic features of these conditions has not yet been firmly established.

Wiskott-Aldrich Syndrome (WAS) (MIM ID #301000)

The Wiskott-Aldrich syndrome (WAS) is a rare X-linked recessive disease characterized by eczema, thrombocytopenia, immune deficiency, and bloody diarrhea caused by a mutation of the WAS gene that normally encodes the Wiskott-Aldrich syndrome protein (WASP), a protein involved in the regulation of actin filament formation. The decreased synthesis of WASP resulting from the mutation in the WAS gene leads to defective actin polymerization (Table 16A-8 in the Annex). The condition is sometimes called eczema-thrombocytopenia-immunodeficiency syndrome in keeping with Aldrich's original description in 1954.

Due to its mode of inheritance, WAS generally becomes symptomatic in children, the overwhelming majority of whom are male. In this condition, the platelets are small, do not function properly, and are removed rapidly by the spleen, which results in easy bruising caused by the thrombocytopenia. Patients also manifest eczema, recurrent infections, and a propensity for autoimmune disorders and malignancies (mainly lymphoma and leukemia) (Figure 16-39 and Figure 16-40).

The diagnosis is made on the basis of clinical parameters, the blood film, and low immunoglobulin levels. Skin testing (allergy testing) may reveal hyposensitivity. It must be remembered that not all patients will have a family history of the disorder, since they may be the first to harbor and manifest the gene mutation. Often, a diagnosis of leukemia may initially be raised on the basis of the low platelets and increased infections and, if suspected, a bone marrow biopsy should be performed. Decreased levels of Wiskott-Aldrich syndrome protein and confirmation of a causative mutation provide the most definitive diagnostic procedures.

In 1994, WAS was linked to mutations in a gene on the short arm of the X chromosome, which encodes WASP. It was later discovered that the disease X-linked thrombocytopenia (**XLT**) was also due to WAS mutations, but different from those that cause full-blown Wiskott-Aldrich syndrome. Furthermore, the rare disorder X-linked neutropenia has been linked to particular mutations of the WAS gene. The WAS gene encodes the WASP, which is 502 amino acids long and is mainly expressed in hematopoietic cells in the bone marrow (Figure 16-39).

The immune deficiency is caused by decreased antibody production, although T cells are also affected (making it a combined immunodeficiency). This leads to increased susceptibility to infections, particularly those caused by high-grade bacterial pathogens affecting the middle ear and sinuses.

The type of mutation affecting the WAS gene correlates significantly with the degree of severity: those mutations that lead to the production of a truncated protein cause significantly more symptoms than those with a missense mutation but a

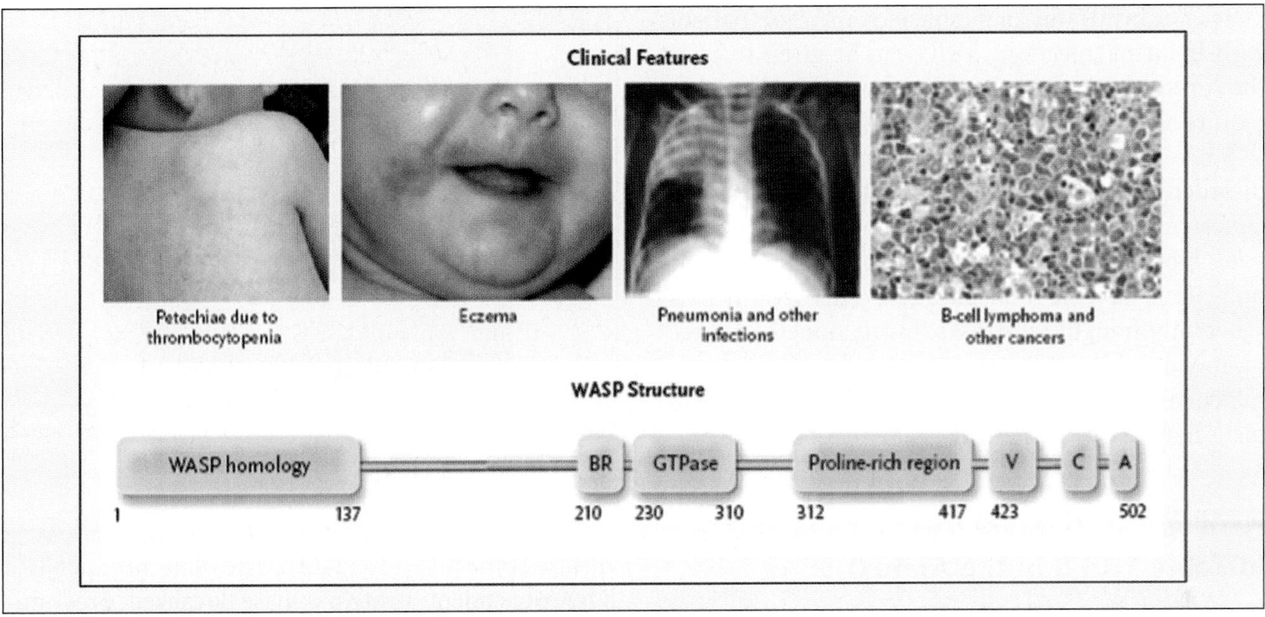

Figure 16-39. Wiskott-Aldrich syndrome. The clinical features of the syndrome (top) include thrombocytopenia, eczema, and respiratory tract infections, and the disease can be complicated by B cell lymphomas that often arise at extranodal sites. The Wiskott-Aldrich syndrome protein (WASP, bottom) has several principal domains: a homology domain found in several related proteins, the basic region (BR) of the guanosine triphosphatase (GTPase) domain, proline-rich region, the verprolin homology domain (V), the central domain (C), and the acidic domain (A) (integers below the domains are the amino acid numbers). (Reproduced with permission from Puck JM, Candotti F. Lessons from the Wiskott-Aldrich syndrome. N Engl J Med. 2006;355:1659–61.)

normal-length WASP. Although autoimmune disease and malignancy occur in both types of mutations, patients with truncated WASP carry a higher risk. The combined incidence of WAS and XLT is about four to 10 in 1 million live births.

Treatment of Wiskott-Aldrich syndrome is based on correcting symptoms. Aspirin and other non-steroidal anti-inflammatory drugs should be avoided, since these may interfere with platelet function. Patients with severely low platelet counts may require

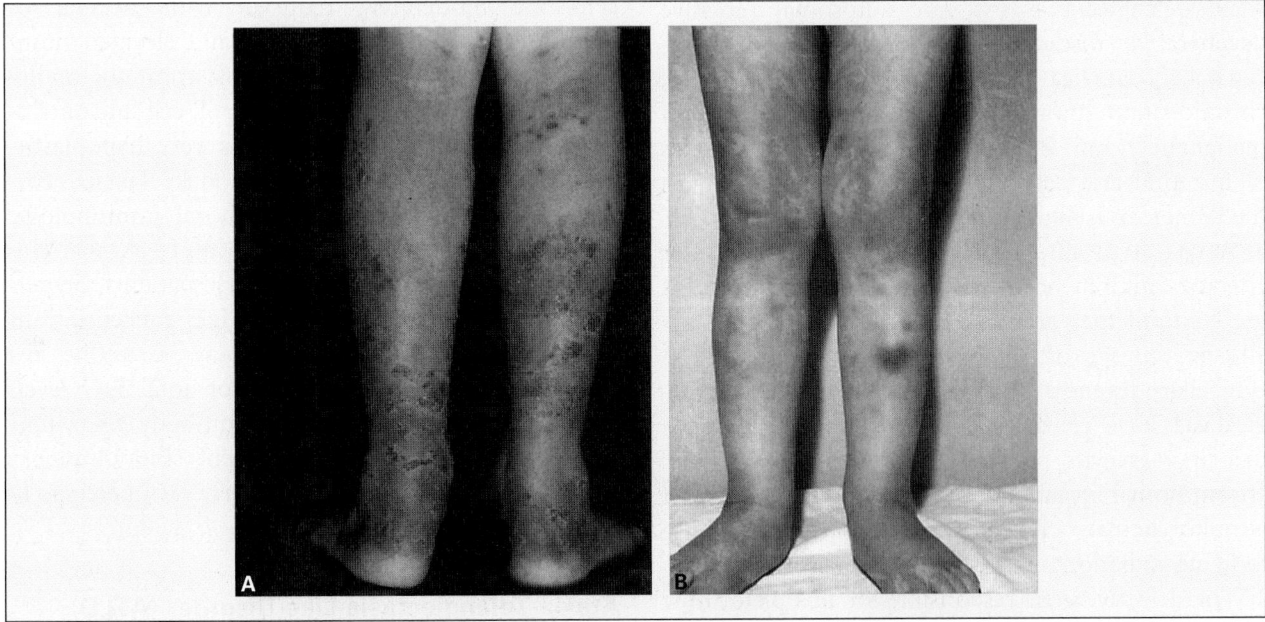

Figure 16-40. Photographs of patients with the Wiskott-Aldrich syndrome. Panel A: Shows eczematoid lesions in a four-year-old boy. Panel B: Shows purpuric lesions in a six-year-old boy.

platelet transfusions or a splenectomy. For patients with frequent infections, IVIG can be given to boost the immune system. Anemia from bleeding may require iron supplementation or blood transfusion.

Since Wiskott-Aldrich syndrome is primarily a disorder of the blood-forming tissues, a hematopoietic stem cell transplant, accomplished through a cord blood or bone marrow transplant, offers the only hope of cure (*Chapter 22*). This treatment is inherently fraught with risks, but is nonetheless recommended for patients with HLA-identical donors, matched sibling donors, or even in cases of incomplete matches if the patient is age five or younger.

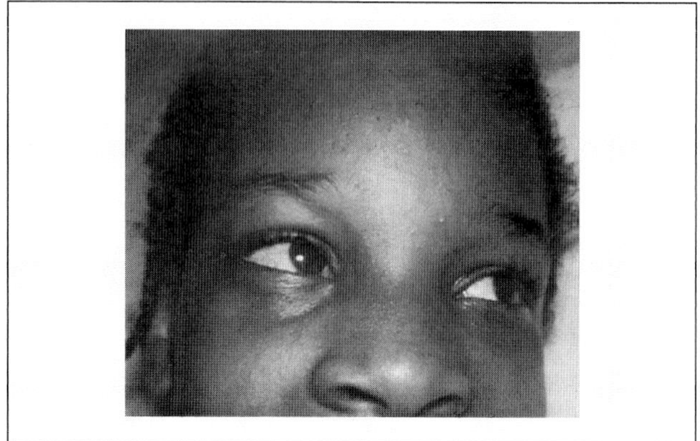

Figure 16-41. Photograph of a 12-year-old girl with ataxia telangiectasia showing the ocular telangiectasis of the conjunctivae. (Courtesy of Dr. Sanford Leiken.)

DNA Repair Defects (Other Than Those in Table 16A-5 in the Annex)

There are a group of well-defined syndromes where immune deficiencies are due to defects in DNA repair mechanisms (Table 16A-8 in the Annex). These disorders comprise ataxia-telangiectasis, ataxia-telangiectasia-like disease (**ATLD**), and a cluster of other rare entities that include Nijmegen breakage syndrome, Bloom syndrome, immunodeficiency with centromeric instability and facial anomalies (ICF), and PMS2 deficiency (CSR deficiency caused by defective mismatch repair).

Ataxia-Telangiectasia (MIM ID #208900)

Ataxia-telangiectasia is a rare autosomal recessive degenerative disease characterized by progressive cerebellar ataxia, oculocutaneous telangiectasis, chronic sinopulmonary disease, a high incidence of malignancy, and various immunologic deficiencies of humoral and cellular immunity (Table 16A-8 in the Annex and Figure 16-41).

Ataxia typically becomes evident soon after affected children begin to walk; the condition progresses until they are confined to a wheelchair, usually by the age of 10 to 12 years. In addition to cerebellar degeneration, patients with ataxia-telangiectasia have elevated levels of serum alpha-fetoprotein, growth retardation, premature aging, chromosomal instability, an increased frequency of lymphoreticular cancers, and hypersensitivity to ionizing radiation and radiomimetic drugs.

The defective gene responsible for this pleiotropic disorder, the ataxia-telangiectasia mutated (**ATM**) gene, was identified in 1995 and was subsequently cloned and mapped to the long arm of chromosome 11 (11q22-23). The gene product is a DNA-dependent protein kinase localized predominantly to the nucleus and involved in mitogenic signal transduction, meiotic recombination, and cell cycle control (Figure 16-42). Cells from patients as well as those of heterozygous carriers have increased sensitivity to ionizing radiation, defective DNA repair, and frequent chromosomal abnormalities and have potential implications for cancer in the general population.

In vitro tests of lymphocyte function have generally shown moderately depressed proliferative responses to T and B cell mitogens (Table 16A-8 in the Annex). Percentages of CD3+ and CD4+ T cells are moderately reduced, with normal or increased percentages of CD8+ and elevated numbers of Tγ/δ T cells. Studies of immunoglobulin synthesis have shown both helper T cell and intrinsic B cell defects. The thymus is very hypoplastic, exhibits poor organization, and lacks Hassall corpuscles. The most frequent humoral immunologic abnormality is the selective absence of IgA, which is present in 50 to 80 percent of these patients. Hypercatabolism of IgA also occurs. IgE concentrations are usually low, and the IgM may be of the low molecular weight variety. IgG2 or total IgG levels may be decreased, and specific antibody titers may be decreased or normal. Recurrent sinopulmonary infections occur in approximately 80 percent of these patients.

Ataxia-Telangiectasia-Like Disorder (ATLD) (MIM ID #604391)

ATLD is an extremely rare condition that could be considered as a differential diagnosis to AT

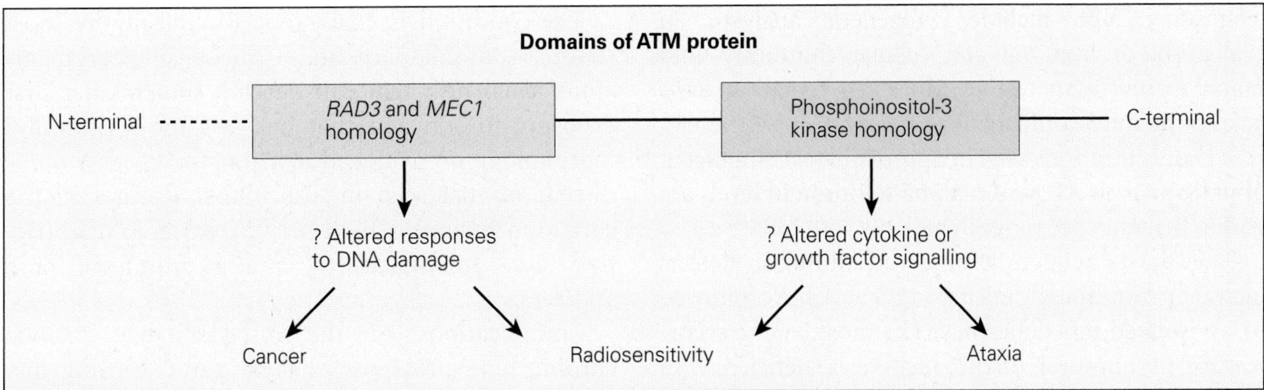

Figure 16-42. Schematic representation of the two domains of the ATM protein affected in ataxia-telangiectasia. The two areas of the ATM protein characterized thus far include a region similar to the DNA-repair/cell-cycle-checkpoint genes found in yeast, RAD3 and MEC1, and another region resembling phosphoinositol-3 kinases. The RAD3-like region could contribute to the altered responses to DNA damage secondary to agents that damage DNA and to genetic instability, which could lead to cancer and increased radiosensitivity. The phosphoinositol-3 kinase region could mediate a number of cytokine or growth factor signals, and defects in this function could be responsible for the increased rate of apoptotic cell death and radiosensitivity as well as death of neuronal cells and ataxia. (Reproduced with permission from Kastan M. Ataxia-telangiectasia—broad implications for a rare disorder. N Engl J Med. 1995;333:662–3.)

(Table 16A-8 in the Annex). ATLD patients are very similar to AT patients in showing a progressive cerebellar ataxia, hypersensitivity to ionizing radiation, and genomic instability. However, ATLD can be distinguished from AT by the absence of telangiectasis, normal immunoglobulin levels, a later onset of the condition, and a slower progression of the disease. It is not known whether ATLD individuals are also predisposed to tumors. The gene mutated in ATLD is hMre11, a gene involved in cell cycle checkpoint and DNA repair in mammals and is located on chromosome 11q21.

Nijmegen Breakage Syndrome, Bloom Syndrome, Immunodeficiency with Centromeric Instability and Facial Anomalies (ICF), and PMS2 Deficiency (Class-Switch Recombination [CSR] Deficiency Caused by Defective Mismatch Repair)

Another group of primary immune deficiency disorders that affect DNA repair include Nijmegen breakage syndrome, Bloom syndrome, immunodeficiency with centromeric instability and facial anomalies (**ICF**), and PMS2 deficiency (CSR deficiency caused by defective mismatch repair) (Table 16A-8 in the Annex).

Nijmegen Breakage Syndrome (NBS) (MIM ID #251260)

Nijmegen breakage syndrome (**NBS**) is a rare autosomal recessive condition of chromosomal instability that is clinically characterized by microcephaly, a distinct "birdlike" facies, growth retardation, immunodeficiency, radiation sensitivity, and a strong predisposition to lymphoid malignancy (Table 16A-8 in the Annex). Ataxia-telangiectasia variant-1 (AT variant-1) is the designation applied to the Nijmegen breakage syndrome and AT variant-2 is the designation for the Berlin breakage syndrome, which differs only in complementation studies. Mutations in the NBS1 (Nibrin) gene located in band 8q21 are responsible for NBS.

More than 40 NBS patients have been diagnosed and molecularly confirmed within North America. The total number of patients diagnosed with NBS (including those in North America) is estimated to be 200 but the number of patients identified worldwide is systematically increasing, probably because physicians are becoming more aware of the disorder. The most common cause of death of patients with the NBS is malignancy with a smaller number due to bone marrow failure and infection.

The diagnosis of NBS should be suspected in a child with a history of psychomotor developmental or somatic growth retardation, recurrent infections due to a combined immune deficiency, and a strongly increased risk of developing cancer, in particular leukemia and lymphoma. The main physical findings of NBS include progressive microcephaly with characteristic facies, growth retardation, and impaired sexual maturation in females. Other frequently observed manifestations include skin pigmentation defects (i.e., café-au-lait and/or vitiligo spots) and minor limb abnormalities. Laboratory studies helpful in diagnosing NBS include cytogenetic analysis, an evaluation of humoral and cellular immunity, and radiation-sensitivity testing. Molecular genetic analysis enables definite confirmation. In contrast to the elevated concentrations seen in approximately 90 percent of patients with AT, serum alpha-fetoprotein levels are within the reference range in patients with NBS.

The most frequently observed humoral defects include a combined deficit of IgG and IgA, followed by an isolated IgG deficiency. The most characteristic feature of humoral disturbances is a deficiency in one or more IgG subclasses, even with total IgG levels in the reference range; selective deficiency of IgG4 and IgG2 are the most common. T cell immunity is impaired in most patients with NBS. The most commonly reported defects are mild-to-moderate lymphopenia, expressed as a low percentage of CD3+ T cells, a low proportion of CD4+ (helper) T cells, and a decreased CD4+/CD8+ ratio. A deficiency of CD4/CD45RA+ (naïve) cells and an excess of CD4/CD45RO+ (memory) cells has been observed, and a high number of natural killer cells have been noted in some patients.

No specific therapy is available for NBS. Replacement immunoglobulin therapy (i.e., IVIG therapy) is indicated in patients with significant reduction of serum IgG or IgG subclass levels and decreased specific antibody responses to protein or polysaccharide vaccines (*Chapter 11*). Antibiotic prophylaxis should be considered in patients with recurrent respiratory tract infections. Cancer treatment must be modified in NBS patients with malignancy because conventional doses of radiotherapy and chemotherapy may lead to severe (even lethal/life-threatening) toxic complications. Bone marrow transplantation can be considered in some patients nonresponsive to these measures.

Bloom Syndrome (BLM) (MIM ID #210900)

Bloom syndrome (also known as Bloom-Torre-Machacek syndrome) is a rare autosomal recessive chromosomal disorder first described by dermatologist Dr. David Bloom in 1954 and characterized by a high frequency of chromosomal breaks and DNA rearrangements (Table 16A-8 in the Annex). The disorder is caused by mutations in the Bloom molecule (**BLM**) gene, which is a member of the DNA helicase family, i.e., enzymes that unwind the two strands of a duplex DNA molecule required for most DNA replicative and repair processes (*Chapter 25*).

The condition is characterized clinically by short stature, a birdlike face, and a sun-sensitive erythematous facial rash that can develop shortly after first exposure to sun and that may assume a butterfly-morphology of reddened skin on the cheeks, reminiscent of that seen in SLE. Other features of the condition include a high-pitched voice, a long, narrow face, micrognathism, and a prominent nose and ears.

Complications of the disorder may include chronic lung problems, diabetes, and learning disabilities and in rare cases mental retardation. Due to an elevated rate of mutation in affected individuals, the most striking complication of the disorder is a high frequency of cancer, including leukemias, lymphomas, and carcinomas.

The diagnosis of Bloom syndrome can be confirmed by chromosome study. Serum immunoglobulin levels often show decreased IgA, IgE, and IgG subclasses, an increased IgM, and a variable reduction of antibodies.

Immunodeficiency with Centromeric Instability and Facial Anomalies (ICF) (MIM ID #242860)

ICF syndrome is a rare autosomal recessive disease characterized by facial dysmorphism, immunoglobulin deficiency, and branching of chromosomes 1, 9, and 16 following phytohemagglutinin (**PHA**) stimulation of lymphocytes (Table 16A-8 in the Annex). The condition is caused by mutations in DNA methyltransferase DNMT3B, resulting in defective DNA methylation. Patients present with facial dysmorphic features, macroglossia, malabsorption, and bacterial and other opportunistic infections.

Affected patients may show decreased or normal numbers of circulating T and B cells and variable degrees of hypogammaglobulinemia and antibody deficiency. Early diagnosis of ICF syndrome is critical since early immunoglobulin supplementation can improve the course of disease. Allogeneic stem cell transplantation should also be considered as a therapeutic option in patients with severe infections or failure to thrive.

PMS2 Deficiency (Class-Switch Recombination [CSR] Deficiency Caused by Defective Mismatch Repair) (MIM ID #276300)

Another very rare defect of DNA repair involves mutations in PMS2 gene resulting in defective CSR associated with low levels of IgG and IgA, elevated IgM, and abnormal antibody responses (Table 16A-8 in the Annex). The condition consists of a constellation of clinical manifestations that include recurrent infections, café-au-lait spots, and increased frequency of lymphoma and colorectal and brain cancer.

Thymic Defects

DiGeorge Syndrome (MIM ID #188400), Chromosome 22q11.2 Deletion Syndrome (MIM ID #611867), Velocardiofacial Syndrome (VCFS) (Shprintzen Syndrome) (MIM ID #192430), and Conotruncal Heart Malformations (CTHM) (MIM ID #217095)

In 1965, Dr. Angelo DiGeorge described a syndrome in four patients with hypocalcemia, thymic, and parathyroid aplasia and congenital outflow tract defects of the heart, which subsequently was named DiGeorge syndrome (**DGS**) (Table 16A-8 in the Annex). This syndrome is due to defective development of the third and fourth pharyngeal pouches, resulting in thymic absence or hypoplasia and associated susceptibility to infection due to a deficit of T cells, conotruncal cardiac defects, and parathyroid hypoplasia (with hypocalcemia) (*Chapter 2* and Figure 16-43).

Children with DiGeorge syndrome have typical features of hypertelorism, antimongoloid slant of the eyes, low-set ears with malformations, and a peculiar "fish mouth" and absent philtrum (Figure 16-44). Although some patients with DiGeorge syndrome demonstrate an autosomal dominant mode of transmission, most cases are sporadic and at least 85 percent of them are associated with deletions of chromosome 22q11.2.

In 1981, Shprintzen reported on 39 patients with a syndrome characterized by cleft palate, cardiac anomalies, typical facies, and learning disabilities that came to be known as velocardiofacial syndrome (**VCFS**) or Shprintzen syndrome. Less frequently encountered features include microcephaly, mental retardation, short stature, slender hands and digits, minor auricular anomalies, and

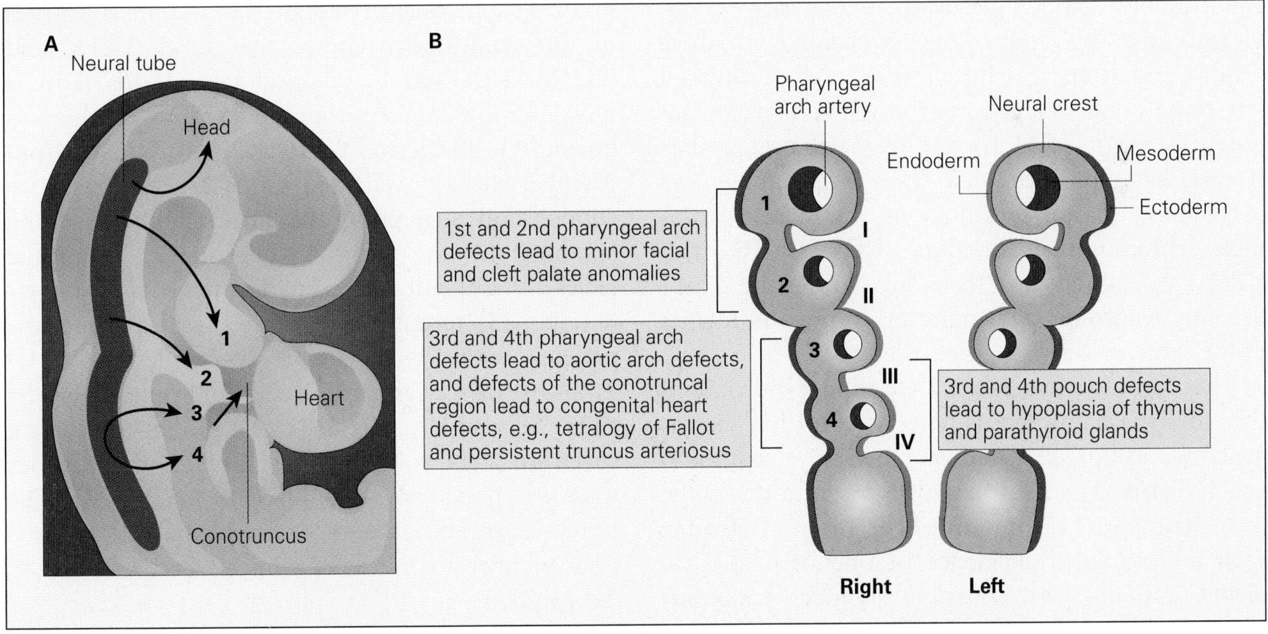

Figure 16-43. Schematic representation of embryonic development of pharyngeal arch structures. Panel A: A lateral right view of the migration of cephalic neural crest cells (indicated by the arrows) derived from the dorsal aspect of the neural tube (neural fold) into the head, pharyngeal arches, and the conotruncal region (outflow tract) of the mouse embryo at approximately 9.5 days (equivalent to about 28 days in a human embryo). Panel B: Coronal section of pharyngeal arches corresponding to a mouse embryo of the same age. Each pharyngeal arch is composed of an outer epithelium of ectoderm (brown), a central core of paraxial mesoderm (red) adjacent to a pharyngeal arch artery, and an inner epithelium of endoderm (lavender), which forms pharyngeal pouches between each pharyngeal arch. Neural crest cells migrate from the caudal hindbrain and form the mesenchyme (red) that surrounds the pharyngeal arch arteries and the mesodermal core. Arabic numerals one to four represent the first to fourth pharyngeal arches, and roman numerals I to IV represent the first to fourth pharyngeal pouches. Note that first and second pharyngeal arch defects lead to minor facial anomalies and cleft palate, third and fourth pouch defects lead to hypoplasia of thymus and parathyroid glands, third and fourth arch artery defects lead to aortic arch defects, and defects of the conotruncal region lead to congenital heart defects such as tetralogy of Fallot and persistent truncus arteriosus. (Adapted from Yamagishi H. The 22q11.2 deletion syndrome. Keio J Med. 2002;51:77–88.)

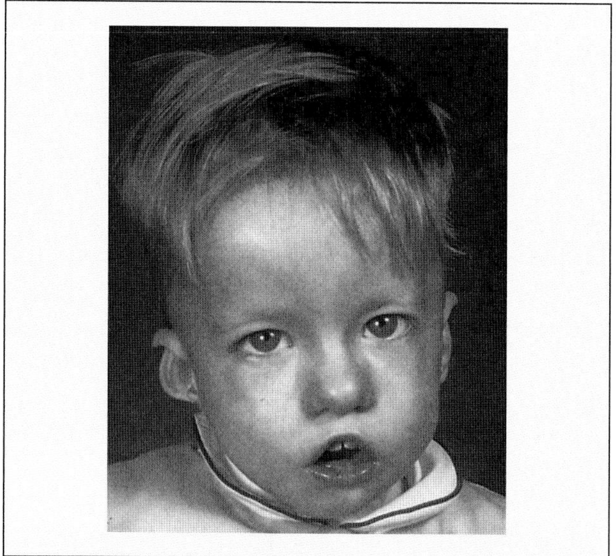

Figure 16-44. A child with DiGeorge syndrome. Note the dysplasia of the ears and mouth and the hypertelorism. (Courtesy of Dr. Fred S. Rosen, reproduced with permission from Kretschmer R, et al. Congenital aplasia of the thymus gland. New Engl J Med 1968;279:1295.)

inguinal hernia. VCFS has also been associated with chromosome 22q11.2 deletions. In the early 1990s, the deletion was reported in association with three distinct syndromes, namely DGS, velocardiofacial syndrome (VCFS), and conotruncal heart malformations (**CTHM**) (MIM ID #217095). Clinical genetic studies have revealed that these syndromes have overlapping clinical presentations and share a common chromosomal deletion. DGS, VCFS, and CTHM café-au-lait are, therefore, part of the 22q11 deletion syndrome (DS) reflecting various outcomes of the same underlying genetic defect.

The chromosome 22q11.2 deletion syndrome is therefore the name that is now given to this heterogeneous group of disorders sharing a common genetic basis. The 22q11.2 deletion syndrome is the most common chromosomal deletion syndrome, with an estimated incidence of one in 4,000 live births. Patients with complete absence of thymus (the so-called "complete" DiGeorge syndrome) account for < 0.5 percent of patients and exhibit a complete T cell immunodeficiency; the majority of patients with 22q11.2 deletion syndrome and immune defects exhibit mild to moderate deficits in T cell numbers and are referred to as the so-called "partial" DiGeorge syndrome. When all patients with chromosome 22q11.2 deletions are considered together, cardiac malformations, speech delay, and immunodeficiency are the most common characteristics. Immune deficiencies due to the lack of thymic development have also been associated with an increased incidence of autoimmune disease; in the 22q11.2 deletion syndrome, autoimmune disease may occur in up to 30 percent of patients. These autoimmune disorders include autoimmune cytopenias, autoimmune arthritis, and autoimmune endocrinopathies such as autoimmune thyroiditis (Hashimoto's thyroiditis). The precise basis for this increased frequency of autoimmunity is unknown but several possibilities have been suggested, including viral infection, deficiency of CD4+CD25+ natural regulatory T cells, or deficiency in the autoimmune regulator (**AIRE**). A mutation affecting the T box-1 (TBX1) gene has been identified as the constellation of thymic and associated defects responsible for the wide variety of clinical manifestations seen in this syndrome (Table 16A-8 in the Annex and Box 16-4).

The acronym "CATCH 22" (cardiac defects, abnormal facies, thymic hypoplasia, cleft palate, hypocalcemia, and 22q11 deletions) was proposed in 1993 as an aid in remembering the main features of the syndrome encompassing DGS, VCFS, and CTHM. However, the clinical use of this term is now considered inappropriate because of the following: (1) the term "CATCH 22" (originally from Joseph Heller's novel titled *Catch-22*) has a negative connotation suggesting the impossibility of doing anything; (2) the term "A" referring to "abnormal facies" is difficult to accept for patients and their families; (3) recent studies have revealed that some patients with Opitz G/BBB syndrome (MIM ID #145410) or Cayler cardiofacial syndrome (MIM ID #125520) also have del 22q11.2 and that the clinical spectrum associated with del 22q11 is much wider than was previously recognized as CATCH 22. The term "22q11DS" is a more appropriate term used now to refer to the wide clinical spectrum due to del 22q11.

A routine test is now available and is based on fluorescence in situ hybridization (**FISH**) using probes (TUPLE1 or N25) from the critical deletion region in 22q11.2 (*Chapter 24*). The test is available in most cytogenetic laboratories to confirm the diagnosis for patients with both typical and atypical clinical presentations. Rarely, deletions are present in 22q11.2 but are not detectable by routine FISH analysis. About 10 cases of such atypical deletions

Box 16-4

T-box 1; TBX1 Gene

The TBX1 gene is a member of a phylogenetically conserved family of genes that share a common DNA-binding domain, the T-box. T-box genes encode transcription factors involved in the regulation of developmental processes. This gene product shares 98 percent amino acid sequence identity with the mouse ortholog. DiGeorge syndrome (DGS)/velocardiofacial syndrome (VCFS), a common congenital disorder characterized by neural-crest-related developmental defects, has been associated with deletions of chromosome 22q11.2 where this gene has been mapped. Studies using mouse models of DiGeorge syndrome suggest a major role for this gene in the molecular etiology of DGS/VCFS. Several alternatively spliced transcript variants encoding different isoforms have been described for this gene.

of 22q11.2 have been reported. Del 22q11 is not detectable by extensive FISH analysis in approximately 10 percent of patients who are clinically diagnosed as having DGS or 22q11DS. These patients include those who have chromosome deletion of 10p or others and those who have undefined genetic etiology. The DiGeorge critical region contains TBX-1 mutations that lead to various manifestations of the disease.

Patients with the "complete" DiGeorge syndrome exhibit a complete T cell immunodeficiency with a severe combined immunodeficiency (SCID) phenotype requiring immune reconstitution by hematopoietic stem cell transplantation (HSCT). Although it appears paradoxical that T cell maturation could occur in the absence of a functional thymus, it appears that immune reconstitution by HSCT in these patients is achieved through peripheral expansion of mature donor T cells brought in by the graft. Thymic transplantation has also been shown to restore normal immune function with the generation of naïve thymic emigrants.

Other Well-Defined Immunodeficiencies

There are a number of other rare, well-defined immunodeficiencies shown in Table 16A-8 in the Annex, which include immunoosseous dysplasias (cartilage-hair hypoplasia syndrome) (MIM ID #250250), immunoosseous dysplasia, Schimke-type (MIM ID #242900), the Netherton syndrome (MIM ID #256500), hepatic veno-occlusive disease with immunodeficiency (VODI) (MIM ID #235550), and X-linked dyskeratosis congenita (DKC) (MIM ID #305000). Previously described are the hyper-IgE syndromes (HIES) (AD-HIES [Job's syndrome], AR-HIES) under phagocytic cell deficiencies (Table 16A-1 in the Annex) and chronic mucocutaneous candidiasis under defects in innate immunity (Table 16A-5 in the Annex).

Diagnosis of the Primary Immunodeficiencies

General Considerations for Diagnosis of the Primary Immunodeficiencies

It may now be possible to construct a unifying summary of the PIDs and offer some practical applications of the information presented in this chapter for improved diagnosis and therapy for patients who present with manifestations of these disorders. As described previously, the majority of PIDs are diagnosed in infancy, where many of the conditions are transmitted with X-linked inherited patterns resulting in a 5:1 male predominance over females. Because of this predominant age distribution in childhood, the PIDs have been thought to be the almost exclusive purview of pediatricians. However, with the improvement and greater availability of easily administered antimicrobial agents, many of the milder cases of PIDs originally seen only in childhood (~ 40 percent) are now living into adolescence or young adulthood, where the distribution between males and females is nearly equal and where the conditions present with slightly different clinical manifestations than classically described in younger children. Therefore, the PIDs are no longer the isolated province of the pediatric immunologist, but must be considered by all health care providers who are entrusted to the care of both children and adults who present primarily with the clinical expressions of immune deficiency with recurrent or an undue susceptibility to infection but also with manifestations of autoimmunity and other clinical forms of immune dysfunction.

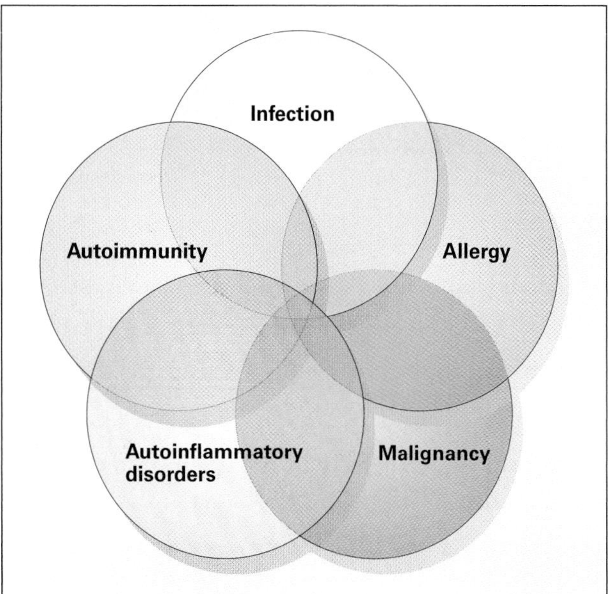

Figure 16-45. Schematic representation of immune system failure leading to a spectrum of disorders of immune dysregulation characterized by susceptibility to infection, allergy, malignancy, autoinflammatory disorders and autoimmunity.

When to Suspect Immune Deficiency: How Many Infections Are too Many Before One Should Consider an Immunodeficiency Workup?

As described in Chapter 1, a decreased defense function of the immune system is the basis for the most common heralding manifestation of immune deficiency seen clinically as an undue susceptibility to recurrent infection. However, the PIDs can also manifest with aberrations of homeostasis presenting clinically as autoimmune disease, e.g., rheumatoid arthritis, or an impaired surveillance function manifesting as malignancy, e.g., lymphoma. The traditional doctrine that patients who have PIDs are defined by their susceptibility to infections has recently been expanded to include a new group of disorders of "immune dysregulation" in which immune system failure in these patients is seen not only by infections, but also by manifestations of allergy, autoimmunity, autoinflammatory disorders, and malignancy (Figure 16-45). These new syndromes of "immune dysregulation" include many of the recently identified immune deficiencies described in this chapter, such as the immune dysregulation, polyendocrinopathy, enteropathy, X-linked (IPEX) syndrome and autoimmune polyendocrinopathy-candidiasis-ectodermal dystrophy (APECED). Recognition of this expanded view has not only helped to increase our understanding of basic immune tolerance mechanisms, but also in turn has led to improved methods of diagnosis and treatment of these disorders. It has also raised awareness and understanding that many disorders of immune dysregulation are caused by the absence of immunoregulatory cells or the failure of normal regulatory lymphocyte apoptosis, which can complicate more traditional immunodeficiency disorders (*Chapters 7* and *9*).

However, since undue susceptibility to infection is by far the most common presenting symptom of the PIDs, the clinician must first decide whether the frequency of infections is significantly excessive or if the types of causative microbial agents responsible for the infections are notably different from those seen in otherwise healthy subjects. A list of useful warning signs has been developed by the Jeffrey Modell Foundation/Immune Deficiency Foundation and provides a valuable basic tool in helping to determine what should be considered abnormal as a basis for further immunologic evaluation in children (Table 16-7).

These include eight or more otitis media infections per year; two or more serious sinus infections per year;

Table 16-7. Basic signs of primary immune deficiency in children and adults

10 Warning Signs of Primary Immunodeficiency in Children	10 Warning Signs of Primary Immunodeficiency in Adults
• Four or more new ear infections within 1 year.	• Two or more new ear infections within 1 year.
• Two or more serious sinus infections within 1 year.	• Two or more new sinus infections within 1 year, in the absence of allergy.
• Two or more months on antibiotics with little effect.	• One pneumonia per year for more than 1 year.
• Two or more pneumonias within 1 year.	• Chronic Diarrhea with weight loss.
• Failure of an infant to gain weight or grow normally.	• Recurrent viral infections (colds, herpes, warts, condyloma).
• Recurrent, deep skin or organ abscesses.	• Recurrent need for intravenous antibiotics to clear infections.
• Persistent thrush in mouth or fungal infection on skin.	• Recurrent, deep abscesses of the skin or internal organs.
• Need for intravenous antibiotics to clear infections.	• Persistent thrush or fungal infection on skin or elsewhere.
• Two or more deep-seated infections including septicemia.	• Infection with normally harmless tuberculosis-like bacteria.
• A family history of PI.	• A family history of PI.

Reproduced with permission from the Jeffrey Modell Foundation/Immune Deficiency Foundation.

Table 16-8. Additional findings suggesting immune deficiency.

• Onset of thrush, chronic diarrhea and failure to thrive in the first months of life
• Recurrent infections • Bacterial pathogens, but also opportunistic organisms such as *Pneumocystis jiroveci, Candida albicans,* and viruses such as varicella, adenovirus, cytomegalovirus, Epstein-Barr virus (EBV), parainfluenza 3
• Pneumonitis that does not clear • PCP, RSV, CMV, and parainfluenza
• Rashes, with erythroderma, or eczema that doesn't resolve with therapy
• Other physical finding; hepatosplenomegaly, lymphadenopathy
• Family history of children dying < 6 months of age
• Lymphopenia, particularly absence of functional T cells, B cells may be present, but do not make specific antibodies • ALC < 3,400 (may be normal); IgM < 20 (may be normal or elevated in some SCID / CID); IgA < 5; lymphocyte proliferation to mitogens < 10% of normal

Adapted with permission from Griffith LM, Cowan MJ, Notarangelo LD, et al. Workshop Participants. Improving cellular therapy for primary immune deficiency diseases: recognition, diagnosis, and management. J Allergy Clin Immunol. 2009; 124:1152–60.

two or more pneumonias per year; recurrent deep infections or infections in unusual areas (e.g., muscle or liver); the need for intravenous antibiotics to clear infections; infection with an opportunistic organism (e.g., *Pneumocystis [carinii] jiroveci* and *giardia*); and persistent thrush in patients older than one year of age. In addition, consanguinity, a family history of primary immune deficiencies in other family members, or early childhood deaths, particularly in males, should raise a high index of suspicion for immune deficiency and should be a basis to consider further immunologic evaluations (Table 16-8). A history of recurrent upper respiratory viral infections, on the other hand, is not a common symptom of PID and should not necessitate an extensive immunologic workup.

Some additional findings suggesting immune deficiency are show in Table 16-15. A history of recurrent upper respiratory viral infections, on the other hand, is not a common symptom of PID and should not necessitate an extensive immunologic workup.

Environmental-Related versus Host-Related Factors: A Useful Clinical Decision-Making Algorithm

After an initial decision is made that the pattern of infections is significantly deviant from the normal and further immunologic investigation is warranted, the next step is to decide whether the susceptibility to infection is related to an increased environmental exposure to infectious agents, i.e., **environmental-related factors,** or to factors within the host that predispose the patient to a vulnerability to infection, i.e., **host-related factors.** Some additional findings suggesting immune deficiency are show in Table 16-15. A history of recurrent upper respiratory viral infections, on the other hand, is not a common symptom of PID and should not necessitate an extensive immunologic workup. (Figure 16-46). Many children and adults experience recurrent infections because of increased exposure to infectious diseases as a consequence of the type of environment in which they are

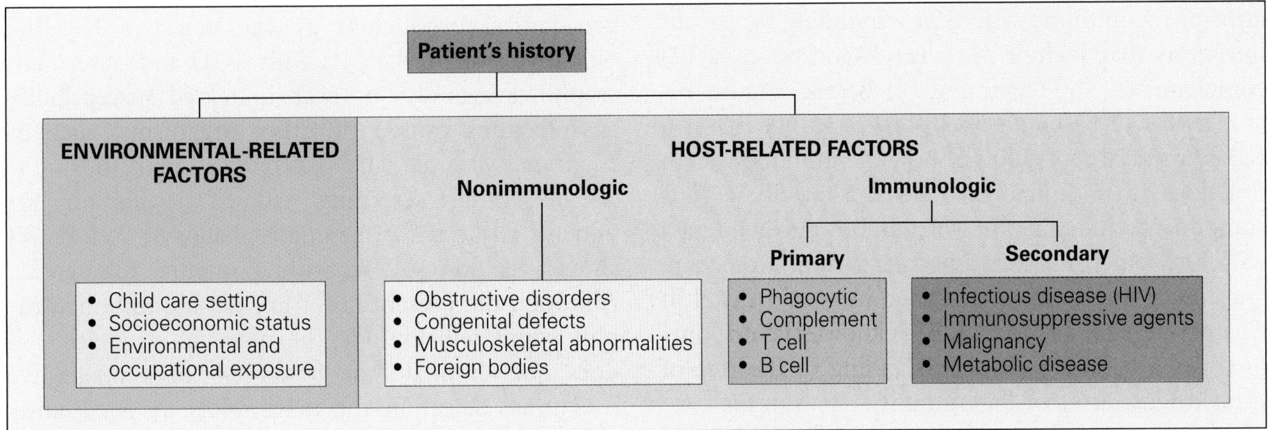

Figure 16-46. Algorithm for workup of patients suspected with immune deficiency exploring environmental-related versus host-related factors.

placed or work. The increased rate of infectious diseases seen in otherwise immunologically normal children placed in child care settings, for example, represents perhaps the most frequent cause of recurrent infections in childhood. Similarly, work-related environmental causes of recurrent infections should be sought in the adult who presents with recurrent infections.

Once environmental-related factors have been excluded, the next step is to determine if the increased susceptibility to infection is related to host-related factors that can be subdivided into **nonimmunologic** and **immunologic** causes. Examples of nonimmunologic entities include obstructive pulmonary disorders, congenital cardiac defects, breaks in the skin barrier, musculoskeletal abnormalities, and foreign bodies. Once these are eliminated, the diagnostic focus should be directed to immunologic causes that include both **primary** and **secondary** causes of immune deficiency. The secondary causes are by far the more frequently encountered and include infectious disease (e.g., HIV), the use of immunosuppressive agents, malignancy, and metabolic disease. Once these have been excluded, the clinician is then left with the challenge of unraveling the least common causes of recurrent infection, the primary immunodeficiency disorders that pose the greatest diagnostic burden because of the complexity and ever-increasing number of clinical entities that comprise this group of disorders.

Evaluation of the Patient with a Suspected Immune Deficiency

For ease of discussion, a useful approach for the evaluation of a patient with a suspected immune deficiency is shown in Table 16-9. This diagnostic scheme is based on an understanding of the role of four different arms of the immune system in responding to various infections that include (1) the phagocytic cells, (2) complement, (3) T cells, and (4) B cells (Figure 16-46). It should be emphasized, however, that this is a rather artificial separation of how the immune system functions in antimicrobial defense since these four components do not act in isolation but rather interact with each other in clearing bacterial, viral, protozoan, and fungal infections as described in greater detail in Chapters 12, 13, 14, and 15. This knowledge not only provides a basis for an understanding of the role of these defense arms of the immune system in the normal host, but also how aberrations in one or more of these components contribute to the unique susceptibilities to certain infections in the immune-deficient host. This then provides a basis for the clinician to choose the most appropriate set of specific clinical tests that will help in determining if the patient has an immune deficiency. A suggested approach to the evaluation of patients using this four-tiered algorithm is summarized in Table 16-9.

Defects in Phagocytic Cell Function

Phagocytes (neutrophils, monocytes, and macrophages) are part of the innate immune system and are critical in quickly providing a first line of defense against invading bacterial organisms (*Chapter 3*). Deficiencies of phagocytic function include two types: (1) **quantitative defects** and (2) **qualitative defects.** Patients with quantitative neutrophil defects, e.g., congenial neutropenia, as described previously, present with a history of recurrent abscesses, abscesses in unusual areas (e.g., the liver, muscle, and/or abdominal cavity), recurrent oral ulcers, severe pneumonias, poor wound healing, or delayed umbilical cord separation (*Chapter 24*). The qualitative defects are those disorders in which the numbers of phagocytes are normal or increased but where their function is impaired. As described previously, the recognition of the rapidly increasing number of genetic mutations affecting the innate immune system and phagocytes has shed considerable light and a better understanding of the molecular basis for increased susceptibility to a variety of microbial agents seen in the patient with defective innate and phagocytic cell function. The defective NADPH pathways, for example, seen in patients with chronic granulomatous disease (CGD), exemplify the qualitative defects. These patients have difficulty clearing catalase-positive organisms (e.g., *Staphylococcus aureus*, *Serratia*, and *Klebsiella*) because of the lack of oxygen radical production by the defective NADPH oxidative system. Patients with CGD and other neutrophil defects also have an increased susceptibility to infections caused by other organisms, such as *Candida*, *Nocardia*, and *Aspergillus* (Table 16-9).

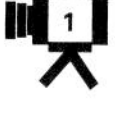

The initial screening clinical evaluation for patients suspected of having a phagocytic cell defect should include a CBC with a manual differential. Although the presence of a normal absolute neutrophil count will exclude the quantitative defects, it does not eliminate the possibility of a qualitative functional defect in the neutrophils. A persistently elevated absolute neutrophil count (> 20,000/μL)

Table 16-9. Suggested workup of a patient for suspected primary immunodeficiencies caused by defects of phagocytic cells, complement, T cells, or B cells

Phagocytic cell defects	
Presentation	Abscesses, deep-seated infections, oral ulcers, pneumonias, poor wound healing, delayed umbilical cord separation
Infections	Caused by catalase positive bacteria (*Staphylococcus aureus, Pseudomonas, Serratia, Klebsiella*), *Candida, Nocardia, Aspergillus*
Examples	
Quantitative defects	Congenital neutropenias
Qualitative defects	Chronic granulomatous disease (CGD)
Laboratory evaluation	
Screening	CBC and differential; DHR assay; serum Ig levels and IgE
Advanced	Dihydrorhodamine test
Specialized	Tests of adherence, chemotaxis, phagocytosis, and microbicidal activity
Complement defects	
Presentation	Recurrent bacterial infections, autoimmune diseases (e.g., systemic lupus erythematosus), and angioedema
Infections	Caused by Gram-positive, e.g., *Staphylococcus*, or Gram-negative, e.g., *Neisseria* bacteria
Examples	Patients with C3 or C567 defects; systemic lupus erythematosus or scleroderma; hereditary angioedema (HAE)
Laboratory evaluation	
Screening	Total hemolytic complement assay (CH50), C3, and C4 levels
Advanced	Quantitation of individual complement components
Specialized	Serum opsonic and chemotactic assays
T cell defects	
Presentation	Failure to thrive, chronic diarrhea, opportunistic infections, polyendocrinopathies, oral thrush
Infections	Viral infections, e.g., herpes simplex, CMV; *Candida*; protozoan, e.g., *Pneumocystis*
Examples	SCID, DiGeorge syndrome
Laboratory evaluation	
Screening	CBC with lymphocyte count and morphology, delayed hypersensitivity testing (candida, trichphyton, and mumps)
Advanced	Determination of quantitative immunoglobulin levels (IgG, IgA, IgM, IgE), and T cell lymphocyte subset enumeration by flow cytometry (CD3, CD4, CD8, CD56, and CD25)
Specialized	Lymphoproliferative responses to mitogens (PHA) Cytokine receptor expression (flow cytometry), cytokine production, measurement of specific molecular deficiencies
B cell defects	
Presentation	Recurrent sinopulmonary infections, diarrhea, GI malabsorption, poor growth, and autoimmunity
Infections	Encapsulated, high-grade bacteria, e.g., *S. pneumonia, H. influenza*, viruses (enteroviruses)
Examples	X-linked agammaglobulinemia, common variable immunodeficiency (CVID)
Laboratory evaluation	
Screening	Determination of quantitative immunoglobulin levels (IgG, IgA, IgM, IgE, and B cell subset enumeration by flow cytometry [CD 19, CD20])
Advanced	Determination of quantitative IgG subclass levels (IgG1, IgG2, IgG3, and IgG4) and specific pre-immunization antibody responses to diphtheria, tetanus toxoids, and pneumococcal and *H. influenza* vaccines; if nonprotective levels, re-vaccinate and check post-immunization titers in three to four weeks and determine lymphoproliferative responses to mitogens (pokeweed) (phytohemagglutinin [PHA], Concanavalin A [ConA], and phorbol myristyl acetate [PMA]/ionomycin)
Specialized	Lymph node biopsy, cytokine analysis, measurement of specific molecular deficiencies

Adapted with permission from Verbsky JW and Grossman WJ. Cellular and genetic basis of primary immunce deficiencies. Pediatr Clin North Am 2006:53:649–84.

may, in fact, be the first clue to other defects of neutrophil function, such as those affecting the ability of neutrophils to migrate from the vasculature (i.e., leukocyte adhesion deficiency, LAD). If the patient has few or no detectable neutrophils, other defects should be considered, e.g., congenital neutropenia (Kostmann's syndrome). Frequently, multiple CBCs with manual differentials performed at periodic intervals, e.g., weekly intervals, are needed to establish fluctuations in neutrophil levels characteristic of other possible causes, such as cyclic neutropenia. In addition to searching for intrinsic causes of neutropenia, the clinician should also consider possible extrinsic causes for the neutropenia, including those caused by a variety of drugs, malignancy, isoimmune/autoimmune disorders, and hypersplenism.

More advanced tests for neutrophil defects focus on possible deficiencies in the NADPH oxidative system as seen in CGD. The traditional functional test used for detection of this system in the past was the nitroblue tetrazolium (**NBT**) test, which determines the ability of activated neutrophils to produce oxygen radicals that reduce NBT to an insoluble blue dye that can be seen microscopically in neutrophils. A more advanced flow-based assay is used by many reference laboratories and is based on the ability of stimulated neutrophils to reduce a nonfluorescent molecule, dihydrorhodamine, to a fluorescent molecule by oxygen radicals (*Chapter 24*). Other more specialized testing for possible neutrophil defects includes examination not only for functional opsonic and chemotactic defects, but also for identification of genetic mutations that underlie these defects. Such deficiencies are quite rare, and their evaluations are conducted primarily in research-based laboratories (*Chapter 24*).

Defects in the Complement Immune System

Although defects in the complement system are rare in comparison to other causes of the PIDs, they should be considered in any patient who presents with recurrent bacterial infections (*Chapter 4*). Some of the most common clinical presentations of patients with complement system defects not only include recurrent infections caused by Gram-positive pyogenic bacteria, as seen with defects of early components, e.g., C3 deficiency, but also those caused by Gram-negative bacteria, e.g., *Neisseria* spp, who have deficiencies of the late components of the complement pathway, e.g., C5, 6, and 7 defects. Patients with defects of early components of the complement cascade may also present an increased prevalence of autoimmune disorders (e.g., systemic lupus erythematosus and scleroderma) and more rarely with hereditary angioedema (**HAE**) (*Chapter 4*).

Screening for most complement defects is accomplished by performing a total hemolytic complement (CH_{50}) assay, C3 and C4 levels (*Chapter 24*). Patients with the clinical presentation of angioedema should be suspected of having a defect in the C1 inhibitor (C1 INH), and a good screening test is the finding of a depressed C4, which should be followed by more precise quantitative measurements of the C1 inhibitor protein and its function. More advanced specialized tests include quantitative determination of individual complement components, as well as serum opsonic and chemotactic assays, which are primarily performed in research-based laboratories (*Chapter 24*).

Defects in the T Cell System

As described previously, T cells play a critically pivotal role in both cellular and humoral expressions of antimicrobial mechanisms of the adaptive immune response (*Chapter 7*). Because T cells are decisive in the killing of intracellular organisms, patients with T cell defects often present with opportunistic intracellular microbial infections and disseminated viral infections. These infections include *Pneumocystis (carinii) jiroveci*, *Cryptococcus*, *Mycobacteria*  spp, *Candida* spp, and a variety of viruses (e.g., cytomegalovirus, Epstein-Barr virus, adenovirus, and varicella). However, since T cells are essential for B cell help and for antibody production by B cells, patients with T cell defects often present with infections caused by deficiencies of antibody that are required for the killing of extracellular bacteria. These are seen primarily in the combined T and B cell deficiencies, such as SCID. Therefore, the diagnostic workup of patients will not only require consideration of tests of T cell function, but also those described below under B cell defects.

Patients with T cell defects commonly present with failure to thrive, refractory diarrhea, and persistent thrush after one year of age. In severely T cell deficient patients, such as the complete DiGeorge syndrome or SCID, infants are occasionally born with evidence of severe graft-versus-host disease (i.e., severe skin rash at birth, liver dysfunction, enteropathy, and reactive pulmonary disease) resulting from the transplacental transfer of maternal lymphocytes that recognize the infant's organs as foreign and begin to attack and destroy them. Patients with T cell defects can also present with a variety of organ specific autoimmune diseases (e.g., type 1 diabetes in infancy, hypothyroidism, and Addison's disease) caused by the attack on these organs by the patient's own immune cells. The basis for these clinical complications is unclear, but are thought to be caused by a breakdown in immune tolerance in which a lack of T regulatory cells or the participation of Th17 cells plays a critical role in the pathogenesis of these disorders (*Chapters 7, 9,* and *19*).

Unlike patients with B cell defects, e.g., agammaglobulinemia, who rarely acquire infections before six months of age resulting from the transient effects of maternally transferred antibodies (*Chapter 2*), infants with T cell defects typically present with opportunistic infections during the first few months of life. Some infants, however, are not diagnosed until much later. It is important, therefore, to carefully monitor the growth of children using standard growth charts to document failure to thrive, an important hallmark of immune deficiency. A significant decrease in weight/height velocity without a clear cause may often provide the first clue to an immune deficiency caused by a T cell defect.

If the initial screening of neonates and infants reveals lymphopenia, a T cell defect should be strongly suspected until proven otherwise. This level of suspicion is critical to obtain a prompt diagnosis of severe combined immune deficiencies before life-threatening infections occur. Early diagnosis is also essential to prevent the administration of live attenuated virus vaccines (e.g., measles, mumps, rubella, varicella, or bacille Calmette-Guérin [**BCG**]) or the administration of blood transfusions containing viable lymphocytes capable of initiating a GVHD, both of which could be lethal in such T cell immunocompromised individuals. It is also vital for physicians to understand that a complete blood cell count (CBC) does not rule out a lymphocyte subset defect. Patients who have specific lymphocyte subset defects often have a normal absolute total lymphocyte count, which is why enumeration of T cell subsets by flow cytometry is required (*Chapter 24*).

Delayed-type hypersensitivity skin testing is another important tool in determining functional defects in T cells (*Chapter 7*). Such testing is functionally informative because it determines the ability of T cells to respond in vivo to foreign antigens to which the patient has been previously sensitized. Typical proteins used to test this response include candida, trichophyton, and mumps antigens.

More advanced testing includes T cell subset analysis (CD3, CD4, CD8, CD56, and CD25) and lymphoproliferative responses to mitogens (PHA) or antigens. Other specialized tests such as measurement of cytokine receptor expression (flow cytometry) and cytokine production may be done to identify specific molecular deficiencies, but these are primarily performed in research-based laboratories.

Defects in the B Cell System

Patients with B cell defects typically present with recurrent sinopulmonary infections caused by encapsulated, high-grade bacteria, e.g., *S. pneumonia, H. influenza,* viruses, and enteroviruses as well as diarrhea, malabsorption, poor growth, and autoimmunity, e.g., common variable immunodeficiency (**CVID**). In severe deficiencies such as X-linked agammaglobulinemia, as described previously, serious bacterial infections caused by high-grade encapsulated bacteria usually occur during the second half of the first year of life because of the protective effects of transplacentally transmitted IgG antibody. In CVID in older patients, the same spectrum of infections is seen but is commonly accompanied by manifestations of autoimmune disease. As described previously, since B cells are functionally dependent on T cell help, B cell defects are often associated with some degree of T cell impairment and therefore testing should include tests of T cell function as described above.

The initial screening clinical evaluation for patients suspected of having a B cell defect should include determination of quantitative immunoglobulin levels (IgG, IgA, IgM, and IgE) and B cell subset enumeration by flow cytometry (CD19 and CD20). More advanced testing includes determination of quantitative IgG subclass levels (IgG1, IgG2, IgG3, and IgG4) and specific pre-immunization antibody responses to diphtheria, tetanus toxoids, and pneumococcal and *H. influenza* vaccines; if nonprotective levels are obtained, vaccination with these vaccines should be performed with evaluation of post-immunization titers in three to four weeks. As described previously, the demonstration of diminished IgG subclasses alone is insufficient for the diagnosis of IgG subclass deficiency as was the usual previous practice; it is now generally accepted, however, that the diagnosis of IgG subclass deficiency should be made only after demonstration of a failure of significant post-immunization antibody responses to the protein and/or polysaccharide vaccines. Other tests include determination of lymphoproliferative responses to mitogens (pokeweed) (phytohemagglutinin [PHA], Concanavalin A [ConA]) and phorbol myristyl acetate (PMA/ionomycin). Specialized tests include lymph node biopsy, cytokine analyses, and measurement of specific molecular moieties or identification of genetic mutations, but these are primarily performed in research-based laboratories.

Management of Patients with Immunodeficiencies

Patients with immunodeficiencies need the same general comprehensive care required of patients with any chronic illness. This should include maintenance of general health and nutrition and emotional well-being as well as particular attention to the management of their infections and rheumatologic and inflammatory conditions.

Control of Infections

Antibiotics are proven lifesavers in the treatment of the many infectious episodes that occur in patients with immunodeficiency. Prior to their availability in the mid-20th century, most patients died in early life from the complications of infection. Because these patients may succumb rapidly to infection, antibiotics should be initiated promptly for treatment and should include primarily bactericidal and not bacteriostatic agents specific for the organism. Continuous prophylactic use of antibiotics may be of benefit; trimethoprim-sulfamethoxazole (TMP-SMX) has been recommended for patients with T cell immunodeficiencies for prevention of pneumonia caused by *Pneumocystis (carinii) jiroveci* (PCP).

Human Immune Globulin

As with many diseases that have been treated successfully by the replacement of an essential missing body protein, e.g., the well-controlled diabetic on insulin therapy, the administration of human immune globulin has proven to be health-restorative in most patients with agammaglobulinemia (*Chapter 11*). Beginning with the initial patient with agammaglobulinemia who was successfully treated by Bruton with injections of human immunoglobulin, the product, administered either by injection or infusion, continues as the preferred method of treatment for most of the severe antibody immunodeficiencies (*Chapter 11*). Two forms of human immunoglobulin are available: (1) 16 percent intramuscular immunoglobulin (Ig) and (2) intravenous immunoglobulin (IVIG). Currently, most antibody-deficient patients with agammaglobulinemia receive IVIG (400 mg/kg) at monthly intervals, although the 16 percent product is used extensively in Europe and in some patients in the United States by subcutaneous infusions at weekly intervals using one-quarter of the monthly dose (100 mg/kg) per week. A notable exception to the use of human immunoglobulin in the antibody deficiencies is in patients with isolated IgA deficiency, where its administration is contraindicated. Serious anaphylactoid reactions caused by anti-IgA antibodies are produced in these patients, resulting from the unavoidable presence of trace amounts of IgA in all human immunoglobulin preparations.

Human Stem Cell Transplantation (HSCT)

Hematopoietic stem cell transplantation (HSCT) is the transplantation of blood stem cells derived from the bone marrow or blood (*Chapter 22*). The procedure was pioneered in the fields of hematology and oncology for treatment of patients with malignant diseases of the hematopoietic system, e.g., leukemia. The procedure was later applied to the treatment of the primary immune deficiencies, and the first successful transplants were performed in 1968 in children with SCID. Human stem cell transplantation from an HLA-identical donor (usually a sibling) has been the treatment of choice for all patients with combined immunodeficiency and Wiskott-Aldrich syndrome (WAS). Most of these transplants have used bone marrow cells aspirated from an anesthetized donor, although peripheral white blood cells enriched for CD34 stem cells have been used as a source for infusion. As genetic testing becomes more widely available and the techniques of HSCT improve (*Chapters 10* and *22*), more patients are being diagnosed with PID and treated with this form of treatment. Shown in Table 16-10 are some of the immunodeficiencies that have been successfully treated by hematopoietic stem cell transplantation. Proper HLA typing is essential to ensure engraftment and to minimize complications of graft-versus-host disease (GVHD), the most frequent complication of HSCT (*Chapters 10* and *22*). Better techniques for identification of latent viral infections, e.g., EBV, the cause of the B cell lymphoma in "David the bubble boy" (*Chapter 7*), have also improved the success of the procedure.

Since umbilical cord blood contains large numbers of HSCs, it is being used as an alternative source of these cells for transplantation. Cord blood has a number of advantages over other sources of HSCs, including greater availability, no medical risk to the donor, and lower risk of latent viral transmission and GVHD. Survival following cord-blood

Table 16-10. Immunodeficiencies that have been successfully treated by hematopoietic stem cell transplantation

Phagocytic deficiencies	Lymphocyte immunodeficiencies
Chronic granulomatous disease	γC deficiency
Severe congenital neutropenias	Janus-associated kinase 3 (JAK3) deficiency
Leukocyte adhesion deficiency 7	Interleukin-7 receptor α (IL7Rα) deficiency
Schwachman-Diamond syndrome	Recombinase-activating gene (RAG) 1/2 deficiency
Chediak-Higashi syndrome	Adenosine deaminase (ADA) deficiency
Griscelli syndrome, type 2	CD45 deficiency
Familial hemophagocytic lymphocytosis (FHL)	CD3δ/CD3ε/CD3ζ deficiency
1. Perforin deficiency (FHL2)	CD3γ deficiency
2. UNC13D deficiency (FHL3)	Reticular dysgenesis
3. Syntaxin 11 deficiency (FHL4)	Artemis deficiency (FHL4)
Interferon-γ receptor (IFN-γR) deficiencies	DNA ligase IV
	Cernunnos/XLF deficiency
Other immunodeficiencies	
Cartilage hair hypoplasia	Purine nucleoside phosphorylase (PNP) deficiency
	Major histocompatibility class II (MHC-II) deficiency
Hyper IgD syndrome	Zeta-chain-associated protein-70 (ZAP70) deficiency
Autoimmune lymphoproliferative syndrome (ALPS) (Fas)	CD8 deficiency
Hyper-IgE syndrome	Winged helix deficiency
Immunodysregulation, polyendocrinopathy, enteropathy X-linked (IPEX) syndrome	Omenn syndrome Ca++ channel deficiency
CD25 deficiency	DiGeorge syndrome
Nuclear factor-κB (NF-κB) essential modulator (NEMO) deficiency	Coloboma, heart anomalies, choanal atresia, retardation of growth and development and genital and ear anomalies (CHARGE syndrome)
NF-κB inhibitor α (NF-κBα) deficiency	
Immunodeficiency, centromeric instability, facial dysmorphism (ICF) Syndrome	Wiskott-Aldrich syndrome
	CD40 ligand deficiency
Nijmegen breakage syndrome	X-linked lymphoproliferative disease
	1. XLP1 (SH2D1A)
	2. XLP2 (XIAP)

Adapted from Gennery AR, Cant AJ. Advances in hematopoietic stem cell transplantation for primary immunodeficiency. Immunol Allergy Clin North Am. 2008;28:439–56.

transplantation in children who have PID has been shown to be as good as transplantation using other stem cell sources, even for rarer conditions such as Omenn syndrome or reticular dysgenesis, for which HSCT results generally are poor. Particular advantages of cord blood include the use of infant HSCs that, when used in infants, may have a longer life than stem cells from older donors.

HSCT, although a risky procedure, is usually highly successful if a genotypically matched family donor or unrelated donor is available. However, for most individuals, this is not the case, and survival from mismatched family (usually parental haplo-identical donor) transplants is substantially lower (approximately 52 percent 10-year survival for all forms of SCID) and associated with predictable toxicity arising from the administration of chemotherapeutic agents to ensure adequate HSC engraftment.

Gene Therapy

Another innovative form of therapy for SCID and some other forms of PID is gene therapy, a procedure in which a defective mutant gene is replaced by the insertion of a normal gene employing a

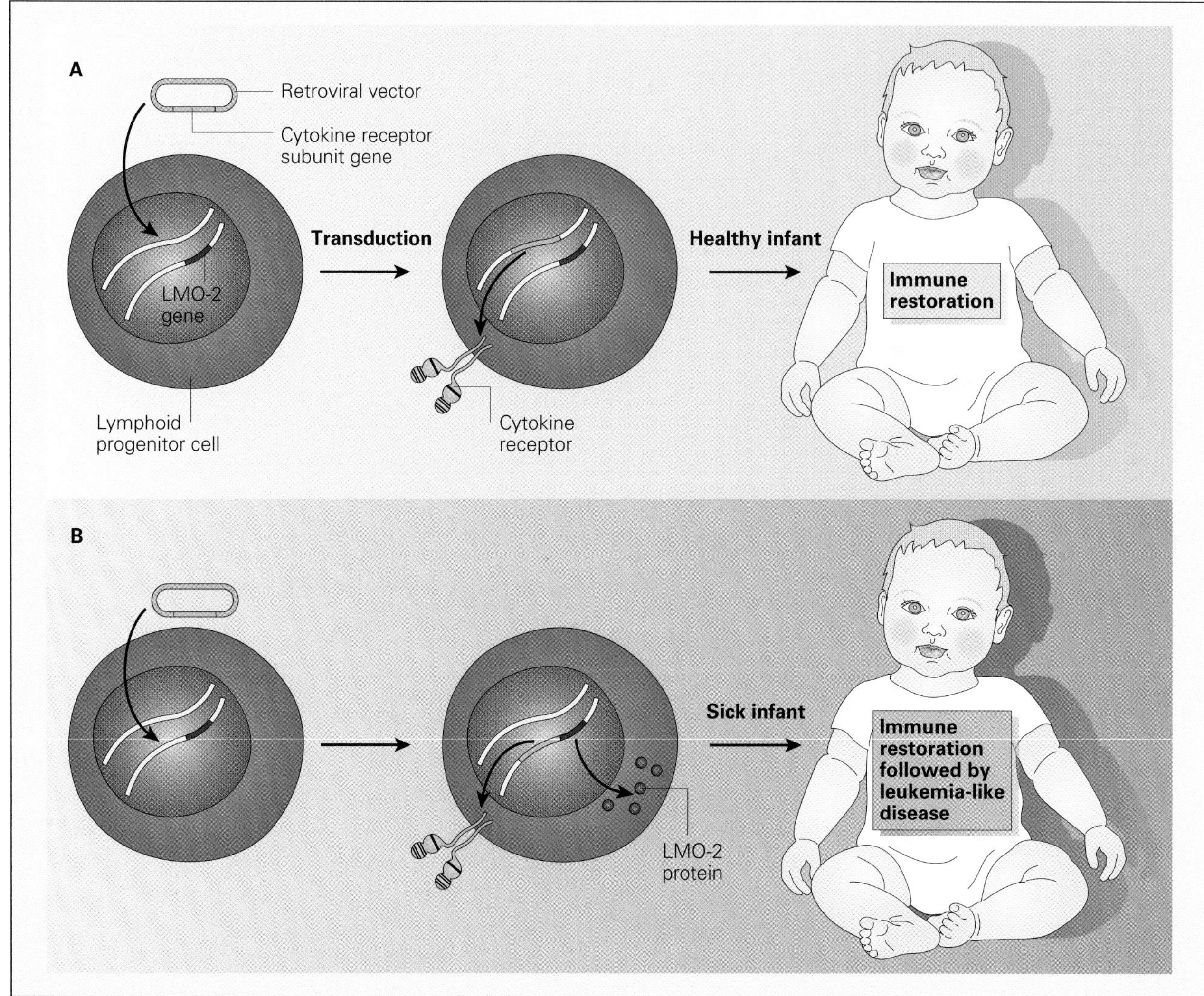

Figure 16-47. Schematic representation of the mechanism of gene therapy in SCID-XL using a retroviral vector to deliver the IL-2 γc gene showing the beneficial as well as the unexpected deleterious outcome of the procedure. Panel A: The insertion of a gene encoding the γc component of the IL-2 receptor into a lymphoid progenitor cell of a patient with SCID-XL with immune restoration. Panel B: Insertion of the gene encoding the cytokine receptor subunit in the immediate vicinity of the LMO-2 gene resulting in the expression of elevated levels of LMO-2 protein (red dots in Panel B) followed by immune restoration by leukemia-like disease. (Adapted with permission from Noguchi P. Risks and benefits of gene therapy. N Engl J Med. 2003;348:193–4.)

carrier called a vector that delivers the therapeutic gene to the patient's target cells. This is a particularly attractive form of therapy because a profound growth and survival advantage is conferred to corrected cells (although this may be variable among different molecular types). The first approved gene therapy procedure for the treatment of a PID was successfully performed in a patient with adenosine deaminase-deficient SCID (**ADA-SCID**). Currently, the types of vectors used in gene therapy are viruses, e.g., retroviruses, adenoviruses, and adeno-associated viruses (**AAV**), and among these, the retrovirus vectors, i.e., mouse leukemia viruses, have been most commonly used. Although the technology is still in its infancy, it has been used with some success in patients with adenosine deaminase deficiency (**ADA-D**), X-linked SCID γc (**SCID-X1**), autosomal recessive SCID (**AR-SCID**) deficiency, X-linked chronic granulomatous disease (**X-CGD**), and Wiskott-Aldrich syndrome (**WAS**).

Risks and Side Effects of Gene Therapy: Insertional Mutagenesis

Although retroviral vectors are potentially useful for gene therapy of PIDs because they are capable of permanently integrating a therapeutic gene into stem cells and achieving long-term expression in differentiating cells, there is, however, a downside. After retrovirus-associated gene therapy, T cell acute lymphoblastic leukemia (**T-ALL**) occurred in five children with SCID-γc. This unanticipated unfortunate outcome is thought to have occurred as a result of insertional mutagenesis, i.e., a leukemogenic mutation caused by the insertion of new genetic material into the normal gene, in which activation of the LMO2 proto-oncogene promoter led to aberrant transcription and expression of the normally suppressed LMO2 gene with resultant uncontrolled T cell proliferation. Shown in Figure 16-47 is a schematic representation of the mechanism of gene therapy in SCID-XL using a retroviral vector to deliver the IL-2 γc gene showing the beneficial as well as the unexpected deleterious outcome of the procedure.

What Is the Status of Gene Therapy for Primary Immunodeficiency?

A general hold was put into place following the initial report of leukemia in the French SCID patients, but that hold only lasted a few months following which clinical trials have been cautiously allowed to resume. There are clinical trials of gene therapy for SCID-γc, WAS, ADA, and CGD currently open and admitting patients in the United States, Europe, and Japan. New approaches such as different gene transfer vectors are being introduced to try to avoid some of the problems seen in the earlier studies. Efforts to find satisfactory treatments for seriously ill patients with primary immunodeficiency have resulted in the development of important new therapeutic procedures with benefits reaching far beyond the relatively small number of patients affected with these rare disorders. Allogeneic bone marrow transplantation, immunoglobulin and enzyme replacement treatments, and more recently gene therapy have all been introduced into clinical medicine as treatments for one or more of the primary immunodeficiency diseases. Beginning in 1990, gene-corrected T cells were first used to treat ADA deficiency SCID. With this demonstration that the gene-transfer procedure could be safely used to introduce functional transgenes into patient cells, clinical trials for a broad range of inherited disorders and cancer were started in the mid-1990s. Of all these early clinical experiments, those addressing primary immunodeficiency have also been the most successful. Both ADA and X-SCID have now been cured using gene insertion into autologous bone marrow stem cells. In addition, some patients with chronic granulomatous disease (CGD) have shown an unexpectedly high level of functionally corrected granulocytes in their blood following infusion of autologous gene-corrected bone marrow. There remain, however, a great many significant challenges to be overcome before gene therapy becomes the treatment of choice for these and other disorders. The use of genes as medicines is the most complex therapeutic system ever attempted, and it may take several more decades of work before the real potential as a treatment for both inherited and sporadic disorders is finally realized.

Conclusions

Immune deficiencies have profoundly guided and shaped our understanding of immunology for the past 50 years. We have moved from having only massive defects in B cells or T cells to having subtle, infection-specific defects that have taught us much about the specific roles of individual molecules and how they interact with organisms and hosts. There are undoubtedly many more specific defects to find, and the tools are ready to be used.

Key Points

- Primary immunodeficiencies (PIDs) comprise more than 150 different disorders that affect the development and/or function of the immune system.
- In most cases, PIDs are inherited as monogenic disorders that follow a simple Mendelian inheritance; however, some PIDs follow a more complex polygenic mode of inheritance.
- With the exception of IgA deficiency (IgAD), which is the most common form of primary immunodeficiency, all other entities of PID are rare and have an overall prevalence of approximately 1:10,000 live births; however, a much higher rate is observed among populations with high consanguinity rates or among genetically isolated populations.
- The PIDs are broadly divided into groups according to the function of the immune system primarily affected; these include (1) defects of innate immunity, including both disorders of immune regulation that present as autoimmune diseases as well as the newly recognized autoinflammatory disorders; and (2) defects in adaptive immune responses,

Case Study: Clinical Relevance

Let us now return to the case study of X-linked agammaglobulinemia (XLA) or Bruton's agammaglobulinemia presented earlier and review some of the major points of the clinical presentation and how they relate to the immune system:

- The history of repeated episodes of pneumonia and otitis media in a male child during the first years of life is a typical presentation of XLA.
- Entirely unusual was the occurrence of the same pneumococcal serotypes during subsequent bouts of infection and the lack of response to pneumococcal vaccine, one of the hallmarks of XLA (Figure 16-2).
- Although this child was studied in the mid-part of the 20th century prior to any knowledge of the immunoglobulin isotypes or the role of B and T cells in protective immunity, a free boundary serum electrophoresis study demonstrated the complete absence of the gamma peak, revealing not only that gamma globulin was the fraction of serum proteins that contained antibody activity, but also establishing the basis for the child's inability to synthesize antibody following immunization as well as the source of his repeated infections.
- These observations led to the successful treatment of the patient with replacement therapy of injectable gamma globulin preparations that established today's usage of replacement gamma globulin therapy in other immune deficiencies by the intravenous and subcutaneous routes as well as its use as an immodulating agent in the therapy of a wide variety of autoimmune disorders (*Chapter 11*).
- The subsequent identification of BTK as the genetic defect of the condition led to the understanding of its role as the signaling molecule involved in the activation of class-switch recombination necessary for the synthesis of the various isotypes of immunoglobulins.
- This case is the first description of agammaglobulinemia and represents a landmark discovery that led not only to the current explosive molecular and phenotypic dissection of the immunodeficiencies that are described in this chapter, but that also set the stage for the subsequent development of clinical immunology as we know it today.

including antibody deficiency syndromes and combined immunodeficiencies (CIDs).

- Defects of innate immunity include disorders of phagocytes, Toll-like receptor (TLR)-mediated signaling, and complement and are all characterized by increased susceptibility to recurrent infections, severe infections, or both, with distinctive susceptibility to various types of pathogens depending on the nature of the immune defect.
- In addition, some forms of PIDs present with immune dysregulation, and others (immunodeficiency syndromes) have a more complex phenotype in which immunodeficiency is only one of multiple components of the disease phenotype.
- The diagnostic workup of the patient suspected of having a PID is based heavily on a carefully taken history to first determine if a true susceptibility to recurrent infections is present. Once established, this is next followed by the determination of whether the susceptibility to infection is related to an increased environmental exposure to infectious agents, i.e., environmental-related factors, or to factors within the host that predispose the patient to a vulnerability to infection, i.e., host-related factors (Figure 16-43).
- Once environmental-related factors have been excluded, the next step is to determine if the increased susceptibility to infection is due to host-related factors, which can be subdivided into nonimmunologic and immunologic causes. Once these are eliminated, the diagnostic focus should be directed to the immunologic causes, which include both primary and secondary causes of immune deficiency.
- The secondary causes are by far the more frequently encountered and include infectious disease (e.g., HIV), the use of immunosuppressive agents, malignancy, and metabolic disease.
- Once these have been excluded, the clinician is then left with the challenge of unraveling the least common causes of recurrent infection, the primary immunodeficiency disorders that pose the greatest diagnostic burden because of the complexity and ever-increasing number of clinical entities that comprise this group of disorders.
- The initial workup can be performed by the primary health care provider, and when appropriate, referred to the specialist for further testing, which is usually only available in specialized research or diagnostic laboratories.

- The treatment of these disorders will be dependent on the specific entity and includes the use of gamma globulin for B cell defects and the use of HSC transplantation for more complex disorders. Gene therapy, while potentially the most effective mode of treatment for many of the PIDs, still must be approached with caution because of the potential adverse effects of malignancy.

Study Questions/Critical Thinking

1. Each of the following is a TRUE statement EXCEPT:
   a. Immunodeficiencies can be divided into primary and secondary immunodeficiencies
   b. Of the primary immunodeficiencies, humoral defects are more common
   c. IgA is the most common primary immune deficiency
   d. IVIG is the treatment of choice for IgA deficiency
   e. HIV infection is a common cause of secondary immunodeficiency
2. Each of the following is a TRUE statement concerning chronic granulomatous disease (CGD) EXCEPT:
   a. The most common pattern of inheritance is the XL form
   b. The disease is caused by an impairment of the NADPH oxidase system
   c. The most common mutation affects the gp91 protein
   d. Granulomata can be seen in the GI and GU tracts
   e. Interferon-alpha is the treatment of choice for the condition
3. Which of the following is a TRUE statement concerning IgG subclass deficiencies?
   a. IgG1 is the most common IgG subclass deficiency
   b. The final diagnosis is made by measurement of individual IgG subclass levels
   c. Post-immunization antibody levels to protein antigens are associated with IgG2 and IgG4 subclasses
   d. The treatment of choice is immunoglobulin replacement
   e. Staphylococcal skin infections are the most common clinical presentation
4. Each of the following is a TRUE statement concerning severe combined immune deficiency (SCID) EXCEPT:
   a. Affected patients suffer from repeated viral, bacterial, and fungal infections
   b. GI manifestations and failure to thrive are common manifestations
   c. Initial infections usually begin after six months of age because of the protection conferred by maternal antibody
   d. The most common molecular defect affects the γc chain of the IL-2 receptor
   e. The treatment of choice in human stem cell transplantation (HSCT)
5. Each of the following is a TRUE statement concerning the chromosome 22q11.2 deletion syndrome EXCEPT:
   a. DiGeorge syndrome was the first entity to be described
   b. Affected infants can present early in the newborn period with hypocalcemic tetany and candidal infection
   c. The genetic mutation of the TBX1 gene is the primary cause of the syndrome
   d. The diagnosis can be always confirmed by demonstration of a deletion in the long arm of chromosome 22q11.2 by FISH analysis

Suggested Reading

OMIM

Amberger J Bocchini CA Hamosh A. A new face and new challenges for Online Mendelian Inheritance in Man. Hum Mutat 2011; In Press

Amberger J Bocchini CA Scott AF Hamosh A. McKusick's Online Mendelian Inheritance in Man (OMIM). Nucleic Acids Res 2009;D7936

McKusick VA. Mendelian Inheritance in Man and its online version, OMIM. Am J Hum Genet 2007; 80:588604

General References

Albert MH, Notarangelo LD, Ochs HD. Clinical spectrum, pathophysiology and treatment of the Wiskott-Aldrich syndrome. Curr Opin Hematol. 2010; 18: 42.

Aldrich RA, Steinberg AG, Campbell DC. Pedigree demonstrating a sex-linked recessive condition characterized by draining ears, eczematoid dermatitis and bloody diarrhea. Pediatrics. 1954; 13: 133–9.

Amberger J, Bocchini CA, Hamosh A. A new face and new challenges for Online Mendelian Inheritance in Man. Hum Mutat. 2011; 32: 564–7.

Amberger J, Bocchini CA, Scott AF, Hamosh A. McKusick's Online Mendelian Inheritance in Man (OMIM). Nucleic Acids Res. 2009; 37 (Database Issue): D793–6.

Arpaia E, Shahar M, Dadi H, et al. Defective T cell receptor signaling and CD8+ thymic selection in humans lacking zap-70 kinase. Cell. 1994; 76: 947–58.

Barbosa MD, Nguyen QA, Tchernev VT, et al. Identification of the homologous beige and Chediak-Higashi syndrome genes. Nature. 1996; 382: 262–5.

Barjaktarevic I, Maletkovic-Barjaktarevic J, et al. Altered functional balance of Gfi-1 and Gfi-1b as an alternative cause of reticular dysgenesis? Med Hypotheses. 2010; 74: 445–8.

Blaese RM, Culver KW, Miller AD, et al. T lymphocyte-directed gene therapy for ADA-SCID: initial trial results after 4 years. Science. 1995; 270: 475–80.

Blume RS, Bennett JM, Yankee RA, et al. Defective granulocyte regulation in the Chediak-Higashi syndrome. N Engl J Med. 1968; 279: 1009–15.

Blume RS, Wolff SM. The Chediak-Higashi syndrome: studies in four patients and a review of the literature. Medicine (Baltimore). 1972; 51: 247–80.

Bordignon C, Notarangelo LD, Nobili N, et al. Gene therapy in peripheral blood lymphocytes and bone marrow for ADA-immunodeficient patients. Science. 1995; 270: 470–75.

Boyle RJ, Le C, Balloch A, et al. The clinical syndrome of specific antibody deficiency in children. Clin Exp Immunol. 2006; 146: 486–92.

Bruton OC. Agammaglobulinemia. Pediatrics. 1952; 9: 722–8.

Buckley RH, Schiff RI, Schiff SE, et al. Human severe combined immunodeficiency: genetic, phenotypic, and functional diversity in one hundred eight infants. J Pediatr. 1997; 130: 378–87.

Buckley RH. Molecular defects in human severe combined immunodeficiency and approaches to immune reconstitution. Annu Rev Immunol. 2004; 22: 625–55.

Casanova JL, Abel L. Genetic dissection of immunity to mycobacteria: the human model. Annu Rev Immunol. 2002; 20: 581–620.

Casanova JL, Jouanguy E, Lamhamedi S, et al. Immunological conditions of children with BCG disseminated infection. Lancet. 1995; 346: 581.

Caudy AA, Reddy ST, Chatila T, et al. CD25 deficiency causes an immune dysregulation, polyendocrinopathy, enteropathy, X-linked like syndrome, and defective IL-10 expression from CD4 lymphocytes. J Allergy Clin Immunol. 2007; 119: 482–7.

Chase NM, Verbsky JW, Routes JM. Newborn screening for T-cell deficiency. Curr Opin Allergy Clin Immunol. 2010; 10: 521–5.

Chiang AK, Chan GC, Ma SK, et al. Disseminated fungal infection associated with myeloperoxidase deficiency in a premature neonate. Pediatr Infect Dis J. 2000; 19: 1027–9.

Coffey AJ, Brooksbank RA, Brandau O, et al. Host response to EBV infection in X-linked lymphoproliferative disease results from mutations in an SH2-domain encoding gene. Nature. 1998; 20: 129–35.

Conley ME, Broides A, Hernandez-Trujillo V, et al. Genetic analysis of patients with defects in early B-cell development. Immunol Rev. 2005; 203: 216–34.

Cosar H, Kahramaner Z, Erdemir A, et al. Reticular dysgenesis in a preterm infant: a case report. Pediatr Hematol Oncol. 2010; 27: 646–9.

Dale DC, Hammond WP. Cyclic neutropenia: a clinical review. Blood Rev. 1988; 2: 168–85.

Dale DC, Person RE, Bolyard AA, et al. Mutations in the gene encoding neutrophils elastase in congenital and cyclic neutropenia. Blood. 2000; 96: 2316–22.

de la Salle H, Hanau D, Fricker D, et al. Homozygous human TAP peptide transporter mutation in HLA class I deficiency. Science. 1994; 265: 237–24.

Devriendt K, Kim AS, Mathijs G, et al. Constitutively activating mutation in WASP causes X-linked severe congenital neutropenia. Nat Genet. 2001; 27: 313–16.

Dong F, Brynes RK, Tidow N, et al. Mutations in the gene for the granulocyte colony-stimulating-factor receptor in patients with acute myeloid leukemia preceded by severe congenital neutropenia. N Engl J Med. 1995; 333: 487–93.

Dorman SE, Holland SM. Interferon-gamma and interleukin-12 pathway defects and human disease. Cytokine Growth Factor Rev. 2000; 11: 321–33.

Dorman SE, Picard C, Lammas D, et al. Clinical features of dominant and recessive interferon gamma receptor 1 deficiencies. Lancet. 2004; 364: 2113–21.

Elder ME. ZAP-70 and defects of T-cell receptor signaling. Semin Hematol. 1998; 35: 310–20.

Ferrari S, Giliani S, Insalaco A, et al. Mutations of CD40 gene cause an autosomal recessive form of immunodeficiency with hyper IgM. Proc Natl Acad Sci USA. 2001; 98: 12614–9.

Feske S, Picard C, Fischer A. Immunodeficiency due to mutations in ORAI1 and STIM1. Clin Immunol. 2010; 135: 169–82.

Fieschi C, Dupuis S, Catherinot E, et al. Low penetrance, broad resistance, and favorable outcome of interleukin 12 receptor beta1 deficiency: medical and immunological implications. J Exp Med. 2003; 197: 527–35.

Filipe-Santos O, Bustamante J, Haverkamp MH, et al. X-linked susceptibility to mycobacteria is caused by mutations in NEMO impairing CD40-dependent IL-12 production. J Exp Med. 2006; 203:1645–59.

Filipovich AH. Life-threatening hemophagocytic syndromes: current outcomes with hematopoietic stem cell transplantation. Pediatr Transplant. 2005; 9 Suppl 7: 87–91.

Foley SC, Préfontaine D, D'Antoni M, et al. Images in allergy and immunology: regulatory T cells in allergic disease. J Allergy Clin Immunol. 2007; 120: 482–6.

Freedman MH. Safety of long term administration of granulocyte colony-stimulating factor for severe chronic neutropenia. Curr Opin Hematol. 1997; 4: 216–24.

Freeman AF, Davis J, Anderson VL, et al. Pneumocystis jiroveci infection in patients with hyper-immunoglobulin E syndrome. Pediatrics. 2006; 118: 1271–5.

Gadola SD, Moins-Teisserenc HT, Trowsdale J, et al. TAP deficiency syndrome. Clin Exp Immunol. 2000; 121: 163–168.

Gallin JI, Alling DW, Malech HL, et al. Itraconazole to prevent fungal infections in chronic granulomatous disease. N Engl J Med. 2003; 348: 2416–22.

Gaspar HB, Bjorkegren E, Parsley K, et al. Successful reconstitution of immunity in ADA-SCID by stem cell gene therapy following cessation of PEG-ADA and use of mild reconditioning. Mol Ther. 2006; 14: 505–13.

Gennery AR, Cant AJ. Advances in hematopoietic stem cell transplantation for primary immunodeficiency. Immunol Allergy Clin North Am. 2008; 28: 439–56.

Genovese G, Friedman DJ, Ross MD, et al. Association of trypanolytic ApoL1 variants with kidney disease in African Americans. Science. 2010; 329: 841–5.

Goldman FD, Ballas ZK, Schutte BC, et al. Defective expression of p56lck in an infant with severe combined immunodeficiency. J Clin Invest. 1998; 102: 421–429.

Gomez L, Le Deist F, Blanche S, et al. Treatment of Omenn syndrome by bone marrow transplantation. J Pediatr. 1995; 127: 76–81.

Griffith LM, Cowan MJ, Notarangelo LD, et al. Workshop participants: improving cellular therapy for primary immune deficiency diseases: recognition, diagnosis, and management. J Allergy Clin Immunol. 2009; 124: 1152–60.

Grimbacher B, Holland SM, Gallin JI, et al. Hyper-IgE syndrome with recurrent infections–an autosomal dominant multisystem disorder. N Engl J Med. 1999; 340: 692–702.

Grunebaum E, Mazzolari E, Porta F, et al. Bone marrow transplantation for severe combined immune deficiency. JAMA. 2006; 295: 508–18.

Hacein-Bey-Abina S, Le Deist F, Carlier F, et al. Sustained correction of x-linked severe combined immunodeficiency by ex vivo gene therapy. N Engl J Med. 2000; 46: 1185–1193.

Hacein-Bey-Abina S, Von Kalle C, Schmidt M, et al. LMO2-associated clonal T cell proliferation in two patients after gene therapy for SCID-X1. Science. 2003; 302: 415–9. Erratum in: Science. 2003; 302: 568.

Hammond WP IV, Price TH, Souza LM, et al. Treatment of cyclic neutropenia with granulocyte colony-stimulating factor. N Engl J Med. 1989; 320: 1306–11.

Henter JI, Horne A, Aricó M, et al. HLH-2004: Diagnostic and therapeutic guidelines for hemophagocytic lymphohistiocytosis. Pediatr Blood Cancer. 2007; 48: 124–31.

Hershfield MS. Enzyme replacement therapy of adenosine deaminase deficiency with polyethylene glycol-modified adenosine deaminase (PEG-ADA). Immunodefecency. 1993; 4: 93–97.

Hershfield MS. New insights into adenosine-receptor-mediate immunosuppression and the role of adenosine in causing the immunodeficiency associated with adenosine deaminase deficiency. Eur J Immunol. 2005; 35: 25–30.

Hofmann SR, Ettinger R, Zhou YJ, et al. Cytokines and their role in lymphoid development, differentiation and homeostasis. Curr Opin Allergy Clin Immunol. 2002; 2: 495–506.

Holland SM, DeLeo FR, Elloumi HZ, et al. STAT3 mutations in the hyper-IgE syndrome. N Engl J Med. 2007; 357: 1608–19.

Horwitz M, Benson KF, Person RE, et al. Mutations in ELA2, encoding neutrophil elastase, define a 21-day biological clock in cyclic haematopoiesis. Nat Genet. 1999; 23: 433–6.

Horwitz ME, Barrett AJ, Brown MR, et al. Treatment of chronic granulomatous disease with nonmyeloablative conditioning and T-cell-depleted hematopoietic allograft. N Engl J Med. 2001; 344: 881–8.

Hubert P, Bergeron F, Ferreira V, et al. Defective p56Lck activity in T cells from an adult patient with idiopathic CD4+ lymphocytopenia. Int Immunol. 2000; 12: 449–57.

International Union of Immunological Societies Expert Committee on Primary Immunodeficiencies, Notarangelo LD, Fischer A, Geha RS, et al. Primary immunodeficiencies: 2009 update. J Allergy Clin Immunol. 2009; 124: 1161-78. Erratum in: J Allergy Clin Immunol. 2010; 125: 771-3.

Introne W, Boissy RE, Gahl WA. Clinical, molecular, and cell biological aspects of Chediak-Higashi syndrome. Mol Genet Metab. 1999; 68: 283–303.

Kostmann R. Infantile genetic agranulocytosis; agranulocytosis infantilis hereditaria. Acta Paediatr Suppl. 1956; 45: 1–78.

Krawczyk M, Reith W. Regulation of MHC class II expression, a unique regulatory system identified by the study of a primary immunodeficiency disease. Tissue Antigens. 2006; 67: 183–97.

Kuhns DB, Alvord WG, Heller T, et al. Residual NADPH oxidase and survival in chronic granulomatous disease. N Engl J Med. 2010; 363: 2600–10.

Kung C, Pingel JT, Heikinheimo M, et al. Mutations in the tyrosine phosphatase CD45 gene in a child with severe combined immunodeficiency disease. Nature Med. 2000; 6: 343–5.

Lekstrom-Himes JA, Dorman SE, Kopar P, et al. Neutrophil-specific granule deficiency results from a novel mutation with loss of function of the transcription factor CCAAT/enhancer binding protein epsilon. J Exp Med. 1999; 189: 1847–52.

Levy J, Espanol-Boren T, Thomas C, et al. Clinical spectrum of X-linked hyper-IgM syndrome. J Pediatr. 1997; 131: 47–54.

Lougaris V, Badolato R, Ferrari S, et al. Hyper immunoglobulin M syndrome due to CD40 deficiency: clinical, molecular, and immunological features. Immunol Rev. 2005; 203: 48–66.

Malech HL, Maples PB, Whiting-Theobald N, et al. Prolonged production of NADPH oxidase-corrected granulocytes after gene therapy of chronic granulomatous disease. Proc Natl Acad Sci USA. 1997; 94: 12133–8.

Marciano BE, Rosenzweig SD, Kleiner DE, et al. Gastrointestinal involvement in chronic granulomatous disease. Pediatrics. 2004; 114: 462–8.

Marciano BE, Wesley R, De Carlo ES, et al. Long-term interferon-gamma therapy for patients with chronic granulomatous disease. Clin Infect Dis. 2004; 39: 692–9.

Masters SL, Simon A, Aksentijevich I, et al. Horror autoinflammaticus: the molecular pathophysiology of autoinflammatory disease. Annu Rev Immunol. 2009; 27: 621–68.

Mazzolari E, Lanzi G, Forino C, et al. First report of successful stem cell transplantation in a child with CD40 deficiency. Bone Marrow Transplant. 2007; 40: 279–81.

McKusick VA. Mendelian Inheritance in Man and its online version, OMIM. Am J Hum Genet. 2007; 80: 588–604.

Minegishi Y, Coustan-Smith E, Rapalus L, et al. Mutation in Igalpha (CD79a) results in a complete block in B-cell development. J Clin Invest. 1999; 104: 1115–21.

Minegishi Y, Coustan-Smith E, Wang YH, et al. Mutations in the human l5/14.1 gene result in B cell deficiency and agammaglobulinemia. J Exp Med. 1998; 187: 71–77.

Minegishi Y, Rohrer J, Coustan-Smith E, et al. An essential role for BLNK in human B cell development. Science. 1999; 286: 1954–1957.

Minegishi Y. Hyper-IgE syndrome. Curr Opin Immunol. 2009; 21: 487–92.

Nagle DL, Karim MA, Woolf EA, et al. Identification and mutation analysis of the complete gene for Chediak-Higashi syndrome. Nat Genet. 1996; 14: 307–11.

Netea MG, van der Meer JW. Immunodeficiency and genetic defects of pattern-recognition receptors. N Engl J Med. 2011; 364: 60–70.

Notarangelo LD, Fischer A, Geha RS, et al. Primary immunodeficiencies: 2009 update. J Allergy Clin Immunol. 2009; 124: 1161–78.

Notarangelo LD, Hayward AR. X-linked immunodeficiency with hyper-IgM (XHIM). Clin Exp Immunol. 2000; 120: 399–405.

Notarangelo LD, Lanzi G, Peron S, et al. Defects of class-switch recombination. J Allergy Clin Immunol. 2006; 116: 855–64.

Notarangelo LD, Mella P, Jones A, et al. Mutations in severe combined immune deficiency (SCID) due to JAK3 deficiency. Hum Mutat. 2001; 18: 255–63.

Notarangelo LD, Santagata S, Villa A. Recombinase activating gene enzymes of lymphocytes. Curr Opin Hematol. 2001; 8: 41–6.

Notarangelo LD. Primary immunodeficiencies. J Allergy Clin Immunol. 2010; 125: S182–94.

O'Shea JJ, Husa M, Li D, Hofmann SR, et al. Jak3 and the pathogenesis of severe combined immunodeficiency. Mol Immunol. 2004; 41:727–37.

Ochs HD, Notarangelo LD. X-linked immunodeficiencies. Curr Allergy Asthma Rep. 2004; 4: 339–48.

Orange JS, Levy O, Brodeur SR, et al. Human nuclear factor kappa B essential modulator mutation can result in immunodeficiency without ectodermal dysplasia. J Allergy Clin Immunol. 2004; 114: 650–6.

Ott MG, Schmidt M, Schwarzwaelder K, et al. Correction of X-linked chronic granulomatous disease by gene therapy, augmented by insertional activation of MDS1-EVI1, PRDM16 or SETBP1. Nat Med. 2006; 12: 401–9.

Ozsahin H, Arredondo-Vega FX, Santisteban I, et al. Adenosine deaminase deficiency in adults. Blood. 1997; 89:2849–55.

Park MA, Li JT, Hagan JB, et al. Common variable immunodeficiency: a new look at an old disease. Lancet. 2008; 372: 489–502.

Parker RI, McKeown LP, Gallin JI, et al. Absence of the largest platelet-von Willebrand multimers in a patient with lactoferrin deficiency and a bleeding tendency. Thromb Haemost. 1992; 67: 320–4.

Person RE, Li FQ, Duan Z, et al. Mutations in proto-oncogene GFI1 cause human neutropenia and target ELA2. Nat Genet. 2003; 34: 308–12.

Pesach IM, Notarangelo LD. Gene therapy for primary immunodeficiencies: looking ahead towards gene correction. J Allergy Clin Immunol. 2011; 127: 1344–50.

Pesach IM, Ordovas-Montanes J, Zhang SY, et al. Induced pluripotent stem cells: A novel frontier in the study of human primary immunodeficiencies. J Allergy Clin Immunol. 2011; 127: 1400–7.

Rao VK, Straus SE. Causes and consequences of the autoimmune lymphoproliferative syndrome. Hematology. 2006; 11: 15–23.

Reeves EP, Lu H, Jacobs HL, et al. Killing activity of neutrophils are mediated through activation of proteases by K^+ flux. Nature 2002; 416: 291–297.

Renner ED, Puck JM, Holland SM, et al. Autosomal recessive hyperimmunoglobulin E syndrome: a distinct disease entity. J Pediatr. 2004; 144: 93–9.

Rigaud S, Fondanèche MC, Lambert N, et al. XIAP deficiency in humans causes an X-linked lymphoproliferative syndrome. Nature. 2006; 444: 110–4.

Roifman CM, Fischer A, Notarangelo LD, de la Morena MT, Seger RA. Indications for hemopoietic stem cell transplantation. Immunol Allergy Clin North Am. 2010; 30: 261–2.

Ross SC, Denson P. Complement deficiency states and infection: Epidemiology, pathogenesis and consequences of neisserial and other infections in an immune deficiency. Medicine. 1984; 63: 243–73.

Routes JM, Grossman WJ, Verbsky J, et al. Statewide newborn screening for severe T-cell lymphopenia. JAMA. 2009; 302: 2465–70.

Seemayer TA, Gross TG, Egeler RM, et al. X-Linked Lymphoproliferative disease: twenty-five years after the discovery. Ped Res. 1995; 38: 471–8.

Segal BH, Barnhart LA, Anderson VL, et al. Posaconazole as salvage therapy in patients with chronic granulomatous disease and invasive filamentous fungal infection. Clin Infect Dis. 2005; 40: 1684–8.

Segal BH, Leto TL, Gallin JI, et al. Genetic, biochemical, and clinical features of chronic granulomatous disease. Medicine (Baltimore). 2000; 79: 160–200.

Shiow LR, Paris K, Akana MC, et al. Severe combined immunodeficiency (SCID) and attention deficit hyperactivity disorder (ADHD) associated with a Coronin-1A mutation and a chromosome 16p11.2 deletion. Clin Immunol. 2009; 131: 24–30.

Sochorová K, Horváth R, Rozková D, et al. Impaired Toll-like receptor 8-mediated IL-6 and TNF-alpha production in antigen-presenting cells from patients with X-linked agammaglobulinemia. Blood. 2007; 109: 2553–6.

Steele RW, Limas C, Thurman GB, et al. Familial thymic aplasia: attempted reconstitution with a fetal thymus in a

Millipore diffusion chamber. N Engl J Med. 1972; 287: 787–91.

Stepp SE, Dufourcq-Lagelouse R, Le Deist F, et al. Perforin gene defects in familial hemophagocytic lymphohistiocytosis. Science. 1999; 286:1957-9.

Straus SE, Jaffe ES, Puck JM, et al. The development of lymphomas in families with autoimmune lymphoproliferative syndrome with germline Fas mutations and defective lymphocyte apoptosis. Blood. 2001; 98: 194–200.

Tchilian EZ, Wallace DL, Wells RS, et al. A deletion in the gene encoding the CD45 antigen in a patient with SCID. J Immunol. 2001; 166: 1308–13.

Torgerson TR. Regulatory T cells in human autoimmune diseases. Springer Semin Immunopathol. 2006; 28: 63–76.

Uzel G. The range of defects associated with nuclear factor kappaB essential modulator. Curr Opin Allergy Clin Immunol. 2005; 5: 513–8.

van der Burg M, van Dongen JJ, van Gent DC. DNA-PKcs deficiency in human: long predicted, finally found. Curr Opin Allergy Clin Immunol. 2009; 9: 503–9.

van der Burg M, van Veelen LR, Verkaik NS, et al. A new type of radiosensitive T-B-NK+ severe combined immunodeficiency caused by a LIG4 mutation. J Clin Invest. 2006; 116: 137–45.

Vanhollebeke B, Truc P, Poelvoorde P, et al. Human Trypanosoma evansi infection linked to a lack of apolipoprotein L-I. N Engl J Med. 2006; 355: 2752–6.

Veillette A. Immune regulation by SLAM family receptors and SAP-related adaptors. Nat Rev Immunol. 2006; 6: 56–6.

Verbsky JW, Grossman WJ. Cellular and genetic basis of primary immune deficiencies. Pediatr Clin North Am. 2006; 53: 649–84.

Villa A, Santagata S, Bozzi F, et al. Partial V(D)J recombination activity leads to Omenn syndrome. Cell. 1998; 93: 885–96.

Vivier E, Raulet DH, Moretta A, et al. Innate or adaptive immunity? The example of natural killer cells. Science. 2011; 331: 44–9.

Vowells SJ, Fleisher TA, Sekhsaria S, et al. Genotype-dependent variability in flow cytometric evaluation of reduced nicotinamide adenine dinucleotide phosphate oxidase function in patients with chronic granulomatous disease. J Pediatr. 1996; 128: 104–7.

Walther MM, Malech H, Berman A, et al. The urological manifestations of chronic granulomatous disease. J Urol. 1992; 147:1314–8.

Winkelstein JA, Marino MC, Johnston RB Jr, et al. Chronic granulomatous disease. Report on a national registry of 368 patients. Medicine (Baltimore). 2000; 79: 155–69.

Worth A, Thrasher AJ, Gaspar HB. Autoimmune lymphoproliferative syndrome: molecular basis of disease and clinical phenotype. Br J Haematol. 2006; 133: 124–40.

Wright DG, Dale DC, Fauci AS, et al. Human cyclic neutropenia: clinical review and long term follow up of patients. Medicine (Baltimore). 1981; 60: 1–13.

Yel L, Minegishi Y, Coustan-Smith E, et al. Mutations in the Mu heavy-chain gene in patients with agammaglobulinemia. N Engl J Med. 1996; 335: 1486–93.

Classification, Characteristic Infections, and Known Genetic Defects Associated with the Primary Immunodeficiencies

All the tables in this annex have been reproduced with permission from Notarangelo LD, Fischer A, Geha RS, et al. Primary immunodeficiencies: 2009 update. J Allergy Clin Immunol. 2009;124:1161–78.

Table 16A-1. Phagocytic cells, number, function, or both

Component	Affected cells	Affected function	Characteristic infections and associated features	Inheritance	Genetic defects
			Disorders of myeloid cells		
1. Severe congenital neutropenia	N	Myeloid differentiation	High-grade bacterial infection due to Gram-positive and Gram-negative bacteria; paronychia, perineal infections. The first subgroup with myelodysplasia, the second with B/T lymphopenia.	AD	ELA2, mistrafficking of elastase (subgroup with myelodysplasia) GFI1: repression of elastase (B/T lymphopenia)
2. Cyclic neutropenia/cyclic hematopoiesis	N	?	Aphthous oral ulcers, gingivitis, lymphadenopathy, pharyngitis, tonsillitis, skin lesions Oscillations of other leukocytes and platelets	AD	ELA2, mistrafficking of elastase
3. Kostmann's syndrome	N	Myeloid differentiation	Aphthous oral ulcers, gingivitis, lymphadenopathy, pharyngitis, tonsillitis, skin lesions Cognitive and neurological defects[a]	AR	HAX-1, impaired neutrophil apoptosis (1q21.3)
4. P14 deficiency	N+L	Endosome biogenesis	Neutropenia Hypogammaglobulinemia ↓CD8 cytotoxicity Partial albinism Growth failure	AR	MAPBPIP: endosomal adaptor protein 14
5. Neutropenia with cardiac and urogenital malformations	N+F	Myeloid differentiation	Structural heart defects, urogenital abnormalities, and venous angiectasias of trunks and limbs	AR	G6PC3: abolished enzymatic activity of glucose-6-phosphatase and enhanced apoptosis of N and F

(Continued)

Table 16A-1. (*Continued*)

Component	Affected cells	Affected function	Characteristic infections and associated features	Inheritance	Genetic defects
6. Glycogen storage disease type 1b	N+M	Killing, chemotaxis, O_2-production	Fasting hypoglycemia, lactic acidosis, hyperlipidemia, hepatomegaly, and neutropenia	AR	G6PT1: glucose-6-phosphate transporter 1
7. X-linked neutropenia/myelodysplasia	N+M	?	Neutropenia and monocytopenia	XL	WAS: regulator of actin cytoskeleton (loss of autoinhibition)
8. β-actin deficiency	N+M	Motility	Mental retardation, short stature	AD	ACTB: cytoplasmic actin
		Defects of granule formation and content			
9. Chediak-Higashi syndrome	N+M		Partial albinism, giant lysosomes, low NK and CTL, acute phase reaction, lymphoma-like "accelerated phase"	AR	Defects in LYST, impaired lysosomal trafficking
10. Griscelli syndrome, type 2	N+M		Partial albinism, low NK and CTL activities, heightened acute phase reaction, encephalopathy in some patients	AR	Defects in RAB27A encoding a GTPase in secretory vesicles
11. Neutrophil-specific granule deficiency	N	Chemotaxis	Recurrent pyogenic infections of the skin, ears, lungs, and lymph nodes caused by Gram-positive cocci and Gram-negative rods N with bilobed nuclei	AR	C/EBPE: myeloid transcription factor
12. Hermansky-Pudlak syndrome, type 2	N		Partial albinism, neutropenia, low NK and CTL activity, increased bleeding	AR	Mutations of AP3B1 gene, encoding for the β subunit of the AP-3 complex
		Defects of oxidative metabolism			
13. Chronic granulomatous disease (CGD)	N+M	Killing (faulty O_2-production)	X-linked and autosomal forms; infections caused by catalase bacteria, *Nocardia*, fungi	XL AR	CYBB: electron transport protein ($gp91^{phox}$) $p22^{phox}$ (16q24) $p47^{phox}$ (7q11.23) $p67^{phox}$ (1q25)
14. Rac 2 deficiency	N	Adherence, chemotaxis, O_2-production	Poor wound healing; defect in adherence	AD	RAC2: regulation of actin cytoskeleton
15. Myeloperoxidase deficiency	N+M		Mucocutaneous, meningeal, bone, and disseminated candidiasis only in the setting of diabetes	AR	MPO; 16q23
		The leukocyte-adhesion deficiencies			
16. Leukocyte adhesion deficiency type 1 (LAD1)	N+M	Adherence, chemotaxis, endocytosis T/NK cytotoxicity	Delayed cord separation, skin ulcers, periodontitis, leukocytosis	AR	Mutations in CD18 or ITGB2: adhesion protein (INTG2; 21q22.3)

Table 16A-1. (*Continued*)

Component	Affected cells	Affected function	Characteristic infections and associated features	Inheritance	Genetic defects
17. Leukocyte adhesion deficiency type 2 (LAD2)	N+M	Rolling chemotaxis	Mild LAD type 1 features plus hh-blood group (Bombay blood group) plus mental and growth retardation; impaired rolling and chemotaxis due to selectin fucosylation defect resulting in infections in childhood	AR	FUCT1, GDP-fucose transporter (11p11.2)
18. Leukocyte adhesion deficiency type 3 (LAD3)	L+NK	Adherence	LAD type 1 plus bleeding tendency	AR	KINDLIN3: Rap1-activation of β1–3 integrins
19. Localized juvenile periodontitis	N	Formylpeptide-induced chemotaxis	Periodontitis only	AR	FPR1: chemokine receptor
20. Papillon-Lefévre syndrome	N+M	Chemotaxis	Periodontitis, palmoplantar hyperkeratosis[b]	AR	CTSC: cathepsin C activation of serine proteases
21. Shwachman-Diamond syndrome	N	Chemotaxis	Pancytopenia, exocrine pancreatic insufficiency, chondrodysplasia	AR	SBDS
			Defects of cytokine-signaling pathways		
22. IFN-γ receptor 1 deficiency	M+L (IFN-γ signaling)	IFN-γ binding and signaling	Susceptibility to *Mycobacteria*, disseminated BCG, and *Salmonella*	AR AD	IFNGR1: IFN-γR ligand binding chain
23. IFN-γ receptor 2 deficiency	M+L (IFN-γ signaling)	IFN-γ signaling	Susceptibility to *Mycobacteria*, disseminated BCG, and *Salmonella*	AR	IFNGR2: IFN-γR accessory chain
24. IL-12p40 deficiency	M (IFN-γ signaling)	IFN-γ secretion	Susceptibility to *Mycobacteria*, disseminated BCG, and *Salmonella*	AR	IL-12B: subunit of IL-12/IL-23 (P40 subunit)
25. IL-12 and IL-23 receptor β1 chain deficiency	L+NK (IFN-γ signaling)	IFN-γ secretion	Susceptibility to *Mycobacteria*, disseminated BCG, and *Salmonella*	AR	IL-12Rβ1: IL-12 and IL-23 receptor β1 chain
26. STAT1 deficiency (2 forms)	M+L (IFN-α/β, IFN-γ, IFN-λ, and IL-27 signaling)	IFN-α/β, IFN-γ, IFN-λ, and IL-27 signaling	Susceptibility to *Mycobacteria*, *Salmonella*, and viruses	AD AR	STAT1 STAT1
27. Type 1 HIES (Job's syndrome; AD HIES)	L+M+N+ epithelial	IFN-γ signaling	Susceptibility to *Mycobacteria* and *Salmonella;* distinctive facial features (broad nasal bridge); eczema; osteoporosis and fractures; scoliosis; failure/delay of shedding primary teeth; hyperextensible joints; bacterial infections (skin and pulmonary abscesses/pneumatoceles) caused by *Staphylococcus aureus*; candidiasis	AD, many *de novo* mutations	STAT3

(*Continued*)

Table 16A-1. (*Continued*)

Component	Affected cells	Affected function	Characteristic infections and associated features	Inheritance	Genetic defects
28. Type 2 HIES (Job's syndrome; AR HIES)	L+M+N+ others	IL-6/10/22/23 signaling IL-6/10/12/23/ IFN-α/IFN-β signaling	Susceptibility to intracellular bacteria (mycobacteria, *Salmonella*), *Staphylococcus*, and viruses.	AR	Tyk2 (most forms unknown)
29. Pulmonary alveolar proteinosis (GM-CSF signaling)	Alveolar macrophages	GM-CSF signaling	Alveolar proteinosis	Biallelic mutations in pseudoautosomal gene	CSF2RA

ACTB = Actin beta; AD = autosomal-dominant; AR = autosomal recessive inheritance; CEBPE = CCAAT/enhancer-binding protein epsilon; CTSC = cathepsin C; CYBA = cytochrome b α subunit; CYBB = cytochrome b β subunit; ELA2 = elastase 2; IFN = interferon; IFNGR1 = interferon-gamma receptor subunit 1; IFNGR2 = interferon-gamma receptor subunit 2; L12B = interleukin-12 beta subunit; IL12RB1 = interleukin-12 receptor beta 1; F = fibroblasts; FPR1 = formylpeptide receptor 1; FUCT1 = fucose transporter 1; GFI1 = growth factor independent 1; HAX1 = HLCS1-associated protein X1; ITGB2 = integrin beta-2; L = lymphocytes; M = monocytes-macrophages; MAPBPIP = MAPBP-interacting protein; Mel = melanocytes; N = neutrophils; NCF1 = neutrophil cytosolic factor 1; NCF2 = neutrophil cytosolic factor 2; NK = natural killer cells; SBDS = Shwachman-Bodian-Diamond syndrome; STAT = signal transducer and activator of transcription; XL = X-linked inheritance.

[a]Cognitive and neurologic defects are observed in a fraction of patients.

[b]Periodontitis may be isolated.

Table 16A-2. Disorders of complement

Component	Examples	Characteristic infections	Inheritance	Genetic defects
C1q deficiency	Absent C hemolytic activity, defective MAC[a]; faulty dissolution of immune complexes; faulty clearance of apoptotic cells	SLE-like syndrome, rheumatoid disease, infections	AR	C1q
C1r deficiency[a]	Absent C hemolytic activity, defective MAC; faulty dissolution of immune complexes	SLE-like syndrome, rheumatoid disease, infections	AR	C1r[a]
C1s deficiency	Absent C hemolytic activity	SLE-like syndrome; multiple autoimmune diseases	AR	C1s
C4 deficiency	Absent C hemolytic activity, defective MAC; faulty dissolution of immune complexes; defective humoral immune response	SLE-like syndrome, rheumatoid disease, infections	AR	C4
C2 deficiency[b]	Absent C hemolytic activity, defective MAC; faulty dissolution of immune complexes	SLE-like syndrome, vasculitis, polymyositis, pyogenic infections	AR	C2[c]
C3 deficiency	Absent C hemolytic activity, defective MAC; defective bactericidal activity; defective humoral immune response	Recurrent pyogenic infections	AR	C3
C5 deficiency	Absent C hemolytic activity, defective MAC; defective bactericidal activity	Neisserial infections, SLE	AR	C5
C6 deficiency	Absent C hemolytic activity, defective MAC; defective bactericidal activity	Neisserial infections, SLE	AR	C6
C7 deficiency	Absent C hemolytic activity, defective MAC; defective bactericidal activity	Neisserial infections, SLE, vasculitis	AR	C7
C8a deficiency[c]	Absent C hemolytic activity, defective MAC; defective bactericidal activity	Neisserial infections, SLE	AR	C8α

Table 16A-2. (*Continued*)

Component	Examples	Characteristic infections	Inheritance	Genetic defects
C8b deficiency	Absent C hemolytic activity, defective MAC; defective bactericidal activity	Neisserial infections, SLE	AR	C8β
C9 deficiency	Reduced C hemolytic activity, defective MAC; defective bactericidal activity	Neisserial infections[d]	AR	C9
C1 inhibitor deficiency	Spontaneous activation of the complement pathway with consumption of C4/C2; spontaneous activation of the contact system with generation of bradykinin from high-molecular-weight kininogen	Hereditary angioedema	AD	C1 inhibitor
Factor I deficiency	Spontaneous activation of the alternative complement pathway with consumption of C3	Recurrent pyogenic infections	AR	Factor I
Factor H deficiency	Spontaneous activation of the alternative complement pathway with consumption of C3	Hemolytic-uremic syndrome, membranoproliferative glomerulonephritis	AR	Factor H
Factor D deficiency	Absent hemolytic activity by the alternate pathway	Neisserial infection	AR	Factor D
Properdin deficiency	Absent hemolytic activity by the alternate pathway	Neisserial infection	XL	Properdin
MBP deficiency[e]	Defective mannose recognition; defective hemolytic activity by the lectin pathway	Pyogenic infections with very low penetrance, mostly asymptomatic	AR	MBP[f]
MASP2 deficiency	Absent hemolytic activity by the lectin pathway	SLE syndrome, pyogenic infection	AR	MASP2
Complement receptor 3 (CR3) deficiency	See LAD1		AR	ITGB2
Membrane cofactor protein (CD46) deficiency	Inhibitor of complement alternate pathway, decreased C3b binding	Glomerulonephritis, atypical hemolytic uremic syndrome	AD	MCP
Membrane attack complex inhibitor (CD59) deficiency	Erythrocytes highly susceptible to complement-mediated lysis	Hemolytic anemia, thrombosis	AR	CD59
Paroxysmal nocturnal hemoglobinuria	Complement-mediated hemolysis	Recurrent hemolysis	Acquired X-linked mutation	PIGA
Immunodeficiency associated with ficolin 3 deficiency	Absence of complement activation by the ficolin 3 pathway	Recurrent severe pyogenic infections mainly in the lungs	AR	FCN3

AD = autosomal dominant inheritance; AR = autosomal recessive inheritance; MAC = membrane-attack complex; MASP-2 = MBP-associated serine protease 2; MBP = mannose-binding protein; PIGA = phosphatidylinositol glycan class A; SLE = systemic lupus erythematosus; XL = X-linked inheritance.

[a]The C1r and C1s genes are located within 9.5 kb of each other. In many cases of C1r deficiency, C1s is also deficient.

[b]Gene duplication has resulted in two active C4A genes located within 10 kb. C4 deficiency requires abnormalities in both genes, usually the result of deletions.

[c]Type 1 C2 deficiency is in linkage disequilibrium with HLA-A25, B18, and -DR2 and complotype, SO42 (slow variant of factor B, absent C2, type 4 C4A, type 2 C4B) and is common in Caucasian subjects (about one per 10,000). It results from a 28-bp deletion resulting in a premature stop codon in the C2 gene; C2 mRNA is not produced. Type 2 C2 deficiency is very rare and involves amino acid substitutions, which result in C2 secretory block.

[d]C8α deficiency is always associated with C8γ deficiency. The gene encoding C8γ maps to chromosome 9 and is normal. C8γ is covalently bound to C8α.

[e]Association is weaker than with C5, C6, C7, and C8 deficiencies. C9 deficiency occurs in about one per 1,000 Japanese.

[f]Population studies reveal no detectable increase in infections in MBP-deficient adults.

Table 16A-3. Defects in innate immunity

Disease	Affected cell	Functional defects	Associated features	Inheritance	Gene defect/presumed pathogenesis
Anhidrotic ectodermal dysplasia with immunodeficiency (EDA-ID)	Lymphocytes + monocytes	NF-κB signaling pathway	Anhidrotic ectodermal dysplasia and specific antibody deficiency (lack of antibody response to polysaccharides) Various infections (mycobacteria and pyogenic bacteria)	XL	Mutations of NEMO (IKBKG), a modulator of NF-κB activation
EDA-ID	Lymphocytes + monocytes	NF-κB signaling pathway	Anhidrotic ectodermal dysplasia, T cell defects, and various infections	AD	Gain-of-function mutation of IKBA, resulting in impaired activation of NF-κB
IL-1 receptor-associated kinase 4 (IRAK4) deficiency	Lymphocytes + monocytes	TIR-IRAK signaling pathway	Bacterial infections (pyogens)	AR	Mutation of IRAK4, a component of TLR and IL-1R signaling pathway
MyD88 deficiency	Lymphocytes + monocytes	TIR-MyD88 signaling pathway	Bacterial infections (pyogens)	AR	Mutation of MYD88, a component of the TLR and IL-1R signaling pathway
WHIM (warts, hypogammaglobulinemia infections, myelokathexis) syndrome	Granulocytes + lymphocytes	Increased response of the CXCR4 chemokine receptor to its ligand CXCL12 (SDF-1)	Hypogammaglobulinemia, reduced B cell numbers, severe reduction of neutrophil count, warts/HPV infection	AD	Gain-of-function mutations of CXCR4, the receptor for CXCL12
Epidermodysplasia verruciformis	Keratinocytes and leukocytes		HPV (group B1) infections and cancer of the skin	AR	Mutations of EVER1, EVER2
Herpes simplex encephalitis (HSE)	Central nervous system resident cells, epithelial cells, and leukocytes	UNC-93B-dependent IFN-α, IFN-β, and IFN-λ induction	Herpes simplex virus 1 encephalitis and meningitis	AR	Mutations of UNC93B1
HSE	Central nervous system resident cells, epithelial cells, dendritic cells, cytotoxic lymphocytes	TLR3-dependent IFN-α, IFN-β, and IFN-λ induction	Herpes simplex virus 1 encephalitis and meningitis	AD	Mutations of TLR3
Chronic mucocutaneous candidiasis	Macrophages, defect of Th16 cells in CARD9 deficiency	Defective Dectin-1 signaling	Chronic mucocutaneous candidiasis	AR AD	Mutations of CARD9 in one family with AR inheritance leading to low number of Th16 cells; defect unknown in other cases
Trypanosomiasis		APOL-I	Trypanosomiasis	AD	Mutation in APOL-I

AD = autosomal dominant; AR = autosomal recessive; EDA-ID = ectodermal dystrophy immune deficiency; EVER = epidermodysplasia verruciformis; HPV = human papilloma virus; IKBA = inhibitor of NF-kB alpha; IRAK4 = interleukin-1 receptor associated kinase 4; MYD88 = myeloid differentiation primary response gene 88; NEMO = NF-κB essential modulator; NF-κB = nuclear factor-κB; SDF-1 = stromal-derived factor 1; TIR = Toll and IL-1 receptor; TLR = Toll-like receptor; XL = X-linked.

[a]Only a few patients have been genetically investigated, and they represented a small fraction of all patients tested, but the clinical phenotype being common, these genetic disorders may actually be more common.

[b]Mutations in CARD9 have been identified only in one family. Other cases of chronic mucocutaneous candidiasis remain genetically undefined.

Table 16A-4. Autoinflammatory disorders

Disease	Affected cells	Functional defects	Associated features	Inheritance	Gene defects
Familial Mediterranean fever	Mature granulocytes, cytokine-activated monocytes	Decreased production of pyrin permits ASC-induced IL-1 processing and inflammation after subclinical serosal injury; macrophage apoptosis decreased	Recurrent fever, serositis, and inflammation responsive to colchicine; predisposes to vasculitis and inflammatory bowel disease	AR	Mutations of MEFV
TNF receptor-associated periodic syndrome (TRAPS)	PMNs, monocytes	Mutations of 55-kD TNF receptor leading to intracellular receptor retention or diminished soluble cytokine receptor available to bind TNF	Recurrent fever, serositis, rash, and ocular or joint inflammation	AD	Mutations of TNFRSF1A
Hyper IgD syndrome		Mevalonate kinase deficiency affecting cholesterol synthesis; pathogenesis of disease unclear	Periodic fever and leukocytosis with high IgD levels	AR	Mutations of MVK
Muckle-Wells syndrome	PMNs, monocytes	Defect in cryopyrin, involved in leukocyte apoptosis and NF-κB signaling and IL-1 processing	Urticaria, SNHL, amyloidosis; responsive to IL-1R/antagonist	AD	Mutations of CIAS1 (also called PYPAF1 or NALP3)
Familial cold autoinflammatory syndrome	PMNs, monocytes	Same as above	Nonpruritic urticaria, arthritis, chills, fever, and leukocytosis after cold exposure Responsive to IL-1R/antagonist (Anakinra)	AD	Mutations of CIAS1 Mutations of NLRP12
Neonatal onset multisystem inflammatory disease (NOMID) or chronic infantile neurologic cutaneous and articular syndrome (CINCA)	PMNs, chondrocytes	Same as above	Neonatal onset rash, chronic meningitis, and arthropathy with fever and inflammation responsive to IL-1R antagonist (Anakinra)	AD	Mutations of CIAS1
Pyogenic sterile arthritis, pyoderma gangrenosum, acne (PAPA) syndrome	Hematopoietic tissues, upregulated in activated T cells	Disordered actin reorganization leading to compromised physiologic signaling during inflammatory response	Destructive arthritis, inflammatory skin rash, myositis	AD	Mutations of PSTPIP1 (also called C2BP1)
Blau syndrome	Monocytes	Mutations in nucleotide binding site of CARD15, possibly disrupting interactions with LPSs and NF-κB signaling	Uveitis, granulomatous synovitis, camptodactyly, rash, and cranial neuropathies; 30% develop Crohn's disease	AD	Mutations of NOD2 (also called CARD15)

(*Continued*)

Table 16A-4. (*Continued*)

Disease	Affected cells	Functional defects	Associated features	Inheritance	Gene defects
Chronic recurrent multifocal osteomyelitis and congenital dyserythropoietic anemia (Majeed syndrome)	Neutrophils, bone marrow cells	Undefined	Chronic recurrent multifocal osteomyelitis, transfusion-dependent anemia, cutaneous inflammatory disorders	AR	Mutations of LPIN2
DIRA (deficiency of the IL-1 receptor antagonist)	PMNs, monocytes	Mutations in the IL-1 receptor antagonist allows unopposed action of IL-1	Neonatal onset of sterile multifocal osteomyelitis, periostitis and pustulosis	AR	Mutations of IL1RN

AD = autosomal dominant inheritance; AR = autosomal recessive inheritance; ASC = apoptosis-associated specklike protein with a caspase-recruitment domain; CARD = caspase-recruitment domain; CD2BP1 = CD2 binding protein 1; CIAS1 = cold-induced autoinflammatory syndrome 1; LPN2 = lipin-2; MEFV = Mediterranean fever; MVK = mevalonate kinase; NF-κB = nuclear factor-κB; PMN = polymorphonuclear cell; PSTPIP1 = proline/serine/threonine phosphatase-interacting protein 1; SNHL = sensorineural hearing loss.

Table 16A-5. Combined T cell and B cell immunodeficiencies

Disease	Circulating T cells	Circulating B cells	Serum immunoglobulin	Associated features	Inheritance	Gene defects/ presumed pathogenesis
T- B+ SCID[a]						
γc deficiency	Markedly decreased	Normal or increased	Decreased	Markedly decreased NK cells; leaky cases may present with low to normal T and/or NK cells	XL	Defect in γ chain of receptors for IL-2, IL-4, IL-7, IL-9, IL-15, IL-21
JAK3 deficiency	Markedly decreased	Normal or increased	Decreased	Markedly decreased NK cells; leaky cases may present with variable T and/or NK cells	AR	Defect in Janus activating kinase 3
IL-7Rα deficiency	Markedly decreased	Normal or increased	Decreased	Normal NK cells	AR	Defect in IL-7 receptor α chain
CD45 deficiency	Markedly decreased	Normal	Decreased	Normal γ/δ T cells	AR	Defect in CD45
CD3δ/CD3ε/ CD3ζ deficiency	Markedly decreased	Normal	Decreased	Normal NK cells; no γ/δ T cells	AR	Defect in CD3δ CD3ε or CD3ζ chains of T cell antigen receptor complex
Coronin-1A deficiency	Markedly decreased	Normal	Decreased	Detectable thymus	AR	Defective thymic egress of T cells and T cell locomotion
T+ B+ NK+ SCID p56Lck deficiency	Normal; CD4 lymphopenia and lack of CD28 expression on CD8+ T cells	Normal	Variable antibody production	Failure to thrive, bacterial, viral, and fungal infection (thrush)	?	Aberrant alternative splicing of exon 7 of the Lck gene resulting in defective TCR signaling

Table 16A-5. (*Continued*)

Disease	Circulating T cells	Circulating B cells	Serum immunoglobulin	Associated features	Inheritance	Gene defects/ presumed pathogenesis
T- B- SCID[a]						
RAG 1/2 deficiency	Markedly decreased	Markedly decreased	Decreased	Defective VDJ recombination; may present with Omenn syndrome	AR	Defect of recombinase activating gene (RAG) 1 or 2
DCLRE1C (Artemis) deficiency	Markedly decreased	Markedly decreased	Decreased	Defective VDJ recombination, radiation sensitivity; may present with Omenn syndrome	AR	Defect in Artemis DNA recombinase-repair protein
DNA PKcs deficiency	Markedly decreased	Markedly decreased	Decreased	Mouse data available only	AR	Defect in DNAPKcs recombinase repair protein
ADA deficiency	Absent from birth (null mutations) or progressive decrease	Absent from birth or progressive decrease	Progressive decrease	Costochondral junction flaring, neurologic features, hearing impairment, lung and liver manifestations; cases with partial ADA activity may have a delayed or milder presentation	AR	Absent ADA, elevated lymphotoxic metabolites (dATP, S-adenosyl homocysteine)
Reticular dysgenesis	Markedly decreased	Decreased or normal	Decreased	Granulocytopenia, deafness	AR	Defective maturation of T, B, and myeloid cells (stem cell defect) Defect in mitochondrial adenylate kinase 2 (AK2)
Non-SCID Defects						
CD3γ deficiency	Normal, but reduced TCR expression	Normal	Normal		AR	Defect in CD3 γ
ZAP-70 deficiency	Decreased CD8, normal CD4 cells	Normal	Normal		AR	Defects in ZAP-70 signaling kinase
CD8 deficiency	Absent CD8, normal CD4 cells	Normal	Normal		AR	Defects of CD8 α chain
ITK deficiency	Modestly decreased	Normal	Normal or decreased		AR	EBV-associated lymphoproliferation
STAT5b deficiency	Modestly decreased	Normal	Normal	Growth-hormone insensitive dwarfism, dysmorphic features, eczema, lymphocytic interstitial pneumonitis, autoimmunity	AR	Defects of STAT5b, impaired development and function of γδT cells, regulatory T and NK cells, impaired T cell proliferation
CD25 deficiency	Normal to modestly decreased	Normal	Normal	Lymphoproliferation (lymphadenopathy, hepatosplenomegaly),	AR	Defects in IL-2Rα chain

(*Continued*)

Table 16A-5. (*Continued*)

Disease	Circulating T cells	Circulating B cells	Serum immunoglobulin	Associated features	Inheritance	Gene defects/ presumed pathogenesis
				autoimmunity (may resemble IPEX syndrome), impaired T-cell proliferation		
CD40 ligand deficiency	Normal	IgM+ and IgD+ B cells present, other isotypes absent	IgM increased or normal, other isotypes decreased	Neutropenia, thrombocytopenia; hemolytic anemia, biliary tract and liver disease, opportunistic infections	XL	Defects in CD40 ligand (CD40L) cause defective isotype switching and impaired dendritic cell signaling
CD40 deficiency	Normal	IgM+ and IgD+ B cells present, other isotypes absent	IgM increased or normal, other isotypes decreased	Neutropenia, gastrointestinal and liver/biliary tract disease, opportunistic infections	AR	Defects in CD40 cause defective isotype switching and impaired dendritic cell signaling
DOCK8 deficiency	Decreased	Decreased	Low IgM, increased IgE	Recurrent respiratory infections. Extensive cutaneous viral and bacterial (staphylococcal) infections, susceptibility to cancer, hypereosinophilia, severe atopy, low NK cells	AR	Defect in DOCK8
Ca++ channel deficiency	Normal counts, defective TCR-mediated activation	Normal counts	Normal	Autoimmunity, anhydrotic ectodermic dysplasia, nonprogressive myopathy	AR AR	Defect in Oral-1, a Ca++ channel component Defect in Stim-I, a Ca++ sensor
MHC- I deficiency	Decreased CD8, normal CD4	Normal	Normal	Vasculitis	AR	Mutations in TAP1, TAP2, or TAPBP (tapasin) genes giving MHC-I deficiency
MHC-II deficiency	Normal number, decreased CD4 cells	Normal	Normal or decreased		AR	Mutation in transcription factors for MHC-II proteins (C2TA, RFX5, RFXAP, RFXANK genes)
Winged helix deficiency (nude)	Markedly decreased	Normal	Decreased	Alopecia, abnormal thymic epithelium, impaired T cell maturation (widely studied nude mouse defect)	AR	Defects in forkhead box N1 transcription factor encoded by FOXN1, the gene mutated in nude mice
Omenn syndrome[b]	Present; restricted heterogeneity	Normal or decreased	Decreased, except increased IgE	Erythroderma, eosinophilia, adenopathy, hepatosplenomegaly	AR (in most cases)	Hypomorphic mutations in RAG1/2, Artemis, IL-7Rα, RMRP, ADA, DNA ligase IV, γc

Table 16A-5. (*Continued*)

Disease	Circulating T cells	Circulating B cells	Serum immunoglobulin	Associated features	Inheritance	Gene defects/ presumed pathogenesis
NHEJ defects						
DNA ligase IV deficiency	Decreased	Decreased	Decreased	Microcephaly, facial dysmorphisms, radiation sensitivity; may present with Omenn syndrome or with a delayed clinical onset	AR	DNA ligase IV defect, impaired nonhomologous end joining (NHEJ)
Cernunnos deficiency	Decreased	Decreased	Decreased	Microcephaly, in utero growth retardation, radiation sensitivity	AR	Cernunnos defect, impaired NHEJ
Purine nucleoside phosphorylase deficiency	Progressive decrease	Normal	Normal or decreased	Autoimmune hemolytic anemia, neurological impairment	AR	Absent purine nucleoside phosphorylase deficiency, T cell and neurologic defects from elevated toxic metabolites (e.g., dGTP)

ADA = adenosine deaminase; AR = autosomal recessive inheritance; ATP = adenosine triphosphate; C2TA = class II transactivator; EBV = Epstein-Barr virus; FOXN1 = forkhead box N1; GTP = guanosine triphosphate; IL (interleukin); JAK3 = Janus-associated kinase 3; NHEJ = non-homologous end joining; RFX = regulatory factor X; RMRP = RNA component of mitochondrial RNA processing endonuclease; NK = natural killer; RAG = recombinase activating gene; SCID = severe combined immune deficiency; STAT = signal transducer and activator of transcription; TAP = transporter associated with antigen processing; TCR = T cell receptor; XL = X-linked inheritance.****Some metabolic disorders such as methylmalonic aciduria may present with profound lymphopenia in addition to their typical presenting features.

[a]Atypical cases of SCID may present with T cells because of hypomorphic mutations or somatic mutations in T cell precursors.

[b]Frequency may vary from region to region or even among communities, i.e., Mennonite, Innuit, and so forth.

[c]Some cases of Omenn syndrome remain genetically undefined.

Table 16A-6. B lymphocytes

Disease	Serum immunoglobulin	Associated features	Inheritance	Genetic defects/presumed pathogenesis
1. Severe reduction in all serum immunoglobulin isotypes with profoundly decreased or absent B cells				
(a) BTK deficiency	All isotypes decreased	Severe bacterial infections; normal numbers of pro-B cells	XL	Mutations in BTK
(b) μ heavy chain deficiency	All isotypes decreased	Severe bacterial infections; normal numbers of pro-B cells	AR	Mutations in μ heavy chain
(c) λ5 deficiency	All isotypes decreased	Severe bacterial infections; normal numbers of pro-B cells	AR	Mutations in IGLL1 (λ5)
(d) Igα deficiency	All isotypes decreased	Severe bacterial infections; normal numbers of pro-B cells	AR	Mutations in Igα

(*Continued*)

Table 16A-6. (*Continued*)

Disease	Serum immunoglobulin	Associated features	Inheritance	Genetic defects/presumed pathogenesis
(e) Igβ deficiency	All isotypes decreased	Severe bacterial infections; normal numbers of pro-B cells	AR	Mutations in Igβ
(f) BLNK deficiency	All isotypes decreased	Severe bacterial infections; normal numbers of pro-B cells	AR	Mutations in BLNK
(g) Thymoma with immunodeficiency (Good's syndrome)	All isotypes decreased	Bacterial and opportunistic infections; autoimmunity	None	Unknown
2. Severe reduction in at least two serum immunoglobulin isotypes with normal or low numbers of B cells				
(a) Common variable immunodeficiency disorders (CVIDs)[a]	Low IgG and IgA and/or IgM	Clinical phenotypes vary: most have recurrent bacterial infections, some have autoimmune, lymphoproliferative, and/or granulomatous disease	Variable	Unknown
(b) ICOS deficiency	Low IgG and IgA and/or IgM		AR	Mutations in ICOS
(c) CD19 deficiency	Low IgG and IgA and/or IgM		AR	Mutations in CD19
(d) TACI deficiency[b]	Low IgG and IgA and/or IgM		AD or AR or complex	Mutations in TNFRSF13B (TACI)
(e) BAFF receptor deficiency[b]	Low IgG and IgM	Variable clinical expression	AR	Mutations in TNFRSF13C (BAFF-R)
3. Severe reduction in serum IgG and IgA with normal/elevated IgM and normal numbers of B cells				
(a) CD40L deficiency[c]	IgG and IgA decreased; IgM may be normal or increased; B cell numbers may be normal or increased	Opportunistic infections, neutropenia, autoimmune disease	XL	Mutations in CD40L (also called TNFSF5 or CD154)
(b) CD40 deficiency[c]	Low IgG and IgA; normal or raised IgM	Opportunistic infections, neutropenia, autoimmune disease	AR	Mutations in CD40 (also called TNFRSF5)
(c) AID deficiency[d]	IgG and IgA decreased; IgM increased	Enlarged lymph nodes and germinal centers	AR	Mutations in AICDA gene
(d) UNG deficiency[d]	IgG and IgA decreased; IgM increased	Enlarged lymph nodes and germinal centers	AR	Mutation in UNG
4. Isotype or light chain deficiencies with normal numbers of B cells				

Table 16A-6. (*Continued*)

Disease	Serum immunoglobulin	Associated features	Inheritance	Genetic defects/presumed pathogenesis
(a) Ig heavy chain mutations and deletions	One or more IgG and/or IgA subclasses as well as IgE may be absent	May be asymptomatic	AR	Mutation or chromosomal deletion at 14q32
(b) κ chain deficiency	All immunoglobulins have lambda light chain	Asymptomatic	AR	Mutation in κ constant gene
(c) Isolated IgG subclass deficiency	Reduction in one or more IgG subclass	Usually asymptomatic; may have recurrent viral/bacterial infections	Variable	Unknown
(d) IgA with IgG subclass deficiency	Reduced IgA with decrease in one or more IgG subclass	Recurrent bacterial infections in majority	Variable	Unknown
(e) Selective IgA deficiency		Usually asymptomatic; may have recurrent infections with poor antibody responses to carbohydrate antigens; may have allergies or autoimmune disease; a few cases progress to CVID, others coexist with CVID in the same family	Variable	Unknown
5. Specific antibody deficiency with normal Ig concentrations and normal numbers of B cells	Normal	Inability to make antibodies to specific antigens	Variable	Unknown
6. Transient hypogammaglobulinemia of infancy with normal numbers of B cells	IgG and IgA decreased	Recurrent moderate bacterial infections	Variable	Unknown

AD = autosomal dominant inheritance; AID = activation-induced cytidine deaminase; AR = autosomal recessive inheritance; BLNK = B cell linker protein; BTK = Bruton tyrosine kinase; ICOS = inducible costimulator; Igκ = immunoglobulin of κ light-chain type; UNG = uracil-DNA glycosylase; XL = X-linked inheritance.

[a]Common variable immunodeficiency disorders; there are several different clinical phenotypes, probably representing distinguishable diseases with differing immunopathogeneses.

[b]Alterations in TNFRSF13B (TACI) and TNFRSF13C (BAFF-R) sequence may represent disease-modifying mutations rather than disease-causing mutations.

[c]CD40L and CD40 deficiency are also included in Table 16A-1.

[d]Deficiency of AID or UNG present as forms of the hyper-IgM syndrome but differ from CD40L and CD40 deficiencies in that the patients have large lymph nodes with germinal centers and are not susceptible to opportunistic infections.

Table 16A-7. Disorders of immune regulation

Disease	Circulating T cells	Circulating B cells	Serum immunoglobulin	Associated features	Inheritance	Genetic defects, presumed pathogenesis
1. Immunodeficiency with hypopigmentation						
(a) Chediak-Higashi syndrome	Normal	Normal	Normal	Partial albinism, giant lysosomes, low NK and CTL activities, heightened acute-phase reaction, late-onset primary encephalopathy	AR	Defects in LYST, impaired lysosomal trafficking
(b) Griscelli syndrome, type 2	Normal	Normal	Normal	Partial albinism, low NK and CTL activities, heightened acute phase reaction, encephalopathy in some patients	AR	Defects in RAB27A encoding a GTPase in secretory vesicles
(c) Hermansky-Pudlak syndrome, type 2	Normal	Normal	Normal	Partial albinism, neutropenia, low NK and CTL activity, increased bleeding	AR	Mutations of AP3B1 gene, encoding for the β subunit of the AP-3 complex
2. Familial hemophagocytic lymphohistiocytosis (FHL) syndromes						
(a) Perforin deficiency	Normal	Normal	Normal	Severe inflammation, fever, decreased NK and CTL activities	AR	Defects in PRF1; perforin, a major cytolytic protein
(b) UNC13D deficiency	Normal	Normal	Normal	Severe inflammation, fever, decreased NK and CTL activities	AR	Defects in UNC13D required to prime vesicles for fusion
(c) Syntaxin 11 (STX11) deficiency	Normal	Normal	Normal	Severe inflammation, fever, decreased NK activity	AR	Defects in STX11, involved in vesicle trafficking and fusion
3. Lymphoproliferative syndromes						
(a) XLP1, SH2D1A deficiency	Normal	Normal or reduced	Normal or low immunoglobulins	Clinical and immunologic abnormalities triggered by EBV infection, including hepatitis, aplastic anemia, and lymphoma	XL	Defects in SH2D1A encoding an adaptor protein regulating intracellular signals
(b) XLP2, XIAP deficiency	Normal	Normal or reduced	Normal or low immunoglobulins	Clinical and immunologic abnormalities triggered by EBV infection	XL	Defects in BIRC4 (XIAP), encoding an inhibitor of apoptosis

Table 16A-7. (*Continued*)

Disease	Circulating T cells	Circulating B cells	Serum immunoglobulin	Associated features	Inheritance	Genetic defects, presumed pathogenesis
				splenomegaly, hepatitis, hemophagocytic syndrome, and lymphoma		
(c) ITK deficiency	Modestly decreased	Normal	Normal or decreased	EBV-associated lymphoproliferation	AR	Mutations in ITK
4. Syndromes with autoimmunity						
(a) Autoimmune lymphoproliferative syndrome (ALPS)						
(i) CD95 (Fas) defects, ALPS type 1a	Increased CD4- CD8- double negative (DN) T cells	Normal	Normal or increased	Splenomegaly, adenopathy, autoimmune blood cytopenias, defective lymphocyte apoptosis, increased lymphoma risk	AD (rare severe AR cases)	Defects in TNFRSF6, cell surface apoptosis receptor; in addition to germline mutations, somatic mutations cause a similar phenotype
(ii) CD95L (Fas ligand) defects, ALPS type 1b	Increased DN T cells	Normal	Normal	Splenomegaly, adenopathy, autoimmune blood cytopenias, defective lymphocyte apoptosis, SLE	AD or AR	Defects in TNFSF6, ligand for CD95 apoptosis receptor
(iii) Caspase 10 defects, ALPS type 2a	Increased DN T cells	Normal	Normal	Adenopathy, splenomegaly, autoimmune disease, defective lymphocyte apoptosis	AR	Defects in CASP10, intracellular apoptosis pathway
(iv) Caspase 8 defects, ALPS type 2b	Slightly increased DN T cells	Normal	Normal or decreased	Adenopathy, splenomegaly, recurrent bacterial and viral infections, defective lymphocyte apoptosis and activation	AR	Defects in CASP8, intracellular apoptosis and activation pathways
(v) Activating N-Ras defect, N-Ras-dependent ALPS	Increased DN T cells	Elevation of CD5 B cells	Normal	Adenopathy, splenomegaly, leukemia, lymphoma, defective lymphocyte apoptosis after IL-2 withdrawal	AD	Defect in NRAS encoding a GTP binding protein with diverse signaling functions, activating mutations impair mitochondrial apoptosis
(b) Autoimmune polyendocrine syndromes (APS)						

(*Continued*)

Table 16A-7. (*Continued*)

Disease	Circulating T cells	Circulating B cells	Serum immunoglobulin	Associated features	Inheritance	Genetic defects, presumed pathogenesis
(i) APECED, autoimmune polyendocrine syndrome type I with candidiasis and ectodermal dystrophy	Normal	Normal	Normal	Autoimmune disease, particularly of parathyroid, adrenal and other endocrine organs plus candidiasis, dental enamel hypoplasia and other abnormalities	AR	Defects in AIRE, needed to establish thymic self-tolerance
(ii) Autoimmune polyendocrine syndrome type II (Schmidt's syndrome)	Normal	Normal	Normal	Addison's disease, type IA diabetes, chronic thyroiditis	Polygenic	?
(c) IPEX, immune dysregulation, polyendocrinopathy, enteropathy (X-linked)	Defects in AIRE, encoding a transcription regulator needed to establish thymic self-tolerance	Normal	Elevated IgA, IgE	Autoimmune diarrhea, early onset diabetes, thyroiditis, hemolytic anemia, thrombocytopenia, eczema	XL	Defects in FOXP3, encoding a T cell transcription factor
(d) CD25 deficiency	Normal to modestly decreased	Normal	Normal	Lymphoproliferation, autoimmunity, impaired T cell proliferation	AR	Defects in IL-2Ra chain

AD = autosomal-dominant; AIRE = autoimmune regulator; AP3B1 = adaptor protein complex 3 beta 1 subunit; AR = autosomal recessive; CASP = caspase; CTL = cytotoxic T lymphocyte; DN = double negative; FOXP3 = forkhead box protein 3; LYST = lysosomal trafficking regulator; NRAS = neuroblastoma Ras protein; PRF1 = perforin 1; RAB27A = Ras-associated protein 27A; SH2D1A = SH2 domain protein 1A; TNFRSF6 = tumor necrosis factor receptor soluble factor 6; TNFSF6 = tumor necrosis factor soluble factor 6; IAP = X-linked inhibitor of apoptosis; XL = X-linked; XLP = X-linked lymphoproliferative disease.

Table 16A-8. Other well-defined immunodeficiencies

Disease	Circulating T cells	Circulating B cells	Serum immunoglobulin	Associated features	Inheritance	Genetic defects/ presumed pathogenesis
1. Wiskott-Aldrich syndrome (WAS)	Progressive decrease, abnormal lymphocyte responses to anti-CD3	Normal	Decreased IgM: antibody to polysaccharides particularly decreased; often increased IgA and IgE	Thrombocytopenia with small platelets; eczema; lymphomas; autoimmune disease; IgA nephropathy; bacterial and viral infections; XL thrombocytopenia is a mild form of WAS, and XL neutropenia is caused by missense mutations in the GTPase binding domain of WASP	XL	Mutations in WAS; cytoskeletal defect affecting hematopoietic stem cell derivatives

Table 16A-8. (*Continued*)

Disease	Circulating T cells	Circulating B cells	Serum immunoglobulin	Associated features	Inheritance	Genetic defects/ presumed pathogenesis
2. DNA repair defects (other than those in 16A-5 in the Annex)						
(a) Ataxia-telangiectasia	Progressive decrease	Normal	Often decreased IgA, IgE, and IgG subclasses; increased IgM monomers; antibodies variably decreased	Ataxia; telangiectasia; pulmonary infections; lymphoreticular and other malignancies; increased α fetoprotein and X-ray sensitivity; chromosomal instability	AR	Mutations in ATM; disorder of cell cycle checkpoint and DNA double-strand break repair
(b) Ataxia-telangiectasia like disease (ATLD)	Progressive decrease	Normal	Antibodies variably decreased	Moderate ataxia; pulmonary infections; severely increased radiosensitivity	AR	Hypomorphic mutations in MRE11; disorder of cell cycle checkpoint and DNA double-strand break repair
(c) Nijmegen breakage syndrome	Progressive decrease	Variably reduced	Often decreased IgA, IgE, and IgG subclasses; increased IgM; antibodies variably decreased	Microcephaly; bird-like face; lymphomas; solid tumors; ionizing radiation sensitivity; chromosomal instability	AR	Hypomorphic mutations in NBS1 (Nibrin); disorder of cell cycle checkpoint and DNA double-strand break repair
(d) Bloom syndrome	Normal	Normal	Reduced	Short stature; bird-like face; sun-sensitive erythema; marrow failure; leukemia; lymphoma; chromosomal instability	AR	Mutations in BLM; RecQ like helicase
(e) Immunodeficiency with centromeric instability and facial anomalies (ICF)	Decreased or normal	Decreased or normal	Hypogammaglobulinemia; variable antibody deficiency	Facial dysmorphic features; macroglossia; bacterial/opportunistic infections; malabsorption; multiradial configurations of chromosomes 1, 9, 16; no DNA breaks	AR	Mutations in DNA methyltransferase DNMT3B, resulting in defective DNA methylation
(f) PMS2 deficiency (class-switch recombination [CSR] deficiency caused by defective mismatch repair)	Normal	Switched and non-switched B cells are reduced	Low IgG and IgA, elevated IgM, abnormal antibody responses	Recurrent infections; café au lait spots; lymphoma, colorectal carcinoma, brain tumor	AR	Mutations in PMS2, resulting in defective CSR-induced DNA double strand breaks in Ig switch regions

(*Continued*)

Table 16A-8. (*Continued*)

Disease	Circulating T cells	Circulating B cells	Serum immunoglobulin	Associated features	Inheritance	Genetic defects/ presumed pathogenesis
3. Thymic defects						
DiGeorge anomaly (chromosome 22q11.2 deletion syndrome)	Decreased or normal	Normal	Normal or decreased	Conotruncal malformation; abnormal facies; large deletion (3Mb) in 22q11.2 (or rarely a deletion in 10p)	*De novo* defect or AD	Contiguous gene defect in 90% affecting thymic development; mutation in *TBX1*
4. Immune-osseous dysplasias						
(a) Cartilage hair hypoplasia	Decreased or normal; impaired lymphocyte proliferation[a]	Normal	Normal or reduced; antibodies variably decreased	Short-limbed dwarfism with metaphyseal dysostosis, sparse hair, bone marrow failure, autoimmunity, susceptibility to lymphoma and other cancers, impaired spermatogenesis, neuronal dysplasia of the intestine	AR	Mutations in RMRP (RNase MRP RNA); involved in processing of mitochondrial RNA and cell cycle control
(b) Immunoosseous dysplasia, Schimke type	Decreased	Normal	Normal	Short stature, spondiloepiphyseal dysplasia, intrauterine growth retardation, nephropathy; bacterial, viral, fungal infections; may present as SCID; bone marrow failure	AR	Mutations in SMARCAL1 involved in chromatin remodeling
5. Netherton syndrome	Normal	Switched and non-switched B cells are reduced	Elevated IgE and IgA; antibody variably decreased	Congenital ichthyosis, bamboo hair, atopic diathesis, increased bacterial infections, failure to thrive	AR	Mutations in SPINK5 resulting in lack of the serine protease inhibitor LEKTI, expressed in epithelial cells
6. Hyper-IgE syndromes (HIES)						
(a) AD-HIES (Job's syndrome)	Normal TH16 cells decreased	Normal	Elevated IgE; specific antibody production decreased	Distinctive facial features (broad nasal bridge), eczema, osteoporosis and fractures, scoliosis, failure/delay of shedding primary teeth, hyperextensible joints, bacterial infections (skin and pulmonary abscesses/pneumatoceles) caused by *Staphylococcus aureus*, candidiasis	AD Often *de novo* defect	Dominant-negative heterozygous mutations in STAT3

Table 16A-8. (*Continued*)

Disease	Circulating T cells	Circulating B cells	Serum immunoglobulin	Associated features	Inheritance	Genetic defects/ presumed pathogenesis
(b) AR-HIES	Normal Reduced Normal	Normal Reduced Normal	Elevated IgE Elevated IgE, low IgM Elevated IgE	No skeletal and connective tissue abnormalities; (1) susceptibility to intracellular bacteria (mycobacteria, *Salmonella*), fungi, and viruses (2) recurrent respiratory infections; extensive cutaneous viral and staphylococcal infections, increased risk of cancer, severe atopy with anaphylaxis (3) CNS hemorrhage, fungal and viral infections	AR	Mutation in TYK2 Mutation in DOCK8 Unknown
7. Chronic mucocutaneous candidiasis	Normal (defect of Th16 cells in CARD9 deficiency)	Normal	Normal	Chronic mucocutaneous candidiasis, impaired delayed-type hypersensitivity to *Candida* antigens, autoimmunity, no ectodermal dysplasia	AD, AR, sporadic	Mutations in CARD9 in one family with AR inheritance; defect unknown in other cases
8. Hepatic veno-occlusive disease with immunodeficiency (VODI)	Normal (decreased memory T cells)	Normal (decreased memory B cells)	Decreased IgG, IgA, and IgM	Hepatic veno-occlusive disease; *Pneumocystis jiroveci* pneumonia; thrombocytopenia; hepatosplenomegaly	AR	Mutations in SP110
9. X-linked dyskeratosis congenita (DKC)	Progressive decrease	Progressive decrease	Variable	Intrauterine growth retardation, microcephaly, nail dystrophy, recurrent infections, digestive tract involvement, pancytopenia, reduced number and function of NK cells	XL	Mutations in dyskerin (DKC1)

AD = autosomal dominant inheritance; AR = autosomal recessive inheritance; ATM = ataxia-telangiectasia mutated; BLM = Bloom syndrome; DNMT3B = DNA methyltransferase 3B; MRE11 = meiotic recombination 11; NBS1 = Nijmegen breakage syndrome 1; TBX1 = T-box 1; TYK2 = tyrosine kinase 2; XL = X-linked inheritance.

[a]Patients with cartilage-hair hypoplasia can also present with typical SCID or with Omenn syndrome.

Chapter 17

Mechanisms of Immunologic Injury

Joseph A. Bellanti, MD
Alejandro Escobar-Gutiérrez, PhD

Classification Systems

The four-group classification system of hypersensitivity reactions causing tissue injury originally proposed by Gell and Coombs in 1963 has provided a valuable taxonomic system for understanding the mechanisms of tissue injury seen in a wide variety of immune-mediated diseases ranging from the allergic diseases to the autoimmune disorders. The system attempted to categorize mechanisms of immunologic injury as they relate to human immunologically-mediated diseases and was restricted to disorders arising from components of adaptive immunity, i.e., B cells and T cells.

Although the classification system continues to serve as a categorization of iconic proportions, it has become increasingly clear that there are other immunologically-mediated diseases that arise from disorders of innate immunity that the original Gell and Coombs classification did not take into consideration. Immunologically-mediated tissue injury is now recognized to derive from the damaging effects of either the innate or the adaptive immune responses.

The adaptive mechanisms of immunologic injury described in this chapter have been clustered into an expanded version of the Gell and Coombs classification of hypersensitivity reactions and are subdivided according to more recently recognized components of the adaptive immune armamentarium responsible for the pathologic sequelae of many immune-mediated clinical disorders. Equally important is the recognition that certain diseases are the consequence of more complex tissue-damaging mechanisms resulting from innate immune-mediated injury. In response to an ever-emerging and constantly widening information pool related to innate immune function in health and disease, a new expanded classification of mechanisms of innate immune tissue injury is presented that may be clinically useful.

LEARNING OBJECTIVES

When you have completed this chapter, you should be able to:

- Understand the Gell and Coombs Type I–IV classification of hypersensitivity reactions and recognize its clinical implications in disease pathogenesis, diagnosis, and treatment of a wide variety of immunologically-mediated conditions
- Recognize the mechanisms of Type I hypersensitivity reactions important in the pathogenesis of allergic (atopic) diseases and asthma
- Differentiate the three types of antibody-mediated Type II hypersensitivity reactions
- Understand the differences between localized and systemic Type III immune complex-mediated hypersensitivity reactions
- Appreciate the new four subtypes of the Type IV T cell-mediated hypersensitivity reactions
- Recognize that the original Gell and Coombs Type I–IV classification is based on abnormalities of the adaptive immune system responsible for tissue injury seen in allergy, chronic infection, and autoimmune disease
- Understand the limitations of the use of the Gell and Coombs classification in defining other types of tissue injury associated with a wide variety of inflammatory disorders that are based on disorders of the innate immune system
- Utilize this information for an understanding of the role these various mechanisms of immunologic injury in the pathogenesis of a wide variety of immunologically-mediated diseases as well as in the maintenance of normal immunologic homeostasis

Introduction: The Concept of Immunologically Mediated Disease

As described in Chapter 1 and throughout this book, the basic function of the immunologic system is to detect and eliminate substances from the body that are recognized as non-self, i.e., reactions to foreign substances or to danger signals. In performing these functions, the host employs a wide variety of cells and cell products derived from both the innate and adaptive immune systems (i.e., cytokines, chemokines, inflammatory mediators, complement, and immunoglobulins), each interacting with one another through a variety of molecular signaling systems to remove these foreign materials or to respond to danger signals. Usually such interactions are efficient and successful without detriment to the host. Occasionally, however, when the type of foreign substance presented to the immune system or the immunologic reactivity of the host to these signals is inappropriate, perturbations occur that lead to harmful sequelae—**the immunologically-mediated diseases.**

In Chapter 1, a model was presented summating the total immunologic reactivity of the host to all foreign material in three phases as a concept of **immunologic balance** (Figure 17-1) in which the ultimate function of the immunologic system is to maintain an equilibrated homeostasis between the external and internal environments. The model is based on the following three assumptions concerning the immune response: (1) the foreign substance drives the system, i.e., active immune responses occur only as long as the foreign substance is present and will cease after its removal; (2) three stages exist through which all foreign substances are removed by the immune system, i.e., the *innate* immune response, the *adaptive* immune response, and the *tissue-damaging* immune responses; and (3) the extent of the progression through these three phases is determined both by the nature of the foreign substance as well as by the genetic constitution of the host and the balance provided by the regulatory mechanisms governing the response. Implicit in this model is that the outcome of the immune encounter can either be **beneficial** or, at times, **detrimental**, and is dependent both on the type and amount of the foreign substance presented as well as on the efficiency of its elimination. As presented in several chapters of this book, if foreignness is successfully eliminated during the first two phases of innate and adaptive immunity, the outcome of the immune encounter will be beneficial and represent the manifestations of the **immune response in health.** If on the other hand the foreign agent persists and cannot be eliminated, the most detrimental expressions of disease are seen in the form of the tissue-damaging immune responses and represent the **immune response in disease.** The duration of this tissue-damaging phase can either be temporary if the foreign insult can be terminated, e.g., cessation of penicillin therapy in a patient with a penicillin reaction, or more protracted if the foreign substance cannot be removed. In this latter scenario, the most serious sequelae of immune injury are manifest in the form of chronic infection (*Chapters 12–15*), autoimmune and autoinflammatory diseases (*Chapter 19*), or cancer (*Chapter 20* and Figure 17-1). This chapter will focus on the mechanisms of immunologic injury contributing to the pathogenesis of a variety of immunologically-mediated diseases.

Mechanisms of Hypersensitivity and Immunologic Injury: Manifestations of the Tissue-Damaging Immune Responses: The Gell and Coombs Classification of Hypersensitivity Reactions

The classical work of Professors Philip George Houthem Gell (1914–2001) and Robert Royston Amos ("Robin") Coombs (1921–2006) is based on a classification of hypersensitivity reactions caused by tissue injury mediated by disorders of the adaptive immune response. The classification divides these hypersensitivity reactions into four major categories (Types I–IV) based not only on the tissue-damaging mechanisms involved in immune injury, but also on the timing and type of immunological component involved, i.e., antibody or cell-mediated. It is important to emphasize that the system is not a disease classification but rather an effort to categorize **mechanisms** of immunologic injury as they relate to human immunologically-mediated diseases and was restricted to disorders arising from components of adaptive immunity, i.e., B and T cells. Consequently, while in some immune-mediated diseases, only one type of mechanism can be causative, in others, more than one type of response may play a role either concurrently or sequentially. Recently, it has become increasingly clear that there are other immunologically-mediated diseases that arise from genetic defects or excessive expression of the

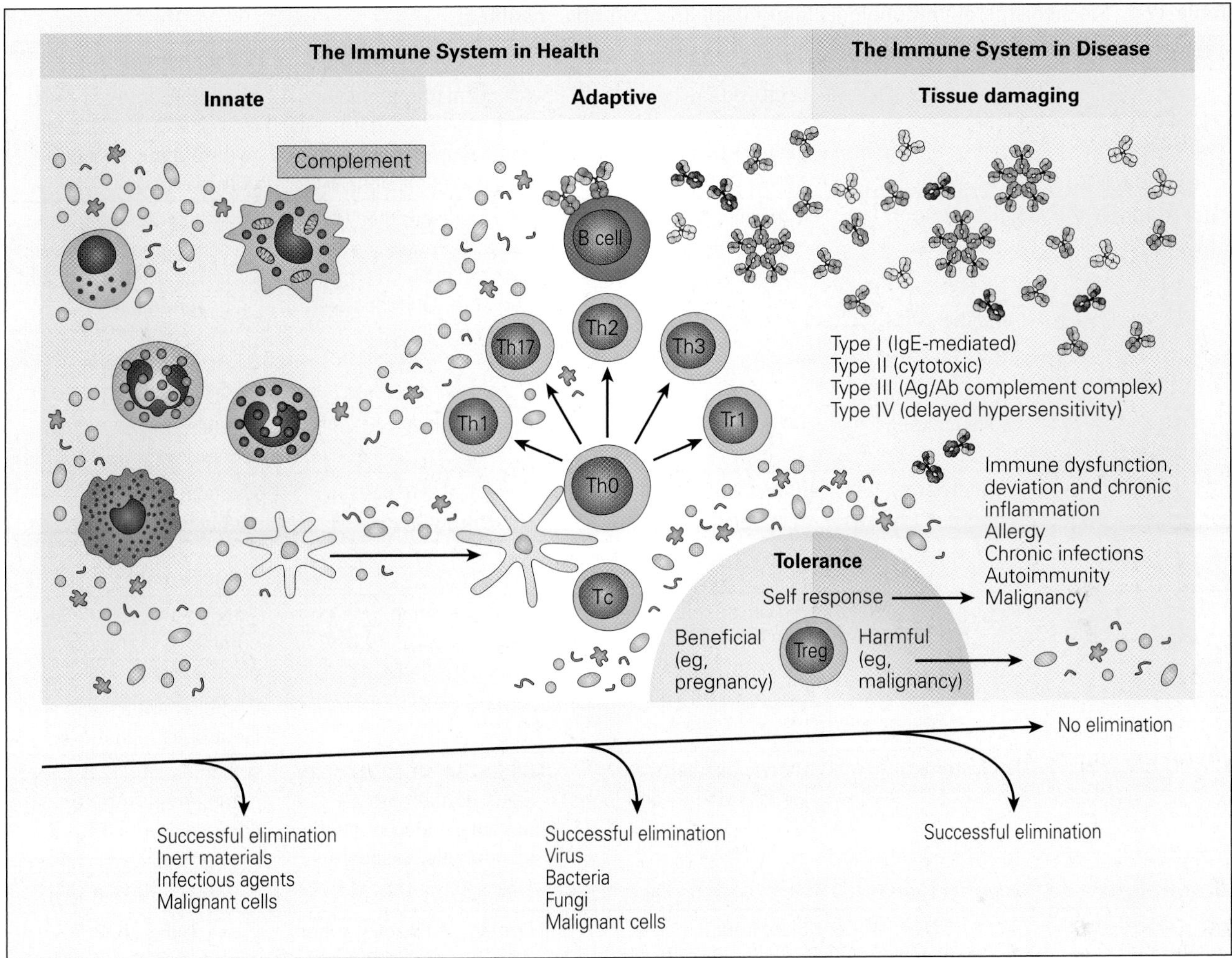

Figure 17-1. Schematic representation of the total immunologic capability of the host based on the efficiency of the elimination of foreign matter. There are three responses through which all foreign substances are removed by the immune system, i.e., the *innate* immune response, the adaptive immune response, and the *tissue-damaging* immune response, the extent of which is determined both by the nature of the foreign substance as well as by the genetic constitution of the host. The outcome of the immune encounter can either be beneficial or detrimental and is dependent on the type and amount of the foreign substance presented and the efficiency of its elimination. If foreignness is successfully eliminated during the first two phases of innate and adaptive immunity, the outcome of the immune encounter will be beneficial and will represent the manifestations of the immune system in health. If the foreign agent persists and cannot be eliminated, the most detrimental expressions of disease are seen in the form of the tissue-damaging immune responses triggered by inflammasome-mediated inflammation or one or more of the Gell and Coombs Type I–IV hypersensitivity reactions that represent the immune system in disease. The duration of the tissue-damaging phase can either be temporary if the foreign insult can be terminated or more protracted if the substance cannot be removed. In this latter scenario, the most serious sequelae of immune injury can manifest in the form of chronic infection, allergic disease, autoimmune disease, or cancer.

inflammasome (recently named inflammasopathies) that the original Gell and Coombs classification does not take into consideration. These include innate response-mediated disorders and autoinflammatory diseases (*Chapter 19* Annex). Nevertheless, the Gell and Coombs classification has unquestionably been extremely important in understanding the mechanisms of tissue injury in several of the infectious diseases (*Chapters 12–15*), adverse reactions to vaccines (*Chapter 23*), the allergic diseases (*Chapter 18*), the autoimmune disorders (*Chapter 19*), and some of the untoward responses to cancer (*Chapter 20*). Since its original description, owing to the recognition of an ever-increasing number of cellular and molecular components involved in adaptive immune injury, the Gell and Coombs classification has been expanded to include subclassifications of the four major originally defined categories that are described in this chapter (Table 17-1).

Table 17-1. Mechanisms of immunologic injury (Gell and Coombs, modified)

Type		Target organs	Clinical manifestations	Mechanisms
I. Anaphylactic		Localized reactions, e.g., skin, respiratory tract, gastrointestinal tract Systemic reactions	Allergic asthma, rhinitis, urticaria, atopic dermatitis (early phase), gastrointestinal allergy, anaphylaxis	IgE bound to mast cells/basophils and mediator release after reaction with allergen
II. Antibody-mediated	A. Cytolytic (cytotoxic)	Circulating blood cells (red cells, white cells, and platelets); basement membrane proteins	Hemolytic anemia, leukopenia, thrombocytopenia, hemolytic disease of the newborn, Goodpasture's syndrome	1. IgG, IgM-mediated complement cytolysis 2. IgG and C3b-mediated opsonization in phagocytes 3. ADCC reactions (NK cells)
	B. Neutralizing	Skeletal muscle cells	Myasthenia gravis	IgG blocking of cellular receptors
	C. Stimulatory	Endocrine and skin cells	Graves' disease Autoimmune urticaria	Overstimulation of cellular receptors with excessive production of hormones or mediators
III. Immune complex-mediated	A. Local	Blood vessels of dermis	Arthus reaction, pneumonitis caused by hypersensitivity	Antigen-antibody (IgG)-complement (Ag-Ab-C) complexes Complement activation Neutrophil recruitment
	B. Systemic	Blood vessels of skin, joints, kidneys, and lungs	Serum sickness, systemic lupus erythematosus, poststreptococcal glomerulonephritis, vasculitis	Antigen-antibody (IgG)-complement (Ag-Ab-C) complexes Complement activation Neutrophil recruitment
IV. Cell-mediated (delayed hypersensitivity)	A. Th1 CD4+ cell-mediated	Skin, lung, GI	Contact dermatitis, tuberculosis, celiac disease	IFN-γ, TNF-α, IL-2 macrophages, NK cells
	B. Th2 CD4+ cell-mediated	Skin, lung, GI	(Chronic) atopic dermatitis (late phase), esophageal GI disorders	IL-4, IL-5, IL-13 eosinophils, B cells
	C. Th17 CD4+ cell-mediated	Skin, lung, GI	Psoriasis, Crohn's disease	IL-17, IL-21, IL-22 neutrophils, fibroblasts, keratinocytes
	D. Cytotoxic CD8+ T cell-mediated	Skin, systemic	Contact dermatitis; celiac disease	CD8+ lymphocytes

The Type I Reaction

The Type I reaction in the human is mediated by IgE antibodies (formerly referred to as "reaginic" antibodies) (Table 17-1 and Figure 17-2). These antibodies are produced by B cells through antigen-presenting cell (**APC**)-Th2 cognate interactions with allergen, display affinity, and specificity for the high-affinity FcεRI receptor on cell membranes of mast cells and basophils (*Chapters 1* and *18*). Following interaction of allergen with these receptor-bound IgE molecules on mediator cells, release of preformed histamine, tryptase, and chymase as well as the generation of cysteinyl leukotrienes (LTC4, LTD4, and LTE4) and prostaglandin D2 occurs within minutes of interaction with allergen and is thus termed the **immediate reaction**. A later subsequent phase, occurring after several hours as a result of the influx of eosinophils mediated by cytokines and chemokines, is termed the **late reaction** and is mediated by a Type IVB reaction described below. Although this IgE response may be seen in the normal individual as a consequence of immunity to parasitic disease (*Chapter 15*), in genetically predisposed (i.e., atopic)

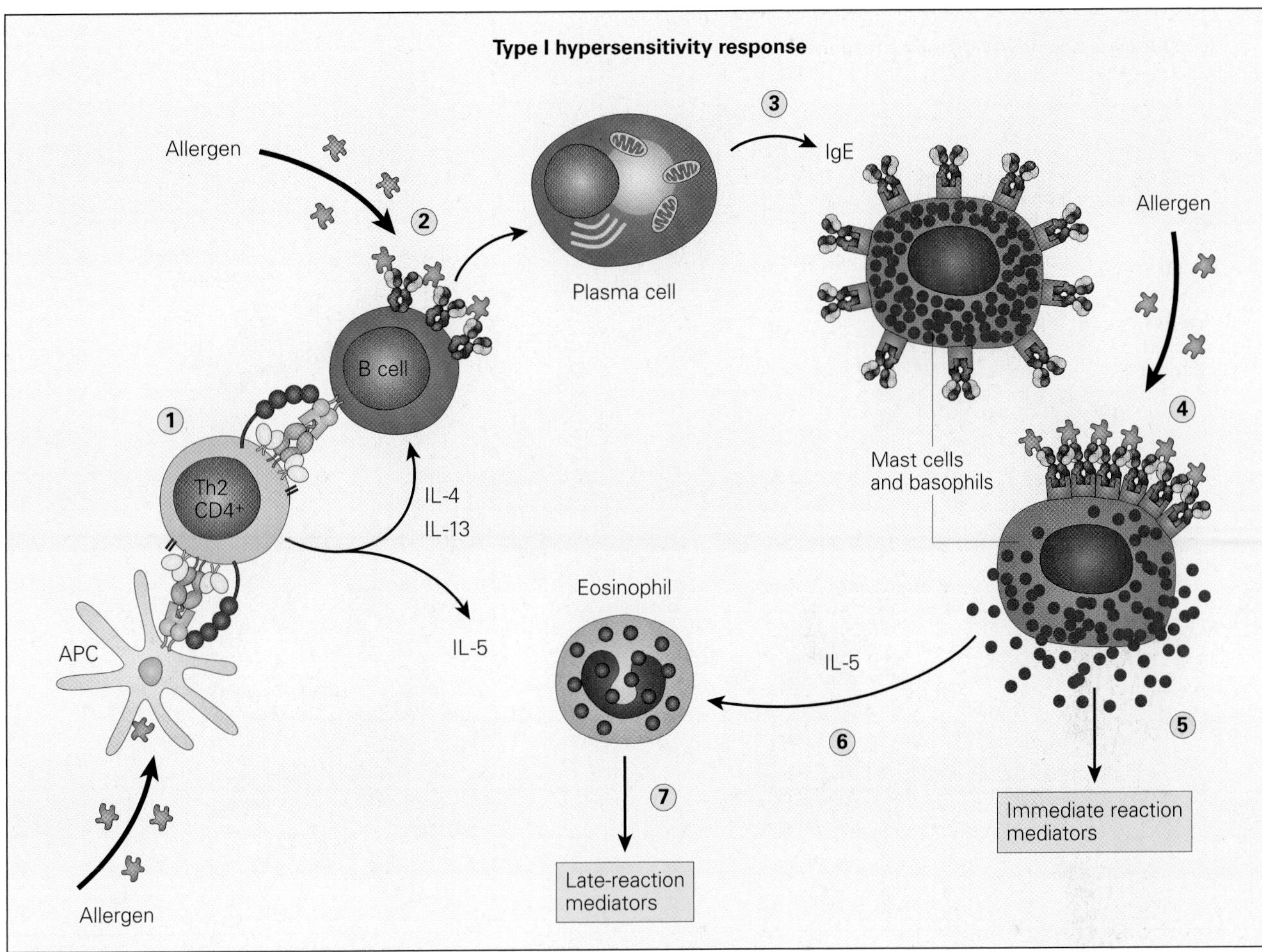

Figure 17-2. Schematic representation of the Type 1 Gell and Coombs hypersensitivity reaction. An initial phase of sensitization takes place where the B cell, i.e., plasma cell (PC), is stimulated by allergen to produce specific IgE antibody either directly or by allergen processed by an antigen-presenting cell (APC)-Th2 cell interaction. These antibodies bind to the high-affinity FcεRI receptor on mediator cells (MCs), i.e., mast cells and basophils, following which the release of pharmacologically vasoactive amines is triggered within minutes of interaction with allergen and is thus termed the immediate reaction. A later phase of the reaction occurs after several hours as a result of the influx of other inflammatory cells, e.g., eosinophils, by cytokines and chemokines and is termed the late reaction.

individuals, this response is often aberrant and excessive and is responsible for the symptoms typically seen with allergic disease (*Chapter 18*). Release of mediators can cause edema, erythema, pruritus, mucus production, smooth cell constriction, and even systemic responses, depending on whether the location of the target organ(s) is localized or more systemically distributed. The target organs most commonly involved in Type I injury are the respiratory tract, the skin, and the gastrointestinal tract, clinically expressed as urticaria/angioedema and atopic dermatitis on skin, allergic rhinitis, and allergic asthma in the respiratory tract, vomiting, abdominal cramping, and diarrhea in the gastrointestinal tract, and the life-threatening expression of systemic involvement known as anaphylaxis (*Chapter 18*).

The Type II Reaction

The Type II reaction or the antibody-target cell reaction is usually brought about by an IgG antibody-mediated response directed against antigens displayed on the surface of a target cell, with or without the participation of complement and/or other cellular elements. There are several origins for the antigens found on target cell surfaces; these include (1) some self-constitutive antigens that are expressed in autoimmune disorders; (2) molecules derived from some intracellular infectious agents, i.e., viruses and bacteria, that are expressed on the host's cell surface; (3) neoantigens resulting from cells transformed by infection, neoplasia, or chemical carcinogens; and (4) some cell surface molecules originating from chemicals (mainly drugs) or extracellular microbial infectious

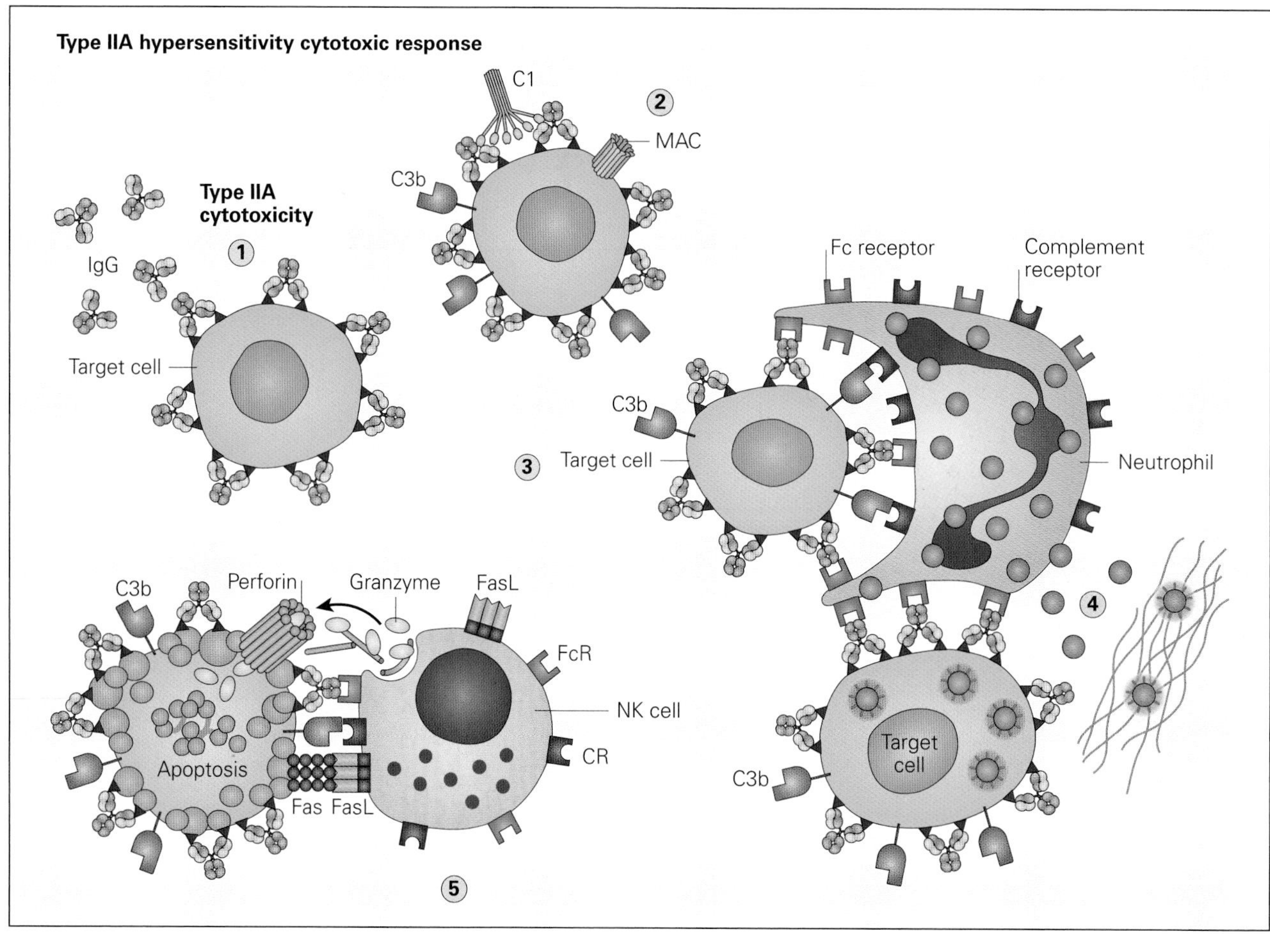

Figure 17-3. Schematic representation of the Type IIA Cell and Coombs cytotoxicity reaction showing four consequences by which a target cell can be killed by various IgG antibody-mediated reactions directed to a surface antigen on a target cell (Panel #1). In the first example (Panel #2), the death of the cell occurs as a result of complement activation with production of the membrane-attack complex and complement-mediated cytotoxicity. The next possibility (Panel #3) results from phagocytosis of the target cell that has been opsonized either by the C3b component of complement or by the Fab fragment of the IgG molecule. Following ingestion of the target cell through complement receptors (CR1, CR2, and CR4 for C3b) or Fc gamma receptors (FcγRI, FcγRIIA, or FcγRIIIA) on the phagocytic cell, respectively, the phagocytosed cell undergoes cell death. If the target cell is too large to be ingested (Panel #4), as in the case of a parasitic organism, cell death can occur through a cytotoxic attack of the target cell mediated by the extracellular release of proteolytic enzymes from the phagocytic cell. A fourth mechanism of cytotoxic cell death (Panel #5) is mediated by a perforin/granzyme mechanism by natural killer cells in an antibody-dependent cellular cytoxicity (ADCC) reaction where the IgG antibody attached to the target cell through its Fab fragment also attaches to the NK cell through its FcγRIIIA receptor, resulting in apoptotic cell death.

agents that are passively (adsorbed) or chemically bound on cell membranes. Collectively, these mechanisms may lead to any of three cell damaging mechanisms or consequences: cell death (i.e., cytotoxicity), cellular neutralization, or cellular stimulation (Table 17-1 and Figures 17-3, 17-4, and 17-5).

Cytotoxicity

In the **cytotoxic subtype** of Type II hypersensitivity (**Type IIA**), the consequences of cell death begin with the binding of antigen-specific antibody with a target cell (Figure 17-3, #1). The target cell is then killed by any of the following mechanisms: (1) antibody (IgM or IgG)-mediated activation of complement on the cell surface leading to cytolysis by the action of the classic pathway of activation and formation of the membrane-attack complex (**MAC**) component (*Chapter 4* and Figure 17-3, #2); (2) opsonization mediated by the binding of C3b fragments on the target cell surface to complement receptors (CR1, CR2, and CR4 for C3b) or with the Fc fragment of IgG target cell-attached antibody through FcγRI, FcγRIIA, or FcγRIIIA (*Chapter 6*), resulting in enhanced uptake and phagocytosis of the target cell by phagocytic cells (neutrophils and macrophages), following which the phagocytosed target cell subsequently undergoes intracellular cell death

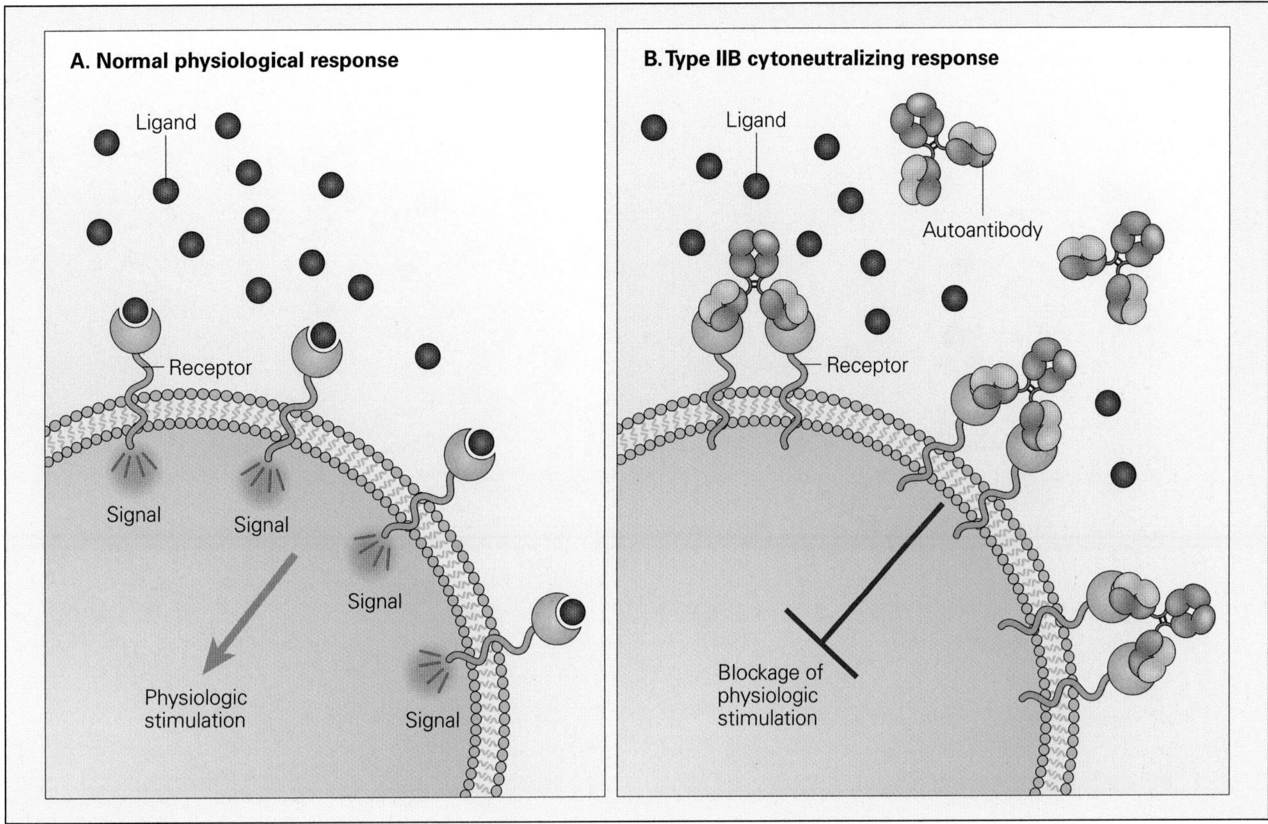

Figure 17-4. Schematic representation of the Type IIB cytoneutralizing response. Panel A: A normal physiologic stimulation of a cell resulting from activation of receptors by ligands. Panel B: Autoantibody directed against the receptor, blocking the binding of the physiologic ligands with the receptors thus preventing normal physiologic stimulation, e.g., anti-acetylcholine receptor antibody, found in myasthenia gravis.

(*Chapter 4* and Figure 17-3, #3); (3) if the target cell is too large to be phagocytosed, cytoxicity can result from the extracellular release of reactive oxygen species and proteolytic enzymes from the phagocytic cell (Figure 17-3, #4); (4) an antibody-dependent cellular cytotoxicity (**ADCC**) reaction (*Chapter 3*) can occur in which either C3b or the Fc fragment of IgG antibodies bound either directly or to cognate antigens on the target cell surface can then interact through C3 receptors or FcγRIIIA, respectively, on a natural killer (**NK**) cell (Figure 17-3, #5).

Examples of diseases mediated by Type IIA cytotoxic reactions are shown in Table 17-1. These include hemolytic disease of the newborn (**HDN**), when transplacentally acquired maternal IgG antibodies directed to a paternal red blood cell (**RBC**) antigen on fetal erythrocytes, e.g., Rh antigen, lead to rapid uptake and destruction of the antibody-coated cells by the fetus with resultant anemia and jaundice; other hemolytic anemias can result from passively acquired antibodies, e.g., blood transfusions or active autoantibody formation in autoimmune diseases, e.g., systemic lupus erythematosus (**SLE**) or complement-mediated destruction of red blood cells; other hematologic pancytopenias can result from innocent bystander cell destruction of platelets, leukocytes, and red blood cells when foreign antigens are nonspecifically coated to their cell surfaces, e.g., usually drugs; and Goodpasture's syndrome, a rare condition characterized by glomerulonephritis and hemorrhaging of the lungs due to autoantibodies targeting self-cell surface antigens on the glomerular basement membrane and the pulmonary alveolus.

Cellular Neutralization

Type IIB hypersensitivity reactions are characterized by **cellular neutralization** as a result of the antagonistic interaction of an autoantibody and a normal cell receptor, resulting in the blockage of a physiologic response of the ligand with its receptor (Figure 17-4). A classic example of this reaction is myasthenia gravis, a disease in which IgG autoantibodies are produced against the acetylcholine receptor in skeletal muscle (*Chapter 19*). These antibodies compete

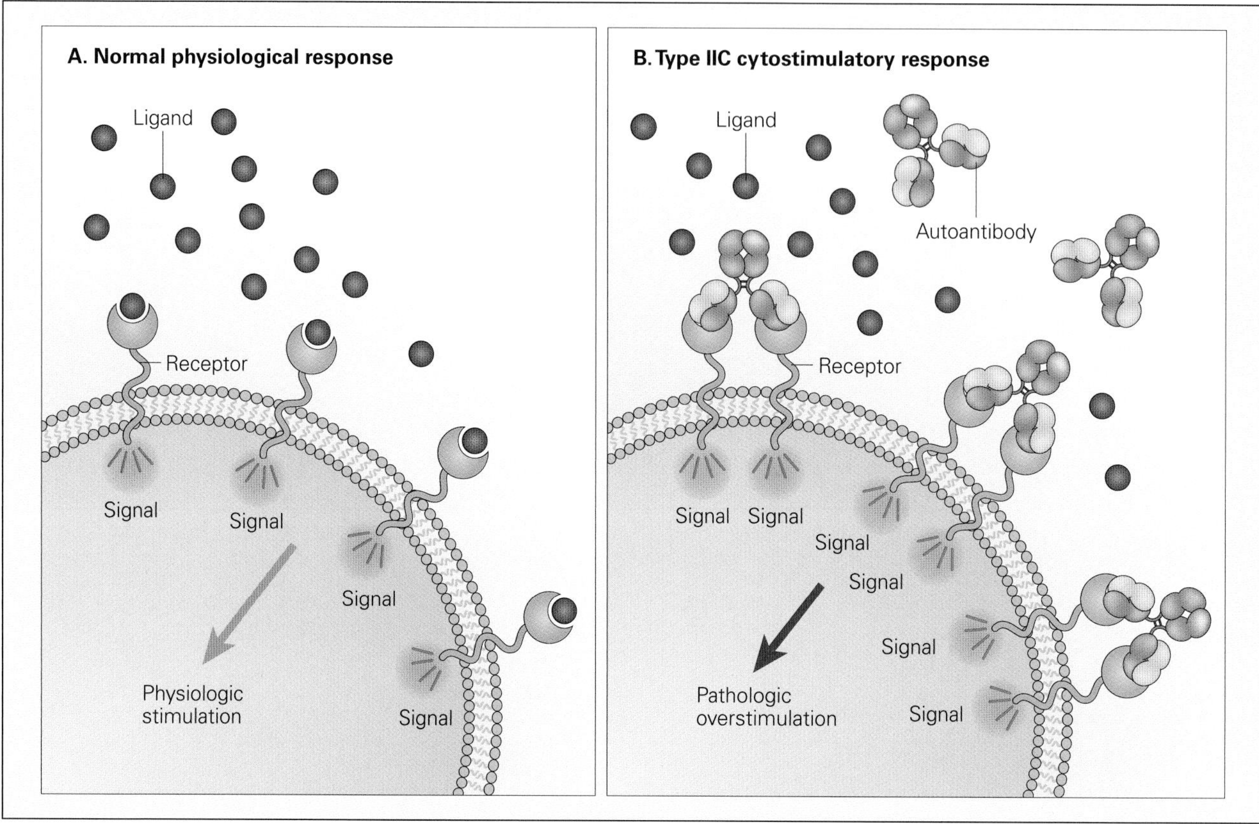

Figure 17-5. Schematic representation of the Type IIC cytostimulatory response. Panel A: A normal physiologic stimulation of a cell resulting from activation of receptors by ligands. Panel B: Autoantibody attached to the receptors, causing excessive pathologic stimulation by the enhancing effect of autoantibody directed against a normal physiologic receptor, i.e., the anti-TSH receptor antibody, responsible for the hyperthyroidism seen in patients with Graves' disease.

with acetylcholine and block or neutralize the effect of acetylcholine at this receptor site, leading to the resultant skeletal muscle weakness characteristic of this disease (Table 17-1).

Cytostimulation

Type IIC hypersensitivity reactions are characterized by **cytostimulation** as a result of the enhancing effect of an autoantibody directed to a normal cell receptor, resulting in the pathologic stimulation of the target cell with a pathologic overproduction of a cell product, e.g., a hormone (Figure 17-5). A disease characterized by this type of hypersensitivity reaction is Graves' disease (thyrotoxicosis), in which autoantibodies, previously referred to as the long-acting thyroid stimulator (**LATS**), directed to the thyrotropin receptor (also known as the thyroid-stimulating hormone [**TSH**] receptor or TSH receptor) lead to the overproduction of thyroid hormones, resulting in hyperthyroidism (*Chapter 19* and Table 17-1). Although this subtype of Type II hypersensitivity has been sometimes classified as a Type V reaction, the assignment of this antibody-mediated reaction to a Type IIB category seems more appropriate.

The Type III Reaction

A third mechanism of immunologic injury is the immune complex, or Type III hypersensitivity reaction. This mechanism of injury is mediated by antigen-antibody-complement (immune) complexes that are formed when the antigen is found in tissues or blood in moderate antigen excess. This mechanism of immunologic injury has great clinical significance and forms the basis for a wide variety of disorders ranging from localized immune complex disease, e.g., Arthus reaction, to more generalized forms of immune complex disorders, e.g., serum sickness, SLE, and poststreptococcal glomerulonephritis (Table 17-1). The basis for these adverse clinical reactions has been clarified by studies of antigen-antibody immune complexes performed both in the classical in vitro quantitative precipitin reaction as well as studies performed in

Box 17-1

A Comparison of the Classical Quantitative Precipitin Reaction Performed in Vitro with Biologic Effects of Antigen-Antibody Immune Complex Formation in Vivo

In the classical in vitro quantitative precipitin reaction, varying amounts of soluble antigen are added to a series of tubes containing a fixed amount of antibody (Figure 17-6A). As the amount of antigen added increases, the amount of precipitate generated also increases up to a maximum and then declines.

In this reaction, the three zones are based on changes in the composition of antigen-antibody complexes formed during the procedure (Figure 17-6A). These include the following:

1. In the first zone of **antibody excess**, each molecule of antigen is bound extensively by antibody, and cross-

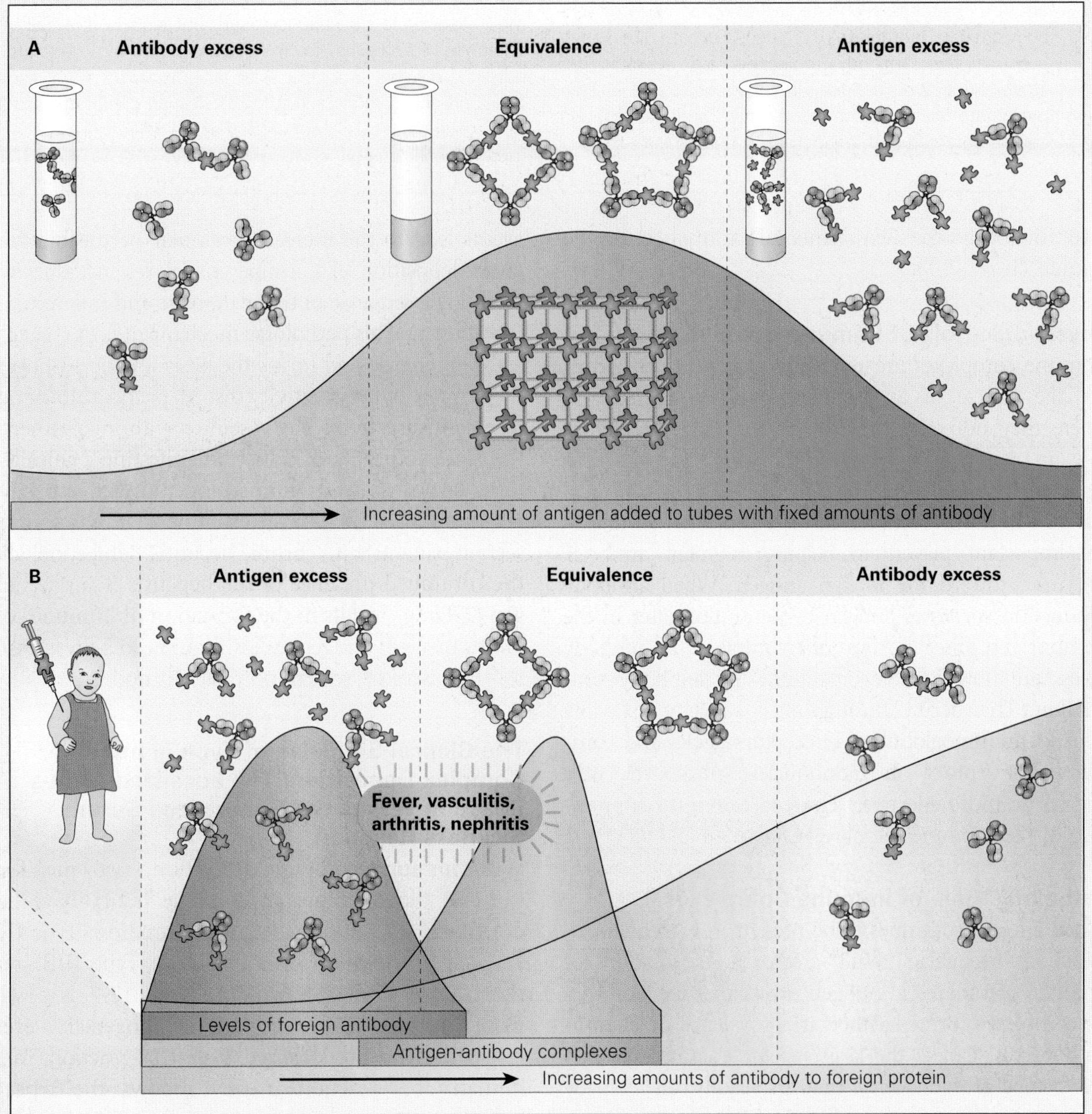

Figure 17-6. Schematic representation of the different sequential consequences of the composition of antigen-antibody immune complexes formed either in vitro or in vivo. Panel A: The classic in vitro quantitative precipitin reaction in which increasing amounts of antigen are added to a series of tubes containing a fixed amount of antibody following which three zones are seen: the zone of antibody excess; the zone of equivalence; and the zone of antigen excess. Panel B: The consequences of in vivo antigen-antibody complexes formation following the injection of a foreign protein into a human following which the adverse effects of tissue injury are mediated by antigen-antibody complex formed in the region of slight antigen excess that are responsible for the symptoms of fever, vasculitis, arthritis, and nephritis seen in many immunopathologic conditions where Type III reactions play a role.

Box 17-1 (continued)

linking between antigen-antibody complexes is rare. This results in the formation of small amount of detectable precipitate at the bottom of the tube and the presence of free antibody in the supernatant fluid.

2. In the second region, the **zone of equivalence**, the binding of antigen with antibody is optimal and extensive lattices are formed by the cross-linking of large antigen-antibody complexes that precipitate in the bottom of the tube with neither antigen nor antibody detected in the supernatant fluid.
3. At higher concentrations of antigen, the third zone of **antigen excess** is seen where the average size of antibody-antigen complexes is once again diminished because few antibody molecules are available for cross-linking with antigen. In this zone, there is little precipitate in the bottom of the tube and free antigen can be detected in the supernatant fluid.

In contrast to the in vitro quantitative precipitin reaction, where the first zone is one of antibody excess progressing to equivalence and antigen excess, in the course of the in vivo immune response, the sequence is reversed, beginning initially with a state of antigen excess followed by equivalence and ending with immune complexes in antibody excess (Figure 17-6B). The small, soluble immune complexes formed in the zone of antigen excess are the cause of many pathological syndromes in vivo. This occurs not only by the soluble nature of antigen-antibody complexes formed in antigen excess that limit their capacity to be phagocytosed, but also by the ability of these complexes to fix complement and generate potent cleavage products with anaphylatoxin (C3a and C5a) and chemotactic activity (C5a), which contribute both to increased vascular permeability and extravascular movement of inflammatory cells, respectively.

vivo in both the experimental animal and the human (Box 17-1).

Physiologic Role of Immune Complexes

Immune complexes are normally formed in vivo during the course of an immune response to antigen, where they not only provide an important regulatory role in augmenting and terminating the immune response, but also participate in the pathologic expressions of immune complex disease. Immune complexes are important players in helping augment antibody responses toward the foreign antigen. When antibody production surpasses antigen concentration later in the immune response, the immune complexes in antibody excess are now capable of suppressing antibody production. This occurs through their capacity to avidly bind to immunoglobulin Fc receptors (**FcR**) and complement receptors on mononuclear phagocytic cells and to be more effectively cleared, leading to suppression of the immune response (*Chapters* 6 and *11*).

Pathologic Role of Immune Complexes

When antigen continues to be present in high quantity, pathologic sequelae result from the formation of immune complexes in antigen excess that are not seen by complexes formed either at equivalence or at antibody excess. Unlike the large insoluble complexes that are formed at equivalence that are readily taken up by phagocytic cells, complexes formed in antigen excess are slightly more soluble, are less likely to be taken up by phagocytic cells, and can fix complement and trigger inflammatory responses with tissue injury resulting from the generation of active anaphylatoxin (C3a and C5a) and chemotactic factors (C5a) (*Chapter 4*). These events lead to the increased vascular permeability and favor deposition of immune complexes in tissues with pathologic sequelae of tissue damage and inflammation (*Chapter 5*). This pathologic mechanism is of great clinical significance and forms the basis for the pathogenesis of many hypersensitivity disorders and autoimmune diseases characterized by vasculitis with involvement of the skin, joints, and kidney, manifesting clinically as rash, arthritis, and glomerulonephritis, respectively (Figure 17-6B). A clinical example of this scenario is seen in patients with chronic hepatitis B infection where the continued presence of the hepatitis B surface antigen (HBsAg) results in the formation of immune complexes in slight antigen excess thought to be responsible for the vasculitis, seen in polyarteritis nodosa.

The Clinical Sequelae of Type III Immune Complex Deposition: The Localized Arthus Reaction versus the Generalized Serum Sickness Reaction

With immune complex deposition, two manifestations of the mechanisms of tissue injury have been described: (1) a localized (Arthus reaction; Type IIIA) and (2) a systemic (serum sickness; Type IIIB) reaction (Table 17-1). Shown in Figure 17-7 is a schematic representation of the pathogenetic events responsible for the localized Type IIIA reaction. In the human, this reaction usually follows the repeated injections of an antigenic substance (e.g., vaccine) into the skin or tissues of a previously immunized individual (*Chapter 23*). The excess antigen forms soluble immune complexes with existing antibody in antigen excess, and these complexes deposit in and around the vascular endothelium of the small blood

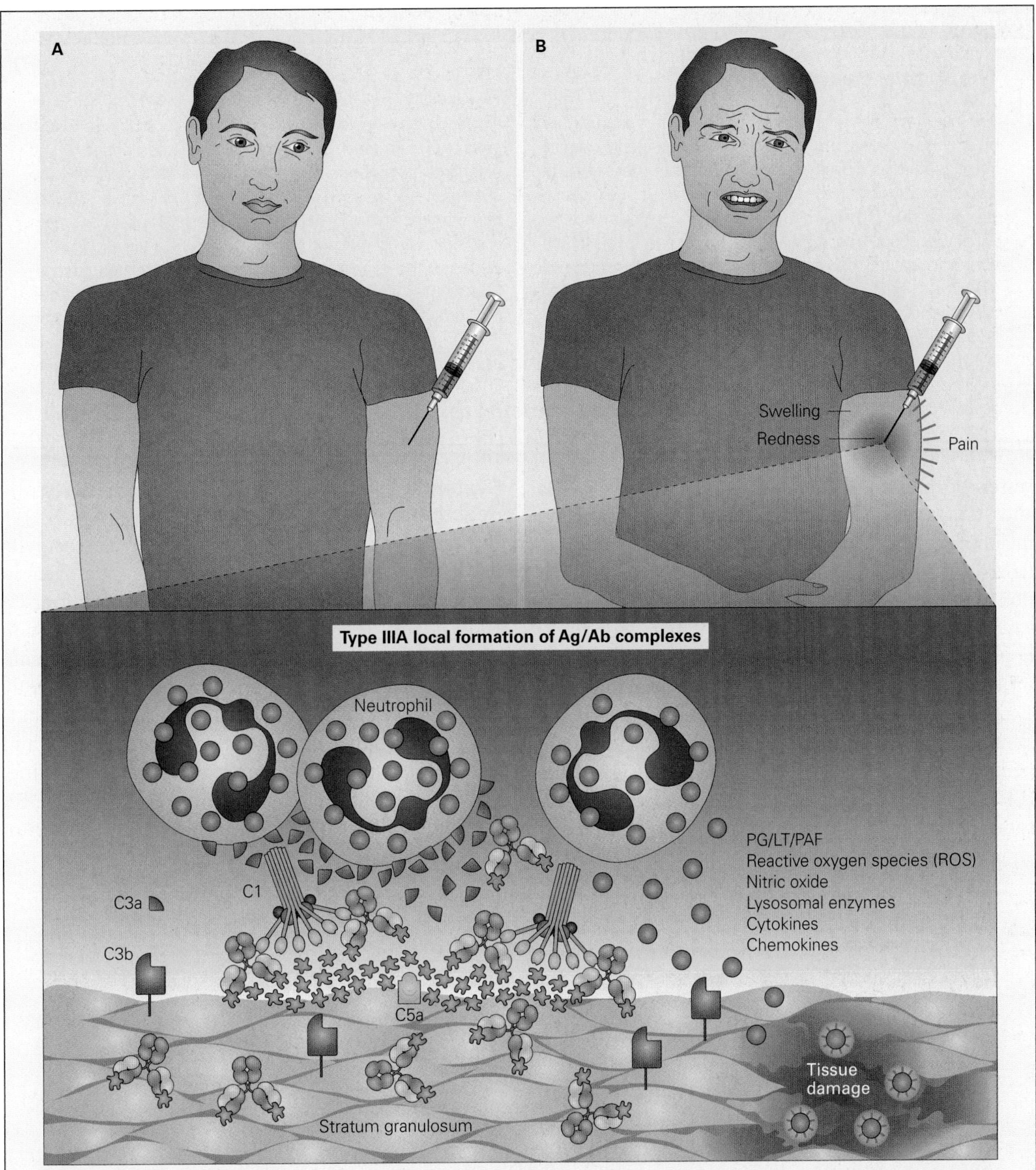

Figure 17-7. Schematic representation of the immune complexes that are responsible for the localized Type IIIA (Arthus) reaction. The pathogenesis of this localized Type III inflammatory reaction results from the following activities of several cleavage products of the complement (C1) cascade: C3b (opsonization and uptake of immune complexes PMNs), C3a, C5a (promotion of tissue deposition of immune complexes by anaphylatoxin activity), C5a (chemotactic emigration of PMNs from blood to tissues), and subsequent release of inflammatory mediators from PMNs (prostaglandins [PGs]/leukotrienes [LTs], reactive oxygen species [ROS], nitric oxide, lysosomal enzymes, cytokines, and chemokines). Although the immune complexes formed in the localized Arthus reaction (shown above) and the systemic reaction (shown in Figure 17-8) are both in antigen excess, note the more compact nature of antigen clustered in the immune complexes that are trapped in tissue in the local reaction in contrast to the more diffuse nature of the complexes formed in the systemic reaction.

Box 17-2

The Arthus Reaction

The local Type IIIA reaction was originally described in 1903 by Nicolas Maurice Arthus, who after repeatedly injecting horse serum subcutaneously into rabbits observed the development of acute local inflammation at the injection site marked by edema, hemorrhage, and necrosis occurring within 24 hours. The Arthus reaction is seen in the human after vaccination of previously immunized and seropositive individuals with tetanus toxoid-containing or diphtheria toxoid-containing vaccines (Figure 17-7A). It was also seen in persons previously immunized with the killed measles vaccine who later were reimmunized with the live measles vaccine (*Chapter 23*). An Arthus reaction is a local vasculitis associated with deposition of immune complexes and activation of complement. Immune complexes form in the setting of high local concentration of injected antigens and high circulating antibody concentration. Arthus reactions are characterized by severe pain, swelling, induration, edema, hemorrhage, and occasionally by necrosis. These symptoms and signs usually occur four to 12 hours after vaccination. Because of the frequency of these vaccine-related adverse effects the Advisory Committee on Immunization Practices (AICP) has recommended that persons who experienced an Arthus reaction after a dose of tetanus toxoid-containing vaccine should not receive Td more frequently than every 10 years, even for tetanus prophylaxis as part of wound management.

vessels of the skin, fix complement (in particular, C3a and C5a), and initiate a sequence of destructive inflammatory reactions within four to 10 hours characterized by a localized vasculitis with neutrophil infiltration and extravasation of fluid and blood cells from the vascular compartment into tissues. Within four to 10 hours, tissue swelling and redness form around the injection site, often called an **Arthus reaction** (Box 17-2). The Type IIIA reaction is initiated by the synthesis and release of many inflammatory mediators from neutrophils, including prostaglandins (PGs)/leukotrienes (LTs), reactive oxygen species (**ROS**), nitric oxide, lysosomal enzymes, cytokines, and chemokines (*Chapter 5*).

Systemic Forms of Type III Hypersensitivity Reactions

In the systemic form of the Type III hypersensitivity reaction, injections of large amounts of antigen in unimmunized persons is typically followed four to 10 days later by antibody production and formation of soluble immune complexes within the circulation. The circulating immune complexes subsequently deposit in the blood vessels of the skin, joints, kidneys, and/or lungs, fix and activate complement, and lead to symptoms of fever, skin rash, swelling, arthritis, and mild organ damage (Figure 17-8). This constellation of symptoms, termed "**serum**

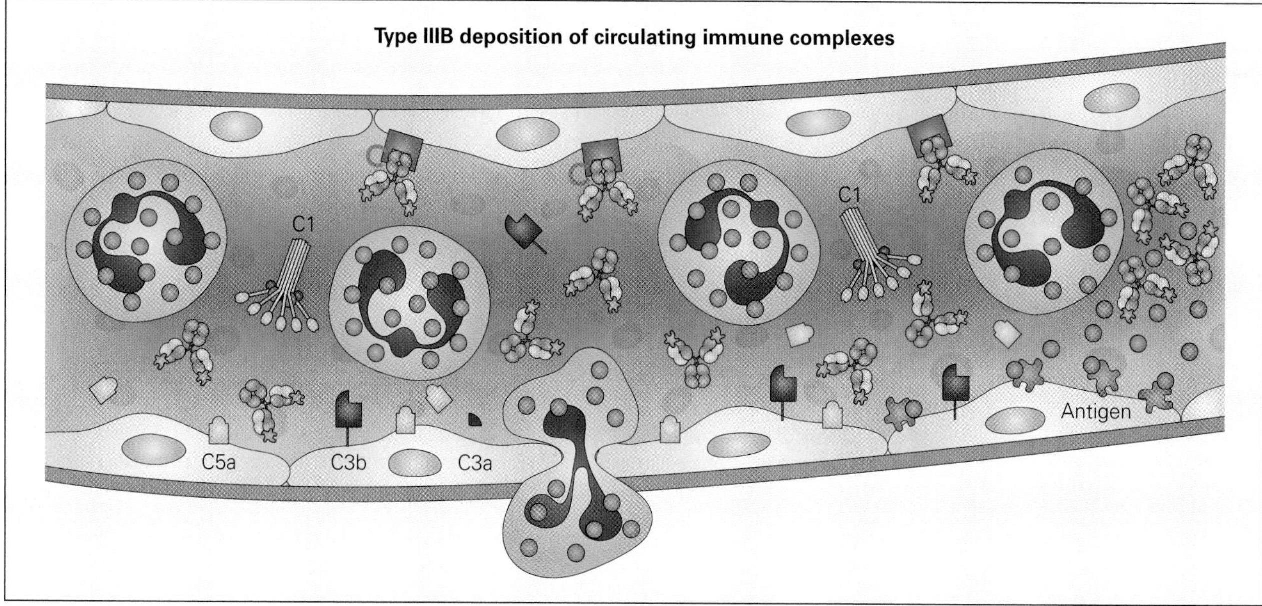

Figure 17-8. Schematic representation of the immune complexes that are responsible for the systemic Type IIIB reactions. In contrast to the local Arthus Type IIIA reaction where the immune complexes form tightly localized in tissue with localized symptoms, the immune complexes in the systemic Type IIIB form in the circulation and deposit more widely on FcγRII receptors on endothelial cells in the blood vessels of the skin, joints, kidneys, and/or lungs, fix complement with generation of cleavage products C3a and C5a, and initiate an inflammatory cascade similar to Type IIIA but with generalized symptoms of fever, skin rash, swelling, arthritis, and organ damage and dysfunction.

Box 17-3

Newer Treatment Modalities for Immune-Complex Mediated Disease

The treatment of immune-complex mediated disease/hypersensitivity has received several novel therapeutic regimens and agents. These include the removal of the offending agent and the use of anti-inflammatory agents (steroids or NSAIDs) in the case of serum sickness. Monoclonal anti-C5 antibody preparations have been evaluated to block the pro-inflammatory effects of C5a in immune complex complement-mediated injury with limited success. Because of its many potential inhibitory effects on immune-complex formation and on numerous steps in complement activation and immune-mediated injury, intravenous immunoglobulin (IVIG) has also been found to be useful (*Chapter 11*). By competing with FcγR, IVIG also prevents immune-complex mediated effects on other cells, such as blockage of platelet destruction in idiopathic thrombocytopenic purpura (ITP) (*Chapter 11*). Rituximab (anti-CD20 antibody) has been studied in autoimmune disease with the intention of depleting B cells, which in turn could suppress production of antibody for immune complex formation.

sickness," was classically described following the administration of horse antiserum used in passive immunization for anti-toxic treatment of bacterial infections, e.g., tetanus and diphtheria (*Chapters 11* and *23*). This classic response to foreign serum is no longer commonly seen since whenever possible, human sources of serum antibody or humanized monoclonal antibody preparations are now used in this form of immunotherapy. However, serum sickness-type reactions continue to be seen following the use of drugs and other biological agents (*Chapter 18*). Symptoms of serum sickness are usually transient and dissipate within weeks once the offending antigen is removed. However, if antigen and immune complex formation continue to persist, important immunopathologic states, such as SLE and certain forms of glomerulonephritis, may result. Shown in Box 17-3 are some of the newer treatment modalities that have been developed for the management of the immune-complex mediated disease/hypersensitivity disorders.

The Type IV Reaction

The fourth major mechanism of immunologic injury is the cell-mediated (delayed hypersensitivity) or Type IV reaction (Table 17-1). Unlike the previous three mechanisms, this response does not involve humoral antibody but is mediated primarily by the action of T lymphocytes. As described in Chapters 1, 7, and 9, the action of T cell subpopulations may involve cytokine production, direct cytotoxic effects, and the recruitment of other cells, e.g., NK cells, eosinophils, neutrophils, and macrophages. Systemic tissue and organ damage involvement has been associated with a variety of CD4+ and CD8+ T cell subtypes and are seen in a variety of clinical conditions with rapid onset and severe consequences, e.g., toxic shock syndrome (**TSS**), resulting from the effects of superantigens, produced by the Gram-positive cocci, *Staphylococcus aureus*, or *Streptococcus pyogenes* (Box 17-4 and *Chapter 3*).

In other T cell-mediated hypersensitivity reactions, the involvement of a variety of T cell subpopulations has been demonstrated, each with differing clinical

Box 17-4

Superantigens

Superantigens are a class of antigens that cause nonspecific activation of T cells, resulting in polyclonal T cell activation and massive cytokine release. These molecules bind directly to conserve regions of MHC-II structures without undergoing any intracellular processing. The superantigen interacts concurrently with the T cell receptor variable region β (TCR Vβ) chain families, independently of the epitope specificities of the T cells (*Chapter 7*). In toxic shock syndrome, many T cells are activated and produce large amounts of cytokines and chemokines, resulting in a sudden rise in the systemic levels of these biological mediators. This process, called systemic inflammatory response syndrome (SIRS), may lead to the multiple organ dysfunction syndrome (MODS), in which several vital organs fail to carry out their vital physiological functions (*Chapter 7*). MODS, if not managed promptly, can progress to irreversible end-stage organ failure culminating in mortality.

expressions. Because Gell and Coombs established their classification long before this growth of expanded knowledge of the T cell response, it is useful to define new subtypes for the Type IV hypersensitivity reaction. There are at least four distinct subtypes of Type IV hypersensitivity reactions that have been described (Table 17-1). These include: (1) Type IVA, Th1 cell-mediated immune responses; (2) Type IVB, Th2 cell-mediated immune responses; (3) Type IVC, Th17 cell-mediated immune responses; and (4) Type IVD, CD8+ cytotoxic cell-mediated immune responses. Although each of these cellular immune mechanisms of immunologic response may provide important beneficial functions in protective immunity, in the context of hypersensitivity, they play major pathogenetic roles in causing detrimental effects to the host.

The Type IVA, Th1 Cell-Mediated Immune Reactions

The Type IVA, Th1 cell-mediated immune reaction is the result of IFN-γ, TNF-α, and IL-2, the main cytokines secreted by Th1 cells (*Chapter 9*). This reaction is best exemplified by the classic delayed hypersensitivity skin reaction (*Chapter 7*). Shown in Figure 17-9 are the sequential steps that lead to the "red bump" that characterizes this archetypal dermal reaction first described in tuberculosis by Koch. Following intracutaneous introduction into a sensitized host, antigen is first taken up by an immature form of a dendritic cell called a Langerhans cell, which is then transported to a draining lymph node where it becomes a mature APC. Antigen processed by the APC is presented to a naïve Th0 CD4+ cell or a memory T cell in the case of a previously sensitized host. These cells then proliferate into an expanded Th1 cell population under the inductive influence of IL-12 (*Chapter 9*). The expanded Th1 cell population then migrates to the initial dermal site where the antigen is located and is activated to release their pro-inflammatory Th1-associated cytokines, IL-2, TNF-α, IFN-γ, and chemokines. After recruitment of macrophages, these cells release additional pro-inflammatory vasoactive mediators, ROS, NO, and other cytokines and chemokines that recruit additional macrophages. These events collectively promote the inflammatory response that characterizes the classic delayed hypersensitivity reaction that demonstrates itself maximally at 48–72 hours.

The release of these mediators from antigen-specific Th1 cells contributes to injury in many different clinical entities such as contact dermatitis (poison ivy), chronic asthma and eczema, drug reactions, primary graft rejection, and, to some degree, many aspects of the autoimmune disorders (Table 17-1). In some cases, i.e., contact dermatitis, which involves both Type 1-mediated and cytotoxic T cell injury, more than one type of T cell immune response may be at play. Although many acute aspects of asthma and eczema are triggered by or involve Type I hypersensitivity responses, it is now recognized that many chronic inflammatory manifestations effects of these diseases involve cellular hypersensitivity (mainly Th2 type) as well as participation of innate immune response-mediated injury (*Chapter 18*).

The chronic persistence of antigen incapable of elimination promotes the development of a prominent Type IVA reaction and subsequent formation of granuloma, a collection of organized cells, mainly macrophages with an infiltrate of lymphocytes or other leukocytes (*Chapter 5*). Granuloma formation is an important component in the pathogenesis of chronic infectious diseases such as tuberculosis, leprosy, histoplasmosis, cryptococcosis, coccidioidomycosis, and blastomycosis, or in non-infectious conditions such as sarcoidosis, Crohn's disease, berylliosis, Wegener's granulomatosis, and Churg-Strauss syndrome.

The Type IVB, Th2 Cell-Mediated Immune Reactions

The Type IVB, Th2 cell-mediated immune reaction is another subtype of the Type IV hypersensitivity reaction in which the cytokines of the Th2 subset play a major role (Figure 17-10). Following activation of the Th2 CD4+ lymphocytes by cognate interaction with APCs, cytokines are released, i.e., IL-13, IL-4, which stimulate expression of adhesion molecules, e.g., VCAM-1 and VLA-4 and eosinophil accumulation (*Chapter 5*). The production of IL-5 promotes activation of eosinophils, and together with chemokines such as CCL11 (eotaxin-1), CCL24 (eotaxin-2), CCL26 (eotaxin-3), CCL2 (MCP-1), and CCL5 (RANTES) produced by endothelial or epithelial cells, enhance the migration of eosinophils into tissues (*Chapter 9*). The production of other cytokines, e.g., GM-CSF and IL-3 with IL-5, promote the maintenance and stability of the eosinophilic-rich localized inflammation. The activated eosinophils subsequently degranulate and release inflammatory mediators (leukotrienes, reactive oxygen species, and cytokines [IL-2, IL-3, IL-4, IL-5, IL-7, IL-13, IL-16, and TNF-α]), cytotoxic molecules (major basic protein [**MBP**], eosinophil

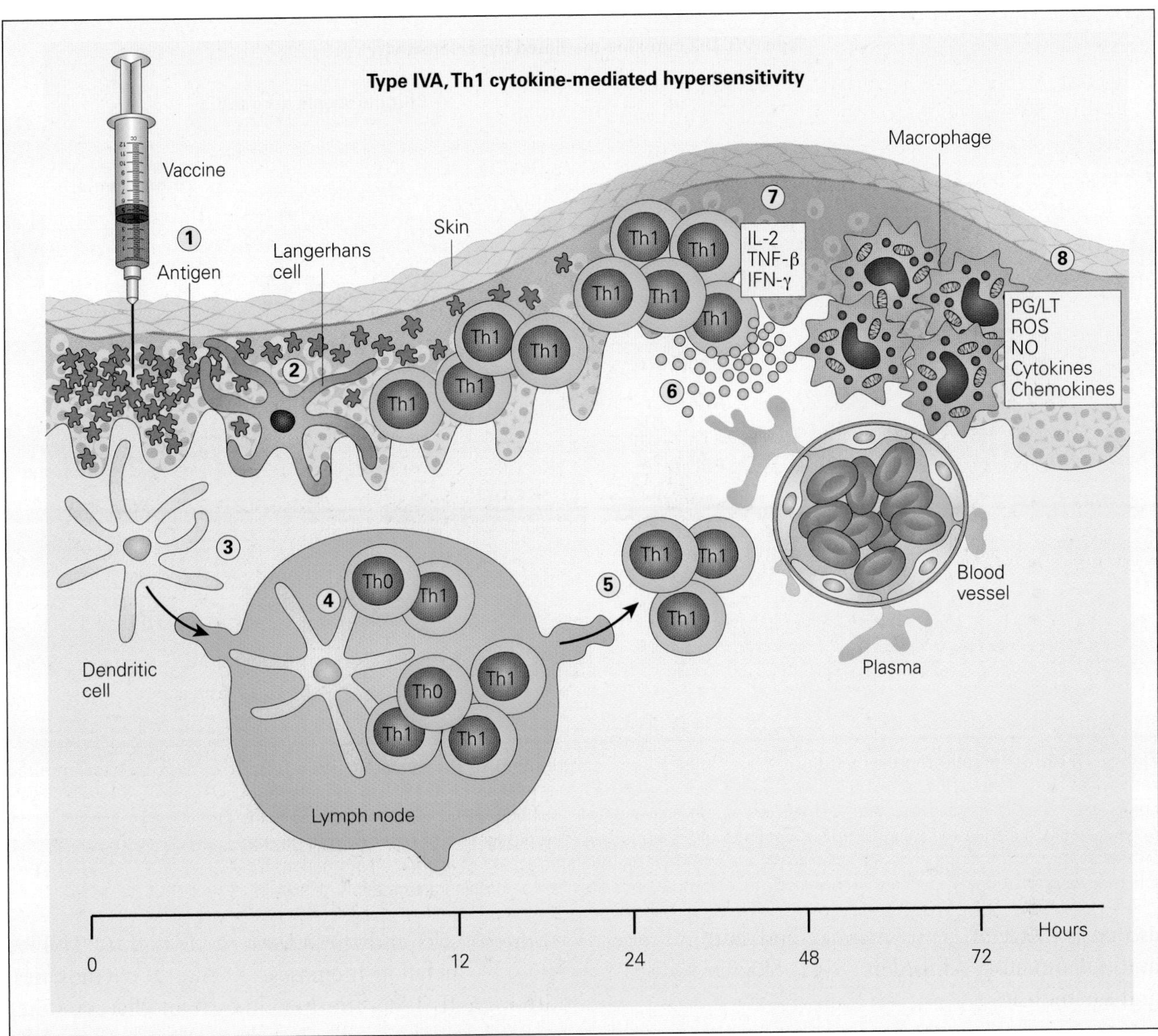

Figure 17-9. Schematic representation of the sequential steps that lead to the development of the Type IVA, Th1 cell-mediated delayed hypersensitivity reaction. Step 1: Antigen is introduced intracutaneously into the skin. Step 2: The Langerhans cell takes up the antigen. Step 3: The Langerhans cell is transported to a draining lymph node where it matures into a dendritic cell (APC). Step 4: The APC presents peptide to a naïve CD4+ Th0 cell or a Th1 memory cell in the case of a previously sensitized patient. Step 5: These cells then proliferate into an expanded Th1 cell population. Step 6: The Th1 cells then migrate back to the dermal site where the antigen is located. Step 7: They release their pro-inflammatory Th1-associated cytokines, IL-2, TNF-α, IFN-γ, and chemokines. Step 8: After recruitment of macrophages, they release additional pro-inflammatory vasoactive mediators, ROS, NO, and other cytokines and chemokines. These events then collectively promote the inflammatory response that characterizes the delayed hypersensitivity reaction.

cationic protein [**ECP**], eosinophil peroxidase [**EPO**], and eosinophil-derived neurotoxin [**EDN**]), and growth factors involved in tissue repair (TGF-β, VDGF, and PDGF) that are responsible for the development of chronic inflammation, tissue injury, and fibrosis. This type of injury is seen in many clinical conditions such as the late reaction observed in allergic patients after immediate skin-prick testing (*Chapter 18*). This late reaction is part of the late component of the dual "early" and "late" IgE-mediated skin reaction that waxes and wanes during the several-hour course of a Type I-mediated reaction. In contrast to the Type I IgE-mediated injury, which contributes to the acute inflammatory features of atopic dermatitis, e.g., redness and pruritus, the Type IVB hypersensitivity reaction is believed to contribute to many of the chronic features of the disease, e.g., thickening of the skin with lichenification caused by fibrotic changes. The Type IVB reaction is also present in many infectious diseases, e.g., cat-scratch fever, aspergillosis, coccidioidomycosis, trichinellosis,

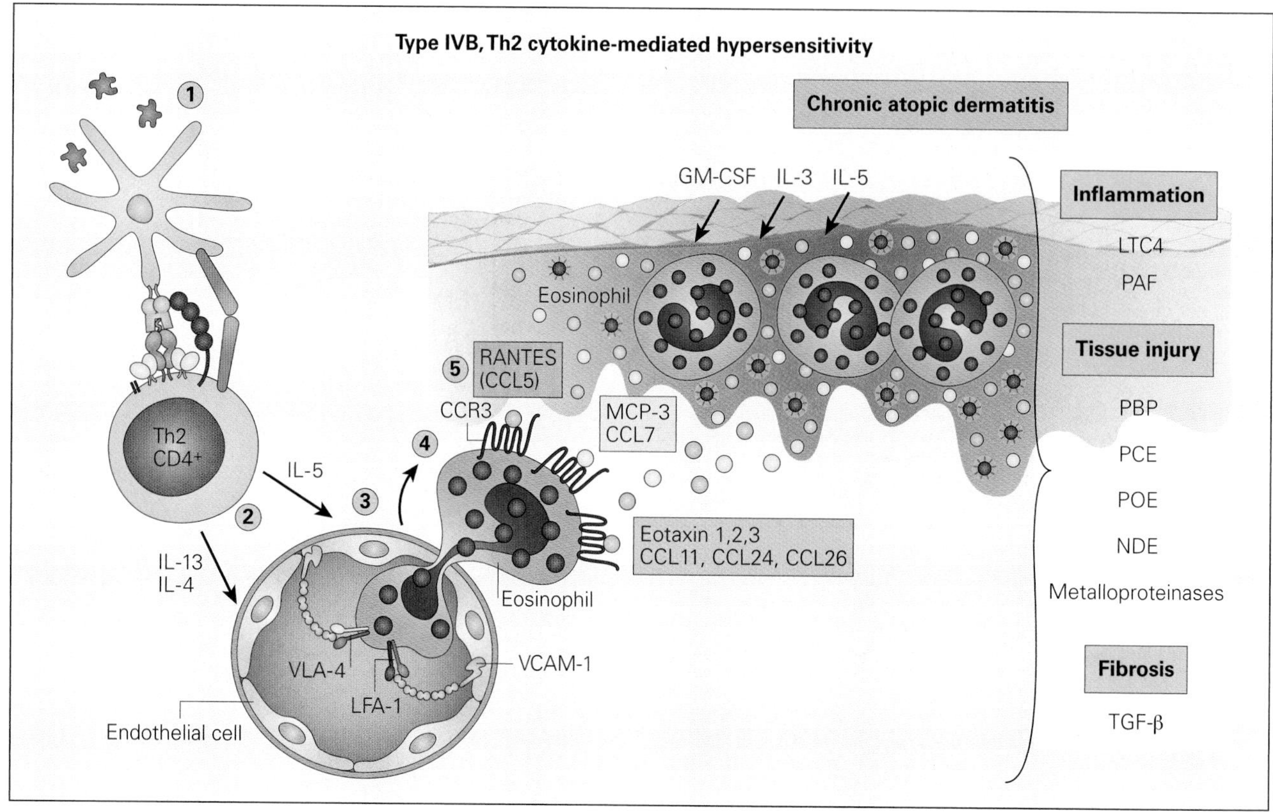

Figure 17-10. Schematic representation of the cellular events contributing to the systemic Type IVB, Th2 cell-mediated immune responses. Following activation of the Th2 CD4+ lymphocytes (#1), the release of IL-13, IL-4 stimulates expression of adhesion molecules, e.g., VCAM-1 and VLA-4, and IL-5 (#2) promotes activation of eosinophils and together with eotaxins produced by endothelial or epithelial cells enhance the migration of eosinophils into tissues (#3). The production of other cytokines, e.g., GM-CSF and IL-3 with IL-5 (#4), promotes the maintenance and stability of the eosinophilia-mediated localized allergic inflammation. Collectively, the release of pro-inflammatory cytokines and inflammatory mediators from eosinophils induce chronic inflammation, tissue injury, and fibrosis (#5).

ascariasis, visceral larva migrans, and autoimmune/autoinflammatory disorders, e.g., Sjögren's disease and sarcoidosis.

The Type IVC, Th17 Cell-Mediated Immune Reactions

A schematic representation of the Type IVC, Th17 cell-mediated immune reaction is shown in Figure 17-11. Following uptake and processing of antigen by DCs, naïve Th0 cells not only undergo maturation to Th17 cells under the influence of the combined actions of IL-1β, IL-6, and TGF-β, but also the stabilization and further expansion of these cells is indirectly provided by the dendritic cell/macrophage-derived IL-23. However, more recent data in humans suggest that IL-23 may directly be involved in the generation of Th17 cells. Th17 cells are present mainly in mucosal compartments and synthesize IL-17, IL-17F, IL-21, and IL-22 (*Chapter 9*). These cytokines promote a series of important events involved in tissue inflammation by the stimulation of fibroblasts, macrophages, endothelial, and epithelial cells and the release of IL-1, IL-6, TNF-α, NOS, metalloproteinases, and chemokines. Although IL-17 is the best known of the cytokines secreted by Th17 cells, it also can be produced by other immune-cell subsets, including NK, CD8+, double negative (CD4-, CD8-), T, and γδ T cells (*Chapter 9*). Among the major activities of IL-17 are its effects on epithelial cells, where it induces the production of neutrophil-attracting chemokines like CXCL1, CXCL2, and CXCL8 (IL-8) that causes the emigration of PMNs from blood vessels into tissues. Additionally, IL-17 upregulates the expression of adhesion molecules on vascular endothelial cells, triggering their secretion of IL-6 and IL-8, which further enhances PMN recruitment. IL-17 also activates macrophages and fibroblasts, the latter together with IL-22 with a role in the increase of collagen production and fibrosis and all of them in the secretion of the pro-inflammatory cytokines IL-6, IL-8, GM-CSF, and TNF-α. IL-21 is an autocrine cytokine that functions as a positive feedback signal for the Th17 cell. Recently, it has become clear that

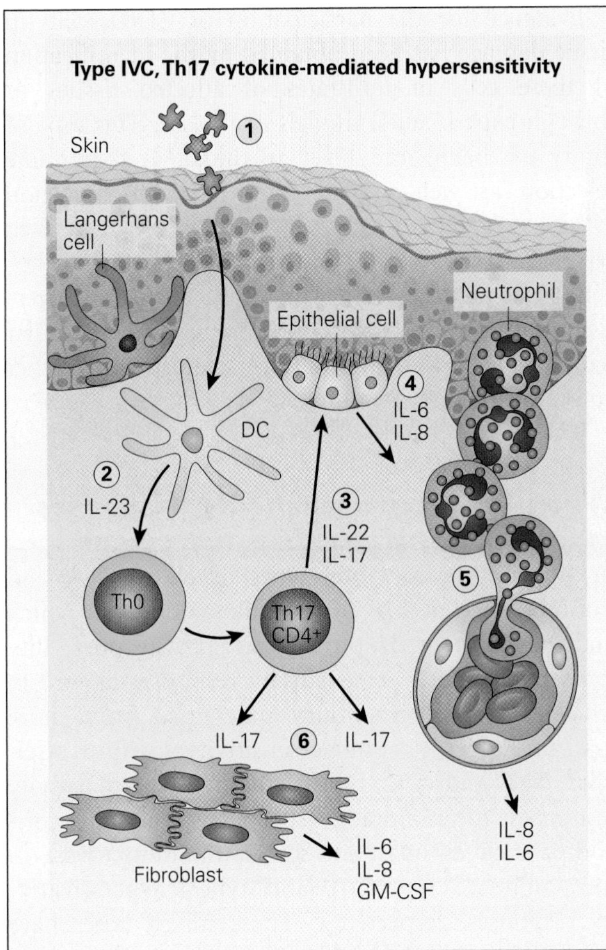

Figure 17-11. Schematic representation of the cellular events contributing to the Type IVC, Th17 type cell-mediated immune responses. Following antigen presentation (#1), IL-23 synthesis by DC (#2) stimulates maturation of a naïve Tho to a Th17 cell, which synthesizes IL-17 and IL-22 (#3), leading to the activation of epithelial cells (#4) to produce IL-6 and IL-8, which leads to the emigration of PMNs from blood vessels into tissues (#5). IL-17 produced by Th17 cells favors endothelial cell expression of adhesion molecules and the production of IL-6, IL-8, and GM-CSF which further enhances PMN recruitment (#6) and also activates fibroblasts to increase collagen production.

Th17 cells display considerable plasticity and can reciprocally modulate and convert into other helper T cell subpopulations, mainly induced Treg cells, i.e., iTreg cells (*Chapter 9*). Moreover, it has been shown that pro-inflammatory cytokines (IL-1β, IL-2, and perhaps IL-6 in humans) may influence the balance between Th17 and iTreg cells. It may therefore be possible to develop a therapeutically novel approach for the treatment of autoimmune diseases through the transformation of Th17 cells toward iTreg cells by the use of monoclonal antibodies or cytokines that affect IL-17.

Th17 cells and their cytokines participate importantly in several chronic inflammatory and autoimmune diseases where their precise pathogenic contribution might vary with the underlying disease (*Chapter 9*). The IL-23/Th17 pathway has been linked to the pathogenesis of some autoimmune diseases not only by the observation that dendritic cells from these patients produce more IL-23 but equivalent amounts of IL-12 compared to healthy controls, but also that Th17 cells from the same patients produce significantly more IL-17 than T cells from healthy donors. Participation of this cell subset has been recognized in the pathogenesis of several autoimmune diseases, e.g., psoriasis and inflammatory bowel disease, as well as several disorders previously classified as Th1 cell-mediated diseases, e.g., rheumatoid arthritis and multiple sclerosis, as well as other conditions such as allergic contact dermatitis, atopic dermatitis, and asthma (*Chapters 18* and *19*).

The Type IVD, CD8+ Cytotoxic Cell-Mediated Immune Responses

A schematic representation of the Type IVD, CD8+ cytotoxic cell-mediated immune reaction is shown in Figure 17-12. Cytotoxic T cells are involved in the elimination of target cells expressing MHC-I molecules charged with peptides from endogenously synthesized proteins of either self- or pathogen-derived origin (*Chapter 10*). These endogenous antigens are first degraded within the cytosol by the proteasome, and the resultant peptides are then transported by the transporter associated with antigen-presentation (**TAP**) complex into the endoplasmic reticulum, where they are loaded onto newly synthesized MHC-I molecules. These peptide-MHC-I complexes are then transported via the Golgi apparatus to the cell surface to be presented to CD8+ T cells. However, exogenous antigens can also be presented in the context of MHC-I by APCs (cross-presentation) when the internalized antigen is exported from the phagosome to the cytosol, where it is degraded by the proteasome. The cytotoxic process is initiated when specific TCRs on the CD8+ T cell membrane recognize cognate epitopes presented in the context of MHC-I molecules. Immediately, there is a redistribution and accumulation of cytoskeletal, adhesion (LFA-1, ICAM-1), and signal-transduction molecules of the CD8+ T cell toward the cell-cell interface, resulting in the formation of an immunological synapse (*Chapter 7*). The synapse enhances the presentation of cognate peptide-MHC-I complexes to cytotoxic T cells and their activation. The cytoskeleton of this activated cell moves the cytoplasmic perforin/granzyme-containing

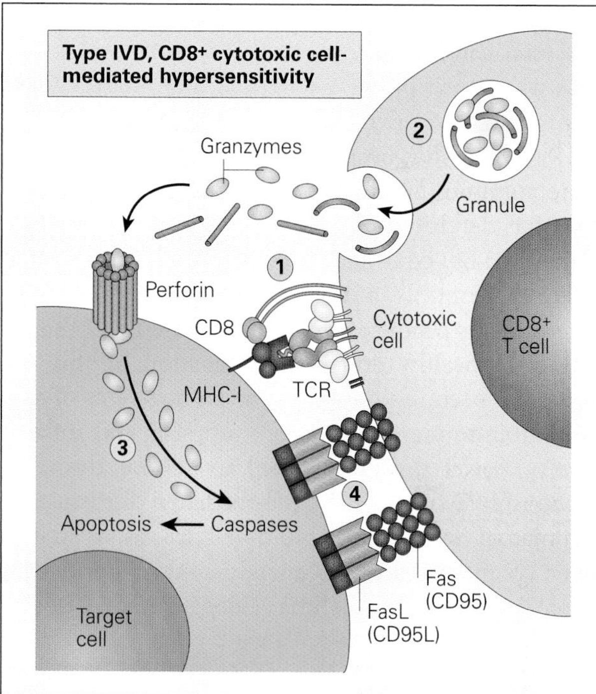

Figure 17-12. Schematic representation of the cellular events contributing to the Type IVD, CD8+ cytotoxic cell-mediated immune responses. Following presentation of a cell-associated antigen on a target cell to a CD8+ T cell in the context of an MHC-I molecule, a CD8+/target cell association is established in which four functional events occur: (#1) The recognition of the relevant epitopes on the antigen by the CD8+ T cell constitutes the first step; (#2) this is followed by the movement of the perforin/granzyme-containing granule toward the cell surface membrane of the CD8+ cytotoxic cell; (#3) after effector/target cell contact is made with the formation of an immunologic synapse, the contents of the granule are discharged into the synapse, resulting in the formation of a perforin-containing cylindrical pore into which the granzymes and other proteolytic proteases are discharged, leading to the apoptotic cell death of the target cell; and (#4), binding of the Fas (CD95) on the cytotoxic cell with the FasL (CD95L) on the target cell augments the apoptotic process.

granules toward the cell surface membrane and the contents of the granules are discharged through the synapse, resulting in the formation of perforin-containing cylindrical pores into which the granzymes and other proteolytic proteases are discharged, leading to the apoptotic cell death of the target cell (Figure 17-12, *Chapters 1* and *9*). Cytotoxicity is also mediated via other pro-apoptotic independent pathways initiated by the interaction of Fas-ligand (CD95L) on the CD8+ cell with the Fas-receptor (CD95) on the target cell surface. High-strength antigen signals promote killing via perforin-granzyme exocytosis, whereas low-antigen signals favor killing via the FasL-Fas pathway. CD8+ T cells are also capable of inducing inflammatory tissue damage by the secretion of other pro-inflammatory cytokines, such as IFN-γ and TNF-α.

Evidence for the participation of CD8+ cells in tissue damage has been obtained by the identification of these cells in infiltrates of affected tissues or through experimental models of disease. This type of injury has being recognized in the allograft immune rejection as well in the graft-versus-host reaction (*Chapter 22*), in the destruction of islet beta cells in type 1 diabetes, as well as participants in the pathogenesis of contact dermatitis, celiac disease, progressive multifocal leukoencephalopathy, large granular lymphocyte leukemia, multiple sclerosis, and other autoimmune diseases (Table 17-1).

Mixed Type Hypersensitivity Responses

In addition to the four types of classic Gell and Coombs' mechanisms of immunologic injury, which may be considered "pure," there is the possibility for **mixed type** hypersensitivity responses as well in which immunologic injury may arise from more than one type of the hypersensitivity reactions. Cellular Th1 and Th2 type cytokine hypersensitivity responses, for example, respectively, elaborate antibodies such as IgG1 and IgE antibodies, which in turn influence Type II/III and Type I hypersensitivity responses, respectively. These mixed types have important clinical significance in such entities as allergic bronchopulmonary aspergillosis (**ABPA**) and extrinsic allergic alveolitis, which are described in greater detail in Chapter 18.

A Proposed Hypersensitivity Classification System for Inflammatory Disorders that Are Based on Abnormalities of the Innate Immune System

Immune-mediated tissue injury may not only result from abnormalities of the adaptive immune system described above upon which the Gell and Coombs Type I–IV hypersensitivity classification is based, but also may be the consequence of tissue injury resulting from hypersensitivity reactions based on abnormalities of the innate immune system. In the Annex to Chapter 19, a new set of autoinflammatory disorders referred to as the inflammasomapathies is presented that is based on a new disease paradigm suggesting that these disorders reflect abnormalities of the innate immune system. In addition to these genetically determined disorders, there are other acquired forms of disturbances of the innate immune system that contribute to

Table 17-2. Mechanisms of innate immune response injury

Modes	Types	Clinical examples	Mechanisms
A. Genetically determined (autoinflammatory diseases) The "inflammasomopathies" (See *Chapter 19* Annex, Table 19A-3 for a more complete list of these disorders)	A1 Monogenic	Familial Mediterranean fever (FMF), pyogenic arthritis, pyoderma gangrenosum, and acne (PAPA)	Single gene mutations encoding molecules involved in innate immune response
	A2 Polygenic	Crohn's disease, Behçet's disease (BD), the seronegative spondyloarthropathies, type 2 diabetes mellitus (T2DM)	Mutations in multiple genes involved in innate immune response
B. PAMP-mediated (infection-associated)	B1 Microbial infections	Herpes, tuberculosis	Innate immune response occurring concomitantly with microbial replication
	B2 Cytokine storm	Influenza, AIDS	Rapid and uncontrolled production and release of cytokines
	B3 Chronic infection	Salmonellosis	Permanent and extended activation of innate response, inflammatory cell activation and release of cytokines
C. Non-infectious exogenous molecules-mediated		Gout, pseudogout, asbestosis, atherosclerosis, type 2 diabetes, silicosis, sarcoidosis (?)	Activation of inflammasomes
D. DAMP-mediated (sterile inflammation)		Inflammation after trauma, stress, ischemia, severe cold exposure	Activation of inflammasomes

clinical disease, e.g., systemic inflammatory response syndrome (**SIRS**). Although the original Gell and Coombs Type I–IV classification of hypersensitivity reactions has provided a most satisfactory system for understanding pathogenetic mechanisms of tissue injury responsible for allergy, chronic infection, and autoimmune disease, it has limitations for its use in defining mechanisms relating to abnormalities of the innate immune system responsible for these newly recognized inflammatory disorders.

The Innate Immune Response as Cause of Tissue Damage

It is now generally recognized that the innate immune response not only functions in the control of viral and microbial infections, but also the same molecular and cellular mechanisms involved in protective immunity may, at times, be a major cause for tissue damage and disease (*Chapter 3*). The pathogen-associated molecular patterns (**PAMPs**) of microbes are recognized as ligands by the main classes of innate immune-signaling receptors referred to as pattern-recognition receptors (**PRRs**) that include the Toll-like receptors (**TLRs**), nucleotide oligomerization domain (**NOD**)-like receptors (**NLRs**), retinoic acid-inducible gene I (**RIG-I**)-like receptors (**RLRs**), and absent in melanoma-2 (**AIM2**) families activate distinct transcriptional programs leading to inflammation, protective antimicrobial responses, and the induction of adaptive immunity (*Chapters 3* and *9*). Shown in Table 17-2 is a proposed grouping of mechanisms of innate immune response injury that is derived from known tissue-injuring mechanisms, which could alone, or in concert, be responsible for the clinical expressions brought about by abnormalities of this system. Because of the molecular complexities of the processes involved in innate immune function, this expansion of the current Gell and Coombs classification is proposed to also include mechanisms involved in innate immune-mediated tissue injury. The use of the term "modes" is proposed in order to differentiate these new categories from those descriptive of adaptive response-mediated hypersensitivity.

Mode A: Genetically-Determined Innate Response Injury

This group of disorders is triggered by dysregulation of the innate immune system and collectively is termed the autoinflammatory diseases (Table 17-2 and *Chapter 19* Annex). They are comprised of a group of clinical disorders originating either from monogenic or polygenic gene mutations that encode proteins involved in inflammasome function (*Chapter 9*). Most of these gene-encoded proteins function as critical enzymes that orchestrate the early inflammatory process via caspase-1 and IL-1β activation. Masters, et al., have offered a comprehensive grouping of these disorders under the heading of the inflammasomopathies (*Chapter 19* Annex).

Monogenic autoinflammatory syndromes are a clinically heterogeneous collection of rare disorders characterized by recurrent episodes of fever, joint symptoms, conjunctivitis, and urticaria-like rash, among others (Table 17-2). Examples of this group of diseases include familial Mediterranean fever (**FMF**), due to mutations on the gene MEFV for pyrin, and hyperimmunoglobulinemia D with periodic fever syndrome (**HIDS**), with mutations in the gene MVK that encodes mevalonate kinase. Also included in this grouping is familial cold autoinflammatory syndrome (**FCAS**), Muckle-Wells syndrome (**MWS**), and neonatal-onset multisystem inflammatory disease (**NOMID**), which are caused by mutations in the gene NOD-like receptor family pyrin domain containing 3 (**NLRP3**), as well as familial juvenile systemic granulomatosis (Blau syndrome) caused by mutations of the NOD2 gene.

The polygenic autoinflammatory conditions are illustrated by the well-known inappropriate responses to bacterial antigenic stimulation of the innate immune system in the gastrointestinal tract, expressed clinically in the protype inflammatory bowel disease (**IBD**) Crohn's disease (**CD**) (Table 17-2). Although CD and ulcerative colitis (**UC**) are the two most common forms of IBD, there are several clinical as well as genetic features that distinguish between them. In CD, inflammation is typically transmural and can be found discontinuously in "skipped regions" throughout the gut, whereas UC primarily affects the mucosal and submucosal layers of the rectum and colon in a continuous pattern. A mutation of the NOD2 locus appears to be the major genetic discriminating factor between the two entities since the mutation is only associated with CD and not UC. This is in contrast to single nucleotide polymorphisms (**SNPs**) (*Chapter 25*) in ECM1 (an intestinal glycoprotein that activates NF-κB) and IL-10 found only with UC and to SNPs in IL-23R and IL-12B encoding the shared p40 subunit of IL-12 and IL-23 (*Chapter 9*) that are associated with IBD in general. These polygenic mutations highlight the complexity of these disorders and illustrate that very often they involve gene mutations of components of both the innate and adaptive immune systems with features of both autoinflammatory and autoimmune disease. Other interesting pathologies in this polygenic category include Behçet's disease (BD), the seronegative spondyloarthropathies, and probably type 2 diabetes mellitus (T2DM).

Mode B: Microbial PAMPs and Tissue Damage

Exogenous PAMPs associated with viruses, bacteria, fungi, protozoa, or helminths have the capacity to trigger the production of multiple cytokines together with activation of NK cells, contributing to the control of microbial replication either by modulating other immune cells, e.g., neutrophils and monocytes/macrophages, or by direct killing of infected cells (Table 17-2). There are three situations described below (Situations B1 to B3) by which such innate immune responses, which are otherwise normally protective, can at times be responsible for deleterious tissue injuring effects on the host.

Situation B-1. In acute microbial infections, the clinical expression of tissue injury can result both from direct injury mediated by the causative agent as well as from the indirect effects of the host innate immune response to a wide variety of microbial PAMPs of the host. The influx of circulating immune cells into the infection-challenged tissue is associated with a rapid release of pro-inflammatory cytokines, reactive oxygen species, proteolytic enzymes, and collateral bystander cellular damage, and not only evokes inflammation and tissue injury, but also stimulates protective innate immune mechanisms. However, these effects are transitory and will endure only until effective resolution of the infection is achieved.

Situation B-2. When the replication of an infectious agent reaches a maximal level in a short period of time or when immune clearance mechanisms are impaired or delayed, the innate immune responses are uncoordinated and result in localized overproduction of reactive cells and pro-inflammatory cytokines. This situation is referred to as cytokine storm, with symptoms of high fever, edema, erythema, extreme fatigue, and nausea, often resulting in fatal outcome. In many infections (influenza, HIV, and viral hepatitis), the effect of this cytokine-induced secondary inflammatory injury can have more deleterious effects than those produced by the invading virus or bacteria themselves.

Situation B-3. In chronic infections, the immune responses generated by the host are incapable of clearing infection and high concentrations of cytokines are locally and continuously produced. If these molecules enter the circulation and are transported to remote sites, they can promote systemic toxic or even lethal effects. Inflammatory cytokines, such as TNF-α and IL-1β, destabilize endothelial cell-cell interactions and lead to vascular dysfunction with capillary leakage, edema, organ failure, and death. These phenomena occur in septic shock, acute lung injury, and acute respiratory distress syndrome (ARDS), all common endpoints seen in patients undergoing serious viral or bacterial infections. Together with these pathophysiologic events, there commonly occurs a special form of cell death accompanied by inflammation, termed "pyroptosis," leading to the destruction of the activated cell with release of cellular contents (*Chapter 5*).

Mode C: Noninfectious Exogenous Molecules and Inflammation

In this mode of innate immune-induced inflammatory reaction, a non-infectious exogenous inert substance can promote the activation of the inflammasome with release of the IL-1 family of proinflammatory cytokines, leading to tissue injury and disease (Table 17-2). Among the wide variety of stimulatory molecules responsible for the pathogenesis of this group of inflammatory disorders are endogenous metabolic products, e.g., monosodium urate crystals in gout or crystals of calcium pyrophosphate dihydrate in pseudogout; environmental pollutants, e.g., asbestos and silica in asbestosis and silicosis; and diagnostic agents, such as gadolinium used in magnetic resonance responsible for the development of nephrogenic systemic sclerosis (*Chapter 3*).

Mode D: Innate Response to Endogenous DAMPs and Sterile Inflammation

The innate immune response can also be activated by damage or danger-associated molecular patterns (**DAMPs**), originating by the host's individual cells themselves as a result of non-infectious injury, e.g., trauma, ischemia, stress, cold exposure, and toxic materials, which in health are important signaling events for tissue and wound repair, but which under exaggerated and abnormal release in disease states can be detrimental to the host (Table 17-2). DAMPs are normally sequestered intracellularly and are therefore hidden from recognition by the immune system under normal physiological conditions. Molecules such as tissue hyaluronate, cytoplasmatic heat shock proteins (HSP), mitochondrial formyl peptides (FP), or nuclear high-mobility group box 1 (HMGB1) are released by dying cells, triggering inflammation and illnesses.

Summary

The four-group classification originally proposed by Gell and Coombs in 1963 has provided a most valuable taxonomic system for understanding the mechanism of injury seen in a variety of adaptive immune-mediated diseases ranging from the allergic diseases to the autoimmune disorders. The system attempted to categorize mechanisms of immunologic injury as they relate to human immunologically mediated diseases and was restricted to disorders arising from components of adaptive immunity, i.e., B and T cells. Although the classification continues to serve a useful purpose, recently it has become increasingly clear that there are other immunologically mediated diseases that arise from disorders of innate immunity that the original Gell and Coombs classification did not take into consideration. Immunologic injury is now recognized to derive both from the damaging effects of either the innate or adaptive immune responses. The adaptive mechanisms of immunologic injury described in this chapter have been clustered into an expanded Gell and Coombs classification of hypersensitivity reactions and are subdivided according to more recently recognized components of the immune armamentarium responsible for the pathologic sequela. Equally important is the recognition that certain diseases are the consequence of more complex mechanisms of tissue damage resulting from innate immune-mediated injury. A proposed classification of mechanisms of innate immune response injury is presented that is derived from known tissue-injuring mechanisms that could alone, or in concert, be responsible for the clinical expressions brought about by abnormalities of this system.

Key Points

- The immunologically-mediated diseases comprise a heterogeneous group of disorders of reactions to environmental agents triggered by either the adaptive or the innate immune systems that lead to the harmful sequelae of the immune response. The Gell and Coombs Type I–IV hypersensitivity reactions are responsible for immunologically mediated diseases where the adaptive immune response is unduly upregulated in the presence of an antigen.

- Type I hypersensitivity is an APC-Th2-B cell interaction mediated by an antibody where the mechanism of immunologic injury is triggered by IgE and, to a lesser extent, by IgG4 antibodies in a chronic state of activation. The major sequelae arise from the release of mediators following the crosslinking of IgE-bound to mast cells or basophils by antigen.
- Two of the four Gell and Coombs hypersensitivity reactions, Type II and Type IV, have been further divided into subtypes to include more specific mechanisms of cellular injury. Type II hypersensitivity reactions include the following cell-damaging mechanisms and their consequences: (1) cell death (i.e., cytotoxicity), (2) cellular neutralization, or (3) cellular stimulation.
- The Type IV hypersensitivity reactions include: (1) Type IVA, Th1 type cytokine-mediated immune responses; (2) Type IVB, Th2 type cytokine-mediated immune responses; (3) Type IVC, Th17 type cytokine-mediated immune responses; and (4) Type IVD, CD8+ cytotoxic cell-mediated immune responses.
- In the cytotoxic subtype of Type II hypersensitivity, the target cell is killed by either an antibody-mediated activation of complement, opsonization of the target cell by phagocytes through C3b or IgG antibody binding of target cells, cytotoxic attack of the target cell by phagocytes, or an antibody-dependent cellular cytotoxicity (ADCC) reaction. Cellular neutralization results from the blockage of a physiologic ligand-receptor interaction by competitive inhibition of a neutralizing IgG antibody with the receptor. Cytostimulation is a result of the enhancing effect of autoantibody bound to physiologic target cell receptors.
- Type III hypersensitivity reactions originated from the former use of heterologous antisera for protective antimicrobial immunity where the production of antibody complexed with the foreign serum protein(s) and complement resulted in either a localized Type IIIA (Arthus) reaction or generalized Type IIIB reactions.
- Allergic bronchopulmonary aspergillosis and extrinsic allergic alveolitis are examples of mixed-type hypersensitivity responses in which the immunologic injury may arise from more than one type of the hypersensitivity reactions.

Study Questions/Critical Thinking

1. Each of the following is a mechanism of immunologic injury that has been associated with Type IV Gell and Coombs hypersensitivity response mechanism EXCEPT:

   a. Contact dermatitis
   b. Atopic dermatitis
   c. Psoriasis
   d. Extrinsic allergic alveolitis
   e. Allergic rhinitis

2. Each of the following is an example of a clinical disease triggered by any of the subtypes of Type II hypersensitivity reactions EXCEPT:

   a. Myasthenia gravis
   b. Graves' disease
   c. Goodpasture's disease
   d. Autoimmune hemolytic anemia
   e. Nickel sensitivity

3. Each of the following cell types are involved in Type IV hypersensitivity reaction EXCEPT:

   a. CD4+ T cells
   b. CD8+ T cells
   c. Neutrophils
   d. Basophils
   e. Eosinophils

4. Each of the following is a disease resulting from the impact of a single mechanism of immunologic injury EXCEPT:

   a. Graves' disease
   b. Extrinsic allergic alveolitis
   c. Psoriasis
   d. Arthus reaction
   e. Idiopathic thrombocytopenia (ITP)

Suggested Reading

Agrawai DK, Shao Z. Pathogenesis of allergic airway and inflammation. Curr Allergy Ashma Rep. 2010; 10: 39–48.

Atassi MZ, Casali P. Molecular mechanisms of autoimmunity. Autoimmunity. 2008; 41: 123–32.

Chen GY, Nunez G. Sterile inflammation: sensing and reacting to damage. Nat Rev Immunol. 2010; 10: 826–37.

Gell PGH, Coombs RRA, eds. Clinical Aspects of Immunology. 1st ed. Oxford, England: Blackwell; 1963.

Hoffman HM, Brydges SD. Genetic and molecular basis of inflammasome-mediated disease. J Biol Chem. 2011; 286: 10889–96.

Kanji S, Chant C. Allergic and hypersensitivity reactions in the intensive care unit. Crit Care Med. 2010; 38 Suppl 6: 162–8.

Lleo A, Invernizzi P, Gao B, et al. Definition of human autoimmunity—autoantibodies versus autoimmune disease. Autoimmun Rev. 2010; 9: 259–66.

Masters SL, Dunne A, Subramanian SL, et al. Activation of the NLRP3 inflammasome by islet amyloid polypeptide provides a mechanism for enhanced IL-1β in type 2 diabetes. Nat Immunol. 2010; 11: 897–904.

Masters SL, Simon A, Aksentijevich I, et al. Horror autoinflammaticus: the molecular pathophysiology of autoinflammatory disease. Annu Rev Immunol. 2009; 27: 621–68.

Pamphilon DH, Scott ML. Robin Coombs: his life and contribution to haematology and transfusion medicine. Br J Haematol. 2007; 137: 401–8.

Pichler WJ. Immune mechanism of drug hypersensitivity. Immunol Allergy Clin North Am. 2004; 24: 373–97

Posadas SJ, Pichler WJ. Delayed drug hypersensitivity reactions—new concepts. Clin Exp Allerfy. 2007; 37: 989–99.

Rajan TV. The Gell-Coombs classification of hypersensitivity reactions: a re-interpretation. Trends Immunol. 2003; 24: 376–9.

Siegrist CA. Mechanisms underlying adverse reactions to vaccines. J Comp Pathol. 2007; 137 Suppl 1: 546–50.

Venuprasad K, Kong YC, Farrar MA. Control of Th2-mediated inflammation by regulatory T cells. Am J Pathol. 2010; 177: 525–31.

Ward CJ. Pathogen sensing in innate immunity. Expert Rev Vaccines. 2010; 9: 19–21.

Chapter 18

Allergic Diseases and Asthma

Stefano Luccioli, MD
Alejandro Escobar-Gutiérrez, PhD
Joseph A. Bellanti, MD

Case Studies

Case Study 1

A 42-year-old female, who is employed as a neonatal care nurse, had recently undergone cholecystectomy following which she developed generalized urticaria, facial angioedema, shortness of breath, wheezing, and hypotension in the surgical recovery room. In the operating room, she had received routine intravenous anesthetics and fluids and her operative course was uneventful. In the surgical recovery room, the patient was receiving a prophylactic beta-lactam antibiotic. History obtained during the preoperative workup revealed no history of cardiac or respiratory disease. She denied a history of drug or latex allergy and allergic history was insignificant except for food allergies to peanuts and tree nuts. On further questioning, she admitted having an itchy rash two years previously following treatment with an antibiotic for tonsillitis.

Given the patient's history and symptoms, an astute surgical resident recognized the early signs of anaphylaxis and stopped the patient's antibiotic infusion. She was given a subcutaneous injection of epinephrine, intravenous fluids, and steroids. Within a short period of time, her blood pressure normalized and her urticaria and difficulty breathing improved. The patient's antibiotic was changed to a non-penicillin (PCN)-containing antibiotic. The remainder of the hospital course was uneventful.

Subsequent skin testing with the PCN major determinant at an allergist's office revealed a large wheal-and-flare reaction that confirmed the suspected allergy to PCN. The patient was instructed to strictly avoid PCN and other beta-lactam drugs in the future.

Case Study 2

A seven-year-old elementary school child was brought to a physician with symptoms of rhinorrhea, frequent sneezing, ocular pruritus (itchiness), and recent dry cough, occurring predominantly at bedtime. Over the past two years, the child's mother had noted a pattern of similar yet less severe symptoms usually occurring during the same season of the year, i.e., spring. Previously, the nasal symptoms, sneezing, and cough had been moderately relieved with over-the-counter allergy medications. Now the cough was fairly persistent and the patient also had recent

LEARNING OBJECTIVES

When you have completed this chapter, you should be able to:

- Define allergy and describe the various types of allergens involved in allergic diseases and asthma
- Understand the major players and pathogenesis of immediate Type I and other hypersensitivity reactions relevant to allergic diseases and asthma
- Understand the gene-environment interactions contributing to the global allergy epidemic and other factors that affect or modify the pathogenesis of allergic diseases and asthma
- Understand the importance of age-related effects of the immune response on expression of allergic disease, including the atopic march
- Recognize the triggers and clinical manifestations of anaphylaxis
- Recognize the acute and chronic clinical manifestations of allergic diseases and asthma
- Discuss the immunologic mechanisms underlying in vivo and in vitro diagnostic allergy tests
- Describe various therapeutic strategies for the treatment of symptoms of allergic diseases and asthma
- Describe various immunomodulatory strategies for the management of allergic diseases, including allergen-specific immunotherapy and the use of monoclonal antibody or anticytokine therapies
- Utilize this information for understanding prevention and management of allergic diseases and asthma

Case Studies (continued)

episodes of difficulty breathing while playing outdoors. The patient had mild to moderate eczema as an infant and there was a paternal family history of asthma.

Evaluation by an allergist revealed positive immediate skin tests predominantly to tree and grass pollens and a few molds, including Alternaria. Spirometry revealed a reduced peak flow and reduced forced expiratory volume (FEV1) that were shown to significantly increase 15 minutes after inhalation of an albuterol nebulization. The patient was started on a course of intranasal and inhaled corticosteroids, antihistamines, and bronchodilators, and the parents were counseled about allergen immunotherapy.

Case Study 3

A 29-year-old female was evaluated for recurrent and pruritic rash of two months' duration. She has had a longstanding history of atopic eczema, mainly involving the antecubital and popliteal fossae. The characteristics of the pruritus and rash were different from her usual presentation of eczema and included daily appearance of "raised bumps" on various areas of her body, including the trunk and limbs. The rash displayed an evanescent pattern of evolution first appearing and then completely disappearing within a few hours with no permanent skin lesions or loss of sensation at the affected skin sites. Initially, the rash was localized to her hands and feet and described at times as painful. More recently, however, the rash has become more widespread and associated with intense pruritus and a more pleomorphic appearance characterized by both small and large raised skin lesions. A similar skin rash has often appeared localized around belt lines or bra straps, and the patient has begun to wear loose clothing. There was no recent illness or history of thyroid or autoimmune disease. There was a strong family history of allergic rhinitis and asthma in several members of the family. She denied taking any medications prior to the event and could not identify any foods or other environmental factors that may have contributed to the appearance of the skin rash. Upon further examination, stroking of the skin elicited the pruritic skin lesions. A diagnosis of chronic urticaria or hives was established. The patient's treatment regimen consisted mainly of antihistamines to control the symptoms of pruritus.

These three cases illustrate the clinical expressions of common allergic diseases, the immunologic basis of which will be described in greater detail in this chapter.

Allergy and Allergic Diseases

Allergic Disease: An Example of Immunologically Mediated Disease

Nowhere are the principles and mechanisms of immunologic injury better illustrated than in the case of the allergic diseases. Allergy represents one of the tissue–damaging immune responses of the immune encounter that involves both a unique foreign substance, i.e., allergen, as well a genetic susceptibility of the affected host to produce a specialized class of antibody, IgE (*Chapter 6*), which gives rise to the allergic manifestations (*Chapter 17*).

In 1906, Clemens von Pirquet (Figure 18-1) coined the term "allergy" (Greek, *allos*, other + *ergon*, action), which referred to a state of altered reactivity to environmental substances. Subsequent modifications of the meaning of the term equated allergy with hypersensitivity. Today, the term "allergy" is sometimes used synonymously with an older term, "atopy" (Gr, *atopia*, from *atopos*, out of place, *a*, not + *topos*, place), which refers to the familial predisposition to what became subsequently known as IgE-mediated allergic disease. Since the concept of immunity presented throughout this book has been one of a reaction to foreignness or to danger signals, allergy is best viewed as a specialized case of immunity in which the reaction to foreign material terminates in a deleterious outcome and may be considered as one of several types of immunologically mediated diseases affecting humans directed at exogenous antigens (*Chapter 17*).

Disease Terminology

Allergy is often considered to be synonymous with hypersensitivity (*Chapter 5*). The allergic condition, however, can be best described as a specific type of hypersensitivity response. **Hypersensitivity** is a general term used to describe objectively reproducible symptoms or signs of tissue injury initiated by exposure to a defined stimulus at a dose tolerated by normal individuals. **Allergy,** on the other hand, is a hypersensitivity reaction initiated by specific immunologic mechanisms that involve antibody-mediated and/or cell-mediated mechanisms to produce distinct disease manifestations (*Chapter 17*). Allergic responses are specific to and typically reproducible upon sufficient, even low level, exposure to

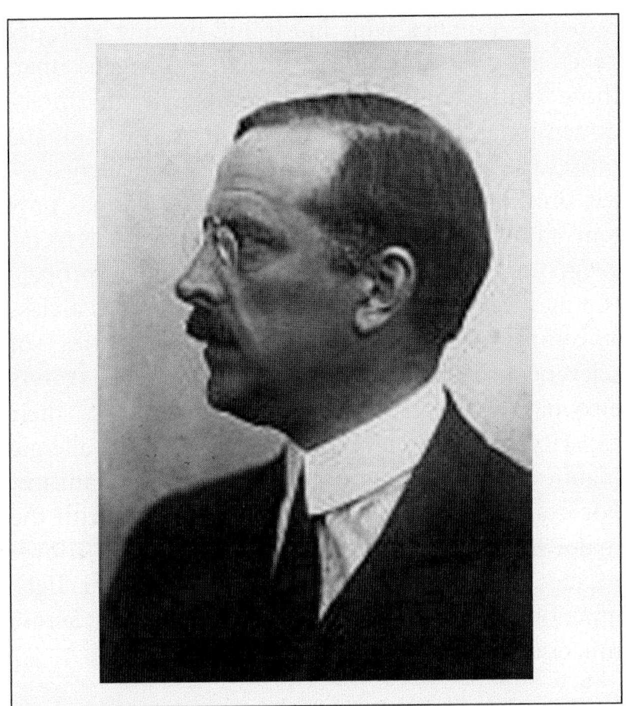

Figure 18-1. Clemens von Pirquet (1874–1929).

the allergenic substance, called an allergen. These manifestations may be clinically divided into those associated with IgE antibody, i.e., **IgE-mediated allergy**, and those not associated with IgE antibody, i.e., **non-IgE-mediated allergy**. Hypersensitivity reactions and/or disease manifestations of hypersensitivity without a defined immunologic mechanism are termed **nonallergic**.

IgE-Mediated Allergy

IgE-mediated allergy is typically divided into two phases: (1) an **early phase** caused by the release of preformed mediators, e.g., histamine and newly synthesized mediators, e.g., leukotrienes and prostaglandins, produced at the site of allergen contact and which typically lead to symptoms of immediate Type I hypersensitivity, i.e., within minutes; and (2) a **late phase** due to the effects of mediator release and the participation of cytokines and chemokines resulting in the recruitment of inflammatory cells, which orchestrate tissue injury responsible for late symptoms (within hours) (*Chapter 17*). It is important to recognize that IgE-mediated allergic symptoms can also be induced or aggravated by nonimmunological factors such as viral infection, irritants, drugs, exercise, and other environmental factors.

Individuals who produce IgE-mediated allergic responses are often termed to be "atopic." As described previously, **atopy** refers to a personal and/or familial tendency, usually in childhood or adolescence, to become sensitized and produce IgE antibodies in response to ordinary exposures to allergens, usually proteins. Atopic individuals are genetically predisposed to be IgE-antibody high-responders and they are identified by skin or blood tests showing IgE sensitization to common allergens and by clinical manifestations of common atopic diseases, such as asthma, eczema, allergic rhinitis, and food allergy. Experimental models to evaluate allergic responses or mechanisms often utilize or create atopic-like conditions in genetically bred animals, i.e., Balb/c mice, which are selected for their high IgE responses to antigens.

Non-IgE-Mediated Allergy

As its name implies, non-IgE-mediated allergy includes a spectrum of hypersensitivity disorders not mediated by IgE antibody. Most patients display IgG antibodies or cell-mediated responses to an allergen and, in some instances, these conditions can manifest immediate symptoms that mimic IgE-mediated allergy. These diseases are differentiated from IgE-mediated allergy by the participation of other hypersensitivity mechanisms leading to tissue injuries that are described in Chapter 17. Examples of disorders involving non-IgE pathogenetic mechanisms include celiac disease (Type IVA), allergic contact dermatitis (Type IVD), and hypersensitivity pneumonitis (Type III and Type IVA) (*Chapter 17*).

In most IgE-mediated allergic disorders, e.g., allergic rhinitis and asthma, acute and/or chronic manifestations of the **allergic response**, are localized to the specific target tissue or organ to which the allergen directly comes in contact. In other allergic conditions, e.g., eczema, reactions to allergen introduced at one site, e.g., the gastrointestinal tract, may manifest acutely or chronically at another tissue or organ site, e.g., the skin or respiratory tract. In yet other allergic disorders, e.g., stinging insect allergy, the injection of the offending venom may lead to more serious generalized allergic manifestations with cardiovascular collapse and respiratory failure in a condition termed "anaphylaxis."

Major Players in Allergic Disease

Allergens

An **allergen** is an immunogenic substance capable of causing allergic disease. All allergens are antigens but not all antigens are allergens. Allergens are environmental, noninfectious, innocuous substances—mostly naturally occurring proteins from plants and animals—that can induce an allergic response in a subpopulation of genetically predisposed individuals. The major routes of exposure to allergens occur by way of skin contact, food or sublingual consumption, inhalation, injection, or intravenous administration. Although allergens are typically identified by their generic source, e.g., peanut, latex, or ragweed pollen, true allergenic substances are specific proteins from these sources and are named by a standardized method of classification, e.g., Ara h 1, Hev b 1, and Amb a 1, respectively (Box 18-1).

Properties of Allergens and Allergenicity

The precise basis of how or why a protein innocuous in a normal host can be capable of inducing powerful IgE antibody responses in a susceptible host is not completely understood. It is generally accepted, however, that certain structural, functional, or biologic properties of the allergen as well as host genetic factors influence the immune responses that are elicited.

An essential requirement for allergenicity is dependent upon structural epitopes found on the allergen that generate a specific IgE antibody capable of binding allergen and initiating the allergic response. Proteins with linear IgE-binding epitopes generally constitute more effective allergens than those with conformational variations in three-dimensional structures. Although most proteins possess structural epitopes necessary for allergenicity, only a small handful of plant and animal protein families are capable of becoming allergens, suggesting that other functional or biologic properties may be operative. Shown in Table 18-1 is a classification of selected functional categories of relevant protein allergens. Some allergens express enzymatic properties that may enhance their capacity to promote IgE sensitization and allergic manifestations through a variety of mechanisms. For example, proteolytic activity associated with the major dust mite allergen, Der p 1, has been shown to digest certain components of intercellular tight junctions that facilitate allergen transfer across mucosal barriers.

Box 18-1

Method of Nomenclature of Allergenic Proteins

The World Health Organization and International Union of Immunological Societies (WHO/IUIS) Allergen Nomenclature Sub-committee has established a generally accepted method for nomenclature of allergens (http//:www.allergen.org). Allergens are named using the first three letters of the genus (space), followed by a single letter for the species (space) and an Arabic number indicating the chronologic order of allergen purification. For example, the peanut allergen *Arachis hypogaea* 1 is Ara h 1; latex allergen *Hevea brasiliensis* 1 is Hev b 1; and giant ragweed allergen *Ambrosia artemisiifolia* 1 is Amb a 1. Some examples of nomenclature of other important allergens include the major cat allergen (*Felis domesticus* allergen 1 or Fel d 1), the major dog allergen (*Canis familiaris* 1 or Can f 1), and the major dust mite allergen (*Dermatophagoides farinae 1* or Der f 1).

Routes of Allergen Entry

Allergens that give rise to allergic diseases access the host through three portals of entry, i.e., the gastrointestinal tract, the respiratory tract, and the skin, and therefore are commonly referred to as ingestants, inhalants, and contactants, respectively (Table 18-2). Although a variety of immunologic mechanisms may be involved in the pathogenesis of allergic conditions, most allergens trigger allergic manifestations through Type I hypersensitivity mechanisms. Allergens can initiate allergic sensitization either as complete immunogens or as low molecular weight molecules referred to as haptens that become fully immunogenic only after combining with a carrier protein, e.g., penicillin (*Chapter 1*).

Allergic Inflammation: The Integrated Response of the Innate and Adaptive Immune Systems

Allergic inflammation results from the sequential activation of a multitude of components of both the constitutive as well as the innate and adaptive immune systems (Figure 18-2). For ease of discussion, these components can be organized into four groups. Prior to activation of the innate and adaptive immune systems, the skin and mucosal surfaces provide a constitutive barrier function (Group 1) to prevent penetration of epithelial surfaces by allergens, microbes, and other foreign and potentially noxious substances. When this system is breached, the innate immune system (Group 2) is then called

Table 18-1. Selected functional categories of relevant protein allergens and their common sources

Functional categories	Proteins	Major allergenic source(s)
Enzyme proteases	Trypsins/chymotrypsins	*Dermatophagoides* (dust mites) feces
	Lysozyme	Egg whites
	Fungal proteases	*Aspergillus fumigatus, Alternaria alternata, Cladosporium herbareum*
	Papain/bromelain/actinidin	Papaya/pineapple/kiwi
	Phospholipase, hyaluronidases	Bee venom
Enzyme inhibitors	Trypsin inhibitors	Soy
	α-amylase inhibitors	Wheat/cereals
Seed storage proteins	Vicilins	Peanut, sesame, tree nuts, legumes
	2S albumins	Mustard, brazil nut, walnut
	Glycinins	Peanut, soybean
	β-conglycinin	Soybean
	Glutens	Wheat/cereals
Pathogenesis-related (PR) proteins (plants) defense against fungi and insects	Bet v 1 (major birch pollen allergen) homologous proteins	Many types of fruits and vegetables (Fagales tree family)
	Lipid transfer proteins (LTP)	Prunoideae fruits, barley, soybean
	Chitinases	Latex, avocado, chestnut, banana
	β-1,3-glucanases	Latex, banana, other fruits and vegetables
	Thaumatin-like proteins	Apple, cherry, bell pepper
Plant virulence factors	Pectate lyases	Pollens (weeds), many fruits and vegetables
Actin-binding proteins	Profilins	Pollens (birch, mugwort, grass), celery, hazelnut, many fruits and vegetables
Calcium-binding proteins	Parvalbumins	Fish
	Caseins	Milk
Lipid-binding proteins	β-lactoglobulin	Milk
	Nonspecific LTP	Wheat
Transport proteins	Lipocalins	Mammalian dander and secretions
	Serum albumins	Milk, mammalian meat
Miscellaneous	β-expansins	Grass pollen
	Uteroglobulin	Cat saliva
	Tropomyosins	Arthropods (shellfish, cockroaches, mites)

upon to respond to signals from the external environment, e.g., PAMPs (*Chapter 3*). Cellular contributors to the innate immune response include the epithelium, endothelial and stromal cells, and other components of the innate immune system, e.g., phagocytic cells (dendritic cells, neutrophils, monocytes/macrophages, and eosinophils), mediator cells (basophils and mast cells), natural killer cells, and the complement system (*Chapter 1*). The dendritic cells provide a key bridge to the adaptive immune system by instructing T lymphocytes and B lymphocytes of the adaptive immune system (Group 3) through a myriad of secreted and cell-bound cytokines. The predominance of Th2-mediated responses favors production of allergen-specific IgE antibodies in allergic inflammation. The cumulative end consequence of these total interactions results in the priming, recruitment, and activation of inflammatory cells and release of inflammatory mediators and cytokines, leading to target cell injury (Group 4). This injury could be of short duration if the allergen can be effectively eliminated

Table 18-2. Routes, types, and mechanisms of common allergens that give rise to allergic disease manifestations

Route	Allergen	Immunologic mechanism	Disease manifestation
Ingestants	Foods	Types I, IV	Food allergy/anaphylaxis, celiac disease
	Drugs	Types I, IV	Allergic drug reactions/anaphylaxis, Steven Johnson's syndrome
Inhalants	Pollens, dust mites, molds, pet dander	Type I	Allergic rhinitis Bronchial asthma
	Aspergillus fumigatus	Types I, III	Allergic bronchopulmonary aspergillosis (ABPA)
	Thermophylic actinomycetes	Types III, IV	Extrinsic allergic alveolitis
Injectants	Drugs (including serum)	Types I, II, III, IV	Allergic drug reaction, hemolytic anemia, serum sickness
	Bee stings	Type I	Venom anaphylaxis
	Vaccines	Type III	Localized Arthus reaction
Contactants	Foods, pet dander, poison ivy, nickel	Types I, IV	Contact urticaria, allergic contact dermatitis

or more protracted with failure of allergen clearance. In the latter case, chronic inflammation and tissue remodeling may result; these represent the most deleterious consequences of the allergic response.

IgE Antibody and Receptors

Properties of IgE

IgE is a monomeric antibody with a molecular weight of 190 kDa and a typical immunoglobulin composition of two light chains and two isotype-specific heavy chains. Each light chain consists of one variable light chain domain (**VL**) and a constant light chain domain (**CL**); each heavy chain consists of one variable heavy chain domain (**VH**) and four constant heavy chain domains: Cε1, Cε2, Cε3, and Cε4 (*Chapter 6* and Figure 18-3).

Of the five immunoglobulin isotypes, IgE displays the lowest serum concentration, with a peak concentration at 10 to 15 years of age in nonatopic individuals (*Chapter 6*). In individuals with allergy, this peak occurs earlier. IgE neither crosses the placenta nor activates complement. Approximately 50 percent of the total IgE resides in the intravascular compartment, with the remaining other half found in tissues bound primarily to mast cells. The half-life of IgE in peripheral blood is approximately one to five days, but IgE can persist in tissues for up to several months when bound to its receptor on mast cells. Elevated IgE levels are generally found in atopic disorders, allergic bronchopulmonary aspergillosis (**ABPA**), and parasitic diseases. A variety of nonparasitic infections, e.g., EBV, HIV, and inflammatory diseases, e.g., Kawasaki disease and malignancies, e.g., Hodgkin's lymphoma and some immunodeficiencies, e.g., hyper-IgE syndrome and Wiskott-Aldrich syndrome, are also associated with elevated IgE levels (*Chapter 16*).

IgE Production

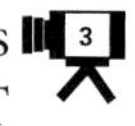

As described in Chapters 1 and 6, IgE synthesis requires the coordinated interaction of APCs, T cells, and B cells. Shown in Figure 18-4 is a schematic representation of the cellular and molecular interactions associated with IgE production. Following uptake and processing of allergen by APCs, e.g., either DCs or B cells, the resultant peptides are presented to T cells in the context of MHC-II molecules (Figure 18-4A). The T/B cell interaction represents a reciprocal stimulatory relationship (Figure 18-4B) where each cell contributes to and then responds to three activation signals generated by each toward the other: **signal 1** occurs when peptides are presented to a naive Tho cell through its TCR in the context of MHC-II with the participation of the CD4 co-receptor; **signal 2** is provided through the interaction of co-stimulatory interactions between upregulated molecules on B cells, e.g., B7.1 (CD80) and B7.2 (CD86) with those on CD4+ T cells, e.g., CD28; and **signal 3** is a cytokine-induced phase brought about initially by the activation of naive T cells by IL-2, IL-4-mediated Th2 differentiation, and the production of IL-4, IL-5, IL-9, and IL-13 that provide additional signals to B cells required to drive IgE synthesis (Figure 18-4A). Recent evidence suggests that basophils may also be an important source for IL-4 and CD40L to further amplify IgE synthesis and drive Th2 cell differentiation.

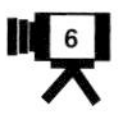

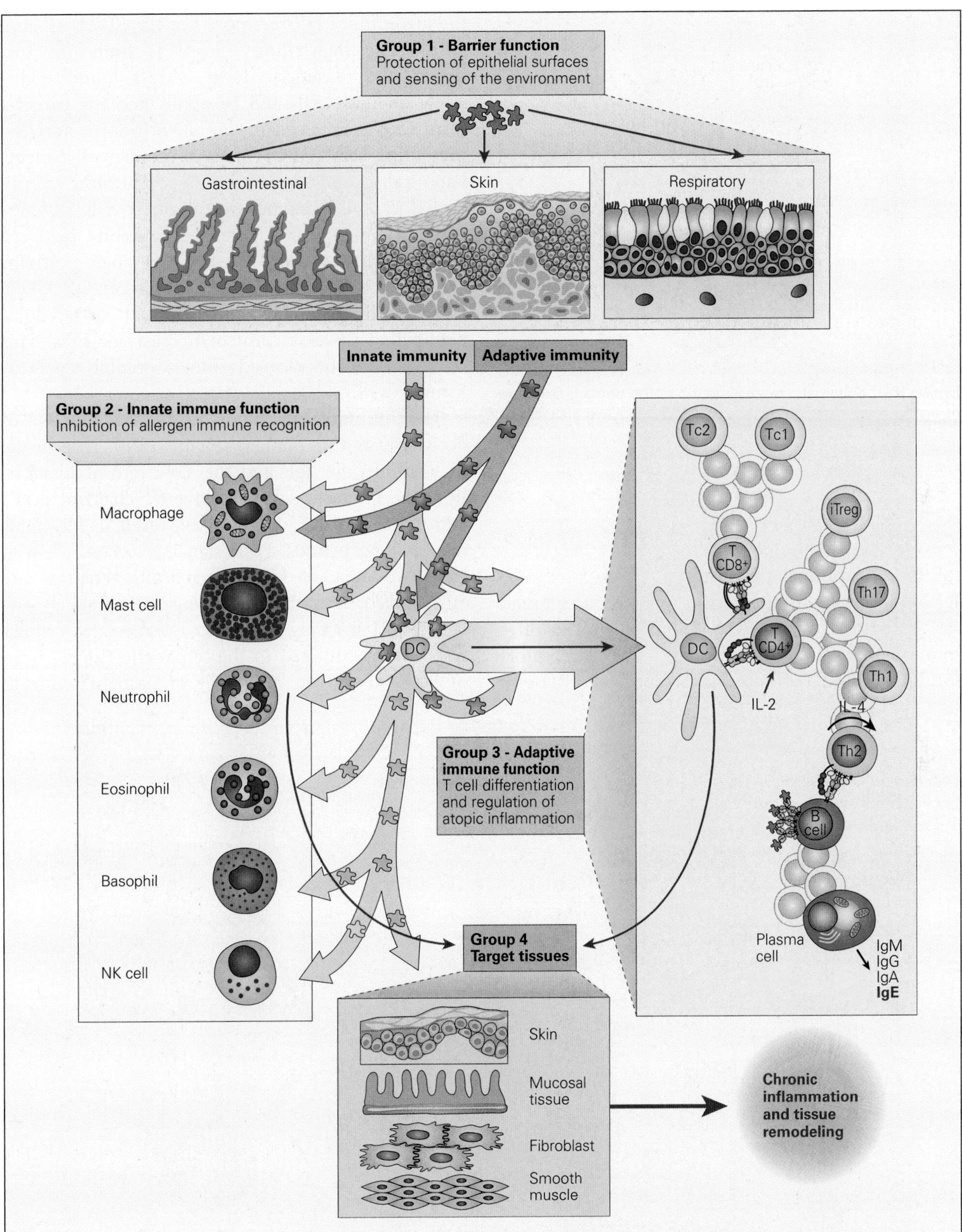

Figure 18-2. Schematic representation of the integrated participation of the constitutive, innate, and adaptive immune responses in allergic inflammation arranged into four groups. Group 1 responses are provided by the protective barrier functions of epithelial surfaces of skin and mucous membranes. Group 2 responses include components of the innate immune system. Group 3 consists of the interactive components of the T and B cells of the adaptive immune system. Group 4 responses represent the cumulative effects of the innate and adaptive immune responses leading to target cell injury. This phase may be of short duration if allergen can be effectively eliminated or more protracted with the failure of allergen clearance resulting in chronic inflammation and tissue remodeling.

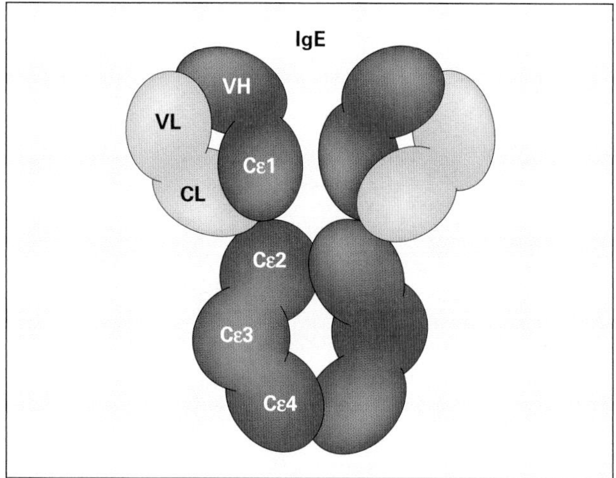

Figure 18-3. Schematic representation of the domain structure of an IgE molecule. An IgE molecule showing two light chains (light green) with one variable light chain domain (VL) and a constant light chain domain (CL) and two isotype-specific heavy chains (red) with five separate domains, one variable heavy chain domain (VH), and four constant heavy chain domains: Cε1, Cε2, Cε3, and Cε4.

IgE Receptors and IgE Binding

IgE antibody binds to specific IgE receptors found on the surface of a variety of innate and adaptive immune cells. There are two distinct cell receptors for IgE: the high-affinity IgE receptor (FcεRI) and the low-affinity IgE receptor (FcεRII; CD23) (Figure 18-5). The high-affinity FcεRI is found in two forms—the tetrameric form ($\alpha\beta\gamma_2$) found exclusively on mast cells and basophils and the trimeric form ($\alpha\gamma_2$) expressed in low quantities on antigen-presenting cells (**APCs**) such as monocytes, Langerhans cells, and dendritic cells. The low-affinity FcεRII receptor can be present on B cells and up-regulated on activated T cells, eosinophils, platelets, and epithelial cells and consists of a single polypeptide chain characterized by an extracellular CD23 lectin-binding domain and a linear extracellular region that serves as proteolytic cleavage sites. This receptor can be cleaved into a soluble (sCD23) form as well.

The IgE molecule binds to the α1 domain of FcεRI via its Cε3 domain (Figure 18-6). Due to the high affinity for IgE and the slow rate of dissociation, the interaction between the α1 chain of FcεRI and the Cε3 of IgE molecule can result in IgE binding for long periods. FcεR signaling occurs when at least two adjacent IgE-bound FcεRI receptors are cross-linked by multivalent allergen on the cell surface. FcεRI signaling leading to IgE-mediated cellular responses is confined to the tetrameric ($\alpha\beta\gamma2$) form of FcεRI found on mast cells or basophils, due to

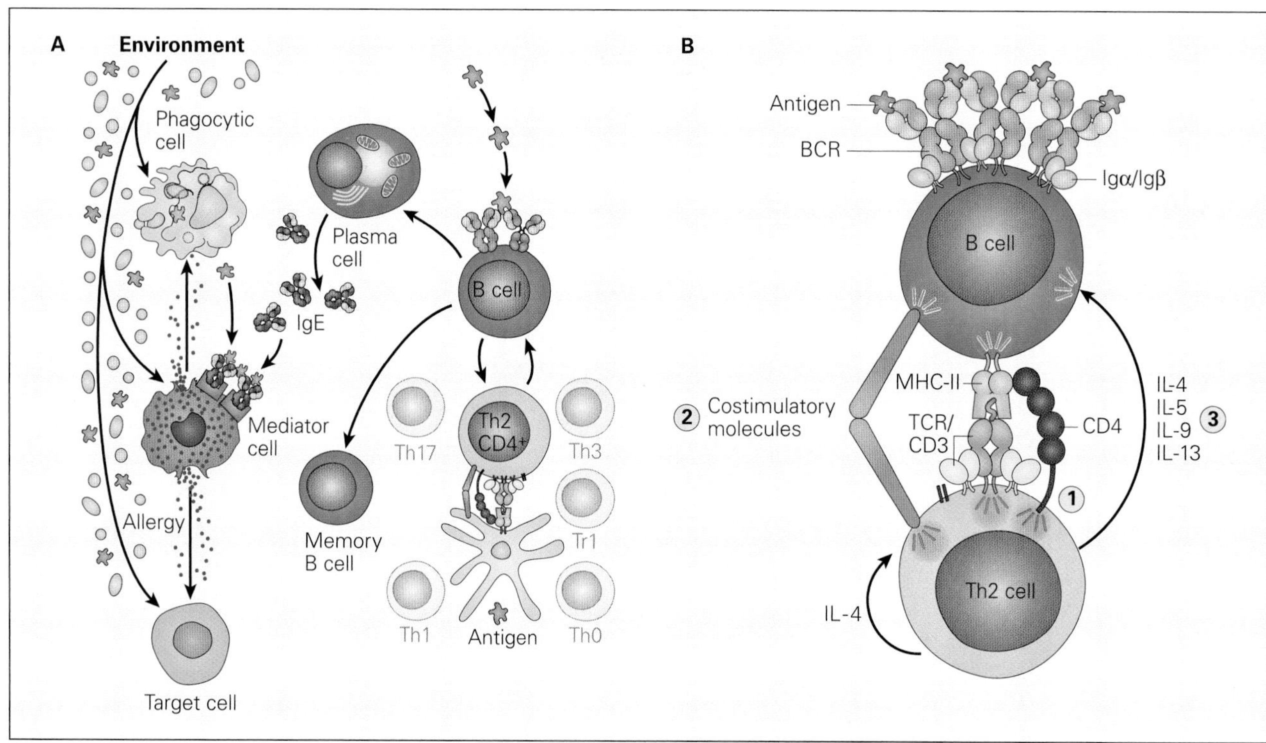

Figure 18-4. Schematic representation of the cellular and molecular events associated with IgE production. Panel A: Uptake and processing of antigen by DCs or B cells that leads to the synthesis of IgE by plasma cells. Panel B: The reciprocal T/B cell activation requiring three stimulatory signals.

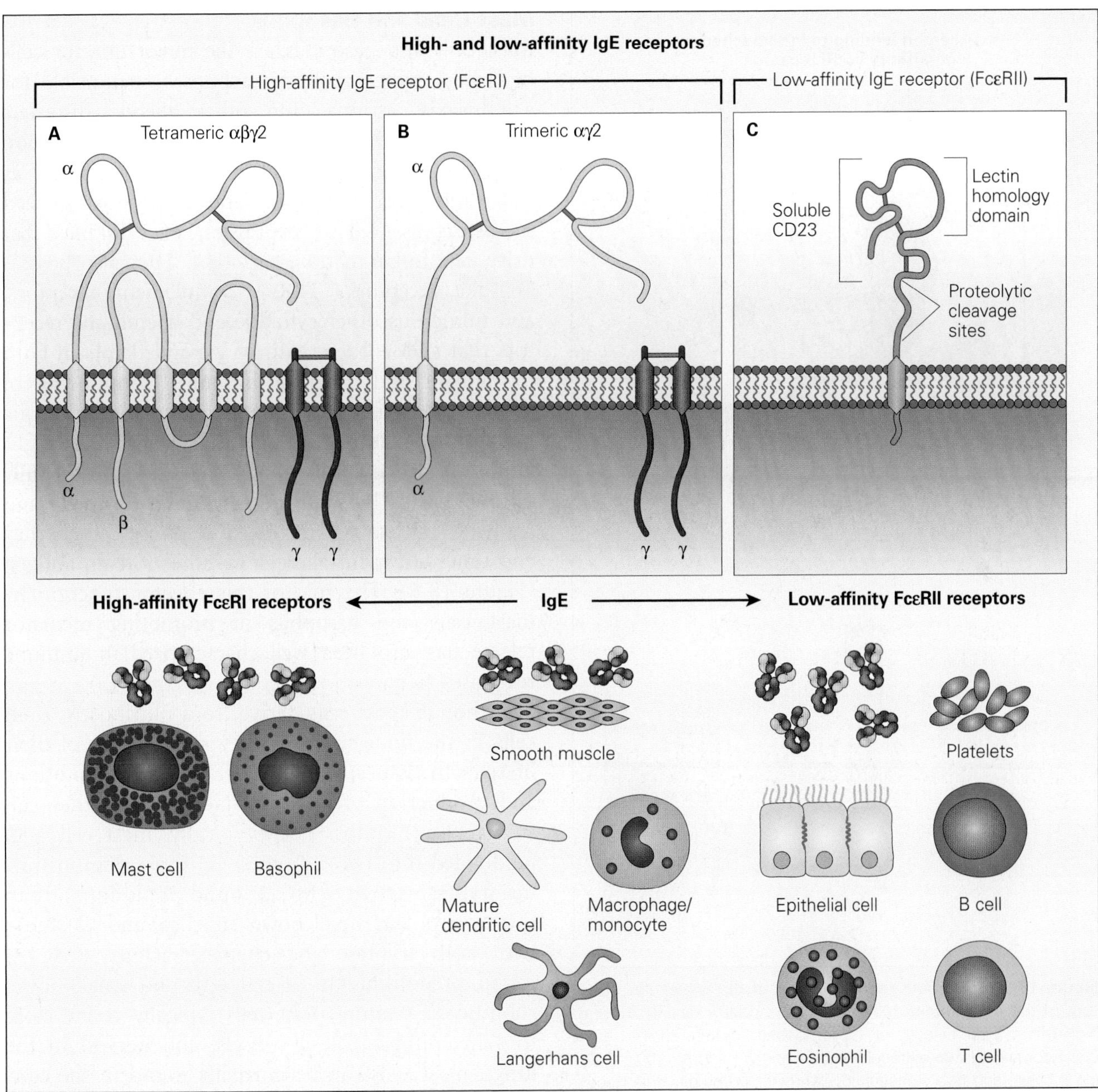

Figure 18-5. Schematic representation of IgE-binding receptors. There are two distinct cell receptors for IgE: the high-affinity IgE receptor (FcεRI) and the low-affinity IgE receptor (FcεRII). Panel A: FcεRI can exist as a tetrameric αβγ2 molecule on mast cells and basophils. Panel B: A trimeric αγ2 molecule on monocytes/macrophages, Langerhans cells, and dendritic cells. Panel C: FcεRII may be found on a wide variety of target cells, e.g., airway smooth and epithelial cells, eosinophils, platelets, and T and B lymphocytes.

the requirement of the β chain for amplifying IgE-mediated intracellular signaling after receptor cross-linking. The β chain is also responsible for amplifying FcεRI cell surface expression on these cells.

Another major regulator of FcεRI cell surface expression on mast cells and basophils is the presence of IgE antibody. For example, the density of FcεRI expression on basophils has been shown to correlate directly with serum IgE levels, and, on mast cells, FcεRI not occupied by IgE has a very short half-life, whereas occupied FcεRI remains expressed on the surface indefinitely. These observations not only explain the high density of these receptors found on mast cells and basophils of individuals with atopic disorders, but also provide a rationale for the use of therapies, e.g., omalizumab that target IgE and/or FcεRI occupation by IgE in preventing FcεRI-mediated allergic responses.

Little is known about the role of the trimeric form ($\alpha\gamma_2$) of the high-affinity FcεRI expressed on

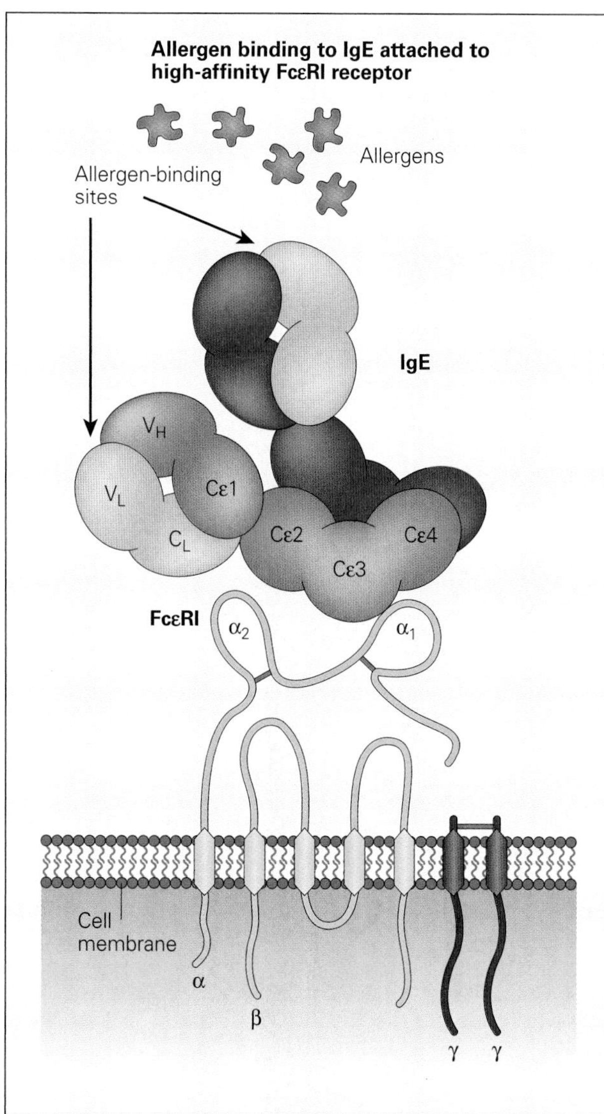

Figure 18-6. Schematic representation of the molecular structure of the high-affinity tetrameric IgE receptor (FcεRI). The IgE high-affinity FcεR1 receptor is composed of four chains: an α chain containing two extracellular domains (α1 and α2), a long single β chain, and two γ chains covalently joined by disulfide bonds. The IgE molecule binds to the α1 domain of the IgE FcεR1 receptor via its Cε3 domain.

the surface of APCs. Since this receptor lacks the critical β chain for signal amplification, it is hypothesized that APCs utilize this receptor as a decoy receptor for sequestration of IgE. The low-affinity FcεRII (CD23) has been shown to have an important regulatory role in IgE synthesis and B and T cell growth and differentiation as well as activation of monocytes. CD23 expression on many cells is upregulated by IgE and IL-4, and both membrane-bound and soluble CD23 expression is increased in allergic disorders. As such, CD23 holds promise as a novel therapeutic target for allergic disorders.

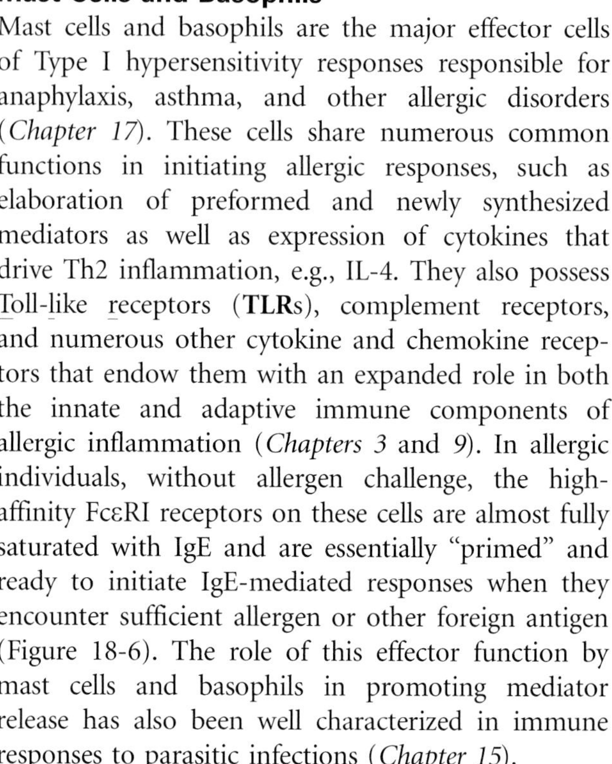

Mast Cells and Basophils

Mast cells and basophils are the major effector cells of Type I hypersensitivity responses responsible for anaphylaxis, asthma, and other allergic disorders (*Chapter 17*). These cells share numerous common functions in initiating allergic responses, such as elaboration of preformed and newly synthesized mediators as well as expression of cytokines that drive Th2 inflammation, e.g., IL-4. They also possess Toll-like receptors (**TLRs**), complement receptors, and numerous other cytokine and chemokine receptors that endow them with an expanded role in both the innate and adaptive immune components of allergic inflammation (*Chapters 3* and *9*). In allergic individuals, without allergen challenge, the high-affinity FcεRI receptors on these cells are almost fully saturated with IgE and are essentially "primed" and ready to initiate IgE-mediated responses when they encounter sufficient allergen or other foreign antigen (Figure 18-6). The role of this effector function by mast cells and basophils in promoting mediator release has also been well characterized in immune responses to parasitic infections (*Chapter 15*).

Although mast cells derive from pluripotent stem cells in the bone marrow, they spend most of their lifespan in tissues, where under the right conditions and production of stem cell factor (**SCF**) they can survive for months. Phenotypically, mast cells can be divided into two subtypes: (1) those demonstrating tryptase activity (MC_T) found predominantly in the airways and small bowel mucosa, and (2) those with both tryptase and chymase activity (MC_{TC}) found predominantly in the skin and small bowel submucosa. Mature mast cells typically reside close to skin epithelia, blood vessels, and nerves. In the lungs, mast cells can be normally found in the connective tissues of the bronchial airway and in the intra-alveolar spaces; in the small bowel, they are typically found in proximity to smooth muscle tissue and mucus-producing glands. Mast cell numbers increase by several-fold in tissues following localized IgE-dependent immediate hypersensitivity responses. This increased mast cell recruitment may be linked to cytokine expression from a recently defined subset of Th2 cells called Th9 cells. These cells favor production of IL-9 over IL-4. IL-9 is a mast cell growth factor that can stimulate mast cell recruitment, protease production, and FcεRI expression.

Basophils, on the other hand, are granulocytes mostly found circulating in the peripheral blood and have a lifespan of a few days. Due to their low numbers in blood (normally < 1 percent of all granulocytes) and fragility in experimental conditions, the clinical role of basophils has only recently been elucidated. They are now recognized to be a major source of early IL-4 and IL-13 production following antigen exposure in both humans and in experimental animal model systems of allergic disease. Basophils also have the capacity to migrate into tissues, providing support for maintaining Th2-induced inflammation and IgE synthesis as well to play an important role as APCs.

Mediator Products of Mast Cells and Basophils

Mast cells and basophils produce a similar mediator profile and express a number of receptors activated by cytokines, chemokines, and growth factors (*Chapters 3* and *9*). The most significant stimulus for activation of these cells in IgE-mediated allergic conditions is achieved by the cross-linking of FcεRI by multivalent allergen, leading to release of preformed and newly synthesized mediators of allergic inflammation, e.g., histamine, leukotrienes, and Th2 cytokines, e.g., IL-4. However, mast cells and basophils can also release mediators through mechanisms independent of IgE. Mast cells have a much larger known repertoire of cytokines and chemokines than basophils and they also produce proinflammatory prostaglandins, e.g., PGD2, and Th1 cytokines, e.g., IFN-γ and TNF-α.

Mast cells and basophils may be activated by additional mechanisms. These include IgG binding to the high-affinity IgG receptor, FcγRI, only present on mast cells, as well as by binding to receptors for complement anaphylatoxins C3a and C5a, present on both mast cells and basophils (*Chapter 4* and Figure 18-18). Enhanced signaling may also result from the binding of PAMPs through TLRs, both of which are expressed on both mast cells and basophils. These activation pathways not only highlight the diverse immune functions of mast cells and basophils in both innate and adaptive immunity, but also provide alternative conduits, independent of IgE, by which other antigens, e.g., parasites, plant lectins, and viral superantigens, can trigger mast cell and basophil responses.

Mast Cell Disorders

Mutations in the tyrosine kinase KIT, the receptor for SCF, can lead to pathologic increases of mast cells in the bone marrow and tissues as part of the clinical disorder of **mastocytosis**. This disease can occur at any age and can be confined to the skin (cutaneous mastocytosis), as evidenced by skin lesions containing dense deposits of mast cells, i.e., urticaria pigmentosa, or involve mast cell infiltrates in the bone marrow and multiple other organs (systemic mastocytosis). In part due to the heightened presence of mast cells in these individuals, clinical symptoms often include flushing and hypotension to a variety of external agents. In severe cases, hematologic malignancies may develop.

Eosinophils

One of the hallmarks of allergen-induced inflammation is the accumulation or infiltration of eosinophils into mucosal tissues. Eosinophils preferentially home to these tissues by the activation of adhesion molecules, i.e., very late antigen-4 (**VLA-4**) and vascu-  lar cell adhesion molecule-1 (**VCAM-1**) (*Chapter 5*), which are upregulated by IL-4, IL-5, chemokines, e.g., eotaxins, and leukotrienes, e.g., LTB4 (Figure 18-7). IL-5 is by far the most important eosinophil-specific factor as it is responsible for both eosinophil growth and differentiation and release of eosinophils from the bone marrow (*Chapter 9*). Since Th2 cells are the major producers of IL-5, eosinophil recruitment is largely dependent on T cell activity. GM-CSF produced by epithelial cells also appears to have a role in the permanence, and possibly activation, of eosinophils in tissues.

Eosinophilic Intracellular Products that Promote Inflammation

Activated eosinophils are equipped with uniquely toxic molecules that they synthesize and store in intracellular granules, many of which can promote allergic inflammation, e.g., major basic protein (**MBP**), which has antihelminth activity and whose levels correlate with bronchial hyperresponsiveness in patients with asthma. Other important eosinophil-derived molecules include neurotoxins and cationic proteins, which also provide RNAse activity against pneumoviruses and peroxidases that generate local tissue damage, as well as proinflammatory leukotrienes, prostaglandins, and platelet-activating factor (**PAF**).

Eosinophilic Disorders

Eosinophilia is a condition characterized by an elevated concentration of eosinophils (eosinophil granulocytes) in the blood. For ease of discussion, it may be useful to classify the eosinophilic disorders

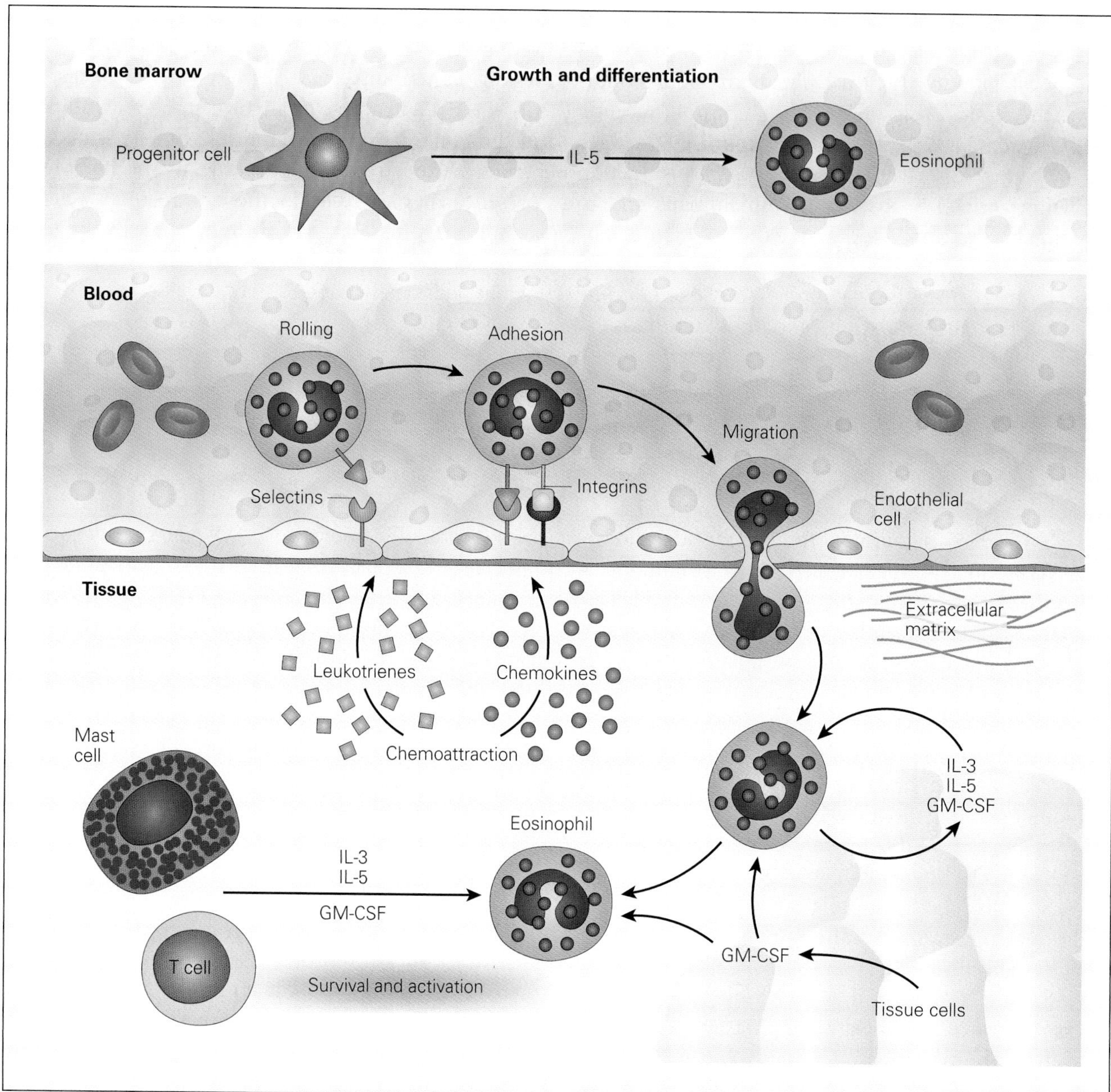

Figure 18-7. Schematic representation of eosinophil maturation in bone marrow, their entry in the blood, and factors that influence their migration into tissue. Eosinophils develop in the bone marrow in response to the stimulation of progenitor cells by interleukin-5. Mature eosinophils in the peripheral blood adhere to endothelial cells through the interaction of selectins and integrins (CD18 and very late antigen-4 [VLA-4]) with endothelial receptors for these molecules. On exposure to chemoattractant mediators, eosinophils undergo diapedesis between endothelial cells and migrate into the tissues. The accumulation and permanence of eosinophils is regulated by the generation of various cytokines e.g., IL-3, IL-5, and GM-CSF, by T cells, and probably mast cells. In response to extracellular-matrix components, eosinophils themselves can also generate the cytokines that prolong their survival.

into those where the primary cause of eosinophilia is located within the eosinophil lineage (**intrinsic eosinophilic disorders**) or those that involve cells or factors outside of the eosinophil lineage (**extrinsic eosinophilic disorders**) (Table 18-3). The intrinsic eosinophilic disorders mainly represent hematologic disorders affecting multipotent or pluripotential hematopoietic stem cells that at least partially involve the eosinophil lineage and are thought to be due mainly to mutational events affecting these lineages. In contrast, the extrinsic eosinophilic disorders are caused by Th2 cytokines released by T cells or tumor cells that either stimulate increased bone marrow production, i.e., "the eosinophil hematopoietins"—IL-5,

Table 18-3. A Pathobiologically-oriented classification of the eosinophilic disorders

Intrinsic eosinophilic disorders	Extrinsic eosinophilic disorders	
	Cell of Origin	
Pluripotent hematopoetic or multipotent myeloid stem cell (mutation)	**T cell (cytokine)***	**Tumor cell (cytokine)**
• Chronic myeloid leukemias • Chronic eosinophilic leukemias • Acute myeloid leukemias • Myelodysplastic syndrome • Other myeloproliferative diseases	• Allergic diseases, e.g. asthma, eosinophilic gastrointestinal disorders, ABPA • Infectious diseases, e.g. helminths, parasites • Autoimmune diseases, e.g. systemic sclerosis • Churg-Strauss syndrome • Graft-versus host diseases • Immunodeficiencies, e.g. Omenn syndrome • Drug-induced hypersensitivity, including drug reactions with eosinophilia and systemic symptoms (DRESS)	• Hodgkin's lymphoma • Cutaneous T cell lymphoma • Acute lymphoblastic/-cytic leukemias • Langerhans cell histiocytosis • Epithelial cancers

Adapted from Simon D, Simon HU. Eosinophilic disorders. J Allergy Clin Immunol. 2007; 119: 1291–300.
*May also include idiopathic hypereosinophilic syndrome

IL-3, and GM-CSF, or recruitment of eosinophils by cytokines with chemoattractant activity, i.e., eotaxin and/or RANTES (*Chapter 9*). Among the extrinsic causes, allergic diseases such as asthma, atopic eczema, eosinophilic GI disorders (**EGID**), and ABPA are prominent causes of tissue or blood eosinophilia. Infectious agents associated with eosinophilia include helminths and other parasitic diseases. It is also important to consider the myriad autoimmune diseases, immune deficiency disorders, malignancies, and drug-induced hypersensitivities that can also present with eosinophilia. Drug reactions with eosinophilia and systemic symptoms (**DRESS**) involve anticonvulsants, antibiotics, and NSAIDs and can be particularly severe and life-threatening.

Dendritic Cells

As described in Chapter 3, dendritic cells (**DCs**) are immune cells of the mammalian innate immune system that provide an important bridge with the adaptive immune system by processing antigen and presenting the resulting peptide to T cells. Two subsets of DCs have been identified: the myeloid and plasmacytoid DCs, i.e., mDCs and pDCs, respectively. These cells are specialized for internalizing foreign antigen and form an important network of sentinels at the interface between the epithelium and the external environment. They are found in an immature state in the upper layers of the epithelium and lamina propria of the skin, lungs, and gastrointestinal tract. In the skin, the immature DCs are referred to as Langerhans cells. Once antigen is internalized and recognized in the context of a "danger" signal (i.e., pathogen- or damage-associated molecular pattern), DCs migrate to draining lymph nodes where they process the antigen in context of the respective MHC for presentation to T cells. In the lymph node, mature DCs synapse with naive T cells and release various cytokines, e.g., IL-4 and IL-12. It appears that the degree of maturation of the DC as well as the intensity of signals generated from these various cellular and cytokine interactions are important factors in driving T cell subset polarization or tolerance. Recent evidence suggests that the pDCs may exert beneficial antiallergic as well as an autoinflammatory effects through their ability to upregulate Treg cells.

Natural Killer Cells

Natural killer (**NK**) cells represent a subgroup of white blood cells that are classified as lymphocytes on the basis of morphology, expression of lymphoid markers, and origin from a common bone marrow lymphoid progenitor cell (*Chapter 2*). These cells are generally considered to be components of the innate immune system because of a lack of antigen-specific cell surface receptors (*Chapter 3*). NK cells were originally described as cytotoxic cells involved in the killing of tumor cells and virus-infected cells and major producers of an array of cytokines with proinflammatory and immunosuppressive properties such as interferon-gamma (IFN-γ), TNF-alpha (TNF-α), and IL–10, respectively.

Another novel lineage of leukocytes, distinct from T cells, B cells, or NK cells, has been identified and is referred to as natural killer T (**NKT**) cells. Since NKT cells are characterized by the expression of a restricted repertoire of T cell receptors (**TCRs**), these cells are also called invariant NKT cells (**iNKT**) cells. Upon activation, iNKT cells produce a large amount of both Type 1 and Type 2 cytokines, i.e., IFN-γ and IL-4/IL-5/IL-13.

The Role of iNKT Cells in Patients with Asthma

Studies of experimentally induced asthma in mice have shown that activated iNKT cells resulted in the development of airway hyperreactivity and airway inflammation, suggesting that these cells could play an additional role in the development of allergic asthma in the human from Th2 cells. Recent studies in the human have shown an increased iNKT cell number in the bronchoalveolar lavage fluid (**BALF**) in patients with asthma. Although initial studies of asthmatic patients showing increased iNKT cells in the BALF were controversial, subsequent studies have confirmed the initial findings of elevated quantities of these cells in BALF.

Despite effective therapies targeting Th2 cytokines for asthma control, many patients with asthma are known to have unrestrained exacerbation of their asthmatic symptoms triggered by viruses, air pollution, and exercise, suggesting that airway hyperreactivity and inflammation may be due to the activation of iNKT cells. Since the invariant TCR of iNKT cells not only recognizes glycolipids from bacteria, e.g., *Sphingomonas*, *Borrelia*, and *Leishmania*, but also by viral antigens, the activation of iNKT cells by theses microbial agents might help to explain the well-known clinical exacerbation of asthma by infectious disease agents.

Pathophysiology

Type I Hypersensitivity and the Allergic Response

As described previously, the Type I hypersensitivity mechanism represents one of the most frequently encountered and clinically important tissue-damaging immune responses (*Chapter 17*). Under the strong influence of Th2 cytokines, e.g., IL-4, IL-5, IL-9, and IL-13, there is preferential IgE antibody production to exogenous allergen(s). The effector cells of Type I hypersensitivity, tissue mast cells and blood basophils, can be characterized as mucosal land mines ready to detonate and disperse their contents of inflammatory mediators when provoked by allergen-bound IgE or other factors. The release of preformed mediators (i.e., histamine, tryptase, and PAF) as well as the elaboration of newly synthesized mediators (i.e., leukotrienes and prostaglandins) by these cells contributes to increased blood flow and

cellular extravasation to the affected tissue(s) as well as spasmogenic effects on smooth muscle and nerve cells. These mediators are not only important in promoting immediate hypersensitivity responses locally but, in some cases, in amplifying the inflammatory response systemically to surrounding tissues and shock organs in a relatively short period of time. Effector cells also release cytokines and chemokines, which further contribute to inflammatory processes by activation and recruitment of inflammatory cells to the site of inflammation. The presence of these inflammatory cells in involved mucosal tissues is a hallmark of allergic inflammation, and their immunostimulatory or immunomodulatory effects contribute to both acute and chronic symptoms experienced by patients with allergic disorders.

The Three Phases of the Allergic Response: Sensitization, Challenge, and Elicitation

The allergic response may be characterized as a cascading set of sequential reactions involving three distinct phases: **sensitization**, **challenge**, and **elicitation** (Figure 18-8). The first phase begins when the genetically predisposed individual is exposed to an allergen via contact (skin), inhalation, ingestion, or intravenous routes. Allergen exposure in a Th2 cytokine-rich environment eventually leads to allergen-specific IgE production. Subsequently, the allergen-specific IgE binds to high-affinity IgE receptors on the surface of basophils and mast cells. These cells now become "primed," and the process and mechanism underlying this specific IgE production is called sensitization. Although the mechanisms underlying allergic sensitization are not completely known, a breakdown in tolerance mechanisms and/or other deficiencies of immunoregulatory function in the host are likely responsible (*Chapter 19*). Shown in Figures 18-9A and 18-9B are descriptions of some of the key T cell subsets and cytokine pathways in allergic inflammation and of the important role Treg cells play in regulating

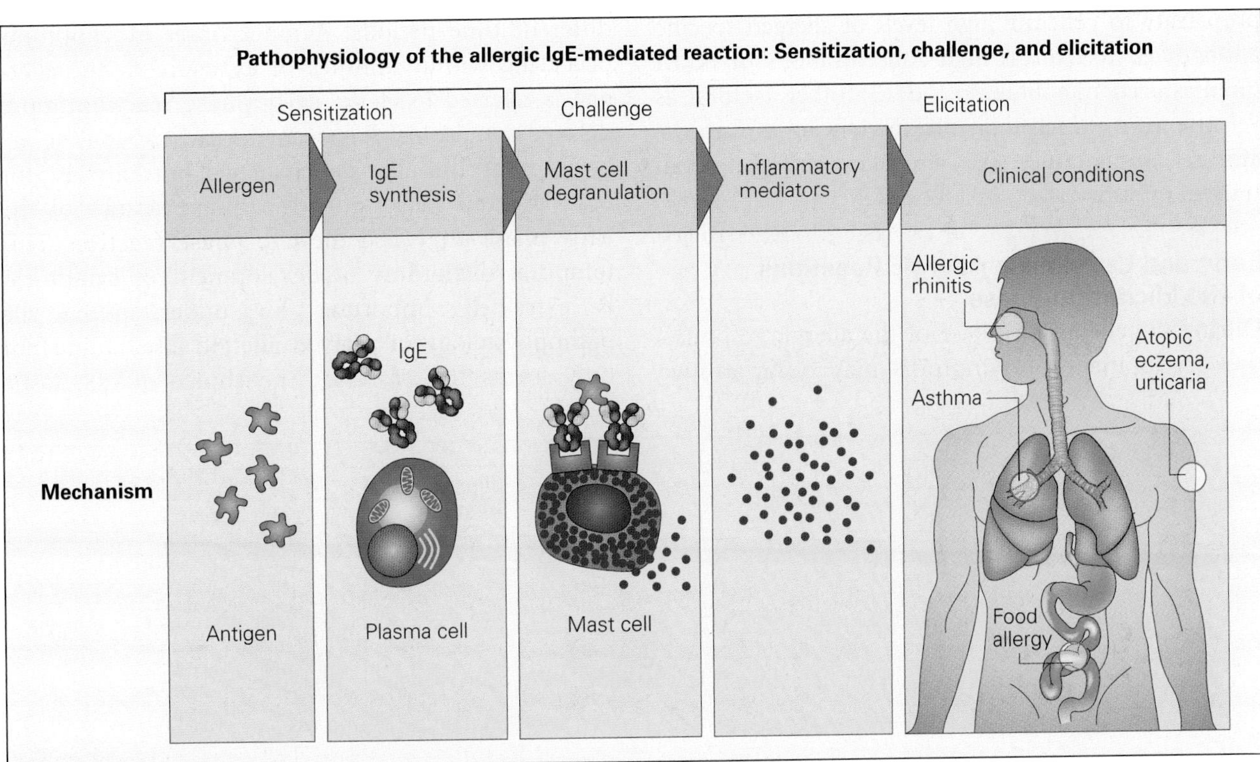

Figure 18-8. Schematic representation of the three phases involved in allergic inflammation: sensitization, challenge, and elicitation of symptoms. (Kindly provided by Thomas B. Casale.)

these subsets and pathways. These figures highlight the many ways in which deficiencies in Treg function could lead to immune imbalances or effects that favor allergic sensitization or inflammation.

Mechanisms of Allergic Sensitization: The Role of T cells

The predominant cell type in allergic disease is the Th2 lymphocyte, and the cytokines released by these cells, i.e., IL-4, IL-5, IL-9, and IL-13, have important roles in driving IgE production and mediating other aspects of allergic inflammation (Figure 18-9A). IL-4 production by Th2 cells and other inflammatory cells has also been recently associated with generation of a novel type of T cell, the Th9 cell, which predominantly releases IL-9. These cells are believed to play important roles in mast cell activation and other aspects of chronic allergic inflammation. Under normal circumstances, Treg cells keep these other T cell lineages in check (Figure 18-9B) and are major players in establishing tolerance to non-noxious foreign antigens. Since Tregs are found in rich supply at mucosal sites where the sensitization process is initiated (*Chapter 8*), a deficiency of Treg function with loss of immunoregulatory activity has been implicated in the pathogenesis of allergic disease. Shown in Figure 18-9B is a schematic representation of the various immunosuppressive pathways that Treg cells exert on cells of the innate and adaptive immune systems and where breakdown in this regulatory function can lead to immunological processes that favor allergic sensitization.

Mechanisms of Allergic Challenge and Elicitation

At any time following the sensitization period, the allergic individual may be re-exposed to the same or a closely related allergen during the second phase of the allergic reaction, referred to as the **challenge phase** (Figure 18-8). During this phase, the allergen interacts with specific IgE molecules bound to the high-affinity FcεRI receptors on mediator cells. Cross-linking of two adjacent FcεRI leads to the degranulation of these cells with the release of mediators that initiate allergic reactions and represents the third phase, referred to as the **elicitation phase**. The clinical symptomatology seen during this phase presents with either localized manifestations, e.g., allergic rhinitis, or more systemic manifestations, e.g., anaphylaxis. Factors that dictate the severity of the allergic reaction include: (1) the concentration and route of allergen exposure; (2) host genetic factors affecting the individual's propensity to generate high levels of allergen-specific antibody or to express high concentrations of FcεRI on mast cell membranes; and (3) other factors, as yet unknown, which influence the efficiency of mediator release at target sites, i.e., skin, gastrointestinal tract, respiratory tract, or blood.

Early and Late Phase Allergic Reactions of the Elicitation Phase

During the elicitation phase of the allergic response, the development of symptoms may occur at two different time periods. A rapid onset of symptoms occurring within minutes of exposure to the allergen is referred to as the **early phase reaction**; more delayed symptoms that occur as early as four to six hours after the allergen challenge but can last for days or even weeks after the disappearance of the early phase are called the **late phase reaction**. This temporal dichotomy of development of symptoms is extremely important for understanding the pathophysiology of a given allergic disease and not only forms the basis for the choice of diagnostic

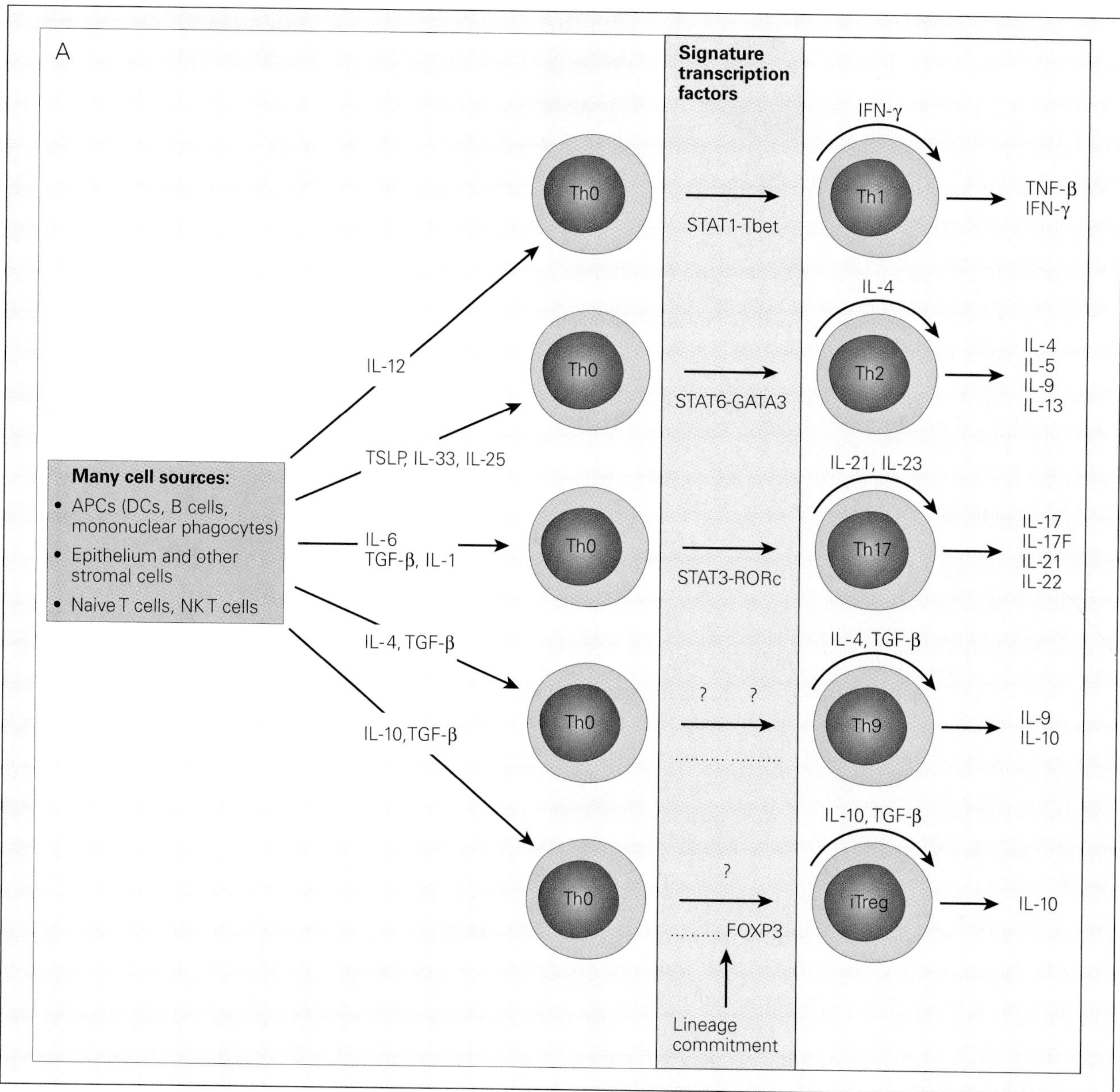

Figure 18-9. Panel A: Schematic representation of the key T cell lineages involved in inflammatory processes together with cytokines affecting their differentiation and cytokines produced by each differentiated T cell. Panel B: Schematic representation of the various immunosuppressive pathways that Treg cells can exert on cells of the innate and adaptive immune systems. (Adapted with permission from Akdis CA, Akdis M. Mechanisms and treatment of allergic disease in the big picture of regulatory T cells. J Allergy Clin Immunol 2009;123:735–46.)

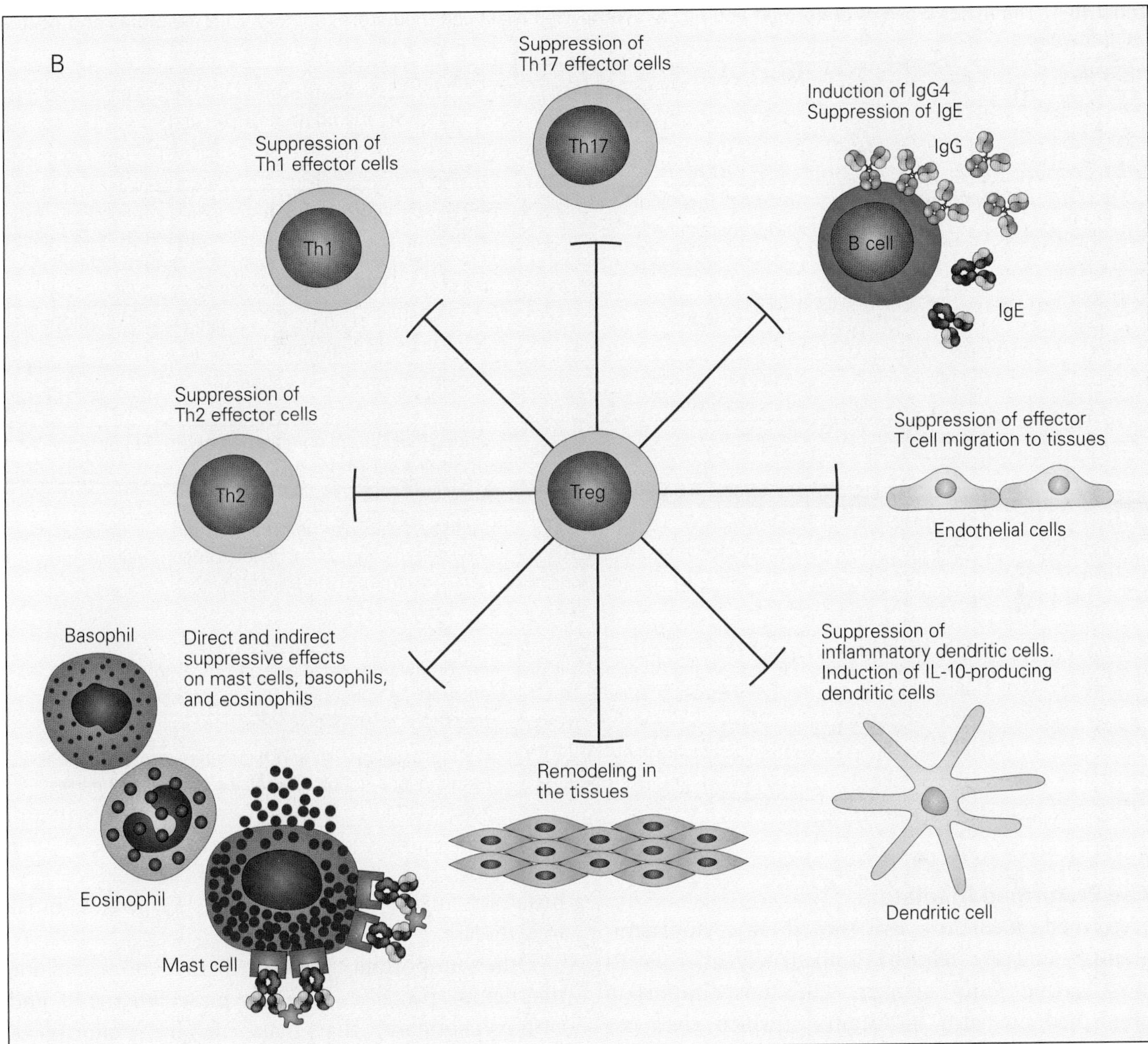

Figure 18-9. (continued)

tests to be employed, but also for the selection of optimal therapy.

Early Phase Reaction

During the early phase reaction, two types of chemical mediators are released by mast cells and basophils: (1) preformed mediators and (2) newly generated mediators. Shown in Table 18-4 are the major mast cell mediators together with examples and postulated functions. The preformed mediators of inflammation are found already synthesized and ready to be released immediately within minutes upon contact with allergen, whereas the newly generated mediators are synthesized de novo and may exert their effects later in the early phase. Upon mediator release, symptoms may include sneezing; an itchy, drippy, or congested nose; wheezing, coughing, or shortness of breath; and even rashes, hives, or skin swelling. When symptoms become more generalized and involve shock organs of the cardiorespiratory tract, the serious condition of anaphylaxis may develop. Mediators induce these symptoms by causing (1) the contraction of smooth muscles of the lung, gastrointestinal tract, and blood vessels; (2) the secretion of mucus by mucous glands in the nose, lungs, and elsewhere; (3) the dilation of blood vessels causing leakage of fluids into tissues; and (4) irritation of nerve endings resulting in either pain or itching.

Table 18-4. The major types of preformed and newly synthesized mast cell mediators together with examples and postulated functions

State	Type	Mediators	Function
Preformed	Biogenic amines	Histamine	Contraction of smooth muscle (lungs and GI tract), mucus secretion, effects on nerve endings, generation of NO (vasodilation)
	Neutral proteases	Tryptase, chymase, carboxypeptidase	Cleavage of complement (C3 and C3a); kallikrein-like activity through generation of angiotensin II; activates fibroblasts; cleave neuropeptides, e.g., substance P; acts with other neutral proteases
	Cytokines and chemokines	TNF-α, eotaxins	Upregulation of adhesion molecules and recruitment of eosinophils and neutrophils
	Acid hydrolases	β-hexosaminidase, β-glucuronidase	Enzymatic activity on epithelium
	Proteoglycans	Heparin	Anticoagulant; anticomplementary; modifies activities of other preformed mediators
		Chondroitin 4 and 6	Unknown functions
Newly synthesized	Arachidonic acid metabolites	Prostaglandins, e.g., PGD_2; cysteinyl leukotrienes, e.g., LTC_4, LTD_4, and LTE_4 (formerly called slow reacting substance of anaphylaxis, i.e., SRS-A)	Increased vascular permeability and coronary vasoconstriction; bronchoconstriction; inflammatory cell recruitment (late phase)
	Cytokines and chemokines	TNF-α, IL-3, IL-4, IL-5, IL-6, IL-10, IL-13, GM-CSF, IL-8, MIP-1α	IgE production; activation and recruitment of eosinophils, mast cells, T cells (late phase); neutrophil chemotaxis, induction of apoptosis
	Other factors	Platelet-activating factor (PAF), Calcitonin gene-related peptide (CGRP)	Platelet aggregation and histamine/serotonin release, bronchoconstriction, depressor effects on heart, vasodilation

The Preformed Mediators

Preformed mediators are stored in cytoplasmic granules and are released immediately after FcεRI cross-linking with allergen. The most important preformed mediator is histamine, which gives rise to the typical acute symptoms of the early phase reaction. Once released, histamine is directed to specific cell surface histamine receptors found in various tissues. Four histamine receptors have been identified, all of which are G protein-coupled receptors expressed on various cell types that work through different intracellular signaling mechanisms (Table 18-5). The binding of histamine with H1 receptors on vascular endothelial and smooth muscle cells in the skin leads to vasodilatation, increased vascular permeability, and the stimulation of axonal reflexes that result in the typical wheal-and-flare response of allergic disease. The recent discovery of H4 receptors on a variety of hematopoietic inflammatory cells has revealed a chemotactic role for histamine on mast cells, eosinophils, and dendritic cells as well as for T cell-associated cytokine responses, suggesting an additional immunomodulatory role of histamine in the pathogenesis of chronic inflammatory disease.

Other important preformed mediators include the neural proteases (e.g., tryptase, chymase, and carboxypeptidase) that make up the majority of protein in the granules (Table 18-4). Their role in inflammation is uncertain but they can cleave complement and fibrinogen and activate fibroblasts. Tryptase levels are frequently elevated following acute episodes of anaphylaxis. TNF-α can be released from mast cells both preformed and newly synthesized and has an important role in upregulating adhesion molecules for inflammatory cell recruitment (e.g., eosinophils and neutrophils).

Newly Synthesized Mediators

Mediators responsible for early (as well as late) phase symptoms of the allergic response include the newly synthesized mediators derived from the metabolism of arachidonic acid (*Chapter 3*) as well as generation of cytokines and chemokines and the potent vasodilator PAF. There are basically two pathways of arachidonic acid metabolism that find

Table 18-5. The four histamine receptors, major tissue locations, and biologic effects

Type	Major tissue locations	Major biologic effects
H1	Smooth muscle, endothelial cells	Induction of acute allergic responses
H2	Gastric parietal cells	Lead to secretion of gastric acid
H3	Central nervous system	Modulate neurotransmission
H4	Mast cells, eosinophils, T cells, dendritic cells	Regulation of immune responses

great clinical application in both the pathogenesis of the allergic diseases as well as a basis for the use of pharmacologic agents for their treatment: (1) the lipoxygenase and (2) the cyclooxygenase pathways (Figure 18-10).

The Lipoxygenase Products: The Leukotrienes

Leukotrienes, or lipoxygenase products, were initially discovered in 1938 as an unidentified group of chemicals released during anaphylaxis, referred to as the "slow-reacting substance of anaphylaxis" (**SRS-A**) because their physiologic effects on smooth muscles were slower than those seen with histamine. Forty years later, SRS-A was characterized as a collection of cysteinyl leukotrienes LTC_4, LTD_4, and LTE_4 due to the presence of cysteine in their structure. The release of histamine activates the enzyme phospholipase A, which in turn releases arachidonic acid from the phospholipid membrane of the mast cell (Figure 18-10). Arachidonic acid is metabolized by 5-lipoxygenase (**5-LO**) to form the various leukotrienes, e.g., LTB_4 (a potent neutrophil chemotactic factor), LTC_4, LTD_4, or LTE_4. Despite their slow onset of action, the leukotrienes, especially LTD_4, are potent inflammatory mediators. In addition to their constricting effect on bronchial smooth muscle, the leukotrienes not only increase the permeability of blood vessels resulting in the swelling of the skin, but are also powerful chemoattractants for eosinophils, thus contributing to chronic allergic inflammation as well.

The Cyclooxygenase Products: The Prostaglandins

The second family of newly synthesized mediators of inflammation generated from arachidonic acid includes the prostaglandins, which are products of the cyclooxygenase (**COX**) pathway acted upon by

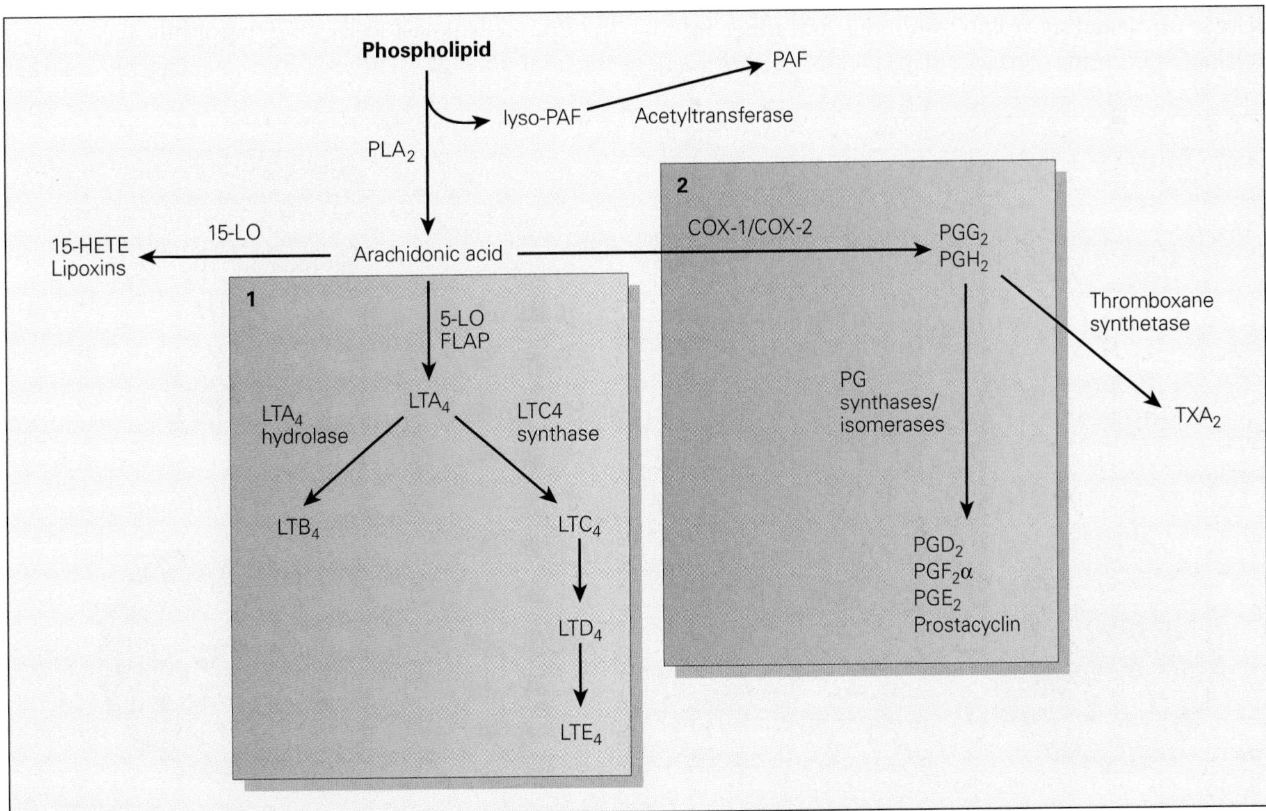

Figure 18-10. Schematic representation of the two major pathways of metabolism of arachidonic acid: (1) the lipoxygenase and (2) the cyclooxygenase pathways.

either of the two cyclooxygenase enzymes, e.g., COX-1 or COX-2 (Figure 18-10). Prostaglandin D_2 (PGD_2) is made only in the mast cells and is a potent bronchoconstrictor. Elevated PGD_2 levels have also been identified in secretions aspirated both from the lungs of patients with asthma as well as from nasal secretions of patients with allergic rhinitis. These effects are not to be confused with the effects of other prostaglandins, e.g., prostaglandin E, which conversely appear to have inhibitory roles on mediator release (Figure 18-11). This latter observation may explain why COX-inhibitor medications have been shown to have little effect in suppressing allergic reactions.

Late Phase Reaction

As the inflammatory response progresses, a late phase reaction may develop within four to six hours and is characterized by an influx of key effector cells, i.e., mast cells, basophils, and eosinophils, but also by a variety of other immune cells, e.g., macrophages, T cells, and NK cells (*Chapter 3*). Although preformed and newly synthesized mediators are also important inductive agents, cytokines and chemokines released during mast cell or basophil activation as well as by endothelial or epithelial cells are largely responsible for this initial inflammatory cell influx. Further release of mediators from eosinophils and other infiltrating immune cells leads to additional inflammation and tissue injury. By virtue of its ability to trigger effector cell mediator release, leading directly to both the early and late phase reactions, IgE plays an instrumental role in the immune system response to allergens.

With the continued presence of the allergic stimulus, uncontrolled progression of both the early and late phases of allergic inflammation eventually leads to activation of multiple cellular responses, e.g., T cells and macrophages, and cytokine pathways that contribute to chronic allergic inflammation and tissue remodeling. In asthmatic lungs, for example, these manifestations include subepithelial fibrosis, goblet cell hyperplasia, myofibroblast hyperplasia, smooth muscle cell hyperplasia, and hypertrophy, which eventually result in thickening of the airway wall and decreased lung function in what is referred to as tissue remodeling.

Role of Cytokines in the Late Phase Reaction and Chronic Allergic Inflammation

Several cytokines have been shown to be important not only in the regulation of IgE synthesis, but also in the accumulation of eosinophils and other inflammatory cells during the allergic reaction (*Chapter 9*). Interleukin-4 (IL-4) produced mainly by Th2 cells, mast cells, and basophils has proven essential for IgE synthesis and the flagship marker

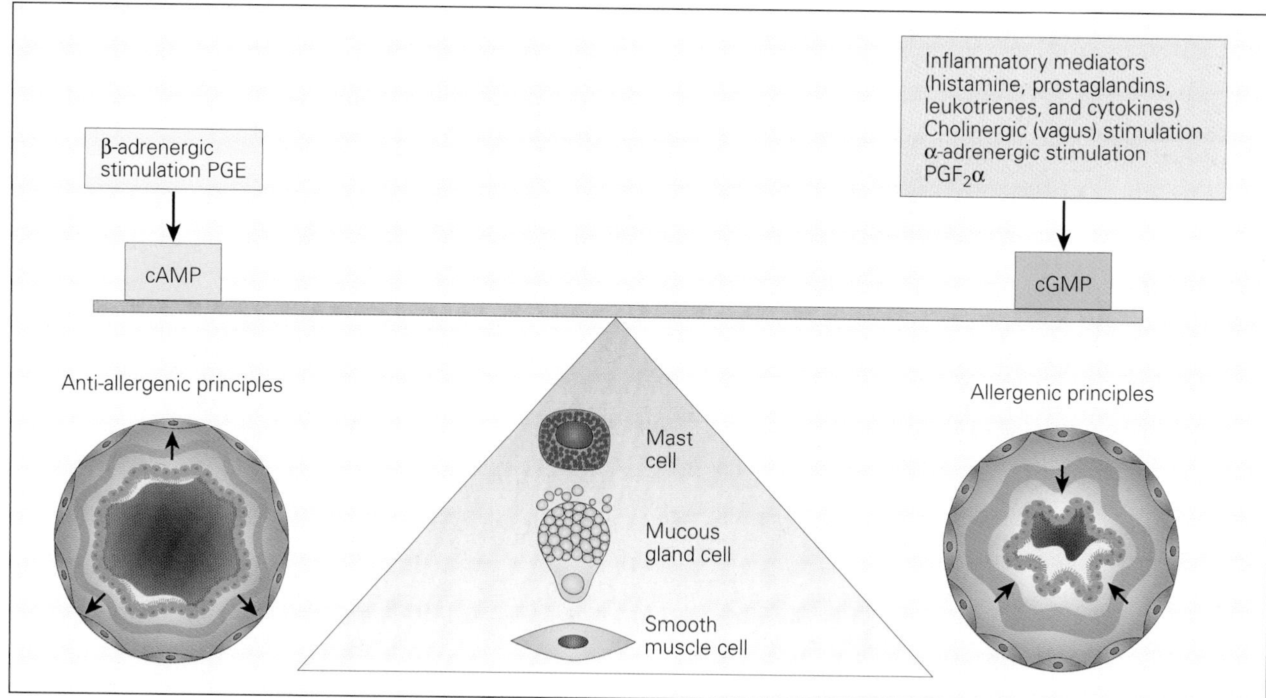

Figure 18-11. Schematic representation of the balance of intracellular cAMP and cGMP and various factors that affect this balance.

of allergic disease. IL-5 plays a key role in the maturation, activation, and survival of eosinophils, and their increased numbers in the blood and tissues is a characteristic feature of allergic disease. TNF-α is also stored preformed within mast cells and is rapidly released after an allergic reaction begins. TNF-α regulates the secretion of two chemokines, RANTES and eotaxin, which together with IL-5 are known to attract and activate eosinophils. TNF-α also promotes the synthesis of cellular adhesion molecules, e.g., VLA-4 (Figure 18-7), crucial for eosinophil and inflammatory cell recruitment to the site of the allergic reaction. In some allergic diseases, such as atopic eczema, recruitment of Th1 cells to inflamed tissues leads to further expression of TNF-α as well as other cytokines, e.g., IFN-γ, IL-1, and chemokines, e.g., IL-8, that lead to further cellular recruitment and tissue injury. There is recent evidence that in some allergic diseases, e.g., asthma and eczema, IL-9 and IL-17 are generated within inflamed tissues by respective Th9 and Th17 cells, and these cytokines contribute to sustaining the chronic inflammatory state in these diseases. Furthermore, the cellular effects of IL-10 and TGF-β help suppress the allergic response and may also stimulate factors, e.g., fibrin and angiogenesis, that promote wound healing and remodeling. In some disease states, such as asthma, this remodeling can be excessive and can promote goblet cell hyperplasia and smooth muscle changes contributing to diminished lung function and chronic lung disease.

The Participation of the Autonomic Nervous System in Allergic Disease

Although the immunologic basis of allergic disease has been highlighted in this section, it should be emphasized that another type of imbalance may exist in the allergic individual. This is an imbalance of the autonomic nervous system upon which the immunologic imbalance may also be superimposed by the neuroendocrine-immune (**NEI**) network described in Chapter 1. The autonomic nervous system is composed of the parasympathetic (cholinergic) and the sympathetic (adrenergic) systems that generally exert opposing effects on various organs. Between these two systems there appears to exist a balance that maintains a homeostatic control over both **mediator cells**, e.g., mast cells and basophils, and **target cells**, e.g., smooth muscle cells and mucus glandular cells. In the mast cell, for example, the release of vasoactive amines (mediators) can be modulated by both adrenergic and cholinergic agonists; similarly, muscle tone in bronchial smooth muscle cells can be modified by the balance between sympathetic and parasympathetic activity (Figure 18-11).

According to current concepts, sympathetic and parasympathetic responses exert their effects through the second messenger system, the cyclic nucleotide system. In the normal resting cell state, a balance appears to exist between intracellular levels of cAMP and those of cGMP, with the effects of cAMP predominating (Figure 18-12A). This balance is not only influenced by both parasympathetic and sympathetic activity, but also by a variety of other reactants, including inflammatory mediators, e.g., histamine, prostaglandins, leukotrienes, and cytokines, as well as the actual levels of cAMP and cGMP.

Following FcεRI cross-linking by antigen, increased intracellular signaling events occur that result in increased cGMP levels, a resultant decrease in cellular levels of cAMP, and eventual release of preformed intracellular mediators (Figure 18-12B). A similar effect may occur with parasympathetic stimulation through the cholinergic receptor as well as sympathetic stimulation through the α-adrenergic receptor. Stimulation of β-adrenergic receptors by epinephrine agonists increases the intracellular levels of camp, leading to decreased mediator release (Figure 18-12C).

The release of mediators also has an effect on the target cell, acting presumably through receptors on the surface of the target cell and secondarily by affecting subepithelial irritant receptors that can exert a cholinergic effect, e.g., through the vagus, on the target cell (Figure 18-13). This interaction disrupts the relative balance of cyclic nucleotides within the target cell and modulates the physiologic state or tone of the cell. The effects of raised levels of cAMP lead to a relaxation of smooth muscle, vasoconstriction of blood vessels, or decreased secretion of mucus from target cells; decreased levels of cAMP have the opposite effect.

The Beta-Adrenergic Theory of the Atopic Abnormality in Bronchial Asthma

In 1968, Szentivany proposed that owing either to a partial β-adrenergic blockade, or to an inefficiency of the β receptor, an imbalance between intracellular levels of cAMP and cGMP exists in the atopic individual, with a tendency toward decreased intracellular levels of cAMP. Such an imbalance would

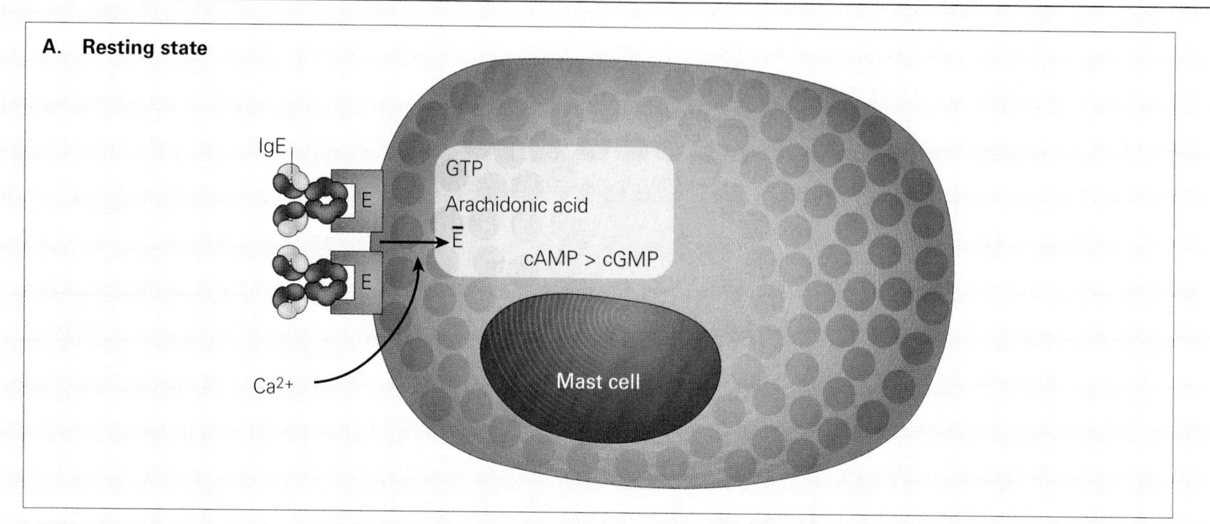
A. Resting state
IgE
E
GTP
Arachidonic acid
Ē
cAMP > cGMP
E
Ca2+
Mast cell

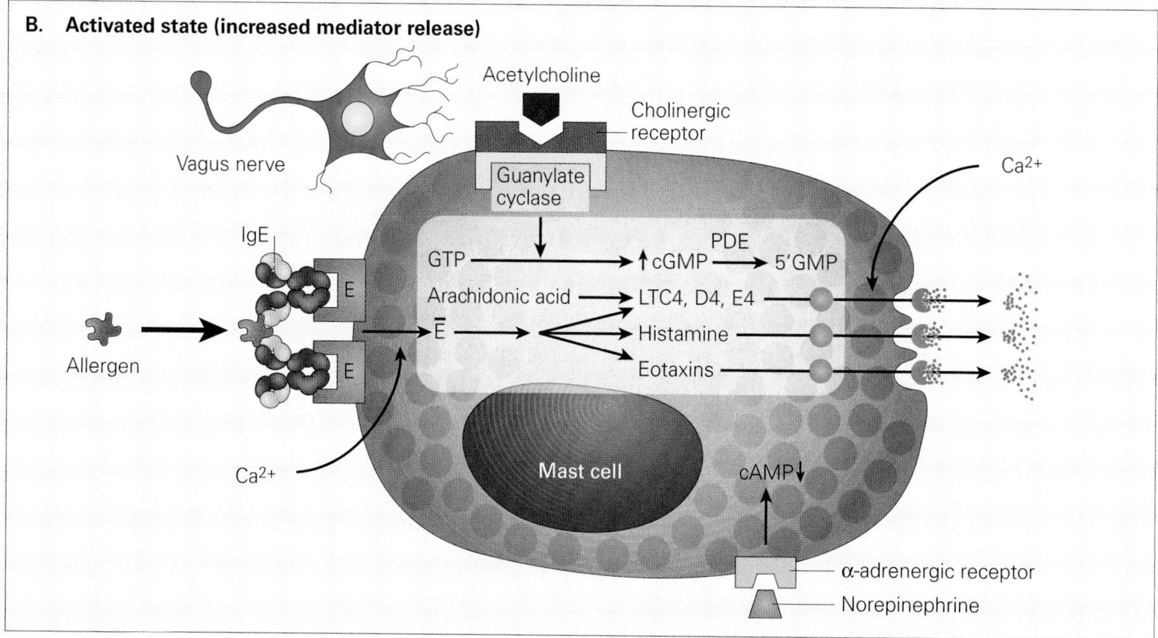
B. Activated state (increased mediator release)
Acetylcholine
Cholinergic receptor
Vagus nerve
Guanylate cyclase
Ca2+
IgE
PDE
GTP
↑cGMP
5'GMP
E
Arachidonic acid
LTC4, D4, E4
Allergen
Ē
Histamine
E
Eotaxins
Ca2+
Mast cell
cAMP↓
α-adrenergic receptor
Norepinephrine

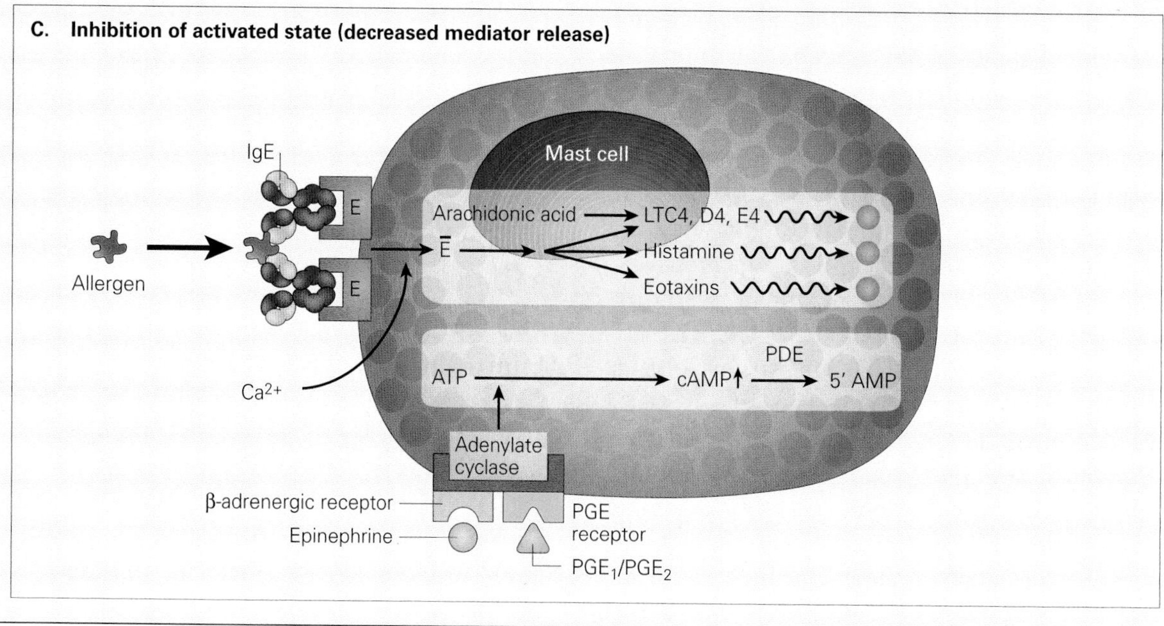
C. Inhibition of activated state (decreased mediator release)
IgE
Mast cell
E
Arachidonic acid
LTC4, D4, E4
Allergen
Ē
Histamine
E
Eotaxins
PDE
ATP
cAMP↑
5' AMP
Ca2+
Adenylate cyclase
β-adrenergic receptor
Epinephrine
PGE receptor
PGE1/PGE2

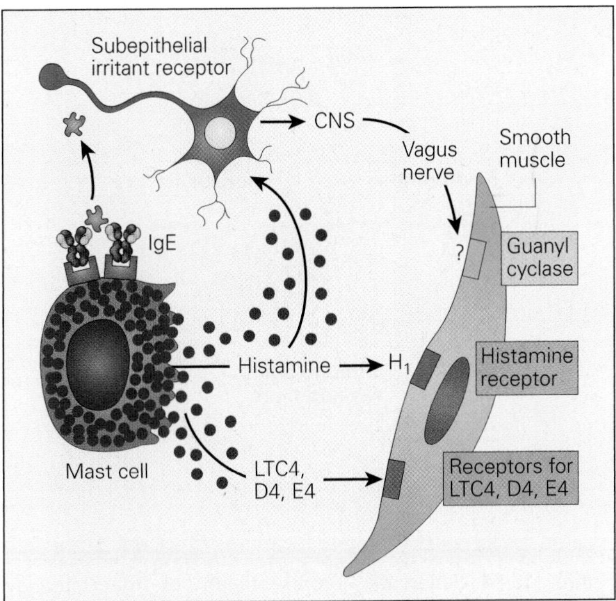

Figure 18-13. Schematic representation of the effects of released mediators on target cells and the indirect effects on irritant receptors.

lead to an aberration in the homeostatic regulation of both mediator and target cells in the atopic individual and a tendency toward hyperactive release of mediators and a hyperresponsiveness of target cells. It is known, for example, that the airways and the skin of the atopic individual are more responsive to a wide variety of both specific and nonspecific stimuli than the airways and skin of the normal individual. In the patient with bronchial asthma, one can see the results of this dual effect. The exaggerated response of the airways of the allergic individual that is known to occur after the inhalation of such nonspecific exogenous irritants as smoke, sulfur dioxide, and drugs, e.g., methacholine, as well as endogenous products, e.g., PGF2α, could be accounted for by this hypothesized autonomic imbalance. The theory of beta-adrenergic blockade is also evidenced clinically by the harmful adverse bronchoconstrictive effects seen in patients with bronchial asthma who receive nonselective β blockers for the control of hypertension.

Nonadrenergic Noncholinergic Airway Inhibitory System and Asthma

As described in Chapter 1, there is extensive cross talk between the nervous system, the endocrine system, and the immune system, referred to as the NEI system. In addition to the pathways of the autonomic system already described, there is another system involved in the neural regulation of the airways consisting of nonadrenergic, noncholinergic (**NANC**) nerves. Although cholinergic nerves form the predominant bronchoconstrictor neural pathway in human airways, the role of adrenergic neural pathways in human airways is unclear. NANC nerves can be either inhibitory or excitatory. In human airways, inhibitory NANC (**i-NANC**) mechanisms are the only neural bronchodilatory mechanisms. The presumed neurotransmitters of the i-NANC system are vasoactive intestinal peptide (**VIP**) and nitric oxide (**NO**). Substance P and neurokinin A have been implicated as the neurotransmitters mediating the excitatory part of the NANC nervous system. Neurokinin-2 (**NK2**) receptors are present on smooth muscle of both large and small airways and mediate part of the bronchoconstrictor effect of tachykinins. Most of the proinflammatory effects of substance P are mediated by the neurokinin-1 (NK1) receptor. Tachykinin receptor antagonists are currently being developed as possible antiasthma therapeutic agents.

Modifying Factors

Introduction: The Allergy Epidemic

In recent decades, there has been an upsurge of epidemic proportions in the prevalence of allergic diseases in various human populations of the

◀**Figure 18-12.** Schematic representation of the effects of the parasympathetic and sympathetic responses in allergic mediator release that are mediated through the cyclic nucleotide system. Panel A: In a resting state, IgE-bound mast cells that do not encounter allergens or other stimuli display a predominance of intracellular cAMP>cGMP and no mediator release. Panel B: An activated state occurs with cross-linking of FcεRI by allergen resulting in increased cGMP levels with conversion to 5′GMP by phosphodiesterase (PDE), a resultant decrease in intracellular levels of cAMP, and eventual release of preformed intracellular mediators e.g., LTC4, D4, E4, histamine, and eotaxins; this process is an energy-requiring step and involves influx of Ca++ ions; activation stimuli may also arise from parasympathetic stimulation, e.g., vagus, leading to the production and interaction of acetylcholine with cholinergic receptors on the cell surface as well as by sympathetic stimulation by agonists, i.e., norepinephrine, interacting with α-adrenergic receptors by directly inhibiting cAMP levels. Panel C: Inhibition of the activated state can occur through stimulation of sympathetic β-adrenergic receptors by agonists, i.e., epinephrine, leading to increased quantities of cAMP resulting from the conversion of ATP to cAMP. The net effect of this intracellular buildup of cAMP is microtubular dissociation and an inhibition of mediator release. A similar increase in cAMP and mediator-release suppression is achieved by stimulation of the prostaglandin E (PGE) receptor by PGE.

world, particularly in pediatric populations. Allergic diseases, such as allergic rhinitis and asthma, are now some of the most common and frequently encountered chronic diseases in medical practice and are responsible for a significant proportion of health care costs and lost days of productivity due to medical illness. Despite the availability of a myriad of therapeutic agents, the morbidity and mortality of allergic diseases, such as asthma and anaphylaxis, have also remained elevated, particularly in disadvantaged populations. Although it is well established that there is a genetic predisposition, e.g., atopy, for the development of allergic diseases, the rapid rise in prevalence of allergic diseases in the past 20 to 30 years is unlikely due to gene alterations in affected populations alone. Rather, different patterns of environmental exposures and other lifestyle changes, such as the "Westernization" effect of shifting populations in recent years from rural to urban settings, that have taken root in more recent years have likely contributed to epigenetic changes in the expression of the allergic phenotype in previously unaffected but genetically susceptible individuals. Also, changes in dietary practices and behaviors, in patterns of exposure and disease complications from infectious agents, and in social rearing habits of children, particularly infants, may have promoted or are continuing to promote effects on immune system development and responsiveness that favor the allergic phenotype.

Recent knowledge concerning the developing human immune system and its interaction with external environmental factors is providing a basis for a clearer understanding of the changing faces of allergic diseases through infancy and childhood in the allergy-prone individual (*Chapter 2*). The allergic diseases, e.g., asthma, are a complex and heterogenous group of immunological disorders that have evolved and become modified by the interplay of genetic factors, development, e.g., age, and the changing environment (Figure 18-14). Although the underlying causes contributing to the development of allergic diseases are still being investigated, there are some important risk factors or features that appear to impact the development and clinical severity of these disorders. These include genetic factors, age and development of the individual, emotional and physical factors, environmental pollutants, altered exposure to common infectious agents, hygienic differences between urban and farm living, i.e., the hygiene hypothesis, and diet or dietary factors and changes in the intestinal microflora.

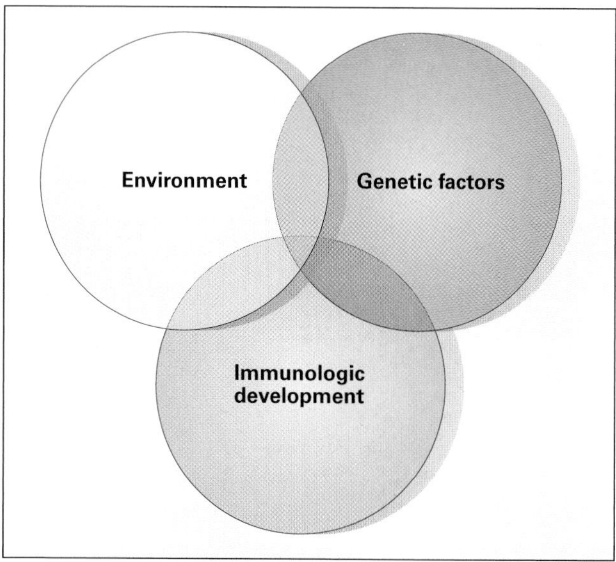

Figure 18-14. Schematic representation of the interplay between environmental, genetic, and developmental factors in the pathogenesis of allergic diseases.

Genetic Factors

There has been increasing study and understanding of the chromosomal regions and genes that regulate IgE synthesis and responsiveness to allergens. It is becoming clear that allergic diseases represent a heterogeneous group of disorders involving multiple genes and pathways. Genetic studies may not only permit early identification of individuals at risk for allergic diseases, but may also facilitate preventive public health measures by understanding gene-environment interactions. They may also unravel novel mechanisms of disease pathogenesis, which could then lead to new drug targets. An equally important area of study is pharmacogenetics, the ultimate goal of which is to understand the genetic basis of the variability of responses and responders to medications.

Genetic factors that affect inflammatory, immunologic, and epithelial structural elements are thought to play a major role in the pathogenesis of allergic disease. Shown in Table 18-6 are some of the major susceptibility genes for allergic diseases according to location and gene function. For ease of discussion, it is possible to group the genes identified as contributing to allergic disease into four broad groups (Table 18-6 and Figure 18-15). Group 1 genes provide a **barrier function** to allergens, microbes, and other foreign potentially noxious substances.

Table 18-6. Susceptibility genes for allergic diseases arranged according to structural level of gene involvement, function, gene products, and examples of consequences with gene aberrations

Group	Structural level of gene involvement	Gene function	Examples of gene products	Consequence(s) of gene aberrations
1	Barrier function	Protection of epithelial surfaces and sensing the environment	FLG, SPINK 5, CTNNA3, COL29A1, ORMDL3/GSDML, PCDH1, Pendrin, IL-13, C11orf30	Increased penetration of microbes and allergens with increased susceptibility to bacterial infection and allergic sensitization
2	Innate immune system	Initiation of allergen recognition	TLR2, TLR4, CD14, IRAKM, GST	Increased risk of microbial exposure and allergic sensitization
3	Adaptive immune system	Regulation of allergic inflammation	IL-13, IL-4RA, STAT6, TBX21, GATA-3, OPN3/CHML, CYF1P2 IRAKM, PHF11, uPAR	T cell differentiation into Th1, Th2, Th9, Th17, Treg cells Promote IgE production and allergic inflammation
			IL-1RL1, IL-33, MYB, WDR36	Increase levels of eosinophils
4	Target tissues	Modulation of consequences of chronic inflammation	Fibroblasts and smooth muscle: ADAM33, PDE4D Skin: COL29A1	Tissue remodeling: GI tract→chronic malabsorption syndrome (celiac disease) Skin→chronic atopic eczema Lung→COPD

A high proportion of these genes are expressed in the epithelium of the three most important portals of entry of foreign substances, i.e., the skin, gastrointestinal, and respiratory tracts. Genes such as filaggrin (FLG), for example, are directly involved in skin barrier function and are associated not only with increased risk of atopic dermatitis, but also with increased atopic sensitization. Other susceptibility genes, such as ORMDL3/GSDML, PCDH1, and C11orf30, are also expressed in the epithelium and may play a role in regulating epithelial barrier function. Group 2 genes sense the foreign substance once it has penetrated the epithelial barriers and comprise the vast array of innate immune system pattern-recognition receptors (**PRRs**) that are found on dendritic cells and other APCs. These genes include PRRs such as TLR2, TLR4, and CD14 that interact with varying levels of allergen and microbial exposure, thereby altering the risk of allergic immune responses. Polymorphisms of other genes including glutathione S-transferase (**GST**) genes have also been shown to modulate the effect of exposures to microbes and allergens that are involved with oxidant stress, such as tobacco smoke and air pollution, important as triggers for asthma susceptibility. Group 3 genes are those of the adaptive immune system that regulate T cell differentiation into Th1, Th2, Th9, Th17, and Treg cells involved in the pathogenesis of allergic inflammation. These genes not only regulate Th1/Th2 differentiation and their effector functions, e.g., IL-13, IL-4RA, and STAT6, TBX21, and GATA-3, but also genes such as IRAKM, PHF11, and uPAR that potentially regulate IgE production and therefore allergic sensitization. This group also includes genes shown to regulate the level of eosinophilia in blood and tissues (IL-1RL1, IL-33, MYB, and WDR36). Group 4 includes genes that modulate the consequences of chronic inflammation on cells of key target tissues, i.e., skin, fibroblasts, and smooth muscle, important in tissue remodeling. These also include ADAM33 and PDE4D, which are expressed in fibroblasts and smooth muscle, and COL29A1, encoding a novel collagen expressed in the skin linked to atopic dermatitis. Some genes can affect more than one disease component. For example, the gene for IL-13 regulates both atopic sensitization through IgE isotype switching but also has direct effects on the airway epithelium and mesenchyme, promoting goblet cell metaplasia and fibroblast proliferation events characteristic of airway remodeling in asthma.

Age

Another set of modifying factors important in allergy is the effect of maturational age. During pregnancy and early infancy, there is a skewing of the Th1/Th2 paradigm toward Th2 dominance. As described in Chapter 2, the decreased Th1 function during pregnancy is consistent with the survival advantage imparted to the fetus during intrauterine existence. After birth, the normal infant continues

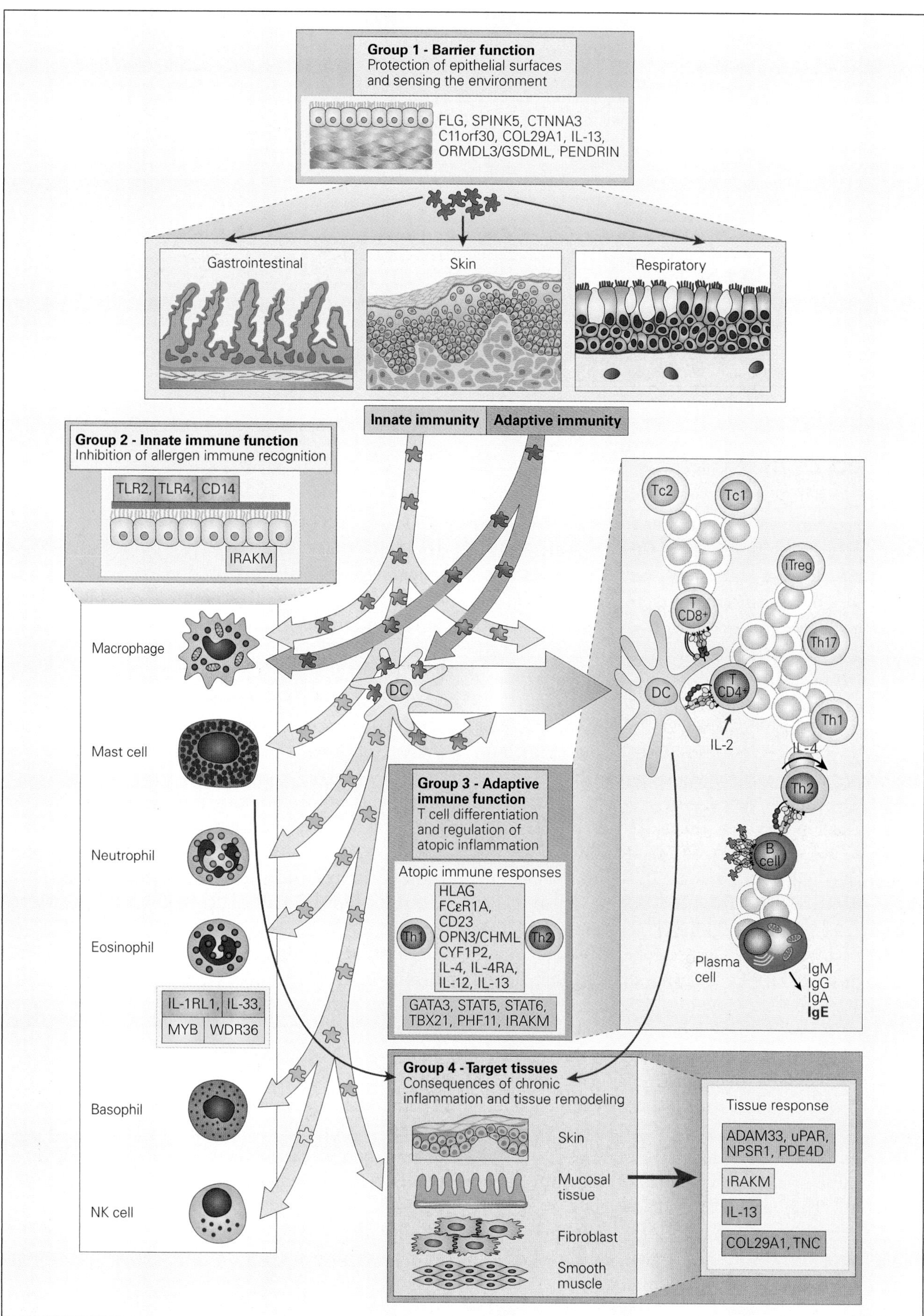
Group 1 - Barrier function
Protection of epithelial surfaces and sensing the environment
FLG, SPINK5, CTNNA3
C11orf30, COL29A1, IL-13,
ORMDL3/GSDML, PENDRIN
Gastrointestinal
Skin
Respiratory
Innate immunity
Adaptive immunity
Group 2 - Innate immune function
Inhibition of allergen immune recognition
TLR2, TLR4, CD14
IRAKM
Macrophage
Mast cell
Neutrophil
Eosinophil
IL-1RL1, IL-33,
MYB WDR36
Basophil
NK cell
DC
Tc2
Tc1
iTreg
T CD8+
Th17
T CD4+
Th1
IL-2
IL-4
Th2
B cell
Plasma cell
IgM
IgG
IgA
IgE
Group 3 - Adaptive immune function
T cell differentiation and regulation of atopic inflammation
Atopic immune responses
HLAG
FCεR1A,
CD23
OPN3/CHML
CYF1P2,
IL-4, IL-4RA,
IL-12, IL-13
Th1
Th2
GATA3, STAT5, STAT6,
TBX21, PHF11, IRAKM
Group 4 - Target tissues
Consequences of chronic inflammation and tissue remodeling
Skin
Mucosal tissue
Fibroblast
Smooth muscle
Tissue response
ADAM33, uPAR,
NPSR1, PDE4D
IRAKM
IL-13
COL29A1, TNC

to show a Th2 skewing during early infancy with the acquisition of normal Th1 by the end of the first year. In contrast, the allergic infant continues to show a prominent Th2 skewing with a delayed acquisition of Th1 function. Recent findings suggest that delayed postnatal maturation of Th1 function is associated with increased risk for early postnatal sensitization to inhalant allergens.

Another area where maturational factors impact the expression of allergic disease is the "atopic march," a clinical term used to describe the evolution of allergic disease manifestations at different ages in infancy and childhood that involve the progressive involvement of three major target organs: (1) the gastrointestinal (GI) tract; (2) the skin; and (3) the respiratory tract (Figure 18-16). The atopic march is notable for manifestations of gastrointestinal allergy, i.e., food allergy, and skin allergy, i.e., atopic eczema, as the earliest clinical manifestations following allergen contact during infancy. This is followed in subsequent years by involvement of the respiratory tract in the form of respiratory allergy, e.g., allergic rhinitis and/or asthma.

Although it is not clear whether food allergy precedes or comes after eczema in this march, they both appear early in infancy and are both risk factors for allergic disease progression to involve the respiratory tract in subsequent years. A defective skin barrier and/or increased intestinal permeability in infants may contribute to development of atopic eczema or food allergy and may also contribute to allergic sensitization to a variety of environmental allergens in the progression of the atopic march. Although implied from these observations is that appropriate skin care to maintain skin barrier function and dietary avoidance of highly allergenic foods during infancy may help to prevent sensitization and the development of allergic disease manifestations, the benefit of these interventions have not been clinically demonstrated.

With the progression of the atopic march, chronic allergic inflammation in skin tissues may lead to the irreversible changes of tissue remodeling, e.g., fibrosis. It is therefore incumbent upon those entrusted to the care of the young patient with allergic disease to identify the antecedents of adult end-stage disease, e.g., the chronic lichenification of skin in atopic eczema or the fibrotic airway changes in asthma leading to chronic obstructive pulmonary disease (**COPD**), and to intervene before the changes become irreversible.

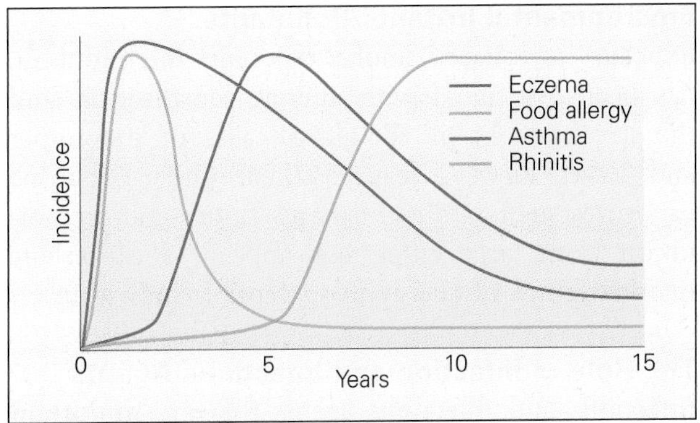

Figure 18-16. **Schematic representation of the appearance of peak prevalences of different types of allergic disease in infancy and childhood during the "atopic march."** (Adapted with permission from Spergel JM. From atopic dermatitis to asthma: the atopic march. Ann Allergy Asthma Immunol 2010;105:99–106.)

Emotional and Physical Factors

An important concept in the management of the allergic individual is consideration of the role of emotional factors and stress as both triggering and exacerbating events in allergic disease. Not only can the morbidity and mortality risk of allergic disease have profound effects on the psychological development of the individual, but it is well observed that the onset of asthma symptoms may be evoked by an emotional upset. Emotional factors exert their effects on mediator cells and target tissues by way of the autonomic nervous system as previously described. Another possible mechanism includes stress-induced release of corticotropin-releasing hormone (**CRH**) that in turn mediates non-IgE dependent mast cell degranulation.

In addition to the aforementioned factors, a variety of physical factors, including heat, cold, exercise, and changes in barometric pressure, may trigger allergic responses. Although the precise mechanism of these factors is not completely understood, they are believed to be mediated primarily through the parasympathetic nervous system and initiated by stimulation of irritant afferent receptors in various shock organs.

◀**Figure 18-15.** **Schematic representation of the susceptibility genes responsible for allergic disease arranged according to their postulated levels of involvement.** Group 1 genes affect barrier function, Group 2 the innate immune system, Group 3 the adaptive immune system, and Group 4 the target tissues. With progression of allergic inflammation, these lead to tissue damage of target tissues with tissue remodeling and irreversible end organ damage.

Environmental Irritants/Pollutants

Exposure to tobacco smoke, especially in childhood, has been associated with allergic sensitization and the development of allergic diseases of the upper and lower airways, e.g., asthma. Other airborne exposures such as diesel exhaust fumes and air pollution from large cities also appear to exacerbate manifestations of allergy in susceptible individuals.

The Role of Infection and Infectious Agents

Infections and infectious agents that are important inducers of Th1 immunity appear to have a dual role in modifying allergic diseases and asthma. On the one hand, certain infections or exposure to antigens from infectious agents may down modulate Th2 responses and diminish the subsequent development of allergic diseases. On the other hand, generation of proinflammatory cytokines from exposures to these microbial antigens can exacerbate existing allergic disease as well. This "double-edged sword" effect on allergic diseases by infectious agents is exemplified by endotoxin, one of the main toxic components of Gram-negative bacteria and a bacterial by-product found in high concentrations in environments contaminated with fecal flora from animals or insects. Levels of endotoxin have been found to be inversely related to allergic sensitization but directly related to asthma manifestations. Endotoxin is synonymous with lipopolysaccharide (**LPS**) that forms the outer cell membrane component of Gram-negative bacteria (*Chapter 12*). LPS has potent immunostimulatory effects mediated through its lipid A moiety, which signals through CD14 on macrophages and Toll-like receptors 2, 4, and 9 found on
5 various cells of the innate immune system (*Chapter 9*). At low levels, LPS is a potent inducer of IL-12 and IFN-γ and other Th1 cytokines that are known to decrease the production of Th2 cytokines such as IL-4, IL-5, and IL-13 thereby providing an explanation for how infections and other exposures to bacterial endotoxin can diminish or abrogate mechanisms necessary for allergic sensitization.

Endotoxin exposures, however, can also potentiate allergic disease manifestations. At high doses, for example, LPS can stimulate the release of inflammatory mediators that override the Th2 suppressing effects at low doses. Since endotoxin has been shown to be a major component of house dust, in which other important allergens, i.e., house dust mite, can be found, the ability of endotoxin to act as an immunoadjuvant for potentiating Th2 responses to these other allergens cannot be ignored. Viral infections, in particular, are well-established inducers of allergic disease manifestations, especially of the upper and lower airways. Severe bronchospasm and wheezing may initially be triggered by a variety of respiratory viruses, e.g., respiratory syncytial virus (**RSV**). Although the precise mechanism of the precipitation of allergic manifestations by these infections is not completely understood, the immunoadjuvant properties on Th2 inflammation by Th1 and/or Th17 immune responses generated by these microorganisms are likely contributing factors. This potentiating effect does not necessarily apply to all microbial by-products, however. Muramic acid, a peptidoglycan found abundantly in Gram-positive bacteria, has been shown to be inversely related with asthma and wheezing in children. More recent evidence suggests that stimulation of the innate immune system by infectious agents may potentiate allergic disease, i.e. asthma (*Chapter 3*).

Urban Lifestyle Factors, "the Hygiene Hypothesis," and Farm Living

How infections modify allergic diseases plays into a well-established hypothesis that attempts to delineate the possible gene-environment changes in recent times that have contributed to the allergy epidemic. The epidemiologic observation that the prevalence of allergic diseases and asthma is much greater in industrialized Western urban societies than in rural or farm communities has formed the basis for the "hygiene hypothesis." In simplified terms, this hypothesis posits that early childhood infections and/or higher levels of exposures to animal filth or by-products, e.g., farm animal antigens and raw milk, more readily present in rural farm settings are important inducers of the Th1 versus the Th2 airway immunologic profile (*Chapter 2*) and help redirect the balance from the predominant Th2 profile in infancy to a more tolerogenic Th1 profile. This redirection is necessary to protect the genetically susceptible host against the allergic diathesis that is characteristic of the Th2 phenotype. Gradual differences in the nature and frequency of exposures to childhood infections or other environmental antigens that induce Th1 immune responses brought about by vaccinations, increased antibiotic use, sanitary practices, and other hygienic features characteristic of urban lifestyles and settings have gradually led to immune imbalances that favor the Th2 phenotype and therefore the increased development of allergic diseases.

Those advancing this hypothesis have relied largely on retrospective comparisons in the prevalence of allergic sensitization or clinical manifestations of allergic diseases in those who live in urban environments versus those living in rural environments, in particular on farms. These studies have also looked at study population differences in relation to a variety of independent factors, such as prevalence of infectious diseases, e.g., hepatitis A, tuberculosis, RSV, etc., frequency of antibiotic use, farm animal exposure, and/or consumption of raw versus pasteurized milk. The most consistent observation associated with increased sensitization and/or allergic disease manifestations has been the loss of inhaled or ingestional antigen exposures from farm living conditions. Infants or children who are raised on farms have consistently more elevated and robust expression of innate immune defense markers such as CD14 and TLR2. They also have higher levels of and more efficient Treg cell populations and enhanced production of IFN-γ and TNF. Since low IFN-γ expression at birth is associated with subsequent development of atopic disease and symptoms, the upregulation of IFN-γ by farming exposure may help restore this immune deviation toward atopy. The finding of elevated levels of IFN-γ in newborns of mothers with farm exposure also provides supportive evidence to timing of exposure, including prenatal antigenic exposures, as an important formative event in subsequent immune system development and reactivity. Family history of atopic disease and lifestyle differences associated with atopy, such as duration of breastfeeding, day care attendance, pet ownership, number of siblings, diet, and education, did not account for these protective farm effects.

Many proponents of this hypothesis believe that allergic diseases can be prevented and/or managed by substituting or modifying the existing environmental, microbial, and dietary conditions found in urban settings with those found in farms or rural environments. To date, however, there has been little demonstration of any direct protective effect or benefit as a result of these interventions.

Dietary Factors and the Intestinal Microflora

With the rising frequency of food allergies, there has also been considerable interest in the role of dietary factors or practices that could be involved in the development of allergic disease. The impact of various food-processing methods and introduction of novel ingredients into the food supply have been suggested as sources of novel food allergens that could overwhelm the normally balanced (tolerant) immune response to foods seen in the healthy individual but that manifest as disease in the genetically susceptible food allergic individual. Also, there is recent evidence that obesity may be linked to various allergic diseases.

A major investigative effort is currently being directed to study the role of the intestinal microflora on the immune response that could either have allergenic or tolerogenic effects. Central to this research is the premise that certain friendly bacterial species in the intestinal tract, i.e., commensal bacteria such as lactobacilli, may have beneficial effects in maintaining a healthy immunologic balance, i.e., symbiosis, important not only in counteracting the growth of harmful disease-producing bacteria, but also in maintaining an equilibrium of both innate and adaptive immune responses that promote intestinal microflora stability and immune tolerance (*Chapter 8*). A selective loss of certain bacterial populations due to frequent antibiotic use or to a host of genetic, dietary, or environmental factors or practices that disturb the normal balanced composition of the microbial flora, e.g., use of infant formula instead of breast milk, may lead to disruption of this intestinal microbial equilibrium referred to as dysbiosis and promote immune dysregulation and allergic inflammation (Figure 18-17).

Based on this premise, the use of supplemental administration of probiotic bacteria has been proposed as a means to correct the altered microbial composition and related immune imbalance to prevent the development or manifestations of allergic diseases. As defined by the World Health Organization (WHO), **probiotics** are "live microorganisms, which when administered in adequate amounts confer a health benefit on the host." To date, although administration of probiotics has shown benefit in reducing the incidence and mortality of severe necrotizing enterocolitis in preterm infants and in the treatment of acute infectious diarrhea and antibiotic-associated diarrhea, evidence supporting a potential health benefit for probiotics on allergic diseases still needs to be elucidated.

Clinical Manifestations of Allergic Disease

As described previously, the clinical manifestations of allergic disease can be the result of either IgE or

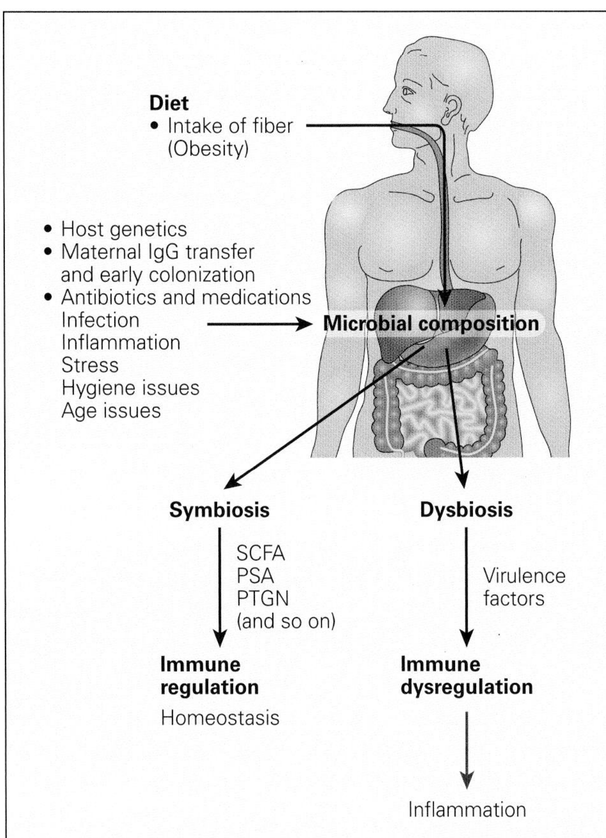

Figure 18-17. Schematic representation of the interaction of diet, microbial composition, and immune system regulation. Diet and other environmental and host factors may have a major effect on gastrointestinal microbiota. A balanced microbial composition is postulated to result in symbiosis promoting the regulation of immune and inflammatory responses through anti-inflammatory and/or immunomodulatory products such as short chain fatty acids (SCFA), polysaccharide A (PSA), and peptidoglycan (PTGN), which helps maintain homeostasis. Dysbiosis would lead to dysregulation of the immune system through lack of beneficial microbial products and an increase in virulence factors, which could leave the host susceptible to inflammation. Dysbiosis could occur through the consumption of a Western diet, as well as through changes induced by factors such as host genetics, maternal transfer, and antibiotic use. (Adapted with permission from Maslowski KM, Mackay CR. Diet, gut microbiota and immune responses. Nat Immunol 2011;12(1):5–9.)

non-IgE-mediated mechanisms. The classic Type I immediate hypersensitivity involving IgE antibody primarily manifests as clinical symptoms that are rapid in onset and duration. This immediate hypersensitivity, however, may also lead to activation of other inflammatory cells or cytokines/mediators, which contribute to the delayed or chronic symptoms seen with many atopic disorders.

A common feature to all allergic manifestations is their exposure to the external environment, which provides a common route of entry for exogenous agents. Allergens have multiple portals of entry, which primarily include the gastrointestinal tract, the skin, and the respiratory tract. In most cases, allergic manifestations are localized to these organ sites. However, in certain circumstances (e.g., when allergens enter the bloodstream by way of subcutaneous, intramuscular, or intravenous injection and bypass the above mentioned portals of entry), allergenic mediators may exert their effects on the cardiovascular system, leading to potentially severe and sometimes fatal clinical consequences of anaphylaxis. In this section, the clinical manifestations of anaphylaxis will be first presented as a prototype of Type I hypersensitivity disease and will be followed by descriptions of disorders primarily localized to the gastrointestinal tract, the skin, and the respiratory tract.

Anaphylaxis

The term "anaphylaxis" is derived from the Greek (*ana*- without, *phylaxis*- protection) and was coined in 1905 by two French investigators, Richet and Portier, during their studies (Box 18-2 and Figure 18-18). Anaphylaxis represents one of the most

Box 18-2

The discovery and coining of the term anaphylaxis by Richet and Portier

Prince Albert I of Monaco (1848–1922), who loved yachting in the Mediterranean Sea, had developed sensitivity to sea anemones. The prince had invited two Parisian scientists, Charles Richet and Paul Portier, to perform studies on the toxin produced by the tentacles of a local jellyfish, *Physalia*, the Portuguese Man of War, for the purpose of developing protective antisera for prevention, i.e., prophylaxis, of these reactions. The scientists were able to isolate the toxin and tried to vaccinate dogs in the hope of obtaining protection, or "prophylaxis," against the toxin. They were horrified to find that subsequent injection of very small doses of the toxin unexpectedly resulted in a new dramatic illness that involved the rapid onset of breathing difficulty and resulted in death within 30 minutes. Richet and Portier termed this "anaphylaxis," or "without protection." They correctly concluded that the immune system first becomes sensitized to the allergen over several weeks and upon re-exposure to the same allergen had resulted in a severe reaction. Although IgE in the human was not discovered until 1968, the antibody in dogs was related to an analogous canine immunoglobulin that resulted in the immediate release of vasoactive amines following subsequent injection of the toxin into the sensitized animals, which caused the anaphylactic reaction. The Nobel Prize in Physiology and Medicine was awarded to Charles Richet in 1913 for this work.

dramatic manifestations of allergic disease mediated by the immediate-Type I hypersensitivity response (*Chapter 17*). Contact of a sensitized individual with even minute amounts of the offending allergen, e.g., penicillin, bee venom, or peanut, can cause sudden and damaging release of mediators from cells of the immune system on various organs of the body. Without prompt medical or emergency care, anaphylaxis can produce life-threatening symptoms of respiratory and cardiovascular compromise in as little as five to 15 minutes.

The important mediators involved in the allergic reaction and anaphylaxis and their biological properties were previously presented in Table 18-4. Release of these mediators in various tissues and end organs of the mucosal immune system (skin, gastrointestinal tract, and lung) contribute to the symptoms of flushing (vasodilation), pruritus (effects on nerve endings), rhinorrhea (mucus hypersecretion), and wheezing (bronchoconstriction) that are typically seen as reactions in other allergic diseases but can also be part of the clinical spectrum of anaphylaxis (Table 18-7). The systemic and rapidly progressive nature of the allergic symptoms affecting primarily the lungs and the cardiovascular system differentiate anaphylaxis from other allergic diseases.

Mechanisms of Anaphylaxis and Severity Factors

In the human, it is generally accepted that anaphylaxis involves the degranulation of mast cells, and to a lesser extent basophils, which collectively lead to the systemic release of mediators, i.e., histamine, that give rise to the condition. Although IgE-dependent responses mediated through the FcεRI receptor are thought to be the primary mechanism for this mediator release, an alternative pathway has been demonstrated, primarily in mouse models, that could also give rise to the condition. The pathway involves antigen-specific IgG antibodies or immune complexes (and complement) mediated through FcγRIII receptors on the surface of macrophages and/or basophils (*Chapters 6* and *17*). This interaction results primarily in the release of platelet-activating factor (**PAF**), a mediator that is known to give rise to smooth muscle contraction and vasodilation (Table 18-4) responsible for symptoms of anaphylaxis. The antigen-antibody dose-response relationships appear to differentiate these mechanisms, as it takes considerably less antigen and specific antibody to trigger IgE-dependent anaphylaxis, in contrast to IgG-dependent anaphylaxis, which requires higher quantities. In the human,

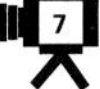

Table 18-7. Clinical signs and symptoms of anaphylaxis.

Cutaneous/subcutaneous/mucosal tissue
Flushing, erythema, hives (urticaria), angioedema, and pilor erection Pruritus of lips, tongue, and palate; edema of lips, tongue, and uvula Periorbital erythema, erythema and edema, conjunctival erythema, and tearing
Respiratory
Nose: erythema, congestion, rhinorrhea, sneezing Laryngeal: erythema and tightness in the throat; dysphagia, dysphonia, and hoarseness; dry staccato cough; stridor; and sensation of erythema in the external auditory canals Lung: shortness of breath, dyspnea, chest tightness, deep cough, and wheezing/bronchospasm (decreased peak expiratory flow)
Cardiovascular
Hypotension Feeling of faintness (near-syncope), syncope, and altered mental status Chest pain Arrhythmia
Gastrointestinal
Nausea and vomiting Crampy abdominal pain Diarrhea
Other
Uterine contractions in women Aura or sense of impending doom

Adapted with permission from Sampson HA, Muñoz-Furlong A, Bock SA, et al. March 2005. Symposium on the definition and management of anaphylaxis: summary report. J Allergy Clin Immunol 2005;115:584–91.

anaphylactic reactions are most likely IgE-dependent since small quantities of antigen are usually involved. However, there is also some evidence that cases of anaphylaxis may be IgG-dependent when large quantities of antigen are introduced.

Agents that Cause Anaphylaxis

Anaphylaxis can be triggered by numerous agents, the most common of which include insect stings, foods, latex, and medications (Table 18-8). For ease of discussion, agents that cause anaphylaxis are broadly classified into those that trigger mediator release from mast cells either by allergic (antibody-mediated) or nonallergic (nonantibody-mediated) stimuli or mechanisms (Figure 18-18). The classic allergic mechanism involves IgE-dependent mediator release, and agents include foods, medications, insect venoms, latex, allergen administered during immunotherapy, natural colorants, and even, though rarely, sensitization through seminal fluid. A second group of agents that elicit anaphylaxis through an allergic mechanism are those that trigger IgE-independent mediator release, presumably through interactions between antigen-specific IgG antibodies or immune complexes and Fc receptors on the surface of mast cells. An example of IgG-dependent anaphylaxis is transfusion-related anaphylaxis seen in patients with IgA deficiency who receive blood or plasma products containing IgA. Since they lack IgA, these individuals mount IgG antibody responses directed to exogenous plasma IgA antibody found in transfused products. Although anti-IgA IgG antibody has been demonstrated in these individuals after receiving these products, the precise pathogenetic mechanism of anaphylaxis remains unclear. Proposed mechanisms have also included the participation of IgG/IgA complexes bound to the Fc gamma receptor or complement pathway activation with the release of anaphylatoxins C3a or C5a (Figure 18-18). Consequently, the use of IgA deficient plasma or washed

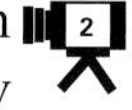

Table 18-8. Agents that cause anaphylaxis and related mechanisms

Type	Mechanism	Example
Allergic (antibody-mediated)	IgE dependent	1. Foods,* e.g., peanuts, tree nuts, milk, crustaceans 2. Medications • Antibiotics, e.g., PCN, sulfa • Hormones, e.g., insulin, progesterone • Monoclonal or chimeric antibodies (likely) • Serum proteins, e.g., antithymocyte globulin • Enzymes, e.g., streptokinase • Chemotherapeutic agents, e.g., cisplatin, asparaginase, etc. 3. Insect venoms, e.g., Hymenoptera 4. Latex 5. Allergen immunotherapy injections 6. Natural colorants, e.g., carmine 7. Seminal fluid
	IgE independent	8. Intravenous immunoglobulin (immune aggregates) 9. Blood and plasma products (IgA containing)
Nonallergic (nonantibody-mediated)	Multimediator complement and kallikrein system activation	10. Angiotensin-converting enzyme inhibitor 11. Dialysis membranes
	Nonspecific degranulation of mast cells and basophils	12. Opioids 13. Muscle relaxants*
	Arachidonic acid metabolism abnormalities	14. Aspirin and other nonsteroidal anti-inflammatory drugs
	Unknown	15. Radiocontrast media (some IgE-mediated reported) 16. Physical factors, e.g., exercise, temperature 17. Idiopathic anaphylaxis

*Increased in atopic individuals.

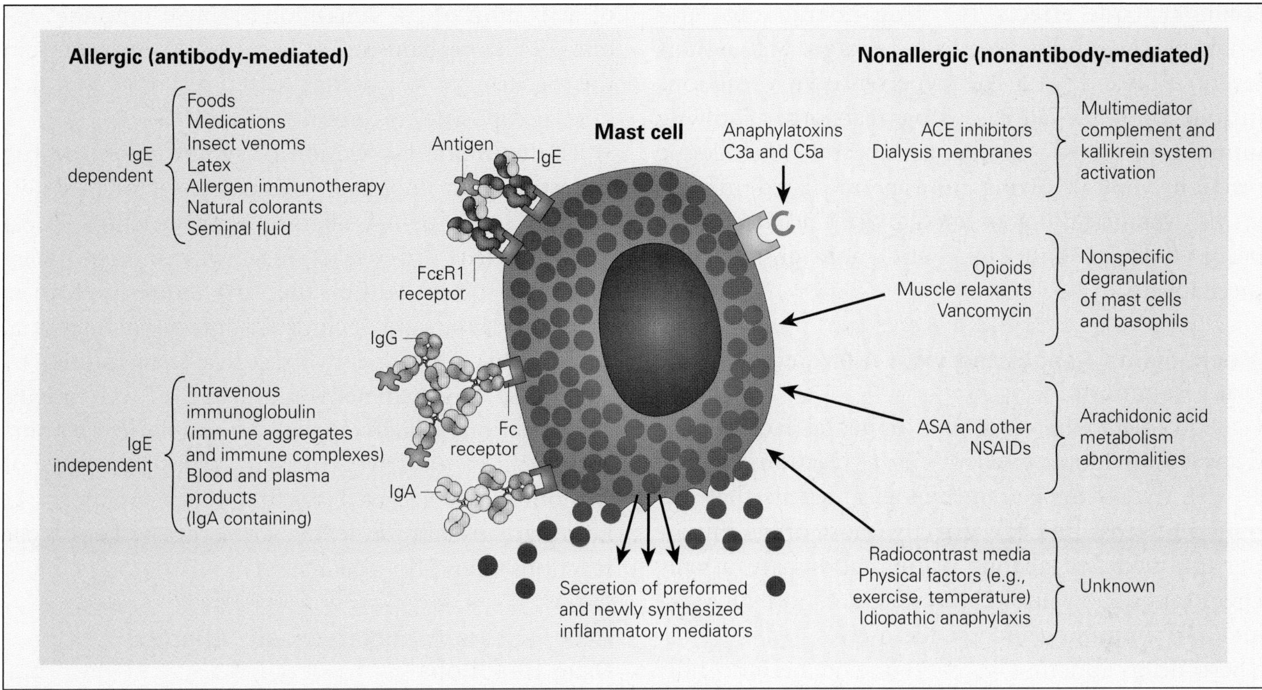

Figure 18-18. Schematic representation of various mechanisms and agents that can induce the release of preformed and newly synthesized mediators from mast cells that can lead to anaphylaxis.

red blood cells significantly reduces the incidence of anaphylaxis in these individuals. Anaphylactic reactions have also been demonstrated following the use of intravenous gamma globulin presumably through immune complexes or aggregates interacting with surface Fc receptors and activating the complement system as well.

A second major group of agents that gives rise to anaphylactic reactions are those that directly induce mast cell degranulation through nonantibody-mediated mechanisms (Table 18-8 and Figure 18-18). Anaphylaxis can occur through activation of the complement and kallikrein-kinin pathways by pharmacologic agents such as angiotensin converting enzyme (**ACE**) inhibitors in patients treated for hypertension or by dialysis membranes in patients undergoing hemodialysis. These anaphylactic reactions can be triggered by the formation of anaphylatoxins, i.e., C3a and C5a, by activation of kallikrein and formation of bradykinin, or by activation of the coagulation cascade through Factor XII (Figure 18-18). Medications such as opiates and muscle relaxants, e.g., succinylcholine, and vancomycin, i.e., the "red man syndrome," are another group of agents that can directly induce mast cell degranulation through nonimmunologic mechanisms. Mediator production by aspirin and nonsteroidal anti-inflammatory drugs (**NSAIDs**) are believed to cause allergic reactions and anaphylaxis through enhanced leukotriene production subsequent to prostaglandin blockade in genetically susceptible individuals. Additional agents that are known to be associated with anaphylactic reactions through unknown mechanisms include radiocontrast media, physical factors, e.g., exercise and variations of temperature, and a group of idiopathic reactions whose etiologic agents have not been identified.

Drugs

Allergic reactions to drugs are responsible for the highest frequency of fatalities from anaphylaxis in humans. The major groups involved in drug allergic reactions include antibiotics, e.g., penicillin, and anti-inflammatory agents, e.g., aspirin, anesthetics, and diagnostic radiocontrast media. Antimicrobial agents used in the prevention of disease, e.g., antisera and vaccines, and monoclonal antibodies are also becoming important causes of drug allergy (*Chapters 11* and *23*).

Classification of Drug Reactions

Adverse drug reactions are commonly divided into the following groups: (1) **overdosage,** (2) **intolerance,** (3) **idiosyncrasy,** (4) **primary side effects,** (5)

secondary side effects, (6) **drug interactions**, and (7) **hypersensitivity reactions** (**allergic** and **nonallergic**) (Table 18-9). The hypersensitivity reactions include both the allergic drug reactions, involving immune-mediated mechanisms, and nonallergic reactions, not involving immune-mediated mechanisms. Manifestations of allergic drug reactions may occur through both IgE- and non-IgE-mediated mechanisms.

Mechanisms Associated with Allergic Drug Reactions

Genetic, metabolic, and environmental factors predispose individuals to allergic drug reactions (Figure 18-19). Except for certain biological agents that can bind and cross-link IgE directly, most drugs initiating IgE-mediated allergic manifestations are usually chemicals of low molecular weight (< 1,000 MW) and not immunogenic by themselves (*Chapter 1*). These drugs function as haptens and become fully immunogenic when a drug component binds with a carrier protein to form a hapten-protein complex recognized by IgE or IgG antibodies. In some cases, the drug has to be metabolized to become immunogenic. In other cases, a direct pharmacological interaction of the drug with T cell receptors may generate a cellular immune response, independent of activation of the innate or adaptive immune systems. This mechanism has been proposed to explain the occurrence of allergic drug reactions on first known exposure to certain medications.

The temporal association of symptoms with drug exposure is an important diagnostic factor in determining the type of allergic drug reaction. Most IgE-mediated drug reactions involve early phase reactions, occur within the first hour after drug administration, and include symptoms of urticaria, angioedema, and anaphylaxis. Reactions caused by late phase IgE-mediated or non-IgE (T cell) mediated reactions usually appear within six to 72 hours and include a variety of skin eruptions with or without fever. Delayed reactions developing > 72 hours are usually indicative of serum-sickness-type reactions (Type III) (*Chapter 17*).

Risk Factors Associated with Allergic Drug Reactions

Although it can appear at any age, drug allergy is seen less frequently in infants and children. This may reflect the developmental immunologic deficiency of the younger patient (*Chapter 2*) or simply the lower degree of exposure to drugs required for sensitization at this age. In fact, an increased risk for allergic drug reactions is associated with

Table 18-9. Classification of drug reactions

Categories	Description	Example(s)
Overdosage	Symptoms that occur after excessive intake or failure of normal metabolism or excretion of a drug	Patient error or nosocomial
Intolerance	Symptoms of overdosage occur at normal pharmacologic doses of the drug	Somnolence from nonsedating antihistamine preparations
Idiosyncrasy	Qualitatively abnormal response after drug administration that differs from its pharmacologic effect but is not immunologically determined	In G-6-PD deficiency, the ingestion of primaquine results in enhanced red cell hemolysis
Primary side effects	Therapeutically undesirable but often unavoidable action of a drug	Drowsiness associated with antihistamine therapy
Secondary side effects	In addition to the primary action of a drug	Candidiasis in patients receiving tetracycline
Drug interactions	The action of one drug upon the effectiveness or toxicity of another	Drugs commonly metabolized by liver p450 enzymatic pathway
Hypersensitivity		
Allergic	Immunologically mediated in sensitive individuals—IgE- and non-IgE mediated	Anaphylaxis to PCN; Steven Johnson's syndrome with sulfa drugs or other drug exanthems
Nonallergic	Nonspecific histamine release, kallikrein, complement, or multimediator pathway alteration	Aspirin-induced asthma, radiocontrast dye-mediated anaphylaxis

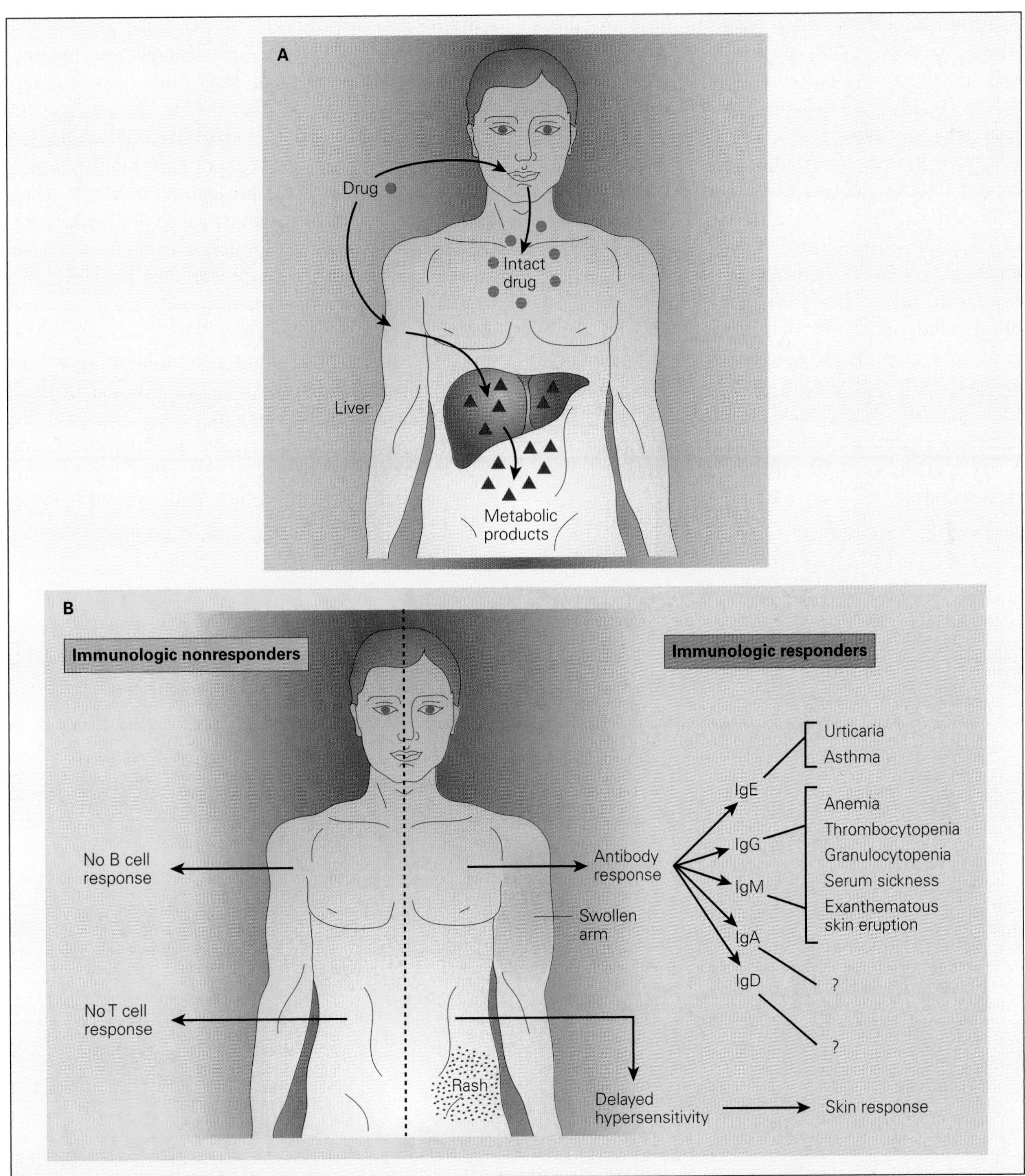

Figure 18-19. Schematic representation of the points at which immune mechanisms may be operative in drug allergy. Panel A: Metabolic degradation of a drug. Panel B: The capacity to respond with the elaboration of components of the immunologic array.

higher dose or prolonged administration of the drug, as well as multiple, intermittent exposures. Another factor influencing drug allergy is the route by which the drug is administered. Topical application of a drug, e.g., the use of antibiotics applied to the skin or conjunctival mucosa, has the greatest capacity for inducing allergic sensitization; oral administration has the least. Thus, strategies to minimize the risk for drug sensitization and allergy may include avoidance of frequent topical use of drugs, e.g., antibiotics that have strong sensitizing potential.

Although allergic drug reactions have not been found to occur with greater frequency in atopic individuals, atopic individuals are at risk for more severe reactions. Increased drug reaction severity in fact may be associated with certain HLA alleles (*Chapter 10*) as supported by the strong association of the development of Steven Johnson's syndrome with certain drugs in Han Chinese individuals with HLA-B*1502. Also, since other allergic drug reactions are often directed against metabolic degradation products of the drug, it is likely that, in the allergic individual, the development of drug allergy may be a function of genetically determined differences in drug metabolism (Figure 18-19). Concomitant use of medications as well as underlying diseases, especially infections, e.g., HIV, could also affect metabolism and immune presentation of the drug antigen.

Antibiotics

The **penicillins** (**PCNs**) cause allergy and anaphylaxis more frequently than any other class of drugs. PCN allergy alone is responsible for nearly 400 deaths per year in the United States. The most frequently used penicillin, benzyl penicillin, produces several distinct metabolic breakdown products. These include a **major determinant**, called the benzylpenicilloyl (BPO) haptenic group, as well as a smaller proportion of minor haptenic determinants that include the benzylpenamaldic acid-mixed disulfide haptenic group (Figure 18-20). As described previously, the major and minor determinants may both act as haptens, and following their binding to tissue proteins, can generate an IgE-mediated penicillin allergy. A clinical paradox is that, although most individuals become sensitized to the major determinant, IgE sensitization to the **minor determinants** confers

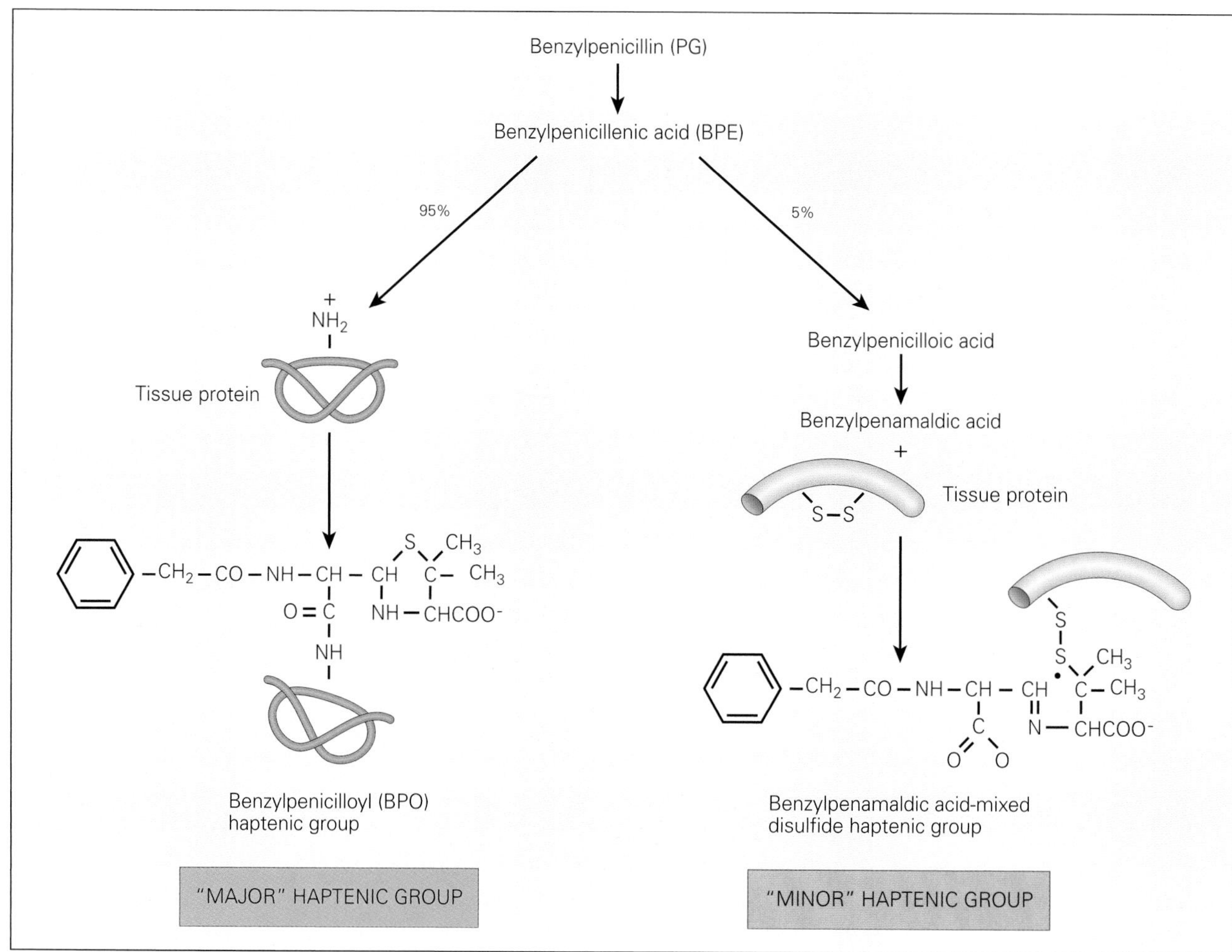

Figure 18-20. Schematic representation of the breakdown products of penicillin thought to be important in penicillin hypersensitivity.

greater risk for severe immediate hypersensitivity reactions to PCNs.

Another relevant clinical issue with PCN allergy concerns cross-reactivity between various types of penicillin derivatives that is related to the common beta-lactam ring structure (Box 18-3 and Figure 18-21). Most semisynthetic penicillins, e.g., oxacillin, nafcillin, ampicillin, and carbenicillin, contain the common beta-lactam ring but vary in the type of side chain attached to this ring. Since most of the immunologic reactivity of the penicillin nucleus is directed to the 6-aminopenicillanic acid (**6-APA**) nucleus of this ring, which is common to all the beta-lactam antibiotics, this explains the high degree of allergic cross-reactivity encountered by these antibiotic homologs. In contrast, with the cephalosporins, side chain cross-reactivity appears to be more important than cross-reactivity with the beta-lactam nucleus. As a result, less than 10 percent cross-reactivity is seen between PCNs and the first-generation cephalosporins and much less cross-reactivity (< 2 percent) is seen with the more distantly related third-generation cephalosporins. Aztreonam, a monobactam, which has a monocyclic beta-lactam ring and poorly organized 6-APA nucleus, has no reported cross-reactivity with other PCNs, and would be a safe antibiotic option for PCN allergic individuals.

Other common classes of antibacterial agents reported to cause IgE-mediated reactions are the **sulfonamides**. Due to their metabolism by hepatic acetylation through the p450 oxidative pathway, certain metabolites containing the sulfanamidoyl determinant have been shown to become haptens that interact with IgE. Some individuals are genetically predisposed to be slow acetylators of sulfonamide-containing drugs, and this contributes to prolonged exposure to metabolites and therefore increased likelihood of developing IgE-mediated allergic reactions. Sulfonamides are also associated with severe T cell-mediated allergic drug reactions involving the skin, such as Steven Johnson's syndrome or toxic epidermal necrolysis. Development of these skin reactions is an absolute contraindication for further use of this drug. Another antibiotic, **vancomycin**, causes a particular dose-dependent adverse response in certain individuals called "red-man syndrome" that is manifested by extreme skin flushing during intravenous drug administration. This reaction is believed to be due to an IgE-independent histamine release. Symptoms are lessened by slowing the rate of intravenous drug infusion.

Box 18-3

The Beta-Lactam Ring (β-lactam)

The beta-lactam ring is part of the structure of several antibiotic families, principally the penicillins, cephalosporins, monobactams, and carbapenems, which are therefore also called beta-lactam antibiotics (Figure 18-21). The beta-lactam ring is a molecule with a heterocyclic ring structure, consisting of three carbon atoms and one nitrogen atom and is a composite of the words lactone (a cyclic ester of an –OH + a–COOH) + amide, and is part of the PCN nucleus referred to as the 6-APA nucleus.

The mechanism of action of these antibiotics is through inhibition of bacterial cell wall synthesis (*Chapter 13*). This has a lethal effect on bacteria, especially the Gram-positive. Certain bacteria, however, have become resistant to beta-lactam antibiotics by expressing beta-lactamase, e.g., methicillin-resistant staphylococcus aureus (MRSA).

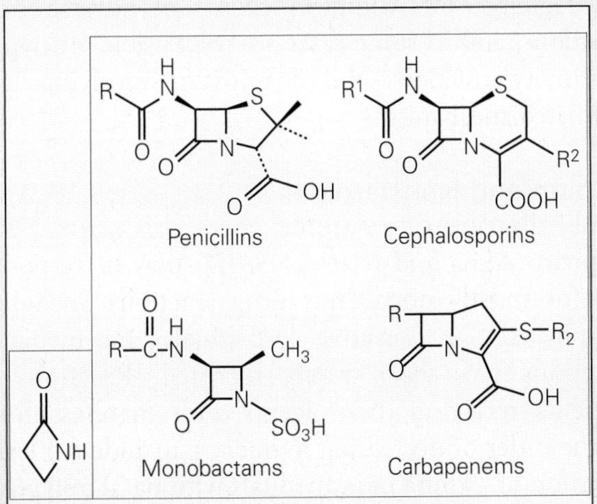

Penicillins — Cephalosporins — Monobactams — Carbapenems

Figure 18-21. Schematic representation of the core beta-lactam structure of several antibiotics. Shown in the left lower insert box is a schematic representation of a beta-lactam ring.

Anesthetics

Drugs used in anesthesia are frequently responsible for allergic drug reactions. The **local anesthetics** are a group of drugs frequently implicated in adverse drug reactions; in some cases, anaphylaxis may result. Local anesthetics are comprised of two groups: esters, e.g., benzocaine, and amides, e.g., lidocaine, based on the presence or absence of the para-aminobenzoic acid (**PABA**) nucleus, respectively (Figure 18-22). Group I, the amino ester group, contains the PABA nucleus and includes such drugs as procaine, benzocaine, and tetracaine; Group II

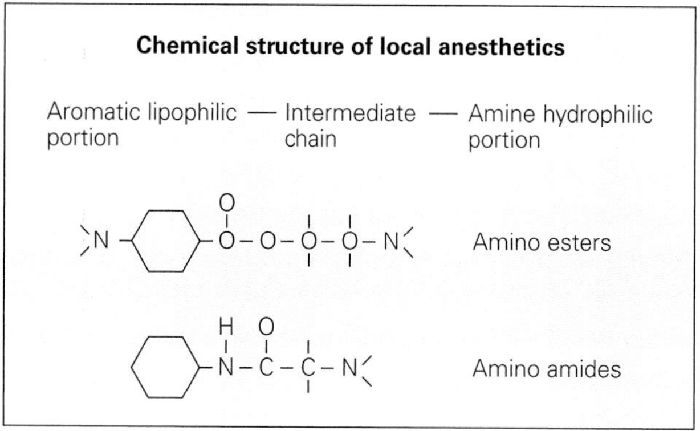

Figure 18-22. Schematic representation of the chemical structure of the two classes of local anesthetics, amino esters and amino amides.

drugs lack the PABA nucleus and include lidocaine, mepivacaine, and dibucaine (Table 18-10). The clinical importance of this division is that patients with allergic reactions to drugs in one group can safely receive drugs in the other.

The cause of allergic reactions is believed to be a breakdown product created by the action of serum pseudocholinesterases leading to the production of PABA, which functions as a hapten. PABA is very antigenic, and following binding to a carrier protein can elicit immediate IgE-mediated reactions, including anaphylaxis, or delayed Type IV reactions manifested by contact dermatitis.

Protein Hormones

Hypersensitivity reactions also result from the use of proteinaceous drugs such as **insulin** and **protamine.** Insulin allergy typically involves an IgE-mediated reaction to nonhuman, porcine, or bovine forms of insulin. Although anaphylaxis has been reported, symptoms of urticaria and angioedema are usually localized to the injection site. Because of the increasing use of humanized insulin, the incidence of insulin allergy has significantly been reduced in recent years. Allergy to protamine, a protein derived from salmon testes and used primarily to reverse heparin

Table 18-10. Classification of local anesthetics

Amino esters (Group I)	Amino amides (Group II)
Procaine	Lidocaine
Benzocaine	Mepivacaine
Tetracaine	Dibucaine
Chloroprocaine	Articaine
Cocaine	Bupivacaine
Proparacaine	Prilocaine
	Ropivacaine

toxicity, has also been reported to result in IgE-mediated anaphylaxis. Interestingly, protamine is also a component of NPH insulin added to prolong its pharmacologic activity. Thus, individuals sensitized to protamine from prior treatment with protamine for heparin toxicity may also manifest cross-reactive allergy to NPH insulin. Conversely, previous allergic sensitization of NPH-treated diabetic patients may also be responsible for subsequent reactions to other protamine-containing drugs.

Monoclonal Antibodies

An increasingly important group of therapeutic agents causing acute anaphylaxis include a wide array of monoclonal antibodies (**mAbs**) being used as targeted therapies for malignancies, transplant rejection, autoimmune disorders, and allergic and infectious diseases (*Chapter 11*). Although all of these genetically engineered products can cause allergic reactions, the chimeric mAbs, e.g., infliximab, that contain > 5 percent residual murine components are particularly prone to induce **human anti-mouse antibody** (**HAMA**) associated with immediate type IgE-mediated reactions. These mAbs may also cause a number of other acute immunologic reactions, such as serum sickness, tumor lysis syndrome, and the more serious and sometimes-fatal cytokine release syndrome (**CRS**) or cytokine storm syndrome.

Chemotherapeutic Agents

Chemotherapeutic agents, e.g., taxanes, cisplatin, and asparaginase, are common causes of adverse drug reactions, and in some cases are responsible for hypersensitivity reactions and anaphylaxis involving IgE-mediated mechanisms.

Aspirin and Nonsteroidal Anti-Inflammatory Agents

Aspirin (**ASA**) and related NSAIDs may be responsible for mostly nonallergic drug reactions, including anaphylaxis, in sensitive individuals; IgE-mediated reactions have been rarely reported. Reactions in patients receiving these agents with manifestations, in the order of decreasing frequency, include (1) exacerbation of asthma in individuals with nasal polyposis, (2) urticaria and angioedema, and (3) anaphylaxis. ASA sensitivity is encountered in 8 to 19 percent of patients with asthma and in 30 percent of individuals with nasal polyps, thus forming the "aspirin triad" of asthma, aspirin sensitivity, and nasal/ethmoidal polyposis, i.e., Samter's syndrome. This sensitivity is believed to be due to the inhibitory effects of ASA on cyclooxygenase activity (Figure 18-10) that results in increased production of inflammatory leukotrienes as well as to indirect effects on mast cell degranulation through inhibition of prostaglandin E_2 (PGE), a mast cell stabilizer (Figure 18-12). NSAIDs with a high degree of cyclooxygenase suppression show a greater potential of adverse drug reactivity with ASA than those NSAIDs with a lower degree of cyclooxygenase suppression. As such, ASA-like agents with poor cyclooxygenase suppressive capacity, e.g., tartrazine and sodium salicylate, do not exhibit this potential for adverse cross-reactivity with ASA.

Radiocontrast Media

Although often mistakenly considered a form of drug allergy, reactions to radiocontrast media (**RCM**) represent the example par excellence of a nonallergic (nonantibody-mediated) drug reaction and an important cause of anaphylaxis in a medical care or diagnostic setting (Table 18-8 and Figure 18-18). Reactions occur within the first few hours after administration of RCM and range from vasomotor reactions, e.g., lightheadedness, syncope, pruritus, and urticaria, to serious sequelae of coma and death. Although the precise mechanism is unknown, RCM is believed to initiate deleterious effects through direct mediator release from mast cells in susceptible individuals. Despite the three- to fivefold greater frequency of RCM reactions in atopic individuals, no IgE-mediated mechanism has consistently been identified, and diagnostic skin testing is nonpredictive of susceptibility to future reactions. Preventive procedures shown to decrease the occurrence and severity of RCM reactions include the use of lower osmolar compared to higher osmolar-iodinated RCM preparations and the preadministration of antihistamines, steroids, and oral adrenergic agents to individuals with a previous history of RCM reactions.

Stinging Insects

A specialized group of systemic IgE-mediated allergic reactions is caused by proteins in venom from stinging insects in the order Hymenoptera. Venom allergy is believed to affect 4 percent of the U.S. population and results in approximately 40 deaths per year. Although the Hymenoptera are comprised of different families, i.e., Apidae (honeybees and bumble bees), Vespidae (hornets, yellow jackets, and wasps), and Formicidae (fire ants and harvester ants), there is a high degree of allergic cross-reactivity to the venoms among these families. Most stings in the United States occur by yellow jackets; however, the most severe reactions occur with honeybees, likely due to the fact that honeybee stings are usually multiple and the stinger with venom is embedded in the skin. Several enzymes have been found in the venom that appear to be potent allergens, e.g., phospholipase A, hyaluronidase, and melittin. Most reactions involve swelling, redness, and pain at the sting site. In some cases, though, venom exposure leads to hypotensive shock without significant skin findings. Age appears to play an important role in reaction severity, as cutaneous systemic reactions are more common in children, while hypotensive shock occurs more frequently in adults. Hymenoptera stings may also result in delayed urticarial complaints and serum-sickness as well as Guillain-Barré syndrome and nephritis. As will be described later, venom allergen immunotherapy provides a very effective management modality to minimize the serious sequela of anaphylaxis caused by insect venom.

Latex Allergy

Latex allergy is exemplary of the direct relationship between frequency of allergen exposure and risk for sensitization (Box 18-4). Individuals with latex allergy make IgE to natural rubber latex protein

Box 18-4

Latex Allergy

In the 1980s, prompted by the universal blood and fluid precautions associated with the AIDS epidemic, the use of latex protection was advocated in health care environments. Prior to this period, latex allergy was relatively rare. With the increased exposure to latex both in occupational and patient care settings, a noticeable increase in the incidence of latex allergy became recognized both in health care workers (5–15 percent) as well as in patients with spina bifida and urogenital abnormalities (24–60 percent) exposed to large amounts of latex in surgical procedures. In recent years, the increased awareness of latex allergy has led to shifts toward reduced use of latex allergens in gloves and other manufactured equipment as well as establishment of latex-free environments in hospital settings. As a result, exposure to environmental latex protein has been greatly minimized and the incidence of latex allergy and anaphylaxis has significantly decreased.

derived from the sap of the rubber tree, *Hevea brasiliensis*. Hypersensitivity to latex may occur via skin contact (Type IV), e.g., gloves, tourniquets, blood pressure cuffs, adhesive tape, and mucosal contact, e.g., condoms and urethral catheters, or via aerosol exposure to latex proteins linked to use of cornstarch powdered gloves. In the latter example, the cornstarch enables release of latex proteins into the air when the gloves are removed and these aerosolized latex proteins are responsible for mild to severe symptoms of allergic rhinitis and asthma. Latex hypersensitivity may also be associated with cross-reactive allergies to certain fruits, e.g., kiwi, banana, and avocado, which share similar hevea-like proteins. Interestingly, because of this cross-reactivity, individuals with allergies to these foods may have a much higher risk for developing latex allergy. Testing for Type I latex allergy is through blood testing, such as specific IgE. Although the standard for allergen testing is the skin prick test, there is no approved skin-testing reagent for latex in the United States.

Clinical Manifestations of Gastrointestinal (Food) Allergy

Most gastrointestinal (**GI**) allergy is manifested by hypersensitivity to certain exogenous substances, usually foods, which gain access to the body via the gastrointestinal tract; it is therefore commonly referred to as **food allergy**. Food allergy is defined as "an adverse health effect arising from a specific immune response that occurs reproducibly on exposure to a given food" (NIH Guidelines, 2010). Food allergy is differentiated from other types of adverse food reactions, which include food intolerances, by its immune-mediated pathogenesis. IgE antibody- and non-IgE antibody-mediated food allergic disorders have been described, as well as a group of disorders that display both IgE and non-IgE-mediated mechanisms (mixed-type) (Table 18-11).

Food allergy encompasses commonly ingested foods and has a higher frequency of occurrence in infants and young children. The underlying mechanisms for the development of food allergies are not fully defined but appear to involve a breakdown in mucosal immunity or oral tolerance. Since food allergy is primarily mediated by the oral route, symptoms typically manifest in the gastrointestinal tract. However, for IgE-mediated food allergy, symptoms more typically involve other organs, such as the skin and lungs, and in some cases the shock organs of the cardiorespiratory tract, leading to anaphylaxis (Figure 18-23).

IgE-Mediated Food Allergy

IgE-mediated food allergy classically presents with immediate hypersensitivity symptoms and can be manifested by **immediate gastrointestinal hypersensitivity** characterized by immediate upper GI symptoms of vomiting and immediate or delayed lower GI symptoms, e.g., diarrhea, cramping, oral allergy syndrome (**OAS**), **acute urticaria**, or **food-induced anaphylaxis**. Essentially any food or food

Table 18-11. Clinical disorders associated with food allergy according to specific MALT system and affected target organs.

Immunologic mechanism	Affected MALT system	Target organ	Clinical disorder
IgE	GALT	GI tract	Immediate GI hypersensitivity; OAS
	SALT	Skin	Acute urticaria; angioedema
	BALT	Respiratory tract	Bronchospasm; asthma; anaphylaxis
Non-IgE (including cell-mediated)	GALT	GI tract	Celiac disease; cow's milk enteropathy; dietary protein enterocolitis; breast milk colitis; proctocolitis; proctitis
	SALT	Skin	Dermatitis herpetiformis
	BALT	Respiratory tract	Heiner syndrome
	NALT	CNS	Behavioral disorders
Mixed IgE and non-IgE	GALT	GI tract	Eosinophilic esophagitis (EOE) Eosinophilic gastroenteritis (EG)
	SALT	Skin	Atopic dermatitis
	BALT	Respiratory tract	FA-induced bronchial asthma

Reproduced with permission from Sabra A, Bellanti JA, Rais JM, Castro HJ, de Inocencio JM, Sabra S. IgE and non-IgE food allergy. Ann Allergy Asthma Immunol 2003;90:71–6.

MALT = mucosal-associated lymphoid tissue; GALT = gastrointestinal lymphoid tissue; GI = gastrointestinal; OAS = oral allergy syndrome; SALT = skin-associated lymphoid tissue; BALT = bronchial-associated lymphoid tissue; NALT = nasal-associated lymphoid tissue; CNS = central nervous system; FA = food allergy.

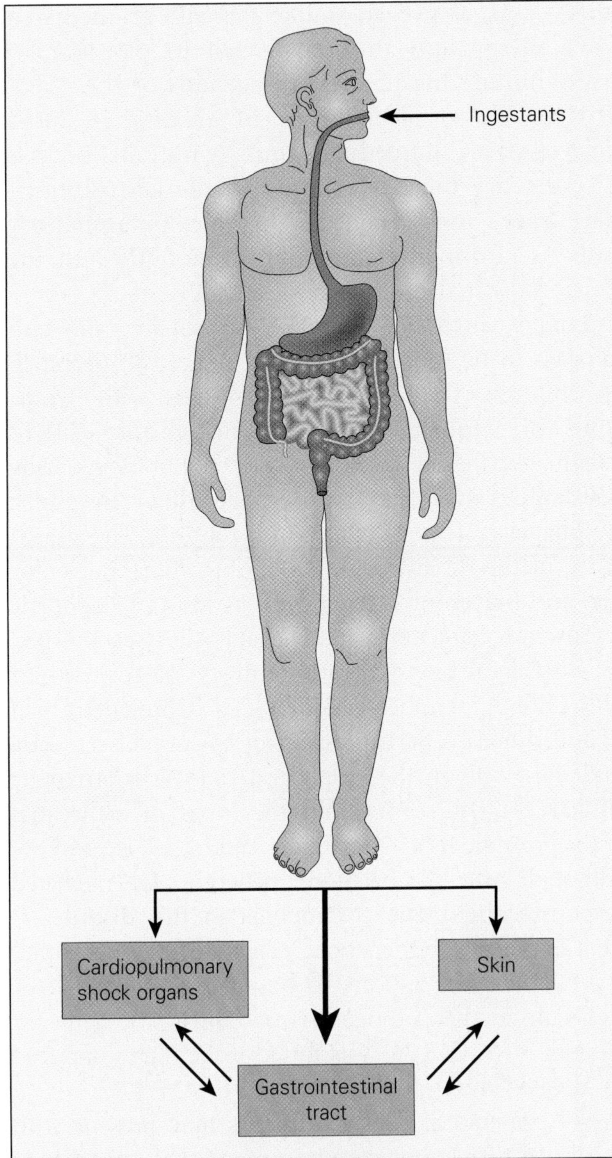

Figure 18-23. Schematic representation of the three target or shock organs responsible for the clinical manifestations of gastrointestinal allergy.

protein ingredient has the capability to elicit an IgE-mediated reaction. Over 170 foods have been implicated in IgE-mediated reactions; however, 90 percent or more of food allergies and serious adverse reactions are limited to a few specific foods or food groups. In the United States, these foods include peanuts, tree nuts, soy, egg, milk, wheat, fish, and shellfish. In Europe, allergies to sesame, mustard, celery, and lupine have also been shown to be important, while buckwheat is a key allergen in Japan and other Asian countries. Today, although a genetic predisposition for food allergy remains paramount, the most clinically important food allergens within populations are largely influenced by environmental factors such as the frequency of exposure to the food and culinary or dietary practices.

Food allergies are currently estimated to affect 3 to 4 percent of the U.S. population, with milk and shellfish allergy being recognized as the most common food allergies in children and adults, respectively. Allergens such as milk and egg are most common in infancy as they are usually outgrown by adulthood, whereas peanut, tree nut, fish, and shellfish allergy are not usually outgrown. Adverse reactions to food allergens are an important cause of emergency room visits and hospitalizations for anaphylaxis and are responsible for an estimated 100 deaths per year.

Clinical Manifestations

Symptoms of IgE-mediated food allergy are similar to those of classic Type I hypersensitivity and anaphylaxis (Table 18-7). Since exposure of allergen is through the gastrointestinal tract, there may be a predominance of early symptoms related to the oral cavity, e.g., swelling and itching of the lip and tongue, and upper gastrointestinal tract, i.e., nausea and/or vomiting. However, the most common manifestations of this food allergy are systemic and involve the skin, i.e., flushing and/or hives, or the respiratory tract, e.g., throat tightness and/or wheezing. The risk for severe reactions is dose-dependent, with the possibility for anaphylaxis occurring with higher the exposure to the offending food. However, there appears to be a wide range of individual sensitivities to food allergen exposures, with a subgroup of sensitive individuals potentially at risk for severe reactions even to low-dose exposures. A pre-existing history of asthma can contribute to reaction severity. Although most food allergic reactions occur immediately within minutes to hours following food ingestion, IgE-mediated food allergy may also manifest with chronic disease symptoms, such as atopic eczema, particularly in children.

Cross-Reactivity and Food Allergens

Another increasingly important area in IgE-mediated food allergy includes the clinical implications of cross-reactive food allergens. A variety of food allergenic proteins and protein families are conserved among plants and animals. As such, IgE antibody specifically directed to protein from one type of food may also react with similar proteins from another food. For example, a patient sensitized to one tree nut, e.g., walnut, could also express allergic cross-reactivity to another tree nut, e.g., pine nut. Shown in Figure 18-24 are examples of the many cross-reactions between foods, plants, fish, and animal proteins important in clinical allergy.

Allergenic cross-reactivity also forms the basis for the previously described localized form of IgE-mediated food allergy referred to as OAS or pollen food allergy syndrome. This syndrome manifests in individuals primarily sensitized to pollen allergens, e.g., birch tree pollen, as immediate reactions of the oral mucosa, i.e., pruritus or edema of the mouth, lips, and palate, upon contact with proteins in raw or uncooked fruits, e.g., apple, peach and/or other plant-based foods that share homology with proteins in these pollens. The food proteins recognized by pollen-specific IgE are highly labile, and cooking or processing of the plant food typically destroys the food's capacity to elicit an allergic response. The lability of these problems may also explain why allergic manifestations to uncooked foods remain confined to the site of oral mucosal contact and rarely involve the gastrointestinal tract or become systemic. The clinical significance of this observation finds application in the type of allergen to be used in diagnostic skin testing. It has been suggested that raw fruits or vegetables be used in addition to conventional commercial food extracts, which may lose some of the important allergic proteins during processing. Similar cross-reactive phenomena to plant foods, i.e., kiwi, banana, and avocado, may be seen in individuals with (rubber tree) latex allergy (Figure 18-24). In these cases, however, both localized as well as generalized allergic symptoms may commonly occur.

Mixed-Type Mediated Food Disorders

Disorders associated with mixed type IgE-mediated forms of food allergy include eosinophilic esophagitis (**EoE**) and eosinophilic gastroenteritis (**EG**), also known as the eosinophilic gastrointestinal disorders (**EGID**) (Table 18-11). Shown in Figure 18-25 is a schematic representation of various pathogenetic mechanisms involved in the various allergenic eosinophilic gastroenteritides together with some proposed treatment regimens. Most affected individuals with these disorders have an atopic history and evidence of serum IgE to specific foods suggestive of a Type I hypersensitivity. Dietary elimination of these food(s), furthermore, prevents or results in resolution of symptoms in most cases. However, unlike typical IgE-mediated food allergy, IgE antibody is felt to play a relatively minor role in the pathogenesis of these disorders. The typical onset of disease is more delayed than immediate, and symptoms of this disorder are mostly localized to the gastrointestinal tract and triggered by an inflammatory response from infiltration of eosinophils into the gastrointestinal mucosa.

EoE is caused by a number of protein foods and appears to be more common in males (80 percent). In children, EoE commonly presents with symptoms of frequent emesis and/or chronic gastroesophageal reflux disease (**GERD**) that is typically resistant to use of antireflux medications. In adults, dysphagia is a more common symptom. The prevalence of the disease is unknown but more individuals are becoming recognized as more diagnostic endoscopies are performed. Diagnosis is established by esophageal biopsy demonstrating > 10 eosinophils/40X HPF. A peripheral eosinophilia is present in half of individuals. The expression of eosinophils, T cells, and mast cells in the esophageal mucosa is strikingly similar to that seen within the lungs of asthmatics with prominent Th2 cytokine and IL-5 expression. 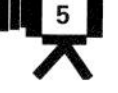
Although the association between IgE-mediated responses and tissue eosinophilia in this disorder is not completely understood, eotaxin-3, an eosinophil chemoattractant, appears to be an important effector molecule in the pathogenesis of EoE as the gene for eotaxin-3 (or CCL26) was found to be highly induced in affected individuals (*Chapter 9*).

EG presents at all ages. Infants may present with failure to thrive, but common manifestations include postprandial nausea and vomiting, abdominal pain, and diarrhea. Evidence of eosinophilic infiltration in the gastric or intestinal mucosa with eosinophils may be localized or diffuse, and food challenge or elimination is often necessary to confirm disease.

In the EGIDs, avoidance of offending food(s) has been shown to relieve most symptoms and allow recovery of gastrointestinal mucosal damage by eosinophils. In some severe cases, however, resolution of symptoms may require strict avoidance of intact food proteins, i.e., elemental amino acid diet. When dietary restriction is difficult, pharmacological therapy with corticosteroids has been shown to ameliorate eosinophilia and symptoms. The EGIDs have also been shown to be good candidates for anti IL-5 cytokine therapy as well (*Chapter 11*). Long-term prognosis of these disorders is unknown.

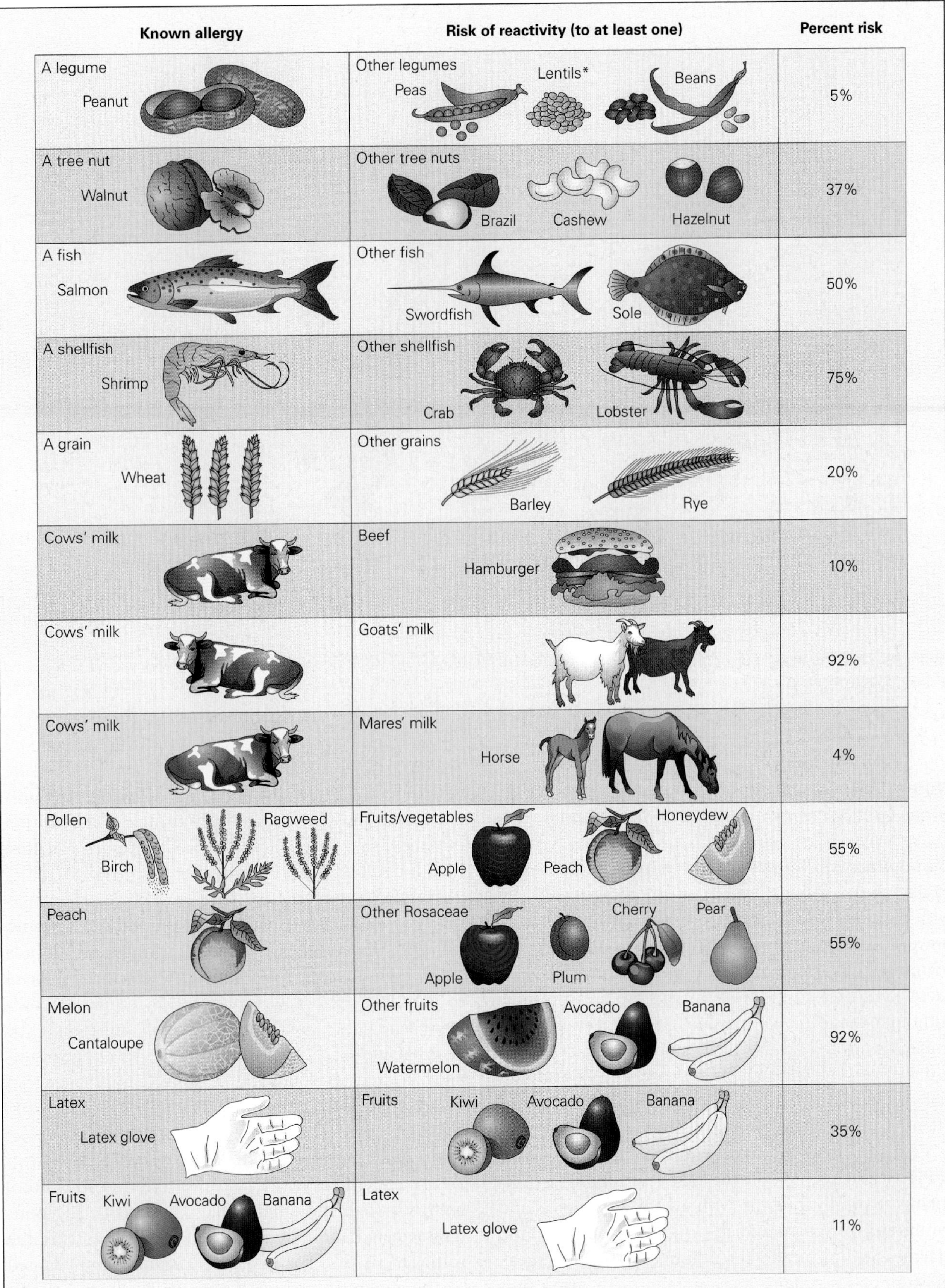

Known allergy
Risk of reactivity (to at least one)
Percent risk
A legume
Peanut
Other legumes
Peas
Lentils*
Beans
5%
A tree nut
Walnut
Other tree nuts
Brazil
Cashew
Hazelnut
37%
A fish
Salmon
Other fish
Swordfish
Sole
50%
A shellfish
Shrimp
Other shellfish
Crab
Lobster
75%
A grain
Wheat
Other grains
Barley
Rye
20%
Cows' milk
Beef
Hamburger
10%
Cows' milk
Goats' milk
92%
Cows' milk
Mares' milk
Horse
4%
Pollen
Birch
Ragweed
Fruits/vegetables
Apple
Peach
Honeydew
55%
Peach
Other Rosaceae
Apple
Plum
Cherry
Pear
55%
Melon
Cantaloupe
Other fruits
Watermelon
Avocado
Banana
92%
Latex
Latex glove
Fruits
Kiwi
Avocado
Banana
35%
Fruits
Kiwi
Avocado
Banana
Latex
Latex glove
11%

Figure 18-24. **Schematic representation of cross-reactions between foods, plants, fish, and animal proteins important in clinical allergy.** The percentage risk estimates the approximate rate of clinical reactivity of one food known be allergenic with at least one other related food in a similar food category. (Adapted with permission from Sicherer SH. Clinical implications of cross-reactive food allergens. J Allergy Clin Immunol. 2001;108:881–90.) *Rates may be higher in patients with multiple legume allergies.

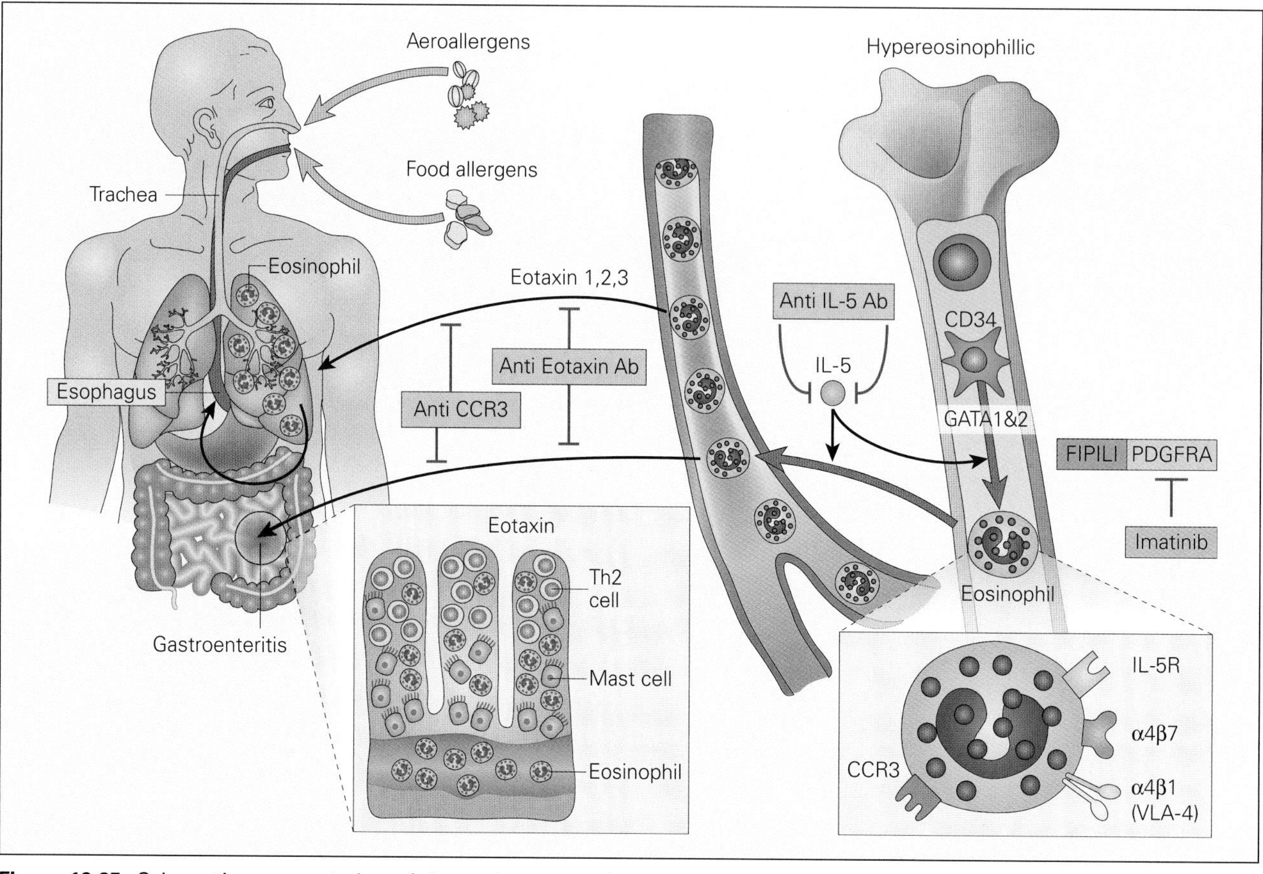

Figure 18-25. Schematic representation of the various causative agents and pathogenetic mechanisms involved in EGIDs and HES together with some treatment strategies based on these considerations. (Adapted with permission from Rothenberg ME. Eosinophilic gastrointestinal disorders (EGID). J Allergy Clin Immunol. 2004;113:11–28.)

Non-IgE Mediated Food Disorders

Some food allergic disorders involve immunological injury without a known IgE-mediated mechanism. **Dietary protein-induced proctitis/proctocolitis** classically affects infants less than six months old fed with cows' milk or soy-based formulas. In some cases, however, symptoms may be triggered by low levels of maternally ingested cows' milk or soy proteins excreted in breast milk while infants are breastfeeding. Although these infants may not appear ill they often present with blood in their stools. Sigmoidoscopy usually shows patchy, friable mucosa, and eosinophils can be detected in stools. Oral tolerance of the offending foods usually develops by two years of age.

Food protein-induced enterocolitis syndrome (FPIES) also presents in the first few months of life. Infants typically present with toxic appearance and symptoms of postprandial projectile vomiting and diarrhea within one to three hours following a meal. In some cases, infants may present with symptoms of shock due to severe dehydration. Causative foods include cows' milk, soy, and cereals. In adults, a similar syndrome has been observed after consumption of shellfish. Symptoms typically resolve within 24 hours after elimination of causative food(s).

Heiner's syndrome is a rare food allergy characterized by growth retardation, gastrointestinal symptoms, iron deficiency anemia, and recurrent pneumonia with hemosiderosis. Most patients also have peripheral eosinophilia. The causative food is primarily cow's milk, and IgG precipitins to cows' milk may be detected in serum, suggesting a Type III antigen-antibody complex response as a possible mechanism of tissue injury in this syndrome (*Chapter 17*).

Celiac disease (also referred to as celiac sprue) is an increasingly prevalent food allergic disorder directed to dietary glutens from wheat, barley, rye, and sometimes oats. Although most individuals make a specific non-IgE-mediated antibody response to gluten proteins, the pathogenesis of celiac disease is predominantly caused by the generation of autoreactive T cells and shares similar characteristics to other autoimmune disorders. In this regard, disease is confined to individuals with distinct genetic HLA haplotypes and involves antibodies generated against an autoantigen, human tissue transglutaminase (**tTG**) (*Chapters 10* and *19*).

Shown in Figure 18-26 is a schematic representation of the sequential molecular events thought to be involved in the pathogenesis of celiac disease. Once gluten is absorbed across the intestinal epithelium, tTG enzymatically deaminates and/or cross-

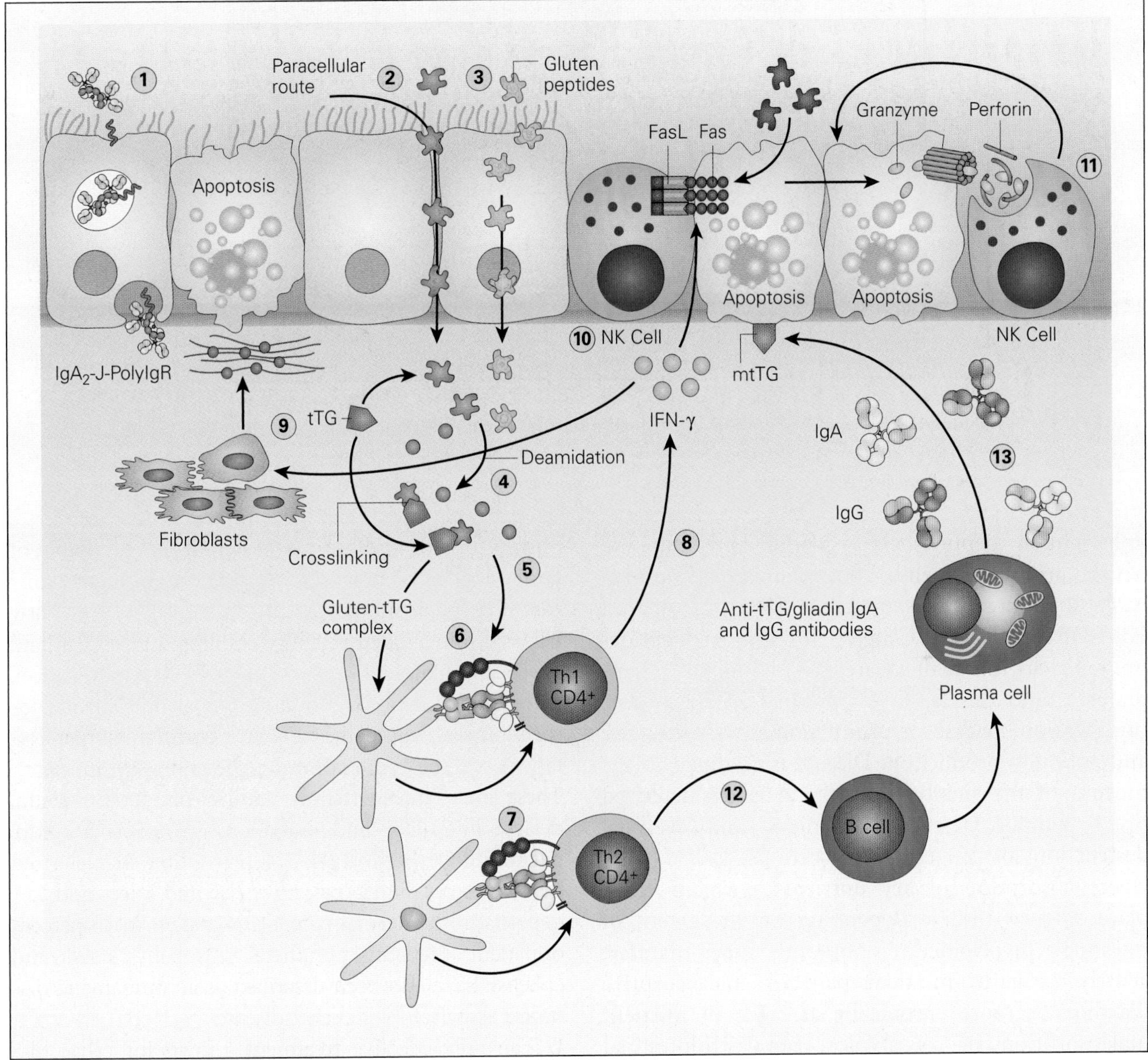

Figure 18-26. Schematic representation of the pathogenesis of celiac disease. Gluten peptides can be transported across the intestinal epithelium by three main mechanisms: retrotranscytosis of secretory IgA (sIgA) (1) through transferrin receptor CD71 paracellularly (2) or transcytosis as a consequence of impaired mucosal integrity attributable to increased release of zonulin (3). Once internalized, deamidation (4) or cross-linking of gluten (5) by tissue transglutaminase (tTG) leads to the production of deamidated gluten or gluten-tTG, respectively. These gluten peptides are taken up and presented by dendritic cells to either CD4+ Th1 (6) or Th2 (7) cells in the context of HLA-DQ2 or HLA-DQ8 molecules. This presentation leads to activated gluten-reactive CD4+ Th1 cells that produce high levels of proinflammatory cytokines (8), with a Th1 cytokine pattern dominated by interferon gamma (IFN-γ). Th-1 cytokines promote inflammatory effects, including fibroblast or lamina propria mononuclear cell (LPMC) secretion of matrix metalloproteinases (MMPs) (9), which are responsible for degradation of extracellular matrix and basement membrane and enhance the cytotoxicity of intraepithelial lymphocytes (IELs) or natural killer (NK) T cells (10). These latter cells facilitate the apoptotic death of enterocytes by the Fas/Fas ligand (FasL) system or interleukin-15 (IL-15)-induced perforin granzyme and NFG2D-MIC signaling pathways (11). Interferon alpha (IFN-α) released by activated dendritic cells further perpetuates the inflammatory reaction by inducing CD4+ T cells to produce IFN-γ. Additionally, through the production of Th-2 cytokines (12), activated CD4+ T cells drive the activation and clonal expansion of B cells, which differentiate into plasma cells and produce antigliadin and anti-tTG antibodies (13). (Adapted with permission from Di Sabatino A, Corazzo GR. Coeliac disease. Lancet. 2009; 373:1480–93.)

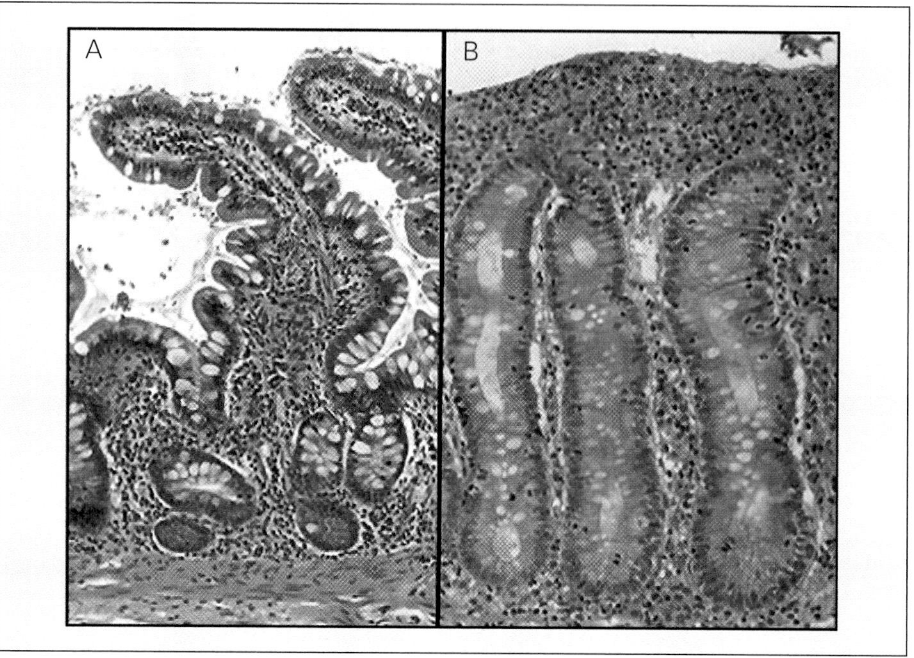

Figure 18-27. Panel A: Photomicrograph of a normal small intestinal villus. Panel B: A villus atrophy with heavy submucosal lymphocyte infiltration seen in celiac disease.

links gluten peptides, i.e., gliadin and glutenin, which are subsequently taken up by intestinal APCs. In individuals expressing MHC-II-associated HLA-DR2 or DR8 (*Chapter 10*), gluten peptides presented in this context are stimulatory to T lymphocytes and this leads to intestinal T lymphocyte proliferation, release of proinflammatory cytokines, and antibody production. Disease is confined to the mucosa of the small intestine and is characterized by T lymphocyte-mediated injury and eventual destruction of fingerlike projections, called villi, where absorption of key nutrients normally takes place (Figure 18-27). Depending on the extent of intestinal involvement, symptoms may manifest acutely as gastrointestinal pain or malabsorptive diarrhea or more chronically as signs of nutrient malabsorption or as atypical nongastrointestinal manifestations. Although antibodies to gliadin and tTG are now routinely measured for screening, the gold standard for diagnosis remains the demonstration of villous inflammation or atrophy on small intestinal biopsy.

Historically, the diagnosis of celiac disease was uncommon and made mostly in infants and young children presenting with sprue-like symptoms of abdominal pain, malabsorptive diarrhea, delayed growth, and, in severe cases, failure to thrive. The disease was not easily distinguished from cystic fibrosis, another condition associated with malabsorption. Recent genetic testing of family members, however, has revealed that celiac disease is a much more prevalent disease than previously believed, often silent in older children and adults, and affects approximately 1.5 percent of the U.S. population. In older populations, complications of nutrient malabsorption (i.e., iron deficiency) or extraintestinal manifestations are the more common presenting symptom(s). These may include short stature or developmental delays, infertility, and osteoporosis/osteopenia. Also, **dermatitis herpetiformis**, a skin eruption characterized by blisters on the elbows, buttocks, and knees and IgA deposits in the dermal papillae, is present in 15 percent of patients. Hepatitis, peripheral neuropathy, ataxia, and epilepsy have also been described as accompanying disorders associated with celiac disease.

The only effective treatment known for celiac disease is avoidance of foods containing gluten. A gluten-free diet has been shown to completely prevent the clinical and pathological complications of celiac disease. Preventing complications and intestinal inflammation is particularly important since, in addition to the manifestations described above, individuals with untreated celiac disease are at increased risk for other serious health conditions, such as autoimmune diseases (i.e., type 1 diabetes mellitus) and certain cancers associated with high mortality, e.g., lymphoma.

Clinical Manifestations of Allergic Diseases of the Skin

The skin is another frequently involved shock organ of allergic diseases. Manifestations of allergic reactions in skin may be classified under two main categories: (1) the immediate, e.g., urticaria and angioedema; and (2) the delayed, e.g., eczema and allergic contact dermatitis (Figure 18-28). These disorders may be induced by inhalants, food, drugs, or contactants. Although the main shock organ is the skin, secondary involvement of the respiratory and gastrointestinal tracts may be seen.

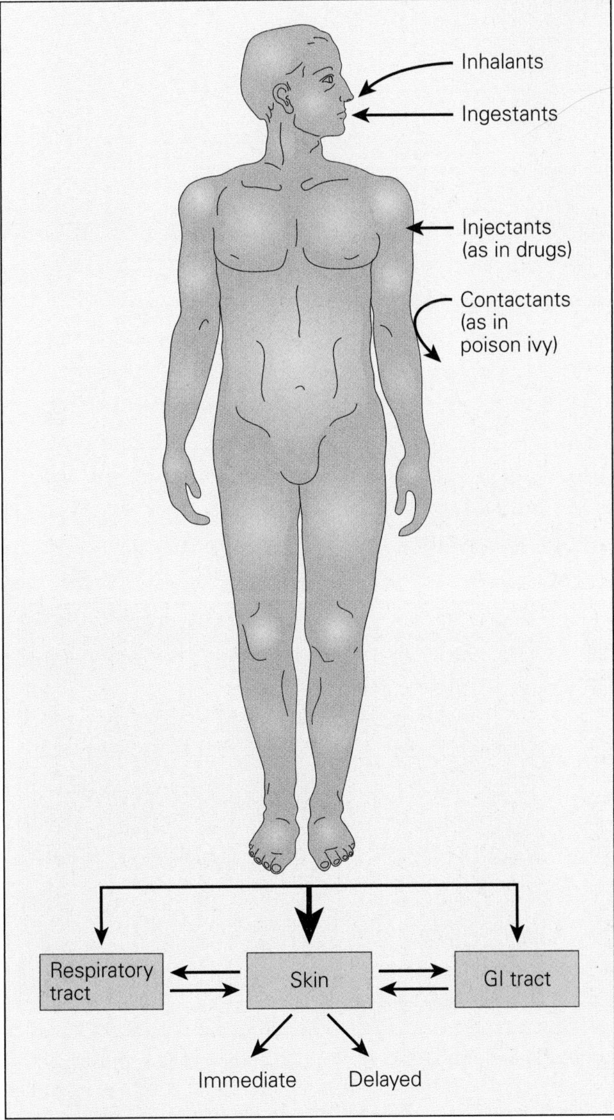

Figure 18-28. Schematic representation of the clinical manifestations of allergy affecting the skin.

Definitions of Allergic Diseases of the Skin

A common umbrella term for localized inflammation of the skin is **dermatitis**. Clinical disorders associated with IgE-mediated Type I hypersensitivity reactions of the skin include **acute urticaria** and **eczema**. These disorders can be localized to certain body parts but are typically systemic. Acute urticaria is usually characterized by sudden onset of skin lesions, i.e., hives, of less than six weeks' duration that resolves rapidly and may have an allergic or nonallergic trigger. In some cases, lesions may become associated with local skin swelling that involves deeper dermal tissues, i.e., **angioedema**, that can persist for hours or days. In contrast, **chronic urticaria**, defined as hives and/or angioedema episodes appearing on and off for longer than six weeks in duration, is seldom IgE-mediated. Some forms of urticaria can occur following skin contact with allergenic substances (**contact urticaria**) or hypersensitivity to insect bites, i.e., from mosquitoes (**papular urticaria**).

Eczema, frequently termed "atopic dermatitis," has a more complex pathogenesis characterized by a skin barrier defect and delayed, chronic inflammatory skin lesions. Patients with eczema can be divided into two major categories: (1) those involving IgE sensitization with high levels of IgE, i.e., **atopic eczema**, and (2) those showing mostly lymphocyte involvement, i.e., **nonatopic eczema**, that may be due to a variety of other mechanisms, e.g., Type IV cell-mediated hypersensitivity. In most cases, a mixed pattern of Type I and Type IV hypersensitivity is likely present (*Chapter 17*). Other disorders associated with delayed reactions of the skin include those triggered by skin contact with low molecular weight chemicals, i.e., haptens or irritants, to produce localized skin lesions, i.e., **contact dermatitis**. When a T cell-mediated immunologic mechanism or typical haptenating substance, e.g., metals, poison ivy, and fragrances, is involved, the reaction is **allergic contact dermatitis**. In rare instances, consumption of certain haptenating substances in food, e.g., coloring agents, may result in generalized skin manifestations and is referred to as **systemic contact dermatitis**.

Urticaria and Angioedema

Urticaria, or hives, is a skin manifestation that has an immediate onset and is characterized by erythema and wheal formation (Figure 18-29A). The urticarial lesion is explained by the triple response of Lewis that includes (1) localized vasodilation (erythema),

(2) transudation of fluid (wheal), and (3) flaring due to a local axon reflex. The lesions are characteristically evanescent, vary in size and shape, and are pruritic. The basic mechanism underlying all of the urticarias involves the localized increase in vascular permeability and the transudation of fluid into surrounding tissues that occurs through the release of vasoactive amines, e.g., histamine, via any of a number of mechanisms described previously (Figure 18-30). Angioedema is a form of urticarial lesion involving the deeper skin layers of the subcutaneous or submucosal tissues leading to swelling characterized by localized edema and giant wheals (Figure 18-29).

Clinical Characteristics of Urticaria

As previously described, urticaria can be clinically classified as (1) acute or (2) chronic, depending on the length of time that the hives persist. Acute

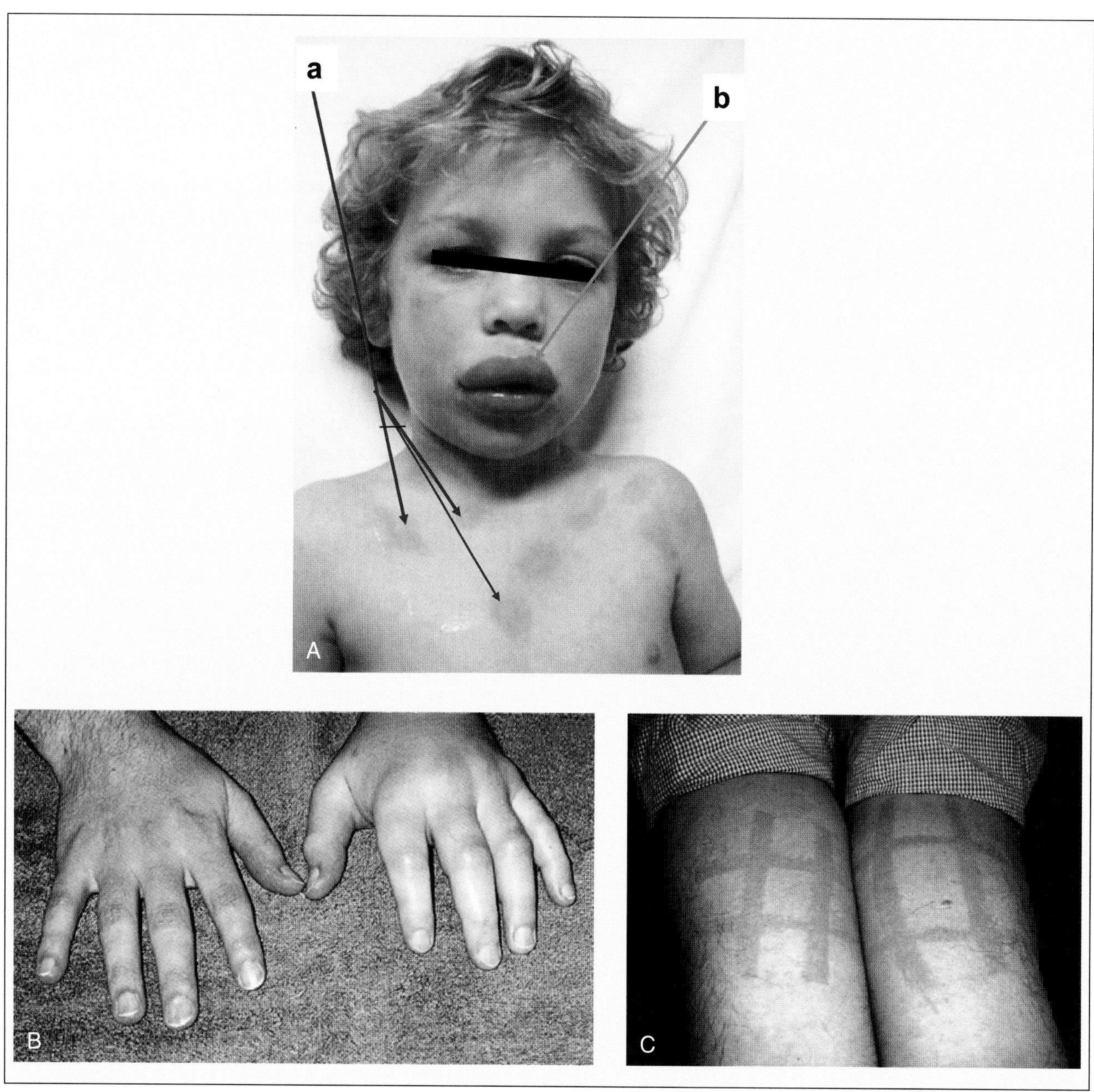

Figure 18-29. Photographs of patients with various forms of urticaria and angioedema. Panel A: Photograph of a child expressing clinical manifestations of urticaria (a) and lip angioedema (b). Panel B: Hand angioedema. The hand on the left in the picture is normal while the one on the right in the picture shows evidence of angioedema. Panel C: Dermatographism. This patient's erythematous skin lesions are caused by stroking or "writing" (i.e., dermatographism) on the skin surface and can be associated with symptoms of chronic urticaria. (Reproduced with permission from Deacock SJ. An approach to the patient with urticaria. Clin Exp Immunol. 2008;153:151–61.)

urticaria is also referred to as allergic urticaria since it is most commonly caused by the release of vasoactive substances from skin mast cells by an IgE-mediated mechanism following oral ingestion of or skin contact with an allergen, e.g., food, pet dander, or insect venom. Other pathogenetic mechanisms for development of urticarial lesions are by way of immune complex-mediated (Type III) mechanisms, e.g., serum sickness drug reaction, or by Type IV contact sensitivity. Clinical entities that should be considered in the differential diagnosis of recurrent urticaria lasting six weeks or greater include **chronic urticaria**, **urticaria pigmentosa**, and **hereditary angioedema**.

Chronic Urticaria

Chronic urticaria can be divided into (1) physical urticaria, (2) urticarial vasculitis, (3) autoimmune chronic urticaria, and (4) chronic idiopathic urticaria (Table 18-12).

Some physical agents (e.g., cold, water [aquagenic], exercise, [delayed skin] pressure, sunlight [solar], and vibration) can induce the direct release of mediators and be associated with chronic urticaria (Table 18-12). **Dermatographism**, or "skin writing," is a physical urticaria triggered in affected individuals by scratching or mild trauma to the skin (Figure 18-29C). **Cholinergic urticaria** represents a group of urticarial responses secondary to sweating, emotion, or exercise. In other cases, moreover, histamine-releasing drugs, e.g., codeine, can exacerbate some forms of physical urticaria or be a direct cause of chronic urticaria complaints.

Urticarial vasculitis is an eruption of inflammatory erythematous wheals that clinically resemble urticaria but histologically show changes of leukocytoclastic vasculitis. It can be divided into normocomplementemic and hypocomplementemic variants. Both subsets can be associated with systemic symptoms, e.g., angioedema, arthralgias, abdominal or chest pain, fever, pulmonary disease, renal disease, episcleritis, uveitis, and Raynaud's phenomenon, i.e., a vasospastic disorder causing vasoconstriction and discoloration of the fingers, toes, and occasionally other areas when subjected to cold. The hypocomplementemic form more often is associated with systemic symptoms and has been linked to connective-tissue diseases, i.e., systemic lupus erythematosus (**SLE**) (*Chapter 4*).

The remainder of the chronic urticarial conditions can be divided into **autoimmune chronic urticaria** and chronic idiopathic urticaria (**CIU**) (Table 18-12). It has been demonstrated that patients with chronic autoimmune urticaria display IgG autoantibodies directed against (1) the alpha chain of the FcεR1 receptor, i.e., anti-FcεR1 antibody, seen in 35 to 40 percent of chronic urticaria cases; and/or (2) the IgE molecule, i.e., anti-IgE antibody, seen in 5 to 10 percent of cases (Figure 18-30). Cross-linking of two or more FcεRI either directly by IgG anti-FcεR1 antibody or indirectly by IgG anti-IgE antibodies directed to IgE bound to FcεRI is proposed as the mechanism for mast cell activation and the release of mediators. There is also evidence that these autoantibody interactions also activate complement, and the interaction of by-products such as C5a with specific receptors on dermal mast cells also results in mediator secretion and symptoms. Since C5a receptors are predominantly found on dermal mast cells and not pulmonary mast cells, this complement-activation phenomenon may explain why symptoms remain localized to the skin and not other allergic mucosal sites, i.e., the lungs.

In patients with chronic autoimmune urticaria, there is higher frequency of HLADR alleles associated with autoimmunity, i.e., HLA DRBI*04, than any of the other chronic urticaria patient groups (*Chapter 10*). Also in many patients there is evidence of autoimmune thyroid (Hashimoto's) disease with presence of circulating IgG anti-thyroid

Table 18-12. Types of chronic urticaria

Type	Pathogenetic mechanism	Example of trigger(s)
Physical urticaria	Direct release of mediators, cholinergic stimuli	Cold, water, exercise, pressure, sunlight, vibration
Urticarial vasculitis	Complement-mediated Non-complement-mediated	Autoimmune diseases
Chronic autoimmune urticaria	Autoantibody-mediated release of inflammatory mediators	IgG anti-IgE IgG anti-FcεR1 (IgG anti-thyroid microsomal, IgG anti-thyroglobulin)
Chronic idiopathic urticaria	?	?

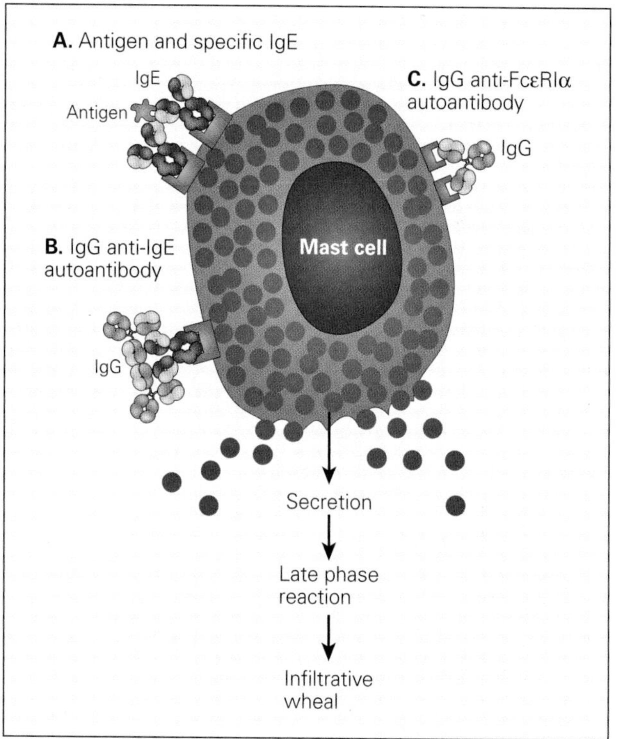

Figure 18-30. Schematic representation of the mechanisms of mast cell activation in chronic autoimmune urticaria. Panel A represents typical antigen cross-linking IgE, while in autoimmune chronic urticaria, Panel B represents IgG anti-IgE antibody, which binds to IgE attached to the FcεR1 receptor; Panel C represents IgG anti-FcεRI directed to the α subunit of FcεRI. In both B and C, cross-linking of two or more FcεRI by these autoantibodies leads to mast cell activation and release of mediators. There is also evidence that complement activation and interaction of C5a with specific receptors on dermal mast cells are responsible for mediator secretion and symptoms. (Adapted with permission from Kaplan AP, Greaves M. Pathogenesis of chronic urticaria. Clin Exp Allergy 2009;39:777–87.)

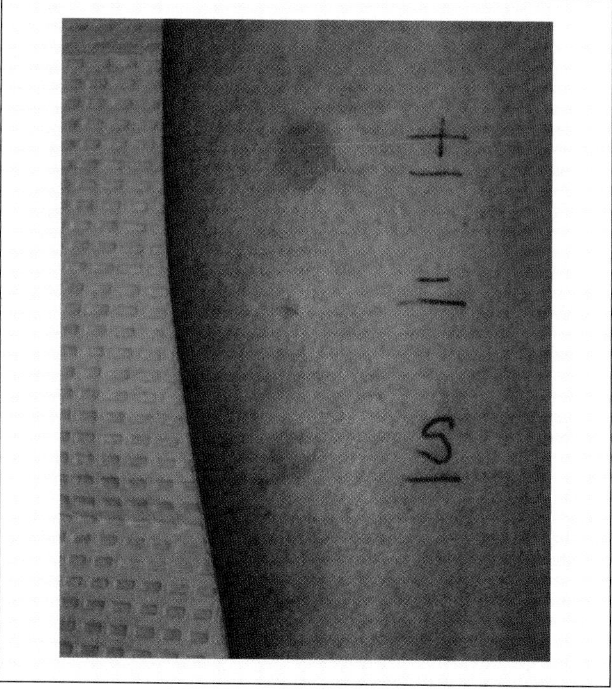

Figure 18-31. Autologous skin test depicting a positive control wheal at the top, a negative saline control at the center, and a positive reaction in a patient with chronic urticaria following the intradermal injection of autologous serum. (Reproduced with permission from Kaplan AP, Greaves M. Pathogenesis of chronic urticaria. Clin Exp Allergy 2009;39:777–87.)

microsomal and/or IgG anti-thyroglobulin antibodies. Although these antibodies are also surmised to have histamine-release properties from mast cells, empiric treatment of the thyroid disorder has not been conclusively shown to improve symptoms of urticaria in these patients.

The diagnosis of chronic autoimmune urticaria usually requires assays performed in specialized research laboratories. However, a practical test that has been employed clinically to approximate the presence of these autoantibodies in patients with chronic urticaria includes the autologous skin test. This test measures for immediate wheal-and-flare reaction upon an intradermal injection of autologous serum (Figure 18-31) and identifies about 30 to 35 percent of chronic urticaria patients with a circulatory histamine-releasing factor (usually but not always associated with antibody).

Despite recurrent symptoms of chronic urticaria that resemble those of autoimmune urticaria, in more than half of these patients, the pathogenesis and triggers are not due to a detectable autoantibody and are unknown, i.e., CIU. Some of these patients may still represent a group of patients with autoimmune chronic urticaria that display no identifiable serum factor(s) associated with histamine release from tissue mast cells. Certain subpopulations of patients with CIU also demonstrate abnormal basophil responsiveness, which could further potentiate disease.

Urticaria Pigmentosa

Urticaria pigmentosa is a rare disease caused by a point mutation at amino acid 816 of the proto-oncogene c-kit and is characterized by excessive numbers of mast cells in the skin that produce hives or lesions on the skin when irritated (Figure 18-32A). The condition is the most common form of cutaneous mastocytosis and is characterized by discrete pink papules that are infiltrated by mast cells. When the lesions are stroked, the presence of these cells causes visible wheal-and-flare formation (Darier's sign) (Figure 18-32B).

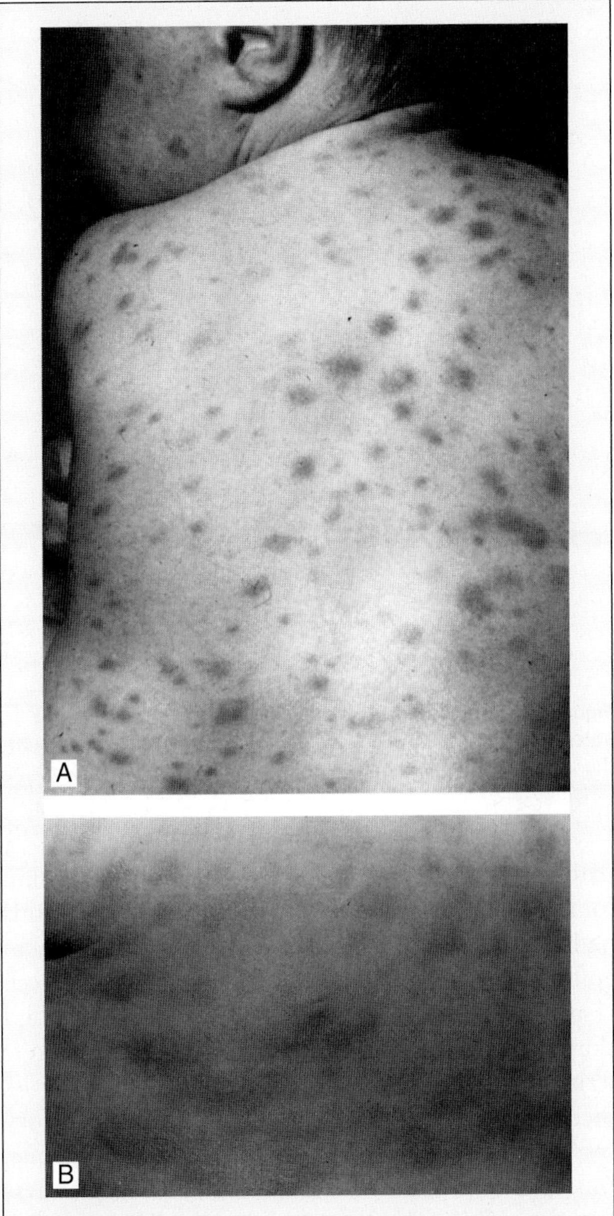

Figure 18-32. Photograph of a patient with urticaria pigmentosa. Panel A: The wide distribution of the lesions. Panel B: The development of visible wheal-and-flare formation after stroking the affected areas (Darier's sign). (Courtesy of Dr. James P. Rotchford.)

Hereditary Angioedema

Hereditary angioedema (**HAE**) is a familial disease transmitted as an autosomal dominant trait (*Chapter 4*). All patients with this disorder present with a sudden onset of large collections of fluid in the subcutaneous tissues (angioedema), which at times can be life-threatening. Three forms of HAE have currently been described. The classic forms are due to mutations in the C1-inhibitor gene (SERPING1), either resulting in deficient levels of antigenic and functional C1-inhibitor (Type I HAE) or intact but dysfunctional mutant protein (Type II HAE). In contrast, Type III HAE (also called estrogen-dependent HAE) is characterized by normal C1-inhibitor activity and has been observed exclusively in women due to an estrogen-dependent overexpression of Factor XII, seen during pregnancy or with the use of oral contraceptives. The diagnosis of HAE is made by demonstration of decreased levels or altered functional activity of C1 esterase or a decrease in C4 with normal C3. Treatment of this disorder has traditionally rested on the use of epsilon-aminocaproic acid and danazol. More recent products have shown quite promising results that include plasma-derived C1-inhibitor concentrate, recombinant C1-inhibitor, ecallantide (DX88, a plasma kallikrein inhibitor), and icatibant (a bradykinin B[2] receptor antagonist). Although each has demonstrated significant efficacy in the treatment of acute attacks, the C1-inhibitor concentrate has also provided a significant benefit in long-term prophylaxis.

Atopic Eczema

Atopic eczema (**AE**) also called atopic dermatitis (AD) is an inflammatory disease of the skin that typically appears in early childhood. The precise etiology of the disorder remains incompletely understood, but is thought to involve a complex interplay of both genetically and environmentally determined factors. The skin manifestations of atopic eczema may be generalized and are characterized by a spectrum of lesions found in different stages of activity. This spectrum may include erythematous, papular vesicular lesions that weep and ooze, particularly in the small infant. In this younger age group, the lesions are usually distributed on the cheeks, forehead, wrists, and the extensor surfaces of the forearms and lower extremities (Figure 18-33). After the age of two years, the skin tends to be thickened, scaly, and lichenified (thickened), and the distribution becomes confined predominantly to the flexural surfaces of the antecubital and popliteal fossae (Figure 18-34).

The condition is strongly associated with atopic diseases such as asthma and allergic rhinitis and generates elevated levels of serum IgE to various antigens. However, it has become clear that many of the clinical features of the disease do not completely fit the picture of a true IgE-mediated or Type I hypersensitivity disorder. For example, high expression of IFN-γ and other Th1 cytokines is found in lesions of atopic eczema, and the typical skin reactions are more insidious and chronic, suggesting the

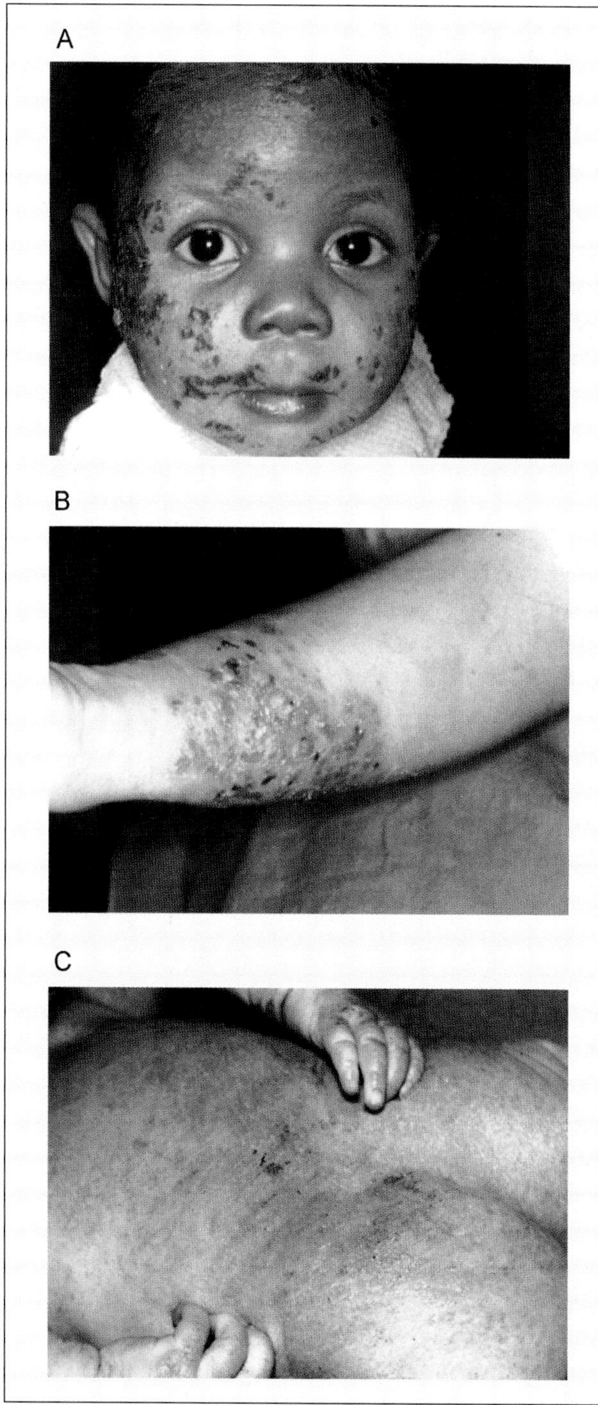

Figure 18-33. Photograph of lesions of atopic eczema in an infant. Panel A: Distribution of the skin eruption on the face. Panel B: On the skin surfaces of the lower forearm. Panel C: On the back. (Courtesy of Dr. James P. Rotchford.)

presence of additional mechanisms of immunologic tissue injury.

Immunopathogenesis of Atopic Eczema

Shown in Figure 18-35 is a schematic representation of the major immunologic events involved in the pathogenesis of atopic eczema from uninvolved skin to the acute and chronic stages of disease. In this pathogenesis, a defective skin barrier and altered skin epithelial cells, i.e., keratinocytes, and dendritic cell responses play key roles. Clinically, the unaffected skin of patients with atopic eczema is abnormal, differing from the skin of normal individuals by its increased dryness and a greater inflammatory responsiveness to irritants. In many affected patients, this dryness is due to a fundamental skin barrier dysfunction (Figure 18-36), which results in loss of fluids and skin moisture. This dysfunction also leads to an increased permeability, permitting a greater penetration of allergens and microbes, e.g., *Staphylococcus aureus*, into the skin. In uninvolved skin, there is a predominance of dendritic-like Langerhans cells (**LC**), which capture IgE molecules through surface FcεRI. Rather than form an innate immune defense to these substances, these LC bind allergen through IgE on their surfaces and migrate to lymph nodes, where they present these allergens to stimulate specific Th2 cell clonal responses. These Th2 cells eventually home to skin and maintain IgE-bound, primed mast cells and LC. Interaction of environmental allergens with IgE-bound mast cells and Th2 cells leads to an early acute stage of skin

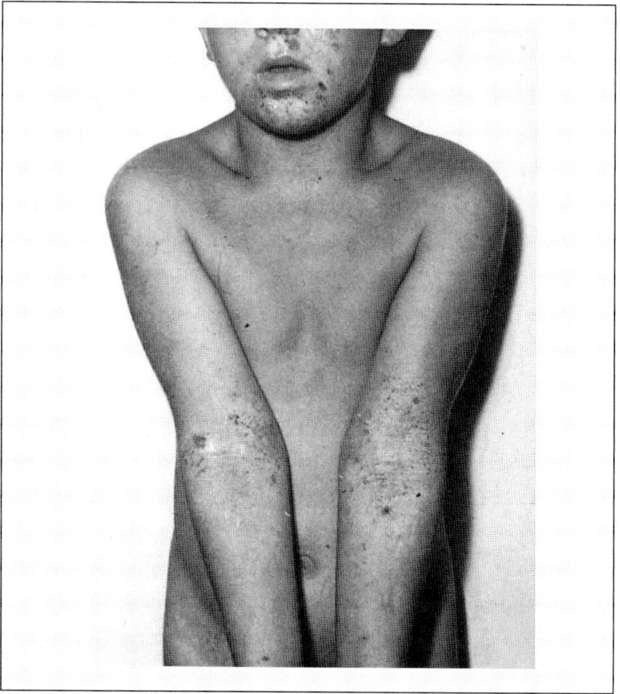

Figure 18-34. Photograph of the lesions of atopic eczema in an older child showing the distribution of the skin eruption on the face and antecubital areas. (Courtesy of Dr. James P. Rotchford.)

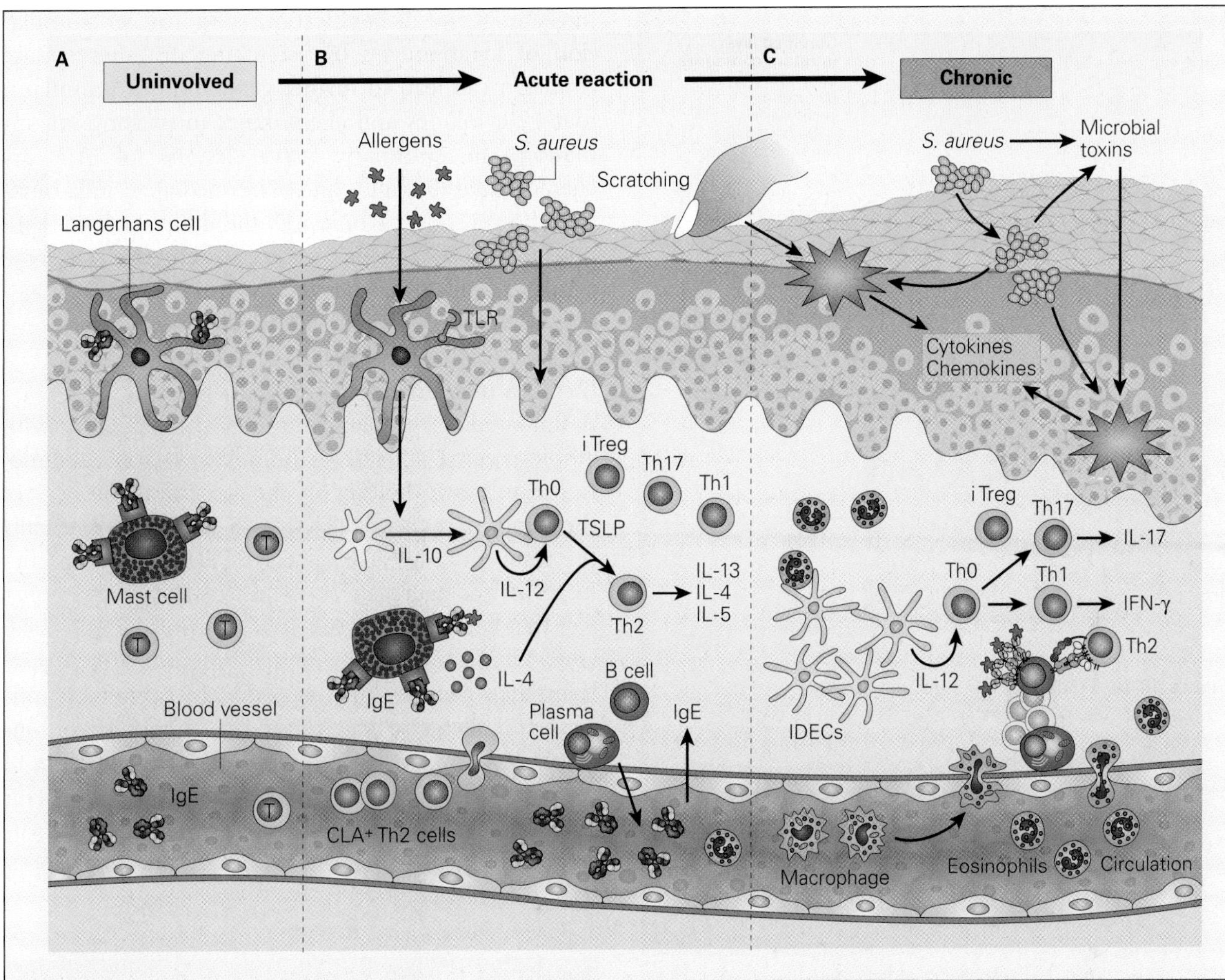

Figure 18-35. Schematic representation of the immunopathogenetic events seen in acute and chronic stages of atopic eczema. Panel A: An underlying Th2 allergic phenotype in atopic eczema leads to elevated serum IgE levels and a predominance of IgE-bound Langerhans cells and primed mast cells in uninvolved skin. Panel B: A defect in barrier function as well as ineffective innate immune system function leads to skin penetration by allergens and microorganisms such as *Staphylococcus aureus*. This penetration is facilitated by environmental allergens, scratching, or microbial toxins that activate keratinocytes to release proinflammatory cytokines and chemokines that induce the expression of adhesion molecules on vascular endothelium and facilitate the extravasation of inflammatory cells into the skin. Keratinocyte-derived thymic stromal lymphopoietin (TSLP) and LC-derived IL-10 also enhance Th2 cell differentiation. Interaction of environmental allergens with IgE-bound LCs leads to uptake, migration, and presentation of allergens to Th2 cells in lymph nodes and eventual homing of CLA+ Th2 cells to the injury site. Interaction of allergen with primed mast cells leads to an early acute stage of skin inflammation characterized by Type I hypersensitivity injury and local stimulation of Th2 cytokines. Panel C: In the chronic stage of skin inflammation, persistence of allergen and microorganisms and/or skin trauma leads to generation of proinflammatory cytokines, e.g., TNF-α, IL-1, and chemokines, e.g., IL-8, from resident keratinocytes into the surrounding tissue. Th2 tissue responses lead to infiltration of activated eosinophils as well as recruitment of FcεRI-expressing, inflammatory dendritic epidermal cells (IDEC), which elaborate high levels of IL-12. This IDEC L-12 production is a key player in the development and recruitment of Th1 cells and the production of a cytokine milieu rich in IFN-γ that favor the recruitment of macrophages and other proinflammatory cells, e.g., Th17 cells. This chronic phase is characterized by skin thickening and lichenification/fibrosis, and the inflammatory contribution of microbial toxins as well as skin trauma by scratching or other physical stimuli that can lead to further generation of proinflammatory cytokines and chemokines by keratinocytes. (Adapted from Leung DYM, Boguniewicz M, Howell M, et al. New insights into atopic dermatitis. J Clin Invest. 2004; 713: 651–7).

inflammation characterized by erythema and pruritus as a result of Type I hypersensitivity injury and a milieu rich in Th2 cytokines. Intertwined with this Th2 inflammation are other innate immune system defects in keratinocyte and dendritic cell (**DC**) function, leading to proinflammatory effects and a susceptibility for skin penetration and infections by bacteria and viruses as well. Due in part to inefficiency in clearing allergens and microbial agents as well as recurring trauma to the skin from scratching or other irritant sources, inflammation persists, leading to recruitment of various inflammatory cells. A

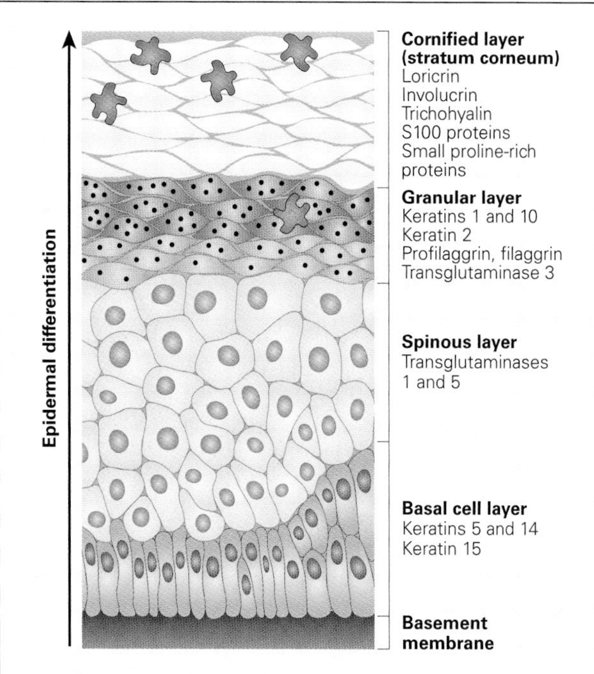

Figure 18-36. Epidermal differentiation and barrier function. The epidermis is the outermost layer of the skin separated from the underlying dermis by the basement membrane and is composed of keratinocytes found at different stages of differentiation within the spinous layer, granular layer, and cornified layer or stratum corneum. Each epidermal layer is characterized by the expression of specific proteins and examples of these are listed in the figure. Profilaggrin and filaggrin molecules are found in the granular layer and perform important regulatory functions in epidermal homeosatsis. Filaggrin monomers are formed by the proteolytic processing of profilaggrin at the transition between the stratum granulosum and the stratum corneum and function by aggregating keratin filaments as well as by undergoing further processing in the upper stratum corneum to release free amino acids that assist in the retention of water. The smaller black dots in the cells of granular layer represent keratohyalin granules composed of filaggrin molecules. (Adapted with permission from McGrath JA, Uitto J. The filaggrin story: novel insights into skin-barrier function and disease. Trends Mol Med. 2008; 14:20–7.)

later chronic phase of disease is orchestrated by local expression of cytotoxins and proinflammatory cytokines, e.g., TNF-α, IL-1, and chemokines, e.g., IL-8, from keratinocytes, recruitment of eosinophils by Th2 cytokines, and also by production of IL-12 and IL-18 from proinflammatory FcεRI-expressing DCs, also called inflammatory dendritic epidermal cells (**IDEC**). This FcεRI-mediated IL-12 expression by IDECs leads to the generation and recruitment of Th1 cells to the skin. Release of Th1 cytokines, e.g., IFN-γ, in turn leads to more proinflammatory effects as well as to the recruitment of macrophages and other cytotoxic cells to the area. There is also evidence that Th17 cells are recruited to the inflamed tissue site. This chronic phase is characterized by skin thickening and lichenification, and further stimulation of keratinocytes by scratching or other surface irritation can lead to further generation of proinflammatory cytokines and chemokines to prolong inflammation. In summary, acute lesions of AD are characterized by IgE- and Th2-mediated inflammation; however, in chronic AD, the infiltration of IL-12 producing IDECs helps lead a switch to a Th1-type cytokine milieu associated with increased IFN-γ expression and related proinflammatory effects.

Defects in Skin Barrier Function

A fundamental problem found in most patients with atopic eczema appears to be a skin barrier dysfunction due to weaknesses in the structural integrity of the stratum corneum (Figure 18-36). This is usually the result of a defect in filaggrin (FLG), which participates in the aggregation of the corneocyte cytoskeleton that produces the cell collapse into corneal scales (Box 18-5). The deficiency in formation of a corneal layer may generate an increased absorption of antigens and allergens that trigger the initial allergic sensitization as well as the extraordinary susceptibility to secondary infections such as *Staphylocoo aureus.* This enhanced skin absorption is also believed to be responsible for IgE sensitization to food and respiratory allergens involved in the atopic march.

Box 18-5

Barrier Dysfunction Associated with Mutations of Profilaggrin and Filaggrin in Patients with Atopic Eczema

Recently, loss-of-function mutations in FLG, the human gene encoding profilaggrin and filaggrin, have been identified as the cause of the common skin condition ichthyosis vulgaris (which is characterized by dry, scaly skin). These mutations, which are carried by up to 10 percent of people, also represent a strong genetic predisposing factor for atopic eczema, asthma, and allergies. Profilaggrin is a major precursor component found within the keratohyalin granules in epidermal granular cells. Loss of profilaggrin or filaggrin leads to a poorly formed stratum corneum (ichthyosis), which is also prone to water loss (xerosis). Recent human genetic studies strongly suggest that perturbation of skin barrier function as a result of the reduction or complete loss of filaggrin expression leads to enhanced percutaneous transfer of allergens. Filaggrin is therefore on the frontline of defense and protects the body from the entry of foreign environmental substances that can otherwise trigger aberrant immune responses.

Defects in Innate Immune and Adaptive Function

Atopic eczema also displays a defect of the innate immune system response to allergens and microbial pathogens due to the impairment of certain antigen presentation and signaling pathways. For example, mutations affecting innate immune PRRs TLR2, NOD1, NOD2, and CD14 on the surface of the skin have been found in patients with atopic eczema (*Chapter 9*); these mutations contribute to the increased susceptibility to infections caused by viruses and bacterial pathogens seen with this disorder. *Staphylococcus aureus* skin infections, for example, occur in over 95 percent of patients. Early susceptibility to these infections is due in part to the predominance of Th2 cell cytokine responses in the skin that lack production of IFN-γ and other cytokines necessary to clear these organisms. Also, there is evidence of defects in production of defensins and other antimicrobial proteins by keratinocytes. This defect results in the loss of effective mechanisms for clearing viral infections as well and may explain the increased frequency of orthopoxvirus (eczema vaccinatum) and herpes (eczema herpeticum) infections in patients with atopic eczema. These pathogens can stimulate the recruitment of other immune effector cells to the skin site that perpetuate the pathogenesis of eczema.

Defects in Adaptive Immune Function and Target Organ Effects

Deficiencies of the epidermal anatomic structures and the innate immune system lead to a dysregulation of adaptive immune system pathways that favor the expression of an exaggerated Th2 response phenotype in atopic eczema patients. Peripheral blood studies in the acute phase of patients with atopic eczema have demonstrated the presence of DCs with low capacity to produce cytokines like IL-12 from deterring the activation of the Th1 lineage and redirecting an initial Th2 response. This response, in turn, results in a vicious cycle of immunologic hyperreactivity to certain allergens. The unremitting inflammation caused by these defects, moreover, favors a chronic irritation of terminal neuronal skin sensors that produces an intense pruritus. Skin scratching as a result of this pruritus leads to further epithelial damage and penetration by allergens and microbes, leading to a vicious and repetitive cycle of inflammation. Shown in Figure 18-37 is a schematic representation of the cycle of pathogenetic events that give rise to and maintain the chronicity of atopic eczema. It has been speculated that Th17 cells participate in the chronic response, augmenting the inflammation through enhanced IL-17 and its capacity to recruit neutrophils. Recent studies have recognized the possible role of IL-31 as the generator of pruritus and chronic inflammation, and the importance of A proliferation-inducing ligand (**APRIL**) as an indicator of disease severity (*Chapter 9*).

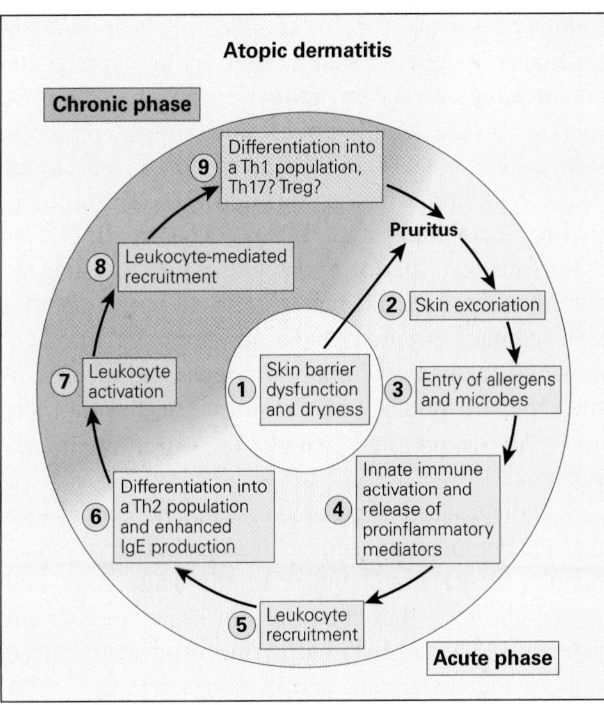

Figure 18-37. Schematic representation of the cycle of pathogenetic events that give rise to the acute and chronic stages of AD and maintain the chronicity of the disorder. AD may be seen as a vicious circle of pathogenetic events in which skin barrier dysfunction is at the center of the cycle (1). Pruritus leads to skin excoriation (2) and entry of allergens and microbes (3), adding to an already existing skin barrier defect. Innate immune mutations of PRRs lead to the release of proinflammatory mediators (4) and recruitment of other immune effector cells of the adaptive immune system (5) with differentiation into a predominant Th2 cell population and enhanced IgE production (6). With more leukocyte activation (7) and leukocyte-mediated recruitment (8), there is further differentiation into a Th1 population, possibly with activation of Th17 cells and modulation by Treg cells (9).

Contact Dermatitis

Although it shares many similar pathologic features with atopic eczema, the immunologic mechanism responsible for contact dermatitis is a Type IV mechanism of delayed hypersensitivity mediated by T lymphocytes. Contact dermatitis is allergic in 20 percent of cases and an irritant in the other 80 percent. In allergic contact dermatitis (**ACD**), etiologic agents include plants (poison ivy), cosmetics, industrial products, detergents, topical medications, clothing, food, and metals, e.g., nickel. The allergens are low molecular weight substances that act as haptens and are preferentially taken upon by skin LC. These LC migrate to the lymph nodes, and antigen presentation generates CD4 and CD8 effector T cell clones. These cells home to the skin and release proinflammatory cytokines, e.g., IFN-γ, TNF-α, IL-2, and cytotoxins, e.g., perforin and granzyme, to cause tissue inflammation and injury 24 to 48 hours after the skin contact occurred. The development of ACD depends on many factors but is mostly influenced by the type and potency of the substance, the skin site, and the degree and length of exposure to the substance.

Pathologically, both atopic eczema and contact dermatitis demonstrate similar features of erythema—papules, vesicles, and bullae in the acute stage and, when chronic, they become thickened, scaly, and lichenified. This is followed by an inflammatory reaction in the underlying dermis and subsequent parakeratosis, scaling, and acanthosis (Figure 18-38). An important differentiating point between the two skin disorders is the distribution of the lesions found in each skin condition; the multiple-area involvement of atopic dermatitis stands in marked contrast to the localization of lesions generally found in contact dermatitis. The anatomic restriction and localization are the key differentiating points between the two entities (Figure 18-39).

Allergic Diseases of the Respiratory Tract

Allergic diseases of the respiratory tract result from exposure of a genetically susceptible host to a variety of noxious agents, the majority of which enter the host by inhalation, e.g., pollens, dust, and pet dander, but others may also access the body by ingestants, e.g., foods and drugs, or injection, e.g., drugs and vaccines (Figure 18-40). These disorders, which include allergic rhinitis and asthma, not only represent the most prevalent allergic diseases, but also represent some of the most commonly encountered chronic illnesses seen in clinical practice. Since the epithelial lining and mucosal barrier components of the nasorespiratory tract (conjunctiva, nasopharynx, and upper and lower respiratory tracts) are contiguous and functionally related, i.e., "the united airways," each and all components may be adversely affected in this allergic attack. Although several of the previously described mechanisms of immunologic injury may be involved, most allergic diseases of the respiratory tract are mediated by Type I hypersensitivity reactions and include conjunctivitis, rhinitis, and asthma. Clinical disorders of the respiratory tract may also involve other mechanisms of immunologic injury. Shown in Table 18-13 are examples of disorders of the respiratory tract mediated by immunologic responses to foreign antigens.

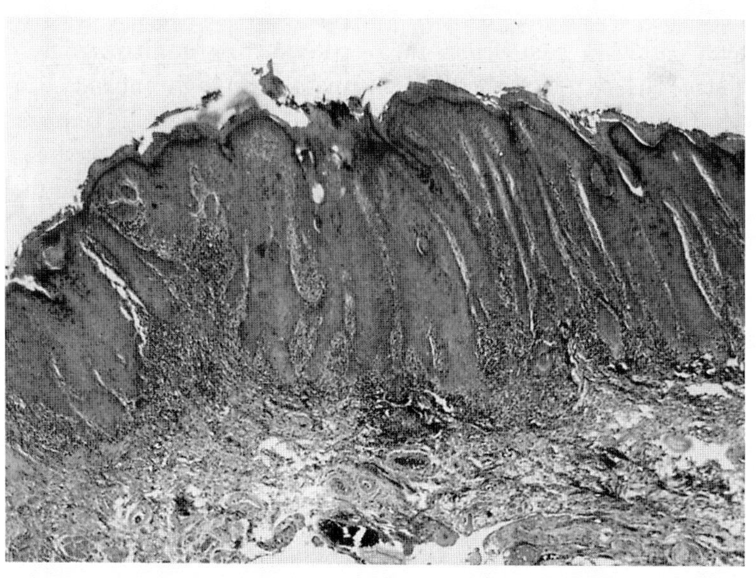

Figure 18-38. Photomicrograph of the skin lesion of atopic dermatitis showing the characteristic inflammatory reaction in the dermis with parakeratosis and acanthosis. H & E stain, x120. (Courtesy of Dr. George H. Green.)

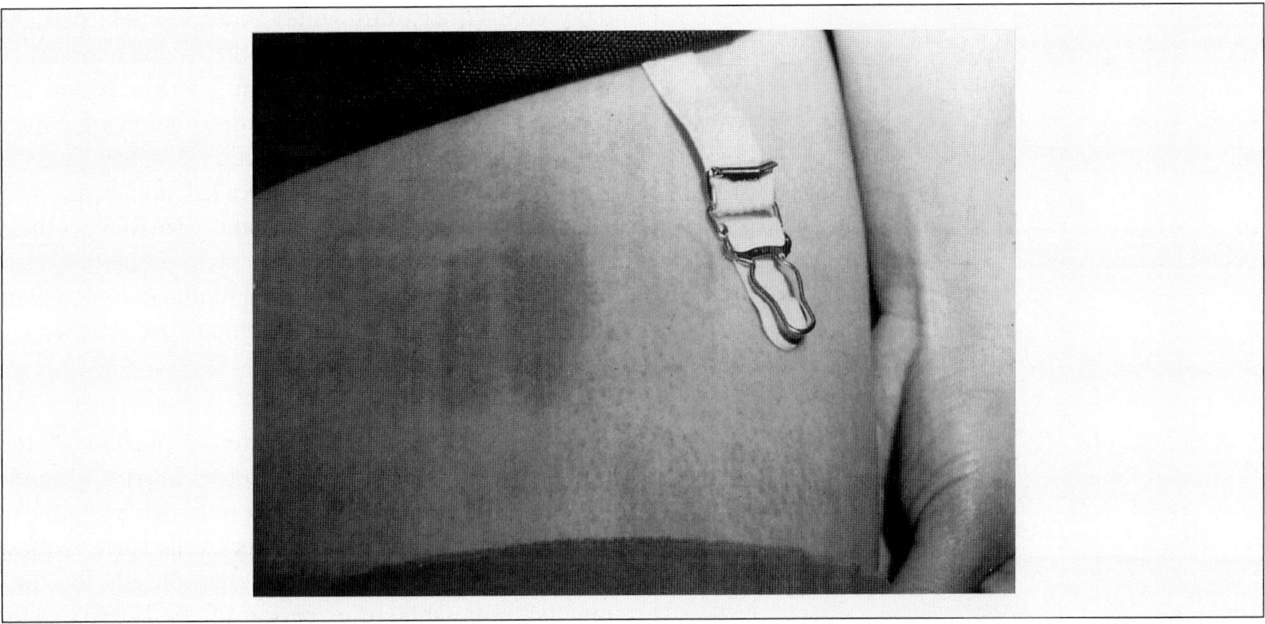

Figure 18-39. Photograph of the thigh of a patient with contact dermatitis due to nickel sensitivity (garter). Note the localization of the lesion to the area in contact with the metallic surface. (Courtesy of Dr. James P. Rotchford.)

Goodpasture's disease is a rare condition characterized by glomerulonephritis and hemorrhage of the lungs triggered by a Type II reaction in which antibody directed against a commonly shared antigen found in the lungs and kidney, i.e., Goodpasture antigen, is involved (Table 18-13). **Allergic bronchopulmonary aspergillosis** (**ABPA**) is a respiratory tract disorder that occurs more commonly in atopic individuals with asthma. In these individuals, the net effect of exposure to various species of *Aspergillus*, e.g., *A. niger*, or *A. fumigatus*, is the production of both IgE nonprecipitating and IgG precipitating antibodies that then contribute to the respective Type I and Type III immunologic reactions and tissue injury characteristic of the clinical entity. ABPA is associated with eosinophilia, and the most characteristic clinical manifestation is obstructive lung disease triggered by IgE-mediated mechanisms. **Hypersensitivity pneumonitis** (also called extrinsic allergic alveolitis, EAA) is an inflammation of the alveoli within the lung caused by hypersensitivity reactions to inhaled organic dusts, e.g., thermophylic actinomycetes, molds, and proteinaceous materials). Sufferers are placed under conditions of intensive exposure to the dust by their occupation or hobbies. The net effect of such exposure is generation of IgG precipitating serum antibodies to these antigens. These antibodies form complexes with the antigen and generate complement in the interstitial tissues of the lung, mediating Type III lung injury. Antigen-specific T cells are also formed in this process, and these cells contribute to delayed hypersensitivity (Type IV) lung injury mechanisms as well. Involvement of the alveoli and bronchioles leads to a restrictive ventilatory defect rather than an obstructive defect seen in ABPA. Delayed hypersensitivity (Type IV) lung injury may also be a prominent feature of many infectious diseases of the respiratory tract, e.g., tuberculosis. Through elaboration of proinflammatory cytokines, e.g., TNF-α, this latter group of respiratory disorders may result in tissue destruction and granuloma formation, which are pathologic features that distinguish these disease entities from the classic allergic diseases of the lung (*Chapter 9*).

Rhinitis

Allergic rhinitis is characterized by immunologically mediated hypersensitivity reactions in the nasal passages with typical symptoms of itching, sneezing, and increased secretions, i.e., rhinorrhea, congestion, and nasal blockage. Most cases are IgE-antibody-mediated and can be differentiated by the type of provoking allergenic substance. For example, seasonal allergic rhinitis often describes allergic rhinitis symptoms triggered by tree or grass pollens, which in temperate climates usually appear only in the spring. Perennial allergic rhinitis refers to symptoms occurring throughout the year and is usually caused by allergens to which individuals have close

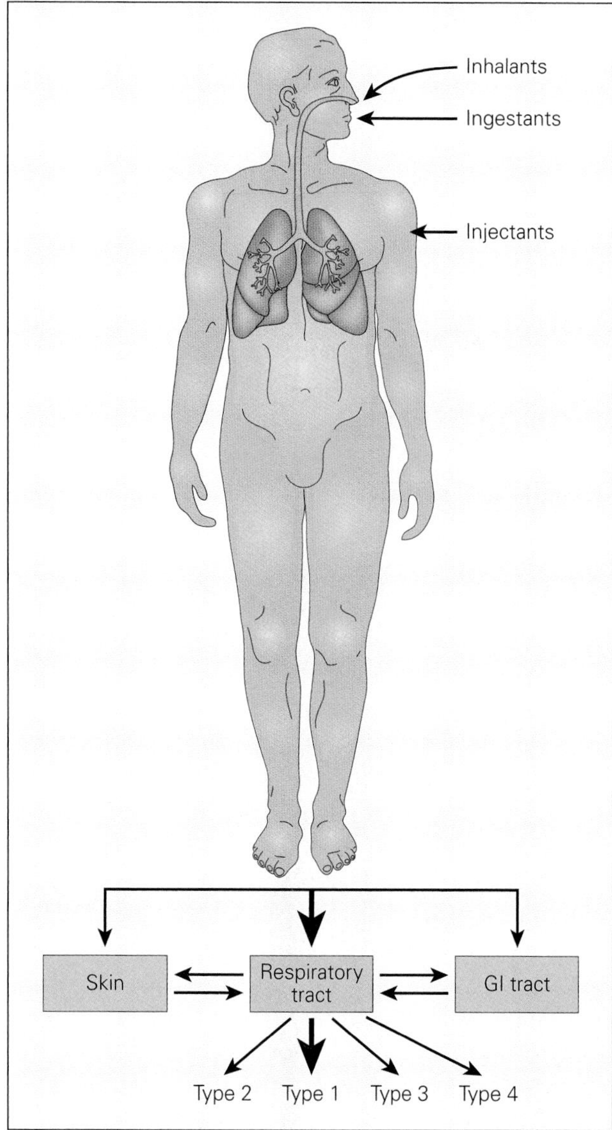

Figure 18-40. Schematic representation of allergic diseases of the respiratory tract.

daily contact, e.g., dust mites and household pets. As described in Table 18-14, a number of different conditions can present with symptoms of rhinitis and are grouped under the nonspecific designation of nonallergic rhinitis. With the exception of a few patients with nasal eosinophilia (the so-called nonallergic rhinitis with eosinophilia syndrome [**NARES**]), these conditions do not typically exhibit immune-mediated nasal inflammation. Nonallergic rhinitis may represent up to 50 percent of all chronic rhinitic complaints.

Conjunctivitis

The conjunctivae form the anterior portion of the eye and represent the eye's primary barrier to environmental antigens, as it is the only ocular epithelia to normally contain inflammatory cells such as mast cells and eosinophils. Although anatomically the conjunctiva represents an extension of the external skin, the major triggering allergens and pathologic pathways are the same as those involving the nasorespiratory tract, and conjunctivitis is often associated with exacerbations of allergic rhinitis. Typical symptoms include itchiness, redness, frequent tearing, and watery discharge from both eyes. In addition to allergic conjunctivitis, there are a number of other conditions that should be considered in the differential diagnosis of conjunctivitis (Table 18-15).

Asthma

Definitions

Asthma (from the Greek, difficulty breathing, panting) is a chronic inflammatory disorder of the airways originally characterized as acute, intermittent, reversible

Table 18-13. Disorders of the respiratory tract mediated by immunologic responses to foreign antigens

Type	Example of disease	Example of antigen	Mechanism
Type I	Allergic rhinitis Asthma	Pollen	IgE antibody
Type II	Goodpasture's syndrome	Goodpasture antigen, which is found in the lung and kidney, e.g., glomerular basement membrane (GBM) antigen	Anti-GBM
Type III	Extrinsic allergic alveolitis (Farmer's lung)	Dust of molding hay	Antigen-antibody complexes (together with Type IV)
Type IV	Tuberculosis	Tuberculoprotein	Sensitized T lymphocytes
Mixed types: I and III	Allergic bronchopulmonary aspergillosis (ABPA); allergic fungal sinusitis	Fungi/molds	IgE and precipitating IgG antibodies
III and IV	Hypersensitivity pneumonitis (i.e., extrinsic allergic alveolitis)	Thermophilic actinomycetes, fungi, animal proteins	Antigen-antibody-complement (Ag-Ab-C) complexes and cell-mediated immunity

Table 18-14. Differential diagnosis of rhinitis

Type	Condition	Triggers
Allergic	Seasonal, "hay fever" (fall weeds)	Pollens: tree, grass (*Florida), weed (*Mediterranean *parietaria*), outdoor molds^
	Perennial	Dust mite, cockroach, indoor molds, animal dander
Infectious		Viral Bacterial
Hormonal		Pregnancy Thyroid disease
Drug-induced	Rhinitis medicomentosa	Topical decongestants
		NSAIDS Cocaine Beta-blockers
Food-induced	Gustatory rhinitis	Spicy foods
Occupational	Allergic and nonallergic causes	Wood dust, grains, laboratory animals, chemicals (i.e., acid anhydrides, glues, and solvents), latex
Atrophic	Primary	Advanced age
	Secondary	Chronic sinusitis, trauma, irradiation
Eosinophilic	Nonallergic rhinitis with eosinophilia (NARES) Aspirin intolerance	
Anatomic/mechanical	Septal deviation Nasal polyposis Adenoidal hypertrophy Foreign body/tumor	
Idiopathic	Vasomotor rhinitis	Nonspecific irritants, e.g., changes in temperature, tobacco smoke, perfumes
Other diseases	Chronic sinusitis	
	Allergic fungal sinusitis	
	Sarcoidosis	
	Sjogren's syndrome	
	Wegener's granulomatosis	
	Gastroesophageal reflux	
	Immotile cilia syndrome	
	Olfactory dysfunction	Parkinson's disease Alzheimer's disease

*Depending on certain climates, some pollens may be present most of the year and thus trigger perennial symptoms,^some outdoor molds occur throughout the year.

obstructive airway disease. A more contemporary definition of asthma emphasizes and places inflammation as the central pathogenetic mechanism. Asthma has been classically divided into extrinsic asthma, in which an exogenous allergen could be identified, and intrinsic asthma, in which no identifiable causative agent could be demonstrated. This classification is no longer adequate, since intrinsic defects may be demonstrated in extrinsic asthma, and extrinsic factors, e.g., respiratory infections, have been suggested to exacerbate intrinsic asthma.

It is now generally accepted that there are both allergic and nonallergic forms of asthma. Asthma resulting from an immunologically mediated reaction should be called **allergic asthma**. Approximately 80 percent of childhood asthma and > 50 percent of adult asthma has been reported to be allergic in origin. Most cases of allergic asthma are initiated by IgE antibodies, i.e., **IgE–mediated allergic asthma**. However, a distinct subset of allergic asthma sufferers has no identifiable IgE-mediated trigger and therefore other non-IgE immunologic

Table 18-15. Differential diagnosis of conjunctivitis

Disorder	Causes	Clinical
Allergic conjunctivitis	Seasonal (grass, ragweed pollens); perennial (dust mite)	Bilateral > unilateral eye involvement; usually associated with rhinitis
Nonallergic conjunctivitis Giant papillary conjunctivitis	Infectious, mechanical (rubbing), contactants Common with contact lens wearers (preservatives or protein-adherent proteins?)	Unilateral > bilateral; may be associated with blepharitis and also rhinitis Large papillae, mostly in upper lid
Atopic keratoconjunctivitis	Associated with allergic eczema	Blepharitis of lower lid common; cataracts; keratoconus; viral infections (i.e., herpes); may cause blindness
Vernal conjunctivitis	Unknown, but seasonal and common in young males	Upper lid involvement-giant papillae; Horner's points; Tranta's dots; corneal ulcers; cataracts and glaucoma

mechanisms may be operative in initiating the inflammation associated with this form of allergic asthma. The mechanisms initiating **nonallergic asthma**, however, are not well defined.

Asthma Pathogenesis and Airway Remodeling

As previously described, inflammation is the central cause of airway hyperreactivity and variable airflow obstruction in asthma and is a universal finding in all asthmatic individuals. Many studies have emphasized the multifactorial nature of asthma, with interactions between neural mechanisms, inflammatory cells (mast cells, macrophages, eosinophils, neutrophils, and lymphocytes), mediators (interleukins, leukotrienes, prostaglandins, and platelet-activating factor), and intrinsic abnormalities of the arachidonic acid pathway and smooth muscle cells. While these types of descriptive studies have revealed a composite picture of asthma, they have failed to provide a basic unifying mechanism.

Shown in Figure 18-41 is a schematic representation of the interrelationships between the inflammatory, immunologic, and epithelial structural elements of the airways that are thought to play a major role in the pathogenesis of asthma. There are three major pathologic processes occurring singularly or simultaneously in the airways of asthmatic individuals. The first process is the acute inflammatory component involving early (histamine and other mediator release) and late phase (recruitment of inflammatory cells and additional cellular damage) responses from the release of mediators triggered by IgE mediated as well as non-IgE mediated processes, i.e., cytokine-mediated. The second process involves the interaction of the acute inflammatory component with the epithelia and smooth muscle receptors of the bronchial wall. This pathology leads to an increase in the existing bronchial hyperresponsiveness to a variety of stimuli. A third process, involving remodeling and excessive repair of damaged tissue, may instead lead to hyperplasia of lung cellular elements as well as stiffening of the bronchioles. These changes could continue to exacerbate pre-existing lung inflammation as well as contribute to decreased lung function and severity of disease.

The above processes also contribute to two stages of airway obstruction: (1) a functional obstruction due to bronchoconstriction of smooth muscle and (2) a structural obstruction with either a reversible phase due to edema or an irreversible phase due to chronic inflammation, i.e., remodeling (Figure 18-42). Thus, there appear to be two major pathways by which exogenous antigens can produce airway obstruction. One is brought on by factors that cause smooth muscle contraction, i.e., **triggers**, and the other by factors that promote inflammation, i.e., **inducers**, allergens, viruses, exercise, or nonspecific irritant inhalation. This dichotomy of responses is clinically important since it forms the basis for treatment with reliever medications, e.g., bronchodilators that address the obstructive lesion, and with controller drugs, e.g., inhaled corticosteroids that are used to reduce airway inflammation in the second stage. Moreover, the type and degree of airway inflammation may not only be variably associated with changes in airway hyperresponsiveness, airflow limitation, and respiratory symptoms, but may also be acutely and chronically associated with the development of airflow limitation as the result of bronchoconstriction, airway edema, and mucus secretion.

Susceptibility Genes for Asthma

Asthma is a disorder with many etiologies rather than a disease of a single cause. As with all allergic diseases,

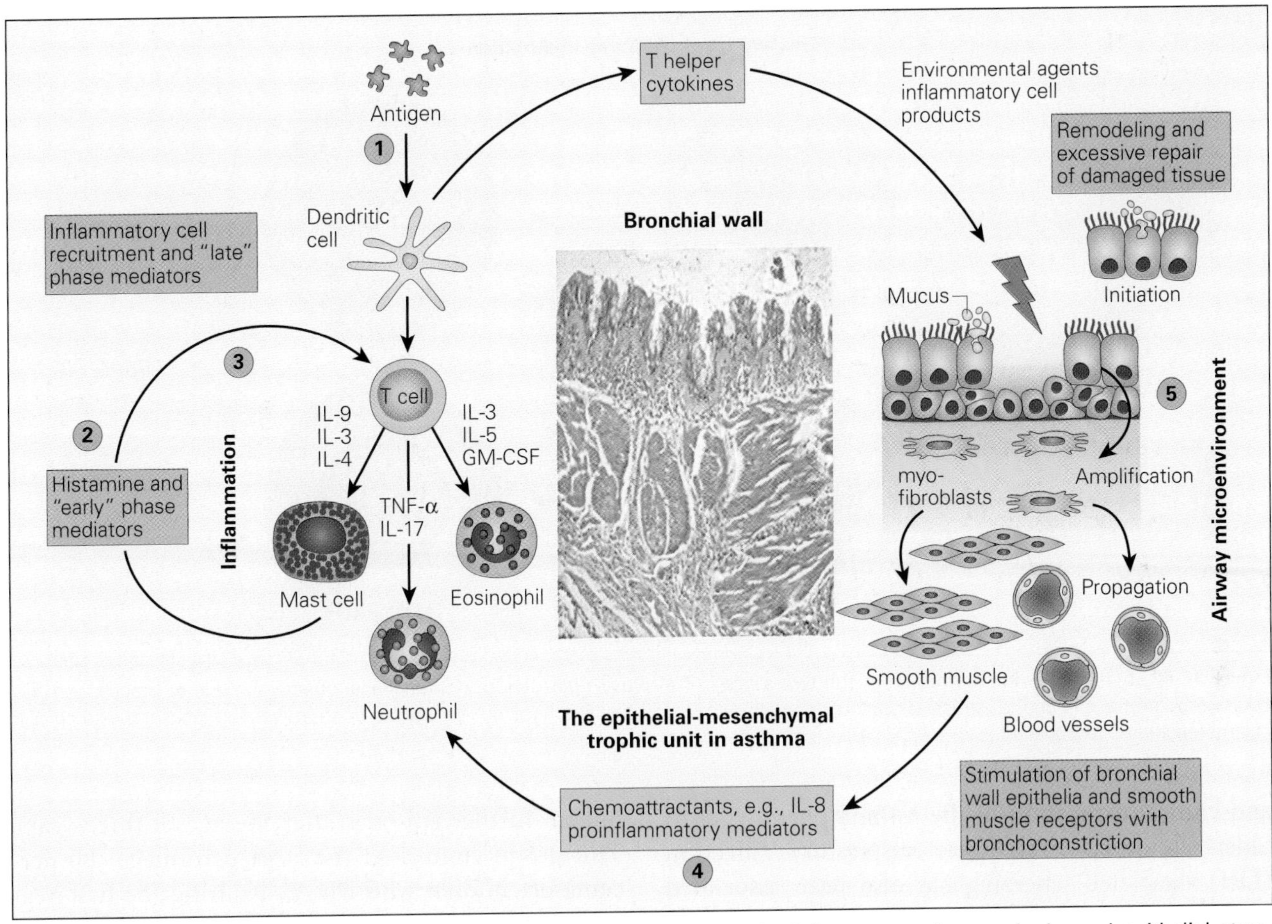

Figure 18-41. Schematic representation of the interrelationships between the inflammatory, immunologic, and epithelial structural elements of the airways that are thought to play a major role in the pathogenesis of asthma. (1) Allergen is introduced to the airways. Allergen presentation in the context of Th2 cytokines favors development of mast cells primed with allergen-specific IgE. (2) Mast cell activation and mediator release, e.g., histamine, leads to early phase response and immediate inflammatory effects. (3) Release of cytokines and other factors in the late phase response leads to inflammatory cell recruitment and further generation of Th2 cytokines involved in maintaining allergic inflammation. (4) Chemoattractants, e.g., IL-8, recruit mast cells as well as neutrophils and eosinophils to the lung, and these cells cause further injury and release of proinflammatory mediators with effects on end target tissues, e.g., smooth muscle. Stimulation of bronchial wall epithelia and smooth muscle receptors results in bronchoconstriction and bronchial hyperresponsiveness to a variety of stimuli. (5) Remodeling and other mechanisms to repair damaged tissue may become excessive and lead to chronic obstructive and inflammatory changes in the lung. These changes are exemplified by the middle photograph, which represents a histologic section through an asthmatic airway. The plate shows that, in addition to the presence of large numbers of inflammatory cells, there are characteristic structural changes, including epithelial goblet cell hyperplasia and metaplasia, thickening of the lamina reticularis, and increased amounts of smooth muscle. (Adapted from Holgate ST. A look at the pathogenesis of asthma: the need for a change in direction. Discov Med. 2010;9:439–47.)

asthma represents the interplay of **environmental**, **genetic**, and **developmental** factors (Figure 18-14). To date, the available genetic linkage studies emphasize significant genetic effects from loci on chromosomes 5, 6, 11, 12, 13, 18, and 20. The heightened Th2 immune activity characteristic of atopy and asthma involves the actions of the cytokines IL-3 IL-4, IL-5, IL-9, and IL-13. Two of these cytokines, IL-4 and IL-13, share a receptor subunit (IL-4Rα) and STAT6 (*Chapter 9*). As described previously, IL-4 is the principal cytokine in inducing Th2 cell growth and IgE synthesis, typical of atopy, whereas IL-13 can also induce IgE synthesis but plays an important role at mucosal sites favoring eosinophilic infiltration, mucus hypersecretion, and bronchial smooth muscle hypertrophy, which are important events in the pathogenesis of asthma. Shown in Table 18-16 are some of the chromosomal locations of candidate genes associated with the pathogenesis of asthma.

Role of Respiratory Viral and Other Microbial Infections and Asthma

Respiratory viral infections have been demonstrated to play an important role in both the development

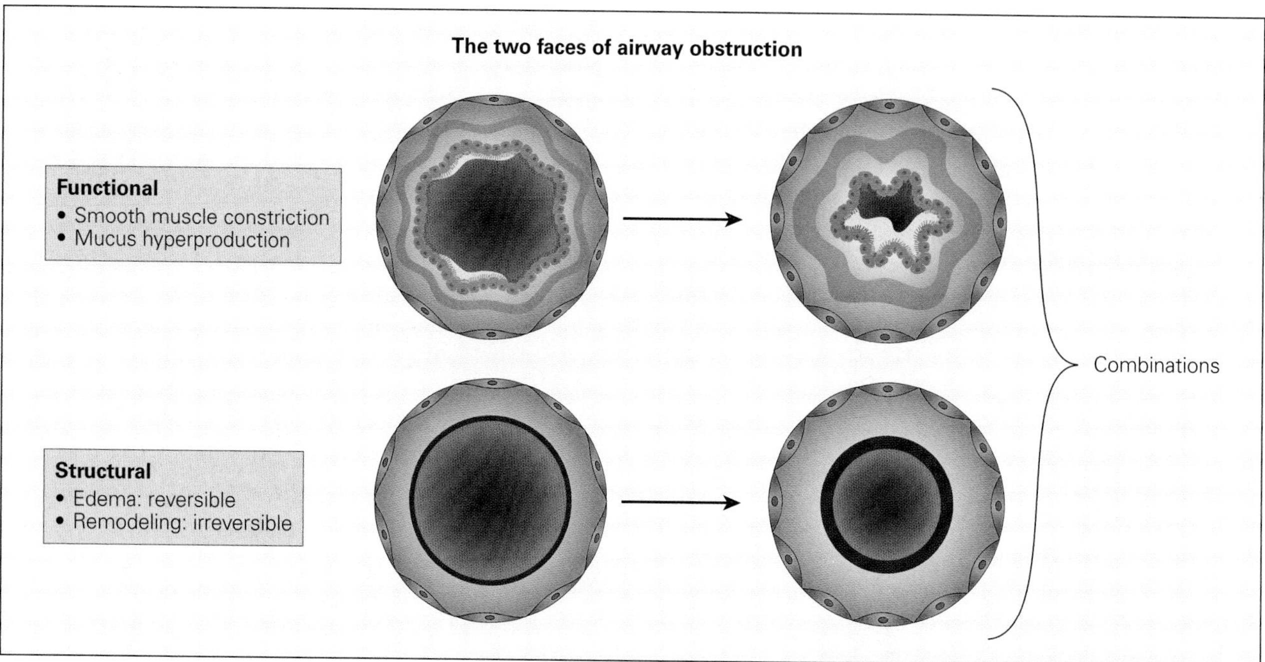

Figure 18-42. Schematic representation of the two stages of airways obstruction. (1) Functional obstruction due to bronchoconstriction of smooth muscle and (2) structural obstruction with either a reversible phase due to edema or an irreversible phase due to chronic inflammation, i.e., remodeling.

and clinical expression of the asthma phenotype. In older children, viral lower respiratory infection (**LRI**)-associated wheezing has also been associated with certain age-related phenotypes. These phenotypes appear to predict both the course and/or development of asthma in these children. The Tucson asthma study has elucidated three patterns of wheezing in children seen during the first six years of life (Figure 18-43 and Table 18-17). The **transient infant wheezers** were children who demonstrated at least one episode of viral LRI-mediated wheeze during the first two to three years of life, but no further episodes after the age of three years. This group comprised the large percentage (80 percent) of children who wheezed during the first year of life, and also included approximately 60 percent of all children wheezing in the second year and 30 to 40 percent of those wheezing in the third year.

Table 18-16. Selected chromosomal locations of candidate genes and gene products associated with the pathogenesis of asthma

Chromosome	Product	Clinical implication
5	IL-13	Involved in bronchoconstriction; may affect responses of bronchodilators
18	IL-4Rα	
12	STAT6	
5	β-2 adrenergic receptor (ADRB2)	
6	HLA-DR	Increased allergen sensitization
20	ADAM33	Variants may influence development of lung remodeling

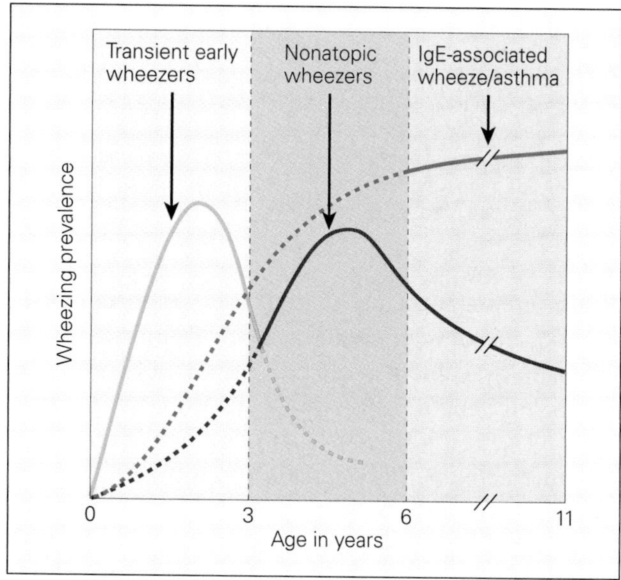

Figure 18-43. Schematic representation of three types of wheezers in childhood. (Adapted with permission from Martinez FD. Respiratory syncytial virus bronchiolitis and the pathogenesis of childhood asthma. Pediatr Infect Dis J. 2003;22(2 Suppl):S76–82.)

Table 18-17. Patterns of wheezing seen during infancy and childhood.

Age of onset of wheezing	Transient	Late onset wheezers	Persistent wheezers
Wheezing at six years	> three years	three to six years	birth to six years
Role of maternal smoking	0	+	+
Male predominance	+	0	0
Role of atopy	0	+	+
Elevated serum IgE levels	0	+	+

Reproduced with permission from Martinez FD. Respiratory syncytial virus bronchiolitis and the pathogenesis of childhood asthma. Pediatr Infect Dis J. 2003;22:S76–82.

A second group, the **nonatopic wheezers**, included children who developed LRI wheezing episodes usually beyond the third year of life (late onset wheezers). This group represented a heterogeneous population with approximately 60 percent of children eventually developing atopic disease and asthma by six years of age, and about 40 percent showing no evidence of atopy. The nonatopic wheezers were postulated to have an alteration in autonomic nervous system control of airway tone and were thus more prone to develop viral-induced acute airway obstruction. A third group, the **atopic wheezers**, represented children who had persistent wheezing during the first six years of life. These children eventually went on to develop atopic asthma. Other characteristics of these three phenotypes are shown in Table 18-17 with maternal smoking and family history of atopic disease being the two greatest risk factors for development of atopic asthma in children.

In children and adults with established asthma, viral upper and lower respiratory tract infections play a significant role in producing acute exacerbations of airway obstruction that may result in frequent outpatient visits or in hospitalizations and are responsible for about 85 percent of exacerbations of asthma in infants. Rhinovirus, the common cold virus, is the most frequent cause of exacerbations, but other viruses, including parainfluenza, RSV, influenza, and coronavirus, also have been implicated, albeit to a lesser extent. The increased tendency for viral infections to produce lower airway symptoms in asthmatic individuals may be related, at least in part, to the interaction between allergic sensitization and allergen exposure; viral infections may then act as cofactors in the induction of acute episodes of airflow obstruction. There is also some evidence that some bacterial infections, such as *Chlamydophila pneumonia* (formerly called *Chlamydia pneumoniae*) and *Mycoplasma pneumoniae*, may play a pathogenetic role in asthma as well.

A Summating General Immunologic Perspective for the Management of the Common Allergic Diseases

In summary, the gastrointestinal tract, the skin, and the respiratory tract constitute the primary target organs of the commonly encountered human allergic diseases. Although the composition of and the route of exposure to exogenous agents may vary, the responses to these agents usually involves IgE-mediated mechanisms. Other Gell and Coombs mechanisms of immunologic injury can occur individually or in combination (*Chapter 17*). There also frequently occurs a sequential evolution of disease expression that is age-dependent with involvement of one target organ progressing sequentially to another, i.e., the "atopic march." In the most severe example of this progression, severe eczema seen initially in the small infant progresses to intractable asthma in the older child. Indeed, higher levels of IgE immunoglobulins are seen in those patients with eczema who also have respiratory tract disease. Factors that foster the progression from one target organ to another may be an expression of the susceptibility genes involving barrier dysfunction, innate and/or adaptive immune dysfunction, or remodeling in the end-target tissues. Much progress has been made in identifying the types and mechanisms of exogenous antigens that evoke allergic responses. However, there are large data gaps in our understanding of the gene-environment-development interactions that are contributing to the allergic sensitization and the allergy epidemic. The future challenge for the management of allergic diseases in the 21st century will be to understand the immune balance that results from these interactions and to intervene before the allergic diathesis can take hold. This may include full-scale environmental interventions to abrogate the necessary stimuli for development of allergic disease or targeting of specific intracellular molecules or pathways that promote and elaborate allergic inflammation.

Management of Allergic Diseases

More than in any other immunologically mediated disease, the causal relationship of persistent antigen to disease expression is best demonstrated in allergic disease (*Chapters 1* and *17*). Symptoms continue precisely as long as the allergen persists. Upon removal of the allergen or blockage of its effects, there is a disappearance of the harmful expressions of the immune response. Thus, when undertaking the management of allergic disease, one of the primary objectives is **identification** and **removal** of the offending allergen by environmental control. If removal of the allergen is not possible or if harmful symptoms have already manifested, then the goal of management focuses on **pharmacologic therapy** targeted to the specific immunologic manifestation or **prevention** of the continued immunologic imbalance by immunomodulation, i.e., specific immunotherapy (*Chapter 11*). The goals of this combined pharmacologic/immunomodulatory therapy are twofold: (1) relief of acute or early phase symptoms and control of chronic disease manifestations by pharmacologic agents and (2) modification of the immunologic responses to subsequent allergen exposure by immunotherapy. In allergic diseases associated with more chronic illnesses such as asthma, in addition to pharmacologic agents that provide relief of symptoms, i.e., relievers, management also relies on the use of therapeutic interventions that are directed to disease control, i.e., controller medications, that minimize risk for future disease exacerbations and prevent the development of irreversible changes of chronic lung impairment, i.e., lung remodeling.

The Diagnosis of Allergic Disease

History and Physical Examination

The diagnostic workup of the patient begins with a thorough history and physical examination. Important components of this evaluation include the identification of risk factors, the recognition of immunologically mediated clinical manifestation(s), and the performance of appropriate diagnostic tests to identify the offending allergen(s). A history of atopic disease in other family members, e.g., allergic rhinitis, asthma, or atopic eczema, is helpful in identifying patterns of allergic disease. Without a family history, about 10 percent of the normal population develops allergic disease. However, this percentage is increased to 20 to 30 percent when there is evidence of allergic disease in one parent or sibling and 40 to 50 percent when both parents manifest allergic disease.

The evaluation should also include a careful review of exposure to potential environmental allergens that may be responsible for the immunologic imbalance. These agents include a panorama of foods, inhalants, contactants, or infecting organisms that may be responsible for the causation or exacerbation of the allergic manifestations. In typical cases, symptoms occur reproducibly each time there is direct exposure to a known allergen or to an environment suspected to contain the putative allergen, e.g., outdoor exposure to ragweed during the pollen season. Sometimes, however, secondary disease manifestations may be the only significant finding. For example, the history of repeated upper respiratory tract infections, e.g., otitis media, may provide the first clue to the diagnosis of allergic disease, particularly in children. Physical examination then confirms what has been elicited by history and will often reveal clinical signs that are age-specific and vary depending on the length and location of exposure to the offending allergen, e.g., acute versus chronic disease manifestations.

Identification of the Allergen

Once a carefully taken history and physical examination suggest an allergic disorder, in vivo and/or in vitro laboratory-based serologic assays for allergen-specific IgE antibody and other inflammatory mediators or markers are the primary testing techniques (Figure 18-44). In some cases, provocation challenges to the suspected allergen may be employed to confirm the suspected diagnosis of allergic disease.

Detection of Allergen-Specific IgE

In Vivo Skin Tests

The most commonly performed technique for the determination of IgE sensitization to a number of offending allergens employs the demonstration of a localized Type I immediate, i.e., wheal-and-flare reaction (*Chapter 17*) when small amounts of the allergen or allergenic extract are applied either into the superficial layers, i.e., **epicutaneous** or skin prick test or into deeper layers of the skin, i.e., **intradermal** skin test (Figure 18-44C). Shown in Figure 18-45 is an immediate typical wheal-and-flare reaction in a ragweed sensitive patient with allergic rhinitis occurring three minutes after epicutaneous injection of ragweed extract.

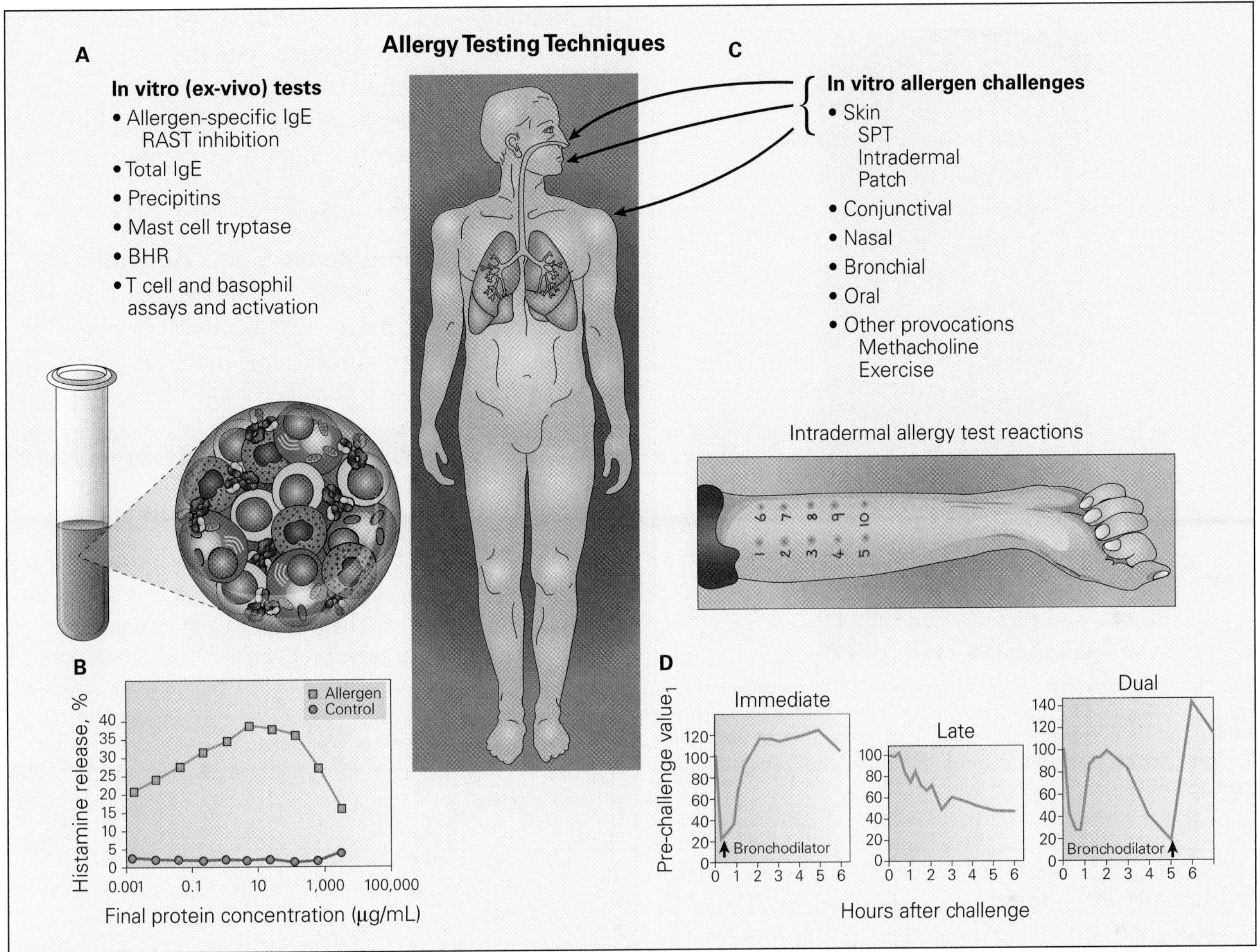

Figure 18-44. **Schematic representation of various in vitro and in vivo diagnostic testing procedures for allergic disease.** Panel A: Various in vitro methods for measurement of total and specific serum IgE. Panel B: A basophil histamine release (BHR) assay. Panel C: Various in vivo methods for IgE-mediated allergy. Panel D: Various bronchial provocation responses, i.e., immediate, late, and dual responses.

Binding of the test allergen with membrane-bound IgE on skin mast cells leads to the release of vasoactive substances, resulting in erythema and induration, e.g., wheal-and-flare reaction, at the site of test application. This response is immediate (within minutes) and its timing assumes diagnostic importance. Occasionally, one encounters late cutaneous allergic reactions (LCAR) that occur four to six hours after the application of the test antigen that is associated with the late phase responses described previously. Other in vivo skin test methods are described in Box 18-6.

In Vitro Immunoassays

Following the discovery and characterization of the IgE molecule in 1967, in vitro immunoassays were developed that measure total IgE or allergen-specific IgE-antibody in serum. The measurement of allergen-specific IgE antibodies in serum is of similar diagnostic value to that of skin tests but has a higher reproducibility that is not influenced by ongoing symptoms, e.g., eczema or urticaria, or treatments, e.g., antihistamines that can blunt immediate hypersensitivity skin test results. The use of in vitro tests also eliminates the small risk for undesirable and sometimes life-threatening systemic allergic reactions that sometimes accompany in vivo skin testing, particularly with certain allergens, e.g., foods. Quantitation of levels of allergen-specific IgE by in vitro immunoassays can also be reliably used to predict the likelihood for a positive oral challenge to food allergen or determine outgrowth of the food allergy.

The radioallergosorbent test (**RAST**), branded and marketed by Pharmacia diagnostics in Sweden in 1974, was one of the first assays for the detection of allergen-specific IgE antibodies. This test employed a solid-phase IgE capture methodology in which the patient's serum is first added to a fixed substrate

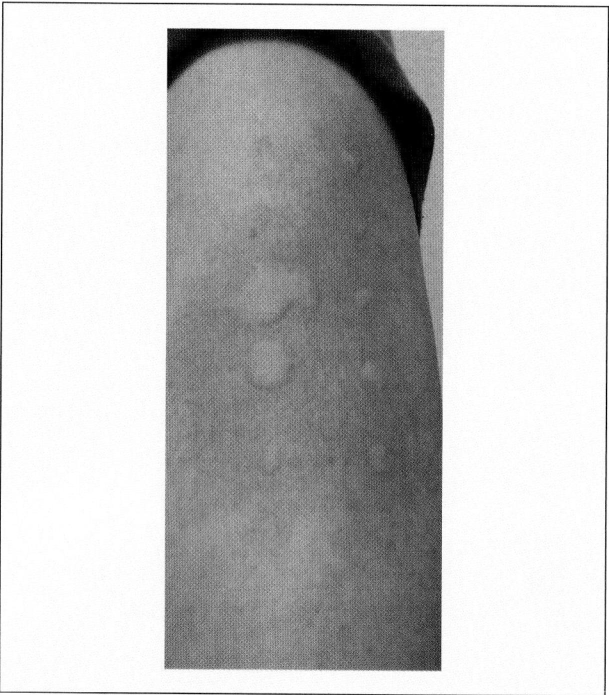

Figure 18-45. A photograph of a positive immediate Type I wheal-and-flare reaction in a ragweed sensitive patient with allergic rhinitis occurring three minutes after epicutaneous injection of ragweed extract.

containing the suspected allergen following which the bound IgE antibodies are detected by the addition of a second radiolabeled anti-IgE antibody. The RAST is no longer in use and has been replaced by several autoanalyzer-based, allergen-specific IgE antibody assays that essentially mimic the RAST's solid-phase capture methodology but eliminate the need for a radioactive marker by incorporating a fluorescent label. Shown in Figure 18-46 is a schematic representation of the general methodology of the measurement of specific IgE antibody by current immunoassays. These newer assays use nonisotypically labeled anti-human IgE and include capture methodologies in which a cellulose sponge matrix is used as an allergosorbent "cap" on which allergen is covalently coupled (ImmunoCAP), or biotinylated allergen bound to an avidin solid phase (the Immulite System), or cellulose wafers covalently coupled allergen (HYTEC-288 system).

Another application of the allergen-specific IgE technology has been used in the measurement of allergen potency using a competitive inhibition assay. In this assay, soluble allergen (typically in an extract) or buffer (sham control) are added to different aliquots of serum before the serum mixture is analyzed in the specific IgE assay. The percentage of inhibition is computed as a semi-quantitative estimate of relative allergen potency. Results may provide useful information to assess the relative allergenicity, in terms of IgE-binding potential, of an allergenic protein or ingredient compared to the native allergenic source.

Basophil Histamine Release and Activation

Although mostly a research tool, basophil histamine release bioassays (**BHR**) can be used to assess the presence of allergen-specific IgE in serum and, since

Box 18-6

In Vivo Skin Tests for Diagnosis of Allergic Diseases

Most in vivo skin tests for the diagnosis of allergic diseases involve commercial, standardized extracts to a variety of allergenic substances. Use of these extracts promotes uniformity in diagnosis. In some diagnostic cases, however, there may be a need to use freshly prepared allergenic sources and apply these directly to the skin. This testing is often employed in diagnosing oral allergy syndrome in which clinical reactivity commonly occurs to relatively labile food proteins. Since conventional commercial food extracts are often processed, they may lose or not contain some or all of the relevant allergenic foods proteins for diagnosis of this condition. Thus, skin test preparations use fresh or raw food samples, as these likely contain the relevant provoking allergens. In addition to the conventional epicutaneous and intradermal skin tests, some physicians utilize **patch testing** where the allergen solution is placed on a pad and taped superficially to the skin. After 24 to 72 hours, an erythematous reaction can be elicited at the site of contact with the offending material. This test is typically used to detect delayed hypersensitivity responses to a variety of dyes, metals, plastics, and organic materials involved in (allergic) contact dermatitis. In these disorders, the offending agents act as haptens that, after conjugation to tissue protein, may activate Th1 cells and cause delayed dermal responses at the test site. Increasing evidence suggests that allergen-specific T cells play also important roles in the late phase of Type I hypersensitivity responses as well. Therefore, patch testing has been proposed and employed for the diagnosis of atopic eczema and food allergy, particularly when allergen-specific IgE testing results are inconclusive. Although studies suggest a strong correlation between results of patch testing and in vivo allergen challenge, the clinical utility of positive results in these applications in the diagnosis of atypical or delayed symptoms of allergic diseases is still debated.

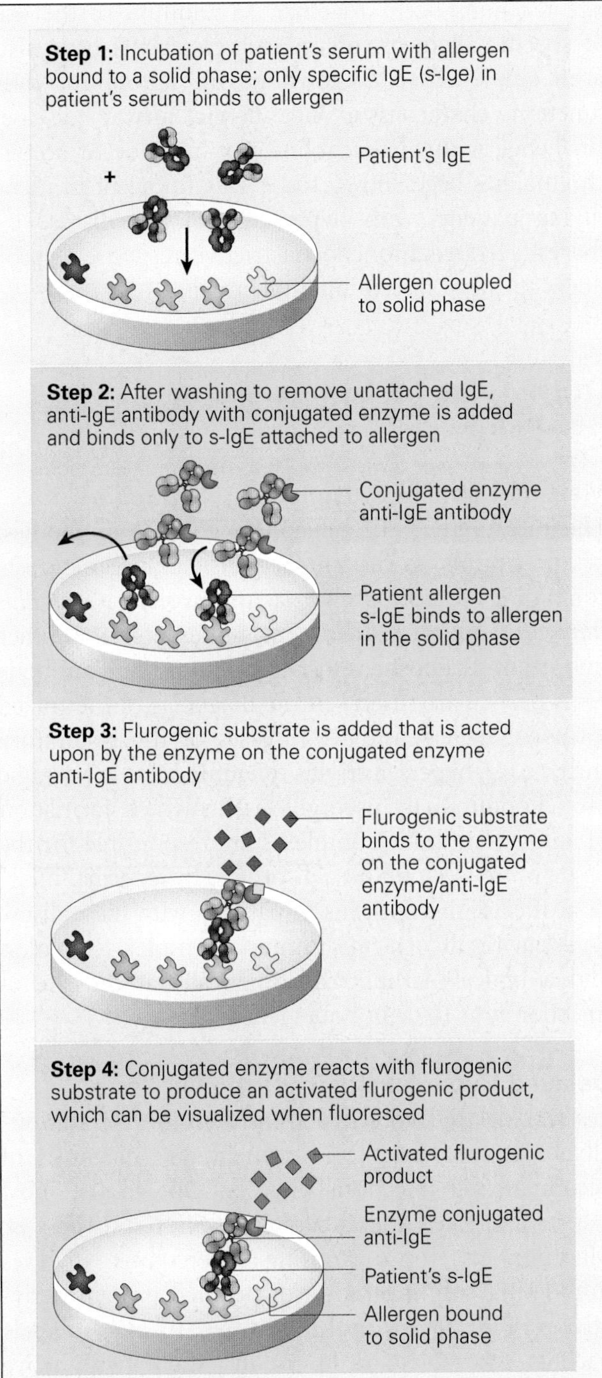

Step 1: Incubation of patient's serum with allergen bound to a solid phase; only specific IgE (s-Ige) in patient's serum binds to allergen
Patient's IgE
+
Allergen coupled to solid phase
Step 2: After washing to remove unattached IgE, anti-IgE antibody with conjugated enzyme is added and binds only to s-IgE attached to allergen
Conjugated enzyme anti-IgE antibody
Patient allergen s-IgE binds to allergen in the solid phase
Step 3: Flurogenic substrate is added that is acted upon by the enzyme on the conjugated enzyme anti-IgE antibody
Flurogenic substrate binds to the enzyme on the conjugated enzyme/anti-IgE antibody
Step 4: Conjugated enzyme reacts with flurogenic substrate to produce an activated flurogenic product, which can be visualized when fluoresced
Activated flurogenic product
Enzyme conjugated anti-IgE
Patient's s-IgE
Allergen bound to solid phase

Figure 18-46. Schematic representation of the general methodology of the measurement of specific IgE antibody by immunoassays used in the detection of specific IgE.

basophils can be stimulated ex vivo, to also predict whether basophil FcεRI-bound IgE has the potential to elicit basophil reactivity following allergen challenge. After basophils are isolated from blood, they are either incubated directly with antihuman IgE and allergen (direct challenge) or initially stripped of IgE, incubated with antihuman IgE, and then challenged with allergen (passive immunization). Histamine, or leukotriene, released into the supernatant is then measured. As incremental doses of allergen are applied to this system, more surface basophil IgE receptors become cross-linked, leading to greater histamine release. This release continues until the receptors become saturated. The percentage of histamine released in relation to the allergen dose can be used to generate a dose-response curve; this curve typically reflects a bell-shaped curve with the maximal histamine release peak of the curve coinciding with the optimal cross-linking allergen concentration (Figure 18-44B). In general, BHR results correlate well with the results of skin testing and allergen challenge. However, the need for freshly obtained blood specimens and difficulties in controlling for spontaneous basophil histamine release limit the routine use of these assays.

In recent years, flow cytometric methods have been used to identify basophils in serum and to measure basophil activation markers as a way to estimate histamine release and reactivity potential following allergen exposure (*Chapter 24*). The measurement of CD63 and CD203c has been employed as activation-linked molecules expressed on basophils following the cross-linking of FcεRI by allergen-bound IgE. Upregulation of CD63 has been shown to correlate with basophil mediator release in patients with atopic dermatitis and food allergy, and CD203c has been found in high levels in these patients. Measuring basophil activity may therefore become a useful marker not only for identifying patients with allergic disorders, but also for monitoring the extent of allergic inflammation and the efficacy of therapy in these patients.

Total Serum IgE

Determination of total serum levels of IgE by competitive (capture and detection) or noncompetitive (labeled antibody) immunoassays (Figure 18-44A) has been shown to be of little value in assessing specific allergenicity. However, determination of elevated total IgE levels is useful in identifying individuals at risk for atopic disease as well as patients with other IgE-producing disorders, e.g., parasitic infections (*Chapter 15*), and patients with hyperimmunoglobulinemia E (Job's syndrome) (*Chapter 16*). Total serum IgE values vary with age, with peak values in the teenage years, and this variation needs to be considered in the diagnostic evaluation.

Mast Cell Tryptase

Another tool to assess allergen-mediated diagnoses, especially following acute reactions consistent with anaphylaxis, is measurement of allergic response end-product mediators in the serum. Common mediators, such as histamine, have a very short half-life (minutes) and are impractical markers for this purpose. Mast cell tryptase, on the other hand, can be detected in the serum up to four hours after a reaction. Two types of tryptase levels, α-tryptase and β-tryptase, give diagnostic information. α-Tryptase estimates mast cell numbers while β-tryptase provides information on mast-cell activation. Elevated levels of β-tryptase correlate highly with systemic mast cell activation and Type I mediator release, especially in cases of venom and drug-induced anaphylaxis; this mediator is not commonly detected in cases of food-induced anaphylaxis. Very high α-tryptase levels in relation to β-tryptase serum levels may signal an underlying mast cell disorder, such as mastocytosis.

Allergen Challenge and/or Provocation Tests

Direct allergen challenge at sites of affected target organs, i.e., the gastrointestinal, skin, or respiratory tracts, is another method of in vivo diagnosis of immediate hypersensitivity states. These procedures include administration of gradually increasing doses of allergen directly applied to mucosae of affected organs, e.g., conjunctiva, nasal passages, bronchial airways, or the oral cavity/gastrointestinal tract, followed by observation and measurement of clinical responses. In food allergy, a well-controlled oral food challenge that is double-blinded and placebo-controlled (**DBPCFC**) is the gold standard for diagnosing a food allergy and determining whether a specific food product or dose will elicit reactions in sensitive individuals.

Bronchial allergen provocation may also provide useful information regarding the characteristics of immune response to an allergen. Three types of responses can be seen following bronchial allergen challenge; these include immediate, late, or dual responses (Figure 18-44D). The immediate responses are characterized by a fall in FEV1, within minutes of challenge, due to the immediate release of preformed mediators in the lung. Symptoms typically normalize within one hour. Late responses, rather, are characterized by a pronounced fall in FEV1 by three to six hours after challenge. In some individuals, dual responses involving both immediate and late reactions occur together. In addition to the use of specific allergens, pharmacologic agents have also been employed to demonstrate the autonomic dysfunction characteristic of allergic airway disease. Challenge with methacholine, an analogue of acetylcholine, has been shown to be a useful agent in identifying patients with hyperactive airway disease by the exaggerated bronchoconstrictive response it produces in these susceptible individuals.

Other Tests for Hypersensitivity Reactions

Measurement of Precipitating Antibodies

The measurement of precipitating (IgG) antibodies, i.e., precipitins, to certain allergens e.g., organic dusts containing thermophilic actinomyces, *Aspergillus fumigatus*, and bird excrement, represents yet another important diagnostic test. Detection of these antibodies is particularly useful in the diagnosis of the mixed forms of hypersensitivity diseases of the respiratory tract, e.g., hypersensitivity pneumonitis or allergic bronchopulmonary aspergillosis, in which formation of antigen-antibody complexes are responsible for the tissue injury seen in these disorders. Intradermal injection of causative antigens in patients with these disorders can result in acute immune complex formation and a typical Arthus reaction locally at the site of injection four to eight hours later.

Delayed Hypersensitivity (Type IV) Tests

Tests of delayed type hypersensitivity have traditionally been used for the assessment and diagnosis of accompanying infectious diseases. One of the most classic tests, i.e., the tuberculin skin test (**TST**) or Mantoux test for diagnosing tuberculosis, involves intradermal administration of purified protein derivative (**PPD**), a glycerol derivative of the tubercle bacillus. After 24 to 72 hours, in patients with active or latent tuberculosis infection (**LTBI**), specifically sensitized Th1 cells home to the skin site and cause release of proinflammatory cytokines that promote the local erythema and induration characteristic of a positive TST. Similar skin delayed hypersensitivity reactions are seen with skin antigens derived from *Histoplasma capsulatum*, *Blastomyces dermatitidis*, *Coccidioides immitis*, *Bartonella henselae*, and atypical mycobacteria. In more recent years, delayed hypersensitivity testing by way of **patch testing** has been performed for diagnosing allergic diseases as well, in particular for diagnosing delayed disease symptoms believed to be mediated by allergen-specific T cells (Box 18-6). In vitro tests of delayed hypersensitivity cellular responses are also available. These tests are described in greater detail in Chapter 7 and rely upon the measurement of cytokines released by a variety of innate and adaptive immune cells.

Prevention of Immunologic Imbalance

The removal of the offending allergen can often lead to prevention of the allergic disorder. The prevention of the expressions of allergic disease focuses on the reduction of allergen exposure and limiting the detrimental effects of immunomodulating factors, e.g., infection, on allergic disease expression. In many cases, this is possible, for example, with the removal of household pets or avoidance of an offending food, drug, or contactant. These avoidance measures can be initiated in the home, school, work, or outdoor environments and may include such simple measures as reading food labels and seeking further information concerning hidden allergenic ingredients in food, drugs, cosmetics, or other consumer products. The control of allergic diseases is particularly important in early infancy and childhood since this is a critical developmental period and window for allergic sensitization. Inappropriate intervention in this period, when the effects of allergic inflammation are still reversible, may result in more chronic and irreversible symptoms of allergic disease later in life. Shown in Table 18-18 are some of the important strategies that have been studied to prevent the development of allergic disease and its sequelae in the young infant and child. It is important to note that although allergen exposure is necessary for development of allergy, environmental allergen avoidance strategies, especially during the formative periods of life, have not consistently been shown to abrogate the future development of allergic diseases.

Therapy

In many cases, such as with household dust mite or seasonal pollen exposure, total elimination of allergen is neither practical nor possible. Moreover, even with strict avoidance measures in place, accidental or unintentional exposures to an allergen remain possible. Thus, when acute and/or chronic symptoms result from allergen exposures, pharmacological management is often necessary to prevent or alleviate these symptoms and severe health consequences. Some of the major pharmacologic agents employed in the treatment and management of

Table 18-18. Primary prevention strategies in allergy

Primary prevention	Rationale	Conclusions
Exclusive breastfeeding (BF)	Avoidance of food allergic sensitization; promotion of antiallergenic factors in breast milk	Generally recommended until six months of age; unclear benefit in allergy prevention
Avoidance of allergens in maternal diet during pregnancy and lactation	Avoidance of food allergic sensitization	No proven benefit in allergy prevention
Delayed introduction of solid allergenic foods in infants until age three	Avoidance of food allergic sensitization	No proven benefit in allergy prevention
Use of hypoallergenic milk formulas versus regular milk formulas	Decreased exposure and sensitization to cows' milk allergen	Some benefit in reducing symptoms of eczema - eHF > pHF; unclear benefit in reducing incidence of allergy; no benefit over BF
Probiotics use	Antiallergenic properties by enhancing Th1 innate responses	Some benefit in reducing symptoms of eczema; no effect on reducing incidence of allergy
Pet ownership in early childhood	Reduced sensitization to pet allergens (due to tolerizing endotoxin exposure)	Benefit demonstrated in reducing pet allergy; unclear benefit in reducing other allergies, although possible synergistic effect seen with cat and dog in adults
House dust mite (HDM) avoidance measures	Reduced sensitizing exposure to HDM	Benefit in reducing clinical manifestations of HDM allergy

Abbreviations: eHF = extensively hydrolyzed formula; pHF = partially hydrolyzed formula.

Table 18-19. Some of major drugs used in the treatment of allergic diseases together with mechanisms of action and examples of clinical use

Drug	Example	Clinical use
Relievers	Loratadine	Allergic rhinitis
Antihistamines	Phenylephrine	Allergic rhinitis
Decongestants	Albuterol	Asthma
β_2-adrenergic agonist	Ipratropium	Asthma
Anticholinergic drug	Epinephrine	Anaphylaxis, asthma
Adrenergic agent		
Controllers		
Corticosteroids	Mometasone, budesonide	Atopic dermatitis, allergic rhinitis,
Topical	Prednisone	Asthma, anaphylaxis
Systemic	Montelukast	Asthma, allergic rhinitis
Leukotriene modifiers	Cromolyn, nedocromil	Asthma
Mast cell stabilizers	Theophylline	Asthma
Phosphodiesterase inhibitors		
Other	Omalizumab (anti-IgE); Mepolizumab	Severe manifestations of allergic diseases/
Biologic response modifiers	(anti-IL-5)	asthma, EGIDs, autoinflammatory disease
Monoclonal abs	Etanercept (anti-TNF-α);	
Anticytokine therapies		

allergic diseases are shown in Table 18-19. Although the specific pharmacologic agents used in the various allergic disorders differ, the general principles of pharmacologic therapy are the same. These include: (1) relief of acute symptoms, (2) control of chronic disease manifestations, and (3) immunomodulation of the immunologic responses to subsequent allergen exposure.

Relief of Acute or Early Phase Symptoms

Drugs that prevent or act on acute symptoms are those that directly block or antagonize preformed and newly synthesized inflammatory mediators; these drugs are commonly referred to as "**relievers**" (Table 18-19 and Figure 18-47). Drugs used in this arsenal vary depending on the nature of complaints, i.e., symptoms localized to specific tissues or organs or those associated with systemic involvement. For example, certain drugs, e.g. beta-adrenergic agonists, counteract and reverse the immediate bronchoconstricting effects of mediators on bronchial smooth muscles.

On the other hand, systemic inflammatory effects or reactions, as seen with anaphylaxis, may produce profound blood vessel vasodilation involving the cardiorespiratory shock organs (Figure 18-47). At this stage, cardiopulmonary support becomes critical and the timely administration of epinephrine, a powerful vasoconstrictor, together with fluid resuscitation and vasopressors are crucial in therapy. Epinephrine can be delivered intramuscularly or subcutaneously either via an epinephrine auto-injector device, e.g., EpiPen, or by direct intramuscular injection. Moreover, since early phase mediator effects are also important in propagating late phase inflammatory responses, e.g., leukotrienes, many of these drugs have important roles in treating, controlling, or preventing the progression of the allergic response to chronicity.

Control of Disease Manifestations

Drugs in this arsenal are typically those that inhibit formation of late phase cellular responses and inflammatory mediators or block their release after allergen exposure. As such, the main function of these drugs is to "**control**" symptoms in an allergen-rich environment by blocking responses that can lead to acute or chronic disease manifestations; they are therefore referred to as "**controller drugs**." Shown in Table 18-19 are some of the major controller drugs and in Figure 18-47 a schematic representation of their mechanisms of action.

A Stepwise Approach for Treatment of Asthma

Asthma provides a useful prototypic allergic disease that exemplifies these pharmacologic principles. Figure 18-48 represents a general schematic stepwise approach for the control of patients with asthma based on disease severity guidelines provided by the 2007 National Asthma and Education Prevention Program (NAEPP). For intermittent asthma, short acting β_2-agonists, such as albuterol, usually suffice for relief of acute symptoms. However, in patients

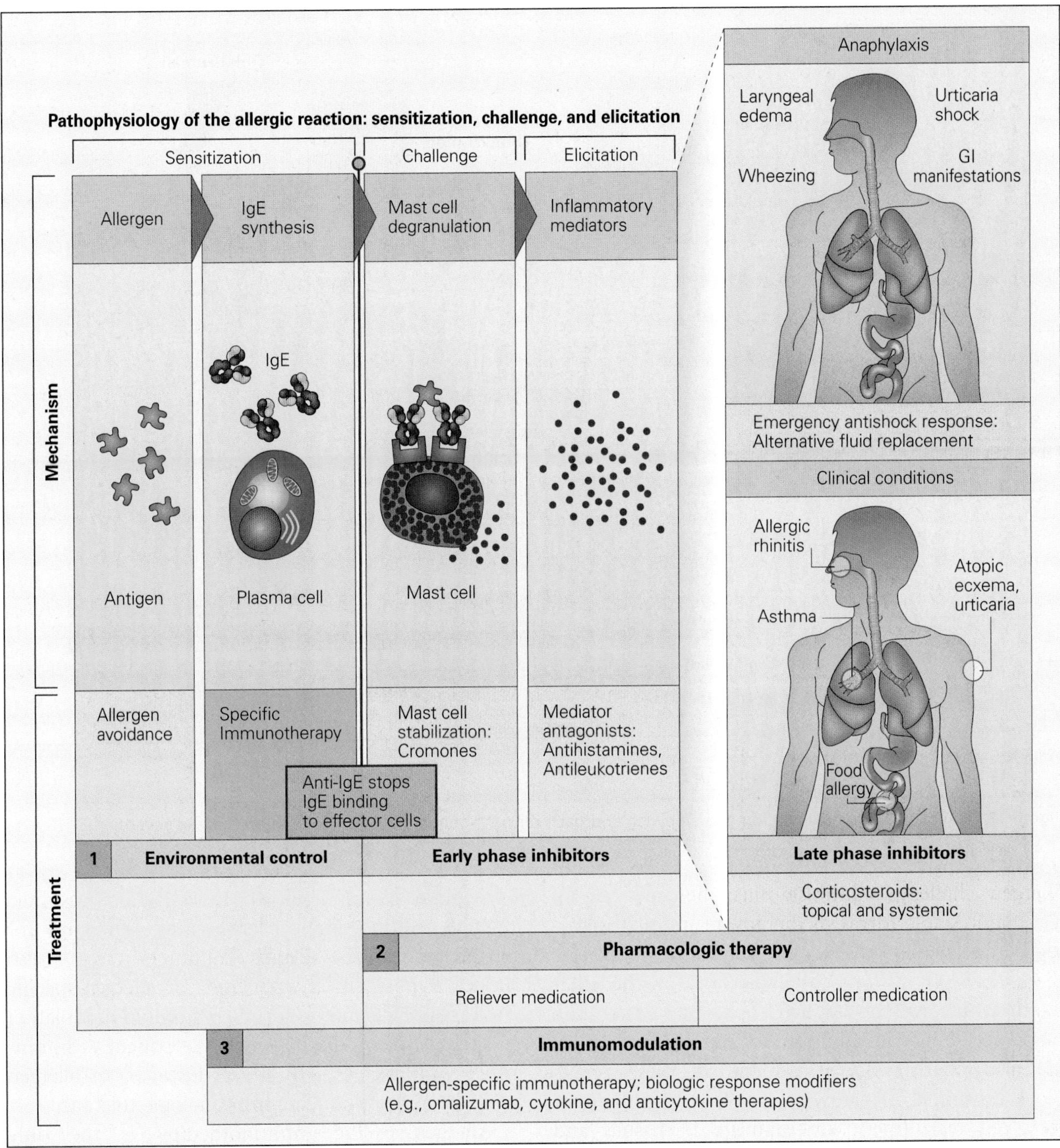

Figure 18-47. Schematic representation of various treatment modalities involved in allergic diseases and anaphylaxis based on pathogenetic mechanisms of allergic disease.

with persistent asthma, inhaled corticosteroids are the mainstay of treatment for the control of symptoms; alternatively, for patients with mildly persistent symptoms, other therapeutic options can be used, i.e., leukotriene receptor antagonists (**LTRAs**), and mast cell stabilizers, e.g., cromolyn or theophylline. Long-acting β_2-agonists, LTRAs, or theophylline are added as symptoms increase in severity. In patients with most severe symptoms, oral corticosteroids (**OCS**) are added, and in patients with severe allergic asthma, other immunomodulator therapy, i.e., anti-IgE (omalizumab), may be considered.

Although not mutually exclusive, each agent can be said to target a specific mechanism or process in the allergic pathway. For example, by targeting histamine—one of the main proinflammatory mediators released during the immediate phase of

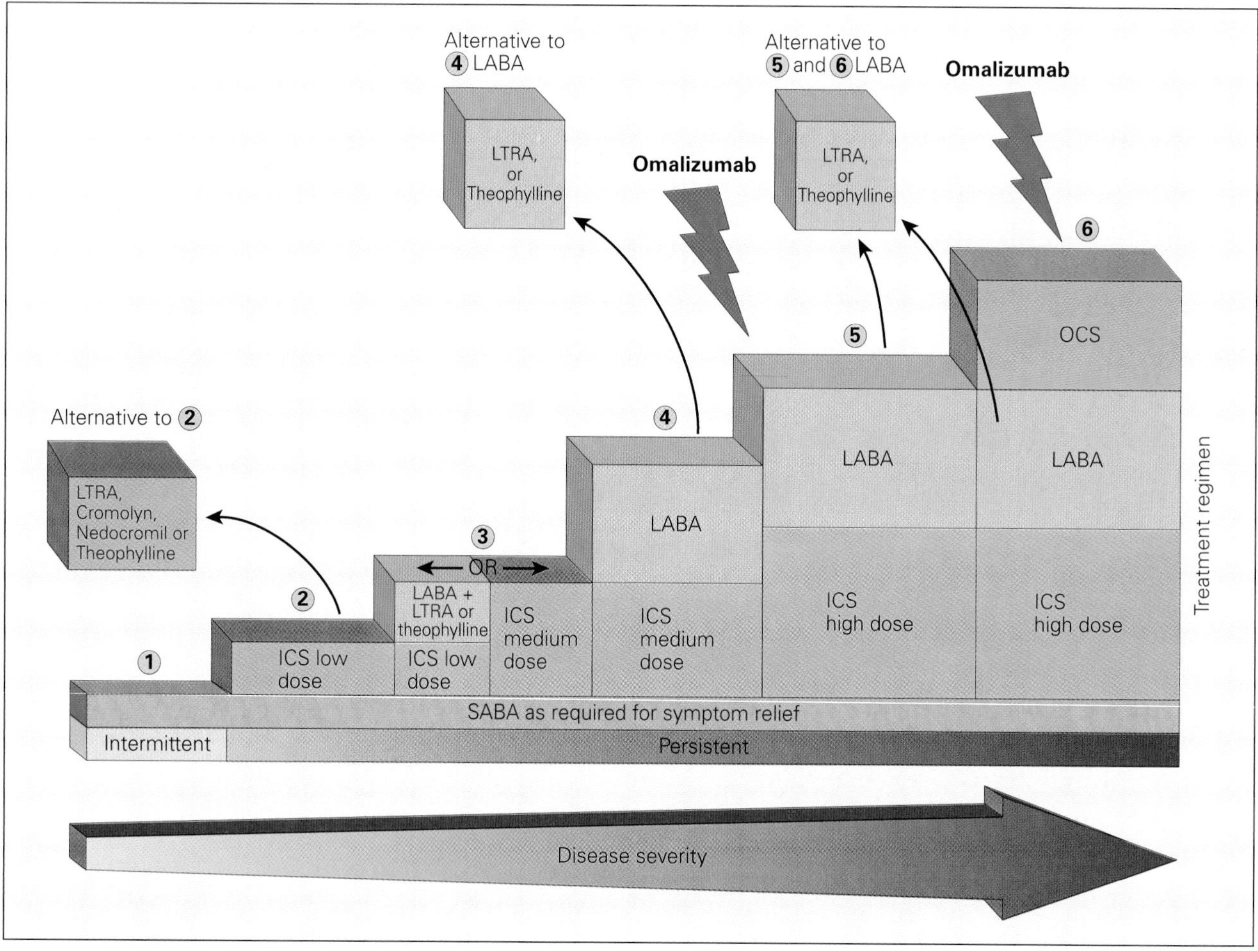

Figure 18-48. Schematic representation of a stepwise approach for treatment of asthma based upon disease severity.

allergen challenge—antihistamines become one of the major staple forms of therapy in the pharmacologic management of acute symptoms of allergic disease. Drugs, such as corticosteroids, on the other hand, which can be applied topically to the skin, nose, and lungs in addition to being taken orally, are also mainstays of treatment, as these agents block a number of pathways that lead to inflammatory cell recruitment and damage in tissues and cause chronic disease symptoms.

Modification of Immunologic Responses to Subsequent Allergen Exposure by Induction of Immune Tolerance: Allergen-Specific Immunotherapy

Immunomodulation was described in Chapter 11 as the process by which the immune response is adjusted or changed to another desired level utilizing three interventive strategies of **immunopotentiation**, **immunosuppression**, or induction of **immunologic tolerance**. Nowhere is the use of immunomodulation to achieve immunologic tolerance better illustrated than its use in specific allergen immunotherapy for allergic diseases. Allergen immunotherapy (also termed hyposensitization therapy or allergen-specific immunotherapy) is a form of immunomodulation for allergic disorders in which the patient is immunized with increasingly larger doses of an allergen with the aim of inducing immunologic tolerance.

Allergen-specific immunotherapy is the only therapeutic strategy that treats the underlying cause of the allergic disorder, whereas other therapies described previously, for the most part, only suppress the symptoms. It is a highly cost-effective therapy that results in an improved quality of life and a reduction in allergic- and allergen-related asthma, as well as a reduction in absenteeism from school or work. Immunotherapy has been shown to produce long-term remission of allergic symptoms in patients with allergic rhinitis, to reduce the severity of associated asthma, and to reduce the chances of developing new sensitizations to allergens and can either reduce the need for medication, reduce the severity of symptoms, or eliminate hypersensitivity altogether. Therapy is usually administered by injections under the skin (subcutaneous) but can be administered under the tongue (sublingually) or orally (oral immunotherapy).

Although subcutaneous injection immunotherapy (**SCIT**) has been shown to be a highly efficacious treatment for allergic disease, its use is largely restricted to specialist centers due to the rare occurrence of serious generalized side effects, i.e., anaphylaxis. As a result, there has been growing interest in the sublingual immunotherapy (**SLIT**), a form of immunotherapy where allergen is introduced beneath the tongue.

When Is Specific Allergen Immunotherapy to Be Considered?

If significant symptoms of allergic disease continue despite environmental control and pharmacotherapy, allergen-specific immunotherapy is often the next modality to be considered in the management of allergic individuals with IgE-mediated allergies. The procedure typically involves administering subthreshold doses of the allergen into the host and gradually increasing the concentrations of allergen until a target concentration of allergen is tolerated clinically, i.e., building up immune tolerance. Immunotherapy is commonly used to reduce the clinical reactivity of individuals with allergic rhinitis and asthma sensitized to common inhalant triggers such as pollens, cat dander, and dust mites. It has also has been employed to reduce the risk for anaphylaxis to venom allergen exposure and for rapid desensitization of patients allergic to drugs that are required for treatment of other diseases, e.g., penicillin desensitization.

Although the precise mechanism(s) of action by which allergen-specific immunotherapy exerts its effects are not completely understood, several mechanisms have been proposed that are shown in Figure 18-49 and Figure 18-50. In rapid desensitization, as sometimes employed in patients with drug allergy in need of desensitization, a full dose of allergen is administered in incremental doses over the course of a few hours. The low-dose allergen administration is believed to provide univalent forms of allergen that occupy IgE bound to its receptor but are not sufficient to cross-link adjacent receptors to trigger degranulation. The gradual administration of these univalent allergenic molecules eventually saturates most IgE-bound receptors on the surface of effector cells (Figure 18-49). Thus, when a fully multivalent

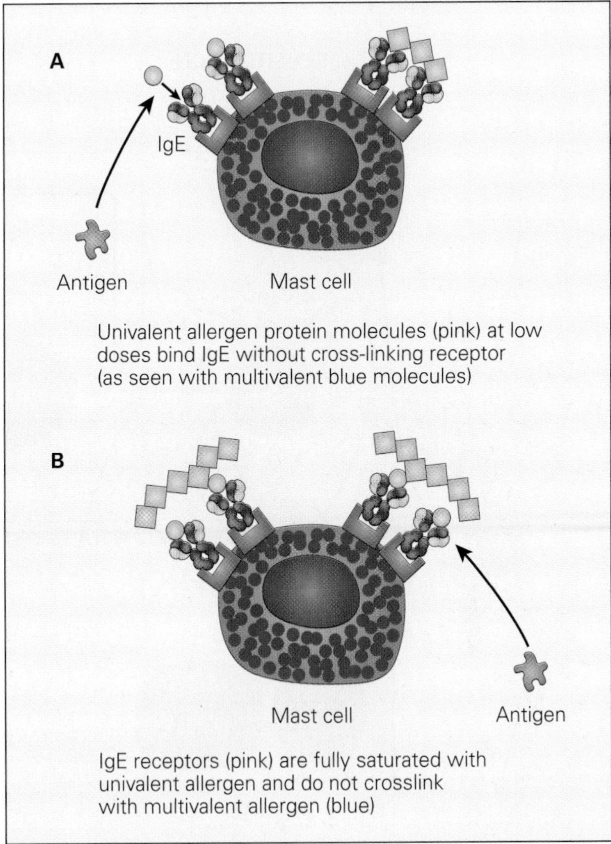

Figure 18-49. Proposed mechanism of rapid allergen desensitization. In this procedure, commonly used for drug desensitization, a full dose of allergenic drug is administered in incremental doses over the course of a few hours. Panel A: Administration of low initial doses of allergen results in univalent forms of allergen that occupy IgE bound to its receptor but are not sufficient to cross-link adjacent receptors to trigger degranulation. The gradual introduction of these univalent allergenic molecules eventually saturates most IgE-bound receptors on the surface of effector cells. Panel B: Due to univalent allergen binding, when a higher, fully multivalent, and potentially reactive allergenic dose is subsequently administered, there are no unoccupied receptors available to cross-link and trigger degranulation.

and potentially reactive allergenic dose is subsequently administered, there are presumably no unoccupied receptors available to cross-link and trigger release of mediators. The oral route of desensitization in this type of desensitization is generally safer and preferred to parenteral routes. The induction of clinical tolerance to the drug by this sensitization method, however, is transient and provides little to no lasting effects; therefore, the desensitization lasts only as long as there is a need for drug treatment or where there is continuing exposure to an allergen. The several proposed mechanisms of action of immunotherapy at several points in the immunologic pathways involved in allergic disease are shown in Figure 18-50.

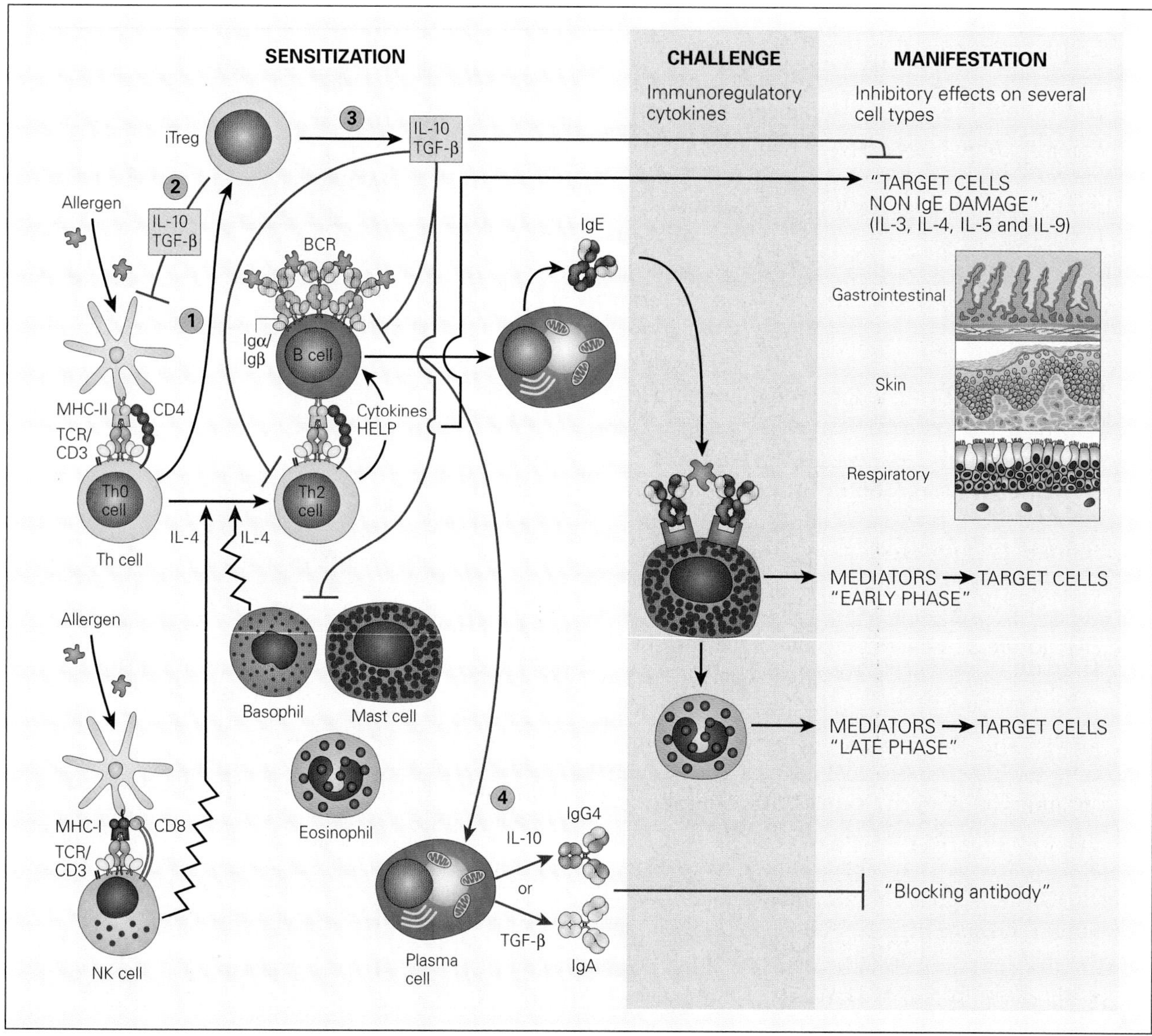

Figure 18-50. Summary of proposed mechanisms of action of immunotherapy. (1) Induction of induced T regulatory (iTreg) cells; (2) production of immunosuppressive IL-10 and TGF-β cytokines to downregulate antigen processing by dendritic cells (DCs); (3) immunomodulation of target cells, B cells, or mast cells/basophils; and (4) modulation of immunoglobulin isotypes by IL-10 and TGF-β with downregulation of IgE production by the production of IgG4 and IgA, which function as "blocking antibodies."

Biological Response Modifiers: Monoclonal Antibody and Anti-Cytokine Therapies for Allergic Diseases

IgE Modulation

In 2003, omalizumab was approved by the U.S. Food and Drug Administration for the treatment of patients with moderate-to-severe or severe allergic asthma. Omalizumab is a recombinant humanized monoclonal anti-IgE antibody comprising a human immunoglobulin G framework onto which is grafted the complementarity-determining region (**CDR**) from an anti-IgE antibody raised in mice (Box 18-7 and *Chapter 11*). Omalizumab selectively binds with high affinity to the Cε3 domain of IgE molecule, the IgE-binding site for the FcεRI receptor alpha chain (Figure 18-51).

Omalizumab inhibits the binding of IgE to the α1 domain of the high-affinity IgE receptor (FcεRI) by binding to the Cε3 epitope on IgE that overlaps with the site to which FcεRI normally binds. This feature is critical to the pharmacological effects of omalizumab since other anti-IgE antibodies that do not share with targeted action can inadvertently cross-link cell surface FcεRI-bound IgE and induce mediator release from basophils and mast cells that could give rise to an

Box 18-7

Omalizumab is a monoclonal antibody identified through conventional somatic cell hybridization techniques. Through this process, researchers identified a murine monoclonal antihuman IgE antibody, MAE11, whose paratope was directed toward the site that binds FcεRI on basophils and mast cells. MAE11 was humanized in a process involving transplantation of the complementarity-determining regions (CDRs; specific areas within the paratope that interact with an antigen—in this instance, human IgE) onto a human IgG1 antibody framework. Additional MAE11 amino acid sequences were also incorporated into the humanized antibody to maintain the proper CDR spatial arrangement. This process resulted in a humanized monoclonal antihuman IgE antibody, rhuMAb-E25 (later named omalizumab), which contained approximately 5 percent nonhuman amino-acid residues.

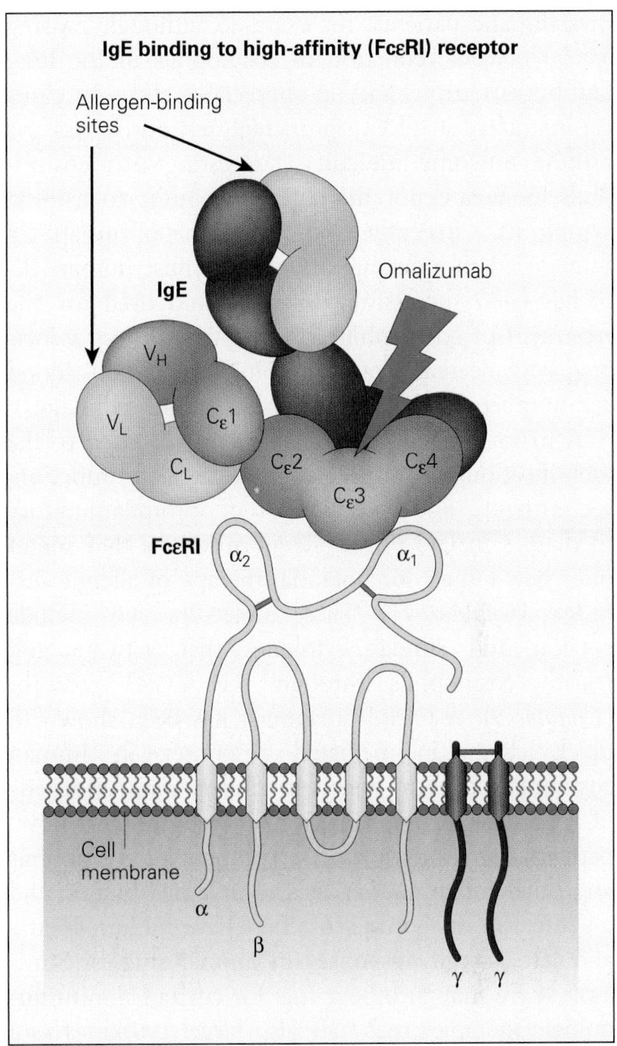

Figure 18-51. Schematic representation of the location of action of omalizumab at the Cε3 domain of IgE molecule, the binding site on IgE for the FcεRI receptor.

inadvertent anaphylactic reaction. Although the binding peptide sequence on IgE that is used to bind to low-affinity IgE receptor (FcεRII) is different from the sequence used to bind to FcεRI, omalizumab, by steric hindrance, also prevents binding of IgE to FcεRII. Treatment with omalizumab also reduces the number of FcεRI receptors on basophils in atopic patients.

Because of its ability to inhibit binding of IgE to its receptor, omalizumab has been shown to reduce the levels of circulating and tissue-bound IgE as well as surface FcεRI receptors on the surface of mast cells, basophils, and dendritic cells. These effects have been shown to decrease the mast cell-dependent early phase responses as well as the late phase inflammatory responses in the lungs of asthmatics. Reduction in eosinophilia observed with omalizumab, presumably through inhibition of the IgE-mediated stimulatory pathway for eosinophil recruitment, is a plausible explanation for the reduction in this late phase inflammation. Targeting IgE may, thus, provide benefit in treating a number of other IgE-mediated allergic disorders, including reduction of anaphylaxis, e.g., peanut food allergy.

Anticytokine and Other Novel Therapies

The goal of most novel cytokine or anticytokine therapies is directed to the blockage or neutralization of the pathologic effects of selected key cytokine molecules (*Chapters 9* and *11*). The major group of cytokines studied in allergic diseases includes those involved in promoting proallergic Th2 responses, e.g., IL-4 or IL-5, or abrogating their effects, e.g., IFN-γ or IL-12. Another area of Th2 response modulation has been directed to DNA-based immunotherapy using CpG oligonucleotide motifs that stimulate innate and Th1-like tolerogenic responses. Therapies such as IL-12 administration or various forms of IL-4 and IL-5 inhibition have shown promise in reducing some forms of allergic inflammation. For example, the administration of soluble IL-4R, a naturally occurring inhibitor of IL-4, to patients with asthma resulted in clinical improvement by downregulating VCAM-1 expression and eosinophil recruitment to tissues. However, reduction in allergic inflammation for these therapies has not always correlated with clinical efficacy and benefits, and, for some therapies, undesirable side effects have limited the clinical use of these therapies. Anti-IL-5 therapy in asthmatic patients, for example, although causing a >50 percent reduction of eosinophils in the lung and bone marrow, had no appreciable effect on clinical markers of FEV1, bronchial responsiveness, or asthma outcome measures, suggesting that eosinophils alone are not the sole contributor to asthma symptoms. Recently, however, mepolizumab, a humanized monoclonal antibody against human IL-5, has been successfully tolerated and used for the treatment of eosinophilic esophagitis and was associated with decreases of eosinophil and CCR3+ blood cell numbers in the peripheral blood and esophagus.

A major research effort is currently directed to the identification of molecules that regulate function, recruitment, and production of proinflammatory mediators in late phase allergic reactions that might offer new targets for potential therapy of allergic disorders (*Chapter 11*). These molecules may include eotaxin and similar cytokines that activate and recruit eosinophils through the CCR3 receptor (*Chapter 9*). A CCR3 antagonist has been shown to block chemokine-mediated responses in human eosinophils in vitro and is in clinical trials. Blockade of VLA-4/VCAM-1 adhesion is yet another novel pathway for inhibition of recruitment of eosinophils and other inflammatory cells to inflamed tissues, and α4 integrin antagonists to VLA4 have inhibited early and late allergic responses in animal studies. Similarly, there may also be a role for current nonimmunologic therapies that may also target cytokines as a secondary pharmacologic effect. For example, lidocaine has been shown to inhibit IL-5-mediated survival and activation of eosinophils, and its use in children with asthma has demonstrated a steroid-sparing effect. There is also a growing body of evidence for the use of anti-TNF-α drugs in the treatment of allergic diseases and asthma. These agents, traditionally developed for the treatment of inflammatory conditions such as rheumatoid arthritis, may also have a role in controlling inflammation in these disorders.

Conclusion

The allergic diseases and asthma represent some of the most common tissue-damaging expressions of the immune response in disease, and their pathogenesis involves both the characteristics of the allergen as well as genetic susceptibility of the affected host. These diseases are, for the most part, caused by a specialized class of antibody, i.e., IgE antibody, which mediates the early and late phases of acute allergic inflammation in conjunction with Th2 cytokine responses. Later stages of allergic inflammation lead to recruitment and participation of Th1 and Th17 and further release of mediators and cytokines, leading to chronic inflammation, sometimes with the irreversible changes of tissue remodeling. A fundamental deficiency of Treg cells has also been recently recognized to play an important role in the pathogenesis of the allergic diseases. The management of these disorders depends upon a carefully taken history, appropriate in vivo and in vitro diagnostic tests, followed by a comprehensive management program beginning with identification and elimination of the offending allergen through environmental control, pharmacotherapy, and, in more refractory cases, the use of immunotherapy. With the continual discovery of novel immunologic mechanisms of allergic inflammation and the multitude of cellular and humoral factors, e.g., IgE, cytokines, and chemokines that collectively contribute to various clinical patterns of allergic disease, the study and management of allergic diseases has been given a more rational approach to the diagnosis and treatment of these clinically perplexing entities that were once diagnostic and therapeutic orphans.

Case Studies: Clinical Relevance

Let us now return to the case studies of anaphylaxis, allergic rhinitis, asthma, and allergic eczema and urticaria presented earlier and review some of the major points of the clinical presentation and how they relate to the immune system.

Case Study 1: Anaphylaxis

- This is a classic example of a drug allergy/anaphylaxis caused by a Type I allergic reaction to penicillin. The symptomatology is caused by an IgE antibody to penicillin, which when fixed to the cell membrane of a mediator cell, e.g., mast cell, and exposed to a penicillin antigen, causes the release of pharmacologically

Case Studies: Clinical Relevance (continued)

vasoactive amines that led to the increased vascular permeability and erythema causing generalized urticaria, facial angioedema, and hypotension.

- This case also illustrates other potential sources of offending environmental antigens (i.e., latex, foods, perioperative medications, etc.) that need to be considered in the differential diagnosis of anaphylaxis. Of note, food ingredients are increasingly becoming recognized as causes of severe allergic reactions, and it may be important to consider low-level exposures from additives derived from these foods that may be found in certain drugs or other therapeutic preparations.
- The skin test introduced a small amount of penicillin antigen and elicited the local allergic reaction of a wheal (localized collection of edema fluid in the dermis) and flare (localized redness) that confirmed the diagnosis. Management of anaphylaxis should include avoidance of the causative agent, prompt administration of epinephrine, and aggressive intravenous fluid administration to combat hypovolemia resulting from extreme vasodilation/third spacing and hypotension.

Case Study 2: Allergic Rhinitis and Asthma

- This patient presented with allergic rhinitis and moderately persistent asthma, most likely allergen-induced.
- The respiratory allergy was the result of allergic inflammation of the nasal mucosa and respiratory epithelia brought about by another Type I reaction, presumably due to tree pollen (since the symptoms of nasal congestion and wheezing were seasonal and occurred primarily in the spring).
- The co-involvement of allergic rhinitis and asthma is well established and illustrates the continuity of the linings of the upper and lower airways, i.e., the "united airways," which can result in an allergic reaction following exposure to an allergen.
- The past history of eczema as a child suggests an atopic predisposition for the production of elevated levels of IgE antibody, which are central to the pathogenesis of both the upper airway involvement (allergic rhinitis) as well as lower airway involvement (allergic asthma).
- This case also illustrates the importance of a carefully taken history. The patient's good therapeutic response to antihistamines is supportive of the diagnosis of allergic disease.
- The involvement in the spring suggests a seasonal pattern consistent with seasonal allergic rhinitis (SAR) in contrast to perennial allergic rhinitis (PAR), where symptoms would occur all year.

Case Study 3: Allergic Eczema and Urticaria

- This case illustrates an allergic reaction involving the skin in two types of diseases caused by a Type I allergic reaction: (1) allergic eczema and (2) urticaria (hives).
- The history elicited different patterns of symptoms seen in allergic eczema that were characterized by chronicity with more protracted involvement of the skin with evidence of chronic inflammation, in contrast to urticaria, which was transitory in nature and with more acute inflammatory responses of edema and pruritus.
- Again, a carefully taken history helped elicit a strong family history of allergic (atopic) disease and consideration of several possible etiologies for acute urticaria, such as drugs, infection, and foods as well as autoimmune disease triggers, i.e., autoimmune thyroiditis commonly seen in females and sometimes a cause of chronic urticaria). As with most cases of urticaria, the etiology is rarely revealed and the management is based upon pharmacologic treatment.

Key Points

- Allergy is best viewed as a specialized case of immunity in which the reaction to foreign material terminates in a deleterious outcome and may be considered as one of several types of immunologically mediated diseases affecting humans directed at exogenous antigens.
- Most, but not all, of the allergic disorders are caused by IgE antibody in a Type I hypersensitivity reaction caused by the release of pharmacologically active preformed and newly synthesized mediators from mediator cells, i.e., mast cells and basophils, following the cross-linking of allergen with membrane-associated IgE fixed to the high-affinity FcεR1 receptor on these cells.
- Anaphylaxis represents the most serious manifestation of allergic disease mediated by the immediate Type I hypersensitivity response and clinically consists of dermatological and mucosal involvement,

e.g., hives and angioedema, respiratory, e.g., wheezing and laryngeal edema, cardiovascular, e.g., hypotension and shock, gastrointestinal, e.g., vomiting and diarrhea, and general symptoms of systemic vasodilation and edema occurring acutely after exposure to an allergen in a specifically sensitized individual.

- The allergic diseases are characterized by high age-related dependency during infancy and childhood associated with maturational effects of the immune response on the expression of allergic disease—i.e., the "atopic march" that shows a progressive development from gastrointestinal, e.g., GI allergy, to dermatologic, e.g., atopic eczema, to respiratory involvement, e.g., asthma.
- The increased prevalence of allergic diseases in recent years has been attributed to the "hygiene hypothesis" that suggests that the increase results from a decrease in the frequency of childhood infection brought about by increased sanitation and more effective antimicrobial control. This, in turn, has decreased the normal inductive stimulus of microbial exposure of Th1 development with a predominance of the allergy pathogenic Th2 influence.
- Several in vivo, e.g., skin tests, and in vitro allergy tests are available for total and specific IgE antibody.
- A variety of therapeutic strategies are now available for treating allergic diseases and asthma, including antihistamines, oral steroids, inhaled and intranasal steroids, leukotriene modifiers, theophylline, anticholinergic agents, bronchodilators, cromones, and adrenaline/epinephrine.
- Several immunomodulatory strategies are now available for the management of allergic diseases, including allergen-specific immunotherapy (subcutaneous and/or sublingual specific allergen immunotherapy) and the use of monoclonal antibody or anticytokine therapies.

Study Questions/Critical Thinking

1. Each of the following is a clinical condition that has been associated with Type III Gell and Coombs hypersensitivity response mechanism EXCEPT:

   a. Post-streptococcal glomerulonephritis
   b. Allergic bronchopulmonary aspergillosis (ABPA)
   c. Graves' disease
   d. Extrinsic allergic alveolitis

2. Choose the IgE molecule domain that binds to the α1 domain of the IgE FcεR1 receptor:

   a. Cε2 domain
   b. VD
   c. Cε3 domain
   d. Cε1 domain

3. Each of the following are antibody allergic reactions EXCEPT:

   a. Peanut allergy
   b. Penicillin allergy
   c. Allergy to Hymenoptera
   d. Opioid allergy

4. A four-year-old child presents to the pediatric clinic with a history of dysphagia and chronic gastroesophageal reflux disease (GERD) with frequent emesis despite use of antireflux medications. Esophageal biopsy reveals an inflammatory reaction confined to the esophagus and characterized by the presence of more than 10 eosinophils per 40X HPF. What is the most likely diagnosis?

   a. GERD
   b. Wegener's syndrome
   c. Crohn's disease
   d. Allergic eosinophilic esophagitis (AEE)

5. Each of the following are mechanisms thought to be involved in the pathophysiology of atopic eczema EXCEPT:

   a. Skin barrier dysfunction
   b. Complement deficiencies
   c. Mutations affecting innate immune pattern-recognition receptors (PRRs)
   d. An exaggerated Th2 response

Suggested Reading

Akdis CA, Akdis M. Mechanisms of allergen-specific immunotherapy. J Allergy Clin Immunol. 2011; 127: 18–27.

Anderson JA, Adkinson NF Jr. Allergic reactions to drugs and biologic agents. JAMA. 1987; 258: 2891–9.

Asarch A, Barak O, Loo DS, et al. Th17 cells. A new therapeutic target in inflammatory dermatoses. J Dermatolog Treat. 2008; 19: 318–26.

Assa'ad A. Eosinophilic gastrointestinal disorders. Allergy Asthma Proc. 2009; 30: 17–22.

Barnes PJ. New therapies for asthma: is there any progress? Trends Pharmacol Sci. 2010; 31: 335–43

Bieli C, Eder W, Frei R, et al. PARSIFAL study group: a polymorphism in CD14 modifies the effect of farm milk consumption on allergic diseases and CD14 gene expression. J Allergy Clin Immunol. 2007; 120: 1308–15.

Boguniewicz M, Leung DY. Recent insights into atopic dermatitis and implications for management of infectious complications. J Allergy Clin Immunol. 2010; 125: 4–13.

Bottema RW, Reijmerink NE, Koppelman GH, et al. Phenotype definition, age, and gender in the genetics of asthma and atopy. Immunol Allergy Clin North Am. 2005; 25: 621–39.

Bourke SJ, Dalphin JC, Boyd G, et al. Hypersensitivity pneumonitis: current concepts. Eur Respir J Suppl. 2001; 32: 81s–92s.

Casale TB, Stokes JR. Future forms of immunotherapy. J Allergy Clin Immunol. 2011; 127: 8–15.

Chahine BG, Bahna SL. The role of the gut mucosal immunity in the development of tolerance against allergy to food. Curr Opin Allergy Clin Immunol. 2010; 10: 220–5.

Chapman MD, Pomés A, Breiteneder H, et al. Nomenclature and structural biology of allergens. J Allergy Clin Immunol. 2007; 119: 414–20.

Cichon S, Martin L, Hennies HC, et al. Increased activity of coagulation factor XII (Hageman factor) causes hereditary angioedema type III. Am J Hum Genet. 2006; 79: 1098–104.

Cochrane Database of Systematic Reviews. Available in Cochrane Library at: www.mrw.interscience.wiley.com/cochrane/probiotics.

Cox L, Nelson H, Lockey R, et al. Allergen immunotherapy: a practice parameter third update. J Allergy Clin Immunol. 2011; 127 Suppl 1: S1–55.

Cox L, Williams B, Sicherer S, et al. Pearls and pitfalls of allergy diagnostic testing: report from the American College of Allergy, Asthma and Immunology/American Academy of Allergy, Asthma and Immunology Specific IgE Test Task Force. Ann Allergy Asthma Immunol. 2008; 101: 580–92.

Creticos PS, Schroeder JT, Hamilton RG, et al. Immune Tolerance Network Group. Immunotherapy with a ragweed-toll-like receptor 9 agonist vaccine for allergic rhinitis. N Engl J Med. 2006; 355: 1445–55.

Creticos PS. The consideration of immunotherapy in the treatment of allergic asthma. J Allergy Clin Immunol. 2000; 105: S559–74.

Davies DE, Wicks J, Powell RM, et al. Airway remodeling in asthma: New insights. J Allergy Clin Immunol. 2003; 111: 215–25.

Deacock SJ. An approach to the patient with urticaria. Clin Exp Immunol. 2008; 153: 151–61.

Dehlink E, Baker AH, Yen E, et al. Relationships between levels of serum IgE, cell-bound IgE, and IgE-receptors on peripheral blood cells in a pediatric population. PLoS One. 2010; 5.

Demain JG, Minaei AA, Tracy JM. Anaphylaxis and insect allergy. Curr Opin Allergy Clin Immunol. 2010; 10: 318–22.

Devereux G. The increase in the prevalence of asthma and allergy: food for thought. Nat Rev Immunol. 2006; 6: 869–74.

Di Sabatino A, Corazzo GR. Coeliac disease. Lancet. 2009; 373: 1480–93.

Durham SR, Leung DY. One hundred years of allergen immunotherapy: time to ring the changes. J Allergy Clin Immunol. 2011; 127: 3–7.

Ebo DG, Verweij MM, De Knop KJ, et al. Hereditary angioedema in childhood: an approach to management. Paediatr Drugs. 2010; 12: 257–68.

Expert Panel Report 3 (EPR-3). Guidelines for the diagnosis and management of asthma—summary report 2007. J Allergy Clin Immunol. 2007; 120: S94–138.

Finegold I, Dockhorn RJ, Ein D, et al. Immunotherapy throughout the decades: from Noon to now. Ann Allergy Asthma Immunol. 2010; 105: 328–36.

Finegold I, Oppenheimer J. Immunotherapy: the next 100 years. Ann Allergy Asthma Immunol. 2010; 105: 394–8.

Gomez MB, Torres MJ, Mayorga C, et al. Immediate allergic reactions to betalactams: facts and controversies. Curr Opin Allergy Clin Immunol. 2004; 4: 261–6.

Gordon BR. Patch testing for allergies. Curr Opin Otolaryngol Head Neck Surg. 2010; 18: 191–4.

Greenhawt MJ, Chernin AS, Howe L, et al. The safety of the H1N1 influenza A vaccine in egg allergic individuals. Ann Allergy Asthma Immunol. 2010; 105: 387–93.

Greenhawt MJ, Li JT, Bernstein DI, et al. Administering influenza vaccine to egg allergic recipients: a focused practice parameter update. Ann Allergy Asthma Immunol. 2011; 106: 11–6.

Gruchalla RS. Drug allergy. J Allergy Clin Immunol. 2003; 111 Suppl 2: S548–59.

Halken S. Prevention of allergic disease in childhood: clinical and epidemiological aspects of primary and secondary allergy prevention. Pediatr Allergy Immunol. 2004; 15: 9–32.

Hamilton RG. Diagnosis and treatment of allergy to hymenoptera venoms. Curr Opin Allergy Clin Immunol. 2010; 10: 323–9.

Harle DG, Baldo BA. Identification of penicillin allergenic determinants that bind IgE antibodies in the sera of subjects with penicillin allergy. Mol Immunol. 1990; 27: 1063–71.

Holgate ST. A look at the pathogenesis of asthma: the need for a change in direction. Discov Med. 2010; 9: 439–47.

Holgate ST. Cytokine and anti-cytokine therapy for the treatment of asthma and allergic disease. Cytokine. 2004; 28: 152–7.

Holloway JW, Yang IA, Holgate ST. Genetics of allergic disease. J Allergy Clin Immunol. 2010; 125: S81–94.

Hsieh MH, Versalovic J. The human microbiome and probiotics: implications for pediatrics. Curr Prob in Pediatr and Adolesc Health Care. 2008; 38: 309–27.

Hu ZQ, Zhao WH, Shimamura T. Regulation of mast cell development by inflammatory factors. Curr Med Chem. 2007; 14: 3044–50.

Irla M, Küpfer N, Suter T, et al. MHC class II-restricted antigen presentation by plasmacytoid dendritic cells inhibits T cell-mediated autoimmunity. J Exp Med. 2010; 207: 1–15.

Iwamura C, Nakayama T. Role of NKT cells in allergic asthma. Curr Opin Immunol. 2010; 22: 807–13.

Johansson SG, Bieber T, Dahl R, et al. Revised nomenclature for allergy for global use: report of the nomenclature review committee of the World Allergy Organization, October 2003. J Allergy Clin Immunol. 2004; 113: 832–6.

Johansson SG, Haahtela T. World Allergy Organization guidelines for prevention of allergy and allergic asthma, condensed version. Int Arch Allergy Immunol. 2004; 135: 83–92.

Jutel M, Akdis M, Akdis CA. Histamine, histamine receptors and their role in immune pathology. Clin Exp Allergy. 2009; 39:1786–800.

Kaplan AP, Greaves M. Pathogenesis of chronic urticaria. Clin Exp Allergy. 2009; 39: 777–87.

Katz Y, Goldberg MR, Stein M, et al. Oral immunotherapy: ready for prime time? J Allergy Clin Immunol. 2011; 127: 289–90.

Kay AB. Allergy and allergic diseases. Second of two parts. N Eng J Med. 2001; 344: 109–13.

Kraft S, Kinet JP. New developments in FcepsilonRI regulation, function and inhibition. Nat Rev Immunol. 2007; 7: 365–78.

Leung DYM, Boguniewicz M, Howell M, et al. New insights into atopic dermatitis. J Clin Invest. 2004; 113: 651–7.

Long A. Aeroallergen sensitization in asthma: genetics, environment, and pathophysiology. Allergy Asthma Proc. 2010; 31: 89–95.

Maggi E. T cell responses induced by allergen-specific immunotherapy. Clin Exp Immunol. 2010; 161: 10–8.

Maleki SJ, Kopper RA, Shin DS, et al. Structure of the major peanut allergen Ara h 1 may protect IgE-binding epitopes from degradation. J Immunol. 2000; 164: 5844–9.

Marshall GD Jr. A centennial anniversary for allergen immunotherapy: pioneering immunomodulation for atopy and beyond. Ann Allergy Asthma Immunol. 2010; 105: 325.

Martinez FD. Respiratory syncytial virus bronchiolitis and the pathogenesis of childhood asthma. Pediatr Infect Dis J. 2003; 22: S76–82.

Maslowski KM, Mackay CR. Diet, gut microbiota and immune responses. Nat Immunol. 2011; 12: 5–9.

McGrath JA, Uitto J. The filaggrin story: novel insights into skin-barrier function and disease. Trends Mol Med. 2008; 14: 20–7.

Minai-Fleminger Y, Levi-Schaffer F. Mast cells and eosinophils: the two key effector cells in allergic inflammation. Inflamm Res. 2009; 58: 631–8.

National Institutes of Health. National Heart, Lung, and Blood Institute. National Asthma Education and Prevention Program. Expert Panel Report 3: guidelines for the diagnosis and management of asthma. August 2007. NIH publication no. 07-4051. Available at: http://www.nhlbi.nih.gov/guidelines/asthma/index.htm.

NIAID-Sponsored Expert Panel: Boyce JA, Assa'ad A, Burks AW, et al. Guidelines for the diagnosis and management of food allergy in the United States: report of the NIAID-sponsored expert panel. J Allergy Clin Immunol. 2010; 126: S1–58.

Nosbaum A, Hennino A, Berard F, et al. Patch testing in atopic dermatitis patients. Eur J Dermatol. 2010 Jul 9.

Ocmant A, Mulier S, Hanssens L, et al. L basophil activation tests for the diagnosis of food allergy in children. Clin Exp Allergy. 2009; 39: 1234–45.

Oh K, Shen T, Le Gros G, et al. Induction of Th2 type immunity in a mouse system reveals a novel immunoregulatory role of basophils. Blood. 2007; 109: 2921–7.

Okada H, Kuhn C, Feillet H, et al. The 'hygiene hypothesis' for autoimmune and allergic diseases: an update. Clin Exp Immunol. 2010; 160: 1–9.

Oyoshi MK, He R, Kumar L, et al. Cellular and molecular mechanisms in atopic dermatitis. Adv Immunol. 2009; 102: 135–226.

Pichler WJ. Immune mechanism of drug hypersensitivity. Immunol Allergy Clin North Am. 2004; 24: 373–97.

Prinz JC, Endres N, Rank G, et al. Expression of Fc epsilon receptors on activated human T lymphocytes. Eur J Immunol. 1987; 17: 757–61.

Riedl MA, Casillas AM. Adverse drug reactions: types and treatment options. Am Fam Physician. 2003; 68: 1781–90.

Sabra A, Bellanti JA, Rais JM, et al. IgE and non-IgE food allergy. Ann Allergy Asthma Immunol. 2003; 90: 71–6.

Sakata D, Yao C, Narumiya S. Prostaglandin E2, an immunoactivator. J Pharmacol Sci. 2010; 112: 1–5.

Sandilands A, Sutherland C, Irvine AD, et al. Filaggrin in the frontline: role in skin barrier function and disease. J Cell Sci. 2009; 122: 1285–94.

Shakir EM, Cheung DS, Grayson MH. Mechanisms of immunotherapy: a historical perspective. Ann Allergy Asthma Immunol. 2010; 105: 340–7.

Shinohara ML, Cantor H. The bridge between dendritic cells and asthma. Nat Med. 2007; 13: 536–8.

Shreffler WG. Evaluation of basophil activation in food allergy: present and future applications. Curr Opin Allergy Clin Immunol. 2006; 6: 226–33.

Simon D, Simon HU. Eosinophilic disorders. J Allergy Clin Immunol. 2007; 119: 1291–300.

Simon HU, Rothenberg ME, Bochner BS, et al. Refining the definition of hypereosinophilic syndrome. J Allergy Clin Immunol. 2010; 126: 45–9.

Simons FE, Frew AJ, Ansotegui IJ, et al. Risk assessment in anaphylaxis: current and future approaches. J Allergy Clin Immunol. 2007; 120: S2–24.

Simons FE. Anaphylaxis. J Allergy Clin Immunol. 2010; 125: S161–81.

Simons FE. Pharmacologic treatment of anaphylaxis: can the evidence base be strengthened? Curr Opin Allergy Clin Immunol. 2010; 10: 384–93.

Singh RK, Gupta S, Dastidar S, et al. Cysteinyl leukotrienes and their receptors: molecular and functional characteristics. Pharmacology. 2010; 85: 336–49.

Solensky R. Drug desensitization. Immunol Allergy Clin North Am. 2004; 24: 425–43.

Solensky R. Hypersensitivity reactions to beta-lactam antibiotics. Clin Rev Allergy Immunol. 2003; 24: 201–20.

Soroosh P, Doherty TA. Th9 and allergic disease. Immunology. 2009; 127: 450–8.

Spergel JM. From atopic dermatitis to asthma: the atopic march. Ann Allergy Asthma Immunol. 2010; 105: 99–106.

Stein ML, Collins MH, Villanueva JM, et al. Anti-IL-5 (mepolizumab) therapy for eosinophilic esophagitis. J Allergy Clin Immunol. 2006; 118: 1312–9.

Stone KD, Prussin C, Metcalfe DD. IgE, mast cells, basophils, and eosinophils. J Allergy Clin Immunol. 2010; 125: S73–80.

Szentivanyi A. The beta adrenergic theory of the atopic abnormality in bronchial asthma. J. Allergy. 1968; 42: 203–32.

Thomsen SF, Ulrik CS, Kyvik KO, et al. Multivariate genetic analysis of atopy phenotypes in a selected sample of twins. Clin Exp Allergy. 2006; 36: 1382–90.

Thurmond RL, Gelfand EW, Dunford PJ. The role of histamine H1 and H4 receptors in allergic inflammation: the search for new antihistamines. Nat Rev Drug Discov. 2008; 7: 41–53.

Till SJ, Francis JN, Nouri-Aria K, et al. Mechanisms of immunotherapy. J Allergy Clin Immunol. 2004; 113: 1025–34.

Torres MJ, Blanca M. The complex clinical picture of beta-lactam hypersensitivity: penicillins, cephalosporins, monobactams, carbapenems, and clavams. Med Clin North Am. 2010; 94: 805–20.

Van der Velden VH, Hulsmann AR. Autonomic innervation of human airways: structure, function, and pathophysiology in asthma. Neuroimmunomodulation. 1999; 6: 145–59.

Vandenbulcke L, Bachert C, Van Cauwenberge P, et al. The innate immune system and its role in allergic disorders. Int Arch Allergy Immunol. 2006; 139: 159–65.

Vivier E, Raulet DH, Moretta A, et al. Innate or adaptive immunity? The example of natural killer cells. Science. 2011; 331: 44–9.

von Mutius E, Vercelli D. Farm living: effects on childhood asthma and allergy. Nat Rev Immunol. 2010; 10: 861–8.

von Mutius E. Asthma and allergies in rural areas of Europe. Proc Am Thor Soc. 2007; 4: 212–6.

Webb LM, Feldmann M. Critical role of CD28/B7 costimulation in the development of human Th2 cytokine-producing cells. Blood. 1995; 86: 3479–86.

Wisniewski JA, Borish L. Novel cytokines and cytokine-producing T cells in allergic disorders. Allergy Asthma Proc. 2011; 32: 83–94.

Wynn TA. Basophils trump dendritic cells as APCs for T(H)2 responses. Nat Immunol. 2009; 10: 679–81.

Chapter 19

Tolerance, Autoimmunity, and Autoinflammation

Vasileios Kyttaris, MD
George C. Tsokos, MD

Case Studies

Case Study 1

A previously healthy thirty-year-old white female was seen in the emergency room with a one-week history of fever, generalized joint pain, and a rash on her face (Figure 19-1A). During the past week, she noticed that she was urinating more frequently than usual but was otherwise healthy prior to this episode. She denied a history of recent illness or contact with any ill persons. Physical examination revealed her to be in mild distress with a temperature of 102° F. She had an erythematous rash over the skin of both cheeks and the chin. Auscultation of her chest revealed a pleural rub over the left anterior chest wall. All the metacarpophalangeal joints of her hands were swollen and tender to palpation. Laboratory examination showed a white blood cell count of 3,000/mm^3, a hemoglobin level of 12 g/dL, a platelet count of 100,000/mm^3, and a serum creatinine level of 1.2 mg/dL. Urinalysis showed significant protein and numerous red blood cell casts. An X-ray

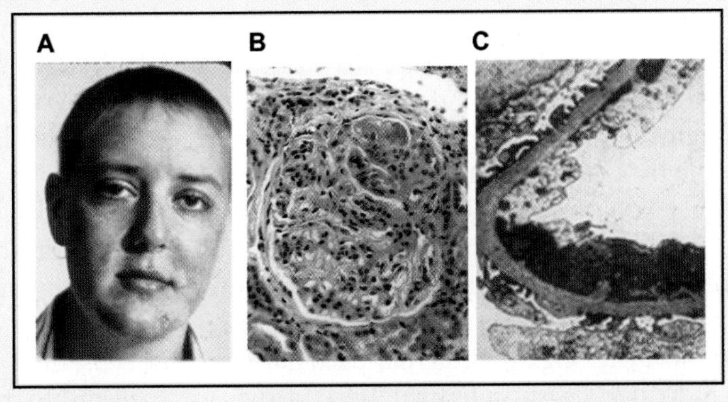

Figure 19-1. Panel A: A young woman with fever, a facial rash, and joint pain. Panel B: Her kidney biopsy showed infiltration of the renal glomeruli with inflammatory cells by light microscopy. Panel C: Electron microscopy showed electron-dense deposits adjacent to the glomerular basement membrane.

LEARNING OBJECTIVES

When you have completed this chapter, you should be able to:

- Understand the concepts and significance of central and peripheral tolerance
- Describe the differences between autoimmunity and autoimmune disease
- List the major systemic and organ-specific autoimmune diseases
- Describe the major theories of pathogenesis of the autoimmune diseases
- Explain the association of autoimmune diseases with MHC
- Describe the major clinical features of the most important autoimmune diseases
- List the current treatment modalities for the autoimmune diseases
- Summarize the clinical applications of tolerance, autoimmunity, and autoinflammation in health and disease

Case Studies: (continued)

of the hands revealed only soft tissue swelling without joint damage. Following hospitalization, a test for antinuclear antibodies (ANAs) was positive with a titer of 1:1280. Complement C3 levels were 50 mg/dl (normal value, 90 to 180 mg/dl) and a test for anti-double-stranded DNA (anti-dsDNA) antibody revealed a positive titer of 1:160. A kidney biopsy performed two days after admission showed cellular infiltration of the glomeruli with crescent formation by light microscopy (Figure 19-1B) and subendothelial electron-dense deposits by electron microscopy (Figure 19-1C).

Case Study 2

A ten-year-old boy was brought to his pediatrician because of increased lethargy and generalized weakness of greater than two weeks duration. His mother noticed that he seemed very hungry, more thirsty than usual, and had increased frequency of urination. She recalled that he had a recent viral infection a few weeks prior to the onset of these symptoms. Physical examination revealed an acutely ill patient, with a rapid pulse of 100/min, decreased skin turgor, a fruity mouth odor, and diffuse abdominal tenderness. Laboratory findings showed a blood glucose level of 350 mg/dL and the presence of glucose and ketones in his urine. He was admitted and intravenous fluids and insulin were administered. Further laboratory testing revealed a positive test for serum anti-islet cell antibodies and anti-insulin antibodies.

Case Study 3

A twenty-five-year-old woman is referred to a neurologist with a chief complaint of difficulty with vision. She is employed as a software developer and stated that the computer screen never really bothered her until recently. Two weeks prior to the visit, she experienced an episode of double vision that was made worse when she turned her head to the left. The double vision persisted for a few days then went away only to return two days later. Although on initial evaluation she did not complain of any other problems, upon further questioning she admitted to having trouble urinating recently with increased frequency and urgency. She also disclosed that her right hand felt numb for the past week. On physical examination, the patient was unable to perform left lateral gaze with her right eye. She also had decreased perception of touch on her right palm and increased bilateral knee reflexes. The remainder of the neurological and general medical examinations was normal. Routine laboratory tests were unremarkable. Analysis of her cerebrospinal fluid showed increased immune globulin and oligoclonal bands on protein electrophoresis. The patient's neurologist ordered an MRI of the brain that showed hyperintense signals in periventricular areas of the brain.

Introduction

For the first half of the twentieth century, the doctrine that formed the central tenet of immunology was that of "horror autotoxicus," the term originally put forth by the brilliant German bacteriologist-immunologist Paul Ehrlich (1854–1915). The term literally referred to the innate aversion of the body to immunological self-destruction and described the belief that the immune system should only be directed to exogenous foreign substances and not to its own tissues. We now know that healthy individuals have a smoldering autoimmune response which at times escapes control and attacks self elements and does so in certain diseases referred to as autoimmune disorders. A major research effort today is being directed to the study of how the immune system is able to discriminate between self and nonself and how to minimize the possibility of autoimmune disease resulting from self-attack while optimizing more effective, beneficial immune responses against foreign, potentially harmful agents, e.g., pathogenic microbes, as well as altered self-constituents, e.g., malignant cells. Moreover, since many antigens encountered by the immune system are not harmful, e.g., commensal bacteria and food substances in the gastrointestinal tract, active mechanisms to prevent an immunologic attack against these innocuous antigens also need to be in place (*Chapter 8*). The immune system, therefore, has devised many checks and balances to circumvent autoimmune disease. These mechanisms induce a state of specific immunologic unresponsiveness referred to as central or peripheral immunologic tolerance, each having a non-redundant function in maintaining antigen receptor diversity (*Chapter 7*) while providing safeguards to effectively curtail self-reactivity.

The concept of tolerance was first described in 1901 when Ehrlich postulated that certain contrivances can prevent the immune reaction against self-antigens. Later, Owen observed that non-identical dizygotic twin calves sharing the same placenta did not react to each other's erythrocytes throughout their lifetime. He hypothesized that exposure of one animal to the other's antigens through their common placenta *in utero* rendered each animal's immune system specifically unresponsive, or tolerant, to the other animal's antigens. Medawar and Brent reached similar conclusions in 1953 when they injected cells from one mouse strain into a neonatal mouse from a different strain and noted that the latter did not react to skin grafts from the former. At about the same time, Burnet put forth the theory of clonal selection that postulated that each antigenic encounter of a host with a foreign substance selects a particular immune cell clone that in turn proliferates and gives rise to a clone of daughter cells with the same specificity. Immunologic (self) tolerance was then thought to be the consequence of a series of mechanisms that deleted the forbidden clones, i.e., lymphocytic clones that recognized non-harmful antigens.

Among the many discoveries in recent years that have elucidated a better understanding of the pathogenetic mechanisms of autoimmune disease is the resurgent interest in suppressor or T regulatory (**Treg**) cells (*Chapters 7* and *9*). This renewed interest in Treg cells has provided the basis to understand how the normal immune system is orchestrated by the endogenous production of this T cell subpopulation that is highly specialized for suppressive function and that when deficient in number or function can be a chief cause of allergic, autoimmune, and other inflammatory diseases specifically due to a loss of immunologic tolerance. This chapter will describe the physiologic processes that are responsible for immunologic tolerance, the pathogenic processes that lead to autoimmune diseases, and the management of these disorders.

Tolerance

One of the most important immunologic principles required for an understanding of autoimmunity and autoimmune disease is the concept of tolerance, which refers to specific immunological unresponsiveness to an antigen resulting from a previous exposure to the same antigen (*Chapters 1* and *7*). Although the most important form of tolerance is non-reactivity to self-antigens, which occurs in the developing fetus during normal ontogeny of the immune system (*Chapter 2*), it is also possible to experimentally induce tolerance to non-self-antigens after birth. When an antigen induces tolerance, it is termed a tolerogen (*Chapter 1*). Tolerance is both antigen and cell clone specific, implying that the immune non-reactivity is not only selective for the tolerogen that induced it, but also that immune responsiveness against other antigens is maintained. It is important to differentiate between tolerance and generalized immune suppression (*Chapter 11*). For example, the lack of response in an otherwise normal host to a potential autoantigen, such as thyroglobulin, reflects tolerance, whereas the lack of response to a panel of antigens brought about by cyclosporine treatment of a patient receiving a kidney transplant reflects immunosuppression (*Chapters 11* and *22*)

Where Does Tolerance Take Place? Central Versus Peripheral Tolerance

For the induction of tolerance, it is critical that both B and T cells become educated (*Chapters 6* and *7*) on how to handle different antigens. The educational process takes place in both the **central** (i.e., the bone marrow and the thymus) and **peripheral** lymphoid organs and tissues (i.e., the spleen and the lymph nodes) (*Chapters 2* and *7*). In these settings, the lymphocytes either become immune competent or tolerant toward the specific antigen that they encounter. There are differences in the mechanisms of tolerance induction and maintenance between T and B cells as well as between central and peripheral lymphoid organs. Shown in Table 19-1 is a classification of the forms of tolerance exhibited by T cells and B cells showing the mechanisms of induction in both of their central and peripheral components.

Table 19-1. Mechanisms of tolerance

T cell tolerance
Central T cell tolerance
Positive selection
Negative selection
Peripheral T cell tolerance
Clonal deletion
Ignorance
Anergy
Lack of co-stimulation
Expression of suppressive molecules
Immune regulation
Direct cell contact
Production of IL-10, TGF-β
B cell tolerance
Central B cell tolerance
Positive selection
Negative selection
Peripheral B cell tolerance
Anergy
Incomplete stimulation
Engagement of suppressor receptors
Receptor editing
Immune regulation

Central T Cell Tolerance: Positive and Negative Selection

Based on the initial hypothesis of Burnet that a central deletion of "forbidden clones" leads to elimination of potentially self-reactive clones, experimental models using transgenic animals provided solid evidence that such mechanisms are of paramount importance for the induction of self-tolerance (*Chapter 25*). After the double negative (**DN**) CD4−CD8− T cell progenitor cells enter the cortex of the thymus, they rearrange their T cell receptors (**TCRs**) and become double positive (**DP**) CD4+CD8+ thymocytes (*Chapters 2* and *7*). From the potential 10^9 different TCR structures found within the thymus, only a fraction can be found in the peripheral tissues, which indicates that many of these cells are eliminated. In the first step of T cell selection within the thymus, called positive selection, only DP cells that bear a TCR that can recognize the self-peptide loaded major histocompatibility (**MHC**) molecule (either MHC-I or MHC-II) on thymic epithelial cells survive (Figure 19-2). T cells with strong affinity to MHC undergo apoptosis and are eliminated. In this initial cell selection, only T cells that display a moderate affinity for MHC survive. T cells that express TCR that do not recognize and fail to interact with a self-peptide loaded MHC are ignored and die by neglect (*Chapter 7*). If the TCR on the DP thymocyte recognizes the peptide-loaded MHC-I molecules and at the same time CD8 interacts with the MHC-I, the T cell receives signals that prevent its death and continued maturation is promoted. During progression along its maturational pathway, the T cell will continue to display the TCR CD8 co-receptor as a single CD8 single positive (**SP**) T cell and will lose expression of its CD4. An entirely analogous process leads to the development of a CD4 SP T cell when the CD4 coreceptors interact with the MHC-II molecule (*Chapter 7*).

In the next step of T cell selection, referred to as negative selection (Figure 19-2), the T cells that bear TCRs that can interact with both the MHC and an antigen come in close proximity with thymic epithelial cells that express on their surfaces MHC-autoantigen complexes. Negative selection may occur either at the DP stage in the cortex or in the newly generated SP T cells in the medulla (*Chapter 7*). In either case, T cells that recognize autoantigens on the surface of the thymic epithelial cells undergo apoptosis, thus preventing peripheral autoimmunity. These autoantigens are proteins derived from a diversity of tissues and organs and are expressed on the thymic epithelial cells at least partly under the regulation of the transcription factor AutoImmune REgulator (**AIRE**). Lack of AIRE in both mice and humans has been shown to result in organ specific autoimmunity; the Autoimmune Polyglandular Syndrome Type 1 (**APS**-1) in patients without AIRE is characterized by immune-mediated damage to the parathyroid and adrenal glands (*Chapter 16*). The key factor in determining positive and negative selection is the strength of the antigen recognition by the maturing T cell; low-avidity recognition leads to positive selection, and high-avidity recognition induces negative selection.

Peripheral T Cell Tolerance

The negative-selection process involved in central T cell tolerance, however, is not foolproof. Not all autoantigens are expressed in the thymus, so mechanisms must be in place in peripheral lymphoid tissues to eliminate or suppress the self-reactive T cell clones that escape from the thymus. In addition to self-antigens, the presentation of nonself-antigens can also result in inappropriate forms of tolerance. In one experimental model of autoimmunity, in

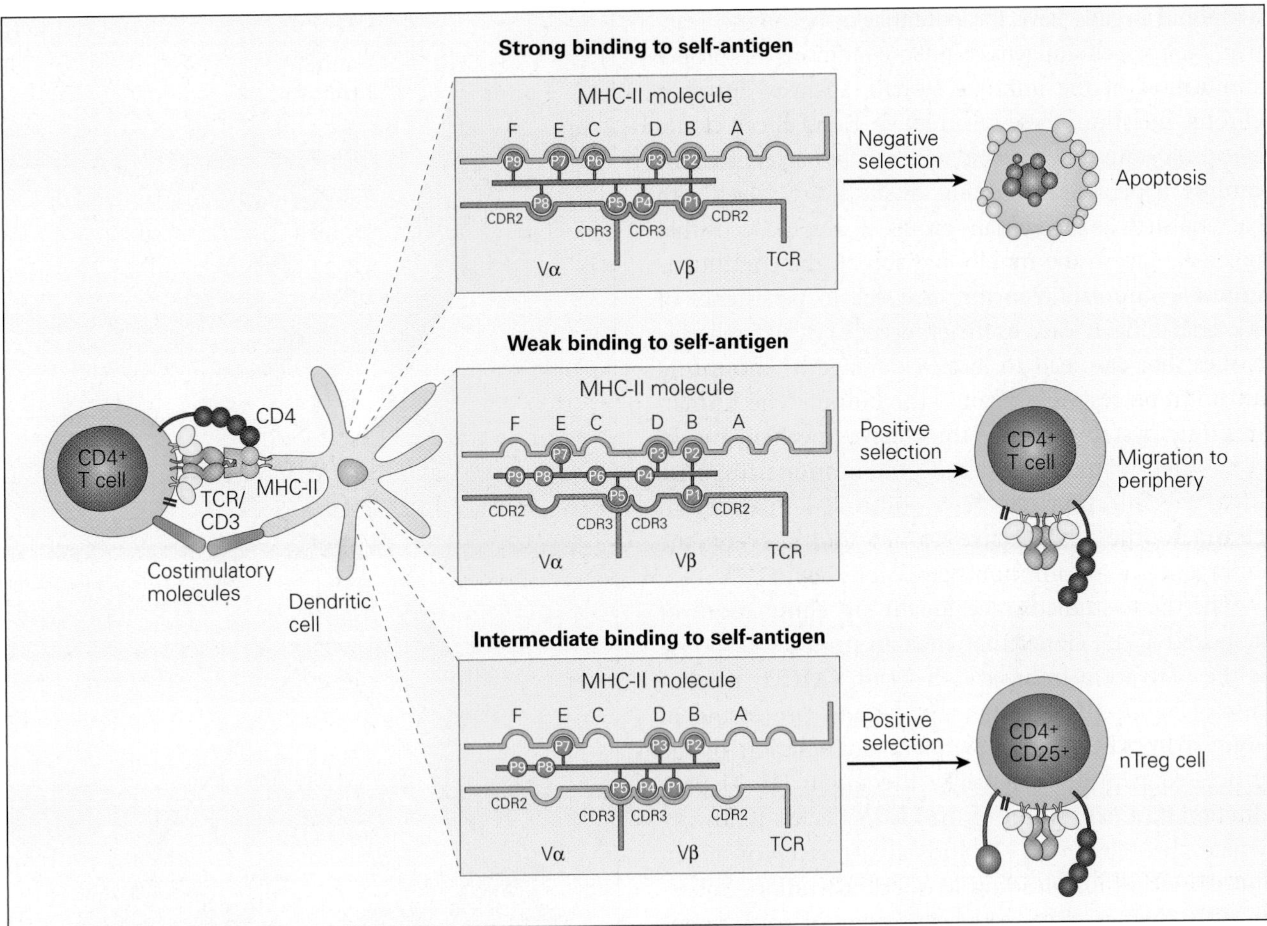

Figure 19-2. Positive and negative selection in the thymus. CD4+ T cells that recognize self-antigens expressed on thymocytes in the context of MHC-II molecules undergo apoptosis. The key factor in determining positive and negative selection is the strength of the antigen recognition by the maturing T cell; low-avidity recognition leads to positive selection, and high-avidity recognition induces negative selection. It is proposed that at this stage, Treg (CD4+CD25+) cells that are autoantigen-specific are generated by intermediate degrees of binding.

which lymphocytic choriomeningitis virus (**LCM**) was inoculated into mice embryos, it was found that those mice later in life were chronically infected with LCM with no immune response to LCM, but paradoxically showed an appropriate immune response to other antigens and were therefore considered tolerant to LCM. In this case, it was presumed that viral antigens were presented to T cells in the thymus and that thymocyte clones that recognized them underwent cell death (negative selection). Thus, in this model system, the LCM antigens that were introduced early in gestation were handled as self-antigens by the maturing immune system and resulted in tolerance. However, in certain congenital intrauterine infections in the human, e.g., **TORCH** infections, an acronym for Toxoplasmosis/*Toxoplasma gondii* Ltd, other infections (Hepatitis B, syphilis, varicella-zoster virus, HIV, and Parvovirus B19), Rubella, Cytomegalovirus, and Herpes simplex, the infected fetus can make antibody, i.e., IgM antibody, and therefore this experimental murine model may not be entirely relevant in the human.

Several self-reactive clones have been isolated from the peripheral blood of healthy people. For example, T and B cells isolated from individuals without multiple sclerosis can react *in vitro* to myelin basic protein (**MBP**), a self-antigen that is one of the targets of the immune response in multiple sclerosis. There have been many proposed mechanisms that contribute to peripheral T cell tolerance. For ease of discussion, these mechanisms can be broadly classified into the following categories: clonal deletion, ignorance, anergy, and immune regulation (Table 19-1).

Clonal Deletion

The self-reactive clones that escape negative selection in the thymus and reach the secondary (peripheral) lymphoid organs have the potential of becoming reactive against self-antigens. Under conditions of proper stimulation of the immune system, such as during a chronic infection, these self-reactive T and B cell clones can proliferate. An example is subacute bacterial endocarditis, a persistent infection of the heart valves with bacteria such as the viridans group of streptococcus that normally live in the mouth and throat; the continuous immune stimulation in this case due to persistence of bacterial antigen leads to the emergence of self-reactive clones that can lead to kidney damage by mounting an immune response against the kidney. The human immune system should, thus, have mechanisms in place that promptly terminate the immune response once the infection has been controlled in order to eliminate the self-reactive clones and prevent the emergence of autoimmunity (*Chapter 12*).

The best studied mechanism of elimination of activated T cell clones that ends an immune response is the Activation-Induced Cell Death (**AICD**) mechanism (Figure 19-3). Upon uptake and processing of antigen by APCs and subsequent presentation of the processed peptide to T cells, interleukin (**IL**-2) production and expression of the IL-2R occurs following which the released IL-2 binds to its receptor in an autocrine fashion, leading to T cell activation. Subsequently, there is an increased expression of death receptors on the surface of the activated T cells that belong to the family of tumor necrosis factor (**TNF**) receptors (*Chapter 9*). The best characterized among these are fragment apoptosis stimulating (**Fas**) (CD95) and its ligand (**FasL**), both of which are expressed on the surface of the activated T cells. The FasL also can be cleaved and released from the T cell as a soluble FasL (s-FasL). The subsequent interaction of the membrane-associated Fas on one T cell with either the soluble or the membrane-associated FasL on another T cell causes apoptosis of the T cell expressing Fas via the caspase pathway (*Chapter 9*). This mechanism leads the activated T cells to undergo AICD, thus ending the immune response. This mechanism is also important for the elimination of self-reactive T cells that expand during repeated activation by an antigenic stimulus.

The importance of the AICD and the Fas pathway in eliminating self-reactive T cell clones has largely been obtained by the study of a strain of mice with defective apoptosis due to a mutation in the Fas gene. The lpr mouse strain (named for the

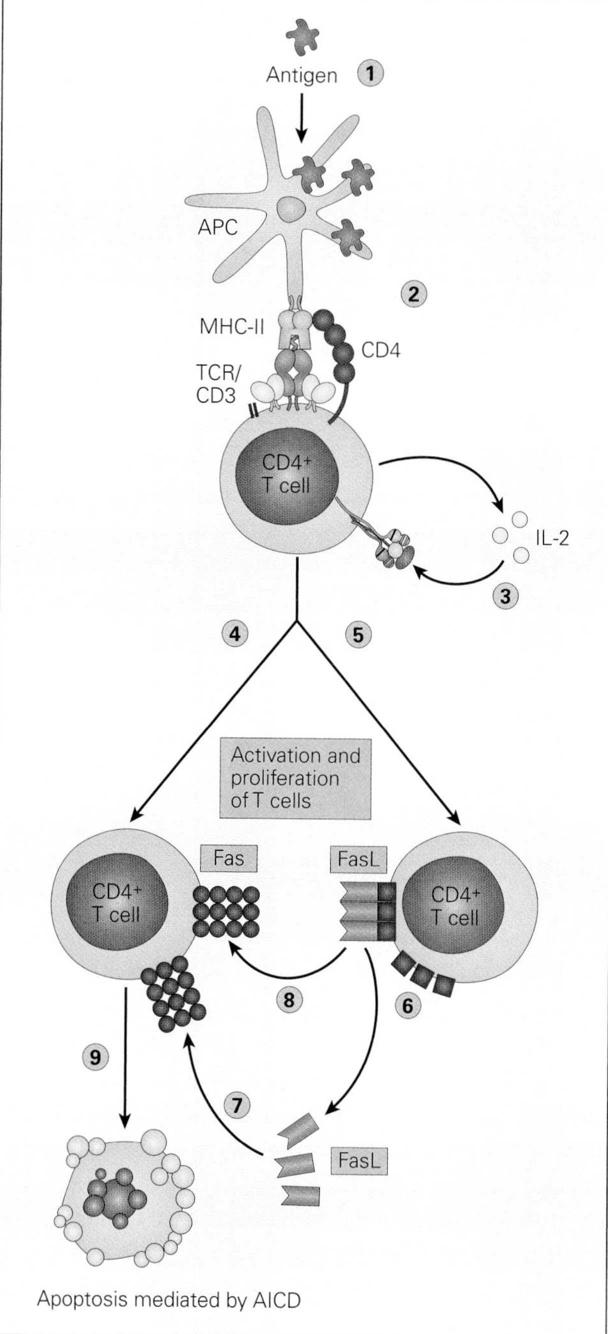

Figure 19-3. Schematic representation of activation-induced cell death (AICD). Upon uptake and processing of antigen by APCs (1) and subsequent presentation of the processed peptide to a CD4+ T cell (2), IL-2 production and expression of the IL-2R occurs followed by their autocrine binding (3), leading to T cell activation. Activated T cells express Fas (4) and FasL (5) on their surfaces or as soluble s-FasL after cleavage of the membrane-associated FasL (6). The interaction of Fas either with s-FasL (7) or with membrane-associated FasL (8) leads to apoptosis (9) by activation-induced cell death (AICD), thus ending the immune response.

lymphoproliferation seen in these mice) does not express Fas on its T cells and therefore displays an expanded lymphocyte population in secondary lymphoid organs that results in profound lymphadenopathy. Furthermore, these Fas-deficient mice exhibit significant self-reactivity and produce a wide variety of autoantibodies. The end result of this dysregulated immune cell expansion is expressed in autoimmune damage of many organs, such as the kidney. The phenotype of lpr mice is evocative of the human disease systemic lupus erythematosus, although the underlying etiologies are different.

There is also another rare human disease called autoimmune lymphoproliferative syndrome (**ALPS**) that is caused by mutations similar to the lpr mouse mutations in either the Fas or the FasL gene (termed ALPS 1a and 1b, respectively) (*Chapter 16*). Patients with these mutations have significant lymphadenopathy and also produce an array of autoantibodies.

The Fas pathway is also affected by interleukin-2 (**IL-2**), the principal cytokine that is responsible for the activation of the T cell after its interaction with antigen (*Chapter 9*). Paradoxically, IL-2 initially helps the T cells proliferate but eventually can lead to AICD by increasing the expression of FasL (Figure 19-3). IL-2 also helps attenuate the immune response by downregulating "survival molecules" such as (FlICE inhibitory protein (**FLIP**) and FADD-like IL-1beta-converting enzyme (**FLICE**), which are proteins that inhibit AICD by preventing the assembly of the Fas death receptor complex referred to as the death-inducing signaling complex (**DISC**) (*Chapter 9*). Thus, IL-2 paradoxically not only acts as a T cell growth factor but also helps downregulate the immune response once it is not required.

Ignorance

Another mechanism that potentially contributes to peripheral T cell tolerance is ignorance. Although T cells found in peripheral lymphoid tissues of healthy individuals have been shown to react with self-antigens *in vitro*, this does not commonly occur *in vivo*. It is thought that the T cells ignore certain self-antigens because either the antigens are located in "privileged" sites or sanctuaries that are inaccessible to recognition by the immune system (e.g., the brain or eye) or have low immunogenicity (i.e., low levels of antigen or low binding affinity of antigen to the TCR).

Sympathetic ophthalmia is an example of an autoimmune disease caused by the release of sequestered ocular self-antigens into the circulation, interacting with self-reactive immune cells that had not been eliminated by negative selection and that progress to autoimmune organ damage. In this disorder, severe inflammatory damage to both eyes occurs a few days to several weeks after an injury to one eye. It is thought that the trauma to one eye releases self-antigens that in turn activate self-reactive immune cells, leading to intense granulomatous inflammation of the injured as well as the unaffected eye. The basis for this hypothesis is supported by the belief that the immune system normally is not exposed to ocular antigens (i.e., the eye is inaccessible). It is unclear, however, if these self-antigens were truly sequestered and were not actually present outside the eye prior to the trauma. When injury occurs, the ocular contents are released into the circulation, and upon interaction of these self-antigens with self-reactive cells, an inflammatory environment is created in and around the eye globe that provides both the antigenic stimulus as well as the resultant deleterious effect in the contralateral eye.

Anergy

One of the major mechanisms that the human body uses to inactivate self-reactive T cell clones that have escaped central and peripheral clonal deletion is anergy (*Chapter 7*). By definition, anergy refers to T cell clones that are unable to respond to an antigenic stimulus. Although they bear a TCR on their surface that recognizes its corresponding antigen, anergic T cells do not produce IL-2 or IL-2 receptor (IL-2R) upon encountering their cognate antigen. Multiple mechanisms have been proposed to explain this apparent block in T cell activation (Figure 19-4).

It is now well established that activation of the T cell during the initiation of an immune response is a two-step process (Figure 19-4). In order for the T cell to mount an effective immune response against its corresponding antigen that is presented by an antigen-presenting cell (**APC**), two signals need to be transmitted (*Chapters 1* and *7*). The first signal is initiated by the cognate interaction between the TCR and the MHC-Ag complex and the second by the pairing of co-stimulatory molecules on the surface of both the T cell and the APC (Figure 19-4A). The interaction of CD28 on the surface of the T cell with its ligand CD80/86 (B7.1/B7.2) surface proteins on

3

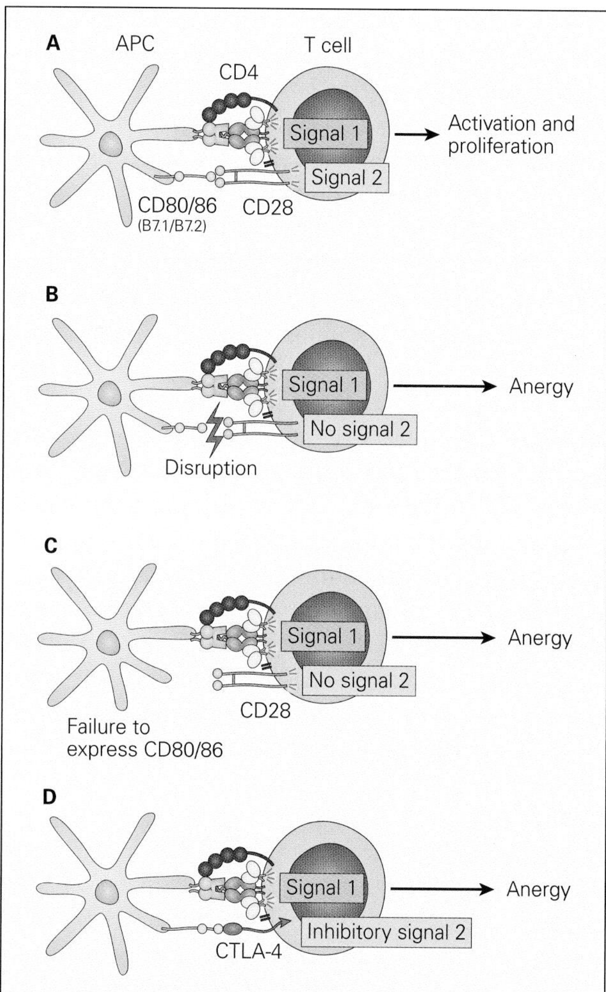

Figure 19-4. Co-stimulation is important for the activation of T cells. Panel A: Following the activation of the 80/86 on the antigen-presenting cell provides the second signal, leading to T cell activation and proliferation. Panel B: Disruption of the CD28/CD80/86 signal or Panel C: Failure to express CD 80/86 can lead to anergy. Panel D: At the same time, the activated T cells upregulate the expression of CTLA-4, a molecule that also interacts with greater affinity to CD80/86, leading to disruption of the costimulatory signal and anergy.

the APC is one of the most important co-stimulatory signals that amplifies the original signal transmitted through the TCR-MHC-Ag interaction. Anergy occurs when disruption of the CD28 CD80/86 interaction leads to insufficient stimulation of the T cell by its cognate antigen (Figure 19-4B), rendering the T cell unresponsive. APCs that express an antigen such as a self-antigen but fail to express CD80/86 also cannot efficiently help activate T cells, providing yet another level of self-tolerance (Figure 19-4C).

Anergy can also result from the interaction between CD80/86 and another molecule, called cytotoxic T lymphocyte–associated (**CTLA**)-4 (or CD152) (Figure 19-4D). CTLA-4, a homologue of CD28, also binds the CD80/86 ligands, but with greater affinity than CD28, resulting in the inhibition and negative regulation of T cell activation (*Chapter 7*). The interaction of CTLA-4 with the B7 molecules provides the T cell with a negative signal, leading to a decrease in the production of IL-2 and IL-2R, causing anergy. Thus, the fate of the interaction between a T cell and an APC is determined by which co-stimulatory molecule the T cell displays on its surface; CD28 will lead to T cell activation and proliferation, while CTLA-4 will lead to anergy. Under physiologic conditions, T cells express CD28 upon initial encounter of the APC, but shortly after stimulation they begin to display CTLA-4 on their surfaces. CTLA-4 helps to terminate the T cell response by sending a downstream negative signal, effectively decreasing the production of IL-2. The significance of CTLA-4 in regulating the immune response in the human is supported by *in vivo* findings in CTLA-4 knockout mice that develop a profound lymphoproliferative disease.

The Clinical Significance of CTLA-4

In humans, CTLA-4 is being used as a biologic response modifier in the treatment of patients with rheumatoid arthritis (**RA**), an autoimmune disease mainly affecting the joints (Box 19-1 and *Chapter 11*). Patients with RA who are treated with these

Box 19-1

Clinical Use of CTLA-4 Preparations in Rheumatoid Arthritis

The comparatively higher binding affinity of CTLA-4 with CD80/86 has made it a potential therapy for patients with autoimmune diseases (*Chapter 11*). Fusion proteins of CTLA-4 with immunoglobulin (Ig) (CTLA-4-Ig) have been used in clinical trials for rheumatoid arthritis. The fusion protein CTLA-4-Ig is commercially available as Orencia (abatacept). A second-generation form of CTLA-4-Ig known as belatacept is currently being tested in clinical trials. Both of these preparations are expected to be also widely used in organ transplantation. In addition, there is increasing interest in the possible therapeutic benefits of blocking CTLA-4 (using antibodies against CTLA, such as ipilimumab) as a means of inhibiting immune system tolerance to tumors and thereby providing a potentially useful immunotherapy strategy for patients with cancer (*Chapter 20*).

CTLA-4 preparations have a significant reduction in joint inflammation. The drug acts by blocking the interaction between CD28 on the self-reactive T cells and CD80/86 on the surface of APCs that present the MHC-self-Ag complex to the T cells (*Chapter 11*).

In recent years, the molecular mechanisms that underlie the induction of anergy have been intensively studied. Insufficient production of key gene transcription activators such as activator protein 1 (**AP-1**, a Jun/Fos heterodimeric protein), NF-κB, and NFAT-1 during T cell activation can lead to a decrease in IL-2 production (*Chapter 9*). It has also been shown that transcriptional suppressors such as the C-AMP response element modulator (**CREM**) can also decrease the transcriptional activity of the IL-2 gene promoter, rendering the T cells anergic. Alterations at multiple other levels of regulation, such as the activity of key kinases (e.g., MAP kinase) and the stability of IL-2 mRNA, can also contribute to decreased IL-2 production in anergic T cells.

Immune Regulation and Treg Cells

Perhaps the most actively studied mechanism of induction and maintenance of tolerance is that mediated by Treg cells, which are involved in immune regulation (*Chapters 7* and *9*). The reactivity of T cells is under the influence of immunoregulatory cells either through direct cell-cell interaction or through the secretion of cytokines, e.g., transforming growth factor (**TGF**)-β and IL-10 (Figure 19-5). Of the multitude of cell-cell interactions that control T cell reactivity, of particular importance are those that comprise a subset of T cells, termed regulatory T or Treg cells, that co-express the CD4 and CD25, i.e., the IL-2 receptor α chain (*Chapters 7* and *9*). These naturally occurring Treg cells inhibit the responses of other T cells and are generated in the thymus, probably during the stage of negative selection, and not only display anergic properties *in vitro*, but also can suppress CD4+CD25− T cells *in vivo*, probably through a cytokine-independent direct cell-cell interaction. Many reports have established that Treg cells

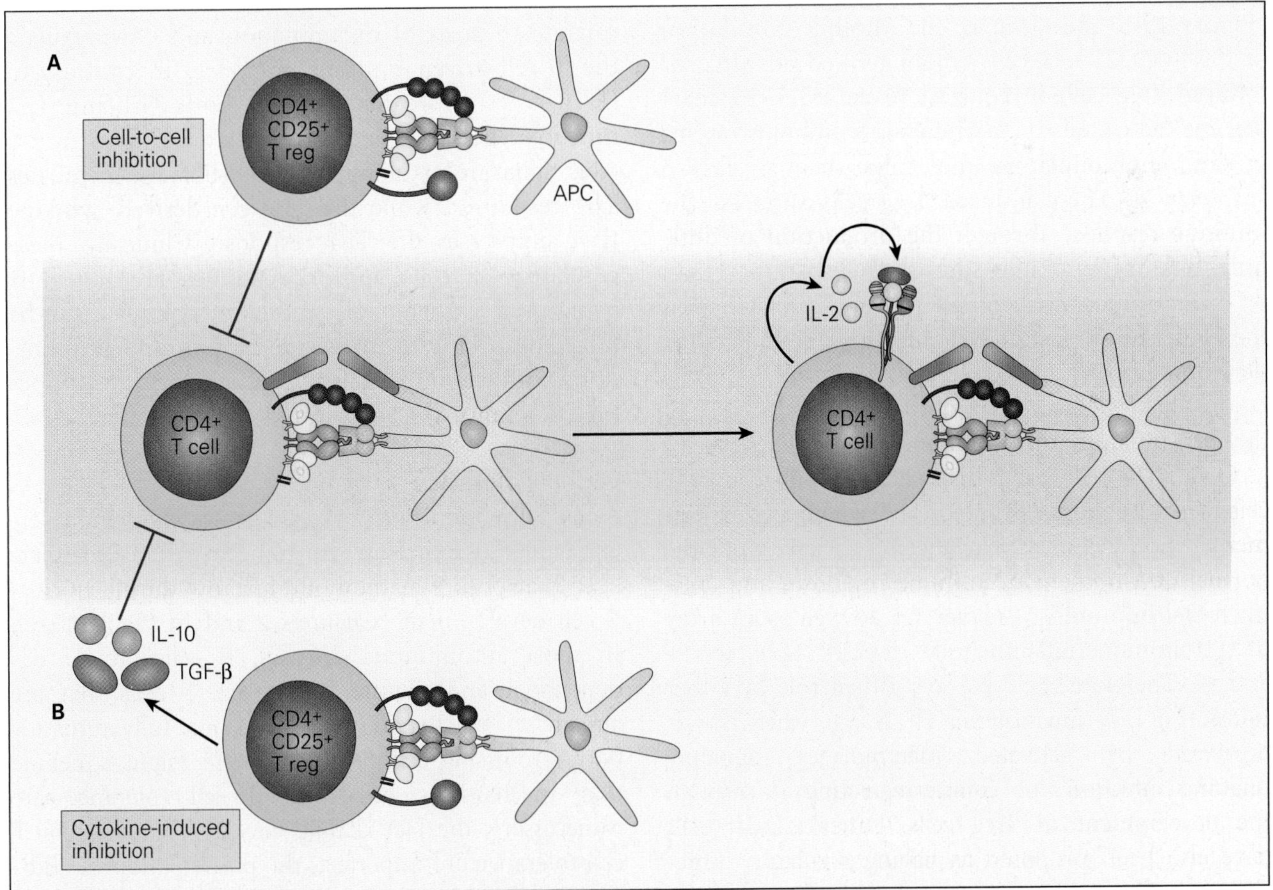

Figure 19-5. Schematic representation of two mechanisms of immune regulation by Treg cells. Panel A: Self-antigen specific CD4+CD25+ T cells can directly suppress the activation of self-reactive T cells through cell-cell interaction. Panel B: Anti-inflammatory cytokines such as IL-10 and TGF-β that are secreted by other immunoregulatory T cells can also suppress the immune response.

are also important in maintaining peripheral tolerance. For example, it has been shown that elimination of these cells in mice leads to various autoimmune diseases; furthermore, a case of a human with a genetic dysfunction of Treg cells has been reported; this patient developed lymphadenopathy and inflammatory infiltrates consisting of self-reactive T cells in multiple organs, including the liver, the intestine, and the lungs.

Once these cells exit the thymus and enter the peripheral lymphoid tissues, they can block the activation of other T cells, thus preventing inflammation. During an active inflammatory process, such as an infection, however, the inhibitory function of these Treg cells can be overcome. Therefore, while the presence of Treg cells is important for the maintenance of tolerance, it does not prohibit the immune system from carrying out its defense function against infectious agents.

Adaptive or Induced Treg Cells

In addition to direct cell-cell interaction, T cell reactivity can also be influenced by cytokines (Figure 19-5 and *Chapter 9*). Another population of CD4+CD25+ T cells (often termed adaptive or induced Treg cells in contrast to natural Treg cells) can be activated in peripheral lymphoid organs by immunomodulatory molecules such as TGF-β (*Chapter 9*). These induced Treg cells suppress the immune response through the production of anti-inflammatory cytokines such as TGF-β rather than by direct contact with other lymphocytes. TGF-β in the presence of IL-6 and IL-23 also can lead to the development of a newly recognized T cell subpopulation that is characterized by the production of the pro-inflammatory cytokine IL-17. These cells, termed Th17 cells, are a distinct subpopulation of T cells separate from Th1 and Th2 which, in experimental mouse models, have been associated with the normal development of immune responses and antimicrobial immunity (*Chapter 12*), as well as an array of autoimmune/inflammatory diseases (*Chapters 7* and *9*). Therefore, TGF-β plays a dual role by either promoting inflammation via Th17 (e.g., when IL-6 is produced by activated macrophages signaling ongoing infection) or counterregulating it through the development of Treg cells. Other CD4+ cells have also been proposed as having regulatory function, such as the Tr1, an IL-10-dependent subpopulation of T cells, which also can downregulate the immune response through the production of anti-inflammatory cytokines. The CD1-restricted natural killer (**NK**) T cells also have been implicated in the regulation of the immune response (*Chapter 3*).

CD8+ Suppressor T Cells

Another example of how T cells are regulated by cytokines is by CD8+ suppressor T cells that can downregulate the T cell-driven response by also producing IL-10 and TGF-β. A particular subset of CD8+ cells that bears the γδ TCR instead of the more prevalent αβ TCR, which are known to populate mucosa-associated lymphoid tissues (**MALT**), is most likely involved in the suppression of immune responses initiated by antigens delivered by the mucosal route of immunization (*Chapter 8*). After the inhalation of small quantities of an antigen, these γδ TCR cells are initially activated in the submucosal areas and become suppressor cells. They then migrate to regional lymph nodes where they suppress the immune response through production of IL-10 and TGF-β. Ingestion rather than inhalation of larger quantities of antigens activates not only CD8+ but also suppressor CD4+ cells that can migrate to areas of inflammation and downregulate the T cell-driven immune response. In contrast to IL-10 and TGF-β that suppress both Th1 and Th2 function, the pro-inflammatory cytokine interferon-γ (the signature cytokine of Th1 cells) downregulates Th2 responses, while the Th2 cell-derived cytokine IL-4 suppresses the Th1 response. Clinically, these regulatory T cells and/or cytokines are not only being used as therapeutic modalities but also can be targeted specifically in various autoimmune conditions with the hope that by influencing T cell function, tolerance will be restored (*Chapter 11*).

B Cell Tolerance

An equally important set of processes involving tolerance are those that are concerned with B cell tolerance that occurs in the bone marrow during normal B cell development (*Chapters 2* and *6*) (Table 19-1). In most autoimmune diseases, B cells are T cell-dependent and require help from T cells that are already self-reactive in order to become fully autoantibody-producing cells. Although one might conclude that mechanisms of direct B cell tolerance are unnecessary, the fact is that since mechanisms for T cell tolerance are imperfect, the participation of additional redundant mechanisms of tolerance are necessary to inhibit the immune systems and help prevent the development of autoimmunity and autoimmune disease. Furthermore, there are instances in which T cell-independent B cells, directly activated by a self-antigen without the participation of T cell help, need to be controlled. For example, a foreign (e.g., microbial) antigen that is structurally similar to a self-antigen can directly activate B cells to produce an antibody that will cross-react with both the foreign and the self-antigen, a phenomenon referred to as molecular mimicry and that is described more fully below. Since B cells also are able to hypermutate their receptors after they mature, the possibility exists that they may become self-reactive later in their development. The immune system, therefore, requires that there be in place mechanisms of B cell tolerance similar to those for the T cell.

Mechanisms of B Cell Tolerance: Central and Peripheral B Cell Tolerance

As with T cell tolerance, B cell tolerance also takes place in central lymphoid tissues in the bone marrow and in peripheral lymphoid tissues (*Chapter 6*). The mechanisms of the education of B cells and the elimination of self-reacting B cell clones, however, differ somewhat from that which control the T cell. B cell maturation is initiated in the bone marrow, but in contrast to T cells, B cells are still immature when they relocate to peripheral lymphoid tissues (*Chapters 2* and *6*). Moreover, although BCR rearrangement in the bone marrow is similar to TCR rearrangement, B cells that bear receptors capable of recognizing self-antigens are not necessarily eliminated in the bone marrow through negative selection. Some of these still-maturing self-reactive B cells exit the bone marrow and relocate peripherally to the spleen, where they reside initially in T cell zones (*Chapter 2*). Negative selection mainly takes place in this phase. The B cells that recognize self-antigens are eliminated through programmed cell death, i.e., apoptosis, or become anergic. The B cells that do not interact with self-antigens survive and migrate into the B cell follicles. During an infection, however, self-reactive B cells can escape negative selection and become part of the immune repertoire, a mechanism that ensures maximal diversity of the antibody spectrum when needed.

The mechanisms of B cell tolerance have been largely explored using transgenic mouse technology (Figure 19-6). In a classic experiment, a mouse strain that is monotransgenic for expression of hen egg lysozyme (after being tolerogenized by fetal exposure to lysozyme and made incapable of anti-lysozyme production) is bred with a second monotransgenic strain carrying the gene for IgM anti-hen egg lysozyme antibody capable of both anti-lysozyme antibody production and also expression of a B cell receptor (**BCR**) capable of specifically recognizing lysozyme on a significant proportion of their B cells. The resulting F1 double transgenic hybrids demonstrated both hen egg lysozyme production and the presence of large numbers of B cells with BCRs that could recognize lysozyme. These F1 hybrids, however, were incapable of anti-lysozyme antibody production following immunization with lysozyme. This experiment demonstrated that the simultaneous presence of lysozyme and B cells bearing B cell receptors specific for lysozyme led to B cell anergy. In a subsequent experiment, B cells from these F1 double transgenic mice when transferred to irradiated, nontransgenic mice of the same strain were capable of anti-lysozyme antibody production after immunization with hen egg lysozyme. This experiment proved that the anergy observed in the B cells from the double transgenic mice was related to the continued presence of and stimulation by lysozyme but could be reversed when the B cells were transferred to a nontransgenic irradiated host devoid of the tolerogenizing effect of lysozyme.

The Clinical Significance of Tolerance

The immune system functions to ensure that self-antigens as well as unharmful antigens do not become targets of the inflammatory response. These mechanisms are in effect both during maturation and in the later stages of the lymphocyte life cycle, resulting in either elimination or functional inactivity (i.e., anergy) of unwanted B and T cell clones. Anergy can be reversed to allow the immune system to recruit the so-called forbidden clones in times of need, such as during an infection, allowing for the generation of diversity, the hallmark aspect of an effective immune response.

The past decades have witnessed a remarkable expansion in our knowledge of lymphocyte physiology, mechanisms that induce and terminate tolerance, and the important role of cytokines in accomplishing these molecular events. This knowledge has, in large part, been derived from studies in experimental animal model systems employing transgenic and knockout mice and molecular studies facilitated by genomics and proteomics. Although some progress has been made in translating these observations to the human using gene mapping and cDNA arrays, additional clinical studies will be

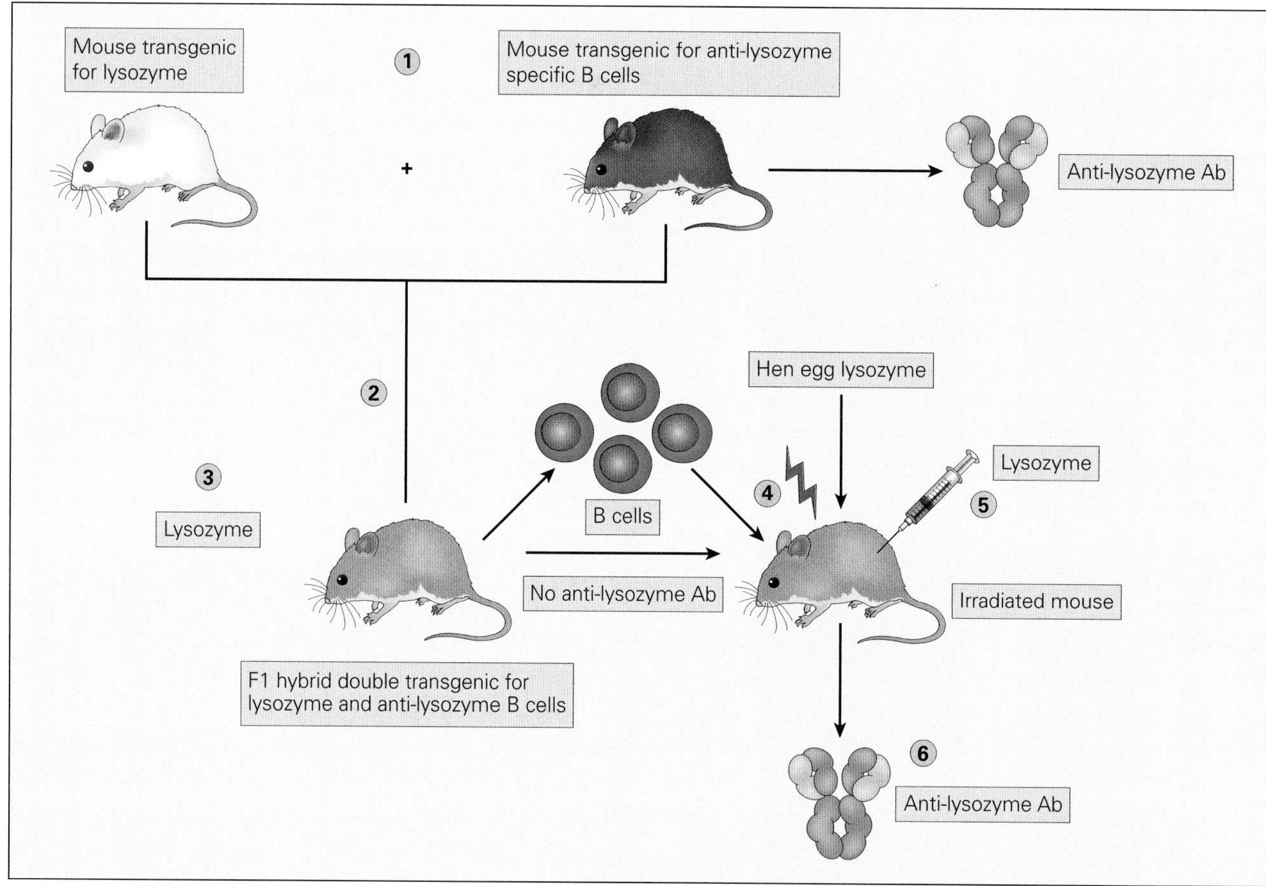

Figure 19-6. Experimental model of B cell anergy. (1) A transgenic mouse expressing hen egg lysozyme (white mouse) was crossed with a mouse transgenic for anti-lysozyme specific B cell production (brown mouse) to produce an F1 hybrid (tan mouse) (2) double transgenic for lysozyme production (3) and anti-lysozymal B cell production; these double transgenic hybrids produced lysozyme but did not produce anti-lysozyme antibody. (4) The B cells from these F1 mice, although unable to react to the lysozyme, when transferred to irradiated mice and immunized with lysozyme (5) resulted in the production of anti-lysozyme antibody (Ab) (6). This proves that the B cells in the F1 mice, although capable of producing anti-lysozyme antibody, if transferred to another mouse were functionally anergized in the presence of endogenously produced lysozyme.

necessary to better understand the pathophysiologic mechanisms involved in autoimmune disease. The challenge will be to make beneficial therapeutic use of this new knowledge for patients suffering from these autoimmune disorders without inducing the detrimental effects of this therapy.

Autoimmunity: A Breakdown of Tolerance

Autoimmunity emerges when the mechanisms of tolerance fail to eliminate or inactivate immune cell clones that react against elements of our own tissues. Although the immune system possesses a vast array of elaborate and sometimes-redundant mechanisms to prevent the emergence of self-reactive lymphocytic clones, about 5 percent of people suffer from autoimmune disease. Autoimmune disease is a term that comprises such different and seemingly unrelated entities as type I diabetes mellitus (**DM**), multiple sclerosis (**MS**), systemic lupus erythematosus (**SLE**), and Hashimoto's thyroiditis (Table 19-2). Epidemiologically, most of these diseases affect predominantly, but not exclusively, women during their reproductive years, with an early peak in incidence during adolescence and a late peak in the fourth through fifth decades of life.

Organ-Specific Versus Systemic Autoimmune Diseases: Autoimmune Response Versus Autoimmune Disease

One can broadly categorize the autoimmune diseases as either **organ-specific**, when autoimmune injury is directed against one organ, or **systemic**, when many different organs and tissues are affected. Shown in Table 19-2 are some of the more common organ-specific and systemic autoimmune diseases

Table 19-2. Partial list of autoimmune diseases

Disease	Main organ affected	Proposed self-antigen(s)	Clinical presentation
Organ-specific autoimmune diseases			
Multiple sclerosis	Central nervous system	Myelin basic protein, myelin oligodendrocyte protein	Loss of vision, weakness of limbs, sensory abnormalities, incontinence
Sympathetic ophthalmia	Eye	Various uveal antigens	Eye pain, loss of vision, sensitivity to light
Graves' disease	Thyroid	Thyrotropin receptor	Hyperthyroidism (weight loss, nervousness, palpitations, diarrhea), exophthalmos
Hashimoto's thyroiditis	Thyroid	Thyroperoxidase, thyroglobulin	Hypothyroidism (weight gain, constipation, skin changes, myxedematous dementia)
Goodpasture's syndrome	Lung, kidney	Glomerular basement membrane (type IV collagen)	Kidney and respiratory insufficiency
Pernicious anemia	Stomach	Intrinsic factor	Anemia, gastritis
Crohn's disease*	Intestine	? microbial antigens	Hemorrhagic diarrhea, abdominal pain, draining fistulas
Ulcerative colitis*	Large Intestine	? microbial antigens	Hemorrhagic diarrhea, abdominal pain
Diabetes mellitus type I	Pancreas	Islet cell, insulin, glutamic acid decarboxylase (GAD)	Polyphagia, polyuria, polydipsia, weight loss
Immune thrombocytopenia	Platelets	Glycoproteins on the surface of platelets	Easy bruising, hemorrhage
Myasthenia gravis	Muscle	Acetylcholine receptor	Muscle weakness, fatiguability
Hemolytic anemia	Red cells	I antigen	Anemia
Systemic autoimmune diseases			
Sjögren's syndrome	Salivary and lacrimal glands	Nuclear antigens (SSA, SSB)	Dry eyes, dry mouth, lung and kidney disease
Rheumatoid arthritis	Joints, lung, nerves	Citrulinated peptides in the joint, IgG	Deforming arthritis, skin nodules, occasional lung and nerve involvement
Wegener's granulomatosis	Lung, kidney	Proteinase 3 (c-ANCA)	Sinusitis, shortness of breath, kidney failure
Systemic lupus erythematosus	Kidney, skin, joints, central nervous system	DNA, histones, ribonucleoproteins	Arthritis, skin rashes, kidney insufficiency, nerve damage

*Although previously considered autoimmune diseases, more recent evidence supports that they are autoinflammatory disorders; see *Chapter 19 Annex*.

seen in the human. Because of the variable pathophysiology of autoimmune disease, it is not unusual for patients to present with symptoms of more than one autoimmune disease, referred to as an overlap or undifferentiated collagen vascular syndrome. In other cases, a patient with one autoimmune disease might have serologic markers but not clinical manifestations of another autoimmune condition.

A clear distinction, therefore, must be made between an autoimmune response and an autoimmune disease. The term autoimmune response refers to the demonstration of an autoantibody or T cell-mediated reactivity directed to a self-antigen. An autoimmune response may or may not be associated with autoimmune disease. For example, many clinically well individuals, particularly women, exhibit an autoimmune response by the presence of serum antinuclear antibodies (**ANAs**) and demonstrate no symptoms. Although the presence of ANA may also be associated with the autoimmune disease SLE, the diagnosis requires the presence of additional clinical features of the disease, e.g., rash, arthritis, or kidney involvement. Although much progress has been made in understanding the pathophysiology of autoimmune

Table 19-3. Etiology of autoimmune diseases

Genetic factors
MHC
Non-MHC genes
Environment
Microorganisms
Viruses
Trauma
UV light
Immune response dysregulation

diseases, the underlying etiopathogenesis remains elusive for most of these disorders. This section will present some of what is currently known about the underlying etiologies and proposed mechanisms that lead to autoimmunity as well as the current understanding of pathophysiology of organ damage in these diseases.

Etiology

It has been postulated that most autoimmune diseases are the result of a complex interplay between genetic factors, environmental triggers, and regulatory aberrations of the immune response (Table 19-3 and Figure 19-7). These factors lead eventually to the loss of self-tolerance, a pivotal mechanism for the emergence of autoimmunity and tissue damage.

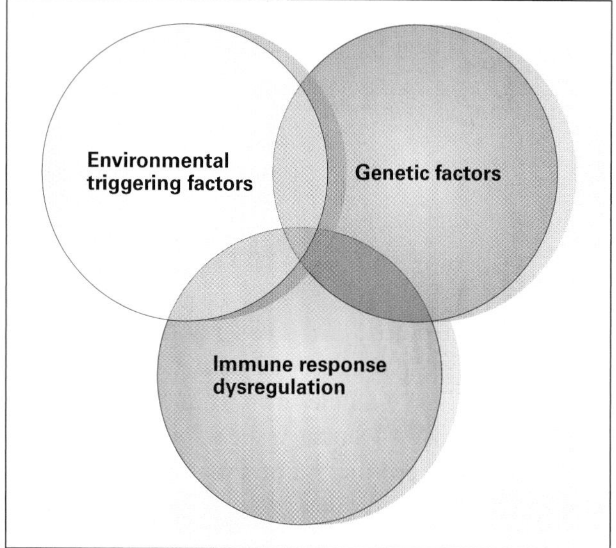

Figure 19-7. Schematic representation of the three etiopathogenic factors involved in autoimmune diseases. The figure illustrates the complex interplay between genetic factors, environmental triggers, and regulatory aberrations of the immune response responsible for the development of autoimmune disease.

Genetic Basis of Autoimmunity

There is now ample evidence for a genetic susceptibility to autoimmune diseases (*Chapter 10*). This is supported not only by the clustering of cases in families but also by the higher concordance rate of autoimmunity in monozygotic versus dizygotic twins, which suggests that autoimmune diseases are, at least, partially inheritable. For example, the concordance rate of systemic lupus erythematosus in monozygotic twins is between 24 percent and 58 percent, while it is only 2 to 5 percent in dizygotic twins. A higher prevalence of certain autoimmune diseases in different ethnic groups (e.g., ankylosing spondylitis [**AS**] in Caucasians and Takayasu's arteritis [i.e., pulseless disease] in Japanese) also supports the conclusion that the genetic makeup of an individual is important for the expression of autoimmunity.

Rarely, mutations in a single gene can lead to the emergence of an autoimmune disease; these are referred to as monogenic diseases. For example, in the monogenic disorder ALPS, referred to previously, mutations in the gene encoding Fas or FasL cause a severe defect in the apoptosis of lymphocytes that results in profound autoimmunity (*Chapter 16*). Most of the autoimmune diseases, however, are polygenic, with as many as thirty or more genes identified that contribute to their pathogenesis and clinical presentation. Moreover, in animal models, it appears that a single gene can predispose to different diseases depending on the genetic makeup of the animal. Extrapolating these observations to the human suggests that the clustering of different autoimmune diseases in a single family may also be attributable to several autoimmunity-predisposing genes.

The first genes that were shown to have a strong association with many autoimmune diseases were found within the MHC locus controlling both MHC-I and MHC-II located on the short arm of chromosome 6 (6p) (*Chapter 10*). Some of the diseases associated with MHC-I and MHC-II are shown in Table 19-4. The MHC-I-associated diseases also include a cluster of newly classified diseases, collectively called autoinflammatory diseases, which are described in the Annex to this chapter and include the spondyloarthropathies, such as AS, reactive arthritis, and psoriasis. Ninety percent of patients with AS have the HLA-B27 gene, although all individuals expressing this gene do not develop the disorder. The precise mechanism by which HLA-B27 can predispose individuals to AS is still under

Table 19-4. Association of autoimmune diseases and MHC

MHC-I association
Ankylosing spondylitis (HLA-B27)
Reactive arthritis (HLA-B27)
Psoriasis (HLA B-13, B-16, B-17)
MHC-II association
Systemic diseases
Systemic lupus erythematosus (HLA-DR2 and DR3)
Rheumatoid arthritis (HLA-DR4)
Organ-specific diseases
Type 1 diabetes mellitus (HLA-DR3 and DR4)
Multiple sclerosis (HLA-DR2)

investigation thirty years after its discovery. One of the most interesting observations is that animals transgenic for the HLA-B27 gene develop spontaneous autoimmunity affecting the gastrointestinal and musculoskeletal systems in a way similar to the human spondyloarthropathies.

There are many more autoimmune diseases associated with MHC-II than with MHC-I; these include SLE (HLA-DR2 and DR3), RA (HLA-DR4), type 1 DM (HLA-DR3 and DR4), and MS (HLA-DR2) (Table 19-4). The alleles HLA-DRB1*0401 and 0404, which are associated with rheumatoid arthritis, are associated with more severe disease. Other genes that are important for the immune response, such as those encoding for components of the complement system (*Chapter 4*) and the pro-inflammatory cytokine TNF family (*Chapter 9*), are also located in the 6p chromosome region and may further account for its association with various autoimmune conditions.

Genetic Associations with Autoimmune Diseases and Autoinflammatory Disorders Outside the MHC Locus

Genetic associations outside the MHC locus also have been found in various autoimmune diseases and more recently with the autoinflammatory disorders described in the Annex to this chapter. Genes encoding different Fc gamma receptors on chromosome 1 that play a role in immune complex clearance, for example, show a moderate association with SLE.

Because of the rapid advances in our recent understanding of the molecular mechanisms of innate immunity (*Chapter 3*), many of the older concepts of diseases originally associated with abnormalities of adaptive immunity are now being reassigned to disorders of the innate immune system and are referred to as autoinflammatory diseases (*Chapter 9*). Crohn's disease, classically referred to as an autoimmune disease, for example, thought previously to be associated with inflammation stimulated by an overactive Th1 cytokine response and more recently with a Th17 response, has now been shown to have a cluster of genetic abnormalities associated with defective innate immune system signaling pathways. Currently, Crohn's disease is more appropriately considered an autoinflammatory disease caused in part by sequence variants in the NOD2/CARD15 gene encoding a protein involved in intracellular signaling associated with innate immunity.

Environmental Triggers of Autoimmunity

There are well-documented differences in the prevalence and severity of many autoimmune diseases seen in different geographic regions which point to the role of environmental factors as potential triggers of autoimmunity in a genetically susceptible individual. In general, a reduced incidence of autoimmune diseases occurs in lower latitudes presumably related to the greater degree of sun exposure and synthesis of vitamin D, which has been shown to have beneficial and important hormonal type immunomodulating properties. On the other hand, conflicting with this hypothesis, one study has shown that the amount of sunlight exposure in different cities around the world was found to correlate positively with the prevalence of dermatomyositis, an autoimmune condition affecting the sun-exposed areas of the skin as well as the muscles. In most cases, however, the causative relationship between an environmental factor and an autoimmune disease has not yet been firmly established.

The most characteristic example of an environmental trigger is the development of rheumatic fever, an autoimmune disease affecting primarily the joints and heart, following an infection with β hemolytic streptococcus group A. This condition is believed to be caused by cross-reactive antibodies between components of the bacteria and tissue antigens found on affected organs. Surface molecules of the microorganism are similar to proteins found in heart muscle and valves. It is likely that the immune cells and antibodies that are directed against these bacterial immunogens also recognize the heart tissue self-antigens. This inappropriate immune response causes autoimmune carditis and valvulitis, leading sometimes to heart block and valvular insufficiency that represent the characteristic clinical findings in patients with rheumatic fever. This phenomenon of antigenic cross-reactivity between a microorganism and self-antigens is called molecular mimicry and has been implicated in the pathogenesis of many autoimmune diseases.

The damage of tissues by exogenous factors, such as viruses, microorganisms, trauma, and ultraviolet light can also lead to the exposure of self-antigens previously hidden from the immune system, i.e., sequestered antigens, resulting in a break in tolerance referred to as immunologic ignorance. The development of persistent myocarditis and hepatitis after infections with Coxsackie and hepatitis C virus, respectively, are thought to be partly due to an autoimmune response directed against previously sequestered antigens of the heart or liver tissues following the viral infection. The same mechanism is thought to underlie sympathetic ophthalmia that was described previously. In systemic lupus erythematosus, exposure to sunlight can lead to disease exacerbation; damage to skin keratinocytes caused by ultraviolet radiation results in nuclear autoantigens being released that exacerbate the immunologic response and worsen the effects of the disease.

Drugs such as hydralazine can also induce a syndrome that is very similar to SLE in a condition that is referred to as drug-induced lupus erythematosus (**DIL**). Of the thirty medications known to cause DIL, the three that most commonly cause the condition are hydralazine, procainamide, and isoniazid. Although the basis for this entity is not entirely clear, these drugs may alter the methylation status of proinflammatory genes, thereby activating them.

Dysregulation of the Immune Response and the Loss of Tolerance

From what has been described thus far, it may now be possible to summarize the pathogenetic events underlying autoimmunity. In carrying out its homeostatic function, the immune system is entrusted with the capacity to suppress or delete autoimmune clones, and it is when these mechanisms fail that autoimmunity arises. The loss of immune regulation most commonly occurs as a series of successive events and rarely as the effect of a single genetic or environmental factor. It may therefore be appropriate to consider the concept of an immunologic milieu that can predispose to autoimmunity once appropriate stimuli have been set in motion to trigger an immunologic response. This milieu is influenced by genetics, prior encounters with antigens, local factors in target-organs, and other endogenous factors, such as the modulating effects of hormones (e.g., estrogens and cortisol).

Under normal circumstances, all of the previously described mechanisms that contribute to tolerance can fail and help give rise to self-reactive clones. Autoreactive T cells after escaping the negative selection in the thymus can persist in the periphery and proliferate during an infection. Defects of apoptosis can also facilitate the development of T cell autoreactivity, including those initiated by decreased Fas-FasL or IL-2–induced AICD, emergence of new, previously sequestered self-antigens, increased co-stimulation (e.g., increased expression of CD28 and decreased expression of CTLA-4), and defects in regulatory T cells. Similar mechanisms can also lead to self-reactive B cell proliferation with or without direct help from T cells. Collectively, these events lead to dysregulation and loss of tolerance, aberrant immune activation, and disease.

Pathophysiology of Autoimmune Diseases

The autoimmune processes can lead to tissue damage via diverse and frequently poorly understood immunologic mechanisms of tissue injury. The classification of immune mechanisms of tissue injury known as the Gell-Coombs classification of tissue injury will be described more completely in Chapter 17. Briefly, there are four major types of hypersensitivity reactions included in this classification: (1) type I, IgE-mediated; (2) type II, cytotoxic reactions; (3) type III, immune complex injury; and (4) type IV, cell-mediated injury. This section will describe some of the better-recognized mechanisms of tissue injury that contribute to autoimmune disease, including the production of pathogenic autoantibodies (type II), the deposition of immune complexes that contain self-antigens (type III), and cellular-mediated cytotoxicity by T cells and NK cells (type IV).

Autoantibodies

Most autoimmune diseases are characterized by the production of antibodies that are directed to self-antigens. As described previously, it is important to determine whether the presence of an autoantibody is causally related to the pathogenesis of an autoimmune disease or represents an autoimmune response epiphenomenon playing no causal role in its development. For example, an antibody directed against the thyroid-stimulating hormone (**TSH**) receptor found in the serum of a patient suffering from palpitations, heat intolerance, and weight loss is central to the pathogenesis and ultimate diagnosis of Graves' disease; without these symptoms, the demonstration of such an antibody has no clinical relevance and plays no role in the causation of disease pathology (*Chapter 17*). Other autoantibodies, such as the Smith (Sm) antibody found exclusively in the serum of patients with systemic lupus erythematosus, likewise play no causative role and simply represent a marker of the disease useful in diagnosis. Although autoantibodies are usually identified in serum, they often are found deposited at the site of inflammation.

It should be emphasized, therefore, that although autoantibodies (especially at low levels) in serum do not predict that an individual has or will develop an autoimmune disease, they may play a physiologic role, such as binding to cellular debris (endogenous antigens or autoantigens), and thus enable its clearance. The physical properties of autoantibody that determine its pathogenicity include:

a. The *affinity* of the antibody to the antigen that plays a role in the formation of immune complexes. These complexes will be more stable if the affinity between the two is high.
b. The *charge* of the antibody that helps the antibody preferentially attach to tissues. In SLE, positively charged autoantibodies (anti-double-strand DNA) associate with the negatively charged basement membrane in the kidney, where they can form complexes *in situ* with DNA and lead to local inflammation (Figure 19-8A).

Mechanisms Involved in Autoantibody-Mediated Damage

There are several proposed mechanisms to explain the pathogenesis of immunologically mediated damage resulting from the direct effects of autoantibody (Figure 19-8). Autoantibodies can exert their effects either by activating or blocking receptors to which they bind. An example of a blocking reaction is seen in a Gell and Coombs type IIB (cytoneutralizing) reaction, where an anti-acetylcholine receptor antibody blocks the binding of the neurotransmitter acetylcholine to its specific receptor at the neuromuscular junction, leading to myasthenia gravis, a disease characterized by muscle weakness (Figure 19-8B) (*Chapter 17*). An example of an activating reaction is seen in a Gell and Coombs type IIB (immunostimulatory) reaction, where an IgG autoantibody binds to the TSH receptor in the thyroid gland, resulting in persistent production of thyroxin seen in a clinical condition called Graves' disease (Figure 19-8C). Another mechanism involved in the pathogenesis of autoimmune disease is carried out by IgG- or IgM-opsonizing autoantibodies that coat cells and prepare them for phagocytosis by phagocytic cells through their Fc receptors. Autoimmune thrombocytopenia and leukopenia, for example, are thought to be mediated by specific anti-platelet or anti-leukocytic antibodies, respectively.

A second major group of mechanisms involved in autoantibody-mediated damage are produced indirectly through a variety of complement-mediated pathways (*Chapter 4*) that involve IgG or IgM complement-fixing antibodies that recognize self-antigens on cells or tissues that lead to tissue damage by mechanisms as shown in Figure 19-9. Cleavage of various components of the complement cascade leads to the production of products that can enhance phagocytosis by opsonins (C3b) and lead to mediator release, increased vascular permeability, and smooth muscle contraction through the production of anaphylatoxins (C3a, C5a), can promote inflammation through the production of chemotactic factors (C5a), or can lead to cytolysis when the membrane attack complex (**MAC**) is activated (C5-9) (*Chapter 17*).

Immune Complexes

Autoantibodies can form complexes with their corresponding self-antigen and deposit in the tissues in a Gell and Coombs type III reaction (*Chapter 17*), leading to the production of chemotactic factors (C5a) (Figure 19-9). The physical properties of the immune complexes, especially size, determine their inflammatory effects on tissues. Small complexes tend to be filtered in the urine while large ones are phagocytosed more readily, and therefore the more soluble intermediate complexes in slight antigen excess are the most pathogenic (*Chapter 17*). The genetic background of the host also plays a role. For example, low levels of Fc receptors on macrophages can lead to decreased clearance of the immune complexes and increased deposition in tissues. This mechanism has been proposed to play

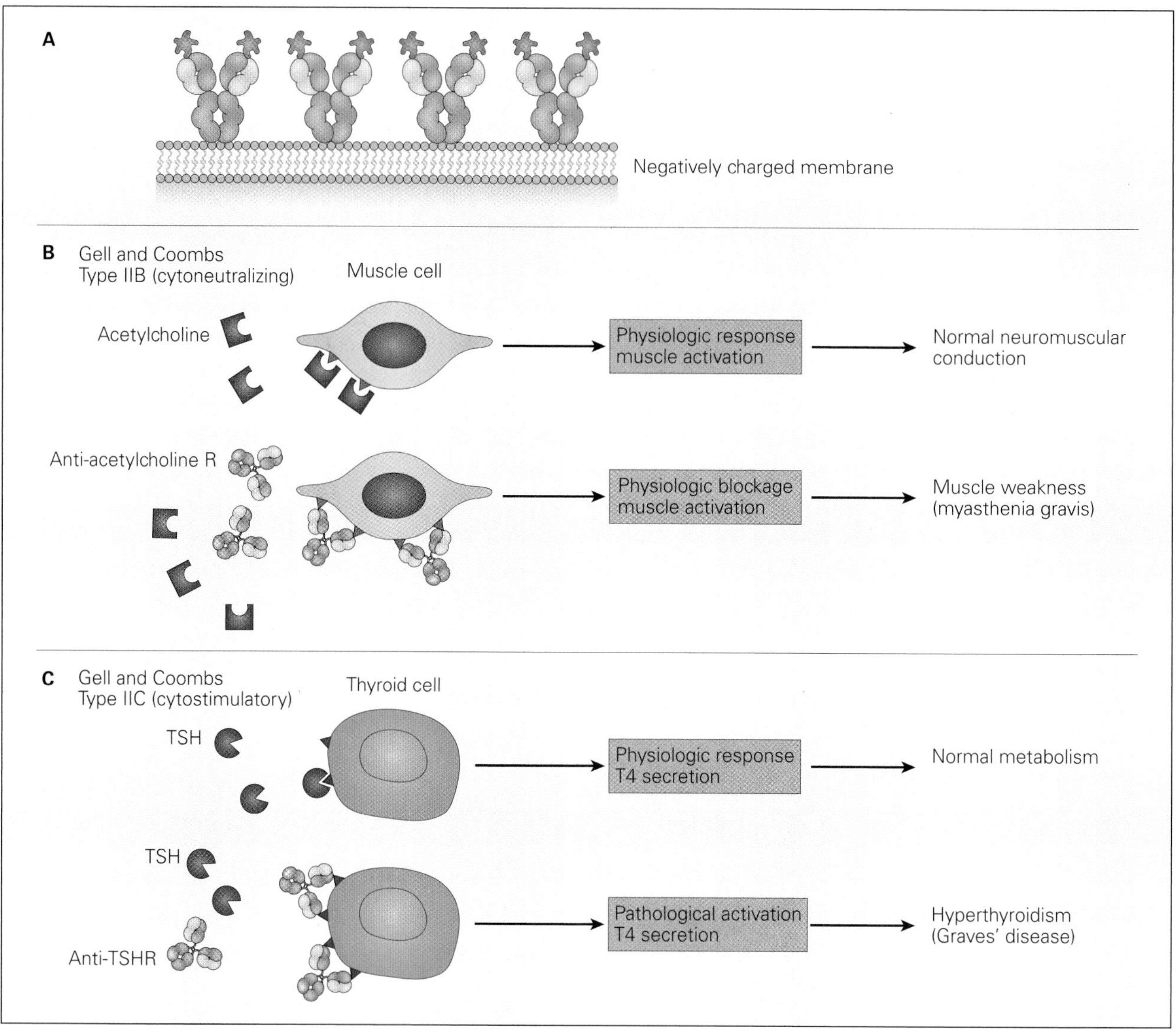

Figure 19-8. Examples of autoantibody-induced damage in autoimmune disease. Panel A: Positively charged autoantibodies can attach to a negatively charged basement membrane. In SLE, positively charged autoantibodies (anti-ds DNA) associate with the negatively charged basement membrane in the kidney, where they can form complexes *in situ* with DNA and lead to local inflammation. Panel B: In a Gell and Coombs type IIB (cytoneutralizing) reaction, anti-receptor, e.g., anti-acetylcholine receptor (R) antibody, can suppress cellular function with blockage of muscle activation and muscle weakness seen in myasthenia gravis. Antibodies can also be involved in the pathogenesis of autoimmune disease by IgG- or IgM-opsonizing autoantibodies that coat cells and prepare them for phagocytosis by phagocytic cells through their Fc receptors. Panel C: In a Gell and Coombs type IIC (immunostimulatory) reaction, anti-receptor, e.g., anti-TSH receptor (R) antibody, can activate cellular function with increased secretion of thyroxin, resulting in hyperthyroidism (Graves' disease).

a role in the pathogenesis of systemic lupus erythematosus.

Cellular-Mediated Cytotoxicity by T Cells and NK Cells

Autoreactive T cells recognize self-antigens or self-antigens that are modified by an infectious agent. T cells can also cause self-tissue damage when appropriately responding to a foreign antigen, leading to a secondary autoimmune response and immunologic injury mediated by a Gell and Coombs type IV reaction (*Chapter 17*). CD8+ cells are involved in these autocytotoxic responses and can directly recognize self-antigens in the context of MHC-I on cellular membranes and cause cellular death. In inflammatory polymyositis, CD8+ cells infiltrate the muscle and are responsible for the observed destruction of the muscle fibers.

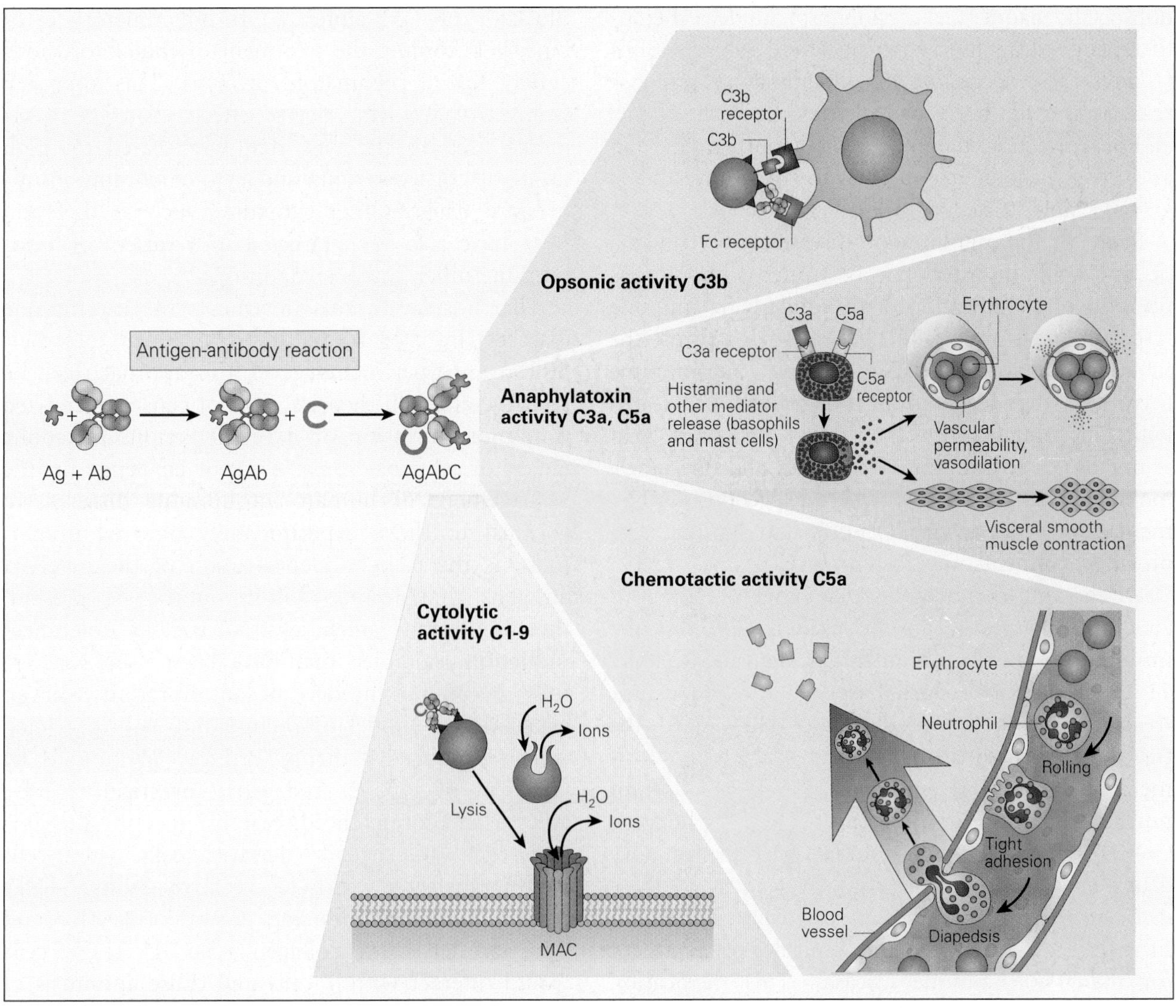

Figure 19-9. Schematic representation of the various actions of complement in an antigen-antibody reaction. The actions can include production of opsonins (C3b), anaphylatoxins (C3a and C5a), chemotactic factors (C5a), and cytolytic activity (C1–9).

CD4+ cells are thought also to play a major role in many autoimmune diseases. They can either direct the cellular autoimmune response or provide help to the B cells to produce autoantibodies. The former is carried out by Th1 cells and is characteristic of many autoimmune organ-specific diseases (i.e., autoimmune diabetes mellitus), while the latter is conducted by Th2 cells and is characteristic of many systemic autoimmune diseases, such as SLE.

Another subpopulation of CD4+ T cells are the Th17 cells that have been recently identified as potentially important in the pathophysiology of a variety of autoimmune diseases (*Chapters 7* and *9*). These pro-inflammatory cells have been shown to play a role in experimental autoimmune encephalomyelitis (the murine equivalent of multiple sclerosis), experimental inflammatory arthritis (the murine equivalent of rheumatoid arthritis), and murine lupus. In addition, although Th17 as a distinct committed T cell subpopulation is not unequivocally proven in humans, T cells that express this cytokine have been found in the joints of patients with rheumatoid arthritis and in the kidneys of those with SLE.

Treatment

Traditionally, the treatment of autoimmune diseases has focused on suppressing the immune system in a nonspecific manner (e.g., cyclophosphamide, a chemotherapeutic drug used to treat severe cases of SLE) (*Chapter 11*), decreasing the inflammatory response (e.g., aspirin has been used to treat rheumatic fever), and/or correcting the functional abnormalities that arise (e.g., cholinergic agents to treat myasthenia gravis) (Table 19-5).

Some of the autoimmune diseases, especially the organ-specific disorders, can be treated without suppression or modification of the underlying immune response and simply with medication to correct the functional abnormality. For example, autoimmune thyroiditis that leads to hypothyroidism is treated with supplementation of the thyroid hormones. That is not the case, however, for diseases affecting single major or multiple organs, where exogenous supplementation is not a viable option and immunosuppressive treatments must be employed.

Often, other medications that have been used as chemotherapeutic agents are used to suppress the immune response and limit organ damage (*Chapter 11*). Methotrexate, which has been used in cancer treatment for many years, has revolutionized the treatment of rheumatoid arthritis. It acts as an antimetabolite that interferes with the production of purines and thus the proliferation of lymphocytes. Corticosteroids and nonsteroidal anti-inflammatory drugs have also been used to treat most of these diseases. Prednisone, since its discovery more than fifty years ago, has been the mainstay of treatment for many autoimmune diseases. This medication has significantly changed the natural history of the disease in patients with systemic lupus erythematosus, despite its significant side effects when used over extended periods of time.

More recently, the underlying mechanisms that contribute to autoimmunity have been targeted, aiming at specifically disrupting the immune response and even reintroducing tolerance. The cytokines that are produced by immune cells at the site of inflammation have been successfully blocked using monoclonal, human, or chimeric (human-mouse) antibodies, or soluble decoy receptors (*Chapter 11*).

Table 19-5. Treatment of autoimmune diseases

Reversal of metabolic effects
Anti-inflammatory medications
Immunosuppression
Cytokine/adhesion molecule targeting
Restoration of self-tolerance

Blockade of TNF-alpha, a pro-inflammatory cytokine, is becoming the treatment of choice for moderately severe rheumatoid arthritis. This approach seems to have less adverse effects than the treatments used in the past that were based on high doses of corticosteroids and cytotoxic/immunosuppressant drugs. Other cytokines, such as IL-1 and IL-6, have also been targeted in a variety of autoimmune/inflammatory conditions.

The most ambitious treatments of autoimmune diseases are attempting to reintroduce tolerance. Still at an experimental level, this approach can be selective and will theoretically not cause generalized immunosuppression or have the serious metabolic effects of corticosteroids. A major challenge for the management of human autoimmune diseases, in contrast to those experimentally induced in animals, is the lack of identification of the involved antigens that induce autoimmunity. At present, this limitation precludes the use of tolerance-induction therapies that have been used successfully in animal models of autoimmunity. In an experimental model of rheumatoid arthritis called collagen-induced arthritis (induced in animals by injection of type II collagen), investigators were able to ameliorate the disease by injecting the animals with "tolerogenic" dendritic cells. These cells were transfected with a vector-encoding TNF-related apoptosis-inducing ligand (**TRAIL**) and then primed with collagen type II. These cells would interact with T cells and cause apoptosis of the collagen II-specific T cells, leading to deletion of the "forbidden clone." Such approaches could be used in the future to induce tolerance in humans if not against the initiating self-antigen, at least against self-antigens in the target organs that perpetuate the autoimmune disease.

Conclusions

Under physiologic conditions, the immune system depends on autoimmune lymphocytic clones that have escaped central tolerance to provide the needed diversity in its struggle with microorganisms. The immune system uses elaborate tolerogenic mechanisms to control those clones when they are not needed. A variety of not well-understood genetic, environmental, and immunoregulatory factors lead to the proliferation of clones that can damage organs and tissues. Since the majority of these mechanisms, including the initiating antigen(s), are elusive, the mainstay of immunologic therapy remains nonspecific immunosuppressants and/or anti-inflammatory drugs. Novel approaches in animals might pave the way for the use of medications aiming at reestablishing tolerance in some of the most serious human autoimmune diseases without the unwanted side effects of the current regimens.

Case Studies: Clinical Relevance

Let us now return to the case studies presented earlier and review some of the major points of the clinical presentation and how they relate to the immune system.

Case Study 1

- This thirty-year-old white female was diagnosed with systemic lupus erythematosus. The disease primarily affects young females and has a higher prevalence in African Americans and Asians than in Caucasians.
- There are many genes that have been associated with the disease, such as those that encode the MHC-II and the Fc gamma receptor (*Chapter 10*).
- Environmental factors that have been implicated in the etiopathogenesis of the disease not only include certain viruses, such as Epstein-Barr virus (EBV), but also physical agents, such as ultraviolet light, which can cause exacerbation of the disease.
- At the cellular level, the disease is characterized by complex functional aberrancies of both B and T cells. Autoreactive B cells give rise to antibody-forming cells that produce an array of autoantibodies directed against proteins and DNA.
- The T cells show a pan-T cell dysfunction with high CD4+ and low CD8+ activity. The T cells provide cognate and noncognate help to the B cells via surface co-stimulatory molecules (e.g., CD40-CD40L interaction) and soluble mediators (e.g., B lymphocyte stimulator [B-lys] or B cell activating factor [BAFF]) and produce cytokines such as IL-6 and IL-10.
- Interestingly, T cells in SLE produce low amounts of IL-2 upon activation; low IL-2 production apparently contributes to decreased activation-induced cell death (AICD) and the persistence of autoreactive T cell clones.
- Although the pathophysiology in SLE is complex, one of the main characteristics of the disease is the production of a diverse array of autoantibodies that either directly kill target cells, e.g., red or white blood cells, in a type II Gell and Coombs reaction, or form immune complexes and deposit on the basement membranes of organs such as the skin and kidney causing tissue damage and inflammation in a Gell and Coombs type III reaction. The result is complement activation (responsible for the low C3 levels) and "homing" of autoreactive cells to various target organs.
- In the skin, the inflammatory cell infiltration is responsible for the rash, while in the kidney, the inflammatory process causes disruption of the basement membrane and damage to the glomeruli, leading to hematuria, proteinuria, and renal insufficiency in a type III Gell and Coombs reaction.
- Shown in Figure 19-10 is a photomicrograph of a skin biopsy from an affected area of skin from a patient with SLE stained by direct immunofluorescence using an anti-IgG antibody showing a band-like IgG deposit in a granular pattern along the epidermal basement membrane (i.e., a positive lupus band test), characteristic of a type III Gell and Coombs reaction.
- Figure 19-11A shows a photomicrograph of a kidney biopsy from a patient with SLE showing a diffusely thickened basement membrane with mild segmental mesangial proliferative changes. In Figure 19-11B, immunofluorescent staining of a glomerulus from this patient shows an irregular, interrupted granular or "lumpy-bumpy" pattern of IgG deposition along capillary walls, supporting the diagnosis of SLE.
- Other manifestations of the disease include nonerosive arthritis, hair loss, mouth ulcers, and various neuropsychiatric syndromes, including psychosis. The current treatment of patients with SLE is still dependent on the use of systemic immunosuppressants such as steroids and cytotoxic drugs (*Chapter 11*).

Case Study 2

- This patient was diagnosed with type I diabetes mellitus and required insulin, the hormone that regulates glucose metabolism. The disease primarily affects young people and is now known to be immunologically mediated.

Case Studies: Clinical Relevance (continued)

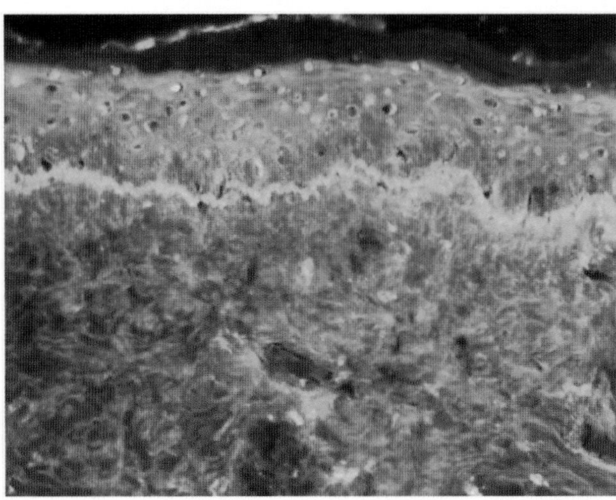

Figure 19-10. Microphotograph of a histological section of a skin biopsy from a patient with SLE prepared for direct immunofluorescence using an anti-IgG antibody showing a band-like IgG deposit in a granular pattern along the epidermal basement membrane (lupus band test is positive), characteristic of immune-complex (Gell and Coombs type III) disease.

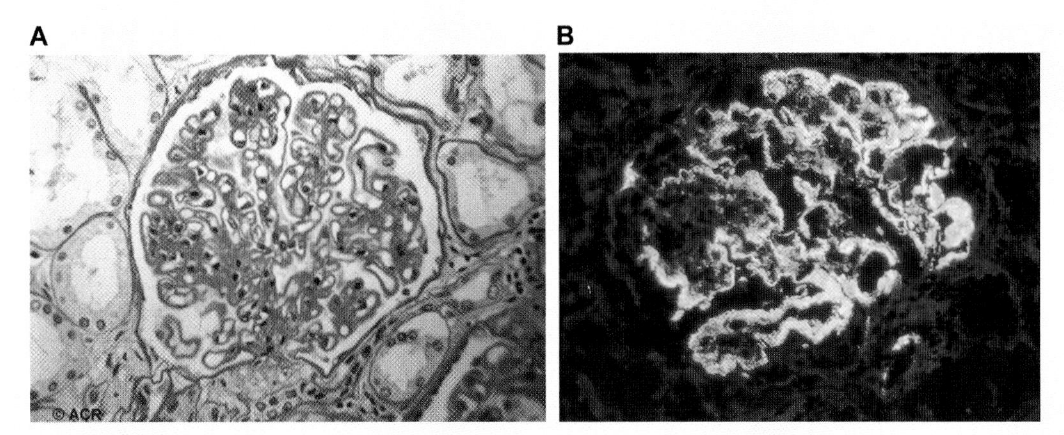

Figure 19-11. Photomicrograph of a kidney biopsy from a patient with SLE. Panel A: Hematoxylin and eosin, ×100, showing a diffusely thickened basement membrane with mild segmental mesangial proliferative changes. Panel B: Immunofluroescent staining of a glomerulus from this patient showing an irregular, interrupted granular or "lumpy-bumpy" pattern of IgG deposition along capillary walls. (Courtesy of Dr. Stephen Ray Mitchell.)

- The initial inciting event was thought to be an environmental trigger, perhaps a virus, superimposed on a genetically susceptible host. More than twenty genes have now been implicated in the pathogenesis of the condition, with certain HLA-DRB and DQA alleles being the most frequently encountered genotypes (*Chapter 10*).
- Both CD4+ and CD8+ T cells infiltrate the pancreas, causing insulitis and eventually destroying the beta cells that produce insulin in a Gell and Coombs type IV reaction. The frequently observed finding of elevated autoantibodies against glutamic acid decarboxylase (GAD), insulin, and islet cells, although useful for diagnosis, do not appear to play a direct pathogenetic role.
- The end result is a severely disrupted metabolism due to lack of insulin that leads initially to hyperglycemia manifesting as polyuria, polydipsia, polyphagia, and weight loss, and eventually causing visual problems, kidney insufficiency, nerve damage, and atherosclerosis.

Case Studies: Clinical Relevance (continued)

- In contrast to SLE, where the immune system directly damages the target organs in a type II and type III Gell and Coombs reaction, diabetes type I is an organ-specific autoimmune disease primarily caused by CD8+ cytotoxic lymphocytes in a type IV Gell and Coombs reaction
- The serious consequences in this disease result from the profound metabolic derangement that is caused by the autoimmune destruction of the pancreatic islet cells. Despite some experimental use of immunosuppression as a treatment modality, the therapeutic interventions in type I diabetes aim at ameliorating its metabolic effects by the administration of insulin.

Case Study 3

- A diagnosis of multiple sclerosis (MS) was made in this young female. The primary pathogenetic mechanism of immunologic injury in this disorder is mediated by autoreactive CD8+ cytotoxic T cells that attack neurons, particularly the myelin and related components of the neuronal axon sheath.
- MS is a disease characterized by Th1 response in the central nervous system, although regulatory T cells and B cells also play a minor role. T cells that express the pro-inflammatory cytokine IL-17 have been implicated in the pathogenesis of experimental encephalomyelitis, the murine equivalent of multiple sclerosis. The immune response leads to demyelination areas in the central nervous system's white matter.
- Patients can have different manifestations depending on the area of the nervous system that has been affected. Symptoms are commonly visual loss due to neuritis of the optic nerve as in the present case, ophthalmoplegia, various paralyses with spasticity, and neurogenic bladder.
- The disease is characterized by either relapses and remissions or a relentless progression leading to significant motor, sensory, and autonomic nervous system damage. The treatment is based on the use of corticosteroids and beta interferons as modulators of the immune response.

Key Points

- Immunologic tolerance is the normal process occurring during normal development of the immune system, which differentiates self from nonself; a breakdown of immunologic tolerance is involved in the development of autoimmune disease
- The mechanisms of tolerance include both T cell and B cell tolerance, which can take place both in central lymphoid tissues in the thymus and bone marrow as well as in peripheral lymphoid tissues.
- The autoimmune disorders are commonly divided into systemic and organ-specific autoimmune diseases.
- The mechanisms of immunologic injury that contribute to the pathogenesis of autoimmune diseases include autoantibody, immune complex formation, and cellular-mediated injury by T and NK cells.
- Current diagnostic and treatment modalities of the autoimmune diseases are based on an understanding of etiopathogenic factors that include genetic and environmental factors and immune response dysregulation.

Study Questions/Critical Thinking

1. Each of the following mechanisms is involved in the induction of peripheral T cell tolerance EXCEPT
   a. deletion
   b. ignorance
   c. anergy
   d. autophagy
   e. immune regulation
2. Which of the following is a TRUE statement concerning transcription factor autoimmune regulator (**AIRE**)?
   a. AIRE is a gene involved in the induction of central tolerance.
   b. Autoantigens expressed on the thymic epithelial cells, at least partly, are under the regulation of the transcription factor AIRE.

c. Lack of AIRE has been described in both mice and humans.
d. Lack of AIRE has been shown to result in central and peripheral tolerance.
e. The autoimmune polyendocrinopathy syndrome type I is associated with a deficiency in AIRE.

3. Which of the following is a FALSE statement concerning activation induced cell death (AICD)?

a. AICD is the best studied mechanism of elimination of activated T cell clones that ends an immune response.
b. Following T cell activation by IL-2, there is an increased expression of death receptors that belong to the TNF superfamily.
c. Fas and its ligand (FasL) are expressed on the surface of the activated T cells.
d. Interaction of Fas with either the soluble or the membrane-associated FasL causes activation of the T cell expressing Fas.
e. Mutations in either the Fas or the FasL gene are associated with autoimmune lymphoproliferative syndrome (ALPS).

4. Which of the following is a FALSE statement concerning the association of autoimmune diseases and MHC?

a. All individuals with the HLA-B27 gene are predisposed to developing ankylosing spondylitis.
b. More autoimmune diseases are associated with MHC-II than with MHC-I.
c. In patients with rheumatoid arthritis the alleles HLA DRB1*0401 and 0404 are associated with more severe disease.
d. The major MHC locus controlling both MHC-I and MHC-II is located on the long arm of chromosome 6.
e. Genes encoding components of the complement system and TNF are also located on chromosome 6.

Suggested Reading

Aoki CA, Roifman CM, Lian ZX, et al. IL-2 receptor alpha deficiency and features of primary biliary cirrhosis. J Autoimmunol. 2006; 27: 50–3.

Brand O, Gough S, Heward J. HLA, CTLA-4, and PTPN22: the shared genetic master key to autoimmunity. Expert Rev Mol Med. 2005; 7: 1–15.

Bueno C, Criado G, McCormick JK, et al. T cell signaling induced by bacterial superantigens. Chem Immunol Allergy. 2007; 93: 161–80.

Crispin J, Kyttaris VC, Juang YT, et al. Signaling and gene transcription aberrations dictate systemic lupus erythematosus T cell phenotype. Trends Immunol. 2008; 29: 110–5.

Frohman EM, Racke MK, Raine CS. Multiple sclerosis: the plaque and its pathogenesis. N Eng J Med. 2006; 354: 942–55.

Goodnow CC, Sprent J, de St Groth BF, et al. Cellular and genetic mechanisms of self tolerance and autoimmunity. Nature. 2005; 435: 590–7.

Jonsdottir T, Gunnarsson I, Risselad A, et al. Treatment of refractory SLE with rituximab plus cyclophosphamide: clinical effects, serological changes, and predictors of response. Ann Rheum Dis. 2008; 67: 330–4.

Kamradt T, Mitchison NA. Tolerance and autoimmunity. N Engl J Med. 2001; 344: 655–64.

Mayadas TN, Tsokos GC, Tsuboi N. Mechanisms of immune complex mediated neutrophil recruitment and tissue injury. Circulation. 2009; 120: 2012–24.

Miossec P, Korn T, Kuchroo VK. Interleukin-17 and type 17 helper T cells. N Eng J Med. 2009; 361: 888–98.

Moisini I, Davidson A. BAFF: a local and systemic target in autoimmune disease. Clin Exp Immunol. 2009; 158: 155–63.

Sakaguchi S. Naturally arising foxp3-expressing CD25+CD4+ regulatory T cells in immunological tolerance to self and non-self. Nat Immunol. 2005; 6: 345–52.

Takahama Y. Journey through the thymus: stromal guides for T cell development and selection. Nat Rev Immunol. 2006; 6: 127–35.

Tsokos GC, Nambiar MP, Tenbrock K, et al. Rewiring the T cell: signaling defects and novel prospects for the treatment of SLE. Trends Immunol. 2003; 24: 259–63.

van Vollenhoven R. The Janus of lupus—benefits and risks with B cell therapy. Lupus. 2008; 17: 447–9.

Weaver CT, Harrington LE, Mangan PR, et al. Th17: an effector CD4 T cell lineage with regulatory T cell ties. Immunity. 2006; 24: 677–88.

Autoinflammatory Disorders Caused by Self-Directed Innate Immune Injury

Joseph A. Bellanti, MD
German A. Benavides, MD

Case Study

A seventy-seven-year-old Caucasian female was referred to an academic center for further evaluation of a positive PPD and a request to perform a QFT-TB Gold test (QFT-TB-G) for tuberculosis. The patient had documented Crohn's disease and had a colectomy and an ileostomy fifteen years previously due to progressive disease and failure of medical therapy.

Biopsy specimens of the resected colon showed chronic inflammation and submucosal and transmural granulomas (Figure 19A-1). QFT-TB-G was negative. In addition, over the past two years, she subsequently developed multiple episodes of chest pain, fever, cough, and shortness

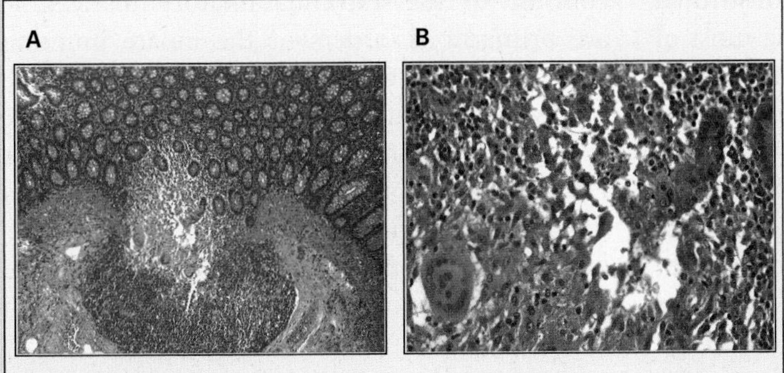

Figure 19A-1. Photomicrograph of a colon biopsy from a patient with regional ileitis (Crohn's disease). Panel A: Low-power view showing granuloma and giant cells infiltrating submucosal tissues. Panel B: High-power view showing granuloma and giant cells. (Courtesy of Dr. Thomas Fleury.)

LEARNING OBJECTIVES

When you have completed this Annex, you should be able to:

- Describe how the autoinflammatory diseases differ from the autoimmune diseases
- Recognize that autoinflammatory diseases are disorders of innate immunity, and autoimmune diseases are disorders of adaptive immunity
- List the major monogenic and polygenic autoinflammatory diseases
- Describe the major theories of pathogenesis of autoinflammatory diseases
- Explain the molecular deficiencies associated with the autoinflammatory diseases
- Describe the major clinical features of the most important autoinflammatory diseases
- List the current treatment modalities for autoinflammatory diseases
- Summarize the clinical applications of autoinflammation in health and disease

Case Study: (continued)

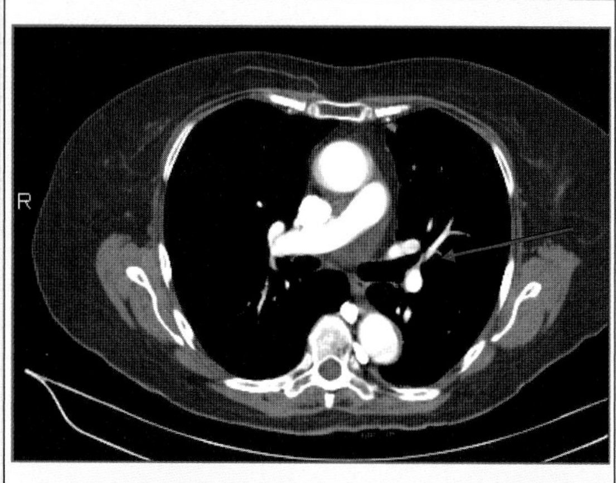

Figure 19A-2. A CT lung scan of a patient showing "tree-in-bud lesions" in the left lung (indicated by the red arrow). (Courtesy of Georgetown University Hospital)

of breath, and was found to have lung infiltrates described as "tree-in-bud" lesions on the CT lung scan (Figure 19A-2). Bronchial alveolar lavage (BAL) specimens did not show growth of *M tuberculosis* or any other significant pathogenic microbes.

Introduction

As described throughout Chapter 19, the concept of diseases in which the host sustains injury as a result of the immune system turning on itself has held a special fascination for immunologists dating back to Paul Ehrlich, who in 1908 first coined the term "horror autotoxicus" to describe this abnormal and abhorrent state wherein the host sustains attack by the immune system on itself—a condition that later formed the basis of what came to be called the autoimmune diseases. Although it was known that the innate and the adaptive immune systems constituted the two arms of the immune system, during most of the twentieth century it was assumed that the highly specialized adaptive immune system carried out the more essential elements concerned with protective and detrimental aspects of immunity, and that the innate immune system played a relatively lesser role. Consequently, during this era, the adaptive limb of immunity dominated scientific thought, including studies of autoimmune diseases that focused on the role of disordered adaptive immune regulation in the pathogenesis of these disorders. Over the past ten years, a group of monogenic diseases, characterized by recurrent inflammation and unexplained fevers, referred to as the autoinflammatory diseases, were shown to result from mutations in cells and proteins of the innate immune system. This seminal discovery has paved the way for a fundamental paradigm shift in our understanding of a wide group of autoinflammatory diseases caused by aberrant self-directed innate immune injury. So much so that a new term, **autoinflammaticus**, was coined as a counterpoint to Ehrlich's horror autotoxicus.

The term autoinflammation is now used interchangeably with innate immune-mediated inflammation, and it is possible to draw a comparison between the autoinflammatory diseases and the autoimmune diseases (Table 19-6). The autoimmune diseases refer to disorders characterized primarily by aberrant adaptive immune responses, in contrast to the autoinflammatory diseases, which are primarily disorders of the innate immune system. The majority of both conditions are transmitted as monogenic and polygenic disorders of either the adaptive or innate immune systems, respectively. Examples of the autoimmune diseases include both the organ-specific and systemic autoimmune diseases described previously, which are characterized both by aberrations of classical major histocompatability complex-based antigen-dependent T cell interactions, as well as injury mediated by activation of CD4 subpopulations (Th1, Th2, Th17, and Treg), together with other innate effector cells (macrophages, mediator cells, and NK cells via cytokine production). Tissue destruction in the autoimmune diseases is primarily mediated directly either by cytotoxic CD8 T cells or by T cell-dependent B cell autoantibody production.

Table 19A-1. Comparison of the features of autoimmune diseases and autoinflammatory diseases

Distinguishing feature	Autoimmune diseases	Autoinflammatory diseases
Arm of immunity affected	Adaptive immunity	Innate immunity
Genetic basis	Monogenic and polygenic disorders of adaptive immune function	Monogenic and polygenic disorders of innate immune function
Specific dysregulated component	Primary dysregulation of classical MHC-based, antigen-dependent T cell responses Resultant secondary contribution of inflammatory responses	Primary dysregulation of innate immune system processing and secretion of pro-inflammatory cytokines, IL-1β, IL-18, and others Resultant primary contribution of inflammatory responses
Effector mechanisms involved	Injury mediated by activation of CD4 subpopulations (Th1, Th2, Th17, and Treg) together with other innate effector cells (macrophages, mediator cells, NK cells via cytokine production) Tissue destruction, mediated directly by cytotoxic CD8 T cells T cell-dependent B cell autoantibody production	The pathological abnormality in autoinflammatory diseases is a failure to control processing and secretion of IL-1β and other pro-inflammatory cytokines in patients with these diseases
Examples of diseases	Organ-specific autoimmune diseases (Celiac disease, Graves' disease, type 1 diabetes, Addison's disease, autoimmune thyroiditis) Systemic autoimmune diseases (SLE, RA)	Familial Mediterranean fever Neonatal-onset multiple system inflammatory disease Systemic-onset juvenile idiopathic arthritis (JIA)
Predominant symptoms	Fever Maculopapular rash Joint involvement (arthritis or arthralgias) Specific organ involvement	Fever Urticarial rash Pyogenic arthritis Pyoderma gangrenosum Neurologic involvement

The autoinflammatory diseases, on the other hand, represent a group of monogenic and polygenic diseases that can present clinically with recurrent inflammation and unexplained fevers as part of their phenotype (Table 19A-1 and Box 19A-1). Examples of the innate-mediated autoinflammatory diseases include familial Mediterranean fever, neonatal-onset multisystem inflammatory disease, and systemic-onset juvenile idiopathic arthritis (**JIA**). Patients with these diseases suffer from chronic fever, urticarial rashes, arthritis, and neurologic involvement. Rapid reversal of disease severity generally occurs after the blocking of IL-1β activity by immune modulating agents (*Chapters 9* and *11*). The pathological abnormality in many of the autoinflammatory diseases appears to be a failure to control processing and secretion of IL-1β and other pro-inflammatory cytokines. The processing and secretion of IL-1β is controlled by caspase-1, an intracellular cysteine protease that cleaves the IL-1β precursor, as well as pro-IL-18, into active cytokines (*Chapter 9*). Caspase-1 functions as part of the inflammasome, a complex of intracellular proteins. The discovery of inflammasomes is one of the hallmarks of cytokine biology; inflammasome-mediated processing regulates the inflammation mediated by IL-1β, IL-18, and potentially other pro-inflammatory cytokines that could be important in these diseases (*Chapter 9*).

A Provisional Classification of Autoinflammatory Diseases

A new classification scheme for autoinflammatory disorders was developed by Masters and colleagues based on the molecular defects associated with a large group of disorders characterized by aberrant innate immune function and inflammation (Table 19A-2). Six categories of autoinflammatory disease were included: (1) IL-1β activation disorders (inflammasomopathies), (2) NF-κB activation syndromes, (3) protein-misfolding disorders, (4) complement-regulatory diseases, (5) disturbances in cytokine signaling, and (6) macrophage-activation syndromes.

Box 19A-1

Autoinflammatory Diseases

Autoinflammatory diseases are linked at the functional level, in which the described mutations are manifested in cells and proteins of the innate immune system. A new classification of the autoinflammatory diseases has been proposed that includes six distinct types of inherited disease categories: IL-1β activation disorders (inflammasomopathies), NF-κB activation syndromes, protein misfolding disorders, complement regulatory diseases, disturbances in cytokine signaling, and macrophage activation syndromes (Table 19A-2). The type 1 IL-1β activation disorders (inflammasomopathies) include mutations within the inflammasomes (intrinsic) and those outside of the inflammasome (extrinsic). The intrinsic defects are due to autosomal-dominant mutations and include three related conditions, collectively termed the cryopyrinopathies or cryopyrin-associated periodic syndromes (CAPS). The cryopyrinopathies consist of familial cold autoinflammatory syndrome (FCAS), Muckle-Wells syndrome (MWS), and neonatal-onset multisystem inflammatory disease/chronic infantile neurologic, cutaneous, and articular syndrome (NOMID/CINCA). The extrinsic defects are due to autosomal recessive mutations and include, among others, familial Mediterranean fever (FMF) and hyperimmunoglobulinemia D with periodic fever syndrome (HIDS) and deficiency of the interleukin-1 receptor antagonist (DIRA) syndrome. An additional group of autosomal-dominant diseases include tumor necrosis factor receptor-associated periodic syndrome (TRAPS), pyogenic arthritis, pyoderma gangrenosum, and acne syndrome (PAPA). Genes responsible for these autoinflammatory HPFS have been identified in the past ten years and include the Mediterranean fever (MEFV) gene (encoding marenostrin/pyrin), responsible for FMF; TNFRSF1A for TRAPS;

Table 19A-2. Provisional molecular/functional classification of autoinflammatory disease

Disease	Example of disease	Gene/(chromosome)/product
Type 1: IL-1β activation disorders (inflammasomopathies)		
Intrinsic	Familial cold autoimmune syndrome (FCAS) NOMID/CINCA	NLRP3/CIAS1 (1q44)
	Muckle Wells	
Extrinsic	FMF	MEFV (16p13.3)/pyrin (marenostrin)
	PAPA	PSTPIP1 (15q24-25.1)
	DIRA	IL1RN/IL1Ra
	CRMO/SAPHO,	Complex
	HIDS	MVK (12q24)/mevalonate kinase
Acquired or complex	Gout	Complex/uric acid
	Type 2 diabetes mellitus	Complex/hyperglycemia
	Fibrosing disorders (silicosis, asbestosis)	Complex/asbestos and silica
Type 2: NF-κB activation disorders	Crohn's disease	NOD2 (16p12)/NOD2(CARD15)
	Blau syndrome	NOD2 (16p12)/NOD2(CARD15)
	Familial cold autoimmune syndrome (FCAS2)	NLRP12 (19q13.4)/NRLP12(NALP12)
Type 3: Protein-folding disorders of the innate immune system	TNF receptor-associated periodic syndrome (TRAPS)	TNFRSF1A (12p13)/TNFR1
		Complex
	Spondyloarthropathies	HLA-B (6p21.3)/HLA-B27
		ERAP1 (5q15)/ERAP1
Type 4: Complement disorders	Acquired hemolytic uremic syndrome (aHUS)	CFH (1q32)/Factor H
		MCP (1q32)/MCP (CD46)
		CFI (4q25)/Factor I
		CFB (6p21.3)/Factor B
	Age-related macular degeneration	CFH (1q32)/Factor H
Type 5: Cytokine-signaling disorders	Cherubism	SH3-binding protein 2/SH3-binding protein 2

(Continued)

Box 19A-1 (continued)

Table 19A-2. (continued)

Disease	Example of disease	Gene/(chromosome)/product
Type 6: Macrophage activation	Familial hemophagocytic lymphohistiocytosis (HLH)	UNC13D (17q21.1)/Munc13-4 PRF1 (10q22)/Perforin 1 STX11 (6q24.2)/Syntaxin 11 Complex/virus
	Chediak-Higashi syndrome	LYST (1q42.3)/ LYST (CHS1)
	Griscelli syndrome	RAB27A (15q21.3)/ RAB27A
	X-linked lymphoproliferative syndrome	SH2D1A (Xq25)/ SAP
	Hermansky-Pudlak syndrome	HPS1-8/ HPS1-8
	Secondary HLH	Complex
	Atherosclerosis	Complex/cholesterol

Reproduced with permission from Masters, S. L., Simon, A., Aksentijevich, I., et al. Horror autoinflammaticus: The molecular pathophysiology of autoinflammatory disease. Annual Review of Immunology 27 (2009): 621–68.

mevalonate kinase for HIDS; NACHT domain-, leucine-rich repeat-, and pyrin domain-containing protein 3 (NLRP3/CIASI/NALP3) gene-encoding NALP3 (cryopyrin/NLRP3) for cryopyrin-associated periodic syndromes; and prolineserine-threonine phosphatase-interacting protein 1 (PSTPIP1) gene-encoding CD2 binding protein (CD2BP1/PSTPIP), responsible for PAPA syndrome. NALP3 and pyrin belong to the same family of pyrin domain-containing proteins, and the CD2-binding protein 1 (CD2BP1), mutated in PAPA patients, binds pyrin.

Recent studies have shown that activation of the IL-1β pathway, which is a common mechanism in the pathogenesis of autoinflammatory diseases, is a unifying factor in these diseases. Constitutive increases in the secretion of IL-1β and IL-18 have been shown in macrophages from NOMID/CINCA and MWS patients, suggesting that mutations in NLRP3 increase production of these pro-inflammatory cytokines. Lipopolysaccharide (LPS) stimulation has been shown to enhance monocytic cell death in peripheral blood mononuclear cells. Impaired pyrin-mediated IL-1β regulation is also implicated in the pathogenesis of PAPA syndrome, as mutations in the PSTPIP1 gene lead to an increased interaction between PSTPIP1 and pyrin, resulting in reduced modulation of the NALP3 inflammasome by pyrin. Thus, there is a common biochemical pathway for both FMF and PAPA, although the precise mechanisms have not been elucidated. The activation of the NALP3 inflammasome leads directly to IL-1β and IL-18 production, and so collectively, some of the autoinflammatory disorders can be therapeutically targeted by IL-1 receptor antagonist (IL-1Ra) or other agents, including MAb and soluble receptors that block IL-1β.

Mutations in other components of the NALP3 inflammasome platform have also been shown to perpetuate excessive IL-1β production. Pyrin interacts with both the NALP3 and apoptosis-associated speck-like protein containing a CARD (ASC) proteins, and it has been proposed that pyrin negatively regulates caspase-1 by competing for binding with ASC. Both the NALP3 and MEFV genes have also been associated with psoriatic JIA, suggesting the potential for shared disease mechanisms between various autoinflammatory syndromes involving abnormal production of IL-1β. Nucleotide-binding oligomerization domain-containing 2 (NOD2/NLRC2), like NALP3, is another member of the NLR family of intracellular proteins involved in innate immune responses by recognition of bacterial components and activation of NF-κB transcription factor. NOD2 mutations are implicated in a number of autoinflammatory disorders, including Crohn's disease (CD), a polygenic autoinflammatory disorder, as described below.

The discovery that Blau syndrome (BS), a rare autosomal dominant disorder, was also associated with NOD2 mutations, arose from clinical observations that granulomata formation, reminiscent of CD, were observed in BS patients. This leads to inflammation of the skin, arthritis, uveitis, and lymphadenopathy. BS has been associated with early-onset sarcoidosis, but it is more likely that such granulomatous inflammation in the young host is part of the intrinsic BS phenotype. A number of complex/acquired autoinflammatory disorders exist whose genetic relations are not known. These include gout, pseudogout, a set of fibrosing disorders, type 2 diabetes mellitus, and Schnitzler syndrome. Although the autoimmune diseases and the autoinflammatory diseases represent distinct polar entities, there are a number of intermediate entities with features of both, including psoriasis, ankylosing spondylitis, reactive arthritis, and Behcet's disease (Figure 19A-3).

Table 19A-3. Diseases caused by self-directed immune injury

	Intermediate diseases	Monogenic autoimmune diseases
Monogenic innate immune diseases CAPS FMF HIDS TRAPS PAPA Blau syndrome	Psoriasis Ankylosing spondylitis Reactive arthritis Behcet's disease	ALPS IPEX APS-1
Polygenic innate immune diseases Crohn's disease Ulcerative colitis Psoriatic arthritis Juvenile idiopathic arthritis		Polygenic autoimmune diseases Celiac disease Graves' disease Type 1 diabetes Addison's disease
Environmentally induced autoinflammatory diseases Gout Asbestosis Silicosis Sarcoidosis (?)		Autoimmune thyroiditis SLE Rheumatoid arthritis
Innate Immune System		**Adaptive Immune System**
AUTOINFLAMMATORY DISEASES		**AUTOIMMUNE DISEASE**

Although the main focus of this new classification of autoinflammatory diseases was directed to IL-1β, it also attempted to broaden the concept of autoinflammatory diseases to include other entities such as diseases that are not primarily mediated by IL-1β. For example, the type 2 diseases are NF-κB-driven, while the type 4 diseases are caused by complement-mediated defects, two other very important pathways of the innate immune system in addition to those triggered by the IL-1-related inflammasomopathies.

The driving force or the genesis of this classification had its origins in the study of a group of relatively rare monogenic disorders but has led to a better understanding of more commonly encountered disorders that heretofore were diagnostic and therapeutic orphans, e.g., sarcoidosis, Crohn's disease, and juvenile idiopathic arthritis. Shown in Table 19A-3 is a schematic representation of the continuum of disorders comprising the autoimmune diseases and the autoinflammatory disorders. The knowledge gained from the study of these rare disorders and the molecular identification of genetic lesions involved in their pathogenesis is providing new tools not only to better diagnose the more commonly encountered polygenic disorders but also to develop new biologic response modifiers to better treat them (*Chapter 11*).

Case Study: Clinical Relevance

Let us now return to the case study presented earlier and review some of the major points of the clinical presentation and how they relate to the immune system:

- This seventy-seven-year-old white female was diagnosed with Crohn's disease. The disease is part of a spectrum of inflammatory conditions known as idiopathic inflammatory bowel diseases (IBD) that comprise two types of chronic intestinal disorders: Crohn's disease and ulcerative colitis.
- The peak onset of IBD is in persons fifteen to thirty years of age, and although it can affect any region of the intestine, Crohn's disease generally involves the

Case Study: Clinical Relevance (continued)

ileum and colon, but it does so in a discontinuous pattern with numerous "skip" areas.

- Ulcerative colitis, on the other hand, involves the rectum and may affect part of the colon or the entire colon (pancolitis) in an uninterrupted pattern.
- In Crohn's disease, the inflammation is often transmural, whereas in ulcerative colitis, the inflammation is typically confined to the mucosa, as in the present case.
- Crohn's disease can be associated with intestinal granulomas, strictures, and fistulas, but these are not typical findings in ulcerative colitis.
- In addition to intestinal manifestations, Crohn's disease can also affect a number of extraintestinal organs such as the eyes, the joints, the central nervous system, and the lung, as seen in this patient, who showed the tree-in-bud pattern seen on the CT scan.
- The tree-in-bud pattern represents bronchiolar luminal impaction with mucus, pus, or fluid, which demarcates the normally invisible branching course of the peripheral airways (Figure 19A-1). It is associated with infection that has spread endobronchially and is classically associated with tuberculosis and bronchopneumonia and is often seen in bronchiectasis and cystic fibrosis.
- Although the finding of a positive TST and a lung lesion on the CT scan in this patient suggested a diagnosis of TB, this possibility was eliminated by a negative QFT-TB-G (an interferon-gamma release assay [IGRA]), suggesting that the positive TST could have been caused by infection with a related mycobacterial organism; the literature has suggested an association between mycobacterium avium paratuberculosis and Crohn's disease in both the human and in a related condition in cattle, i.e., Johne's disease or paratuberculosis.
- Accumulating evidence suggests that Crohn's disease results from an inappropriate or unrelenting inflammatory response to an as-yet-unidentified intestinal microbe(s) in a genetically susceptible host owing to a deficiency of innate immune processing and consequently persistent antigen-driven inflammation.
- This eventually leads to a deficiency in the number, or function, of T regulatory (Treg) cells in gut mucosa, which then unleashes an uninhibited immune response characterized by the production of the pro-inflammatory cytokines, TNF-α, IL-1β, IL-12, IL-2, IFN-γ, and IL-17 responsible for the chronic inflammation associated with the clinical manifestations of Crohn's disease.
- Genetic studies have highlighted the importance of key molecular sensors of the innate immune system that control normal host-microbial interactions in the healthy host and that, when deranged, contribute to the pathogenesis of Crohn's disease. Prominent among these genetic abnormalities are mutations found in the nucleotide oligomerization domain 2 (NOD2), autophagy genes 4, 7, 8, 10, and components of the interleukin-1 and interleukin-23-type 17 helper T cell (Th17) pathway.
- The NOD2 protein is an intracellular innate immune sensor of bacterial peptidoglycan that activates the inflammatory cascade through activation of NF-κB and MAP kinase-signaling systems.
- These findings open up new avenues for better diagnosis and treatment of Crohn's disease and other autoinflammatory disorders.

Key Points

- The autoinflammatory diseases refer to a group of disorders originally identified in a cluster of monogenic chronic or periodic inflammatory syndromes but that now have been broadened to include an increasing number of related polygenic and complex disorders that have as their common pathway inflammation initiated through the innate immune system, where supranormal synthesis of pro-inflammatory mediators, such as IL-1β, generates inflammation-induced tissue injury after exposure to a variety of both exogenous and endogenous stimuli. These stimuli range from a wide variety of external activators which include cold, asbestos, silica, and alum adjuvants, to endogenous substances such as uric acid, glucose, and other endogenous metabolic products.
- A clear distinction should be made between the autoinflammatory diseases, which reflect defects of the innate immune system, and the autoimmune diseases, which express defects in the adaptive immune system.
- Although inflammation is the hallmark manifestation that distinguishes autoinflammatory diseases from autoimmune disorders, the two entities represent a continuing spectrum of disorders with considerable overlap between them.

- The etiology of the autoinflammatory disorders has been biologically linked with several gene mutations involving key signaling pathways of the innate immune system that has provided the basis for a functional classification into six groups: IL-1β activation disorders (i.e., inflammasomopathies), NF-κB activation disorders, protein-folding disorders, complement disorders, signaling disorders in cytokine pathways, and macrophage disorders.
- A knowledge of the molecular mechanisms involved in the pathogenesis of the autoinflammatory disorders forms the basis for their current management with biologic modifying agents, e.g., IL-1β antagonists and TNF-α inhibitors, as well other emerging therapeutic modalities (*Chapter 11*).

Study Questions/Critical Thinking

1. Each of the following mechanisms is involved in the pathogenesis of autoinflammatory disorders, EXCEPT
   a. IL-18 overproduction
   b. IL-1β receptor antagonist deficiency
   c. mevalonate kinase deficiency
   d. NADPH oxidase deficiency
   e. UNC 13 mutation
2. Each of the following are TRUE statements concerning the autoinflammatory disorders, EXCEPT
   a. Some may respond positively to anti IL-1β treatment.
   b. The presence of autoantibody is a basic requirement for their diagnosis.
   c. Granulomas can be found in tissue biopsies in some of the disorders.
   d. Most are characterized by fever, urticarial rash, and pyogenic arthritis.
   e. They include disorders in the activation of NF-κB.
3. Which of the following entities is not considered part of the monogenic autoinflammatory disorders?
   a. FMF
   b. Muckle-Wells syndrome
   c. PAPA
   d. DIRA
   e. gout
4. Each of the following is a TRUE statement concerning Crohn's disease, EXCEPT
   a. NOD2 mutations have been shown in affected patients.
   b. Overexpression of pro-inflammatory cytokines are thought to play a role in submucosal lesions.
   c. Patients have shown increased susceptibility to infections caused by intracellular bacteria, e.g., *M tuberculosis.*
   d. Manifestations are restricted to the gastrointestinal tract.
   e. Anti-TNF-α biologic preparations are effective in management.

Suggested Reading

Abbott GF, Rosado-de-Christenson ML, Rossi SE, et al. Imaging of small airways disease. J Thorac Imaging. 2009; 24: 285–98.

Aksentijevich I, Masters SL, Ferguson PJ, et al. An autoinflammatory disease with deficiency of the interleukin-1-receptor antagonist. N Engl J Med. 2009; 360: 2426–37.

Dinarello CA. Interleukin-1beta and the autoinflammatory diseases. N Engl J Med. 2009; 360: 2467–70.

Glaser RL, Goldbach-Mansky R. The spectrum of monogenic autoinflammatory syndromes: understanding disease mechanisms and use of targeted therapies. Curr Allergy Asthma Rep. 2008; 8: 288–98.

Lachmann HJ, Kone-Paut I, Kuemmerle-Deschner JB, et al. Canakinumab in CAPS study group: use of canakinumab in the cryopyrin-associated periodic syndrome. N Engl J Med. 2009; 360: 2416–25.

Masters SL, Simon A, Aksentijevich I, et al. Horror autoinflammaticus: the molecular pathophysiology of autoinflammatory disease. Annu Rev Immunol. 2009; 27: 621–68.

McGonagle D, Aziz A, Dickie LJ, et al. An integrated classification of pediatric inflammatory diseases, based on the concepts of autoinflammation and the immunological disease continuum. Pediatr Res. 2009; 65: 38–45.

Reddy S, Jia S, Geoffrey R, Lorier R, et al. An autoinflammatory disease due to homozygous deletion of the IL1RN locus. N Engl J Med. 2009; 360: 2438–44.

Rossi SE, Franquet T, Volpacchio M, et al. Tree-in-bud pattern at thin-section CT of the lungs: radiologic-pathologic overview. Radiographics. 2005; 25: 789–801.

Chapter 20

Immune Responses to Cancer

Jimmy Hwang, MD
John L. Marshall, MD
Doru T. Alexandrescu, MD
Louis M. Weiner, MD
Joseph A. Bellanti, MD

Case Study

A 52-year-old male was found to have bilateral axillary lymphadenopathy during a follow-up medical visit. Sixteen months previously, the patient was diagnosed with a 3-mm Breslow depth ulcerated cutaneous melanoma on the right shoulder blade. (Breslow's depth is used as a prognostic factor in melanoma of the skin. It is a description of how deeply tumor cells have invaded.) Despite surgical excision of the primary dermatologic malignancy and administration of one year of adjuvant interferon, the patient now experiences a life-threatening relapse as demonstrated by the presence of multiple metastatic pulmonary nodules visualized by CT imaging, with the largest one measuring 4 cm in diameter. Because of the progressive nature of the malignancy, immunotherapy with ipilimumab, a fully human antibody that binds to cytotoxic T lymphocyte-associated antigen 4 (CTLA-4), was initiated once monthly at a dosage of 3 mg/kg (*Chapter 11*). During the first two months of treatment, the rate of tumor growth appeared to diminish, and after the third and fourth doses, a marked tumor regression was seen. After six months of treatment, there was almost complete disappearance of the lung lesions originally seen on the CT scan without development of new lesions. This favorable therapeutic response has continued for 36 months of currently follow-up evaluation. This case presentation demonstrates that immunotherapy can be a very effective adjunctive treatment of cancer in some patients manifesting tumors refractory to conventional therapies. It also raises the following questions: What are the antitumor immune responses? How do these antitumor immune responses work? What segments of the immune response can be triggered or augmented by immunotherapy? What are the current and emerging immunotherapeutic modalities for treatment of cancer?

Introduction

As described in Chapter 1, a third recognized function of the immune system is *surveillance*, a function that normally provides the host with the ability to recognize and destroy altered self, e.g., cell mutants that

LEARNING OBJECTIVES

When you have completed this chapter, you should be able to:

- Understand the general concepts of immunologic surveillance and tumor antigenicity
- Describe the differences between carcinogen-induced and viral-induced tumors
- Explain the differences in the concept of immunoediting
- Give some examples of the clinical applications of tumor antigenicity
- Describe the important relationships of immune tolerance with the malignant state
- Understand the different roles of Th1, Th2, Th17, and Treg cells in antitumor immunity
- Outline the different mechanisms used by the malignant cell to evade the immune response
- List the most current immunologic strategies used in the immunotherapy of malignant diseases
- Utilize this knowledge for the prevention of cancer in the healthy host and for the management of patients with malignant disease

have undergone malignant transformation and are recognized as "non-self." A hypofunctioning of this role has been thought to be associated with a propensity for development of malignant disease. The idea that there may be immune responses to tumors is based upon the immunologic surveillance theory as described below. This theory is supported by both evidence from the experimental animal as well as the human and has led to an intensive research effort to develop practical modalities to prevent or treat cancer in the human by exploitation of an enhanced immune system. In the past decade, there have been significant advances in the field of tumor immunotherapy, which are grounded in the idea that the immune system can selectively recognize and subsequently destroy cancer cells. This chapter will describe the major basic concepts of tumor antigenicity, normal immune mechanisms directed against cancer cells, the possible survival mechanisms used by the cancer cell to evade the immune system, and some of the recent clinical applications of immunotherapy of human malignancies.

The Concept of Immunologic Surveillance and Tumor Antigenicity

The Immunologic Surveillance Theory

The immunologic surveillance theory was originally put forth independently by Burnet and Thomas, who suggested that the immune system continually surveyed the body for the presence of malignant cells, which were continuously arising as a result of mutations. Because such cells were recognized as foreign, they were postulated and, in some cases, have subsequently been shown to be eliminated by similar innate and adaptive immune mechanisms as those marshaled in response to any other foreign configuration, e.g., bacteria, viruses, fungi, and parasites (*Chapters 12, 13, 14,* and *15*). While this concept has some validity, it has also become apparent that immune surveillance is but one mechanism of host tumor immunity. Its potential strength is based on the knowledge that cancer cells do indeed express tumor-associated antigens (**TAA**s) or tumor-specific antigens (**TSA**s) that can be recognized by the immune system as foreign following which malignant cells expressing these antigens are destroyed and eliminated. The logical corollary to this theory is that development of cancer can be explained by the ability of the tumor to evade immune recognition either by the failure of the immune system to be adequately generated or by the induction of immune tolerance or other inhibitory mechanisms used by the tumor to escape immune detection and elimination.

Tumor Antigenicity: Carcinogen-Induced versus Viral-Induced Tumors

Shown in Figure 20-1 is a schematic representation of how the development of tumor antigens induced by carcinogens differs from those brought about by viral infection (Figure 20-2). In the case of carcinogen-induced tumors, regardless of morphologic similarity, each new tumor induced by the same agent possesses a different TAA specificity unique to that tumor (Figure 20-1). In contrast, the tumor-specific antigens in tumors induced by viruses cross-react with those on tumors induced by the same or similar viruses even though their morphologic appearance may differ (Figure 20-2).

Tumor-Specific Antigens

Based upon studies in the experimental animal, immune surveillance, in the classical sense, appears to be restricted mainly to virally-induced tumors.

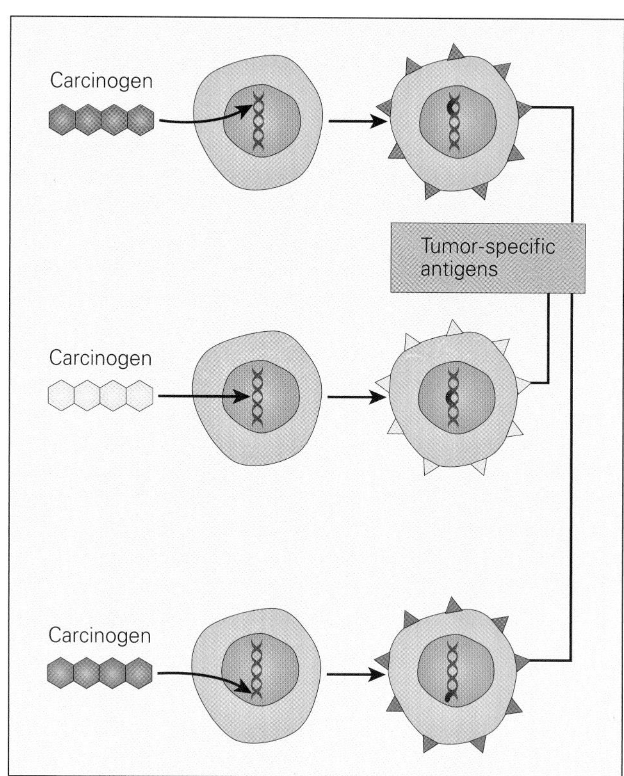

Figure 20-1. Schematic representation of development of tumor-specific antigens by a chemical carcinogen. Note that when cells of identical genetic identity are transformed by the same chemical carcinogen, each new tumor has its own unique antigenic specificity regardless of morphologic appearance.

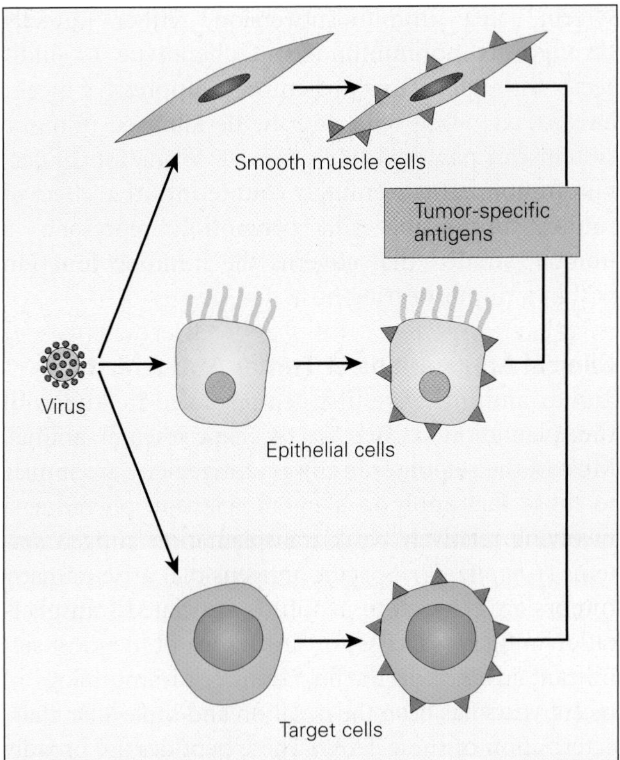

Figure 20-2. Schematic representation of development of tumor-specific antigens by a tumor virus. Note that although the morphologic appearance may vary, each tumor induced by a single virus retains the same TSA on the cell surface.

Moreover, some tumors may be devoid of these foreign antigens and may not express these antigens. Thus, they would be recognized as self components and continue to grow by evading the immune response.

Clinically, both the validity as well as the limitation of the immune surveillance concept has been elucidated by observations made in immunosuppressed patients, such as those infected with the human immunodeficiency virus (HIV) or allogeneic transplant recipients who require intense immunosuppressive therapy to prevent graft rejection. Although the incidence of some malignancies, such as some lymphomas, Kaposi's sarcoma, and squamous cell carcinomas, which may be virally mediated by HTLV, HHV-8, and human papilloma virus (**HPV**), respectively, are increased in these patients, the incidence of other epithelioid malignancies, such as adenocarcinomas, does not seem significantly changed. Thus, it is likely that the immunologic surveillance theory addresses but one aspect of the body's defenses against malignancy.

Cancer Immunosurveillance versus Immunoediting

More contemporary thinking about tumorigenesis focuses on the principles of "immune shaping and editing" pioneered by the studies of Robert Schreiber and others. The cancer immunoediting process is envisaged to consist of three phases: elimination, equilibrium, and escape, which have been termed the "three Es of cancer immunoediting" (Figure 20-3). The initial elimination phase corresponds to the original concept of cancer immunosurveillance in an immunologically competent host, whereby nascent tumor cells are successfully recognized and eliminated

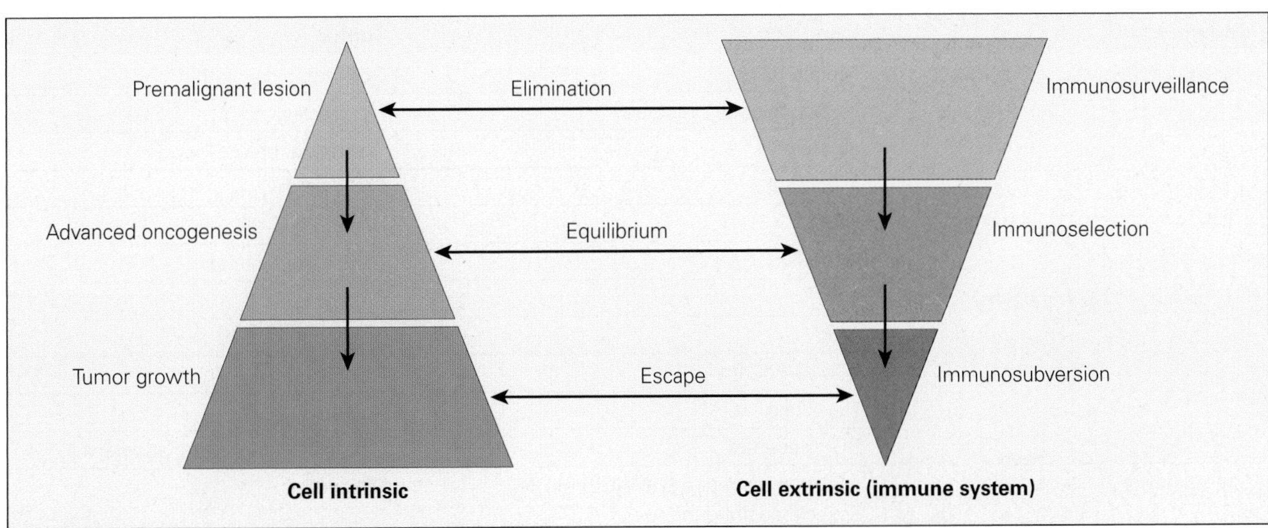

Figure 20-3. Schematic representation of the immunoediting process consisting of three phases: elimination, equilibrium, and escape, termed the "three Es of cancer immunoediting." Carcinogenesis is envisaged as a multistep process resulting from cross talk of cancer-cell–intrinsic factors and host immune system (cell-extrinsic) effects. (Adapted with permission from Zitvogel L, Tesniere A, Kroemer G. Cancer despite immunosurveillance: immunoselection and immunosubversion. Nat Rev Immunol. 2006;6:715–27.)

by the immune system, thus returning the tissues to their normal state of function. In this premalignant phase, there is no clinically discernible tumor growth and no clinical symptoms.

Tumor cells that elude the immunosurveillance phase will progress to the second phase of immune editing, called the equilibrium phase of advanced oncogenesis, where tumor expansion and metastasis are minimal (tumor dormancy) and usually occur without symptoms. This phase of equilibrium is a poorly understood process where the immune system is envisaged to control tumor cell growth but not completely eliminate the transformed cells. It is hypothesized that in this equilibrium phase, two outcomes may occur. In the first, the immune system may eventually eliminate all tumor cells, in essence leading to an outcome that is not physiologically distinct from the first phase of elimination. In the second scenario, the constant interaction of the immune system with tumors over a long period of time may actually "edit" or sculpt the phenotype of the developing tumor, resulting in the immunoselection of a tumor that has been shaped into a less-immunogenic state that survives.

Tumors that are no longer susceptible to immune attack then progress into the third phase of the immunoediting process, termed "escape." It is thought that the emergence of clinical symptoms of cancer generally correlates with this stage. During this escape phase, the tumor subverts the immune system, i.e., immunosubversion, either directly through its nonimmunogenic phenotype or indirectly through a variety of immunosuppressive mechanisms, e.g., Treg cells, and the destabilized immune system can paradoxically promote formation of certain tumors. This seemingly counterintuitive effect of tumor suppression and promotion represents a unique paradox that governs the immune function within a tumor bearing host.

Clinical Applications of Tumor Antigenicity

Tumor antigens were first demonstrated in studies of transplantation models in the experimental animal. Most of the responses in tumor antigenicity are similar to those that apply to allograft rejection phenomena involving relatively weak transplantation antigen systems (*Chapter 22*). Specific antigens that arise in many tumors are referred to as tumor-associated transplantation antigens (**TATAs**) or TAAs. One of the most significant advances in the field of tumor immunology in recent years has been the isolation and molecular characterization of these TAAs. These peptides are broadly categorized in four groups: (1) unique antigens specific for an individual tumor; (2) overexpressed peptides or proteins that are found to a variable degree on normal tissue; (3) shared tumor antigens; and (4) viral antigens that may be shared among different cells, but confined to malignancy (Table 20-1).

The first category of TAAs consists of unique antigens that are specific to an individual tumor, e.g.,

Table 20-1. Various types of tumor-associated antigens (TAAs) identified in the human

Category	Examples	Tumor
Unique tumor-specific antigens	Mutant p21/ras	Colorectal, pancreatic
	Immunoglobulin idiotype	B cell malignancy
	β-catenin	Colorectal, breast
	Mutant p53	Pancreatic
	CDK4	Melanoma
	Mutant EGFR VIII	Glioblastoma, lung
Overexpressed self-antigen peptides	CEA	Colorectal
	Muc-1	Colorectal
	GA733/EpCam	Colorectal
	Her-2/neu	Breast
	EGF Receptor	Colorectal, lung, head, and neck
Shared tumor antigens	Melanoma antigen E (MAGE) tumor-associated antigen	Melanoma
Viral-associated antigens	Human papilloma virus (HPV)	Cervical
	Hepatitis B virus (HBV)	Hepatocellular
	Epstein–Barr virus (EBV)	B cell malignancy

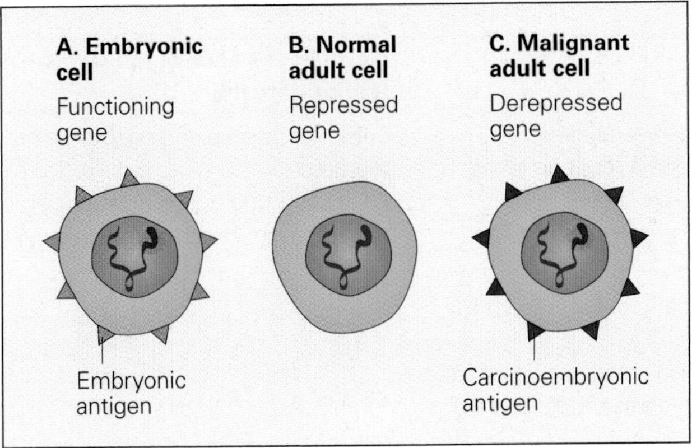

Figure 20-4. Postulated mechanism of emergence of carcinoembryonic antigens. Panel A: A normal embryonic antigen produced by a functioning gene within an embryonic cell. Panel B: Repression of the gene with no further elaboration of the embryonic antigen in the adult cell. Panel C: Derepression of the gene in the malignant cell with reappearance of the embryonic antigen (e.g., carcinoembryonic antigen, CEA) on the surface of the cell.

mutant p53 found in pancreatic cancer. These peptides are derived from mutated proteins that are not found in normal host tissues. The second category of antigens includes those that are overexpressed in tumor cells but that are also present in normal tissues. This category includes the carcinoembryonic antigen (**CEA**) associated with colorectal cancer. This antigen is expressed primarily during embryonal development, and then is less commonly found in the adult (Figure 20-4). The third category includes those antigens shared among different tumors but confined to malignancies, e.g., melanoma antigen E (**MAGE**) tumor-associated antigen. These are usually transcriptionally reactivated genes not expressed in normal host tissues. This category is variably referred to as embryonic antigens, developmental antigens, or cancer testis antigens. Finally, viral antigens from viral-associated antigens, such as those induced by the human papilloma virus (**HPV**), hepatitis B virus (**HBV**), and Epstein–Barr virus (**EBV**), which may also be tumorigenic, could serve as tumor-specific targets for the immune system. Other tumor markers that relate to the development of malignant tumors have been identified (Box 20-1). Although useful in diagnosis, their relevant role in tumor immunity has not been established.

Tolerance and the Malignant State

The principles of tumor immunity are grounded both in an understanding of the polymorphism of the MHC-peptide interaction (*Chapter 10*) as well as the intrathymic acquisition of T cell development and tolerance (*Chapters 3, 7,* and *19*). Autoreactive T cells that recognize dominant self-antigen, for example, are deleted in the thymus by a process called *negative selection* (*Chapters 7* and *19*). Moreover, autoreactive T cells with weak MHC recognition are neglected. These two processes are known as *central tolerance.* Some T cells escape thymic selection and can recognize self under specific conditions in

Box 20-1

Tumor Marker Tests

Definition

Tumor markers are a group of proteins, hormones, enzymes, receptors, and other cellular products that are overexpressed and produced in higher than normal amounts by malignant cells. Tumor markers are usually normal cellular constituents that are present at normal or very low levels in the blood or tissues of healthy persons, but if the substance in question is produced by the tumor, its levels will be increased either in the blood or in the tissue of origin. Shown in Table 20-2 are some of the tumor markers in common clinical use.

Purpose

The majority of tumor markers are used to monitor patients for recurrence of tumors following treatment. In addition, some markers are associated with a more aggressive course and higher relapse rate and have value in staging and prognosis of the cancer. Most tumor markers are not useful for screening because levels found in early malignancy overlap the range of levels found in healthy persons.

Precautions and Limitations of the Use of Tumor Markers

Not every tumor will cause a rise in the level of its associated marker, especially in the early stages of some cancers. When a marker is used for cancer screening or diagnosis, the physician must confirm a positive test result by using imaging studies, tissue biopsies, and other procedures. False positive results may occur when the patient has cross-reacting antibodies that interfere with the test or other nonmalignant conditions, e.g., elevated PSA in urinary tract infection or benign prostatic hypertrophy, elevated CA-125 antigen in fallopian tube inflammatory conditions, elevated alpha fetoprotein in liver regeneration, and elevated CEA and/or CA-20-9 in inflammatory bowel disease.

Table 20-2. Tumor markers in common clinical use

Name	Type of tumor marker	Clinical use	Normal reference range levels (varies with lab)
Alpha-fetoprotein (AFP)	Oncofetal antigen	Prenatal diagnosis of spina bifida Diagnosis and monitoring of patients with non-seminoma testicular cancer Elevated in almost all yolk sac tumors and 80% of malignant liver tumors	< 15 ng/L in men and nonpregnant women Levels > 1,000 ng/L indicate malignant disease (except in pregnancy)
CA (Cancer)125	Protein antigen	Diagnosis and monitoring of women with ovarian cancer May also be elevated in malignancies of the liver, colon, pancreas, breast, lung, and digestive tract	< 35 U/mL
Carcinoembryonic antigen (CEA)	Oncofetal antigen	Colorectal cancer May also be elevated in persons with breast, colon, lung, gastric, ovarian, pancreatic, and uterine cancer	< 3 μg/L for nonsmokers; < 5 μg/L for smokers
Estrogen receptor (ER)	Tissue receptor for estrogen	The level of ER in the tissue is used to determine whether a person with breast cancer is likely to respond to estrogen therapy with tamoxifen, which binds to the receptors blocking the action of estrogen. May also be expressed in ovarian cancer, uterine cancer.	< 6 fmol/mg protein is negative; > 10 fmol/mg protein is positive
Progesterone receptor (PR)	Tissue receptor for progesterone	PR has the same prognostic value as ER and is measured by similar methods	Tissues with no express PR receptor expression are less likely to bind estrogen analogues used in tumor treatment Persons with negative ER and PR have < 5% chance of responding to endocrine therapy. Those positive for both markers have > 60% chance of tumor shrinkage when treated with hormone therapy.
Human chorionic gonadotropin (hCG)	Hormone produced by cells of the trophoblast and developing placenta	Trophoblastic tumors and choriocarcinoma. About 60% of testicular cancers secrete hCG. hCG is also produced less frequently by a number of other tumors.	< 20 IU/L for males and non--pregnant females; > 100,00 IU/L indicates trophoblastic tumor
Prostate specific antigen (PSA)	Small glycoprotein with protease activity that is specific for prostate tissue; found in bound and free form	Present in low levels in all adult males High levels are seen in prostate cancer, benign prostatic hypertrophy, and inflammation of the prostate	< 4 ng/L
CA-20-9		Pancreatic cancer	< 37 U/mL

peripheral tissues. Peripheral tolerance concerns mature lymphocytes once they have exited primary lymphoid organs and are circulating in the periphery.

T cells can recognize nonmutated self antigens on tumor cells and therefore represent anti-self responses. T cell activation requires two distinct signals. Signal 1 is delivered by the interaction between the T cell receptor (**TCR**) and the antigenic peptides presented on MHC molecules. Signal 2 is provided by one of several nonspecific co-stimulatory molecules such as the binding of CD28 on T cells with B7 family molecules on antigen-presenting cells (**APCs**). Another molecule that binds to the B7 family, cytotoxic T lymphocyte antigen 4 (**CTLA-4**), also known as CD152, transmits an inhibitory signal to T cells in contrast to CD28, which transmits a stimulatory signal. CTLA-4 is also found in regulatory T cells and may be therefore important to their suppressive function.

Cross-presentation and Cross-priming of Tumor Antigens

Cancer cells frequently stimulate Signal 1 alone, and inefficiently stimulate Signal 2. Accordingly, cancer cells may preferentially induce tolerance. Hence, tumor antigens must be presented through antigen-presenting cells to initiate and sustain anti-tumor immune responses. This is achieved by a process called *cross-presentation*, namely, tumor cells or tumor antigens are taken up by APCs, which process the antigens and present them on the APC cell surface restricted for this on MHC-I and MHC-II molecules. APCs such as dendritic cells (**DCs**) can efficiently prime T cells, where they display MHC antigen complexes (Signal 1) together with co-stimulatory molecules (Signal 2), which activate naive T cells in a process called *cross-priming*. This process can also cause T cell unresponsiveness or cross-tolerance (*Chapters 7* and *11*).

Since individual B and T lymphocytes are antigenically committed to a specific unique antigen, their clonal expansion upon recognition of foreign antigens is required to obtain sufficient antigen-specific B and/or T lymphocytes to achieve an appropriate immune response. Although the kinetics of primary adaptive immune responses are slower than innate immune responses, the differentiation of lymphocyte subsets into long-lived and short-lived memory cells

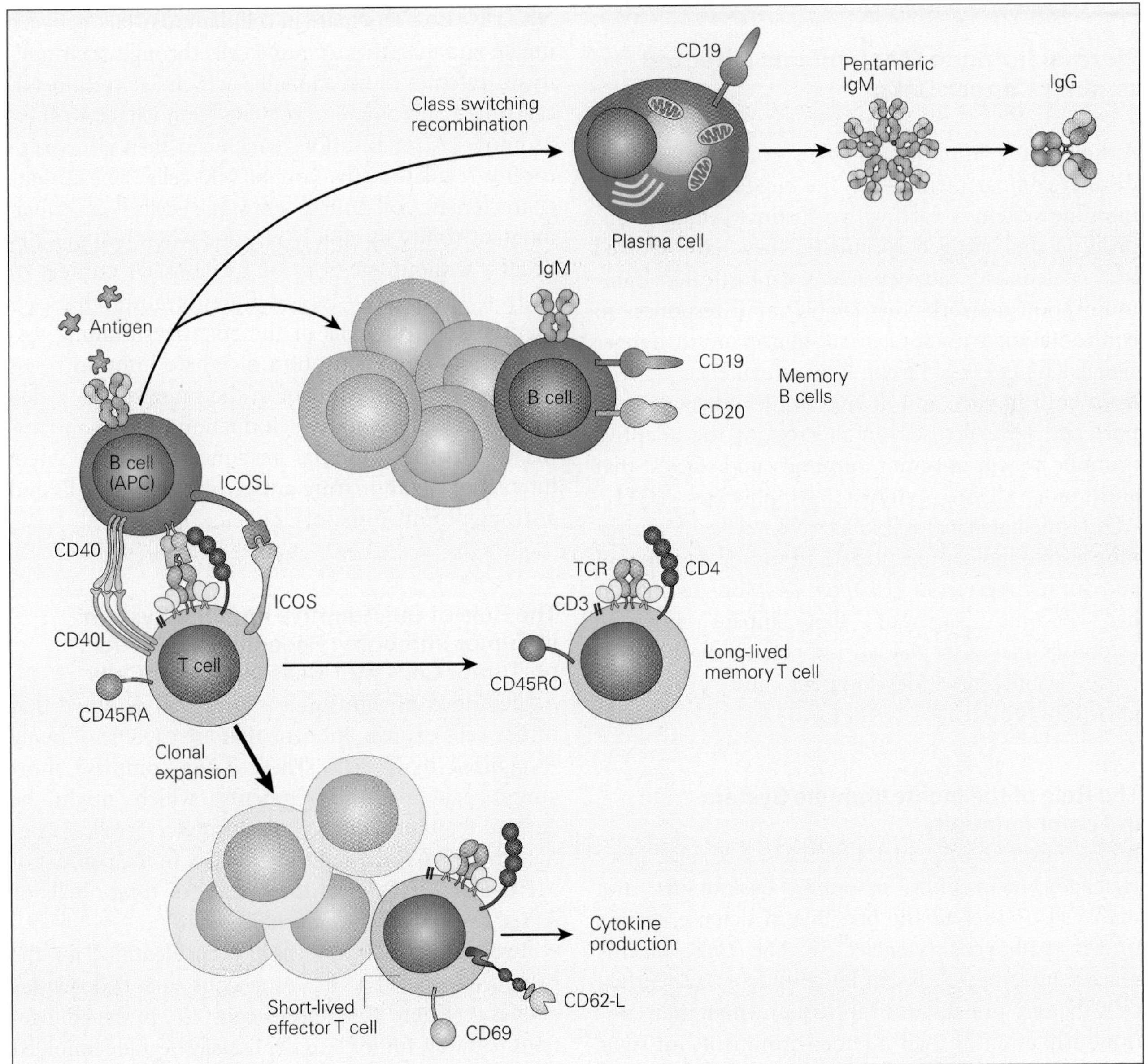

Figure 20-5. Schematic representation of the clonal expansion and generation of subsets of lymphocytes differentiating into long-lived and short-lived memory cells during the course of a primary adaptive immune response, resulting in larger T and B cell responses upon subsequent exposure to the same antigen.

during the primary immune response results in larger responses upon subsequent exposure to the same antigen (Figure 20-5 and *Chapter 6*).

Because of their enormous plasticity, immune cells exert multiple effector functions that are continually fine-tuned by cytokine and chemokine alterations in tissue microenvironments (*Chapter 9*). Therefore, the immune system is not only involved in the maintenance of tissue homeostasis between the internal and extracellular environments, but also in the pathogenesis of many chronic diseases related to chronic infection, autoimmune disease, and malignancy. Now let us examine how these components of immune defense are marshaled in the attack of tumor cells.

Normal Immune Mechanisms Directed against Cancer Cells

Although the immune system is composed of two distinct compartments—i.e., the innate and adaptive immune systems—each with a distinct cellular composition and antigen specificity, they have evolved interrelated and interdependent sophisticated communication networks that enable rapid responses to confrontation with foreign substances or to danger signals (*Chapter 5*). Several lines of evidence, derived from both in vitro and in vivo studies, strongly support and have focused on the role of the adaptive immune system in tumor immunity and suggest that antitumor CD8+ cytotoxic lymphocytes (**CTL**), ADCC-mediated natural killer (**NK**) cells, or antitumor antibodies can participate in tumor destruction and tumor regression (*Chapter 1*). More recently it has become apparent that innate immune responses may also play an important role in resistance against the development and progressive growth of tumors.

The Role of the Innate Immune System in Tumor Immunity

Innate immune cells, including DCs, NK cells, macrophages, neutrophils, basophils, eosinophils, and mast cells, represent the first line of defense against foreign pathogens (*Chapter 1*). The DCs, macrophages, and mast cells can be considered as sentinel cells that are pre-stationed in tissues where they continuously monitor their microenvironments for signs of invasion. When tissue homeostasis is perturbed, these sentinel cells immediately release soluble mediators, such as cytokines, chemokines, matrix remodeling proteases, and reactive oxygen species (**ROS**), as well as bioactive mediators such as histamine and prostaglandin metabolites that induce mobilization and infiltration of additional leukocytes into damaged tissue as part of the inflammatory response (*Chapter 5*). Macrophages and mast cells can also activate vascular and fibroblast responses in order to orchestrate the elimination of the malignant cell and to initiate local tissue repair. DCs, on the other hand, take up tumor antigens and migrate to lymphoid organs, where they present processed peptides to T cells for the induction of specific antibody and CMI responses. DCs are, therefore, key players in the interface between innate and adaptive immunity. NK cells also participate in cellular cross-talk between innate and adaptive immune cells through their ability to interact bidirectionally with DCs; certain NK cell subsets eliminate immature DCs, whereas others promote DC maturation, which can then also reciprocally regulate activation of NK cells. The unique characteristic of innate immune cells—i.e., their inherent ability to rapidly respond when tissue injury occurs, without memory of previous encounters or antigen specificity—is a defining feature that sets them apart from cells of the adaptive immune system. Thus, acute activation of innate immunity sets the stage for establishment of the more sophisticated adaptive immune system. Induction of efficient primary adaptive immune responses requires direct interactions with mature antigen-presenting cells and a strong proinflammatory milieu.

The Role of the Adaptive Immune System in Tumor Immunity: Recognition of TAAs on Tumor Cells by T Cells and Other Cells

As described previously, it is now well accepted that tumor cells express antigens that are capable of being recognized by T cells. These TAAs comprise short amino acid peptide segments, which might be derived from any intracellular protein. T cells recognize these TAAs through their TCRs in the context of MHC-I or MHC-II on the surface of tumor cells or APCs, respectively (*Chapters 7* and *10*).

Two distinct pathways have been identified for the processing of TAAs, the exogenous and endogenous pathways (Figure 20-6 and *Chapter 10*). In the endogenous pathway, tumor cells continually degrade unfolded intracellular proteins within the proteosome into short peptide fragments. Following transport through several

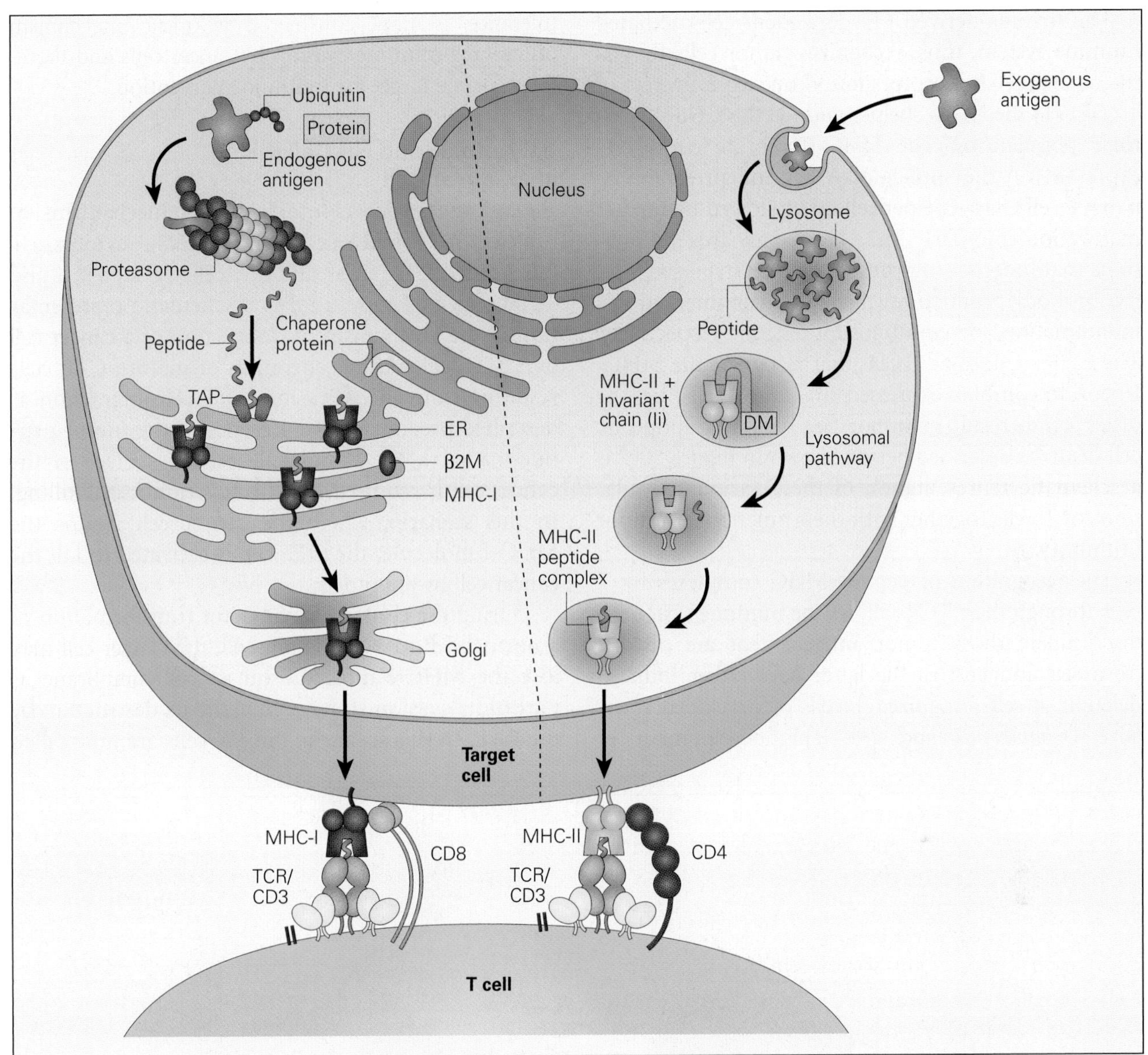

Figure 20-6. Tumor-associated antigen processing. Abbreviations: ER = endoplasmic reticulum; MHC = major histocompatibility complex; TCR = T cell receptor.

pathways in the endoplasmic reticulum, these fragments are then loaded onto the MHC-I. The final MHC-I/peptide complexes are then transported to the tumor cell surface through the Golgi apparatus for presentation to CD8+ T cells (Figure 20-6).

In the exogenous pathway, professional APCs,
3 including dendritic cells and macrophages, through a variety of endocytic pathways, take up intracellular proteins that have been released from damaged or injured tumor cells (*Chapter 10*). These intracellular proteins can then be degraded in lysosomal pathways to peptides that, when complexed with MHC-II on the cell surfaces, are presented to CD4+ T cells. Alternatively, the APCs may also process the tumor proteins through the endogenous pathway. In this way, APCs are able to prime both MHC-I and MHC-II responses and give rise to specific antibody and cell-mediated immune responses important in tumor immunity.

Adaptive immune cells, such as B lymphocytes, 6
CD4+ helper T lymphocytes, and CD8+ CTLs, distinguish themselves from innate leukocytes by expression of somatically generated, diverse antigen-specific receptors, which are formed as a consequence of random gene rearrangements that allow a more flexible and broader repertoire of responses than those conducted by innate immune cells, which express germline-encoded and more stereotyped receptors (*Chapters 6* and *7*).

The thymus-derived (T) dependent cell-mediated immune system, thus, recognizes tumor cells by virtue of their TCR receptors found on two universes of T cells: (1) the CD4+ helper and (2) the CD8+ cytotoxic populations. The MHC-II/peptide complexes expressed on the surface of APCs and presented to naive T cell CD4+ helper cells are followed by further maturation into Th1, Th2, Th17, and Treg populations that function to promote delayed hypersensitivity, antibody production (through B cell interaction), inflammation, or immunosuppression, respectively. The CD8+ cytotoxic T cells that recognize the MHC-I/peptide complex expressed on tumor cells, on the other hand, result in tumor cell lysis and apoptotic cell death as described below. Shown in Figure 20-7 is a schematic representation of these various populations of T cells together with their functions in tumor immunity.

The recognition of peptide-MHC complexes by T cells through their TCRs allows the immune system to discriminate those tumor antigens that are distinct from self antigens, as the latter have either induced deletion of self-recognized T cells or developed tolerance (*Chapters 7* and *19*). This development of tolerance is now considered a prime mechanism underlying immune evasion by cancer cells and therefore a prime target for immune intervention.

T Cytotoxic and NK Cell Killing of a Cancer Cell

Two of the major cytotoxic killing mechanisms of tumors are carried out by either CD8+ cytotoxic T (also called CTL cells) and NK cells (*Chapters 1* and *3*). Shown in Figure 20-8 is a schematic representation of the mechanism of destruction of a cancer cell by a CTL cell. After generation of mature CTL cells resulting from the APC-antigen/T cell interaction as described previously, the presence of the tumor peptide-loaded MHC-I molecule on the surface of the cancer cell is required for effective tumor cell killing. In this scenario, where the cancer cell retains the MHC-I molecule, the CTL cell is activated to kill the cancer cell by apoptosis.

During the course of malignant transformation of a normal cell to a malignant cell, the cancer cell may lose the MHC-I molecule on its cell membrane as part of its evasion strategy to elude its destruction by the CTL. In this scenario, the NK cells are now called

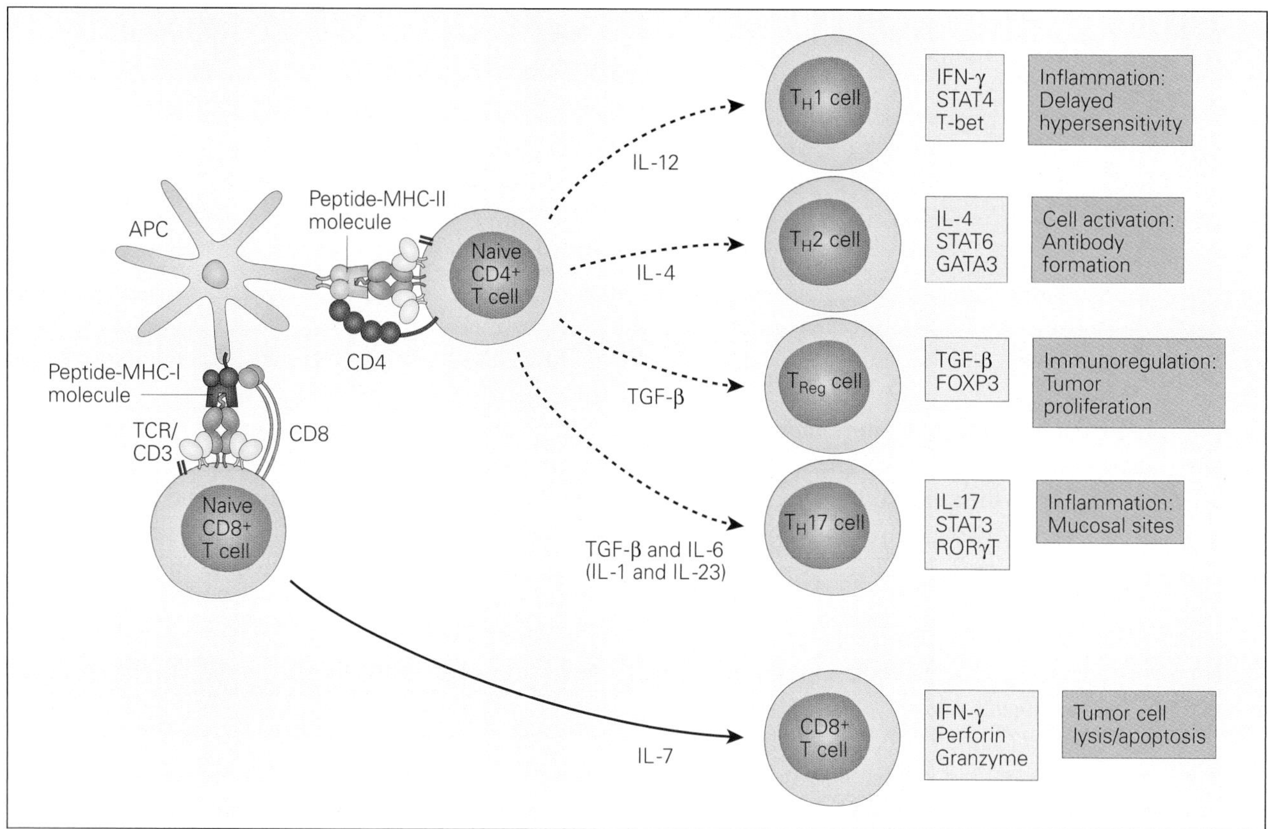

Figure 20-7. Schematic representation of various populations of CD4+ and CD8+ T cells together with their functions in tumor immunity.

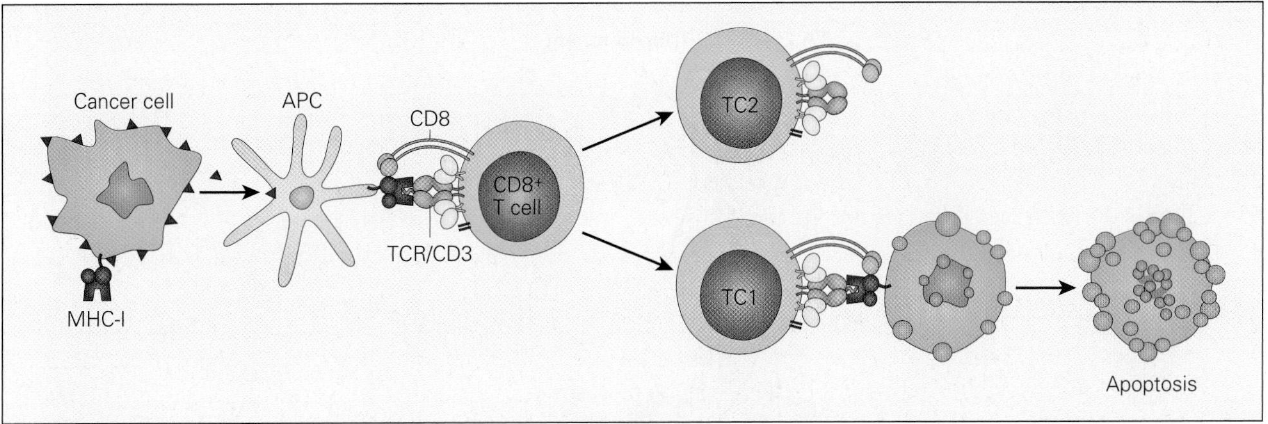

Figure 20-8. Schematic representation of the role of T cytotoxic cells in the killing of a cancer cell that retains the MHC-I receptor. The tumor-specific antigen (TSA) is processed by an APC following which the processed TSA is then displayed on a MHC-I molecule and presented to the CTLR of a CTL cell, which is then activated to kill the cancer cell by apoptosis.

into play. Shown in Figure 20-9 is a schematic representation of the mechanisms of killing of a tumor cell by the NK cell. Normally, NK cells display two types of receptors: (1) a killer-activating receptor (**KAR**) with specificity for a number of cell surface ligand molecules; and (2) a killer-inhibiting receptor (**KIR**) with specificity for a MHC-I ligand. The interaction of a NK cell with a normal cell consists of the binding of both of these receptors with their respective ligand molecules, which are found on the cell membrane of a normal cell; the binding of the KAR with an KAR activation ligand (L) on a cell leads to an activation signal that enhances the killing activity of the cell, and conversely the binding of the KIR with an MHC-I molecule ligand results in an inhibitory signal restraining the killing activity of the cell. Since the inhibitory activity of the KIR-MHC-I interaction is greater than the killing activity of the KAR-L interaction, no reaction is seen when a NK cell encounters a normal cell. In the event of the loss of expression of a MHC-I molecule by the cancer cell, since the NK interaction with the cancer cell now can only occur through the KAR ligand, the cancer cell will be killed by the unopposed KAR activation pathway. As described previously, the apoptotic killing mechanism involves the assembly of a membrane-associated perforin cylindrical structure into which the granzymes deliver their death-dealing blow (*Chapters 1* and *3*).

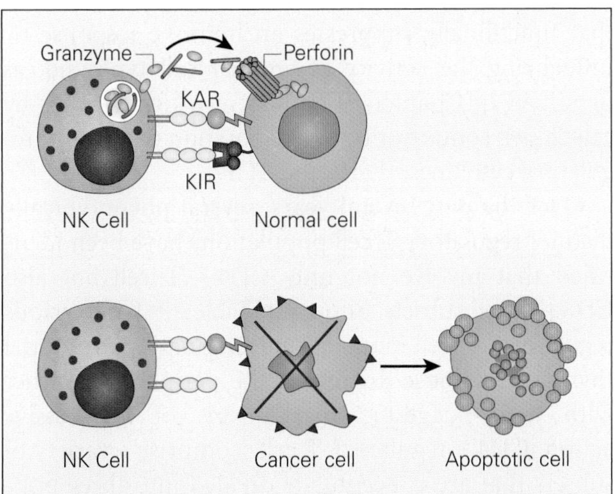

Figure 20-9. Schematic representation of the mechanisms by which the NK cell discriminates between the nonkilling of a normal cell and the killing of a cancer cell that has lost its MHC-I receptor. In the NK cell interaction with a normal cell, the inhibitory activity of the KIR-MHC-I interaction overrides the killing activity of the KAR-L interaction, and no NK killing of a normal cell occurs. In the cancer cell interaction, since there is no opposing KIR-MHC-I binding, the unopposed enhanced killing activity by the KAR-L interaction leads to successful NK cell killing of the cancer cell by apoptosis.

An alternative mechanism of destruction of the tumor cell by an NK cell can occur by an ADCC mechanism where the Fab portion of an IgG antibody produced by B cells binds to the surface TSA and bridges to an Fc receptor on the NK cell by attachment through its Fc portion of the antibody molecule (*Chapters 1* and *3*). Shown in Figure 20-10 is comparison of these two mechanisms of killing of a cancer cell by a NK cell.

The Role of Th17 Cells in Tumor Immunity

T helper 17 (**Th17**) cells play important roles in either antimicrobial protection at mucosal surfaces (*Chapters 8, 13,* and *15*) or in the promotion of inflammation involved in the pathogenesis of a

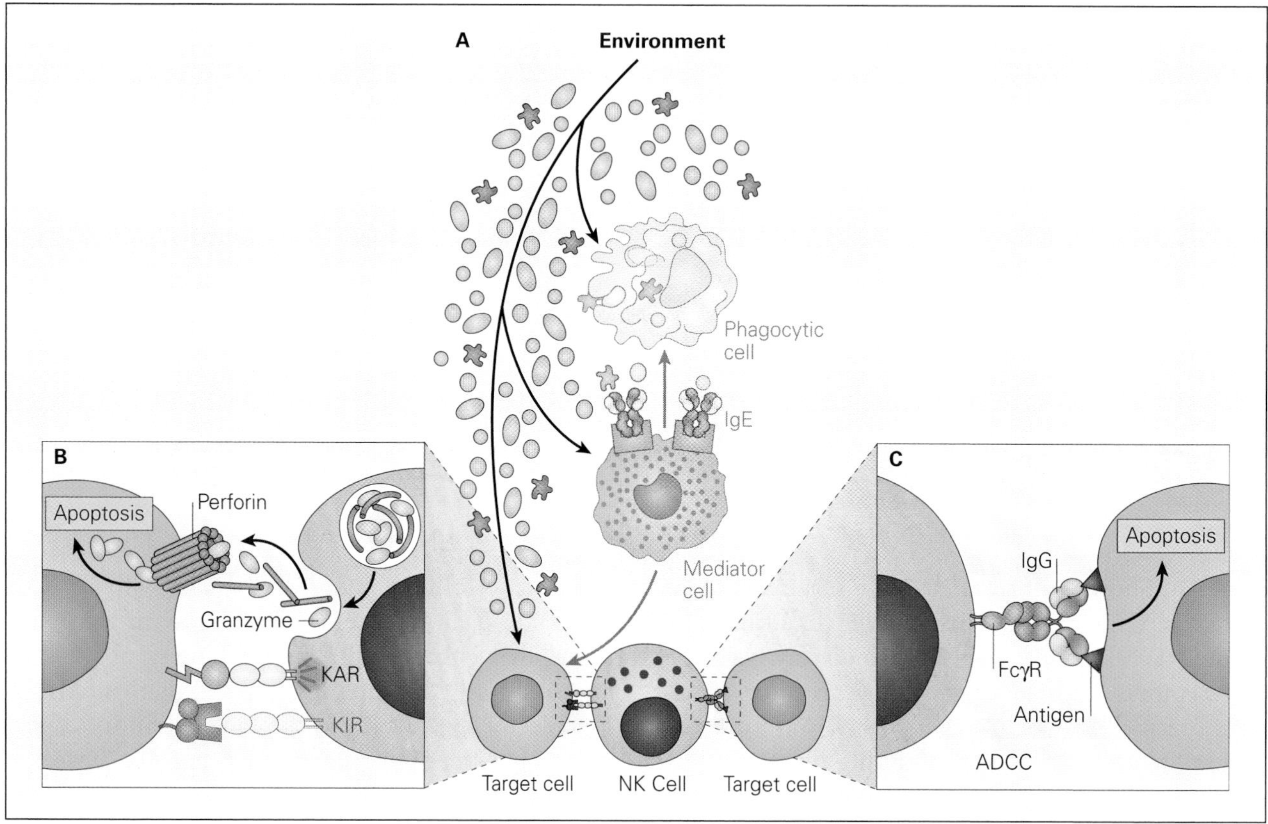

Figure 20-10. Panel A: Comparison of the two mechanisms of killing target cells by NK cells. Panel B: Direct NK cell killing of a cancer cell by a perforin/granzyme mechanism. Panel C: In contrast to NK killing by an ADCC mechanism.

number of autoimmune diseases (*Chapter 19*). Recent studies in the experimental animal have also shown their active participation in tumor immune responses. Shown in Figure 20-11 is a schematic representation of the various pathways that Th17 cells play in antitumor immunity.

The Role of Treg Cells in Tumor Immunity

As described previously, there are two types of tolerance: central tolerance and peripheral tolerance (*Chapter 7*). Central tolerance concerns immature lymphocytes as they differentiate in the primary lymphoid organs, i.e., the thymus and the bone marrow. The main mechanisms of inducing central tolerance are clonal deletion and inactivation of self-reactive lymphocytes. Peripheral tolerance concerns itself with the acquisition of immune unresponsiveness (i.e., tolerance) in peripheral lymphoid tissues. It has been suggested that regulatory T cells are responsible for the induction and maintenance of both central and peripheral tolerance and, in the case of tumor immunity, are thought to be recruited in the periphery by the tumor cells themselves (*Chapters 7* and *9*). Regulatory T cells can be defined as a T cell population that functionally suppresses an immune response by influencing the activity of another cell type and, as described in Chapters 9 and 19, can occur either by cell-to-cell contact or by the elaboration of immunoregulatory cytokines, IL-10, and TGF-β.

Over the past several years, several phenotypically distinct regulatory T cell populations have been identified that involve not only CD4+ T cell but also CD8+ T cell subsets. Shown in Table 20-3 are various regulatory T cell populations originating from the thymus and those arising in the periphery together with their suggested mechanisms of suppressive action. CD4+ regulatory T cells comprise a variety of subsets that are conceptually divided into three populations: (1) the classic regulatory CD4+CD25+ FOXP3+ T cells are thought to be thymus derived, and are termed naturally occurring regulatory T cells (nTreg cells); (2) CD4+IL-10+FOXP3- regulatory T cells that are induced in vitro with various protocols or in vivo in response to exogenous antigen challenge and are termed adaptive regulatory T cells, induced regulatory (iTreg) T cells, or T regulatory 1 cells (TR1

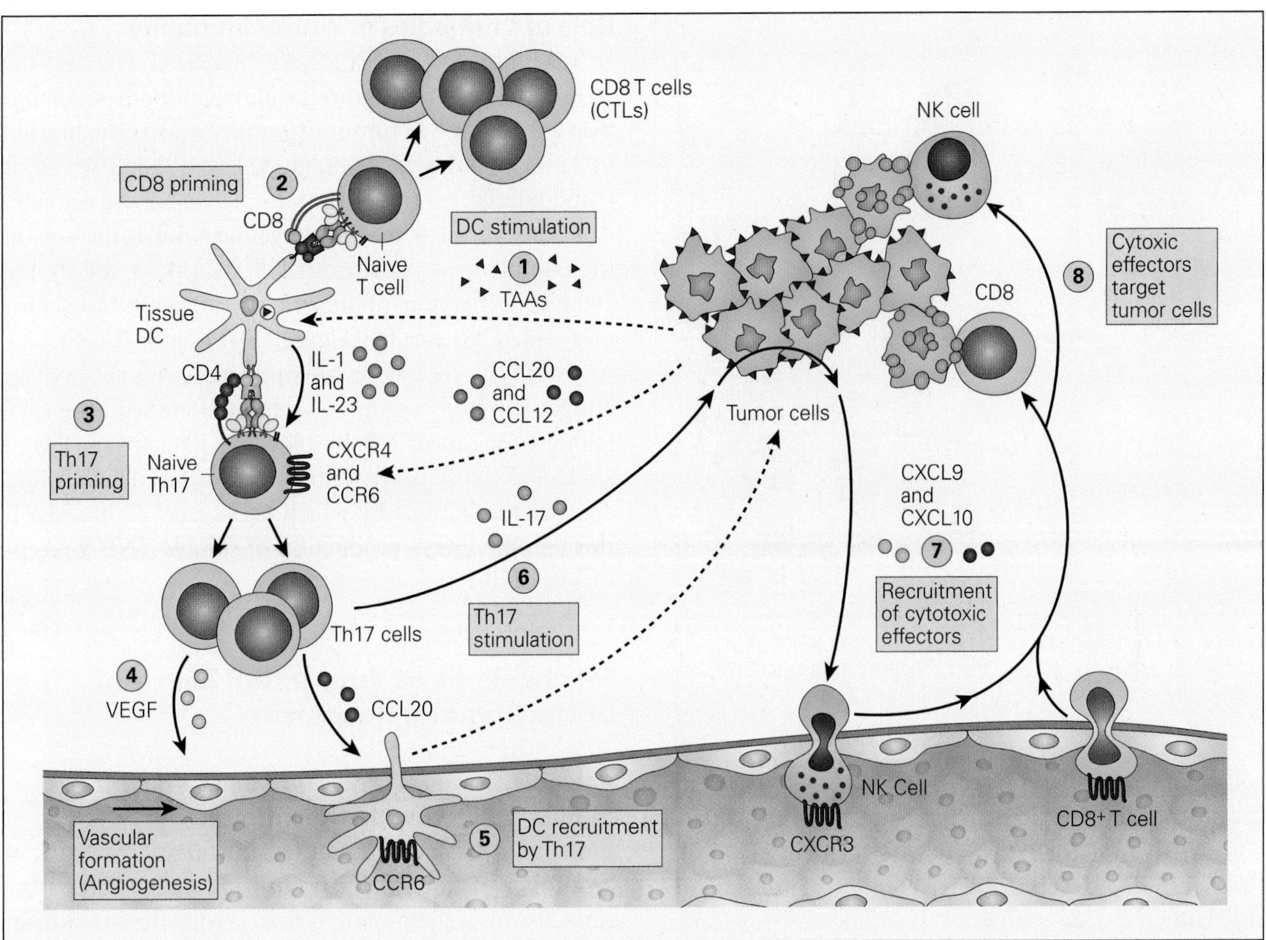

Figure 20-11. **Schematic representation of the various pathways that Th17 cells play in antitumor immunity.** Tumor-associated antigens (TAAs) shed from tumor cells are taken up by resident tissue dendritic cells in the tumor microenvironment (1) and following cognate presentation of MHC-I/peptide or MHC-II/peptide to CD8 (2) or Th17 cells (3), respectively, there is clonal expansion of antitumor CTLs as well as Th17 activation that secretes angiogenic factors, i.e., VEGF (4) and chemotactic factors for the recruitment of DCs (5). Following the stimulation of Th17 cells and their synthesis of IL-17 (6) induces the tumor cells to secrete chemotactic factors, e.g., CXCL9 and CXCL10 (7), leading to the recruitment of additional cytotoxic effectors, i.e., NK and CD8+ cells (8).

Table 20-3. Various regulatory T cell populations

Cell subset	Suggested origin	Suggested mechanism of suppressive action
CD4+ T cell subset		
CD4+CD25+FOXP3+ (nTreg) cells	Thymus	Cell-cell contact
CD4+IL-10+FOXP3- (iTreg or TR1) cells	Periphery	IL-10
CD4+TGF-β+ (TH3) cells	Periphery	TGF-β
CD8+ T cell subset		
CD8+CD25+ T cells	Thymus	TGF-β, CTLA-4
CD8+CD28- T cells	Periphery	Targeting ILT3* and ILT4**
CD8+CD62L+CD122+ T cells	ND	ND
CD8+IL-10+ T cells	Periphery	IL-10

*ILT3 = immunoglobulin-like transcript 3; **ILT4 = immunoglobulin-like transcript 3.

The dual role of antibody directed to tumor specific antigen: antibody-complement killing of the cancer cell or enhancement of tumor growth by blocking antibody.

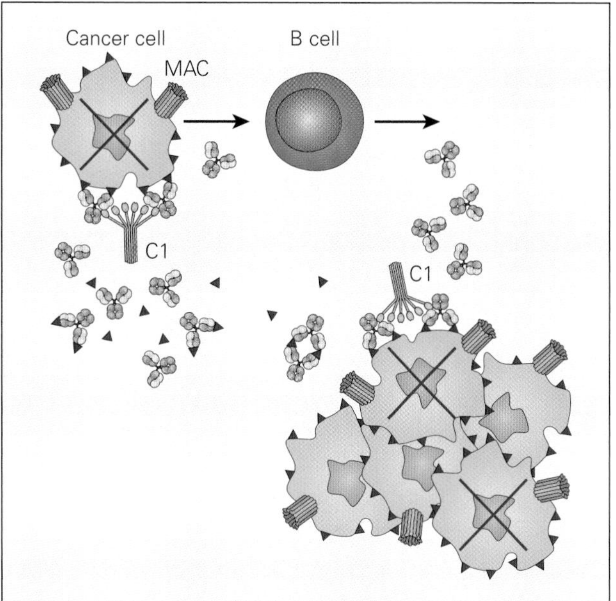

Figure 20-12. Schematic representation of the killing of a cancer cell, which expresses a TSA by an antibody-complement mediated reaction by antibody directed to a TSA molecule.

cells); and (3) CD4+TGF-β+ T cells that are also induced Treg cells activated in the periphery in the context of oral tolerance and are termed TH3 cells. As will be described in greater detail below, regulatory T cell-mediated immunosuppression is one of the crucial tumor immune-evasion mechanisms and the main obstacle to successful tumor immunotherapy.

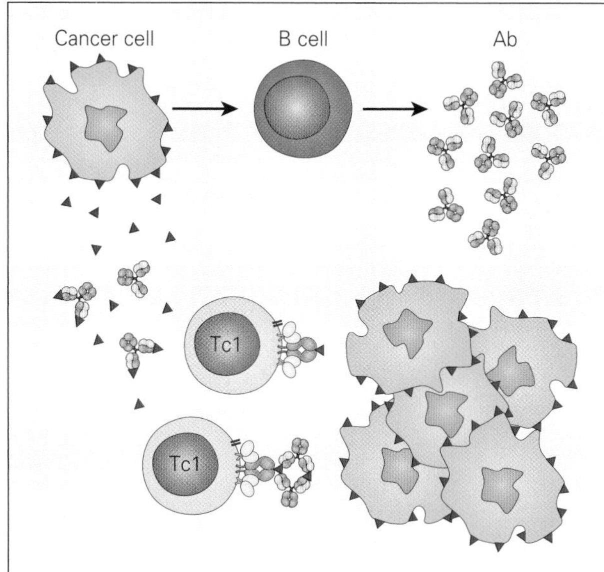

Figure 20-13. Schematic representation of the inhibitory effects of antibody or TSA-antibody complexes on the killing of a cancer cell by a CTL killing (blocking antibody).

Role of Antibodies in Tumor Immunity

In addition to their indirect beneficial role in the ADCC mechanism of tumor killing, antibodies can also play a direct role in tumor immunity. Antibody directed to TAA can either facilitate the killing of a tumor cell or paradoxically be responsible for its enhanced growth. Antibody directed to TAA together with activation of the complement system can kill the cancer cell by the cytolytic activation of the membrane-activation complex (**MAC**) cascade (Figure 20-12 and *Chapter 4*). Alternatively, TAA alone or complexed with antibody as antigen-antibody complexes can interfere with the CTL killing of a cancer cell by blocking its activity (Figure 20-13). As will be described in greater detail below, another mechanism by which CTLs may be blocked is through the excess production of soluble TNF-α receptors (s-TNF-Rs).

Mechanisms of Tumor Cell Evasion of the Immune Response

Possible Survival Mechanisms Used by the Cancer Cell to Evade the Immune System

From what has been presented thus far, it is clear that a number of potential mechanisms may underlie the capacity of a malignant cell to avoid destruction at the hands of the immune system. As described earlier, the immune system is unlikely to be the only defense bulwark against malignancy, so that tumor growth might not be exclusively related to evasion of the tumor by the immune system. The countermeasures that a tumor may employ include downexpression of potential target antigens and inhibition of the T cell response and direct modulation of proinflammatory cytokines, as will described below. These evasion mechanisms may serve as novel targets for cancer therapy.

Tumor Necrosis Factor (TNF)

Tumor necrosis factor-alpha (**TNF-α**) and lymphotoxin (**LT-α** or TNF-β) are two interrelated members of the TNF family that, in native form, are homotrimers of 17 and 17.5 kDA peptides, respectively (*Chapter 9* and Figure 20-14). Their genes are located adjacent to one another within the class III major histocompatibility complex (MHC) region in mammals (*Chapter 10*). While LT-α is predominantly produced by lymphocytes, TNF-α is produced by macrophages, lymphocytes, and other cells in selected situations. These cytokines have many in vitro effects that

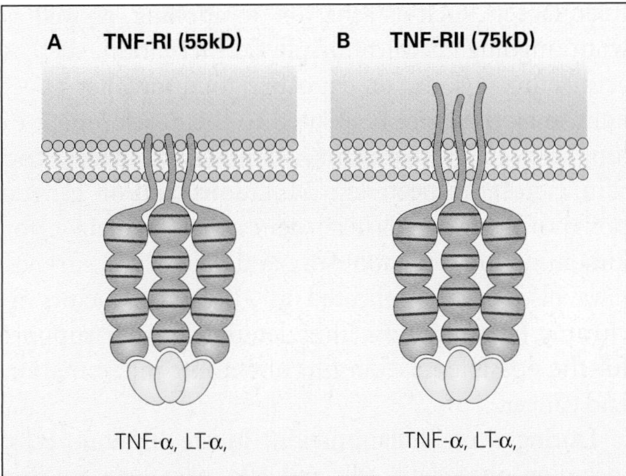

Figure 20-14. Schematic representation of the general structures of the various members of the TNF cytokine family. TNF-α and TNF-β (LT-α) are the best-recognized forms that exist in trimeric form and that attach to their respective trimeric receptors (TNF-R and LTR). There are two receptors that bind TNF-α, called TNF-RI and TNF-RII.

include growth inhibition or lysis of transformed cells, activation of phagocytic cells, upregulation of various cell surface proteins, particularly growth factors, and control of the development and expression of cell-mediated antitumor immune responses. They also display a wide spectrum of reactions in vivo, some of which include necrosis of tumors, leukocytosis and inflammation, cachexia, and shock. Their biologic effects are induced by their engagement with their specific cell surface receptors (*Chapter 9*). The activities attributed to these cytokines have evoked considerable interest for their potential use as anticancer agents. A human recombinant interleukin-2 product, aldesleukin, for example, has been licensed for the treatment of adults with metastatic renal cell carcinoma (**RCC**) and metastatic melanoma (*Chapter 11*). Although TNF-α would seem to be a potentially optimal antitumor therapy, clinical trials to date indicate that systemically administered TNF-α so as to achieve biologically effective supraphysiologic concentrations in blood has at best limited clinical efficacy and considerable unacceptable toxicity.

TNF Receptors/Inhibitors

Of the more than 20 proteins that comprise the TNF receptor (**TNF-R**) family, two clinically important TNF receptors are TNF-RI (55 kD), expressed by most cell types, and TNF-RII (75 kD), restricted to lymphoid cells (*Chapter 9* and Appendix 2). These two distinct families of TNF receptors are found either on cell surfaces or, when released, as extracellular soluble TNF Receptors (**sTNF-Rs**). The soluble form of the receptor is a truncated version of the membrane TNF-R consisting of its extracellular binding domain and is found in blood and in body fluids. These sTNF-Rs are expressed constitutively and, when released by the malignant cell, are thought to be another form of tumor evasion by their capacity to bind to TNF-α and to inhibit its activity in the surrounding microenvironment of an immune target. Both of these soluble receptors are present in increased levels in the sera of patients with malignancies. There is now evidence that this increase in serum levels above normal constitutive levels is due to their excessive production by cancer cells and/or tumor vasculature and that inhibition of TNF-α/LT by these soluble receptors may be a mechanism by which tumors escape the immunosurveillance system. The removal of soluble cytokine inhibitors present in the plasma of patients with a variety of cancers, might, therefore, be a unique therapeutic intervention leading to tumor regression by increasing local tumor destructive inflammatory responses while sparing systemic effects. The prospective clinical studies by Langkopf and Atzpodien support this putative tumor protective effect and have demonstrated an inverse relationship between patient survival and levels of soluble TNF receptors in blood. More recent clinical studies by Lentz, employing immunoadsorbent methods of TNF-R removal from plasma, have provided further evidence that a variety of tumor types are susceptible to immunologic destruction mediated by TNF-α after the removal of these sTNF-Rs surrounding the tumor (Figure 20-15). The overproduction of TNF-α (originally called "cachexin") and other proinflammatory cytokines may also be the mechanism for the systemic effects of fever, weight loss, malaise, and cachexia seen in cancer patients with extensive disease.

General Concepts of the Role of the Immune System and Inflammation in Tumor Immunity or Progression: Beneficial or Detrimental Outcomes

The immunologic events involved in tumor immunity in many respects are the same as those marshaled in response to infectious agents. Acute activation of innate immunity sets the stage for subsequent activation of the more sophisticated adaptive immune responses. Induction of efficient primary adaptive immune responses requires direct interactions with

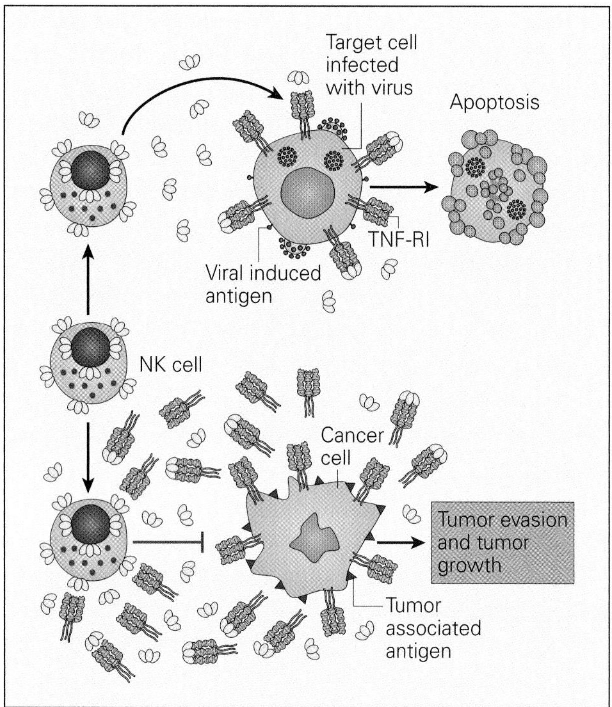

Figure 20-15. Schematic representation of the proposed normal killing mechanisms of a tumor cell by a TNF-producing activated CTL compared to inhibition of TNF killing resulting from its neutralization by excessive production of sTNF-Rs in the surrounding microenvironment of the tumor cell. (Adapted with permission from Dr. M. Rigdon Lentz, MD.)

mature antigen-presenting cells and a proinflammatory milieu. Nonetheless, there is accumulating evidence to suggest that a perturbed innate/adaptive immune balance as seen in chronic inflammation or chronic infection may also enhance conditions for tumorigenesis. The molecular mechanisms that underlie harmful, excessive stimulation of immune cell responses are numerous and complex. Genetic predisposition underlies some disorders, such as pancreatitis, ulcerative colitis, and some rheumatoid diseases. Others are associated with infectious disease pathogens that are able to evade natural tissue immune clearance mechanisms and persist. For example, *Helicobacter pylori*, a Gram-negative bacterium, causes chronic gastritis in infected hosts and in some patients may be associated with gastric cancer, e.g., adenocarcinoma and lymphoma, whereas infection with hepatitis B or hepatitis C virus (HBV and HCV, respectively) is linked to chronic hepatitis, cirrhosis, and in some patients with subsequent development of hepatocellular carcinoma. Similarly, infection with HPV has been associated with vulvar squamous cell carcinomas and adenocarcinomas. Unresolved inflammation resulting from exposure to toxic factors such as asbestos or smoking, as well as from ongoing chemical or physical irritation, such as acid-reflux disease or exposure to ultraviolet (UV) light, may therefore be related to the development of lung cancer, gastroesophageal junction cancer, and skin cancer, respectively. Mutations and/or genetic polymorphisms in crucial genes that regulate cytokine function, metabolism, and leukocyte survival have also been implicated as etiological factors in chronic inflammation, thus lending further support for the possible relationship of chronic inflammation and cancer.

During acute inflammation, innate immune cells, including phagocytic cells and NK cells, form the first line of immune defense and regulate subsequent activation of adaptive immune responses. By contrast, during chronic inflammation, these roles can be reversed—i.e., adaptive immune responses can cause ongoing and excessive activation of innate immune cells. In arthritis, for example, activation of T and B lymphocytes results in antibody deposition into affected joints, prompting recruitment of innate immune cells into tissue. Once within the tissue, activation and/or degranulation of mast cells, granulocytes, and macrophages, in combination with humoral immune responses, leads to joint destruction. By contrast, whereas acutely activated innate immune cells contribute to efficient T cell activation, chronically activated innate immune cells can cause T cell dysfunction through the production of reactive oxygen radicals.

Regardless of the underlying initiating cause or pathogenetic mechanism, if an infectious or assaulting agent is inadequately cleared and persists in tissue, or a tissue is subjected to ongoing insult and damage that fails to heal in a timely manner, host inflammatory responses can persist and exacerbate chronic tissue damage, which can cause primary organ dysfunction and systemic complications.

Shown in Figure 20-16 is a schematic representation of the hypothetical sequelae of progressive pathogenetic events that occur during the emergence of a cancer. It is the same sequence of events described previously in other chapters for failure of elimination of an infectious agent or foreign substance now applied to a malignancy. In this general synthesizing scheme, failure of elimination of the foreign substance leading to its persistence resulted in inflammation, immunopathology seen in chronic microbial infection (*Chapters 12, 13, 14,* and *15*), or autoimmune disease (*Chapter 19*); in the case of cancer, this failure of elimination would lead to further malignant progression and cancer expansion. It may

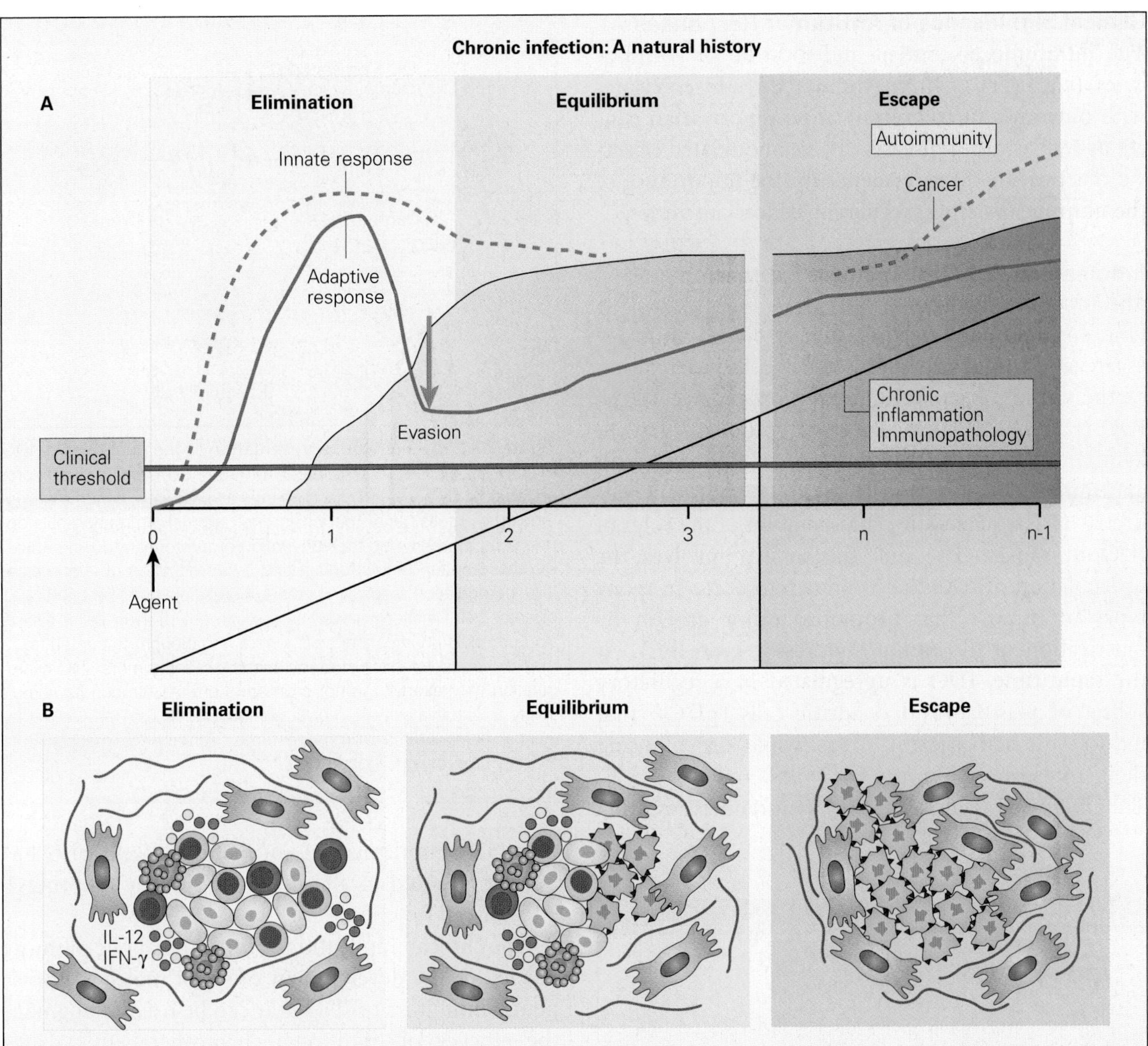

Figure 20-16. Panel A: Schematic representation of the sequelae of pathogenetic events that follow from failure of elimination of an infectious agent or foreign substance, leading to persistence of the foreign configuration with resultant inflammation, immunopathology in the form of autoimmune disease, or malignancy. Panel B: The three phases of cancer immunoediting: elimination, equilibrium, and escape correlated with the morphologic assessment of emerging cancer cells during these various stages. During the first phase of elimination, only normal cells are seen (red); the few malignant cells that emerge are removed by apoptosis; during equilibrium, both normal cells (red) are seen as cancer cells appear (green); during escape, a predominance of cancer cells are seen (green), with no normal cells evident.

now be possible to superimpose the "three Es of cancer immunoediting," i.e., elimination, equilibrium, and escape, upon the three progressive stages of the immune response evolving from innate and adaptive immunity and terminating in the chronic irreversible phase of cancer. During the first phase of immunoediting, i.e., **elimination**, the innate immune response would play the primary role in eliminating the greater part of emergent cancer cells through apoptotic cell death; in the second phase of **equilibrium**, the adaptive immune response would be partially effective in containing tumor progression and would result in one population of tumor cells capable of being detected by an effective T and B cell response as well as a second emerging population of tumor cells that has learned how to escape immune detection and is being "sculpted" by a futile attempt of an ineffective adaptive immune response; the failure of the immune struggle with the cancer cell would be seen in the third phase of **escape** of immunoediting during which no immune killing would be possible and only further cancer expansion would be seen (Figure 20-16).

Clinical Significance of Antitumor Responses

The intratumoral content and location of lymphocytes (e.g., CTL) within tumors directly correlates with outcomes in colorectal cancer and ovarian cancer as well as other diseases. These and related observations provide direct evidence for the importance of the immune system in regulating cancer outcomes.

Indoleamine-2,3 Dioxygenase Expression and Immune Escape

One of the many factors that promote immune escape and tumor growth in cancer cells is activation of the enzyme indoleamine 2,3-dioxygenase (**IDO**). IDO is an enzyme that converts tryptophan (Trp) to kynurenine (Kyn) and is involved in tumor growth and immune suppression (Box 20-2). Shown in Figure 20-17 is a schematic representation of the roles of IDO in cancer. The first mechanism involves the upregulation of IDO that is known to occur in many types of tumors that promotes tumor growth by inactivation of the tumor suppressor gene Bin1. At the same time, IDO is upregulated in a regulatory subset of plasmacytoid dendritic cells (**pDCs**) that induces the activation of Tregs, while also blunting their interconversion to Th17 inflammatory cells. The increased generation of kynurenine resulting

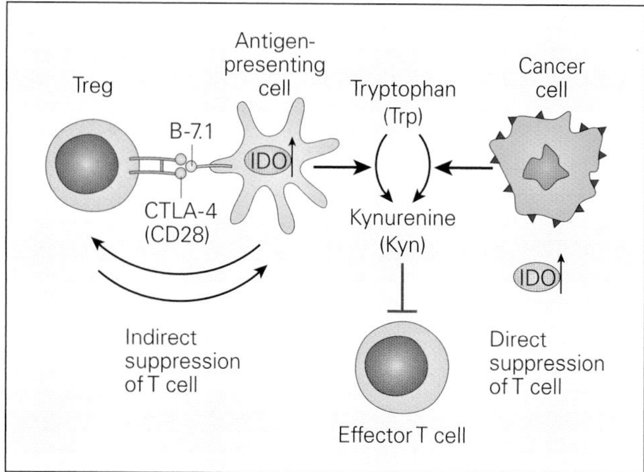

Figure 20-17. Schematic representation of the dual roles of IDO in cancer. IDO is an important immunomodulatory enzyme produced both by activated macrophages as well as by other immunoregulatory cells and performs its normal immunoregulatory functions by catalyzing the conversion of tryptophan to kynurenine. By consumption of tryptophan and overproduction of kynurenine, IDO upregulation leads to T cell suppression both by blunting T effector cell function as well as recruitment of Treg cells. IDO is also upregulated in cancer cells where it is thought to contribute to the immune subversion strategy used by many tumors. IDO dysregulation may exert its tumor promoting effects through its known ability to inactivate the tumor suppressor gene Bin1 as well as by incapacitating effective immune tumor surveillance mechanisms, thereby promoting tumor growth.

from IDO upregulation in T effector cells also has been implicated in T cell suppression by blunting T effector cell function.

The clinical implications of this metabolic pathway has led to the development of small molecule therapeutic inhibitors of IDO that can be used to augment the efficacy of traditional chemotherapeutic drugs used to treat various forms of human cancer. By promoting antitumor immune responses in combination with cytotoxic chemotherapy, IDO inhibitors may offer a drug-based strategy to more effectively attack systemic cancer.

Box 20-2

IDO Pathway

Indoleamine-pyrrole 2,3-dioxygenase (IDO) is an immunomodulatory enzyme produced by some alternatively activated macrophages and other immunoregulatory cells that catalyses tryptophan through the generation of kynurenine and has been associated with mechanisms of cancer escape and expansion. Originally, activated Treg cells would induce the expression of IDO in DCs that will translate signals promoting T cell anergy and apoptosis. This state of anergy would be expanded by the arrival of these dysfunctional DCs expressing high cytoplasmic concentration of IDO into the draining lymph nodes. Their subsequent interaction and suppression of local effector T cells, like CTL, would reduce immunosurveillance in the lymph node favoring uncontrolled metastasis of tumor cells to these converted sites. Additionally, IDO has been linked to the inactivation of the tumor suppressor gene Bin1 that has been implicated in the genesis of uncontrolled growth in cancer cells. So, IDO plays a dual role favoring cancer; it promotes cancer growth and suppresses immunosurveillance.

Specific Immunosuppressive Mechanisms that Have Been Identified in Recent Years: Treg Cells, IDO Expression, Gr1+ Myelocytes, and Elaboration of Immunosuppressive Cytokines such as TGF-β and IL-10

Detrimental Role of Treg Cells in Human Malignancies

Regulatory T cells play an important role in suppressing the effector mechanisms directed against TAAs resulting from the myriad of factors produced within the tumor microenvironment. As described previously, there are four potential sources of Treg cells recruited in the tumor microenvironment: (1) the thymus, (2) the bone marrow, (3) the blood, and (4) the lymph node. The most common postulated mechanism of Treg cell incitement is by the tumor expression of chemokines, such as CCL22, that bind to specific chemokine receptors, such as CCR4, on Treg cells. Shown in Figure 20-18 are various mechanisms that the tumor microenvironment uses in suppressing the antigen-presenting capacity and function of resident DCs. These dysfunctional APCs induce Treg cell activation and expansion into more powerful suppressive phenotypes. Moreover, the presence of TGF-β itself converts CD4+CD25- T cells into iTreg cells by their synthesis of CD25 and FOXP3.

Mechanism(s) of Immunosuppressive Action of Treg Cells

Shown in Figure 20-19 is a schematic representation of the various proposed mechanisms of immunosuppressive action of Treg cells based primarily on data derived from studies in experimental animals. The induction

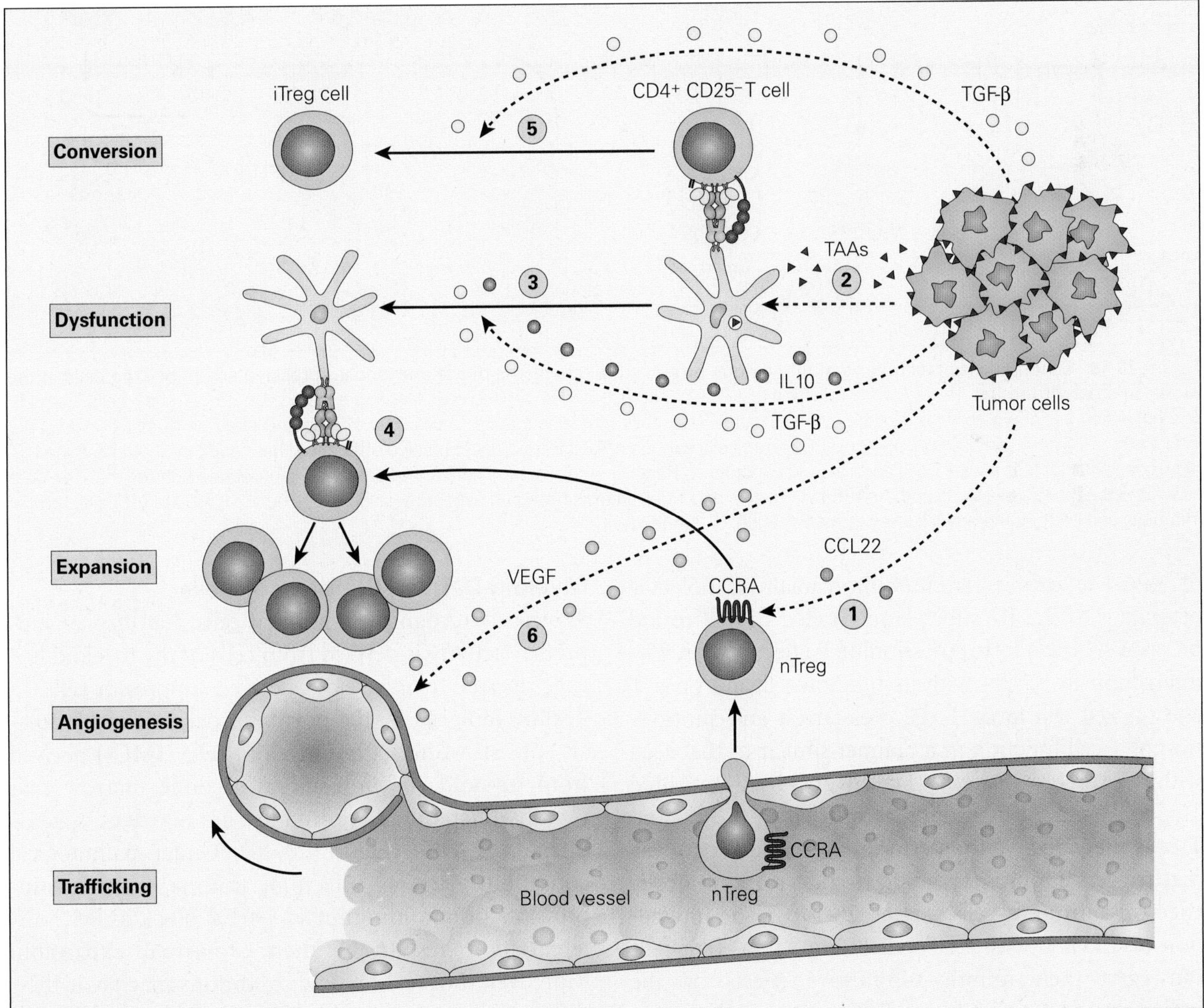

Figure 20-18. **Schematic representation of the various mechanisms that the tumor microenvironment uses in suppressing the antigen-presenting capacity and function of resident DCs.** Following tumor production of chemokines (e.g., CCL22), nTreg cells are expressing CCR4 and are recruited from the vascular compartment (1). Following their release from the tumor, TAAs are normally taken up by DCs (2) leading to the activation of CD4+CD25- T effector cells. The subsequent release of the immunoregulatory cytokines IL-10 and TGF-β from the tumor suppresses DC differentiation and function, resulting in a dysfunctional DC (3). The nTregs recruited by the tumor are stimulated by the dysfunctional DCs to expand (4) leading to immunosuppressive activity in the tumor environment. The TGF-β released from the tumor cells can also lead to the conversion of the CD4+CD25- T effector cells into CD4+CD25+ Treg cells, leading to further immunosuppressive activity (5). The tumor production of VEGF stimulates angiogenesis (6).

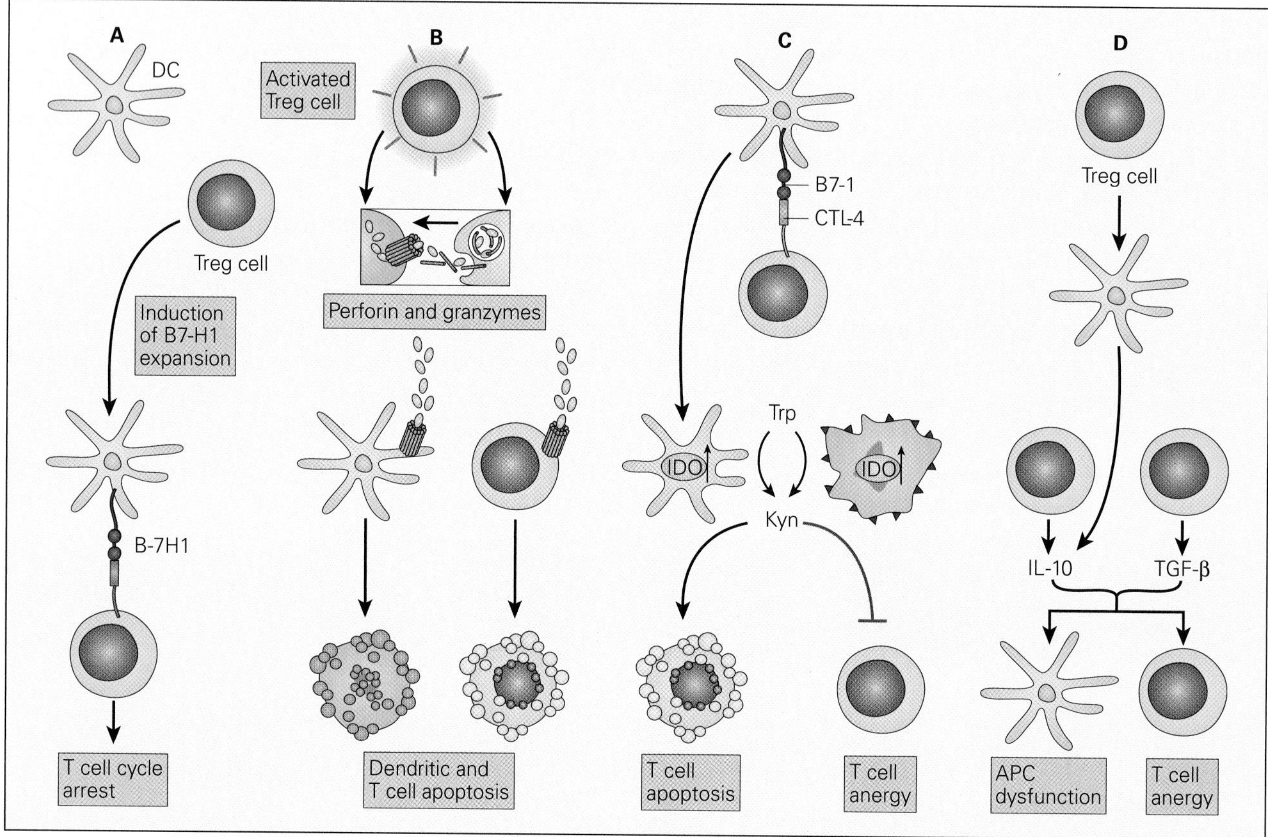

Figure 20-19. Schematic representation of the various proposed mechanisms of the immunosuppressive action of Treg cells in the tumor microenvironment. Panel A: The induction of APCs to express B7-H4 by Treg cells leads to suppression of T effector cells. Panel B: The enhanced perforin/granzyme B pathway by activated Treg cells may also induce cytotoxicity of DCs and effector T cells. Panel C: The interaction of CTLA-4 with CD80/CD86 on APCs, Treg cells can exert their immunosuppressive effects by the induction of indoleamine 2,3-dioxygenase (IDO) that favors T cell anergy and/or apoptosis. Panel D: An increased concentration of TGF-β produced both by the Treg cells as well as the tumor cells leads both to APC dysfunction and T cell anergy. (Adapted with permission from Zou W. Regulatory T cells, tumour immunity and immunotherapy. Nat Rev Immunol. 2006; 6: 295-307.)

of APCs to express an immunoregulatory molecule belonging to the B7 super family called B7-H4 found on an APC leads to suppression of T-effector cells. The interaction of B7-H4 with its unknown ligand on a T effector cell will favor T cell cycle arrest and suppression of T cell function in a manner similar to that seen with CTLA-4 activation (Figure 20-19A). Activated Treg cells may also induce cytotoxicity of DCs and T cells mediated by the perforin/granzyme B pathway that triggers apoptosis, leading to a decrease of locally effective antitumor cells (Figure 20-19B). The interaction of CTLA-4 with CD80/CD86 on APCs, Treg cells can exert their immunosuppressive effects by the induction of IDO that favors T cell anergy and/or apoptosis (Figure 20-19C). A recently proposed immunosuppressive mechanism of Treg cells is mediated by the action of an increased concentration of TGF-β produced both by the Treg cells as well as the tumor cells that leads both to APC dysfunction and T cell anergy (Figure 20-19D).

Myeloid-Derived Suppressor Cells

A recently recognized source of cells that display suppressor activity is derived from cells of the myeloid lineage referred to as myeloid-derived suppressor cells. In healthy individuals, the normal process of myelopoiesis consists of immature myeloid cells (**IMCs**) derived from myeloid cell progenitors in bone marrow that rapidly differentiate into mature granulocytes, macrophages, or DCs (Figure 20-20). Under pathological conditions such as infection, trauma, immunosuppression, or autoimmunity, a partial block in IMC differentiation results in their abnormal expansion. Moreover, those pathologic conditions may favor their differentiation into myeloid-derived suppressor cells (**MDSCs**) expressing STAT-induced immune suppressive factors, such as arginase 1, inducible nitric oxide synthase (**iNOS**), and reactive oxygen species (**ROS**), with a reduced expression of surface cell molecules like MHC-I and a consequent suppression of antigen-specific T cell activation.

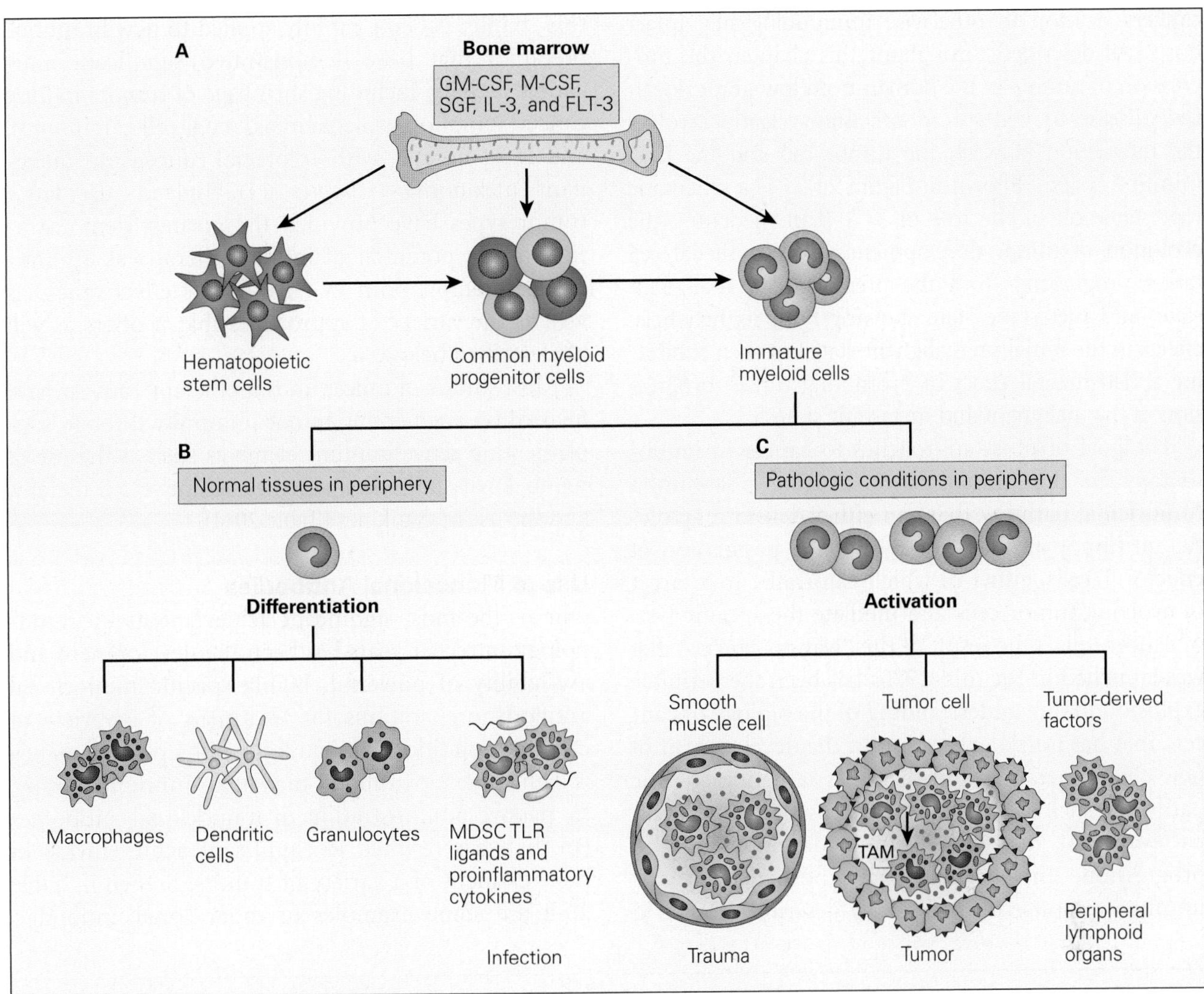

Figure 20-20. Schematic representation of the normal and pathological differentiation of myeloid cells. Panel A: In the bone marrow, hematopoietic stem cells can progressively differentiate into common myeloid progenitor and then to immature myeloid cells under the inductive influence of several growth factors, including GM-CSF, M-CSF, SCF, IL-3, and FLT-3. The immature myeloid cells migrate into peripheral tissues where they can differentiate and participate in either physiologic or pathologic conditions according to the local environment. Panel B: Shows the normal differentiation of myeloid precursors into macrophages, dendritic cells, granulocytes, and myeloid-derived suppressor cells (MDSCs) in peripheral tissues in response to infection. Panel C: Shows the progressive changes of trauma, tumor development peripheral lymphoid infiltration induced by tumor derived factors. In response to tumor-derived factors, MDSCs exhibit the capacity to differentiate into tumor-associated macrophages (TAMs) and contribute to antigen-non-specific T cell suppression in cancer. SCF = stem cell factor; FLT3 = FMS-related tyrosine kinase 3. (Adapted with permission from Gabrilovich DI, Nagaraj S. Myeloid-derived suppressor cells as regulators of the immune system. Nat Rev Immunol. 2009;9:162-74.)

In humans, MDSCs are a heterogeneous population of cells derived from IMCs and immature macrophages that are commonly defined as CD14– CD11b+ (αM integrin) cells expressing the common myeloid marker CD33 but lacking the expression of markers found on mature cells such as MHC-II HLA-DR (in mice they are recognized by the expression of CD11b+GR1+). In response to tumor derived factors, MDSCs have exhibited the capacity to differentiate into tumor-associated macrophages (**TAMs**) distinguished by the absence of GR1 concurrent to the absence of any of the IMC-specific proteins such as arginase 1 or iNOS, depending on tumor microenvironment. TAMs contribute to antigen-non-specific-T cell suppression in cancer and are capable of producing IL-1β, IL-6, IL-10, and TGF-β.

Recent Clinical Applications of Immunotherapy of Human Malignancies

With few notable exceptions, as in the case of patients with immune deficiency (*Chapter 16*), most human cancers develop in otherwise immunologically intact hosts. As described throughout this chapter, the progression of tumors in the human from low-grade, localized disease to widespread metastasis clearly involves the interaction between the tumor cell and the host immune system. Shown in Figure 20-21 is a schematic representation of the role of TGF-β in mediating the evolution of tumor development in an epithelial cell target progressing from the premalignant, malignant state, and metastatic state showing both its beneficial effects in the initial premalignant state but then exhibiting a detrimental effect in promoting tumor progression in the malignant and metastatic states.

The goal of most approaches to cancer immunotherapy in the human is to activate a common tumoricidal pathway that can either deliver a cytolytic antitumor antibody or mobilize a population of effector T cells, either of which can traffic to a target of evolving tumor cells and mediate the specific lysis of cancer cells. One result of the "war on cancer" that was launched in the mid-1970s has been the veritable explosion in our understanding of the biology of cancers that has found expression in the development of new chemotherapies and therapies targeting specific pathways, such as the epidermal growth factor (EGF) pathway that may drive tumor development and progression. In addition, the knowledge of the immune response to malignancy described earlier in this chapter is being rapidly applied to new immunotherapies that have demonstrated significant anticancer activity, including shrinkage of tumors in lung cancer, lymphomas, leukemias, renal cell carcinomas, and most notably with colorectal cancer and malignant melanoma (*Chapter 11*). Indeed, the latter tumor types have provided the greatest demonstration of the potential of immunotherapy as an anticancer therapy, both in terms of its effectiveness as well as the variety of approaches that it offers as will be described below.

Most studies of cancer immunotherapy thus far have focused on augmenting tumor immunity through supplementing active immune elements such as the use of monoclonal antibodies, vaccines, adoptive cell therapy, and the use of cytokines (Table 20-4).

Use of Monoclonal Antibodies

One of the most significant achievements in immunology in recent years has been the development and availability of powerful, highly specific monoclonal antibody preparations for treatment of a variety of clinical conditions, including human malignancy (*Chapter 11*). Antibody-mediated immunotherapy, by passive administration of monoclonal antibodies (mAbs), has resulted in significant achievements in the treatment of a variety of tumors. Shown in Table 20-4 are some examples of monoclonal antibodies

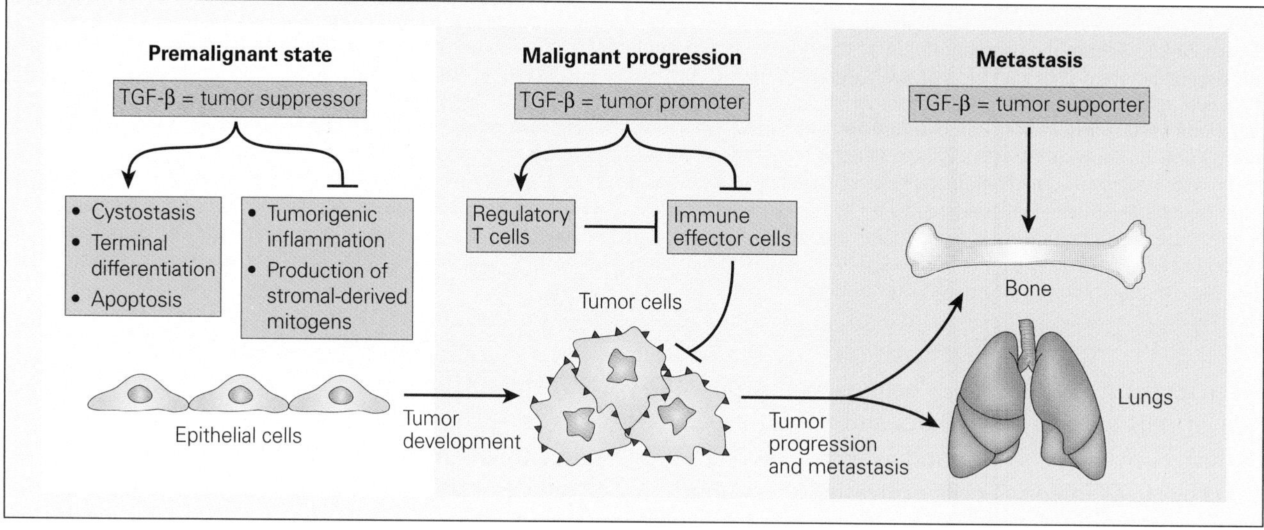

Figure 20-21. Schematic representation of the role of TGF-β in mediating the tumor development in an epithelial cell target progressing from the premalignant to the malignant state and terminating in the metastatic state. In the premalignant state, TGF-β functions as a tumor suppressor by blocking the expression of stromal-derived mitogens and suppressing protumorigenic inflammation. In this initial state, TGF-β supports the cytostasis, terminal differentiation, and apoptosis of premalignant cells, which have either an overexpressed oncogene or suppressed tumor-suppressor gene. Once the epithelial cells become fully malignant, TGF-β has the opposite effect by blocking the antitumor immune response either directly or through Treg cells. Once a tumor is established, TGF-β further supports the formation of metastases to several distal sites, including bone and lung tissues. (Adapted with permission from Flavell RA, Sanjabi S, Wrzesinski SH, Licona-Limon P. The polarization of immune cells in the tumour environment by TGF beta. Nat Rev Immunol. 2010;10:554–67.)

Table 20-4. Some examples of modes of conventional immunotherapy

- Use of monoclonal antibodies
- Vaccines directed against tumor-associated antigens (tumor peptides)
- Adoptive T cell transfusion (T effector cells)
- Use of cytokines (IL-7, IL-15, and IL-21) or inhibitors of cytokines (TGF-β) or their signaling pathways (CTLA-4)

that are most advanced in development and that are or are becoming available for clinical use in cancer immunotherapy. Most recently with the increasing recognition of the importance of Treg cells, Th17 cells, and the pivotal role of TGF-β in directing the balance and plasticity of these CD4+ T cell subsets, a major investigative effort has been directed to the development of products that may inhibit TGF-β signaling pathways.

Although the precise effector mechanisms of these antibody agents is unclear, their postulated mechanisms of action are varied and include perturbation of growth factor-related signaling, antibody-complement mediated toxicity and ADCC, and inhibitory effects on growth factors that result in blockage of angiogenesis (Table 20-5). Other theories have also been demonstrated, e.g., the non-ADCC-mediated apoptosis effects of cetuximab. Other advances of monoclonal antibody therapy include conjugation of radioactive or other cytotoxic ligands to the antibody thus allowing the antibody to serve as a carrier molecule for other cytotoxic molecules, e.g., iodine-131 tositumomab and lutetium-177 (^{177}Lu) for the treatment of CD20+, follicular non-Hodgkin's lymphoma and prostatic cancer, respectively, thus achieving the "magic bullet" aspiration of Ehrlich, made famous in the 1940 film about Paul Ehrlich, a physician and father of immunology who pioneered the concept of chemicals as medicines.

Augmentation of Cell-Mediated Immune Responses to Tumors

Because of the importance of cell-mediated immunity in tumor defense, there has also been increased interest in procedures that augment the generation of antitumor cytotoxic responses. Such strategies include the adoptive transfer of in vitro expanded patients' blood leukocytes or tumor-infiltrating lymphocytes (**TILs**), vaccines to immunize against TAAs, gene therapy, and others.

These various strategies have resulted in the proof of principle of the role of immunotherapy in the treatment of malignancies (i.e., the ability to generate antitumor cytotoxic T lymphocytes in vitro and in vivo in cancer patients). However, the clinical responses of all these techniques have not been optimal and it may require further modification, including combination chemotherapy and immunotherapy. Furthermore, it is becoming evident that even in the presence of an adequate antitumor cytotoxic response, the resistant cancer cells may develop mechanisms to resist killing by the cytotoxic lymphocytes as described previously. In such cases, sensitizing agents in the form of adjuvants may be required to reverse the resistance of the tumor cells to killing

Table 20-5. Some monoclonal antibody preparations available for clinical use in cancer immunotherapy

Product	Target	Postulated mechanism of action	Clinical use
Cetuximab Panitumumab Matuzumab	Human epidermal growth factor receptor (EGFR)	Growth inhibition of EGF by binding to EGFR	EGFR-expressing, metastatic colorectal carcinoma, head and neck cancer
Trastuzumab	Growth factor receptor protein (HER2)	Neutralization by binding with HER2	Breast cancer
Rituximab	CD20 antigen on the surface of B cells	Complement-dependent and ADCC mediated cytotoxicity	Diffuse large B cell lymphoma (DLBCL), CD20+, non-Hodgkin's lymphoma, rheumatoid arthritis
Iodine-131 tositumomab and yttrium-90 ibritumomab tiuxetan	CD20 antigen on the surface of B cells	Same as rituximab, and ionizing radiation from the radioisotope	B cell non-Hodgkin's lymphoma (NHL)
Bevacizumab	Human vascular endothelial growth factor (VEGF)	Antiangiogenesis effects by binding VEGF and preventing its interaction with its receptors	Metastatic carcinoma of the colon or rectum, lung cancer, breast cancer, renal cell carcinoma

and thus facilitate the cytotoxic activity mediated by immunotherapy. Clearly, significant advances have been made in cancer immunotherapy and will undoubtedly continue to be developed to achieve an improved clinical response and greater tumor elimination. Further advances in deciphering the interplay between the tumor and the host immune system and the microenvironment in which this occurs will undoubtedly lead to the development of new classes of immunotherapeutics.

Use of Cytokines and Chemokines

The use of recombinant IFN-α originated in early studies of "natural" interferon extracted from human leukocytes, which produced occasional beneficial responses in renal cell carcinoma and malignant melanoma. The mechanism of interferon, although not known with certainty, is believed to occur through the generalized enhancement of both innate and adaptive immune responses (*Chapter 13*). Although clinical trials using IFN-α to date have demonstrated resolution of disease in only limited numbers (< 10 percent) of patients, the clinical responses may be long-lasting, up to decades in duration. The toxicities of IFN-α regimens, however, may be considerable, and most commonly consist of flu-like symptoms, depression, cytopenias (leukopenia, anemia), abnormal liver function tests, and weight loss and the development of autoimmune disorders. These adverse effects have limited the use of interferons in these diseases. Although the use of other cytokines and/or chemokine administration (IL-7, IL-15, and IL-21) have shown promise, they are largely investigational at present.

Shown in Table 20-6 are some general concepts of the beneficial or detrimental outcomes of the tumor cell/ immune system interaction

Table 20-6. General concepts of the beneficial or detrimental outcomes of the tumor cell/immune system interaction

- Adaptive and innate immune cells regulate tissue homeostasis and efficient wound healing.
- Altered interactions between adaptive and innate immune cells can lead to chronic inflammatory disorders.
- In cancers, an abundance of infiltrating innate immune cells, such as macrophages, mast cells, and neutrophils, correlates with increased angiogenesis and/or poor prognosis.
- In cancers, an abundance of infiltrating lymphocytes correlates with favorable prognosis.
- Chronic inflammatory conditions enhance a predisposition to cancer development.
- Long-term usage of nonsteroidal anti-inflammatory drugs and selective cyclooxygenase-2 inhibitors reduces cancer incidence.
- Polymorphisms in genes that regulate immune balance influence cancer risk.
- Immune status in humans and in mouse models affects the risk of cancer development in an etiology-dependent manner.
- Genetic elimination or depletion of immune cells alters cancer progression in experimental models.
- Activation of antitumor adaptive immune responses can suppress tumor growth.

Adoptive Cell Therapy

Adoptive cellular therapy is defined as the infusion of immune effector cells for the treatment and/or prevention of disease. The development of successful strategies for treating human tumors requires an understanding of the effector mechanisms that participate in the control of tumor growth and progression as described in this chapter. The arsenal of host cellular immune responses to tumors includes the complete array of nonspecific effector cells of the innate immune system, i.e., natural killer cells and macrophages, as well as effector cells of the adaptive immune system, which include those with limited diversity for antigen recognition, such as the CD4+ γδ+T cells, and highly specific effector cells with vast diversity for antigen recognitions, such as antibody-producing B cells and CD4+ αβ+ T cells.

The idea that lymphocytes extracted from a tumor environment may be sensitized and therefore may have the potential to induce tumor regression has led to the use of TILs in clinical trials. In this procedure, lymphocytes are grown ex vivo directly from tumors in the presence of the interleukin 2 (IL-2), the classic T cell growth factor (*Chapter 9*). Following expansion in culture for several weeks, the TILs are reinfused into the patient (Figure 20-22). More recently, an exciting development has been a modification of adoptive cellular therapy by the use of gene-modified lymphocytes. Genes encoding TCRs isolated from high avidity T cells that recognize cancer antigens have been inserted into circulating human lymphocytes using retroviral or lentiviral vectors to redirect lymphocyte specificity to these cancer antigens.

Current clinical protocols for adoptive cell therapy are depicted in Figure 20-22. Adoptive cell therapy (**ACT**) requires the generation of highly avid tumor-antigen-reactive T cells. Tumor specific T cells,

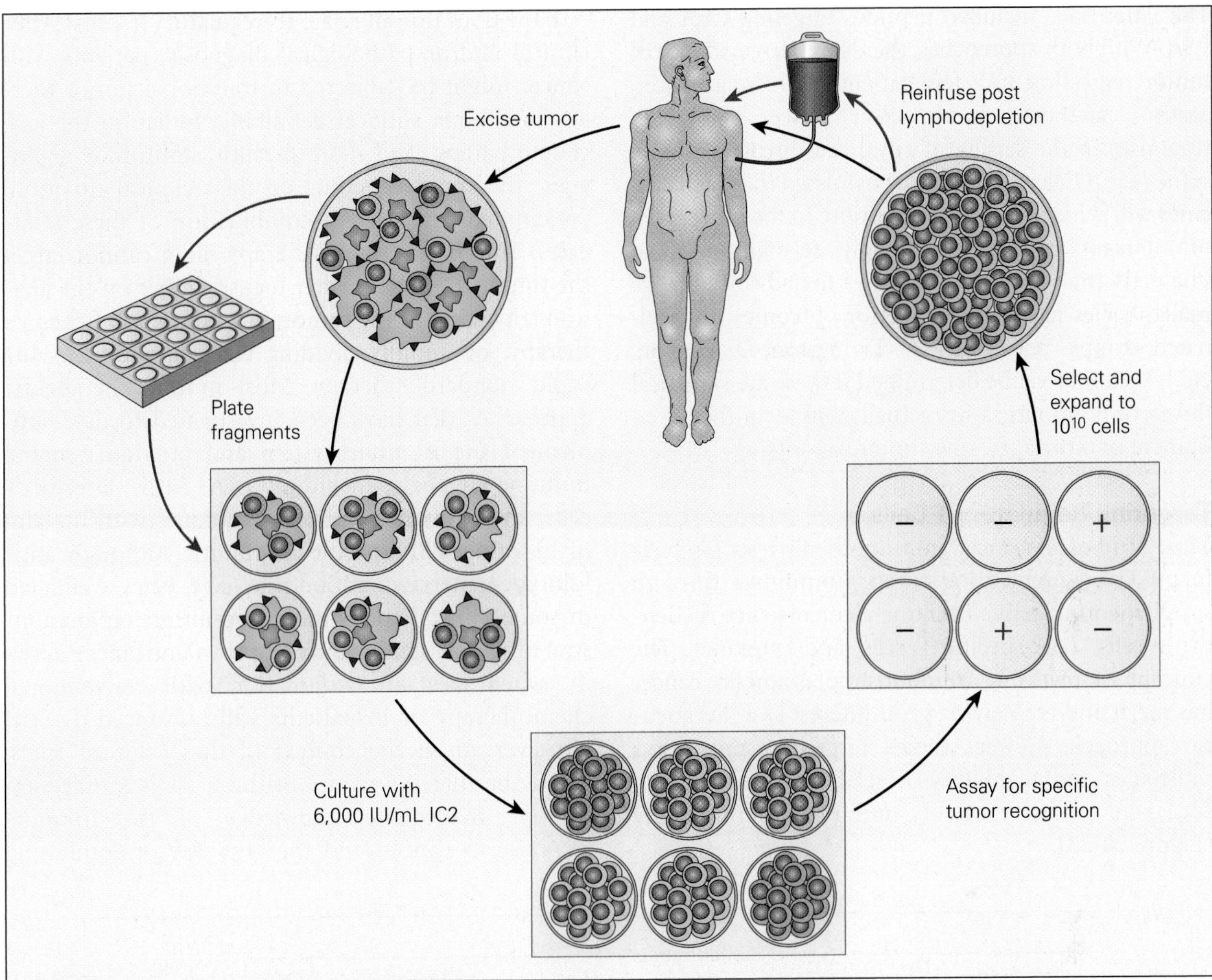

Figure 20-22. Current clinical protocols for adoptive cell therapy (ACT). (Adapted with permission from Rosenberg SA, Restifo NP, Yang JC, et al. Adoptive cell transfer: a clinical path to effective cancer immunotherapy. Nat Rev Cancer. 2008;8:299–308.)

derived from TILs, can be efficiently isolated ex vivo from melanoma lesions using high levels of interleukin-2 (IL-2). TILs are successively selected for their ability to secrete high levels of interferon-γ (IFN-γ) when cultured with autologous or allogeneic MHC-matched tumor-cell lines. Alternatively, cell-mediated lysis has been used to identify tumor-reactive T cells for transfer. Highly avid, tumor-antigen-reactive T cell populations selected for ACT are rapidly expanded (to up to 10^{10} cells) using CD3-specific antibody, exogenously supplied IL-2, and irradiated allogeneic peripheral-blood mononuclear "feeder" cells and are validated for activity before transfer. Patients now receive systemic immunosuppression before the adoptive transfer of antitumor lymphocytes. Although cyclophosphamide and fludarabine have been traditionally used for lymphodepletion methods, newer, as-yet-unpublished regimens also include total body irradiation. Clinically, these approaches have been explored in melanomas with clear evidence of tumor shrinkage and suggestions of improved survival in patients treated with these therapies. In the largest clinical TIL trial to date, 60 percent of metastatic melanoma patients who had not previously received any immunotherapy showed objective responses, although the characteristics of the tumor environment that produces TILs in vivo remain unclear.

Antitumor Vaccines

A number of vaccine approaches have been evaluated over the years that have ranged from the preparations of whole autologous tumor cells with or without adjuvants to more specific genetically prepared engineered products to cross-react with tumor-associated antigens.

The latter have included peptides targeting CEA and PSA. With both approaches, there has been evidence of tumor regression in a few patients with lung cancer, gastric carcinoma, and colon cancer. However, responses in the setting of advanced disease are rare; some (e.g., Olivera Finn) have postulated that such vaccines will achieve their greatest utility in the prevention or adjuvant setting. Disturbingly, several published Phase III trials of cancer vaccines for advanced stage malignancies have shown inferior outcomes in vaccinated groups (reference P. O. Livingston, D. Morton, etc.). It cannot yet be determined if these are statistical flukes, or if immunization actually selects for the development of more aggressive tumor variants.

Targeting Regulatory T Cells

Most studies of cancer immunotherapy so far have focused on augmenting tumor immunity through supplementing active immune elements such as dendritic cells, TAA-specific T cells, and cytokines. The concept of reversing immunosuppression in cancer has merit and is receiving great interest as a therapeutic approach. Newer studies targeting suppressive molecules and regulatory T cells point the way to successful application of tumor immunotherapy (Figure 20-23).

How does this all relate to regulatory T cells? After clinical and/or pathological diagnosis, patients with cancer might be subjected to traditional tumor therapy, including surgical debulking, radiation therapy, chemotherapy, and more recently, antitumor angiogenic therapy. Depending on their clinical situation, patients could receive a combination of these strategies. Traditional tumor therapy often cannot target the tumor itself, but rather focuses either on the anatomic location of the tumor, or in the case of chemotherapy, on rapidly dividing cells, but remains the "gold standard" therapy. Most immunotherapeutic approaches that have been investigated to date supplement the immune system and provide essential immune elements, including TAA, APCs, effector T cells, and cytokines and/or chemokines with the aim of boosting TAA-specific immunity. Although anti-idiotype-generated antibodies have been evaluated in some clinical trials, they have ultimately demonstrated to not significantly improve anticancer activity when used in conjunction with conventional chemotherapy or in patients with advanced disease. However, given the context of these clinical trials, it may be that the failure of the trials is a reflection of our inadequate knowledge of the immune response to cancer, and the best way of combining

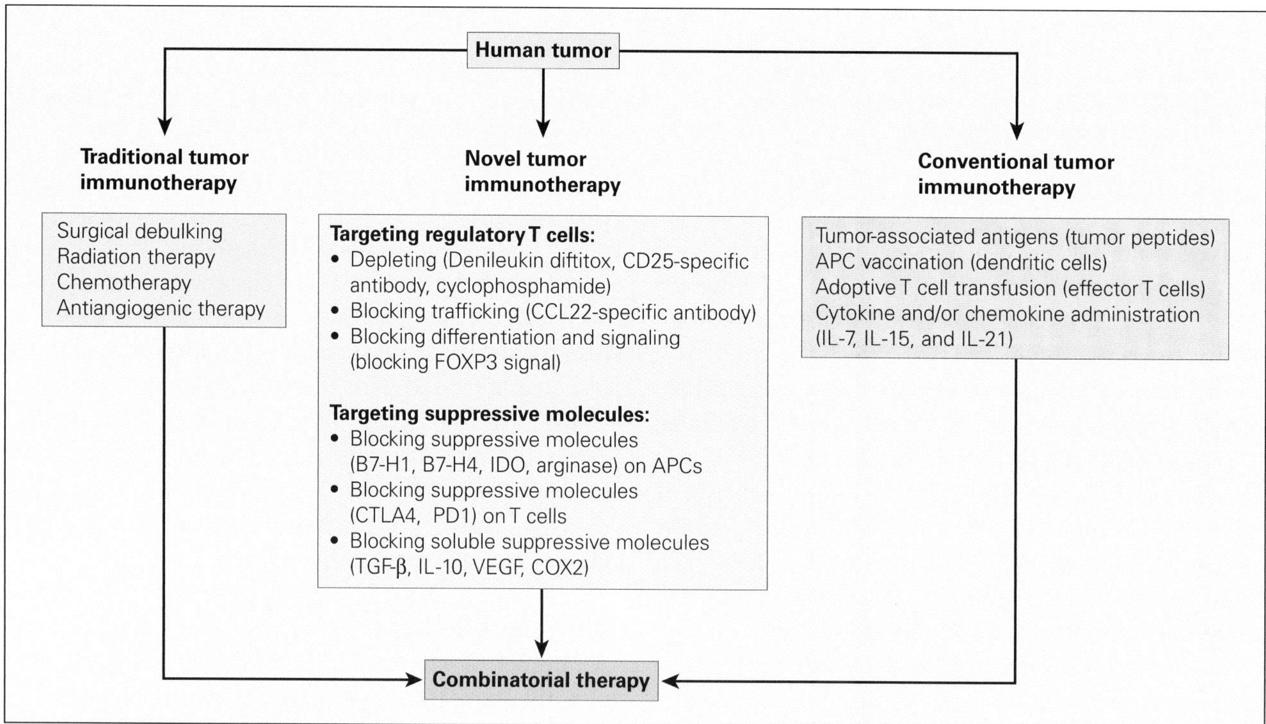

Figure 20-23. Comparison of traditional tumor therapy, conventional immunotherapy, and novel forms of immunotherapy, including therapeutic targeting of suppressive mechanisms, including regulatory T cells. (Adapted from Zou W. Regulatory T cells, tumour immunity and immunotherapy. Nat Rev Immunol. 2006;6:295–307.)

immunological and chemotherapy, rather than a failure of the principle of immunotherapy in cancer. Two additional approaches have demonstrated promise in gastrointestinal cancers, including colorectal and pancreatic: the use of APC and autologous tumors and the use of viral therapy, e.g., vaccinia vectors, modified to bear TAAs with additional co-stimulatory molecules. Large confirmatory studies are ongoing, with the results eagerly awaited.

Summary

Our understanding of the immune response to cancer has come a long way since the original descriptions of the immunologic surveillance theory of Burnet and Thomas, who put forth the concept that the immune system continually surveyed and subsequently eliminated the malignant cells that were continuously arising as a result of mutations. Although there is evidence for both a viral and chemical mutational etiology, the precise basis for the malignant transformation in the human is not well understood, and most malignancies are considered spontaneous in their origin. While the immunologic surveillance concept had limited validity, it gave rise to a more complete concept of immune editing in which the immune response initially eliminated the majority of malignant cells but that later struggled to maintain an equilibrium phase during which the tumor adapted to a less recognizable phenotype but later progressed to a more evasive stage during which the tumor succeeded to escape immune surveillance. The immune response to cancer has been thwarted not only by the low immunogenicity of the cancer cell, but also by the ability of the cancer cell to divert the immune response from an effective effector T cell cytolytic response to an ineffective immune tolerant or anergic state mediated primarily by the host's Treg system and associated immunosuppressive cytokines, especially TGF-β. In addition to the classic therapeutic modalities of chemotherapy, surgery, and radiation, the application of these immunologic principles is finding great therapeutic promise in tumor immunotherapy, including the use of monoclonal antibody, adoptive cell transfer, and tumor vaccines.

Case Study: Clinical Relevance

Let us now return to the case study of malignant melanoma presented earlier and review some of the major points of the clinical presentation and how they relate to the immune system:

- Melanoma is a malignant tumor of melanocytes, which are found predominantly in skin but also in other sites such as the bowel and the eye.
- Although it is one of the less common types of skin cancer, it causes the majority (75 percent) of skin cancer-related deaths.
- Whether it is called malignant melanoma or simply melanoma, this cancer can metastasize (spread) rapidly. With early detection and proper treatment, however, melanoma has a high cure rate.
- Around 60,000 new cases of invasive melanoma are diagnosed in the United States each year, more frequently in males and in Caucasians, particularly those living in sunny climates. There also is evidence that excessive exposure to UV radiation from indoor tanning equipment increases the risk of melanoma.
- The conventional treatment of melanoma has included surgical removal of the tumor, adjuvant treatment, chemotherapy, or radiation therapy. More recently, immunotherapy has been added to the therapeutic regimen.
- Immunotherapy of cancer originated in large part from investigations of melanoma immunobiology. The characterization of tumor melanoma antigens and the study of immune responses directed to these antigens provided the rationale and justification for the use of immunotherapy in augmenting antitumor immune responses for melanoma and other malignancies.
- The understanding that MAGE-1 represented a tumor antigen specifically recognized by the cytotoxic CD8+ lymphocytes gave support to the idea that the immune system could respond to the tumor antigens, which, in turn, provided further stimulus in identifying other immune therapeutic targets and biomarkers predicting response.
- These advances have contributed to the development of vaccines, biological agents (interferon, interleukins), cellular therapies, and antibodies currently in use to treat melanoma and other malignancies (*Chapter 11*).
- The anti-CTLA-4 treatment administered in the case presentation was used to block the cytotoxic T

Case Study: Clinical Relevance (continued)

lymphocyte antigen 4 (CTLA-4), the T cell regulatory molecule that transmits an inhibitory signal to T cells and acts as a counterbalance to CD28, which transmits a stimulatory signal (*Chapter 7*). Intracellular CTLA-4 is also found in regulatory T cells and may be important to their antitumor function.

- Anti-CTLA-4 treatment alone or in combination with vaccines has been shown to induce long-term regression in therapy-resistant melanoma. Although the precise mechanism of action of anti-CTLA-4 treatment is unknown, binding of CTLA-4 to its APC CD80/86 ligand induces the APCs to generate high amounts of indoleamine 2,3 dioxygenase, an immune suppressive enzyme. Thus, preventing the CTLA-4 inhibitory loop was shown to enhance antitumor responses by a reversal of tumor-induced immune tolerance.
- Although immune therapy approaches are promising, Phase III randomized studies have yet to confirm a survival advantage with any immune therapy procedure and improvement in long-term survival. In the setting of advanced Stage IV melanoma, CTLA-4 blockade with the CTLA-4 antibody tremelimumab has shown restoration of effector and memory CD4+ and CD8+ T cells and generation of transient T cell resistance to Treg-mediated suppression. These effects correlated with clinical results.
- Other immunotherapeutic approaches consist of modulation of Toll-receptor signaling and adoptive cellular therapies, where the immune cells are primed and expanded in an extracorporeal environment in order to better recognize the antigen and to avoid the endogenous immunosuppressive effects of the tumor.
- The recent cutting-edge method of direct transfer of tumor-specificity to non-tumor-specific T cells through specific retroviral transfer of alpha and beta chains of a particular T cell receptor are quite promising. Such investigational approaches being performed at the National Institutes of Health (NIH) have resulted in objective cancer regressions in 30 percent of patients, higher than with conventional therapy.

Key Points

- The immune response to cancer is best viewed as a specialized case of immunity in which the malignant cell has adapted and learned how to persist by co-opting the host's immunosuppressive apparatus through a skewing of the T cell cytolytic bulwark from an effective Th1/Th2, CD8, and NK system to a less effective immunosuppressive state mediated by Treg cells and immunosuppressive cytokines, e.g., TGF-β.
- Tumors express both tumor-specific antigens (TSAs) and through gene activation, the emergence of previously suppressed embryonic antigens, e.g., CEA.
- In contrast to tumors induced by carcinogens in which each new tumor has its own unique antigenic specificity regardless of morphologic appearance, each tumor induced by viruses consistently expresses specific antigens that cross-react with other tumors induced by the same or similar viruses even though their morphologic appearance may differ.
- The traditionally accepted immunologic surveillance concept has been modified by the more current immunoediting theory consisting of the "three Es" (elimination, equilibrium, and evasion).
- Current immunologic strategies used in the immunotherapy of malignant diseases include monoclonal antibody, adoptive cell transfer, and tumor vaccines.

Study Questions/Critical Thinking

1. Each of the following are components of the "three Es of cancer immunoediting" EXCEPT:
   a. Elimination
   b. Extinction
   c. Evasion
   d. Equilibrium
2. Each of the following are examples of tumor-associated antigens (TAAs) identified in the human EXCEPT:
   a. Overexpressed self-antigen peptides
   b. Unique tumor-specific antigens
   c. Shared tumor antigens
   d. Bacterial-associated antigens
3. The following are mechanisms and immune cells that actively participate in cancer evasion by suppressing the immune response EXCEPT:
   a. Dysfunctional dendritic cells
   b. Myeloid-derived suppressor cell
   c. NKT cell

   d. Excessive production of sTNF-R
   e. The indoleamine 2,3-dioxygenase (IDO) pathway

4. Each of the following events are associated with the activation of indoleamine-2,3 dioxygenase EXCEPT:
   a. Increased tryptophan metabolism
   b. Increased synthesis of kynurenine
   c. Induction of cancer cell mitosis
   d. Shift from a Th17 to a Treg phenotype
   e. Increased expression of KIR receptors on NK cells

5. The following homeostatic immune actions are favored in the premalignant state by TGF-β EXCEPT:
   a. Apoptosis of premalignant cells
   b. Downregulation of tumorigenic inflammation
   c. Cytostasis
   d. Inhibition of effector cells
   e. Blockage of stromal antigen expression

Suggested Reading

Bird L. Regulatory T cells: Nurtured by TGFbeta. Nat Rev Immunol. 2010; 10: 466.

Bonavida B. Principles of Tumor Immunology. In Nutritional Oncology. 2nd Edition. Heber D, Blackburn GL, Go VLW, Milner J, eds. Burlington, MA: Academic Press; 2006.

Boon T, Coulie PG, Eynde BJV. T cell responses against melanoma. Ann Rev Immunol. 2006; 24: 205–8.

Bui JD, Schreiber RD. Cancer immunosurveillance, immunoediting and inflammation: independent or interdependent processes? Curr Opin Immunol. 2007; 20: 203–8.

de Visser KE, Eichten A, Coussens LM. Paradoxical roles of the immune system during cancer development. Nat Rev Cancer. 2006; 6: 24–37.

Drake CG. Prostate cancer as a model for tumour immunotherapy. Nat Rev Immunol. 2010; 10: 580–93.

Emens and Jaffe. Leveraging the activity of tumor vaccines with cytotoxic chemotherapy. Cancer Res. 2005; 65: 8059–64.

Flavell RA, Sanjabi S, Wrzesinski SH, et al. The polarization of immune cells in the tumour environment by TGFbeta. Nat Rev Immunol. 2010; 10: 554–67.

Gattinoni L, Powell DJ Jr, Rosenberg SA, et al. Adoptive immunotherapy for cancer: building on success. Nat Rev Immunol. 2006; 6: 383–93.

Hippen KL, Merkel SC, Schirm DK, et al. Massive ex vivo expansion of human natural regulatory T cells (Tregs) with minimal loss of in vivo functional activity. Sci Transl Med. 2011; 3: 1–9.

Johnson LA, Morgan RA, Dudley ME, et al. Gene therapy with human and mouse T-cell receptors mediates cancer regression and Blood. 2009; 114: 535–46.

Klein G, Klein E. Surveillance against tumors–is it mainly immunological? Immunol Lett. 2005; 100: 29–33.

Koebel CM, Vermi W, Swann JB, et al. Adaptive immunity maintains occult cancer in an equilibrium state. Nature. 2007; 450: 903–7.

Kurts C, Robinson BW, Knolle PA. Cross-priming in health and disease. Nat Rev Immunol. 2010; 10: 403–14.

Lake RA, Robinson BW. Immunotherapy and chemotherapy-a practical partnership. Nat Rev Cancer. 2005; 5: 397–405.

Lewis JD, Reilly BD, Bright RK. Tumor associated antigens: from discovery to immunity. Int Rev Immunol. 2003; 22: 81–112.

McDermott U, Downing JR, Stratton MR. Genomics and the continuum of cancer care. N Engl J Med. 2011; 364: 340–50.

Ménard C, Ghiringhelli F, Roux S, et al. Ctla-4 blockade confers lymphocyte resistance to regulatory T-cells in advanced melanoma: surrogate marker of efficacy of tremelimumab? Clin Cancer Res. 2008; 14: 5242–9.

Ribas A, Antonia S, Sosman J, et al. Results of a phase II clinical trial of 2 doses and schedules of CP-675,206, an anti-CTLA-4 monoclonal antibody, in patients (pts) with advanced melanoma. J Clin Oncol. 2007; 25:118s.

Rosenberg SA, Restifo NP, Yang JC, et al. Adoptive cell transfer: a clinical path to effective cancer immunotherapy. Nat Rev Cancer. 2008; 8: 299–308.

Smyth MJ, Dunn GP, Schreiber RD. Cancer immunosurveillance and immunoediting: the roles of immunity in suppressing tumor development and shaping tumor immunogenicity. Adv Immunol. 2006; 90: 1–50.

Swann JB, Vesely MD, Silva A, et al. Demonstration of inflammation-induced cancer and cancer immunoediting during primary tumorigenesis. Proc Natl Acad Sci USA. 2008; 105: 652–6.

Zeh HJ, Stavely-O'Carroll K, Choti MA. Vaccines for colorectal cancer. Trends Mol Med. 2001; 7: 307–13.

Zitvogel L, Tesniere A, Kroemer G. Cancer despite immunosurveillance: immunoselection and immunosubversion. Nat Rev Immunol. 2006; 6:715–27.

Zou W. Regulatory T cells, tumour immunity and immunotherapy. Nat Rev Immunol. 2006; 6: 295–307.

Chapter 21

Lymphoproliferative Disorders: Monoclonal Gammopathies and Neoplasms of the Immune System (Lymphomas, Leukemias)

Blanche Mavromatis, MD
Khaled El-Shami, MD, PhD
Joseph A. Bellanti, MD

Case Studies

Case Study 1

A 55-year-old female horseback rider was evaluated by her primary care physician before undergoing surgery for a back-related injury. On routine preoperative evaluation, she was found to be mildly anemic with a hematocrit of 34. Evaluation of the anemia included measurement of serum iron, folic acid, and vitamin B12 concentrations, all of which were normal. A serum protein electrophoresis revealed a protein monoclonal spike and a borderline elevated IgG serum concentration of 2 gm/dL. A bone marrow biopsy showed 5 percent plasma cells. No lytic lesions were seen on a skeletal survey.

Case Study 2

A 40-year-old man presented with back pain. Initial laboratory evaluation revealed a hematocrit of 28 percent. Further investigation of the anemia disclosed a monoclonal gammopathy with IgG levels elevated at 4,500 mg/dL. A skeletal survey showed lytic lesions in the skull and pelvis and a sharply circumscribed osteolytic lytic lesion in the vertebra at the level of L4-L5, which on biopsy was diagnosed as a plasmacytoma, i.e., a neoplasm of malignant plasma cells growing within soft tissue or the skeleton (Figure 21-1).

A bone marrow biopsy was performed and showed 60 percent plasma cells. The aspirate was also sent for cytogenetic study and FISH analysis for chromosome 13 deletion and his siblings were also tested for HLA compatibility.

LEARNING OBJECTIVES

When you have completed this chapter, you should be able to:

- Understand the several malignant neoplasms that comprise the lymphoproliferative disorders
- Appreciate the differences between B and T cell lineages of the lymphoproliferative disorders
- Be able to describe the spectrum of disorders characterized by abnormal proliferation of B cells: monoclonal gammopathy of undetermined significance (MGUS), smoldering multiple myeloma (SMM), and multiple myeloma (MM)
- Recognize that the lymphomas and lymphocytic leukemias are examples of lymphoproliferative diseases in which clonal production of immunoglobulin is less readily apparent and nonexistent and although they include disorders of abnormal proliferation of either B cell or T cell origin, the B cell disorders predominate
- Understand the techniques of immunoelectrophoresis and immunofixation used in the diagnosis of the gammopathies and principles of immunotyping for classification of all groups of the lymphoproliferative disorders
- Utilize this knowledge for a better understanding of benign lymphoproliferative tissue conditions in the normal host as well as the management of malignant lymphoproliferative disorders

Case Studies (continued)

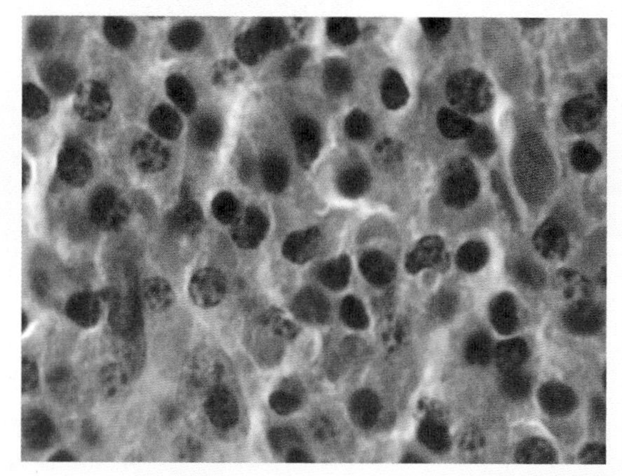

Figure 21-1. Photomicrograph of a histologic section of a plasmacytoma found within the vertebra at L4-L5 (Case 2).

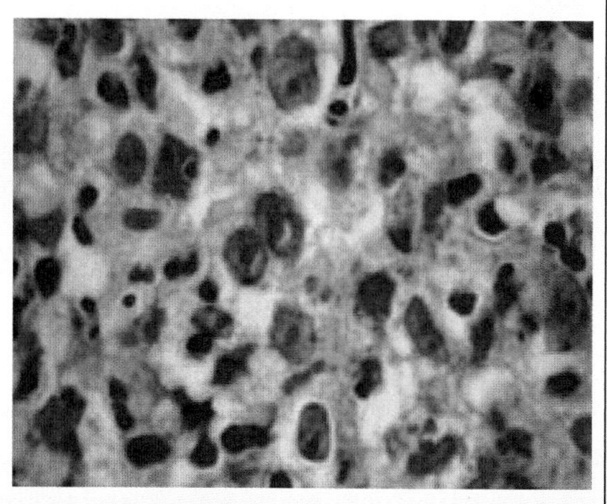

Figure 21-2. Photomicrograph of a histologic section of a nodule from the left lower bronchus of the patient, showing a typical owl's eye appearance (Case 3).

Case Study 3

A 12-year-old girl presented with a six-month history of dry cough, breathlessness, an episode of hemoptysis, intermittent low-grade fever, and a 12 kg weight loss. She had been treated with several courses of antibiotics and had been started on antituberculosis treatment after a chest radiograph revealed nonhomogeneous opacities with cavitary lesions in the left hemithorax. A contrast computed tomography (CT) of the chest revealed several enlarged mediastinal lymph nodes suggesting necrotic lymphadenopathy. Despite four months of antituberculosis treatment, she failed to show any clinical or radiological improvement. On examination, she was a thin, 12-year-old female in no acute respiratory distress. There were several audible wheezes over the left anterior and posterior lung fields. A lymph node measuring two by three cm was palpable in the left supraclavicular space. Laboratory investigation revealed an anemia with hemoglobin of 7.4 g/dL, a leukocytosis of 29,260/mm^3, and an elevated platelet count of 832,000/mm^3. Erythrocyte sedimentation rate was 140 mm/hr. Bronchoscopy revealed a nodule in the left lower lobe bronchus that on biopsy revealed several histiocytes with a bilobed nuclei with prominent eosinophilic inclusion-like nucleoli thus resembling an "owl's eye" appearance (Figure 21-2).

Introduction

The lymphoproliferative diseases represent a set of disorders characterized by the abnormal proliferation of a clone of lymphocytes resulting in a monoclonal lymphocytosis. Most commonly the term is used to define a group of malignant neoplasms arising from the abnormal proliferation of lymphoid cells at different stages of maturation and include, among others, the plasma cell neoplasms, Hodgkin's and non-Hodgkin's lymphomas, and lymphocytic leukemias. Classically, when such proliferation involves cells that synthesize and secrete immunoglobulin, i.e., B lymphocytes and plasma cells, the disorder is associated with excessive production of serum immunoglobulins and is exemplified by immunosecretory myelomas, e.g., multiple myeloma, Waldenström's macroglobulinemia, and a polyneuropathy/organomegaly/endocrinopathy/edema/M-protein (a monoclonal protein)/skin abnormalities (**POEMS**) syndrome, among others.

The lymphoproliferative disorders commonly involve the two major cell types of the adaptive immune system, i.e., the B cells and T cells, which are derived from pluripotent hematopoietic stem cells in the bone marrow (*Chapters 2, 6,* and *7*). Although the precise pathogenetic basis for development of the lymphoproliferative disorders is not entirely clear, individuals with immune dysregulation, e.g., immune deficiency, are known to have an increased propensity to manifest these conditions (*Chapter 16*). This occurs when any of the numerous control points of the immune system become dysfunctional, and immunodeficiency or deregulation of lymphocytes is more likely to occur. Several inherited gene mutations have been identified to cause lymphoproliferative disorders (*Chapter 16*), as have acquired causes, e.g., HIV infection, and iatrogenic causes, e.g., organ transplantation and immunosuppressive therapies (*Chapters 11* and *22*).

In contrast to the B cell lymphoproliferative disorders characterized by abnormal synthesis of a monoclonal immunoglobulin product, e.g., multiple myeloma, the lymphomas and lymphocytic leukemias, on the other hand, have been considered as examples of lymphoproliferative diseases in which clonal production of immunoglobulin is less readily apparent or nonexistent and in which distinctive features are often found only in the proliferative cells themselves. As a result of recent advances in molecular biology and genetics, these disorders have been more precisely classified and better understood. The technology, referred to as "molecular profiling" (Box 21-1), has not only permitted a clearer definition of the lymphoproliferative disorders themselves, but has also provided the scientific proof of their ancestral cellular origins by identification of specific molecular markers. Furthermore, advances in molecular profiling have also allowed more detailed subclassification of these diseases into more discernible clinical entities (*Chapter 25*). This chapter will focus on the immunologic aspects of selected lymphoproliferative diseases, which range from the more indolent low-grade monoclonal gammopathies of B cells to more devastating diseases of lymphocytes such as the aggressive lymphomas and acute leukemias.

Box 21-1

Molecular Profiling

Molecular profiling is a new discipline that uses a variety of molecular biology techniques for the study of the lymphoproliferative diseases to generate a semiquantitative assessment of genomic alterations, transcription, mRNA, and protein expression in various cell types (*Chapter 25*). These techniques have been made possible by basic science advances in molecular biology and have been propelled by the sequencing of the human genome, and include restriction enzyme analysis, polymerase chain reaction (PCR), hybridization techniques, and microarray platforms. They have not only had particular relevance for the clinical characterization of the gammopathies, the leukemias, and lymphomas, but also have led to the identification of molecular risk markers predicting progression, treatment response, and survival. Thus, molecular profiling of disease processes, such as the lymphoproliferative diseases, has not only allowed a clearer understanding of their molecular origins and fundamental relationships, but also has opened new therapeutic approaches tailored to these molecular profiles.

Abnormal Proliferation of B Cells: The Monoclonal Gammopathies of Undetermined Significance (MGUS), Smoldering Multiple Myeloma (SMM), and Multiple Myeloma (MM)

Introduction

The spectrum of disorders characterized by clonal proliferation of fully differentiated postgerminal center B cells, i.e., plasma cells, is broad and includes the monoclonal gammopathies of undetermined significance (**MGUS**), smoldering multiple myeloma (**SMM**), and multiple myeloma (**MM**). As shall be described below, the severity of these diseases ranges from the benign entities, MGUS and SMM, which are asymptomatic disorders characterized by monoclonal plasma cell proliferation localized in the bone marrow in the absence of end-organ damage, to multiple myeloma, a more generalized and malignant disorder that is characterized by a distinct pattern of end-organ damage and is often fatal.

The Concept of Monoclonal Gammopathy

As described in Chapter 6, the immunoglobulins are a family of heterogeneous glycoprotein molecules produced in plasma cells, the terminally differentiated B cells, in response to a myriad of antigens to which these cells may be exposed. The heterogeneity of these molecules reflects those variations in primary amino acid sequences that contribute to antibody specificity and function and are readily demonstrated by electrophoresis of serum (Figure 21-3 and *Chapter 6*). Shown in Figure 21-3A are the broad gamma globulin peaks seen in both the healthy individual with normal concentrations of gamma globulin (in blue) and in patients with elevated gamma globulin concentrations (in red) as seen in patients with chronic infections, autoimmune diseases, or chronic liver disease, e.g., cirrhosis. These both represent polyclonal production of gamma globulin by multiple families of plasma cell-producing clones in the normal individual and in patients with hypergammaglobulinemia, respectively. In Figure 21-3B is shown the typical M "spike" in the gamma region of the serum electrophoretic pattern in a patient with multiple myeloma that is also seen as a "blip" in the gamma arc by immunoelectrophoresis (Figure 21-3C).

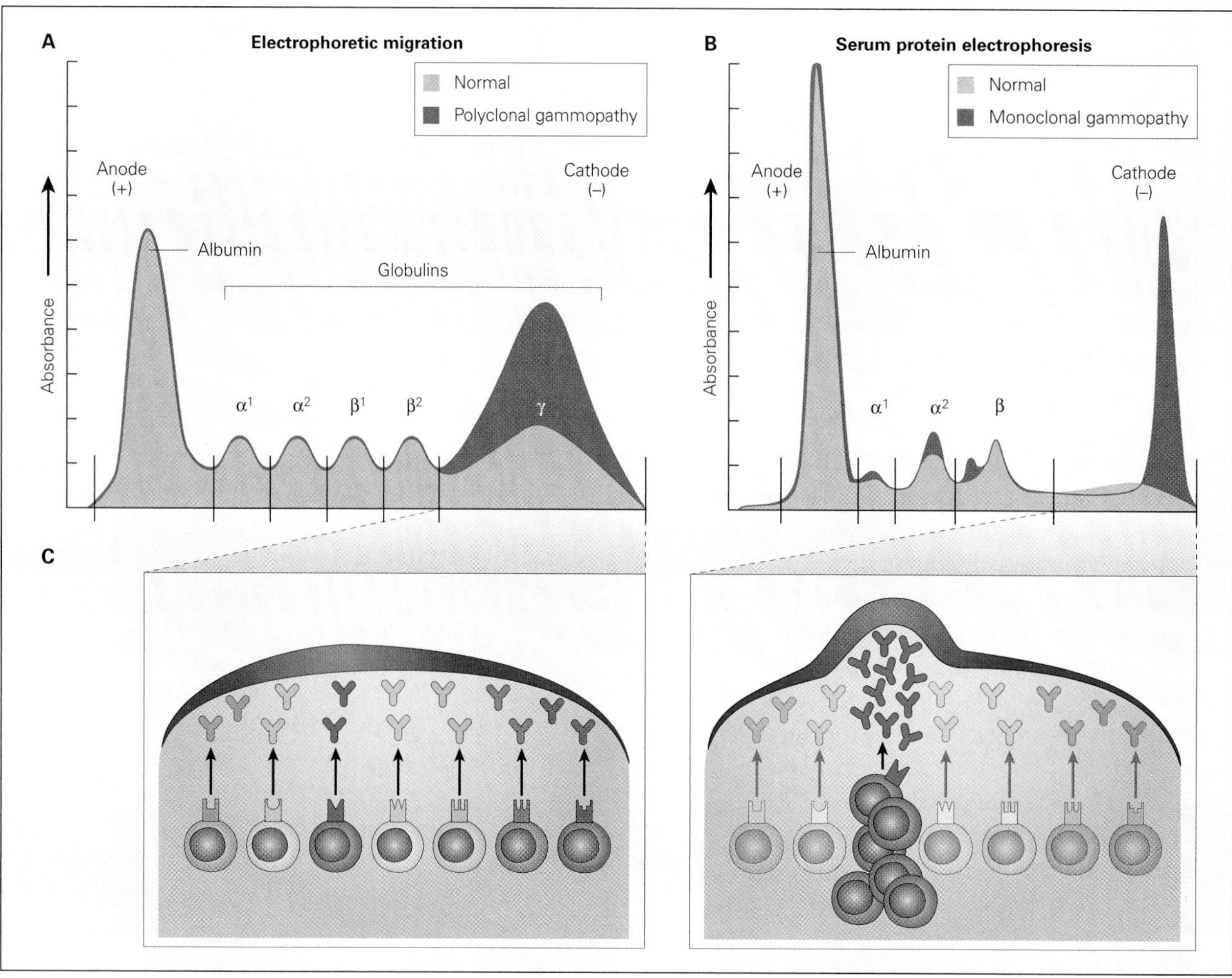

Figure 21-3. Typical patterns of the distribution of serum proteins as determined by protein electrophoresis. Panel A: A normal serum electrophoretic pattern (blue) in a healthy individual compared to an elevated gamma globulin pattern (red) seen in a patient with chronic infection, autoimmune disease, or chronic liver disease. Panel B: An abnormal serum electrophoretic pattern seen in a patient with multiple myeloma showing the typical monoclonal M "spike" in the gamma region of the serum proteins. Panel C: Schematic representation of the wide, long, polydispersed immunoelectrophoretic IgG arc (as described in Box 21-2) consisting of several families of immunoglobulins produced by several clones of B cells in the normal individual (left) in contrast to the truncated arc if one clone is selected for proliferation that gives rise to a restricted increase of monoclonal IgG product that is visualized as a "blip" in the immunoelectrophoretic pattern in a patient with multiple myeloma (right).

Monoclonal Gammopathies of Undetermined Significance

MGUS, formerly called benign monoclonal gammopathy, is an asymptomatic condition characterized by an abnormal proliferation of a single clone of plasma cells that produces a monoclonal immunoglobulin product or its component parts, i.e., light and heavy chains, and that has no evidence of end organ damage. These abnormal products can be detected in the serum or urine either by serum or urine protein electrophoresis (Figure 21-3), immunoelectrophoresis (Box 21-2), or immunofixation (Box 21-3). MGUS is considered a premalignant condition for which close clinical follow-up is required because of the risk of progression to multiple myeloma or evolution to another lymphoproliferative disorder, e.g., chronic lymphocytic leukemia (**CLL**).

Epidemiology

The prevalence of MGUS varies from 0.5 to 3.6 percent depending on the population being studied. The incidence increases with age as observed in a large study from the Mayo Clinic in which 21,463 patients over the age of 50 were evaluated. In this study, an incidence of 5.3 percent was found among patients 70 years of age or older in contrast to 3.2 percent for those over 50 years. The incidence was slightly higher in men than in women (3.7 versus 2.9 percent). The most common MGUS subtype was IgG (69 percent), followed by IgM (17.2 percent),

Box 21-2

Immunoelectrophoresis

Immunoelectrophoresis is a technique by which antigens are separated on the basis of electrophoretic mobility, usually in gels (*Chapter 6*). This is followed by the immunoprecipitation of the separated proteins by a specific antiantigen antibody that is diffused into the gel. Shown in Figure 21-4 is a schematic representation of how immunoelectrophoresis of normal and myeloma serum is performed.

Step 1: The sera are applied to wells punched out of agar-coated slides (Panel A).

Step 2: The agar slide is placed in an electric field and proteins migrate; albumin to the anode (+) and the gamma globulins to the cathode (–) (Panel B).

Step 3: An antiserum containing several families of antibodies to the serum proteins is applied into the central trough. These antibodies diffuse into the agar toward the separated serum proteins that have also diffused into the agar (as indicated by the arrows) (Panel C).

Step 4: Where the serum proteins and their specific antibodies meet, precipitation arcs develop (Panel D). Each arc has a characteristic position and shape for the particular protein that is related to the extent of its migration and amount of its concentration. In this illustration, the serum is depicted as being composed of five proteins when, in fact, most antisera directed to whole human serum result in precipitin arcs of at least 25 or more components. The IgG in the normal serum forms a long sweeping arc; the IgG in the myeloma serum is distorted because of the high concentration of a monoclonal protein and forms a "bleb" on the IgG arc as demonstrated in Figure 21-3C.

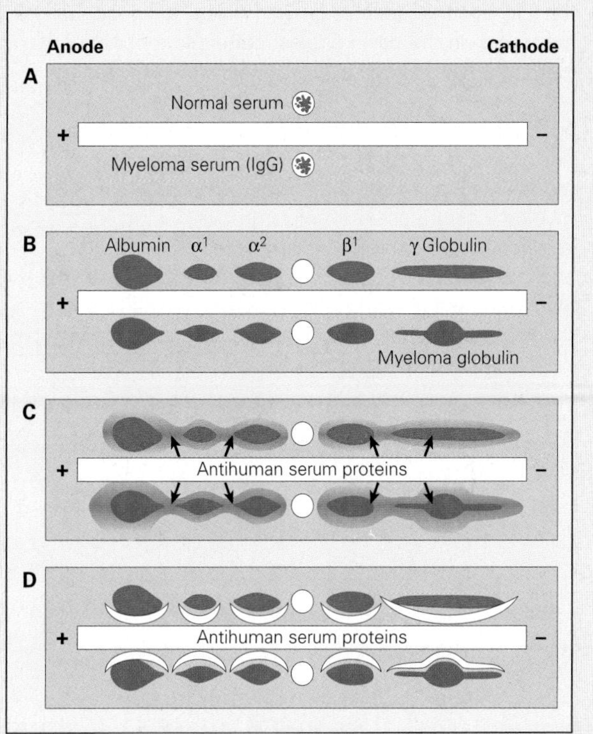

Figure 21-4. Schematic representation of immunoelectrophoresis of normal and myeloma serum.

and IgA (10.8 percent). The incidence also appeared to be slightly higher in African Americans (AAs) when compared to Caucasians. Another study of 2,046 veterans with MGUS comparing racial differences showed that the risk of progression to multiple myeloma at 10 years was the same in both subgroups, i.e., 17 percent in AAs compared to 15 percent in Caucasians. These findings emphasize both the need for a better understanding of the natural history of MGUS, as well as factors linked to the pathogenesis of the disease. In addition to an increased risk of development of myeloma, patients with MGUS have a greater likelihood of developing primary amyloidosis, Waldenström's macroglobulinemia, CLL, and plasmacytoma. Several conditions have been associated with MGUS and are listed in Table 21-1.

Genetics

Translocations involving the immunoglobulin heavy chain gene, located on chromosome 14 at band 14q 32-33 (*Chapter 6*), are seen in up to 50 percent of patients with MGUS and SMM, an entity that clinically falls between MGUS and overt multiple myeloma. Other abnormalities include deletion of chromosome 13 seen in up to 50 percent of patients with MGUS as well as mutations of Ras, p16, Myc, and p53 (*Chapter 6*). Less common, nonrandom genetic abnormalities include 11q13, 6p21, 16q23, and 20q11.

Progression

Because of their susceptibility to progressive disease, patients with MGUS need to be followed indefinitely since the risk of progression persists throughout their lives with an average frequency of 1 percent per year (Figure 21-6). Recent efforts have focused on attempts to identify those patients with MGUS at higher risk of transformation, either for closer follow-up or for consideration for chemopreventive trials. The measurement of free kappa and lambda

Box 21-3

Immunofixation Electrophoresis (IFE)

IFE is another technique by which antigens are separated on the basis of electrophoretic mobility and identified by immunoprecipitation as with immunoelectrophoresis except that the antisera is overlaid onto the agar and the resulting precipitins appear as bands and not arcs (Figure 21-5). Shown below is a schematic representation of how IFE is performed using a myeloma serum as an example. In this illustration, the serum is depicted as being composed of six proteins, and the M band reacts only with the anti-IgG serum and with the anti-kappa antiserum, thus identifying the myeloma protein as an IgG protein comprised of only kappa light chains (*Chapter 6*).

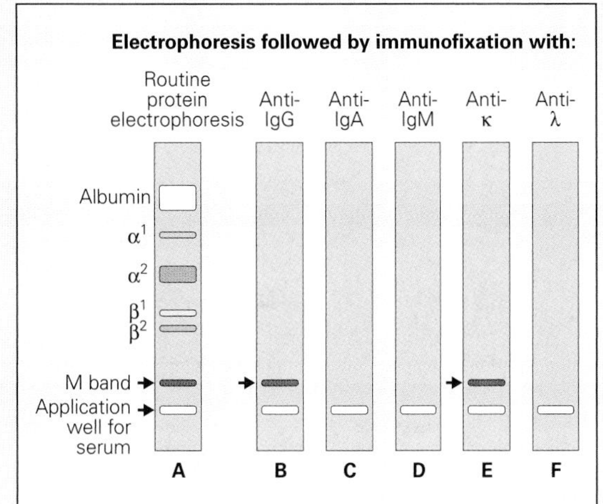

Figure 21-5. Schematic representation of immunoelectrophoresis of normal and myeloma serum.

Table 21-1. Conditions other than plasma cell dyscrasias or lymphoproliferative disorders associated with MGUS disorders

Chronic infections
Tuberculosis
Osteomyelitis
CMV
Hepatitis C virus
HIV virus
Autoimmune diseases
Chronic active hepatitis
Primary biliary cirrhosis
Nonmalignant hematologic conditions, e.g., von Willebrand's disease
Pure red cell aplasia
Hematologic and nonhematologic malignancies
Neurologic disorders
Peripheral neuropathy
POEMS syndrome (Box 21-4)
Dermatologic disorders, e.g., prurigo nodularis

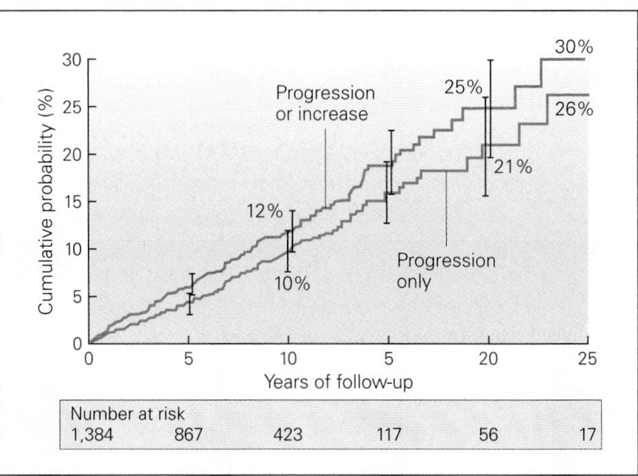

Figure 21-6. Probability of progression among 1,384 residents of southeastern Minnesota in whom monoclonal gammopathy of undetermined significance was diagnosed from 1960 through 1994. The top curve shows the probability of progression to a plasma cell cancer (115 patients) or of an increase in the monoclonal protein concentration to more than 3 grams per deciliter or the proportion of plasma cells in bone marrow to more than 10 percent (32 patients). The bottom curve shows only the probability of progression of MGUS to multiple myeloma, IgM lymphoma, primary amyloidosis, macroglobulinemia, chronic lymphocytic leukemia, or plasmacytoma (115 patients). The bars show 95 percent confidence intervals. (Adapted with permission from Kyle RA, Therneau TM, Rajkumar SV, et al. A long-term study of prognosis in monoclonal gammopathy of undetermined significance. N Engl J Med. 2002;346:564–9.)

chains in serum and urine, measured by a free light chain (**FLC**) assay and commonly expressed as the free kappa/lambda ratio, quantifies the light chains secreted by the abnormal plasma cell. The normal mean free kappa, free lambda, and kappa/lambda ratios in serum and urine are shown in Table 21-2. The free kappa/lambda ratio has been proven to be a good predictive tool for progression to MM with a higher incidence for those with an abnormal ratio of either < 0.26, or > 1.65 (Figure 21-7).

A new model developed at the Mayo Clinic as a predictive marker of progression incorporates measurements of the serum FLC ratio, the serum M spike size, and the type of immunoglobulin produced. Those patients with non-IgG MGUS and a high serum M protein who lack these predictive markers had a 5 percent risk of progression at 20 years compared to a risk of 58 percent for those with an abnormal ratio. Another study suggested that the presence of circulating plasma cells may serve as another predictive marker of transformation. Patients with circulating plasma cells were twice as likely to progress compared to those who did not. The usefulness of these markers will require further studies to confirm their predictive value.

Table 21-2. Normal mean free kappa, free lambda, and kappa/lambda ratios in serum and urine

	Mean free kappa mg/L (range)	Mean free lambda mg/L (range)	Mean free kappa/free lambda ratio (range)
Serum	7.3 (3.3–19.4)	12.7 (5.7–26.3)	0.6 (0.26–1.65)
Urine	5.5 (0.41–15.1)	3.2 (0.8–10.1)	1.87 (0.46–4.00)

The clonal plasma cells can evolve from that of an MGUS to MM as they acquire additional genetic or epigenetic abnormalities. Although the precise mechanism for this transformation is not understood, it appears to involve a two-hit genetic model of malignancy (Figure 21-8). The first hit includes primary translocations involving the immunoglobulin heavy chain (**IgH**) locus on chromosome 14q32 together with sites that include 11q13 (CCND1 [cyclin D1 gene]), 4p16.3 (FGFR-3 and MMSET), 6p21 (CCND3 [cyclin D3 gene]), 16q23 (c-Maf), and 20q11 (MafB). These mutations likely occur during infections or immune dysregulation when IgH switch recombination or somatic hypermutation is taking place (*Chapter 6*). The second hit appears to be a random event involving Ras mutations, p16 methylation, myc oncogene changes, secondary translocations, and p53 mutations.

How Benign Is the Plasma Cell of MGUS?

Because patients with MGUS do not show the full-blown malignant phenotype seen in patients with MM, its corresponding plasma cell was considered to be closer to the normal plasma cell than that seen in myeloma. Recent studies using microarray technology, however, have shown this is not the case and have revealed that there are differences between normal plasma cells and those found in patients with MGUS or MM (*Chapter 25*). Shown in Figure 21-9 are the results of studies of plasma cells from five healthy volunteers, seven patients with MGUS, and 24 patients with multiple myeloma. Using hierarchical clustering of 125 genes, two distinct molecular profiles were identified: normal samples and MGUS/MM samples. Supervised analysis identified 263 genes differentially expressed between N and MGUS and 380 between N and MM of which 197 were observed in the progression from N to MGUS. When MGUS was compared to MM, however, only 74 genes were differentially expressed. The results of these studies suggested that by the time a patient had developed MGUS, a large part of the malignant transformation had already occurred. These patterns have provided further insight into the pathogenesis of the transformation process. Shown in Figure 21-10 are the genes that are expressed during B cell differentiation showing gene expression profiling at various stages of B cell differentiation and in several types of mature B cell lymphoma (*Chapter 6*).

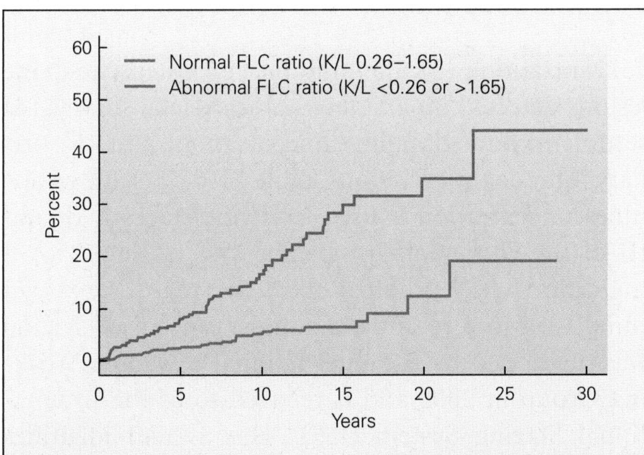

Figure 21-7. Risk of progression to MM based on the FLC ratio. Those with an abnormal FLC ratio (upper curve) are compared to those with a normal FLC ratio (lower curve). (Adapted with permission from Rajkumar SV, Kyle RA, Therneau TM, et al. Serum free light chain ratio is an independent risk factor for progression in monoclonal gammopathy of undetermined significance. Blood. 2005;106:812–7.)

Standardizing the Definition of MGUS

The diagnostic criteria for MGUS have recently been revised by a group of experts and are listed in Table 21-3. The availability of standard criteria is clearly very important to better determine the incidence and risk of disease progression in MGUS.

Smoldering Multiple Myeloma

SMM refers to a clinical entity characterized by its indolent nature and with a significantly higher probability of evolving into a frank multiple myeloma when compared to MGUS (Figure 21-11). It is estimated to account for 15 percent of newly diagnosed plasma cell neoplasms, although a true estimate is difficult to establish. The diagnostic criteria are listed in Table 21-4. The risk of evolving into multiple myeloma is estimated to be between 10–20 percent

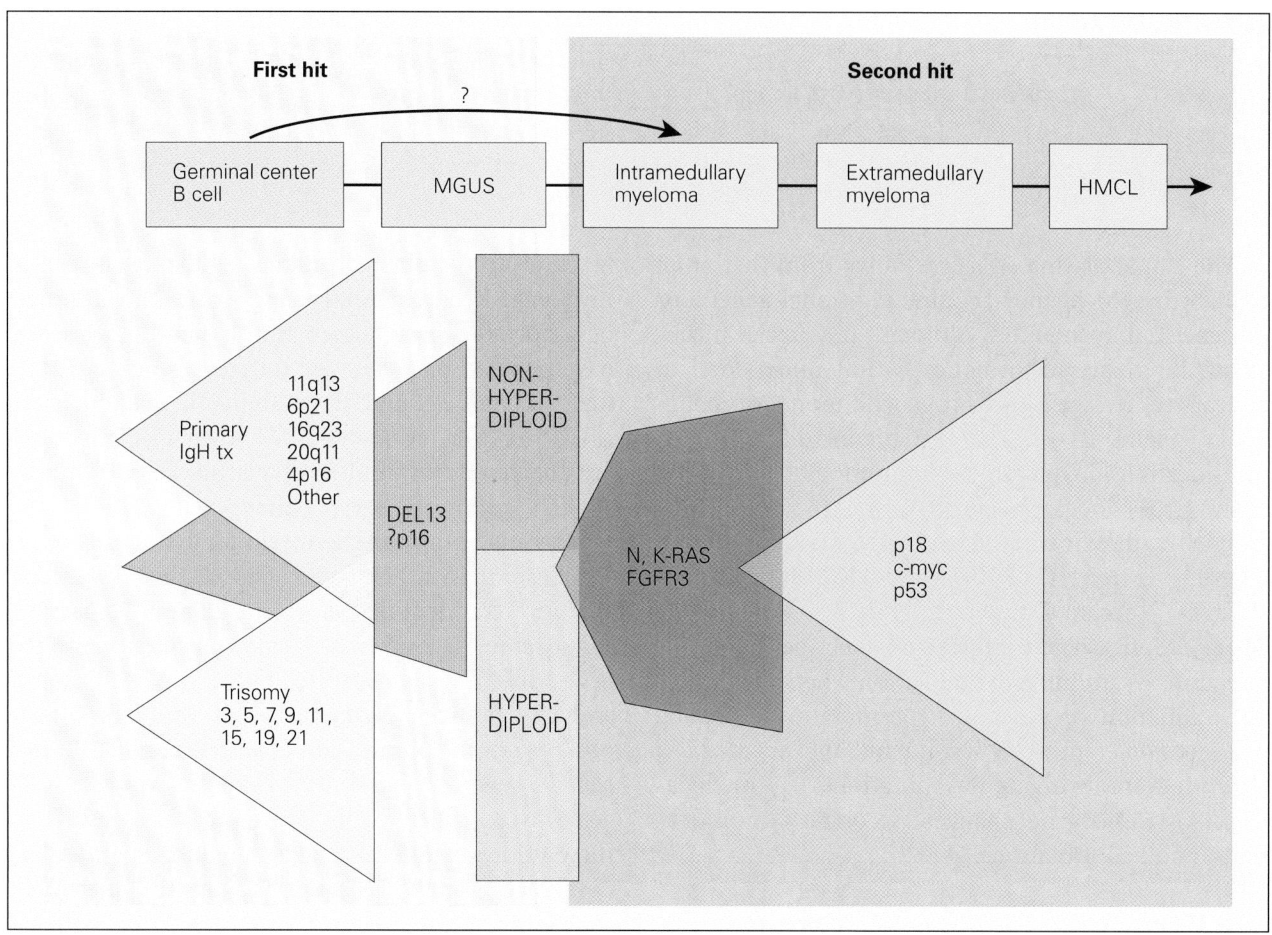

Figure 21-8. **Schematic representation of two pathways of progression to plasma cell neoplasia.** Two defined stages of pathogenesis are depicted, with shaded triangles indicating the possible timing and frequency of known oncogenic events. The earliest changes ("first hit") include two partially overlapping pathways, indicated by primary IgH translocations (tx) and multiple trisomies. Deletion 13 (most often in nonhyperdiploid tumors) and p16 methylation might be included among the earliest changes, but could sometimes be involved in progression. Activating mutations of N- and K-Ras appear to mark, if not cause, the MGUS to MM transition in some tumors, but can also occur as later progression events. Late oncogenic changes ("second hit") include inactivation of p18 and p53, and also translocations that dysregulate c-Myc. Inactivation of Rb, PTEN, and secondary translocations not involving c-Myc are not depicted. (Adapted with permission from Hideshima T, Bergsagel PL, Kuehl WM, et al. Advances in biology of multiple myeloma: clinical applications. Blood. 2004;104:607–18.)

per year depending on the study and the definitions used. Consequently, these patients require closer follow-up compared to those with MGUS and may be candidates for preventive therapy studies. No treatment is otherwise recommended.

Multiple Myeloma

MM is a neoplastic disorder characterized by the malignant proliferation of plasma cells in the bone marrow, affecting close to 19,000 individuals in the United States and with a median survival of five years and that, to this day, remains an incurable disease. Diagnostic criteria for the disease are listed in Table 21-5. There are two staging systems for the diagnosis of multiple myeloma. First published in 1975, the Durie-Salmon staging system relies on five factors: (1) hemoglobin concentration; (2) serum calcium concentration; (3) the number of osteolytic bone lesions detected on a radiographic skeletal survey; (4) serum immunoglobulin concentration; and (5) urinary light chain excretion (Table 21-6). Serum creatinine concentration is used to divide stages I, II, and III of the Durie-Salmon staging system into A (< 2 mg/dL or < 177 umol/L) or B (> 2 mg/dL or > 177 umol/L). More recently, a simpler system of staging was developed by the International Myeloma Working Group in 2005 and is referred to as the International Staging System (ISS). This system identifies two simple yet powerful prognostic markers: (1) β2 microglobulin, which is a surrogate marker for disease burden; and (2) serum albumin, whose expression is negatively regulated by IL-6, a prototypical growth factor for myeloma cells (*Chapter 9*); the use of these markers allows the division of patients into

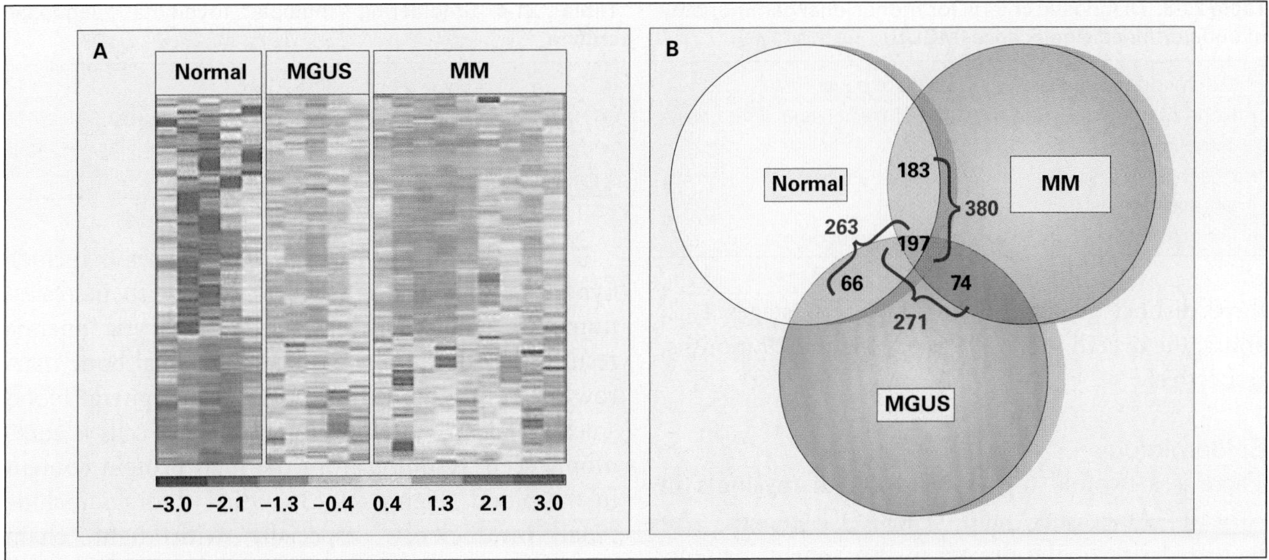

Figure 21-9. Gene array analysis demonstrating the differences between normal and malignant plasma cells found in normal (N), MGUS, and MM. Panel A: Specific genes differentially expressed between N and MGUS; 263 genes were identified, most of which were downregulated (shown in blue). Panel B: Schematic summary of data showing 380 genes differentially expressed between the normal plasma cell and the multiple myeloma plasma cell. Of those, 197 are also differentially expressed in MGUS. The progression to MM from MGUS involves only 74 additional genes. (Adapted and reproduced with permission from Davies FE, Dring AM, Li C, et al. Insights into the multistep transformation of MGUS to myeloma using microarray expression analysis. Blood. 2003;102:4504–11.)

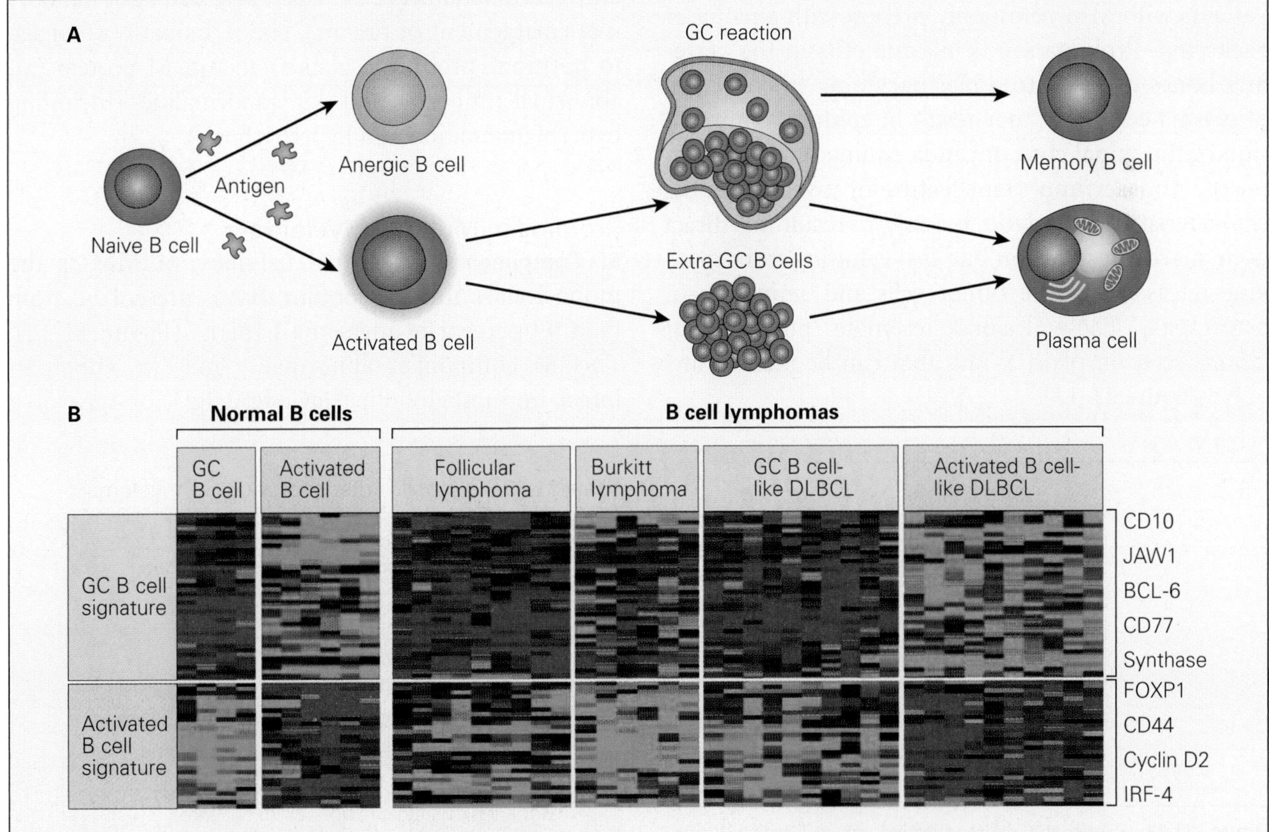

Figure 21-10. Mature B cell lymphomas: cell of origin. Panel A: When naive B cells encounter antigen, they become activated and face three cell fates: clonal expansion and selection in a germinal center (GC), clonal expansion and differentiation at extra-GC sites, or anergy. Eventually, B cells either die or differentiate to memory B cells or antibody-secreting plasma cells. Panel B: Gene array analysis showing a relationship between stages of B cell differentiation and several types of mature B cell lymphomas. (Adapted and reproduced with permission from Shaffer AL, Rosenwald A, Staudt LM. Lymphoid malignancies: the dark side of B cell differentiation. Nat Rev Immunol. 2002;2:920–32.)

Table 21-3. Diagnostic criteria for monoclonal gammopathy of undetermined significance (MGUS)

- Serum monoclonal protein < 3 g/dL or equal
- None or only moderate amounts of monoclonal light chains in the urine
- Absence of end organ damage such as lytic bone lesions, anemia, or renal insufficiency
- Less than 10 percent plasma cells in the bone marrow

three distinct groups (Table 21-7). For stages 1, 2, and 3, the overall survival was 62, 44, and 29 months, respectively.

Epidemiology

There is a twofold higher incidence of myeloma in African Americans and Pacific Islanders. An increased risk of the disease is also seen in patients with MGUS, in those exposed to irradiation or petroleum products, and in certain occupations, including farming, paper production, furniture manufacturing, and woodworking.

Clinical Features

Patients with MM commonly present with anemia or back pain. Proliferation of plasma cells in the vertebral bones can lead to a plasmacytoma (a collection of plasma cells) that may result in epidural compression of the spinal cord or cauda equina if left undiagnosed. Another important feature of myeloma is the characteristic bony lytic lesions, a result of direct bone marrow expansion but also resulting from cytokine release from the tumor cells and activation of osteoclasts. These lesions resemble punched-out lesions seen on plain X-rays that can be seen in any bone (Figure 21-12).

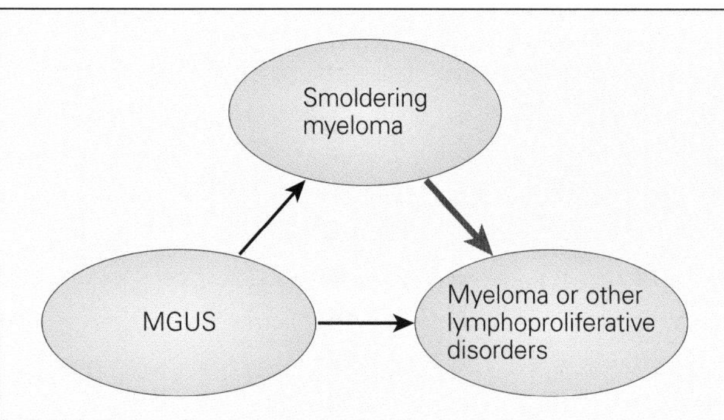

Figure 21-11. Schematic representation of the interrelationships of monoclonal gammopathy of underdetermined significance (MGUS), smoldering multiple myeloma (SMM), and multiple myeloma (MM). Although both MGUS and SMM can progress to MM, SMM shows a higher probability of transformation into frank myeloma or other lymphoproliferative diseases.

Table 21-4. Smoldering multiple myeloma diagnostic criteria

- Serum M protein > or equal to 3 g/dL
- Bone marrow plasma cells > or equal to 10 percent
- Absence of anemia, hypercalcemia, lytic bone lesions, renal insufficiency

The hematologic features of the disease include hypercellularity of the bone marrow with increased numbers of plasma cells and normocytic anemia resulting from the replacement of normal bone marrow by infiltrating tumor cells. On peripheral blood smear, rouleaux formation of red blood cells is commonly seen, resulting from the high protein content in the blood (Figure 21-13). Other findings include renal insufficiency, especially with light chain myeloma, hyperviscosity syndrome, increased risk of infections, and bleeding diathesis.

POEMS syndrome (Box 21-4) (also known as **Crow-Fukase syndrome**, **Takatsuki disease**, or **PEP syndrome**) is a rare syndrome whose acronym reflects its main clinically recognizable features: polyneuropathy (peripheral nerve damage), organomegaly (abnormal enlargement of organs), endocrinopathy (damage to hormone-producing glands)/edema, M-protein (an abnormal antibody), and skin abnormalities (including hyperpigmentation and hypertrichosis).

Proteins in Multiple Myeloma

M Components. A virtual hallmark of MM is the monoclonal immunoglobulin that is present in more than 99 percent of myeloma patients (Figure 21-14). This M component abnormality may be either an intact immunoglobulin (IgG, IgA, IgD, or IgE) or a

Table 21-5. Diagnostic criteria for multiple myeloma

1. Clonal plasma cells > 10 percent on bone marrow biopsy or (in any quantity) in a biopsy from other tissues (plasmacytoma)
2. A monoclonal protein (paraprotein) in either serum or urine
3. Evidence of end-organ damage (related organ or tissue impairment, ROTI):
   - Hypercalcemia (corrected calcium > 2.75 mmol/L)
   - Renal insufficiency attributable to myeloma
   - Anemia (hemoglobin < 10 g/dL)
   - Bone lesions (lytic lesions or osteoporosis with compression fractures)
   - Frequent severe infections (> two a year)
   - Amyloidosis of other organs
   - Hyperviscosity syndrome

Table 21-6. Durie-Salmon staging system

- Stage 1: all of
  - Hb > 10g/dL
  - Normal calcium
  - Skeletal survey: normal or single plasmacytoma or osteoporosis
  - Serum paraprotein level < 5 g/dL if IgG, < 3 g/dL if IgA
  - Urinary light chain excretion < 4 g/24h
- Stage 2: fulfilling the criteria of neither 1 nor 3
- Stage 3: one or more of
  - Hb < 8.5 g/dL
  - High calcium > 12 mg/dL
  - Skeletal survey: three or more lytic bone lesions
  - Serum paraprotein > 7 g/dL if IgG, > 5 g/dL if IgA
  - Urinary light chain excretion > 12g/24h

Stages 1, 2, and 3 of the Durie-Salmon staging system can be divided into A or B, depending on serum creatinine:
  - A: serum creatinine < 2 mg/dL (< 177 umol/L)
  - B: serum creatinine > 2 mg/dL (> 177 umol/L)

Bence-Jones protein (free kappa [κ] chain or free lambda [λ] chain), or both. The frequency of the different paraproteinemias in several large series of myeloma patients is indicated in Table 21-8. The most common finding is a serum monoclonal immunoglobulin by itself. Bence-Jones proteins with a serum myeloma globulin and Bence-Jones proteins alone are somewhat less common. A monoclonal gammopathy cannot be demonstrated in less than 1 percent of myeloma patients, even though the remainder of the clinical, laboratory, and radiological findings (except for the absence of renal function impairment) are entirely consistent with the disease. In many of these cases, the cells synthesize an immunoglobulin but fail to secrete it; in other cases, however, neither extracellular nor intracellular immunoglobulin can be detected by the highly sensitive techniques used, and one must conclude that these cells are making proteins with no discernible markers.

Bence-Jones Proteins. In multiple myeloma, the disproportionate synthesis of the immunoglobulin myeloma proteins is frequently associated with an excessive production of its individual parts, e.g., light and heavy chains (*Chapter 6*). Bence-Jones proteins, which are homogeneous free light chains, were first recognized almost 160 years ago and have provided a valuable tool in the diagnosis of multiple myeloma. These urinary proteins have peculiar heat precipitability properties. When the urine is heated at pH 5, Bence-Jones proteins will precipitate at temperatures in the range of 48° to 56°C and will redissolve on boiling. When the urine is allowed to cool, the proteins reprecipitate.

Immunologic and electrophoretic techniques are usually employed for the recognition of Bence-Jones proteins and, at present, provide the most definitive tests for their detection. An electrophoretically homogeneous protein that reacts with an antiserum to a κ chain or λ chain but does not react with an antiserum to the heavy chain of any immunoglobulin is, by present-day criteria, a Bence-Jones protein.

Approximately 50 percent of myeloma patients are found to have detectable Bence-Jones proteinuria if the added precaution of concentrating the urine is taken. Under some conditions, particularly in the presence of renal failure, Bence-Jones proteins may also be found in the serum.

Table 21-7. International Staging System (ISS)

- Stage I: β_2-microglobulin (β2M) < 3.5 mg/L, albumin ≥ 3.5 g/dL
- Stage II: β2M < 3.5 and albumin < 3.5; or β2M between 3.5 and 5.5
- Stage III: β2M > 5.5

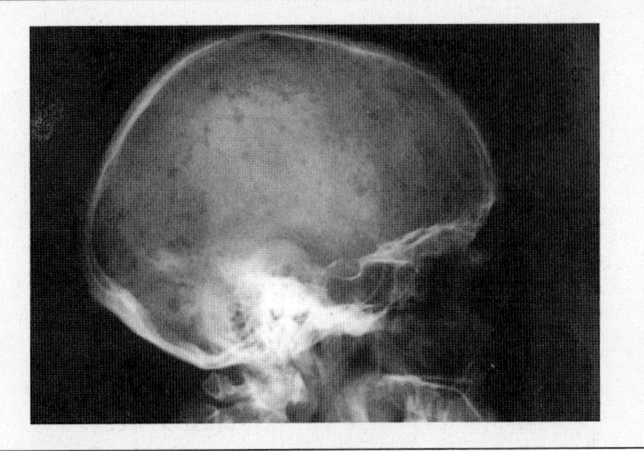

Figure 21-12. Skull X-ray of a patient with multiple myeloma showing many well-demarcated osteolytic lesions in the calvarium.

Management of Multiple Myeloma

There are two components in the management of the patient with MM: (1) supportive care and (2) therapy. Supportive care includes proper hydration to protect the kidneys from obliterative obstruction, avoidance of radiographic procedures using contrast media, and use of bisphosphonates to prevent the development of osteoporosis and fractures. The more conventional chemotherapeutic drugs include the alkylating agents cyclophosphamide and

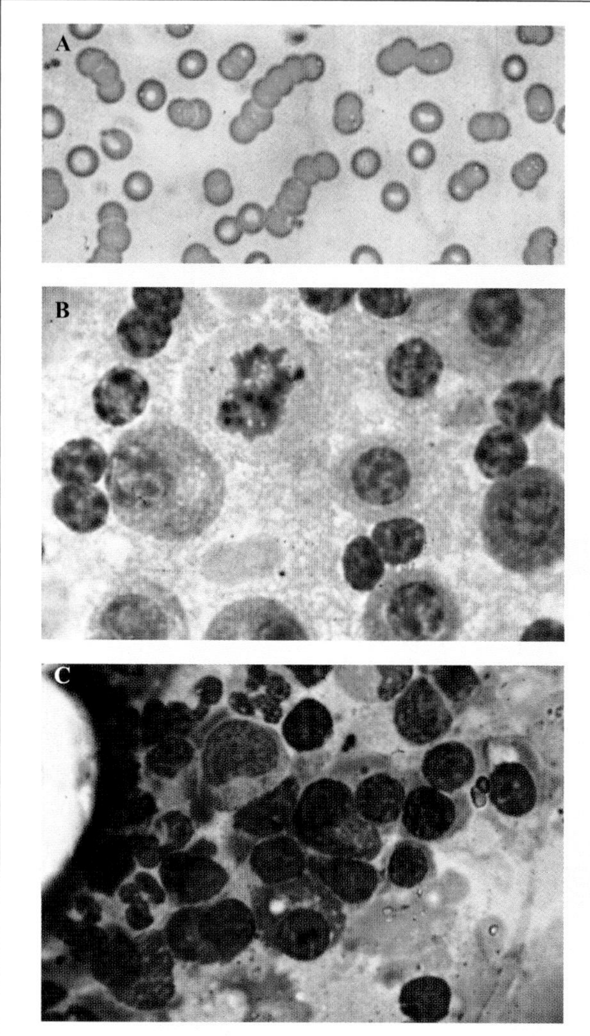

Figure 21-13. Hematologic findings in multiple myeloma. Panel A: Peripheral blood smear showing rouleaux (side-to-side stacking of red blood cells with the typical "stack of coins" appearance) and diffuse staining of the background, indicating high protein content. Smear is from a patient with IgA myeloma. Panel B: Comparison of condensed nuclear chromatin and mature cytoplasm, markers of developed cells. The myeloma cells show large, primitive nuclei in the presence of well-developed cytoplasm (nuclear-cytoplasmic asynchrony). Panel C: Bone marrow from a patient with macroglobulinemia showing cells of the lymphocytic-plasmatic type.

Box 21-4

POEMS Syndrome

POEMS syndrome is a condition characterized by peripheral neuropathy (P), a monoclonal plasma cell disorder (M), and other paraneoplastic conditions, including organomegaly (O), endocrinopathy (E), skin changes (S), papilledema, edema, effusions, ascites, and thrombocytosis. These patients are unique in that their bony features are sclerotic. The syndrome is associated also with Castleman's disease. Distinction should be made between chronic inflammatory demyelinating polyneuropathy (CIDP) and monoclonal gammopathy of underdetermined significance (MGUS)-associated peripheral neuropathy. Suspicion for the disease should be raised in the setting of thrombocytosis and sclerotic bone lesions on plain skeletal radiographs. Therapy involves irradiation, steroids, and chemotherapy.

Castleman's disease is a rare disorder characterized by clonal or monoclonal B cell lymphoproliferative disorder that may develop in the lymph node tissue throughout the body (i.e., systemic disease [plasma cell type]). Most often, they occur in the chest, stomach, and/or neck (i.e., localized disease [hyaline-vascular type]). Less common sites include the armpit (axilla), pelvis, and pancreas. Usually the growths represent abnormal enlargement of the lymph nodes normally found in these areas (lymphoid hamartoma). There are two main types of Castleman's disease: hyaline-vascular type and plasma cell type. The hyaline-vascular type accounts for approximately 90 percent of the cases. Most individuals exhibit no symptoms of this form of the disorder (asymptomatic) or they may develop noncancerous growths in the lymph nodes. The plasma cell type of Castleman's disease may be associated with fever, weight loss, skin rash, early destruction of red blood cells leading to unusually low levels of circulating red blood cells (hemolytic anemia), and/or abnormally increased amounts of certain immune factors in the blood (hypergammaglobulinemia).

melphalan, adriamycin, vinca alkaloids, and corticosteroids such as dexamethasone or combinations such as vincristine, adriamycin, or dexamethasone (**VAD**) (Table 21-9).

Recently, several new classes of drugs have been added to the antimyeloma armamentarium (Table 21-9). The first of these include thalidomide, a drug used for its hypnotic properties and previously popular among pregnant women in Europe, but later found to be responsible for the catastrophic cases of fetal limb abnormalities, i.e., phocomelia (an extremely rare malformation in which babies are born with limbs that look like flippers on a seal). It was quickly withdrawn from the market until the 1990s, when, because of its antiangiogenic properties, testing in patients with multiple myeloma revealed significant antitumor properties. Several single-agent Phase II studies confirmed its anti-myeloma activity with response rates of up to 47 percent in previously treated individuals leading to the approval of the drug in 1998 by the FDA for patients with multiple myeloma. Mechanisms of action of thalidomide

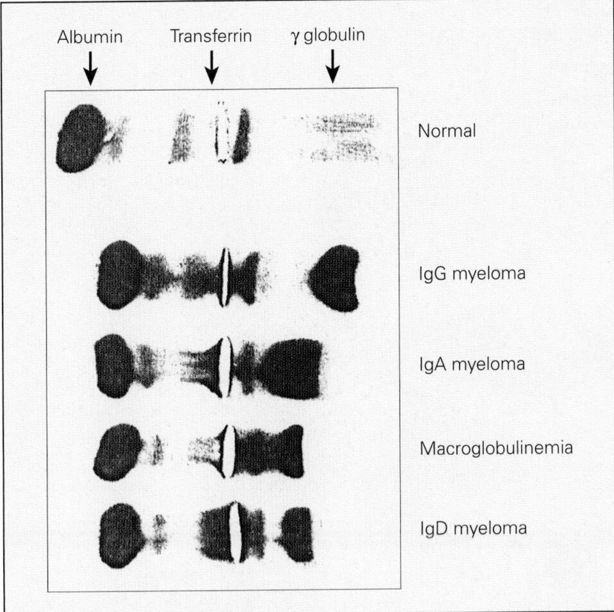

Figure 21-14. Agar gel electrophoresis of human sera. At the top is a normal serum with the albumin, transferrin, and gamma globulin fractions indicated. The four sera below are from patients with monoclonal gammopathy, and the type of monoclonal immunoglobulin is indicated at the right.

include inhibition of IL-6, activation of apoptotic pathways, and activation of T cells (Figure 21-15). Combination trials with thalidomide and corticosteroids revealed even higher response rates up to 64 and 78 percent, especially in previously untreated patients. It is now used as the initial therapy of MM either alone or in combination with other drugs. The first-line therapy of choice for newly diagnosed patients is thalidomide with dexamethasone. After attaining some degree of remission, the next step is to proceed with autologous bone marrow transplantation, which is now a well-established therapeutic modality (Table 21-9).

Other analogues of thalidomide include lenalidomide, a novel, orally administered immunomodulatory drug (IMiD), which is 10,000 times more potent than the parent drug. Shown in Figure 21-16, IMiD was recently approved by the FDA for treatment of a myelodysplastic syndrome (MDS) subtype. Lenalidomide has also recently been combined with prednisone and melphalan in ongoing studies of patients with relapsed disease and has shown very high response rates.

Table 21-8. Frequency of various M components in multiple myeloma

Finding	Percent occurrence
Serum myeloma globulin alone	48
Serum myeloma globulin plus Bence-Jones protein	31
Bence-Jones protein alone	20.5
No monoclonal immunoglobulin	0.5

Table 21-9. First-line therapy of myeloma

- Dexamethasone + thalidomide +/– autologous transplant
- Melphalan + prednisone +/– thalidomide +/– autologous transplant
- VAD +/– cyclophosphamide
- Allogeneic transplantation
- Tandem transplant
- Radiation therapy for plasmacytoma

Bortezomib, a new class of drugs known as proteasome inhibitors (*Chapter 11*), was approved by the FDA in 2003 for patients with relapsed disease (Table 21-10). In one clinical trial, 2.7 percent of patients had a complete remission, with a total response rate of 27.7 percent. It is now being studied as a first-line therapy in newly diagnosed patients in combination with other agents.

The Lymphomas

Malignant transformation of lymphocytes gives rise to another diverse group of malignancies known as lymphomas. The origin of the lymphocytes from within the lymph node compartment, as well as accompanying genetic abnormalities, determines the disease biology of the subtype that develops. The American Cancer Society estimates that in 2009, the number of new non-Hodgkin's lymphoma cases in the United States was 65,980 and Hodgkin's lymphoma was 8,220, representing the sixth most common cancers for men, and fifth for women.

Lymphomas are commonly divided between Hodgkin's and non-Hodgkin's lymphomas and include over 40 different subsets, each with unique immunologic properties, clinical manifestations, therapy, and outcomes. Over the years, a number of classifications have been developed to help differentiate between the various lymphomas. The earlier classifications relied primarily on morphology. With advances in genetics and molecular biology, they are now grouped based on the specific disease entity. Shown in Table 21-11 is the 2008 updated World

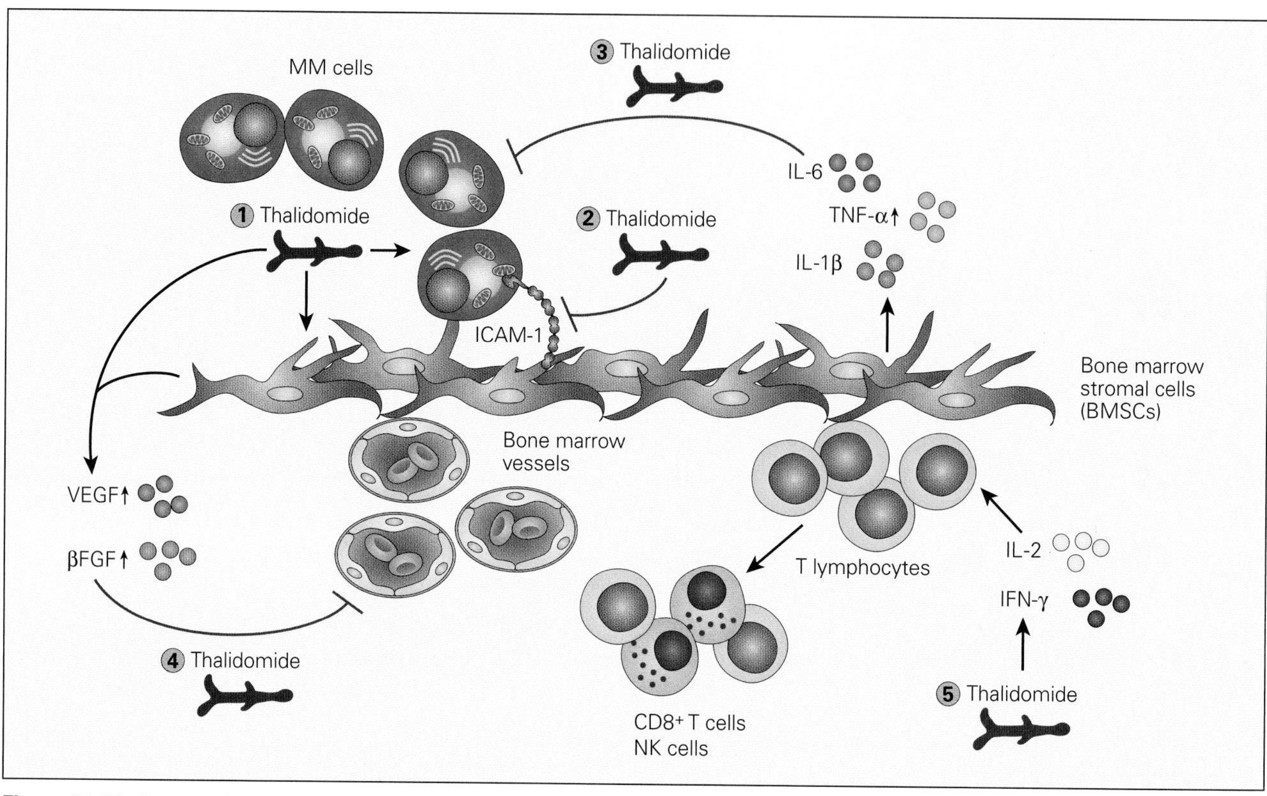

Figure 21-15. Proposed mechanism of action of thalidomide in multiple myeloma. Step 1: Thalidomide directly inhibits myeloma cell growth. Step 2: Thalidomide inhibits myeloma cell adhesion to BMSCs. Step 3: Thalidomide blocks IL-6, TNF-α, and IL-1β secretion from BMSCs. Step 4: Thalidomide blocks the ability of VEGF and β-FGF to stimulate neovascularization of bone marrow. Step 5: Thalidomide induces IL-2 and INF-γ secretion from T cells. (Adapted with permission from Richardson P, Hideshima T, Anderson K. Thalidomide: emerging role in cancer medicine. Ann Rev Med. 2002;53:629–57.)

Health Organization (WHO) classification that is now accepted as standard. It classifies lymphomas primarily into three large groups: the B cell, T cell, and natural killer cell tumors. Other less common groups are also recognized. Hodgkin's lymphoma, although considered separately within the WHO (and earlier) classifications, is now recognized as being a tumor of, albeit markedly abnormal, lymphocytes of mature B cell lineage. Also included in this new classification are the previously described plasma cell neoplasms. Shown in Table 21-12 is a comparison of the frequency of occurrence of the various lymphomas with histopathologic findings and clinical features.

Newer Techniques for the Identification of Lymphoma Subtypes

Although pathologists have traditionally relied solely on morphologic appearances of lymphomas to categorize them, a variety of molecular techniques are now available for better delineation of these lymphocytic malignancies (Box 21-5 and *Chapter 25*). These newer methods include immunophenotyping, cytogenetics, fluorescent in situ hybridization (**FISH**) and a variety of new molecular procedures such as microarray techniques, which have greatly helped delineate the subtype of the lymphoproliferative disorder. Lymphocytes express immunoglobulins on their cell surface, consisting of heavy and light chains. Because of clonality, the cells express either kappa or lambda light chain. The lymphocytes also express various cell surface markers identified using monoclonal antibodies, and characterized by their cluster designation (**CD**) number. These markers are used both diagnostically and as targets for therapeutic intervention. Immunophenohistochemistry and flow cytometric analysis are both used to determine the particular cell profile. Table 21-13 and Table 21-14 review some of the surface lymphocyte markers that distinguish normal from abnormal lymphocytes and which may provide additional assistance in the diagnosis of the lymphoproliferative disorders. Other important tools include cytogenetic changes detected by routine cytogenetics or by PCR analysis.

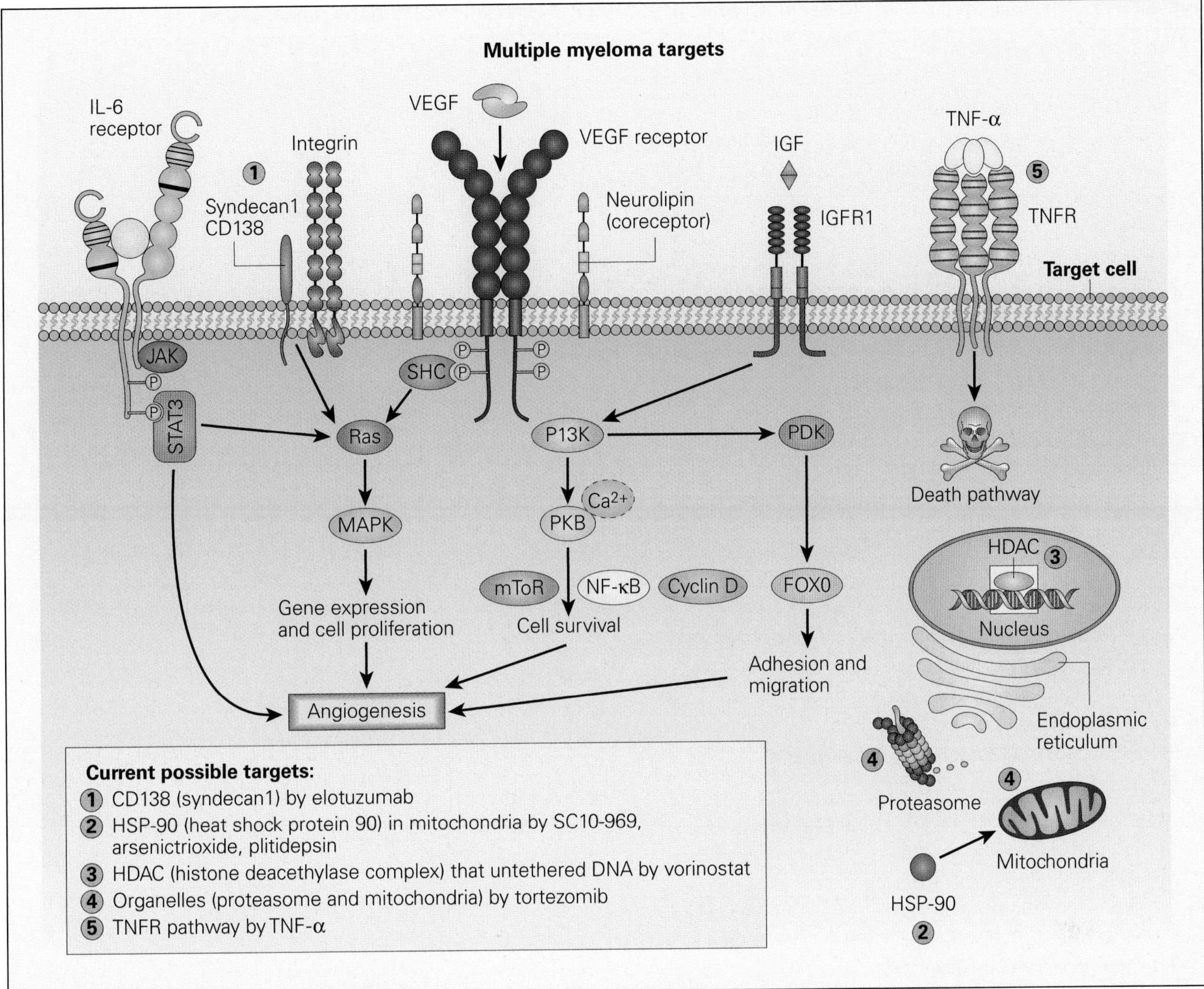

Figure 21-16. Schematic representation of new biological therapies for the treatment of multiple myeloma showing points at which signaling pathways may be targeted. Step 1: Drugs that target surface ligands, e.g., elotuzumab that targets syndecan 1 (CD138). Step 2: Drugs that target HSP-90, e.g., arsenic trioxide. Step 3: drugs that target HADC, e.g., vorinostat. Step 4: Drugs that target mitochondria and the proteasome, e.g., bortezomib. Step 5: Drugs that target TNFR e.g., TNF or anti-TNFR. (Adapted with permission from Chanan-Khan AA, Borrello I, Lee KP, et al. Development of target-specific treatments in multiple myeloma. Br J Haematol. 2010;151:3–15.)

Mechanisms of Lymphomagenesis

Lymphocyte homeostasis is governed by a balance of cell growth and proliferation, typically in response to antigenic stimulation, and programmed cell death, i.e., apoptosis, following eradication of the antigen in question. Accelerated lymphocyte expansion during and after antigen encounter increases the likelihood of random genetic errors that may result in clonal expansion of malignant lymphoid cells.

This paradigm of antigen-driven lymphoid tumors is a unifying theme in a number of conditions that are associated with increased incidence of lymphoid

Table 21-10. Drugs for relapsed multiple myeloma and their mechanisms of action

Drug	Mechanism of action	Status
Bortezomib	Proteosome inhibitor	FDA approved
Lenalidomide	Antiangiogenic	Phase III
Arsenic trioxide	Antiapoptotic	Phase II
Tubacin	HDAC6 inhibitor	Preclinical

Table 21-11. The 2008 updated World Health Organization (WHO) classification of lymphoid neoplasms

Mature B cell neoplasms

- Chronic lymphocytic leukemia/small lymphocytic lymphoma
- B cell prolymphocytic leukemia
- Lymphoplasmacytic lymphoma (such as Waldenström macroglobulinemia)
- Splenic marginal zone lymphoma
- Plasma cell neoplasms:
  - Plasma cell myeloma
  - Plasmacytoma
  - Monoclonal immunoglobulin deposition diseases
  - Heavy chain diseases
- Extranodal marginal zone B cell lymphoma, also called MALT lymphoma
- Nodal marginal zone B cell lymphoma (NMZL)
- Follicular lymphoma
- Mantle cell lymphoma
- Diffuse large B cell lymphoma
- Mediastinal (thymic) large B cell lymphoma
- Intravascular large B cell lymphoma
- Primary effusion lymphoma
- Burkitt lymphoma/leukemia

Mature T cell and natural killer (NK) cell neoplasms

- T cell prolymphocytic leukemia
- T cell large granular lymphocytic leukemia
- Aggressive NK cell leukemia lymphoma
- Extranodal NK/T cell lymphoma, nasal type
- Enteropathy-type T cell lymphoma
- Hepatosplenic T cell lymphoma
- Blastic NK cell lymphoma
- Mycosis fungoides/Sezary syndrome
- Primary cutaneous CD30-positive T cell lymphoproliferative disorders
  - Primary cutaneous anaplastic large cell lymphoma
  - Lymphomatoid papulosis
- Angioimmunoblastic T cell lymphoma
- Peripheral T cell lymphoma, unspecified
- Anaplastic large cell lymphoma

Hodgkin's lymphoma

- Classical Hodgkin's lymphomas:
  - Nodular sclerosis
  - Mixed cellularity
  - Lymphocyte-rich
  - Lymphocyte depleted or not depleted
- Nodular lymphocyte-predominant Hodgkin's lymphoma

Immunodeficiency-associated lymphoproliferative disorders

- Associated with a primary immune disorder
- Associated with the human immunodeficiency virus (HIV)
- Posttransplant
- Associated with methotrexate therapy
- Primary central nervous system lymphoma occurs most often in immunocompromised patients, in particular those with AIDS, but it can occur in the immunocompetent as well. It has a poor prognosis, particularly in those with AIDS. Treatment can consist of corticosteroids, radiotherapy, and chemotherapy, often with methotrexate.

Table 21-12. Comparison of the frequency of occurrence of the various lymphomas with histopathologic findings and clinical features

Lymphoma type	Relative incidence	Histopathology	Cell markers	Overall five-year survival	Clinical features
Precursor T cell leukemia/ lymphoma	40% of lymphomas in childhood	Lymphoblasts with irregular nuclear contours, condensed chromatin, small nucleoli and scant cytoplasm without granules.	TdT, CD2, CD7		It often presents as a mediastinal mass because of involvement of the thymus. [16] It is highly associated with NOTCH1 mutations. Most common in adolescent males.
Follicular lymphoma	40% of lymphomas in adults	Small "cleaved" cells (centrocytes) mixed with large activated cells (centroblasts). Usually nodular ("follicular") growth pattern.	CD10, surface Ig	71–77%	Occurs in older adults. Usually involves lymph nodes, bone marrow, and spleen. [16] Associated with t(14;18) translocation overexpressing Bcl-2. Indolent.
Mantle cell lymphoma	3–4% of lymphomas in adults	Lymphocytes of small to intermediate size growing in diffuse pattern.	CD5	50–70%	Occurs mainly in adult males. Usually involves lymph nodes, bone marrow, spleen, and GI tract. Associated with t(11;14) translocation overexpressing cyclin D1. Moderately aggressive.
B cell chronic lymphocytic leukemia/ lymphoma	3–4% of lymphomas in adults	Small resting lymphocytes mixed with variable number of large activated cells. Lymph nodes are diffusely effaced.	CD5, surface immunoglobulin	50%	Occurs in older adults. Usually involves lymph nodes, bone marrow, and spleen. Most patients have peripheral blood involvement. Indolent.
MALT lymphoma	~ 5% of lymphomas in adults	Variable cell size and differentiation. 40% show plasma cell differentiation. Homing of B cells to epithelium creates lymphoepithelial lesions.	CD5, CD10, surface Ig		Frequently occurs outside lymph nodes. Very indolent. May be cured by local excision.
Diffuse large B cell lymphoma	40–50% of lymphomas in adults	Variable. Most resemble B cells of large germinal centers. Diffuse growth pattern.	Variable expression of CD10 and surface Ig	60%	Occurs in all ages, but most commonly in older adults. Often occurs outside lymph nodes. Aggressive.

(continued)

Table 21-12. Comparison of the frequency of occurrence of the various lymphomas with histopathologic findings and clinical features (continued)

Lymphoma type	Relative incidence	Histopathology	Cell markers	Overall five-year survival	Clinical features
Burkitt's lymphoma	< 1% of lymphomas in the United States	Round lymphoid cells of intermediate size with several nucleoli. Starry-sky appearance by diffuse spread with interspersed apoptosis.	CD10, surface Ig	50%	Endemic in Africa, sporadic elsewhere. More common in immunocompromised and in children. Often visceral involvement. Highly aggressive.
Mycosis fungoides	Most common cutaneous lymphoid malignancy	Usually small lymphoid cells with convoluted nuclei that often infiltrate the epidermis, creating Pautrier microabscesses.	CD4	75%	Localized or more generalized skin symptoms. Generally indolent. In a more aggressive variant, Sezary's disease, there is skin erythema and peripheral blood involvement.
Peripheral T cell lymphoma, unspecified	Most common T cell lymphoma	Variable. Usually a mix small to large lymphoid cells with irregular nuclear contours.	CD3		Probably consists of several rare tumor types. It is often disseminated and generally aggressive.
Nodular sclerosis form of Hodgkin's lymphoma	Most common type of Hodgkin's lymphoma	Reed-Sternberg cell variants and inflammation. usually broad sclerotic bands that consists of collagen.	CD15, CD30		Most common in young adults. It often arises in the mediastinum or cervical lymph nodes.
Mixed-cellularity subtype of Hodgkin's lymphoma	Second most common form of Hodgkin's lymphoma	Many classic Reed-Sternberg cells and inflammation.	CD15, CD30		Most common in men. More likely to be diagnosed at advanced stages than the nodular sclerosis form. Epstein-Barr virus involved in 70% of cases.

tumors, especially B cell non-Hodgkin's lymphomas (**NHL**). Such conditions include states of chronic inflammation following infection with a number of organisms that neither possess any oncogenes nor display the ability to integrate into the host cell genome. Such organisms include: (1) *Helicobacter pylori*, which plays a pivotal role in gastric lymphoma, particularly the mucosa-associated lymphoid tissue (**MALT**); (2) *Chlamydia psittaci*, which is closely linked to extranodal marginal zone lymphomas; (3) *Campylobacter jejuni*, which is present in rare small intestinal lymphomas; and, (4) *Borrelia burgdorferi* that has recently been linked to primary cutaneous B cell lymphomas. Hepatitis C virus is a RNA virus without known oncogenic potential that has also been epidemiologically linked to a number of NHL including splenic marginal zone lymphoma and lymphoplasmacytic lymphoma.

Additionally, increases in NHL have also been noted among patients with autoimmune diseases. Patients with Sjogren's syndrome, systemic lupus erythematosus, and rheumatoid arthritis have a lifetime risk of lymphomas that ranges from 4–19 percent. This latter observation suggests that autoreactive lymphocytes are similarly prone to undergo malignant transformation during the sustained

Box 21-5

Newer Techniques for the Diagnosis of Lymphoproliferative Disorders

Pathologists have traditionally depended heavily on the morphologic appearances of lymphomas to categorize them. Thirty years ago, morphology was the only tool available. Suspicious lymphoid tissue was (and still is) fixed in formalin, embedded in paraffin, sliced very thinly (five microns or less), placed on a glass slide, and stained with hematoxylin and eosin. The earliest attempts to categorize lymphomas relied solely on this method.

Starting in the 1970s, additional molecular techniques were developed to study the nature of both benign and malignant lymphoid cells that are described more fully in Chapter 25.

Immunophenotyping: Different types of lymphoid cells express different antigenic molecules on their surface cell membrane that can be detected by antibodies that will adhere specifically to these molecules.. The antibodies are commonly altered in special ways so their presence can be detected by certain marker molecules attached to the antibodies (e.g., fluorescent markers), so that the technique can be used to assess what kinds of antigens are located on the cell membrane. These antibodies can detect "cluster designation" or "CD" numbers (Appendix 3). Immunophenotyping has become important in evaluating (1) the malignancy of a lymphoid proliferation and (2) the lymphoma category to which it belongs.

Three methods of immunophenotyping that yield comparable information are:

1. immunohistochemistry
2. immunofluorescence
3. flow cytometry

Cytogenetics: Malignant lymphoid cells, like all cells, can be made to proliferate in vitro, and their metaphase chromosomes can be examined for characteristic translocations (called "karyotyping"). Morphological microscopic observations very frequently can be correlated to correspond to genetic abnormalities detected by molecular techniques.

Fluorescent in situ hybridization (FISH): In addition to the technique of karyotyping, which displays whole chromosomes from metaphase spreads of dividing cells, FISH can be used to search for specific chromosomal abnormalities in the DNA of interphase cells. The advantages of this technique are its ability to utilize nondividing cells, to examine 200 or so cells at a time rather than the 20 of conventional karyotyping, and to identify subtle defects undetectable by karyotyping.

Molecular techniques: A variety of basic molecular techniques are becoming available for detecting clonal (neoplastic) rearrangements of the immunoglobulin gene in B cell malignancies or of the T cell receptor gene in T cell malignancies. These rearrangements are too subtle to be detected by conventional cytogenetics. The last several years have seen an explosion of interest in cDNA or oligonucleotide **microarray techniques,** in which the expression levels of thousands of messenger RNAs are simultaneously measured (*Chapter 25*). This creates a genome-wide portrait of the cell's gene activity, a global perspective that has yielded many fresh insights. Although not yet a technique used in diagnostic laboratories, it soon may become readily available.

lymphoproliferative response associated with chronic autoantigen stimulation.

At the other end of the spectrum, immune deficiency states, whether congenital, iatrogenic, or AIDS-related, are associated with dramatic increases in the risk of lymphoma (*Chapter 17*). It is noteworthy, however, that immune deficiency-associated lymphomas are typically induced by infectious pathogens with transforming abilities. EBV is the prototypical example of a DNA virus that is capable of transforming B lymphocytes both in vitro and in vivo and has been linked to a number of lymphoid tumors, both Hodgkin's and non-Hodgkin's lymphomas.

Table 21-13. Some of the surface lymphocyte markers that distinguish normal from abnormal lymphocytes

All lymphoid cells	CD45+ (leukocyte common antigen)
B cell	CD19+, CD20+, CD22+
Low-grade lymphomas	CD19+, CD20+, CD22+, occasionally CD5+, CD43+
Follicular center cell	CD19+, CD20+, CD22+, CD10+
T cell	CD2+, CD3+, CD5+, CD7+, CD4+ or CD8+
Natural killer cells	CD16+, CD56+, CD57+

Treatment of the Lymphomas

Chemotherapy

Various chemotherapeutic regimens are used in the treatment of lymphomas. These drugs are used either as single agents or in combination. Rituximab (as described below) is frequently added for the treatment of B cell malignancies (*Chapter 11*). Commonly used chemotherapeutic drugs include alkylating

Table 21-14. Antigen expression during B cell development

	Central lymphoid tissues (antigen-independent differentiation)				Peripheral lymphoid tissues (antigen-dependent differentiation)		
	CD19 CD38 CD10 Pre B cell	CD22 Immature B cell	CD20 Mature B cell	CD52 Mature activated B cell	GCB (germinal center B cell)	Memory B cell	Plasma cell
CD19	+	+	+	+	+	+	–
CD10	+	+/–	–	–	+	?	–
CD20	–	–/+	+	+	++	+	–
CD38	++	+	+	+	++	?	++
CD22	–	+	+	+	+		
CD52				+			
CD80	–						

(Adopted from Janeway CA. *Immunobiology. The immune system in health and disease.* Garland Publishing; 1997).

agents, antimetabolites such as nucleoside analogues, anthracyclines, plant alkaloids, antitumor antibiotics, topoisomerase inhibitors, biologic agents, and steroids. The most commonly encountered side effects of these agents include myelosuppression, nausea, vomiting, mucositis, and susceptibility to infection. Certain agents can also cause cardiac toxicity, bladder, irritation, or neuropathy. Antiemetic agents are effective in minimizing nausea, and growth factors help maintain peripheral blood counts and are often used in conjunction with chemotherapy.

Immunotherapy: Rituximab, Targeting Anti-CD20

Rituximab is a genetically engineered chimeric anti-CD20 immunoglobulin G1 (IgG1) monoclonal antibody consisting of human IgG-1 and κ constant regions linked to murine variable domains (Figure 21-17A and *Chapter 11*). It was the first chimeric monoclonal antibody approved by the FDA in 1997 to treat cancer. Its mechanism of action includes the induction of ADCC (antibody-dependent cell-mediated cytotoxicity) by NK cells or cytotoxic T lymphocytes with resultant apoptosis or cell destruction of the malignant cell mediated by complement-mediated cytolysis (Figure 21-17B). The polymorphisms of the leukocyte Fcγ receptors, i.e., FcγR, (*Chapter 6*) required to link the IgG bound antigen to activate the cytotoxic lymphocyte may not only provide an explanation for the variability of responsiveness to this agent but also may offer a predictive marker of those most likely to benefit from this treatment.

Indolent B Cell Lymphomas

There is a group of relatively slow-growing B cell lymphomas referred to as indolent B cell lymphomas originally classified with the non-Hodgkin's lymphomas (Table 21-15). This group of slow growing B cell non-Hodgkin's lymphomas includes follicular lymphomas (**FL**), MALT lymphomas, small lymphocytic lymphoma (**SLL**), lymphoplasmacytoid type, splenic marginal zone lymphoma (**MZL**), and nodal MZL lymphoma. These lymphomas are often considered chronic diseases that are incurable with current therapies. The newly introduced follicular lymphoma international prognostic index (**FLIPI**) score (Box 21-6) can help risk-stratify patients with this disease. Shown in Figure 21-18 is a photomicrograph

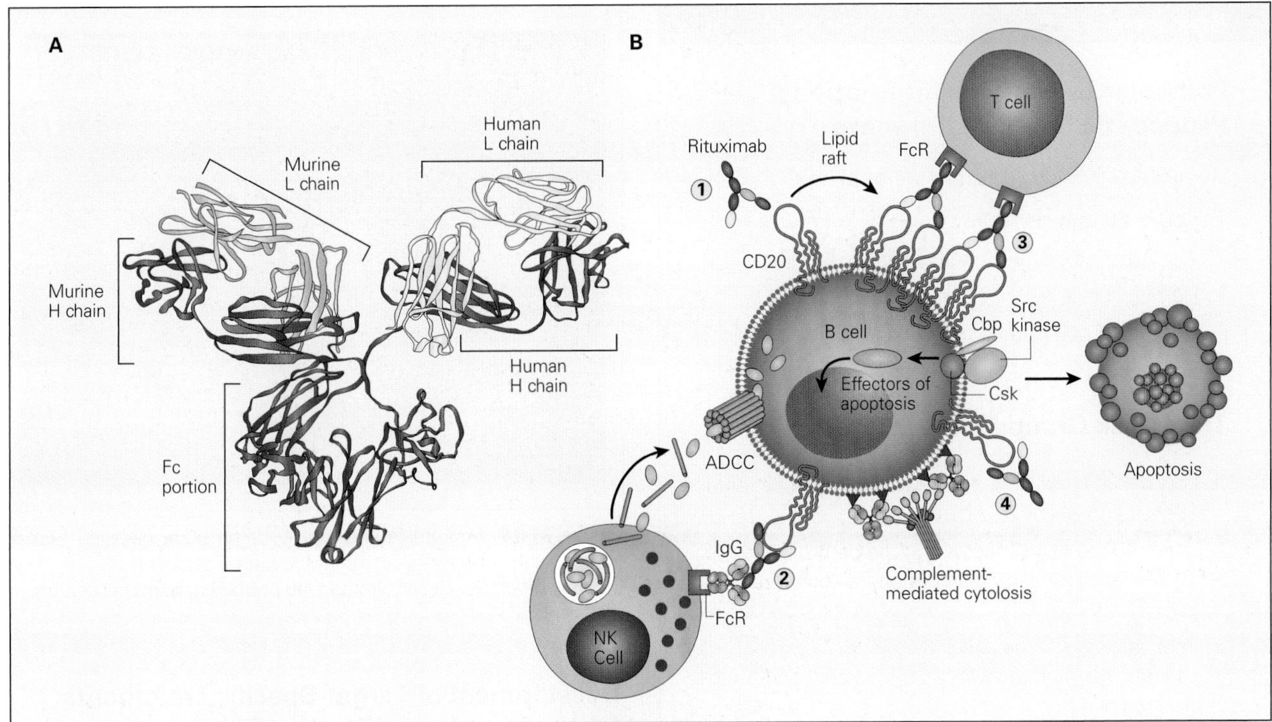

Figure 21-17. Panel A: The molecular structure of rituximab. Panel B: A schematic representation of the postulated mechanisms of action of rituximab with the CD20 molecule: a transmembrane protein expressed by 95 percent of mature B cells. Following binding of rituximab with the CD20 receptor on the B cell (1), cell destruction can occur by ADCC (antibody-dependent cell-mediated cytotoxicity) by NK cells (2) or cytotoxic T lymphocytes (3) with resultant apoptosis or by complement-mediated cytolysis (4). (Adapted with permission from Olszewski AJ, Grossbard ML. Empowering targeted therapy: lessons from rituximab. Sci STKE. 2004 Jul 13;2004(241):pe30.)

of a typical histologic morphology of a follicular lymphoma showing prominent germinal centers, the hallmark feature of this malignancy.

Until recently, little progress was made in improving the overall survival of these patients despite therapeutic intervention. Studies now suggest that newer therapeutic approaches may have finally succeeded in making an impact on survival, most likely as a result of the introduction of the monoclonal antibody rituximab and the use of radioimmunoconjugates (Table 21-16). In vitro studies showed that rituximab can sensitize lymphoma cells to subsequent chemotherapy. Treatment is generally initiated with the development of systemic symptoms, e.g., fever, night sweats, weight loss, severe pain, or when there is evidence of significant palpable adenopathy, organ dysfunction, or radiologic evidence of significant tumor growth and continued until these findings resolve; treatment is resumed if there is recurrence of the disease. Numerous therapeutic options are available, including watchful waiting, treatment with rituximab alone, combination treatment with rituximab and

Table 21-15. Immunologic and genetic characteristics of indolent B cell lymphomas

Lymphoma subtype	
Follicular lymphoma	CD 20+, CD10+/Bcl-6, t(14;18)
MALT lymphoma	CD20+, light chain restriction, absence of CD5/CD10
SLL	CD20+, co-expression of CD5 and CD23, absence of t(11;14)
Splenic MZL	CD20+, lack of expression of CD5, CD10, CD23, CD43
Nodal MZL	CD20+, no co-expression of CD5 or CD10
Mantle cell lymphoma	CD20+CD5+, CD23−, expression of cyclin D1, t(11:14)
Lymphoplasmactoid lymphoma	CD20+, CD52 expression, monoclonal immunoglobulin light chain

Adapted from Gascoyne RD. Hematopathology approaches to diagnosis and prognosis of indolent B-cell lymphomas. Hematology Am Soc Hematol Educ Program. 2005;299–306.

Box 21-6

Follicular Lymphoma International Prognostic Index (FLIPI) score

Five adverse prognostic factors were selected:

1. Age (> 60 versus ≤ 60)
2. Ann Arbor stage (III–IV versus I–II)
3. Hemoglobin level (< 12 g/dL versus ≥ 12 g/dL)
4. Number of nodal areas (> 4 versus ≤ 4)
5. Serum LDH level (> normal versus ≤ normal)

Three Risk Groups Were Defined

1. Low risk (0–1 adverse factor, 36 percent of patients, 10-year survival of 70.7 percent)
2. Intermediate risk (2 factors, 37 percent of patients, 10-year survival of 51 percent and a hazard ratio of 2.3)
3. Poor risk (≥ 3 adverse factors, 27 percent of patients, 10-year survival of 35.5 percent and a hazard ratio of 4.3)

One Point Is Given for Each Factor Present at Diagnosis

Patients with zero to one factor are classified as low-risk patients and have five- and 10-year survivals of 90 percent and 71 percent, respectively.

Patients with two factors are classified as intermediate risk and they have five- and 10-year survivals of 78 percent and 51 percent, respectively.

High-risk disease patients have three to five factors and five- and 10-year survivals of 53 percent and 36 percent, respectively. The relative frequencies of the three risk categories are 36 percent, 37 percent, and 27 percent, which is a significant improvement over the IPI distribution in follicular lymphoma.

chemotherapy, or radioimmunoconjugates. Other therapeutic agents currently studied include other monoclonal antibodies such as those targeting CD22, CD52, and CD80, anti-bcl-2 antisense therapies, histone deacetylase inhibitors, proteasome inhibitors, rapamycin analogues, and anti-idiotype vaccines (given either after conventional chemotherapy or after rituximab therapy alone).

Staging Hodgkin's and Non-Hodgkin's Lymphomas

The staging of Hodgkin's and non-Hodgkin's lymphomas is based on the Modified Ann Arbor Staging Classification (Box 21-7).

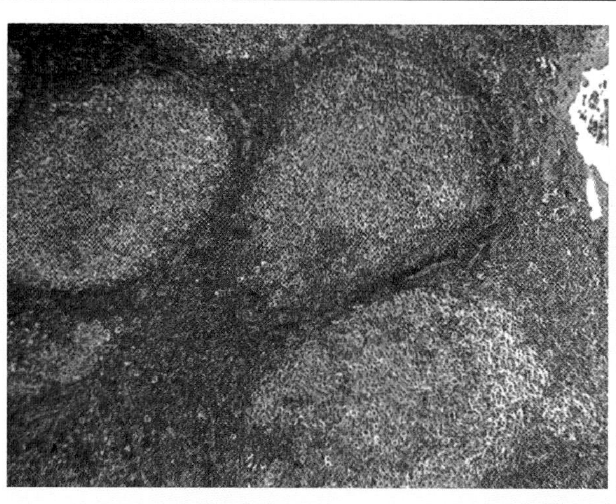

Figure 21-18. Photomicrograph of a lymph node biopsied from a patient with follicular lymphoma showing a typical histologic morphology of a follicular lymphoma with prominent germinal centers.

Development of Target-Specific Treatments for the Lymphoproliferative Diseases

Over the past decade, several novel agents have been developed for the treatment of the lymphoproliferative diseases that have dramatically improved outcomes for patients with these disorders. As described previously for new drug targets for the treatment of multiple myeloma, several new therapeutic targets are being developed for the treatment of the other lymphoproliferative disorders. Shown in Figure 21-19 and Table 21-17 are some of the new biological therapies together with their mechanisms of action and clinical applications. These include (1) **anti-idiotypic antibody for vaccine development**, e.g., anti-idiotype antibody; (2) **cell surface**

Table 21-16. Therapeutic approaches used in low-grade lymphomas

Conventional	Investigational*
1. Watchful waiting 2. Chemotherapy a. Nucleoside analogues b. Alkylating agents c. Combinations with anti-CD20 (rituximab + fludarabine, rituximab + CVP, rituximab + CHOP)	1. Chemotherapy bendamustine 2. Monoclonal antibodies a. Anti-CD22 (epratuzumab) b. Anti-CD80 (galiximab) c. Anti-Hu1D10 (apolizumab) d. Anti-VEG-F (bevacizumab)
3. Monoclonal antibodies Anti-CD20	3. Vaccines Anti-idiotype vaccines
4. Radioimmunoconjugates Anti-CD20 radiolabeled	4. Bcl-2 antisense oblimersen

Box 21-7

Staging Hodgkin's and Non-Hodgkin's Lymphomas

Stage Involvement

- I Single lymph node region (I) or one extralymphatic site (I_E).
- II Two or more lymph node regions, same side of the diaphragm (II) or local extralymphatic extension plus one or more lymph node regions same side of the diaphragm (II_E).
- III Lymph node regions on both sides of the diaphragm (III) that may be accompanied by local extralymphatic extension (III_E).
- IV Diffuse involvement of one or more extralymphatic organs or sites.

Symptoms

A = no B symptoms
B = presence of at least one of these:

1. Unexplained weight loss > 10 percent baseline during six months prior to staging
2. Drenching night sweats
3. Otherwise unexplained febrile episodes (> 38°C)

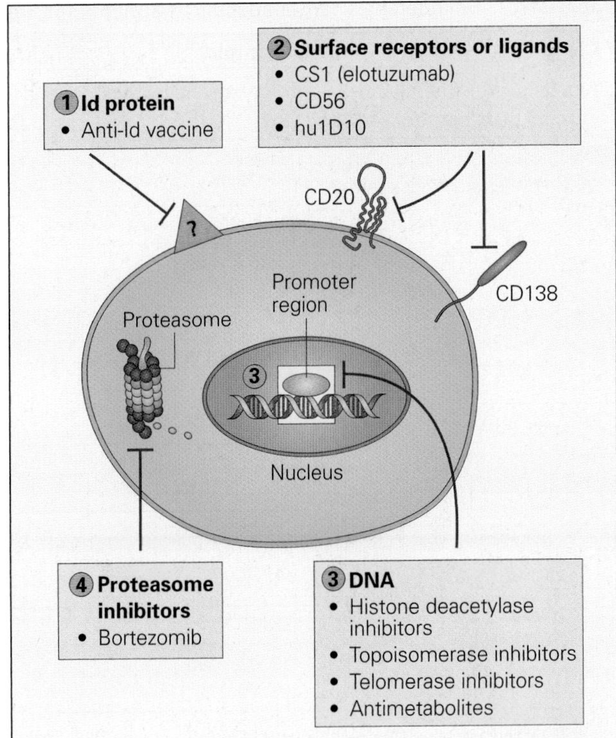

Figure 21-19. Schematic representation of the cellular and signaling receptors and pathways that are targeted by some of the new biological therapies for the lymphoproliferative diseases. These include (1) anti-idiotypic vaccine development, (2) cell surface receptors as targets for new agents that modulate signaling pathways e.g., CD20 (Rituxan), CD138 (EGF-R) inhibitors, IL-6 (CNTO328), CS1 (elotuzumab), and CD56 (anti-NK R antibody [huN901-DM1]); (3) DNA targets, e.g., histone deacetylase inhibitors (vorinostat), topoisomerase inhibitors (doxorubicin), telomerase inhibitors (GRN163L), and HLA-DR antibody (apolizumab); (4) pro-apoptotic targets that are directed to blocking angiogenesis by the use of cytokines or anticytokines, e.g., anti-VEGF (*Chapter 11*); and (5) proteasome inhibitors (bortezomib).

receptors as targets for new agents that modulate signaling pathways, e.g., CD20 (rituximab), CD138 (EGF-R) inhibitors, IL-6 (CNTO328), CS1 (elotuzumab), and CD56 (anti-NK R antibody [huN901-DM1]); (3) **DNA targets**, e.g., histone deacetylase inhibitors (vorinostat), topoisomerase inhibitors (doxorubicin), telomerase inhibitors (GRN163L), and HLA-DR antibody (apolizumab); (4) **pro-apoptotic targets** that are directed to blocking angiogenesis by the use of cytokines or anticytokines, e.g., anti-VEGF (*Chapter 11*); and (5) **proteasome inhibitors** (bortezomib).

Aggressive Lymphomas

Aggressive non-Hodgkin's lymphomas (**NHLs**) are fast-growing forms of lymphoma that include the formerly called high-grade lymphomas as well as some categories of intermediate-grade NHL. Aggressive NHLs are generally responsive to conventional cancer therapies such as chemotherapy and radiation therapy. Shown in Table 21-18 is a list of these aggressive lymphomas and in Figure 21-20 is a photomicrograph of a lymph node biopsy from a patient with diffuse large B cell lymphoma.

The standard therapy of these aggressive lymphomas includes the use of rituximab, in combination with chemotherapy, usually cyclophosphamide, doxorubicin, vincristine, and prednisone, i.e., CHOP. Several studies have confirmed the superiority of combination therapy over chemotherapy alone as measured by response rate and duration of disease-free survival. The addition of rituximab to the CHOP regimen has been shown to increase the complete-response rate and prolongs event-free and overall survival in elderly patients with diffuse large B cell lymphoma, without a clinically significant increase in toxicity. Similar to chemotherapy alone, the use of autologous stem cell transplantation (**SCT**) has been shown to produce clinical remission in patients with relapsed disease. Allogeneic SCT may also be

Table 21-17. Selected new target-specific treatments for the lymphoproliferative disorders

Class	Example	Mechanism of action	Clinical condition
Anti-idiotypic antibody for vaccine development	Idiotypic anti-idiotypic vaccine	Tumor-associated antigens (TAA)	Multiple myeloma, Hodgkin's lymphoma
Cell surface receptors that modulate signaling pathways	Rituxan	Monoclonal anti-CD20 antibody	Multiple myeloma, NHL
	CNT0328	Inhibition of EGF-R	Multiple myeloma
	Elotuzumab	Monoclonal antibody to CS1, cell surface glycoprotein highly expressed in myeloma cells	Multiple myeloma
	HuN901-DM1	AntiCD56 (NK-R)	Multiple myeloma and other CD56-expressing solid tumors
DNA targets	Apolizumab	hu1D10	Multiple myeloma, NHL
	Vorinostat	Histone deacetylase inhibitor	Multiple myeloma, cutaneous T cell lymphoma
	Doxorubicin	Topoisomerase inhibitors	Multiple myeloma, ovarian cancer, AIDS-related Kaposi's sarcoma
	GRN163L	Telomerase inhibitor	Multiple myeloma
	Apolizumab	HLA-DR antibody	Multiple myeloma, non-Hodgkin's lymphoma
Proapoptotic, antiangiogenic	Thalidomide	Multiple antiproliferative actions (proapoptotic, antiangiogenic)	Multiple myeloma and other cancers
Proteasome inhibitors	Bortezomib	Proapoptotic inhibitor of the proteasome, a multicatalytic enzyme that mediates many cellular regulatory signals by degrading regulatory proteins or their inhibitors	Multiple myeloma

considered an appropriate option for patients with more advanced disease.

Prognostic markers traditionally have included the LDH, age, stage, the presence of extranodal sites, and advanced stage (International Prognostic Index, IPI). The most effective therapy for those with higher IPI score has yet to be determined, and the role of transplantation in this setting remains controversial. More recent advances in molecular profiling have shown that this group represents three different subtypes with different responses and survival rates.

Evaluating Response to Therapy

Standardized guidelines for response assessment have been developed to ensure comparability among clinical trials in NHL (Table 21-19). These have not only facilitated comparisons between different trials, but have also have assisted in the evaluation of new agents. Revised guidelines will soon include the use of newer technologies such as PET scans in their criteria.

EBV-Associated Lymphomas

The EBV virus, originally described in 1964, was the first human virus to be implicated in malignant transformation in humans. During primary infection in the oropharynx, EBV establishes lifelong latency in B cells that are preferentially infected through the CD21 receptor and subsequently programmed to persist in the B memory cell compartment. The virus persists as an episome in infected B cells, establishing a latent infection where only a limited array of subdominant EBV antigens is expressed (*Chapter 13*). Since its original description, EBV has been associated with a heterogeneous group of malignant diseases. One of the earliest recognitions of the oncogenic potential of EBV was unfortunately observed in David Vetter (*Chapter 7*), the "bubble boy" with SCID who developed a B cell lymphoma after receiving a bone marrow transplant from his sister containing latently EBV-infected B cells that progressed to the emergence of a B cell lymphoma.

Table 21-18. A list of aggressive non-Hodgkin's lymphomas (NHLs)

B cell types
AIDS-associated lymphoma
• Large noncleaved cell lymphomas
• Large cell immunoblastic, plasmacytoid
• Small noncleaved cell
lymphoma/lymphoma (HTLV-1+)
Primary mediastinal large B cell
• Diffuse large cell lymphoma
• Diffuse mixed cell
Diffuse large cell
Burkitt's lymphoma/diffuse small noncleaved cell lymphoma
Central nervous system (CNS) lymphoma
Large cell immunoblastic
Lymphoblastic lymphoma
Mantle-cell lymphoma (sometimes behaves indolently)
Posttransplantation lymphoproliferative disorder
T cell types—also see T cell subtypes
Adult T cell leukemia/lymphoma
Angioimmunoblastic
Anaplastic large cell (T cell/null cell)
Lymphoblastic lymphoma/leukemia
Precursor T cell
Peripheral T cell

All EBV-positive malignancies are associated with the virus's latent cycle, and three distinct types of EBV latency have been characterized (Figure 21-21). The number of latently infected B cells within an individual remains stable over years unless the individual receives immunosuppressive therapy. Healthy individuals mount a vigorous humoral and cellular immune response to primary EBV infection. Although antibodies to the viral membrane proteins neutralize virus infectivity, the cellular immune response, consisting of CD4+ and CD8+ T cells, is essential for controlling both primary infection and latent EBV-infected cells. Three types of EBV latency have been described as shown in Figure 21-21. Latency type III is expressed in lymphoblastoid cell lines (LCL) and is characterized by expression of the entire array of nine EBV latency proteins, i.e., EBNAs 1, 2, 3A, 3B, 3C, LP, BARF0, and the two viral membrane proteins LMP1 and LMP2. These cells would normally be highly susceptible to killing by EBV-specific T cells, and this pattern of EBV gene expression is only seen in the EBV-associated lymphoproliferative diseases (EBV-LPD) that occur in individuals with congenital immunodeficiency (*Chapter 16*) or acquired immunodeficiency such as the human immunodeficiency virus (HIV) infection or who are receiving intensive immunosuppression after solid organ or hematopoietic stem cell transplantation (HSCT). In latency type II EBV infection, a more restricted array of viral proteins is expressed, i.e., EBNA-1, BARF0, LMP1, and LMP2, and is observed in EBV-positive Hodgkin's disease, some types of T and NK cell lymphomas, and some cases of B cell lymphoma. In latency type I, found in EBV-positive Burkitt lymphoma, only EBNA-1 and BARF0 are expressed.

These EBV-associated lymphomas represent a spectrum of conditions starting from polyclonal hyperplasia to aggressive lymphoma (Table 21-12). In addition to the emergence of EBV-associated lymphoma seen in the wide array of congenital and

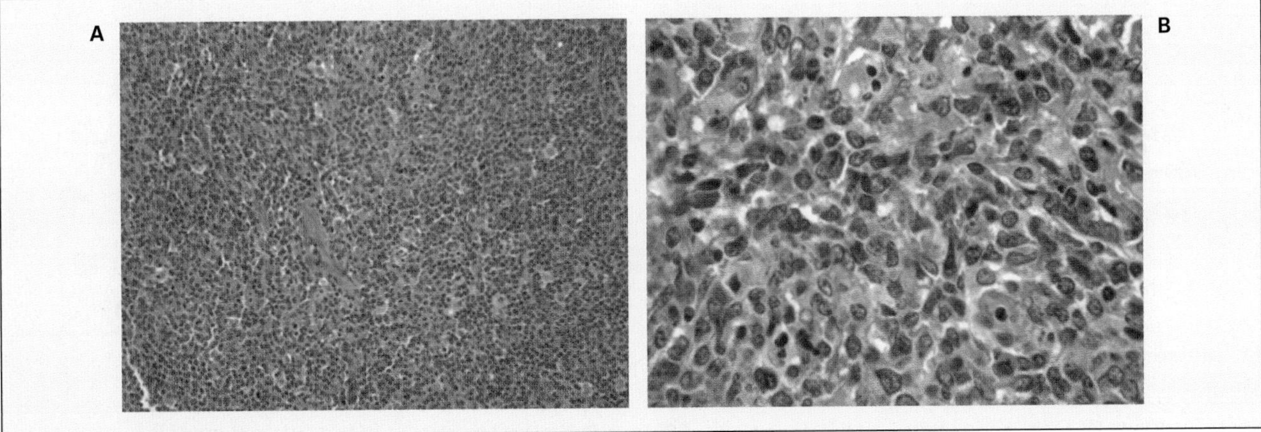

Figure 21-20. Photomicrograph of a lymph node biopsy from a patient with diffuse large B cell lymphoma. Panel A: A low power (x 10) magnification showing a diffuse pattern of confluent lymphocytes with loss of normal lymphosis organization. Panel B: A higher (x 40) magnification. (Courtesy Victor Nava MD, Georgetown University Medical Center.)

Table 21-19. Drugs being studied in non-Hodgkin's lymphoma (Cheson CA Journal, 2005)

Drug	Mechanism of action	Phase of clinical testing in lymphoma
Bortezomib	Proteasome and NF-κB inhibition	Phase II
Bendamustine	Alkylating/antimetabolite	Phase II
Oblimersen sodium	Bcl-2 antisense	Phase II
SAHA and depsipeptide	Histone deacetylase inhibition	Phase II
CCI-779	Inhibits mTOR	Phase II/III

acquired forms of immunosuppression, EBV infection has also been implicated and holds a special place in the pathogenesis of HIV-related lymphoma because of a decrease of EBV-targeting lymphocytes and an increase in the EBV viral load in the patient infected with HIV (*Chapter 13*). EBV expression is seen in all cases of primary HIV-related central nervous system lymphomas as well as in 30–60 percent of HIV-related Burkitt's and diffuse large B cell lymphomas.

EBV-related lymphomas can also be seen in immunocompetent patients and include the high-grade Burkitt's lymphoma, where 95 percent of endemic cases from Africa express the virus. These cases are associated with type I latency. EBV-positive B cell lymphomas occurring in the immunocompetent host include some cases of diffuse large B cell lymphoma and CD30+ Ki-1+ anaplastic large cell lymphoma of B cell type. Between 10 and 35 percent of these tumors are EBV positive expressing a type II latency pattern with a higher frequency seen in oral cavity lymphomas.

Classical Hodgkin's Lymphoma (Disease)

Classical Hodgkin's lymphoma (**cHL**) is a B cell neoplasm characterized by a minority of neoplastic cells, the Reed-Sternberg (**RS**) cells, which are located within an extensive infiltrate of reactive cells, such as T cells, B cells, plasma cells, stromal cells, eosinophils, and macrophages. The RS cells shape their microenvironment by attracting specific favorable T cell subsets, e.g., regulatory (Treg) and T helper 2 (Th2) cells and producing factors such as CC-chemokine ligand 17 (CCL17 or TARC), TGF-β, and IL-10. Recently, the presence of invariant NKT cells has been detected in lymph node suspensions from patients with cHL. The RS cells, thus, secrete various cytokines that together with those secreted by this wide array of immune cells collectively shape the extensive and pleomorphic inflammatory infiltrate characteristic of classic Hodgkin's lymphoma.

The diagnosis of Hodgkin's lymphoma is based on the recognition of RS cells (Box 21-8) and/or Hodgkin's cells in an appropriate cellular background in tissue sections from a lymph node or extralymphatic organ, such as the bone marrow, lung, or bone. Core needle or excision biopsy is required to establish the diagnosis unequivocally and to determine the histologic subtype. RS cells (Figure 21-22) represent postgerminal center B cells with unsuccessful immunoglobulin gene rearrangement that survive by a

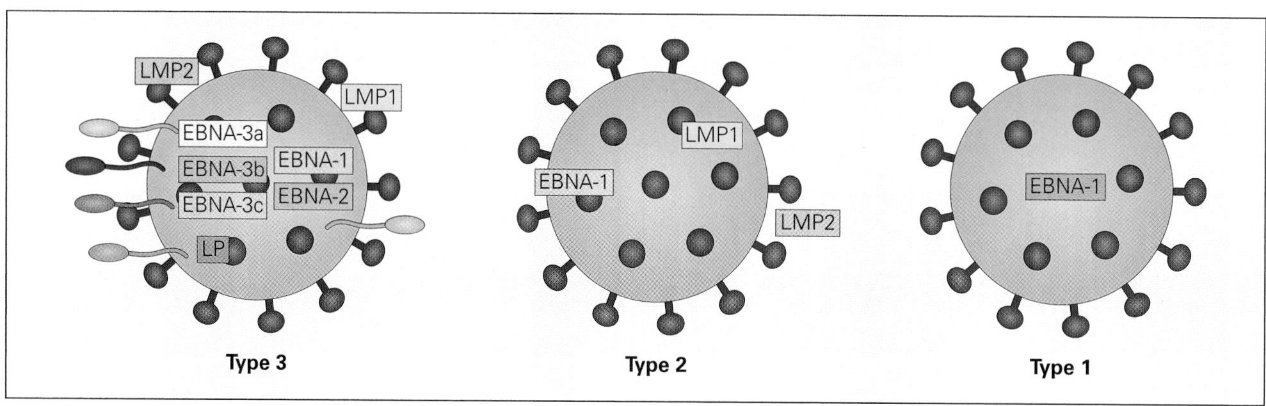

Figure 21-21. Schematic representation of the three types of Epstein-Barr virus latency. The various types of EBV latency proteins are seen in each of the three patterns of EBV latent infections. Abbreviations: EBV = Epstein-Barr virus; LP = leader protein; LMP = latent membrane protein; EBNA = EBV nuclear antigen. (Adapted with permission from Heslop HE. Biology and treatment of Epstein-Barr virus-associated non-Hodgkin lymphomas. Hematology Am Soc Hematol Educ Program. 2005;260–6.)

Box 21-8

Reed-Sternberg (RS) cells are large and are either multinucleated or have a bilobed nucleus (thus resembling an "owl's eye" appearance) with prominent eosinophilic inclusion-like nucleoli (Figure 21-22).

Reed-Sternberg cells are CD30 and CD15 positive, usually negative for CD20 and CD45. The presence of these cells is necessary, but not sufficient, for the diagnosis of classical Hodgkin's lymphoma. They can also be found in reactive lymphadenopathy (such as infectious mononucleosis, carbamazepine-associated lymphadenopathy) and rarely non-Hodgkin lymphomas.

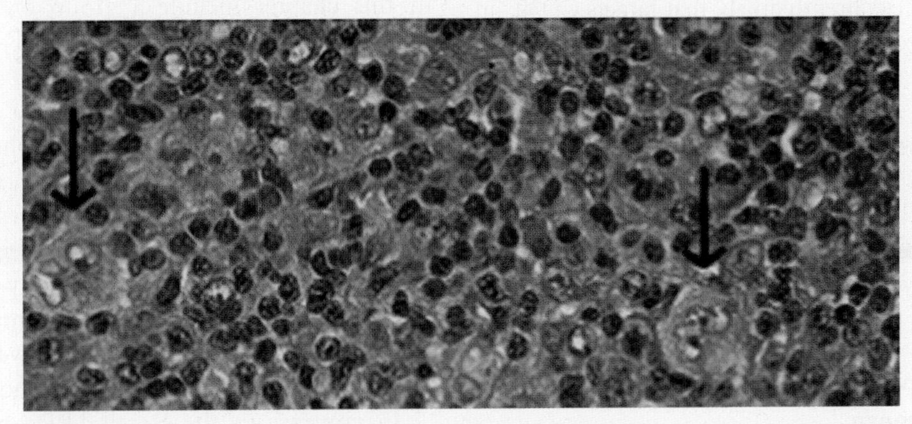

Figure 21-22. Reed-Sternberg cells with typical "owl's eye" appearance.

variety of mechanisms, including type II latent infection by the EBV virus. Proteins expressed by the EBV virus such as EBNA1, LMP1, and LMP2 play an important role in upregulating key genes in the RS cell.

Staging

The staging for Hodgkin's lymphomas and non-Hodgkin's lymphoma is similar and is based on a series of tests and procedures to determine what areas of the body are affected. These procedures include documentation of the histology, physical examination, blood tests, chest X-ray radiographs, computed tomography (**CT**) scans or magnetic resonance imaging (**MRI**) scans of the chest, abdomen, and pelvis, and a bone marrow biopsy. Positron emission tomography (**PET**) scan is now used instead of the gallium scan for staging. In the past, a lymphangiogram or surgical laparotomy (which involves opening the abdominal cavity and visually inspecting for tumors) were performed. Lymphangiograms or laparotomies are very rarely performed, having been supplanted by improvements in imaging with the CT scan and PET scan.

On the basis of this staging, the patient will be classified according to the previously described Ann Arbor staging classification scheme and include the following stages:

- **Stage I** is involvement of a single lymph node region (**I**) (mostly the cervical region) or single extralymphatic site (**Ie**);
- **Stage II** is involvement of two or more lymph node regions on the same side of the diaphragm (**II**) or of one lymph node region and a contiguous extralymphatic site (**IIe**);
- **Stage III** is involvement of lymph node regions on both sides of the diaphragm, which may include the spleen (**IIIs**) and/or limited contiguous extralymphatic organ or site (**IIIe, IIIes**);
- **Stage IV** is disseminated involvement of one or more extralymphatic organs.

The absence of systemic symptoms is signified by adding "A" to the stage; the presence of systemic symptoms is signified by adding "B" to the stage. For localized extranodal extension from mass of nodes that does not advance the stage, subscript "E" is added.

Therapy

Early Stage Disease

Until recently, therapy for limited stage Hodgkin's disease consisted of brief courses of chemotherapy with

Adriamycin (doxorubicin), Bleomycin, Vinblastine, and Dacarbazine (**ABVD**), followed by irradiation of the involved field. Newer clinical trials are evaluating different combinations of chemotherapeutic agents, e.g., gemcitabine, a deoxycytidine analogue, to determine their efficacy in the treatment of refractory or relapsed Hodgkin's lymphoma. Several monoclonal antibody preparations are being evaluated including an antibody-drug conjugate, i.e., brentuximab, that targets CD30, an antigen expressed on the surface of RS cells in Hodgkin's lymphoma and anaplastic large-cell lymphoma.

Advanced Disease

Although 80–85 percent of patients with advanced HD treated with ABVD experienced complete remission, the overall five-year survival was 73 percent. More aggressive combination chemotherapy regimens are being evaluated.

Lymphocyte-Predominant Hodgkin's Disease

Lymphocyte-predominant Hodgkin's disease (**LPHD**) is a rare subtype of Hodgkin's lymphoma, comprising 3–5 percent of all patients with Hodgkin's disease. The pathognomonic feature is the lymphocytic and histiocytic cell, rather than RS cell of cHL. Unlike the RS cells, the lymphocytic and histiocytic cells express both CD20 and CD45 and are negative for CD15 and CD30. EBV has been detected in association with cHL but not in LPHD, indicating that the triggering molecular events between these subtypes may differ. In one long-term study, rituximab in combination with chemotherapy was shown to result in durable remission. Although autologous transplants have been performed in limited numbers of patients with LPHD, the results have been equivocal and some patients experienced relapse after transplant, requiring subsequent chemotherapy.

Summary

The lymphoproliferative disorders (**LPDs**) described in this chapter include a group of malignant neoplasms arising from the abnormal proliferation of lymphoid cells at different stages of maturation and include, among others, the plasma cell neoplasms, Hodgkin's and non-Hodgkin's lymphomas, and lymphocytic leukemias. These disorders represent a set of conditions characterized by the abnormal proliferation of a clone of lymphocytes resulting in a monoclonal lymphocytosis. The LPDs commonly involve the two major cell types of the adaptive immune system, i.e., the B cells and T cells, which are derived from pluripotent hematopoietic stem cells in the bone marrow.

In contrast to the B cell LPDs characterized by abnormal synthesis of a monoclonal immunoglobulin product, e.g., multiple myeloma, the lymphomas and lymphocytic leukemias, on the other hand, have been considered as examples of LPDs in which clonal production of immunoglobulin is less readily apparent or nonexistent and in which distinctive features are often found only in the proliferative cells themselves. As a result of recent advances in molecular biology and genetics, these disorders have been more precisely classified and better understood. These advances have also allowed more detailed sub-classification of these diseases into more discernible clinical entities that have led to improved diagnosis and therapy of these disorders.

Case Studies: Clinical Relevance

Let us now return to the case studies of presented earlier and review some of the major points of the clinical presentation and how they relate to the immune system.

Case Study 1. Monoclonal Gammopathy of Undetermined Significance (MGUS)

- In the case presented, the patient was found to be mildly anemic with a protein monoclonal spike on serum protein electrophoresis, a borderline elevated IgG serum concentration < 3 g/dL, < 10 percent plasma cells on bone marrow biopsy, and no lytic lesions on skeletal survey. These findings are consistent with monoclonal gammopathy of undetermined significance (MGUS).
- Monoclonal gammopathy of undetermined significance, formerly known as **benign monoclonal**

Case Studies: Clinical Relevance (continued)

gammopathy and smoldering multiple myeloma (SMM), are characterized by an expansion of monoclonal plasma cells and both can progress to symptomatic multiple myeloma (MM) at the rate of 1–2 percent a year.

- MGUS is the most frequent plasma cell disorder and its incidence increases markedly with age, reaching approximately 3 percent in subjects over 70 years old.
- MGUS is defined by a serum M-protein concentration of less than 30 g/L and fewer than 10 percent of plasma cells in the bone marrow, while patients with SMM meet the diagnostic criteria for MM but are asymptomatic.
- SMM resembles MGUS in that end-organ damage is absent, but clinically it is far more likely to progress to active MM or amyloidosis.
- Patients may be diagnosed with MGUS if they fulfill the following three criteria:
  - A monoclonal paraprotein band < 30 g/L (< 3 g/dL);
  - Plasma cells < 10 percent on bone marrow examination; and
  - No evidence of bone lesions, anemia, hypercalcemia, or renal insufficiency related to the paraprotein.
- Management of MGUS includes the following:
  - A protein electrophoresis should be repeated annually
  - A rise in the level of monoclonal protein, should prompt referral to a hematologist.
  - The hematologist will perform a skeletal survey (X-rays of the proximal skeleton), check the blood for hypercalcemia and deterioration in renal function, evaluate the urine for Bence-Jones protein, and complete a bone marrow biopsy.
- The patient was referred to a hematologist who recommended follow-up at yearly intervals.

Case Study 2. Multiple Myeloma

- In this case, the patient presented with back pain and was found to be anemic; upon further evaluation, a protein monoclonal spike was found with elevated serum IgG concentrations of 4.5 g/dL; in contrast to the patient presented in Case 1, a bone marrow biopsy performed in this patient showed 60 percent plasma cells and several lytic lesions were detected on skeletal survey, thus confirming the diagnosis of multiple myeloma.
- Multiple myeloma, also known as MM, myeloma, or plasma cell myeloma, is a malignant proliferation of plasma cells, the terminally differited cells of the B cell lineage; B cells are a crucial part of the adaptive immune system responsible for the production of antibodies in humans and other vertebrates (*Chapter 6*).
- B cells are produced in the bone marrow from precursor cells and once differentiated are transported throughout the lymphatic system and populate the lymph nodes, spleen, and other lymphoid structures.
- Due to the ubiquitous nature of the system affected, multiple myeloma manifests itself with systemic symptoms that are often difficult to diagnose.
- The diagnostic criteria for multiple myeloma include the following:
  - Clonal plasma cells > 10 percent on bone marrow biopsy or (in any quantity) in a biopsy from other tissues (e.g., plasmacytoma)
  - A monoclonal protein (paraprotein) in either serum or urine (except in cases of true nonsecretory myeloma)
  - Evidence of end-organ damage felt related to the plasma cell disorder (related organ or tissue impairment, ROTI, commonly referred to by the acronym CRAB):
    - Hypercalcemia (corrected calcium > 2.75 mmol/L)
    - Renal insufficiency attributable to myeloma
    - Anemia (hemoglobin < 10 g/dL)
    - Bone lesions (lytic lesions or osteoporosis with compression fractures)
- Interphase fluorescence in situ hybridization (FISH) may provide an additional approach to investigate chromosomal aberrations in tumor cells; using this technique, deletions of chromosome 13 (del[13]) have been used as predictive markers of patients with MM as high risk.
- The condition is generally thought to be incurable, but remissions may be induced with steroids, chemotherapy, thalidomide, and stem cell transplants.
- The patient received four weeks of radiation therapy to the spine and was initiated on dexamethasone and thalidomide treatment. His siblings were tested for HLA compatibility for the possibility of a future bone marrow transplant.

Case Study 3: Hodgkin's Disease: Nodular Sclerosing Type

- The patient presented with cough, hemoptysis, intermittent fevers, and weight loss. The enlarged mediastinal and supraclavicular lymph nodes with an anemia, leukocytosis, thrombocytosis, and elevated ESR are commonly seen features of Hodgkin's disease. A biopsy of the bronchial nodule confirmed the

Case Studies: Clinical Relevance (continued)

diagnosis of Hodgkin's disease, nodular sclerosing type.

- Hodgkin's disease, or Hodgkin's lymphoma, originates from lymphocyte proliferation that spreads from one lymph node to another and can affect the lymph nodes, spleen, bone marrow, and other internal organs.
- The condition is characterized by the presence of a specific type of B cell-derived histiocyte known as a Reed-Sternberg (RS) cell. These cells have bilobed nuclei and prominent microscopic eosinophilic inclusion-like nucleoli, appearing as "owl's eyes."
- The age-related disease occurrence is bimodal, with two age peaks: the first in young adulthood (age 15–35 years) and the second in adults over 55 years.
- Risk factors may include male sex, a positive family history for Hodgkin's disease, history of Epstein-Barr virus infection, or an immunocompromised state, such as that seen in HIV infection.
- Symptoms most often include a painless swelling in the neck, axilla, or groin accompanied by night sweats, fevers, weight loss, fatigue, cough, dyspnea, and/or pruritus.
- Hodgkin's disease can categorized into two primary classifications: classic Hodgkin's disease and lymphocyte-predominant Hodgkin's disease based on RS cell morphology and the composition of the reactive cell infiltrate seen in the lymph node biopsy specimen.
- The definitive diagnosis of HD is made by lymph node biopsy. The bilobed, multinucleated RS cells are the characteristic histopathologic finding.
- Staging of HD, as described previously, is based on documentation of tumor histology, a physical examination, blood tests, chest X-ray radiographs, computed tomography (CT) scans or magnetic resonance imaging (MRI) scans of the chest, abdomen, and pelvis, and a bone marrow biopsy. Positron emission tomography (PET) scans may also be used in the staging process. On the basis of these findings, the patient will be classified according to a staging classification. The absence of systemic symptoms is signified by adding "A" to the stage; the presence of systemic symptoms is signified by adding "B" to the stage.
- Patients with early stage disease (IA or IIA) are effectively treated with radiation therapy or chemotherapy. The choice of treatment depends on the age, sex, bulk, and the histological subtype of the disease. Patients with later disease (III, IVA, or IVB) are treated with combination chemotherapy alone. Patients of any stage with a large mass in the chest are usually treated with combined chemotherapy and radiation therapy. The survival rate is generally over 90 percent when the disease is detected early. Even in the later stages, HD has a very high cure rate. Most patients are successfully treated and enter remission.
- The patient presented was started on chemotherapy, with adriamycin, bleomycin, vincristine, and dacarbazine (ABVD), and showed excellent clinical and radiological response. She was declared cured after six cycles of chemotherapy.

Key Points

- The lymphoproliferative disorders comprise a wide assortment of malignant neoplasms arising from the abnormal proliferation of lymphoid cells at different stages of maturation and include, among others, the plasma cell neoplasms, Hodgkin's and non-Hodgkin's lymphomas, and lymphocytic leukemias.
- Advances in our understanding of T and B cell lineages as well as new developments in molecular biology and genetics have permitted better methods of classification of these disorders by molecular profiling and have led to better diagnosis and treatment.
- The disorders of B cells that involve excessive clonal proliferation and production of abnormal quantities of immunoglobulin include monoclonal gammopathy of undetermined significance (MGUS), smoldering multiple myeloma (SMM), and multiple myeloma (MM).
- The lymphomas and lymphocytic leukemias are examples of lymphoproliferative diseases in which clonal production of immunoglobulin is less readily apparent and nonexistent and although they include disorders of abnormal proliferation of either B cell or T cell origin, the B cell disorders predominate.
- There are a variety of classification systems for categorizing and staging the various lymphomas that utilize immunologic principles and techniques.

Study Questions/Critical Thinking

1. Each of the following are examples of lymphoproliferative disorders EXCEPT:

a. Multiple myeloma
b. Smoldering multiple myeloma
c. Chronic lymphatic leukemia
d. Hodgkin's lymphoma
e. Systemic lupus erythematosus

2. Each of the following are examples of techniques used to diagnose the monoclonal gammopathies EXCEPT:

a. Immunoelectrophoresis
b. Immunofixation
c. Determination of urinary protein
d. FISH assays
e. Determination of relative amounts of kappa and lambda chains

3. Which of the following triggers are thought to be important in the pathogenesis of the lymphoproliferative disorders:

a. Dysfunctional dendritic cells
b. Myeloid-derived suppressor cell
c. EBV infection
d. Excessive production of TNF
e. The indoleamine 2,3-dioxygenase (IDO) pathway

4. Each of the following examples of drug targets for treatment of the lymphoproliferative disorders EXCEPT:

a. Anti-CD20 monoclonal antibody
b. Thalidomide
c. Anti-idiotypic antibody
d. NADPH oxidase enzymes
e. Proteasome inhibitors

5. Each of the following are classic components of Hodgkin's lymphoma EXCEPT:

a. Reed-Sternberg (RS) cells
b. Pleomorphic cellular involvement
c. Eosinophilia
d. Bence-Jones protein
e. Fibrosis

Suggested Reading

Anderson KC. Lenalidomide and thalidomide: mechanisms of action—similarities and differences. Semin Hematol. 2005; 42: S3–8.

Bartlett JB, Dredge K, Dalgleish AG. The evolution of thalidomide and its IMiD derivatives as anticancer agents. Nat Rev Cancer. 2004; 4: 314–22.

Bergsagel DE, Wong O, Bergsagel PL, et al. Benzene and multiple myeloma: appraisal of the scientific evidence. Blood. 1999; 94: 1174–82.

Borowitz M, Bray RA, Gascone R, et al. Immunophenotypic analysis of hematologic neoplasia by flow cytometry. Cytometry. 1997; 30: 236–44.

Cartron G, Dacheux L, Salles G. Therapeutic activity of humanized anti-CD20 monoclonal antibody and polymorphism in IgG Fc receptor FcγRIIIa gene. Blood. 2002; 99: 754–8.

Cesana C, Klersy C, Barbarano L, et al. Prognostic factors for malignant transformation in monoclonal gammopathy of undetermined significance and smoldering multiple myeloma. J Clin Oncol. 2002; 20: 1625–34.

Chanan-Khan AA, Borrello I, Lee KP, et al. Development of target-specific treatments in multiple myeloma. Br J Haematol. 2010; 151: 3–15.

Cheson BD, Horning SJ, Coiffier B, et al. Report of an international workshop to standardize response criteria for non-Hodgkin's lymphomas: NCI Sponsored International Working Group. J Clin Oncol. 1999; 17: 1244.

Cheson BD, Leonard JP. Monoclonal antibody therapy for B-cell non-Hodgkin's lymphoma. N Engl J Med. 2008; 359: 613–26.

Cheson BD What is new in lymphoma? CA Cancer J Clin. 2004; 54: 260–72.

Christian F, Anthony DF, Vadrevu S, et al. p62 (SQSTM1) and cyclic AMP phosphodiesterase-4A4 (PDE4A4) locate to a novel, reversible protein aggregate with links to autophagy and proteasome degradation pathways. Cell Signal. 2010; 22: 1576–96.

Coiffier B, Lepage E, Briere J, et al. CHOP chemotherapy plus rituximab compared with CHOP alone in elderly patients with diffuse large-B-cell lymphoma. N Engl J Med. 2002; 346: 235–42.

Cortelazzo S, Ponzoni M, Ferreri AJ, et al. Lymphoblastic lymphoma. Crit Rev Oncol Hematol. ePub Jan 25 2011.

Davies FE, Dring AM, Li C, et al. Insights into the multistep transformation of MGUS to myeloma using microarray expression analysis. Blood. 2003; 102: 4504–11.

Dimopoulos MA, Moulopoulos LA, Maniatis A, et al. Solitary plasmacytoma of bone and asymptomatic multiple myeloma. Blood. 2000; 96: 2037–44.

Dispenzieri A. POEMS syndrome. Blood Rev. 2007; 21: 285–99.

Durie BG, Salmon SE. A clinical staging system for multiple myeloma: correlation of measured myeloma cell mass with presenting clinical features, response to treatment and survival. Cancer. 1975; 36: 842–54.

Eichholz A, Merchant S, Gaya AM. Anti-angiogenesis therapies: their potential in cancer management. Onco Targets Ther. 2010; 3: 69–82.

Fonseca R, Bailey RJ, Ahmann GJ, et al. Genomic abnormalities in monoclonal gammopathy of undetermined significance. Blood. 2002; 100: 1417–24.

Fonseca R, Barlogie B, Bataille R, et al. Genetics and cytogenetics of multiple myeloma: a workshop report. Cancer Res. 2004; 64: 1546–58.

Gascoyne RD, Rosenwald A, Poppema S, et al. Prognostic biomarkers in malignant lymphomas. Leuk Lymphoma. 2010; 51 Suppl 1: 11–9.

Gascoyne RD. Hematopathology approaches to diagnosis and prognosis of indolent B-cell lymphomas. Hematology Am Soc Hematol Educ Program. 2005; 299–306.

Greenlee RT, Hill-Harmon MB, Murray T, et al. Cancer statistics, 2001. CA Cancer J Clin. 2001; 51: 15–36.

Greipp PR, San Miguel J, Durie BG, et al. International staging system for multiple myeloma. J Clin Oncol. 2005; 23: 3412–20.

Heslop HE. Biology and treatment of Epstein-Barr virus-associated non-Hodgkin lymphomas. Hematology Am Soc Hematol Educ Program. 2005; 260–6.

Hideshima T, Bergsagel PL, Kuehl WM, et al. Advances in biology of multiple myeloma: clinical applications. Blood. 2004; 104: 607–18.

International Myeloma Working Group. Criteria for the classification of monoclonal gammopathies, multiple myeloma and related disorders: a report of the International Myeloma Working Group. Br J Haematol. 2003; 121: 749–75.

Jackson C, Sirohi B, Cunningham D, et al. Lymphocyte-predominant Hodgkin lymphoma: clinical features and treatment outcomes from a 30-year experience. Ann Oncol. 2010; 21: 2061–8.

Kuehl WM, Bergsagel PL. Multiple myeloma: evolving genetic events and host interactions. Nature Rev Cancer. 2002; 2: 175–87.

Kumar S, Rajkumar SV, Kyle RA, et al. Prognostic value of circulating plasma cells in monoclonal gammopathy of undetermined significance. J Clin Oncol. 2005; 23: 5668–74.

Kumar S, Rajkumar SV. Thalidomide and dexamethasone: therapy for multiple myeloma. Expert Rev Anticancer Ther. 2005; 5: 759–66.

Kyle RA, Greipp PR. Smoldering multiple myeloma. N Engl J Med. 1980; 302: 1347–9.

Kyle RA, Rajkumar SV. Monoclonal gammopathy of undetermined significance and smoldering multiple myeloma. Curr Hematol Malig Rep. 2010; 5: 62–9.

Kyle RA, Rajkumar SV. Multiple myeloma. N Engl J Med. 2004; 351: 1860–73.

Kyle RA, Therneau TM, Rajkumar SV, et al. Prevalence of monoclonal gammopathy of undetermined significance. N Engl J Med. 2006; 354: 1362–9.

Kyle RA, Therneau TM, Rajkumar SV, et al. A long-term study of prognosis in monoclonal gammopathy of undetermined significance. N Engl J Med. 2002; 346: 564–9.

Kyle RA, Vincent Rajkumar S. Treatment of multiple myeloma: an emphasis on new developments. Ann Med. 2006; 38: 111–5.

Kyle RA. Monoclonal gammopathy of undetermined significance: natural history in 241 cases. Am J Med. 1978; 64: 814–26.

Kyle RA. 'Benign' monoclonal gammopathy after 20 to 30 years of follow-up. Mayo Clini Proc. 1993; 68: 26–36.

Landgren O, Rajkumar SV. Development of early treatment strategies for high-risk myeloma precursor disease in the future. Semin Hematol. 2011; 48: 66–72.

Landgren O, Gridley G, Turesson I, et al. Risk of monoclonal gammopathy of undetermined significance and subsequent multiple myeloma among African American and white veterans in the United States. Blood. 2006; 107: 904.

Laubach J, Richardson P, Anderson K. Multiple myeloma. Annu Rev Med. 2011; 62: 249–64.

Laubach JP, Schlossman RL, Mitsiades CS, et al. Thalidomide, lenalidomide and bortezomib in the management of newly diagnosed multiple myeloma. Expert Rev Hematol. 2011; 4: 51–60.

Pfreundschuh MG, Rueffer U, Lathan B, et al. Dexa-BEAM in patients with Hodgkin's disease refractory to multidrug chemotherapy regimens: a trial of the German Hodgkin's Disease Study Group. J Clin Oncol. 1994; 12: 580–6.

Poppema S. Immunobiology and pathophysiology of Hodgkin lymphomas. Hematology Am Soc Hematol Educ Program. 2005; 231–8.

Rajkumar SV, Blood E, Vesole D, et al. Phase III clinical trial of thalidomide plus dexamethasone compared with dexamethasone alone in newly diagnosed multiple myeloma: a clinical trial coordinated by the Eastern Cooperative Oncology Group. J Clin Oncol. 2006; 24: 431–6.

Rajkumar SV, Dispenzieri A, Kyle RA. Monoclonal gammopathy of undetermined significance, Waldenstrom macroglobulinemia, AL amyloidosis, and related plasma cell disorders: diagnosis and treatment. Mayo Clin Proc. 2006; 8: 693–703.

Rajkumar SV, Kyle RA, Therneau TM, et al. Serum free light chain ratio is an independent risk factor for progression in monoclonal gammopathy of undetermined significance. Blood. 2005; 106: 812–7.

Rajkumar SV, Kyle RA. Multiple myeloma: diagnosis and treatment. Mayo Clin Proc. 2005; 80: 1371–82.

Rajkumar SV. MGUS and smoldering multiple myeloma: update on pathogenesis, natural history, and management. Hematology Am Soc Hematol Educ Program. 2005; 340–5.

Rech J, Repp R, Rech D, Stockmeyer B, et al. A humanized HLA-DR antibody (hu1D10, apolizumab) in combination with granulocyte colony-stimulating factor (filgrastim) for the treatment of non-Hodgkin's lymphoma: a pilot study. Leuk Lymphoma. 2006; 47: 2147–54.

Richardson P, Hideshima T, Anderson K. Thalidomide: emerging role in cancer medicine. Annu Rev Med. 2002; 53: 629–57.

Richardson P. Management of the relapsed/refractory myeloma patient: strategies incorporating lenalidomide. Semin Hematol. 2005; 42 Suppl 4: S9–15.

Richardson PG, Barlogie B, Berenson J, et al. Clinical factors predictive of outcome with bortezomib in patients with relapsed, refractory multiple myeloma. Blood. 2005; 106: 2977–81.

Richardson PG, Barlogie B, Berenson J, et al. A phase 2 study of bortezomib in relapsed, refractory myeloma. N Engl J Med. 2003; 348: 2609–17.

Richardson PG, Barlogie B, Berenson J, et al. Extended follow-up of a phase II trial in relapsed, refractory multiple myeloma: final time-to-event results from the SUMMIT trial. Cancer. 2006; 106: 1316–9.

Richardson PG, Sonneveld P, Schuster MW, et al. Bortezomib or high-dose dexamethasone for relapsed multiple myeloma. N Engl J Med. 2005; 352: 2487–98.

Schmitz N, Trümper L, Ziepert M, et al. Treatment and prognosis of mature T-cell and NK-cell lymphoma: an analysis of patients with T-cell lymphoma treated in studies of the German High-Grade Non-Hodgkin Lymphoma Study Group. Blood. 2010; 116: 3418–25.

Sehn LH, Donaldson J, Chhanabhai M, et al. Introduction of combined CHOP plus rituximab therapy dramatically improved outcome of diffuse large B-cell lymphoma in British Columbia. J Clin Oncol. 2005; 23: 5027–33.

Shaffer AL, Rosenwald A, Staudt LM. Lymphoid malignancies: the dark side of B-cell differentiation. Nat Rev Immunol. 2002; 2: 920–32.

Witzig TE, Kyle RA, WM OF, Greipp PR. Detection of peripheral blood plasma cells as a predictor of disease course in patients with smoldering multiple myeloma. Br J Haematol. 1994; 87: 266–72.

Xu C, de Vries R, Visser L, et al. Expression of CD1d and presence of invariant NKT cells in classical Hodgkin lymphoma. Am J Hematol. 2010; 85: 539–41.

Chapter 22

Transplantation Immunity and Clinical Applications

Sandra Rosen-Bronson, PhD

Case Study

A 40-year-old African American female with end-stage renal failure secondary to diabetes and hypertension was in need of a kidney transplant. Upon initial evaluation by the transplant center, the patient was HLA typed and her serum was tested for the presence of HLA antibody. Her HLA type was found to be HLA A23, 33; B44, 58; DR7, 13. HLA antibody assays indicated that she had broadly reacting antibodies against both HLA class I and class II antigens and her panel reactive antibody (PRA) was 85 percent (Box 22-1). Additional studies indicated that the antibody specificities in the patient's serum included A74, B53, and DR15, which are three of the antigens expressed by the patient's husband. Although the patient's husband was willing to donate a kidney, he was found to be ABO-incompatible with the patient. Since her two children were also willing to be considered as possible kidney donors, they were both HLA typed and crossmatched with the patient. The children were found to be HLA identical with each other (HLA A23, 74; B44, 53; DR7, 15) and, as expected, one haplotype matched with the patient. Flow cytometric and CDC crossmatches were preformed using each of the children's cells and their mother's serum. The crossmatches with both children were found to be strongly positive and therefore they were excluded as potential donors. Subsequently, the patient was listed in the OPTN/UNOS registry in the hope that she would be offered an organ from a deceased donor. Her "unacceptable antigens" were listed as A74, B53, and DR15. No donor offers were received over a three-year period during which her clinical condition not only continued to deteriorate, but also her vascular access for hemodialysis was progressively being compromised.

Fortuitously, a friend from the patient's church became aware of her illness and offered to donate a kidney. The friend was found to be ABO-compatible and her HLA type was A2, 68; B44, 51; DR7, –. However, the crossmatch was found to be positive using the flow cytometric method. In view of the patient's deteriorating clinical condition, the transplant program enrolled the patient in a desensitization protocol where she received plasmapheresis four times along with a dose of IVIG after each treatment. At the completion of the desensitization regimen, the crossmatch with the donor's cells was repeated and found to be negative. After receiving a single dose of intraoperative thymoglobulin, the patient was successfully transplanted with her friend's kidney.

LEARNING OBJECTIVES

When you have completed this chapter, you should be able to:

- Define the terms autologous, syngeneic, allogeneic, and xenogeneic grafts used in transplantation
- Classify the different types of graft rejection reactions into first and second set graft rejection
- Understand the different components of the histocompatibility antigens HLA-A, HLA-B, HLA-C, HLA-DR, HLA-DQ, and HLA-DP and their relationships to MHC-I and MHC-II
- Recognize the importance of identification of parental HLA haplotypes in HLA matching and ABO blood group types to determine compatibility of potential donors with recipients of solid organ transplants
- Understand what is meant by the degree of antigen mismatch in solid organ transplantation and the importance of allele level matching in hematopoietic stem cell transplantation
- Define hyperacute, acute, and chronic graft rejection
- Explain the basis of graft-versus-host disease (GVHD) and its application in graft-versus-leukemia (GVL)
- Classify the various classes of currently available immunosuppressive agents commonly used in transplantation and their mechanisms of action
- Summarize the various tissue typing and crossmatching methods performed prior to transplantation to assess donor-recipient compatibility for human leukocyte antigen (HLA) and ABO blood group compatibility
- Recognize the clinical applications of transplantation immunity in health and disease

Box 22-1

Panel reactive antibody (PRA). The percentage PRA value is a measure of a patient's level of sensitization to donor antigens. It is the percentage of cells from a panel of blood donors against which a potential recipient's serum reacts. The higher the PRA, the more sensitized a patient is to the general donor pool, and thus the more difficult it is to find a suitable donor. A patient may become sensitized as a result of pregnancy, a blood transfusion, or a previous transplant.

Introduction

In a clinical setting, the term transplantation generally refers to the transfer or replacement of cells, tissues, or organs from one individual to another. The source of the transplant can either be a person's own body, another human, or another species. Once an esoteric science, transplantation now enjoys a wide variety of clinical applications as a major therapeutic option for a growing list of diseases, including end-stage organ failure, a variety of malignancies, immune deficiency and other genetic disorders, and autoimmune syndromes. In the human, with the exception of transplantation of one's own tissues, where the recognition of "self" components evokes no immune response, the transplantation of all other tissues, i.e., from another human or another species, triggers immune responses that are similar to those mounted against foreign substances and that can be complex and at times evoke severe complications.

Although by definition even a simple blood transfusion is a transplant, which usually evokes no reaction in a recipient with a normal immune system, in an immunosuppressed patient, it can have severe immune consequences as a result of immune reactivity of immunologically active lymphocytes in the transfused blood, which can react against the tissues of the immunoincompetent recipient, i.e., the graft-versus-host (**GVH**) reaction, which is described more fully below. In general, transplants are broadly classified as solid organ or hematopoietic stem cell transplants and within these classifications are categorized according to the relationship of the donor and the recipient.

Transplant Immunity

Definitions

A variety of terms are used to define antigens and immune responses stimulated in a transplant setting according to the relationship of the donor and the recipient (*Chapter 10*). Shown in Table 22-1 are examples of terms used to define grafts employed in transplantation together with immune responses stimulated by them. The tissues transplanted from the same individual (i.e., **autografts**) are termed autologous transplants since they contain autoantigens or "self" antigens and under normal circumstances evoke no immune responses. As the term implies, an autograft is a transplant of self-tissue or cells, e.g., skin or hematopoietic stem cells (**HSC**). Autologous skin transplants are often performed on burn patients, and autologous HSC transplantation is commonly used as a means of rescuing cancer patients subsequent to myeloablative chemotherapy (*Chapter 20*).

Another term used to define a transplant involving a donor and a recipient who are genetically identical is a **syngeneic** graft. The term **isograft** is sometimes used when referring to a syngeneic transplant between two different genetically identical individuals. In humans, only a transplant involving identical twins would be a true syngeneic isograft. In an animal model, a syngeneic transplant would involve two animals derived from the same inbred strain. The term **allogeneic** graft refers to a transplant that involves the transfer of an **allograft** containing **alloantigens**, which are genetically controlled characteristics that differentiate one member of a given species from another (*Chapter 10*). The vast majority of transplants carried out in humans are allogeneic. However, due to the serious shortage of donor organs, researchers are actively investigating ways to successfully perform **xenotranplantation**, which involves the transfer of organs or tissues, i.e., a **xenograft**, containing **xenoantigens** between members of two different species.

The Immune Responses Involved in Transplantation

The immune responses involved in transplantation are governed by the laws that are based on the genetics of the donor and recipient (*Chapter 10*). Shown in Figure 22-1 is a schematic representation of the genetic controls affecting transplantation in a mouse model system in which a variety of transplants are conducted either between members of two genetically

Table 22-1. Examples of terms used in transplantation

Type of graft	Source of graft	Name of graft	Type of antigen	Type of immune response stimulated
Autologous	Same individual	Autograft	Autoantigen	Normally none; abnormally stimulated in autoimmune disease, e.g., autoimmunization
Syngeneic	Genetically identical individual; e.g., identical twin	Isograft	Isoantigen	Isoimmunization
Allogeneic	Genetically different member of the same species	Allograft	Alloantigen	Alloimmunization
Xenogeneic	Genetically different member from another species	Xenograft	Xenoantigen	Xenoimmunization

identical (syngeneic) mouse strains, or from one member of one inbred species (allogeneic) to another or from a foreign species (**xenogeneic**) to one of the inbred mouse strains. In this model, there are the following participants: (1) a genetically inbred white mouse strain (**Strain A**) containing homozygous MHCa; (2) a genetically inbred black mouse strain (**Strain B**) containing homozygous MHCb; (3) an **F1 hybrid** offspring (**F1 Strain A/B**) resulting from the crossmating of the two parental types, the offspring of which contain genetic characteristics from both parents as a heterozygote MHCa,b; and (4) a guinea pig representing a member of a foreign species. A skin graft from a member of Strain A to another member of Strain A (or from Strain B to Strain B) will be accepted. A skin graft from a member of Strain B to a member of Strain A, or vice versa, will be rejected. A skin graft from Strain A transferred to the F1 hybrid will be accepted because the hybrid recognizes, at least in part, one half of the genetic makeup of the transplant as self antigen and will not evoke rejection. A skin graft from the F1 hybrid to either parental strain, on the other hand, will be rejected since the recipient will recognize only one half of the genetic identity of the donated tissue as self and one half as foreign. Finally, a skin graft from a guinea pig to either parental strain will be rejected as a foreign graft (xenograft).

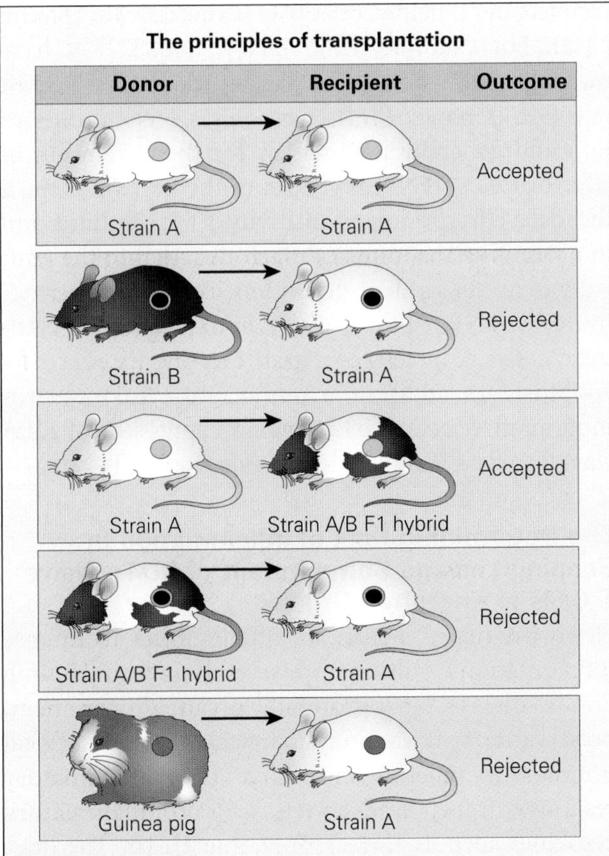

Figure 22-1. Schematic representation of the genetic controls affecting transplantation in a mouse model system.

As shown in Table 22-1, depending on the relationship of the donor and the recipient, a variety of terms are used to describe the immune response to a transplant, i.e., autoimmunization, isoimmunization, alloimmunization, and xenoimmunization, and as described previously in the human, the most important of these is alloimmunization or an alloimmune response. An alloantigen can be any molecule that is encoded by a polymorphic gene and, therefore, is expressed in different forms in genetically different individuals of the same species. The term "alloimmunity" is also used to refer to the immune response stimulated by an alloantigen. An alloimmune response can involve the two modes of antigen processing described in Chapter 10, i.e., either the direct recognition of nonself human leukocyte antigen (**HLA** nonself) (the "exogenous" pathway; ie, MHC-II) or the indirect recognition of an alloantigen-derived peptide presented by self-HLA (the "endogenous" pathway; ie, MHC-I). Sensitization to alloantigens can occur in a variety of clinical settings, including transplantation, pregnancy, and blood transfusions. Once sensitized, many individuals develop potent antibodies and cell-mediated immune responses specific for HLA antigens.

In a transplant recipient who has never been previously sensitized to histocompatibility antigens, the first step of the immune response requires the recognition of the donor's (nonself) HLA antigens by the T cell receptor on the recipient's alloreactive T lymphocytes (*Chapter 7*). This interaction triggers a cascade of specific and nonspecific immune events that ultimately lead to rejection of the transplanted organ. Transplant rejection is caused primarily by a cell-mediated immune response to HLA antigens expressed on donor antigen-presenting cells (**APCs**) transferred along with the transplanted organ. The process of graft rejection can be divided into two phases: (1) a **sensitization phase** in which antigen reactive lymphocytes in the recipient's lymph node proliferate in response to the donor's alloantigens and (2) an **effector phase** in which the recipient's sensitized effector cells mediate immune destruction of the graft. For initial sensitization to take place, CD4+ and CD8+ T cells must proliferate as a result of the recognition of nonself HLA antigens. The response to major histocompatibility antigens involves recognition of both the HLA molecule and an associated peptide ligand in the cleft of the HLA molecule (*Chapter 7*).

Activation of host CD4+ T helper cells requires interaction with an APC expressing an appropriate peptide-HLA molecule complex along with a requisite co-stimulatory signal (Figure 22-2). Recognition of donor HLA antigens on the cells of the graft induces vigorous T cell proliferation in the recipient. Both dendritic cells and vascular endothelial cells from the donor organ induce vigorous proliferation of recipient T cells in this reaction. The major proliferating cell is the CD4+ T cell, which recognizes HLA class II antigens directly or HLA peptides presented by host APCs. This amplified population of activated T helper cells plays a central role in the induction of the various effector mechanisms involved in graft rejection.

A variety of effector mechanisms participate in allograft rejection, which are shown in the various numbered pathways in Figure 22-2. The most common of these are cell-mediated reactions involving delayed-type hypersensitivity and cytotoxic T lymphocyte (**CTL**) mediated cytotoxicity (*Chapter 7*). In addition, complement-dependent antibody lysis or natural killer (**NK**) destruction by antibody-dependent cell-mediated cytotoxicity (**ADCC**) can occur (*Chapter 3*). The hallmark of cell-mediated graft rejection is an influx of T cells and macrophages into the graft. Histologically, the infiltration often resembles that seen during a delayed-type hypersensitivity response in which cytokines produced by Th1 cells promote macrophage infiltration. Recognition of donor HLA class I antigens on the graft by recipient CD8+ cells can lead to CTL-mediated killing. In some cases, graft rejection can also be mediated by CD4+ T cells that function as HLA class II restricted cytotoxic cells.

In each of the effector mechanisms, cytokines secreted by T helper cells play a central role (Figure 22-2). For example, IL-2, IFN-γ, and TNF-α have each been shown to be important mediators of graft rejection (*Chapter 9*). IL-2 promotes T cell proliferation and generally is necessary for the generation of effector CTLs. IFN-γ is central to the development of the delayed-type hypersensitivity Th1 response and in promoting the influx of macrophages into the graft with their subsequent activation into more destructive cells. TNF-α has been shown to have direct cytotoxic activity on cells of a graft exerting its effects by apoptosis. In addition, a number of cytokines promote graft rejection by inducing expression of HLA class I or class II molecules on engrafted cells.

The Determining Role of Inflammation in Shaping Lineage Commitment of CD4+ Naive T Cells in Engrafted Organs

Newly engrafted organs are often subject to intense inflammation resulting from several causes, including donor disease, inappropriate organ procurement, preservation in nonphysiological fluids, surgical trauma, or reperfusion injury. The inflammatory response, in turn, leads to release of proinflammatory cytokines such as IL-6, TNF-α, and IL-1β. The lineage commitment of naive recipient CD4+ T cells in

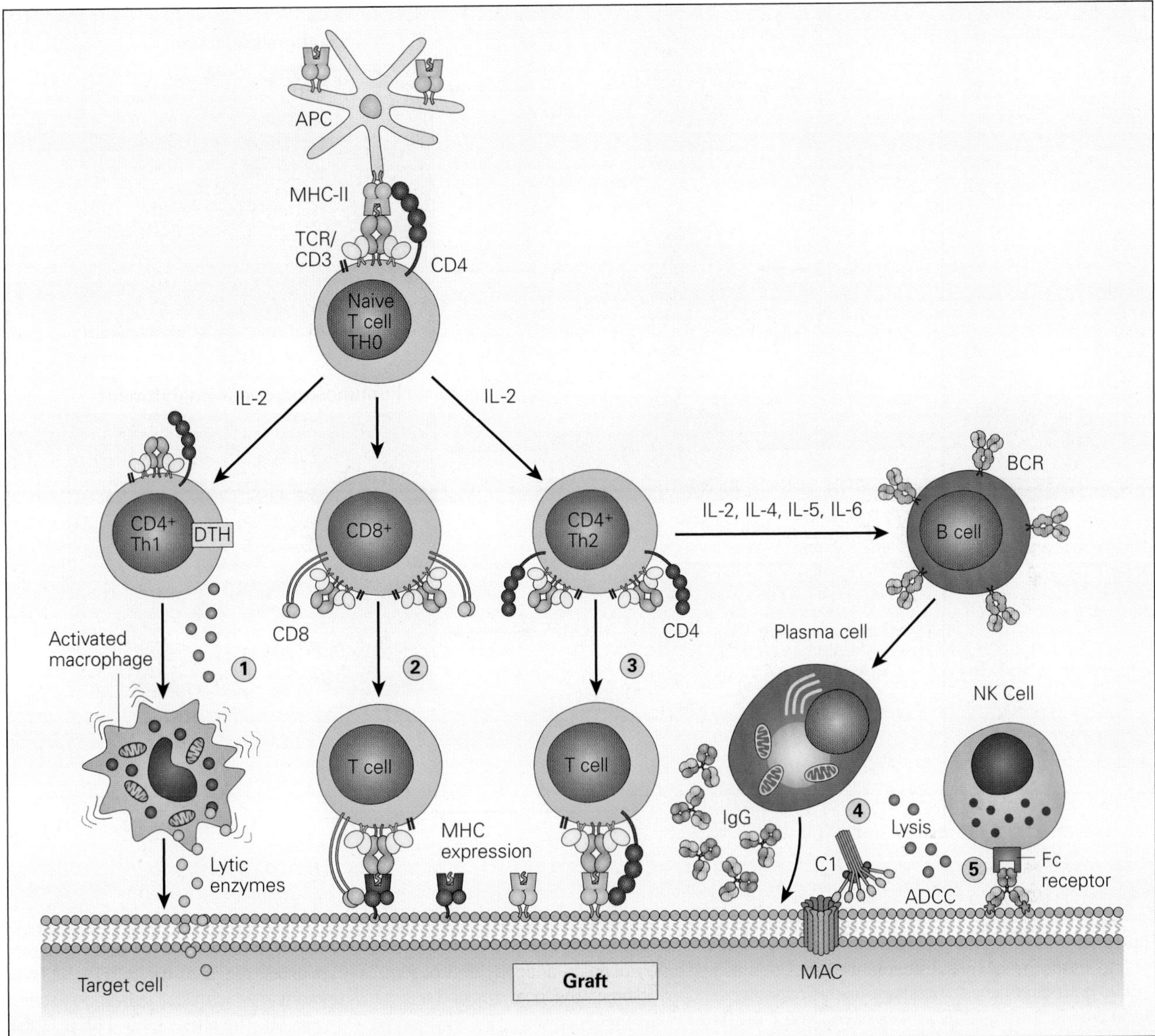

Figure 22-2. Schematic representation of the cellular events involved in antigen recognition and immune reactivity associated with graft recognition.

the graft is determined by the cytokine environment in which these cells recognize donor antigens. Thus, depending on the nature of the cytokine milieu present when antigen activation occurs, naive recipient CD4+ helper T cells can differentiate along diverse developmental cellular pathways with either cytopathic and/or immunoregulatory functions (Figure 22-3). When CD4+ T cells are activated in the presence of IL-12, usually produced by activated, mature DCs, they differentiate into IFN-γ-producing Th1 cells. In contrast, when CD4+ naive T cells are activated in the presence of IL-4, they differentiate into Th2 cells, which produce IL-4, IL-5, and IL-13. In the absence of proinflammatory cytokines, TGF-β induces differentiation of CD4+ T cells into expression of FOXP3+ Tregs. In contrast, expression of TGF-β with IL-6 or IL-21 prevents development of the transplant-protective effects of Tregs; instead, the antigen-reactive CD4+ T cells become IL-17-producing Th17 cells, which are highly cytopathic (Figure 22-3).

Relative Balance Between Rejection-Prone Effector T Cells and Rejection-Blocking, Immunosuppressive Tregs

Until recently, it was believed that recipient naive T cells activated by donor antigens became terminally differentiated Th1 or Th2 cells that had opposing effects, i.e., Th1-dependent responses were thought

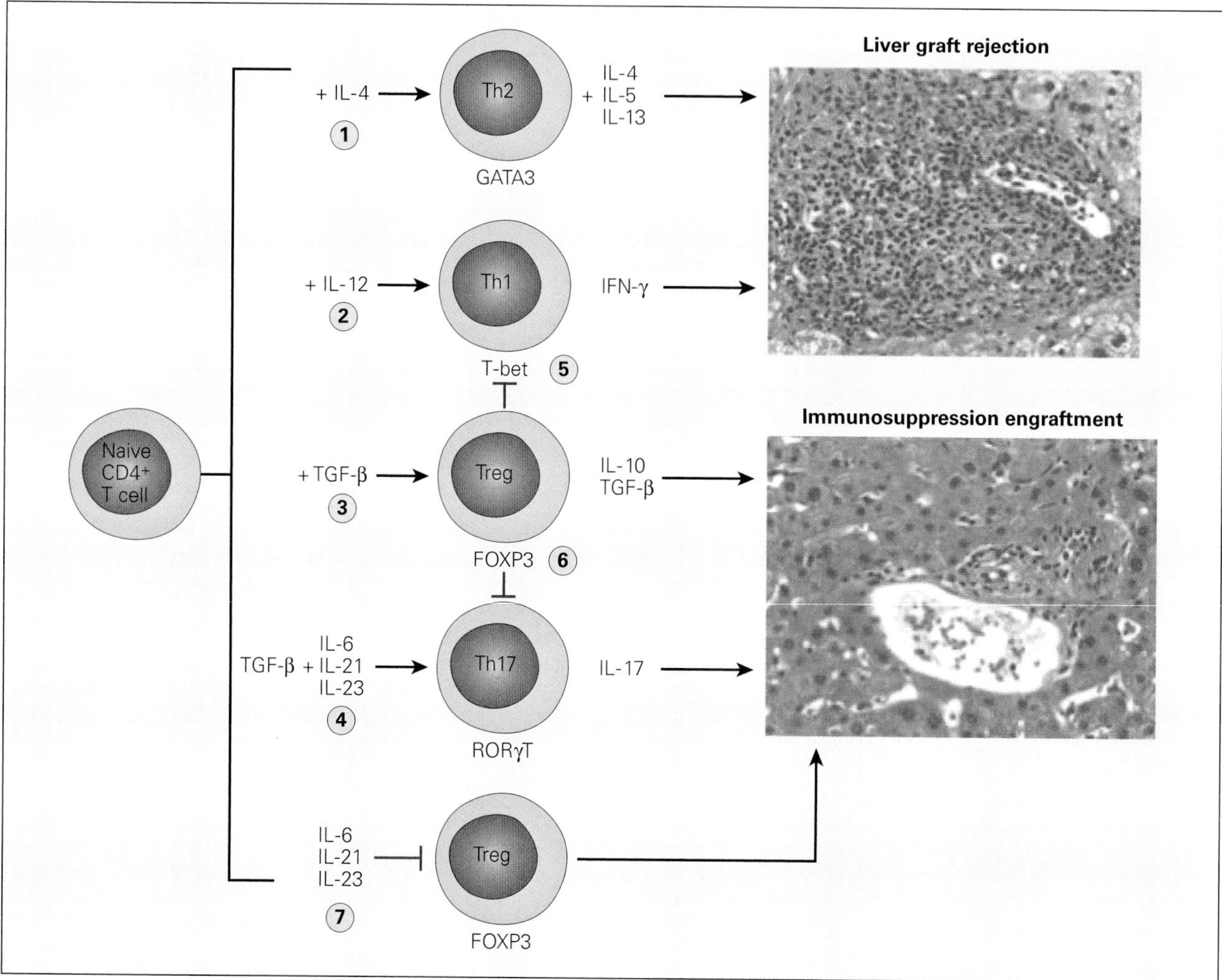

Figure 22-3. Schematic representation of the effects of cytokine environment on lineage commitment of naive CD4+ T cells in determining outcome of liver transplantation. Upon activation by cognate antigens and costimulatory signals, recipient naive CD4+ T cells acquire graft-destructive or graft-protective phenotypes, depending on the local cytokine microenvironment in which T cell activation occurs. In the presence of IL-4, CD4+ T cells become Th2 **(1)** and in the presence of IL-12 they become Th1 cells **(2)**. The presence of TGF-β, in the absence of proinflammatory cytokines, induces differentiation of recipient CD4+ T cells into tissue-protective FOXP3+ Treg cells **(3)**; in contrast, TGF-β in the presence of IL-6, IL-21, or IL-23 induces the differentiation of CD4+ naive T cells into the Th17 phenotype **(4)**. The Treg cells can inhibit the induction of tissue-destructive Th1 **(5)** or Th17 **(6)** cells. The presence of IL-6, IL-21, or IL-23 blocks the generation of Tregs **(7)** that can further enhance graft rejection. (Adapted and reproduced with permission from Sánchez-Fueyo A, Strom TB. Immunologic basis of graft rejection and tolerance following transplantation of liver or other solid organs. Gastroenterology. 2011;140:51–64.)

to generate cytopathic graft rejection and Th2-dependent responses cytoprotective effects. However, this previously held Th1/Th2 paradigm was incorrect since it was subsequently shown that both Th1 and Th2 can each mediate graft rejection (Figure 22-3). Treg cells are now accepted as the key arbiters of immunologic tolerance that determine whether a graft will undergo cytopathic graft rejection or be maintained in a tolerant cytoprotective state (*Chapter 19*). The currently accepted paradigm is that the outcome of rejection or graft acceptance is ultimately determined by the relative balance between cytopathic Th1 and Th17 CD4+ T cells versus rejection-blocking, cytoprotective regulatory T cells (Figure 22-4). This balance, in turn, depends on the qualitative levels of cytokines in the inflammatory microenvironment in which T cell activation takes place.

Although the specific role of Th17 cells in allograft rejection is currently being evaluated, events that block T cell commitment to the graft-protective Treg phenotype appear to prevent the development of transplant tolerance. The presence of Th17 cells in the allograft may, in fact, become a biomarker of its indirect detrimental effects through tissue inflammation leading to graft rejection rather than

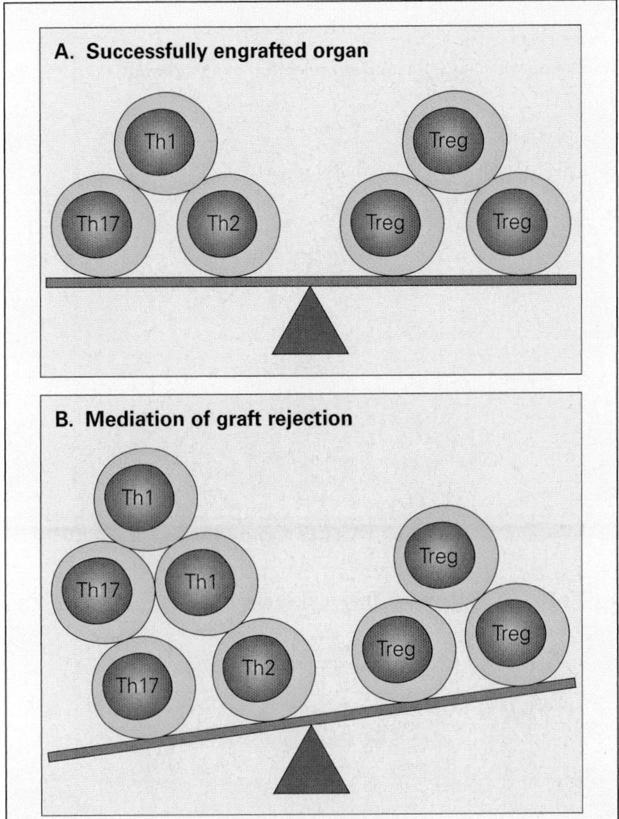

Figure 22-4. **Schematic representation of the balance between cytopathic Th1, Th2, and Th17 cells versus cytoprotective regulatory T cells in the outcome of organ transplant.** The ultimate outcome of graft rejection or tolerance depends on the relative balance between rejection-prone effector T cells and rejection-blocking, immunosuppressive Tregs. Panel A: Shows how organ engraftment is promoted by a balanced Treg/effector cell ratio preventing the destructive effects of Th1, Th2, and Th17 cells that mediate graft rejection. Panel B: Shows how an excessive number of rejection-prone effector T cells unbalanced by a sufficient number of Treg cells can mediate graft rejection. Tolerogenic therapeutic strategies differ in their capacity to directly affect this ratio by deleting rejection-prone effector T cells and/or promoting the function and number of immunosuppressive Tregs. (Adapted with permission from Sánchez-Fueyo A, Strom TB. Immunologic basis of graft rejection and tolerance following transplantation of liver or other solid organs. Gastroenterology. 2011;140:51–64.)

a direct mechanism of graft destruction. Moreover, the production of proinflammatory cytokines such as IL-6, TNF-α, IL-12, and IFN-γ promote the acquisition of cytodestructive Th1 and Th17 cells, but not FOXP3+ immunoregulatory cytoprotective Treg cells. As described in Chapter 9, Th17 and Tregs have remarkable plasticity and are closely interlinked. Thus, Tregs can differentiate into IL-17-producing cells in the presence of IL-2 and IL-1β, whereas in the presence of IL-27, Th17-producing cells also produce IL-10, an immunosuppressive cytokine that prevents them from functioning as destructive effector cells. Thus, new drug targets that prevent inflammation in the graft and draining lymph nodes might facilitate graft retention by promoting tolerance through their effects on these immunoregulatory cytokines.

First and Second Set Graft Rejection

Like all immune responses, allospecific immunity demonstrates both specificity and memory and therefore patients who have been previously sensitized to HLA antigens are at a greater risk of developing more rapid and more severe forms of graft rejection. Shown in Figure 22-5 is a schematic representation of the two prototypes of graft rejection of an allograft referred to as *first set* and *second set* reactions compared to graft acceptance of an autograft; these responses are based on the classic principles of immune responses following either initial encounter with a self or foreign antigen, respectively. In allograft rejection, there is a relatively longer temporal requirement in first set rejection in contrast to a subsequent encounter characterized by a more rapid recall of immune events in the so-called second set reaction mediated by the classic secondary or anamnestic booster responses (Figure 22-5B, first set rejection, and Figure 22-5C, second set rejection). As shown in Figure 22-5A, during the acceptance of an autograft, revascularization occurs in 3–7 days followed by healing, which occurs between 7–10 days, terminating in resolution at 12–14 days. The same initial events occur during a first set rejection within the first 3–7 days; however, at 7–10 days, cellular infiltration is seen followed by thrombosis and necrosis at 12–14 days, replacing the normal healing process and resolution, which occurs during autograft acceptance. The same events occur during second set rejection but at a more accelerated rate, with cellular infiltration occurring at 3–4 days and terminating in more rapid onset of thrombosis and necrosis at 5–6 days.

Sensitization to HLA antigens plays a critical role in graft rejection, which can occur through transfusion, pregnancy, or a previous transplant. HLA antibody production by a sensitized patient can be restimulated through reexposure to nonself HLA antigens or by unrelated immune events such as a viral infection or an inflammatory process. Although uncommon, antibodies with specificity for HLA

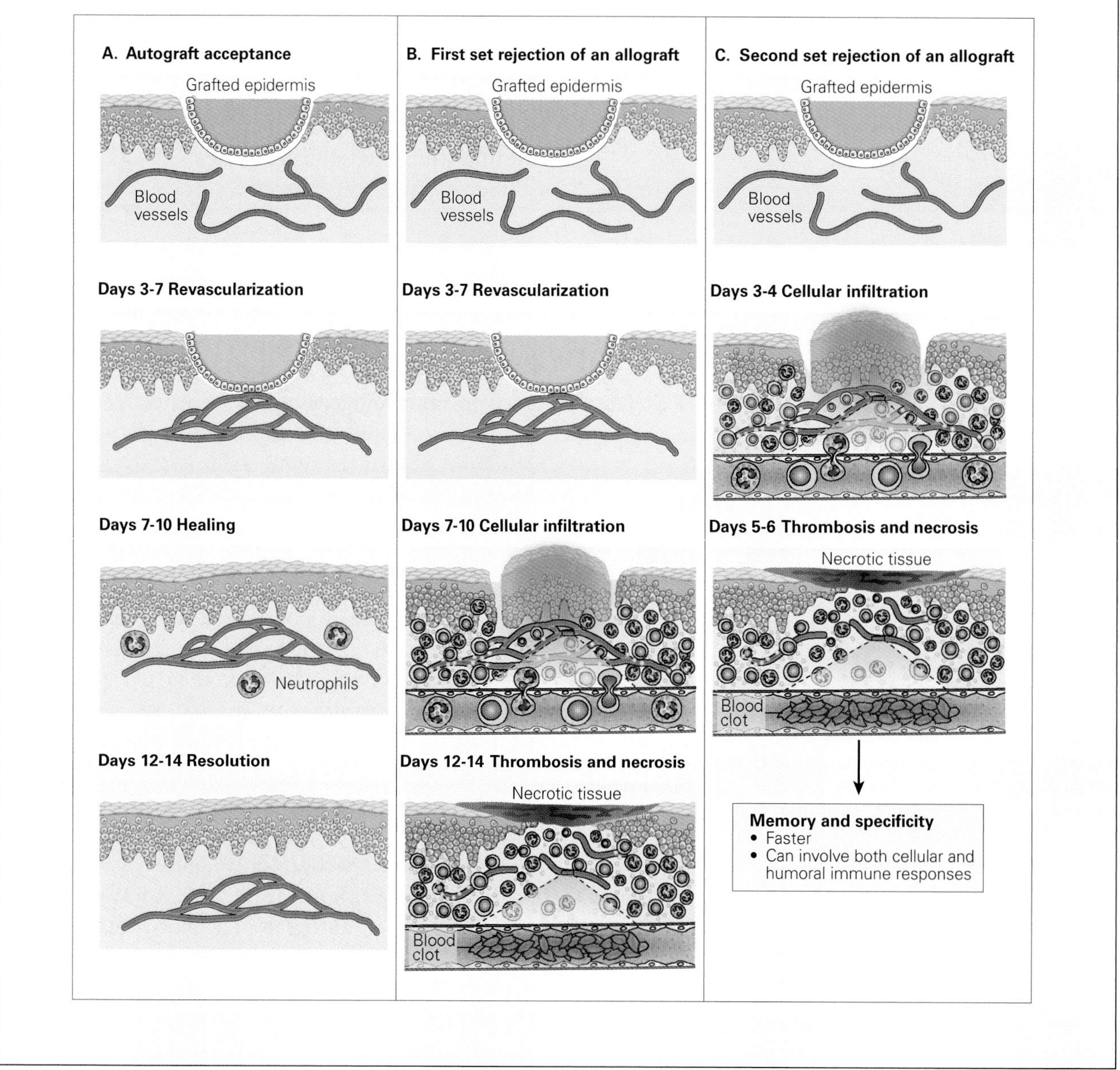

Figure 22-5. Schematic representation of prototype concepts. Panel A: Acceptance of an autograft. Panel B: First set rejection of an allograph. Panel C: Second set rejection of an allograph.

antigens have been reportedly generated through stimulation by certain bacterial antigens in the phenomenon referred to as molecular mimicry (*Chapter 19*).

Histocompatibility Antigens

In general, the acceptance or rejection of a transplanted tissue or organ by an individual depends on the laws of transplantation that are dictated by whether or not the recipient shares all or most of the donor's histocompatibility antigens (Figure 22-1). In humans, histocompatibility antigens include the major blood group antigens, HLA antigens, and a variety of minor histocompatibility antigens.

ABO antigens. The antigens that determine blood types are glycoproteins and glycolipids and there are three major types of blood-group antigens, O, A, and B, that differ only slightly in the composition of their carbohydrate structures. ABO antigens are expressed on the surface of red blood cells and are best known for their role in determining blood compatibility in the transfusion setting where infusing a patient with blood from a donor with the incorrect

ABO group may cause a transfusion reaction that can have fatal consequences. When this occurs, the donor red cells are destroyed by strongly reactive naturally occurring or acquired antibodies circulating in the recipient's bloodstream that are reactive against the major blood group antigens expressed on the surface of the donor's red blood cells.

ABO antigens are important histocompatibility antigens not only because they are expressed on the surface of red blood cells, but also on the endothelial surfaces lining all blood vessels and therefore are prime targets for immunologically mediated injury (*Chapter 17*). If an ABO incompatible organ, for example, is transplanted, it is rapidly and irreversibly rejected due to these antibodies circulating in the recipient's bloodstream.

HLA antigens. Another group of histocompatibility antigens, particularly important in HSC transplantation, are the highly polymorphic major histocompatibility antigens, which in humans are referred to as human leukocyte antigens or the HLA (*Chapter 10*). Individuals express as many as 14 different classical HLA molecules encoded by alleles at different genetic loci (Table 22-2) and inherit the genes for one set of seven HLA molecules from each parent. Therefore, heterozygous individuals express two different HLA-A molecules, two different HLA-B molecules, two different HLA-C molecules, two different HLA-DR molecules, two different HLA-DQ molecules, and two different HLA-DP molecules. In addition, some haplotypes include a second DR beta chain locus, DRB3, DRB4, or DRB5. The DR beta chains encoded by the alleles at these loci form heterodimers with DR alpha chains and the DR molecules are referred to as DR52, DR53, and DR51, respectively.

Solid Organ Transplantation

In the solid organ transplant setting, the degree of HLA compatibility is usually described in terms of the number of mismatches at HLA-A, -B, and DR antigens (Table 22-3). A perfect match is described as a zero antigen mismatch, and when a donor and recipient share no antigens, the term six-antigen mismatch is used. Although the HLA types of the donor and recipient are typically derived using DNA-based typing methods, the degree of matching is evaluated based on antigen or serologic level typing information and C, DQ, and DP antigens are ignored.

Modern therapies have made it possible to sufficiently suppress an organ transplant recipient's immune system so that HLA matching is no longer critical (*Chapter 10*). However, recipients who receive a well-matched donor organ, in general, have fewer episodes of rejection and better long-term graft survival. In addition, better-matched transplants require

Table 22-2. Major histocompatibility complex (MHC) molecules

Antigen	Class	Molecular composition of heterodimer	MHC gene(s)	Originally defined by	Currently typed by
HLA-A	I	MHC-encoded heavy chain + β 2-microglobulin	A	Antibodies	DNA-based assays
HLA-B	I	MHC-encoded heavy chain + β 2-microglobulin	B	Antibodies	DNA-based assays
HLA-C	I	MHC-encoded heavy chain + β 2-microglobulin	C	Antibodies	DNA-based Assays
HLA-DR	II	MHC-encoded α chain + MHC-encoded β chain	DRA + DRB1	Cellular assays	DNA-based assays
HLA-DR51	II	MHC-encoded α chain + MHC-encoded β chain	DRA + DRB5	Cellular assays	DNA-based assays
HLA-DR52	II	MHC-encoded α chain + MHC-encoded β chain	DRA + DRB3	Cellular assays	DNA-based assays
HLA-DR53	II	MHC-encoded α chain + MHC-encoded β chain	DRA + DRB4	Cellular assays	DNA-based assays
HLA-DQ	II	MHC-encoded α chain + MHC-encoded β chain	DQA1 + DQB1	Cellular assays	DNA-based assays
HLA-DP	II	MHC-encoded α chain + MHC-encoded β chain	DPA1 + DPB1	Cellular assays	DNA-based assays

Table 22-3. HLA matching for solid organ transplantation

	HLA TYPE		
Recipient:	A1, 2	B7, 8	DR15, 17
Donor A	A1, 1	B8, 8	DR17, 17
			0 antigen mismatch
Donor B	A2, 29	B13, 44	DR7, 15
			4 antigen mismatch
Donor C	A3, 3	B7, 8	DR15, 17
			2 antigen mismatch
Donor D	A1, 3	B7, 8	DR15, 17
			1 antigen mismatch

less immunosuppressive drugs and therefore patients experience less drug toxicity and the overall cost of lifelong immunosuppression is less.

Hematopoietic Stem Cell Transplantation

In the HSC transplant setting, because the patient's immune system is nonfunctional either as a result of the underlying disease or chemotherapy, the need for precise HLA matching is much greater and the degree of matching is described in terms of number of HLA alleles matched (Table 22-4). Recent studies have clearly demonstrated that hematopoietic stem cell transplant recipients have improved overall survival with bone marrow or peripheral blood stem cell (**PBSC**) transplants from donors who are HLA-allele matched. Typically clinicians prefer donors who are a 10/10 allele match with the recipient at HLA-A, -B, -C, -DRB1, and -DQB1.

Minor Histocompatibility Antigens

Minor histocompatibility antigens (**mHA**) are immunogenic peptides from polymorphic cellular proteins. They can be derived from any endogenous cellular protein that is present in different allelic forms in different individuals. In a transplantation setting, individual mHA mismatches between donor and recipient typically trigger a weak immune response that is manifested as a slow and less severe rejection process. In humans, mHAs have been shown to play a role in the development of graft-versus-host disease, and multiple mHA mismatches can induce strong T cell responses in patients receiving an HSC transplant. Several mHAs with broad or limited tissue expression have been described in humans and have been shown to be target antigens for both graft-versus-host and graft-versus-leukemia immune responses.

In 2004 in the United States, approximately 16,000 patients with end-stage renal disease received a kidney transplant and more than 6,000 patients with liver failure received a liver transplant. Although the overall numbers are much smaller, heart, lung, and small bowel transplants are becoming increasingly common (to learn more, go to http://www.ustransplant.org).

Generally speaking, the ideal donor for a transplant would be HLA-matched with the recipient.

Table 22-4. HLA matching for HSC transplantation

	HLA type				
Recipient:	A*01:01, *02:01	B*07:02, *08:01	C*07:01, *07:02	DRB1*03:01, *15:01	DQB1*02:01, *06:01
Donor A	A*01:01, *02:01	B*07:02, *0:801	C*07:01, *07:02	DRB1*03:01, *15:01	DQB1*02:01, *06:01
					= 10/10 Match
Donor B	A*01:01, *03:01	B*07:02, *08:01	C*07:01, *07:02	DRB1*03:01, *15:01	DQB1*02:01, *06:01
					= 9/10 Match
Donor C	A*01:01, *02:01	B*07:02, *44:02	C*05:01, *07:02	DRB1*03:01, *15:01	DQB1*02:01, *06:01
					= 8/10 Match

However, with the exception of kidneys and to a smaller degree livers and lungs, donor organs are generally recovered from deceased individuals and very few patients receive well-matched organs. In the United States, patients who are in need of an organ transplant are placed on a nationwide waiting list and as donor organs become available, they are allocated to patients based on a complex algorithm that includes ABO compatibility, the degree of HLA matching, the strength and specificity of preexisting donor specific HLA antibody, and time on the waiting list (to learn more, go to http://www.unos.org).

Since there is a severe shortage of deceased donor organs available, each year there are many more patients awaiting transplants than those who receive transplants. For this reason, minimizing death on the waiting list is a major concern, and the overriding goal of organ allocation is to be fair and equitable to all patients. In recent years, particularly for liver, heart, and lung transplants, allocation systems have focused on the development of objective criteria for evaluation of the clinical status and the urgency of an individual patient's need for a life-saving transplant. The algorithm for the allocation of donated kidneys is currently under review in the United States. Although the new system is likely to continue to take into account factors such as ABO compatibility, HLA matching, and presensitization, additional criteria are being evaluated that would facilitate the derivation of an objective net lifetime benefit score for each patient.

Types of Solid Graft Rejection: Hyperacute, Acute, and Chronic Rejection

Rejection of transplanted organs remains the main barrier to transplantation today. It occurs as a result of humoral and cell-mediated immune responses by the recipient to specific antigens present in the donor tissue and can be categorized based on the time frame in which it occurs.

Hyperacute Rejection

Hyperacute rejection is a form of a complement-mediated type III hypersensitivity response (*Chapter 17*) in recipients with preexisting antibodies to the donor (for example, ABO blood type antibodies). Hyperacute rejection occurs within minutes after transplantation with rapid agglutination of the blood, and the transplant must be immediately removed to prevent a severe systemic inflammatory response (*Chapter 3*). This is a particular risk in kidney transplants, and so a prospective cytotoxic cross-match is performed prior to kidney transplantation to ensure that antibodies to the donor are not present. Hyperacute rejection is analogous to a blood transfusion reaction as it is a humoral-mediated immune response. Hyperacute rejection occurs within the first 24 hours after transplantation but can develop rapidly within minutes after an organ is transplanted and it is usually severe and irreversible (Figure 22-6). This type of rejection occurs when there are preexisting high-titer antibodies in the recipient's blood that have specificity for donor

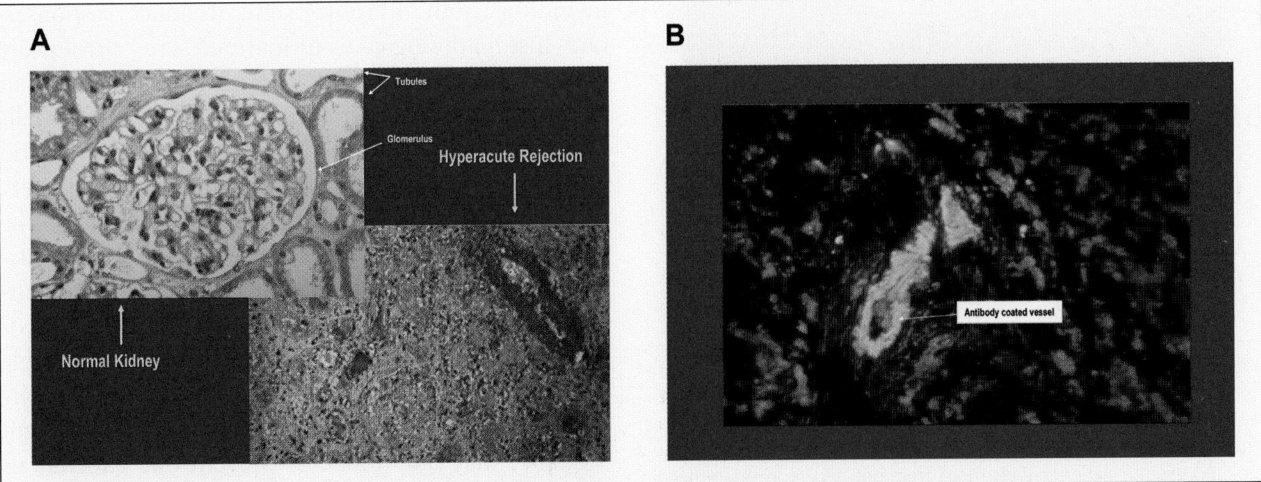

Figure 22-6. A photomicrograph of a kidney undergoing hyperacute graft rejection. Panel A: Light micrograph comparing a normal kidney with a kidney undergoing hyperacute rejection with thrombosis of a renal arteriole. Panel B: A section of a kidney undergoing hyperacute rejection stained by immunofluorescence showing an antibody-coated blood vessel.

histocompatibility antigens. Shown in Figure 22-6 is a photomicrograph of a kidney undergoing hyperacute graft rejection.

The donor-specific antibodies bind rapidly to target antigens on the vascular endothelium of the donor organ and, subsequently, the complement system is activated along with a cascade of immune processes that stimulate coagulation, inflammation, and an influx of neutrophils into the graft. The kidney and heart are most susceptible to hyperacute rejection, but the liver is relatively resistant. Renal histology shows fibrin thrombi-occluded glomerular capillaries and small vessels with extensive necrosis. Hyperacute rejection can be prevented by careful prescreening of transplant candidate serum for the presence of antibodies directed at donor histocompatibility antigens.

Acute Rejection

Acute rejection is the most common form of rejection and is recognized as a sudden decline in graft function (Figure 22-7). Acute rejection can begin within days or weeks after transplantation (as opposed to hyperacute rejection, which is immediate). The risk of acute rejection is highest in the first three months after transplantation. However, acute rejection can also occur months to years after transplantation. Although the causes and clinical course of acute rejection can vary, factors that contribute to the development of acute rejection include the degree of HLA mismatch, retransplantation, broadly reactive anti-HLA antibody, and, in particular, antibody specific for donor HLA antigens. In addition, the recipient's genetic makeup and age can also affect the nature and severity of acute rejection. The immune response involved in acute rejection includes both cellular and humoral mechanisms. The most reliable method for diagnosis of acute rejection is a percutaneous needle biopsy of the allograft. Shown in Figure 22-7 is a photomicrograph of a kidney undergoing acute rejection showing the histologic hallmarks of dense mononuclear cell infiltrates and varying degrees of tubulitis.

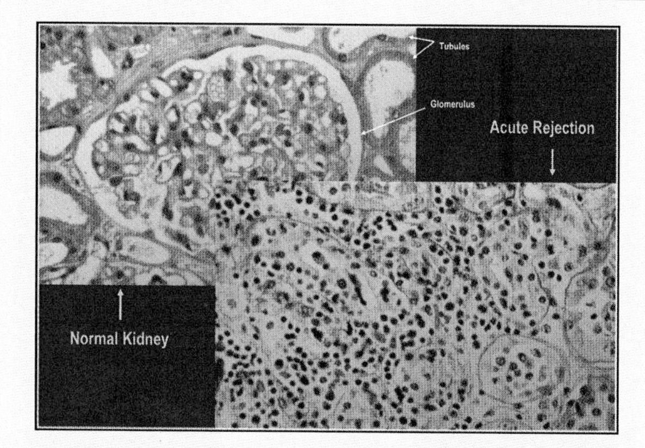

Figure 22-7. A photomicrograph of a kidney undergoing acute rejection showing the histologic hallmarks of dense mononuclear cell infiltrates and varying degrees of tubulitis. Although in most instances acute rejection is reversible with increased immunosuppression, patients with more frequent and more severe episodes of acute rejection have been shown to be more likely to develop chronic graft rejection.

Chronic Rejection

Chronic rejection is less well defined than either hyperacute or acute rejection and remains a major obstacle to long-term graft survival. The term chronic rejection was initially used to describe a long-term loss of function in transplanted organs associated with fibrosis of the internal blood vessels of the transplanted tissue. But this pathology is now termed chronic allograft vasculopathy. The term chronic rejection is reserved for cases of transplant rejection where the rejection is due to a poorly understood chronic inflammatory and immune response against the transplanted tissue. It occurs after an extended period of time that can vary from a few months to several years and is characterized by gradual loss of function of the graft. Chronic rejection is thought to be most likely caused by a mosaic of concurrent processes involving different cell types and immune mechanisms, including both humoral and cellular responses. On histopathologic examination, the chronically rejected organ shows mononuclear cell infiltration predominantly of the T cell line, although B cells may also be involved. How rapidly it develops and how severe it manifests are dependent on a variety of factors, including the underlying disease of the patient, whether or not donor-specific HLA antibodies are present, and the degree of HLA matching. One of the reasons that chronic rejection is particularly difficult to treat is that the multiple contributing pathogenetic factors are not necessarily interdependent. Therefore, any one treatment modality may only block or prevent one pathway or mechanism while other treatment regimens may cause the chronic rejection to progress. Although the process may be slowed or delayed, it is extremely difficult to totally prevent this insidious progressive deterioration of graft function.

The definitive diagnosis of chronic rejection is again generally made by biopsy of the organ in question. Kidneys with chronic rejection have fibrosis (scarring) and damage to the microscopic blood vessels in the parenchyma of the kidney (Figure 22-8). Livers with chronic rejection have a decreased number of bile ducts on biopsy. This is referred to as the "vanishing bile duct syndrome." Transplanted lungs with chronic rejection are said to have "bronchiolitis obliterans," a scarring problem in the substance of the lung. Chronic rejection in heart grafts is felt to be manifest by accelerated graft atherosclerosis.

Hematopoietic Stem Cell Transplantation

A growing list of malignancies and genetic disorders are being successfully treated with HSC transplantation (to learn more, go to http://www.nmdp.org or http://www.bmdw.org). In general, the preferred HSC donor is an HLA-identical sibling; however, for many patients, a matched related donor is not available. For this reason, there is a growing network of donor registries all over the world, and many patients are successfully transplanted with matched or minimally mismatched unrelated donors.

Historically, the most common source of donor stem cells has been **bone marrow**, which is the spongy tissue in the medulla. Bone marrow was the source first used for stem cell transplants because it

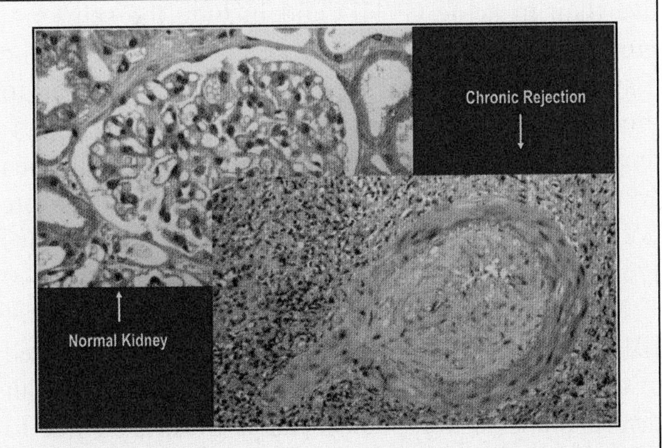

Figure 22-8. A photomicrograph of a kidney undergoing chronic rejection showing fibrosis (scarring) and damage to the microscopic blood vessels in the substance of the kidney.

has a rich supply of stem cells. Marrow donation is a surgical procedure performed in a hospital under general anesthesia. Bone marrow from the donor's pelvic bones is aspirated using a special hollow needle. Many donors receive an autotransfusion with a unit of their own previously donated blood.

The source of hematopoietic stem cells for transplant has expanded to include not only bone marrow, but also **peripheral blood stem cells** (**PBSC**). Although normally the quantity of hematopoietic stem cells in the peripheral circulation is low, the number can be greatly increased by treating the donor for five to seven days prior to donation with growth factors that stimulate the release of stems cells from the bone marrow into the peripheral circulation (*Chapter 9*). When enough stem cells are present in the bloodstream, the donor undergoes a process called apheresis during which the blood stem cells are separated from the donor's blood while the remaining blood is infused back into the donor's bloodstream. The donation process is relatively easy and donor complication rates are lower than with bone marrow. The advantages of PBCS as a stem cell source for transplant include a shorter time to engraftment with a more rapid recovery of neutrophil and platelet counts. In addition, extra donor stem cells can often be collected and stored frozen for potential donor lymphocyte infusion (**DLI**) if the patient relapses. Nevertheless, recent studies suggest that PBCS may not be the best option for all patients and there may be a significantly increased risk of severe chronic graft-versus-host disease (**GVHD**) and transplant-related mortality.

A third source of hematopoietic stem cells is blood recovered from the umbilical cord of a newborn baby. Umbilical cord blood contains high concentrations of hematopoietic stem cells. The advantages of this stem cell source include rapid availability because units are collected and stored frozen. In addition, umbilical cord blood stem cell transplants are less prone to rejection than either bone marrow or peripheral blood stem cells. This is probably because the cells have not yet developed the features that can be recognized and attacked by the recipient's immune system. Also, because umbilical cord blood lacks mature T cells, there is less chance that the transplanted cells will attack the recipient's body causing GVHD. For these reasons, there is a decreased need for precise HLA matching. Although a growing number of multiple cord transplants are being performed, the disadvantages of cord blood are that many units are small and do not provide an adequate cell dose for larger patients and engraftment is typically slower than with bone marrow or PBSC.

The differential risks and benefits of the three stem cell sources are currently an important area of investigation. Ultimately the optimal donor and stem cell source for an individual patient depends on multiple factors, including their diagnosis, disease status, and the availability of a fully HLA-matched donor.

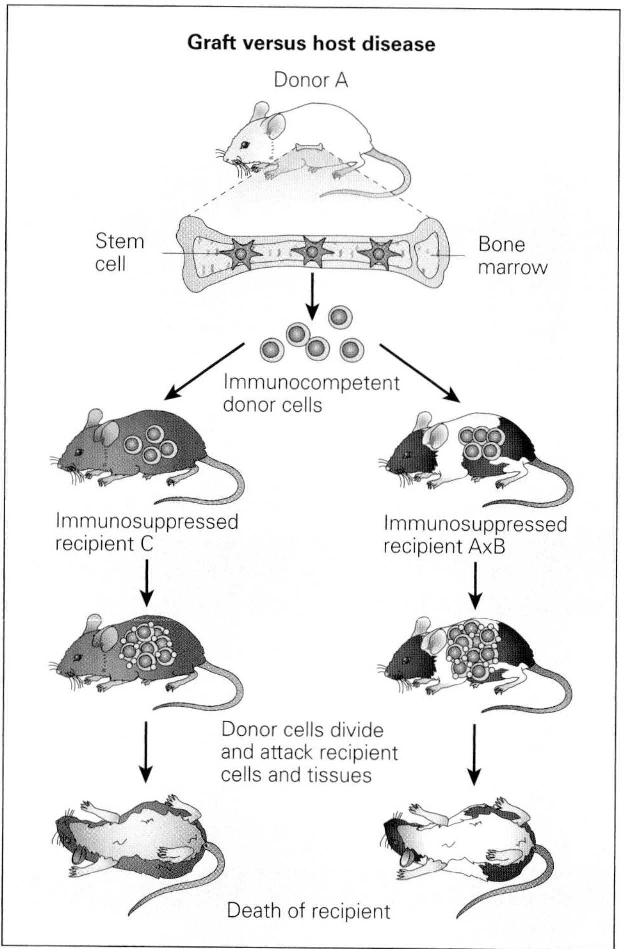

Figure 22-9. A schematic representation of graft-versus-host disease.

Graft-versus-Host Disease

Unlike solid organ transplantation, where rejection poses the greatest danger, for HSC transplant patients the greatest risk is GVHD. The immune response involved in GVHD is very similar to that observed in graft rejection and involves the same effector mechanisms observed in graft rejection. However, in GVHD, the donor's T cells are recognizing the recipient's histocompatibility antigens as nonself (Figure 22-9).

Although GVHD is most often thought of as a complication of HSC transplantation, other patient groups are also at risk of developing the syndrome, including recipients of small bowel transplants and any immune-compromised patient receiving non-irradiated blood transfusions.

The primary targets of the immune response in GVHD are the skin, liver, and intestinal tract of the transplant recipient. The severity of acute GVHD can range from very mild to severe and is categorized as grade I (mildest) through IV (most severe), (Table 22-5). The mildest form, grade I, typically involves a relatively mild skin rash and diarrhea with slightly elevated liver enzymes. Patients with the most severe form of GVHD have generalized erythroderma with bullous formation and desquamation. Patients have severely elevated liver enzymes (bilirubin > 15 mg/100 mL) with extensive diarrhea and abdominal pain. The overall grade of acute GVHD is predictive of the patient's outcome, with the highest rates of mortality in those with grade IV, or severe, GVHD.

Chronic Graft-versus-Host Disease

The term chronic GVHD, a more diverse form of the syndrome generally developing after day 100 posttransplant, is classified as either limited or extensive. Chronic GVHD can occur either de novo in patients who never manifested clinical evidence of acute GVHD or it may emerge after a quiescent interval following resolution of the acute GVHD. The organs and systems involved can be more extensive than in acute GVHD and include the skin, oral mucosa, eyes, lungs, liver, and intestinal tract. The manifestations of chronic GVHD can be similar to those of systemic progressive sclerosis as well as systemic autoimmune disorders such as systemic lupus erythematosus and rheumatoid arthritis. As in acute GVHD, the stage and classification of the patient's symptoms are predictive of their prognosis.

Multiple factors affect the occurrence and severity of GVHD. The incidence of GVHD is increased in unrelated matched donor transplants compared with related matched transplants. This is most likely due to the increased genetic disparity and additional mismatched minor histocompatibility antigens. Likewise, patients who receive HLA-mismatched transplants are at an even greater risk of developing severe

Table 22-5. Clinical staging of acute GVHD by organ system

Stage	Skin	Liver	Intestinal tract
I	Maculopapular rash < 25% of body surface	Bilirubin 2–3 mg/100 mL	Diarrhea > 280 mL/m^2 body surface area
II	Maculopapular rash 25–50% body surface	Bilirubin 3–6 mg/100 mL	Diarrhea > 555 mL/m^2 body surface area
III	Generalized erythroderma	Bilirubin 6–15 mg/100 mL	Diarrhea > 833 mL/m^2 body surface area
IV	Generalized erythroderma with bullous formation and desquamation	Bilirubin > 15 mg/100 mL	Severe abdominal pain with or without ileus

Reproduced with permission from Thomas ED, Storb R, Clift RA, et al., Bone marrow transplantation (second of two parts). N Engl J Med. 1975;292:895–902.

GVHD. Other risk factors are increased age of either the donor or the recipient and the stem cell source.

Prevention and Treatment of GVHD

The incidence and severity of GVHD increases with increasing HLA disparity between donor and recipient. For this reason, every effort is made to identify a donor who is 10/10 allele matched with the recipient and, if this is not possible, the least mismatched donor is selected. Overall survival is also improved and GVHD decreased when the HCS donor is young, optimally less than 30 years old.

To prevent GVHD, most patients receive prophylactic immunosuppressive drug therapy posttransplant (*Chapter 11*). Another strategy for minimizing GVHD is the selective depletion of mature T lymphocytes from the stem cell product prior to infusion. While patients who receive T cell depleted grafts experience less GVHD, they also have a significantly increase rate of relapse or recurrence of malignancy.

The conventional preparative regimen for HSC patients includes myeloablative doses of chemotherapy aimed at eliminating malignant cells and creating an environment in the patient's bone marrow that will allow engraftment of donor hematopoietic stem cells. However, high-dose chemotherapy often results in increased levels of circulating cytokines. This "cytokine storm" is thought to increase the ability of graft immune cells to recognize host antigens. In addition, high-dose therapy can lead to localized tissue damage and may cause the exposure of cryptic antigens in susceptible organs such as the skin, liver, or intestine. Recently, immunosuppressive but nonmyeloablative protocols are often used to prepare patients for transplant. Such nonmyeloablative approaches not only minimize GVHD, but also reduce the overall toxicity of the transplant procedure and often allow sicker and more elderly patients to be successfully transplanted.

Graft versus Leukemia

Since it is known that patients with leukemia who experience GVHD have a lower relapse rate of their disease, some degree of GVHD may be beneficial for a patient's overall survival. It is thought that this happens because while attacking the tissues of the patient, the donor immune cells often also attack residual tumor cells remaining after transplant. This graft-versus-leukemia (**GVL**) phenomenon was first documented in acute leukemia. However, similar effects have also been observed in malignant lymphoma, myeloma, and possibly solid tumors. For certain diseases, such as chronic myelogenous leukemia (**CML**), the GVL effect may well be the most important reason that allogeneic transplants are successful in curing the disease. Learning more about the mechanism of GVL and developing ways to separate the negative effects of GVHD from the beneficial and potentially curative effects of GVL are areas of intense research.

Immunosuppression

There is a growing arsenal of immunosuppressive drugs used to inhibit or control the immune response against transplanted organs and tissues (*Chapter 11*). Although there are multiple targets and mechanisms of action, the overriding goal of all immunosuppression is to avoid triggering an alloimmune response by preventing T cell activation with subsequent cytokine release and cell proliferation (Figure 22-10). Shown in

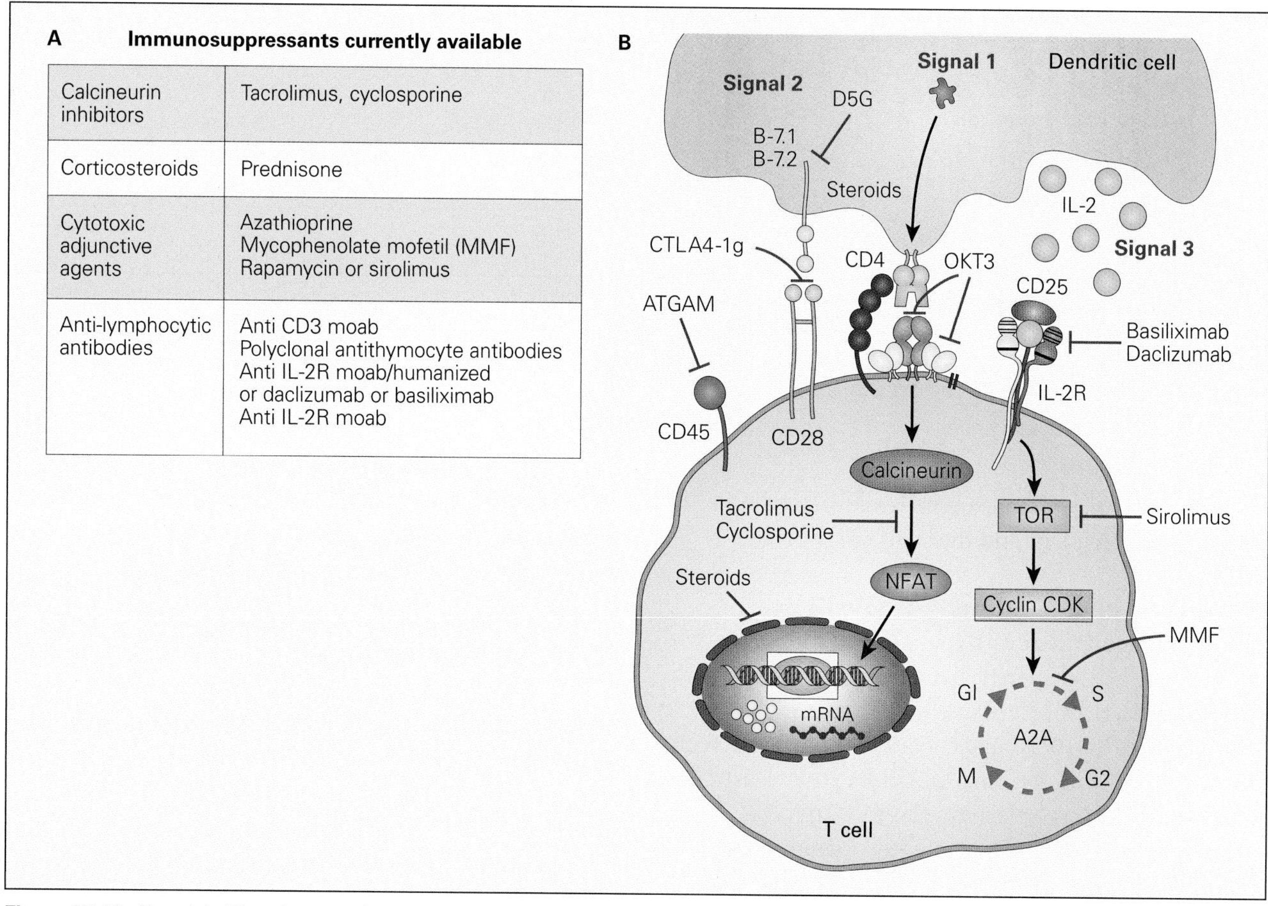
A Immunosuppressants currently available

Calcineurin inhibitors	Tacrolimus, cyclosporine
Corticosteroids	Prednisone
Cytotoxic adjunctive agents	Azathioprine Mycophenolate mofetil (MMF) Rapamycin or sirolimus
Anti-lymphocytic antibodies	Anti CD3 moab Polyclonal antithymocyte antibodies Anti IL-2R moab/humanized or daclizumab or basiliximab Anti IL-2R moab

Figure 22-10. Panel A: The classes of some of the currently available immunosuppressive agents commonly used in transplantation. Panel B: Their sites of action.

Figure 22-10A are the classes of some of the currently available immunosuppressive agents and in Figure 22-10B their sites of action.

Calcineurin Inhibitors

The two primary immunosuppressive drugs used in transplantation today, cyclosporine and **tacrolimus** (**FK506**), both function through the inhibition of calcineurin, which is a protein phosphatase responsible for activating the transcription of IL-2 (Figure 22-11). The mode of action of cyclosporine involves its binding to the cytosolic protein, cyclophilin, which is an immunophilin present in a variety of cells including T lymphocytes (*Chapter 11*). Similarly, tacrolimus binds to another immunophilin referred to as FKBP-12. The immunophilin-drug complex formed by either drug subsequently binds to calcineurin and prevents it from dephosphorylating a critical transcription factor called nuclear factor of activated T cells (**NFAT**). This prevents NFAT from migrating into the cell nucleus and initiating the synthesis of a variety of interleukins including IL-2.

Both cyclosporine and tacrolimus are potent immune suppressors and most immunosuppressive regimens contain one or the other of these two drugs. However, both drugs also have numerous serious side effects, including hypertension, nephrotoxicity, and hepatotoxicity. Both drugs also interact with a wide variety of other drugs and other substances, including grapefruit juice.

Adjunctive Agents

Sirolimus (also known as **rapamycin**) is a relatively new immunosuppressant drug especially useful in kidney transplants (Figure 22-10). Originally developed as an antifungal agent, sirolimus is a macrolide antibiotic ("-mycin") first discovered as a product of the bacterium *Streptomyces hygroscopicus* isolated in a soil sample from Easter Island. Despite its similar name, sirolimus it is not a calcineurin inhibitor like tacrolimus or cyclosporine. However, it has a similar suppressive effect on the immune system. Although tacrolimus and sirolimus bind to the same immunophilin, FKBP-12, the sirolimus-FKBP12

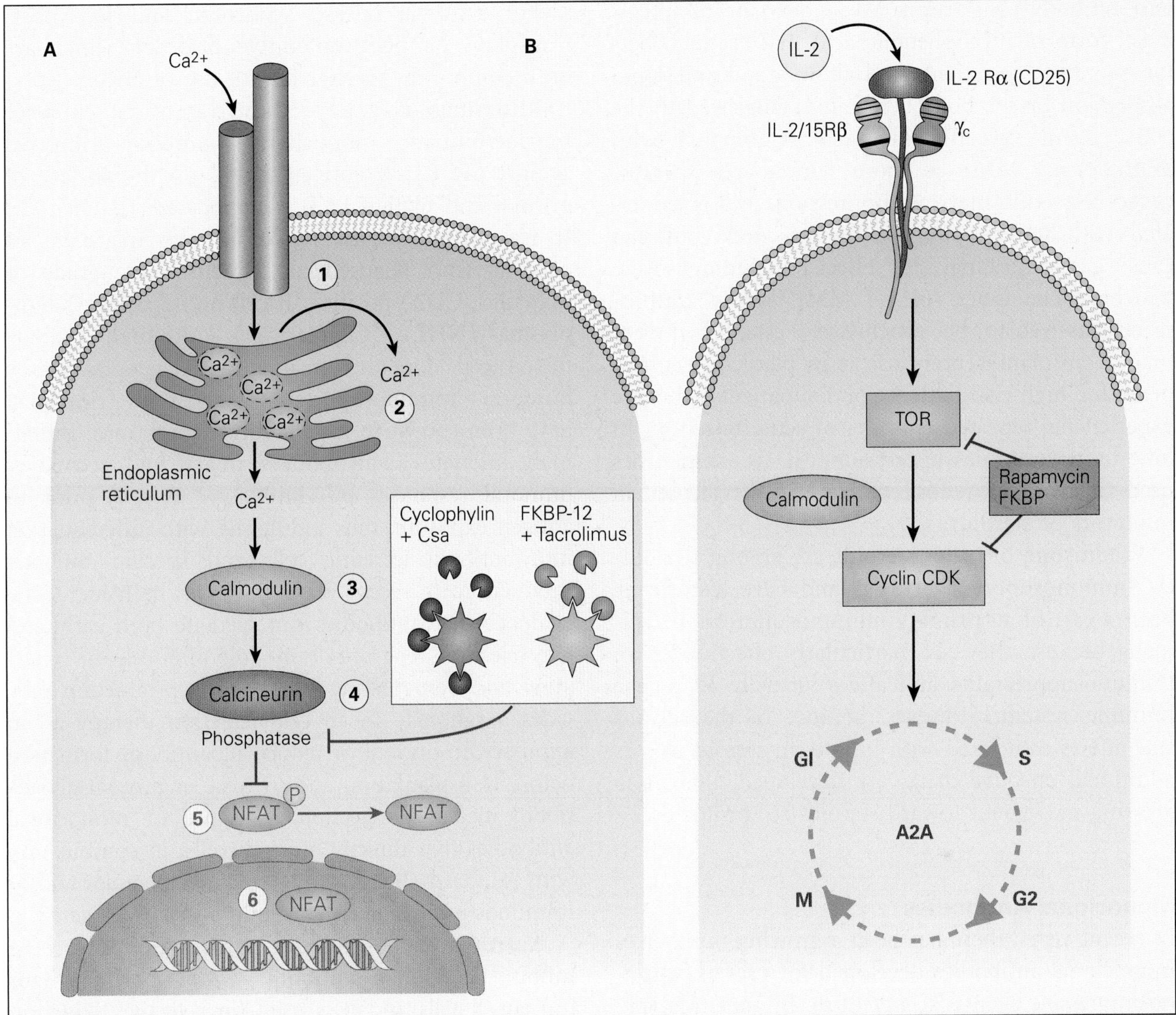

Figure 22-11. The sites of action of two classes of calcineurin inhibitors. Panel A: Tacrolimus forms an immunophilin-drug complex that subsequently binds to calcineurin and prevents it from dephosphorylating a critical transcription factor call NFAT (nuclear factor of activated T cells). Panel B: Although tacrolimus and sirolimus bind to the same immunophilin, FKBP-12, the sirolimus-FKBP12 complex acts through a different pathway and inhibits a serine/threonine kinase called mTOR that regulates translation and cell division, thus inhibiting lymphocyte proliferation.

complex acts through a different pathway and inhibits a serine/threonine kinase called mTOR that regulates translation and cell division. Thus, sirolimus inhibits lymphocyte proliferation (Figure 22-11). The chief advantage of sirolimus over calcineurin inhibitors is that it is not toxic to kidneys and therefore sirolimus is often used in conjunction with calcineurin inhibitors and/or mycophenolate mofetil to provide steroid-free immunosuppression regimens.

Azathioprine is a chemotherapeutic drug, now rarely used for chemotherapy but more for immunosuppression in organ transplantation and autoimmune disease such as rheumatoid arthritis, inflammatory bowel disease, or Crohn's disease. It is a pro-drug, converted in the body to the active metabolite 6-mercaptopurine. Azathioprine acts to inhibit purine synthesis necessary for the proliferation of cells, especially leukocytes and lymphocytes. It is a safe and effective drug used alone in certain autoimmune diseases, or in combination with other immunosuppressants in organ transplantation. Its most severe side effect is bone marrow suppression.

Mycophenolate mofetil (MMF) is similar to azathioprine in that is inhibits de novo purine synthesis therefore inhibiting lymphocyte proliferation and antibody production. Mycophenolate mofetil is a salt form of mycophenolic acid that is much better tolerated by patients and allows good and rapid absorption by the body before it is converted to the active agent mycophenolic acid. Compared with azathioprine, MMF is more lymphocyte specific, causes less bone marrow suppression, and is associated with fewer opportunistic infections but can cause gastrointestinal side effects, including severe diarrhea. The exact role of MMF versus azathioprine has yet to be conclusively established, but many transplant centers use it in place of azathioprine for high-risk patients or for patients who are experiencing repeated episodes of acute rejection. In long-term immunosuppression, it is sometimes used to avoid or reduce the dosage of calcineurin inhibitors or steroids.

Prednisone or other steroids are among the oldest immunosuppressive drugs and have historically been a part of all primary immunosuppression regimens because they are particularly effective as an immunosuppressants and affect virtually all of the immune system. However, because of the serious side effects associated with long-term steroid use, as additional effective drugs are developed, there is a growing movement toward steroid-free protocols.

Monoclonal Antibodies

In recent years, there has been a growing number of monoclonal antibodies developed for uses as immunosuppressive agents (*Chapter 10*). By targeting specific cell surface receptors, monoclonal antibodies are designed to affect different aspects of T cell activation, including intracellular signaling, cell adhesion, and co-stimulation.

Basiliximab and **daclizumab** are both chimeric mouse-human monoclonal antibodies that bind to the IL-2 receptor on T cells. Multiple doses of these antibodies are administered over a period of time. The antibody saturates the IL-2 receptors and prevents T cell activation. These drugs reduce the incidence and severity of acute rejection in kidney transplantation without increasing the incidence of opportunistic infections.

OKT3 is specific for the T cell marker CD3. It was one of the first monoclonal antibodies developed for use as an immunosuppressive agent. It was formerly used in the prevention of rejection and is occasionally used in treatment of severe acute rejection, but has fallen out of common use due to the severe cytokine release syndrome and late post-transplant lymphoproliferative disorder, which are both commonly associated with use of OKT3.

Rituximab is a genetically engineered chimeric murine/human monoclonal antibody directed against the CD20 antigen found on the surface of normal and malignant B lymphocytes (*Chapter 11*). It was originally developed for the treatment of patients with relapsed or refractory, low-grade or follicular, CD20-positive, B cell non-Hodgkin's lymphoma (**NHL**) (*Chapter 21*). Although initially introduced for the treatment of neoplasm, the humoral immunosuppressant effects of rituximab have been shown to have clinical significance. Rituximab interferes with both primary and secondary humoral responses by eliminating B cells prior to antigen exposure, thus interfering with differentiation into antibody-secreting cells and specific antibody production. In recent years, there has been increasing evidence that antibodies can mediate both early and late rejection. The important role of B cells in generating and perpetuating alloantibody production provides a rationale for B cell depletion therapy as an approach to prevent or reduce alloantibody formation before transplantation and to treat or prevent alloantibody-mediated rejection. The use of monoclonal antibodies that directly target B cells, in combination with standard alloantibody-depleting therapies and/or immunosuppression, is currently being investigated.

Antithymocyte globulin (thymoglobulin) is a rabbit polyclonal antibody with specificity for human T cells and it is used for selective depletion of T cells. It is used for the prevention and treatment of acute rejection in organ transplantation and therapy of aplastic anemia. It is frequently given at the time of the transplant to prevent rejection, but is typically reserved for patients who have a high risk of acute rejection such as those who have been previously sensitized to HLA antigens. Thymoglobulin is associated with cytokine-release syndrome when it is used, and in the longer term, may increase the risk of posttransplant lymphoproliferative disorder.

Summary of Mechanisms of Action and Side Effects of Immunosuppressive Drugs

Shown in Table 22-6 is a summary of the mechanisms of action of some of the major induction immunosuppressive biologic agents that include polyclonal and monoclonal antibody preparations showing the

Table 22-6. Summary of the mechanisms of action of some of the major induction immunosuppressive biologic agents that include polyclonal and monoclonal antibody preparations showing the target cells and postulated effects

Agent	Type	Target	Effect
ATG/ALG	Polyclonal	Bind multiple antigens on lymphoid cells	Complement-mediated cytolysis; opsonization and clearance
OKT3	Monoclonal	Binds CD3 on T cells	Complement-mediated cytolysis; opsonization and clearance; modification of CD3 receptor
Diclizumub Basiliximab	Monoclonal	Binds to the α-subunit (CD25) of the IL-2 receptor	Downregulation of the IL-2 receptor; CD4+ T cell depletion
Rituximab	Monoclonal	Binds to the CD20 surface molecule on B cells	Downregulation of mature B cells

target cells and postulated effects. The major classes of maintenance immunosuppressive agents and their major side effects are shown in Table 22-7. These agents include the corticosteroids, cyclosporine, tacrolimus, azathioprine, MMF, and sirolimus.

Intravenous immune globulin (**IVIG**) is a plasma product prepared from a large pool of normal donors; it has a wide range of immunomodulatory and immunoprotective properties (*Chapter 11*). Although it has been used for more than 20 years to treat primary immunodeficiency disorders, IVIG products have also long been known to be effective in the treatment of autoimmune and inflammatory disorders. The true mechanisms of IVIG action are still poorly understood, however, interference with antibody-binding sites and/or inhibition of antibody production possibly though anti-idiotypic antibody has been suggested.

Most recently, it has been demonstrated that in some patients, IVIG treatment can greatly reduce anti-HLA antibodies. This was an important finding because one of the most difficult groups of patients to successfully transplant are those who have been previously sensitized to HLA antigens through either a prior transplant, pregnancy, or transfusion and who have strong, broadly reacting HLA antibodies. Many transplant programs have developed protocols designed to temporarily "desensitize" patients in order to create a window of opportunity during which antibody titers are reduced to a level where a transplant can be carried out without danger of hyperacute rejection. Desensitization protocols typically utilize either high-dose IVIG alone or multiple cycles of plasmapheresis combined with a lower dose of IVIG with or without Rituximab. While it remains to be known whether IVIG treatment can induce a lasting modulation or tolerance, it is clear that this approach is providing many more highly sensitized patients with the opportunity to receive a transplant.

Histocompatibility Testing

The role of the histocompatibility laboratory has evolved in recent years from that of simply "tissue typers" to an integral part of the transplant team. While HLA typing is still an important function of the laboratory, with the development of advanced HLA antibody detection assays, there has come a greater appreciation of the clinical importance of donor-specific antibody and there

Table 22-7. Summary of the major maintenance immunosuppressive agents and their major side effects

Agent	Major side effects
Corticosteroids	Hypertension, glucose imbalance, dyslipidemia, osteoporosis
Cyclosporine	Nephrotoxic effects, hypertension, dyslipidemia
Tacrolimus (FK506)	Similar to cyclosporine but less hirsutism and gum hypertrophy; IDDM is seen with an incidence up to 20%
Azathioprine	Bone marrow suppression
Mycophenolate mofetil (MMF)	Diarrhea/GI upset, increased frequency of CMV infection
Sirolimus	Hyperlipidemia, thrombocytopenia

has been a shift in the role of the histocompatibility laboratories. Since the presence of antibody directed against HLA antigens in the serum of a prospective transplant recipient is now recognized as an important deterrent to the success of a transplanted organ, the detection of these antibodies by these advanced techniques offers an important predictive marker in transplant medicine. Most laboratories are more and more involved in aiding the transplant surgeon in assessing the risk of a transplant by identifying clinically relevant donor-specific antibodies (Figure 22-12).

For patients in need of an HSC transplant, the laboratory not only provides HLA typing for the patient and potential donors, but it also often provides expertise and advice for donor search strategies and final donor selection (Figure 22-13).

HLA typing was historically preformed using a method referred to as a complement-dependent lymphocytoxicity (**CDC**) assay (Figure 22-14).

The CDC assay (sometimes also called a microlymphocytotoxicity assay) is a two-stage, complement-dependent reaction in which recipient lymphocytes are first incubated with known panels of antisera and then with fresh frozen rabbit serum as a source of complement. The binding of antibody to specific HLA antigens on the lymphocyte's surface activates complement leading to membrane damage and eventually cell death. The membrane damage is visualized microscopically as uptake of a dye by the injured cells. When more than 50 percent of the cells in a test well have membrane damage, it is assumed that the cells express the HLA antigen targeted by the HLA antisera contained in the test well. Commercially available HLA class I typing trays contain panels of antisera for the identification of the HLA-A, -B, and -C antigens. HLA class II typing trays contain panels of antisera with specificity for HLA-DR and -DQ antigens. Typically, HLA class I typing is carried out using unseparated lymphocytes or purified T lymphocytes, and HLA class II typing is done using purified B lymphocytes.

Antibody Monitoring and Specificity Analysis: Private versus Public HLA Epitopes

The crossmatch is the final diagnostic tool used to detect incompatibility and provides antibody screening and specificity analysis that are essential components of the ultimate decision of whether or not to transplant using a particular donor organ. Historically, the gold standard measure of the degree of sensitization to HLA antigens has been the percentage panel reactive antibody (**PRA**). The

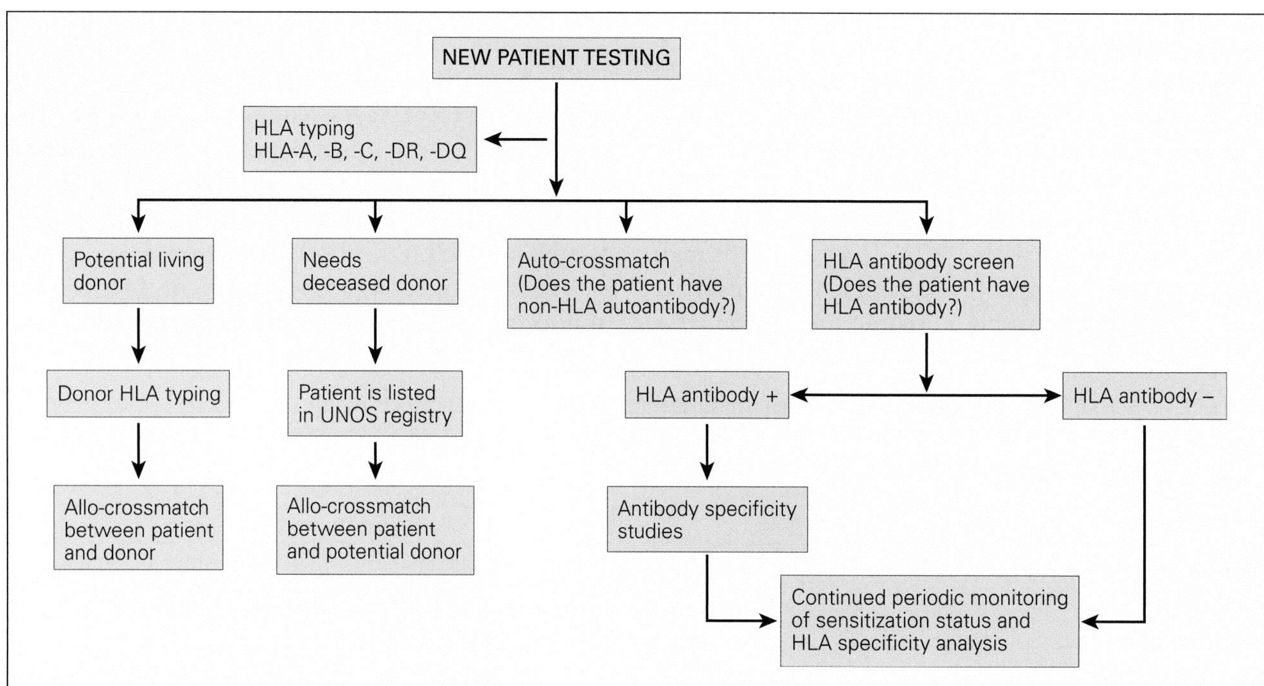

Figure 22-12. Histocompatibility testing for solid organ transplant candidates.

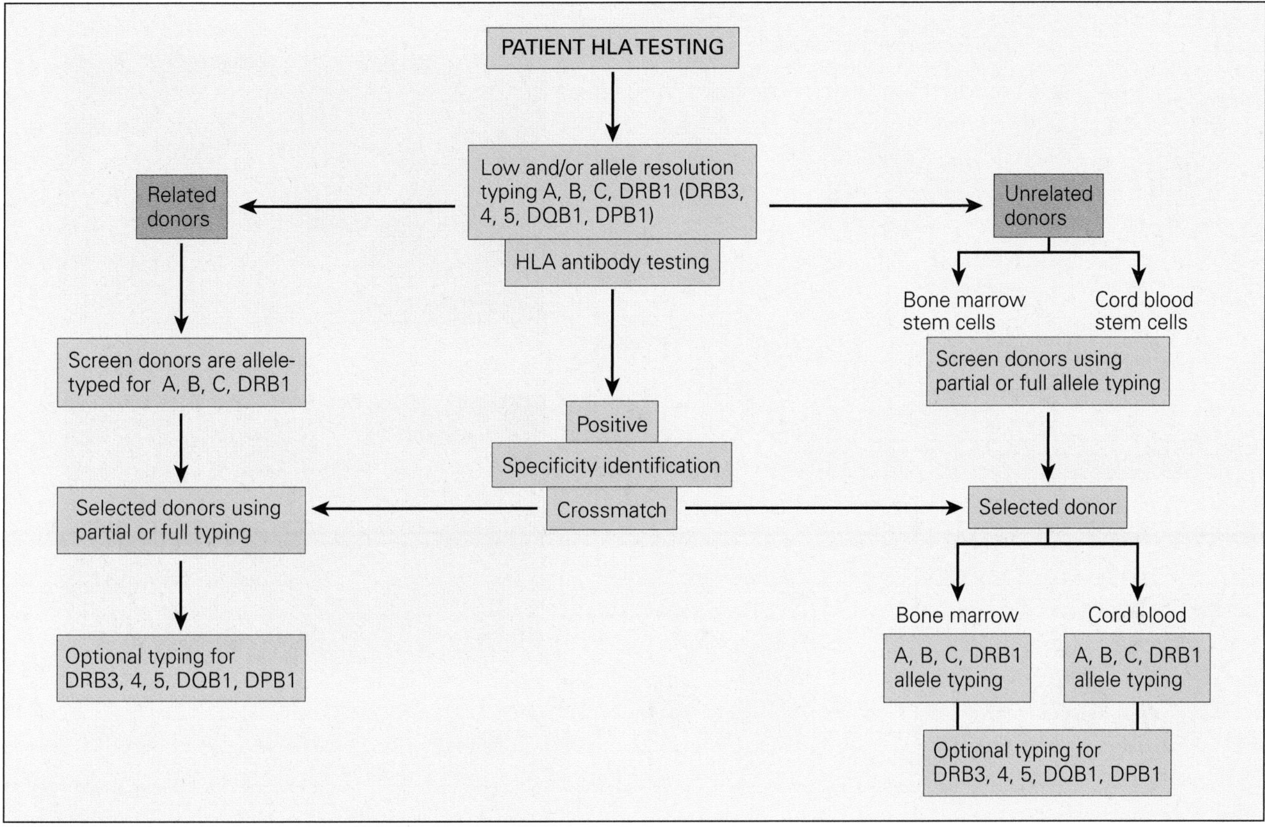

Figure 22-13. Histocompatibility testing for HSC transplant candidates.

name of the test is derived from the fact that patient's serum is tested with a panel of cells with known HLA types. The percentage PRA reflects the number of different cells with which the antisera reacts. Therefore, the percentage PRA is not a reflection of antibody titer, but rather a reflection of the nature of antibody specificity.

In transplantation immunology, the terms private and public HLA epitope determinants are commonly used. The unique epitope configuration on one HLA antigen represents what is referred to as a private epitope of the specific HLA antigen, while epitopes shared by more than one HLA antigen represent the public determinants. In some HLA antigens, e.g., HLA-A1, more than one private epitope has been defined, while in others, e.g., HLA-B35, -B51, the private epitopes have not yet been identified. For example, a patient with an antibody directed at a private epitope on a single low-frequency HLA antigen could have a very low PRA of approximately 15 percent. On the other hand, a patient with an antibody directed at a high-frequency public epitope could have a PRA of > 80 percent. Both patients, however, would be equally likely to experience hyperacute rejection if transplanted with an incompatible organ. The selection of the PRA screening method and the frequency of the screening differ based on the clinical needs and immunologic profile of the individual recipient. Highly sensitized individuals typically require more extensive and frequent screening than those who are not sensitized, and patients are routinely retested following potential sensitizing events such as transfusion, pregnancy, or graft rejection. There are currently two general types of assays used for antibody characterization and crossmatching: (1) **cell-based assays** using either a CDC or flow cytometric method (Figures 22-14 and 22-15); and (2) **solid-phase assays** using either flow cytometric or ELISA-based methods (Figure 22-16).

Cell-Based Assays

Complement-Dependent Lymphocytotoxicity Assays

The original CDC antibody screening and crossmatch methods were essentially identical to that

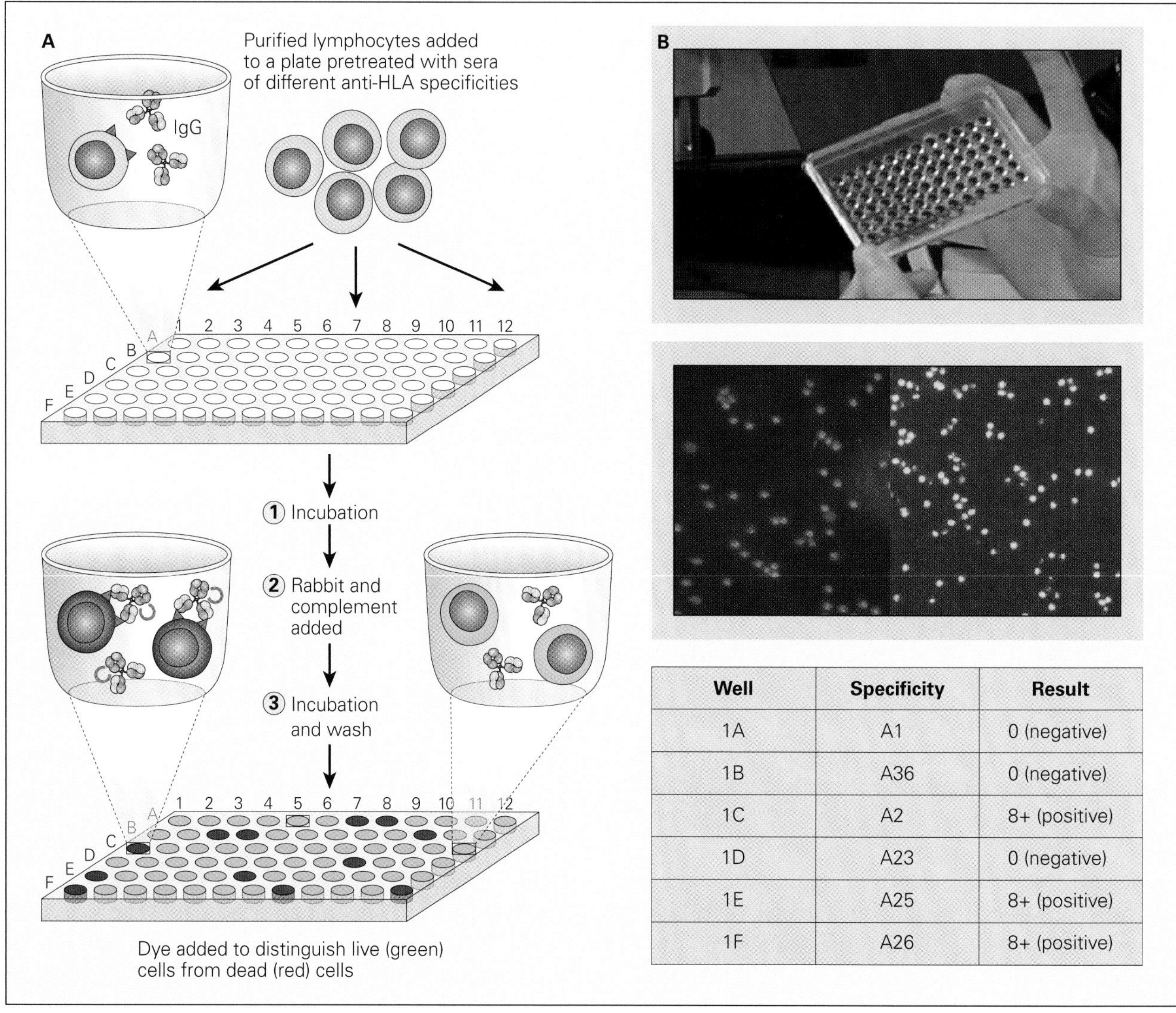

Well	Specificity	Result
1A	A1	0 (negative)
1B	A36	0 (negative)
1C	A2	8+ (positive)
1D	A23	0 (negative)
1E	A25	8+ (positive)
1F	A26	8+ (positive)

Figure 22-14. Schematic representation of a complement-dependent lymphocytotoxicity assay for the determination of HLA typing. Panel A: The various steps in the test procedure. Panel B: A representative example of the test results.

described above for serologic HLA typing by the microlymphocytotoxicity method. The basic difference between the two is that in HLA typing, the recipient's lymphocytes are tested with a known panel of anti-HLA antibodies, whereas in the CDC crossmatch, the recipient's serum is tested for antibody directed against HLA antigens on donor lymphocytes. The basic principle of both the microlymphocytotoxicity method and the CDC assay is complement-mediated lymphocyte membrane injury initiated by antibody bound to its specific antigen. For a CDC crossmatch, donor lymphocytes are incubated with diluted and undiluted recipient serum prior to the addition of complement. The original or standard CDC assay has undergone various modifications over time to increase test sensitivity and specificity.

Antihuman Globulin Augmented Cytotoxicity Technique

The antiglobulin modification of the basic CDC was introduced to increase the sensitivity of the assay and it can be used for PRA assays or a donor-recipient crossmatch. Antihuman immunoglobulin is used in a manner similar to the Coombs reagent in red cell serology. In this assay, diluted antiglobulin is added to the PRA or crossmatch trays immediately before the addition of complement. It is thought that the binding of the antiglobulin to the antibody previously attached to the HLA antigens gives the complement a greater number of binding sites and can enhance the strength of reactions.

The CDC assay has been used for many years for detection of HLA antibody. However, this test is limited by the requirement for viable lymphocytes, by the high variability of the test's complement component, and by the inability to detect all HLA-specific antibodies (i.e., noncomplement fixing antibodies). Another disadvantage of CDC antibody analysis is that HLA antibodies are not the only antibodies detected in a CDC assay. Non-HLA autoantibodies can also be cytotoxic and therefore detected in a complement-dependent lymphocytotoxic assay. These autoantibodies are not clinically relevant, as they do not impact graft survival. In addition, CDC assays designed to be more sensitive to HLA antibodies are also more often sensitive to non-HLA autoantibodies.

Flow cytometric crossmatch. A flow cytometric crossmatch, like a CDC crossmatch, begins with the incubation of donor cells with patient serum (Figure 22-15). Subsequently, the method uses a combination of direct and indirect immunofluorescence to detect patient-antibody binding and to distinguish between T cell and B cell binding. Patient-antibody binding is detected indirectly using a secondary antibody such as an FITC-conjugated goat antihuman IgG. Simultaneously, T cells and B cells are distinguished through differential direct immunofluorescent staining with fluorescently labeled CD3 and CD19 or CD20, respectively. The flow cytometer renders an electronic histogram of increased fluorescence intensity on donor T cells and B cells in the presence of test serum containing putative HLA antibodies compared to HLA antibody-negative control serum (Figure 22-15B).

Solid Phase Assays

In recent years, a variety of solid phase methods have been developed for the detection and specificity analysis of HLA antibodies. A common feature of the solid phase assays is that they all utilize affinity purified HLA class I or purified HLA class II antigens attached to a solid support such as a microtiter tray or a microparticle (Figure 22-16). Both flow cytometric and ELISA-based tests are commercially available with variations that include the use of pooled, soluble antigens from multiple phenotypes for screening purposes, a panel of soluble antigens from single phenotypes, or single purified HLA antigens. Shown in

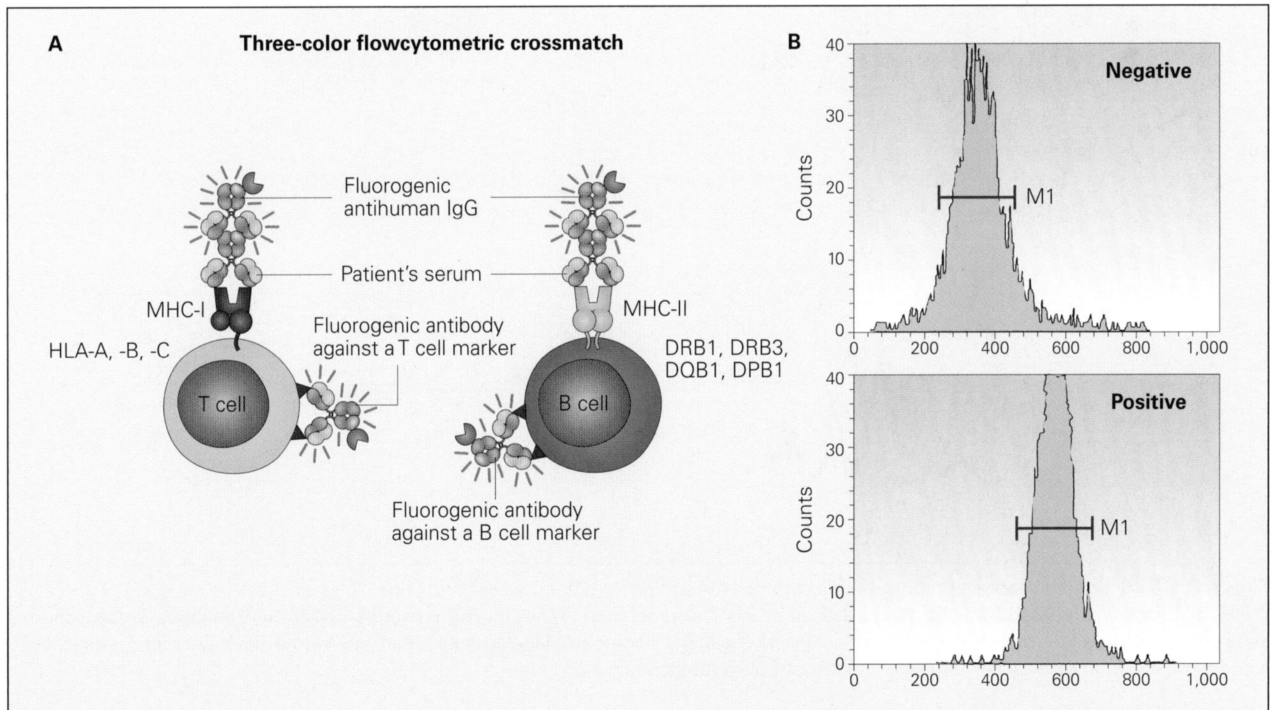

Figure 22-15. Schematic representation of direct and indirect immunofluorescence used in a flow cytometric crossmatch. Panel A: The cells of the donor are separated by direct immunofluorescence using specific fluorogenic-labeled antibody to T and B cell markers; the presence of donor-specific antibody in the patient's serum is detected by indirect immunofluorescence using a fluorogenic-labeled antihuman IgG. Panel B: Flow cytometer histograms show positive and negative crossmatch results.

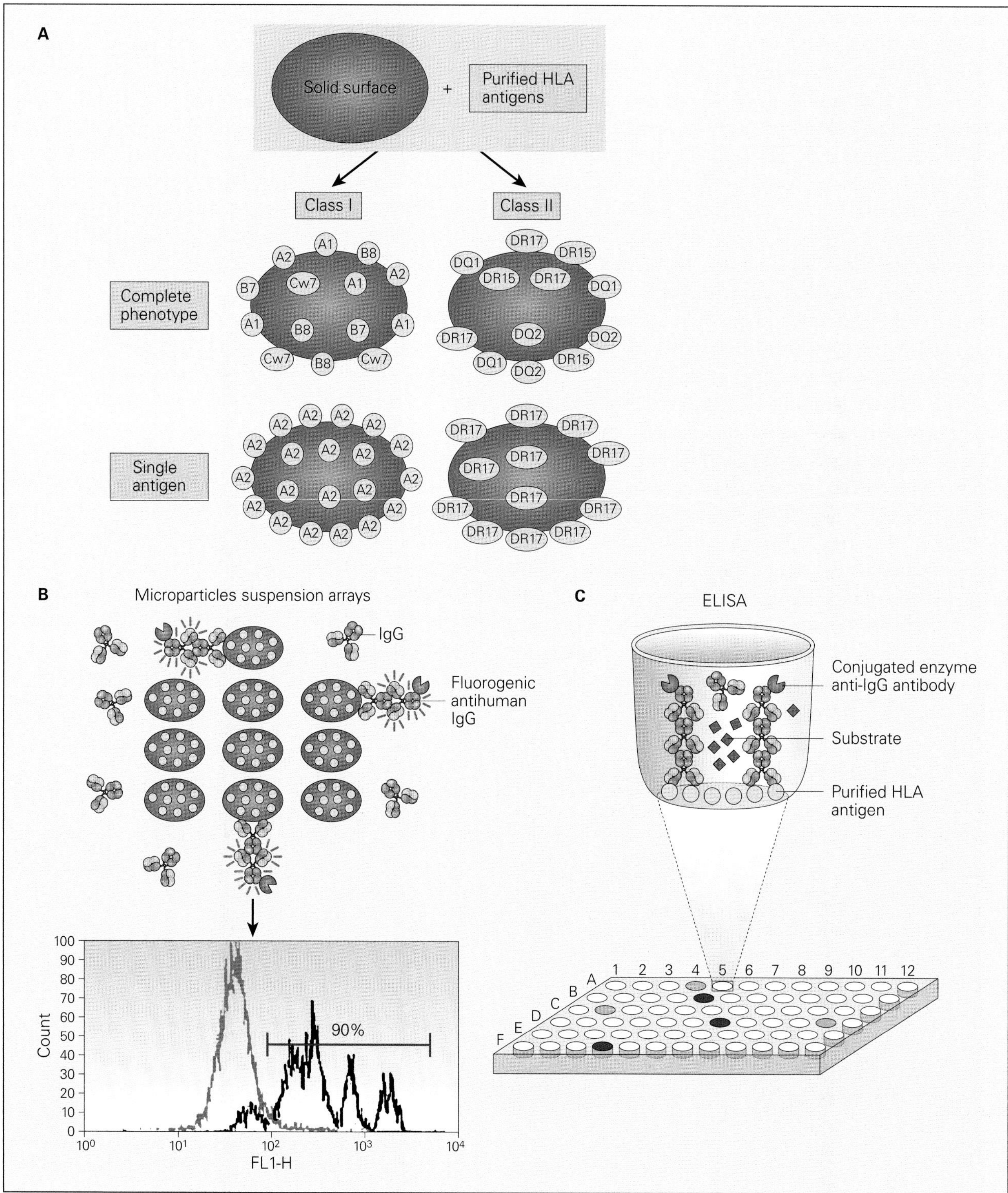

Figure 22-16. Schematic representation of solid phase HLA antibody detection assays. Panel A: Shows the various class I and class II HLA molecules expressed on solid surfaces used in the test procedure. Panel B: The presence of anti-HLA antibody in the patient's serum is detected either by indirect immunofluorescence using a fluorogenic-labeled antihuman IgG with a flow cytometric-based technique or by a colorimetric technique using an indirect ELISA methodology.

Figure 22-16 is a schematic representation of two of the solid phase assays; in panel A, a solid surface, e.g., a latex particle, is coated either with soluble antigens of multiple types used in identifying the complete HLA phenotypic pattern of antibody or with soluble antigens from single phenotypes used to identify antibody to single HLA antigens. Used in concert with cellular crossmatch assays, modern solid phase assays are a critical component of antibody monitoring, specificity analysis, and the overall histocompatibility evaluation of a patient and a potential transplant donor.

DNA-Based Molecular Methods

Today, virtually all HLA typing is performed by DNA-based molecular methods using genomic DNA isolated from nucleated cells. The most common methods include amplification of the HLA genes using the polymerase chain reaction (**PCR**) and utilize either HLA allele-specific PCR primers (SSP) or oligonucleotide probes (SSO) (*Chapter 25*).

Sequence-specific primers (SSP). For SSP typing, PCR primer pairs are designed to anneal only to a specific allele or set of alleles. The HLA type of the target gene is determined by analyzing with which sequence-specific primer pairs amplification occurs. This technique is very rapid since typing involves only SSP-PCR amplification of purified genomic DNA followed by visualization of the amplified products on an agarose gel stained with ethidium bromide. Typically a positive (amplification) control primer pair is included with each specific primer pair to monitor for amplification failures that can result in the misinterpretation of typing results.

Sequence-specific oligonucleotide probes (SSO). This method of HLA DNA typing involves an initial PCR amplification of the gene of interest (e.g., HLA-A or HLA-B) using a locus-specific primer set designed to amplify the relevant polymorphic sequences of the gene of interest (e.g., exon 2 of HLA-A). The resulting amplified target DNA is subsequently spotted onto replica membranes (*Chapter 25*). Each membrane is then probed using a different labeled antigen group or allele-specific oligonucleotide probe. Following hybridization of the specific probes, the HLA type is determined by analyzing the pattern of specific hybridization obtained with the panel of probes designed to detect different polymorphic sequences within the target gene. A variation of SSO typing, sometimes referred to as reverse SSO, involves linking a panel of specific probes to a membrane, different wells of a microtiter plate, or fluorescent microparticles. Thus, for reverse SSO HLA typing, the amplified target DNA from one person is tested with a single "probe-strip," microtiter tray microparticle panel.

Sequence-based typing (SBT). This method involves the direct DNA sequencing of HLA genes. As in SSO typing, SBT includes an initial PCR amplification of the gene of interest followed by direct DNA sequencing using a specific nested sequencing primer.

Summary

Transplantation of organs between genetically different individuals of the same species, once a formidable task, now is performed more readily as a result of great advances in immunology and in better techniques used both for the identification of suitable donors of organs and tissues as well as improved surgical techniques that permit more successful and safer engraftment. The field of transplantation now enjoys a wide variety of clinical applications and has provided major therapeutic options for a growing list of diseases, including end-stage organ failure, a variety of malignancies, immune deficiency and other genetic disorders, and autoimmune syndromes. The primary obstacle to successful transplantation is the cell-mediated immune response directed by the recipient host to the allogenic response to donor tissue that, if left unchecked, results in rejection and graft destruction. A greater understanding of the immunologic mechanisms that control the expression of proinflammatory and immunosuppressive cytokines in the early period after transplantation and the development of more effective chemotherapeutic and biologic products has contributed greatly to the success of the procedure in recent years. The ultimate goal of these immunologic interventions is to induce transplantation tolerance, a state in which the allograft is specifically accepted without the need for chronic immunosuppression. The recent identification of regulatory Treg cells and Th17 cells has provided a greater understanding of graft rejection and engraftment than was provided by the traditional Th1/Th2 paradigm. Until routine transplantation tolerance becomes fully attainable, patients who receive transplanted organs will still require nonspecific immunosuppressant drugs, many of which possess undesirable toxic side effects as well as manifestations of excessive immunosuppression such as opportunistic infections and cancers. Continued research in the field of transplantation immunology will continue to provide better tools for successful and safer transplantation of tissues and organs as well as more effective and safer therapeutic modalities.

Case Study: Clinical Relevance

Let us now return to the case study of a patient in need of a kidney transplant that illustrates both the utilization of immunologic techniques to identify prospective donors as well as the use of immunomodulating agents (described in Chapter 11) to achieve successful transplantation when there is no HLA-identical donor.

- Matching a patient in need of a transplanted solid organ with a prospective donor is a three-step process that includes: (1) the identification of the patient's HLA haplotypes; (2) the screening for potential HLA antibodies in the patient's serum directed to any of the donor's HLA haplotypes; and (3) ABO typing and crossmatching of donor and patient for detection of ABO incompatibility that may result in rejection of the transplanted organ.
- The first step in matching the patient identified her HLA phenotype as HLA A23, 33; B44, 58; DR7, 13.
- Screening for the antibodies to HLA antigens revealed the presence of broadly reactive serum antibody to both HLA class I and class II antigens by the panel reactive antibody (PRA) assay (85 percent), which could have resulted either from previous isoimmunization from a previous transplant or pregnancy.
- This was followed by more specific testing that revealed the presence of serum antibody to A74, B53, and DR15. Since these antibodies were reactive with three of the antigens expressed by the patient's husband, this suggested that the patient's HLA antibodies were probably the result of prior pregnancies. A more carefully taken history revealed that in addition to the two pregnancies that resulted in her two living children, the patient also had two additional pregnancies that had resulted in miscarriages providing additional support for a causative role in the induction of the patient's anti-HLA antibodies.
- The patient's husband was excluded as a possible donor because of an ABO incompatibility and the two children were similarly excluded because of incompatible HLA crossmatches, and the patient's unacceptable antigens were identified as A74, B53, and DR15. This would mean that any prospective donor would be excluded if an antibody to these HLA haplotypes existed in the donor serum as detected by an incompatible crossmatch. Despite a three-year listing on a nationwide registry, no donor offers were received.
- Although the patient's friend was a mismatch donor, the positive crossmatch detected by the flow cytometric method called into question the donor suitability of this individual.
- Due to the deteriorating condition of the patient, this interfering anti-HLA antibody was overcome through a desensitization procedure in which the deleterious antibody in the patient's serum was first removed by four plasmapheresis procedures supplemented by the immunomodulating effects of IVIG received after each treatment.
- This case study illustrates the application of the immunologic and genetic principles underling the proper management of patients in need of transplanted organs.
- Although the general health care provider usually will not be directly involved in the specifics of donor selection and laboratory aspects of organ transplantation, a thorough understanding of the principles and mechanisms of transplantation immunology will provide the clinician powerful diagnostic and therapeutic tools for the total management of all patients with immunologically mediated diseases whose pathogeneses are based on the same immunologic principles and mechanisms underlying organ transplantation.

Key Points

- There are four types of terms used to classify grafts used in transplantation immunology: autologous (within the same individual), syngeneic (between two genetically identical individuals), allogeneic (between genetically different members of the same species), and xenogeneic grafts (between members of different species).
- First set rejection usually occurs within 10 days when a graft is placed into a different allogeneic host for the first time; second set rejection occurs within one week after a second graft of the same antigeneic specificity is placed into the same allogeneic host for the second time.
- The human leukocyte antigen (HLA) classification is the name of the major histocompatibility complex (MHC) system in humans.
- HLA-A, HLA-B, and HLA-C correspond to MHC-I; HLA-DR, HLA-DQ, and HLA-DP correspond to MHC-II.
- Matching a patient in need of a transplanted solid organ with a prospective donor is a three-step process that includes: (1) the identification of the

patient's HLA haplotypes; (2) the screening for potential HLA antibodies in the recipient's serum directed to any of the donor's HLA haplotypes; and (3) ABO typing and crossmatching of donor and recipient for detection of ABO incompatibility.

- Hyperacute rejection is a form of a complement-mediated type III hypersensitivity response in graft recipients with preexisting antibodies to the donor (for example, ABO blood type antibodies) (*Chapter 17*). Hyperacute rejection occurs within minutes after transplantation with rapid agglutination of the blood requiring removal of the transplanted organ to prevent a severe systemic inflammatory response.

- Acute rejection is the most common form of graft rejection and is recognized as a sudden decline in graft function. Acute rejection usually begins one week after transplantation (as opposed to hyperacute rejection, which occurs within minutes and is the result of a cell-mediated immune attack of the donor graft by the recipient).

- The term "chronic rejection" is reserved for cases of transplant rejection where the rejection is due to a poorly understood chronic inflammatory and immune-mediated response of the recipient against the transplanted tissue. It occurs after an extended period of time that can vary from a few months to several years and is characterized by gradual loss of function of the transplanted graft.

- Graft-versus-host disease (GVHD) is a common complication of allogeneic bone marrow transplantation in which functional immune cells in the transplanted marrow recognize the recipient as "foreign" and mount an immunologic attack. In the classical sense, acute GVHD is characterized by selective damage to the liver, skin and mucosa, and the gastrointestinal tract. Newer research indicates that GVHD can target other organs including the immune system (the hematopoietic system, e.g., the bone marrow and the thymus) itself, and the lungs in the form of idiopathic pneumonitis.

- Graft-versus-leukemia (GVL) is a major component of the overall beneficial effects of allogeneic bone marrow transplantation (BMT) in the treatment of leukemia. It results from a reaction of the transplanted bone marrow against the leukemic cells.

- The various classes of currently available immunosuppressive agents commonly used in transplantation include: (1) the cytotoxic chemotherapeutic agents, e.g., the calcineurin inhibitors, e.g., tacrolimus, cyclosporine, the corticosteroids, adjunctive cytotoxic agents, e.g., azathioprine, mycophenolate mofetil (MMF), rapamycin (sirolimus); and (2) the immunosuppressive biologic agents, e.g., ATG/ALG, OKT3, diclizumub, basiliximab, and rituximab; intravenous immunoglobulin (IVIG) has recently been used as an immunomodulatory agent.

- A variety of new tissue typing and crossmatching methods based on DNA-based genomic technology are currently in use to assess donor-recipient compatibility for human leukocyte antigen (HLA) and ABO blood group compatibility that have largely replaced older serologic and functional assays that were used previously.

Study Questions/Critical Thinking

1. A graft transferred from one individual to that same individual is called a:

   a. Syngeneic graft
   b. Xenogeneic graft
   c. Allogeneic graft
   d. Autologous graft (autograft)

2. Complement activation, endothelial damage, inflammation, and thrombosis occurring within minutes are characteristic of:

   a. Acute rejection
   b. Hyperacute rejection
   c. Delayed rejection
   d. Chronic rejection

3. Methods used to reduce the likelihood of graft rejection include all of the following EXCEPT:

   a. HLA matching for HLA-A, HLA-B, and HLA-C
   b. Crossmatching
   c. Screening for preformed antibodies
   d. Measurement of quantitative serum levels of IgG

4. Each of the following statements regarding GVHD is correct EXCEPT:

   a. GVHD is one of the principal limitations to the success of BMT
   b. The principal organs involved in GVHD include the skin, liver, and intestines
   c. Chronic GVHD is characterized by fibrosis and atrophy
   d. Elimination of T cells from the marrow inoculum has increased the success of engraftment

5. Which immunosuppressive blocks lymphocyte proliferation by inhibiting IL-2 signaling?

   a. Cyclosporin
   b. Azathioprine
   c. Mycophenolate mofetil
   d. Rapamycin

Suggested Reading

Bluestone JA, Auchincloss H, Nepom GT, et al. The immune tolerance network at 10 years: tolerance research at the bedside. Nat Rev Immunol. 2010; 10: 797–803.

Flomenberg N, Baxter-Lowe LA, Confer D, et al. Impact of HLA class I and class II high-resolution matching on outcomes of unrelated donor bone marrow transplantation: HLA-C mismatching is associated with a strong adverse effect on transplantation outcome. Blood. 2004; 104: 1923–30.

Gebel HM, Bray RA, Nickerson P. Pre-transplant assessment of donor-reactive, HLA-specific antibodies in renal transplantation: contraindication vs. risk. Am J Transplant. 2003; 3: 1488–500.

Hurley CK, Baxter Lowe LA, et al. National Marrow Donor Program HLA-matching guidelines for unrelated marrow transplants. Biol Blood Marrow Transplant. 2003; 9: 610–5.

Moll S, Pascual M. Humoral rejection of organ allografts. Am J Transplant. 2005; 5: 2611–8.

Morishima, et al. The clinical significance of human leukocyte antigen (HLA) allele compatibility in patients receiving a marrow transplant from serologically HLA-A, HLA-B and HLA-DR matched donors. Blood. 2002; 99: 4200.

Norman DJ, Turka LA. Primer on transplantation. 2nd Edition. Mt Laurel, NJ: American Society of Transplantation; 2001.

Petersdorf EW, Anasetti C, Martin PJ, et al. Limits of HLA mismatching in unrelated hematopoietic cell transplantation. Blood. 2004; 104: 2976–80.

Petersdorf EW, Anasetti C, Martin PJ, et al. Tissue typing in support of unrelated hematopoietic cell transplantation. Tissue Antigens. 2003; 61: 1–11.

Rodey G.E. HLA beyond tears. Atlanta: De Novo; 1991.

Sánchez-Fueyo A, Strom TB. Immunologic basis of graft rejection and tolerance following transplantation of liver or other solid organs. Gastroenterology. 2011; 140: 51–64.

Thomas ED, Storb R, Clift RA, et al., Bone marrow transplantation (second of two parts). N Engl J Med. 1975; 292: 895–902.

Chapter 23

The Use of Vaccines and Antibody Preparations

Maria Lattanzi, MD
Rino Rappuoli, PhD
Konrad Stadler, PhD

LEARNING OBJECTIVES

When you have completed this chapter, you should be able to:

- Describe the differences between active immunization involving the use of vaccines and passive immunity involving the use of antibody preparations prepared in other hosts or in vitro systems
- Understand the differences between live, attenuated, and inactivated vaccines
- Describe the differences between the classic Pasteur method of vaccine development and the newer genomic method of reverse vaccinology
- Explain the basic role of host immune responses in development of protective immunity to vaccines
- Outline the various schedules of vaccine administration recommended for various age groups and for different clinical situations
- Recognize the various adverse effects of vaccines and understand the various immunologic mechanisms responsible for these
- Gain an appreciation for the future of vaccine development through research and its importance for development of therapies for emerging diseases
- Describe various antibody preparations used in passive immunization
- Understand the vast contributions of vaccines to public health and disease prevention during the last century
- Utilize this knowledge for a better understanding of antimicrobial immunity in the normal host as well as in individuals with immune disorders

Case Study

A previously healthy 18-year-old Caucasian male was hospitalized for a five-day illness characterized by fever, malaise, myalgia, nausea, vomiting, earache, and photophobia, accompanied by coryza and nonproductive cough. On the day prior to admission, a rash erupted on his wrists and the dorsa of his feet. He had previously received a series of three killed measles vaccines at monthly intervals when he was five years old. Upon admission, he was acutely ill with fever of 39°C. His conjunctivae and posterior pharynx were erythematous but without exudate. Clear nasal discharge was present and shotty anterior and posterior cervical nodes were palpable. He had rales and decreased breath sounds at the base of his right lung. His heart revealed a regular rhythm and a grade II/'VI systolic ejection murmur at the base; no gallops were heard. The rash gradually progressed upward and became mostly concentrated on his upper extremities with major involvement of his trunk, arms, and hands but spared his face; a few scattered lesions remained on his feet and legs. The rash was maculopapular, erythematous, and nonpruritic, and some of the lesions became petechial and raised with a papular appearance after 24 hours (Figure 23-1).

Laboratory data on admission revealed a hemoglobin concentration of 11.2 g/dL; a leukocyte count of 5,000/mm^3 with 63 percent neutrophils, 8 percent band forms, 11 percent lymphocytes, 1 percent atypical lymphocytes, 15 percent monocytes, and 2 percent eosinophils; a platelet count of 107,000/mm^3; and lactic dehydrogenase (LDH) 242 IU/mL. Cold agglutinins, VDRL, heterophil, and proteus OX-19 titer were negative. A chest X-ray showed an infiltrate in the right middle lobe (Figure 23-2).

By the third hospital day, the patient became afebrile. The heart murmur could no longer be heard. A chest X-ray on the fourth day showed normal heart size and clearing of the pulmonary infiltrate. The patient was discharged on the sixth hospital day after substantial clearing of his rash. Acute and convalescent measles complement fixation titers were both 1:512.

Case Study (continued)

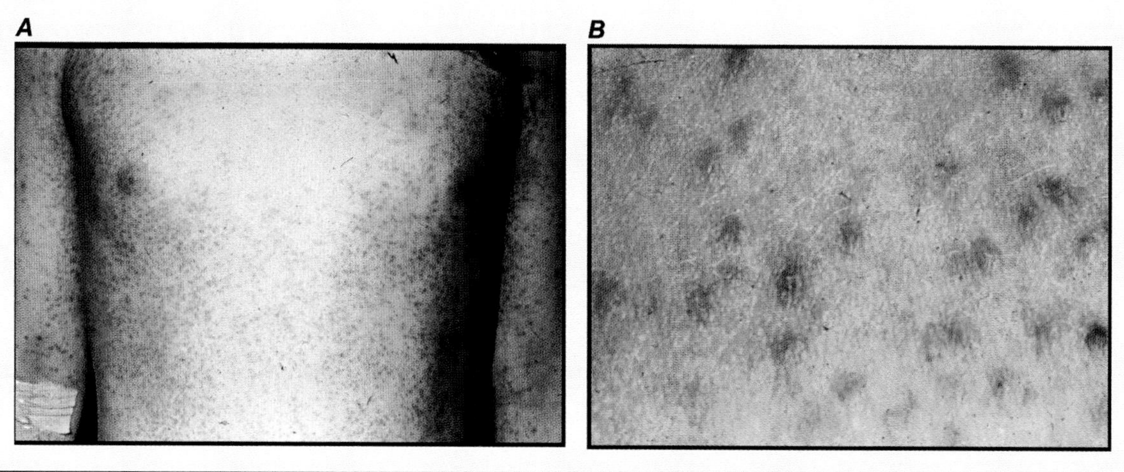

Figure 23-1. Atypical measles rash. **Panel A:** A petechial hemorrhagic rash in the patient localized to the trunk and upper extremities. **Panel B:** A closer view of the petechial rash showing a raised papular pattern. (Courtesy of Dr. Vincent A. Fulginiti.)

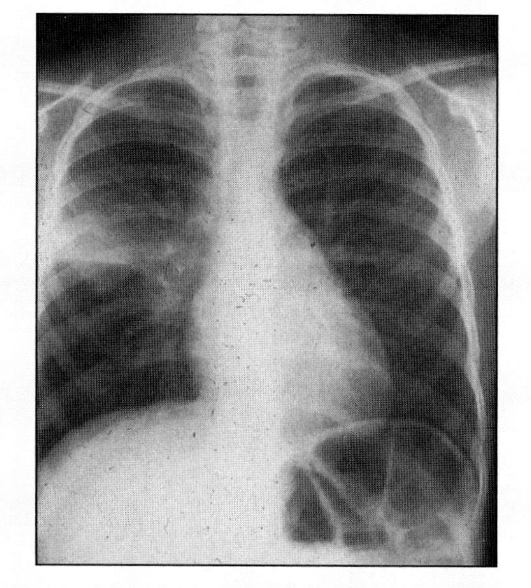

Figure 23-2. Chest roentgenogram of the patient showing right middle lobe infiltrate. (Courtesy of Dr. Vincent A. Fulginiti.)

This patient manifests a clinical entity referred to as atypical measles, a condition characterized by an altered immunologic expression of infection by measles virus that occurred in persons who had been given the old killed measles virus vaccine (which did not provide complete immunity and is no longer available). These subjects were paradoxically not only incompletely immunized against measles, but also became sensitized to the virus so that when they were later exposed to natural measles infection, the expression of the disease was altered in the form of the condition referred to as atypical measles.

Introduction

The use of vaccines is an example of active immunization where the initiation of immunity occurs after exposure of the host to an antigen following which humoral and cell-mediated components are stimulated in the recipient in the form of B cell and T cell immune responses. In contrast, passive immunization involves the transfer of antibody or gamma globulin formed in other hosts or in ex vivo systems to an unimmunized host to achieve protective immunity to an infectious disease or immunosuppression of an immunologically mediated disorder (*Chapter 11*). From time immemorial, the basic principles of protective immunity were elucidated from the study of infectious diseases. The use of vaccines for the prevention of infectious disease, also referred to as immunoprophylaxis, developed from the observation that individuals who recovered from a specific infectious disease did not contract that disease again. This notion of natural protective immunity can be traced back to the ancient Greeks who in the 5th century BC observed that individuals who had recovered from the plague of Athens were protected from subsequent attacks. This protective immune function that accompanied natural infection also led to an appreciation of the memory function of the immune system and the ability to boost immune responses. This forms the basis of vaccine usage through the capacity of the immune response to be greatly augmented following subsequent exposure to a previously experienced antigen (*Chapter 6*). However, it took hundreds of years to exploit and translate these ancient principles of protective immunity following natural infection to the prevention of infectious disease by vaccines.

The first successful efforts in the field of immunoprophylaxis evolved from a series of observations that ultimately led to the eradication of smallpox. The ancient Chinese had for centuries used powdered crusts taken from the skin lesions of patients with smallpox to immunize individuals by inhalation. Subsequently, the intradermal application of powdered smallpox crusts, a process referred to as **variolation**, was practiced in the Middle East and was brought to the Western world by Lady Mary Montagu (Figure 23-3). Both the Chinese and the Middle Eastern procedures, while effective in inducing protective immunity, were not without undesirable side effects since some of the subjects who received these primitive vaccines developed full-blown smallpox that was often fatal. Nonetheless, the practice of variolation was adopted in England since the morbidity and mortality of smallpox contracted by the procedure was considerably lower than that from natural infection.

The birth of the science of immunology was ushered in by Edward Jenner who, at the end of the 18th century, observed that milkmaids who came in contact with cattle infected with a virus related to smallpox, i.e., vaccinia (from the Latin *vacca*, for cow), were solidly protected against smallpox (Figure 23-4).

Jenner used the less dangerous vaccinia material obtained from a pustular lesion on the skin of a milkmaid to inoculate an eight-year-old boy and made the amazing observation that the child was immune to subsequent challenge to smallpox (Figure 23-5).

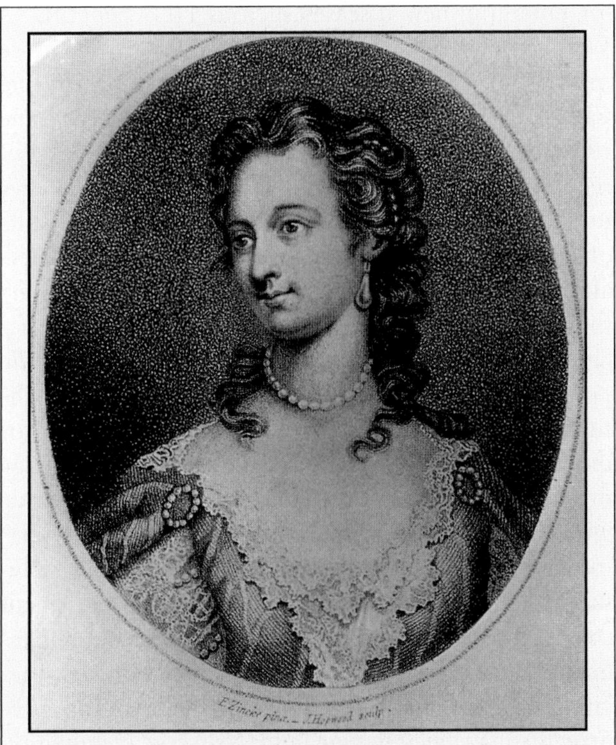

Figure 23-3. Lady Mary Wortley Montagu (1689–1762). (Courtesy of National Library of Medicine.)

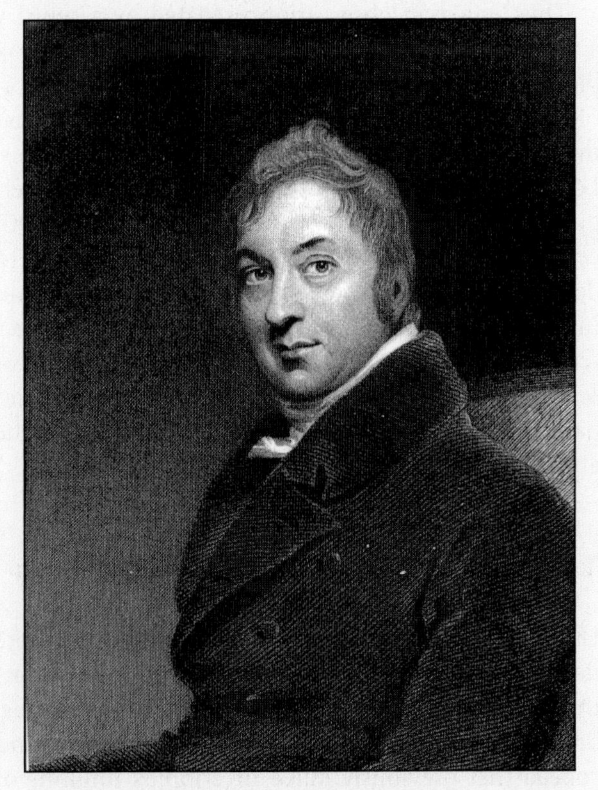

Figure 23-4. Edward Jenner (1749–1823). (Courtesy of National Library of Medicine.)

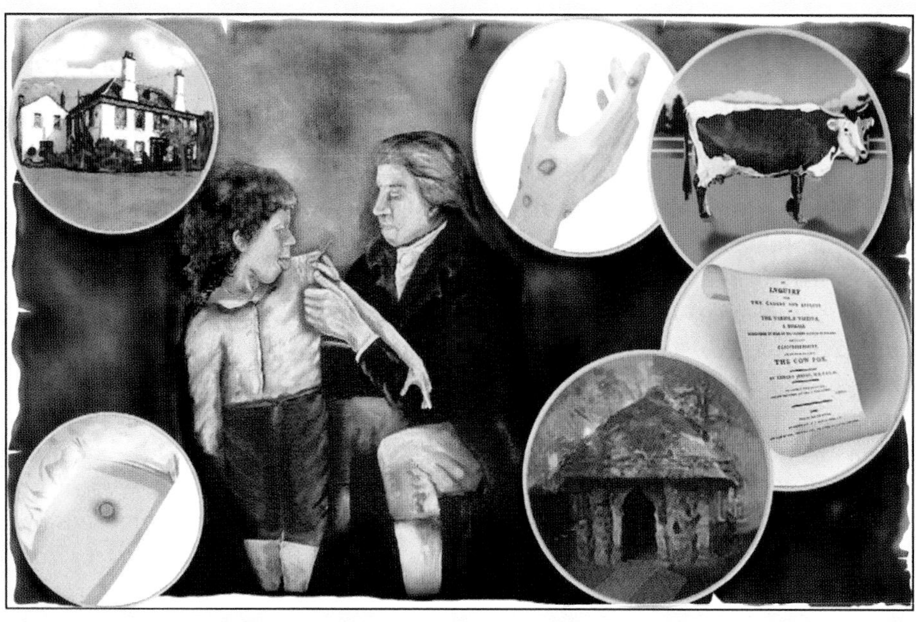

Figure 23-5. **Center: Edward Jenner inoculating eight-year-old James Phipps with cowpox.** Clockwise from upper left: Jenner's home, the Chantry, in Berkeley, United Kingdom (now the Edward Jenner Museum); lesions of cowpox on the hand of Sarah Nelmes, a dairymaid; Blossom, the cow that was a source of cowpox; Jenner's manuscript, "An Inquiry into the Causes and Effects of the Variolae Vaccinae, a Disease Discovered in Some of the Western Counties of England—Particularly Gloucestershire—and Known by the Name of the Cow Pox"; the "Temple of Vaccinia," where Jenner provided free vaccination to the people of Berkeley; and vaccinia lesions after inoculation. (Reproduced with permission from Mullin D. Prometheus in Gloucestershire: Edward Jenner, 1749–1823. J Allergy Clin Immunol. 2003; 112: 810–4.)

This Jennerian observation predated by a century a more scientific approach to vaccination that took place in the 19th century with the birth of microbiology and the discovery by Koch and Pasteur that infectious diseases were caused by microorganisms. Louis Pasteur and his coworkers succeeded in developing the first rabies vaccine at the end of the 19th century and thus established the basic principles to develop vaccines by "isolating, inactivating, and injecting infectious agents" (Figure 23-6). Large-scale vaccination came only after the discovery of safe and reproducible ways to inactivate toxins and pathogens by heat or formaldehyde or by the attenuation of pathogens by passage in vitro.

Technologies Used to Produce Vaccines

Using these simple basic technologies, vaccines were developed from 1920 to 1980 for the successful control of many infectious diseases, such as tetanus, diphtheria, poliomyelitis, pertussis, measles, and rubella that previously killed or crippled millions of people throughout the world. However, by the mid-1970s, these basic technologies were inadequate to address the need for development of newer vaccines for emerging new diseases such as HIV, hepatitis C, West Nile virus, and avian influenza, and more modern approaches were required. Thus, beginning with the 1980s, renewed enthusiasm in vaccine research was catapulted both by the advent of recombinant DNA technology as well as by a better understanding of the immune system. The results of these developments spawned a whole new generation of efficacious recombinant vaccines, including the rotavirus vaccine, the hepatitis A and B vaccines, and the acellular vaccine against *Bordetella pertussis.* Progress in the field of conjugation technology also provided a critical method for the production of more effective vaccines. This technology provided a method for joining a polysaccharide with a protein carrier that converted a thymic-independent antigen, i.e., polysaccharide, to a polysaccharide/protein hybrid with thymic-dependent properties. These polysaccharide/protein conjugates enabled the production of more highly effective vaccines against *Haemophilus influenzae* type b (**Hib**), *Streptococcus pneumoniae,* and *Neisseria meningitidis* than older vaccines made from purified polysaccharides alone.

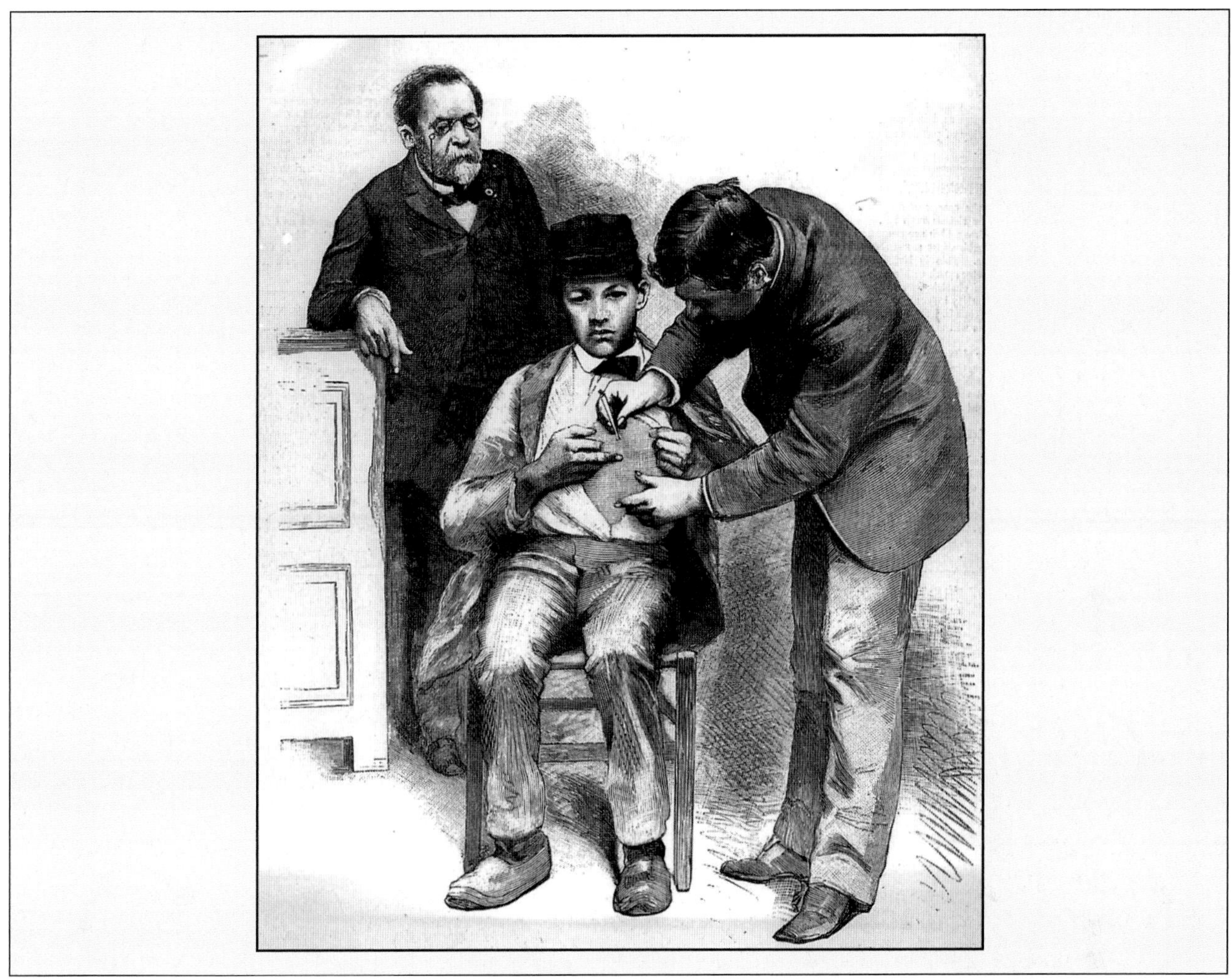

Figure 23-6. Louis Pasteur, at left, watches as an assistant inoculates a boy for "hydrophobia" (rabies). Wood engraving in "L'Illustration" for *Harper's Weekly*. 1885; 29: 836. (Courtesy of the National Library of Medicine.)

The Genomic Revolution of Vaccine Development

The availability of the first complete genome sequence of a free-living organism, i.e., *H. influenzae,* in 1995 marked the beginning of the "genomic era" that launched a totally new approach to vaccine design for the treatment of microbial infections that improved upon the classic Pasteur method. This methodology, called "reverse vaccinology," was not based on the more time-consuming classic method of isolating and growing microorganisms but rather on the use of algorithms to mine the genomic information encased within the DNA blueprint of the bacterium itself. This technologic revolution allowed for the first time the capacity to move beyond the confines imposed by the Pasteur method to a more modern computer-assisted technology. This, in turn, enabled the more rapid production of rationally designed vaccine candidates starting with information encoded within the microbial genome and then progressing to the identification and production of structural proteins for inclusion in vaccines. Shown in Figure 23-7 is a schematic representation comparing the Pasteur method with the reverse vaccinology method of vaccine development. The reverse vaccinology approach has been able to produce vaccine candidates, currently undergoing clinical trials, against *N. meningitidis* group B, a pathogen that could not be addressed by several decades of conventional vaccine development (Box 23-1).

Many novel antigens with properties that could overcome the limits of previous vaccine candidates were discovered and are now being tested in clinical trials. Today, the genome-based approach is routine

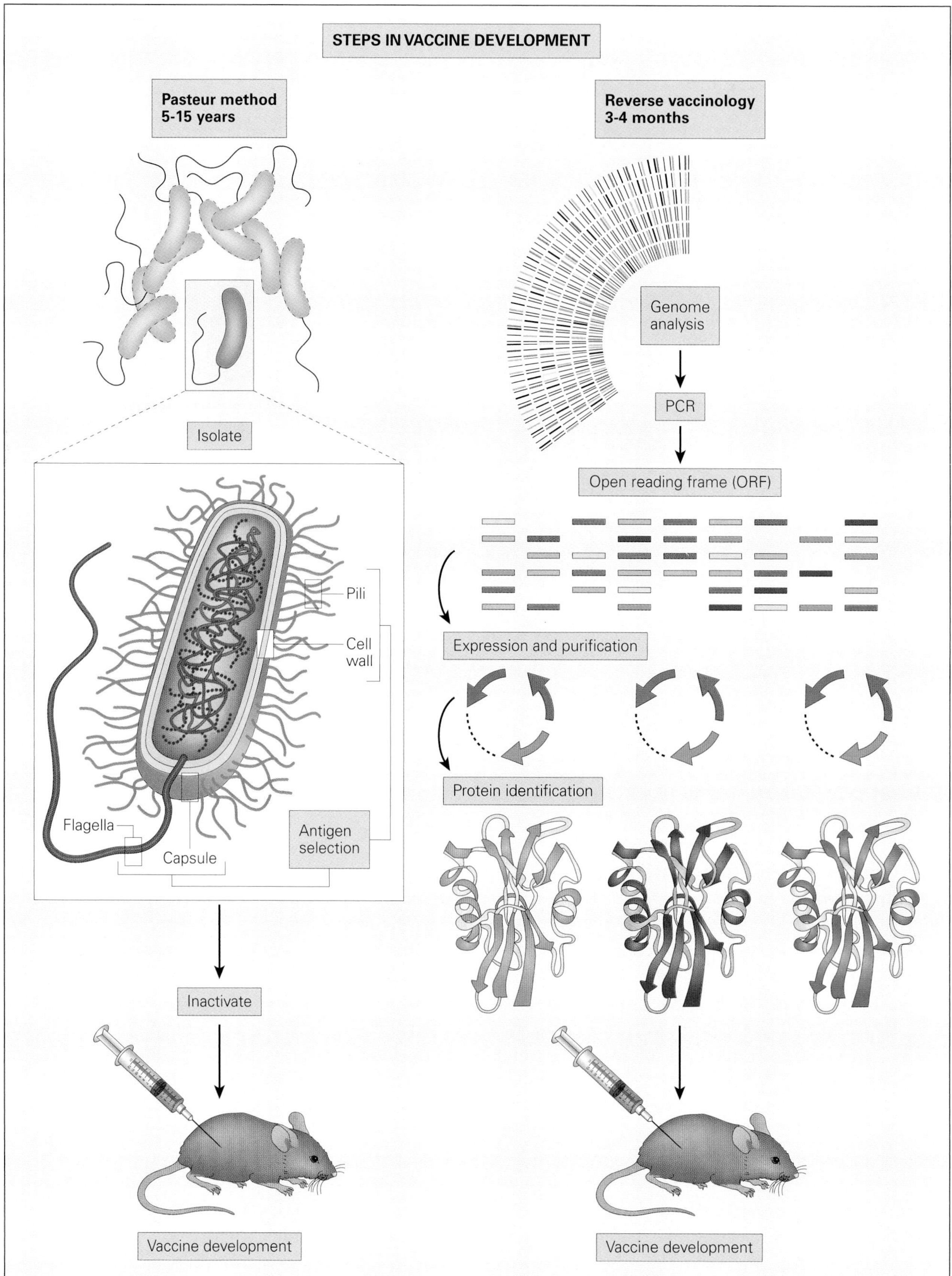

Figure 23-7. Schematic comparison of the Pasteur method with the reverse vaccinology method of vaccine development.

Box 23-1

The Development of the Meningococcal B Vaccine: The First Achievement of the Reverse Technology Technique.

The first pathogen addressed by the reverse vaccinology methodology was meningococcus serotype B (MenB), a pathogen that is responsible for 50 percent of meningococcal meningitis worldwide. This bacterium had been refractory to vaccine development because its capsular polysaccharide is structurally identical to a human polysaccharide "self-antigen" and therefore was not capable of evoking the reaction of foreignness essential for immune reactivity. The power of the reverse vaccinology technique allowed the identification of more than 90 previously unidentified surface antigens, 29 of which were capable of eliciting protective bactericidal antibody following immunization.

in vaccine development and is being applied to streptococci, *Chlamydiae*, staphylococci, *Plasmodium falciparum*, and other pathogens. The genomic revolution has been made possible by the rapidly evolving use of computers in biological research, i.e., biocomputing, which currently has become a powerful and crucial tool for vaccine development.

Benefits of Vaccinations

Vaccination represents one of the greatest triumphs of public health interventions ever made, sparing millions of people from the mortality and ravages of infectious diseases. It has been estimated that the use of currently available vaccines prevents the death of more than eight million lives annually, which translates into one person saved every five seconds. During the 20th century, vaccination, together with clean water, improved sanitation, and antimicrobial therapies, brought about the control of most infectious diseases, making it one of the greatest achievements of civilization.

The eradication of smallpox virus in 1977 represents one of the most brilliant successes of vaccination (Figure 23-8). It has been estimated that from the time of the development of the vaccine to the present, smallpox eradication has spared the global community some 350 million new smallpox victims and some 40 million deaths from the disease. The cost-benefit advantages of vaccination are equally impressive. The discontinuation of routine smallpox immunization and conversion of resources to other health needs has been estimated to have resulted in a savings of greater than $2 billion annually.

Vaccination has also resulted in the elimination of poliovirus from the Americas since 1994, the Western Pacific since 2000, and Europe since June 2002. Moreover, the incidence of seven other serious infectious diseases in the United States (diphtheria, measles, rubella, mumps, pertussis, Hib, and tetanus) has fallen by more than 98 percent (Table 23-1).

However, despite these outstanding achievements, the value of vaccines has been frequently ignored, often for economic reasons. Currently, although the production processes and costs of vaccine development are similar to those of other pharmaceuticals, the profitability for industry is relatively very low. In fact, the economic value associated with vaccines is considered less significant when compared with that of pharmaceuticals. Studies performed to evaluate economic benefits of vaccines have demonstrated significant cost-effectiveness when compared to cumulative costs of treatment, hospitalization, and lost working days. Although recent studies have demonstrated the cost-effectiveness of pediatric vaccination programs with diphtheria, tetanus, acellular pertussis (**DTaP**), measles, mumps, rubella (**MMR**), and Hib vaccines in the United States, a question may be raised: Are these the correct parameters to measure the value of vaccines? Although vaccines unquestionably are able to prevent death, disability, suffering, pain, and illness, how is it possible to quantify the value of a human life and the value of health? If these "intangible" values were to be included in a cost-benefit analysis, the present cost/benefit ratio would be grossly underestimated by a factor between 10 and 100, thus highlighting the real value of prevention.

Types of Vaccines

Vaccination has come a long way since Edward Jenner's first experiments with cowpox and smallpox in 1796, but its general concept is still the same—the induction of protective immunity and therefore prevention from disease. Immunity can be achieved either actively or passively. Active immunity is characterized by protection against a pathogen generated by a person's own immune system, which can be acquired either by natural infection or by active vaccination. In contrast, passive immunity is distinguished by

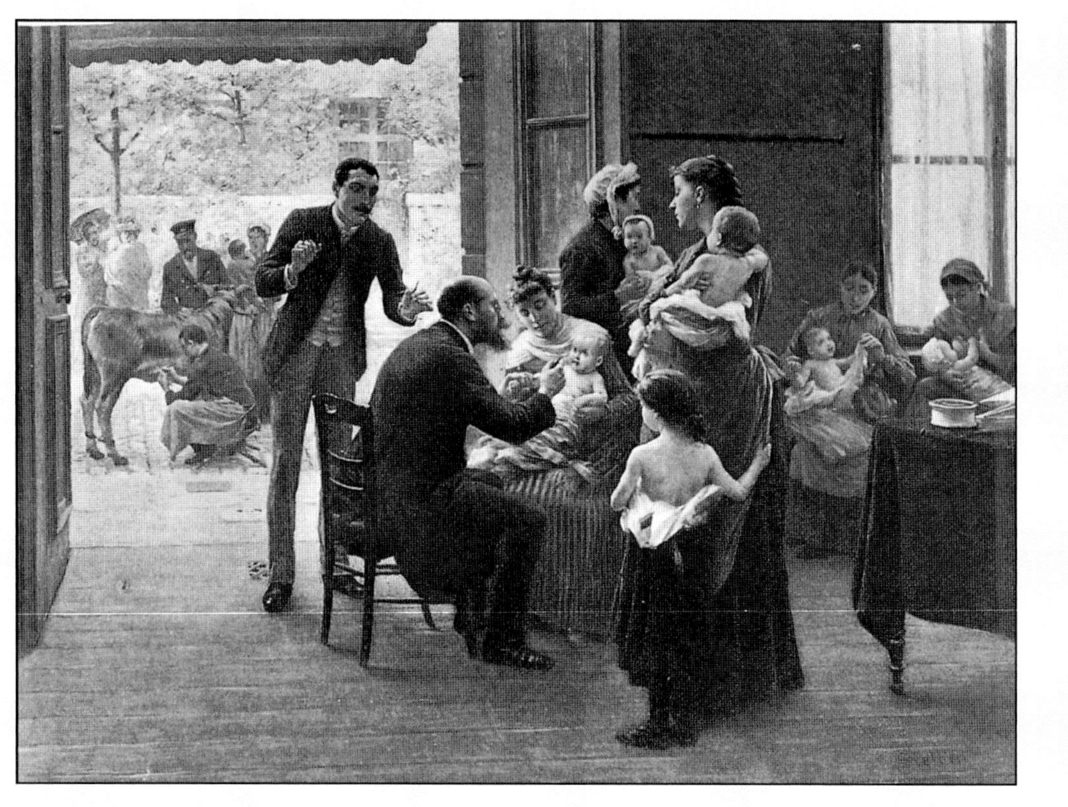

Figure 23-8. Administration of live smallpox vaccine by Scalbert. (Courtesy of the National Library of Medicine.)

protection provided by antibodies that are not produced by the recipient but rather by antibodies produced in other hosts or in vitro systems that can be transferred artificially by injection, or naturally, e.g., during pregnancy or by breast-feeding, resulting in transfer of antibody from the mother to the offspring.

For ease of discussion, vaccines can be broadly divided into three classic categories: live attenuated microorganisms, inactivated (killed) whole microorganisms, or purified subunit vaccines. Nucleic acid-based vaccines represent a newly emerging fourth category.

Table 23-1. Universal routine vaccination reduced by more than 98 percent the incidence of nine harmful diseases from the United States and eradicated two of them (smallpox and polio)

Disease	Maximum number of cases (year)	Number of cases in 2002	Reduction (%)
Smallpox	48,164 (1901–1904)	0	<100.0
Poliomyelitis	21,269 (1952)	0	100.0
Diphtheria	206,939 (1921)	1	99.99
Measles	894,134 (1941)	44	99.90
Rubella	57,686 (1969)	18	99.78
Mumps	152,209 (1968)	270	99.86
Pertussis	265,269 (1934)	9771	98.20
H. influenzae type b	20,000 (1992)	<100	98.79
Tetanus	1,560 (1923)	25	98.44

Source: CDC 1998. Impact of vaccines universally recommended for children—U.S., 1990–98. *MMWR* 48: 577–81; modified.

Live Attenuated Vaccines

Live attenuated vaccines are prepared by modifying disease-producing ("wild") viruses or bacteria in a manner whereby they lose almost or all of their pathogenic properties. As a result, the vaccine organism retains the ability to replicate in humans but to such a low extent that it usually does not cause illness. Over a limited period of time, it provides a continuous antigenic stimulation to the immune system. The immune response to the vaccine virus is virtually identical to that produced by natural infection because the immune system does not differentiate between an infection with a weakened vaccine pathogen and an infection with the wild type. Therefore, live attenuated vaccines induce both humoral and cell-mediated immunity and generally are effective after a single dose, except those administered orally. There are many examples of highly successful vaccines that have been developed using live attenuated pathogens. Historically, those widely used vaccines were generated either by exposure of the pathogen to an environmental insult like chemicals or elevated temperatures, or by repeated in vitro passage of the pathogens. The molecular mechanisms of their attenuation were poorly understood; today, such noncharacterized vaccines would be difficult for their introduction into the marketplace. However, today's available genomic technology permits a more rational creation of live attenuated bacterial and viral strains by modification of their genome. Live attenuated vaccines available in the United States include live viruses and live bacteria.

There are several limitations for the use of live attenuated vaccines: (1) pregnancy of the recipient (although there are no solid scientific data available for a contraindication and more research is required to definitively address this concern); (2) circulating antibody to the vaccine pathogen, e.g., maternally derived antibodies that can make the vaccine ineffective by interference with replication of the vaccine organism, which would result in a poor or no response to the vaccine. Measles vaccine virus seems to be most sensitive to blockage by circulating antibody; poliovirus and rotavirus vaccine viruses are least affected. Maternally derived serum IgG antibodies are less efficient at restricting replication of attenuated viral vaccines administered mucosally rather than those systemically; (3) live attenuated pathogens can theoretically replicate to a relatively higher degree in immunocompromised persons (e.g., patients with leukemia, or those treated with immunosuppressive drugs, or with HIV infection or with primary immunodeficiencies) and therefore are more susceptible to severe or fatal reactions; (4) the vaccine pathogen can lose its attenuation during manufacture or during replication in vaccine recipients by reversion or second-site compensatory mutations, resulting in serious disease. This was known to occur with the live (oral) poliovirus vaccine (**OPV**) that led to its replacement with the safer inactivated poliovirus vaccine (**IPV**) in industrialized countries; (5) the potential risk for contamination of the vaccine with live adventitious pathogens during manufacturing; and (6) anything that damages the live organism like heat and light can cause the vaccine to be ineffective so it must be handled and stored very carefully.

Inactivated Vaccines

The easiest method to prepare an inactivated vaccine is through the use of heat and/or chemical treatment of the bacteria or viruses. The chemicals used for inactivation include formaldehyde or beta-propiolactone. Since inactivated vaccines do not contain living microbes and therefore do not replicate in the host, these vaccines cannot cause disease from infection by the given pathogen, even in immunocompromised persons. Another advantage is that all antigens present in the pathogen are also included in the vaccine. On the other hand, some of the antigens retained in the vaccine may have toxic properties and may be responsible for undesirable adverse side effects. Since inactivated vaccines are nonreplicative, to be effective, they must contain relatively much more antigen than live vaccines that exert their effects through amplification in the immunized host. The inactivated vaccines, therefore, always require multiple or booster dose administration. In general, the first dose does not produce protective immunity, but primes the immune system. A protective immune response develops after the second, or third, or even fourth dose of vaccine. This is particularly important during the routine immunization of infants and children where a protective and durable immune response may require several booster doses of vaccines. Unlike live attenuated vaccines, inactivated antigens are usually not affected by circulating antibody. Thus, inactivated vaccines may be given when antibody is present in the blood (e.g., in infancy, or following receipt of antibody-containing blood products). Another distinguishing feature from live attenuated vaccines is the quality of the immune response; inactivated vaccines induce mostly humoral and little or no cellular immunity. The antibody titers against inactivated antigens diminish with time, and as a result, most inactivated vaccines require periodic supplemental doses to increase or boost antibody titers. Shown in Table 23-2 is a comparison of the properties of live attenuated and inactivated vaccines together with characteristics of the immunization responses to these vaccines related to the status of the antigen.

Subunit Vaccines

Subunit vaccines consist of one or more of the purified components of the microbial antigens encompassing the major antigenic sites of a pathogen. Therefore, it is critical to identify the correct immunogen(s) of the pathogen that are involved in inducing protective immunity before developing subunit vaccines. A striking advantage of subunit vaccines is that antigens causing undesirable side effects could be theoretically excluded from the vaccine preparation, thereby increasing their safety. Moreover, some proteins, if included in the vaccine, may paradoxically suppress the immune response, whereas other proteins may actually enhance disease. Since fewer components are usually included in subunit vaccines, there is less antigenic competitive inhibition than in vaccine preparations containing whole microbial constituents. Unfortunately, subunit vaccines are generally less efficacious than whole inactivated vaccines and most of them require adjuvants to give a solid protective immune response. The decreased protective immunogenicity might be a result of nonnative conformation of the antigens, so that the antibodies produced against the subunit may not recognize the same protein on the surface of the intact pathogen. Antigens, from which subunit vaccines are produced, are purified either directly from the pathogen or are expressed in prokaryotic or eukaryotic cells of mammalian, yeast, or insect origin using recombinant DNA technology (*Chapter 25*).

The first subunit vaccines were developed in the 1920s and included diphtheria and tetanus bacterial toxoids, i.e., formalin-inactivated toxins. The rationale for development of these toxoids derived from the observation that since the clinical manifestations of diphtheria or tetanus were caused largely by toxins produced by their respective disease-causing bacteria, it followed that the production of antitoxin neutralizing antibodies was the essential component of protective immunity (*Chapter 12*). The discovery of an effective method to detoxify tetanus and diphtheria toxin by formaldehyde treatment retaining the beneficial immunogenic but eliminating the pathogenic properties allowed the introduction of mass immunization

Table 23-2. Comparison of the properties of live attenuated and inactivated vaccines together with characteristics of the immunization responses related to the status of the antigen

Property	Nonreplicative (killed or inactivated vaccines)	Replicative (live attenuated vaccines)
Example	Bacterial diphtheria, tetanus, acellular pertussis (DTaP) Some viral (inactivated poliovirus [IPV], influenza, hepatitis B)	Viral (rubeola, rubella, mumps [MMR], oral poliovirus [OPV], yellow fever, rotavirus, influenza)
Route of administration	Systemic: subcutaneous	Systemic: subcutaneous (MMR, yellow fever); mucosal: oral (OPV, rotavirus); nasal (influenza)
Immunization principle	Preformed antigenic mass	Self-replicative
Effect of passive serum antibody	No inhibitory effect	May prevent successful immunization, i.e., systemic vaccines; less effect with mucosal vaccines
Duration of immunity	Relatively short; requires "boosters"	Relatively long (mimic natural infection); do not usually require boosters
Prime immunity mechanism(s)	Humoral (IgG)	Humoral (IgG, IgA); cellular immunity

that led to the almost complete elimination of both diseases from developed countries.

Another group of subunit vaccines include polysaccharide vaccines directed against encapsulated bacteria. As described previously in Chapter 12, capsular polysaccharide is the major virulence factor for many important pathogens, e.g., *Streptococcus pneumoniae*. The well-known susceptibility of patients with humoral immune deficiencies to infections caused by these encapsulated bacteria (*Chapter 16*) is supported by the observation that nonencapsulated mutants are nonpathogenic due to their high susceptibility to serum complement. Thus, capsular polysaccharides have been used to develop subunit vaccines against *N. meningitidis* group A (**MenA**), group C (MenC), group Y (MenY), and group W135 (MenW135), against 23 serotypes of *S. pneumoniae*, against *H. influenzae* type b (Hib), and against *Salmonella typhi*.

Despite their clinically proven effectiveness, these vaccines have several disadvantages. Since capsular polysaccharides are T-independent antigens (*Chapter 6*), they are able to induce only short-lived antibody responses, mainly of IgM and IgG_2 isotypes in adults. Moreover, their immunogenicity and efficacy are very poor or absent in children, especially those below two years of age. In addition, polysaccharides do not induce immunological memory, and repeated immunization does not augment specific antibody titers. Paradoxically, the induction of immune tolerance has been described in adults following immunization with these capsular polysaccharides. The resolution of many of these obstacles was provided by the conjugation technology described previously that allows the generation of semi-synthetic conjugated vaccines, as described more fully below.

Recombinant DNA Technology and New Subunit Vaccines

The subsequent progress of recombinant DNA technology in the late 1970s allowed the further development of new subunit vaccines, exemplified by recombinant vaccines against hepatitis B (**HBV**), the acellular vaccines against *B. pertussis*, and most recently against the human papillomaviruses (**HPV**). The observation that serum antibodies elicited by the surface protein of the HBV (HBsAg) were able to neutralize the virus and to generate protective immunity led to the development of plasma-derived HBsAg subunit vaccines. However, this early vaccine could not be produced in sufficient quantities since the virus could only be purified from the plasma of infected patients, raising safety concerns about possible transmission of plasma-derived infections. The application of the recombinant DNA technology allowed the production of safer yeast- and mammalian cell-derived vaccines, which rapidly replaced the older plasma-derived vaccine. In 1992, the Global Advisory Group of the World Health Organization recommended that all countries integrate hepatitis B vaccine into their national immunization programs. So far, more than 160 countries have followed this recommendation (WHO, 2004). The main objective of hepatitis B immunization strategies is to prevent chronic HBV infection and its serious consequences, including liver cirrhosis and hepatocellular cancer. Studies performed in Taiwan have clearly demonstrated a reduction in the incidence of primary liver cancer in children born after the implementation of routine infant hepatitis B vaccination programs. The recombinant HBV vaccine is thus the first successful vaccine preventing cancer.

The genetically detoxified pertussis toxin (**PT**) was the first recombinant bacterial subunit vaccine that was developed. A vaccine composed of the whole, inactivated *B. pertussis* cells had been available for mass vaccination since the late 1940s. Although this vaccine was very efficacious in preventing the disease, the severe adverse reactions, although never proven to be caused by the vaccine, not only contributed to a fall in vaccine compliance during the 1970s, but raised a need for a new, safer vaccine. Since the pertussis toxin represents one of the primary virulence factors of *B. pertussis*, a major investigative effort was directed to the development of acellular pertussis vaccines containing the purified chemically inactivated PT. However, it was subsequently recognized that the formaldehyde and glutaraldehyde treated PT was susceptible to reversion to a more pathogenic form. To overcome these problems, Pizza and coworkers developed a mutant PT by genetic engineering, having the same antigenic properties as the wild type, but without toxicity. Several clinical trials were initiated in children and adults using a monovalent vaccine or a combination of the mutant PT with other pertussis antigens, demonstrating the safety of the nontoxic PT mutant. Moreover, the safety profile of the mutant PT vaccine was found to be superior to a whole cell pertussis vaccine. Furthermore, all formulations of the mutant PT vaccine induced high titers of long-lasting anti-PT neutralizing antibodies and very strong antigen-specific T cell responses.

The repertoire of effective viral subunit vaccines became enormously expanded by the observation that protective antigens of a large number of enveloped and nonenveloped RNA and DNA viruses can self-assemble into virus-like particles (**VLPs**). As the name implies, VLPs are three-dimensional structures that mimic the appearance of native virions. They are formed when one or more viral structural proteins are co-expressed in eukaryotic or prokaryotic cells and self-assemble into virus-like structures. Unlike the whole virus, they are not infectious because of a lack of the viral genome. Generally, VLPs are highly immunogenic because they display a large number of antigenic sites and conformational epitopes in the same way that native virus particles do. There are two VLP-derived vaccines directed against certain HPV subtypes. One vaccine is directed against two subtypes, i.e., 16 and 18, which are associated with cervical cancer; the other vaccine is directed against four subtypes and not only contains subtypes 16 and 18, but also subtypes 6 and 11, which cause genital warts. After having been shown to be highly efficient in clinical trials, both vaccines have been licensed and are available for clinical use.

The Future of Subunit Vaccine Development: The Genomic Approach

The possibility to have access to the whole genome sequences of the vast majority of microorganisms has completely revolutionized the prospects and the idea of vaccine development. The genomic approach or "reverse vaccinology" did not arise from microbiology, but rather from the comprehensive genomic sequence of the pathogen made possible by rigorous computer analysis that can predict those antigens that are most likely to be vaccine candidates. The comprehension of the genome of a microorganism now makes unnecessary the cultivation and human handling of the pathogen itself, in marked contrast to the earlier conventional approach. The analysis of the microbial genome allows the simultaneous visualization of all the protein antigens encoded within its structure irrespective of the degree of in vitro and in vivo expression or the specific phase of microbial growth. This technology not only avoids exposure to dangerous pathogens, but also offers the unique possibility for vaccine development even for those pathogens that cannot be cultured. Moreover, the process allows the identification not only of all the antigens selected using the conventional biochemical, serological, and microbiological methods, but also the discovery of novel, unknown antigens. The availability of suitable animal models of infection and the knowledge of immunological correlates of protection, however, are still essential to identify good vaccine candidates. Unfortunately, as good correlates of protection are infrequent, this may limit the speed and the effectiveness of the approach. Another limit of the genomic approach is its inability to identify nonprotein antigens, such as polysaccharides, which are currently considered important components of successful vaccines, and to identify CD1-restricted antigens such as glycolipids, which represent new promising vaccine candidates, as in the case of tuberculosis (Box 23-2).

As described previously, the first successful application of the reverse vaccinology approach is represented by the meningococcus serotype B (**MenB**), for which for more than 40 years of research with conventional approaches have failed. The screening and the analysis of the complete genome of the virulent strain MenB MC58 has provided several conserved, surface-exposed, immunogenic antigens that are now undergoing clinical trials in humans. After the successful experience with MenB, many other important bacterial pathogens are being addressed using the genomic approach (*Streptococcus agalactiae*, *Streptococcus pyogenens*, *Porphyromonas gingivalis*, and *Chlamydia trachomatis*). Moreover, better vaccines directed against parasites and viruses could be developed by the use of the reverse vaccinology.

Conjugated Vaccines

In 1996, the prestigious Laskey prize was awarded for the development of conjugated vaccines, created by the chemical coupling of a polysaccharide to a carrier protein. As described previously, this procedure converts T-independent antigens (like polysaccharides) into T-dependent antigens by providing a source of appropriate T cell epitopes (located on the carrier protein) capable of priming carrier specific T cells, which will then provide help to B cells

Box 23-2

CD1-Restricted Antigens and New TB Vaccines

In recent years, many efforts have focused on the identification of new vaccine candidates against *Mycobacterium tuberculosis*. These vaccine candidates include live attenuated DNA and subunit vaccines. However, most vaccine candidates against TB, including the BCG vaccine, are thought to protect the host by augmenting cell-mediated immunity to control mycobacterial replication (*Chapter 12*). This mechanism of protection differs substantially from that of most vaccines currently used in humans against many extracellular pathogens that generally confer protection by eliciting protective antibody (Ab) responses. For many decades, the scientific paradigm was that Ab plays little or no role in the host defense against intracellular pathogens such as *M. tuberculosis*. However, in recent years, studies from several laboratories using monoclonal Abs (mAbs) have demonstrated beneficial effects of Abs on various aspects of *M. tuberculosis* infection. CD1 represents one member of a family of five nonpolymorphic MHC-I molecules in humans (CD1a to -e) that present lipid-associated carbohydrate structures to CD1-restricted T cells. The *M. tuberculosis* virulence factors LAM and PIM are glycolipid antigens that bind CD1b and CD1d, leading to activation of CD1b-restricted αβ Th cells and CD1d-restricted natural killer-like T (NKT) cells, respectively. Other *M. tuberculosis* Abs, such as those directed against mycolic acid, also stimulate CD1b-restricted T cells. These studies suggest that Abs can have beneficial effects on the course of *M. tuberculosis* infection and provide a new rationale for the development of Ab-inducing vaccine candidates. Learning how to appropriately stimulate CD1-restricted T cell responses may be, therefore, critical in the successful development of such new TB vaccines.

for the production of polysaccharide-specific antibodies. The carrier proteins utilized in the development of conjugate vaccines included tetanus toxoid, diphtheria toxoid, and the nontoxic mutant of the diphtheria toxin, referred to as the cross-reacting material (**CRM**) 197. This technology has been successfully applied to the development of conjugated vaccines, which now represent a powerful tool replacing the pure polysaccharide vaccines.

The first conjugate vaccines developed were directed against Hib. Conjugated Hib vaccines were shown to be highly immunogenic and efficacious, to induce immune memory, immunoglobulin isotype switching, and antibody affinity maturation in children less than 18 months, all properties that were not manifested by the pure polysaccharide vaccines. These conjugate vaccines have not only been introduced in several industrialized countries throughout the world (often in combination with the diphtheria, tetanus, and pertussis vaccines), but their use is also now being implemented in developing countries. In the countries where it has been used to immunize infants, often starting at the age of two months, the conjugated Hib vaccine has contributed to a dramatic reduction in the incidence of invasive Hib diseases. In addition, vaccination has resulted in a reduction of Hib carriage that has resulted in a reduced transmission of the bacteria to unimmunized subjects, a phenomenon referred to as herd immunity.

The success of Hib conjugate vaccines prompted several groups to consider the development of conjugated vaccines against the other two capsulated pathogens that are the most frequent cause of bacterial meningitis: *N. meningitidis* and *S. pneumoniae.*

The first conjugated vaccines against meningococcus C (**MenC**) were licensed in the United Kingdom in 1999–2000 and used in national immunization campaigns. The results were impressive: within a few months, cases of MenC meningitis almost disappeared in the vaccinated population. Moreover, the vaccine provides some evidence of herd immunity, as there is also a reduction of MenC disease in unvaccinated individuals.

The first conjugated vaccine against serogroup A, C, Y, and W135 was licensed in the United States in 2005 and a second in 2010. These conjugated vaccines have been recommended by the U.S. Advisory Committee on Immunization Practices (ACIP) for all persons 11–18 years of age, as well as for anyone 2–55 years of age who is at increased risk of meningococcal disease. Revaccination is also recommended for individuals starting college who had received a polysaccharide vaccine five or more years previously.

In 2000, a heptavalent-conjugated vaccine against pneumococcus (PCV7) was licensed in the United States containing polysaccharides from seven serotypes (4, 6B, 9V, 14, 18C, 19F, and 23F) conjugated to the CRM197 as a carrier protein. This vaccine was shown to be safe, highly immunogenic in all age groups, and efficacious to prevent invasive diseases caused by *S. pneumoniae* strains covered by the vaccine. A 13-valent version of the vaccine

(PCV13) containing polysaccharides from 13 serotypes (the same contained in the licensed heptavalent vaccine plus 1, 3, 5, 6A, 7F, and 19A) was licensed by the U.S. Food and Drug Administration (FDA) for prevention of invasive pneumococcal disease (IPD) caused by the 13 pneumococcal serotypes covered by the vaccine and for prevention of otitis media caused by serotypes in the 7-heptavalent pneumococcal conjugate vaccine formulation (PCV7). PCV13 is approved for use in the United States among children aged six weeks to 71 months and succeeds PCV7, which was licensed by the FDA in 2010.

A similar approach is now under consideration for the development of subunit vaccines against other pathogens. For example, a conjugate vaccine consisting of the capsular polysaccharide Vi of *S. tyhpi* conjugated to a nontoxic recombinant *Pseudomonas aeruginosa* exotoxin A was more than 90 percent efficacious against typhoid fever after two immunizations, six weeks apart, in two- to five-year-old children in a highly endemic area. Other conjugate vaccines are under development against various serotypes of group B streptococci using the type-specific capsular polysaccharides and against *Shigella sonnei* and *S. flexneri* using the O-specific polysaccharide of LPS.

Next-Generation Vaccines

DNA Vaccines

DNA vaccines represent a relatively new and potentially useful fourth category of vaccine development. The concept is relatively simple; plasmid DNA that encodes a protective antigen under the control of a powerful promoter active in eukaryotic cells is directly administered into the vaccinees. The most important advantage of DNA vaccines is that the antigen is expressed in cells of the vaccinated person and is presented to the immune system in its native conformation. Therefore, this strategy sidesteps the purification process of vaccine antigens, which is costly and can adversely affect vaccine efficacy. The expressed vaccine antigen is processed by the cell and epitopes are presented efficiently to the immune system by both the MHC-I pathway for CTL induction and the MHC-II restricted pathways for the induction of T helper (T_H) cells and B cells. In this way, a very balanced immune response is induced more similar to infection-induced immunity than by an inactivated pathogen. Another advantage is that the DNA does not interfere with existing antibodies. The first-generation DNA vaccines have been shown to be effective in small animals but they show only very limited effectiveness in large animals and humans. This might be due to inefficient transfection of DNA into cells and low expression level of the vaccine antigen. However, the technology has improved considerably by the use of various adjuvants and by optimizing the DNA vectors and their delivery.

Vector Vaccines

The use of live viral or bacterial vectors to deliver DNA or RNA encoding antigens into cells is another promising approach for vaccination. Some bacterial delivery systems (e.g., *Shigella* and *Listeria* monocytogenes) have been developed that are able to release plasmid DNA encoding the antigen from the bacteria into the cytosol of cells, where the genes are translated, processed, and presented to the immune system. In contrast to the DNA delivery systems of bacteria, viral vectors have the gene encoding the antigen integrated in their genome (*Chapter 13*). Either attenuated or replication-defective viruses are being employed to construct viable recombinants that express the protective antigen. Poxviruses (e.g., vaccinia virus, modified vaccinia virus Ankara [MVA], and Avipoxvirus) contain a large genome in which foreign genes can be integrated. These viruses are highly attenuated in humans but still replication competent and therefore bear a potential safety risk, especially for immunocompromised persons. In contrast, replication-defective virus vectors do not cause a productive infection because genes essential for the virus life cycle are deleted from the viral genome; genes encoding the vaccine antigen replace them. Therefore, the viral vectors undergo only an abortive infection in vivo; the virus enters cells, where the viral genome containing the antigen is expressed, processed, and presented to the immune system. Generally, vector vaccines are able to induce very potent humoral and cellular immune responses. As in the case of live attenuated vaccines, preexisting humoral immunity against the virus vector, mediated by maternal antibodies, previous infection, or vaccination, can decrease the efficacy of the vaccine. Many different virus vectors have been engineered and some of them, such as the vaccinia virus vector, adenovirus, or alphavirus vector systems, have been already tested in clinical trials but are not yet approved for human use.

Standard Vaccines for Industrialized Countries and Recommendations for Their Usage

Recommendations for immunization practices are based on scientific knowledge of vaccine characteristics, the principles of immunization, the epidemiology of specific diseases, and host characteristics. In addition, the experience and judgment of public health officials and specialists in clinical and preventive medicine play a key role in developing recommendations that maximize the benefits and minimize the risk and costs associated with immunization.

Principles of Vaccine Scheduling

Optimal responses to a vaccine depend on multiple factors, including the nature of the vaccine as well as the age and immune status of the recipient (Figure 23-9). Recommendations for the age at which vaccines are administered are influenced by age-specific risks for disease, age-specific risks for complications, capacity of persons of a certain age to respond to the vaccine, and potential interference with the immune response by passively transferred antibody. Vaccines that have demonstrated efficacy and safety are recommended for members of the youngest age group at risk for experiencing the disease for which the vaccine is being administered.

Measles vaccine provides a good example of this concept. The optimal timing for administration of this vaccine depends on both the rate of disappearance of passively acquired maternal antibodies and the risk of exposure to measles virus. At birth and in the first six months of life, most infants have passively acquired serum antibody to measles virus because of transplacentally acquired maternal specific antibodies. These antibodies limit both wild type and vaccine viral replication, thus interfering with the immune response. In many developing countries, where measles is highly epidemic and frequently affects infants, routine measles vaccination is recommended at the age of nine months. However, in developed countries, where measles is less common, measles vaccine is recommended routinely at age 12 to 15 months.

As described previously, mucosal immunization offers a potential advantage to this age-related limitation of measles immunization. The pioneering studies of Sabin established the utility of aerosol methods of measles immunization in a set of classic studies in Mexican children. In contrast to immunization with live vaccines administered by the parenteral route where efficacy is limited by the presence of the maternally derived serum antibody, the aerosol route appears to be less affected by the presence of transplacentally acquired serum antibody, thus allowing the successful vaccination of younger infants, e.g., six to seven months of age, when measles has the greatest morbidity and mortality. Studies of measles vaccines administered by aerosol immunization continue and in the near future may provide additional advantages similar to those seen with other vaccines developed for mucosal immunization, e.g., influenza vaccine live, intranasal vaccine.

Spacing of Vaccines

Most vaccines, particularly the inactivated vaccines such as the toxoids, recombinant subunit, and polysaccharide conjugate vaccines, require the administration of greater than two doses for development of an adequate and durable antibody response. Tetanus and diphtheria toxoids require periodic reinforcement or booster doses to maintain protective antibody concentrations. In contrast, a single dose of a live attenuated virus vaccine is generally considered sufficient for the induction of a prolonged, often lifelong protective immune response. However, since vaccine-induced antibody titers have been shown recently to decline temporally more rapidly than those induced by natural infection, durable and long-lasting protective immunity may require an adult booster dose of live attenuated vaccine. Approximately 90–95 percent of recipients of a single dose of a parenterally administered live vaccine at the recommended age (i.e., MMR, varicella, and yellow fever) develop protective antibodies within two weeks. However, because a limited proportion of recipients (< 5 percent) of MMR vaccine fail to respond to one dose, a second dose is recommended to provide another opportunity to develop immunity. The majority of persons who fail to respond to the first dose of MMR respond to a second dose. In the same way, if approximately 20 percent of persons aged > 13 years fail to respond to the first dose of varicella vaccine, 99 percent of recipients seroconvert after two doses. These

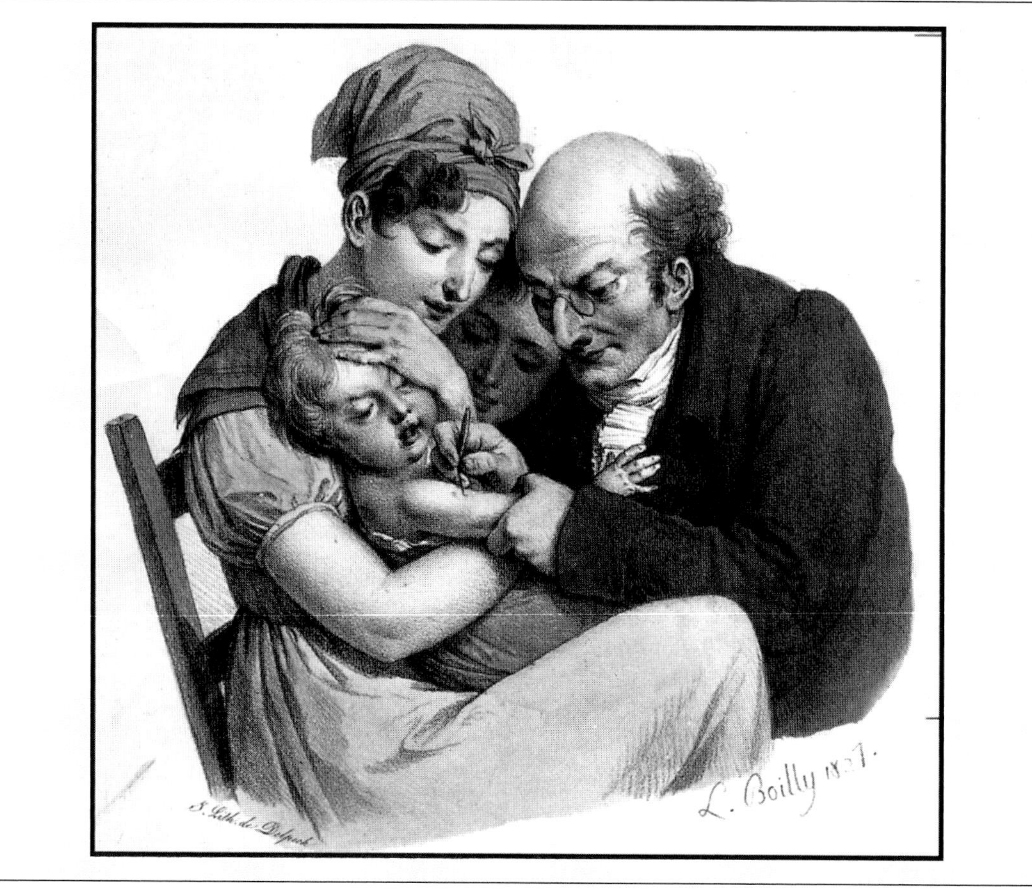

Figure 23-9. Vaccination of an infant with smallpox vaccine illustrating the effect of age on vaccine effectiveness. (From L. L. Boilly, 1827; courtesy of the National Library of Medicine.)

multiple doses constitute a primary vaccination series and are not "booster" doses.

Clinical studies confirm that recommended ages and intervals between doses of multidose antigens provide optimal protection or have the best evidence of efficacy. Shown in Table 23-3 are the recommended vaccines and minimum ages and intervals between vaccine doses. Because of immunological memory, longer than recommended intervals between doses do not diminish the immunologic responses to live attenuated vaccines as well as to the inactivated vaccines that usually require more than one dose to achieve primary immunity. Similarly, delayed administration of recommended booster doses does not reduce the antibody response to such doses. Thus the interruption of a recommended primary series or an extended lapse between booster doses does not require reinitiation of the whole vaccination series.

In certain circumstances, administering doses of a multidose vaccine at shorter than the recommended intervals might be necessary. This can occur when a person is behind schedule and needs to be brought up-to-date as quickly as possible or when international travel is impending. In these situations, an accelerated schedule can be used with intervals between doses shorter than those recommended for routine vaccination. Although the effectiveness of all accelerated schedules has not always been evaluated in clinical trials, immune response induced by accelerated intervals is believed to induce adequate protection.

However, vaccine doses should not be administered at intervals less than the minimum intervals or earlier than the minimum age. Administration of doses of a vaccine at intervals less than the minimum intervals or earlier than the minimum age may result in a reduced immune response with reduced vaccine efficacy and should be avoided (Table 23-2). Conversely, too-frequent administration of some inactivated vaccines, such as tetanus toxoid, can result in increased rates of localized

Table 23-3. Recommended and minimum ages and intervals between vaccine doses

Vaccine and dose number	Recommended age for this dose	Minimum age for this dose	Recommended interval to next dose	Minimum interval to next dose
Hepatitis B-1	Birth	Birth	1–4 months	4 weeks
Hepatitis B-2	1–2 months	4 weeks	2–17 months	8 weeks
Hepatitis B-3	6–18 months	24 weeks	—	—
Diphtheria-tetanus-acellular pertussis (DTaP)-1	2 months	6 weeks	2 months	4 weeks
DTaP-2	4 months	10 weeks	2 months	4 weeks
DTaP-3	6 months	14 weeks	6–12 months	6 months
DTaP-4	15–18 months	12 months	3 years	6 months
DTaP-5	4–6 years	4 years	—	—
Haemophilus influenzae, type b (Hib)-1	2 months	6 weeks	2 months	4 weeks
Hib-2	4 months	10 weeks	2 months	4 weeks
Hib-3	6 months	14 weeks	6–9 months	8 weeks
Hib-4	12–15 months	12 months	—	—
Inactivated poliovirus (IPV)-1	2 months	6 weeks	2 months	4 weeks
IPV-2	4 months	10 weeks	2–14 months	4 weeks
IPV-3	6–18 months	14 weeks	3.5 years	6 months
IPV-4	4–6 years	4 years	—	—
Pneumococcal conjugate (PCV)-1	2 months	6 weeks	8 weeks	4 weeks
PCV-2	4 months	10 weeks	8 weeks	4 weeks
PCV-3	6 months	14 weeks	6 months	8 weeks
PCV-4	12–15 months	12 months	—	—
Measles, mumps, rubella (MMR)-1	12–15 months	12 months	3–5 years	4 weeks
MMR-2	4–6 years	13 months	—	—
Varicella (Var)-1	12–15 months	12 months	3–5 years	12 weeks
Var-2	4–6 years	15 months	—	—
Hepatitis A (HepA)-1	12–23 months	12 months	6–18 months	6 months
HepA-2	18–41 months	18 months	—	—
Influenza, inactivated (TIV)	6 months and older	6 months	1 month	4 weeks
Influenza, live attenuated (LAIV)	24 months–49 years	24 months	1 month	4 weeks
Meningococcal conjugate (MCV)	11–12 years	2 years	—	—
Meningococcal polysaccharide (MPSV)-1	—	2 years	5 years	5 years
MPSV-2	—	7 years	—	—
Tetanus-diphtheria (Td)	11–12 years	7 years	10 years	5 years
Tetanus-diphtheria-acellular pertussis (Tdap)	≥11 years	10 years	—	—
Pneumococcal polysaccharide (PPSV)-1	—	2 years	5 years	5 years
PPSV-2	—	7 years	—	—

(continued)

Table 23-3. Recommended and minimum ages and intervals between vaccine doses (continued)

Vaccine and dose number	Recommended age for this dose	Minimum age for this dose	Recommended interval to next dose	Minimum interval to next dose
Human papillomavirus (HPV)-1	11–12 years	9 years	2 months	4 weeks
HPV-2	11–12 years (+ 2 months)	109 months	4 months	12 weeks
HPV-3	11–12 years (+ 6 months)	114 months	—	—
Rotavirus (RV)-1	2 months	6 weeks	2 months	4 weeks
RV-2	4 months	10 weeks	2 months	4 weeks
RV-3	6 months	14 weeks	—	—
Herpes zoster	60 years	60 years	—	—

Source: *The Pink Book*, CDC, 2009.

reactions in some vaccines, e.g., Arthus reactions, as will be described below. Such reactions probably result from formation of circulating antigen-antibody-complement complexes that initiate type III immunologic reactions (*Chapter 17*).

As in developed countries, where children receive vaccines against more than 15 severe infectious diseases, the problem of spacing the administration of many different vaccines should be addressed. Guidelines are given in Table 23-4. Inactivated vaccines do not interfere with the immune response to other inactivated vaccines or to live vaccines. An inactivated vaccine can be administered either simultaneously or at any time before or after a different inactivated or live vaccine.

Live attenuated vaccines behave differently. The immune response to one live virus vaccine might be impaired if administered within 30 days of another live virus vaccine, as shown by both animal and human studies. To minimize the potential risk for interference, parenterally administered live vaccines should not be administered on the same day but rather greater than four weeks apart from one another whenever possible (Table 23-4). If parenterally administered live vaccines are separated by less than four weeks, the second vaccine administered should not be counted as a valid dose and should be repeated at four weeks or more after the last, invalid dose. Yellow fever vaccine can be administered at any time after single-antigen measles vaccine. Oral live bacterial vaccines (Ty21a typhoid vaccine) and parenteral live virus vaccines (i.e., MMR, varicella, and yellow fever) can be administered simultaneously or at any interval before or after each other, if indicated.

Simultaneous administration of all indicated vaccines is an essential component of vaccination programs because it increases the probability that a child will be fully immunized at the appropriate age. Simultaneous administration of different vaccines is particularly important when return of the recipient for further vaccination is uncertain, when imminent exposure to several vaccine-preventable diseases is expected, or when preparing for international travel on short notice. Currently, several combined vaccines do exist to facilitate vaccination process, reduce the number of injections, and help reach expected vaccination coverages: e.g., MMR and measles, mumps, rubella, varicella (**MMRV**) vaccine. Administering combined MMR and

Table 23-4. Guidelines for spacing of live attenuated and inactivated vaccines

Antigen combination	Recommended minimum interval between doses
Two or more inactivated[a]	Can be administered simultaneously or at any interval between doses
Inactivated and live	Can be administered simultaneously or at any interval between doses
Two or more live intranasal or injectable[b]	Four-week minimum interval, if not administered simultaneously

Source: CDC, 2006.

a. The American Academy of Pediatrics suggests a one-month interval between tetanus toxoid, reduced diphtheria toxoid, and reduced acellular pertussis vaccine and tetravalent meningococcal conjugate vaccine if these vaccines are not administered on the same day (AAP, 2006).

b. Live oral vaccines (e.g., Ty21a typhoid vaccine and rotavirus vaccine) can be administered simultaneously or at any interval before or after inactivated or live injectable vaccines.

MMRV vaccine yields results similar to administering individual measles, mumps, rubella, and varicella vaccines at different sites. Responses to MMR and varicella vaccines administered on the same day are identical to vaccines administered a month apart. Therefore, no medical basis exists for administering these vaccines separately for routine vaccination instead of the preferred combined vaccine. In Western Europe, hexavalent combination vaccines are now available for the primary immunization of children against diphtheria, tetanus, pertussis, polio, hepatitis B, and *H. influenzae* type b (DTaP-IPV-HBV-Hib). If similar combinations were available in the United States, it would facilitate vaccination practice dramatically by reducing the number of injections and improving vaccine compliance.

Unless specifically recommended for injection in the same syringe, different vaccines administered simultaneously should be injected separately and at different anatomic sites. If both upper and lower limbs are used for simultaneous administration of different vaccines, the anterolateral thigh is often chosen for intramuscular injections and the deltoid region for subcutaneous injections. If more than one injection must be administered in a single limb of an infant or a child, the thigh usually is preferred because of its large muscle mass. The distance separating two injections in the same limb should be sufficiently extended (e.g., one to two inches) to minimize the chance of overlapping local reactions. Although simultaneous administration of vaccines known to be associated with frequent local or systemic reactions could theoretically accentuate these reactions, increased severity or frequency of adverse reactions has not been observed after simultaneous administration of the most widely used vaccines.

U.S.-Recommended Vaccination Schedules

The recommended routine childhood immunization schedule for infants, children, and adolescents in the United States is revised annually and is approved by the Advisory Committee on Immunization Practices (ACIP), the American Academy of Pediatrics (AAP), and the American Academy of Family Physicians (AAFP) (Tables 23-5, 23-6, and 23-7). A vaccine schedule for adults is also available for routine use (Table 23-8) as well as for immunocompromised and high-risk persons (Table 23-9).

Physicians and other health care providers should always ensure that they are following the most up-to-date schedules, which are available from the CDC's National Immunization Program Web site at http://www.cdc.gov/nip/.

Shown in Table 23-7 are catch-up schedules and minimum intervals between doses for children whose vaccinations have been delayed. A vaccine series does not need to be restarted regardless of the time that has elapsed between doses.

Interferences by Immune Globulins

As described previously, passively acquired antibodies can hamper the immune response to certain vaccines, both live and inactivated, and to toxoids. The result can be either the absence of seroconversion or a blunting of the immune response with lower final antibody concentration in the vaccinee. Not all vaccines, however, are affected equally by immune globulin administration. Generally, live virus vaccines, which have the requirement of self-replication within the recipient to elicit adequate immune responses, are the most affected, with some exceptions. The probable mechanism by which passively acquired immune globulin blunts the immune response is neutralization of vaccine virus, resulting in inhibition of viral replication leading to an insufficient antigenic mass. The most affected live virus vaccines are measles, mumps, rubella, and varicella, which are neutralized by the administration of blood (e.g., whole blood, packed red blood cells, and plasma) and other antibody-containing products (e.g., immune globulin, hyperimmune globulin, and intravenous immune globulin) available in the United States and other developed countries that contain antibodies to these viruses. Antibody-containing products can inhibit the immune response to measles and rubella vaccines for more than three months. Recommended intervals between receipt of various blood products and measles containing vaccine and varicella vaccine are listed in Table 23-10.

Blood products available in developed countries are unlikely to contain a substantial amount of antibody to yellow fever vaccine virus. This is why yellow fever vaccines can be administered at any time before, concurrent with, or after administering any immune globulin or hyperimmune globulin (e.g., hepatitis B immune globulin and rabies immune globulin). The length of time that interference with parenteral live vaccination (except yellow fever vaccine) can persist after administration of the antibody-containing product is a function of the amount of antigen-specific antibody contained in

Table 23-5. Recommended immunization schedule for persons aged zero through six years—United States, 2010

Vaccine ▼ Age ►	Birth	1 month	2 months	4 months	6 months	12 months	15 months	18 months	19–23 months	2–3 years	4–6 years
Hepatitis B[1]	HepB	HepB			HepB						
Rotavirus[2]			RV	RV	RV[2]						
Diphtheria, Tetanus, Pertussis[3]			DTaP	DTaP	DTaP	see footnote[3]	DTaP				DTaP
Haemophilus influenzae type b[4]			Hib	Hib	Hib[4]	Hib					
Pneumococcal[5]			PCV	PCV	PCV	PCV				PPSV	
Inactivated Poliovirus[6]			IPV	IPV	IPV						IPV
Influenza[7]					Influenza (Yearly)						
Measles, Mumps, Rubella[8]						MMR		see footnote[8]			MMR
Varicella[9]						Varicella		see footnote[9]			Varicella
Hepatitis A[10]						HepA (2 doses)				HepA Series	
Meningococcal[11]										MCV	

Light shading: Range of recommended ages for all children except certain high-risk groups. Dark shading: Range of recommended ages for certain high-risk groups.

Source: CDC, 2010.

the product. Therefore, after an antibody-containing product is received, parenteral live vaccines (except yellow fever vaccine) should be delayed until the passive antibody has degraded (Table 23-11). If a dose of parenteral live virus vaccine (except yellow fever vaccine) is administered after an antibody-containing product but at a shorter interval than recommended, the vaccine dose should be repeated unless serologic testing indicates a response to the vaccine. The repeat dose or serologic testing should be performed after the interval indicated for the antibody-containing product (Table 23-10). Following the same principles, as vaccine virus replication with stimulation of immunity occurs one to two weeks after vaccination, the interval of administering any of these vaccines and subsequent administration of an antibody-containing product is < 14 days, vaccination should be repeated after the recommended interval, unless serologic testing indicates that antibodies were produced.

Interference with current inactivated vaccines, toxoids, recombinant subunit, and polysaccharide vaccines is less marked than with live vaccines. Therefore, administering inactivated vaccines either simultaneously with or at any interval before or after receipt of an antibody-containing product should not substantially impair development of a protective antibody response (Table 23-10). The vaccine and antibody preparation should be administered at different sites by using the standard recommended dose. Increasing the vaccine dose volume or number of administrations is not indicated or recommended.

A humanized mouse monoclonal antibody product (palivizumab) is available for prevention of respiratory syncytial virus infection among infants and young children. This product contains only antibody to respiratory syncytial virus; hence, it will not interfere with immune response to live or inactivated vaccines.

Vaccine Safety

The main goal of vaccination is to protect mankind from vaccine-preventable infectious diseases,

Table 23-6. Recommended immunization schedule for persons aged seven through 18 years—United States, 2010

Vaccine ▼ Age ►	7–10 years	11–12 years	13–18 years
Tetanus, Diphtheria, Pertussis[1]		Tdap	Tdap
Human Papillomavirus[2]	see footnote 2	HPV (3 doses)	HPV series
Meningococcal[3]	MCV	MCV	MCV
Influenza[4]	Influenza (Yearly)		
Pneumococcal[5]	PPSV		
Hepatitis A[6]	HepA Series		
Hepatitis B[7]	Hep B Series		
Inactivated Poliovirus[8]	IPV Series		
Measles, Mumps, Rubella[9]	MMR Series		
Varicella[10]	Varicella Series		

Range of recommended ages for all children except certain high-risk groups. Range of recommended ages for catch-up immunization. Range of recommended ages for certain high-risk groups.

Source: CDC, 2010.

Table 23-7. Catch-up immunization schedule for persons aged four months through 18 years who start late or who are more than one month behind in the United States, 2010

Persons aged four months to six years					
		MINIMUM INTERVAL BETWEEN DOSES			
Vaccine	**Minimum age for dose 1**	**Dose 1 to dose 2**	**Dose 2 to dose 3**	**Dose 3 to dose 4**	**Dose 4 to dose 5**
Hepatitis B	Birth	4 weeks	8 weeks (and at least 16 weeks after first dose)	–	–
Rotavirus	6 weeks	4 weeks	4 weeks	–	–
Diphtheria, tetanus, pertussis	6 weeks	4 weeks	4 weeks	6 months	6 months[3]
Haemophilus influenza type b	6 weeks	4 weeks If first dose administered at younger than age 12 months **8 weeks (as final dose)** If first dose administered at age 12–14 months **No further doses needed** If previous dose administered at age 15 months or older	4 weeks If current age younger than 12 months **8 weeks (as final dose)** If current age is 12 months or older and first dose administered at younger than age 12 months and second dose administered at younger than 15 months **No further doses needed** For healthy children if previous dose administered at age 24 months or older	8 weeks (as final dose) This dose only necessary for children aged 12 months through 59 months who received 3 doses before age 12 months or for high-risk children who received 3 doses at any age	–
Pneumococcal	6 weeks	4 weeks If first dose administered at younger than age 12 months **8 weeks (as final dose for healthy children)** If first dose administered at age 12 months or older or current age 24 through 59 months **No further doses needed** For healthy children if first dose administered at age 24 months or older	4 weeks If current age is younger than 12 months **8 weeks (as final dose for healthy children)** If current age 12 months or older **No further doses needed** For healthy children if previous dose administered at age 24 months or older	8 weeks (as final dose) This dose only necessary for children aged 12 months through 59 months who received 3 doses before age 12 months or for high-risk children who received 3 doses at any age	–
Inactivated poliovirus	6 weeks	4 weeks	4 weeks	6 months	–
Measles, mumps, rubella	12 months	4 weeks	–	–	–
Varicella	12 months	3 months	–	–	–
Hepatitis A	12 months	6 months	–	–	–

(continued)

Table 23-7 Catch-?show up immunization schedule for persons aged four months through 18 years who start late or who are more than one month behind in the United States, 2010 (continued)?>

Persons aged seven through 18 years					
		MINIMUM INTERVAL BETWEEN DOSES			
Vaccine	**Minimum age for dose 1**	**Dose 1 to dose 2**	**Dose 2 to dose 3**	**Dose 3 to dose 4**	**Dose 4 to dose 5**
Tetanus, diphtheria/tetanus, diphtheria pertussis	7 years	4 weeks	4 weeks If first dose administered at younger than age 12 months 6 months If first dose administered at 12 months or older	6 months If first dose administered at younger than age 12 months	–
Human papillomavirus	9 years	ROUTINE DOSING INTERVALS ARE NOT RECOMMENDED			
Hepatitis A	12 months	6 months	–	–	–
Hepatitis B	Birth	4 weeks	8 weeks (and at least 16 weeks after first dose)	–	–
Inactivated poliovirus	6 weeks	4 weeks	4 weeks	6 months	–
Measles, mumps, rubella	12 months	4 weeks	–	–	–
Varicella	12 months	3 months If person is younger than 13 years 4 weeks If person is aged 13 years or older			

Source: CDC, 2010.

Table 23-8. Recommended adult immunization schedule, by vaccine and age group in the United States, 2010

VACCINE ▼ AGE GROUP ▶	19–26 years	27–49 years	50–59 years	60–64 years	≥65 years
Tetanus, diphtheria, pertussis (Td/Tdap)[1,*]	Substitute one-time dose of Tdap for Td booster; then boost with Td every 10 years				Td booster every 10 years
Human papillomavirus[2,*]	3 doses (females)				
Varicella[3,*]	2 doses				
Zoster[4]				1 dose	
Measles, mumps, rubella[5,*]	1 or 2 doses		1 dose		
Influenza[6,*]			1 dose annually		
Pneumococcal (polysaccharide)[7,8]	1 or 2 doses				1 dose
Hepatitis A[9,*]	2 doses				
Hepatitis B[10,*]	3 doses				
Meningococcal[11,*]	1 or more doses				

* Covered by the Vaccine Injury Compensation Program.

For all persons in this category who meet the age requirements and who lack evidence of immunity (e.g., lack documentation of vaccination or have no evidence of prior infection)

Recommended if some other risk factor is present (e.g., based on medical, occupational, lifestyle, or other indications)

No recommendation

Source: CDC, 2010.

Table 23-9. Vaccines that might be indicated for adults, based on medical and other indications in the United States, 2010

INDICATION ▶ VACCINE ▼	Pregnancy	Immunocompromising conditions (excluding human immunodeficiency virus [HIV])[3-5,12]	HIV infection[3-5,12,13] CD4+ T lymphocyte count <200 cells/μL	HIV infection[3-5,12,13] CD4+ T lymphocyte count ≥200 cells/μL	Diabetes, heart disease, chronic lung disease, chronic alcoholism	Asplenia[13] (including elective splenectomy and persistent complement component deficiencies)	Chronic liver disease	Kidney failure, end-stage renal disease, receipt of hemodialysis	Health-care personnel
Tetanus, diphtheria, pertussis (Td/Tdap)[1,*]	Td	Substitute one-time dose of Tdap for Td booster; then boost with Td every 10 years							
Human papillomavirus[2,*]		3 doses for females through age 26 years							
Varicella[3,*]	Contraindicated			2 doses					
Zoster[4]	Contraindicated				1 dose				
Measles, mumps, rubella[5,*]	Contraindicated			1 or 2 doses					
Influenza[6,*]	1 dose TIV annually								1 dose TIV or LAIV annually
Pneumococcal (polysaccharide)[7,8]		1 or 2 doses							
Hepatitis A[9,*]	2 doses								
Hepatitis B[10,*]					3 doses				
Meningococcal[11,*]	1 or more doses								

*Covered by the Vaccine Injury Compensation Program.

Light shading: For all persons in this category who meet the age requirements and who lack evidence of immunity (e.g., lack documentation of vaccination or have no evidence of prior infection)

Dark shading: Recommended if some other risk factor is present (e.g., based on medical, occupational, lifestyle, or other indications)

White: No recommendation

reducing, as much as possible, the incidence of adverse events. Although vaccines are broadly considered to be the safest and most effective medical intervention strategy, and have been responsible, in conjunction with antibiotics and modern hygiene, for the steady decline in the mortality and morbidity caused by infectious diseases, the issue of vaccine safety has been with us since vaccination was first established in the 19th century (Figure 23-10). Although the occurrence of severe adverse events could be tolerated for a "life-saving" drug given to a patient for treatment of a disease, this is not the case for vaccines, which are given for the prevention of infectious disease to healthy individuals who want to remain healthy. As a consequence, incidence and severity of side effects should always be considered as a cost-benefit ratio in the context of disease treatment or prevention.

Contraindications and Precautions

A contraindication indicates that a vaccine should not be administered, while a precaution specifies a situation in which vaccine may be indicated if the benefit of vaccination to the individual is judged to outweigh the risk. The vast majority of both contraindications and precautions are temporary, so vaccination could be performed subsequently. The only real contraindication applicable to all vaccines is a history of a severe allergic reaction after a prior dose of vaccine or to a vaccine constituent.

Other true contraindications are:

- administration of live attenuated vaccines to subjects with severe immunosuppression;
- administration of subsequent doses of pertussis-containing vaccines to children who experienced an encephalopathy less than seven days after administration of a previous dose of DTP or DTaP vaccines;
- administration of a live attenuated vaccine to a pregnant woman because of a theoretical risk to the fetus;
- administration of a live attenuated vaccine in a child with evolving neurological disease.

A precaution is a condition in a recipient that might increase the risk for a serious adverse reaction or that might compromise the ability of the vaccine to produce immunity. Under normal circumstances, vaccinations should be deferred when a precaution is present. Moderate or severe acute illness, regardless of the absence or presence of fever, is a general precaution to vaccination. Health care providers sometimes inappropriately consider a condition to be a contraindication or precaution to vaccination. Withholding vaccine in such instances results in a missed opportunity to administer needed vaccine.

A concise summary of true and false contraindications, as of December 2006, is given in Table 23-12.

Current Vaccines and Safety Concerns

Assuring the safety of each vaccine is essential to the continued integrity of vaccination programs.

Table 23-10. Suggested intervals between administration of antibody-containing products for different indications and measles-containing vaccine and varicella vaccine

Product/indication	Dose, including mg immunoglobulin G (IgG)/kg body weight	Recommended interval before measles or varicella vaccination (months)
Respiratory syncytial virus immune globulin (IG) monoclonal antibody (Synagis)	15 mg/kg intramuscularly (IM)	None
Tetanus IG	250 units (10 mg IgG/kg) IM	3
Hepatitis A IG		
Contact prophylaxis	0.02 mL/kg (3.3 mg IgG/kg) IM	3
International travel	0.06 mL/kg (10 mg IgG/kg) IM	3
Hepatitis B IG	0.06 mL/kg (10 mg IgG/kg) IM	3
Rabies IG	20 IU/kg (22 mg IgG/kg) IM	4
Measles prophylaxis IG		
Standard (i.e., nonimmunocompromised) contact	0.25 mL/kg (40 mg IgG/kg) IM	5
Immunocompromised contact	0.50 mL/kg (80 mg IgG/kg) IM	6
Blood transfusion		
Red blood cells (RBCs), washed	10 mL/kg negligible IgG/kg intravenously (IV)	None
RBCs, adenine-saline added	10 mL/kg (10 mg IgG/kg) IV	3
Packed RBCs (hematocrit 65%)	10 mL/kg (60 mg IgG/kg) IV	6
Whole blood (hematocrit 35–50%)	10 mL/kg (80–100 mg IgG/kg) IV	6
Plasma/platelet products	10 mL/kg (160 mg IgG/kg) IV	7
Cytomegalovirus intravenous immune globulin (IGIV)	150 mg/kg maximum	6
IGIV		
Replacement therapy for immune deficiencies	300–400 mg/kg IV	8
Immune thrombocytopenic purpura treatment	400 mg/kg IV	8
Postexposure varicella prophylaxis	400 mg/kg IV	8
Immune thrombocytopenic	1,000 mg/kg IV	10
Kawasaki's disease	2 g/kg IV	11

Source: CDC, 2006.

Both proven and discredited safety issues are of concern to the public and to public health authorities, because even mistaken beliefs about vaccines can impact vaccine acceptance. In developed countries, children currently routinely receive vaccines against 16 important infectious diseases shown in Table 23-3, and every vaccination usually requires multiple doses. Given the number of injections required and the close temporal relationship between vaccinations and the onset of many childhood diseases, it is not surprising that there has been considerable speculation about the possible links between other diseases and childhood vaccinations. Nevertheless, when detailed studies have been undertaken, the possibility of a causative link with vaccination has mostly been eliminated or not proven (Table 23-13).

Although a claim of complete safety is impossible for any medical intervention, with more than a century of experience involving many billions of doses worldwide, it can be stated with confidence that vaccines have an enviable and exemplary safety profile. Moreover, in recent years, the safety of vaccines has improved enormously while the tolerance of side effects has declined. What was acceptable 20 years ago is not tolerable today.

Regulation of Vaccines in the United States

The development and use of vaccines in the United States from the safety perspective is highly regulated and subject to intensive oversight. To reduce liability and respond to public health concerns, Congress passed the National Childhood Vaccine Injury Act (NCVIA) in 1986. This act was influential in

Table 23-11. Guidelines for administering antibody-containing products and vaccines

Simultaneous administration	
Combination	**Recommended minimum interval between doses**
Antibody-containing products and inactivated antigen	Can be administered simultaneously at different sites or at anytime between doses
Antibody-containing products and live antigen	Should not be administered simultaneously. If simultaneous administration of measles-containing vaccine or varicella vaccine is unavoidable, administer at different sites and revaccinate or test for seroconversion after the recommended interval (see Table 23-10)

Nonsimultaneous administration		
Product administered		
First	**Second**	**Recommended minimum interval between doses**
Antibody-containing products	Inactivated antigen	N/A
Inactivated antigen	Antibody-containing products	N/A
Antibody-containing products	Live antigen	Dose-related
Live antigen	Antibody-containing products	Two weeks

Source: CDC, 2006.

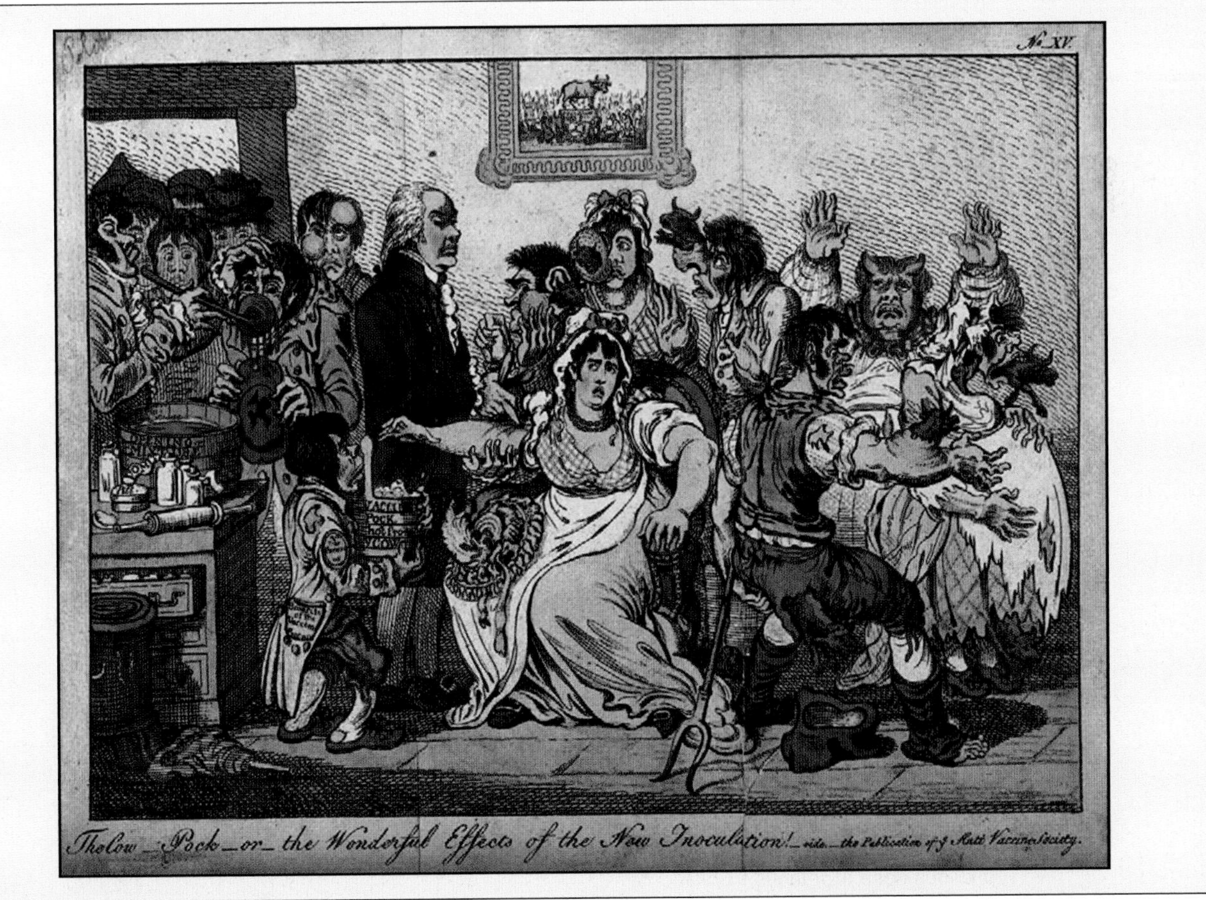
Nº XV.
The Cow-Pock—or—the Wonderful Effects of the New Inoculation!

Figure 23-10. Vaccines have been met with skepticism since they were first introduced. (Reproduced with permission from the Wellcome Library; London, UK; http://library.wellcome.ac.uk.)

Table 23-12. Guide to contraindications and precautions to commonly used vaccines

Vaccine	True contraindications and precautions	False (vaccines can be administered)
General for all vaccines	**Contraindications** – Serious allergic reaction (e.g., anaphylaxis) after a previous vaccine dose or to a vaccine component **Precautions** – Moderate or severe acute illness with or without fever	• Mild acute illness with or without fever • Mild to moderate local reaction (i.e., swelling, redness, soreness); low-grade or moderate fever after previous dose • Lack of previous physical examination in well-appearing person • Current antimicrobial therapy • Convalescent phase of illness • Premature birth (hepatitis B vaccine is an exception in certain circumstances) • Recent exposure to an infectious disease • History of penicillin allergy, other nonvaccine allergies, relatives with allergies, receiving allergen extract immunotherapy • Lactation/breast-feeding
DTaP	**Contraindications** – Severe allergic reaction after a previous dose or to a vaccine component – Encephalopathy (e.g., coma, decreased level of consciousness, prolonged seizures) not attributable to another identifiable cause within seven days of administration of previous dose of DTP or DTaP – Progressive neurologic disorder, including infantile spasms, uncontrolled epilepsy, progressive encephalopathy; defer DTaP until neurologic status clarified and stabilized **Precautions** – Temperature of ≥ 104°F (≥ 40.5°C) within 48 hours after vaccination with a previous dose of DTP or DTaP that is not attributable to another identifiable cause – Collapse or shock-like state (i.e., hypotonic hyporesponsive episode) within 48 hours after receiving a previous dose of DTP/DTaP – Seizure within three days of receiving a previous dose of DTP/DTaP – Persistent, inconsolable crying lasting three hours or more within 48 hours after receiving a previous dose of DTP/DTaP Guillain-Barré syndrome ≤ 6 weeks after previous dose of tetanus toxoid-containing vaccines – Moderate or severe acute illness with or without fever	• Temperature of < 104°F (< 40.5°C), fussiness or mild drowsiness after a previous dose of diphtheria toxoid-tetanus toxoid-pertussis vaccine (DTP)/DTaP • Family history of seizures • Family history of sudden infant death syndrome • Family history of an adverse event after DTP or DTaP administration • Stable neurologic conditions (e.g., cerebral palsy, well-controlled convulsions, developmental delay)
DT, Td	**Contraindications** – Severe allergic reaction after a previous dose or to a vaccine component **Precautions** – Guillain-Barré syndrome ≤ 6 weeks after previous dose of tetanus toxoid-containing vaccine	Allergic or other severe reaction following administration of equine tetanus antitoxin

Table 23-12. Guide to contraindications and precautions to commonly used vaccines (continued)

Vaccine	True contraindications and precautions	False (vaccines can be administered)
	– Moderate or severe acute illness with or without fever	
Tdap	**Contraindications** – Severe allergic reaction after a previous dose or to a vaccine component – Encephalopathy (e.g., coma, decreased level of consciousness, prolonged seizures) within seven days of administration of previous dose of DTP, DTaP, or Tdap **Precautions** – Moderate or severe acute illness with or without fever – Guillain-Barré syndrome (GBS) $\leq$ 6 weeks after previous dose of tetanus toxoid-containing vaccine – Progressive or unstable neurologic disorder, uncontrolled seizures, or progressive encephalopathy until a treatment regimen has been established and the condition has stabilized – History of Arthus-type hypersensitivity reactions following a prior dose of tetanus toxoid-containing vaccine; defer vaccination until at least 10 years have elapsed since last tetanus toxoid-containing vaccine	• Temperature of > 104°F (> 40.5°C), within 48 hours after vaccination with a previous dose of DTP/DTaP that is not attributable to another identifiable cause • Collapse or shock-like state (i.e., hypotonic hyporesponsive episode) within 48 hours after receiving a previous dose of DTP/DTaP • Seizure within three days after receiving a previous dose of DTP/DTaP • Persistent, inconsolable crying lasting three hours or more within 48 hours after receiving a previous dose of DTP/DTaP • History of extensive limb swelling after DTP/DTaP/Td that is not an Arthus-type reaction • Stable neurologic disorder • History of brachial neuritis • Latex allergy that is not anaphylactic • Immunosuppression
IPV	**Contraindications** – Severe allergic reaction (e.g., anaphylaxis) after a previous vaccine dose or vaccine component **Precautions** – Pregnancy – Moderate or severe acute illness with or without fever	• Previous receipt of one or more doses of oral polio vaccine
MMR	**Contraindications** – Severe allergic reaction (e.g., anaphylaxis) after a previous vaccine dose or to a vaccine component – Pregnancy – Known severe immunodeficiency (e.g., hematologic and solid tumors; receiving chemotherapy; congenital immunodeficiency; long-term immunosuppressive therapy; or patients with human immunodeficiency virus [HIV] infection who are severely immunocompromised) **Precautions** – Recent ($\leq$ 11 months) receipt of antibody-containing blood product (specific interval depends on product)	• Positive tuberculin skin test • Simultaneous TB skin testing • Breast-feeding • Pregnancy of recipient's mother or other close or household contact • Recipient is child-bearing-age female • Immunodeficient family member or household contact • Asymptomatic or mildly symptomatic HIV infection • Allergy to eggs

(continued)

Table 23-12. Guide to contraindications and precautions to commonly used vaccines (continued)

Vaccine	True contraindications and precautions	False (vaccines can be administered)
	– History of thrombocytopenia or thrombocytopenic purpura – Moderate or severe acute illness with or without fever	
Hib	Contraindications – Severe allergic reaction (e.g., anaphylaxis) after a previous vaccine dose or to a vaccine component – Age < 6 weeks Precaution – Moderate or severe acute illness with or without fever	
Hepatitis B	Contraindication – Severe allergic reaction (e.g., anaphylaxis) after a previous vaccine dose or to a vaccine component Precautions – Infant weighing < 2,000 grams – Moderate or severe acute illness with or without fever	• Pregnancy • Autoimmune disease (e.g., systemic lupus erythematosus or rheumatoid arthritis)
Hepatitis A	Contraindications – Severe allergic reaction (e.g., anaphylaxis) after a previous vaccine dose or to a vaccine component Precautions – Pregnancy – Moderate or severe acute illness with or without fever	
Varicella	Contraindications – Severe allergic reaction (e.g., anaphylaxis) after a previous vaccine dose or to a vaccine component – Substantial suppression of cellular immunity – Pregnancy Precautions – Recent (≤ 11 months) receipt of antibody-containing blood product (specific interval depends on product) – Moderate or severe acute illness with or without fever	• Pregnancy of recipient's mother or other close or household contact • Immunodeficient family member or household contact • Asymptomatic or mildly symptomatic HIV infection • Humoral immunodeficiency (e.g., agammaglobulinemia)
PCV	Contraindication – Severe allergic reaction (e.g., anaphylaxis) after a previous vaccine dose or to a vaccine component Precaution – Moderate or severe acute illness with or without fever	

Table 23-12. Guide to contraindications and precautions to commonly used vaccines (continued)

Vaccine	True contraindications and precautions	False (vaccines can be administered)
Trivalent inactivated influenza vaccine (TIV)	**Contraindication** – Severe allergic reaction (e.g., anaphylaxis) after a previous vaccine dose or to a vaccine component **Precautions** – Moderate or severe acute illness with or without fever	• Nonsevere (e.g., contact) allergy to latex or thimerosal • Concurrent administration of Coumadin or aminophylline
LAIV	**Contraindications** – Severe allergic reaction (e.g., anaphylaxis) after a previous vaccine dose or to a vaccine component – Pregnancy – Known severe immunodeficiency (e.g., hematologic and solid tumors; receiving chemotherapy; congenital immunodeficiency; long-term immunosuppressive therapy; or patients with human immunodeficiency virus infection who are severely immunocompromised) – Previous history of GBS – Certain chronic medical conditions **Precaution** – Moderate or severe acute illness with or without fever	
PPV	**Contraindication** – Severe allergic reaction (e.g., anaphylaxis) after a previous vaccine dose or to a vaccine component **Precaution** – Moderate or severe acute illness with or without fever	History of invasive pneumococcal disease or pneumonia
MCV4	**Contraindications** – Severe allergic reaction (e.g., anaphylaxis) after a previous vaccine dose or to a vaccine component **Precautions** – Moderate or severe acute illness with or without fever – History of Guillain-Barré syndrome (if not at high risk for meningococcal disease)	
MPSV	**Contraindications** – Severe allergic reaction (e.g., anaphylaxis) after a previous vaccine dose or to a vaccine component **Precautions** – Moderate or severe acute illness with or without fever	

(continued)

Table 23-12. Guide to contraindications and precautions to commonly used vaccines (continued)

Vaccine	True contraindications and precautions	False (vaccines can be administered)
HPV	Contraindications – Severe allergic reaction (e.g., anaphylaxis) after a previous vaccine dose or to a vaccine component Precautions – Moderate or severe acute illness with or without fever – Pregnancy	
Rotavirus	Contraindications – Severe allergic reaction after a previous dose or to a vaccine component Precautions – Moderate or severe acute illness with or without fever – Immunosuppression – Receipt of an antibody-containing blood product within six weeks – Preexisting gastrointestinal disease – Previous history of intussusception	

Source: CDC, 2006.

creating the National Vaccine Program Office (NVPO) that coordinates immunization-related activities between all Department of Health and Human Services (DHHS) agencies, including the Centers for Disease Control and Prevention (CDC), the Food and Drug Administration (FDA), the National Institutes of Health (NIH), and the Health Resources and Services Administration (HRSA). Currently, the development of new vaccines in the United States requires FDA regulation and approval in conjunction with continued surveillance of risk/benefit considerations by the CDC and these other federal organizations. Industry is now also required to expand its Phase II, III, and IV human clinical trials prior to vaccine licensure to document even rare adverse vaccine reactions. In addition to these regulations of government and industry, large health maintenance organizations (HMOs) are subject to postmarketing screening for potential previously unrecognized adverse vaccine reactions. Following the recognition and reporting of any adverse vaccine reactions, the CDC performs case control analyses to define any possible causal relationships. The National Childhood Vaccine Injury Act of 1986 requires health care providers to report certain adverse events that occur following vaccination to the Vaccine Adverse Event Reporting System (**VAERS**) established by the CDC and FDA in 1990. VAERS provides a mechanism for the collection and analysis of adverse events (side effects) associated with vaccines currently licensed in the United States. Adverse events are defined as health effects that occur after immunization that may or may not be related to the vaccine. VAERS data are monitored continually to detect unknown adverse events or increases in known side effects. Academic and other appropriate institutions are eligible for NIH-grant support for research studies of these suspected adverse vaccine reactions for a better understanding of their pathogenesis. Finally, adverse vaccine effects found to be causally related to a vaccine can be awarded compensation through the National Vaccine Injury Compensation Program.

Immunologically Mediated Complications of Vaccines

Part of our knowledge on vaccine safety comes from past experience. When vaccines have shown safety problems, important lessons have been learned and approaches have been modified to avoid repeating the problem. Shown in Table 23-14 are some of the safety issues that were seen in the past, some of which had an immunologic basis.

For ease of discussion, these immunologically mediated adverse effects to vaccines may be divided

Table 23-13. Suspected links between vaccines and adverse effects that have been disproved or are unsubstantiated by research

Vaccine	Safety issues	Outcome
MMR	Autism Inflammatory bowel disease	Disproved Disproved
Pertussis	Chronic encephalopathy	Disproved
Polio	Contracting HIV	Disproved
Thimerosal (a preservative)	Autism Neurodevelopmental delays	Disproved Unsubstantiated
Hepatitis B	Multiple sclerosis Diabetes	Disproved Disproved
Hib conjugate	Diabetes	Disproved
Lyme[a]	Autoimmune disorders	Unsubstantiated
Bovine serum (used to culture virus-comprising vaccines)	Prion disease	Unsubstantiated
Anthrax	Gulf War syndrome	Unsubstantiated
Aluminum products as vaccine adjuvant	Macrophagic myofascitis Asthma	Unsubstantiated Unsubstantiated
DTP	Atopy Sudden infant death syndrome	Unsubstantiated Unsubstantiated
IPV	Cancer due to SV40 contamination	Disproved

a. Vaccine no longer available.

into: (1) those effects that are seen in immunologically compromised hosts; (2) those hypersensitivity reactions that are seen predominantly in allergic (atopic) individuals (*Chapter 18*); and (3) those effects that are seen in normal hosts and appear to be related to the vaccine antigen or the route of administration.

Adverse Effects of Vaccines Seen in Immunologically Compromised Hosts

Not only does the status of the immune response affect the success of primary immunization, but it also may contribute to its adverse effects. These are usually seen after the use of live attenuated vaccines and predominantly in individuals with depressed immune function (*Chapter 16*). For example, progressive vaccinia (vaccinia necrosum or vaccinia gangrenosa) has been observed in children with defects in T cell immunity, e.g., severe combined immunodeficiency (**SCID**) (Figure 23-11). This rare but highly fatal complication of smallpox immunization consists of a failure of the primary lesion to heal normally with progressive spread to adjacent areas of skin (Figure 23-11B). With necrosis of tissue (Figure 23-11C), new lesions develop over a period of months, often involving metastatic lesions to other parts of the body such as bone and viscera. This complication, which fortunately is no longer seen owing to the cessation of routine smallpox immunization, carried a high mortality (*Chapter 16*). It was also seen in immune deficiencies secondary to other conditions, e.g., leukemia, lymphoma, and patients receiving immunosuppressive therapy. Since the basis of this tragic complication was a specific deficiency of cell-mediated immunity (**CMI**), the recommended treatment of the condition with vaccinia immune globulin (**VIG**) alone, therefore, was not totally satisfactory, and human stem cell (**HSC**) immunologic reconstitution was the more suitable and preferable treatment.

Another example of a vaccine complication related to an underlying immune deficiency is a condition in which the Bacillus Calmette-Guérin (**BCG**) vaccine (directed against tuberculosis) becomes disseminated (*Chapter 16*). As with progressive vaccinia, the condition is not only seen in children with primary T cell immune deficiencies, but also in individuals with secondary immune deficiencies related to disease or treatment, e.g., leukemia, lymphoma, and patients receiving immunosuppressive therapy. If BCG is accidentally given to an immunocompromised patient (e.g., an infant with SCID), it can cause disseminated or life-threatening infection. The documented incidence of this occurring is less than one per million administered immunizations. In 2007, the WHO stopped recommending BCG for infants with HIV, even if there is a high risk of exposure to TB, because of the risk of disseminated BCG infection in these patients (which is approximately 400 per 100,000).

Pregnancy also constitutes an altered physiologic state in which the general status of cell-mediated immunity is known to be decreased and therefore the use of live attenuated vaccines, e.g., MMR, is contraindicated because of the possibility of enhanced viral disease in the mother as well as the detrimental effects of infection of the fetus. In the case of rubella immunization, although virus shedding of vaccine virus has been reported, no reports

Table 23-14. Safety issues associated with the use of vaccines

Vaccine	Problem	Comment	Outcome
Killed respiratory syncytial virus	Enhanced disease after exposure to virus		Vaccine was never introduced onto the market
Oral polio virus	Reversion to virulence with paralytic disease in vaccinees and contacts	Despite adverse effects, the vaccine is responsible for the eradication of polio	Live vaccines now require larger and more stable deletions before approval
Live oral rotavirus (RotaShield)	Intussusception		Vaccine removed from the market and the required safety database has been expanded for future products
Inactivated measles	Atypical measles; localized Arthus reaction		Vaccine removed from the market
Measles (high dose)	Increased mortality from all causes in females		Never licensed
MMR	Anaphylaxis	Resulted from rare allergic reactions to gelatin in the vaccine	
Intranasal inactivated flu with bacterial toxin adjuvant	Bell's palsy (facial paralysis)		Vaccine removed from the market
Subcutaneous inactivated flu vaccine containing trace egg protein	Allergic reactions	Resulted from rare allergic reactions in egg sensitive recipients	Vaccine can be safely given except if history of severe anaphylactic reactions to egg
Whole-cell pertussis vaccine	Febrile seizures; encephalopathy	Apparently due to the whole cell pertussis component	Removed from market in the majority of the developed world
Anthrax—cell-free filtrate product (anthrax vaccine adsorbed)	Reactogenic		Purified recombinant protein will be available in the near future
1976 Swine flu	Guillain-Barré syndrome	Molecular mimicry of a component in the swine flu vaccine that cross-reacted with neural tissue	Vaccination discontinued
Smallpox	Generalized vaccinia, encephalitis, myocarditis, and eczema vaccinatum	Despite adverse events, the vaccine was responsible for eradication of smallpox	Use stopped after eradication of smallpox

Source: Vaccine Development: Current Status and Future Needs. October 2005. The American Academy of Microbiology.

of congenital rubella syndrome in a previously immunized woman have been verified. It is apparent from these unfortunate clinical experiences that individuals with impaired immunologic reactivity, on the basis of either the primary or acquired causes of immune deficiencies, should not receive live attenuated vaccines.

Adverse Hypersensitivity Reactions Seen Predominantly in Allergic (Atopic) Individuals

Since many vaccines are grown in tissue culture or eggs, e.g., viral vaccines, there is an opportunity for contamination with heterologous tissues, proteins, or other foreign substances that can lead to immunologically mediated (allergic) reactions in a genetically susceptible (atopic) host (*Chapter 18*). The possible allergens in viral vaccines that could give rise to allergic reactions include: (1) culture media in which the virus is grown, e.g., egg protein; (2) components of media or its additives, e.g., gelatin; and (3) foreign antigens that may be added during the preparation and purification of the vaccine, e.g., antibiotics. Most hypersensitivity reactions are seen in atopic individuals and are associated with egg protein or antibiotics, e.g., penicillin. Newer techniques in vaccine preparation, such as zonal

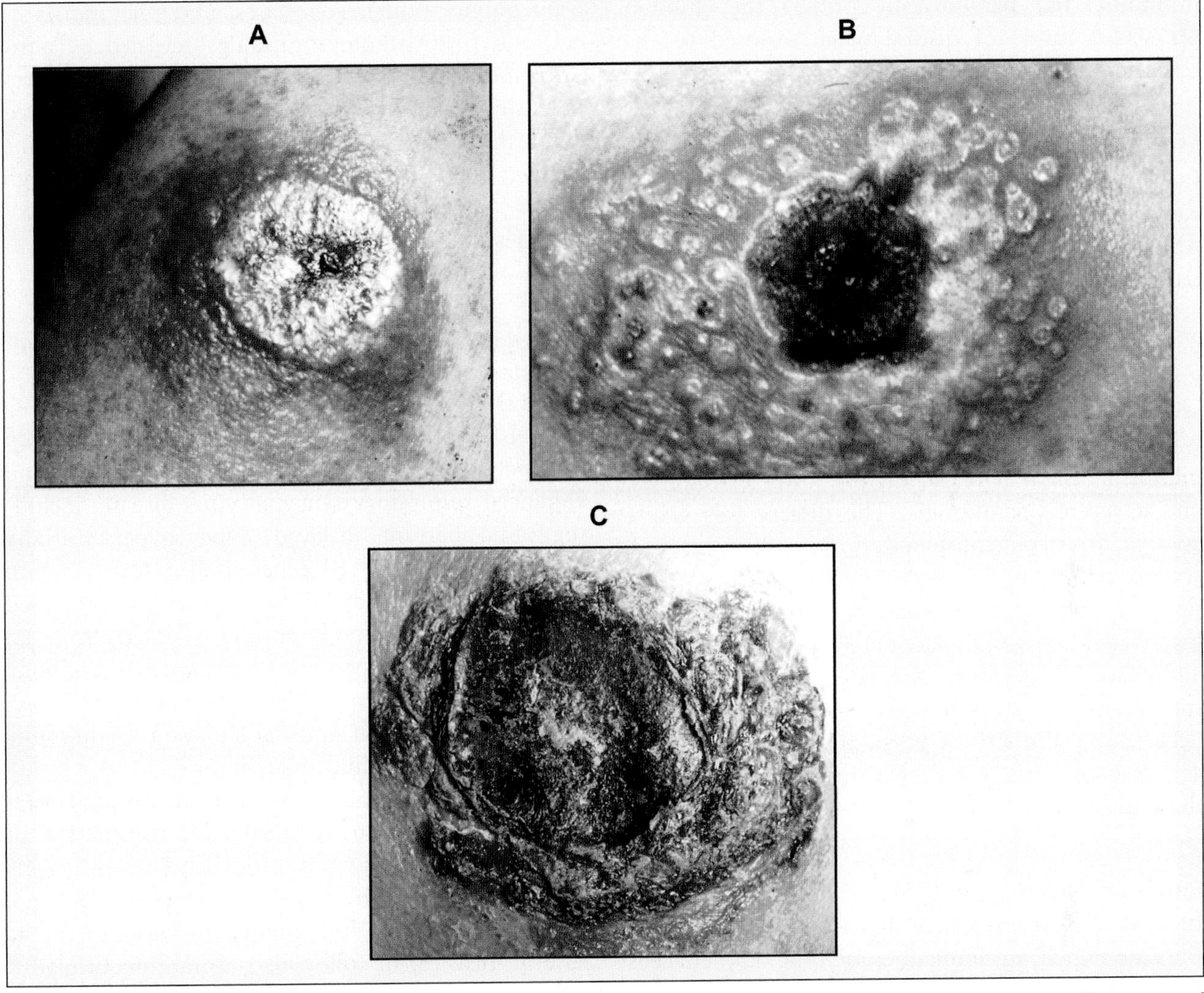

Figure 23-11. Photographs of vaccinia gangrenosa occurring in a patient with a T cell immunodeficiency. Panel A: Early stage of the lesion. Panel B: Progressive stage showing satellite lesions surrounding the primary lesion. Panel C: The necrotic phase. (Courtesy of Dr. Vincent A. Fulginiti.)

centrifugation, appear to have reduced the frequency of severe anaphylactic reactions to these contaminating materials.

Debate over the safety of giving egg-containing immunizations to egg-allergic (EA) children once again occurred during the recent global pandemic of the H1N1 influenza A virus. Recent studies evaluating the practice of vaccinating egg-allergic patients with egg-containing H1N1 influenza A vaccine indicate the safety irrespective of past reaction history, including egg anaphylaxis or high level of egg sensitization, and it is recommended that administration of H1N1 vaccine to egg-allergic children can be performed without prior skin testing or graded challenge dosing.

Adverse Effects of Viral Vaccines Seen in Normal Hosts that Appear to be Related to the Nature of the Vaccine Antigen or the Route of Administration

Of all the paramyxoviruses, measles virus (**MV**) and respiratory syncytial virus (**RSV**) have been recognized for decades as two of the major viral causes of pediatric illnesses associated with significant morbidity and mortality. In the 1960s, formalin-inactivated vaccines against both of these agents were developed and administered to infants and children in the United States. Two unfortunate episodes of severe adverse hypersensitivity reactions occurred in children receiving these vaccines. The vaccines not only failed to produce protective immunity, but paradoxically primed the children for severe forms of disease when exposed to the respective wild-type viruses.

Measles Virus

In the 1960s, formalin-inactivated measles virus vaccines were introduced in the United States. Although the vaccines were immunogenic, serum antibody levels waned within months to a couple of years. Ironically, 15 to 60 percent of immunized children subsequently exposed to wild-type measles virus during community outbreaks developed a severe form of disease called atypical measles that was characterized by high fever, a petechial or morbilliform rash that began on the lower extremities, and a severe pneumonitis. The disease was severe enough to warrant hospitalization in many cases. A second related problem was that when these children who had been previously immunized with the inactivated measles vaccine were subsequently administered the live attenuated measles vaccine subcutaneously, an Arthus-like swelling and redness occurred at the site of injection within 12 hours. The vaccine was withdrawn in 1967 because of these problems.

Respiratory Syncytial Virus

In 1961, a formalin-inactivated vaccine against RSV was developed in human embryonic kidney cells and monkey kidney cells. During 1966, the inactivated vaccine was administered in one to three doses to RSV-seronegative and RSV-seropositive infants and children, and a formalin-inactivated parainfluenza vaccine was administered to control groups of children. Although the RSV vaccine was found to be immunogenic, it elicited mainly nonprotective antibodies. During the winter of 1966–1967, immunized children were exposed to RSV in the community, and those who were seronegative for the virus prior to vaccination experienced a significant greater increase in the frequency and severity of lower respiratory illness and a greater incidence of hospitalization compared to the control children. This clinical entity has been referred to as enhanced respiratory syncytial virus disease. The main clinical manifestations in these children included bronchoconstriction and pneumonia, and tragically two immunized infants died as toddlers as a consequence of subsequent RSV infection. Autopsy findings in these two children showed bronchopneumonia, atelectases, and pneumothoraces, and histopathologic findings revealed a "peribronchiolar monocytic infiltration with some excess in eosinophils." High titers of RSV were recovered from the lungs of the two children. No vaccine against RSV has been licensed since, although efforts are now under way to develop new RSV vaccines.

Pathogenetic Mechanisms Underlying Atypical Measles and Enhanced Respiratory Syncytial Virus Disease

Several hypotheses have been advanced to explain the pathogenesis of both atypical measles and enhanced respiratory syncytial virus disease, including an aberrant delayed type hypersensitivity response and a type III generalized Arthus reaction (*Chapter 17*). Perhaps the most widely accepted hypothesis is that both entities resulted from an imbalance in the systemic and mucosal antibody responses elicited in response to inactivated vaccines, establishing an unusual situation for immune complex formation and tissue injury.

Following immunization with inactivated vaccine there appears to be a selective stimulation of serum IgG antibody but little mucosal IgA antibody in the respiratory tract (Figure 23-12A). Immunization with live attenuated vaccine (in the case of measles) or following natural infection with either virus, on the other hand, stimulates a more balanced production of both serum (IgG) and mucosal (IgA) antibody (Figure 23-12B). Following immunization with inactivated vaccines, therefore, the respiratory tract is not fully immunized and there is produced the anomalous situation of compartmentalization with selective stimulation of the humoral serum compartment without immunization of the respiratory IgA secretory component, a situation of immunologic imbalance. Following natural infection with either measles or RSV, there is abnormal replication of virus within the respiratory tract and an accelerated anamnestic serum antibody response with the creation of a favorable condition for formation of immune complexes of viral antigen, IgG antibody, and complement within the lung, with subsequent tissue injury mediated by a type III mechanism (Figure 23-13A). In support of this mechanism of accelerated antibody responses is the finding that subsequent exposure of the previously killed viral vaccine

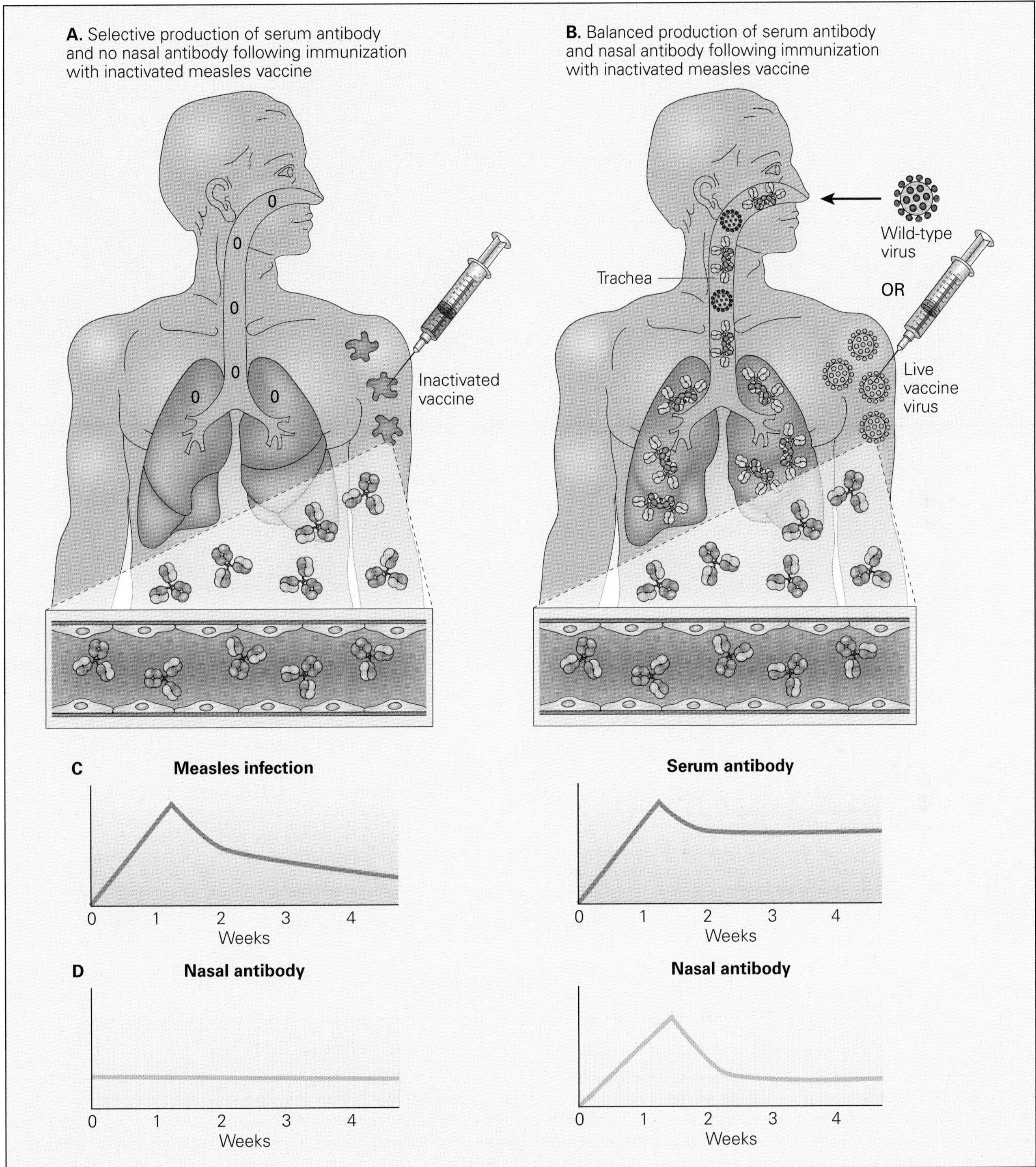

Figure 23-12. Schematic representation of the development of nasal mucosal and serum antibody following immunization with inactivated measles vaccine compared to responses seen after live measles vaccine or natural infection. Panel A: Note the selective production of serum antibody and the absence of nasal antibody following immunization with inactivated vaccine. Panel B: Note the balanced production of nasal and serum antibody following either natural infection or immunization with live attenuated vaccine.

recipients to either of the wild-type viruses led to strong Th2 polarization and enhanced antibody production in both diseases. A similar type III mechanism has been proposed for the localized Arthus-type reaction observed in children previously immunized with killed measles vaccine and who subsequently received the live attenuated measles vaccine (Figure 23-13B).

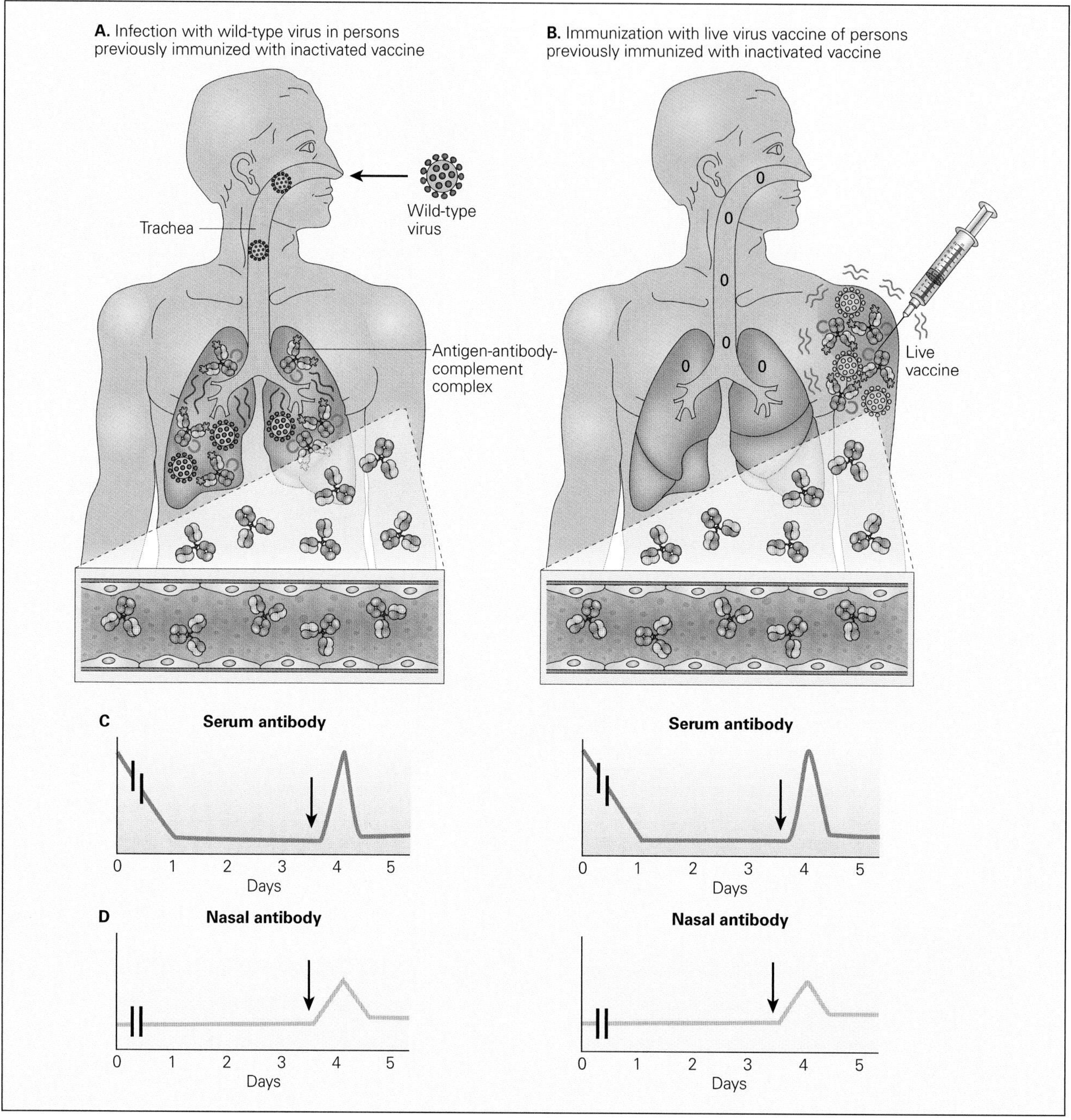

Figure 23-13. Schematic representation of the development of the proposed type III immune complex-mediated injury seen in atypical measles or enhanced respiratory syncytial virus disease. Panel A: Note the anomalous viral replication in the unprotected respiratory tract coupled with selective stimulation of the humoral serum compartment, creating a situation of immunologic imbalance favoring immune complex formation within the respiratory tract. Panel B: Note a similar type III mechanism proposed for the localized Arthus-type reaction in children previously immunized with killed measles vaccine and who subsequently received the live attenuated measles vaccine with conditions of viral replication and anamnestic antibody formation, favoring immune complex formation and localized tissue injury.

Passive Immunotherapy

Introduction

Classically, immunotherapy referred to passive immunization, i.e., the use of serum antibody or gamma globulin in the treatment or prevention of infectious diseases by transferring to one host antibodies actively produced in another. A specialized use of the term "immunotherapy" is its use in immunosuppression in a variety of immunologically mediated disorders (*Chapter 11*). The term immunotherapy has been broadened to include the use of immunologic applications in the hyposensitization therapy of allergic disease (*Chapter 18*) and in the treatment of cancer (*Chapter 20*). The complexity of the term has been increased by the extension of immunotherapy to the adoptive transfer of immunologically competent tissues or cells, e.g., bone marrow stem cells, thymus, and their products for the replacement therapy of immune deficiency disorders (*Chapter 16*), cancer (*Chapter 20*), or the lymphoproliferative disorders (*Chapter 21*). This section of the chapter will focus primarily on those applications of passive immunotherapy in the prevention or therapy of infectious diseases.

Historical Aspects of Passive Immunotherapy

In the late 19th century, it was discovered that immune serum from animal and human origin could be useful in the treatment of infectious diseases. The practice of administering polyclonal immunoglobulins isolated from hyperimmune sera of animal or human origin, introduced by Von Behring and Kitasato, has been used extensively in prophylactic as well as therapeutic settings (Figure 23-14). However, in the mid-1930s, penicillin and other antimicrobials were discovered and serum therapy was rapidly abandoned because antimicrobials were more effective and less toxic. Moreover, a high percentage of persons who received heterologous serum showed side effects of serum sickness (*Chapters 17* and *18*) that consisted of fever, chills, and immediate allergic reactions, e.g., hives, bronchospasm, and wheezing. Nevertheless, in relatively few situations, immune serum globulin is still indicated for postexposure prophylaxis against some viruses (rabies, measles, hepatitis A, hepatitis B, and varicella) and for treatment of toxin-dependent diseases (diphtheria, tetanus, and botulism) (Tables 23-15 and 23-16).

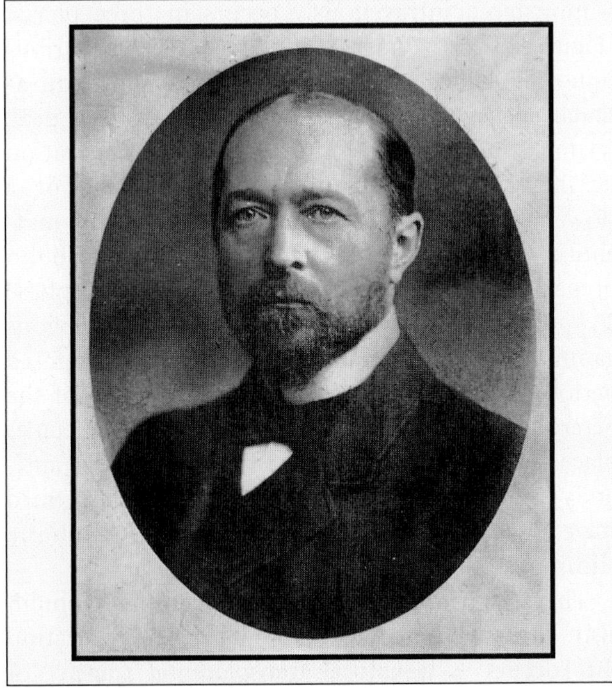

Figure 23-14. Emil Adolf von Behring (1854–1917). (Courtesy of the National Library of Medicine.)

Principles of Passive Immunization

As described previously, passive immunization is defined as the transfer of antibodies from an immune host into a nonimmune host to attain a desired prophylactic or therapeutic effect. Currently, in most cases, passive immunization is achieved with immunoglobulin preparations derived from pooled human plasma (*Chapter 11*). In industrialized countries, virtually all such products are derived from human plasma or serum. Products of human origin are preferred over those obtained from the originally used animal sources because these proteins do not elicit an immune response that could have an adverse effect, i.e., serum sickness. There are several principles underlying the use of passive immunization.

Immediacy of Action

The most important principle guiding the use of passive immunization is its immediacy of action, i.e., the ability of a preformed antibody to exert its effects immediately following its interaction with antigen. The delay of the latent period required by an active immune response is therefore avoided, which provides the great practical advantage of passive immunization over active immunization by its superiority in emergency situations when there is insufficient time to achieve active immunity or when vaccine may not be available. In general, the efficacy of passive immunization is directly related to the length of time between exposure to the pathogen and administration of the antibody product; the shorter the time interval, the greater the likelihood of success. In some instances, the antibody may be given prior to exposure, as in the use

Table 23-15. Antibody preparations available per passive immunity against infectious diseases in the United States

Product	Abbreviation/ brand name	Principal use
Standard human immune serum globulins (HISG, gamma globulin)		
Immune globulin, intravenous	IVIG, IGIV	Treatment of antibody deficiencies, Kawasaki disease
Immune globulin, intramuscular	IG, ISG	Treatment of antibody deficiency; prevention of measles, hepatitis A
Specific human immune serum globulins for intramuscular or subcutaneous use		
Hepatitis B immune globulin	HBIG	Prevention of hepatitis B
Varicella-zoster immune globulin	VZIG	Prevention or modification of chickenpox
Rabies immune globulin	RIG	Prevention of rabies
Tetanus immune globulin	TIG	Prevention or treatment of tetanus
Vaccinia immune globulin	VIG	Prevention or treatment of vaccinia, prevention of smallpox
Botulinum immune globulin	BIG	Treatment of newborn botulism
Specific human intravenous immune globulins		
Cytomegalovirus immune globulin	CMV-IVIG, CMVIG, CytoGam	Prevention of treatment of CMV infection
Respiratory syncytial virus immune globulin	RSV-IVIG, RSVIG, RespiGam	Prevention of RSV infection
Animal serum and globulins		
Tetanus antitoxin (equine)	TAT	Prevention or treatment of tetanus (when TIG unavailable)
Diphtheria antitoxin (equine)	DAT	Treatment of diphtheria
Botulinum antitoxin (equine)		Treatment of botulism
Monoclonal antibodies		
Palivizumab (anti-RSV-F)	Synagis	Prevention of RSV infection

of gamma globulin for prevention of hepatitis A infection in individuals traveling to high-risk areas. In addition, passive immunization is the treatment of choice in individuals with primary or secondary humoral immune deficiencies (*Chapter 16*).

Metabolism of Gamma Globulin

Also critically important in the use of passive immunization are the physicochemical and biologic factors that govern the metabolism of gamma globulin (*Chapter 6*). It is now generally accepted that once antibody molecules are synthesized, they, like all other protein molecules, have a limited biologic half-life. There is a continual loss by catabolism and anabolic replacement of these molecules in a dynamic state referred to as "turnover." By the very nature of the passive immunization procedure itself, the passive introduction of gamma globulin molecules into a host ensures that the duration of antibody activity will be finite and related to the biologic half-life of the particular isotype. For example, if homologous (human) IgG is administered to a healthy human, the mean biologic half-life ($t^1/_2$) is 23 days. More rapid rates of degradation are observed with other isotypes, e.g., mean $t^1/_2$IgA = six days and mean $t^1/_2$IgM = five days (*Chapter 6*). The half-life of gamma globulin from other species, i.e., heterologous (horse) gamma globulin, is much shorter, with a mean $t^1/_2$horse gamma globulin = six days. These events are represented schematically in Figure 23-15 together with patterns of elimination of both homologous (human) and heterologous (horse) gamma globulin.

The pattern of elimination of gamma globulin administered intravenously occurs in three phases (Figure 23-15). **Phase 1** is a period of redistribution or equalization between vascular and extravascular spaces that results in a striking drop in peak serum concentration shortly after administration of the gamma globulin. **Phase 2** consists of a slower, steady drop in serum levels due to the metabolic (catabolic) half-life of the gamma globulin preparations. These patterns for phase 1 and phase 2 apply to both homologous and heterologous gamma globulin. **Phase 3** represents an accelerated period of degradation occurring in the case of the heterologous (horse) gamma globulin that takes place simultaneously with the development of antibody to the foreign gamma globulin. This third stage is referred to as the phase of **immune elimination.**

These metabolic properties of gamma globulin also have relevance to the passive immunization that occurs as a natural transplacental transfer of IgG in the human infant (*Chapter 2*). The gradual

Table 23-16. Summary of the efficacy of antibody in the prevention and treatment of infectious diseases

Infection	Prophylaxis	Treatment
Bacterial infections		
Respiratory infections (streptococcus, *Streptococcus pneumoniae, Neisseria meningitidis, Haemophilus influenzae*)	Proven (NR)[a, b]	Proven (NR)[b]
Diphtheria	Unproven (NR)	Proven
Pertussis	Unproven (NR)	Unproven (NR)
Tetanus	Proven	Proven
Other clostridial infections:		
C. botulinum	Proven	Proven
C. difficile	Unproven (NR)	Probable benefit
Staphylococcal infections		
Toxic shock syndrome	Unproven (NR)	Probable benefit
Antibiotic resistance	Unproven (NR)	Possible benefit
S. epidermidis in newborns	Possible benefit	Not studied
Invasive streptococcal disease (toxic shock syndrome)	Unproven (NR)	Probable benefit
High-risk newborns	Possible benefit (NR)	Probable benefit
Shock, intensive care, and trauma	Possible benefit (NR)	Unproven
Pseudomonas infection		
Cystic fibrosis	Unproven (NR)	No benefit
Burns	Unproven (NR)	No benefit
Viral diseases		
Hepatitis A	Proven	No benefit
Hepatitis B	Proven	No benefit
Hepatitis C	Unproven (NR)	No benefit
HIV infection	Unproven (NR)	Unproven (NR)
RSV infection	Proven	Unproven (NR)
Herpesvirus infections		
CMV	Proven	Possible benefit
EBV	Unproven (NR)	Unproven (NR)
HSV	Unproven (NR)	Unproven (NR)
VZV	Proven	Unproven (NR)
Parvovirus infection	Unproven (NR)	Proven (NR)[b]
Enterovirus infection	Proven (NR)[b]	Proven (NR)[b]
In newborns	Unproven	Possible benefit
Ebola	Possible benefit	Unproven
Rabies	Proven	No benefit
Measles	Proven	No benefit
Rubella	Unproven (NR)	No benefit
Mumps	Unproven (NR)	No benefit
Tick-borne encephalitis virus (TBEV)	Possible benefit	No benefit
Vaccinia	Proven	Proven

Reproduced with permission from Keller MA, Stiehm ER. Passive immunity in prevention and treatment of infectious diseases. Clin Microbiol Rev. 2000;13:602-14.

a. NR, not recommended.

b. Except for immunodeficient patients.

degradation and diminished serum IgG concentrations following birth contributes to the physiologic hypogammaglobulinemia seen in normal human infancy (*Chapter 16*).

Immunosuppressive Properties of Gamma Globulin

Another principle of passive immunization is manifest by the immunosuppressive effects of gamma

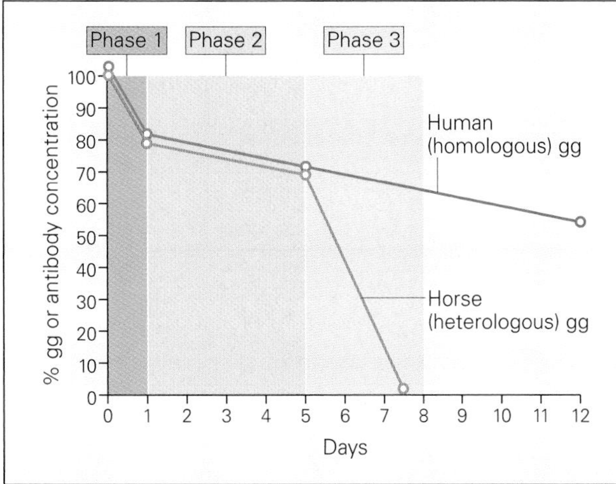

Figure 23-15. Schematic comparison of the catabolism of human gamma globulin with horse gamma globulin showing the three phases of catabolism. Phase 1: Shows a period of equalization or redistribution. Phase 2: Shows a metabolic phase related to the biologic half-life ($t^1/_2$). Phase 3: Shows immune elimination, which is more accelerated with horse gamma globulin owing to the development of antibody to the foreign gamma globulin.

globulin (*Chapter 11*). The passive administration of gamma globulin or specific antibody will inhibit active production of antibody by means of negative feedback inhibition. As described in Chapter 11, a variety of mechanisms have been proposed to explain the immunosuppressant actions of IVIG, including: Fc receptor blockade or modulation, enhancement of T cell regulatory function, inhibition of B cell function, anti-idiotypic antibodies, complement inhibition, cytokine inhibition, accelerated catabolism of autoantibodies, and an inhibition of Fas-mediated cell death by Fas-blocking antibodies. Shown in Figure 23-16 is a schematic representation of some of these immunosuppressive mechanisms of IVIG. These are also elaborated upon in Box 23-3.

Two clinical applications of the immunosuppressive effects of specific antibody are shown in Figure 23-17. These include the use of anti-Rh_0 antibodies for the prevention of erythroblastosis fetalis and the use of anti-lymphocyte serum (**ALS**) in the prevention of graft rejection in solid organ transplantation. If red blood cells from an Rh_0-positive individual are coated with anti-Rh_0 antibody prior to injection into an Rh_0-negative individual (as in the case of an Rh_0 mother carrying an Rh_0-positive infant), the formation of anti-Rh_0 antibodies is prevented. This use of antibody-induced immune suppression is thought to primarily affect the "afferent" limb of the immune response by preventing the production of antibody. A second clinical application of the immunosuppressive actions of gamma globulin in solid organ transplantation by the use of ALS is thought to inhibit the immune response by interfering with the "efferent" limb of immunity (Figure 23-17).

The Use of Monoclonal Antibodies in Passive Immunotherapy

Due to the enormous progress made in the field of monoclonal antibodies (**mAbs**), the reintroduction of antibody-based therapies against a wide spectrum of pathogens is under investigation (*Chapter 11*). Currently, the availability of human and humanized mAbs is no longer a limiting factor and these products can be developed theoretically against any pathogen by the hybridoma technology (*Chapter 6*). By using recombinant DNA technologies, mAbs can be produced within a short time in large quantities, which makes them a valuable tool against emerging and reemerging infectious diseases. Furthermore, mAbs circumvent many of the problems linked to polyclonal sera, including risks related to the use of human or animal blood products, low content of specific antibodies, and lot-to-lot variation. Additionally, mAbs with high activity against a given pathogen can be selected, which not only translates into higher therapeutic efficacy, but also into marked reduction of the quantity required for therapy. Several mAb preparations directed against pathogens are currently being tested in clinical studies and one is already approved for the prevention of serious lower respiratory tract disease caused by RSV in pediatric patients at high risk of RSV disease.

One limitation of the use of mAbs therapy is their high pathogen specificity; by definition, a mAb is recognizing only one single epitope, but most pathogens are circulating in nature in antigenically diverse forms. Therefore, prior to initiating therapy for a given infectious disease, the exact identification of the pathogen is mandatory, which requires rapid and reliable diagnostic tools. Rapid identification becomes even more important owing to the fact that antibody therapy is most effective in a preventive setting or at very early time points of disease. For pathogens, which are antigenically variable, the use of an antibody cocktail active against the most common antigenic types might offer a

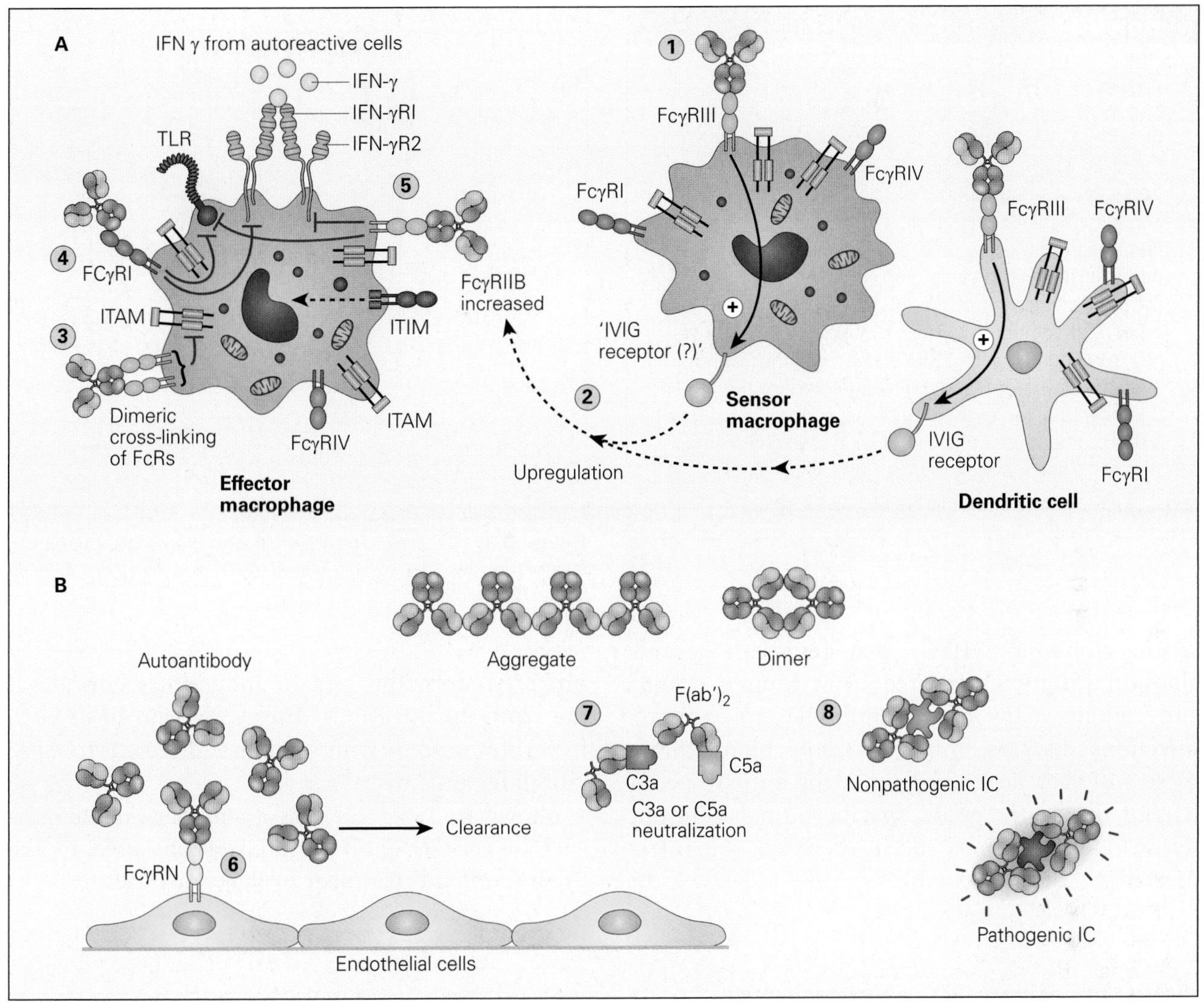

Figure 23-16. Schematic representation of the immunosuppressive mechanisms of IVIG. Panel A: IVIG can actively suppress the inflammatory response by any of the following mechanisms: (1) the binding of IVIG with FcγR receptors (FcγRI, FcγRIII, or FcγRIV) on sensor macrophages and/or DCs followed by the expression and activation of an as-yet-unknown IVIG receptor (2) can subsequently suppress activation of effector macrophages via upregulation of FcγRIIB; (3) the cross-linking of dimeric FcR by IVIG can result in blockage of subsequent ITAM-mediated activation responses; (4) inhibition of the activating effects of either FcγRI or (5) FcγRIII-signaling by IVIG can lead to blockage of TLR or IFN-γ activation, respectively. Inhibition of the IFN-γ response is due to PU.1-mediated transcriptional repression of IFN-γR2. Panel B: IVIG can suppress the inflammatory responses passively by competing for occupancy of the FcγR IgG receptors or by induction of immunosuppression through inhibition of cellular activation. Passive inhibition can occur by any of the following mechanisms: (6) competition for occupancy of FcRn receptors by IgG monomers with soluble autoantibody and enhanced clearance of pathogenic autoantibodies; (7) binding of F(ab)2 fragments with complement fragments C3a and C5a with neutralization of their proinflammatory activity; (8) competition of IVIG-derived Ig aggregates, dimers, or ICs with pathogenic ICs for occupancy of activating FcγRs with blockage of immune activation. (Adapted from and reproduced with permission from Clynes R. IVIG therapy: interfering with interferon-gamma. Immunity. 2007;26:4-6.)

solution. RNA viruses have a particularly high mutation rate and a broad spectrum of virus mutants (quasispecies) are circulating in an infected organism at the same time. Against those viruses like human immunodeficiency virus (HIV) or hepatitis C virus (**HCV**), it will be difficult to define a mAb cocktail since virus escape-mutants will be formed readily and the therapy will become ineffective (*Chapter 13*). However, also in those cases, mAbs might be useful as supportive therapy to antivirals.

Types of Preparations Used in Passive Immunization for Infectious Diseases

The various antibody preparations currently available in the United States for use in passive immunity against infectious diseases are shown in Table 23-15. These include human immune

Box 23-3

Classes of Fc Receptor

Fc receptors are specific protein molecules found on the surface of certain cells—including macrophages (monocytes), neutrophils, eosinophils, dendritic cells, Langerhans cells, mast cells, natural killer cells, platelets, epithelial cells, endothelial cells, hepatocytes, and B cells—that provide the membrane-binding sites for the Fc fragment of the IgG, IgA, IgM, and IgE isotypes that contribute to the many protective and overall immunomodulating functions of the immune system (*Chapters 6* and *11*). A summary of the major Fc receptors for each of the major immunoglobulin isotypes together with their binding affinities, cell distribution, and biologic effects following binding to their specific ligands is presented in Chapter 6.

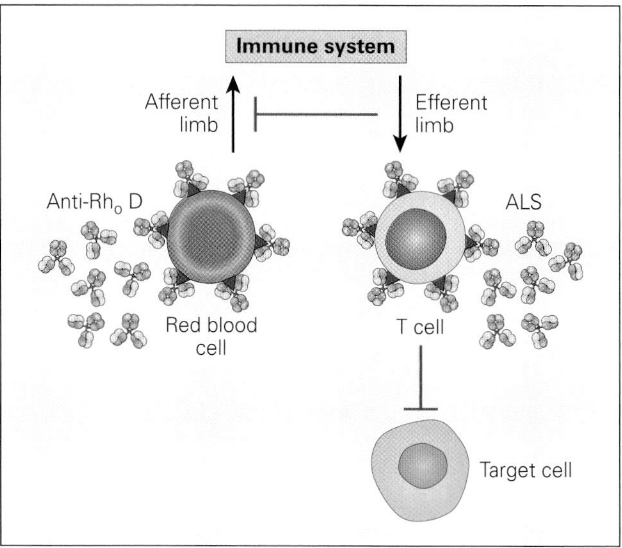

Figure 23-17. Schematic representation of the modes of immunosuppression by specific anti-Rh_0 antibody and by antilymphocyte serum (ALS).

serum globulins (HISG) that represent gamma globulin products prepared from human donors and contain many of the antibodies to common infectious diseases found in whole blood. Since these will vary depending upon the antibody content in the donor pools, specific human immune serum globulins have been prepared for intramuscular or subcutaneous use. These are prepared from the sera of individuals convalescing from an infectious disease or who have been hyperimmunized with vaccines directed to specific infectious diseases.

Shown in Table 23-16 is a summary of the efficacy of various antibody preparations used in the prevention and treatment of infectious diseases.

Case Study: Clinical Relevance

Let us now return to the case study of atypical measles presented earlier and review some of the major points of the clinical presentation and how they relate to the immune system.

- Several years following the immunization of children with killed measles vaccine, two types of reactions were seen: (1) a systemic reaction that occurred following exposure to natural measles, and (2) localized reaction that occurred at the site where a subsequent live measles virus vaccine was administered.
- The systemic or generalized form was referred to as atypical measles and was characterized by the development of high fever, toxicity, and skin lesions that took an atypical form and distribution similar to those described in the case study. In contrast to the skin eruption seen in natural measles that begins on the face and has a tendency to spread caudally, the atypical lesions began on the lower extremities and spread upward with sparing of the face. In addition, a high incidence of pneumonia and pleural effusion was reported in these children.
- As described previously, another atypical form of viral infection was seen in children previously immunized with killed respiratory syncytial virus (RSV) vaccines who when later were exposed to natural RSV developed a more severe form of the disease in a condition referred to as enhanced respiratory syncytial virus disease.
- Two major explanations have been suggested for the pathogenesis of both of these atypical diseases. One theory holds that humoral immunity, in the form of antigen-antibody complexes, was responsible for the atypical rash and the altered bronchiolitic disease and other manifestations of the syndrome. A second theory is that of enhanced cell-mediated immunity.

Case Study: Clinical Relevance (continued)

- In support of the first possibility was the finding that the localized indurated erythematous reactions were observed in children usually within the first 24 hours, a finding characteristic of the classic Arthus reaction (*Chapter 17*).
- Histopathologic examination of biopsies of these localized lesions revealed the presence of mixed-type inflammatory infiltrate consisting of lymphocytes, monocytes, and neutrophils clustered around blood vessels. Examination by immunofluorescence revealed deposition of immunoglobulins (IgG, IgA, and IgM), measles antigen, and β1 C-globulin (C3 or the third component of complement).
- More recently, the studies of Polack have confirmed the immune complex theory of immunologic injury and have concluded that atypical measles and the enhanced respiratory syncytial virus disease were serious diseases that resulted from immunization of children with inactivated vaccines against measles and RSV.
- Both vaccines failed to elicit protective antibody and, in both cases, postvaccination exposure to wild-type virus led to immune complex deposition in affected tissues, vigorous anamnestic CD4+ T lymphocyte proliferative responses, and a Th2 bias of the immune response.
- Although the clinical manifestations of both illnesses were different and were related to individual target tissue tropism of each virus, the similarities in immune responses elicited and primed for by the vaccines suggest that atypical measles and the enhanced respiratory syncytial virus disease shared a common general mechanism of illness, namely that of immune complex formation.
- Furthermore, these diseases resulted from an imbalanced and disproportionate response of a primed immune system exposed to wild-type virus in the absence of protective antibody.
- These experiences, although now only of historic interest, highlight the importance of understanding the requirements of vaccines for the production of protective immunity against these agents and the future development of new, safe, and effective vaccines for the protection of young infants.

Key Points

- Active immunity is characterized by protection against a pathogen generated by a person's own immune system, which can be acquired either by natural infection or by active vaccination.
- Passive immunity is protection provided by antibodies that are not produced by the recipient but rather by antibodies produced in other hosts or in vitro systems that can be transferred artificially by injection, or naturally, e.g., during pregnancy or by breast-feeding, resulting in transfer of antibody from the mother to the offspring.
- The use of vaccines for the prevention of infectious disease developed from the observation that individuals who recovered from a specific infectious disease did not contract that disease again.
- The classic method of vaccine development by the Pasteur method by "isolating, inactivating, and injecting infectious agents" has been replaced in modern times by a genomic approach referred to as "reverse vaccinology" starting with genome analysis with information encoded within the microbial genome and then progressing to the identification and production of structural proteins for inclusion in vaccines.
- Vaccines can be broadly divided into three classic categories, live attenuated microorganisms, inactivated (killed) whole microorganisms, or purified subunit vaccines. Nucleic acid-based vaccines represent a newly emerging fourth category.
- Live attenuated vaccines retain the ability to replicate in humans at a low extent that usually does not cause illness but that provides a continuous antigenic stimulation to the immune system with an immune response virtually identical to that produced by natural infection. Since these vaccines are dependent on sufficient replication to induce protective immunity, they may be inhibited by preformed antibody.
- Inactivated vaccines because of their nonreplicative nature rely on a preformed antigenic mass to induce an adequate immune response and, unlike live attenuated vaccines, are not affected by preformed antibody.
- Subunit vaccines are a type of inactivated vaccine consisting of one or more of the purified components of the microbial antigens found within the major antigenic sites of a pathogen.

- Recombinant DNA technology has permitted the development of several new subunit vaccines, including recombinant vaccines against hepatitis B (HBV), the acellular vaccines against *B. pertussis*, and most recently against the human papillomaviruses (HPVs).
- Conjugated vaccines are created by the chemical coupling of a polysaccharide to a carrier protein, which converts T-independent antigens (like polysaccharides) into T-dependent antigens (located on the carrier protein), which will then provide help to B cells for the production of polysaccharide-specific antibodies. Examples of conjugated vaccines include those directed against *Haemophilus influenzae* type b (Hib), *N. meningitides*, and *S. pneumoniae*.
- DNA vaccines and vector vaccines that use live viral or bacterial vectors to deliver DNA or RNA encoding antigens into cells represent new-generation vaccines.
- There are contraindications of vaccine use where vaccines should not be given, as in the case of administration of live attenuated vaccines to subjects with severe immunosuppression; there are also precautions of vaccine use that include conditions where a recipient might have an increased risk of a serious adverse reaction or where there may be compromise of the vaccine to produce immunity, as in the case of a severe acute illness or inhibition by maternally acquired antibody with early immunization with a live attenuated vaccine before the age of 12 months, respectively.
- There are several types of immunologically mediated adverse effects to vaccines that include: (1) those that are seen in immunologically comprised hosts; (2) those that are seen predominantly in allergic (atopic) individuals; and (3) those seen in normal hosts and appear to be related to the vaccine antigen or the route of administration.
- Atypical measles and the enhanced respiratory syncytial virus disease were serious diseases that resulted from immunization of children with inactivated vaccines against measles and RSV.
- The use of serum therapy for prevention or treatment of infectious diseases, i.e., passive immunization, represents one of immunology's earliest applications.
- There are two major gamma globulin preparations used in passive immunization: (1) standard human immune serum globulins (HISG, gamma globulin); and (2) special human immune serum globulins for intramuscular or subcutaneous use.
- The development of monoclonal antibodies (mAbs) against a wide spectrum of pathogens by hybridoma technology represents one of the great new applications of passive immunization.

Study Questions/Critical Thinking

1. Each of the following is a TRUE statement concerning vaccines EXCEPT:
   a. The oral poliovirus vaccine is an example of a live attenuated vaccine
   b. The duration of immunity is generally longer for inactivated vaccines than for live attenuated vaccines
   c. *Haemophilus influenzae* type b (Hib) is an example of a conjugate vaccine
   d. Inactivated vaccines usually require booster injections
   e. Immunization of a patient with a live attenuated vaccine is an example of a contraindication to vaccine usage
2. Each of the following is a TRUE statement concerning the MenB vaccine EXCEPT:
   a. An example of one of the great triumphs of reverse vaccinology
   b. A major cause of meningococcal meningitis worldwide
   c. A type of live attenuated vaccine
   d. Development was impeded because the capsular polysaccharide of MenB is structurally identical to human polysaccharide
   e. Indicated for high-risk populations, e.g., the military
3. Which of the following is a TRUE statement concerning hepatitis B:
   a. Hepatitis B immune globulin is effective in the prevention of hepatitis B infection
   b. 10–15 percent of recipients of hepatitis B vaccine fail to respond with antibody production
   c. Hepatitis B vaccine consists of the hepatitis B surface antigen
   d. Treatment of choice for active hepatitis B infection is immunoglobulin replacement
   e. Hepatitis B vaccine is an inactivated vaccine
4. Each of the following is a TRUE statement concerning atypical measles EXCEPT:
   a. Affected patients presented with a rash that began on the face and progressed caudally

b. Seen in children who received the killed measles vaccine
c. Characterized by a high incidence of pulmonary infiltrates
d. Caused by immune complex formation
e. The localized lesion seen at a site of subsequent live vaccine in a prior killed vaccine recipient is a type of Arthus reaction

5. Each of the following is a TRUE statement concerning passive immunization EXCEPT:
   a. The use of animal sera carries a risk of serum sickness
   b. Intravenous immune globulin is indicated for replacement therapy of humoral immune deficiencies
   c. Special human intravenous immune globulin has been an effective treatment of infants with RSV infection
   d. Efficacy of antibody in the prevention and treatment of HIV has been proven
   e. Efficacy of antibody in the prevention but not the treatment of measles has been proven

Suggested Reading

American Academy of Pediatrics, Committee on Infectious Diseases. Prevention of pertussis among adolescents: recommendations for use of tetanus toxoid, reduced diphtheria toxoid and acellular pertussis (Tdap) vaccines. Pediatrics. 2006; 117: 965–78.

Ashkenazi S, Passwell JH, Harlev E, et al. Safety and immunogenicity of Shigella sonnei and Shigella flexneri 2a O-specific polysaccharide conjugates in children. J Infect Dis. 1999; 179: 1565–8.

Atkinson WL, Pickering LK, Watson JC, et al. General immunization practices. In Vaccines 4th ed. Philadelphia: Saunders; 2004.

Ballow M. The IgG molecule as a biological immune response modifier: mechanisms of action of intravenous immune serum globulin in autoimmune and inflammatory disorders. J Allergy Clin Immunol. 2011; 127: 315–23.

Bellanti JA. Biologic significance of the secretory A immunoglobulins. Pediatrics. 1971; 48: 715–29.

Black S, Shinefield H, Fireman B, et al. Efficacy, safety, and immunogenicity of heptavalent pneumococcal conjugate vaccine in children: Northern California Kaiser Permanente Vaccine Study Center Group. Pediatr Infect Dis J. 2000; 19: 187–95.

Center for Disease Control and Prevention (US). General recommendations on immunization: recommendations of the Advisory Committee on Immunization Practices (ACIP) and the American Academy of Family Physicians (AAFP). MMWR. 2006; 55.

Center for Disease Control and Prevention (US). Haemophilus b conjugate vaccines for prevention of Haemophilus influenzae, type b disease among infants and children two months of age and older: recommendations of the ACIP. MMWR. 1991; 40: 1–7.

Center for Disease Control and Prevention (US). Impact of vaccines universally recommended for children – US, 1990–98. MMWR. 1998; 48: 577–81.

Center for Disease Control and Prevention (US). Measles, mumps, and rubella—vaccine use and strategies for elimination of measles, rubella, and congenital rubella syndrome and control of mumps: recommendations of the Advisory Committee on Immunization Practices (ACIP). MMWR. 1998; 47: 1–57.

Center for Disease Control and Prevention (US). Preventing pneumococcal disease among infants and young children: recommendations of the Advisory Committee on Immunization Practices (ACIP). MMWR. 2000; 49: 1–35.

Centers for Disease Control and Prevention (US). Prevention and control of meningococcal disease: Recommendations of the Advisory Committee on Immunization Practices (ACIP). MMWR Recomm. 2005; 54: 1–21.

Center for Disease Control and Prevention (US). Prevention of pneumococcal disease: recommendations of the Advisory Committee on Immunization Practices (ACIP). MMWR. 1997; 46: 1–24.

Center for Disease Control and Prevention (US). Prevention of varicella: recommendations of the Advisory Committee on Immunization Practices (ACIP). MMWR. 1996; 45: 8.

Center for Disease Control and Prevention (US). Recommended adult immunization schedule–United States. 2010. MMWR. 2010; 59(1) quick guide.

Center for Disease Control and Prevention (US). Recommended immunization schedule for persons aged 0 through 18 years–United States. 2010, MMWR. 2010; 58(51 & 52) quick guide.

Center for Disease Control and Prevention (US). Updated recommendations from the Advisory Committee on Immunization Practices (ACIP) for revaccination of persons at Prolonged Increased Risk for Meningococcal Disease. MMWR. 2009; 58: 1042–3.

Centers for Disease Control and Prevention (US). Vaccine Development: current status and future needs: The Pink Book. 2005 11th ed. Atlanta: CDC.

Can be accessed at http://www.cdc.gov/vaccines/pubs/pinkbook/downloads/appendices/A/age-interval-table.pdf.

Clynes R. IVIG therapy: interfering with interferon-gamma. Immunity. 2007; 26: 4–6.

Cohen D, Ashkenazi S, Green MS, et al. Double-blind vaccine-controlled randomised efficacy trial of an investigational Shigella sonnei conjugate vaccine in young adults. Lancet. 1997; 349: 155–9.

Del Gudice G. Towards the development of vaccines against Helicobacter pylori: status and issues. Curr Opin Investig Drugs. 2001; 2: 40–4.

Ehreth J. The global value of vaccination. Vaccine. 2003; 21: 596–600.

Eskola J. Immunogenicity of pneumococcal conjugate vaccines. Pediatr Infect Dis J. 2000; 19: 388–93.

Eskola J, Kilpi T, Palmu A, et al. Efficacy of a pneumococcal conjugate vaccine against acute otitis media. N Engl J Med. 2001; 344: 403–9.

Fleischmann RD, Adams MD, White O, et al. Whole-genome random sequencing and assembly of Haemophilus influenzae. Rd Science. 1995; 269: 496–512.

Garland SM, Smith JS. Human papillomavirus vaccines: current status and future prospects. Drugs. 2010; 70: 1079–98.

Glenny AT, Hopkins BE. Diphtheria toxoid as an immunizing agent. Brit J Exp Pathol. 1923; 4: 283–88.

Granoff D, Feavers I, Borrow R. Meningococcal vaccines. In Vaccines, 4th ed. Philadelphia: Saunders, 2004.

Gréco M. The future of vaccines: an industrial perspective. Vaccine. 2002; 20: S101–S103.

Greenhawt MJ, Chernin AS, Howe L, et al. The safety of the H1N1 influenza A vaccine in egg allergic individuals. Ann Allergy Asthma Immunol. 2010; 105: 387–93.

Ipp MM, Gold R, Goldbach M, et al. Adverse reactions to diphtheria, tetanus, pertussis-polio vaccination at 18 months of age: effect of injection site and needle length. Pediatrics. 1989; 83: 679–82.

Jansen KU, Shaw AR. Human papillomavirus vaccines and prevention of cervical cancer. Annu Rev Med. 2004; 55: 319–31.

Kao JH, Chen DS. Global control of hepatitis B virus infection. Lancet Infect Dis. 2002; 2: 395–403.

Keller MA, Stiehm R. Passive immunita in prevention and treatment of infectious diseases. Clin Microbiol Rev. 2000; 13: 602–14.

Kelso JM, Li JT, Nicklas RA, et al. Adverse reactions to vaccines. Ann Allergy Asthma Immunol. 2009; 103: S1–14.

Kendrick PL, Eldering G, Dixon MK. Mouse protection tests in the study of pertussis vaccine: a comparative study using intracerebral route for challenge. Am J Publ Health. 1947; 37: 803.

Lang ML. Glatman-Freedman A. Do CD1-restricted T cells contribute to antibody-mediated immunity against Mycobacterium tuberculosis? Infect Immun. 2006; 74: 803–9.

Lin FY, Ho VA, Khiem HB, et al. The efficacy of a Salmonella typhi Vi conjugate vaccine in two-to-five-year-old children. N Engl J Med. 2001; 344: 1263–9.

Martin DB, Weiner LB, Nieburg PI, et al. Atypical measles in adolescents and young adults. Ann Intern Med. 1979; 90: 877–81.

Miller E, Salisbury D, Ramsay, M. Planning, registration, and implementation of an immunization campaign against meningococcal serogroup C disease in the UK: a success story. Vaccine. 2001; 20(Suppl 1) S58–67.

Murphy TV, Pastor P, Medley F, et al. Decreased Haemophilus colonization in children vaccinated with Haemophilus influenzae type b conjugate vaccine. J Pediatr. 1993; 122: 517–23.

Myers MG, Beckman CW, Vosdingh RA, et al. Primary immunization with tetanus and diphtheria toxoids: reaction rate and immunogenicity in older children and adults. JAMA. 1982; 248: 2478–80.

National Bacteriological Laboratory, Sweden. A clinical trial of acellular pertussis vaccine in Sweden. Technical Report. 1988.

O'Hagan D, Rappuoli R. The safety of vaccines. DDT. 2004; 9: 846–54.

Paoletti LC, Kasper DL. Conjugate vaccines against group B Streptococcus types IV and VII. J Infect Dis. 2002; 186: 123–6.

Paoletti LC, Madoff LC, Kasper DL. Surface structures of group B Streptococcus important in human immunity. In VA Fischetti, RP Novick, JJ Ferretti, DA Portnoy JI Rood Gram-Positive Pathogens. Washington, DC: American Society for Microbiology, 2000.

Passwell JH, Harlev E, Ashkenazi S, et al. Safety and immunogenicity of improved Shigella O-specific polysaccharide-protein conjugate vaccines in adults in Israel. Infect Immun. 2001; 69: 1351–7.

Peltola H. Worldwide Haemophilus influenzae type b disease at the beginning of the 21st century: global analysis of the disease burden 25 years after the use of the polysaccharide vaccine and a decade after the advent of conjugates. Clin Microbiol Rev. 2000; 13: 302–17.

Petralli JK, Merigan TC, Wilbur JR. Action of endogenous interferon against vaccinia infection in children. Lancet. 1965; 2: 401–5.

Petralli JK, Merigan TC, Wilbur JR. Circulating interferon after measles vaccination. N Eng J Med. 1965; 273: 198–201.

Pizza M, Covacci A, Bartoloni A, et al. Mutants of pertussis toxin suitable for vaccine development. Science. 1989; 246: 497–500.

Pizza M, Scarlato V, Masignani V, et al. Identification of vaccine candidates against serogroup B meningococcus by whole-genome sequencing. Science. 2000; 287: 1816–20.

Polack FP. Atypical measles and enhanced respiratory syncytial virus disease (ERD) made simple. Pediatr Res. 2007; 62: 111–5.

Poland GA. Prevention of meningococcal disease: current use of polysaccharide and conjugate vaccines. Clin Infect Dis. 2010; 50(Suppl 2): S45–53.

Poland GA, Jacobson RM. The age-old struggle against the antivaccinationists. N Engl J Med. 2011; 364: 97–9.

Ramon G. Sur le pouvoir floculant et sur les propriétés immunisantes d'une toxine diphthérique rendue anatoxique (anatoxine). CR Acad Sci (Paris) 1923; 177: 1338–40.

Ramon G. Sur la production des antitoxins. CR Acad Sci (Paris). 1925; 181: 157–9.

Ramsay M, Andrews NJ, Trotter CL, et al. Herd immunity from meningococcal serogroup C conjugate vaccination in England: database analysis. Br Med J. 2003; 326: 365–6.

Rappuoli R, Reverse vaccinology. Curr Opin Microbiol. 2000; 3: 445–50.

Rappuoli R. Reverse vaccinology, a genome-based approach to vaccine development. Vaccine. 2001; 19: 2688–91.

Rappuoli R, Covacci A. Reverse vaccinology and genomics. Science. 2003; 302: 602.

Rappuoli R, Miller H, Falkow S. The intangible value of vaccination. Science. 2002; 297: 937–8.

Sabahi F, Rola-Plesczcynski M, O'Connell S, et al. Qualitative and quantitative analysis of T lymphocytes during normal human pregnancy. Am J Reprod Immunol. 1995; 33: 381–93.

Salmaso S, Mastrantonio P, Tozzi AE, et al. Sustained efficacy during the first 6 years of life of 3-component acellular pertussis vaccines administered in infancy: the Italian experience. Pediatrics. 2001; 108: E81.

Schaible UE, Kaufmann SHE. CD1 molecules and CD1-dependent T cells in bacterial infections: a link from innate to acquired immunity? Semin Immunol. 2000; 12: 527–35.

Scheifele D, Bjornson G, Barreto L, et al. Controlled trial of Haemophilus influenzae type b diphtheria toxoid conjugate combined with diphtheria, tetanus and pertussis vaccines, in 18-month-old children, including comparison of arm versus thigh injection. Vaccine. 1992; 10: 455–60.

Shinefield HR, Black SB, Staehle BO, et al. Safety, tolerability and immunogenicity of concomitant injections in separate locations of M-M-R® II, VARIVAX® and TETRAMUNE® in healthy children vs. concomitant injections of M-M-R® II and TETRAMUNE® followed six weeks later by VARIVAX®. Pediatr Infect Dis J. 1998; 17: 980–5.

Vaccine Development: current status and future needs. A report from the American Academy of Microbiology. 2005.

Villa LL. Prophylactic HPV vaccines: reducing the burden of HPV-related diseases. Vaccine. 2005.

Villa LL, et al. Prophylactic quadrivalent human papillomavirus (types 6, 11, 16, and 18) L1 virus-like particle vaccine in young women: a randomised double-blind placebo-controlled multicentre phase II efficacy trial. Lancet Oncol. 2005; 6: 271–8.

Wenger JD, Ward JI. Haemophilus influenzae vaccine. In Vaccines, 4th ed. 2004.

World Health Organization. Hepatitis B vaccines. Weekly Epidemiological Record. 2004; 28: 253–64.

Yeh SH, Gurtman A, Hurley DC, et al. Immunogenicity and Safety of 13-Valent Pneumococcal Conjugate Vaccine in Infants and Toddlers. Pediatrics. 2010; 126: e493–e505.

Chapter 24

Clinical Applications of Laboratory Diagnostic Immunology

Susan M. Orton, PhD
James D. Folds, PhD
Joseph A. Bellanti, MD

Case Study

A seven-year-old white male patient was referred for evaluation of recurrent bouts of paranasal sinusitis, streptococcal pharyngeal tonsillitis, lower respiratory tract infections, and continuous low-grade fever requiring frequent use of antibiotics for the past two years. During the previous year, he developed intermittent ocular swelling and redness but had no complaints of visual problems, light sensitivity, or tearing. Review of systems revealed a six-month history of joint pain in both knees, elbows, and hands without swelling of the joints, which often limited his daily activities without any direct relationship to any known cause. The mother also related episodes of a generalized, nonpruritic, salmon-red erythematous rash consisting of localized discrete lesions, measuring 1 × 1 cm in size, most prominently seen on the face and trunk, and that were exacerbated by fever.

A detailed review of the patient's family pedigree of his past five generations revealed a strong genetic predisposition for autoimmune diseases (Figure 24-1).

The following disorders were elicited in the family history: immunodeficiency, polyarteritis nodosa (PAN), rheumatoid arthritis (RA), Raynaud's phenomenon, systemic lupus erythematosus (SLE), and bronchial asthma (BA). A remarkably increased prevalence of juvenile idiopathic arthritis (JIA) (formerly referred to as juvenile rheumatoid arthritis, JRA) was found in several family members, including the mother. The family pedigree consisted of 76 relatives spanning five generations, with 41 male and 35 female relatives. Of the male relatives, 12 (34.2 percent) had one or more of the following conditions: immunodeficiency, 6 (54.5 percent); PAN, 0 relatives; RA, 1 (9 percent); Raynaud's phenomenon, 1 (9 percent); SLE, 0; bronchial asthma, 5 (45.4 percent); and JIA, 3 (27.2 percent). Of the 35 female relatives, 11 (31.4 percent) had one or more of the following: immunodeficiency, 9 (81.8 percent); PAN, 1 (9 percent); RA, 1 (9 percent); Raynaud's phenomenon, 2 (18.2 percent); SLE, 3 (27.2 percent); bronchial asthma, 3 (27.2 percent); and JIA, 2 (18.2 percent).

LEARNING OBJECTIVES

When you have completed this chapter, you should be able to:

- Understand the differences in the use of immunologic techniques for diagnosis of immunologically mediated diseases from those used as assessment tools for diseases with no immunologic basis
- Comprehend the principles underlying the immunologic procedures used in laboratory diagnostic immunology
- Describe the clinically relevant immunologic techniques that measure various parameters of the innate and adaptive immune systems organized into screening, functional, and specialized tests
- Identify the diagnostic use of immunologic procedures required for specific clinical conditions including the immune deficiency disorders, allergic diseases, and autoimmune disorders
- Gain an appreciation for the future of diagnostic immunology testing and its importance for early diagnosis and appropriate therapy
- Utilize this knowledge for a better understanding of immunologic mechanisms involved in disease pathogenesis and maintenance of health

Case Study (continued)

The patient's older sister was subsequently evaluated for recurrent otitis media as well as hearing and speech impairment (Figure 24-1). In addition, she has a history of recurrent bouts of sore throats, bronchitis, two episodes of pneumonia, and mild bronchial asthma, which is treated with inhalers. At the age of six years, she contracted fifth disease (erythema infectiosum) and a few weeks later developed joint pain and morning stiffness, predominantly in the knees and ankles, which later led to limping. A year later, she developed recurrent bouts of generalized rash, most prominent on the face in the malar area and upper thorax, which was accentuated by fever. Moreover, she began to experience several episodes of Raynaud's phenomenon. Her physical examination revealed no lymphadenopathy, organomegaly, or evidence of swollen joints, although she complained of having joint pain on movement. Because of her medical history and clinical presentation, she currently is being evaluated for possible JIA evolving into a SLE-like presentation.

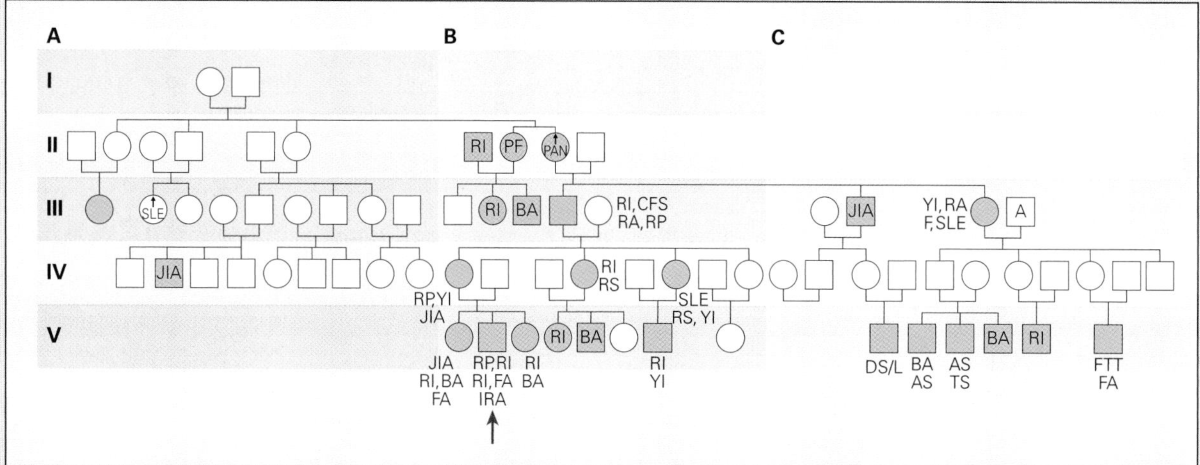

Figure 24-1. Patient's family pedigree. Arrow indicates patient. Panel A: Extension of patient's maternal great-grandmother's pedigree (generation II). Panel B: Patient's immediate pedigree (generations II–V). Panel C: Extension of patient's maternal grandfather's pedigree (generations III–V). A = alopecia; AS = Asperger's syndrome; BA = bronchial asthma; CB = chronic bronchitis; CFS = chronic fatigue syndrome; DS/L = Down's syndrome/leukemia; F = fibromyalgia; FA = food allergy; JIA = juvenile idiopathic arthritis; PAN = polyarteritis nodosa; PF = pulmonary fibrosis; RA = rheumatoid arthritis; RI = recurrent infections; RP = Raynaud's phenomenon; RS = recurrent sinusitis; SLE = systemic lupus erythematosus; TS = Tourette's syndrome; YI = yeast infection; † = dead of; O = female; = male. (Adapted from Bueso MB, Caballero R, Castro HJ, et al. Recurrent infections and joint pain. Allergy Asthma Proc 2006; 27: 164–71.)

Introduction

Immunologically based techniques of laboratory diagnosis are used in conjunction with other clinical and laboratory procedures for the assessment of immunologic function in the diagnosis of various disease states. In recent decades, there has been an explosive growth of these diagnostic immunologic procedures that have resulted from advances in many areas of science and medicine and from new technologies. These new techniques have expanded the scope of diagnostic laboratory immunology from their historical origins in infectious diseases to the diagnosis of other disorders whose pathogenetic etiologies are now better understood. Serologic diagnostic testing for infection, for example, while still important, is no longer the mainstay of laboratory immunology testing. Autoimmune diseases, allergy and asthma, organ and bone marrow transplantation, lymphoid and plasma cell and solid malignancies, and primary and secondary immune deficiencies have all provided new challenges and opportunities to advance the wide range of immunologic laboratory procedures that clinicians have at their disposal. For ease of discussion, it may be possible to divide the diagnostic applications of immunology into two major categories: (1) the use of immunologic techniques for the diagnosis of diseases in which altered immunologic function occurs; and (2) the use of immunologic procedures as assessment tools employed in the diagnosis of diseases that have no immunologic basis.

Immunologic Techniques for Diagnosis of Diseases with Altered Immunologic Function

General Considerations

The clinically relevant immunologic techniques for evaluation of diseases with altered immunologic function can be divided into the two major divisions of the immune system: (1) **tests of innate immune function** (that measure phagocytic cell, mediator cell, natural killer (**NK**) cell functions, and complement); and (2) **tests of adaptive immune function** (that measure the many activities of T and B cells). These procedures have been arbitrarily arranged into three levels of diagnostic testing that include **screening tests**, **functional tests**, and **specialized tests**, as shown in Table 24-1. This classification attempts to provide a practical diagnostic algorithm for the clinician that groups testing into levels of increasing complexity beginning initially with screening assays that are performed in most routine service laboratories and then progressing into functional and later more specialized tests that are usually only performed in specialty or research laboratories, respectively. The more sophisticated tests of immune function used by research laboratories are referenced in the reading list that provide descriptions of more complex diagnostic techniques organized into phases of activation, functional output, or complexities of the immune system

Table 24-1. Clinically relevant techniques used for evaluation of immunologic function organized according to major categories found within the innate and adaptive immune systems

Category	Component	(Primary) screening	(Secondary) functional	(Tertiary) specialized
Innate immune system Phagocytic cell	Monocyte/macrophage Neutrophil Eosinophil Dendritic cell	CBC and differential	Adherence Chemotaxis Phagocytosis Bactericidal activity	Adhesion molecules Chemokines Particle uptake NADPH oxidase Reactive oxygen species (ROS)
Mediator cell	Mast cell Basophil	Tissue CBC and differential	Tryptase	Histamine, prostaglandins, leukotrienes
Natural killer (NK) cell	Perforin/granzyme ADCC	CD3−/ CD16+CD56+	Cytolytic activity	Perforin
Complement function	C1–C9	CH50, C3, C4	Opsonic (C3b) Anaphylatoxin (C3a, C5a) Chemotactic (C5a) Cytolytic (C5–9)	
Adaptive immune system B cell function	Lymphocyte	CBC and differential IgM, IgG, IgA, IgE IgG1, IgG2, IgG3, IgG4	Immunophenotyping CD19, CD20	Pre- and postspecific antibody responses
T cell function	Lymphocyte	CBC and differential immunophenotyping CD3+/CD4+ CD3+/CD8+ In vitro delayed hypersensitivity testing	In vivo antigen and mitogen lymphoproliferation assays	Cytokine analysis Cytolytic activity

that define its normal (or abnormal) function, which are beyond the scope of this textbook.

General Procedures Used in Diagnostic Immunologic Testing

Two of the major immunologic developments of the 20th century that have had the greatest impact on diagnostic immunology are (1) the hybridoma technology developed by Kohler and Milstein in 1975 that provided a method for the in vitro production of large quantities of homogenous antibody to a single antigenic specificity, i.e., monoclonal antibody (*Chapter 6*); and (2) flow cytometry (**FCM**), also referred to as fluorescent activated cell sorting (**FACS**), a technology of molecular identification dependent on the use of monoclonal antibody that permitted the detection and characterization of various cells and molecules of the immunologic system. The FACS technology was driven by the occurrence of the AIDS epidemic in 1981 (*Chapter 13*) and the recognition that measurement of absolute CD4 T cell counts was a critical measure for disease assessment for diagnosis, treatment, and follow-up of patients infected with the human immunodeficiency virus (**HIV**). Flow cytometry applied in the monitoring of HIV infection was subsequently followed by the routine application of this technology to the evaluation of lymphoproliferative disorders, and more recently to the study of immunodeficiency disorders and other immune-mediated diseases.

Enumeration of Cells by FCM Immunophenotyping and Functional Analysis

FCM is a technique for separating and examining cells and molecules, and when used in the characterization of lymphocyte populations and subpopulations, the method is referred to as **immunophenotyping**. The technique involves the utilization of an electronic monochromatic light source detection system (typically lasers) that provides the excitation energy permitting the measurement of cell types, which in the case of immunotyping involves the fluorescent labeling of monoclonal antibodies (i.e., fluorochromes) attached to the surface of various cell populations. Each cell emits nonfluorescent forward and side scatter as well as fluorescent signals if one or more fluorochrome conjugated monoclonal antibodies is bound to the cell (Figure 24-2). The cell size is measured by the side scatter and the granularity of each cell is measured by the forward scatter.

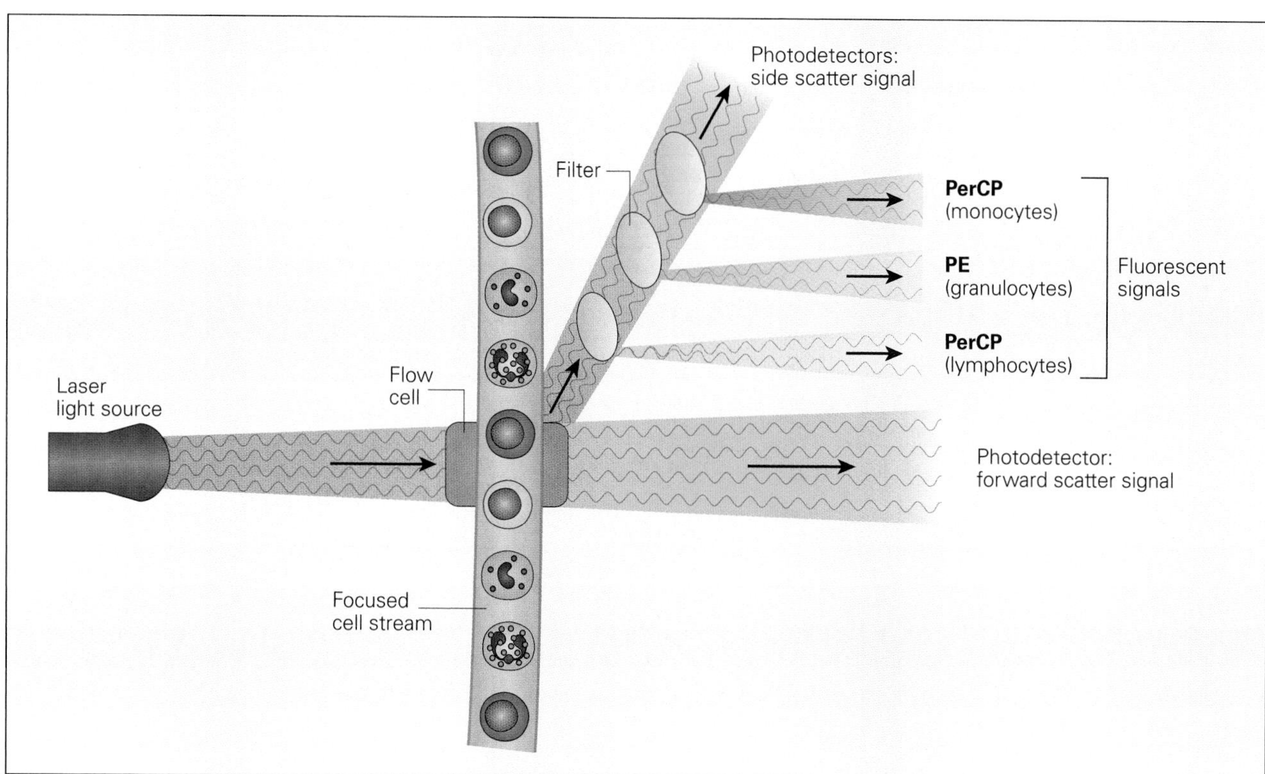

Figure 24-2. Schematic representation of a flow cytometer with one illumination light source (laser) set up to collect five parameters. These include the two forward and side scatter nonfluorescent parameters as well as three fluorescent parameters, green (FITC), orange (PE), and red (PerCP) light. FITC = fluoroscein isothiocyanate; PE = phycoerythrin; PerCP = peridin chlorophyll protein.

Flow cytometry provides a useful diagnostic tool for the clinician to evaluate the immune system by determining the proportion and subsequently the absolute numbers of lymphocyte subsets and other cell types. It has found several uses including the detection or absence of a specific cell population or subpopulation, the screening for altered expression of a specific extracellular or intracellular protein, the assessment of biological changes associated with specific immune defects, and the evaluation of certain functional immune characteristics. The advantage of FCM lies in its ability to precisely analyze a large number of cells rapidly and objectively. Shown in Figure 24-3 is an example of an immunophenotypic analysis of a whole blood sample showing the separation of cellular components into lymphocytes, monocytes, and granulocytes.

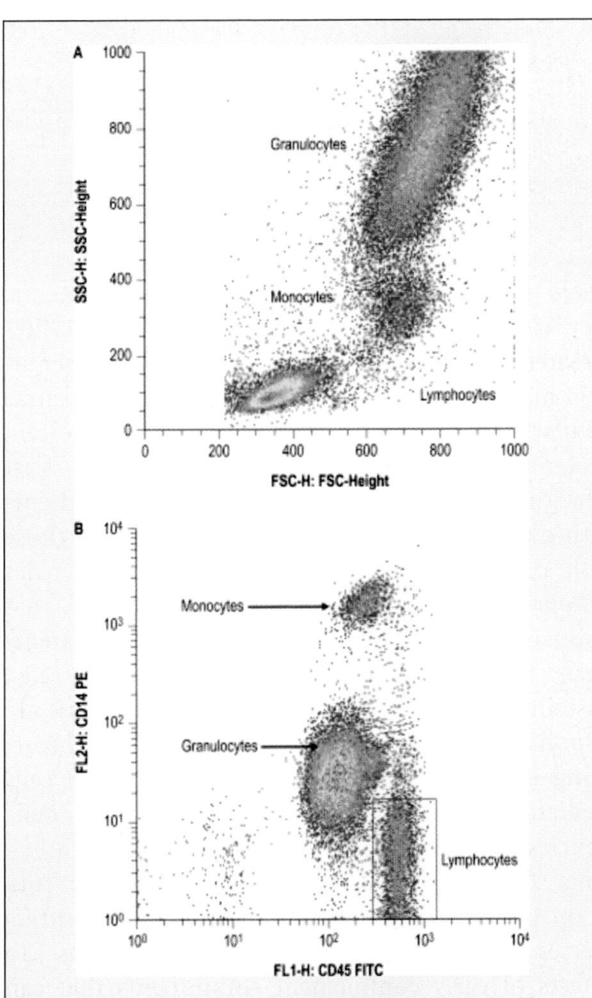

Figure 24-3. An immunophenotypic analysis of a whole blood sample showing the separation of lymphocytes, monocytes, and granulocytes. (Reproduced with permission from Fleisher T, de Oliveira JB. Flow cytometry. 3rd. ed. In: *Clinical Immunology: Principles and Practice.* Philadelphia, PA: Elsevier Limited; 2008:1436.)

General Considerations for the Workup of Patients Suspected to Have a Primary or Secondary Immune Deficiency

One of the major indications for diagnostic immunologic testing is in the assessment of patients suspected with primary or secondary immune deficiencies (*Chapter 16*). Shown in Table 24-2 is a list of some of the important clinical clues that indicate the need for an immunodeficiency workup. The patient's clinical history and family history represent the keystone determinants to begin an immunodeficiency evaluation. Since many of the primary immunodeficiency disorders (**PID**s) are X-linked, a particularly relevant clue in making a diagnosis is obtained by eliciting a history of similar infections occurring in other family members, particularly males, who may have died early in life, possibly due to recurrent or fulminant infections. In many cases, the infections may be caused by unusual or opportunistic agents (*Chapter 12*). Even if a detailed family history cannot be obtained, every attempt should be made to carefully document the other important clinical clues shown in Table 24-2.

A history of recurrent infections is the hallmark for initiating an immunodeficiency workup. As described in Chapter 16, infants or children who develop multiple bouts of otitis media ($\geq$ eight in one year) or several serious sinus infections should be highly suspected of having a PID. Serious pneumonia, deep-seated infections (i.e., meningitis, osteomyelitis, cellulitis, or sepsis), skin abscesses, or infections that fail to clear after appropriate antibiotic therapy are other signs of a PID (Table 24-3). Although aberrations of the defense function of the immune system responsible for recurrent infection are the

Table 24-2. Clues leading to a suspicion of a primary immunodeficiency disorder (PID)

Family history
Infections Types of organisms Site and frequency of infections Failure to clear infections with oral antibiotics Severity of infections
Birth anomalies
Laboratory values
Autoimmunity
Increased occurrence of malignancies

Table 24-3. Clinical conditions frequently associated with PID

Infections Unusually severe Recurrent Unusual organisms
Sinus infections Malabsorption
Autoimmunity Rheumatoid diseases Lupus-like syndromes
Abscesses, skin lesions
Chronic diarrhea
Failure to thrive
Oral thrush
Incomplete healing of wounds
Adverse reactions to live vaccines
Absent lymph nodes or tonsils
Absent thymic shadow on X-ray

Table 24-4. Infectious agents associated with PID

Antibody deficiencies *Hemophilus influenzae* *Streptococcus pneumonia* *Giardia lamblia* *Cryptosporidium* species Enteroviruses
Cellular or combined deficiencies *Candida albicans* *Pneumocystis carinii* (now called *Pneumocystis jiroveci*) *Mycobacterium* species Cytomegalovirus Epstein-Barr virus Varicella virus Enteroviruses
Phagocyte or phagocytosis deficiencies *Pseudomonas* species *Klebsiella* species *Staphylococcus aureus* *Serratia marcescens* *Candida albicans* *Nocardia* species *Aspergillus* species
Complement or complement component deficiencies *Neisseria meningitides* *Neisseria gonorrhoeae*

most common heralding signs of PID, defects of the homeostatic and surveillance immune functions are becoming increasingly recognized, and patients with PID may also present initially with manifestations of immune dysregulation, i.e., autoimmunity or defective surveillance, i.e., malignancy, respectively (*Chapters 1* and *16*). Clinical presentations other than infection, therefore, such as autoimmune disorders, lymphoreticular malignancy, failure to thrive, or adverse reactions to live vaccines may also be clues for the initiation of a PID workup. Although the PIDs have been traditionally considered the exclusive purview of pediatricians, since most of these disorders were traditionally first recognized in children, with improvement in treatment with intravenous gamma globulin and antibiotics, many of the patients, particularly those with milder defects, may continue to survive and remain undiagnosed even into adulthood. Therefore, immunodeficiency is no longer the isolated province of the pediatric immunologist and must be seriously considered even by those entrusted to the care of the adult patient.

Particular types of microorganisms are associated with certain immunodeficiencies (Table 24-4). Because of the dependence of opsonizing antibody for uptake and killing of encapsulated bacteria, bacterial infections caused by *Streptococcus pneumoniae* and *Hemophilus influenzae* type b are often seen in patients with B lymphocyte disorders (*Chapters 12* and *16*). It should be noted, however, that although these organisms are common pathogens of childhood where they are causative agents of otitis media, they are also involved in more serious, severe life-threatening diseases such as septicemia or meningitis both in children and adults with PID. Intracellular infections caused by viruses and certain bacteria, e.g., mycobacteria, as well as certain yeast infections are more commonly seen in patients with defects of T cell–mediated immunity, or those with combined T and B cell immunodeficiencies (*Chapters 12, 13,* and *16*). Viruses, moreover, that result in benign self-limiting, localized (i.e., latent) viral infections in healthy individuals (e.g., Epstein-Barr, varicella, and cytomegalovirus) are responsible for serious and sometimes life-threatening infection in individuals with impaired cell-mediated immune function. Phagocytic cell deficiencies, on the other hand, often result in infections caused by bacterial (Gram negative and Gram positive) or fungal organisms (e.g., *Nocardia* species and *Aspergillus* species). In contrast to defects of early complement components that can be associated with autoimmune disorders, e.g., systemic lupus erythematosus (**SLE**) (C1qrs defects) or with Gram-positive infections (C3 defects), in late complement component deficiencies (C5-9 defects), more serious infections caused by Gram-negative bacteria, e.g., *Neisseria meningitidis* and *Neisseria gonorrheae*, are often seen (*Chapters 4* and *16*).

Shown in Figure 24-4 is a schematic representation of the sequence of various tests that are used for measurement of PMN, complement, and T and B cell function commonly used in the workup of patients who present with recurrent infections suspected to have immune deficiency.

Assessment of Innate Immunity

Phagocytic Cell Function

The measurement of phagocytic cell function is most commonly carried out in the assessment of patients suffering from recurrent bacterial infection (Table 24-5). As described in Chapter 16, cells of the phagocytic cell system include circulating monocytes and tissue macrophages as well as circulating myeloid cells, particularly neutrophils. Abnormalities of phagocytic cells include both **quantitative** deficiencies in which the numbers of these cells are diminished (Table 24-5) as well as a variety of **qualitative** or functional deficiencies where the numbers may be normal but where they manifest intrinsic functional defects (Table 24-6). Phagocytic cells participate not only in *innate* immunity through phagocytosis, intracellular microbicidal activity, and inflammation, but also are intimately involved in linkage to *adaptive immunity* and function as antigen-presenting cells (**APCs**) through antigen processing and presentation of resultant peptides to T cells with subsequent activation of effector T cells and B cells.

When to Suspect Phagocytic Cell Dysfunction

The clinical presentations of patients with neutrophil disorders usually share common features, i.e., cutaneous infections, gingivitis, periodontal disease, and oral

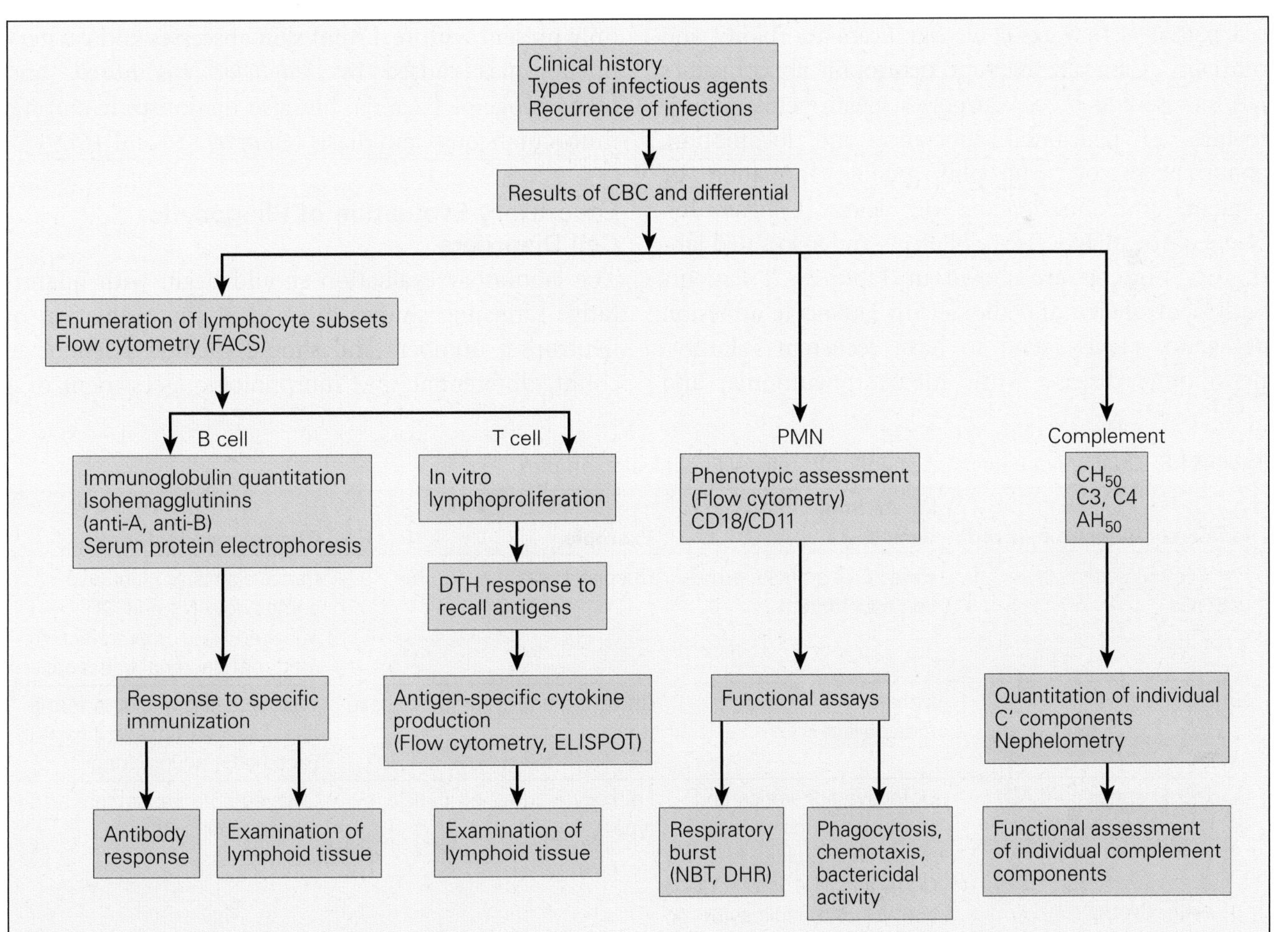

Figure 24-4. **Schematic representation of an algorithm of various immunologic tests used in the workup of patients who present with recurrent infections suspected to have immune deficiency.** The tests are organized into tests of PMN, complement, and T and B cell function. PMN = polymorphonuclear or neutrophil assays; NBT = quantitative nitroblue tetrazolium (NBT) test; DHR = dihydrorhodamine 123 assay; AH50 = alternative pathway hemolytic activity.

Table 24-5. Quantitative defects of phagocytic cells with clinical examples

Innate cell involved	Innate immunologic defect	Example	Clinical manifestation
Defects in numbers of neutrophils	Neutropenia	Congenital, infectious, malignant, autoimmune disease	Increased susceptibility to bacterial infection
Defects in numbers of macrophages	Splenectomy Functional splenectomy	Surgical removal following trauma Sickle-cell anemia	Increased susceptibility to bacterial infection

ulceration. Cutaneous infections with *S. aureus* are often recurrent and can be severe. Neutrophils are major cellular components of blood and are important in mediating acute inflammatory responses. Their ability to respond and clear infections is the result of a series of well-organized reactions, including migration to sites of infections (chemotaxis), recognition and uptake of invading organisms, metabolic upregulation, and killing of the microbe (*Chapter 5*). Quantitative or qualitative deficiencies resulting in neutropenia or a marked decrease in functional activity of any of the phagocytic cell pathways may result in significant morbidity and mortality. Clinically relevant neutrophil abnormalities fall into several broad categories: neutropenia, abnormalities of neutrophil adherence and locomotion, abnormalities of neutrophil granule formation or content, and abnormalities of killing (*Chapter 16*). Some of the phagocytic cell defects and associated laboratory findings are shown in Table 24-7. Patients with neutropenia and those with leukocyte adhesion deficiency (**LAD**) tend to have recurrent cellulitis, periodontal disease, otitis media, pneumonia, and rectal or gastrointestinal infections with diminished inflammation and lack of pus formation. In contrast, patients with chronic granulomatous disease (**CGD**) have significant problems with liver and bone abscesses, as well as pneumonias with selected organisms, including *Staphylococcus aureus*, *Serratia marcescens*, *Burkholderia cepacia*, and *Nocardia* and *Aspergillus* species. Furthermore, they tend to have a lower frequency of *Escherichia coli* and streptococcal species infections compared with patients with neutropenia or LAD. Patients with hyper-IgE syndrome not only present with recurrent skin abscesses and cavitary pneumonias caused by *Staphylococcus aureus* and other pyogenic bacteria, but also demonstrate chronic mucocutaneous candidiasis (*Chapters 14* and *16*).

Laboratory Evaluation of Phagocytic Cell Disorders

The laboratory evaluation should begin with quantitative screening studies directed at the evaluation of neutrophil numbers and should include a leukocyte count, differential, and morphologic assessment of a

Table 24-6. Qualitative defects of phagocytic cells with clinical examples

Innate component involved	Innate immunologic defect	Example	Clinical manifestation
Primary and secondary granules	Defects of granule formation and content	Chediak-Higashi syndrome	Partial albinism, giant lysosomes, low NK and CTL; impaired lysosomal trafficking, recurrent bacterial infections
NADPH oxidase	Defects in oxidative metabolism	Chronic granulomatous disease (CGD)	Widespread granuloma formation, increased susceptibility to bacterial infection, fungi
Leukocyte adhesion (LAD) defects	Defective adherence and chemotaxis from integrin mutations resulting in CD18 and CD15 defects, and failure of leukocyte adhesion and emigration of cells	Leukocyte adhesion deficiency type 1 (LAD1)	Delayed cord separation, skin ulcers, periodontitis, leukocytosis
Interferon-γ/IL-12	Interferon-γ/IL-12 pathway defects	BCGosis	Susceptibility to salmonella and mycobacteria

Table 24-7. Differential diagnosis of selected phagocyte cell defects and associated laboratory findings

Phagocytic cell defect	Example	Associated laboratory findings
Disorders of myeloid cells	Severe congenital neutropenia	Persistent neutropenia and maturation arrest detected by bone marrow studies
	Cyclic neutropenia	Intermittent neutropenia requiring serial measurements (at two- to three-week intervals)
	X-linked neutropenia	Altered WASP expression by means of FCM or mutation analysis
Defects of granule formation and content	Chediak-Higashi syndrome	Giant lysosomal inclusion bodies seen in granulocytes (with partial albinism)
	Griscelli syndrome type 2	Neutropenia without inclusion bodies (with partial albinism)
Defects of oxidative metabolism	Chronic granulomatous disease	Defective oxidative burst by means of DHR assay or NBT
Leukocyte adhesion deficiency (LAD)	LAD1	Low/absent CD18 and CD11 expression by means of FCM; persistent leukocytosis
	LAD2	Bombay phenotype; absent CD15 (Sialyl-Lewis X) expression
	LAD3	Mutation analysis only
Defects of cytokine-signaling pathways	Hyper-IgE syndrome	IgE level > 2,000 IU/mL; low Th17 cell numbers; some with STAT3 deficiency
	Interferon-γ/IL-12	Several molecular defects of the interferon-γ/IL-12 pathway assessed by FCM

WASP = Wiskott-Aldrich syndrome protein.

stained blood smear (Table 24-1). Neutropenia, as assessed by a CBC, is clinically significant when polymorphonuclear neutrophil (**PMN**) numbers fall below 1,000/μL and, when below 500/μL, have a very high incidence of susceptibility to serious bacterial infection. Because of the episodic recurring pattern of cyclic neutropenia, the performance of multiple absolute neutrophil counts two to three times a week is required for at least a four- to six-week period.

After quantitative and morphologic abnormalities have been ruled out, the evaluation should next proceed to functional assessment of PMN activity by tests that may include assessment of any of the steps in PMN function described above (Table 24-1). Although most of these tests are not routinely available in many clinical laboratories, they can be performed in specialty laboratories. Cell surface adhesion molecule expression and the assessment of the respiratory burst activity are more frequently encountered than defects in chemotaxis or phagocytosis. Of the various adhesion molecules on the surface of PMNs, defects in the expression and upregulation of beta-2 integrins (CD18, CD11a-c) are the most frequently encountered and can be assessed by FCM (*Chapter 5*). These surface adhesion molecules promote adhesion to ligands on vascular endothelial cells, and defects in their expression result in LAD (*Chapter 16*). FCM phenotyping is used to determine cell surface basal levels of expression as well as upregulated levels after appropriate stimulation.

The neutrophil oxidative burst pathway can be assessed by a number of assays that measure the biochemical activity of the hexose monophosphate pathway (*Chapter 5*). Upon recognition and ingestion of foreign material, PMNs undergo metabolic changes that result in the generation of reactive oxygen species and hydrogen peroxide (respiratory burst). These molecules, in addition to other non-oxidative mechanisms, are responsible for the killing of ingested microbes. The importance of the respiratory burst is best illustrated by the morbidity and mortality associated with defects in this system as seen in CGD. Several mutations in genes of the nicotinamide adenine dinucleotide phosphate-reduced (**NADPH**) oxidase system have been described in this disorder that are responsible for both an X-linked (the most common) as well as several autosomal forms (*Chapter 16*). The frequency of CGD in the United States is at least one in 200,000 live births, and may be higher in certain populations. Although the majority of patients are diagnosed as toddlers and young children with recurrent infections or granulomatous lesions, the disease may also have its initial clinical presentation in adults.

The lung, skin, lymph nodes, and liver are the most frequent sites of infection. The majority of infections in CGD in North America and Europe are due to five microorganisms: *Staphylococcus aureus*, *Burkhoderia cepacia*, *Serratia marcescens*, *Nocardia* species, and *Aspergillus* species.

Respiratory burst activity can be assessed by several methods, including the nitroblue tetrazolium (**NBT**) dye reduction test, chemiluminescence, and FCM. The NBT test is an older test that was based on uptake of the NBT dye by PMNs in the presence or absence of a stimulus, such as latex beads. As a result of the oxidative burst generated by the neutrophils, the NBT is converted from its colorless oxidized form to its blue reduced formazan form. The change in color is measured photometrically or spectrophotometrically. A more sensitive flow cytometric assay has been developed that has largely replaced the NBT test that relies upon the change in fluorescence of dihydrorhodamine 123 from a nonfluorescent resting state to a fluorescent-emitting state in cells that have been stimulated and can be detected by FCM. Both methods, NBT and flow cytometry, are used to detect CGD patients and carriers (Figure 24-5).

Mediator Cell Function

As described in Chapters 1, and 18, the major mediator cells with clinical applicability are the basophils and the mast cells and, to a large degree, the eosinophils (that also show phagocytic activity). Two types of mast cells have been identified in skin, respiratory, and digestive tract connective tissues based on the types of neutral proteases present in their secretory granules. One group found in intestinal mucosa and lung alveolar wall tissue contains only tryptase [MC(T)], whereas the other predominates in normal skin and intestinal submucosa and contains both tryptase and chymase [MC(TC)] (*Chapter 3*). Tryptase is elevated in anaphylaxis and mastocytosis and therefore has important diagnostic value as a marker of these conditions.

Histamine is a potent vasoactive mediator stored as a preformed molecule in the cytoplasmic granules of both basophils and mast cells and released along with other mediators of inflammation, e.g., leukotrienes, in response to both immunologic and nonimmunologic stimuli in several allergic conditions where immediate hypersensitivity (type I) plays a pathogenetic role (*Chapter 18*). The basophil histamine release (**BHR**) assay has been shown to be useful as a quantitative assay of allergen potency and as an in vitro model for the study of triggers of mediator release from basophils. Peripheral blood leukocytes isolated from a donor are incubated with varying concentrations of allergen extract or anti-human IgE as a positive control. Histamine release is measured by enzymatic, radiometric, or spectrophotofluorometric techniques and is complete within 30 minutes. Measurement of elevated blood histamine has been reported in several

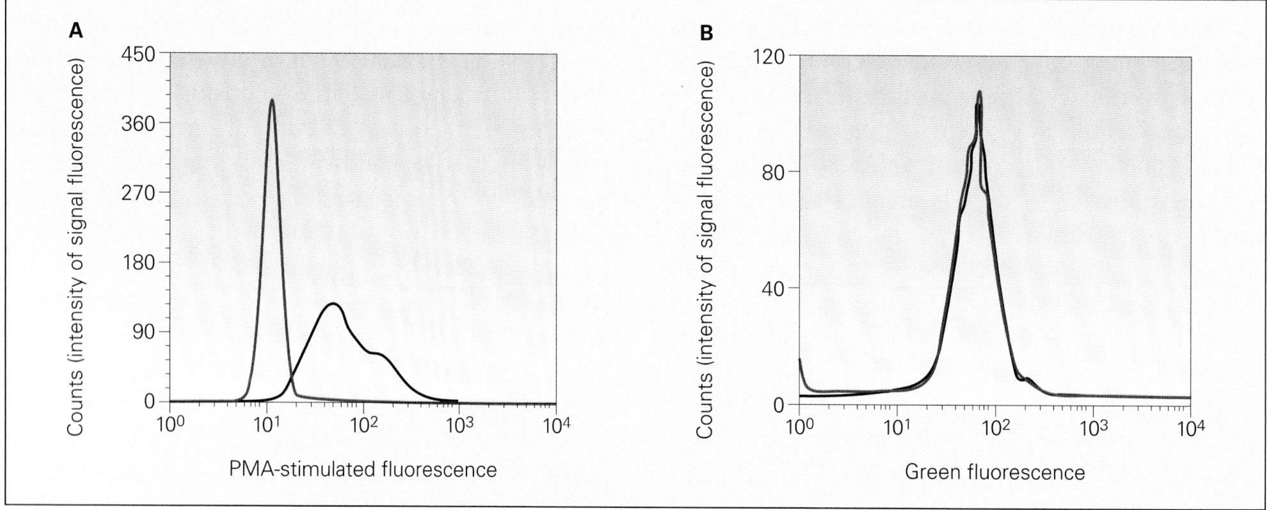

Figure 24-5. **Schematic representation of the technique of flow cytometric analysis of oxidative function of PMNs by dihydrorhodamine staining.** Panel A: A nonfluorescent red peak of dihydrorhodamine 123 at the left and a black peak shifted to the right with increased fluorescence in PMA-stimulated cells from a normal individual. Panel B: Overlapping of both peaks with no shift in the fluorescent emission peak in stimulated PMNs from a patient with CGD. PMA = Phorbol-12-myristate-13-acetate.

allergic conditions, e.g., following ingestion of a food allergen in food allergic subjects, but the blood specimen requires special handling to prevent its degradation by plasma histaminases.

Mediators released from eosinophils are also important in promoting inflammation in many infections, e.g., parasitic infections, and allergic conditions, e.g., allergic rhinitis and asthma (*Chapter 18*). Eosinophil cationic peptide (**ECP**) is a basic protein present in eosinophil granules and is involved in tissue injury in allergic diseases where eosinophils play a significant role. Elevated levels of ECP have been detected in the serum, sputum, and nasal secretions of individuals undergoing a late-phase allergic reaction (usually 6 to 24 hours after exposure) where eosinophil influx is found at the reactive site. ECP measurements, however, have shown limited clinical utility for monitoring patients with asthma and other allergic diseases. Despite their unquestioned value in research studies, these assays are rarely used clinically in the routine diagnosis of human allergic disease.

Natural Killer Cells

Natural killer cells (or NK cells) are a type of cytotoxic lymphocyte that constitutes another important component of the innate immune defense system (*Chapter 3*). NK cells play a major role in the rejection of tumors and virally infected cells. They kill cells by apoptosis either directly by releasing small cytoplasmic granules of proteins called perforin and granzyme or indirectly by the participation of an IgG molecule by the bridging effect of its Fab portion to the target cell and its Fc fragment to an Fc receptor on the NK cell by antibody-dependent cellular cytoxicity (**ADCC**). They are also the source of a variety of cytokines (*Chapter 9*).

When to Suspect NK Cell Dysfunction

NK cell defects are uncommon entities that manifest clinically with an increased susceptibility to viral infection. Although the numbers of circulating NK cells have been shown to be depressed in studies of patients with AIDS compared to normal uninfected controls, the quantitative differences in levels between groups were not statistically significant. Deficiency in NK cell function has also been described in a limited number of patients with recurrent herpes virus infections and, together with defects in T cytotoxic lymphocytes, have been demonstrated to be associated with the uncontrolled infection-induced inflammatory response that produces multiple organ damage (hemophagocytic lymphohistiocytosis [**HLH**] *Chapter 16*). One of these disorders is X-linked lymphoproliferative syndrome (**XLP**), an inherited disorder characterized by an abnormal immune response to infection with the Epstein-Barr virus (**EBV**) (*Chapter 13*). XLP, which is usually an asymptomatic disorder until EBV infection is encountered, manifests as an uncontrolled lymphoproliferative disorder that is usually fatal unless bone marrow transplantation is performed. Other disorders caused by defective intracellular vesicle trafficking, such as Chediak-Higashi syndrome and Griscelli syndrome type 2, can also commonly manifest with a secondary lymphohistiocytic syndrome.

Laboratory Evaluation of NK Cell Disorders

Testing of NK cell function includes immunophenotyping by means of flow cytometry and assays of cytotoxicity using standard in vitro assays including a four-hour ^{51}Cr-release assay. NK cell function is assessed by the ability of peripheral blood lymphocyte preparations to lyse ^{51}Cr-labeled NK-sensitive tumor target cells, releasing the ^{51}Cr into the culture supernatant. The amount of radioactive chromium released from the target cells is proportional to the NK cell lytic activity. There is also an FCM method to measure NK cell lytic activity, but it also requires the use of a susceptible target cell line. In addition, intracellular flow cytometry can be used to evaluate the expression of certain molecules defective in XLP1 and XLP2, i.e., SLAM-associated protein (**SAP**) and X-linked inhibitor of apoptosis (**XIAP**), respectively (*Chapter 16*).

Complement Function

The complement system is another major component of the innate immune system (*Chapter 4*). It works in concert with other components of innate immunity and the adaptive immune system to provide pathways and mechanisms for removing foreign microorganisms or damaged cells. The complement system consists of more than 40 proteins that are primarily glycoproteins that become activated to help remove any unwanted microorganisms or other affected material through various pathways. The complement system is under strict regulation to prevent uncontrolled activation that could cause host tissue damage.

Complement proteins work in a cascading fashion and they exist as precursors in plasma. After activation, the proteins interact with the next protein in the system and ultimately end with a lytic event (or lysis of the cell). There are several pathways whereby the complement cascade can become activated and produce profound results as a result of its activation. The complement system, its various pathways, and active products provide a formidable first line of defense for the host. At least three pathways, classical, alternative, and mannose-binding lectin, have been defined, and they all contribute to an intact immune system.

The complement cascade consists of three separate pathways that converge in a final common pathway (*Chapter 4*). The pathways include the classical pathway (C1qrs, C2, and C4), the alternative pathway (C3, factor B, and properdin), and the lectin pathway (mannose-binding lectin). The classical pathway is triggered by interaction of the Fc portion of an antibody (IgM, IgG1, IgG2, and IgG3) or C-reactive protein with C1q. The alternative pathway is activated in an antibody-independent manner. Lectins activate the lectin pathway in a manner similar to the antibody interaction with complement in the classical pathway. These three pathways converge at component C3. Although each branch is triggered differently, the common goal is to deposit clusters of C3b on a target. This deposition provides for the assembly of the membrane-attack complex (**MAC**), components C5b-9. The MAC exerts powerful killing activity by creating perforations in cellular membranes. Deficiencies in complement predispose patients to infection via two mechanisms: (1) ineffective opsonization and (2) defects in lytic activity (defects in MAC). Specific complement deficiencies are also associated with an increased risk of developing autoimmune disease such as SLE (*Chapter 16*).

When to Suspect Complement Dysfunction

Complement defects should be suspected in basically three types of clinical settings: (1) patients with autoimmune diseases, e.g., SLE; (2) in patients who present with recurrent infection; and (3) in patients with chronic recurrent angioedema. The clinical presentation in which a complement defect should be suspected is determined by the specific site at which the complement defect is located. Abnormalities in the early components of the classical complement pathway (C1q, C1r, C4, and C2) typically manifest as systemic lupus erythematosus-like autoimmunity, but recurrent sinopulmonary infections are also seen, especially in C2 deficiency. The first individual with a deficiency of a component of the complement system (C2 deficiency) was identified in 1960 in a patient with SLE. Since that original description, genetically determined deficiencies of most of the other components of the complement system have been identified in humans. Because of the opsonic-promoting effects of C3b in facilitating uptake and intracellular killing of high grade, virulent encapsulated bacteria, e.g., *Streptococcus pneumoniae*, defects in C3 produce a clinical phenotype of recurrent bacterial infection that is indistinguishable from an antibody defect, although this complement deficiency is markedly less frequent than humoral immunodeficiencies. Deficiencies of the third complement-activation pathway, initiated by mannose-binding lectin (**MBL**), appear to be associated with recurrent acute respiratory tract infections in young children due to various organisms (*S. pneumonia* and *N. meningitidis*) as well as increased incidence of rheumatic diseases. Patients lacking the alternative pathway components, factor D, and properdin have also been reported to have recurrent *N. meningitidis* infections. Lack of C3, the central complement component, as well as factor I and factor H, has been associated with recurrent infectious complications similar to that seen in antibody deficiencies. Inherited deficiencies of the later components of the cascade (C5–C9) are usually associated with a greater susceptibility to infections with *Neisseria* species, usually *N. meningitidis* that might not manifest until adolescence or young adulthood. Clinically, these patients manifest *Neisserial* meningitis, sepsis, or gonococcal arthritis. Alternative complement-pathway defects, including properdin, factor B, and factor D deficiencies, also present with severe *Neisserial* and other bacterial infections. Factor H deficiency is associated with atypical (not associated with diarrhea) hemolytic uremic syndrome or glomerulonephritis and also with secondary C3 deficiency that can result in recurrent pyogenic infections. Finally, C1 esterase inhibitor deficiency causes hereditary angioedema, whereas DAF (decay-accelerating factor) and CD59 defects are seen in patients with paroxysmal nocturnal hemoglobinuria. Patients lacking the alternative pathway components, factor D, and properdin have also been reported to have recurrent *N. meningitidis* infections. Lack of C3, the central complement component, as well as factor I and factor H, have been associated with recurrent infectious complications similar to that seen in antibody deficiencies. Membranoproliferative glomerulo-nephritis and vasculitis have also been associated with C3 deficiency.

Laboratory Evaluation of Complement Defects

Two basic screening tests are used for assessing complement activity (Figure 24-4). The total hemolytic complement (CH50) test measures the function of the classic complement cascade, whereas the AH50 measures the function of the alternative pathway (*Chapter 4*). It measures the complement activity in dilutions of the patient's plasma with sheep erythrocytes that have been coated with anti-sheep erythrocyte antibody. The antibody-coated sheep-erythrocyte immune complex activates the complement cascade. If all components are present and functioning, the sheep erythrocytes are lysed and the hemolysis can be measured. A patient with a total defect in one of the components of the classic pathway would show no hemolysis. Patients with mild (heterozygous) defects of C1, C4, C2, or C3 may not show a decrease in hemolysis because of redundancy in the system.

To confirm the specific complement component defect, an immunochemical method would be used to quantitate the individual component. Nephelometry is commonly used for quantitation of complement components. Nephelometry or immunochemical assays can only measure the presence and quantity of a component and will not detect an altered or dysfunctional complement component. If one suspects that a deficiency in complement activation may be a result of activation of the complement system, split components such as C4a, C4d, or Bb can be quantitated. Their presence suggests activation of the complement system.

There are reference laboratories offering functional assays for specific component deficiencies. These assay systems assess the ability of the patient's serum to lyse antibody-coated sheep erythrocytes in the presence of reagents lacking specific complement components. By using a process of elimination, it may be possible to identify the missing or dysfunctional components in the patient's sample. Overall, detection of inherited deficiencies of complement is available and can detect most of the possible defects. Complement deficiencies are rare, about 0.03 percent of the population, and the patient's history and clinical presentation are important in making the correct diagnosis.

Assessment of Adaptive Immunity

Quantitative Enumeration of T and B Cells; Immunophenotyping by FCM

As described previously, the technology of immunophenotyping by FCM has provided a major advance in the assessment of both humoral and cellular components of the adaptive immune system. A wide variety of monoclonal antibodies are now available for the quantitative enumeration of B cell, T cell, and NK cell subsets. These include antibodies to CD3, CD4, and CD8 that can identify the T helper (CD4+) and T cytotoxic (CD8+) subsets; CD19 to enumerate B cells; and CD16 and CD56 to enumerate NK cells (Table 24-8 and *Appendix 3*). This remarkable achievement has provided techniques to assess the proportion of these major cell subsets in peripheral blood as an initial screening test to evaluate patients suspected of T cell, B cell, or combined T and B cell immunodeficiencies as well as a number of other clinical entities, e.g., lymphoproliferative and autoimmune endocrine disorders (Table 24-8).

B Cell Function: Tests of Humoral Immunity

When to Suspect B Cell Dysfunction

The flagship immune deficiency that ushered in many of the subsequent developments in clinical immunology was X-linked agammaglobulinemia (**XLA**) described by Bruton in 1952 (*Chapter 16*). Evaluation of patients with defects in the B cell compartment, as with all four categories of the common immunodeficiency disorders, follows the same diagnostic strategy of linking clinical observation with laboratory investigation. The antibody deficiencies, also referred to as B cell or humoral immunodeficiencies, include both the inherited genetic defects as well as the acquired or secondary defects. In either case, the final pathogenetic determinant responsible for recurrent infection is defective antibody production or function.

During normal gestation, the full-term fetus acquires adult levels of immunoglobulin G (IgG) from the mother during the third trimester. After

Table 24-8. Common lymphocyte markers and their normal distributions on T, B, and NK cells in adult subjects determined by FCM

Surface antigens	Target cell recognized	Percent positive	Cells/mm^3
T cells			
CD3	Pan T lymphocyte	57–86	650–2108
CD5	Pan T lymphocyte (plus some B cells)	56–84	638–2099
CD2	Pan T lymphocyte (plus some NK cells)	76–93	876–2258
CD3/CD4	Helper/regulatory T lymphocyte	29–57	358–1259
CD3/CD8	Cytotoxic/effector T lymphocyte	13–47	194–836
CD4/CD45RO	Memory CD4 T lymphocyte	12–34	203–976
CD4/CD45RA	Naive CD4 T lymphocyte	2.5–25	31–533
CD8/CD45RO	Memory CD8 T lymphocyte	3–14	34–309
CD8/CD45RA	Naive CD8 T lymphocyte	7–28	101–636
CD3/CD8/CD57	Immune activation	≤ 16	≤ 249
CD3/HLA-DR	Activated T lymphocyte	≤ 15.1	≤ 291
CD3/CD25	Activated T lymphocyte	≤ 37.4	≤ 756
B cells			
CD19	Pan B lymphocyte	3.5–15.5	49–424
CD20	Pan B lymphocyte	3.5–17	47–409
CD20/CD5	B lymphocyte subset	1.5–8.5	13–145
CD20/CD24	Fc epsilon RII expressing B cell	1.6–13.2	38–360
CD20/CD27	Memory B lymphocyte	0.7–6.3	16–118
NK cells			
CD3−/CD16+CD56+	NK cells	4.5–30	87–505
Lymphocytes	Total lymphocytes	17–41	1173–2640

Adapted from data generated in the Flow Cytometry Section, Immunology Service, DLM, CC, NIH, Bethesda, MD. The 95 percent confidence interval for the WBC is 4300–9200/mm^3. (Reproduced with permission from Fleisher T, de Oliveira JB. Flow cytometry. (In: *Clinical Immunology: Principles and Practice* 3rd ed. Philadelphia, PA: Elsevier Limited; 2008:1436.)

birth, levels of maternal IgG decrease significantly during the first six months of postnatal life resulting from the normal catabolism of maternal IgG (t$^1/_2$ life = 24 days), following which the production of endogenous IgM, IgG, IgA, and IgE begins (*Chapter 2*). As a consequence of this transient protection of the infant by passively acquired maternal immunity, the development of infections in an infant with an antibody deficiency typically does not become evident until the later six months of postnatal life. The B lymphocyte deficiency may either be relatively mild and create only rare problems, or may result in a severe deficiency with serious bacterial infection due to a complete inability to synthesize and secrete antibodies, as seen in classic XLA (*Chapter 16*).

Repeated infections caused by common encapsulated, pyogenic organisms, such as *Streptococcus pneumoniae*, *Staphylococcus aureus*, *Haemophilus influenzae* type b (**Hib**), and *Neisseria meningitidis* may serve as significant indicators for evaluation of most inherited immunodeficiencies but is particularly prominent in the case of B cell immunodeficiency. Diarrhea affects up to 25 percent of these patients and is often associated with *Giardia lamblia* infection. Another clue to consider in humoral deficiencies is failure to clear an infection even after appropriate antimicrobial therapy. Typically, patients with severe agammaglobulinemia do not respond to specific immunization with tetanus/diphtheria toxoid or polysaccharide pneumococcal or *Hemophilus influenzae* type b vaccines and may develop serious infections when given attenuated viral vaccines, e.g., vaccine-associated polio paralysis (**VAPP**) following administration of the live oral poliovirus vaccine (**OPV**) (*Chapter 23*).

Laboratory Assessment for Defective Humoral Immunity

Shown in Box 24-1 are some general considerations for B cell testing. In contrast to the

Box 24-1

General Considerations for B cell Testing

B cell testing is done primarily by in vivo (vaccination) studies.

General considerations for vaccination studies are:

- protein vaccines (e.g., tetanus toxoid) measure T cell–dependent responses;
- polysaccharide vaccines (e.g., Pneumovax) measure T cell-independent responses;
- recall antigens: antigen has been experienced previously; antibody produced is typically isotype-switched subclass (e.g., IgG) when (booster) vaccine is given;
- neoantigens: antigen is new to immune system; antibody production is of non-isotype-switched subclass (IgM) following primary (first) vaccination, and of isotype-switched (IgG) subclass following secondary vaccination e.g., bacteriophage Phi X174.

Box 24-2

Nephelometry is a technique that measures the amount of light scatter of a suspension of small particles when a light source is passed through the suspension at an angle. The technique is commonly used in diagnostic immunology for the quantitative measurement of serum IgM, IgG, and IgA.

laboratory evaluation of patients with defective T cell, phagocytic cell, or complement function, which is performed largely by in vitro testing, B cell testing is done primarily by in vivo (vaccination) studies. An algorithm of laboratory tests for assessing various PIDs, including B lymphocyte immunocompetence, was shown previously in Figure 24-4 and Table 24-1. Shown in Table 24-9 are tests used in the evaluation of patients with suspected antibody deficiency.

Screening Tests Used in the Evaluation of Suspected Antibody Deficiency

The initial B cell testing can be performed in most clinical laboratory settings. Although in most B lymphocyte immunodeficiencies, the lymphocyte count may be normal to slightly decreased, the initial screening evaluation usually begins with a complete blood count (**CBC**) and differential. The next step in evaluation of a humoral immunodeficiency involves quantitation of immunoglobulin levels, which, in most clinical laboratories, is performed by some form of nephelometry (Box 24-2).

Normal immunoglobulin levels depend on a number of factors, including age and sex of the individual as well as ethnic and genetic background. The principal immunoglobulins routinely measured in serum are IgG, IgA, and IgM. Quantitation of IgE is useful in supporting some diagnoses (e.g., allergic disease and hyper-IgE syndrome), while IgD is not routinely helpful since it is primarily a membrane-associated immunoglobulin and not found in appreciable levels in serum (*Chapter 6*). It is important to compare the quantitative levels of serum immunoglobulins with age-adjusted reference values in order to avoid incorrect diagnosis owing to errors in interpretation, particularly in children in whom levels vary considerably with age (Tables 24-10 and 24-11). Although there are no rigid standards for absolute values of immunoglobulins to make a diagnosis of an immunoglobulin deficiency, an IgG value of less than 300 mg/dL in an adolescent or adult or values clearly below the 95 percent confidence interval for age-adjusted reference values in children should prompt further evaluation. Serum protein electrophoresis and immunofixation are qualitative methods and, although useful for the diagnosis of gammopathies (*Chapter 21*), are not adequate for the workup of patients suspected with immune deficiency.

Another initial screening method for evaluation of humoral immune function is the measurement of natural anti-blood group antibodies (e.g., isohemagglutinins) or antibodies acquired from previous immunizations or infections (Table 24-9). Values of serum anti-A and anti-B isohemagglutinins (except in type AB positive patients) are dependent on the age and blood group of the patient and are predominantly associated with IgM-class antibodies, whereas those resulting from previous immunizations or infections are IgG. Low or absent isohemagglutinin titers would be indicative of poor IgM synthesis and would suggest further studies.

The definitive method to evaluate in vivo antibody production involves immunizing a patient with a protein-derived vaccine (e.g., tetanus and diphtheria toxoid) and a polysaccharide-derived vaccine (e.g., pneumococcal vaccine) and comparing

Table 24-9. Tests used in the evaluation of suspected antibody deficiency

Diagnostic testing level	Assays to be performed
Screening tests	CBC and differential Quantitative determination of immunoglobulin levels (IgG, IgA, IgM, IgE) Specific antibody levels: 1. Circulating specific antibody levels to prior vaccines; and 2. Blood group antigens (isohemagglutinins) Pre- and postimmunization antibody levels directed to: 1. Protein antigens 2. Carbohydrate antigens Quantitative determination of IgG subclasses (IgG1, IgG2, IgG3, IgG4)
Secondary tests	B cell immunophenotyping In vitro functional studies (Table 24-12)
Tests to exclude rare and secondary causes	Thoracic computed tomography to exclude thymoma (particularly useful if patient is > 50 years old with low B cell numbers) Intracellular FCM or genetic evaluation for BTK (XLA) or SAP/XIAP (XLP) Genetic evaluation of NEMO to rule out anhydrotic ectodermal dysplasia with immune deficiency Fecal α1-antitrypsin, urinary protein, serum albumin, absolute lymphocyte count to exclude gastrointestinal or urinary protein loss or lymphatic loss HIV testing to exclude AIDS Complement function (CH50, AP50) to exclude complement deficiency Karyotype to exclude immunodeficiency, centromeric instability, facial anomalies syndrome Sweat chloride or genetic evaluation to exclude cystic fibrosis

BTK = Bruton tyrosine kinase; XLA = X-linked agammaglobulinemia; SAP/XIAP = SLAM-associated protein/X-linked inhibitor of apoptosis; NEMO = NF-kappa-B essential modulator.

preimmunization and three- to four-week postimmunization antibody levels. The now-routine use of conjugate vaccines has not only been of great benefit in providing protective immunity against certain organisms such as the pneumococcus, but also should be taken into consideration in the laboratory diagnosis of immunodeficiency (Box 24-3).

Depending on the age and vaccination history of a patient suspected of having a B cell immunodeficiency, one can measure antigen-specific antibody responses to the agents used for vaccination. Most infants will have received a battery of vaccinations by the time they are one year of age. It is important to evaluate the patient's ability to develop an antibody response to both protein and carbohydrate antigens. These vaccinations usually include tetanus and diphtheria toxoids (protein antigens), common viral vaccines, and Hib and pneumococcal polysaccharide vaccines. The presence of antibodies elicited by one or more of these vaccinations should be indicative of an intact humoral immune system. However, abnormally low levels of one or more of the antibodies

Table 24-10. Immunoglobulin levels (age-related reference ranges)

	Immunoglobulin levels (mg/mL)		
	IgG	IgM	IgA
Cord blood	6.36–16.06	0.06–0.25	0.01–0.03
1 month	2.51–9.06	0.20–0.87	0.01–0.53
2 months	2.06–6.01	0.17–1.05	0.02–0.46
3 months	1.76–5.81	0.24–0.89	0.04–0.46
4 months	1.96–5.58	0.27–1.01	0.04–0.73
5 months	1.72–8.14	0.33–1.09	0.08–0.68
6 months	2.15–7.04	0.35–1.02	0.08–0.68
7–9 months	2.17–9.04	0.34–1.26	0.11–0.90
10–12 months	2.94–10.69	0.41–1.49	0.16–0.84
1 year	3.45–12.13	0.43–1.73	0.14–1.06
2 years	4.24–10.51	0.48–1.68	0.14–1.24
3 years	4.41–11.35	0.47–2.00	0.22–1.59
4–5 years	4.63–12.36	0.43–1.96	0.25–1.54
6–8 years	6.33–12.80	0.48–2.07	0.33–2.02
9–10 years	6.08–15.72	0.52–2.42	0.45–2.36
Adult	6.39–13.49	0.56–3.52	0.70–3.12

Table 24-11. Total serum IgE (IU/mL)

Age	Gender	Geometric mean	Upper 95 percent confidence limit
6–14 years	M	42.7	527
	F	43.3	344
15–24 years	M	33.6	447
	F	18.6	262
25–34 years	M	16.8	275
	F	16.6	216
35–44 years	M	21.7	242
	F	19.3	206
45–54 years	M	19.2	254
	F	13.3	177
55–64 years	M	21.3	354
	F	11.7	148
65–74 years	M	21.2	248
	F	11.5	122
> 75 years	M	18.4	219
	F	9.2	124
6–75 years	All M	22.9	317
	All F	14.7	189

(Reproduced with permission from Barbee RA, Halonen M, Lebowitz M, et al. Distribution of IgE in a community population sample: correlations with age, sex, and allergen skin test reactivity. J Allergy Clin Immunol. 1981;68:106–11.)

against the vaccines might support a diagnosis of B cell deficiency. Paired serum samples should be obtained before and three to four weeks after the standard dose of vaccine is administered and assayed for antigen-specific immunoglobulins. In specific IgG subclass deficiencies, individuals do not respond adequately to certain microorganisms with pronounced polysaccharide capsules and may be related to a specific IgG2 subclass deficiency.

Guidelines for normal responses, which are usually provided by the testing laboratory, typically consist of finding at least a fourfold increase in antibody levels and/or protective antibody levels after immunization. An alternative strategy to assess humoral immunity, particularly useful in patients already receiving immunoglobulin replacement therapy, involves immunization with a neoantigen, such as the bacteriophage Phi X174. This procedure, however, is only available in certain specialized centers.

An additional test that is sometimes performed in conjunction with immunoglobulin determination is quantification of IgG subclass levels. Although the diagnosis of IgG subclass deficiency was previously made solely on the basis of diminished IgG subclass levels, this is no longer considered adequate. The complete evaluation of an IgG subclass deficiency now requires documentation of an abnormality in specific antibody production before initiating immunoglobulin therapy, making the value of this test of more limited utility. As described previously, measurement of pre- and postimmunization-specific antibody levels is the most useful test to confirm defective antibody production and is essential in making a diagnosis of humoral deficiency particularly

Box 24-3

The Use of Conjugate Vaccines in the Workup of the Patient Suspected with Humoral Immunodeficiency

Conjugate vaccines are created by covalently attaching a poorly immunogenic polysaccharide antigen to a carrier protein, thereby conferring the immunological attributes of the carrier on the attached antigen (*Chapter 23*). This technique for the creation of an effective immunogen is most often applied to bacterial polysaccharides for the prevention of invasive bacterial disease and has been particularly effective in children younger than two years who respond poorly to purified polysaccharide vaccines but who respond well to conjugate vaccines developed from polysaccharide antigens such as *Hemophilus influenzae* type b (Hib) and pneumococcus combined with either tetanus toxoid or diphtheria toxoid. However, from an immunologic perspective, it should be emphasized that these conjugate-generated antibodies are predominantly IgG1- (and IgG3)-mediated responses, while age-dependent anti-polysaccharide antibody production in children older than two years is characterized by the development of an IgG2-mediated response. Nonconjugate versions of purified polysaccharide-specific vaccines, e.g., the 24-valent pneumococcal polysaccharide vaccine (PPSV), are sometimes used to immunize children older than two years to distinguish immaturity of the immune system in the healthy child from more serious humoral immunodeficiency disorders, e.g., specific antibody deficiency (SAD) or isolated IgG2 deficiency (*Chapter 16*). Nonconjugate vaccines can, in general, be administered to children older than two to three years, keeping in mind that immunologic maturity is not reached at the same age by every child. The recent availability of the pneumococcal 13-valent conjugate vaccine that has replaced the heptavalent version should further clarify the diagnostic dilemma surrounding the laboratory investigation of humoral immune deficiencies in infants and young children.

when the total immunoglobulin levels are only modestly decreased (or even normal) in the setting of recurrent bacterial infection.

Secondary Tests Used in the Evaluation of Suspected Antibody Deficiency

B Cell Immunophenotyping

Once screening tests have been performed, additional secondary testing focuses on determining the presence or absence of B cells by using flow cytometry (Tables 24-1 and 24-9). This is particularly useful for diagnosis of congenital forms of agammaglobulinemia because this group of disorders typically is characterized by absent or extremely decreased circulating B cell numbers resulting from underlying defects that block B cell development (*Chapter 16*). More recently, characterization of B cell subsets, particularly directed at memory and immature B cells, has been suggested as a means to further characterize patients with common variable immunodeficiency (**CVID**). Studies that test in vitro B cell signaling and immunoglobulin biosynthesis are generally performed only in research centers.

As described previously, FCM has also been useful for the subset analysis of T and B lymphocyte populations and should be included in the evaluation of all patients suspected of immune deficiency to help clarify the particular defect causing the immunodeficiency (Figure 24-4). The most commonly used B cell-specific markers are CD19 and CD20. Normal peripheral blood B lymphocytes (as defined by anti-CD19, anti-CD20, or both) make up between 4 percent and 10 percent of lymphocytes. A marked decrease or absence in the number of B cells in peripheral blood may suggest a possible immunodeficiency relating to lack of B cell differentiation, and this would be supported by decreases in B cell lymphoid tissue such as the tonsils. Monoclonal antibodies and flow cytometry are used to define and quantitate populations of helper and cytotoxic T lymphocytes. T helper cells are defined as CD3+ and CD4+, while cytotoxic T cells express CD3 and CD8 (*Chapter 7*). Decreased numbers of CD4+ T lymphocytes, often associated with HIV infection, may contribute to an inability to mount a primary immune response.

In Vitro Functional Studies

Once the quantities of lymphocytes have been measured, one of the classic methods of measuring the functional status of humoral immunity is to assay B cell lymphocyte function following stimulation by a variety of nonspecific mitogens, antibody directed to CD markers, or stimulation by specific antigens to which the patient has been immunized (Table 24-12).

Tests to Exclude Rare and Secondary Causes

Depending on these initial test results, more specific testing can be initiated for a more detailed investigation. Shown in Table 24-9 are additional tests and procedures used to exclude rare and secondary causes of recurrent infection, which enter into the differential diagnosis of the primary and secondary humoral immune deficiency disorders. Even if immunodeficiency is diagnosed using routine laboratory studies, it is important that the clinician seek additional studies to define the precise genetic basis for the defect, if possible, to acquire as much information as possible for proper diagnosis, genetic counseling, and treatment.

T Cell Function: Tests of Cell-Mediated Immune Function

Cell-mediated immune responses result from complex interactions between antigen-presenting cells,

Table 24-12. In vitro lymphocyte activators

Name of lymphocyte activator	T cells	B cells
Mitogens		
Phytohemagglutinin (PHA)	Yes	No
Concanavalin A (ConA)	Yes	No
Lipopolysaccharide (LPS)	No	Yes
Pokeweed mitogen (PWM)	Yes	Yes
Antibodies directed to cell surface molecules		
Anti-CD3	Yes	No
Anti-CD28	Yes	No
Anti-IgM	No	Yes
Anti-CD40	No	Yes
sCD40L	Yes	No
Microbial antigens		
Staphylococcal enterotoxin B (SEB)	Yes	No
Staphylococcus aureus Cowan strain (SAC)	No	Yes
Allogeneic cells	Yes	No
Recall antigens		
Tetanus	Yes	No
Candida	Yes	No

T cells, and cytokines (*Chapter 7*). As described previously, antigen is taken up and processed by APCs, and peptide is presented to the T lymphocytes attached to major histocompatability complex (**MHC**) antigens on the surface of the antigen-presenting cell that are specific for the antigen being presented (*Chapter 10*). The T cell receptor (**TCR**) on the surface of T lymphocytes is also specific to the antigen presented on the MHC molecule, but the T cell must first recognize the MHC molecule itself. Thus, cell-mediated immune responses are considered MHC-restricted; this prevents nonspecific immune responses from developing (*Chapter 7*). This recognition phase is followed by cell activation, elaboration of soluble mediators, proliferation, and cytotoxic activity. Defects in any one of these broad pathways of cellular processes may lead to increased susceptibility to infections or cancers. T lymphocyte disorders rarely occur as isolated T cell deficiencies; more often, T lymphocyte deficiencies are a component of a combined T and B lymphocyte deficiency.

As with defects in humoral immunity, cell-mediated defects are also associated with frequent and/or serious infections, usually of the respiratory system, skin, or gut that may be difficult to treat with standard therapies. However, defects in cell-mediated immunity are often associated with infections caused by intracellular organisms, particularly viral and fungal organisms that, in an immunocompetent host, are not considered virulent. Since the passive transfer of maternal antibody does not influence the manifestations of cell-mediated defects as in the case of the humoral immune deficiencies, congenital defects in cell-mediated immunity generally are associated with clinical manifestations within the first six months of life and may manifest as a failure to thrive in addition to susceptibility to recurrent infection. Allergy, autoimmunity, and lymphomas are other important hallmarks of T cell mediated immunodeficiencies and occur more frequently in immunodeficient patients than in healthy individuals. Assessment of cell-mediated immune function, therefore, is not only important for the diagnosis of infectious disease, but also has found application in monitoring the effects of immunomodulatory therapy in the allergic diseases, the autoimmune disorders, and cancer as well as the assessment of vaccine effectiveness.

When to Suspect T Cell Dysfunction

Some of the more common T cell and combined immunodeficiencies are shown in Table 24-13 together with their distinctive features. Patients with T cell deficiency usually manifest failure to thrive, diarrhea, and recurrent infections caused by opportunistic pathogens, such as *Candida albicans* (thrush), *Pneumocystis jiroveci*, or cytomegalovirus very early in life (Table 24-13). On physical examination, patients with T cell deficiency may show paucity of lymph nodes and during infancy will demonstrate absence of a thymic shadow on a chest X-ray, although a decreased thymic shadow can also be observed in response to stress and may not be visualized in up to 50 percent of normal infants. Other common findings are chronic diarrhea, recurrent bacterial infections affecting multiple sites, and persistent infections despite adequate conventional treatment. SCID is a pediatric emergency because early diagnosis can dramatically improve the clinical

Table 24-13. Some common T cell and combined immunodeficiencies together with distinctive clinical features

T cell defect	Associated clinical/laboratory findings
SCID	Failure to thrive, chronic diarrhea, oral thrush, recurrent or severe bacterial, viral and/or fungal infections
CD40 and CD40 ligand deficiency	Recurrent sinopulmonary and opportunistic infections with low IgG and IgA levels and variable IgM levels
Wiskott-Aldrich syndrome	Easy bruisability, eczema, recurrent otitis media, diarrhea, thrombocytopenia with small platelets
DiGeorge syndrome	Hypoparathyroidism, cardiac malformations, dysmorphic features, variable T and B cell defects
Anhydrotic/hypohidrotic ectodermal dysplasia with immunodeficiency (NEMO or IkBa deficiency)	Recurrent mycobacterial or pyogenic infections, with or without skin, hair, and nail abnormalities; poor fever responses
X-linked lymphoproliferative disease (XLP)	Hypogammaglobulinemia, persistent or fatal EBV infection
Chronic mucocutaneous candidiasis	Recurrent oral, esophageal, or skin infection caused by *Candida* species

outcome. Skin rashes are common, particularly with specific T cell disorders, including Omenn and Wiskott-Aldrich syndromes (*Chapter 16*). Other severe cellular or combined defects present with a variety of clinical findings (Table 24-13).

Laboratory Evaluation of T Cell Function

Screening Tests

The diagnostic workup of patients with suspected T cell and combined immunodeficiency can be performed according to the tiered level of screening tests shown in Tables 24-1 and 24-14. The initial screening should include careful analysis of the white blood cell count and differential. The absolute lymphocyte count should be compared with age-matched control ranges for proper interpretation. Severe lymphopenia in an infant (< 3,000/mm^3) is a critical finding that should prompt immediate immunologic evaluation if confirmed by a repeat CBC. Since transfusion of nonirradiated blood products to a patient with severe cellular immune defect can produce a potentially fatal graft-versus-host disease (*Chapters 7* and *22*), any blood product considered for use in an infant with a suspected T cell deficiency should therefore be irradiated. Patients with symptoms of cellular immunodeficiency typically should have testing for the presence of HIV (i.e., HIV viral load assay) rather than serologic testing for anti-HIV antibody since immunoglobulins produced by HIV-infected infants are non-functional and, if detected, may be of maternal origin.

Part of the initial T cell screening tests should also include quantitative assessment of cellular immunity by immunophenotyping of T cells using FCM. Shown in Table 24-8 are the distributions of CD markers on T, B, and NK cells from normal adult subjects. In infants and children, it is equally important to carefully review subsets, comparing them with age-appropriate reference ranges. Shown in Tables 24-15, 24-16, and 24-17 are the age-dependent changes in naïve, memory, and activated lymphocyte populations and subpopulations for CD3, CD4, and CD8 T cells in infants and children.

Delayed-Type Hypersensitivity Skin Testing

Another screening assay of cellular immunity is the classical in vivo test of cutaneous delayed-type hypersensitivity (**DTH**), which is the in vivo correlate of the in vitro Th1/macrophage interaction (*Chapter 7*). This test measures the recall response to an intradermal injection of an antigen to which an individual previously has been exposed and sensitized. Three antigens are commonly used: (1) purified protein derivative (**PPD**), (2) *Candida albicans*, and (3) mumps; tetanus toxoid and trichophyton antigens may also be used. The use of several antigens decreases the chance of a false negative response that could result from a lack of prior exposure to an antigen. The injection site is monitored for the presence of induration 48 to 72 hours after administration of antigen. A positive result is characterized by induration of at least 2 mm greater than a positive control site.

Although skin testing is a sensitive indicator of intact cellular immunity, negative results must be interpreted with caution. Responses are very unreliable

Table 24-14. Tests used in the evaluation of suspected T cell and combined immunodeficiency

Diagnostic testing level	Assays to be performed
Screening tests	CBC and differential HIV testing Lymphocyte immunophenotyping Delayed-type hypersensitivity skin testing
Secondary tests	T cell proliferation (mitogens, alloantigens, recall antigens) T cell cytokine production Flow cytometric evaluation of surface or intracellular proteins, such as CD40 ligand (CD154 on activated T cells), IL-2 receptor g chain (CD132), MHC-I and II, IL-7 receptor a chain (CD127), CD3 chains, WASP Enzyme assays: adenosine deaminase, PNP FISH for 22q11 deletion TREC numbers TCR repertoire analysis Mutation analysis

WASP = Wiskott-Aldrich syndrome protein; PNP = purine nucleoside phosphorylase; FISH = fluorescence in situ hybridization; TREC = T cell receptor excision circle.

Table 24-15. Age-dependent changes in lymphocyte populations and subpopulations for CD3, CD4, and CD8 T cells expressed as immunophenotypic reference range (80 percent confidence interval)

	T cells					
	CD3		CD4		CD8	
Age	% positive	Cells/mm^3	% positive	Cells/mm^3	% positive	Cells/mm^3
0–3 mo	53–84	2500–5500	35–64	1600–4000	12–28	560–1700
3–6 mo	51–77	2500–5600	35–56	1800–4000	12–24	590–1600
6–12 mo	49–76	1900–5900	31–56	1400–4300	12–24	500–1700
1–2 yr	53–75	2100–6200	32–51	1300–4300	14–30	620–2000
2–6 yr	56–75	1400–3700	28–47	700–2200	16–30	490–1300
6–12 yr	60–76	1200–2600	31–47	650–1500	18–35	370–1100
12–18 yr	56–84	1000–2200	31–52	530–1300	18–35	330–920

Table 24-16. Age-dependent changes in lymphocyte populations and subpopulations for naïve CD4/CD45RA cells, memory CD3/CD4/CD45RO cells, and activated CD4/HLA-DR helper T cells expressed as immunophenotypic reference range (80 percent confidence interval)

	CD4 T cell subpopulations					
	CD4/CD45RA		CD3/CD4/CD45RO		CD4/HLA-DR	
Age	% CD4 positive	Cells/mm^3	% CD3/CD4 positive	Cells/mm^3	% CD4 positive	Cells/mm^3
0–3 mo	64–95	1200–3700	2–22	60–900	2–6	40–180
3–6 mo	77–94	1300–3700	3–16	120–630	2–10	60–280
6–12 mo	64–93	1100–3700	5–18	160–800	2–11	50–260
1–2 yr	63–91	1000–2900	7–20	210–850	2–11	70–280
2–6 yr	53–86	430–1500	9–26	220–660	3–12	50–180
6–12 yr	46–77	320–1000	13–30	240–630	3–13	40–120
12–18 yr	33–66	240–770	18–38	240–700	4–11	30–100

Table 24-17. Age-dependent changes in lymphocyte populations and subpopulations for naïve CD8/CD45RA cells, memory CD3/CD4–/CD45RO cells, and activated CD8/HLA-DR cytotoxic T cells expressed as immunophenotypic reference range (80 percent confidence interval)

	CD8 T cell subpopulations					
	CD8/CD45RA		CD3/CD4–/CD45RO		CD8/HLA-DR	
Age	% CD8 positive	Cells/mm^3	% CD3/CD4- positive	Cells/mm^3	% CD8 positive	Cells/mm^3
0–3 mo	80–99	450–1500	1–9	30–330	2–20	20–160
3–6 mo	85–98	550–1400	1–7	30–290	3–17	30–170
6–12 mo	75–97	480–1500	1–8	40–330	4–27	40–290
1–2 yr	71–98	490–1700	2–12	60–570	6–33	60–600
2–6 yr	69–97	380–1100	4–16	90–440	7–37	70–420
6–12 yr	63–92	310–900	4–21	70–390	6–29	40–270
12–18 yr	61–91	240–710	4–24	60–310	5–25	30–180

in children younger than one year of age, even with prior antigen exposure. In addition, cell-mediated immunity is often suppressed, resulting in a lack of DTH response, i.e., anergy, during some viral (e.g., HIV) and bacterial infections, cancer, and immunosuppressive therapy as well as following immunization with a live attenuated viral vaccine. A practical clinical application of this inhibitory effect of live vaccines has led to the recommendation to perform PPD testing prior to the routine immunization of infants with live attenuated viral vaccines, i.e., measles, mumps, rubella, or varicella vaccines (*Chapter 23*). The limited availability of suitable purified recall antigens, however, has further diminished the use of DTH testing, and many institutions have abandoned the technique. A negative DTH, if performed, should be followed up either with repeated testing or with appropriate in vitro assays of T cell function, as described below.

Secondary Tests

In Vitro T Cell Proliferation Assays (Mitogens, Alloantigens, and Recall Antigens)

The standard in vitro test of lymphocyte function is the lymphocyte proliferation assay (**LPA**), which measures peripheral blood T cell proliferation in response to nonspecific mitogens (phytohemagglutinin, concanavalin A, or pokeweed mitogen) or to specific antigens such as tetanus and diphtheria toxoids or *C. albicans* (Table 24-12). Proliferation is assessed by the incorporation of ^{3}H-thymidine into replicating DNA by lymphocytes as they divide in response to the mitogen or the antigen. Quantitation of incorporated ^{3}H-thymidine allows one to assess the proliferative capacity of the cells, since the amount of ^{3}H-thymidine incorporated is directly proportional to the degree of proliferation.

The various types of stimulants used in LPA can provide distinct information on the functional capacity of the cellular immune system. Mitogens, including plant lectins such as phytohemagglutinin or anti-CD3 antibodies, are potent stimulators for proliferation. They are polyclonal activators and stimulate most T lymphocytes in culture to proliferate. An absent or poor mitogen response suggests a severe defect in cell-mediated immunity. As in the case of the in vivo DTH responses, positive in vitro proliferative responses to recall antigens, such as tetanus toxoid, *C. albicans* antigens, and streptokinase, are seen only in subjects who have been previously exposed to the antigens, and a positive response is indicative of intact cellular responsiveness.

Mitogen/Antigen-Induced Cytokine Production

In addition to proliferation and cytotoxicity, one of the other major functions of T cells is to produce soluble mediators, such as cytokines, that are involved in various aspects of the immune response (*Chapter 9*). The plasma levels of these various mediators can be quantitatively measured and their variations assessed in normal and disease states. However, since many of these mediators are consumed rapidly soon after they are produced, measurement of plasma levels of certain cytokines may not be clinically relevant. The assessment of relative ratios of cytokines produced by individual cell types can also be used to qualitatively evaluate the nature of an immune response, e.g., Th1/Th2 analysis. The ability to assess cytokine secretion on a cellular level in vitro from whole blood or peripheral blood mononuclear cell (PBMC) culture can also provide more clinically relevant information to assess whether the cytokine of interest is produced in detectable amounts in a disease state or to assess the response to vaccination in a normal subject. For these applications, cytokine levels are measured by an enzyme-linked immunosorbent assay (**ELISA**) (Box 24-4).

The technique of cytokine measurement has permitted the determination of antigen-induced cytokine production at the cellular level as a marker for enumeration of antigen-specific cells. Detection at the single cell level allows the identification and enumeration of antigen-specific CD4 and CD8 T cells. Two approaches most commonly used for single cell cytokine production are the enzyme-linked immunospot (**ELISPOT**) and FCM-based detection of intracellular cytokine production.

ELISPOT assays use wells that contain a membrane to which an anti-cytokine antibody has been attached (Figure 24-6). Cells are added to the wells together with an antigen or mitogen and, after an appropriate period of incubation (ranging from a number of hours to days), they secrete cytokines that bind to the "capture antibodies" attached to the membrane. The cells are removed, the membranes washed, and the bound cytokines are detected by using a color development step that utilizes a second antibody, i.e., the "detection antibody," directed to the captured antigen. The number of spots, indicative of cytokine secretion, is counted in each well and is divided by the input cell number to yield a ratio of number of spot-forming cells per input cell number. A number of clinically useful assays have been developed for the diagnosis of active or latent tuberculosis that utilize the in vitro measurement of IFN-γ released from lymphocytes stimulated by purified synthetic mycobacterial peptides, i.e., the interferon-gamma release assays (**IGRAs**). One of the IGRAs employs a modification of the ELISPOT technology and has been clinically utilized in PPD skin test positive individuals to

Box 24-4

Principles of the Enzyme-Linked Immunosorbent Assay (ELISA)

The enzyme-linked immunosorbent assay (ELISA), also known as an enzyme immunoassay (EIA), is an immunologic technique used to detect the presence of an antibody or an antigen in a sample. The ELISA has become an important diagnostic tool in medicine not only because of its simplicity and accuracy, but also because of its safety over other techniques that employ radioactive materials.

Performing an ELISA involves at least one antibody that displays specificity for a particular antigen. An unknown amount of antigen is immobilized by a "capture antibody" attached to a solid surface (usually a polystyrene microtiter plate). After the antigen is immobilized, a second antibody called the "detection antibody" is added, forming a complex with the antigen. The detection antibody can be covalently linked to an enzyme or can itself be detected by a secondary antibody, which is linked to an enzyme. Between each step, the plate is typically washed with a mild detergent solution to remove cells, proteins, or antibodies that are not specifically bound. After the final wash, a chemical substrate is added to the plate that allows the enzyme to convert the substrate to a detectable signal, most commonly a visible color change. The intensity of the color correlates with the quantity of antigen in the sample.

ELISPOT is a variant of standard ELISA technology commonly used for the detection of cytokine-producing cells. Cytokines produced by cultured antigen-specific T cells are allowed to be secreted and bind to primary antibodies that have been immobilized in ELISPOT wells. Secondary antibodies conjugated to color-producing enzymes bind to the "captured" cytokines and addition of the substrate identifies each cell producing the cytokine(s) of interest. ELISPOT technology seems the most sensitive technique to detect antigen-specific T cells and is particularly useful for the measurement of interferon-γ (IFN-γ) and tumor necrosis factor-α (TNF-α).

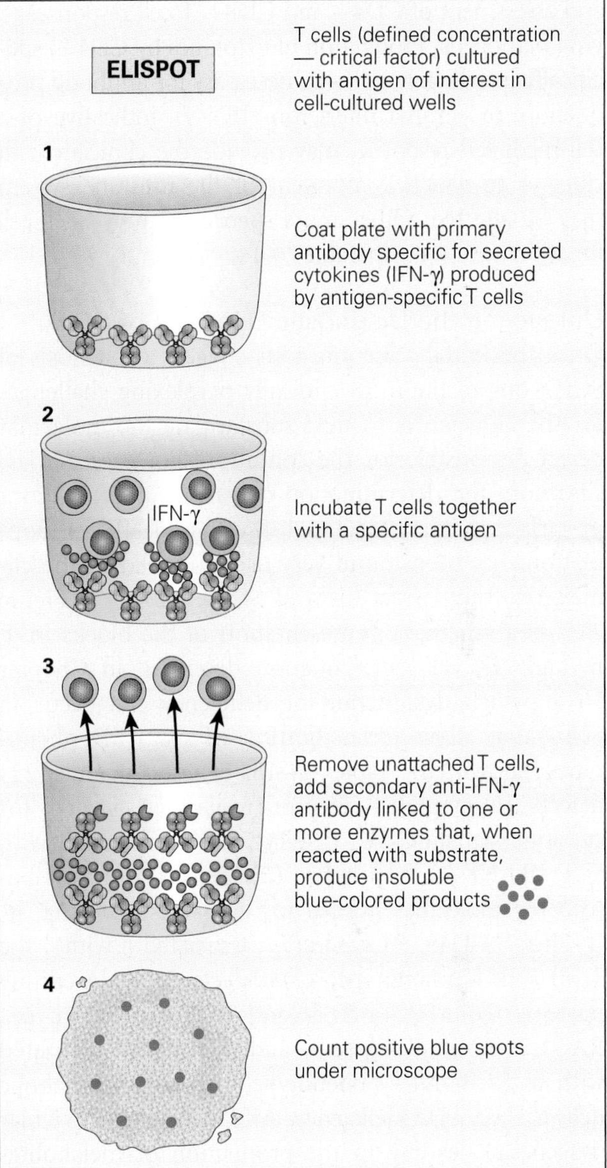

Figure 24-6. The principle of the ELISPOT assay used for assay of interferon-gamma. Panel 1: Wells are first coated with anti-IFN-γ antibody. Panel 2: Defined concentrations of purified peripheral blood mononuclear cells (PBMC), mostly T cells, are added to the anti-IFN-γ antibody-coated wells together with a specific antigen. Panel 3: Following an appropriate incubation period, usually 20 hours, the activated T cells synthesize IFN-γ that is captured by the membrane-bound antibody. After washing to remove cells and proteins, an enzyme-conjugated detection antibody is added, followed by the addition of substrate for color development in the form of insoluble blue colored spots. Panel 4: The number of spots correlates with the quantity of IFN-γ in the sample as determined by an ELISA.

differentiate active or latent tuberculosis from other mycobacterial infections or BCG immunization. The ELISPOT can be used to enumerate antigen-specific T cells in vitro, for example, in response to infection or vaccination. A predetermined number of T cells are cultured in vitro for a number of hours to days (depending on the type of responding cells of interest). The quantity of the cytokine produced is determined by the number of spots.

Detecting cytokine production by FCM is a simpler alternative. Cells of interest are incubated with a specific antigen and co-stimulatory antibody, followed by treatment with an agent to prevent secretion of cytokines from the cell. After several hours, the cells can be stained for surface markers, such as CD4 and CD8, and for intracellular cytokine production. This assay has been particularly useful to study the response to antigens and assessment of CD4+ and CD8+ T cell responses to viral pathogens. Production of cytokines by CD4+, specifically interleukin-4 (IL-4), necessary for antibody production, or gamma interferon (IFN-γ), indicative of a cell-mediated response, may provide the clinician with clues as to which component of the immune system may be affected. Other more specialized tests of T cell function are shown in Table 24-14.

Unraveling the Diagnostic Dilemma of SCID

Once the initial screening tests suggest a diagnosis of SCID, one of the most clinically perplexing challenges for the clinician is to next substantiate the molecular defect responsible for the condition. For ease of classification, the determination of various combinations of surface markers for T cell, B cell, and NK cell populations has been found very useful in leading the clinician to the correct form of SCID. Shown in Figure 24-7 is a schematic representation of the blocks in T, B, and NK cell differentiation described in Chapter 16 at which dysfunction or deficiency can occur in SCID that allow a classification of six SCID phenotypes shown in Table 24-18. These include: (1) defects in cytokine receptor molecules needed for cytokine signaling, i.e., IL-2Rγc, JAK3 associated with a T−B+NK− phenotype; (2) defects in cytokine-receptor molecules needed for cytokine signalling, ie, IL-7Rα, CD45, CD3δ/ε/ζ associated with the T−B+NK+ phenotype; (3) defects in DNA-editing proteins required for TCR and BCR expression, i.e., RAG1/2, Artemis, ligase-4, and Cerunnos, associated with a T−B−NK+ phenotype; (4) severe metabolic defects, i.e., ADA deficiency, AK2 deficiency (reticular dysgenesis), leading to the production of metabolites toxic for all lymphocyte types, resulting in a T−B−NK− phenotype; and (5) defects in TCR signaling, i.e., MHC-II (bare lymphocyte syndrome) and defect in p56lck (expressed on the CD4 co-receptor) associated with a CD8+CD4−B+NK+ phenotype; and (6) defects in ZAP70 (expressed in the zeta chain) associated with a CD4+CD8−B+NK+ phenotype.

Other useful tests in special circumstances include fluorescence in situ hybridization for the 22q11 microdeletion found in the majority of patients with DiGeorge syndrome and the velocardiofacial syndrome and specific enzyme assays to evaluate for adenosine deaminase and purine nucleoside phosphorylase (**PNP**) deficiencies. Evaluation for intracellular Wiskott-Aldrich syndrome protein (**WASP**) expression by means of flow cytometry can be performed in selected centers to screen for possible Wiskott-Aldrich syndrome (*Chapter 16*). Direct evaluation of T cell function, as assessed by the proliferative response to mitogens, recall antigens, and/or alloantigens, is an important part of evaluating cellular immunity. The same sort of culture conditions can also be used to evaluate for cytokine production using the culture supernatant (alternatively, one can evaluate cytoplasmic cytokine expression using flow cytometry). Quantification of T cell receptor excision circles (**TRECs**) and evaluation of the T cell repertoire can be used for additional evaluation of immune status. TRECs are formed during the normal editing of the TCR genes during T cell differentiation and maturation within the thymus and persist within the cell as extragenomic circular pieces of DNA. TREC copies are diluted over time as the T cells proliferate after antigen encounter. Therefore, naïve T cells that have recently emigrated from the thymus will present relatively high TREC levels compared with those of aged, antigen-experienced T cells. TREC evaluation (also CD41, CD45RA1, and CD311T cells by flow cytometry) can be used as a diagnostic confirmation of low thymic output that would be found in DiGeorge syndrome or to monitor immune reconstitution after bone marrow transplantation. More recently, the quantification of TRECs on blood derived from the Guthrie card obtained from infants after delivery has been initiated as a neonatal screening tool for SCID (and other significant T cell defects) in both Wisconsin and Massachusetts. The finding of low TREC levels in neonates should prompt immediate follow-up with immunophenotyping by means of flow cytometry. A recent report from Wisconsin suggests that this test has a very low rate of false positive or inconclusive results (approximately 0.00009 percent and 0.0017 percent, respectively).

Laboratory Diagnosis of Allergic Diseases

In Vivo and In Vitro Diagnostic Assays for the Allergic Diseases

Allergic diseases are among the most common disorders of human immune regulation (*Chapter 18*). The allergic or immediate hypersensitivity response was first described by Von Piquet at the turn of the 20th century, but it was not until 1968 that IgE, the immunoglobulin responsible for immediate type I hypersensitivity, was elucidated as the antibody class responsible for the allergic diseases. The presence of specific IgE against common environmental aeroallergens,

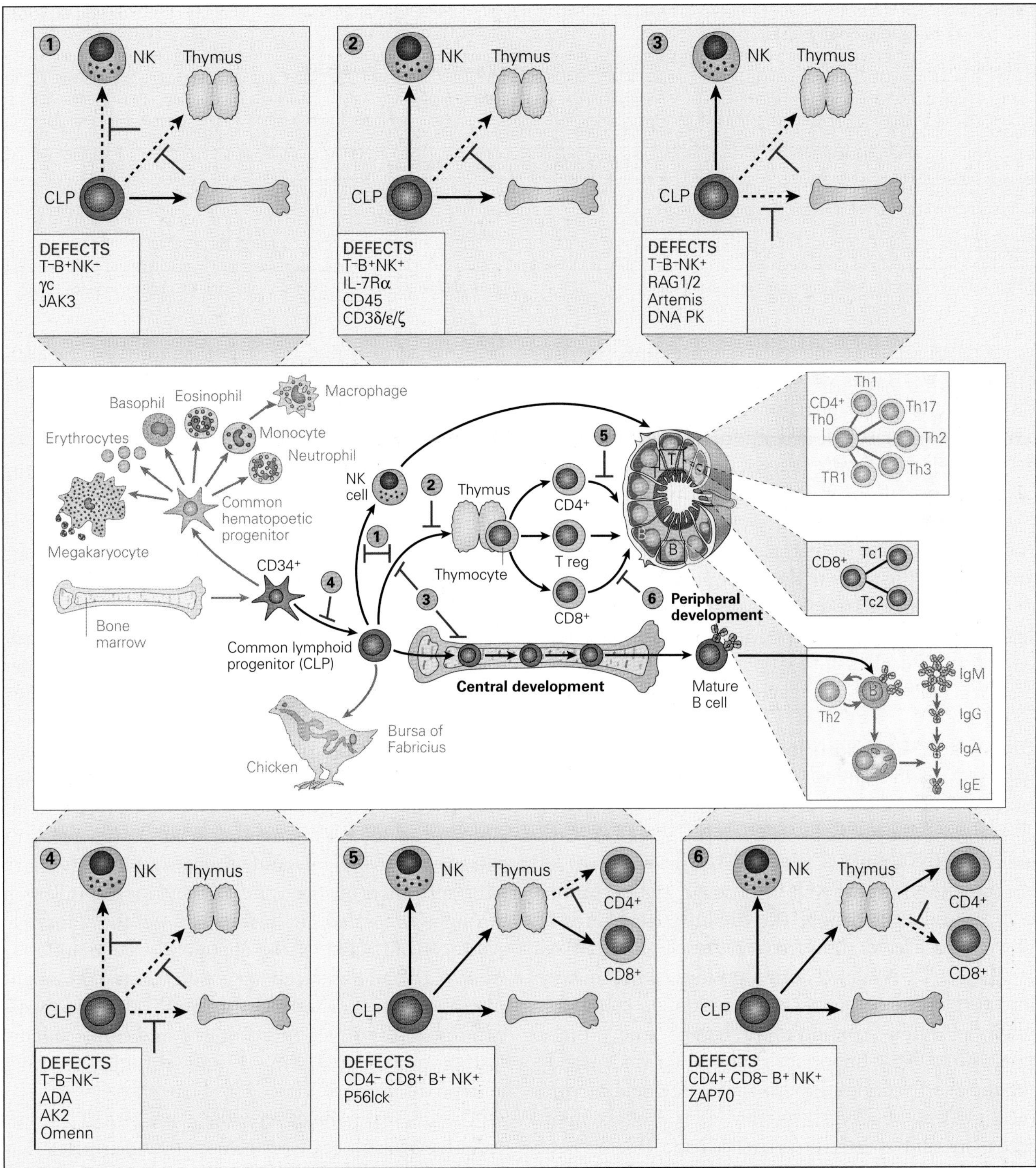

Figure 24-7. Schematic representation of the blocks in T, B, and NK cell differentiation at which dysfunction or deficiency can occur in SCID. Upper panel shows the location of the blocks; lower panel shows a more detailed representation of specific blocks in T, B, or NK cell differentiation in each of the types of SCID shown in Table 24-18.

therefore, now represents the classical mechanism of allergic tissue injury in the atopic individual and the basis for both in vivo and in vitro diagnostic testing.

There are a myriad of diseases associated with an IgE-mediated response ranging from well characterized systemic diseases such as an anaphylactic reaction associated with stinging insects, e.g., hymenoptera, to those localized allergic diseases that manifest at mucosal surfaces that include allergic rhinitis, asthma, atopic dermatitis, and gastrointestinal disorders associated with food hypersensitivities. As described in Chapter 18, the primary molecular

Table 24-18. Various immunophenotypic types of SCID correlated with genetic/molecular defects, cellular localization, and points of ontogenetic blocks

Phenotype	Pathway affected and genetic defect(s)
#1 T−B+NK−	Cytokine signaling: IL-2Rγc, JAK3
#2 T−B+NK+	Cytokine signaling: IL-7Rα, CD45, CD3δ/ε/ζ
#3 T−B−NK+	DNA editing: RAG1/2, Artemis, DNA PK
#4 T−B−NK−	Metabolic defects: adenosine deaminase (ADA), AK2, Omenn syndrome
#5 CD4−CD8+ B+ NK+	Positive selection/signaling: p56lck
#6 CD4+CD8− B+ NK+	Signaling: ZAP70

JAK3 = Janus kinase 3; RAG = recombination-activating gene; AK2 = adenylate kinase 2; ZAP70 = zeta-chain associated protein kinase, 70 kD.

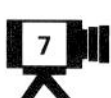
mechanism of these allergic responses involves the cross-linking of allergen with specific IgE antibodies on the surface of mediator cells, e.g., mast cells. This leads to mast cell activation and degranulation and the release of various mast cell mediators, complement activation, deposition of immune complexes, and infiltration of activated T cells into susceptible tissues. While accurate detection of IgE antibody in the skin as demonstrated by an immediate wheal and flare reaction is important for confirmation of allergic disease, it is the accurate and complete clinical history of the patient, as with all diseases, that drives the diagnosis of allergic disease.

Diagnostic Algorithm for Allergic Disease

Diagnosis of the specific allergenic response, which is essential for institution of allergen immunotherapy or allergen avoidance, can be determined by both in vitro and in vivo testing (*Chapter 18*). The diagnosis of allergic disease begins with a thorough clinical history and physical examination. The clinical presentations of the various allergic disorders are extensively described in Chapter 18. A subject with a positive clinical history for allergic disease and a positive skin or blood test result for IgE is considered to have a true positive result (Box 24-5). Important measures for understanding the effectiveness of in vivo skin testing and in vitro measurement of allergen-specific IgE are based upon sensitivity and specificity as well as the positive and negative predictive powers of the test (Box 24-5). In general, in vivo tests are more sensitive but less specific since nonspecific irritants in the in vivo preparations and technique can occasionally give rise to false positive results.

In vitro methods of allergen testing include allergen-specific IgE assays, basophil histamine release, or lymphocyte-stimulation tests. In vivo testing involves controlled allergen challenge (most commonly intradermal skin testing, followed by respiratory, gastric, or ocular challenge) that is closely monitored by the allergist for signs of an acute allergic reaction (*Chapter 18*).

In Vitro Allergen Testing

The most common in vitro assay for allergy testing is the detection and quantitation of allergen-specific IgE antibody. Total serum IgE and measurement of other vasoactive mediators, cytokines, and markers of inflammation are also measured to help the clinician assess an allergic response in the patient. In vitro measurement of histamine release from basophils coated with allergen-specific IgE is another alternative method to in vivo intradermal skin testing, although this test is usually performed only in specialized research laboratories. Allergen-specific IgE immunoassays are used as an alternative when skin testing is not practical or possible. These conditions include: (1) patients in whom skin prick or intradermal testing is equivocal or negative; (2) lack of availability or licensure of a skin test allergen strongly suggested by history to be the causative pathogenetic agent of the allergic disease manifestations; (3) patients receiving medications that might interfere with skin testing, e.g., antihistaminic medications; and (4) requirement for additional allergy testing in patients with asthma, rhinitis, or other allergic diseases.

The original radioallergosorbent test (**RAST**) as initially developed and performed by Pharmacia has been substituted with more modern immunoassays that have replaced radiolabeled reagents with ELISA assays. The current assays use allergenic materials bound to a solid matrix to which the patient's serum is added, and following incubation and a wash step, an enzyme-labeled anti-human IgE antibody is added (*Chapter 18*). After a second incubation and another wash step, enzyme substrate is added, the response is measured, and the results are calculated and reported. The majority of assays are quantitative rather than

Box 24-5

Sensitivity and Specificity Parameters of Diagnostic Allergy Tests

Sensitivity and **specificity** are statistical parameters that measure the effectiveness of either in vitro or in vivo tests of allergic disease for determining the capacity of either test to correctly distinguish between true positives and true negatives. **Sensitivity** measures the proportion (percentage) of actual positives that are correctly identified (i.e., the percentage of truly allergic patients who are correctly identified by the test as having the condition and not incorrectly including those who do not have allergy). **Specificity** measures the proportion (percentage) of negatives that are correctly identified as negative (i.e., the percentage of nonallergic individuals who are correctly identified as not having the condition and excluding those who do have allergic disease). Shown in Table 24-19 is an example of a study of 465 individuals comparing the sensitivity and specificity of an in vitro allergen-specific IgE test; 345 subjects were considered to be nonallergic as determined by history and negative skin testing and 120 were considered allergic on the basis of history and skin test positivity.

Table 24-19. Comparison of sensitivity and specificity of allergen-specific IgE testing

Results of allergen-specific IgE testing	Allergic sensitization (SPT-positive) n = 120	No allergic sensitization (SPT-negative) n = 345
Positive n = 117	True positive (TP): n = 85	False positive (FP): n = 32
Negative n = 348	False negative (FN): n = 35	True negative (TN): n = 313

Diagnostic sensitivity of the IgE antibody test was determined as follows: percentage positivity in patients with allergic disease = TP/[TP + FN] × 100; 85/[85 + 35] = 85/120 = **71%**

Diagnostic specificity of the IgE antibody test was determined as follows: percentage negativity in patients with no allergic disease = TN/[TN + FP] × 100; 113/[113 + 32] = 113/145 = **78%**

Positive predictive value of an IgE antibody test: percentage of patients with a positive IgE antibody test result who have allergic disease = TP/[TP + FP] × 100; 85/[85 + 32] = 85/117 = **73%**

Negative predictive value of an IgE antibody test: percentage of patients with a negative IgE antibody test result who have no allergic disease = TN/[TN + FN] × 100; 313/[313 + 35] = 313/348 = **90%**

qualitative. Unfortunately, there is a lack of uniform standardization of the various assays available for measuring total and allergen-specific IgE, even though there are published guidelines for assay design, performance, standardization, and quality assurance. Therefore, it is important for the clinician to be aware of which assay the referral laboratory is performing as well as any changes in assay format or procedure that may have been instituted. Results of properly performed and interpreted intradermal skin testing usually agree with the results of modern allergen-specific IgE assay, but the two methods differ in relative sensitivity and specificity, as described previously. Recently, purified recombinant allergens have become attractive for in vivo skin testing not only because their availability in pure form simplifies reagent preparation, but also because of their reproducibility and standardization. When there are discrepant results between the in vivo and in vitro tests, e.g., a positive skin test and a negative immunoassay, it is generally assumed to be a limitation of the immunoassay rather than problems with the skin test. It is, therefore, more prudent for the clinician to rely on the skin test rather than the immunoassay because of the greater dependence of the in vitro test on purity and heterogeneity of the allergen. However, with the promising availability and future use of certain purified recombinant allergens as diagnostic reagents in both in vivo and in vitro IgE antibody testing, these difficulties may be obviated.

In Vivo Allergen Testing

The epicutaneous or skin prick/puncture and intradermal skin tests are the two most common clinically used in vivo methods for diagnosis of allergic response. The skin test is considered the reference method for determining an IgE-specific allergic response, while the bronchial provocation test is more commonly used to evaluate asthmatic conditions. The clinical indication for skin testing is any reasonable suspicion that the origin of the patient's symptoms is caused by an allergic response. There are a multitude of allergens available for testing, and the physician, through thorough patient questioning and evaluation of symptoms, can decide which allergens are more likely to be the cause of the patient's problems and test for those particular allergens. It is important to use well-characterized allergen extracts that contain known amounts of allergen. Purified recombinant allergens are now available and are prepared as diagnostic and therapeutic extracts with known quantities of allergen standardized by protein purity in order to maintain consistency of content and to reduce lot-to-lot variation. The skin test should not be performed if the patient is receiving allergen immunotherapy or any medications at the time of testing, such as antihistamines, which might interfere with the development of the wheal-and-flare reactions and may give rise to false negative skin tests (*Chapter 18*). Briefly, the skin prick technique consists of placing a drop of allergen onto the surface of the skin with a single, dual, and multiple-point standardized device to introduce the allergen into the epidermis; the intradermal method is performed by injecting a small amount of allergen directly under the skin. Following either technique, the injected sites are inspected for the development of a wheal and erythematous reaction after about 15 minutes. If there is no response, the sites are reinspected after 30 minutes. If there are reactions at 15 minutes, they are read again at 30 minutes, and if larger, the 15-minute response is discarded. The diameter of the wheal and the amount of erythema are measured to the nearest millimeter. Rather than a single-dose injection, a skin test titration can be performed that involves the intradermal injection of three- or tenfold serial dilutions of the same extract into different sites in the skin. The purpose of skin test titration is to determine the degree of patient sensitivity; the greater the patient's sensitivity to the allergen extract, higher the serial dilution and lower concentration of the test allergen will be required. A tenfold dilutional series of allergens can provide much more information compared to a single concentration that gives a positive result. A histamine control should always be placed to assure skin reactivity and to provide a reference (i.e., positive control) together with a diluent to ensure there is no response to the diluent itself (i.e., negative control). In reading skin prick or intradermal skin test results, the following points should be taken into consideration for proper interpretation and accurate diagnosis.

- Presence of a positive skin test does not necessarily mean that the patient has an allergic disease due to that particular reaction. This is where serial skin titration can help, since a higher end point dilution that is still positive increases the likelihood that the allergen is responsible for the patient's symptoms.
- Tests may be falsely negative when the patient is actually sensitive. This is most likely due to the allergen preparation; lack of stability, low potency, and/or variability between lots of allergens. Also, the amount of actual allergen in relation to the amount of protein in the extract may be very small. Again, a series of varying concentrations of the allergen tested may be beneficial in this case as well.
- The use of in vivo testing for allergic disease by itself is not considered to be good clinical practice. Studies have shown that intradermal skin test results alone may not indicate clinically significant sensitivity to some allergens, but intradermal skin testing and allergen-specific IgE values were much more efficient together in diagnosing certain allergies.

Laboratory Diagnosis of Autoimmune Disorders

Introduction

The autoimmune disorders are characterized by the loss of normal immune homeostatic function seen in genetically susceptible hosts that results in an abnormal immune response directed to their own tissues (*Chapter 19*). As described in Chapter 19, a clear distinction must be made between an autoimmune response and an autoimmune disease (Box 24-6).

The hallmark of the autoimmune disorders is the presence of self-reactive T cells, autoantibodies, and inflammation. In recent years, a major investigative effort has been directed to the study of why the

Box 24-6

Autoimmune Disease versus Autoimmune Response

The term "autoimmune response" refers to the demonstration of an autoantibody or T cell–mediated event directed to a "self-antigen." An autoimmune response may or may not be associated with autoimmune disease. For example, many clinically well individuals, particularly women, exhibit an autoimmune response to the presence of serum antinuclear antibodies (ANAs) and demonstrate no symptoms. Although the presence of ANA may also be associated with the autoimmune disease, e.g., systemic lupus erythematosus (SLE), the diagnosis requires the presence of additional clinical features of the disease, e.g., rash, arthritis, or kidney involvement.

immune system turns against itself (*Chapter 19*). This has resulted not only in a greatly advanced understanding of the mechanisms of tissue injury seen in the autoimmune disorders, but has also provided the basis for the creation of new clinical laboratory technologies useful for the diagnosis of these clinically perplexing conditions.

The use of these new diagnostic tests, however, is fraught with some difficulty since no single laboratory test can unequivocally establish a diagnosis of an autoimmune disorder but rather requires multiple laboratory tests together with a carefully taken medical history. The diagnosis of autoimmune disease in patients, therefore, is based primarily upon clinical history and physical examination and is supported by appropriate laboratory tests. For ease of discussion, the laboratory tests commonly used for the diagnosis of the autoimmune diseases can be divided into three levels based upon the complexity of the test procedure: (1) **level A** (**first-line diagnostics**) includes generalized tests of innate immune dysfunction that measure various nonspecific markers of the inflammatory response commonly available in most clinical laboratories; (2) **level B** (**second-line diagnostics**) includes tests of adaptive immune dysfunction that measure a variety of specific autoantibodies directed against cellular and extracellular protein and nucleic acid components; and (3) **level C** (**third-line diagnostics**) includes various tests of molecular genetics that may serve useful for the diagnosis of many inflammatory syndromes that characterize the autoimmune disorders (Table 24-20).

Level A (First-Line Diagnostics) Testing

After a detailed history and physical examination, the initial laboratory assessment of the patient suspected with autoimmune disease should consist of a complete blood cell count, including a white blood cell and differential count, and the determination of acute-phase reactants, e.g., CRP, and an erythrocyte sedimentation rate (**ESR**). Acute-phase reactants are proteins found in serum that are increased during the acute phase of inflammation and, in addition to CRP, include the less commonly measured proteins shown in Table 24-21. The majority of these are produced in the liver in response to stimulation by inflammatory cytokines such as interleukin-6 (IL-6), interleukin-1β (IL-1β), and tumor necrosis factor-α (TNF-α) released from monocytes and macrophages (*Chapter 9*). The ESR is a major clinically useful monitoring test for acute-phase inflammation and correlates with increased levels of the acute-phase reactants, in particular, fibrinogen. The ESR is higher in women than in men and, in healthy individuals, displays an upper limit of 15 mm/hr in men and 20 mm/hr in women $\leq$ 50 years of age.

A relatively new level A acute-phase diagnostic test measures procalcitonin (**PCT**), a prohormone of calcitonin produced in the C cells of the thyroid gland. In healthy subjects, PCT levels are less than 0.10 ng/mL. Several studies have shown that PCT is

Table 24-20. Immunodiagnostic tests used in the autoimmune diseases

Level	Immunologic target	Example of diagnostic tests
Level A (first-line diagnostics)	Innate immune dysfunction	CBC, comprehensive metabolic panel, measurement of acute-phase reactants (CRP); erythrocyte sedimentation rate (ESR), complement activity (CH50, C3, C4) Less common markers: (ceruloplasmin, ferritin, fibrinogen, haptoglobin, albumin)
Level B (second-line diagnostics)	Adaptive immune dysfunction	Antinuclear antibodies (ANAs) levels and patterns (see Table 24-22) Specific cellular autoantibodies (see Table 24-23) Rheumatoid factor (RF) Anticyclic citrullinated peptide antibodies Antiphospholipid antibodies Antineutrophil cytoplasmic autoantibodies (ANCAs) Cryoglobulins Lupus anticoagulant/anticardiolipin/aPL autoantibodies
Level C (third-line diagnostics)	Molecular and genetic studies	HLA studies Single gene defects in the inflammasomopathies

Table 24-21. Examples of acute-phase reactants

C-reactive protein (CRP)
Fibrinogen
Plasminogen
Ferritin
Ceruloplasmin
Complement factors
Haptoglobin
Hemopexin
Granulocyte colony-stimulating factor (G-CSF)
Serum amyloid A
Alpha-1 antitrypsin
Interleukin-1 receptor antagonist (IL-1RA)

mainly produced during severe bacterial infections where its levels are increased up to 200 times greater than normal, in contrast to low levels found during viral infections, autoimmune illnesses, and graft-versus-host disease. In patients with autoimmune disease, such as SLE or immunodeficiency, PCT has not only been found useful in distinguishing a bacterial infection from a disease flare, but also is a useful aid for the early diagnosis of osteomyelitis.

Serum Amyloid A (SAA)

Serum amyloid A (**SAA**) is another cytokine-induced acute-phase protein produced in the liver that has been used diagnostically in some of the autoimmune and autoinflammatory disorders. Although its precise function is incompletely understood, several investigations have suggested that SAA plays a role in the inflammatory process through its cytokine-like property and by its capacity to induce other proinflammatory cytokines. Median normal plasma concentration of SAA in healthy persons is 3 mg/L, but it can increase to more than 2,000 mg during the acute-phase response. SAA is the serum precursor of the amyloid A protein, which, when overproduced, is the principal component of the amyloid deposits found in inflammation-associated reactive amyloidosis. Clinical amyloidosis occurs not only in up to 10 percent of patients with chronic infections, but also in several autoinflammatory conditions, including RA, JIA, and Crohn's disease. Although the kidneys are most often affected, any organ may be involved. Amyloidosis is the most severe complication of familial Mediterranean fever (FMF) with manifestations of the nephrotic syndrome and eventually uremia. Since amyloid beta (Aβ) peptides play a pivotal role in the development of Alzheimer's disease, it is tempting to speculate on the relationship of inflammation-induced stimulation of SAA in the pathogenesis of this clinically perplexing disorder.

Complement

As described in Chapter 4, the complement proteins consist of a set of more than 40 cascading serum proteins that can be activated in a variety of clinical conditions by several agents, including immune or antigen-antibody complexes. Complement components are synthesized in the liver and increased levels are frequently found in inflammatory disorders. The most frequently analyzed components for clinical assessment are CH50, C3, and C4. Depressed complement levels (C3 and/or C4), in contrast, are commonly present in SLE, particularly with renal involvement, acute postinfectious glomerulonephritis, and membranoproliferative glomerulonephritis (due to immune complex formation and complement consumption *Chapter 17*) as well as in hepatic disease and several congenital deficiencies of complement components (*Chapter 4*). Hereditary complement deficiencies of C1q, C4, and C2 have been associated with an increased risk of autoimmune disease, especially SLE.

In addition to the more commonly measured CRP, elevated levels of serum ferritin (SF) have been shown to be a useful nonspecific marker of a large number of inflammatory diseases such as adult-onset Still's disease and systemic-onset juvenile idiopathic arthritis (JIA), where high levels of SF have been shown to reflect disease activity. Highly elevated ferritin levels are also a laboratory hallmark of hemophagocytic lymphohistiocytosis (**HLH**), a condition characterized by pathologic proinflammatory activity of T cells and macrophages (*Chapter 16*). Genetic (primary) HLH is one group of disorders of immune regulation, inherited as autosomal-recessive or X-linked disorder, which frequently develops early in life. Acquired (secondary) HLH occurs in all age groups and may be triggered by severe infection, malignancy, or autoimmune disease.

Level B (Second-Line Diagnostics) Testing

Antinuclear Antibodies

Level B (second-line diagnostics) testing usually begins with detecting the presence of antinuclear autoantibodies (**ANA**). Detection and identification of ANAs are essential for the assessment of systemic and organ-specific autoimmune diseases. This test has been used for several decades and has proven very useful. It combines the detection of a wide range of autoantibodies with good sensitivity, reproducibility, economy, and ease of use. The initial screening usually employs an indirect fluorescent assay, where patient's serum is incubated with a target cell containing a source of the nucleic acid and associated protein antigens. Following incubation and appropriate washing, the slide is incubated with a fluorescent-labeled antihuman antibody, and after a final incubation and washing, the slide is visualized using a fluorescent microscope. Two items of information can be gained by measuring ANAs this way: (1) the titer at which the patient's serum is positive; and (2) the particular fluorescent-staining pattern observed, both of which are dependent upon the specificity of the autoantibody for the particular nuclear antigenic component being measured. Some staining patterns are not antigen specific and may reflect reactivity of several different autoantibodies with various components of the nuclear content, while others are antigen specific and are directed to specific components such as centromere patterns. Further level B testing is then performed to determine the antigen specificity of the autoantibodies present.

Although the ANA assay has also been developed in an ELISA format, it does not reveal the staining pattern information provided by the IFA procedure important for the clinician. It has been shown that certain autoantibody subsets are associated with certain systemic autoimmune diseases, e.g., SLE. Therefore, it is important to identify the antigenic target of the ANA. There have also been some cases where disease-specific autoantibodies are present prior to the onset of clinical symptoms. Detection of these disease-specific autoantibodies in asymptomatic individuals may permit early diagnosis and preventative treatment.

The ANAs are nuclear, nucleolar, or perinuclear autoantibodies that are not only found in low levels in healthy individuals, but, when elevated, are a characteristic finding in patients with a variety of autoimmune disorders. The ANAs represent the flagship autoimmune disease-screening test frequently performed in the initial workup of the patient suspected with autoimmune disease. Although their pathogenetic role is not clear, ANAs are suggestive of autoimmunity when they are persistently present in high titers together with the clinical features of the disease. Positive ANA testing is associated with several inflammatory rheumatic diseases, including SLE, mixed connective tissue disease (**MCTD**), and Sjögren's syndrome. ANAs can also be helpful for the diagnosis of several nonrheumatic autoimmune diseases, such as autoimmune hepatitis, autoimmune thyroiditis, and drug-induced autoimmune syndromes.

Laboratory Assays for ANA

The IFA-screening tests for ANA are performed by indirect immunofluorescence using either frozen sections of animal tissue or, more appropriately, cultured cell lines (e.g., human epithelial Hep-2 cells). Shown in Figure 24-8 are different patterns of nuclear localization of ANA immunofluorescence that include the following: (1) peripheral (rim), (2) homogeneous (diffuse), (3) speckled, (4) centromere, and (5) nucleolar patterns; the homogeneous and the speckled patterns are more common. Shown in Box 24-7 are some clinical associations of IFA patterns with clinical autoimmune diseases. Although the patterns of IFA are neither specific nor diagnostic of an autoantibody or an autoimmune disease entity, they can guide the clinician in the choice of additional diagnostic tests, such as the double-immunodiffusion assays, the immunoblot test, or ELISA to detect specific antibodies (ANA profile). ELISA technology is now the most commonly used technique but tends to produce more false positive and true weak positive results. When necessary, laboratories use more reliable and sensitive assays such as the immunoprecipitation (Farr) technique to confirm dubious ELISA results. The Farr technique is superior to the ELISA in detecting anti-double-stranded DNA (anti-dsDNA) antibodies in patients with SLE; indeed, Farr correlates with global disease activity as well as renal and vascular involvement.

Measurement of Specific Antinuclear Autoantibodies

Shown in Table 24-22 are the specific antinuclear autoantibodies seen in systemic autoimmune diseases together with their antigenic determinants and clinical disease associations.

Anti-dsDNA Antibody

Since their discovery in 1957, attention has focused on anti-dsDNA antibodies and their role in pathogenesis of certain autoimmune diseases, i.e., SLE. Detection of autoantibodies against double-stranded DNA (**dsDNA**) are the prototypic autoantibodies found most often in patients with SLE. Anti-dsDNA antibodies are a major component of ANA specificity, serving as a serological marker of diagnostic

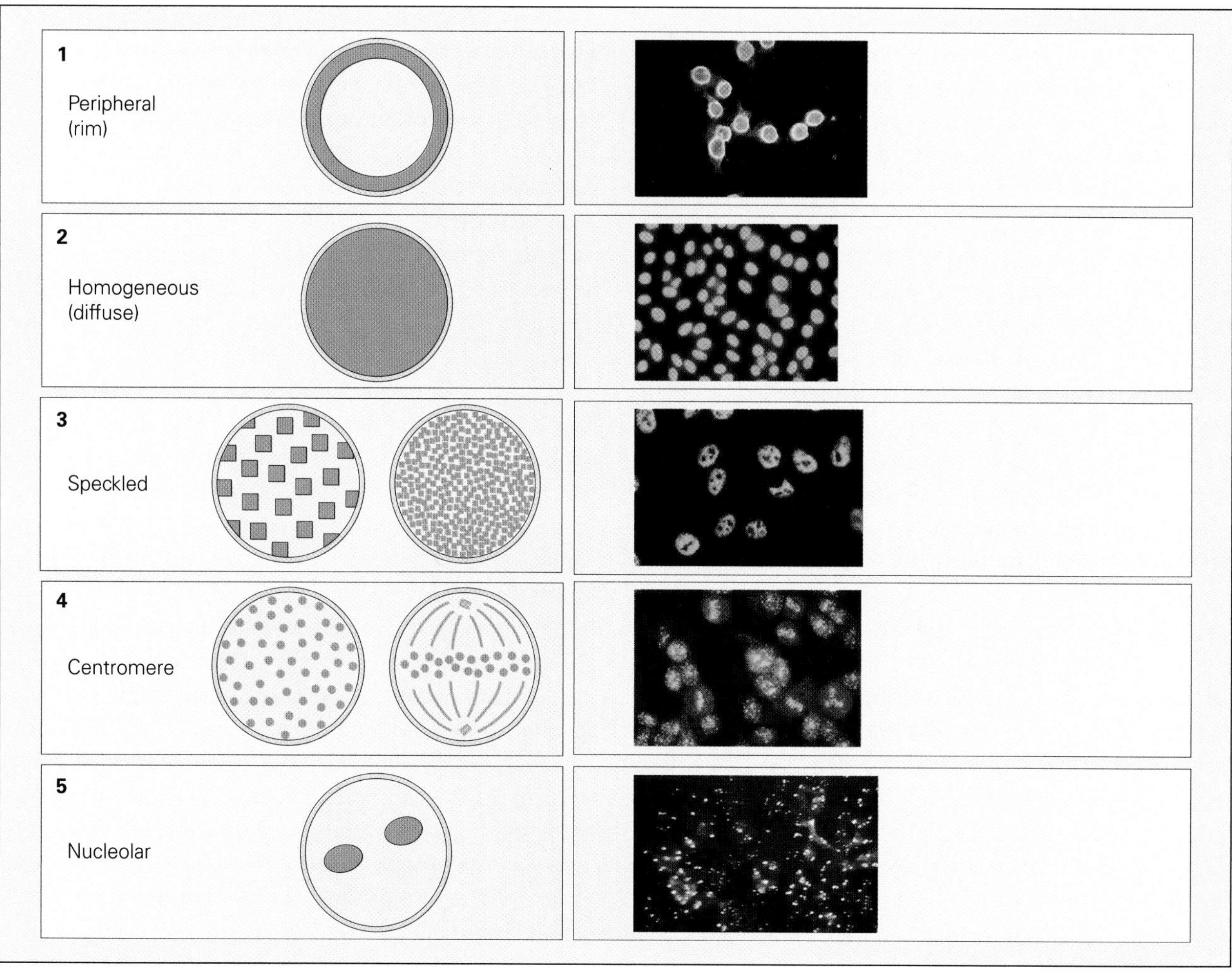

Figure 24-8. Different immunofluorescent patterns that have been identified by indirect immunofluorescence following incubation of sera of patients with a variety of autoimmune diseases with various target cells that include the following patterns: (1) peripheral (rim), (2) homogeneous (diffuse), (3) speckled, (4) centromere, and (5) nucleolar pattern.

and prognostic significance. The close association of anti-dsDNA with SLE has suggested that anti-dsDNA antibodies can signal critical events in SLE pathogenesis and can guide the clinician in managing these patients. The term anti-DNA antibody in common usage refers to antibodies that bind specifically to dsDNA. Tests for antibodies to single-stranded DNA (**ssDNA**) are available; however, their performance characteristics and clinical associations are quite distinct from anti-dsDNA antibodies and are therefore of no clinical utility and should not be ordered outside of research settings.

Typically, the technique most often used for detection of anti-dsDNA is by indirect immunofluorescence (IFA) using the hemoflagellate *Crithidia luciliae*, whose kinetoplast contains DNA as the substrate for binding of the anti-DNA antibodies in patients' serum. There are also ELISA assays and multiplex bead assays for detection of anti-dsDNA antibodies. Positive anti-dsDNAs antibodies are rarely encountered in healthy individuals and appear highly specific of SLE; they are observed in 84 to 95 percent of children and in about 50 to 70 percent of untreated adults with this disease. The titer of anti-dsDNA antibodies is clinically important for monitoring disease activity, and a rise in anti-dsDNA antibodies usually precedes SLE exacerbation by a few weeks. High titers have been identified in lupus nephritis and their levels tend to rise and fall with disease activity. In addition to anti-dsDNA autoantibodies, other autoantibodies have been demonstrated that bear the names of patients found to have these antibodies, e.g., anti-Sm ("Smith") antibodies. Anti-Sm antibodies are antibodies directed against the LSm proteins, a family of RNA-binding proteins found in virtually every cellular organism; the anti-Sm antibodies were first described in a patient with SLE

Box 24-7

Some Clinical Associations of IFA Patterns with Clinical Autoimmune Diseases

The **homogeneous pattern** of ANA is due to the presence of anti-histone and/or anti-dsDNA antibodies that are highly specific of SLE; the presence of anti-dsDNA may also result in a **peripheral** or **rim** pattern. The **speckled pattern** is associated with anti-Sm (anti-Smith antigen), anti-SSA, and anti-SSB antibodies of Sjögren's syndrome and MCTD. The **nucleolar** pattern is related to anti-Scl70 antibodies in systemic sclerosis, and the **centromere** pattern is seen with antibodies to the kinetochore in the CREST (calcinosis, Raynaud's phenomenon, esophageal disease, sclerodactyly, telangiectasia) syndrome and in primary biliary cirrhosis. Cytoplasmic fluorescence reveals different patterns and is indicative of the distinct antigens involved: antimitochondrial autoantibodies display a granular pattern; autoantibodies to the Golgi organelle show granules arranged in clusters at one or both cell poles; the anti-keratin antibody pattern is characterized by a fibrous network that spreads out from the perinuclear region while autoantibodies to nonmuscle myosin decorate the stress fibers of the cytoskeleton.

and the Sm protein antigens and their specific antibodies were named in honor of this patient, Stephanie Smith. Related to autoantibodies that have been found to be clinically useful in the diagnosis of the systemic autoimmune diseases, others have been helpful for the diagnosis of the organ-specific autoimmune disorders (Table 24-23).

Assays for Extractable Nuclear Antigens

A particular class of ANAs specific for extractable nuclear antigens (**ENA**) was initially described in 1959 (Table 24-23). Since that time, many different ENA antibodies have been described but the two most commonly performed ENA assays measure anti-Sm and anti-RNP autoantibodies. The detection of these autoantibodies and the identification of their specificity have become well-established tools for the laboratory diagnosis of several autoimmune diseases. In most cases, ENA testing is ordered after an initial ANA screen. The indications for use are to establish a diagnosis in patients with suggestive clinical symptoms, to exclude a diagnosis of autoimmune disease in patients with few or uncertain clinical signs, to subclassify patients with a known diagnosis, and to monitor disease activity. One of the major clinical uses of measurement of the anti-ENA autoantibodies is separating MCTD (which usually has greater anti-RNP positivity) from SLE (which usually has greater anti-Sm reactivity) (Table 24-23).

Testing for anti-ENA antibodies has historically relied on gel-based immunoprecipitation techniques such as double immunodiffusion (**DID**) and counterimmunoelectrophoresis. The association of specific types of ENA antibodies with rheumatological diseases was established using these gel-based immunoassay techniques. However, autoantibody testing is an evolving field, and the older gel-based immunodiffusion assays are being replaced with the less specific, more sensitive ELISA and fluorescent-based bead assay systems.

The widespread use of autoantibody testing has greatly improved the ability to diagnose both the complex systemic autoimmune diseases, e.g., SLE, as well as the more targeted organ-specific autoimmune disorders, e.g., autoimmune thyroiditis, both of which can often be very difficult to recognize. That being said, one must interpret the results of such testing with the understanding that the newer assay methods, e.g., ELISA, for detection of autoantibodies may give false positive results due to increased sensitivity compared to older methodologies, such as DID (also called Ouchterlony precipitin) methods. It is important to interpret results of autoantibody testing in light of both the clinical context and the methodology employed.

Level C (Third-Line Diagnostics) Testing

With the discovery of the genome, Level C (third-line diagnostics) testing is emerging as the major area for development of new diagnostic technologies for the autoimmune and autoinflammatory disorders. Nowhere has the translation of basic molecular biology and immunology into clinical applicability been better exemplified than by the great diagnostic and therapeutic advances that have been made in rheumatoid arthritis.

Rheumatoid arthritis (**RA**) is a chronic, systemic disorder characterized by inflammation and synovial proliferation that results in joint destruction, disability, and increased morbidity that affects up to 1 percent of the global population, predominantly women. Other organ systems such as pulmonary, ocular, and cardiovascular systems may also be affected. Early diagnosis of RA is beneficial to help avoid rapid progression and complications resulting in decreased mobility, deformity, and

Table 24-22. Specific antinuclear autoantibodies seen in systemic autoimmune diseases together with their antigenic determinant and clinical disease associations

Autoantibody	Indirect immuno-fluorescent pattern	Antigenic determinant	Clinical associations
Antinuclear antibodies			
Anti-dsDNA	Peripheral Rim	dsDNA	High specificity for SLE; often correlates with active severe disease
Anti-extractable nuclear antigens (anti-ENA) Anti-Sm Anti-RNP	Speckled	Smith (Sm) Proteins containing U1-RNA	High specificity for SLE MCTD, SLE, RA, scleroderma, Sjögren's syndrome
Anti-SSA (anti-Ro)	Speckled	RNPs	Sjögren's syndrome, SLE (subacute cutaneous lupus), neonatal lupus
Anti-SSB (anti-LA)	Speckled	RNPs	Sjögren's syndrome, SLE, neonatal SLE
Anticentromere	Centromere	Centromere/kinetochore region of chromosome	Limited scleroderma (CREST), pulmonary hypertension, primary biliary cirrhosis
Anti-Scl 70	Speckled	DNA topoisomerase I	Diffuse scleroderma
Anti-Jo-1 (anti-synthetase antibodies)	Speckled	Histadyl tRNA synthetase (other tRNA synthetases)	Inflammatory myopathies with interstitial lung disease, fever, and arthritis
Anti-SRP	Speckled	Antibody to signal recognition protein	Inflammatory myopathies with poor prognosis
Anti-PM/Scl	Speckled	Antibody to nucleolar granular component	Polymyositis/scleroderma overlap syndrome
Anti-Mi-2	Speckled	Antibodies to a nucleolar antigen of unknown function	Dermatomyositis
Anti-histone antibody	ELISA	Histones	SLE and drug-induced SLE
Other autoantibodies seen in systemic autoimmune disorders			
Lupus anticoagulant antibody: Anti-thrombin	Coagulation assays	Thrombin	SLE
Lupus anticoagulant antibody: Anti-PL	ELISA	Phospholipid (PL)	Antiphospholipid syndrome
Anti-cytoplasmic antibodies			
Anti-neutrophil cytoplasmic antibody (ANCA): pANCA	Perinuclear	Myeloperoxidase	Polyarteritis nodosa Churg-Strauss
Anti-neutrophil cytoplasmic antibody (ANCA): cANCA	Cytoplasmic	Proteinase 3	Wegener's granlomatosis Microscopic polyangiitis

MCTD = mixed connective tissue disease.

disability that have been prevented by the successful development and availability of the new anti-TNF agents (*Chapter 11*).

Genetic and environmental risk factors have been identified to be associated with RA and have formed the basis for some of the level C testing. These include the association with RA of specific HLA-DR4 haplotypes, in particular certain alleles such as DRB1*0401, DRB1*0404, DRB1*0405, and DRB1*0408. The presence of "shared epitope" confers an even greater relative risk of disease development and illustrates the concepts of "molecular mimicry" and "epitope spreading" contributing to autoimmune disease pathogenesis described in Chapter 19. The role of an infectious etiology has also been suggested in the development of RA. It has been suggested that infection

Table 24-23. Specific cellular autoantibodies seen in some of the organ-specific autoimmune diseases together with their antigenic determinant and clinical disease associations

Organ-specific antibodies			Example of clinical disease
Anti-liver	Anti-mitochondrial antibody	Mitochondria	Primary biliary cirrhosis
	Anti-smooth muscle antibody	Smooth muscle	Autoimmune hepatitis
Anti-thyroid	Anti-TSH-R	Thyroid stimulating hormone receptor (TSH-R)	Graves' disease
	Anti-TPO Anti-TG	Thyroid peroxidase (TPO) (microsomal) Thyroglobulin (TG)	Hashimoto's thyroiditis
Anti-stomach	APCA	Parietal cell (PC)	Perncious anemia Gastric cancer
	AHPA	*Helicobacter pylori*	Gastric cancer
Anti-neuronal	Anti-NAR	Nicotinic acetylcholine receptor (NAR)	Myasthenia gravis
	Anti-MUSK	Muscle-specific kinase (MUSK)	Myasthenia gravis

may serve as an environmental trigger in the genetically susceptible individual. The precise mechanism(s) and specific infectious agents responsible for this phenomenon, however, have yet to be described.

Rheumatoid Factor

The American College of Rheumatology established criteria for the diagnosis of RA in 1987. Rheumatoid factor (**RF**) is an IgM antibody directed to the Fc portion of human IgG that forms immune complexes with IgG resulting in some of the tissue damage seen in RA. IgM RF has been a major target of most laboratory testing for RF. The sensitivity of RF in the diagnosis of RA is 75 percent, but its specificity is low. RF may also be found in other non-RA conditions, such as chronic infections (bacterial endocarditis, tuberculosis, leprosy, infectious mononucleosis, and hepatitis C), other autoimmune diseases (primary Sjögren's syndrome, SLE, vasculitis, and idiopathic pulmonary fibrosis), and some malignancies (Waldenström's macroglobulinemia, non-Hodgkin's lymphoma, or chronic lymphocytic leukemia).

The presence of RF can be detected using a variety of different assays. The initial assay that was developed for the measurement of RF employed sheep erythrocytes coated with rabbit immunoglobulins that agglutinated in the presence of RF. A latex agglutination assay was later developed, as well as ELISA, and recently nephelometry has been adapted to measure RF. The nephelometric technique is considered superior because of its ability to detect changes in absolute levels at earlier stages of disease as well as greater assay precision.

Anti-Citrullinated Protein Antibodies (ACPA) or Anti-Cyclic Citrullinated Protein Antibodies (anti-CCP)

The lack of specificity of RF has led to the development of newer assays based upon the measurement of antibodies directed against citrullinated peptides found in the sera of patients with RA. Anti-CCP antibodies are directed against citrulline residues formed in posttranslational modifications of arginine. The main epitope for these antibodies is filaggrin (a filament-associated protein that binds to keratin fibers in the stratum corneum to build a dense matrix of cytoskeleton fibrils, which, with other structures, forms a functional barrier at the skin surface), and there is cross-reactivity between ACPA and anti-keratin and anti-perinuclear factor. It has been suggested that the inflamed synovial tissue is the site of anticitrullinated protein production in patients with RA. During inflammation, arginine residues in proteins such as vimentin can be enzymatically converted into citrulline ones (a process called citrullination) and, if their shapes are significantly altered, the proteins may be seen as antigens by the immune system and an immune response generated. Anti-CCPs have proven to be powerful biomarkers of disease activity in RA that not only allow the diagnosis of RA to be made at an earlier stage, but also are believed to be important predictive markers of the worst outcomes of RA, i.e., joint erosion and deformity, and that, therefore, may be useful in identifying those patients requiring more aggressive treatment.

Anti-Neutrophil Cytoplasm Antibodies

Autoimmune diseases of the vascular system or autoimmune vasculitis vary extensively depending upon the initial organ involved. These patients may often be misdiagnosed by the primary care physician or even left undiagnosed due to a wide array and level of symptoms. The presence of anti-neutrophil cytoplasm antibodies (**ANCA**) is most often associated with small vessel vasculitis (**SVV**), such as Wegener's granulomatosis, microscopic polyangiitis, or locally limited such as "renal limited" or "upper airway limited" focal necrotizing vasculitis (Table 24-22). The diagnosis of a primary vasculitic condition again requires an extensive history of the patient's condition and evaluation of a more or less characteristic group of symptoms and features, some of which are more specific for vasculitis, while others are more indicative of a general inflammatory condition (fever, fatigue, arthralgias, loss of appetite, increased erythrocyte sedimentation rate, etc.). The organs most often affected by vasculitis include the kidneys, lungs, and upper airways. Biopsy specimens showing defined histopathological changes are considered the gold standard, but this may not always work since some biopsy specimens, e.g., nasal biopsy specimens, frequently indicate nonspecific inflammation anyway. The most common neutrophil granule components that are the targets of ANCA are proteinase 3 (**PR3**) or myeloperoxidase (**MPO**). These target antibodies tend to be unique to patients with SVV. Detection of ANCA is by IFA of neutrophils fixed to microscope slides and a more specific PR3 and MPO ELISA assay. The IFA provides information regarding the presence and titer of anti-neutrophil antibodies, while the ELISA assay detects PR3- and MPO-specific antibodies indicative of a vasculitic syndrome. So, strongly positive results for neutrophil-specific antibodies by IFA combined with positive results for PR3- or MPO-ANCAs strongly support a diagnosis of necrotizing SVV.

Immunologic Procedures as Assessment Tools Employed in the Diagnosis of Diseases that Have No Immunologic Basis

In addition to the use of immunologic techniques for evaluation of diseases with altered immunologic function, there are innumerable applications of immunologic procedures that are used in virtually all of the clinical disciplines of medicine for diagnosis of diseases that have no immunologic basis. Examples of these include the measurement of hormones by radioimmunoassay, the immunotyping of lymphomas and leukemias (*Chapter 21*), identification of tumor markers in several solid tumors, and a myriad of other applications that are beyond the scope of this textbook.

Summary

The common theme in diagnosis of both primary immunodeficiencies and other immune-mediated diseases such as allergy and autoimmune disease involves a thorough documentation of the patient's signs and symptoms, family history, etc., followed by appropriate laboratory testing. In most cases, congenital immune defects result in frequent and sometimes serious infections that may become apparent in infancy or early childhood. However, some defects may not be detected until adulthood. Defects may occur in the T cell system, the B cell system, the phagocytic system, or the complement system and usually result in an increased number of infections. In some cases, infections occur due to unusual infecting agents. Regardless of the age of onset or the exact nature of the immune defect, the sinopulmonary system, skin, and intestinal tract are most commonly infected; however, any organ or location may become involved. Diagnostic immunology has come a long way since its early origins in infectious diseases and undoubtedly will continue to find application in all branches of medicine in the future.

Case Study: Clinical Relevance

Let us now return to the case study of JIA presented earlier and review some of the major points of the clinical presentation and how they relate to the immune system:

- JIA is one of the most common rheumatic diseases of children and is a major cause of chronic disability.

The diagnosis of JIA is based on the physical finding of arthritis (or synovitis) in at least one joint that persists for at least six weeks, with other causes being excluded and with an onset occurring in individuals < 16 years of age.

Case Study: Clinical Relevance (continued)

- Arthritis usually is defined as either joint swelling, limited motion with pain, or a combination of both. The usual presentation of JIA often includes an insidious or abrupt onset, with morning stiffness and arthralgia during the day; easy fatigability in the early afternoon, which can lead to absenteeism from school; limping; and joint swelling. Unlike the arthritis of SLE and RA, the arthritis is nonmigratory, affects selected joints, and in severe cases can lead to joint deformity.
- The involved joint often is warm, lacks full range of motion, and occasionally is painful on motion but usually not erythematous. Our patient presented a limitation in his writing skills because of the stiffness and pain in his hand joints. Another of his major complaints was arthralgia in both knees, which sometimes resulted in limping.
- Shown in Table 24-24 are three categories of JIA: (1) oligoarthritis or pauciarticular disease, (2) polyarthritis or polyarticular disease, and (3) systemic disease.
- Oligoarthritis predominantly affects the joints of the lower extremities, such as the knees and ankles. Involvement of upper extremity large joints, although seen, is not characteristic of this type of onset. Involvement of the hip is almost never a presenting sign of a deteriorating functional course.
- The polyarticular disease generally affects at least five joints; both large and small can be involved, often in symmetric bilateral distribution. Usually it resembles the usual presentation of adult RA.
- The systemic-onset disease is manifested by arthritis and prominent visceral involvement including hepatosplenomegaly and lymphadenopathy. Another characteristic is spiking fevers (as demonstrated by both the patient and his sister) typically occurring several times each day, with temperature returning to the reference range or below the reference range. Each febrile episode is often accompanied by characteristic faint, erythematous, and macular rash; these evanescent salmon-colored lesions may be linear or circular and are distributed most commonly over the trunk and proximal extremities.
- After a thorough evaluation of the patient, the diagnosis of JIA, the systemic-onset type, was established.
- Because of the patient's susceptibility to recurrent infections, an additional diagnosis of immune deficiency was considered.

Table 24-24. Categories of JIA

Onset type and course subtype	Subsequent clinical manifestations	Outcome
Polyarthritis		
RF, seropositive	Female Older age Hand/wrist Erosions Nodules Unremitting	Poor
ANA, seropositive	Female Young age	Good
Seronegative	—	Variable
Oligoarthritis		
ANA, seropositive	Female Young age Chronic anterior uveitis (iridocyclitis)	Excellent (except uveitis)
RF, seropositive	Polyarthritis Erosions Unremitting	Poor
HLA-B27, positive	Male Older age	Good
Seronegative	—	Good
Systemic disease		
Oligoarthritis	—	Good
Polyarthritis	Erosions	Poor

RF = rheumatoid factor; ANA = antinuclear antibodies; HLA = human leukocyte antigen.

Case Study: Clinical Relevance (continued)

- The results of postvaccine responses to protein (i.e., tetanus and diphtheria) were normal; the booster vaccine response to pneumococcal vaccine, however, showed a complete lack of response to all serotypes tested and therefore, a specific antibody deficiency (SAD) was diagnosed (*Chapter 16*).
- Based on these findings, treatment with intravenous gamma globulin (IVIG) 400mgm/kg every four weeks was initiated. Prior to each infusion, the child was pretreated with oral diphenhydramine to avoid any side effects of the infusion and to promote a good tolerance to the treatment.
- Since initiation of IVIG therapy, the patient has shown significant clinical improvement (Figure 24-9). The frequency of his recurrent upper and lower respiratory infections, as well as the rash on the trunk and the joint pain, have diminished. However, on some occasions, the use of antibiotics and nonsteroidal anti-inflammatory drugs has been required. His daily activities also have been resumed, although he still requires homebound education. Occasionally, he still manifests low-grade fever with baseline temperatures of 98–99°F and occasional febrile peaks of approximately 100°F, associated with abdominal pain, redness of the eyes, and facial rash (Figure 24-9).
- A diagnosis of juvenile rheumatoid arthritis of the systemic onset type was established, and, based upon his humoral immune deficiency, treatment with intravenous immunoglobulin was initiated with remarkable improvement in his symptomatology.

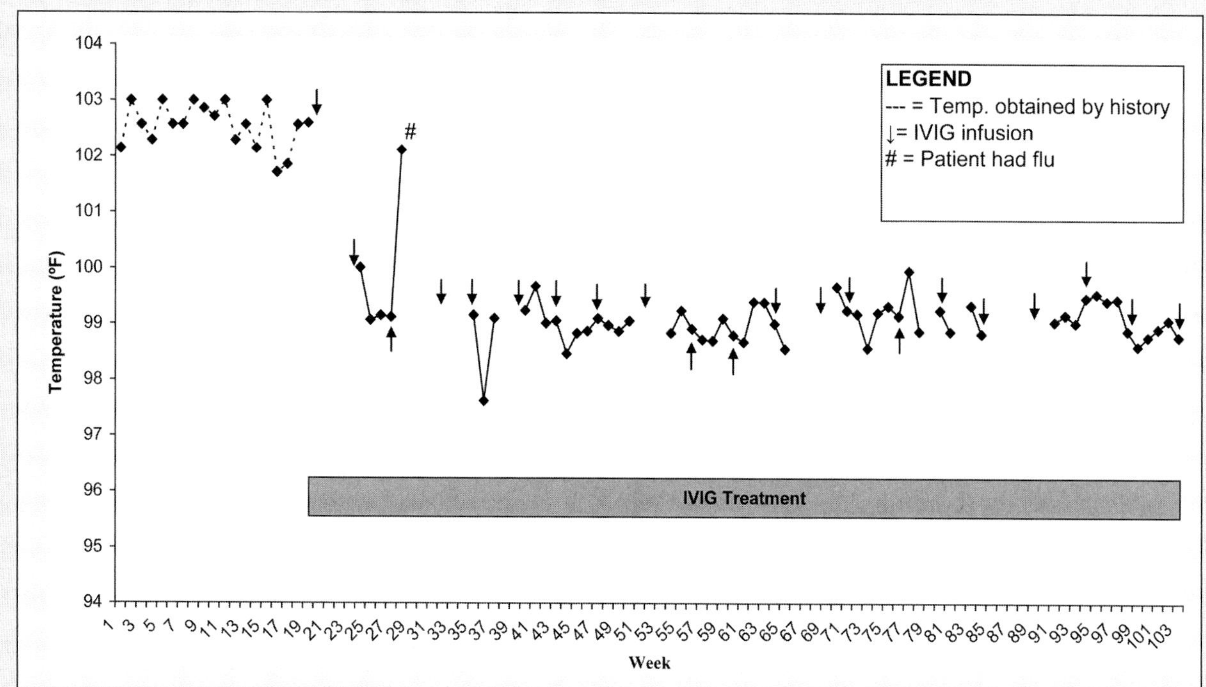

Figure 24-9. Average weekly temperatures of our patient's pre- and post-IVIG treatment. (Reproduced with permission from Bueso MB, Caballero R, Castro HJ, et al. Recurrent infections and joint pain. Allergy Asthma Proc. 2006;27:164–71.)

Key Points

- The diagnostic applications of immunology can be divided into two major categories: (1) the use of immunologic techniques for the diagnosis of diseases in which altered immunologic function occurs; and (2) the use of immunologic procedures as assessment tools employed in the diagnosis of diseases that have no immunologic basis.
- The clinically relevant immunologic techniques for evaluation of diseases with altered immunologic function can be divided into the two major divisions of the immune system: (1) tests of innate immune function (that measure phagocytic cell, mediator cell, NK functions, and complement); and (2) tests of adaptive immune function (that measure the many activities of T and B cells).

- Abnormalities of each cell or cellular product of the innate and adaptive immune systems include both quantitative deficiencies in which the numbers of cells or levels of cell product are diminished as well as a variety of qualitative or functional deficiencies where the numbers may be normal but where they manifest intrinsic functional defects.
- It is important to identify the appropriate diagnostic immunologic test procedures required for specific clinical conditions for their use in immune deficiency disorders, allergic diseases, and autoimmune disorders.
- The appropriate utilization of this knowledge will lead to a better understanding of immunologic mechanisms involved in disease pathogenesis as well as the maintenance of health.

Study Questions/Critical Thinking

1. Each of the following have been associated with chronic granulomatous disease EXCEPT:
   a. Underlying defect is a deficiency of the NADPH oxidase system
   b. Can be diagnosed by flow cytometric analysis of PMN function by dihydrorhodamine staining
   c. Defective delayed hypersensitivity skin responses
   d. Increased susceptibility to opportunistic bacterial microbes of low virulence that are characteristically catalase positive
   e. Several systems such as the lung, gastrointestinal, and genitourinary tracts are frequently affected by granulomata

Answer = c

2. Each of the following have been associated with X-linked agammaglobulinemia EXCEPT:
   a. Usually not clinically apparent until after transplacental maternal antibody has waned after six months of age
   b. Infections are typically caused by Gram-positive, highly pathogenic encapsulated organisms such as *Streptococcus pneumonia* and *Haemophilus influenza* type b
   c. Flow cytometry of peripheral blood lymphocytes shows the absence of B cells
   d. The disease is now known to be due to defects in a tyrosine kinase, Bruton tyrosine kinase (BTK)
   e. There is a high incidence of allergic disease in affected patients

Answer = e

3. Each of the following have been associated with X-linked SCID EXCEPT:
   a. A T−B+NK- pattern is seen
   b. Deficiencies of IL-2R γc, JAK3
   c. Human stem cell transplantation from an HLA-identical donor (usually a sibling) has been the treatment of choice for all patients
   d. A chromosome 22q11.2 deletion
   e. Graft-versus-host reactions are a potential problem

Answer = d

4. Each of the following should be considered in a four-year-old patient presenting with eczema and wheezing EXCEPT:
   a. An elevated IgE
   b. Eosinophilia
   c. Positive immediate skin tests
   d. Positive delayed skin tests
   e. Positive allergen-specific serum IgE responses

Answer = d

5. A 24-year-old African American lady gives a history of migratory arthralgias, skin sensitivity to sun, and alopecia. Each of the following is helpful in diagnosis EXCEPT:
   a. Positive ANA titer
   b. Positive anti-dsDNA antibody
   c. Positive anti-Sm antibody
   d. Positive ANCA
   e. Urinary albuminuria and RBC casts

Answer = d

Suggested Reading

Arnett FC, et al. The American Rheumatism Association 1987 revised criteria for the classification of rheumatoid arthritis. Arthritis Rheum. 1987; 31: 315–24.

Barbee RA, Halonen M, Lebowitz M, et al. Distribution of IgE in a community population sample: correlations with age, sex, and allergen skin test reactivity. J Allergy Clin Immunol. 1981; 68: 106–11.

Bender JM, Rand TH, Ampofo K, et al. Family clusters of variant X-linked chronic granulomatous disease. Pediatr Infect Dis J. 2009; 28: 529–33.

Bonilla FA, and Geha RS. Primary immunodeficiency diseases. J Allergy Clin Immunol. 2003; 111: S571–581.

Breda L, Nozzi M, De Sanctis S, et al. Laboratory tests in the diagnosis and follow-up of pediatric rheumatic diseases: an update. Semin Arthritis Rheum. 2010; 40: 53–72.

Bueso MB, Caballero R, Castro HJ, et al. Recurrent infections and joint pain. Allergy Asthma Proc. 2006; 27: 164–71.

Castro C, Gourley M. Diagnostic testing and interpretation of tests form autoimmunity. J Allergy Clin Immunol. 2010; 125: S238–47.

Chapel HM, Webster ADB. Assessment of the immune system. In H. D. Ochs, C. I. E. Smith, and J. M. Puck (eds.), Primary immunodeficiency Diseases: a Molecular and Genetic Approach. New York: Oxford University Press; 1999.

Conley ME, ER Stiehm. Immunodeficiency disorders: general considerations. In E. R. Stiehm (ed.), Immunologic Disorders of Infants and Children. Philadelphia: W. B. Saunders; 1996.

Dolen WK, et al. Immunoassay of specific IgE: low levels require measurement of allergen specific background. Ann Allergy. 1992; 69: 151–6.

Fleisher T, de Oliveira JB. Flow cytometry. In Clinical immunology: principles and practice. 3rd ed. Philadelphia, PA: Elsevier Limited; 2008.

Folds JD, Schmitz JL. Clinical and laboratory assessment of immunity. J Allergy Clin Immunol. 2003; 111: S702–11.

Hamilton RG, Williams PB. Specific IgE Testing Task Force of the American Academy of Allergy, Asthma & Immunology. Human IgE antibody serology: a primer for the practicing North American allergist/immunologist. J Allergy Clin Immunol. 2010; 126: 33–8.

Hamilton RG. Clinical laboratory assessment of immediate-type hypersensitivity. J Allergy Clin Immunol. 2010; 125: S284–96.

International Union of Immunological Societies. Primary immunodeficiency diseases: report of an IUIS Scientific Committee. Clin Exp Immunol. 1999; 118: 1–28.

Mackay IR, Rose NR. The autoimmune diseases, 4th ed. St. . Louis, MO: Elsevier Academic Press; 2006.

Nelson HS, Oppenheimer J, Buchmeier A, et al. An assessment of the role of intradermal skin testing in the diagnosis of clinically relevant allergy to timothy grass. J Allergy Clin Immunol. 1996; 97: 1193–201.

Oliveira JB, Fleisher TA. Laboratory evaluation of primary immunodeficiencies. J Allergy Clin Immunol. 2010; 125: S297–305.

Orton SM, Peace-Brewer A, Schmitz JL, et al. Practical evaluation of methods for detection and specificity of autoantibodies to extractable nuclear antigens. Clin Diagn Lab Immunol. 2004; 11: 297–301.

Rosen FS, Cooper MD, Wedgewood RJP. The primary immunodeficiencies. N Engl J Med. 1995; 333: 431–40.

Steele RW, Metz JR, Bass JW, et al. Pneumothorax and pneumomediastinum in the newborn. 1971; 98: 629–32.

Tan EM, Cohen AS, Fries JF, et al. The 1982 revised criteria for the classification of systemic lupus erythematosus. Arthritis Rheum. 1982; 25: 1271–7.

Vowells SJ, Fleisher TA, Sekhsaria S, et al. Genotype-dependent variability in flow cytometric evaluation of reduced nicotinamide adenine dinucleotide phosphate oxidase function in patients with chronic granulomatous disease. J Pediatr. 1996; 128: 104–7.

Wood RA, Phipatanakul W, Hamilton RG, et al. A comparison of skin prick tests, intradermal skin tests, and RASTs in the diagnosis of cat allergy. J Allergy Clin Immunol. 1999; 103: 773–9.

Chapter 25

Basic Molecular Biology for Immunology

Alejandro Escobar-Gutiérrez, PhD
Joseph A. Bellanti, MD
Catalin Marian, MD, PhD

LEARNING OBJECTIVES

When you have completed this chapter, you should be able to:

- Differentiate the characteristics between DNA and RNA
- Explain the differences between nucleosides and nucleotides
- Define the terms genome, transcriptome, and proteome
- Understand the concept of the genetic code and DNA and RNA base pairing
- Describe the mechanisms of signal transduction, transcription, and translation
- Define the following examples of DNA technology: restriction enzyme analysis, hybridization techniques, polymerase chain reaction (PCR), and genetic transformation of mice
- Summarize the general principles of DNA technology and give examples of each
- Recognize the rapid uses of DNA technology and their clinical applications in health and disease

Not a day passes without a new article appearing in the clinical literature that does not contain a perplexing and often confusing description of a basic molecular technique. The use of the Western blot in Lyme disease, a microarray for diagnosis of lymphoma, a knock-out mouse used to evaluate a new primary immunodeficiency disorder, or a hybridization technique to identify a new autoimmune disease all serve as examples of the importance of a general understanding of molecular biology to the management of patients entrusted to the care of the busy health care provider. The technology that propelled the success of the Human Genome Project and that launched the successful comprehensive sequencing of the human genome is revolutionizing and finding great application in medicine and will continue to do so in the years ahead. The applications of DNA technology hold particular relevance to the field of clinical immunology since many of the immunologically mediated diseases that were described previously as phenomenological entities are now being better understood by discoveries elucidated in molecular terms.

In recent years, a new field of systems biology has emerged in which the study of the human genome is being increasingly applied to diagnostic testing in routine laboratories. This practice is not only replacing the more obsolete and less accurate diagnostic procedures used previously, but is also providing a molecular basis for a clearer understanding of the pathogenesis of diseases that were once diagnostic and therapeutic orphans. Although the general health care provider will not usually be directly involved in the performance of these molecular procedures, an understanding of the principles and mechanisms upon which they are based will be helpful in providing the clinician with powerful diagnostic and therapeutic tools for improved management of patients with immunologically mediated diseases far beyond our present dreams and expectations.

Introduction

In recent years, the explosive increase in the number of basic science advances made possible by discoveries in molecular biology and propelled by the sequencing of the human genome are transforming every aspect of clinical medicine. These advances have particular relevance to the clinical applications of immunology in health and disease since the whole of the immune response is genetically controlled (*Chapter 2*). The pace with which these advances are being made, however, is so rapid and their content so complex that it is often difficult for the clinically oriented health care provider interested in the clinical applications of immunology to keep current. The purpose of this chapter is to briefly elucidate some of the key aspects of basic molecular biology and to illustrate their use in diagnosis and therapy of immunologically mediated disease states as well as in the maintenance of health. An understanding of the structure of the DNA molecule and the techniques used to measure its functions are, therefore, necessary for a clear comprehension of the applications of these advances to the clinical aspects of immunology in health promotion and disease control.

Nucleic Acids (DNA, RNA): Nucleobases, Sugars, and Phosphate Groups; Nucleosides versus Nucleotides

The term nucleic acids is generally used for the designation of deoxyribonucleic acid (DNA) and ribonucleic acid (RNA), the biological macromolecules essential for life. These molecules are made up of three components: (1) a purine or pyrimidine nucleobase; (2) a pentose sugar; and (3) a phosphate group. The nucleobases found in DNA consist of cytosine (C), guanine (G), adenine (A), and thymine (T); the nucleobases found in RNA are cytosine (C), guanine (G), adenine (A), and, substituting for thymine, uracil (U) (Figure 25-1).

A useful mnemonic for distinguishing which of the nucleobases are purines from those that are pyrimidines is shown in Box 25-1.

The pentose sugar found in DNA is a 2′-deoxyribose molecule (i.e., a ribose without an oxygen) and in RNA is a ribose moiety. The presence or absence of a phosphate group in the nucleic acid structure distinguishes nucleosides from nucleotides. A nucleoside consists of a nucleobase plus a sugar, and a nucleotide is composed of a nucleobase, a sugar, and a phosphate group (Figure 25-2).

The Genome, the Transcriptome, and the Proteome

It is now well established that in all life forms, the information for cellular function is stored and encoded within the DNA molecule. The total content of genetic material in a cell is called the **genome**, and all the encoded proteins are known as the **proteome**. In recent years, an entire field of biology has emerged, referred to as systems biology, in which the study of the genome, i.e., genomics, together with the study of the proteome, i.e., proteomics, is being increasingly applied to unraveling complex pathways underlying all biological processes. Genomics and proteomics are closely related emerging basic science fields that not only focus on the identification and characterization of the

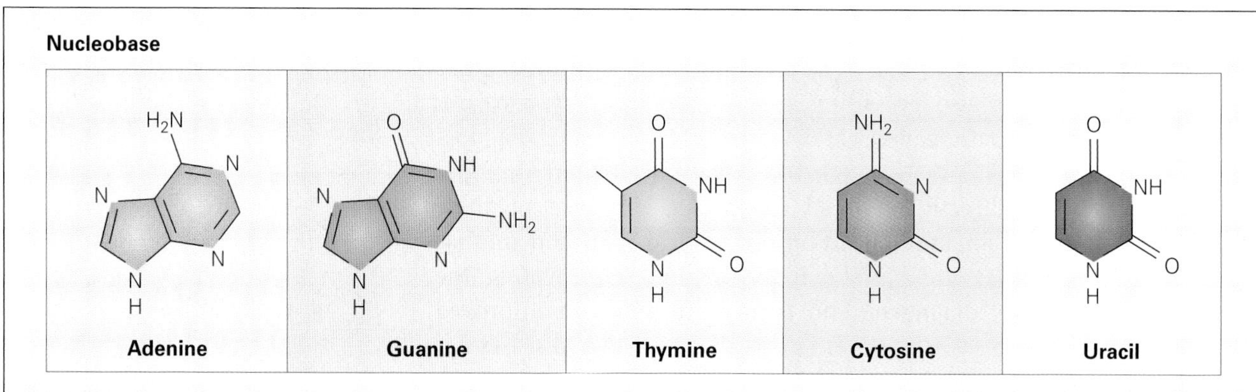

Figure 25-1. Chemical structures of the nucleobases.

Box 25-1

A Mnemonic for Purines and Pyrimidines

Of the various nucleobases found in DNA (A, G, C, and T) and in RNA (A, G, C, and U), the first two in each molecule are purines (the double-ringed class of molecules) and the last two are pyrimidines (the single-ringed class of molecules) and can be remembered by the mnemonic "pure as gold", i.e., purines, adenine, and guanine, and by default the remaining two nucleobases in either DNA, i.e., C and T, or RNA, i.e., C and U, are pyrimidines.

genome and proteome of a given cell or entire organism, but also demonstrate clinical application in many of the disorders of immune function. Associated with these concepts, another very useful area of study in molecular biology is the study of the **transcriptome**, a collective term that includes all species of RNA molecules such as messenger RNA (mRNA), ribosomal RNA (rRNA), and the transfer RNAs (tRNAs) as well as other noncoding RNA molecules transcribed from the genome.

The Structure of the DNA Molecule

DNA is a double-stranded structure consisting of two intertwining long chains composed of repetitive nucleotides with backbones made of sugars and phosphate groups joined by ester bonds. As described previously, each nucleotide is a three-membered molecule formed by deoxyribose with the phosphate group attached to one end and a nitrogen-containing molecule (nucleobase) linked to the other end (Figure 25-3).

Nucleotides are polymerized one to another through a covalent bond (phosphodiester bond) between the phosphate group in the deoxyribose of one nucleotide and the only free hydroxyl group on the pentose (in the position 3′) of the next nucleotide (Figure 25-3). The two strands of a DNA molecule run in an antiparallel manner to each other and are held together in a characteristic double helix, which resembles a ladder that has been twisted into a spiral (Figure 25-4). The sides of the "ladder" are formed by a backbone of deoxyribose-phosphate molecules, and the "rungs" consist of the nucleotide bases of each strand, which are joined together by hydrogen bonds. Nucleotide pairing in DNA molecules occurs in complementary fashion where G binds only to C and A pairs only with T (Figure 25-4). The term single nucleotide polymorphism (**SNP**) refers to the situation when the pairing of a single nucleobase—A, T, C, or G—with its complementary partner differs between members of a biological species or between one DNA chain with another.

The strands of individual DNA molecules can be pulled apart enzymatically or by heating without breakage of the strand itself; likewise, the double helix can be rejoined again without any change due to the strict complementarity of both strands. During DNA replication or amplification, each strand can be used as a template for de novo synthesis of two identical new double helixes, a very important characteristic that guarantees the accurate transmission of the encoded information in the DNA molecule from one cell or organism to their descendants.

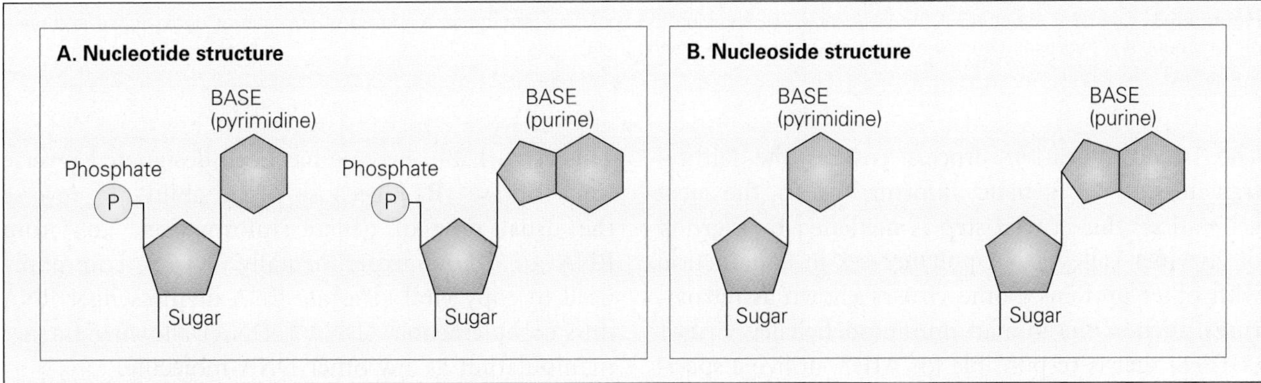

Figure 25-2. Schematic comparison of the tri-component nucleotide (nucleobase, sugar, and phosphate) of a nucleotide with the bi-component (nucleobase and sugar) structure of a nucleotide.

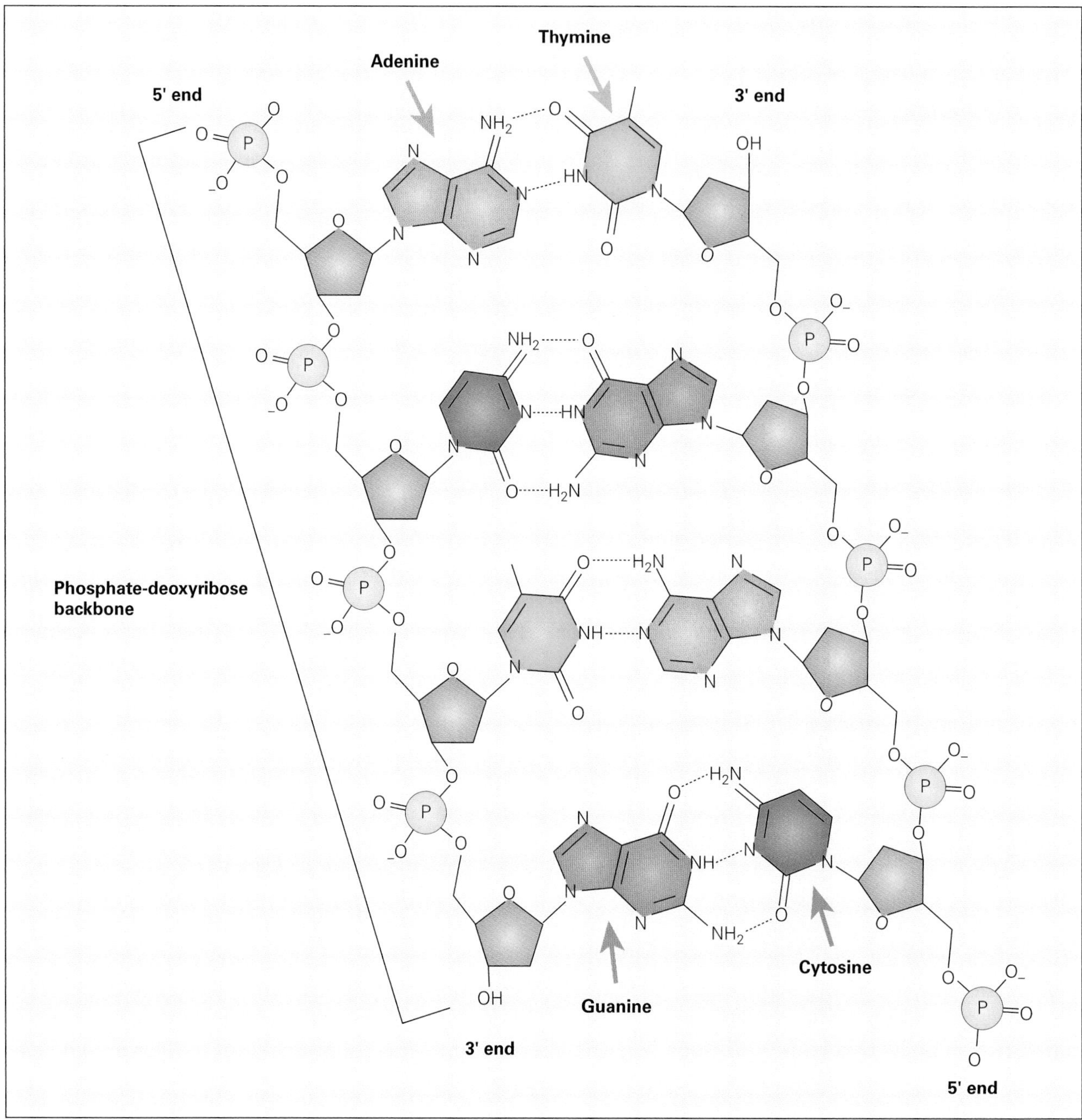

Figure 25-3. Chemical structure of the DNA molecule showing the backbone structures made up of linkages of deoxyribose and phosphate groups and hydrogen bonding of the nucleobases A → T and G → C.

The DNA replication process ensures the faithful transmission of genetic information to the next generation; this crucial step is mediated by a group of enzymes called DNA-polymerases in conjunction with other proteins. Some viruses known as retroviruses, such as the human immunodeficiency virus-1 (HIV-1) that is responsible for AIDS, utilize a specialized RNA-dependent DNA-polymerase that uses RNA as a template instead of DNA (*Chapter 13*). This remarkable enzyme has been designated reverse transcriptase (**RT**) because of its ability to reverse the usual flow of genetic information, i.e., from RNA to DNA. Experimentally, RT is commonly used to copy viral genomic RNA or messenger RNA into complementary DNA (cDNA) allowing further manipulation as any other DNA molecule.

RNA displays a structure similar to DNA with the exception of a backbone chain that contains

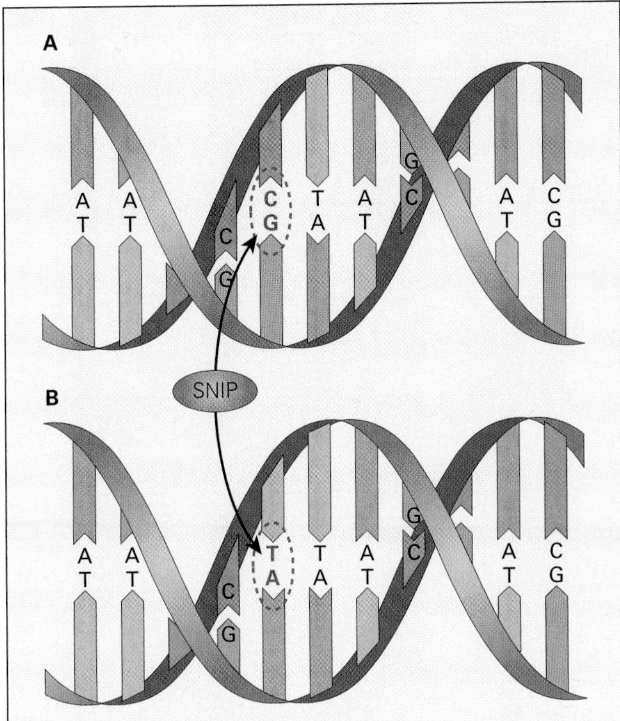

Figure 25-4. Schematic representation of the two intertwining double helix chain structures of the DNA molecule showing the characteristic nucleobase pairing of A → T and G → C. The DNA sequence variation occurring when a single nucleobase—A, T, C, or G—in the nucleotide genomic structure differs between members of a biological species or between the pairing of one DNA chain with another is referred to as a single nucleotide polymorphism (SNP).

ribose as the five-carbon sugar linked to the corresponding phosphate group. As described previously, in the RNA molecule, thymine is replaced by uracil (U), another pyrimidine, resulting in A-U base pairing. In contrast to the double-stranded structure of DNA, RNA molecules are usually single stranded and can fold up internally into distinctive shapes. In contrast to its use in viruses, where RNA can store genetic information similar to DNA, the RNA molecule is used by prokaryotic and eukaryotic cells in many other ways, such as protein synthesis. There are at least three forms of RNA with specific activities: (1) **messenger RNA (mRNA)**, a complimentary copy of one of the DNA strand molecules formed during transcription and, after translocation to the ribosomes within the endoplasmic reticulum, serves as the "blueprint" for the synthesis of protein by a process referred to as translation; (2) **ribosomal RNA (rRNA)**, the essential component of the ribosome responsible for protein synthesis; and (3) **transfer RNA (tRNA)**, a small RNA molecule whose main role is to transfer specific amino acids to a growing polypeptide chain. Transfer RNA comprises a family of 61 molecules, each one with a three-base structure, i.e., an anticomplementary codon (anticodon), which specifically carries out base pairing with the corresponding codon structure found on the mRNA. Each tRNA transports individual amino acids to the ribosome and arranges them in the correct order according to the messages encoded by the mRNA.

The Genetic Code

The **genetic code** is the set of rules by which information encoded in genetic material (DNA or mRNA sequences) is translated into the amino acid sequences of proteins by living cells. The code is provided by a set of three nucleotide sequences called a codon that specifies a single amino acid in the nascent polypeptide chain. The primary amino acid structure of a given protein, therefore, is encoded by a specific sequence of contiguous triplets that are collectively called **genes**. Since there are four different nucleotide bases in each DNA or RNA molecule, there are only 64 possible triplet/codon combinations. However, because there are only 20 amino acids, a single amino acid can be encoded by more than one triplet, resulting in the characteristic redundancy of the genetic code (Table 25-1). It is important to highlight that there are three codons that have no significant productive genetic function and cannot be used to encode amino acids. These include UAA, UAG, and UGA, which are referred to as nonsense triplets or stop codons since, when they appear, their function is to terminate the synthesis of the nascent polypeptide chain.

Protein Biosynthesis

Within the nucleus, the DNA serves as an "instruction manual" providing all of the information needed for the cell to work properly. As described previously, the translation of all genomic information into a "language" that can be used directly by the cell is performed by the three different RNA species. In eukaryotic (nucleated) cells, the encoding gene sequences are referred to as **exons** but are not contiguous and are regularly "interrupted"

Table 25-1. The genetic code

First position	Second position: U	C	A	G	Third position
U	UUU Phenylalanine (Phe, F)	UCU Serine (Ser, S)	UAU Tyrosine (Tyr, Y)	UGU Cysteine (Cys, C)	U
	UUC Phenylalanine (Phe, F)	UCC Serine (Ser, S)	UAC Tyrosine (Tyr, Y)	UGC Cysteine (Cys, C)	C
	UUA Leucine (Leu, L)	UCA Serine (Ser, S)	UAA STOP	UGA STOP	A
	UUG Leucine (Leu, L)	UCG Serine (Ser, S)	UAG STOP	UGG Tryptophan (Try, W)	G
C	CUU Leucine (Leu, L)	CCU Proline (Pro, P)	CAU Histidine (His, H)	CGU Arginine (Arg, R)	U
	CUC Leucine (Leu, L)	CCC Proline (Pro, P)	CAC Histidine (His, H)	CGC Arginine (Arg, R)	C
	CUA Leucine (Leu, L)	CCA Proline (Pro, P)	CAA Glutamine (Gln, Q)	CGA Arginine (Arg, R)	A
	CUG Leucine (Leu, L)	CCG Proline (Pro, P)	CAG Glutamine (Gln, Q)	CGG Arginine (Arg, R)	G
A	AUU Isoleucine (Ile, I)	ACU Threonine (Thr, T)	AAU Asparagine (Asn, N)	AGU Serine (Ser, S)	U
	AUC Isoleucine (Ile, I)	ACC Threonine (Thr, T)	AAC Asparagine (Asn, N)	AGC Serine (Ser, S)	C
	AUA Isoleucine (Ile, I)	ACA Threonine (Thr, T)	AAA Lysine (Lys, K)	AGA Arginine (Arg, R)	A
	AUG Methionine (Met, M)	ACG Threonine (Thr, T)	AAG Lysine (Lys, K)	AGG Arginine (Arg, R)	G
G	GUU Valine (Val, V)	GCU Alanine (Ala, A)	GAU Aspartic acid (Asp, D)	GGU Glycine (Gly, G)	U
	GUC Valine (Val, V)	GCC Alanine (Ala, A)	GAC Aspartic acid (Asp, D)	GGC Glycine (Gly, G)	C
	GUA Valine (Val, V)	GCA Alanine (Ala, A)	GAA Glutamic acid (Glu, E)	GGA Glycine (Gly, G)	A
	GUG Valine (Val, V)	GCG Alanine (Ala, A)	GAG Glutamic acid (Glu, E)	GGG Glycine (Gly, G)	G

by noncoding intervening sequences called **introns**, which represent DNA regions within a gene that are not translated into protein. These noncoding regions are transcribed to precursor mRNA (pre-mRNA) and some other RNAs (such as long noncoding RNAs) and are subsequently removed by a process called splicing as they progress to mature mRNA. After intron splicing (i.e., removal), the mRNA consists only of exon-derived sequences, which are translated into a protein. Thus, protein biosynthesis requires the elimination of such introns, as will be described below.

The sequence of molecular events involved in protein synthesis is summarized schematically in Figure 25-5 (*Chapter 9*). For ease of discussion, these include: (1) **signal transduction**, (2) **transcription**, and (3) **translation**, i.e., the "**three Ts.**"

The first step in the process of protein synthesis is referred to as **signal transduction** (from the Latin for leading across or initiating a signal). This step includes the cascade of events that takes place following cell membrane activation after a ligand interacts with its specific receptor followed by dimerization of its constituent parts (Figure 25-4). Dimerization can take two forms: (1) if the dimer is composed of two identical molecules, it is referred to as homodimerization; (2) when dimerization occurs between two different molecules, the

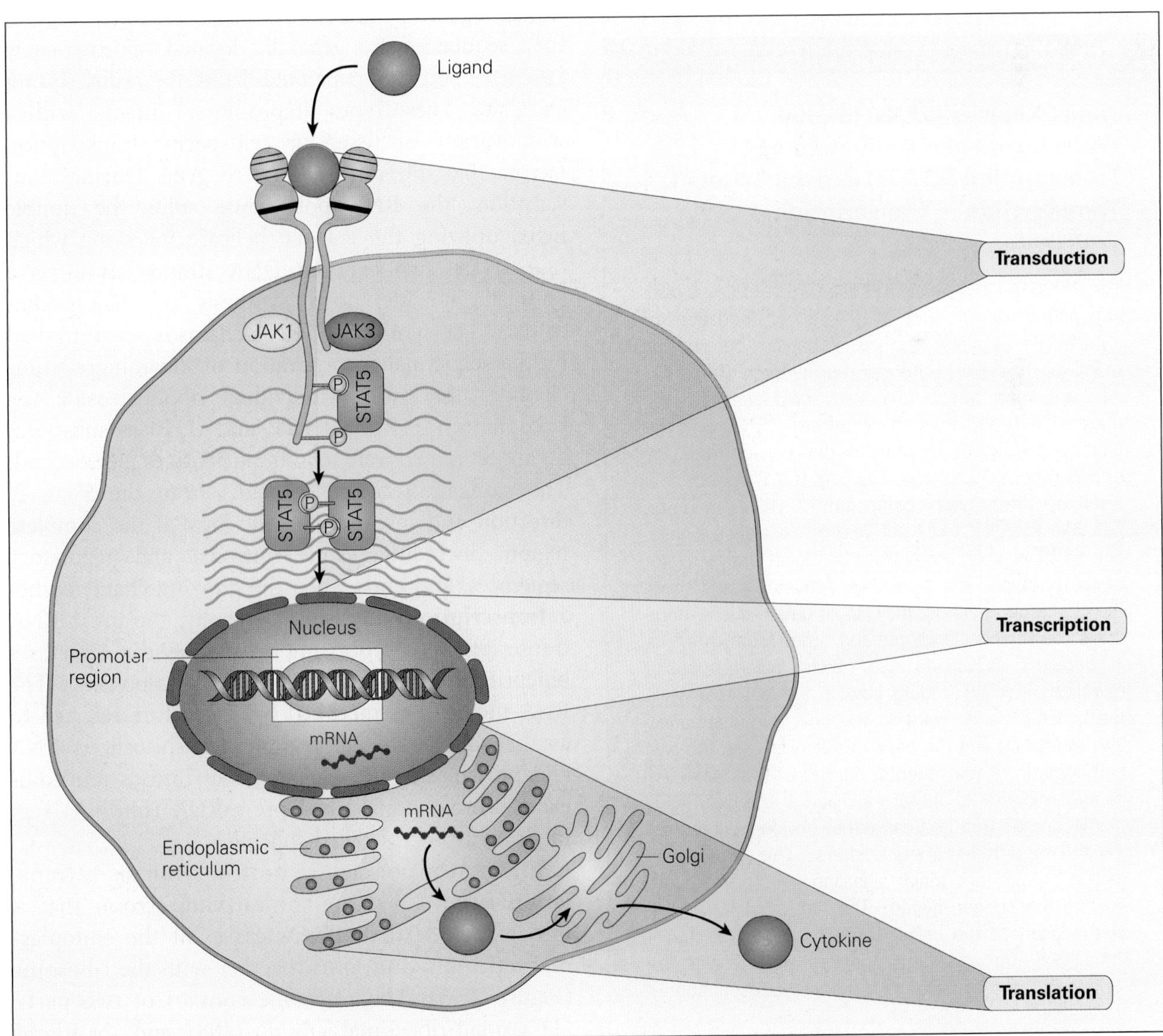

Figure 25-5. Schematic representation of the three steps involved in protein synthesis. Transduction → transcription → translation, i.e., the "three Ts."

process is called heterodimerization. Following dimerization, a series of kinase (i.e., a phosphorylase) reactions occur that phosphorylate cytoplasmic substrates that are then activated and can phosphorylate other substrates, leading eventually to a final product called a transcription factor that initiates the second "T" of the process referred to as **transcription** (Figure 25-5). As described in Chapter 9, this is exemplified by the ubiquitous occurrence of tyrosine kinase reactions in the JAK-STAT pathway leading to final activation factors (Box 25-2).

During the next step, **transcription**, the encoding sequences of the DNA are enzymatically transcribed into a pre-mRNA transcript following the dictum of complementary base pairing as described above. The resulting mRNA is a mirror image of the DNA.

Box 25-2

Janus Kinases (JAKs) (Signal Transducers and Activators of Transcription (STATs) and the "Triple T," Transduction → Transcription → Translation

The JAK-STAT pathways comprise a set of key signaling pathways involved in the accommodation of extracellular signals that are received by specific receptors located on the cell membranes. These signals are then transmitted, i.e., transduced, to the nuclear DNA and then to cytoplasmic RNA with the ultimate production of proteins that can perform any of a number of functions. The JAK-STAT system consists of three main components: (1) a receptor, (2) JAK, and (3) STAT. JAK is short for Janus kinase, and STAT is short for signal transducer and activator of transcription. The term JAK derives, in part, from the Roman god Janus, the god of gates, doors, doorways, beginnings, endings, and time. Most often he is depicted as having two heads facing opposite directions; one head looks back at the last year while the other looks forward to the new, simultaneously into the future and the past. In a similar way, the two components of the receptor portion of the JAK-STAT pathway (Figure 25-5) make allusion to the two heads of the Roman god and can either be identical (homodimers) or different (heterodimers). This set of cascading events is a major signaling alternative to the second messenger system. The JAK-STAT system is at the heart of the cellular and molecular biology of virtually all immunologic responses and involves the "triple Ts," a triad of transduction → transcription → translation.

The transcription is catalyzed by enzymes called RNA polymerases and starts at specific sites on the DNA called **promoter regions**. RNA polymerase and several transcription factors bind to the promoter regions and influence the rate that transcription can occur from that gene. There are two different types of promoters: proximal (basal or core) and distal (upstream). The **proximal promoters** are found in all protein-coding genes, separated approximately 30 to 50 base pairs (bps) from the coding region, contain a sequence of seven bases (TATAAAA) called the **TATA box**, and are the "target" of a large complex of some 50 different proteins. In addition to the proximal promoters, there are distal sequences referred to as **distal promoters** located upstream from a given gene that have additional regulatory functions. These "remote" regulatory sequences are generally located approximately 200 to 1,000 bps separated from the transcription start site. These types of promoters interact with a wide variety of tissue or cell-specific transcription factors that differ from gene to gene. During transcription, the RNA polymerase splits the double helix, utilizing the enzyme helicase following which one of the two exposed DNA strands serves as a template for de novo synthesis of the nascent mRNA. The synthesis of RNA chains is accomplished by the sequential incorporation of incoming ribonucleotides that utilize individual ribonucleoside triphosphates (GTP, CTP, ATP, and UTP) as substrates at an estimated rate of 20 nucleotides per second. The elongation of mRNA runs from the 5′ to 3′ direction and involves the full copy of the complete region, including exons, introns, and regulatory sequences, and ends when the growing chain reaches a **transcription stop site**. Generally, the pre-mRNA transcripts need processing before they can serve as a blueprint for a given protein at the ribosome. The RNA molecule is modified by a structure referred to as the spliceosome, a complex of specialized RNA and protein subunits that removes introns and joins exons from a transcribed pre-mRNA (hnRNA) segment by a process called splicing.

The next major step in protein synthesis is **translation** (from the Latin for carrying across) that is initiated when the mRNA arrives at the endoplasmic reticulum and joins together with the ribosome (Figure 25-5). The ribosome consists of two parts: (1) a small ribosomal subunit (40S), and (2) a large ribosomal subunit (60S). The first step involves the union of the mRNA with the small ribosomal subunit near the open reading frame (**ORF**) and begins at the initiation or start codon, usually AUG, the triplet coding for methionine. The large ribosomal subunit (60S) then binds to the complex to complete the assembly of the ribosome. The mRNA then emerges from the ribosome in between its two subunits with the codons exposed, allowing protein synthesis to begin. Next, the aminoacyl-tRNA is called to participate by the nucleotide sequence of the next codon on the mRNA blueprint. Adjacent amino acids establish a permanent junction through the enzymatic formation of a peptide bond between them, i.e., the reaction of a carboxyl (−COOH) group with an amino ($-NH_2$) group to form the peptide bond ($-\overset{O}{\overset{\|}{C}}-\underset{|}{N}-H$). Each individual tRNA carries a specific amino acid to the ribosomes, enabling their assembly into the nascent protein until a termination codon is reached, thus ending the synthesis process. The synthesized protein can exist in three forms: (1) secreted as an extracellular product, (2) retained in a soluble form inside the cytoplasm, or (3) expressed on the surface of intracellular organelles or on cellular membranes as receptors (Table 25-2). A schematic representation of the total transfer of information from DNA → RNA → to synthesis of a protein is shown in Figures 25-6 and 25-7.

DNA Technology: Techniques for DNA Analysis

The knowledge of the structural and biochemical characteristics of DNA has allowed a greater understanding of gene expression and regulation and has provided the basis for the development of highly reliable techniques for DNA analysis and clinical applications known collectively as **DNA technology.** The technology has been propelled immensely by the success of the Human Genome Project, which was completed in 2003 by achieving the epochal feat of comprehensive sequencing of the human genome. Probes and other materials are now available for use in techniques for DNA analysis often derived from fragments of DNA that were isolated, purified, and amplified for use in the Human Genome Project.

This scientific field has not only revolutionized the basic studies of immunology, but has also allowed the large-scale production of immunological products, e.g., cytokines and modified monoclonal antibodies, and the development of novel recombinant vaccines for the treatment of a wide variety of diseases (*Chapters 12* and *23*). Indeed, a large number of industries have focused their research and development efforts on DNA-technology-based production of immunologically relevant molecules for research, diagnosis, and therapeutics.

Some of the major advances in research and clinical applications that have been achieved through DNA technology are summarized in Table 25-3. For ease of discussion, the techniques have been divided into five categories based upon five molecular techniques of DNA analysis: (1) restriction enzyme analysis; (2) polymerase chain reaction (**PCR**); (3) hybridization techniques; (4) DNA nucleotide sequence analysis; and (5) genetic transformation of mice.

Table 25-2. The three forms of expression of ribosomal-synthesized proteins together with examples of their immunological function

Location	Examples of immunologic function
Cell membrane	Antigen receptors (TCR, BCR); epitope presentation (MHC-I and -II, CD1); adhesion molecules (ICAM, selectins); co-stimulatory molecules (CD40, ICOS); pattern-recognition receptors (TLR, SR)
Cytosol	Signaling molecules (IRAK, NF-κB); pattern-recognition receptors (NLR, RIG-1)
Extracellular	Cytokines, secreted immunoglobulins

Restriction Enzyme Analysis

Individual genes can be cleaved at specific sites by **restriction enzymes** (Table 25-3). These enzymes are bacterial nucleases or endonucleases that result in cleavage through sugar-phosphate linkages of double-stranded DNA at specific sites (named restriction sites) depending upon the local nucleotide sequence, resulting in formation of DNA fragments of different but defined lengths.

The location of **restriction sites** in particular genes or the entire genome differ from person to person based on individual- or population-based sequence variations resulting from single base changes in DNA known as **single nucleotide polymorphisms** (**SNP**). Since the distance between

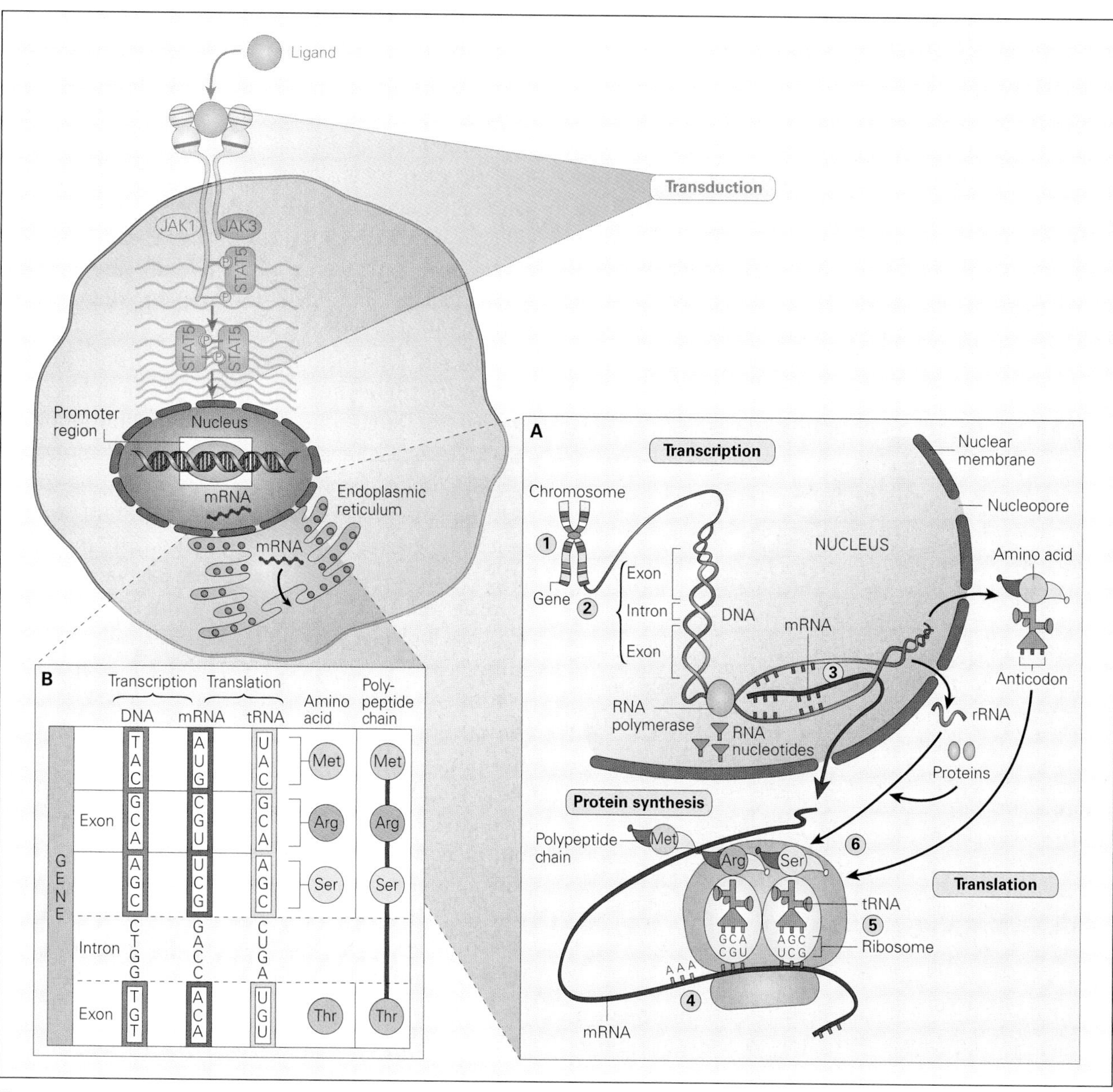

Figure 25-6. Schematic representation of the total transfer of genetic information from DNA → RNA → to synthesis of a protein. Panel A: The uncoiling of a gene located in a chromosomal locus (1), following which DNA genomic information is transcribed into mRNA by an RNA polymerase (2). The mRNA is translocated from the nucleus (3) to its cytoplasmic location on a ribosome within the endoplasmic reticulum (4), where each codon of the mRNA binds to the anticodon template-recognition site of a tRNA (5) carrying an attached amino acid. The activated contiguous amino acids are joined during protein synthesis translation following which the newly synthesized proteins are released from their ribosomal location (6). Panel B: Summarizes various steps involved in the transfer of genetic information from transcription, translation, to protein synthesis.

individual SNPs on a given individual DNA molecule might vary depending on the distribution of such SNPs along the particular gene of study, the DNA fragments resulting from restriction enzyme digestion will give rise to restriction fragments of varying length sizes. This variation, called restriction fragment length polymorphism (**RFLP**), permits the identification of particular genotypes, individuals, or species, producing a characteristic DNA fingerprinting for each individual.

Applications of Restriction Enzyme Analysis

Isolated restriction enzymes have been used to manipulate DNA in a variety of scientific applications utilizing a variety of laboratory procedures. In one technique called **Southern blotting**, DNA

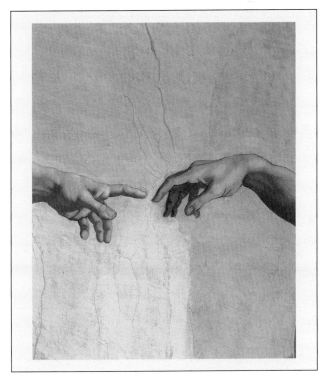

Figure 25-7. A conceptual view of the transfer of information from DNA → RNA → to synthesis of a protein. (Reproduced with the permission from the Director of the Vatican Museums.)

fragments generated by restriction nuclease treatment are first separated according to their molecular size by agar electrophoresis and then transferred ("blotted") onto a membrane of nitrocellulose paper or nylon paper, to which they adhere firmly, mirroring the pattern on the gel (Figure 25-8). Alkaline denaturation of the DNA fragments permits the separation of the DNA chains, allowing their hybridization with a specific DNA probe labeled with either a radioactive isotope (which can be analyzed by radioautography) or an enzyme, such as alkaline phosphatase or horseradish peroxidase (which can later be used to enzymatically cleave a colorless chromogen-linked substrate into a colored and readily measurable product). The size of the DNA fragments in each band can then be determined by reference to bands of molecules of DNA standards with known sizes (molecular weight markers).

An adaptation of this technique to detect specific sequences in RNA is called **Northern blotting**. In this case, RNA molecules instead of DNA molecules are separated by their sizes on gel electrophoresis and then detected by hybridization with a probe that is usually a labeled, single-stranded DNA molecule.

Restriction enzymes react with substrates usually comprised of specific sequences of four to eight nucleotides to generate products characterized either with sharp "blunt" ends or with staggered ends, which leave short single-stranded tails at the two ends of the fragment (**cohesive ends**). Any two different DNA samples treated with the same restriction enzyme generate fragments with the same cohesive ends, allowing the permanent fusion of each other through the complementary base pairs in their tails via an enzymatic reaction mediated by the ligase enzyme. Mixed DNA molecules produced this way are called **recombinant DNA**. DNA sequences can be amplified in vitro and artificially "inserted" into host living cells, both prokaryotes and eukaryotes, by using expression vectors, usually bacterial plasmids (Figure 25-9), or viruses (e.g., lambda phage, bacteriophage M13). The host cell with a single recombinant vector will divide into a colony with millions of cells with identical DNA inserts, forming a population called a **clone**. Examples of technological applications of DNA cloning in immunology include the manufacture of hepatitis B vaccine or human cytokines for therapeutic purposes (*Chapter 23*).

Although Western blot technology is not an example of a restriction enzyme analytical technique, it is included in this section because of its clinical importance in diagnosis of many diseases. The Western blot (also referred to as the protein immunoblot) is an analytical technique for the detection of specific proteins in a given sample of tissue homogenate or extract using gel electrophoresis to separate the native or denatured proteins (*Chapter 6*). The proteins are then transferred to a membrane, e.g., nitrocellulose, where they are probed using antibodies specific to the target protein. There are several clinical applications of Western blotting, including its use for the diagnosis of several infectious diseases. The confirmatory HIV test, for example, employs a Western blot to detect anti-HIV antibody in a human serum sample. Proteins from known HIV-infected cells are separated and blotted onto a membrane following which the patient's serum is applied to the membrane during the primary antibody incubation step. Free antibody is then washed away, and a

Table 25-3. Some major advances of research and clinical applications of DNA-based technologies

Technique	Mechanism	Example of clinical application
Restriction enzyme analysis • Restriction fragment length polymorphism (RFLP) • Southern blotting • Northern blotting • Recombinant DNA • Western blotting*	• Cleavage of DNA or RNA into fragments by restriction enzyme • DNA/DNA analysis • RNA/DNA analysis • Construction of mixed DNA molecules • Gel electrophoresis of proteins	• Allows the identification of particular genotypes, individuals, or species, i.e., DNA fingerprinting • Production of recombinant molecules for vaccine and cytokine production and a variety of other clinically useful products • Diagnosis of HIV infection and Lyme disease
Polymerase chain reaction (PCR) • Reverse-transcriptase-PCR (RT-PCR) • Real-time PCR	• Amplification of DNA or RNA using thermophilic Taq-polymerase	• Identification of DNA or RNA for diagnosis of infectious disease agents, tissue typing for transplantation, genetic diseases
Hybridization techniques • DNA hybridization • Fluorescence in situ hybridization (FISH) • Nucleic acid microarray	• Use of complementary DNA probes for the identification of nucleic acid sequences	• Identification of DNA for diagnosis of infectious disease agents, tissue typing for transplantation, genetic diseases
DNA nucleotide sequence analysis	• DNA sequencing using the dideoxy nucleotide method • Next generation sequencing (pyrosequencing, reversed terminator-based, sequencing by ligation) • Third-generation sequencing	• Identification of mutations and single nucleotide polymorphisms (SNPs) involved in immunodeficiencies and autoimmune and allergic diseases • Indirect determination of the amino acid sequence of proteins
Genetic transformation of mice • Transgenic mouse • Knock-out mouse	• Insertion of a gene into an inbred mouse • Deletion of a gene in an inbred mouse	• Allows the study of function of a gene and/or its product and provides an animal model of human disease

* Although Western blotting is not an example of a restriction enzyme analytical technique, it is included for methodological completeness.

secondary antihuman antibody linked to an enzyme signal is added. The stained bands then indicate the proteins to which the patient's serum contains antibody. Western blot testing is also commonly performed using a two-test protocol for the serologic diagnosis of Lyme disease (LD). Samples drawn from patients within four weeks of disease onset usually undergo testing for IgM and IgG antibody; samples drawn more than four weeks after disease onset are tested for IgG only. The determination of IgM and IgG antibody in patients' acute and convalescent sera is assessed by the number of bands detected. In the two-test protocol, a positive IgM immunoblot is defined by reactivity to two or more of the following bands: 25 (OspC), 39 (BmpA), and 41 (Fla) kDa. An IgG immunoblot is considered positive if five or more of the following bands are observed: 21, 25 (OspC), 28, 30, 39 (BmpA), 41 (Fla), 45, 58, 66, and 93 kDa. Western blot can also be used as a confirmatory test for hepatitis B infection.

Polymerase Chain Reaction

The PCR is a technique used to amplify, or make many copies of, small segments of DNA and is based on the ability of a DNA polymerase enzyme to synthesize a strand of DNA complementary to a targeted segment of DNA called the template DNA. PCR requires a sample that contains at least one DNA molecule of the region to be amplified and one set of **primers**, short segments of nucleotides (oligonucleotides) that have sequences complementary to areas adjacent to each side of the target sequence flanking both ends of the specific region that will be amplified in the reaction. Using this technique, DNA molecules can be copied into billions of identical molecules,

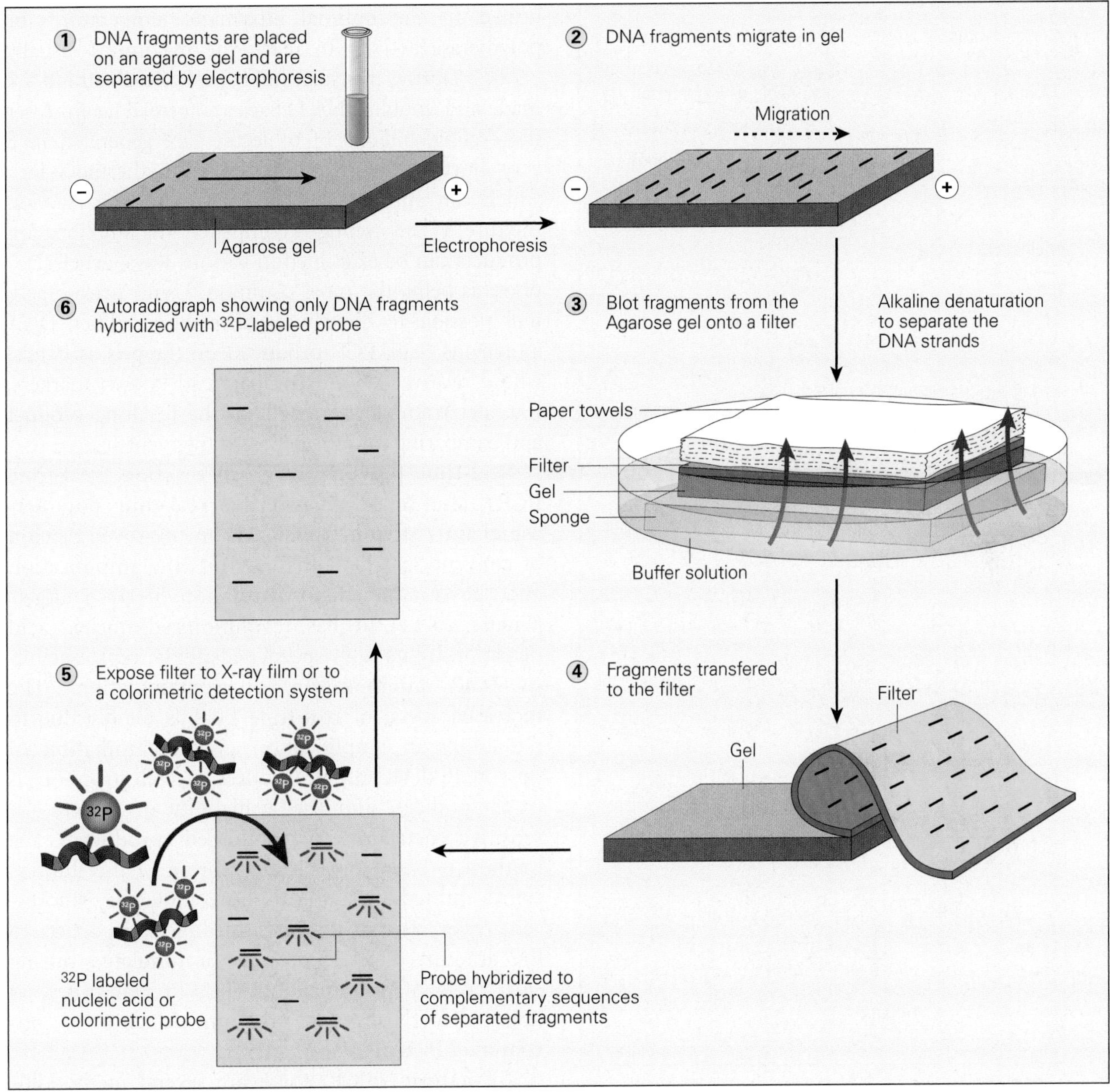

Figure 25-8. Schematic representation of the Southern blot technique. (1) DNA fragments generated by restriction nuclease treatment are separated by agarose gel electrophoresis and fragments are transferred to the filter (2); the electrophoretically separated DNA fragments are transferred ("blotted") onto a membrane (3); the membrane-imprinted DNA bands are alkaline treated to separate DNA chains (4); the isolated DNA chains are hybridized with a specific radioactively labeled or enzyme-linked DNA probe (5); the DNA bands bound to the probe are detected by (6) radioautographic or colorimetric methods (6).

allowing the replication of specific DNA regions in a very large number of DNA copies from a very small quantity of the template DNA. The amplification of RNA molecules (viral or mRNA) is also possible, and this requires the transcription of the RNA molecule of interest into DNA (complementary DNA or cDNA) by using the enzyme reverse transcriptase, as described earlier in this chapter, through a procedure known as reverse-transcriptase-PCR **(RT-PCR).** PCR provides enough material as starting template for further sequencing or for the identification of known genes (or mRNA) by their specific nucleotide sequences.

There are three stages that take place during the PCR, usually requiring 30–40 repeated cycles of amplification in order to achieve **exponential** increases in the number of DNA molecules (Figure 25-10). These include: (1) a **denaturation stage,**

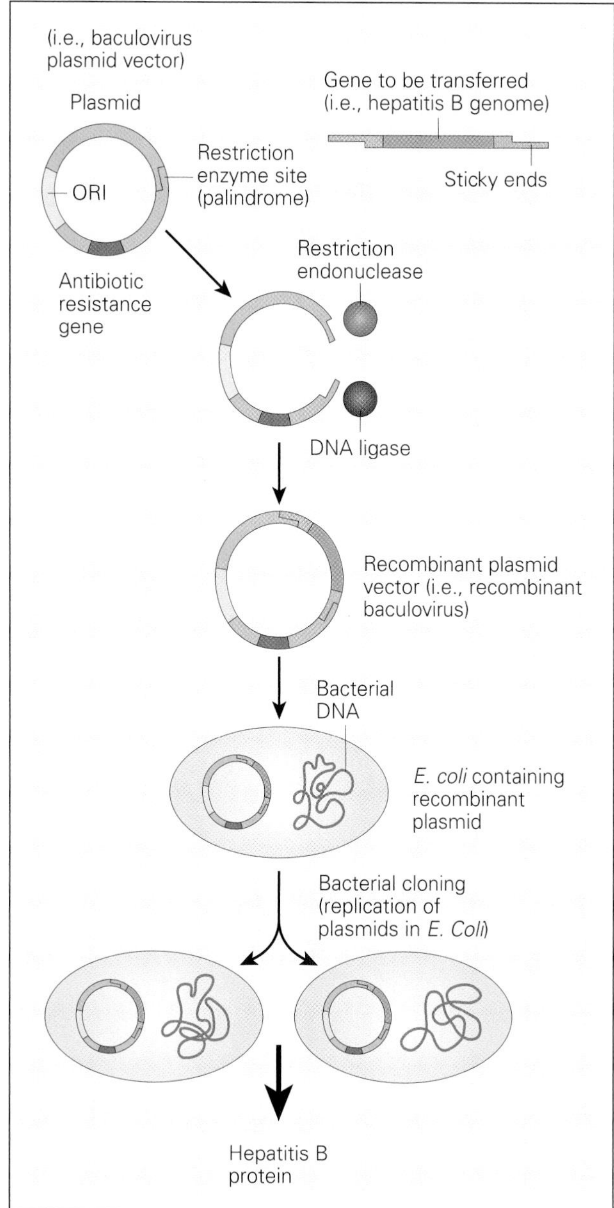

Figure 25-9. Schematic representation of a plasmid showing several restriction enzyme sites and its use in the production of hepatitis B protein in the manufacture of hepatitis B vaccine.

during which the DNA is heated at a temperature of approximately 95°C; during this step, the DNA double helixes are opened and single strands are melted apart; and (2) **annealing**, during which the DNA is brought to a lower temperature of approximately 50–60°C depending on the melting temperatures of the primers, allowing the primers to bind their complementary regions on both DNA strands. At this stage, the DNA polymerase, known as **Taq polymerase**, initiates the extension of the nascent DNA molecule. (3) **Elongation** is the final stage, where the material is heated to the optimal enzymatic temperature for polymerase activity to reach the maximum, usually ~72°C. During this step, full copies of each strand are made and double DNA helixes are formed again. After the cycling, billions of molecules are generated in a very short time in an automated cycler (thermocycler), which can automatically heat and cool the reaction mixture. When cycling is completed, the amplification products can be examined in various ways, gel electrophoresis being the most common. Using agarose gels, it is possible to directly visualize the amplified DNA amplicons (e.g., PCR products) on the gels as bands, whose relative size are compared to known markers, thus determining the length of the resulting product and comparing it to the expected fragment size.

Real-time polymerase chain reaction (**real-time PCR**), also called **quantitative real-time polymerase chain reaction** (**qPCR**), is an improved version of conventional PCR that permits the amplification and the simultaneous quantitation of DNA targets (Figure 25-11). It has revolutionized nucleic acid detection by its high speed, sensitivity, reproducibility, and minimization of contamination. The increased speed of real-time PCR is mainly due to reductions in amplification cycles, elimination of post-PCR detection procedures (gel electrophoresis or any other), and the availability of devices for sensitive detection of amplified products. The method is based on the monitoring of the fluorescence emitted by a fluorophore molecule (fluorescent reporter) that increases in direct proportion to the amount of PCR product accumulated during each cycle of amplification (i.e., in real time), as opposed to the product endpoint detection in conventional PCR.

To perform qPCR, there are several methodologies (platforms) available, each one with advantages and disadvantages; therefore, a comprehensive evaluation should be performed when deciding which platform to use.

Molecular beacons are single-stranded oligonucleotide hybridization probes that have a stem-and-loop (hairpin-like) structure that are used to detect or "report" the presence of specific nucleic acids in homogenous solutions (Figure 25-12). In the loop structure, there is a probe sequence complementary to a target sequence, and the stem is formed by the annealing of short complementary sequences at both ends of the probe sequence. A fluorophore, also referred to as a reporter molecule, is covalently

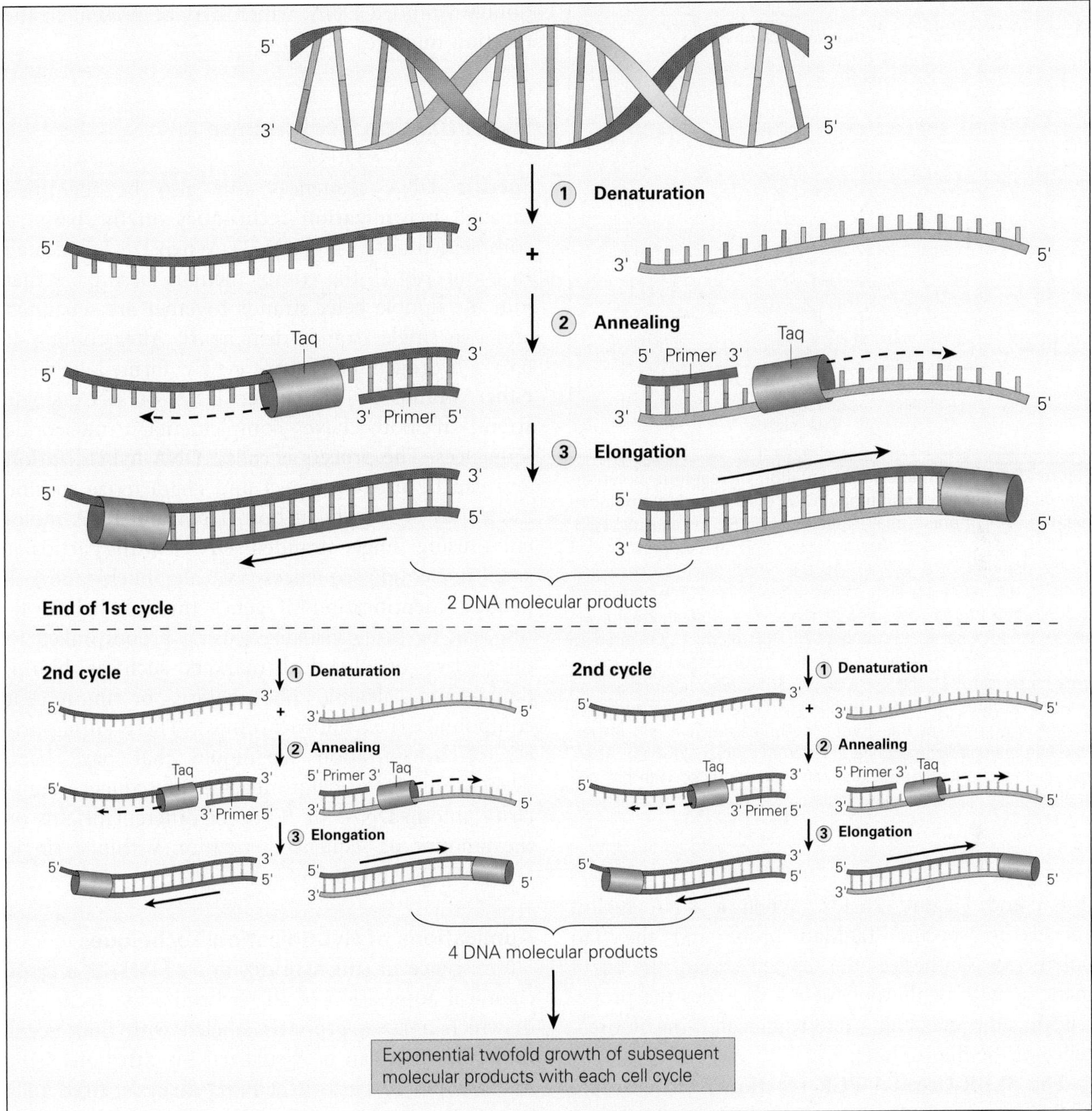

Figure 25-10. Schematic representation of the polymerase chain reaction (PCR) technique showing the three stages of the assay: denaturation, annealing, and elongation stages. The separation of the two single DNA strands in the (1) denaturation stage is followed by binding of primers to the isolated template DNA during the (2) annealing stage and terminates the first cycle with the (3) elongation phase initiated by the Taq polymerase. The assay is repeated sequentially during several subsequent cycles during which there is an exponential production of subsequent molecular copies of descendant molecules.

linked to the end of one arm of the probe and a quencher molecule that decreases the fluorescence intensity of the fluorophore is covalently linked to the other end of the probe. Molecular beacons do not fluoresce when they are free in solution; however, when they hybridize to a DNA strand containing a target sequence, they undergo a conformational change, resulting in the dissociation of the quencher initiating the fluorescence of the fluorophore.

The **TaqMan-based qPCR** is an example of the sequence-specific DNA probe method that utilizes the 5′ exonuclease activity of Taq DNA polymerase to cleave a oligonucleotide probe with a fluorophore covalently attached to the 5′-end and a quencher at

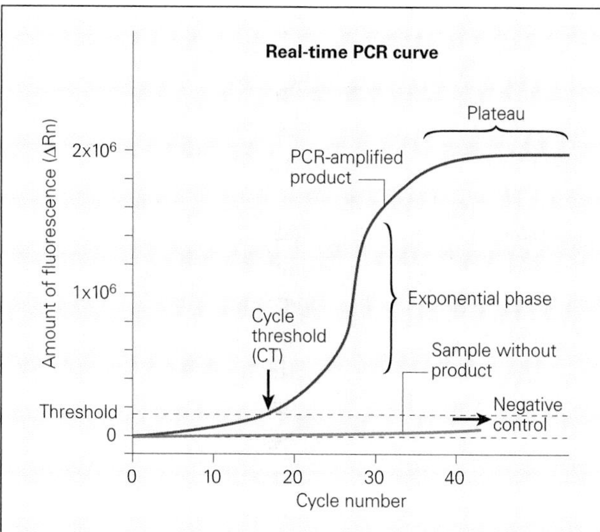

Figure 25-11. **Schematic representation of real-time polymerase chain reaction (real-time PCR), also called quantitative real-time polymerase chain reaction (qPCR).** In real-time PCR, specific dyes are used that fluoresce only in the presence of double-stranded DNA (y-axis). As the amplification process progresses, the result is a shift of the sigmoid curve. The amount of fluorescence (Rn) is measured at the end of each thermal cycle and is proportional to the amount of PCR product generated to that point of time. Relative quantitation is expressed in terms of cycle threshold (CT), the cycle at which fluorescence crosses an established threshold value. Samples without the target template do not incorporate or transform the fluorescent dye and do not generate enough fluorescence to reach the threshold value. Absolute quantitation (copy numbers) can be determined with the use of appropriate quantitative standards.

the 3′-end (Figure 25-13). When a DNA region anneals to specific TaqMan probe and the Taq polymerase synthesizes the nascent strand, the enzymatic activity of the polymerase degrades the probe, relieving the quenching effect, and allowing fluorescence of the fluorophore.

The SYBR-Green I PCR reaction is an example of the nonspecific fluorescent intercalator dye-based method that uses of a fluorophore that fluoresces only when bound directly to double-stranded DNA (Figure 25-13). When the SYBR-Green fluorophore is present in the PCR reaction mixture, it binds to the newly synthesized double-stranded amplicons and the intensity of the fluorescent emissions increases proportionally. The SYBR-Green assay is able to detect highly variable genome regions for which probe design is often difficult, its relative simplicity making it easy to implement and its cost is comparatively lower than other platforms. The major disadvantage of this reaction is the nonspecific binding of the intercalator dye to any double-stranded DNA, which may be present in the reaction mixture.

Hybridization Techniques

Specific DNA sequences can also be identified through **hybridization techniques** on the basis of complementarity (Table 25-3). When DNA is heated to about 100°C, the complementary base pairs that join the double helix strands together are separated and two single strands drift apart. After cooling at 65°C, hydrogen bonds are newly formed between either strands or any other DNA or RNA single strand if both have complementary nucleotide sequences. The process is called **DNA hybridization** and can be used to detect and characterize specific nucleotide sequences in both DNA and RNA molecules using single-stranded DNAs with particular small nucleotide sequences (i.e., oligonucleotides) as **probes.** Identification of genes through hybridization can be easily visualized using probes linked to radioactive or chemical markers such as biotin, digoxigenin, alkaline phosphatase, or fluorescent compounds (i.e., fluorochromes). There are a variety of hybridization techniques that have been developed for the determination of sequence similarity among DNAs or RNAs of different origins or the amount of sequence repetition within a single DNA or RNA motif.

Applications of Hybridization Techniques

Fluorescence in situ hybridization (**FISH**) is a cytochemical application of the hybridization technique in which a DNA probe is labeled with fluorescent molecules that can be visualized by ultraviolet light microscopy. To perform a FISH analysis, fixed cells mounted on a microscope slide are heated to allow the separation of the chromosomal DNA and the subsequent hybridization with a fluorogenic-labeled DNA probe (Table 25-3 and Box 25-3). After cooling, the cell preparations are observed by fluorescence microscopy that identifies the chromosomal location of the hybridized target DNA. Shown in Figure 25-14 is an example of the use of FISH for the identification of a 22q11.2 deletion in a patient with the 22q11.2 deletion syndrome (*Chapter 16*). A variety of fluorochromes can be simultaneously used for labeling different DNA probes (multiplex), which can detect many types of genes or genetic changes.

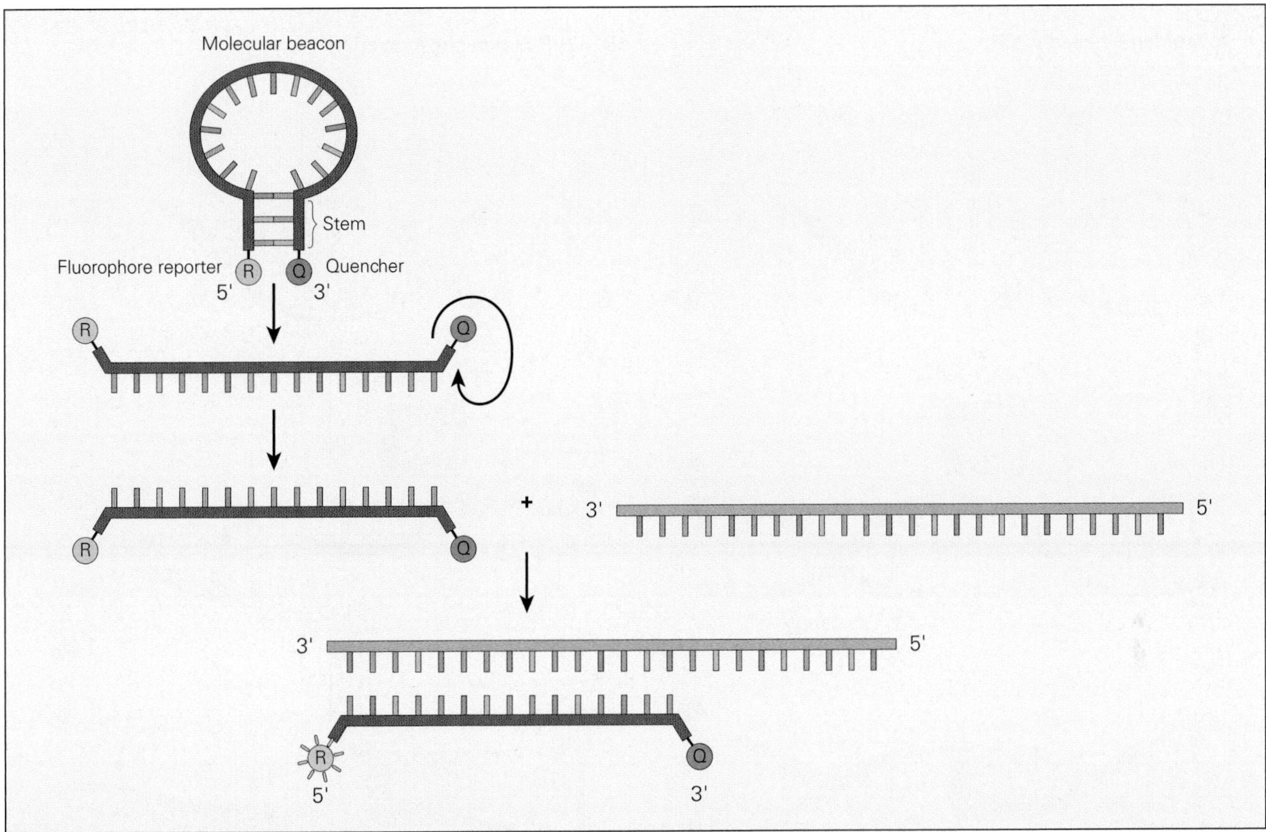

Figure 25-12. Schematic representation of a molecular beacon. Molecular beacons are hairpin-shaped molecules with an internally quenched fluorophore whose fluorescence is restored when they bind to a target nucleic acid sequence. This is a novel nonradioactive method for detecting specific sequences of nucleic acids.

DNA Nucleic Acid Microarray

One of the more recent applications of hybridization techniques is the **DNA nucleic acid microarray** analysis (Table 25-3). Microarray technology evolved from Southern blotting, where fragmented DNA attached to a substrate is probed with a known gene or fragment and hybridization between the two DNA strands occurs, utilizing the property of complementary nucleic acid sequences to specifically pair with each other by forming hydrogen bonds between complementary nucleotide base pairs (Figure 25-15).

In this method, thousands of marker complementary DNA (cDNA) probes specific for selected genes or the entire transcriptome are fixed onto solid supports (glass, plastic, or silicon chips) in miniaturized arrays in order to perform multiple hybridizations simultaneously (Figure 25-15). The microarray is exposed to a solution containing a mixture of single-stranded cDNAs derived from mRNA, each one with a different fluorochrome label. Since a high number of complementary base pairs in a nucleotide sequence is associated with tighter noncovalent bonding between the two strands, after removal of nonspecific binding sequences by washing, only strongly paired strands will remain hybridized. After hybridization, the microarray is observed for the presence of fluorescent spots by fluorescence or laser microscopy. Fluorescently labeled target sequences that bind to a probe sequence generate a signal that depends on the strength of the hybridization determined by the number of paired bases, allowing the measurement of hybridization levels (i.e., fluorescence intensity) in spots that are compared to levels of hybridization under control conditions (Figure 25-15). DNA microarrays are being used in a variety of immunologic disorders to measure the expression level of large variety of **genes** of immunologic importance, e.g., cytokines, growth factors, or to **genotype** multiple regions of a genome to identify the location of possible genetic defects, e.g., the absence of BTK in X-linked agammaglobulinemia (*Chapter 16*).

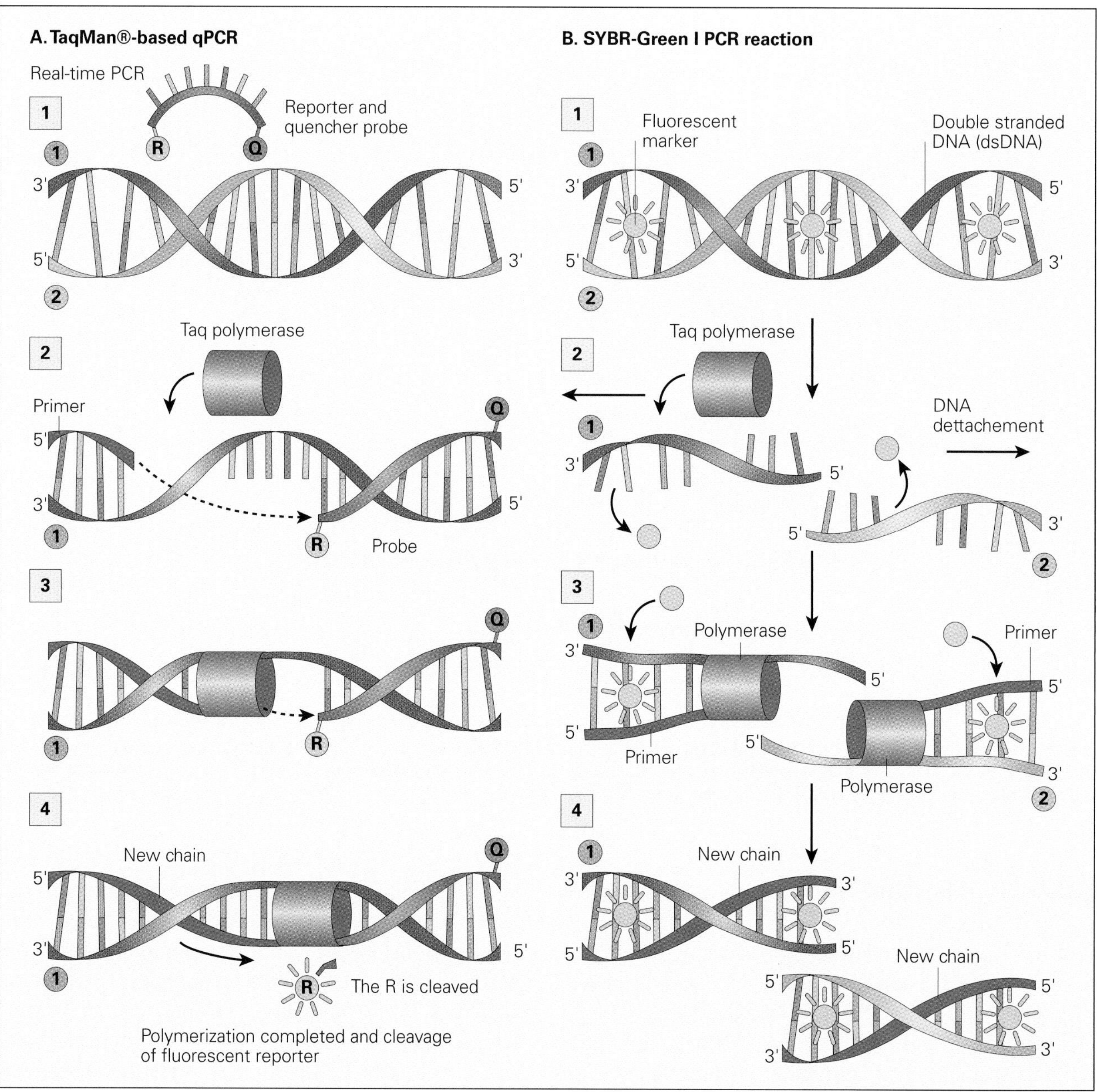

Figure 25-13. Schematic representation of real-time polymerase chain reaction (real-time PCR), also called quantitative real-time polymerase chain reaction (qPCR). Panel A: Shows the sequence-specific DNA probe method using the TaqMan-based qPCR that utilizes the Taq DNA polymerase to release the 5′-end-attached fluorophore from its detection-inhibiting quencher at the 3′-end of the probe. Panel B: Shows a nonspecific fluorophore-based assay that illustrates the use of the SYBR-Green I real-time PCR reaction as an intercalator-based method with the use of a dye that only fluoresces when bound to double-stranded DNA.

DNA Sequencing

DNA sequencing is the term used to determine the order of the nucleotide bases—adenine, guanine, cytosine, and thymine—in a molecule of DNA. Knowledge of DNA sequences has not only become indispensable for basic biological research, but also is finding great clinical application in numerous applied fields of immunology such as in the diagnosis of infectious diseases, autoimmunity, and cancer. The advent of DNA sequencing has been instrumental in the sequencing of the human genome in the Human Genome Project that has launched a molecular revolution in medicine.

Although historically several methods of DNA sequencing have been developed, the chain-termination method developed by Sanger and coworkers in 1975 soon became the classic method of choice,

Box 25-3

Probes Used for FISH Assays

Probes are now available for use in FISH assays often derived from fragments of DNA that were isolated, purified, and amplified for use in the Human Genome Project. The size of the human genome, however, is so large compared to the length that could be sequenced directly that it was necessary to divide the genome into fragments. These fragments were then put into a library by digesting a copy of each fragment into still smaller fragments using sequence-specific endonucleases, measuring the size of each small fragment using size-exclusion chromatography, and using that information to determine where the large fragments overlapped one another. To preserve the fragments with their individual DNA sequences, the fragments were added into a system of continually replicating bacterial populations. Clonal populations of bacteria, each population maintaining a single artificial chromosome, are stored in various laboratories around the world. These bacterial artificial chromosomes (BACs) have been created as DNA constructs utilizing plasmid technology for transforming and cloning in bacteria, usually *E. coli*. The artificial chromosomes (BACs) can be grown, extracted, and labeled, and are the most common sources of probes used in FISH assays.

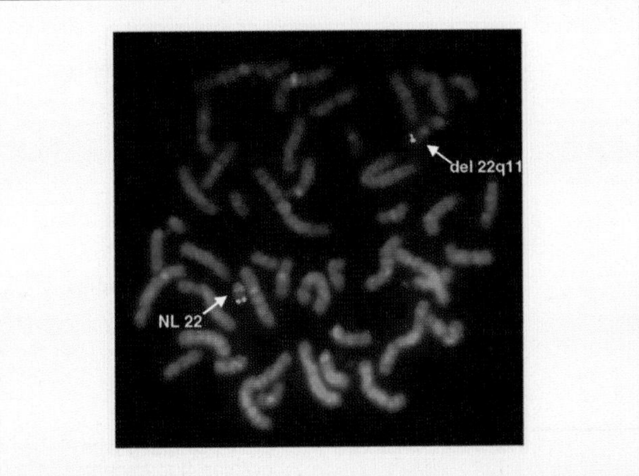

Figure 25-14. FISH of metaphase chromosomes with fluorescently labeled probes to detect a deletion of chromosome 22q11. The green signal control is seen at the distal end of both homologues of chromosome 22; note the presence of the red signal for the test probe on one homologue of chromosome 22 (NL 22) and the absence of the test probe on the other homologue (del 22q11), implying a deletion of that locus on one chromosome. (Courtesy of Beverly Emanuel, PhD, Philadelphia, PA.) (Reproduced with permission from Goldmuntz E. DiGeorge syndrome: new insights. Clin Perinatol. 2005; 32: 963–978.)

owing to its relative ease of performance as well as its reliability and reproducibility (Figure 25-16). The method relies on the fundamental differences in the chemical structure between two basic DNA building-block chemical moieties: (1) the deoxyribonucleotides (dNTPs) that contain a 3′-OH group in the deoxyribose moiety that can be normally used for DNA synthesis, and (2) the dideoxyribonucleotides (ddNTPs) that lack the 3′-OH group required for the formation of a phosphodiester bond needed to construct the phosphate-deoxyribose backbone structure of the DNA molecule and without which DNA strand extension terminates (Figure 25-3).

The chain-termination method requires a single-stranded DNA template, a DNA primer, a DNA polymerase, normal deoxynucleotide phosphates (dNTPs), and the DNA-terminating modified nucleotides (dideoxyNTPs) (Figure 25-16). These ddNTPs can be radioactively or fluorescently labeled for detection in automated sequencing instruments. The DNA sample is divided into four separate sequencing reactions containing all four of the standard deoxynucleotides (dATP, dGTP, dCTP, and dTTP) and the DNA polymerase. To each reaction is added only one of the four dideoxynucleotides (ddATP, ddGTP, ddCTP, or ddTTP), which are the chain-terminating nucleotides, thus terminating DNA strand extension and resulting in DNA fragments of varying length. Thus, after 30 to 40 PCR cycles, the mixture will contain a number of fragments of differing lengths depending on the number of bases that had been added to the chain before its growth was arrested. When the mixture is subjected to gel electrophoresis to separate the components, the different DNA strands migrate separated by length from longest to shortest. Because each dideoxyribonucleotide is labeled with a different fluorochrome, each one will give a particular signal when illuminated by a laser beam. The resolution is good enough that a difference of one nucleotide is able to establish a distance of that strand from the next shorter and next longer strand. The automatic scanning provides a record of each wavelength of light and a computer generates an image with colored peaks representing each wavelength in the sequence as it passes through the beam (Figure 25-16).

Next-generation sequencing. The high demand for low-cost sequencing has driven the development

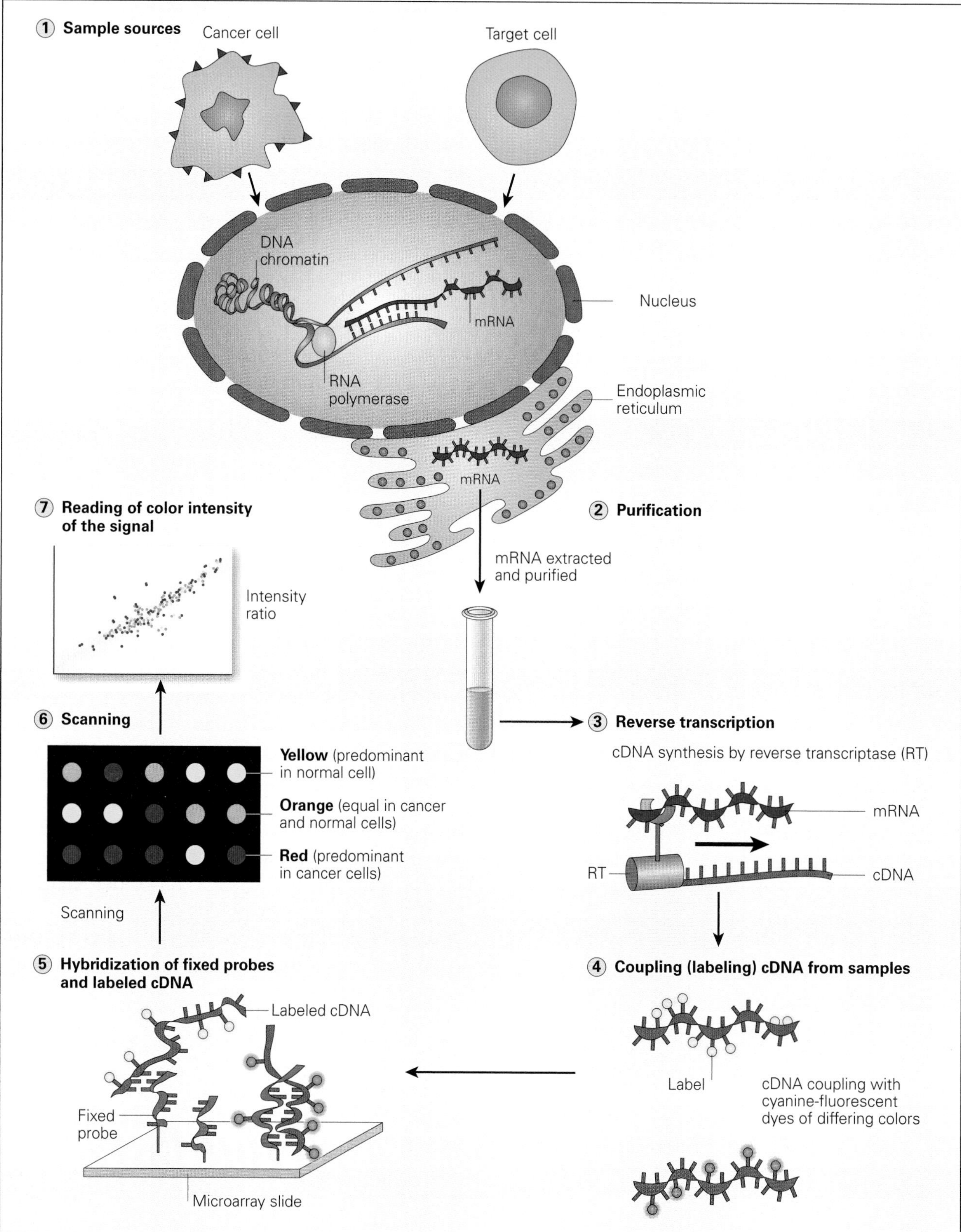

Figure 25-15. Schematic representation of the use of cDNA microarrays to distinguish tumor from normal tissue (1); samples of each tissue are processed and mRNA extracted and purified (2); cDNA is synthesized from the mRNA by reverse transcription (3); the cDNA from each sample is labeled with cyanine-fluorescent dyes of differing colors (4); the labeled cDNA molecules are hybridized to fixed probes containing complementary strands of DNA (5); after washing to remove unattached strands, the microarray is scanned (6) and read to determine fluorescent intensities emitted by the attached labeled cDNA strands that correspond to each gene (7); yellow spots correspond to genes more strongly expressed in the normal cell, red spots correspond to genes with higher expressed in both the cancer and normal cells.

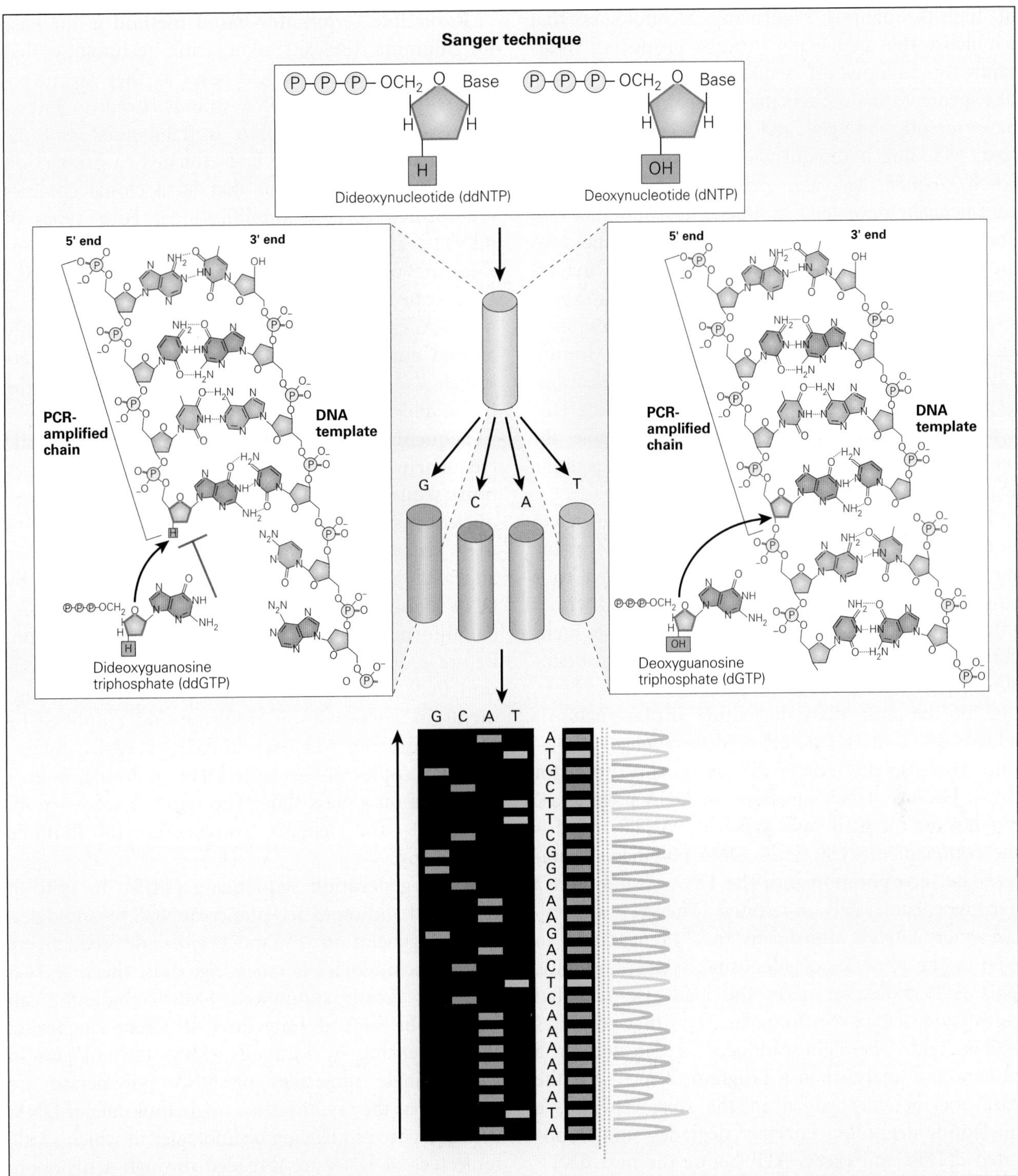

Figure 25-16. Schematic representation of DNA sequencing by the chain-termination method (Sanger method). Chemical structures of dideoxynucleotides and deoxynucleotides are shown at top. The chain-termination method requires a single-stranded DNA template, a DNA primer, a DNA polymerase, normal deoxynucleotide phosphates (dNTPs), and the DNA-terminating modified nucleotides (dideoxyNTPs) (pink tube). The DNA sample is divided into four separate sequencing reactions, containing all four of the standard deoxynucleotides (dATP, dGTP, dCTP, and dTTP) and the DNA polymerase. To each reaction is added only one of the four dideoxynucleotides (ddATP, ddGTP, ddCTP, or ddTTP), which are the chain-terminating nucleotides, thus terminating DNA strand extension and resulting in DNA fragments of varying length. These are then subjected to size separation by electrophoresis. An example is given of the sequence readout produced by exposing the separated DNA fragments to laser excitation and recording the signal corresponding to each fragment as they pass through the laser beam during electrophoresis. Because each ddNTP is labeled with a different fluorescent dye, the color and the succession of DNA fragments that are recorded can be used to reconstitute the DNA sequence.

of high-throughput sequencing technologies that parallelize the sequencing process, producing thousands or millions of sequences at once. Several next-generation sequencing (NGS) technologies have recently emerged and have been commercialized, including pyrosequencing, reversed terminator-based sequencing, and sequencing by ligation, commercially developed by Roche 454, Illumina GA, and ABI SOLiD, respectively. These technologies are able to generate three to four orders of magnitude more sequence and are considerably less expensive than the Sanger method. To date, these new technologies have been successfully applied toward ChIP-sequencing (chromatin immunoprecipitation-sequencing) to identify binding sites of DNA-associated proteins, RNA-sequencing to profile the mammalian transcriptome, and whole human genome sequencing.

Pyrosequencing method is based on the detection of pyrophosphate release on nucleotide incorporation. A sequencing primer is hybridized to a single stranded DNA template and incubated with a mixture of DNA polymerase, ATP sulfurylase, luciferase, and apyrase, as well as the substrates, adenosine 5′phosphosulfate (APS), and luciferin. Next, one of the four deoxynucleotide triphosphates is added: dGTP, dCTP, dTTP, or deoxyadenosine alfa-thio triphosphate (dATPαS) as a substitute for dATP, because it is a substrate for DNA polymerase but not for the luciferase. When the dNTP added is the complementary one, the DNA polymerase catalyzes its incorporation into the DNA strand, and a pyrophosphate (PPi) is released. The ATP sulfurylase quantitatively transforms the PPi produced to ATP in the presence of adenosine 5′phosphosulfate. This ATP molecule drives the luciferase-mediated conversion of luciferin to oxyluciferin that generates visible light. The light produced is detected by a camera and analyzed in a program, detecting if the base was actually added in the step. Apyrase, a nucleotide-degrading enzyme, degrades unincorporated dNTPs and excess ATP, before the next dNTP is added (addition of dNTPs is performed one at a time). Among pyrosequencing commercialized platforms, 454 (Roche) relies on the amplification of DNA inside water droplets in an oil solution (emulsion PCR), with each droplet containing a single DNA template attached to a single primer-coated bead or clonal colony.

Reversible terminator-based method is the base for Illumina (Solexa) sequencing technology that enables detection of single bases as they are incorporated into growing DNA strands based on reversible dye-terminators. DNA is fragmented and the generated molecules are first attached to primers on a slide and amplified so that local clonal colonies are formed (bridge amplification). Four types of ddNTPs are added, and nonincorporated nucleotides are washed away. Unlike pyrosequencing, the DNA can only be extended one nucleotide at a time. A camera takes images of the fluorescently labeled nucleotides then the dye along with the terminal 3′ blocker is chemically removed from the DNA, allowing a next cycle.

Sequencing by ligation corresponds to SOLiD (sequencing by oligonucleotide ligation and detection) sequencing. Here, a pool of all possible oligonucleotides of a fixed length is labeled according to the sequenced position. Oligonucleotides are annealed and ligated; the preferential ligation by DNA ligase for matching sequences results in a signal informative of the nucleotide at that position. Before sequencing, the DNA is amplified by emulsion PCR, i.e., compartmentalization of DNA fragments in a water-in-oil emulsion and amplified by PCR in isolation. The resulting bead, each containing only copies of the same DNA molecule, is then deposited on a glass slide. The result is sequences of quantities and lengths comparable to Illumina sequencing.

Third-generation sequencing (TGS). In spite of the recent and rapid acceptance of NGS technologies, a new generation of single-molecule sequencing (**SMS**) technologies is emerging; thus, the first TGS has been already announced. SMS technologies can roughly be binned into three different categories: (1) sequencing by synthesis (**SBS**) technologies in which single molecules of DNA polymerase are observed as they synthesize a single molecule of DNA; (2) nanopore-sequencing technologies in which single molecules of DNA are threaded through a nanopore or positioned in the vicinity of a nanopore, and individual bases are detected as they pass through the nanopore; and (3) direct imaging of individual DNA molecules using advanced microscopy techniques. Each of these technologies provides novel approaches and has advantages and disadvantages with respect to specific applications.

Genetically Transformed Mice

The use of genetically transformed mouse models has provided unique tools for the study of human disease and immune responses. These models have not only permitted the identification and expression of genes involved in innate and adaptive immune responses, but also have provided the capability to analyze many cell functions and effector molecules (e.g., cytokines, antibodies) controlled by these genes. As intact organisms, they also offer a much more complete and physiologically relevant picture of immune responses than those provided by in vitro systems. Also, genetically engineered mice have been used to generate chimeric or humanized monoclonal antibodies for clinical use (*Chapter 11*) that eliminate or minimize many of the murine components of these molecules that are recognized as foreign by the human immune system and that are responsible for adverse effects associated with the use of these products.

A **transgenic mouse** (or any other animal model) is one that carries a foreign DNA (called a transgene) that has been artificially inserted into its genome. The transgene is constructed using recombinant DNA technology and usually includes the structural DNA and other sequences to enable it to be incorporated into and expressed by the DNA of the host mouse (Figure 25-17). Transgenic mice have been obtained in one of the three ways shown in Box 25-4.

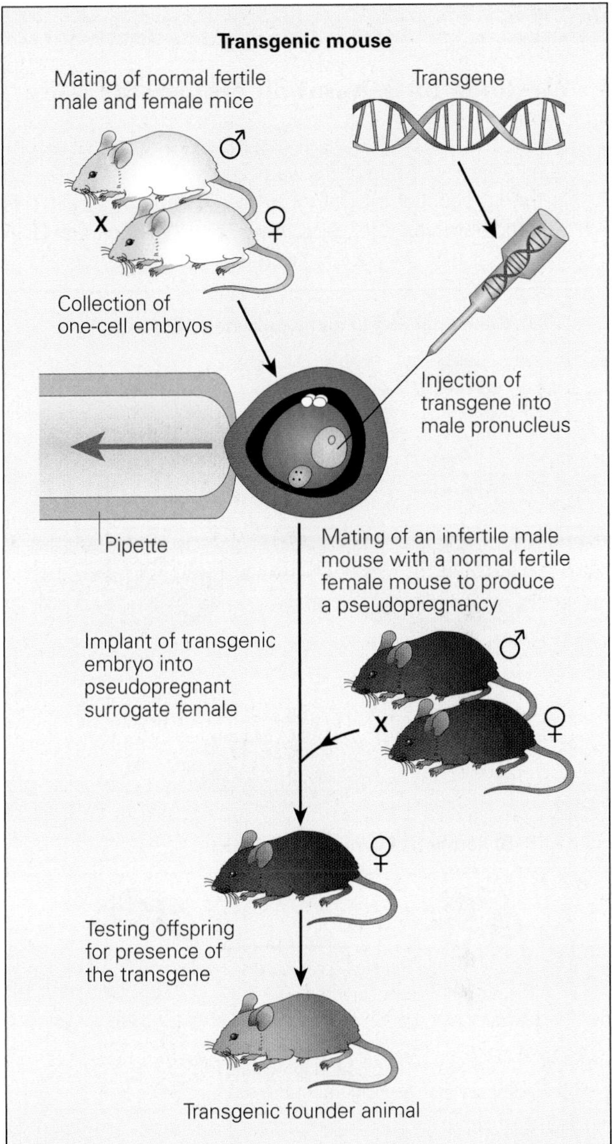

Figure 25-17. Schematic representation of the construction of a transgenic mouse. Restriction enzymes are used to cleave the gene of interest at the restriction sites. The gene is inserted into the host DNA with the help of DNA ligase. Along the embryo development, the inserted gene will become part of the mouse's DNA and will be found in all cells of the host. The embryo is implanted into a pseudopregnant female. After several weeks of age, each newborn mouse is tested for the presence of the gene of interest and selected.

Clinically Relevant Applications of Molecular Biologic Techniques to Immunology in Health and Disease

The past decade has seen an explosive development and use of DNA-based genomic assays that are finding clinical application to many immunology related fields. Shown in Table 25-4 are some of the clinical fields where DNA-based genomic assays are yielding important clinical applications.

The first suggestion that genomic studies could have clinical applications came in 1999, when microarray-based transcriptional profiling was proposed for the differential diagnosis of acute myeloid and lymphocytic leukemias. These studies later resulted in the identification of gene expression signatures correlating clinical outcomes with genetic signatures in both the hematological malignancies and solid tumors. In several of these malignancies, microarray studies, for example, have not only facilitated new drug development for the treatment of cancer, but also have helped identify subgroups of patients who may benefit from adjuvant therapy. Shown in Table 25-5 are some of the new adjuvant therapies for hematologic and solid tumors together

Box 25-4

Methods of Generating Transgenic Mice

Transgenic mice have been generated using three techniques. The most straightforward and widely used method is the introduction of DNA into the nucleus of a cell. This method involves the microinjection of exogenous DNA into the male pronuclei of fertilized eggs as shown in Figure 25-17. The injected eggs are then transferred to the oviduct of a pseudopregnant female and allowed to develop to term. The integration of the exogenous DNA into the genome of the fertilized egg is believed to occur through the normal process of chromosomal breakage and repair, occurring randomly in the genome. The exogenous DNA is often integrated as multiple copies into a single site in a head-to-tail array; however, multiple integrations also can occur. In this method of producing transgenic mice, it is important that the random integration occurs at the single-cell stage so that the exogenous DNA is integrated into the genome of all cells in the organism, especially the germ cells. When integration occurs at later stages, mosaic animals are produced in which the exogenous DNA is confined to specific developmental compartments or cell lineages.

A second method for producing transgenic mice takes advantage of the pluripotential capacity of embryo-derived stem (ES) cells (Figure 25-18). In this method, the ES cells in culture are transformed using conventional gene-transfer techniques, and the transformed cells are reintroduced in early blastocysts, which are transferred to appropriately timed pseudopregnant females. The transformed ES cells contribute to the development of a chimeric offspring; one can identify chimeric mice in which the ES cells have contributed to the germ line. This method allows the selection of the desired genotype or phenotype in the cultured ES cells prior to implantation. Although ES cells have been used to produce transgenic mice that express specific genes, this method is used primarily to target a transgene construct to a predetermined chromosomal locus through homologous recombination, thus producing

A. Gene targeting of embryonic stem (ES) cells
Mouse blastocyst
Embryonic cell
Transgene introduced into the ES cells by electroporation
The transgenic ES cells are selected and expanded in tissue culture
Pure population of targeted ES cells
B. Generation of gene-targeted mice
Targeted ES cells are injected into blastocysts
Which are implanted into pseudopregnant surrogate mothers
Which give rise to a chimeric mouse with germ cells containing the transgene
A chimeric male mouse is then bred with a normal female mouse to generate either a gene-targeted or a normal mouse
♂
♀
Egg
Sperm
"Knock-in" or "knock-out" gene-targeted mice
Normal mice

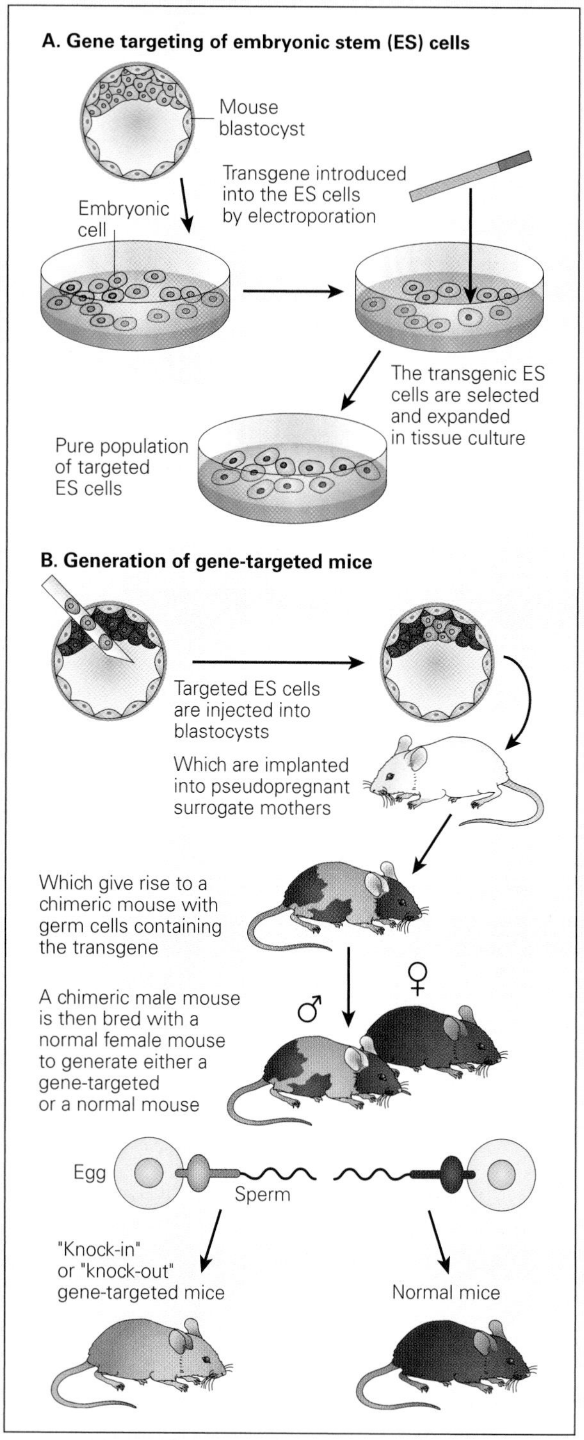

Figure 25-18. **Schematic representation of the embryonic stem (ES) cell culture method for the generation of "knock-in" or "knock-out" transgenic mice.** Panel A: Embryonic stem cells are obtained from a mouse blastocyst and cultured in vitro. A transgenic vector is introduced into the ES cells by electroporation (a method using electricity to transfer the DNA across a cell membrane), following which the ES cells that either express or exclude the targeted gene are selected in the cultured ES cells. Panel B: The selected transgenic ES cells are injected into blastocysts and then implanted into the uterus of foster mothers to complete the pregnancy and to generate chimeric mice capable of transmitting the mutant gene to their progeny. The chimeric mice are then bred with normal female mice to generate either gene-targeted or normal mice. Those transgenic mice that express a gain-of-function gene are referred to as "knock-in" transgenic mice; those transgenic mice that fail to express the normal gene function are referred to as "knock-out" transgenic mice.

Box 25-4 (continued)

transgenic mice that carry a mutation in a specific gene. These mutations can produce "gain-of-function" or "loss-of-function" transgenic animals that are referred to as "knock-in" and "knock-out" transgenic animals, respectively, which can inactivate the gene or alter the function of the corresponding protein. Thus, the ES cell method has several advantages over the other techniques for producing transgenic mice, although the technique is technically demanding.

Transgenic mice also have been produced by the infection of early embryos with recombinant retroviruses carrying an exogenous gene. This method has an advantage in that only a single copy of the provirus is found at the chromosomal integration site; however, the technique has several limitations. For example, since the retroviruses may not uniformly infect all cells in early embryos, the frequency of germ line transmission is relatively low. In addition, the expression of genes introduced in retroviral vectors is often low, and only a relatively small fragment of the DNA (smaller than 10 kb) can be cloned into the retroviral vector.

with the genetic alterations that were discovered on the basis of genomic studies.

In the case of infectious diseases, the development of new rapid diagnostic assays for the identification of pathogens has been enhanced by the availability of techniques for genetic sequencing of DNA motifs followed by comprehensive, comparative analysis with genomic sequences available in currently accessible databases. The development of new vaccines has also witnessed the genomic revolution that has not only led to the development of more effective, easily deployable vaccines through "reverse vaccinology" (*Chapter 23*), but also holds great promise for the development of effective currently unavailable vaccines in the future for TB, malaria, and HIV/AIDS. These genomic techniques have also resulted in the production of highly effective new monoclonal antibody therapies, e.g., palivizumab for RSV. The use of genomic assays and technology has also contributed to the molecular understanding of the molecular defects that are responsible for the myriad immune deficiency disorders that often present clinically as an undue susceptibility to recurrent and persistent infections as well as a propensity to the autoimmune disorders and malignancy (*Chapter 16*).

The management of patients with autoimmune disease has been greatly enhanced by the study of transcriptional biomarkers important in the pathogenesis, diagnosis, and assessment of disease severity, as well as the development of new therapeutic agents for the treatment of these clinically perplexing disorders, e.g., anti-TNF-α products (*Chapters 11* and *19*). Beginning with the discovery of the blockbuster anti-TNF-α medications for the treatment of rheumatoid arthritis, the genomic techniques are being rapidly applied to the development of other products for the diagnosis and treatment of the autoimmune disorders.

The fields of allergic diseases and asthma have likewise been enhanced through the study of these genomic assays and have led to a better understanding of genetic susceptibility to and diagnosis of

Table 25-4. Some clinical applications of DNA-based genomic assays to immunology related diseases

Field	Clinical applications
Cancer	Drug discovery Predictive markers of response to new cancer drugs
Infectious diseases and immune deficiency disorders	New rapid diagnostic assays
	New techniques for rapid development of more effective vaccines, e.g., reverse vaccinology (*Chapter 23*)
	New treatments, e.g., palivizumab for RSV
Autoimmune diseases	Identifying therapeutic targets Biomarkers for diagnosis, assessment of disease activity, and response to treatment
Allergic diseases and asthma	Genetic susceptibility diagnostics
	New treatment modalities, e.g., cytokines, anticytokine monoclonal, e.g., omalizumab

Table 25-5. Some examples of new adjuvant therapies for malignant diseases based upon molecular targets and related genetic alterations

Tumor type	Therapeutic agent	Molecular target	Genetic alteration
Hematologic malignancies			
Acute myeloid leukemia	Lestaurtinib	Receptor tyrosine kinase	FLT3
Chronic myelomonocytic leukemia	Sunitinib, imatinib	Receptor tyrosine kinase	PDGFRB
Chronic myeloid leukemia	Lestaurtinib	Nonreceptor tyrosine kinase	JAK2
Solid tumors			
Breast cancer	Lapatinib	Receptor tyrosine kinase	ERBB2
Lung cancer, glioblastoma	Gefitinib, erlotinib	Receptor tyrosine kinase	EGFR
Breast, ovarian cancer	Olaparib	DNA damage or repair	BRCA1, BRCA2

these disorders as well as to the development of new pharmaceutical agents based on pharmacogenetics. Genomic-engineering techniques based upon genomic studies have also resulted in new treatment modalities for the allergic diseases and asthma, e.g., cytokines, anticytokine monoclonal, e.g., omalizumab (*Chapters 11* and *18*).

Acknowledgment. The authors thank Dr. Gilberto Vaughan for his excellent critical review of the chapter.

Key Points

- **DNA** is a double-stranded structure, consisting of two intertwining long chains composed of repetitive nucleotides with backbones made of a 2′-deoxyribose molecule and phosphate groups joined by ester bonds.
- **RNA** displays a similar structure to DNA except that it contains ribose as the 5-carbon sugar linked to the corresponding phosphate group and is usually found as a single-strand structure.
- The nucleobases found in DNA consist of cytosine (C), guanine (G), adenine (A), and thymine (T); the nucleobases found in RNA are cytosine (C), guanine (G), adenine (A), and, substituting for thymine, uracil (U).
- A nucleoside consists of a nucleobase plus a sugar and a nucleotide is composed of a nucleobase, a sugar, and a phosphate group.
- Nucleotide pairing in DNA molecules occurs in complementary fashion where G only binds to C, and A only pairs with T; in RNA, although G-C pairing is maintained as in DNA, since thymine is replaced by uracil (U), A-U base pairing occurs.
- The genome, transcriptome, and proteome are terms that define the flow of genetic information from DNA (the genome) initiated after induction of signals by ligand/membrane-receptor binding to transcription of genetic information from DNA to mRNA (transcriptome), terminating in translation leading to protein synthesis (the proteome).
- The **genetic code** is the set of rules by which information encoded in the genome is translated into the amino acid structure provided by a set of three nucleotide sequences called a codon that specifies a single amino acid in the nascent polypeptide chain.
- Restriction enzyme analysis, hybridization techniques, polymerase chain reaction (PCR), and genetic transformation of mice are all techniques of the new DNA technology that are finding application in diagnosis and treatment of many immunologically related disorders including the infectious diseases, the allergic diseases, the autoimmune disorders, and cancer.

Study Questions/Critical Thinking

1. Each of the following is a true statement concerning the DNA molecule EXCEPT:

   a. A double-stranded structure
   b. Composed of four bases (A, T, C, and G)
   c. Transcribes to mRNA
   d. Activity is inhibited by protein

2. Which of the following is an example of the use of a molecular technique in the diagnosis of Lyme disease:

a. Southern blotting
b. Northern blotting
c. PCR
d. Western blotting

3. The diagnosis of the 22q11.2 deletion syndrome has been facilitated by which of the following DNA-based technologies:

a. Fluorescence in situ hybridization (FISH)
b. Reverse-transcriptase-PCR (RT-PCR)
c. Nucleic acid microarray
d. Southern blotting

4. Each of the following statements regarding the genetic code is correct EXCEPT:

a. Set of rules by which information is encoded in the genome
b. Information is translated into the amino acid structure
c. Transmits information by a triplicate nucleotide sequence
d. The genetic code is identical for each synthesized protein product

5. Each of the following is a true statement concerning DNA technology EXCEPT:

a. Reverse transcriptase involves flow of genetic information from RNA to DNA
b. DNA sequencing involves use of the dideoxy nucleotide method
c. Knock-out mouse is an example of a highly sedated animal
d. Amplification of DNA or RNA involves use of the thermophilic Taq-polymerase

Suggested Reading

Bottema RW, Nolte IM, Howard TD, et al. Interleukin 13 and interleukin 4 receptor-α polymorphisms in rhinitis and asthma. Int Arch Allergy Immunol. 2010; 153: 259–67.

Bouzigon E, Forabosco P, Koppelman GH, et al. Meta-analysis of 20 genome-wide linkage studies evidenced new regions linked to asthma and atopy. Eur J Hum Genet. 2010; 18: 700–6.

Broadhead ML, Clark JC, Dass CR, et al. Microarray: an instrument for cancer surgeons of the future. ANZ J Surg. 2010; 80: 531–6.

Brown JR, Magid-Slav M, Sanseau P, et al. Computational biology approaches for selecting host-pathogen drug targets. Drug Discov Today. 2011; 16: 229–36.

Davis MM. A prescription for human immunology. Immunity. 2008; 29: 835–8.

Hawkins GA, Lazarus R, Smith RS, et al. The glucocorticoid receptor heterocomplex gene STIP1 is associated with improved lung function in asthmatic subjects treated with inhaled corticosteroids. J Allergy Clin Immunol. 2009; 123: 1376–83.

Ishmael FT, Stellato C. Principles and applications of polymerase chain reaction: basic science for the practicing physician. Ann Allergy Asthma Immunol. 2008; 101: 437–43.

Koppelman GH, Meyers DA, Howard TD, et al. Identification of PCDH1 as a novel susceptibility gene for bronchial hyperresponsiveness. Am J Respir Crit Care Med. 2009; 180: 929–35.

Ledue TB, Collins MF, Craig WY. New laboratory guidelines for serologic diagnosis of Lyme disease: evaluation of the two-test protocol. J Clin Microbiol. 1996; 34: 2343–50.

Lehman HK, Hernandez-Trujillo VP, Ballow M. The use of commercially available genetic tests in immunodeficiency disorders. Ann Allergy Asthma Immunol. 2008; 101: 212–8.

Leonardo SM, Harnett MM, Lerch-Gaggl AF, Gauld SB. Fluorescence-based assays as tools for understanding immunologic processes. Ann Allergy Asthma Immunol. 2009; 102: 84–90.

Lipkin WI. Microbe hunting. Microbiol Mol Biol Rev. 2010; 74: 363–77.

Malherbe L. T-cell epitope mapping. Ann Allergy Asthma Immunol. 2009; 103: 76–9.

McDermott U, Downing JR, Stratton MR. Genomics and the continuum of cancer care. N Engl J Med. 2011; 364: 340–50.

Meyers DA. Genetics of asthma and allergy: what have we learned?. J Allergy Clin Immunol. 2010; 126: 439–46.

Moloney M, Shreffler WG. Basic science for the practicing physician: flow cytometry and cell sorting. Ann Allergy Asthma Immunol. 2008; 101: 544–9.

Pang T. Germs, genomics and global public health: How can advances in genomic sciences be integrated into public health in the developing world to deal with infectious diseases? Hugo J. 2009; 3: 5–9.

Pascual V, Chaussabel D, Banchereau J. A genomic approach to human autoimmune diseases. Annu Rev Immunol. 2010; 28: 535–71.

Patel AC. Basic science for the practicing physician: gene expression microarrays. Ann Allergy Asthma Immunol. 2008; 101: 325–32.

Reisdorph NA, Reisdorph R, Bowler R, et al. Proteomics methods and applications for the practicing clinician. Ann Allergy Asthma Immunol. 2009; 102: 523–9.

Rotimi CN, Jorde LB. Ancestry and disease in the age of genomic medicine. N Engl J Med. 2010; 363: 1551–8.

Sanger F, Coulson AR. A rapid method for determining sequences in DNA by primed synthesis with DNA polymerase. J Mol Biol. 1975; 94: 441–8.

Sanger F, Nicklen S, Coulson AR. DNA sequencing with chain-terminating inhibitors. Proc Natl Acad Sci U S A. 1977; 74: 5463–7.

Schuster SC. Next-generation sequencing transforms today's biology. Nat Methods. 2008; 5: 16–8.

Sigal LH. Molecular biology and immunology for clinicians: electrophoresis and western blot/immunoblot analysis. J Clin Rheumatol. 1996; 2: 209–14.

Sigal LH. Molecular biology and immunology for clinicians: DNA polymerase and the polymerase chain reaction. J Clin Rheumatol. 1997; 3: 135–9.

Sigal LH. Molecular biology and immunology for clinicians: electrophoresis and Western blot/immunoblot analysis. J Clin Rheumatol. 1996; 2: 209–14.

Sigal LH. Molecular biology and immunology for clinicians: Nucleic acid electrophoresis techniques: Southern and n blot and restriction fragment length polymorphisms. J Clin Rheumatol. 1996; 2: 331–5.

Sigal LH. Molecular biology and immunology for clinicians: T-cell signal transduction. J Clin Rheumatol. 2002; 8: 113–6.

Slager RE, Hawkins GA, Ampleford EJ, et al. IL-4 receptor α polymorphisms are predictors of a pharmacogenetic response to a novel IL-4/IL-13 antagonist. J Allergy Clin Immunol. 2010; 126: 875–8.

Su HC. The technological transformation of patient-driven human immunology research. Immunol Res. 2009; 43: 167–71.

Thomas DM, Fleming NI, Holloway AJ, et al. Molecular medicine: a clinician's primer on microarrays. Intern Med J. 2004; 34: 565–9.

Appendix 1: Memory Hooks and Acronyms

Memory Hooks

The term "memory hook," as used in this textbook, is arbitrarily defined as a type of mnemonic or device using a pattern of letters that assists the reader in remembering a key event important in immunologic function.

The "Rule of Eights"

A useful mnemonic in remembering the relationship of MHC molecules on antigen-presenting cells (APCs) to either a CD4 or a CD8 T cell is the "rule of eights." Molecules processed by APCs through the "exogenous" pathway present peptides in association with MHC-II and CD4 lymphocytes ($2 \times 4 = 8$). Peptide fragments of proteins that have been processed within the cell through the "endogenous" pathway present peptide in association with MHC-I and CD8 lymphocytes ($1 \times 8 = 8$).

The "Three T's" of Cellular Signaling: Transduction, Transcription, and Translation

The three steps in signaling pathways involved in protein synthesis beginning with the binding of a ligand with a cell surface receptor initiates the first "T," **transduction**, to lead across. This then proceeds to the phosphorlyation of a number of cascading substrate molecules by kinases (i.e., phosphorylases) that result in the ultimate production of a transcription factor that binds to a promoter region of DNA within the nucleus. This then initiates the second "T," **transcription**, to write across, during which messenger RNA (mRNA) is formed. After leaving the nucleus, the mRNA sits on a ribosome within the endoplasmic reticulum and acts as a "blueprint" to initiate the third "T," **translation**, to carry across, culminating in the assembly of amino acids into a final protein

The "A's and C's" (A's for the Fab and C's for the Fc Fragments, Respectively)

This memory hook is designed to help associate specific functions of the **Fab** fragment of the immunoglobulin molecule with the **A's** (amino-terminal half of a heavy chain and one light chain, aberrated amino acid sequence, and antigen-binding or antibody active fragment); and the **Fc** fragment with the **C's** (carboxyl-terminal half of a heavy chain, carbohydrate, crystallizable, constant amino acid sequence, complement fixation, crosses the placenta, and cellular attachment through Fc receptors).

The "Three E's" of Cancer Immunoediting: Elimination, Equilibrium, and Escape

The cancer "immune shaping and editing" process, pioneered by the studies of Robert Schreiber, consists of three phases: **elimination**, **equilibrium**, and **escape.** In the initial **elimination** phase, nascent tumor cells are successfully recognized and eliminated by the immune system. In the **equilibrium** phase, tumor cell growth is controlled but the tumor is not completely eliminated. In this phase, the constant interaction of the immune system with the tumor actually "edits" or "sculpts" the developing tumor, resulting in immunoselection of a tumor that has been shaped into a less immunogenic state that survives. During the **escape** phase, the tumor subverts the immune system either directly through its nonimmunogenic phenotype or indirectly through a variety of immunosuppressive mechanisms, e.g., Treg cells that can paradoxically promote tumor growth.

A mnemonic for purines and pyrimidines

Of the various nucleobases found in DNA (A, G, C, and T) and in RNA (A, G, C, and U), the first two in each molecule are purines (the double-ringed class of molecules) and the last two are pyrimidines (the single-ringed class of molecules) and can be remembered by the mnemonic "**pu**re **a**s **g**old", i.e., **pu**rines, **a**denine, and **g**uanine, and by default the remaining two nucleobases in either DNA, i.e., C and T, or RNA, i.e., C and U, are pyrimidines.

Acronyms That Can Drive You Crazy But That You Will Need to Know

An acronym (Greek, acro, peak, nym, name) is an abbreviation formed from the first letter of a series of words, used since ancient times to construct a quick reference for a more complicated series of words. Throughout this book, each time an acronym is introduced, the full set of words is defined and each initial letter is underlined. Although acronyms at times can be frustrating, particularly when they are not defined, a familiarity with their meanings should facilitate a better understanding of immunology when these acronyms are encountered in other vehicles of communication.

Alphabetized Acronyms in *Immunology IV*

5-LO: F-lipoxygenase
6-APA: 6-aminopenicillanic acid
7TM: seven transmembrane

ABPA: allergic bronchopulmonary aspergillosis
ABVD: adriamycin, bleomycin, vinblastine, dacarbazine
ACE: angiotensin-converting enzyme
ACIP: Advisory Committee on Immunization Practices
ACL: American cutaneous leishmaniasis
ACT: adoptive cell therapy
AD-EDA-ID: autosomal-dominant form of EDA-ID
ADA: adenosine deaminase
ADCC: antibody-dependent cellular cytotoxicity
Ag-Ab: antigen-antibody complex
Ag-Ab-C: antigen-antibody-complement
AGIF: adipogenesis inhibitory factor
AID: activation-induced cytidine deaminase
AIDS: acquired immunodeficiency syndrome
AIM2: absent in melanoma-2
AIRE: autoimmune regulator
AK2: adenylate kinase 2
ALPS: autoimmune lymphoproliferative syndrome
AMD: age-related macular degeneration
ANA: anti-nuclear antibodies
ANC: absolute neutrophil count
ANCA: anti-neutrophil cytoplasm antibody; p-ANCA is a protoplasmic-staining antineutrophil cytoplasmic antibody that shows a perinuclear staining pattern; c-ANCA, or classical antineutrophil cytoplasmic antibody, shows a diffusely granular, cytoplasmic-staining pattern.
Anti-HER: anti-human epidermal growth factor receptor
AP: adapter protein
AP-1: activation protein-1 transcription factor complex
AP-1: activator protein 1
AP3: adaptor-related protein 3
APACHE II: acute physiology and chronic health evaluation II
APAF-1: apoptotic peptidase activating factor
aPC: activated protein C
APC: antigen-presenting cell
APE: apurinic/apyrimidinic endonuclease
APECED: autoimmune polyendocrinopathy-candidiasis-ectodermal dystrophy
APOL1: apolipoprotein L-1
Apo−1 or CD95 or APT 1 or apoptosis antigen 1 or TNFRSF6
ART: antiretroviral therapy
AS: ankylosing spondylitis
ASC: apoptosis-associated speck-like protein containing a CARD
ATLD: ataxia-telangiectasia-like disease
ATM: ataxia telangiectasia mutated
AVP: antiviral proteins

B-CLL: B cell chronic lymphocytic leukemia
BAD: BCL-xL/BCL-2-associated death promoter
BAFF: B cell-activating factor
BAFF-R: B cell-activating factor
BALF: bronchoalveolar lavage fluid
BALT: bronchus-associated lymphoid tissue
BAX: BCL-2-associated X protein
BB: mid-borderline
BCG: Bacille Calmette-Guérin vaccine for tuberculosis
BCL-2: B cell lymphoma 2
BCL-xL: B cell lymphoma extra large
BCR: B cell receptor
BID: baculovirus inhibitor of apoptosis repeat domain
BID: BCL-2-interacting domain
BIRC4: baculoviral IAP repeat-containing protein 4
BL: borderline lepromatous
BLyS: B lymphocyte stimulator
BM: basement membrane
BPA: bronchopulmonary aspergillosis
BPD: bronchopulmonary dysplasia
BPI: bactericidal permeability-increasing protein
BS: Blau syndrome
BSAP: B cell lineage-specific activator protein
BSE: bovine spongiform encephalopathy
BT: borderline tuberculoid
BTK: Bruton's tyrosine kinase

C: constant
c-FLIPs: cellular FLICE-inhibitory proteins
C/EBPε: CCAAT enhancer binding protein epsilon
C1 INH: C1 inhibitor
C4bp: C4-binding protein
CAPS: cryopyrin-associated periodic syndromes
CARD: caspase-recruiting domain
Caspase: cysteine-aspartate proteases
CATCH-22: cardiac defects, abnormal facies, thymic hypoplasia, cleft palate, hypocalcemia, and 22q11 deletions
CBC: complete blood count
CCL: CC chemokine ligand
CCR5: CC chemokine receptor type 5
CD: cluster of differentiation
CD: Crohn's disease
CD2BP1: CD2-binding protein 1
CDC: complement-dependent lymphocytoxicity
cDNA: complementary DNA
CDR: complementarity-determining regions
CEA: carcinoembryonic antigen
CF: complement fixing
CFS: chronic fatigue syndrome
CG: cathepsin G
CGD: chronic granulomatous disease
CH: constant heavy
cHL: classical Hodgkin's lymphoma
CHO: Chinese hamster ovary
CHS: Chediak-Higashi syndrome
cIAPs: cellular inhibitors of apoptosis proteins
CJD: Creutzfeldt-Jacob disease
CL: constant light
CLD: chronic lung disease
CLL: chronic lymphocytic leukemia
CLP: common lymphocyte precursor
CLR: C-type lectin receptors
CMC: chronic mucocutaneous candidiasis
CMI: cell-mediated immunity
CMIS: common mucosal immune system
CML: chronic myelogenous leukemia
CMV: cytomegalovirus
CNS: central nervous system
CNTF: ciliary neurotrophic factor
COPD: chronic obstructive pulmonary disease
COX: cyclooxygenase
CpG: cytosine and guanosine dinucleotide
CpG ODN: synthetic oligodeoxynucleotides containing immunostimulatory CpG motifs
CR: complement receptor
CR3: complement receptor 3
CR4: complement receptor 4
CRAC: Ca++ release-activated Ca++
CRD: carbohydrate-recognition domain
CREM: C-AMP response element modulator
CRH: corticotropin-releasing hormone
Chromosome 22q11.2 deletion syndrome: a syndrome caused by the deletion of a small piece of chromosome 22 which has several presentations, including DiGeorge syndrome (DGS), DiGeorge anomaly, velo-cardio-facial syndrome, Shprintzen syndrome, conotruncal anomaly face syndrome, Strong syndrome, congenital thymic aplasia (CTA), and thymic hypoplasia
CRP: C-reactive protein
CRS: cytokine-release syndrome
CsA: cyclosporine
CSF: colony-stimulating factor
CSF-1: colony-stimulating factor 1
CSF-1-R: macrophage colony-stimulating growth factor 1 receptor precursor
CSP: circumsporozoite surface protein
CSR: class-switch recombination
CT: cholera toxin
CT-B: cholera toxin B

CTHM: conotruncal heart malformations
CTL: cytotoxic T lymphocytes
CTLA: cytotoxic T lymphocyte antigen
CTLA4: cytotoxic T lymphocyte antigen 4
CVID: common variable immunodeficiency
CXCR4: CXC chemokine receptor type 4

DAF: decay-accelerating factor
DAI: DNA-dependent activator of IFN-regulatory factor
DAMP: danger- or damage-associated molecular pattern
DC: dendritic cell
DC-SIGN: dendritic cell-specific intercellular adhesion molecule 3 grabbing non-integrin
DC-SIGN: dendritic cell-specific ICAM3 grabbing non-integrin
DD: death domain
DGS: DiGeorge syndrome
DHR: dihydrorhodamine
DID: double immunodiffusion
DIL: drug-induced lupus erythematosus
DIRA: deficiency of the interleukin-1 receptor antagonist
DISC: death-inducing signaling complex
DLI: donor lymphocyte infusion
DLP: diacyl lipopeptides
DM: diabetes mellitus
DMARD: disease-modifying anti-rheumatic drug
DN: double negative
DNA-PK: DNA-dependent protein kinase
DNA-PKcs: DNA-PK catalytic subunit
DNT: double-negative T cells
DOCK8: dedicator of cytokinesis 8
DP: double positive
DRESS: drug reactions with eosinophilia and systemic symptoms
DSB: double-strand break
dscDNA: double-stranded, complementary DNA
dsRNA: double-stranded RNA
dsSMAC: distal SMAC
DTH: delayed hypersensitivity
DTH: delayed-type hypersensitivity

EA: early antigen
EAE: experimental autoimmune encephalomyelitis or experimental autoimmune encephalitis ; sometimes called experimental allergic encephalomyelitis (EAE)
EBI3: Epstein-Barr virus induced 3
EBNA: EBV nuclear antigen
EBV: Epstein-Barr virus
EC: epithelial cell
ECP: eosinophil cationic protein
ECP: eosinophil cationic peptide
EDN: eosinophil-derived neurotoxin
EGF: epidermal growth factor
EGID: eosinophilic GI disorders
ELISA: enzyme-linked immunosorbent assays
ELISPOT: enzyme-linked immunospot
ENA: extractable nuclear antigens
EPO: eosinophil peroxidase
EPO: erythropoietin
ER: endoplasmic reticulum
ES: excrete or secrete
ESR: erythrocyte sedimentation rate
ETEC: enterotoxigenic *E. coli*
EV: epidermodysplasia verruciformis

Fab: antigen-binding fragment of an immunoglobulin molecule
FACS: fluorescence-activated cell sorter
FADD: Fas-associated death domain
FAE: follicle-associated epithelium
Fas: fragment, apoptosis stimulating
FasL: Fas ligand
Fc: crystallizable fragment of an immunoglobulin molecule
FCAS: familial cold autoinflammatory syndrome
FCM: flow cytometry
FcR: Fc receptors
FGF: fibroblast growth factor
FGFR-1: fibroblast growth factor receptor 1 precursor
FHL: familial hemophagocytic lymphohistiocytosis
FISH: fluorescence in situ hybridization
FL: follicular lymphomas
FLC: free light chain
FLICE: FADD-like IL-1 beta-converting enzyme
FLIP: FLICE inhibitory protein
FLIPI: follicular lymphoma international prognostic index
FLT3-L: FMS-like tyrosine kinase 3 ligand
FMF: familial Mediterranean fever
fMLF: N-formylmethionyl-leucyl-phenylalanine residues receptor
FOXP3: forkhead box P3
FPR1: formyl peptide receptor 1
FSGS: focal segmental glomerulosclerosis

GALT: gut-associated lymphoid tissue
GAS: (IFN) gamma-activated site
GAS: group A streptococci

GC: glucocorticosteroids
GE: granulocyte elastase
GF: growth factor
GH: growth hormone
GI: gastrointestinal
GM-CSF: granulocyte-macrophage colony-stimulating factor
GP: glycoproteins
GPCR: G-protein coupled receptors
GPI: glycophosphatidylinositol
GR: glucocorticoid receptor
Graves' disease: an autoimmune disease caused by autoantibodies (i.e., TSH receptor antibody [TSHR-Ab], also previously called long-acting thyroid stimulator [LATS]) that activate the TSH-receptor (TSHR), thereby stimulating thyroid hormone synthesis and secretion, and thyroid growth, causing a diffusely enlarged goiter
GRE: glucocorticosteroid regulatory element
GU: genitourinary
GVH: graft versus host
GVHD: graft-versus-host disease
GVL: graft versus leukemia

H: hemagglutinin
H-ESKD: hypertension-attributed end-stage kidney disease
HAART: highly active antiretroviral therapy
HAE: hereditary angioedema
HAMA: human anti-mouse antibody
HBsAg: hepatitis B surface antigen
HBV: hepatitis B virus
HC: heavy chain
HDN: hemolytic disease of the newborn
HEV: high endothelial venules
HHV6: human herpes virus 6; causative agent of roseola infantum or sixth disease
HHV8: human herpes virus 8; also known as Kaposi's sarcoma-associated herpesvirus (KSHV), the causative agent of Kaposi's sarcoma (KS)
Hib: *Haemophilus influenzae* type b
HIDS: hyperimmunoglobulin D with periodic fever syndrome
HIGM: hyperimmunoglobulinemia M syndrome
HIV: human immunodeficiency virus
HLA: human leukocyte antigen
HLH: hemophagocytic lymphohistiocytosis also known as hemophagocytic syndrome,
HGM-1: high-mobility group protein B1 encoded by HMGB1; HGM-1 is a cytokine mediator of inflammation secreted by activated macrophages and monocytes HMGB1: high-mobility group box 1, a gene that encodes high-mobility group protein B1 (HGM-1)
HMP: hexose monophosphate pathway or shunt; also known as the pentose phosphate pathway
HPA: hypothalamic-pituitary
HPSII: Hermansky-Pudiak syndrome type II
HPV: human papilloma virus
HPV: hypervariable regions
HRF: homologous restriction factor
HSC: hematopoietic stem cells
HSC/P: hematopoietic stem cell and progenitor
HSCT: human stem cell transplantation
HSP: heat shock proteins
HSP90: heat shock protein 90
HSV: herpes simplex virus
HSV-1 and -2: herpes simplex types 1 and 2
HTLV-1: human T cell leukemia virus-1

i-NANC: inhibitory NANC
i-NOS- inducible nitric oxide synthetase gene
IAP: inhibitor of apoptosis proteins
IBD: inflammatory bowel disease
ICAM: intercellular adhesions molecule
ICAM-3: intercellular adhesion molecule-3
ICF: immunodeficiency with centromeric instability and facial anomalies
ICOS: inducible co-stimulator molecule
IDO: indoleamine 2,3-dioxygenase
IDU: intravenous drug user
IEC: intestinal epithelial cell
IEL: intraepithelial T lymphocytes
IFN: interferon
IFN-γ: interferon-gamma
IFNGR: IFN-gamma receptor
IFNR: interferon receptor
Ig: immunoglobulin
IgD: immunoglobulin D
IgE: immunoglobulin E
IgG- immunoglobulin G
IgH: immunoglobulin heavy chain
IGH@: immunoglobulin heavy chain locus
IgM: immunoglobulin M
IGRA: interferon-gamma release assay
IgSF: immunoglobulin superfamily
IKK: IκB kinase (IKK) is an enzyme complex that inhibits NF-κB kinase; IKK is composed of a heterodimer of the catalytic IKK alpha and IKK beta subunits and a "master" regulatory protein termed NEMO (NF-κB essential modulator) or IKK gamma

IL: interleukin
IL-1: interleukin-1
IL-10: interleukin-10
IL-10 receptor, beta: a subunit for the interleukin-10 receptor; IL10RB is its human gene; L10RB has also recently been designated CDW210B
IL-12: interleukin-12
IL-1β: interleukin-1 beta
IL-1RA: IL-1 receptor antagonist
IL-1RI, -RII: IL-1 type I and II
IL-22BP: interleukin-22 binding protein
IL-2R: interleukin-2 receptor; three protein chains (α, β, and γ) are non-covalently associated to form the IL-2R. The α and β chains are involved in binding IL-2, while signal transduction following cytokine interaction is carried out by the γ-chain, along with the β subunit.
IL-2Ra: IL-2 receptor alpha chain; also called CD25
IL-4: interleukin-4
IL-6: interleukin-6
IL-6R: interleukin-6 receptor, also known as CD126; composed of IL6RA and the shared signaling receptor gp130
IL-6RA: interleukin-6 receptor alpha
IL-8: interleukin-8
ILF: isolated lymphoid follicles
IMC: immature myeloid cell
iNKT: invariant natural killer T cells
iNOS: inducible nitric oxide synthase
IPEX: immune dysregulation, polyendocrinopathy, enteropathy, X-linked
IRAK: IL-1R-associated kinase
IRAK-4: interleukin-1 receptor activated kinase 4
IRF9: IFN-regulatory factor 9
IRIS: immune reconstitution inflammatory syndrome
IRS-1: insulin receptor substrate-1
IS: immunological synapse
ISCOM: immunostimulating complexes
ISRE: IFN-response elements
ITAM: immunoreceptor tyrosine-based activation motifs
ITIM: immunoreceptor tyrosine-based inhibitory motifs
ITK: IL-2-inducible T cell kinase
ITP: idiopathic thrombocytopenic purpura
IVIG: intravenous gamma globulin

J: joining chain
JAK: Janus kinase
JIA: juvenile idiopathic arthritis; formerly called juvenile rheumatoid arthritis (JRA)
JNK: c-Jun N-terminal kinase
JRA: juvenile rheumatoid arthritis; now called juvenile idiopathic arthritis (JIA)

KAR: killer-activating receptor
KD: Kawasaki disease
KIR: killer inhibitory receptors also called killer-cell immunoglobulin-like receptors (KIRs)
KIT: receptor for stem cell factor (SCF)
KSHV-IL6: Kaposi's sarcoma-associated herpes virus interleukin-6-like protein

LAD: leukocyte adherence deficiency
LAD I: leukocyte adhesion deficiency type I
LAD II: leukocyte adhesion deficiency type II
LAD III: leukocyte adhesion deficiency type III
LAM: lipoarabinomannan
LAT: linker for activated T cells
LATS: long-acting thyroid stimulator that is now known as TSH receptor antibody (TSHR-Ab) and is a thyroid-stimulating autoantibody associated with Graves' disease; the autoantibody is reactive against thyroid cell receptors for thyroid-stimulating hormone (TSH) and thus mimics the effects of the hormone.
LBP: LPS-binding protein
LC: light chain of an immunoglobulin molecule
LCF: lymphocyte chemoattractant factor
LCK: leukocyte-specific protein tyrosine kinase
LCM: lymphocytic choriomeningitis virus
LFA: leukocyte function-associate antigens
LFA-1: lymphocyte function-associated antigen-1
LIF: leukemia inhibitory factor
LL: lepromatous leprosy
LMF: lymphocyte mitogenic factor
LOX: lipooxygenase
LP: lamina propria
LPA: lymphocyte proliferation assay
LPG: lipophosphoglycan
LPHD: lymphocyte-predominant Hodgkin's disease
LPS: lipopolysaccharides
Lptn: lymphotactin
LPV: lamina propria venules
LRR: leucine-rich repeat
LT: heat-labile enterotoxin
LT: labile enterotoxin
LT: lethal toxin
LT: leukotrienes
LT: lymphotoxin previously known as tumor necrosis factor-beta
LT-α: lymphotoxin alpha

LT-β: lymphotoxin beta
LTA: lipoteichoic acid
LTBI: latent tuberculosis infection
LTR: lymphotoxin-a receptor
LYST: lysosomal trafficking

M: microfold; usually referring to M cells (or microfold cells) that are found in the follicle-associated epithelium of the Peyer's patch
M cells: also called microfold cells are cells found in the follicle-associated epithelium of the Peyer's patch; they transport organisms and particles from the gut lumen to immune cells across the epithelial barrier, and thus are important in stimulating mucosal immunity
M-CSF: macrophage-CSF
mAb: or moAb, monoclonal antibody
MAC: membrane-attack complex
Mac-1: macrophage-1
MAD proteins: Mothers Against Decapentaplegic, originally defined in Drosophila, are essential components of the signaling pathways of the transforming growth factor-beta receptor family (e.g., TGFBR)
MAdCAM-1: mucosal addressin cell adhesion molecule-1
MAGE: melanoma antigen E
MAIT: mucosal-associated invariant T cells
MALT: mucosa-associated lymphoid tissues
MAMP: microbe-associated molecular pattern
MAP: mitogen-activated protein
MAPK: mitogen-activated protein kinase
MARCO: macrophage receptor with collagenous structure
MASP: MBL-associated proteins
MASP: MBL-associated serine proteases
MBL: mannan-binding lectin, also called mannose-binding lectin
MAVS: mitochondrial antiviral signaling protein
MBP: mannose-binding protein
MC: mast cells
MCP: macrophage chemotactic protein
MCP-3: monocyte chemoattractant protein-3
mda-7: melanoma differentiation-associated-7
MDC: macrophage-derived chemokine
mDC: myeloid dendritic cell
MDSC: myeloid-derived suppressor cells
MEC: mammary-enriched chemokine
MEFV: (Mediterranean fever), a human gene that encodes a protein called pyrin (also known as marenostrin); various mutations of this gene lead to familial Mediterranean fever (FMF)
MGUS: monoclonal gammopathies of undetermined significance
mHA: minor histocompatibility antigen
MHC: major histocompatibility complex
MIF: macrophage migration inhibitory factor
MIP: macrophage inflammatory protein
MLN: mesenteric lymph nodes
MM: multiple myeloma
MMF: mycophenolate mofetil
MMP: matrix metalloproteinases
moAb or mAb: monoclonal antibody
MPO: myeloperoxidase
MR: mannose receptor
MS: multiple sclerosis
MSD: myelodysplastic syndromes, a diverse collection of hematological conditions associated with ineffective production (or dysplasia) of the myeloid class of blood cells
MSM: men who have sex with men
MSP: merozoite surface proteins
MSR: macrophage scavenger receptor
MSU: monosodium urate
MT: microtubules
MTP: metatarsophalangeal
MWS: Muckle-Wells syndrome
MyD88: myeloid differentiation primary-response protein 88
MYO5A: myosin VA
MZ: marginal zone
MZL: marginal zone lymphoma

N: neuraminidase
NACHT: neuronal apoptosis inhibitory protein (NAIP), MHC-II transcription activator (CIITA), incompatibility locus from *P. anserina* (heterokaryon)(HET-E), telomerase-associated protein (TPI)
NAD: nicotinamide adenine dinucleotide
NADPH: nicotinamide adenine dinucleotide phosphate
NAIP: neuronal apoptosis inhibitory protein
NALP: NACHT-LRR and pyrin domain-containing proteins
NALT: nasopharyngeal-associated lymphoid tissue
NANC: nonadrenergic, noncholinergic
NBS: Nijmegen breakage syndrome
NBT: nitroblue-tetrazolium (NBT), an older colorimetric test used previously for the diagnosis of chronic granulomatous disease
NEI: neurologic endocrine immune
NEMO: NF-kB essential modulator

neo: neomycin
NET: neutrophil extracellular traps
NF: nuclear factor
NF-κB: nuclear factor-kappa B, also called nuclear factor kappa-light-chain-enhancer of activated B cells, a protein complex that controls the transcription of DNA
NFAT: nuclear factor of activated cells
NGF: nerve growth factor
NHEJ: nonhomlogous end joining, a pathway that repairs double-strand breaks in DNA; it is referred to as "non-homologous" because the break ends are directly ligated without the need for a homologous template, in contrast to homologous recombination, which requires a homologous nucleotide sequence to guide repair
NHL: non-Hodgkin's lymphoma
NIF: neutrophil inhibitor factor
NK: natural killer cell
NLR: NOD-like receptor
NLRP3: NOD-like receptor (NLR) family, pyrin domain containing 3
NO: nitric oxide
NOD: nucleotide-binding oligomerization domain
NOMID: neonatal onset multisystem inflammatory disease
NOS: nitric oxide synthase
NP: genome nucleoprotein
NSAIDs: non-steroidal anti-inflammatory drugs

OAS: 2',5-oligoadenylate synthetase
OPV: oral poliovirus vaccine
ORF: open reading frame
OS: Omenn syndrome
OSM: oncostatin M

P: properdin
PABA: paraminobenzoic acid
PAF: platelet-activating factor
PALS: periarterial lymphatic sheath
PAMP: pathogen-associated molecular pattern
PAN: periarteritis nodosa
PAN: pyrin and NACHT domain-containing proteins
PANDAS: pediatric autoimmune neuropsychiatric disorders associated with streptococcal infection
PAPA: pyogenic arthritis, pyoderma gangrenosum, and acne
PAX: paired box (PAX) genes, a family of tissue-specific transcription factors
PBSC: peripheral blood stem cells
PC: plasma cell
PCN: penicillin
PCR: polymerase chain reaction
PCT: procalcitonin
pDC: plasmacytoid dendritic cell
PDGF: platelet-derived growth factor
PDGFR: platelet-derived growth factor receptor
PECAM-1: platelet endothelial cell adhesion molecule-1
PEG: polyethylene glycol
PG: prostaglandin
PHA: phytohemagglutinin
PI3P: phosphatidylinositol 3-phospoate
PID: primary immunodeficiency disorders
PIGA: phosphatidylinositol N-acetylglucosaminyltransferase subunit A
PIGR: polymeric immunoglobulin receptor
PKR: interferon-inducible double-stranded RNA-dependent protein kinases
PLCG1: phospholipase C, gamma-1
PLGF: placental growth factor
PMA: phorbol myristate acetate
PMN: polymorphonuclear neutrophils
PNAd: peripheral lymph node addressin
PNH: paroxysmal nocturnal hemoglobinuria
PNP: purine nucleoside phosphorylase
POEMS: polyneuropathy/organomegaly/endocrinopathy/edema/M-protein/skin
Pol II: polymerase II
poly-A: polyadenylation
polyIgR: polymeric Ig receptor
PP: Peyer's patch
PPD: purified protein derivative
PR3: proteinase 3
PRA: panel-reactive antibody
PRR: pattern-recognition receptor or pathogen-recognition receptor
PSTPIP1: porlineserine-theronine phosphate-interacting protein 1
PTB: phosphotyrosine-binding
PTLD: post-transplantation lymphoproliferative disorder
PTX3: pentraxin-related protein
PV: parasitophorous vacuole
PYD: pyrin domain
PYPAF: pyrin domain-containing Apaf1-like proteins

RA: retinoic acid
RA: rheumatoid arthritis
RAB27A: A gene belonging to the small GTPase superfamily, Rab family that encodes a membrane-bound protein, Ras-related protein

Rab-27A that is involved in protein transport and small GTPase-mediated signal transduction. Mutations in this gene are associated with Griscelli syndrome type 2.
RAG: recombinase-activating gene
RAG1 and RAG2: recombination activating gene-1 and -2
RANTES: regulated upon activation normal T cell expressed and secreted
RAR: retinoic acid-binding receptor
RAST: radioallergosorbent test
RBC: red blood cell
RCA: regulators of complement activation
RCC: renal cell carcinoma
REV: regulator of virion
RF: rheumatoid factor
RFLP: restriction fragment length polymorphism
rhG-CSF: recombinant human G-CSF
RIG-I: retinoic-acid-inducible gene I
RLH: RIG-like helicases
RLR: RIG-I-like receptors
RNI: reactive nitrogen intermediates
ROI: reactive oxygen intermediates
RORγ: RAR-related orphan receptor gamma, a transcription factor encoded by the RORC (RAR-related orphan receptor C) gene
ROS: reactive oxygen species
RR: reversal reaction
RS: Reed-Sternberg
RSS: recombination signal sequences
RSV: respiratory syncytical virus
RSV-IGIV: respiratory syncytial virus immune globulin, a sterilized soluble preparation of specific antibody to respiratory syncytial virus (RSV), a virus responsible for serious illness in children
RT: reverse transcriptase
RT-PCR: reverse transcriptase PCR
RTK: receptor tyrosine kinase

SAA: serum amyloid A
SAD: specific antibody deficiency, a primary antibody deficiency disorder that is characterized by normal levels of IgG, IgA, and IgM but an inability to make specific antibodies, most commonly in response to polysaccharide antigens
SALT: skin-associated lymphoid tissue
SAP: serum amyloid P component
SAP: signaling lymphocytic activation molecule (SLAM)-associated protein
SARS: severe acute respiratory syndrome
SBDS: Shwachman-Bodian-Diamond syndrome
SBS: sequencing by synthesis
SBT: sequence-based typing
SC: secretory component
SC: subcutaneous
SCF: stem cell factor
SCFR: mast/stem cell growth factor receptor precursor
SCID: severe combined immunodeficiency
SCIT: subcutaneous immunotherapy
SCN: severe congenital neutropenia
SCT: stem cell transplantation
SED: subepithelial dome
SFK: Src family kinases
SH: Src homology
SH-2: Src homology 2
SHM: somatic hypermutation
SIgA: secretory form of IgA
SIgG: surface IgG
sIL-6R: soluble form of IL-6 receptor
SIRS: systemic inflammatory response syndrome
SLAM: signaling lymphocyte-activation molecule
SLE: systemic lupus erythematosus
SLIT: sublingual immunotherapy
SLL: small lymphatic lymphoma
SLP-76: SH2-containing linking protein of 76 kDa
SMAC: supramolecular activation complexes
SMM: smoldering multiple myeloma
SMS: single molecule sequencing
SNP: single nucleotide polymorphisms
SOCS3: suppressors of cytokine-signaling 3
SOD: superoxide dismutase
SP: single positive T cell; the development of T lymphocytes in the thymus proceeds through multiple, defined steps, each of which is characterized by expression and/or downregulation of distinct cell surface markers, the most prominent of which are double positive (DP) thymocytes that are later positively selected to survive and committed either to CD4 SP or CD8 SP thymocytes as they leave the thymus and populate peripheral lymphoid tissues
SR: scavenger receptors, a group of receptors that recognize modified low-density lipoprotein (LDL) by oxidation or acetylation.
SRS-A: slow-reacting substance of anaphylaxis; now characterized as a mixture of the leukotrienes LTC4, LTD4, and LTE4
ssDNA: single-stranded DNA
SSO: sequence-specific oligonucleotide
ssRNA: single-stranded RNA
ST: heat-stable enterotoxin
STAT: signal tranducer and activator of transcription

STAT3: signal transducer and activator of transcription 3
STAT4: signal transduction and activator of transcription 4
STIM1: stromal interaction molecule 1
sTNF-R: soluble TNF receptor
SVV: small vessel vasculitidities

T1: transitional 1
T1DM: type 1 diabetes mellitus
TAA: tumor-associated antigens
TAB: TAK-1-binding proteins
TACI: transmembrane activator and calcium-modulator and cyclophilin-ligand interactor
TAF: transciption-associated factor
TAK-1: TGF-B-activated kinase-1
TAM: tumor-associated macrophages
TAP: transporter associated with antigen presentation
TAT: transactivator
TATA: tumor-associated transplantation antigens
TBI: total body irradiation
tBID: truncated BID
Tc: T cytotoxic cell, also called CD8+ T cell
TCR: T cell receptor
TD: T-dependent
TEC: thymic epithelial cell
TECK: thymus-expressed cytokine
TEN: toxic epidermal necrolysis
TF: tissue factor, also called platelet tissue factor, factor III, thrombokinase, or CD142; a protein present in subendothelial tissue, platelets, and leukocytes necessary for the initiation of thrombin formation from the zymogen prothrombin
TFII: transcription factor II
TGF-β: transforming growth factor beta
TGS: third-generation sequencing; a method for sequencing single DNA molecules without the need to halt between read steps
Th: T helper cell
Th1: T helper 1 cell
Th17: T helper 17 cell
Th2: T helper 2 cell
TI: T-independent
TIL: tumor-infiltrating lymphocytes
TIMP: tissue inhibitors of metalloproteinase
TIR: Toll-IL-1 related
TK: tyrosine kinase
TKY2: tyrosine kinase 2
TL: tuberculoid leprosy
TLP: triacyl lipopeptides
TLR: Toll-like receptor
Tm: memory T
TMP/SMX: trimethoprim/sulfamethoxazole
TNF: tumor necrosis factor; usually refers to tumor necrosis factor-alpha
TNF-α: tumor necrosis factor-alpha
TNF-R: TNF receptor
TORCH: toxoplasma, rubella, cytomegalovirus, and herpes viruses
TR1: Treg1 cell
TRADD: TNFR-associated death domains
TRAF: TNF receptor-associated factors
TRAF2: TNF receptor-associated factor 2
TRAF6: TNF receptor-associated factor 6
TRAIL: TNF-related apoptosis-inducing ligand
TRAIL-R: TNF-related apoptosis-inducing ligand receptor
TRAPS: TNFR1-associated periodic syndromes
TREC: T cell receptor-excision circle
Treg: T regulatory cell
TRIF: Toll/IL-1 receptor domain-containing adaptor protein-inducing IFN
TSA: tumor-specific antigens
TSE: transmissible spongiform encephalopathies
TSH: thyroid-stimulating hormone
TSHR-Ab: TSH receptor antibody
TSI: thyroid-stimulating immunoglobulins; these antibodies formerly called LATS are found in patients with Graves' disease and activate thyroid cells by binding to the thyroid cells in a longer and slower way than the normal thyroid-stimulating hormone (TSH), leading to an elevated production of thyroid hormone
TSLP: thymic stromal-derived lymphopoietin
TSLS: toxic shock-like syndrome
TSS: toxic shock syndrome
TST: tuberculin skin test

UC: ulcerative colitis
UNC: mutations, originally described in the nematode *Caenorhabditis elegans*, causing locomotory defects, i.e., uncoordinated or UNC mutants
UNC-93B deficiency: an autosomal-recessive defect in innate immunity that results in increased susceptibility to herpes simplex (HSV) encephalitis
UNG: uracil DNA glycosylase

V: variable
V(D)J: variable (diversity) joining
VAD: vincristine adriamycin dexamethasone
VAHS: virus-associated hemophagocytic syndrome

VAPP: vaccine-associated paralytic poliomyelitis
VCA: viral capsid antigen
VCAM: vascular cell adhesion molecules
VCAM-1: vascular cell adhesion molecule-1
VCFS: velo-cardio-facial syndrome; also called Shprintzen syndrome (see chromosome 22q11.2 deletion syndrome)
vCJD: variant CJD
VEGF: vascular endothelial growth factor
VH: variable heavy chain of an immunoglobulin molecule
VIP: vasoactive intestinal peptide
VL: variable light chain of an immunoglobulin molecule
VLA: very late antigen
VLA-4: very late antigen-4
VSG: variant surface glycoproteins
VSP: variant surface protein
VZV: varicella zoster virus

WAS: Wiskott-Aldrich syndrome
WASP: Wiskott-Aldrich syndrome protein
WBC: white blood cell
WHIM: warts, hypogammaglobulinemia, infections caused by HPV and myelokathexis
WSXWS: tryptophan-serine-X-tryptophan-serine motif

X-HIM: X-linked hyper-IgM syndrome
XIAP: X-linked inhibitor of apoptosis protein
XL-EDA-ID: X-linked anhydric ectodermal dysplasia with immunodeficiency
XLA: X-linked agammaglobulinemia; also called Bruton type agammaglobulinemia
XLF: XRCCR-like factor, also known as Cernunnos, a protein encoded by the human NHEJ1 gene required for the non-homologous end-joining (NHEJ) pathway of DNA repair
XLN: X-linked form of severe congenital neutropenia
XLP: X-linked lymphocyte proliferative syndrome
XLT: X-linked thrombocytopenia
XMRV: xenotropic murine leukemia virus-related virus

ZAP-70: zeta-associated protein of 70 kDa

Appendix 2: Common Cytokines and Chemokines

Table A2.1 Growth factors

Growth Factors	MW (KDa)	Receptors	Chromosome location	Cell sources	Property/function	Disease association
G-CSF	19	G-CSFR	17q21	Fibroblasts, macrophages, endothelial cells, and BM stromal cells	Stimulates neutrophil development and release from BM	Elevated in acute infections and produced by various tumors
GM-CSF	22	CD116 and βc subunit	5	Macrophages, T cells, and endothelial cells	Differentiation of myeloid DC and other myeloid cells	Idiopathic pulmonary alveolar proteinosis due to GM-CSF deficiency
M-CSF/CSF1	44	CSF-1R/ c-Fms	5	T cells, osteoblasts, BM stroma, monocytes, endothelial cells, fibroblasts, and smooth muscle cells	Stimulates monocyte and myocyte development	Deficient in osteopetrosis; elevated in chronic inflammation
TGF-β1	25	TGF-βR I and II	19q13	Chondrocytes, Treg and Th3 cells, and monocytes	Anti-inflammatory; inhibits immune cells; switch to IgA production	
MIF	12.5	MIF-R	22q11.2	Pituitary cells, T cells, monocytes, and eosinophils	Inhibits macrophage migration; activates macrophages; proinflammatory	
SCF/c-kit ligand		c-kit	12q22-q24	Stromal cells, fibroblasts, endothelial cells, epithelial cells, smooth muscle cells, mast cells, and eosinophils	Stimulates germ cells, melanocytes, BM progenitor cells, mast cells, and eosinophils	Elevated in allergic and asthmatic inflammation
Flt3 ligand	31/45	Flt3	19q 13.3	Myeloid cells, endothelial cells, stromal cells, and by most tissues	Stimulates pluripotent hematopoietic stem cells, lymphoid, and myeloid progenitor cells	Elevated and mutated in leukemia

Table A2.2. Lists of cytokines and chemokines

Interleukins				
Family	**Structure**	**MWkDa**	**Members**	**Other names**
IL-1 family	Heterodimers and homodimer	17	IL-1F1 IL-1F2 IL-1F3 IL-1F4 IL-1F5 IL-1F6 IL-1F7 IL-1F8 IL-1F9 IL-1F10 IL-1F11	IL-1α IL-1β IL-1Ra IL-18, IFN-γ-inducing factor IL-36RA = IL-36Ra IL-36α, IL-1Rrp2 See IL-37 IL-36β, IL-1Rrp2 IL-36γ, IL-1Rrp2 IL-1H (IL-38) IL-1ε, IL-1Hy2, IL-33
IL-1Ra (antagonist)	Heterodimer	16.1-20 kd		
IL-2	Monomer	15.5 kd		
IL-3	Monomer	15 kd		
IL-4	Monomer	15 kd		
IL-5	Homodimer	15 kd		
IL-6 family	Homodimer	19-26 kd	IL-6, See LIF See OSM See CT-1 See IL-11 See IL-31 and CLC	
LIF	Monomer			
OSM (oncostatin M)	Monomer			
IL-7	Monomer	25 kd	IL-7 See TSLP	

Receptors	Cell sources	Property/function	Disease association
IL-1RI, IL-1RII IL-18R IL-36R IL-36R IL-18R(?) IL36R IL-36R ? ST-2	Macrophages, monocytes, lymphocytes, keratinocytes, microglia, megakaryocytes, neutrophils, fibroblasts, synovial lining cells, epithelial cells	Agonist Agonist Receptor antagonist (IL1R1) Agonist IL-36R antagonist Agonist Anti-inflammatory Agonist Agonist Receptor antagonist (?) Agonist	Wide range of autoimmune, e.g., RA, IBD, psoriasis, and febrile autoinflammatory diseases, e.g., FMF, gout, type II diabetes
IL-1RI	Monocytes, macrophages, fibroblasts, neutrophils, endothelial and epithelial cells, keratinocytes	Antagonism of IL-1	Deficient in a wide range of autoimmune and inflammatory diseases, e.g., RA, IBD, psoriasis
IL-2Rα, β, γ (CD25, CD122β) CD132 (γ)	CD4 and CD8 activated T cells, DCs, NK cells, NKT cells	Proliferation of effector T and B cells, development of Treg cells, differentiation and proliferation of NK cells and growth factor for B cells	Deficient in T cell-mediated autoimmune and inflammatory diseases, X-linked severe combined immunodeficiency
IL-3Raβ = IL-3Raβc (CD123)	T cells, macrophages, NK cells, mast cells, eosinophils, stromal cells	Hematopoietic growth factor, activation of basophils and eosinophils	Role in allergic diseases, different types of cancers, lymphocytic and acute myeloid leukemias
IL-4R type I, IL-4R type II (CD124, CD132γ)	Th2 cells, basophils, eosinophils, mast cells, NKT cells, g/d T cells	Induction of Th2 differentiation, IgE class switch, upregulation of class II MHC expression on B cells, upregulation of CD23 and IL-4R, survival factor for B and T cells, role in tissue adhesion and inflammation	Inflammatory and autoimmune diseases (allergy/asthma and diabetes mellitus), chronic lymphocytic leukemia
IL-5R (CD125, βc)	Th2 cells, activated eosinophils and mast cells, Tc2 cells, g/d T cells, NK and NKT cells, CD4- ckit- CD3e-IL2Ra- (Peyer's patches)	Differentiation and function of eosinophils, remodeling and wound healing	Allergy/asthma, hypereosinophilic syndrome
IL-6R, (sIL-6R) (CD126, gp130)	Endothelial cells, fibroblasts, monocytes/ macrophages, T cells	Liver: synthesis of acute phase proteins; leukocytes: trafficking, activation; T cell: differentiation, activation, survival; B cell: differentiation, and growth, production of IgG, IgM, IgA hematopoiesis	Autoimmune disease, chronic inflammatory disease, B cell malignancy, SLE, JRA, Castleman disease, plasmacytoma/ multiple myeloma Fever
LIFR with gp130	Bone marrow stroma, fibroblasts	Maintains embryonic stem cells	
OSMR or LIFR with gp130	T cells, macrophages	Stimulates Kaposi's sarcoma	Kaposi's sarcoma
IL-7R and sIL-7R (CD127, CD132γ)	Epithelial cells, keratinocytes, DCs, B cells, and monocytes/ macrophages, stromal cells	Proliferation of pre-T, T, pre-B and pro-B cells (mice), megakaryocytes maturation, VDJ recombinations, naïve T cell survival, synthesis induction of inflammatory mediators in monocytes	Allergy/autoimmunity and psoriasis

(continued)

Table A2.2. Lists of cytokines and chemokines (continued)

Interleukins				
Family	**Structure**	**MWkDa**	**Members**	**Other names**
TSLP	Monomer	15kd		
IL-8	Homodimer	16 kd		
IL-9	Monomer	14 kd		
IL-10	Homodimer	20.5 kd		
IL-11	Monomer	19 kd		
IL-12 (p35/p40)	Heterodimer	35 kd and 40 kd		
IL-13	Monomer	10 kd		
IL-14 (Since no studies have identified the IL-14 gene, IL-14 is nonexistent at the present time.)				
IL-15	Monomer	14–15 kd		

Receptors	Cell sources	Property/function	Disease association
IL7Rα and TSLP-R	Epithelial cells, especially lung and skin	Stimulates hematopoietic and somatic cells, activates dendritic cells; Th2 polarizing	Elevated in Netherton syndrome and atopic disease Inducer of allergic diseases
CXCR1 and CXCR2	Monocytes, macrophages, neutrophils, lymphocytes, endothelial cells, epithelial cells, fibroblasts, keratinocytes, chondrocytes, synovial cells, hepatocytes	Chemoattractant for neutrophils, NK cells, CD8 T cells, basophils, eosinophils; mobilization of hematopoietic stem cells; angiogenesis	Increased levels during Inflammatory diseases (RA, psoriasis, bacterial and viral infections)
IL-9R (CD132γ)	Th2, Th9, mast cells, eosinophils	Th2 and mast cells, growth factor, inhibition of Th1 cytokines, IgE production, chemokine and mucus production in bronchial epithelial cells	Helminth infections, Hodgkin lymphoma, asthma, food allergy
IL-10R1/IL-10R2 complex (IL-10Rα, IL-10Rβ)	T cells, B cells, monocytes, macrophages, DCs	Immune suppression	Cancer, allergy, deficient in autoimmune and autoinflammatory disorders
IL-11Ra 1 (IL-11R, CD130)	Stromal cells: fibroblasts, epithelial cells, endothelial cells, vascular smooth muscle cells, synoviocytes, osteoblasts	Growth factor for myeloid, erythroid, and megakaryocyte progenitors; bone remodeling; protects epithelial cells and connective tissue; induction of acute-phase protein; inhibition of macrophage activity; promotion of neuronal development	Increased during allergic asthma
IL-12Rb1 and IL-12Rb2	Monocytes, macrophages, neutrophils, microglia, DCs, B cells	Induce Th1 cell differentiation and cytotoxicity; activation of NK cells, polarization to Th1 cells	In deficiency, there is Impaired Th1 response with higher susceptibility to intracellular pathogens; used as a potential anticancer agent
IL-13R1a1 and IL-13R1a2	T, NKT, and mast cells, basophils, eosinophils	Switching to IgG4 and IgE, Th2 polarization, upregulation of CD23, MHC-II on B cells, induction of CD11b, CD11c, CD18, CD29; CD23 and MHC-II on monocytes, activation of eosinophils and mast cells, recruitment and survival of eosinophils	Asthma, allergic rhinitis, fibrosis, defense against parasite infections
IL-15Rα, IL2Rβ (CD122, CD132γ)	Monocytes, keratinocytes, skeletal muscle cells, non-T cells	T cell activation, proliferation and activation of NK cells, differentiation of g/d T cells, suppression of IL-2 induced AICD of T cells, homeostasis of CD8 memory T cells, NK and NKT cells, enhancement of Th2 differentiation, and suppression of allergic rhinitis	Autoimmune and inflammatory diseases

(continued)

Table A2.2. Lists of cytokines and chemokines (continued)

Interleukins				
Family	**Structure**	**MWkDa**	**Members**	**Other names**
IL-16	Homotetramer	56 kd		
IL-17A	Cysteine knot, homodimer, or heterodimer	35 kd		
IL-17B, C, D	Cysteine knot, homodimer	41 kd, 40 kd, 52 kd		
IL-17F	Cysteine knot, Homodimer, or heterodimer	44 kd		
IL-18	Heterodimer	22.3 kd	IL-1F4	
IL-19	Monomer	20.5 kd		
IL-20	Monomer	17.5 kd		
IL-21	4-helix bundle, monomer	15 kd		
IL-22	6 antiparallel ahelices, monomer	23 kd		
IL-23 (p19p40)	Heterodimer	IL-12b p40, 40 kd; IL-23 p19, 19 kd		
IL-24	Homodimer and monomer	18 kd, unglycosylated mature protein; 35 kd, observed size of secreted IL-24, glycosylated		
IL-25 (IL-17E)	Homodimer	17 kd		

Receptors	Cell sources	Property/function	Disease association
CD4	T cells, mast cells, eosinophils, monocytes, DCs, fibroblasts, epithelial cells	Chemotaxis of CD4+ T cells, modulation of T cell response	Increased during various inflammatory and infectious diseases including atopic eczema, allergic asthma, Crohn's disease, RA, hepatitis C infection, and tuberculosis; inhibits HIV infection
IL-17RAR (sIL-17R) (CD217)	Th17 cells, CD8+ T cells, NK cells, NKT cells, g/d T cells, neutrophils	Induction of proinflammatory cytokines, chemokines, and metalloproteases; recruitment of neutrophils	RA, MS, IBD, psoriasis, allergic asthma, atopic dermatitis, contact hypersensitivity
For IL-17B, IL-17RB (sIL-17H1, IL25R); for IL-17C and D, not known	IL-17B: neuronal cells, chondrocytes; IL-17C: immune cells under certain conditions; IL-17D; resting B and T cells	Induction of proinflammatory cytokines, chemokines, and metalloproteases; IL-17B: chondrogenesis and osteogenesis	RA, allergic asthma, inflammatory cardiomyopathy, Wegener's granuloma
IL-17RA (5IL-17R) (CD217) and IL-17RC (sIL-17RL)	Th17 cells, CD8+ T cells, NK cells, NKT cells, g/d T cells, neutrophils	Induction of proinflammatory cytokines, chemokines, and metalloproteases; recruitment of neutrophils	IBD, psoriasis, allergic asthma
IL-18R	Mainly macrophages, Kupffer cells, keratinocytes, osteoblasts, astrocytes, DCs	Induction of IFN-γ in synergy with IL-12, enhances NK cell cytotoxicity, promoting Th1 or Th2 cell responses depending on cytokine milieu; inhibits Tregs	Autoimmune diseases or inflammatory disorders, RA, psoriasis, MS, type I diabetes
IL20Rα, IL-10Rβ	Monocytes, keratinocytes, airway epithelial cells, and B cells	Proinflammatory activator of monocytes; favors Th2 immunity	Psoriasis
IL-20R1/IL-10Rβ and IL-22R1/IL-10Rβ	Monocytes, fibroblasts, keratinocytes, epithelial and endothelial cells	Keratinocyte proliferation and TNF production; expands hematopoietic progenitors	Psoriasis, RA, atherosclerosis
IL-21R, CD132γ	T cells (predominantly Th17), NKT cells	Regulation of T, B, and NK cell proliferation, differentiation, apoptosis, antibody isotype balance, cytotoxic activity	Cancer, SLE, RA
IL-10R2 chain and IL-22R1 chain	Activated T cells (predominantly Th17), NKT cells, macrophages; also Th22 cells	Pathogen defense, wound healing, epithelial tissue reorganization, stimulates non-leukocytes	Psoriasis, IBD, cancer
IL-12Rb1 and IL-23R	Macrophages, activated DCs	Stimulates production of proinflammatory IL-17 and promotes memory Th17 T cell proliferation	Susceptibility to extracellular pathogens, exacerbate organ-specific autoimmune inflammation
IL-20R1/IL-20R2 and IL-22R1/IL-10Rβ	Melanocytes, T cells, monocytes, keratinocytes	Tumor suppression, wound healing; stimulates non-hematopoietic tissues	Melanoma, psoriasis
IL-17RA and IL-17RB	Th2 cells, mast and epithelial cells, eosinophils and basophils from atopic individuals	Induction of Th2 responses, IgE, IgG1, IL-4, IL-5, IL-13, and IL-9 production	Gastrointestinal disorders, asthma

(continued)

Table A2.2. Lists of cytokines and chemokines (continued)

Interleukins				
Family	**Structure**	**MWkDa**	**Members**	**Other names**
IL-26	6 α-helices, homodimer	38 kd		
IL-27 (p28 and EBI3)	Heterodimer	IL-27a p28, 28 kd; IL-27b EBI3, 25.4 kd		
IL-28A/B/IL-29 (IFNIλ family)	Monomer	IL-28A, 22.3 kd; IL-28B, 22.2 kd; IL-29, 21.9 kd		
IL-30 (p28 subunit of IL-27)		28Kd		
IL-31	4-helix bundle	24 kd		
IL-32	Unknown	14.9–26.6 kd		
IL-33	β-trefoil fold	30 kd (active form, 18 kd)		IL-1F11
IL-34	Homodimer	39 kd monomers		
IL-35 (p35 and EBI3)	Heterodimer	60 kd		
IL-36α IL-36β IL-36γ				IL-1F6, 8 of 9
IL-36Ra				IL-1F5
IL-37	Homodimer	17–24 kd		IL-1F7

Receptors	**Cell sources**	**Property/function**	**Disease association**
IL-10R2 chain and IL-20R1 chain	Activated T cells (predominantly Th17), NKT cells, mast cells	Activation and regulation of epithelial cells, proinflammatory	
WSX-1 and gp130	Activated DCs, macrophages, epithelial cells	Induction of Tbet promoting Th1 cell differentiation, inhibition of Th17-cell response via STAT1; also induces IL-10	Immune pathology because of uncontrolled inflammatory response
IL-28R1/IL-10R2	Monocyte-derived DCs	Antiviral immunity	Role in allergic, autoimmune, and infectious diseases
	Dendritic cells	Th1 polarizing	
IL-31RA/OSMRb	Activated CD4 T cells (mainly Th2) and CD8 T cells	Induction of IL-6, IL-8, CXCL1, CXCL8, CC chemokine ligand 2, and CC chemokine ligand 8 production in eosinophils, upregulates chemokine mRNA expression in keratinocytes, expression of growth factors and chemokines in epithelial cells, inhibition of proliferation and apoptosis in epithelial cells	Atopic dermatitis, allergic contact dermatitis, prurigo nodularis, chronic spontaneous urticaria, nonatopic eczema, asthma, other inflammatory disorders
Unknown	Monocytes, macrophages, NK cells, T cells, fibroblasts, epithelial cells	Induction of TNF-a, IL-8, and IL-6, by macrophage and T cells, apoptosis	RA, IBD, autoimmune diseases
ST2	Necrotic cells and nuocytes (innate effector leukocyte that mediates type 2 immunity), endothelial cells, and other somatic cells	Transcriptional repressor activity, induction of Th2 inflammation by mast cells and eosinophils	Autoimmune and cardiovascular diseases, asthma, gastrointestinal tract
CSF1R	Heart, brain, liver, kidney, spleen, thymus, testes, ovary, small intestine, prostate, colon; most abundant in spleen	Proliferation of myeloid progenitor cells	
Unknown	Treg cells	Proliferation of Treg cells and inhibition of Th17 cell function, suppression of inflammatory responses	IBD, collagen-induced arthritis
IL-1Rrp2 and accessory protein (AcP)	Skin and monocytes	Macrophages and dendritic cells	Elevated in skin inflammation
IL-1Rrp2 and accessory protein (AcP)		Antagonist of IL-36	
IL-18Ra ?	Monocytes, tonsil plasma cells, breast carcinoma cells, dendritic and epithelial cells	Suppression of proinflammatory cytokines and inhibition of DC activation; synergizes with TGF-β	RA

(continued)

Table A2.2 Lists of cytokines and chemokines (continued)

Chemokines				
Family	**Structure**	**MWkDa**	**Members**	**Receptors**
C	Cysteine-rich proteins (C-C)	8–14 KD	Lymphotactin XCL1 XCL2	XCR1
CC	Cysteine-rich proteins (C-CC-C)	8–14 KD	CCL1 (I-309)	CCR8
			CCL2 (MCP-1	CCR2
			CCL3 (MIP-1α)	CCR1, 5
			CCL4 (MIP-1β)	CCR5>1
			CCL5 (RANTES)	CCR1, 3, 5
			CCL6 (MRP-1 of mice)	CCR1
			CCL7 (MCP-3)	CCR1, 2, 3, 5, 10
			CCL8 (MCP-2)	CCR2, 3, 5>1
			CCL9/CCL10 (MRP-2)	CCR1
			CCL11 (eotaxin)	CCR3>5
			CCL12 (MCP-5 in mice)	CCR2
			CCL13 (MCP-4)	CCR1, 2, 3>5
			CCL14a (HCC-1)	CCR1, 5
			CCL14b (HCC-3)	?
			CCL15 (HCC-2)	CCR1, 3
			CCL16 (HCC-4; LEC)	CCR1, 2, 5
			CCL17 (TARC)	CCR4>8
			CCL18 (PARC)	?
			CCL19 (ELC)	CCR7
			CCL20 (LARC)	CCR6
			CCL21 (SLC)	CCR7
			CCL22 (MDC)	CCR4
			CCL23 (MPIF-1)	CCR1, 5
			CCL24 (Eotaxin 2)	CCR3
			CCL25 (TECK)	CCR9
			CCL26 (Eotaxin 3)	CCR3
			CCL27(CTACK)	CCR10
			CCL28(MEC)	CCR10>3
CXC	Cysteine-rich proteins (C-CXC-C)	8–14 KD	CXCL1 (Groα) CXCL2 (Groβ) CXCL3 (Groγ)	CXCR2
			CXCL4 (PF4)	CXCR3β
			CXCL5 (ENA78)	CXCR2>1
			CXCL6 (GCP2)	CXCR2>1
			CXCL5 (NAP2)	CXCR2
			CXCL8 (IL-8)	CXCR1, 2

Cell sources	Property/function	Disease association
	Attracts T cell (CD4+) and precursors; homeostatic function	
Monocytes, Th2>Th1 cells, neutrophils	Induce the migration of monocytes and other cell types such as NK cells, dendritic cells, T and B cells, eosinophils, and basophils	Proinflammatory; RANTES, MIP-1α, and MIP-1β can suppress HIV infection
Monocytes, DCs, Th2>Th1, NK cells		
Monocytes, DCs, Th1>Th2, NK cells, basophils, eosinophils, fibroblasts		
Monocytes, DCs, Th1>Th2, NK cells basophils, eosinophils, B cells		
Monocytes, DCs, Th1>Th2, NK cells, basophils, eosinophils		
T, B lymphocytes, macrophages, NK cells		
Monocytes, Th2>Th1 cells, NK cells, eosinophils, basophils, DCs	Inflammatory	
	Inflammatory	
Monocytes, PMNs, T cells, adipocytes	Allergic reactions	
Th2 T cells, eosinophils, basophils, mast cells		
Monocytes, T and B cells, eosinophils	Inflammatory	
Monocytes, Th2>Th1 cells, basophils, eosinophils, DCs		
Monocytes, T cells, eosinophils	Homeostatic	
Monocytes	Inflammatory	
Monocytes, T cells, eosinophils, DCs	Homeostatic	
Monocytes, T cells, NK cells, DCs	Homeostatic	
Th2 cells, Treg cells, thymocytes, DCs	Anti-inflammatory	
B cells, naïve T cells, DCs	Inflammatory	
T and B cells, NK cells, mature DCs	Activation of T cells, inflammatory	
Immature DCs, Th17 cells, NK and B cells		
T and B cells, NK cells, mature DC cells	Inflammatory	
Th2 cells, Treg cells, DCs, thymocytes	Activation of T cells, inflammatory	
PMNs, macrophages, T cells		
T cells, eosinophils, basophils, monocytes	Anti-inflammatory	
Thymocytes, T cells and monocytes, DCs	Allergic reactions	
Eosinophils, basophils	Mucosal inflammation, homeostatic in thymus	
CLA+ memory T cells, B cells		
Naïve T cells, eosinophils, IgA+ B cells	Allergic reaction	
	Skin inflammation	
Effects mainly on neutrophils and to a lesser extent on monocytes, lymphocytes, ECs, basophils, eosinophils, fibroblasts, melanocytes	Inflammatory, angiogenic	
	Inflammatory, angiogenic	
	Inflammatory, angiogenic	
Inhibits PMN adherence to ECs	Homeostaic and anti-angiogenic	
PMNs, epithelial cells, endothelial cells	Inflammatory, angiogenic	
PMNs, epithelial cells, endothelial cells	Inflammatory, angiogenic	
PMNs, epithelial cells, endothelial cells, mast cells	Inflammatory, angiogenic	
PMNs, basophil, CD8 T cell, epithelial cells (macrophage adhesion), endothelial cells	Inflammatory, angiogenic	

(continued)

Table A2.2 Lists of cytokines and chemokines (continued)

Chemokines				
Family	**Structure**	**MWkDa**	**Members**	**Receptors**
			CXCL9 (MIG) CXCL10 (IP10) CXCL11 (I-TAC)	CXCR3
			CXCL12 (SDF-1)	CXCR4, 7
			CXCL13 (BLC/BCA1)	CXCR5>3
			CXCL14 (BRAK)	?
			CXCL15 (Lungkine)	?
			CXCL16 (SEXCKINE)	CXCR6
CX_3 C	Cysteine-rich proteins (C-CXXXC-C)	8–14 KD	CX3CL1 (fractalkine)	CX3 CR1

Interferons					
Family	**Structure**	**MWkDa**	**Members**	**Other names**	**Receptors**
IFN-γ	Homodimer	34 kd			Interferon-gamma receptor is a heterodimer of IFNGR1 (CD119) and IFNGR2
IFN-α	Monomer	19–26 kDa	IFNA1, IFNA2, IFNA4, IFNA5, IFNA6, IFNA7, IFNA8, IFNA10, IFNA13, IFNA14, IFNA16, IFNA17, IFNA21		Interferon-α/β receptor (IFNAR) is a heteromeric receptor composed of one chain with two subunits referred to as IFNAR1 (CD118) and IFNAR2
IFN-β	Monomer in vivo, homodimer in vitro	20 kDa			Interferon-α/β receptor (IFNAR) is a heteromeric receptor composed of one chain with two subunits referred to as IFNAR1 (CD118) and IFNAR2

Cell sources	Property/function	Disease association
Th1>Th2 cells, NK cells (inhibit epithelial cells), B cells	Inflammatory, lymphocyte attractants, anti-angiogenic	
Most leukocytes, T and B lymphocytes, bone marrow progenitor cells, epithelial cells, cerebellar cells, thymocytes, pDCs, iDCs, endothelial cells	Inhibits HIV-1, retention of BM cells, pro-angiogenic, WHIM syndrome warts	
B cells and some T cells, DCs	Homeostatic	
Monocytes, T cells, B cells		
Neutrophils, epithelial, endothelial cells	Pulmonary inflammation	
NKT cells, T cells, endothelial cells		
Acts on monocytes, NK and T cells, PMNs, DCs, astrocytes, and neurons	Homeostatic in CNS; inflammatory elsewhere	

Cell sources	Property/function	Disease association
NK and NKT cells, Th1 cells, CD8 T, and B cells	Weak antiviral properties, promotes cytotoxic activity, Th1 differentiation, upregulation of MHC-I and II, inhibition of cell growth, proapoptotic effects and control of AICD, regulation of local leukocyte endothelial interaction, and enhancement of microbial killing ability by activating macrophages	Promotes antitumor and antibacterial effects and is expressed in autoimmune diseases
Monocytes/macrophages, lymphoblastoid cells, fibroblasts, and a number of different cell types following induction by viruses, nucleic acids, glucocorticoid hormones, and low-molecular-weight substances	Stimulates the production of two enzymes: a protein kinase and an oligoadenylate synthetase; increases MHC-I	Antiviral, antiparasitic, antiproliferative activities; elevated in autoimmune diseases, e.g., SLE
Fibroblasts	p53 is activated in virally infected cells to evoke an apoptotic response and is critical for antiviral defense of the host; increases MHC-I expression	Treatment for multiple sclerosis (MS); antiviral

Table A2.3 The tumor necrosis factor (TNF) superfamily

TNF ligand	Receptor (TNFRSF)	Chromosome location	Cell sources	Property/function	Disease association
Lymphotoxin α1/ TNFβ2 (LTα1β2)	LTβR HVEM	6	T cells, B cells	Cell killing, endothelial cell activation; lymph node development	?
TNF (TNF-α)	TNFR1 (CD120a)/DR2 TNFR2 (CD 120b)		Macrophages, NK cells, T cells	Local inflammation, cytotoxicity, endothelial and Treg cell activation	?
Lymphotoxin (LTα)	TNFR1 TNFR2 HVEM		T cells, B cells	Lymphoid organogenesis	?
LIGHT	LTβR HVEM DcR3	19	Activated T cells, monocytes, NK cells, and DCs	Activates DCs; co-stimulatory of CD8+ T cells	?
CD27L/CD70	CD27		T cells, B cells, NK cells, and BM stem cells	Stimulates T cell and B cell proliferation during the CD70-CD27 interaction with DCs	?
4-1BBL	4-1BB/CD137		DCs, B cells, macrophages	Co-stimulates B cells, mast cells, T cells, and Treg cells	?
FasL	Fas (CD95)/DR1 DcR3	1	T cells, stroma (?)	Proapoptotic, $Ca2^{+}$-independent cytotoxicity, proinflammatory	?
OX40L	OX40/CD134		DCs, macrophages, B cells, EC, NK cells	Co-stimulates activated Teff and Treg cells	?
AITRL /GITRL	AITR/GITR		?	?	?
TL1A (TNFSF15)	DcR3 DR3	9	Endothelial cells, myeloid and T cells	?	IBD (Crohn's disease)
CD30L	CD30		Activated T and B cells, and DCs	Stimulates T and B cell proliferation	?
TRAIL	DR1 DR2 DR3 DR4 OPG	5	T cells, monocytes	Apoptosis of T cells and tumor cells	Antitumor effects
RANKL/OPG-L/ TRANCE	OPG/RANK	13q	Activated T cells and B cells	Stimulated DCs and T cells; activates osteoclasts and resultant bone resorption	Role in bone loss; deficiency results in osteopetrosis
BTLA	HVEM			Coinhibitor of T and B cells	

Table A2.3 The tumor necrosis factor (TNF) superfamily (continued)

TNF ligand	Receptor (TNFRSF)	Chromosome location	Cell sources	Property/function	Disease association
GITRL	GITR		DCs, B cells	Activated T and B cells, Tregs	
BAFF/BLys	TACI BAFFR or BR3 BCMA	13q	Macrophages, DCs, neutrophils, astrocytes	B cell proliferation	Rheumatoid arthritis, SLE, Sjogren's syndrome
APRIL	TACI BCMA	17p	T cells	B cell proliferation	?
TWEAK	TWEAKR/Fn14		Macrophages	Angiogenesis	?
CD40L	CD40	Xq26	T cells, mast cells	B cell activation, class switching	Deficiency results in hyper-IgM syndrome
EDA (A1) EDA (A2)	EDAR XEDAR	Xq12	Ectodermal organs (hair and teeth)	Development of hair, teeth, and exocrine gland	Hypohydrotic ectodermal dysplasia*
B-amyloid precursor protein (APP)	DR6	21	Neurons, axons, hepatocytes	Neuronal death	Alzheimer's disease
NGF (myelin inhibitory factors)	Trk A coupled with p75(NTR)	1p13.1	Neuronal cells, muscle cells, and immune cells	Survival of neurons; proinflammatory	Deficiency results in congenital insensitivity to pain with anhydrosis (CIPA)
BD-NF	Trk B coupled with p75(NTR)	11p13	EC, fibroblasts, epithelial cells	Stimulates neurons and promotes pruritus	Asthma and rhinitis; atopic dermatitis
NT-3	Trk C coupled with p75(NTR)	19q13.3	EC, fibroblasts, epithelial cells	Stimulates neurons and promotes pruritus	Involved in allergies
PGRN (progranulin)/ GEP (granulin-epithelin precursor)/ PCD GF (platelet-derived growth factor)	TNFR1 TNFR2		Epithelial cells, leukocytes, neurons, chondrocytes	Anti-inflammatory; blocks TNF-TNFR-signaling pathways	Inhibits collagen-induced arthritis

* This form of ectodermal dysplasia is seen in two clinical forms of the disease called hypohydrotic ectodermal dysplasia caused by mutations in the ectodysplasin A (EDA) gene (EDA A1 and EDA A2). These clinical entities are not associated with immune deficiency and differ from the X-linked and AD forms of ectodermal dysplasia associated with immune deficiency that is caused by NEMO and IκBα mutations, respectively. All forms of these genetic diseases, however, ultimately lead to defective NF-κB signaling that is responsible for the defective ectodermal development that characterizes these disorders.

Appendix 3: Cluster of Differentiation (CD) Molecules

To access this site, which contains continuously updated information on CD molecules, click on the following link, http://prow.nci.nih.gov/, or access the Web site by the following quick response (QR) code:

PROW Protein Reviews On The Web NCI NCBI

Table A3.1 Common CD molecules

Index of information available from PROW					
Current guides: expanded format including summary sentence and abstract **Past guides:** older guides with excellent information; some data may be dated					
CD molecule	**Alternate names**	**Current guides**	**Past guides**	**Entrez gene**	**Assigning workshop**
CD1a	R4; HTA1	—	CD1a	909	
CD1b	R1	—	CD1b	910	
CD1c	M241; R7	—	CD1c	911	
CD1d	R3	—	CD1d	912	
CD1e	R2	—	CD1e	913	
CD2	CD2R; E-rosette receptor; T11; LFA-2	—	CD2	914	
CD3delta	CD3d	—		915	
CD3epsilon	CD3e	—		916	
CD3gamma	CD3g	—		917	
CD4	L3T4; W3/25	—	CD4	920	
CD5	Leu1; Ly1; T1; Tp67	—	CD5	921	
CD6	T12	—	CD6	923	
CD7	gp40	—		924	
CD8alpha	Leu2; Lyt2; T cell co-receptor; T8	—		925	
CD8beta	Leu2; CD8; Lyt3	—		926	
CD9	DRAP-27; MRP-1; p24	—	CD9	928	
CD10	EC 3.4.24.11; neprilysin; CALLA; enkephalinase; gp100; NEP	—		4311	

(continued)

Reproduced with permission from the National Institute of Health.

Table A3.1 Common CD molecules (continued)

Index of information available from PROW					
Current guides: expanded format including summary sentence and abstract **Past guides:** older guides with excellent information; some data may be dated					
CD molecule	**Alternate names**	**Current guides**	**Past guides**	**Entrez gene**	**Assigning workshop**
CD11a	Alpha L integrin chain; LFA-1 alpha	—	CD11a	3683	
CD11b	Alpha M integrin chain; alpha M-beta 2; C3biR; CR3; Mac-1; Mo1	—	CD11b	3684	
CD11c	Alpha X integrin chain; Axb2; CR4; leukocyte surface antigen p150, 95	—	CD11c	3687	
CDw12	p90-120	—	CDw12	23444	
CD13	APN; EC 3.4.11.2; gp150	—	CD13	290	
CD14	LPS-R	—	CD14	929	
CD15u	Sulphated CD15				HLDA7
CD16a	FCRIIIA	—		2214	
CD16b	FCRIIIB	—		2215	
CDw17	LacCer		CDw17		
CD18	CD11a beta subunit; CD11b beta subunit; CD11c beta subunit; beta 2 integrin chain	—	CD18	3689	
CD19	B4	—	CD19	930	
CD20	B1; Bp35	—		931	
CD21	C3d receptor; CR2; EBV-R	—	CD21	1380	
CD22	BL-CAM; Lyb8	—	CD22	933	
CD23	B6; Blast-2; FceRII; Leu20; low-affinity IgE receptor	—	CD23	2208	
CD24	BA-1; HSA	—	CD24	934	
CD25	IL-2R alpha chain; IL-2R; Tac antigen	—	CD25	3559	
CD26	EC 3.4.14.5; ADA-binding protein; DPP IV ectoenzyme	—	CD26	1803	
CD27	S152; T14	—	CD27	939	
CD28	T44; Tp44	—	CD28	940	
CD29	Platelet GPIIa; VLA-beta chain; beta 1 integrin chain	—		3688	
CD30	Ber-H2 antigen; Ki-1 antigen	—	CD30	943	
CD31	GPiia'; endocam; PECAM-1	—	CD31	5175	
CD32	FCR II; Fc gamma RII	—		2212	
CD33	gp67; p67	—	CD33	945	
CD34	gp105-120	—	CD34	947	
CD35	C3bR; C4bR; CR1; immune adherence receptor	—	CD35	1378	
CD36	GPIIIb; GPIV; OKM5-antigen; PASIV	—	CD36	948	
CD37	gp52-40	—	CD37	951	
CD38	T10; cyclic ADP-ribose hydrolase	—	CD38	952	
CD39		—		953	
CD40	Bp50	—	CD40	958	
CD41	GPIIb; alpha IIb integrin chain	—		3674	
CD42a	GPIX	—	CD42a	2815	
CD42b	GPIb-alpha; glycocalicin	—	CD42b	2811	
CD42c	GPIb-beta	—	CD42c	2812	
CD42d	GPV	—	CD42d	2814	

Table A3.1 Common CD molecules (continued)

Index of information available from PROW					
Current guides: expanded format including summary sentence and abstract **Past guides:** older guides with excellent information; some data may be dated					
CD molecule	**Alternate names**	**Current guides**	**Past guides**	**Entrez gene**	**Assigning workshop**
CD43	gpL115; leukocyte sialoglycoprotein; leukosialin; sialophorin	—	CD43	6693	
CD44	ECMR III; H-CAM; HUTCH-1; Hermes; Lu, In-related; Pgp-1; gp85	—	CD44	960	
CD44R	CD44v; CD44v9	—	CD44R	960	
CD45	B220; CD45R; CD45RA; CD45RB; CD45RC; CD45RO; EC 3.1.3.4; LCA; T200; Ly5	—	CD45	5788	
CD46	MCP	—	CD46	4179	
CD47R	Rh-associated protein; gp42; IAP; neurophilin; OA3; MEM-133; formerly CDw149	—	CD47	961	
CD48	BCM1; Blast-1; Hu Lym3; OX-45	—	CD48	962	
CD49a	Alpha-1 integrin chain; VLA-1 alpha chain	—		3672	
CD49b	Alpha-2 integrin chain; GPIa; VLA-2 alpha chain	—		3673	
CD49c	Alpha-3 integrin chain; VLA-3 alpha chain	—		3675	
CD49d	Alpha-4 integrin chain; VLA-4 alpha chain	—	CD49d	3676	
CD49e	Alpha-5 integrin chain; FNR alpha chain; VLA-5 alpha chain	—		3678	
CD49f	Alpha-6 integrin chain; platelet GPI; VLA-6 alpha chain	—		3655	
CD50	ICAM-3	—	CD50	3385	
CD51	VNR alpha chain; alpha V integrin chain; vitronectin receptor	—		3685	
CD52		—	CD52	1043	
CD53		—	CD53	963	
CD54	ICAM-1	—	CD54	3383	
CD55	DAF	—	CD55	1604	
CD56	Leu19; NKH1; NCAM	—	CD56	4684	
CD57	HNK1; Leu7	—		964	
CD58	LFA-3	—	CD58	965	
CD59	1F-5Ag; H19; HRF20; MACIF; MIRL; P-18; protectin	—	CD59	966	
CD60a	GD3		CDw60		HLDA7
CD60b	9-O-acetyl-GD3		CDw60		HLDA7
CD60c	7-O-acetyl-GD3		CDw60		HLDA7
CD61	CD61A; GPIIb/IIIa; beta 3 integrin chain	—		3690	
CD62E	E-selectin; ELAM-1; LECAM-2	—	CD62E	6401	
CD62L	L-selectin; LAM-1; LECAM-1; Leu8; MEL-14; TQ-1	—	CD62L	6402	
CD62P	P-selectin; GMP-140; PADGEM	—	CD62P	6403	
CD63	LIMP; MLA1; PTLGP40; gp55; granulophysin; LAMP-3; ME491; NGA	—	CD63	967	
CD64	FC gamma RI; FCR I	—	CD64	2209	
CD65	Ceramide-dodecasaccharide; VIM-2				
CD65s	Sialylated CD65; VIM2				
CD66a	NCA-160; BGP	—	CD66a	634	

(continued)

Table A3.1 Common CD molecules (continued)

Index of information available from PROW					
Current guides: expanded format including summary sentence and abstract **Past guides:** older guides with excellent information; some data may be dated					
CD molecule	**Alternate names**	**Current guides**	**Past guides**	**Entrez gene**	**Assigning workshop**
CD66b	CD67; CGM6; NCA-95	—	CD66b	1088	
CD66c	NCA; NCA-50/90	—	CD66c	4680	
CD66d	CGM1	—	CD66d	1084	
CD66e	CEA	—	CD66e	1048	
CD66f	Pregnancy-specific b1 glycoprotein; SP-1; PSG	—	CD66f	5669	
CD68	gp110; macrosialin	—	CD68	968	
CD69	AIM; EA 1; MLR3; gp34/28; VEA	—	CD69	969	
CD70	CD27 ligand; Ki-24 antigen	—		970	
CD71	T9; transferrin receptor	—	CD71	7037	
CD72	Ly-19.2; Ly-32.2; Lyb-2	—		971	
CD73	Ecto-5′-nucleotidase	—	CD73	4907	
CD74	Class II-specific chaperone; Ii; invariant chain	—	CD74	972	
CD75	Lactosamines				HLDA7
CD75s	Alpha-2,6-sialylated lactosamines (formerly CDw75 and CDw76)		CDw75; CDw76		HLDA7
CD77	Pk blood group antigen; BLA; CTH; Gb3		CD77		
CD79a	Ig alpha; MB1	—		973	
CD79b	B29; Ig beta	—		974	
CD80	B7; BB1	—	CD80	941	
CD81	TAPA-1	—	CD81	975	
CD82	4F9;C33;IA4;KAI1; R2	—	CD82	3732	
CD83	HB15	—	CD83	9308	
CD84		—	CD84	8832	
CD85	ILT/LIR family	—	CD85	10859	HLDA7
CD86	B7-2;B70	—	CD86	942	
CD87	uPAR	—	CD87	5329	
CD88	C5aR	—	CD88	728	
CD89	Fc alpha-R; IgA Fc receptor; IgA receptor	—	CD89	2204	
CD90	Thy-1	—	CD90	7070	
CD91	ALPHA2M-R; LRP	—		4035	
CD92	CTL1; formerly CDw92	—	CD92	23446	
CDw93		—	CDw93	23447	
CD94	Kp43	—	CD94	3824	
CD95	APO-1; Fas; TNFRSF6; APT1	—	CD95	355	
CD96	TACTILE	—		10225	
CD97		—	CD97	976	
CD98	4F2; FRP-1; RL-388	—	CD98	4198	
CD99	CD99R; E2; MIC2 gene product	—		4267	
CD100	SEMA4D	—	CD100	10507	
CD101	IGSF2; P126; V7	—	CD101	9398	
CD102	ICAM-2	—	CD102	3384	
CD103	ITGAE; HML-1; integrin alpha E chain	—	CD103	3682	

Table A3.1 Common CD molecules (continued)

Index of information available from PROW					
Current guides: expanded format including summary sentence and abstract **Past guides:** older guides with excellent information; some data may be dated					
CD molecule	**Alternate names**	**Current guides**	**Past guides**	**Entrez gene**	**Assigning workshop**
CD104	Beta 4 integrin chain; TSP-1180; beta 4	—		3691	
CD105	Endoglin	—	CD105	2022	
CD106	INCAM-110; VCAM-1	—		7412	
CD107a	LAMP-1	—	CD107a	3916	
CD107b	LAMP-2	—	CD107b	3920	
CD108	SEMA7A; JMH human blood group antigen; formerly CDw108	—	CD108	8482	
CD109	8A3; E123; 7D1				
CD110	MPL; TPO-R; C-MPL	CD110		4352	HLDA7
CD111	PVRL1; PRR1; HevC; nectin-1; HIgR	CD111		5818	HLDA7
CD112	HVEB; PRR2; PVRL2; nectin-2	CD112		5819	HLDA7
CDw113	PVRL3, nectin-3; poliovirus receptor-related 3; nectin-3	—		25945	HLDA8
CD114	CSF3R; HG-CSFR; G-CSFR	—	CD114	1441	
CD115	c-fms; CSF-1R; M-CSFR	—	CD115	1436	
CD116	GM-CSF receptor alpha chain	—	CD116	1438	
CD117	c-KIT; SCFR	—	CD117	3815	
CD118	LIFR; leukemia inhibitory factor receptor	—		3977	HLDA8
CDw119	IFNgR; IFNgRa	—		3459	
CD120a	TNFRI; p55	—		7132	
CD120b	TNFRII; p75; TNFR p80	—		7133	
CD121a	IL-1R; type 1 IL-1R	—		3554	
CDw121b	IL-1R, type 2	—		7850	
CD122	IL-2R beta	—	CD122	3560	
CD123	IL-3R alpha	—		3563	
CD124	IL-4R	—	CD124	3566	
CDw125	IL-5R alpha	—	CDw125	3568	
CD126	IL-6R	—	CD126	3570	
CD127	IL-7R; IL-7R alpha; p90 Il7 R	—	CD127	3575	
CDw128a	CXCR1; IL-8RA	—		3577	
CDw128b	CXCR2; IL-8RB	—		3579	
CD129	Reserved				
CD130	gp130	—	CD130	3572	
CD131	Common beta subunit	—	CDw131	1439	
CD132	IL2RG; common cytokine receptor gamma chain; common gamma chain	—	CD132	3561	
CD133	PROML1; AC133; hematopoietic stem cell antigen; prominin-like 1	—	CD133	8842	HLDA7
CD134	OX40	—		7293	
CD135	flt3; Flk-2; STK-1	—	CD135	2322	
CDw136	MSP receptor; ron; p158-ron	—	CDw136	4486	
CDw137	4-1BB; ILA	—	CDw137	3604	
CD138	heparan sulfate proteoglycan; syndecan-1	—		6382	

(continued)

Table A3.1 Common CD molecules (continued)

Index of information available from PROW					
Current guides: expanded format including summary sentence and abstract **Past guides:** older guides with excellent information; some data may be dated					
CD molecule	**Alternate names**	**Current guides**	**Past guides**	**Entrez gene**	**Assigning workshop**
CD139		—	CD139	23448	
CD140a	PDGF-R; PDGFRa	—		5156	
CD140b	PDGFRb	—		5159	
CD141	fetomodulin; TM	—	CD141	7056	
CD142	F3; coagulation factor III; thromboplastin; TF	—	CD142	2152	
CD143	EC 3.4.15.1; ACE; kininase II; peptidyl dipeptidase A	—	CD143	1636	
CD144	Cadherin-5; VE-cadherin	—	CD144	1003	
CDw145					
CD146	MCAM; A32; MUC18; Mel-CAM; S-endo	—	CD146	4162	
CD147	5A11; basigin; CE9; HT7; M6; neurothelin; OX-47; EMMPRIN; gp42	—	CD147	682	
CD148	HPTP-eta; DEP-1; p260	—	CD148	5795	
CDw149	New designation is CD47R				
CD150	SLAM; IPO-3; formerly CDw150	—	CDw150	6504	
CD151	PETA-3; SFA-1	—	CD151	977	
CD152	CTLA-4	—	CD152	1493	
CD153	CD30L	—		944	
CD154	CD40L; T-BAM; TRAP; gp39	—		959	
CD155	PVR	—		5817	
CD156a	ADAM8; MS2 human; formerly CD156	—	CD156a	101	
CD156b	ADAM17; TACE; cSVP	CD156b		6868	HLDA7
CDw156C	ADAM10; a disintegrin and metalloproteinase domain 10	—		102	HLDA8
CD157	BP-3/IF-7; BST-1; Mo5	—	CD157	683	
CD158	KIR family		KIR Family		HLDA7
CD159a	NKG2A	—		3821	HLDA7
CD159c	NKG2C; killer cell lectin-like receptor subfamily C, member 2	—		3822	HLDA8
CD160	BY55 antigen; NK1; NK28	CD160		11126	HLDA7
CD161	KLRB1; NKR-P1A; killer cell lectin-like receptor subfamily B, member 1	—	CD161	3820	
CD162	PSGL-1, PSGL	—	CD162	6404	
CD162R	PEN5 (a post-translational modification of PSGL-1)	—		6404	HLDA7
CD163	GHI/61; M130; RM3/1	—		9332	
CD164	MUC-24; MGC-24v	—		8763	
CD165	AD2; gp37	—	CD165	23449	
CD166	BEN; DM-GRASP; KG-CAM; Neurolin; SC-1; ALCAM	—	CD166	214	
CD167a	TRKE; TRK6; CAK; EDDR1; DDR1; MCK10; RTK6; NTRK4	CD167a		780	HLDA7
CD168	HMMR; IHABP; RHAMM	CD168		3161	HLDA7
CD169	Sialoadhesin; SIGLEC1	CD169		6614	HLDA7
CD170	SIGLEC5			8778	HLDA7

Table A3.1 Common CD molecules (continued)

Index of information available from PROW					
Current guides: expanded format including summary sentence and abstract **Past guides:** older guides with excellent information; some data may be dated					
CD molecule	**Alternate names**	**Current guides**	**Past guides**	**Entrez gene**	**Assigning workshop**
CD171	L1; L1CAM; N-CAM L1	CD171		3897	HLDA7
CD172a	SIRP alpha	—		8194	HLDA7
CD172b	SIRP beta; signal-regulatory protein beta 1	—		10326	HLDA8
CD172g	SIRP gamma; signal-regulatory protein beta 2	—		55423	HLDA8
CD173	Blood group H type 2				HLDA7
CD174	Lewis y	—		2525	HLDA7
CD175	Tn				HLDA7
CD175s	Sialyl-Tn				HLDA7
CD176	TF				HLDA7
CD177	NB1				HLDA7
CD178	FasL; TNFSF6; APT1LG1; CD95-L	CD178		356	HLDA7
CD179a	VpreB; VPREB1; IGVPB	CD179a		7441	HLDA7
CD179b	IGLL1; lambda5; immunoglobulin omega polypeptide; IGVPB; 14.1 chain	CD179b		3543	HLDA7
CD180	LY64; RP105	CD180		4064	HLDA7
CD181	CXCR1 (was CDw128A); IL8R alpha	—		3577	HLDA8
CD182	CXCR2 (was CDw128B); IL8R beta	—		12765	HLDA8
CD183	CXCR3; GPR9; CKR-L2; IP10-R; Mig-R	CD183		2833	HLDA7
CD184	CXCR4; fusin; LESTR; NPY3R; HM89; FB22	CD184		7852	HLDA7
CD185	CXCR5; chemokine (C-X-C motif) receptor 5, Burkitt's lymphoma receptor 1	—		643	HLDA8
CDw186	CXCR6; chemokine (C-X-C motif) receptor 6	—		10663	HLDA8
CD191	CCR1; chemokine (C-C motif) receptor 1, RANTES receptor	—		1230	HLDA8
CD192	CCR2; chemokine (C-C motif) receptor 2, MCP-1 receptor	—		1231	HLDA8
CD193	CCR3; chemokine (C-C motif) receptor 3, eosinophil eotaxin receptor	—		1232	HLDA8
CD195	CCR5	—		1234	
CD196	CCR6; chemokine (C-C motif) receptor 6	—		1235	HLDA8
CD197	CCR7 (was CDw197); chemokine (C-C motif) receptor 7	—		1236	HLDA8
CDw198	CCR8; chemokine (C-C motif) receptor 8	—		1237	HLDA8
CDw199	CCR9; chemokine (C-C motif) receptor 9	—		10803	HLDA8
CDw197	CCR7	—		1236	HLDA7
CD200	OX2	—		4345	HLDA7
CD201	EPC R	—		10544	HLDA7
CD202b	Tie2; Tek	CD202b		7010	HLDA7
CD203c	NPP3; PDNP3; PD-Ibeta; B10; gp130RB13-6; ENPP3; bovine intestinal phosphodiesterase	CD203c		5169	HLDA7
CD204	Macrophage scavenger R			4481	HLDA7
CD205	DEC205			4065	HLDA7
CD206	MRC1; MMR	CD206		4360	HLDA7
CD207	Langerin			50489	HLDA7

(continued)

Table A3.1 Common CD molecules (continued)

Index of information available from PROW					
Current guides: expanded format including summary sentence and abstract **Past guides:** older guides with excellent information; some data may be dated					
CD molecule	**Alternate names**	**Current guides**	**Past guides**	**Entrez gene**	**Assigning workshop**
CD208	DC-LAMP			27074	HLDA7
CD209	DC-SIGN			30385	HLDA7
CDw210	IL-10 R			3587; 3588	HLDA7
CD212	IL-12 R			3594	HLDA7
CD213a1	IL-13 R alpha 1	CD213a1		3597	HLDA7
CD213a2	IL-13 R alpha 2			3598	HLDA7
CDw217	IL-17 R			23765	HLDA7
CDw218a	IL-18R alpha; IL-18R alpha				HLDA8
CDw218b	IL-18R beta; IL-18R beta				HLDA8
CD220	Insulin R			3643	HLDA7
CD221	IGF1R			3480	HLDA7
CD222	Mannose-6-phosphate/IGF2R	CD222		3482	HLDA7
CD223	LAG-3	CD223		3902	HLDA7
CD224	GGT; EC2.3.2.2	CD224		2678	HLDA7
CD225	Leu13			8519	HLDA7
CD226	DNAM-1; PTA1; TLiSA1	CD226		10666	HLDA7
CD227	MUC1; episialin; PUM; PEM; EMA; DF3 antigen; H23 antigen	CD227		4582	HLDA7
CD228	Melanotransferrin			4241	HLDA7
CD229	Ly9			4063	HLDA7
CD230	Prion protein			5621	HLDA7
CD231	TM4SF2; A15; TALLA-1; MXS1; CCG-B7; TALLA	CD231		7102	HLDA7
CD232	VESP R			10154	HLDA7
CD233	Band 3; erythrocyte membrane protein band 3; AE1; SLC4A1; Diego blood group; EPB3	CD233		6521	HLDA7
CD234	Fy-glycoprotein; Duffy antigen	CD234		2532	HLDA7
CD235a	Glycophorin A	—		2993	HLDA7
CD235b	Glycophorin B	—		2994	HLDA7
CD235ab	Glycophorin A/B cross-reactive mAbs				HLDA7
CD236	Glycophorin C/D				HLDA7
CD236R	Glycophorin C	—		2995	HLDA7
CD238	Kell	—		3792	HLDA7
CD239	B-CAM	—		4059	HLDA7
CD240CE	Rh30CE	—		6006	HLDA7
CD240D	Rh30D	—		6007	HLDA7
CD240DCE	Rh30D/CE cross-reactive mAbs				HLDA7
CD241	RhAg	—		6005	HLDA7
CD242	ICAM-4	—		3386	HLDA7
CD243	MDR-1	—		5243	HLDA7
CD244	2B4; NAIL; p38	—		51744	HLDA7
CD245	p220/240				HLDA7
CD246	Anaplastic lymphoma kinase	—		238	HLDA7
CD247	Zeta chain	—		919	HLDA7

Table A3.1 Common CD molecules (continued)

Index of information available from PROW					
Current guides: expanded format including summary sentence and abstract **Past guides:** older guides with excellent information; some data may be dated					
CD molecule	**Alternate names**	**Current guides**	**Past guides**	**Entrez gene**	**Assigning workshop**
CD248	TEM1, endosialin; CD164 sialomucin-like 1, tumor endothelial marker 1	—		57124	HLDA8
CD249	Aminopeptidase A; APA, gp160	—		2028	HLDA8
CD252	OX40L; TNF (ligand) superfamily member 4, CD134 ligand	—		7292	HLDA8
CD253	TRAIL; TNF (ligand) superfamily member 10, APO2L	—		8743	HLDA8
CD254	TRANCE; TNF (ligand) superfamily member 11, RANKL	—		8600	HLDA8
CD256	APRIL; TNF (ligand) superfamily member 13, TALL2	—		8741	HLDA8
CD257	BLYS; TNF (ligand) superfamily, member 13b, TALL1, BAFF	—		10673	HLDA8
CD258	LIGHT; TNF (ligand) superfamily, member 14	—		8740	HLDA8
CD261	TRAIL-R1; TNFR superfamily, member 10a, DR4, APO2	—		8797	HLDA8
CD262	TRAIL-R2; TNFR superfamily, member 10b, DR5	—		8795	HLDA8
CD263	TRAIL-R3; TNFR superfamily, member 10c, DCR1	—		8794	HLDA8
CD264	TRAIL-R4; TNFR superfamily, member 10d, DCR2	—		8793	HLDA8
CD265	TRANCE-R; TNFR superfamily, member 11a, RANK	—		8792	HLDA8
CD266	TWEAK-R; TNFR superfamily, member 12A, type I transmembrane protein Fn14	—		51330	HLDA8
CD267	TACI; TNFR superfamily, member 13B, transmembrane activator and CAML interactor	—		23495	HLDA8
CD268	BAFFR; TNFR superfamily, member 13C, B cell-activating factor receptor	—		115650	HLDA8
CD269	BCMA; TNFR superfamily, member 17, B cell maturation factor	—		608	HLDA8
CD271	NGFR (p75); nerve growth factor receptor (TNFR superfamily, member 16)	—		4804	HLDA8
CD272	BTLA; B and T lymphocyte attenuator	—		151888	HLDA8
CD273	B7DC, PDL2; programmed cell death 1 ligand 2	—		80380	HLDA8
CD274	B7H1, PDL1; programmed cell death 1 ligand 1	—		29126	HLDA8
CD275	B7H2, ICOSL; inducible T cell co-stimulator ligand (ICOSL)	—		23308	HLDA8
CD276	B7H3; B7 homolog 3	—		80381	HLDA8
CD277	BT3.1; B7 family: butyrophilin, subfamily 3, member A1	—		11119	HLDA8
CD278	ICOS; inducible T cell co-stimulator	—		29851	HLDA8
CD279	PD1; programmed cell death 1	—		5133	HLDA8
CD280	ENDO180; uPARAP, mannose receptor, C type 2, TEM22	—		9902	HLDA8
CD281	TLR1; Toll-like receptor 1	—		7096	HLDA8
CD282	TLR2; Toll-like receptor 2	—		7097	HLDA8
CD283	TLR3; Toll-like receptor 3	—		7098	HLDA8

(continued)

Table A3.1 Common CD molecules (continued)

Index of information available from PROW					
Current guides: expanded format including summary sentence and abstract **Past guides:** older guides with excellent information; some data may be dated					
CD molecule	**Alternate names**	**Current guides**	**Past guides**	**Entrez gene**	**Assigning workshop**
CD284	TLR4; Toll-like receptor 4	—		7099	HLDA8
CD289	TLR9; Toll-like receptor 9	—		54106	HLDA8
CD292	BMPR1A; bone morphogenetic protein receptor, type IA	—		657	HLDA8
CDw293	BMPR1B; bone morphogenetic protein receptor, type IB	—		658	HLDA8
CD294	CRTH2; PGRD2; G protein-coupled receptor 44	—		11251	HLDA8
CD295	LEPR; leptin receptor	—		3953	HLDA8
CD296	ART1; ADP-ribosyltransferase 1	—		417	HLDA8
CD297	ART4; ADP-ribosyltransferase 4; Dombrock blood group glycoprotein	—		420	HLDA8
CD298	ATP1B3; Na+/K+ -ATPase beta 3 subunit	—		483	HLDA8
CD299	DCSIGN-related; CD209 antigen-like, DC-SIGN2, L-SIGN	—		10332	HLDA8
CD300a	CMRF35 family; CMRF-35H	—		11314	HLDA8
CD300c	CMRF35 family; CMRF-35A	—		10871	HLDA8
CD300e	CMRF35 family; CMRF-35L1				HLDA8
CD301	MGL; CLECSF14, macrophage galactose-type C-type lectin	—		10462	HLDA8
CD302	DCL1; Type I transmembrane C-type lectin receptor DCL-1	—		9936	HLDA8
CD303	BDCA2; C-type lectin, superfamily member 11	—		170482	HLDA8
CD304	BDCA4; neuropilin 1	—		8829	HLDA8
CD305	LAIR1; leukocyte-associated Ig-like receptor 1	—		3903	HLDA8
CD306	LAIR2; leukocyte-associated Ig-like receptor 2	—		3904	HLDA8
CD307	IRTA2; immunoglobulin superfamily receptor translocation-associated 2	—		83416	HLDA8
CD309	VEGFR2; KDR (a type III receptor tyrosine kinase)	—		3791	HLDA8
CD312	EMR2; EGF-like module containing, mucin-like, hormone receptor-like 2	—		30817	HLDA8
CD314	NKG2D; killer cell lectin-like receptor subfamily K, member 1	—		22914	HLDA8
CD315	CD9P1; prostaglandin F2 receptor negative regulator	—		5738	HLDA8
CD316	EWI2; immunoglobulin superfamily, member 8	—		93185	HLDA8
CD317	BST2; bone marrow stromal cell antigen 2	—		684	HLDA8
CD318	CDCP1; CUB domain-containing protein 1	—		64866	HLDA8
CD319	CRACC; SLAM family member 7	—		57823	HLDA8
CD320	8D6; 8D6 antigen; FDC	—		51293	HLDA8
CD321	JAM1; F11 receptor	—		50848	HLDA8
CD322	JAM2; junctional adhesion molecule 2	—		58494	HLDA8
CD324	E-cadherin; cadherin 1, type 1, E-cadherin (epithelial)	—		999	HLDA8

Table A3.1 Common CD molecules (continued)

Index of information available from PROW					
Current guides: expanded format including summary sentence and abstract **Past guides:** older guides with excellent information; some data may be dated					
CD molecule	**Alternate names**	**Current guides**	**Past guides**	**Entrez gene**	**Assigning workshop**
CDw325	N-cadherin; cadherin 2, type 1, N-cadherin (neuronal)	—		1000	HLDA8
CD326	Ep-CAM; tumor-associated calcium signal transducer 1	—		4072	HLDA8
CDw327	SIGLEC6; sialic acid binding Ig-like lectin 6	—		946	HLDA8
CDw328	SIGLEC7; sialic acid binding Ig-like lectin 7	—		27036	HLDA8
CDw329	SIGLEC9; sialic acid binding Ig-like lectin 9	—		27180	HLDA8
CD331	FGFR1; fibroblast growth factor receptor 1	—		2260	HLDA8
CD332	FGFR2; fibroblast growth factor receptor 2 (keratinocyte growth factor receptor)	—		2263	HLDA8
CD333	FGFR3; fibroblast growth factor receptor 3 (achondroplasia, thanatophoric dwarfism)	—		2261	HLDA8
CD334	FGFR4; fibroblast growth factor receptor 4	—		2264	HLDA8
CD335	NKp46; NCR1 (Ly94); natural cytotoxicity triggering receptor 1	—		9437	HLDA8
CD336	NKp44; NCR2 (Ly95); natural cytotoxicity triggering receptor 2	—		9436	HLDA8
CD337	NKp30; NCR3	—		259197	HLDA8
CDw338	ABCG2; ATP-binding cassette, subfamily G (WHITE), member 2	—		9429	HLDA8
CD339	Jagged1; Jagged1 (Alagille syndrome)	—		182	HLDA8
CD340	ERBB2 v-erb-b2 erythroblastic leukemia viral oncogene homolog 2, neuro/glioblastoma-derived oncogene homolog (avian) (Homo sapiens)			ERBB2 (CD340)	

For additional information, contact: mpr@mail.nih.gov.

Index

Visual Glossary

Environment

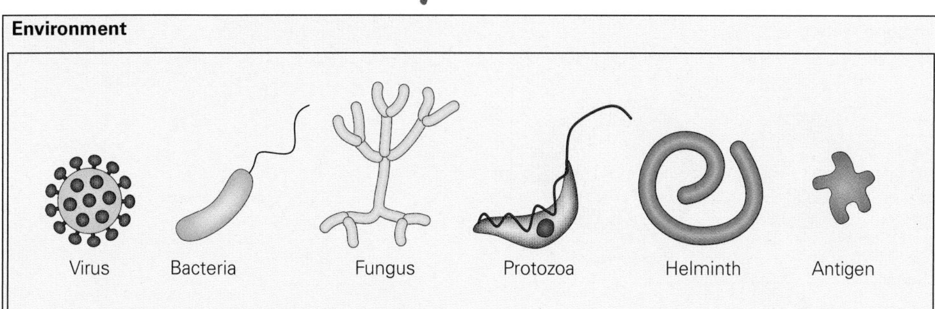

Target cells

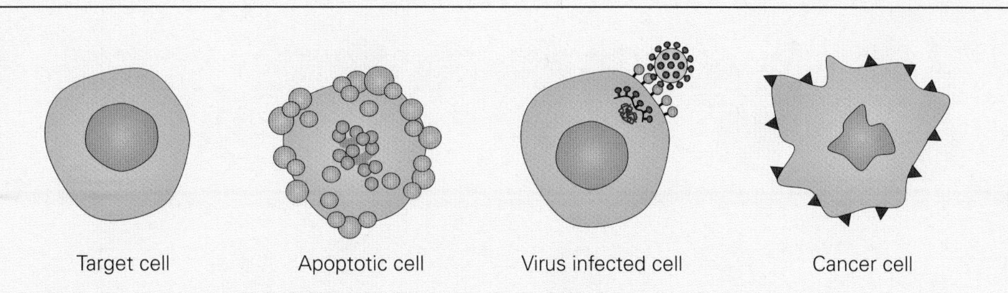

Cells of the innate immune system and complement

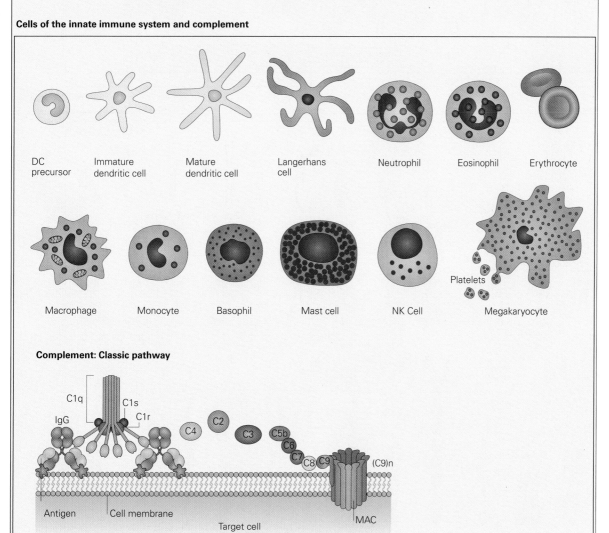

DC precursor
Immature dendritic cell
Mature dendritic cell
Langerhans cell
Neutrophil
Eosinophil
Erythrocyte

Macrophage
Monocyte
Basophil
Mast cell
NK Cell
Platelets
Megakaryocyte

Complement: Classic pathway

C1q
C1s
C1r
IgG
C4
C2
C3
C5b
C6
C7
C8
C9
(C9)n
Antigen
Cell membrane
Target cell
MAC

Cells and cell products of the adaptive immune system

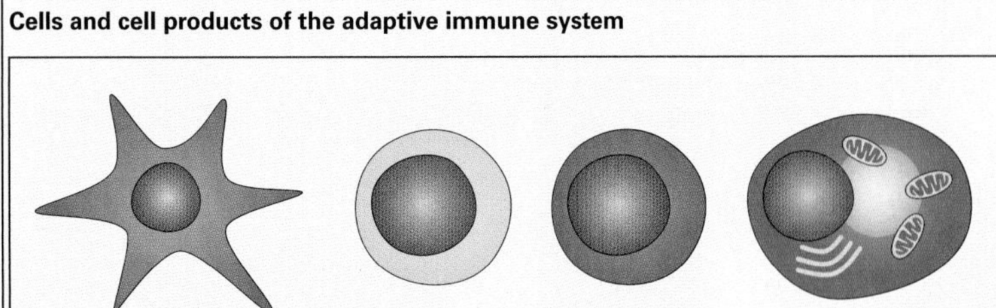

Immunoglobulins

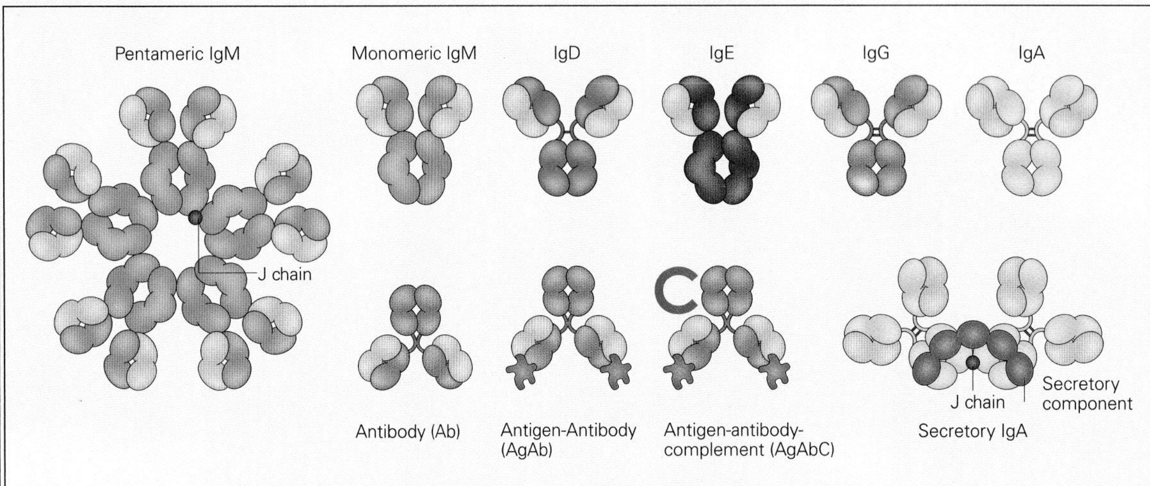

Cell receptors

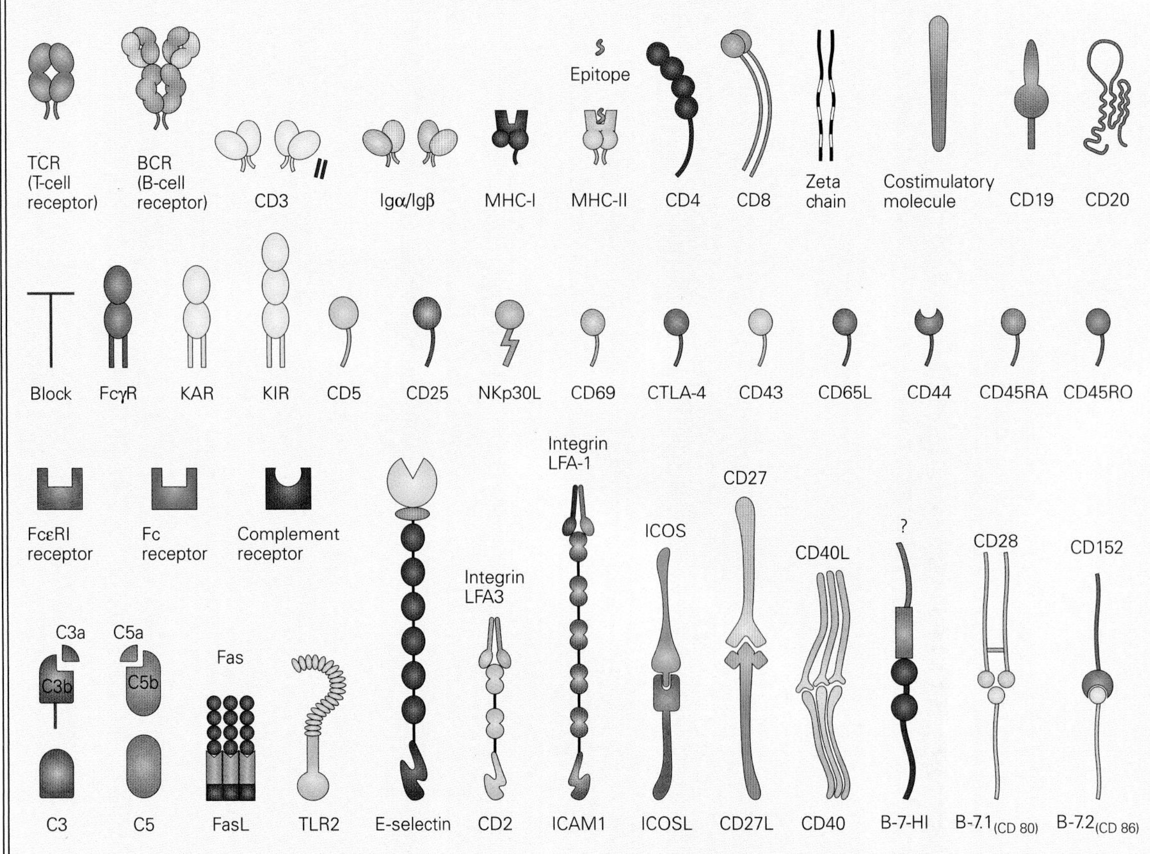